Student Resource CD-ROM for *Aschenbrenner:* Drug Therapy In Nursing, Second Edition

This reliable resource accompanies the text and provides additional tools to help you succeed!

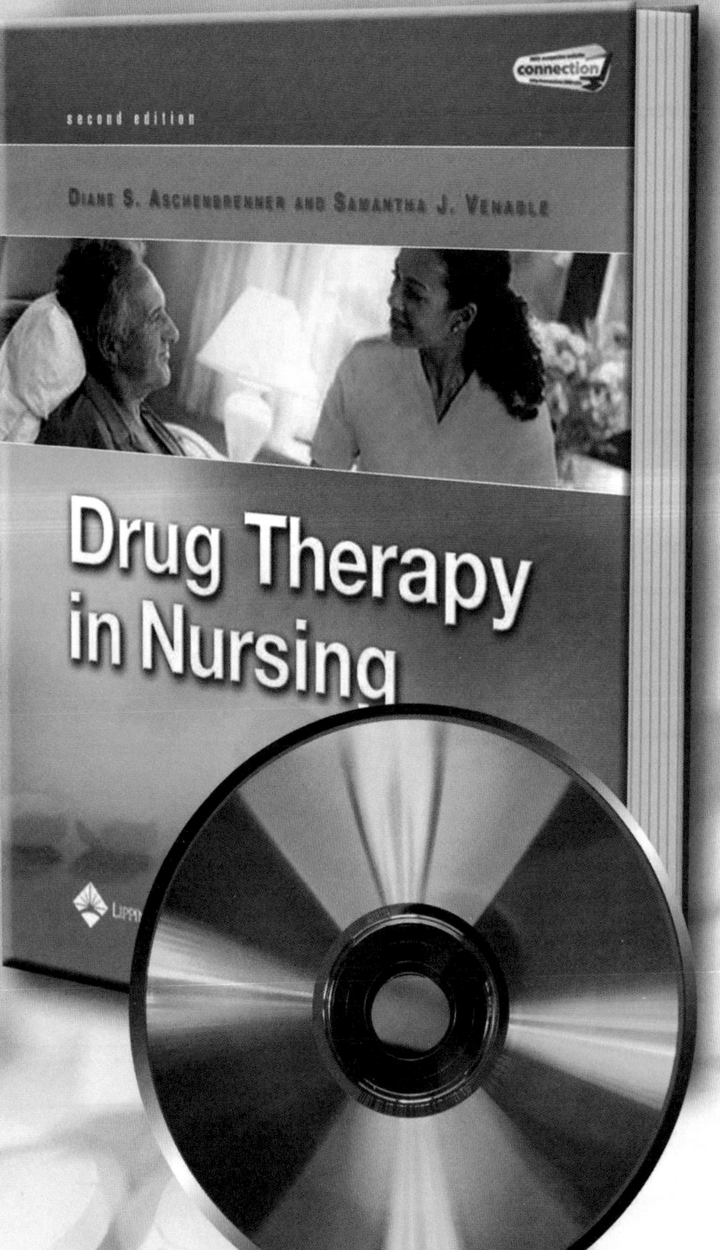

NCLEX-style Review Questions

Ten NCLEX-style Student Review Questions per chapter, including alternate-format questions, provide rationales to facilitate your understanding.

Concept Map Exercises

Over 40 interactive "drag and drop" review exercises assist you through visual learning. Concept maps based on those in the text help you to identify drugs by their drug class and understand their relationship to one another. Features audio pronunciations of all drug names.

Animations

Animations help you understand concepts including:

- The Cell Cycle
- Absorption
- Distribution
- Drug Binding
- Excretion
- Intramuscular Medication
- Intravenous Medication

Self-Study Dosage Calculation

Questions and Dosage Calculator

- Nearly 100 dosage calculation problems!

Preventing Medication Errors Video

Reviewing all aspects of medication error prevention. Topics include:

- Interpreting Medication Orders
- Transcribing Medication Orders
- Reviewing Medication Orders
- Preparing Medications
- Administering Medications
- Assessing Patient Response
- Procedural Safeguards
- Reporting Medication Errors

And Don't Forget...Connection Student Resource Center http://connection.lww.com

In addition to your FREE CD-ROM, Connection's exclusive resource centers for students provide dynamic book-specific supplements such as content updates, web links, downloadable images, review questions and more! Connect today. **http://connection.lww.com/go/aschenbrenner.**

For more information...

Call TOLL FREE 1-800-399-3110

Visit us on the Web at LWW.com/nursing or nursingcenter.com

Lippincott Williams & Wilkins

A5G120F

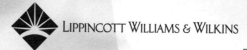

Drug Therapy in Nursing

Drug Therapy in Nursing

edition 2

Diane S. Aschenbrenner, MS, APRN, BC
Course Coordinator
Johns Hopkins University
School of Nursing
Baltimore, Maryland

Samantha J. Venable, MS, RN, FNP
Professor
Saddleback College
Mission Viejo, California

Lippincott Williams & Wilkins
A **Wolters Kluwer** Company
Philadelphia • Baltimore • New York • London
Buenos Aires • Hong Kong • Sydney • Tokyo

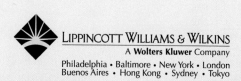

Senior Acquisitions Editor: Margaret Zuccarini
Senior Developmental Editor: Melanie Cann
Editorial Assistant: Delema Caldwell-Jordan
Senior Production Editor: Debra Schiff
Director of Nursing Production: Helen Ewan
Senior Managing Editor/Production: Erika Kors
Art Director: Carolyn O'Brien
Interior Design: BJ Crim
Cover Designer: Vasiliky Kiethas
Senior Manufacturing Manager: William Alberti
Compositor: Circle Graphics
Printer: RRD-Willard

2nd Edition

9 8 7 6 5 4 3 2

Library of Congress Cataloging-in-Publication Data

Aschenbrenner, Diane S.
Drug therapy in nursing / Diane S. Aschenbrenner, Samantha J. Venable.—2nd ed.
p. ; cm.
Includes bibliographical references and index.
ISBN 0-7817-4839-9 (alk. paper)
1. Chemotherapy. 2. Pharmacology. 3. Nursing. I. Venable, Samantha J. II. Title.
[DNLM: 1. Drug Therapy—Nurses' Instruction. 2. Pharmaceutical Preparations—Nurses' Instruction. 3. Pharmacology—Nurses' Instruction. WB 330 A813d 2005]
RM125.N83 2005
615.5'8—dc22
2004027103

LWW.com

To my children, John, Emily, and Allison, for their continuing patience and support, and to my students for all that they have taught me.

DSA

To my husband, Ben, who continues to be the rock that keeps me grounded, my family who graciously support me in all my professional efforts, and the students who consistently remind me that the best part of teaching is the student.

SV

contributors

Delia C. Baquiran, MSN, MSB, RN
Vice President, Health Services
Atlantis Health Plan
New York, New York

Andrew R. Benson, BS, RN
Nurse Clinician I, Cardiology Care Unit
Johns Hopkins Hospital
Baltimore, Maryland

Steven D. Glow, MSN, RN, FNP, CEN, EMT-P
Adjunct Assistant Professor, College of Nursing
Montana State University-Bozeman, Missoula Campus
Bozeman, Montana

Kathie Judy Guth, MS, RN
Instructor
Johns Hopkins University School of Nursing
Baltimore, Maryland

Bernard Vincent Keenan, MSN, RN, BC
Clinical Instructor
Johns Hopkins University School of Nursing
Baltimore, Maryland

Shari J. Lynn, MSN, RN
Clinical Faculty
Johns Hopkins University School of Nursing
Baltimore, Maryland

Barbara E. Prescott, BSN, MA, ND, RNC, FNP
Nursing Faculty
Salish Kootenai College
Pablo, Montana

Brenda K. Shelton, MS, RN, CCRN, AOCN
Clinical Nurse Specialist
The Sidney Kimmel Comprehensive Cancer Center at Johns Hopkins
Baltimore, Maryland

Joyce B. Vazzano, MS, RN
Instructor
Johns Hopkins University School of Nursing
Baltimore, Maryland

Barbara Van de Castle, MSN, RN
Instructor
Johns Hopkins University School of Nursing
Baltimore, Maryland

reviewers

Kim Baily, PhD, RN
Associate Professor of Nursing
Cerritos College
Norwalk, California

Sandra Drozdz Burke, PhD (c), MSN, ANP, CS
Teaching Associate; Nurse Practitioner
University of Illinois College of Nursing at Urbana
Urbana, Illinois

Shirley A. Dinkel, PhD (c), APRN
Assistant Professor
Washburn University
Topeka, Kansas

Michelle M. Frost, MSN, BSN-H, RN, SANE, WHCNP
Assistant Professor of Nursing
Columbia Gorge Community College
The Dalles, Oregon

Charlene Beach Gagliardi, MSN, BSN, RN
Faculty—Department of Nursing
Mount St. Mary's College
Los Angeles, California

Stephen Gilliam, PhD, FNP, APRN, BC
Assistant Professor
Medical College of Georgia, School of Nursing
Athens, Georgia

Lynn R. Grommet, MNSc, RNC
Nursing Faculty
East Arkansas Community College
Forrest City, Arkansas

Susan C. Immelt, PhD, RN
Assistant Professor
Towson University
Towson, Maryland

Patricia Meehan Jones, MSN, BSN, RN
Instructor, Adult Health Nursing
Pensacola Junior College
Pensacola, Florida

Clair Kaplan, MSN, APRN (WHNP), MHS, MT (ASCP)
Assistant Professor
Saint Joseph College
West Hartford, Connecticut

Patricia Lange-Otsuka, EdD, MSN, APRN, BC
Graduate Nursing Program Chair and Associate Professor of Nursing
Hawaii Pacific University
Kaneohe, Hawaii

Tara J. Latto, MS, RN
Instructor in Nursing
Morton College
Cicero, Illinois

Margaret McEntee, PhD, RN
Associate Professor
University of Maryland School of Nursing
Baltimore, Maryland

Tara McMillan Queen, MN, BSN, RN, ANP-C, GNP
Faculty/Nurse Practitioner
Mercy School of Nursing
Charlotte, North Carolina

Winnie Pickering, PhD (c), MSN, BSN, ADN
Associate Professor in Nursing, Second Year Nursing Faculty Member
James A. Rhodes State College
Lima, Ohio

Deanna L. Reising, PhD, RN, CS
Assistant Professor
Indiana University School of Nursing
Bloomington, Indiana

Sally P. Scavone, MS, BS, RN
Professor, Nursing
Erie Community College, City Campus
Buffalo, New York

Suzanne E. Tatro, MS, RN
Instructor of Nursing and Coordinator of the Computer Assisted Instruction Lab
York Technical College
Rock Hill, South Carolina

Gail Vitale, MS, APRN, BC
Assistant Professor
Lewis University College of Nursing and Health Professions
Romeoville, Illinois

Linda B. Wheeler, MSN, RN, CCRN
Lecturer
University of North Carolina Greensboro School of Nursing
Greensboro, North Carolina

Shirley K. Woolfe, MSN, RN, CCRN, CNRN, PN
Clinical Assistant Professor
Indiana University School of Nursing
Indianapolis, Indiana

"How will I ever learn all of this?" and "Where do I begin?" are questions that nursing students frequently ask themselves and their faculty when beginning to study pharmacology. The subject is indeed vast for novices in the profession who lack the skills to organize drug information appropriately. Students feel overwhelmed by all of the isolated pieces of drug information they must learn. Consequently, they lose sight of "the forest for the trees."

PROTOTYPE APPROACH

For years, many pharmacology faculty have favored a prototype approach to teaching pharmacology. This method encourages identification of "the trees" and facilitates recognition of "the forest." Use of a prototype, a drug that is representative of a class (or group) of drugs, helps students because it offers a systematic approach to grouping drug data, while beginning to recognize individual drug names. It gives students a "method" of learning and organizing large amounts of information. *Drug Therapy in Nursing, Second Edition,* is designed and written by faculty who themselves teach nursing pharmacology using the prototype approach. At last, nursing pharmacology faculty have a text that matches the way they teach. *Drug Therapy in Nursing, Second Edition,* is that text!

CLINICAL JUDGMENT AND CLINICAL APPLICATION

Drug Therapy in Nursing, Second Edition, is unique in that it presents a totally nursing-focused framework to support the teaching and learning of nursing pharmacology. Learning the pharmacology facts about different drug prototypes is only half of the knowledge nursing students need. Because they're learning to be nurses, they must understand how to apply this knowledge to patient care. Nurses must learn to think critically, evaluate information, and make decisions. However, this essential aspect of knowledge application has never been thoroughly addressed in nursing pharmacology texts. Frequently, students view *nursing application* of drug knowledge as less important than learning the hard drug facts. This thinking is fostered when the pharmacology textbooks they use present the nursing process after or apart from drug knowledge in a brief paragraph or chart. *Drug Therapy in Nursing, Second Edition,* fully integrates core drug knowledge with core patient information, appropriately stressing, as no other text does, the relationship between the two bodies of information.

As with all other factual, scientific, or medical information utilized by nurses, the student must learn to integrate this knowledge into their practice and apply it to patient care. Applying drug information to patient care may overwhelm students because every patient is different, with different responses, positive or negative, to the same drug therapy. If the student sees each patient situation as an isolated case, learning is again hampered. This text provides a systematic framework for assessing and evaluating patient responses that change in accord with health, age, gender, lifestyle, and other factors. This important *patient focus* is strengthened by use of the nursing process framework. Pharmacologic facts are integrated into nursing, to help the student apply knowledge to practice, safely administer drugs, educate patients, and begin to make the journey from novice to expert.

USE OF A SYSTEMATIC FRAMEWORK

The authors of *Drug Therapy in Nursing, Second Edition,* present a systematic framework for drug therapy with every prototype drug. The framework consists of two basic areas of information: first, core drug knowledge and core patient variables; and second, actions of the nurse utilizing this knowledge.

Core Drug Knowledge highlights the important drug facts about a prototype drug. Core drug knowledge includes pharmacotherapeutics, pharmacokinetics, pharmacodynamics, contraindications and precautions, adverse effects, and drug interactions.

Core Patient Variables identify the major topics that should be assessed in every patient to determine special considerations that need to be taken into account when administering a drug to a patient. Core patient variables include health status; lifespan and gender; lifestyle, diet, and habits; environment; and culture and inherited traits. The relevant variables for each particular prototype are presented in the text.

The nurse utilizes knowledge about the drug and knowledge about the patient to maximize the therapeutic effect of the drug, minimize the adverse effects of the drug, or provide patient and family education. The authors of this text call what the nurse does with knowledge about the drug and the individual patient "nursing management in drug therapy."

ORGANIZATION

Drug Therapy in Nursing, Second Edition, has 13 units and 10 appendices. The first three units address the principles and process of nursing management in drug therapy, and the basics of core drug knowledge and patient-related variables. The next ten units present the nursing management of drugs affecting various body systems and disease states. The text concludes with 10 appendices.

Unit 1, Foundations for Drug Therapy in Nursing, consists of three chapters. Chapter 1 explains the framework for the text and how this framework relates to the application of drug knowledge to clinical practice. **This is a crucial chapter for students to read so that they will best understand the content in the rest of the text.** The remaining chapters address basic pharmaceutical knowledge, drug development and its related safeguards, and drug delivery, and the modes of drug administration.

Unit 2, Core Drug Knowledge, includes two chapters that present the basics of pharmacology: pharmacotherapeutics, pharmacokinetics, and pharmacodynamics; and adverse effects and drug interactions.

Unit 3, Core Patient Variables, includes seven chapters that highlight information pertinent to patient assessment relevant to drug therapy. This is not an exhaustive list of every aspect that can be considered by these variables. The topics include lifespan issues (children, pregnant or breast-feeding women, and older adults); lifestyle, diet, and habits issues (substance abuse, dietary considerations, and complementary medication use); environment (influences on drug therapy); and culture and inherited traits (influences on drug therapy). The core patient variable of health status is not presented as this includes all physiology, pathophysiology, disease states, and their related treatments.

Units 4 through 12 present drugs affecting the various body systems, and drugs used to treat diseases and their symptoms.

The Appendices present essential information on Canadian drug information, diagnostic and imaging agents, enzymes and débridement therapy, enteral nutrition, parenteral nutrition, antidotes, immunizations, antiemetic drugs, therapeutic and toxic levels of selected drugs, and drugs causing photosensitivity. Emphasis is given in the appendixes to the nursing management of these drug therapies.

PEDAGOGY

- **Chapter Learning Objectives** identify key content within the chapter to help direct student learning.
- **Key Terms** identify terms that are key to understanding each chapter's contents.
- **Chapter Summaries** highlight the most important information presented in the chapter.
- **Questions for Study and Review** encourage the student to reflect on the important aspects of the chapter. Answers are provided in the back of the text.

NEW FEATURES WITH THIS EDITION

- More pathophysiology information relevant to drug therapy to assist with understanding and critical thinking
- Featured website(s) on the opening page of each chapter provides additional chapter-related information on disease processes, drug information sources, patient education, or professional organizations. Additional websites are found on the Connection companion website for the text (*http://www.connection.lww.com/go/aschenbrenner*).
- Separate chapters on drugs affecting hematopoiesis and drugs affecting the immune response with revised expanded content
- Significantly revised chapters on pharmacokinetics, adverse effects, substance abuse, drugs relieving anxiety and producing sleep, drugs treating mood disorders, drugs treating psychotic disorders and dementia (with emphasis to differentiate the two conditions), drugs treating seizure disorders, and drugs affecting glucose levels.

KEY FEATURES

- **Concept Maps** introduce the student to all drugs that will be mentioned in the chapter. Each map identifies the drug class, its prototype, and drugs in the class that are similar to or different from the prototype.
- **Physiology Figures** illustrate physiologic processes relevant to the drug class and link drug actions to physiology.
- **Memory Chips** assist students in studying and preparing for clinical practice, providing a quick reference of key points for each prototype drug.
- **Focus on Research** boxes highlight current research in pharmacology. The implications for nursing practice are addressed for each article.
- **Community-Based Concerns** highlight nursing issues related to drug therapy carried out in patients' homes and communities.
- **Critical Thinking Scenarios** challenge students to develop critical thinking skills for applying pharmacology knowledge to patient care.
- **Drug Summary Tables** relate pharmacotherapeutics and general dosage data to pharmacokinetic parameters.
- **Drug Interaction Tables,** for every prototype drug, highlight known drug-drug and drug-food interactions. When diagnostic and laboratory test values are affected by drug use, this information is pointed out as well.

ANCILLARY PACKAGE

These excellent ancillary materials make teaching and learning even easier!

Instructor's Resource CD. The Instructor's Resource CD contains the following items:

- A thoroughly revised and updated **Instructor's Manual,** featuring lecture outlines and teaching strategies, suggestions for in-class activities and discussion points, case studies for small group discussion or assignments, and answers to the critical thinking scenarios in the textbook
- **PowerPoint Lecture Slides** for each chapter in the textbook, designed to complement the lecture outlines in the Instructor's Manual and featuring art from the text
- A thoroughly revised and augmented **Test Generator,** containing more than 800 NCLEX-style questions
- An **Image Bank,** containing illustrations from the book in formats suitable for printing and incorporating into PowerPoint presentations and Internet sites

Student Resource CD. Packaged with the textbook at no additional charge, this CD contains the following items:

- **Interactive Concept Maps,** based on those in the text, allow the student to place the drugs in their appropriate drug classes, and hear the drug names pronounced.
- **Quizzes for every chapter, featuring traditional and alternative-format NCLEX-style questions**

- **In-depth animations** illustrating pharmacologic and pharmacokinetic mechanisms bring the text to life
- **Video on Preventing Medication Errors** reinforces safety issues, teaching students habits for careful clinical practice
- **Dosage Calc Challenge** provides review of dosage calculation concepts to further promote patient safety

Study Guide to Accompany Drug Therapy in Nursing, Second Edition. Authored by Diane Aschenbrenner and Samantha Venable, this study guide has been carefully designed to complement the textbook. Information is reviewed according to the types of knowledge presented in each textbook chapter (e.g., key terms, physiology and pathophysiology, core drug knowledge, core patient variables). The *Study Guide* provides students further study and learning opportunities through various techniques, such as multiple-choice questions, matching, decision trees, and case studies, that encourage critical thinking and the application of knowledge. Students are moved through the levels of learning, beginning with knowledge of terms and acquisition of facts, and progressing to the application of knowledge in each chapter. Answers for all of the exercises are provided at the end of the study guide to assist students with independent study.

Connection Companion Website. Log on to *http://connection.lww.com/go/aschenbrenner* for additional student and faculty resources: case studies, drug update links, and links to websites that support content in the book.

How to Use *Drug Therapy in Nursing*

LOOK AHEAD!

Before reading the chapter content, read the **Learning Objectives.** These objectives help you to understand what is important and why. Review the **Key Terms** lists to become familiar with new vocabulary presented throughout the narrative. Finally, take a look at the **Concept Map.** The concept map introduces you to all of the drugs that will be mentioned in the chapter and shows you how they are related to one another.

Drugs That Affect Cholinergic Function

(C) Cholinergic agonists

- (C) Direct-acting muscarinic agonists
  - [P] **pilocarpine**
  - acetylcholine
  - bethanechol
  - carbachol
  - cevimeline
  - methacholine
- (C) Direct-acting nicotine agonists
  - [P] **nicotine**
- (C) Indirect-acting cholinergic agonists
  - [P] **neostigmine**
  - ambenonium chloride
  - demecarium
  - edrophonium
  - physostigmine
  - pyridostigmine
  - tacrine
  - irreversible cholinesterase inhibitors

(C) Cholinergic antagonists

- [P] **atropine**
- antisecretory anticholinergics
- benztropine
- hyoscyamine
- ipratropium
- scopolamine
- trihexyphenidyl
- urinary tract relaxants

The symbol (C) indicates the **drug class.**
Drugs in **bold type** marked with the symbol [P] are prototypes.
Drugs in blue type are closely related to the prototype.
Drugs in red type are significantly different from the prototype.
Drugs in black type with no symbol are also used in drug therapy; no prototype

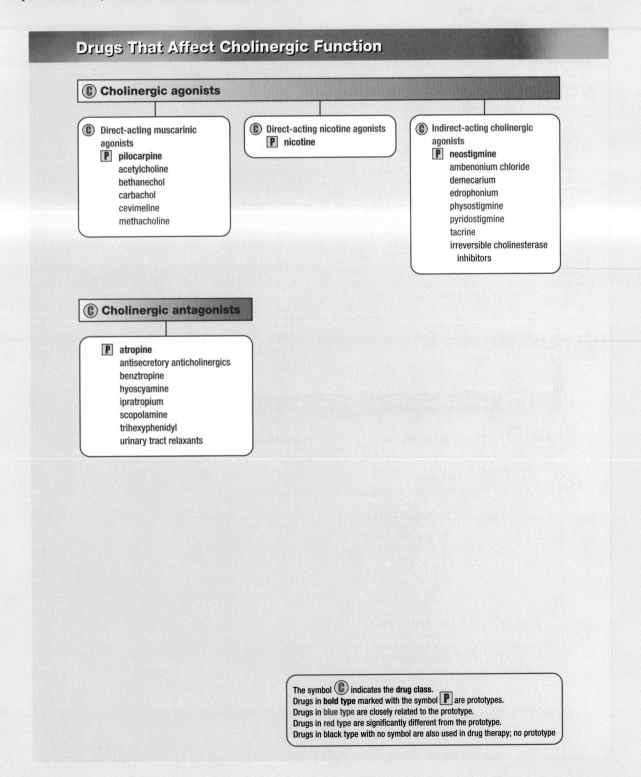

PREPARE FOR CLINICAL PRACTICE!

Learn the pharmacologic facts about each drug prototype; then understand how to apply this knowledge to patient care. The **Core Drug Knowledge/Core Patient Variables framework** gives you a method for organizing and remembering large amounts of information!

NURSING MANAGEMENT OF THE PATIENT RECEIVING [P] NEOSTIGMINE

Core Drug Knowledge

Pharmacotherapeutics

The most significant indication for neostigmine therapy is myasthenia gravis. In this disease, the neuromuscular junction is affected by an autoimmune process that diminishes the number of functional nicotinic receptors at the junction. The result is the characteristic weakness and fatigue that accompany exercise in people with this disease. The use of neostigmine effectively increases the amount of acetylcholine available at the myoneural junction, resulting in enhanced strength of muscle contraction.

Other clinical indications include urinary retention and paralytic ileus. Neostigmine is also used as an antidote for nondepolarizing neuromuscular blocking agents.

Pharmacokinetics

Neostigmine is administered both orally and parenterally. It is poorly absorbed when given orally. Onset of action occurs within 2 to 4 hours when taken orally, and within 10 to 30 minutes when given parenterally. The drug is metabolized by microsomal liver enzymes and hydrolyzed by cholinesterases. Duration of effect varies considerably among patients. Approximately 80% of neostigmine is excreted in the urine within 24 hours as unaltered drug and metabolites (see Table 14.2).

Pharmacodynamics

Neostigmine is a reversible inhibitor of postsynaptic cholinesterase and therefore acts as a cholinergic agent by increasing the synaptic presence of acetylcholine.

You can review key facts about each prototype drug by reading its **Memory Chip.**

MEMORY CHIP

[P] Neostigmine

- An indirect-acting cholinoceptor stimulant used in the management of myasthenia gravis
- Major contraindications: GI obstruction or ileus, urinary tract obstruction, peritonitis
- Most common adverse effects: nausea or vomiting, diarrhea, abdominal pain, miosis, salivation, diaphoresis, sinus bradycardia
- Most serious adverse effects: cholinergic crisis, cardiac arrest
- Maximizing therapeutic effects: Administer at regular intervals throughout the day to ensure adequate blood levels.
- Minimizing adverse effects: availability of atropine, the antidote for cholinergic crisis
- Most significant nursing responsibility: Differentiate between cholinergic crisis and myasthenic crisis.
- Most important patient education: symptoms of cholinergic crisis and need for immediate medical attention

Drug Summary Tables summarize selected indications, route and dosage information, and pharmacokinetics for the drugs under discussion.

TABLE 14.6 Summary of Selected (C) Cholinergic Antagonists

Drug (Trade) Name	Selected Indications	Route and Dosage Range	Pharmacokinetics
[P] atropine (Atropine Sulfate; *Canadian:* Apo-Benztropine)	Anesthesia induction, premedication for surgery Bradycardia Biliary spasm, GI radiography, irritable bowel syndrome, peptic ulcers, urinary incontinence, asthma, bronchitis, reversal of bronchospasm, hiccups, organophosphate poisoning, arrhythmias (e.g., angiography induced, postmyocardial infarction, succinylcholine induced), myelodysplasia, neuromuscular blockade reversal, hyperhidrosis, hypothermia, rhinorrhea, tetanus asystole, dental procedures	*Adult:* SC, IM, or IV, 0.3–0.6 mg 60 min before inducing anesthesia *Adult:* IV, 0.5–2.0 mg *Adult:* 0.3–1.2 mg q4–6h any route for GI or anticholinergic uses	*Onset:* SC, varies; IM, 10–15 min; IV, immediate *Duration:* 4 h $t_{1/2}$: 2.5 h
benztropine (Benztropine Mesylate, Cogentin)	Drug-induced extrapyramidal symptoms, akathisia, dystonic reactions, haloperidol-induced acute dystonic reaction, parkinsonism, drooling, myoclonus, priapism	*Adult:* PO, IM, IV, 1–4 mg daily or bid	*Onset:* PO, 1 h; IM, IV, 15 min *Duration:* PO, IM, IV 6–10 h $t_{1/2}$: 4–8 h
flavoxate (Urispas)	Urinary incontenence	*Adult:* PO, 100–200 mg tid–qid *Children:* Safety not demonstrated	*Onset:* Rapid *Duration:* 24 h $t_{1/2}$: 6 h

(continued)

And **Drug Interaction Tables** summarize known drug–drug and drug–food interactions.

TABLE 14.5 Agents That Interact With P Neostigmine

Interactants	Effect and Significance	Nursing Management
aminoglycoside antibiotics (neomycin, streptomycin, kanamycin)	Mild nondepolarizing blocking action	Monitor for increased neuromuscular blockade.
corticosteroids	Decreases effect of anticholinesterase therapy in myasthenia gravis	Ensure respiratory support if needed.
depolarizing muscle relaxants (succinylcholine) and mivacurium	Increased, prolonged neuromuscular blockade	Avoid use if possible. If not, administer these drugs only as directed and only if indicated. Provide emergency respiratory support.
magnesium	Antagonizes and counteracts beneficial effects of neostigmine	Avoid magnesium-containing drugs and foods.
anticholinesterase drugs	Excessive GI stimulation and symptoms of cholinergic crisis or underdosage in patients with myasthenia gravis	Have antidote (atropine or belladonna) available to treat overdosage.

Focus on Research boxes highlight current research in pharmacology. The implications for nursing practice are addressed for each article.

Community-Based Concerns boxes highlight nursing issues related to drug therapy carried out in patients' homes and communities.

FOCUS ON RESEARCH

Box 8.2 Can Adverse Drug Effects Be Prevented?

Gurwitz, J. H., Field, T. S., Harrold, L. R., et al. (2003). Incidence and preventability of adverse drug events among older persons in the ambulatory setting. *Journal of the American Medical Association, 289*(9), 1107–1116.

The Study

All Medicare enrollees cared for by a multispecialty group practice in an ambulatory setting were assessed over a 1-year period to determine whether they had incurred adverse drug effects. The medical records and all relevant institutional records of the patients were reviewed. The overall rate of adverse drug events was found to be 50.1 per 1,000 person-years; more than one fourth of events were identified as preventable. The adverse drug effects that were considered to be serious, life-threatening, or fatal composed 38% of the total adverse effects. The more serious adverse effects were more likely to be preventable than the less serious adverse effects. Preventable adverse effects were associated with errors in prescribing and monitoring as well as older patient errors in self-administration of medications. The drug classes most frequently associated with preventable adverse drug effects were cardiovascular agents, diuretics, nonopioid analgesics, hypoglycemics, and anticoagulants.

Nursing Implications

Adverse effects from drug therapy cause substantial morbidity and mortality in older adults. Although many adverse effects cannot be prevented, nurses should be vigilant to help protect patients from those that are preventable. Nurses should question any medication order in which the wrong drug or dose appears to have been ordered for the patient. Nurses also need to recognize the importance of patient education concerning proper administration of prescribed drug therapy. Multiple teaching sessions and the use of various teaching techniques, including written information, role play, and return demonstration, should be used when providing the older adult with drug information. Special attention should be given when the patient is prescribed one of the drug classes highly associated with preventable adverse effects.

COMMUNITY-BASED CONCERNS

Box 8.3 Identification and Management of Polypharmacy Problems

- Question the patient about any and all drug therapy that he or she is taking or has taken in the past. Remember to ask about any nonprescribed, over-the-counter (OTC) preparations.
- Ask to see the drug bottles to verify the physician's or nurse practitioner's orders and evaluate the patient's knowledge about the drugs. Frequently, patients will pull out plastic bags or boxes full of drugs.
- Read the labels carefully. Attempt to identify drugs unknown to the patient or unclear prescriptions. If the prescriptions have changed frequently, or the patient has a long history of chronic health problems, the drug labels may be worn, faded, or difficult to read.
- Determine which drug prescriptions and OTC preparations are for current use. Some patients keep drugs for problems they no longer have.
- Determine whether therapy can be simplified. Consult with the physician or nurse practitioner as indicated.
- Assist the patient in creating a time schedule to take all prescribed drugs appropriately but in accordance with the patient's lifestyle. Use memory aids as needed.

Featured Weblinks direct you to additional sources of information about the chapter topic.

FEATURED WEBLINK

http://www.healthcentral.com/mhc/top/000185.htm

Adrenergic agents are used for many diseases and disorders. For information on using adrenergic agents for shock, visit the Health Central website.

DEVELOP CRITICAL THINKING SKILLS!

Learn how critical thinking can change patient outcomes. Challenge yourself! Use the new knowledge you've gained to "think through" the situations presented in the **Critical Thinking Scenarios.**

CRITICAL THINKING SCENARIO

Neostigmine therapy

Amy Rose, a 27-year-old legal assistant, has been admitted to your unit with a diagnosis of myasthenia gravis. She has been started on neostigmine therapy, and you are wondering how to differentiate between undermedication with the possibility of a myasthenic crisis, and overmedication with the possibility of a cholinergic crisis.

1. Explain the key differences between the two situations, and propose a nursing management strategy that you could use for either situation.
2. Discuss the implications of a health care provider–ordered edrophonium test. Why do you think this test would be ordered?

REVIEW WHAT YOU HAVE LEARNED!

Read the **Chapter Summary** to review the most important information presented in the chapter. Finally, answer the **Questions for Study and Review** to check your understanding and retention of the new information you have learned.

acknowledgments

The author team would like to acknowledge the contributions of the entire Lippincott Williams & Wilkins publishing staff for their hard work on this text. Special thanks to Melanie Cann, Senior Developmental Editor, and Debra Schiff, Senior Production Editor, for in-house editing; Alison Darrow, for freelance editing; and to Margaret Zuccarini, for overall cheerleading and faith that we could do it again.

Leah W. Cleveland, RN, MSN, EdD, CS, was a founding member for the text *Nursing Management in Drug Therapy* and participated in the development of the text now known as *Drug Therapy in Nursing*. Due to prior professional commitments, she was unable to participate in this Second Edition of *Drug Therapy in Nursing*. We thank her for all her prior contributions.

contents

Appendices

features index

CRITICAL THINKING SCENARIOS

COMMUNITY-BASED CONCERNS

FOCUS ON RESEARCH

PHYSIOLOGY FIGURES

MEMORY CHIPS

DRUG SUMMARY TABLES

DRUG INTERACTION TABLES

Foundations for Drug Therapy in Nursing

unit 1

Nursing Management in Drug Therapy

chapter 1

Learning Objectives

At the completion of this chapter the student will:

1 Identify the defining components of core drug knowledge.
2 Identify the defining components of core patient variables.
3 Define nursing management of drug therapy.
4 Describe how the prototype approach to drugs is a helpful learning tool.
5 Differentiate the three main sources of data used in assessment of core drug variables.
6 Describe how core drug knowledge and core patient variables are used in nursing management in drug therapy.
7 Explain general strategies for maximizing the therapeutic effects of drug therapy.
8 Explain general strategies for minimizing adverse effects of drug therapy.
9 Identify the importance of patient and family education in drug therapy.
10 Discuss how to evaluate drug therapy and its nursing management.
11 Describe the varied settings in which nurses use nursing management techniques to assist patients receiving drug therapy.

KEY TERMS

adverse effects
contraindications and precautions
core drug knowledge
core patient variables
culture and inherited traits
drug interactions
drug response
environment
health status
life span and gender
lifestyle, diet, and habits
nursing management in drug therapy
pharmacodynamics
pharmacokinetics
pharmacotherapeutics
prototype drug

FEATURED WEBLINK

http://www.usp.org/information/behav_00.htm
Nurses play a key role in educating patients and their families about drug therapy. Interested in finding out more? Visit the United States Pharmacopeia site for medication counseling behavior guidelines.

CONNECTION WEBLINK

Additional Weblinks are found on Connection:
http://www.connection.lww.com/go/aschenbrenner.

Nurses have a vital role in managing drug therapy of people with medical conditions. The nurse uses knowledge about the drug (core drug knowledge) and knowledge about the individual patient (core patient variables) to maximize the therapeutic effects of the drug, minimize the adverse effects of the drug, and provide patient and family education. The term *patient* is used in this text to identify the person who is taking the drug. It should not be interpreted to mean that drug therapy or the nursing management involved occurs solely in an acute, inpatient setting. Most drug therapy now occurs outside of hospitals.

Nurses apply pharmacology (i.e., the scientific body of drug knowledge) to meeting the assessed care needs of the patient. The pharmacologic facts relevant to each drug, termed **core drug knowledge,** are:

- **Pharmacotherapeutics:** the desired, therapeutic effect of the drug
- **Pharmacokinetics:** the changes that occur to the drug while it is inside the body
- **Pharmacodynamics:** the effects of the drug on the body
- **Contraindications and precautions:** conditions under which the drug should not be used or must be used carefully with monitoring
- **Adverse effects:** unintended and usually undesired effects that may occur with use of the drug
- **Drug interactions:** effects that may occur when the drug is given along with another drug, food, or substance

These components of core drug knowledge are discussed in more depth in Chapters 4 and 5.

In addition to knowing the pharmacologic facts about each drug that a patient receives, nurses assess the patient for factors that may or will interact with drug therapy. These areas of assessment, termed **core patient variables,** are:

- **Health status:** the presence of disease, illness, and allergy; chronic conditions causing system or organ dysfunction; diminished memory or mental capacity
- **Life span and gender:** age, physiologic development, reproductive stage, and gender
- **Lifestyle, diet, and habits:** amount of activity and exercise; sleep–wake patterns; occupation; financial resources or access to health insurance coverage to offset the cost of the drug, or both; eating preferences and patterns; use or abuse of substances (e.g., nicotine, alcohol, and illegal drugs); use of over-the-counter (OTC) drugs; use of alternative health practices (e.g., herbal medicine, folk remedies); and ability to read and write
- **Environment:** location in which the drug therapy will be administered, such as hospital, home, or long-term care facility; properties of the physical environment that may alter a drug's action or effect, induce adverse effects from a drug, or set limitations on whether the drug may be administered in that setting; and exposure to potentially harmful substances, or a pathology induced from a harmful environmental substance, that requires drug therapy for treatment
- **Culture and inherited traits:** religious, social, and ethnic backgrounds that may affect the individual's receptiveness to drug therapy; also, genetic traits that affect a drug's pharmacokinetic and pharmacodynamic properties

The nurse considers the core drug knowledge and the core patient variable categories and determines potentially important interactions between them. An important interaction is an area in which key elements of the drug overlap—or potentially may overlap—with specific patient factors, thus requiring nursing management. **Nursing management in drug therapy** is the process of planning and implementing actions that will maximize the therapeutic effects and minimize the adverse effects of a drug. The nurse also considers these important interactions when planning and providing patient and family education relevant to the drug therapy. Finally, the nurse evaluates the effectiveness of both the drug therapy and the nursing interventions. Thus, the nurse applies knowledge in an individualized manner to meet the care needs of a particular patient receiving a particular drug therapy. Figure 1.1 shows how the interactions between core drug knowledge and core patient variables can be used to manage therapy.

Nursing management in drug therapy helps ensure quality and comprehensive nursing care. It occurs in all settings, including hospitals, long-term care facilities, outpatient centers and clinics, health care providers' offices, and patients' homes. Some aspects of nursing management are more relevant to a particular setting than others are; for example, considering the patient's lifestyle is more important for the nurse when drug therapy occurs in the home than when it occurs in a hospital.

MANAGING DRUG THERAPY THROUGH THE NURSING PROCESS

The nurse uses the nursing process when managing the care of a patient receiving drug therapy. The nursing process is a series of steps in which the nurse assesses and identifies a patient's response to health-related problems and then plans and implements interventions to manage the problem and promote a healthful outcome. The six steps of the nursing process are assessment, diagnosis, outcome identification, planning, intervention, and evaluation. Figure 1.2 shows how the nursing process corresponds to the phases of nursing management in drug therapy.

Assessment

Assessment of Core Drug Knowledge

Nurses need to know about all drugs a patient is taking, including prescribed and OTC drugs. The first step for a nurse is to identify the core drug knowledge relevant to a patient's drug therapy. The nurse needs to be familiar with every drug the patient is taking, to determine whether interactions with core patient variables are likely to occur and consider what nursing management is required. Although memorizing information on every available drug would be difficult, if not impossible, the nurse is responsible for using available, current drug references to review unfamiliar data before administering the drug or instructing the patient to self-administer the drug.

In the assessment phase, the nurse identifies the drug to be administered and its prototype. Currently, more than 3,800 prescription and nonprescription drugs and nutritional and

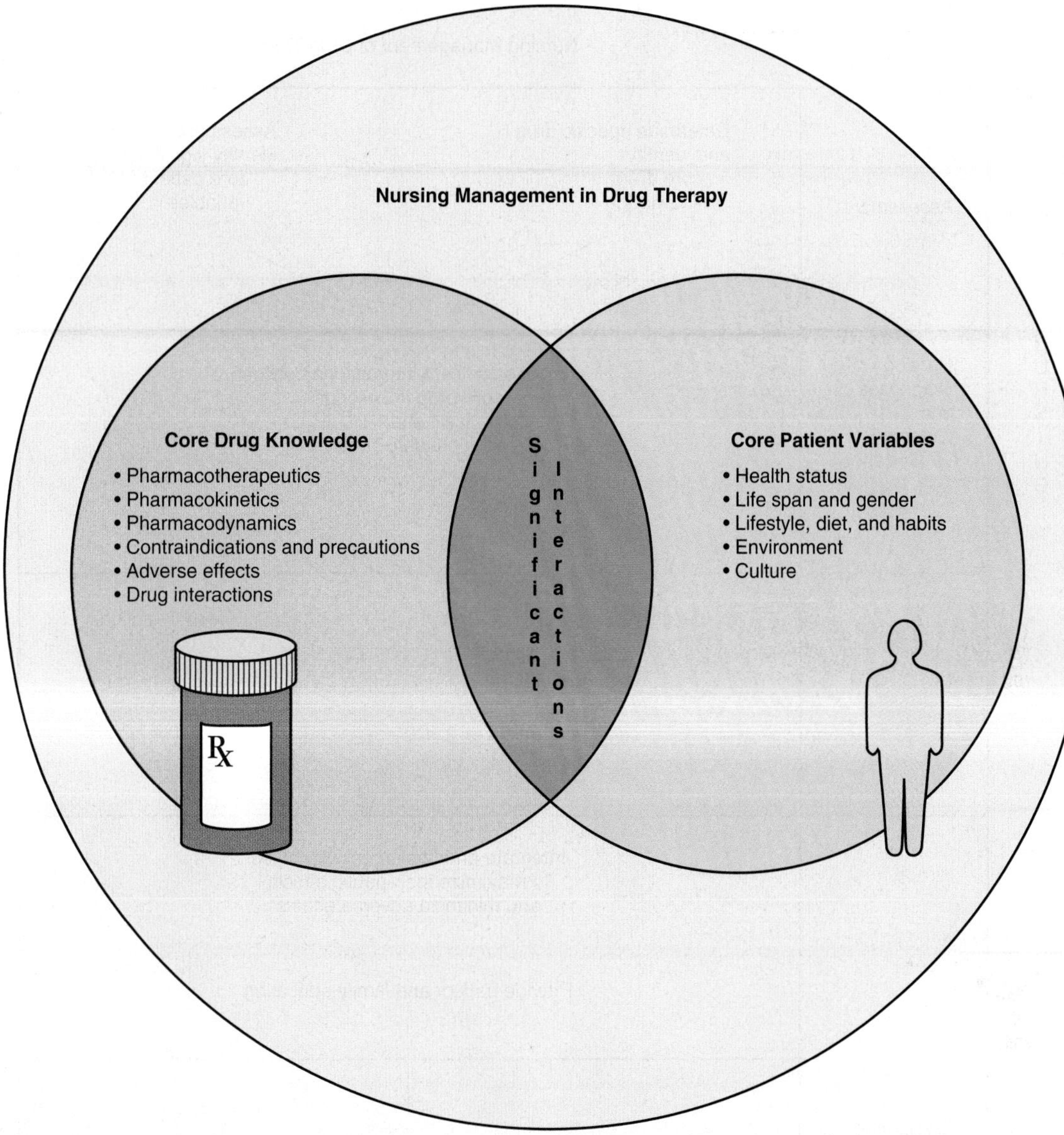

FIGURE 1.1 Relationships among core drug knowledge, core patient variables, and nursing management in drug therapy. The nurse considers both the core drug knowledge and the core patient variables to provide appropriate nursing management in drug therapy.

dietary supplements are listed in the *United States Pharmacopeia* (U.S. Pharmacopeia website). Thousands of combination drugs, both prescription and OTC, as well as brand new drugs are added every year. The sheer volume of drug forms makes it impossible for the nurse to memorize up-to-date information regarding nursing management of every drug. An efficient way to learn and understand as much as possible of the vast information about drugs is to use a prototype approach. A **prototype drug** is typical of a group of drugs within a drug class. For example, hydrochlorothiazide is a prototype drug that represents all of the thiazide diuretics. By learning the core drug knowledge about the prototype, the nurse then knows something about related drugs. Prototypes are typically the first drug of a class. Occasionally, as other drugs in a class are developed, the "original" is not used as frequently in practice. The preference for one particular drug over another is also influenced by regional patterns and trends. This text generally uses the original, or classic, drug in a class as the prototype drug. If this drug is not widely used anymore, another representative drug of the class is used.

Assessment of Core Patient Variables

In drug therapy, the nurse assesses the current health status of the patient and gathers data on other core patient variables to identify those that are relevant to the individual patient. Assessment of the core patient variables also allows the nurse to predict (to some degree) the future needs of the patient. Data for this assessment come from three sources: (1) the patient interview and history, (2) the physical examination, and (3) the medical record, which includes current laboratory and other diagnostic findings. Pertinent findings are then assimilated to form a current, accurate picture of the patient's needs regarding drug therapy. These facts establish a baseline for the patient's treatment and care.

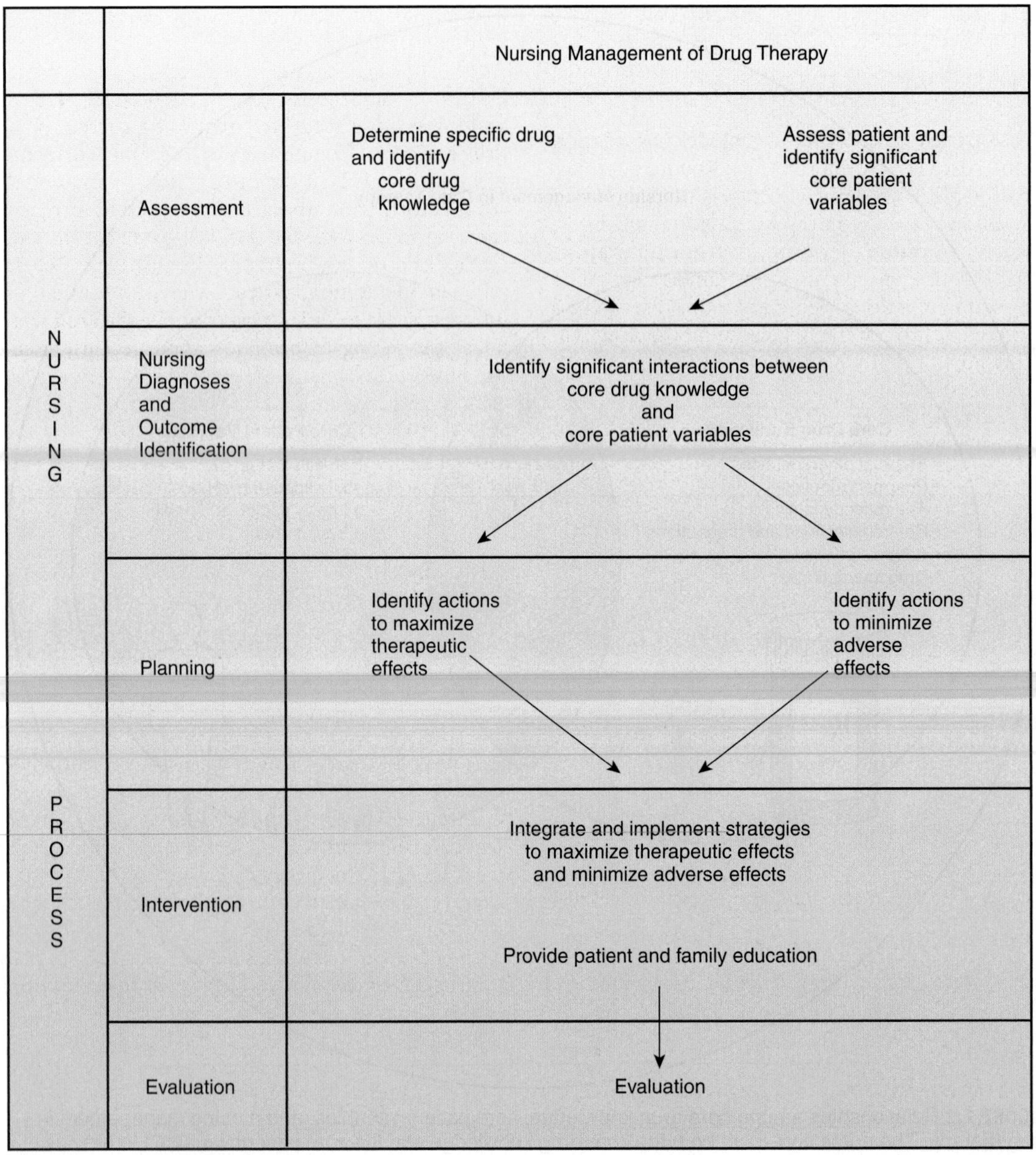

Nursing Management of Drug Therapy
NURSING PROCESS
Assessment
Determine specific drug and identify core drug knowledge
Assess patient and identify significant core patient variables
Nursing Diagnoses and Outcome Identification
Identify significant interactions between core drug knowledge and core patient variables
Planning
Identify actions to maximize therapeutic effects
Identify actions to minimize adverse effects
Intervention
Integrate and implement strategies to maximize therapeutic effects and minimize adverse effects
Provide patient and family education
Evaluation
Evaluation

FIGURE 1.2 Relationship of nursing management in drug therapy to the nursing process.

THE PATIENT INTERVIEW AND HISTORY

Most assessment data come from an assessment interview, in which the patient responds to questions. To be most effective, the nurse asks open-ended questions. Open-ended questions allow the patient to give details and explanations, whereas closed-ended questions require a single or particular response. Although closed-ended questions are a quick way to obtain information, they limit the depth of a response.

An example of an open-ended question is, "What kind of drug allergies do you have, if any?" An example of a closed-ended question is, "Are you allergic to penicillin?" The second question limits the patient's response to "Yes" or "No." Although this response answers the immediate question, important information can be missed. Open-ended questions may elicit the information that the patient is allergic to ampicillin. This fact is important to know because people who are allergic to ampicillin may also be allergic to penicillin. Closed-ended questions are most useful in emergency situations and when particular information must be determined quickly. An open-ended approach is preferable during the assessment interview if time and the patient's physical state permit.

Follow-up questions must be asked whenever the patient responds in a closed-ended manner. If, for example, the patient identifies an allergy to a particular drug, the nurse asks the patient to describe the allergic event. Using this technique, the nurse gains additional information with which to evaluate the patient's response. The patient may believe an event or response is a sign of an allergy, when in fact it may be a normal response to or an adverse effect of the drug. For example, if the patient describes a rash occurring on the third day of taking a drug, this may indicate a true allergy. However, if the patient describes a rash that occurred 6 weeks after completing a drug, a drug allergy is unlikely.

The nurse seeks information on several topics during the assessment interview (Box 1.1) and then determines which core patient variables are relevant to the drug therapy being planned for the individual.

Health Status. A patient's health status includes information about illnesses, diseases, chronic conditions, and allergies. This information allows the nurse to assess functioning of body systems and organs. Impaired functioning may interact with or alter the action of a drug. Pharmacotherapeutics, pharmacokinetics, and pharmacodynamics may all be affected. For example, if the patient has kidney disease, and the drug is excreted through the renal system, the drug will not be eliminated as rapidly as it would in someone with normal kidney function. Because the drug is not eliminated as quickly, the drug levels may remain higher than normally expected. The patient may then exhibit increased therapeutic effect from the drug or be at increased risk for adverse effects. Patients with impaired functioning of a body system or organ may have special educational needs for drug therapy. For example, patients with impaired vision, hearing, or dexterity or those with decreased memory or mental capacity need educational materials tailored to meet their particular needs.

A complete drug history is necessary to assess the health status of the patient adequately and to assess a patient's needs and knowledge accurately regarding current or proposed drug regimens. Components of a complete drug history are given in Box 1.2. In the drug history interview, the nurse seeks information about current drug therapy, including the drug name, dose, and time last given. Any new drugs prescribed should not interact adversely with a current drug regimen. In addition, patients who are admitted to acute or long-term care facilities must continue the drug therapy they have been taking. Information about recently used drugs is also important because some drugs have long-lasting effects that may interact with a newly administered drug. Finally, the patient's drug therapy may have direct bearing on the understanding and interpretation of data obtained from physical assessment and laboratory findings. The data may indicate an expected therapeutic effect, an adverse effect, or an interaction between drugs. For example, knowing that a patient regularly takes the anticoagulant warfarin (Coumadin) would explain why the patient's clotting time is prolonged. Knowing that a patient is currently taking digoxin (Lanoxin), a drug that slows the heart rate, may explain why that person is experiencing adverse drug effects, such as extreme bradycardia with nausea and weakness.

Asking a patient to describe why he or she is taking the drug provides a great deal of information about the learning needs of that patient. The nurse may find that the patient has an excellent knowledge base or, conversely, that the patient has inadequate information or misconceptions concerning drug therapy. One patient may state that the drug is a diuretic to treat hypertension; another patient may state that the drug is a fluid pill; and another patient may have no understanding of what the drug does or why it was prescribed. Patients have different learning needs that require different approaches from the nurse.

Lack of adherence to prescribed drug therapy is very important to determine. However, merely confirming lack

BOX 1.1 Components of the Patient Interview

Health Status

- Presence of acute or chronic disease
- Drug history

General Function and Activity Level

- Developmental level
- Ability to see, read, and write
- Ability to hear and understand spoken instruction
- Occupation
- Activity and exercise patterns
- Sleep and rest patterns
- Dietary patterns: frequency of meals and snacks, foods usually eaten, foods avoided, medical dietary supplements, including vitamins, minerals, and herbal or folk remedies
- Female patients: reproductive status (e.g., pregnant or planning pregnancy, lactating), premenopausal, postmenopausal

Lifestyle and Drug Use

- Insurance and other economic resources to pay for drug therapy
- Street (illegal) drugs used: frequency and route of street drugs, last time street drugs were used
- Alcohol used: amount of alcohol consumed daily, last time alcohol consumed
- Cigarettes or other nicotine-containing products used: amount used daily
- Caffeine used: amount of daily caffeine consumption

Environment

- Description of home setting or living accommodations
- Location of home (city, industrial, suburban, rural)

Culture

- Religious beliefs
- Ethnic practices

BOX 1.2 Components of a Complete Drug History

- Currently prescribed medications
- Prescribed dosages and routes of the medications
- When each medication was last taken
- Patient's description of why the medication was prescribed
- Other prescribed medications taken in the recent past but not currently
- Reason the medications were stopped
- Known drug allergies
- When allergic effect occurred
- Description of specific allergic effects that occurred
- Known food or environmental allergies
- Over-the-counter (OTC) medications used, such as cough and cold remedies, vitamins and minerals, and headache remedies
- Frequency of OTC drug use
- Last time the OTC medications were used

of adherence is not enough; the nurse needs to explore the reason the patient has stopped taking drug therapy as ordered. A patient may have stopped taking a drug for a variety of reasons. The patient may no longer have a medical indication for the drug, or the patient may have had an adverse reaction. The drug may have been discontinued on the advice of the prescriber, or the patient may have discontinued it independently. People may independently stop taking a drug because they think they no longer need it, they think it is not effective, they are experiencing unpleasant adverse effects, the prescription ran out and they cannot get to the pharmacy, or they cannot afford the drug.

Allergies are another aspect of the drug history that must be identified correctly and documented carefully in the medical record. Drug, food, and environmental allergies should be noted. Although allergies are an individual aspect of health status, they are usually considered part of the complete drug history and thus are discussed as part of the drug history rather than as a separate element. Health care providers need to know the patient's allergies so that they do not prescribe or administer drugs to which the individual is allergic. Ask the patient to describe the symptoms of the allergic reaction and note them in the appropriate area of the patient's record. True allergic reactions include formation of rash or hives, itching, redness, swelling, difficulty breathing, and anaphylactic shock. Descriptions of nausea or vomiting, however, are adverse effects of drug therapy. In addition to drug allergies, food or environmental allergies must be identified and documented. Elements of some foods are found in some drugs; for example, iodine is an element of many contrast media used in radiologic studies. Environmental allergens, if present, may complicate the health status of the individual. The nurse also gathers data about the patient's use of OTC drugs; these preparations may interact with prescribed drugs and alter their effect or produce adverse effects.

Life Span and Gender. During assessment, the nurse determines the patient's developmental level, ability to read and write, and ability to understand directions. This information is needed to plan patient education on drug therapy, including the nurse's approach and teaching methods.

Determining the stage of the reproductive cycle of female patients is important. If a drug is extremely toxic to the fetus, women of childbearing age need to be cautioned not to become pregnant while taking the drug. If a woman is past childbearing age (postmenopausal), a drug that is toxic to the fetus may be used. Certain drugs may cross the placenta, affecting fetal growth and development and sometimes causing birth defects or teratogenic effects. Therefore, if the woman is already pregnant, alternative drug therapy is usually indicated. Additionally, assessment for breast-feeding is important because some drugs cross into breast milk and will have some effect on the infant and the mother.

Lifestyle, Diet, and Habits. The nurse asks questions about a patient's lifestyle because of its potential effect on drug therapy. For example, the patient's levels of exercise and general activity may influence drug effect. Patients who are very active and who exercise are likely to have better circulatory systems than those who are inactive. These lifestyle choices affect the distribution of drugs within the body. People who are very active may also be more likely to incur accidental injury than other, less active people. Their increased incidence of injury would put them at greater risk than their more sedentary peers for certain adverse drug effects, such as prolonged bleeding with warfarin, an anticoagulant.

The patient's use of street drugs, alcohol, cigarettes, and caffeine must be determined because these substances can affect some drug actions or alter the health or physiologic functioning of the patient. For example, a cigarette smoker may have respiratory disease. Cigarette smoking also alters the pharmacokinetics of some drugs, such as theophylline, a bronchodilator.

Information on normal dietary intake is useful because food or food elements interact with certain drugs. For example, monoamine oxidase inhibitors (a class of antidepressants) interact with tyramine-rich foods (e.g., aged cheese, red wine) and can induce a hypertensive crisis. Some foods affect the absorption and action of a drug; for example, milk interferes with the absorption of tetracycline, an antibiotic. Many drugs can increase or decrease appetite or alter taste sensations. The nurse needs to assess the patient for these potential effects.

Because instructions for taking many drugs include whether they should be taken with food, the nurse needs to know how frequently and regularly the patient eats. If a drug is to be taken three times a day with food and the patient eats three meals a day, the patient may be instructed to take the drug with meals. However, if the patient normally eats only one or two meals a day or eats five or six meals a day, and this pattern was not assessed, the patient will not receive the correct dosage if the instruction to take with meals is followed.

Sleep and rest patterns and occupation are important to assess because they also have a bearing on drug therapy. People who work nights and sleep during the day will need the timing of their drug dosages varied because a daytime schedule is usually recommended for taking drugs, to enable uninterrupted sleep at night. Knowledge of the patient's customary rest patterns provides a baseline to determine whether drug therapy is therapeutic (e.g., a drug given to induce sleep) or whether an adverse drug effect (e.g., insomnia) is occurring. Certain occupations may place the patient at risk for injury and consequently at risk for adverse effects from some drugs.

Economic factors may determine whether the patient will adhere to prescribed drug therapy; therefore, these factors should be assessed. If the drug is very expensive and the patient cannot afford the drug or health insurance to offset or defray drug costs, the patient's inability to purchase the drug may preclude his or her adherence to therapy.

Environment. The home setting or living environment is assessed because it may give clues to the patient's adherence to the drug regimen or to potential risks from the therapy. For example, if a patient is receiving a drug that causes dizziness as an adverse effect, stairs in the house may pose a risk for falls. If the home does not have running water, a patient may be unable to adhere to handwashing instructions that precede self-injection of insulin. General factors to assess include cleanliness, lighting, adequate heat, water, and refrigeration. A home visit by a visiting or home health nurse may be the most accurate way to obtain this information.

Environmental factors outside of the home may also affect drug therapy. Environmental elements or substances in the environment may predispose the patient to adverse drug

effects. Direct sunlight, for example, may cause sunburn when the patient is prone to photosensitivity from tetracycline, an antibiotic.

The nurse needs to determine the environment in which the drug will be administered. Some drug therapy occurs only in certain environments or settings (e.g., general anesthetics are only given in an operating room). Other drugs, such as oral antibiotics, may be used in all health care settings, including the patient's home. The strategies selected to maximize therapeutic effect or minimize adverse effects may depend on the drug administration environment. Materials selected for patient and family teaching may also depend on the environment in which drug therapy occurs. Patients may start drug therapy in one environment and continue therapy in another—for example, the hospital and then the home—or therapy may be lifelong, as with antidiabetic agents. The patient may begin taking a drug in a hospital and continue taking it in a subacute care center before concluding therapy in the center or continuing therapy at home. Planning for discharge of a patient from an acute care setting begins the day of admission. Therefore, during assessment, the nurse must gather data that will be important in meeting the goals of drug therapy once the patient is discharged. Where the patient will go after discharge will alter the education required. If the patient will receive drug therapy at home, the nurse needs to assess the home as previously described.

Some home drug therapies, such as intravenous (IV) therapy, may require special equipment, technologies, or skills. In these cases, the nurse assesses the ability of the patient or responsible caregiver to administer drug therapy safely and effectively. Additional assessments are made about the ability to take appropriate actions if a problem occurs. For example, the nurse needs to know whether the patient or caregiver can describe the actions he or she would take if an infection occurred as a result of IV therapy. The nurse can assess this information by asking hypothetical questions about typically encountered problems and having the patient or caregiver describe how to handle the problem described.

Culture and Inherited Traits. Culture and inherited traits is the last core patient variable to include in the health history and drug assessment. This text uses the term *culture* in its broadest interpretation, which may not directly reflect the definition given by some sociologists or anthropologists. Religious restrictions or cultural practices may affect the patient's acceptance of prescribed drug therapy. Christian Scientists, for example, who believe in healing through prayer, may not accept drug therapy to manage hypertension. Patients with some ethnic backgrounds may have altered responses to particular drug therapies. African Americans, for example, exhibit a diminished therapeutic response to antihypertensive agents, such as angiotensin-converting enzyme inhibitors.

Recently, it has been determined that there may be individual variation to drug therapy. These variations are inherited but are not related to racial or ethnic backgrounds. Instead, they are caused by genetic variations. These unique genetic variations may not be evident until a patient begins therapy with a particular drug; that is, they cannot be predicted ahead of time. Many of these variations are related to the P-450 isoenzyme system. Specific knowledge about the effects of genetic variation on drug therapy is currently in its infancy. Genetic research is being conducted to identify the presence or absence of various isoenzymes in individuals. Knowing whether a patient lacks a specific isoenzyme used in metabolizing a particular drug before starting drug therapy would enable the therapy to be tailored to the patient's needs, preventing possible adverse effects.

THE PHYSICAL EXAMINATION

After completing the health history interview, the nurse performs the second part of the assessment—the physical examination. The physical examination focuses on the core patient variables of health status and life span and gender and should be comprehensive. The patient's history and present complaints (the main reason for seeking health care) usually dictate which body systems require in-depth assessment.

General observation will provide some information on health status. Approximate age and, depending on the stage, pregnancy, can be determined by general observation as well. Physical assessment of the systems (e.g., the respiratory system) will provide information about disease or illness.

Baseline data, such as vital signs, height, and weight, must be measured. Ideally, the height and weight are taken directly by the nurse or someone delegated by the nurse (rather than asking the patient for this information). An accurate measurement of body size is an important factor in computing the correct dose of many drugs. During emergencies, this information may be estimated.

The nurse closely inspects the skin of all patients for rashes and document their appearance and location. Failure to do so could result in the rash being misinterpreted as a drug reaction. If IV drugs may be ordered, other areas to inspect closely are the peripheral blood vessels. If a history of IV drug abuse is reported, scarring or inflammation of the vessels may be present. In such cases, the nurse can anticipate potential problems with IVs.

All gathered data must be analyzed in terms of the specific current and proposed drugs, identifying any actual and potential problems related to providing drug therapy.

THE MEDICAL RECORD

In addition to the patient interview and history and physical examination, complete assessment data for the core patient variables are also derived from a review of the patient's medical record and test results. The medical record provides information about the patient's health status, lifestyle, diet, habits, and environment.

Areas of the medical record that are specifically important include laboratory and other diagnostic test results. For drug therapy, pertinent findings may include blood levels of a drug or test results related to drug action. For example, blood glucose levels are pertinent findings in diabetic patients receiving insulin to control hyperglycemia. A computed tomography scan report indicating the tumor burden of a patient receiving chemotherapy is also a relevant finding. The nurse reviews all diagnostic findings, paying special attention to those findings relevant to body systems at risk for adverse effects from currently used drugs (Table 1.1).

Past medical records may be used to verify the patient's drug history. Moreover, they may provide details relevant to the patient's current treatment. Patients may forget previous drug reactions, past illnesses, family histories, and other essential baseline information, but these data may be available in previous medical records. Review of the med-

TABLE 1.1 General* Laboratory Test Values: Normal Ranges

System Tested	Diagnostic Test	Normal Values
Hepatic	Bilirubin (total)	0.3–1.0 mg/dL
	Indirect unconjugated bilirubin	0.2–0.7 mg/dL
	Direct conjugated bilirubin	0.1–0.4 mg/dL
	AST (formerly SGOT)	7–27 U/L
	ALT (formerly SGPT)	1–21 U/L
	PTT	20–30 s
	PT	12–14 s
Renal	BUN	8–25 mg/dL
	Serum creatinine	0.6–1.5 mg/dL
	Creatinine clearance	Women: 120–180 L/d
Hematologic	Hct	Men: 140–200 L/d Women: 36%–48%
	Hgb	Men: 42%–52% Women: 12–16 g/dL
	WBC count	Men: 14–18 g/dL
	Platelets	5,000–10,000/mm^3 150,000–400,000/mm^3

*Ranges for normal laboratory test values may vary according to health care setting, the laboratory performing the test, and the testing equipment. This information should be considered a basic guide. Nurses need to be familiar with normal ranges used in the facility or agency in which they work.

Fischbach, F.T. (2001). *Nurses' quick reference to common laboratory and diagnostic tests (3rd ed.).* Philadelphia: Lippincott Williams & Wilkins.

ical record is important regardless of whether the drug is administered in a hospital, extended care facility, outpatient center, or the patient's home. This part of the assessment can be done either before or after the interview and physical examination.

See the accompanying display, Identifying Core Patient Variables, for a critical thinking approach to identifying the core patient variables discussed in the previous sections.

CRITICAL THINKING SCENARIO

Identifying core patient variables

1. Propose questions to ask patients who tell you that they are allergic to a drug.
2. Your patient, a 75-year-old man living on a fixed income from a Social Security pension, is to be discharged on a new drug for hypertension. In assessing core drug knowledge for the patient's drug therapy, you identify adverse effects of dizziness and dry mouth. Identify the core patient variables that you would evaluate most carefully for relevance to this patient's drug therapy.

Nursing Diagnoses and Outcome Identification

Data that have been gathered throughout the patient's assessment are interpreted by the nurse according to their relevance to drug therapy. The nurse reviews the core drug knowledge and the core patient variables from which significant interactions may be generated. The nursing diagnoses and patient outcomes are names or labels given to these interactions.

Nursing diagnoses are based on classifications proposed by the North American Nursing Diagnosis Association (NANDA). The diagnosis may reflect a current, actual problem or the risk for developing a problem related to drug therapy. A patient may be receiving a drug that addresses a current problem, yet use of this drug may put the patient at risk for developing other problems. For example, a patient has a nursing diagnosis of Chronic Pain related to cancer. If the patient is taking morphine to control the pain, the diagnoses related to the drug therapy would be Risk for Injury related to sedation from narcotic drug use and Constipation related to adverse effects of morphine. Selected nursing diagnoses pertaining to drug effects are given in Box 1.3.

In addition to diagnoses that reflect current or potential problems from effects of drugs, many other types of drug-related diagnoses may be appropriate. The diagnosis of Deficient Knowledge may be appropriate if a new drug has been prescribed. Ineffective Therapeutic Regimen Management may be appropriate if the individual has not been taking drug therapy as prescribed because he or she has misunderstood the directions. Ineffective Coping may be a nursing diagnosis for a patient who continually forgets to take a prescribed drug for a chronic condition (e.g., insulin for diabetes). Nursing diagnoses are highly individualized and cannot be predicted from prescribed drug therapy alone. Reputable textbooks devoted specifically to nursing diagnosis contain additional information.

BOX 1.3 Selected Nursing Diagnoses Pertaining to Drug Effects

- Constipation
- Diarrhea
- Acute Pain
- Chronic Pain
- Fatigue
- Risk for Infection
- Risk for Injury
- Disturbed Sensory Perception
- Ineffective Sexuality Patterns
- Disturbed Sleep Pattern
- Disturbed Thought Processes
- Interrupted Breast-feeding
- Acute Confusion
- Deficient Fluid Volume
- Excess Fluid Volume
- Imbalanced Nutrition: More than Body Requirements
- Imbalanced Nutrition: Less than Body Requirements
- Impaired Urinary Elimination
- Urinary Retention

The next phase of the nursing process is outcome identification—that is, determining the desired results of nursing interventions. Outcomes develop from the data gained in assessment, and the diagnosis selected. A plan for a patient receiving drug therapy would identify outcomes related to the patient's specific drug regimen.

Planning

Once the important interactions between the core drug knowledge and the core patient variables have been identified, the nurse devises strategies to maximize the therapeutic effects and minimize the adverse effects of the drug therapy. The nursing process step of planning is used. Planning begins with identifying interventions necessary to reach the desired outcome. Planning continues by defining what needs to be done to achieve the identified outcomes.

Maximizing Therapeutic Effects

To maximize the therapeutic effects of any given drug therapy, the nurse must know what the desired therapeutic effects are and how they are achieved. Strategies appropriate for the patient are then used to promote these effects. Although these strategies are drug specific, a few general principles exist:

- Administer the drug in a manner that will promote its absorption. A drug administered orally may be given with meals or on an empty stomach, depending on the drug. When giving a drug parenterally, use the appropriate administration technique for the desired route. A route different from that prescribed may alter absorption and the desired effect. For example, if an intramuscular injection is accidentally given subcutaneously, absorption will be slower and the onset of the therapeutic effect delayed.
- Administer the drug at the appropriate time to maintain blood levels of the drug that will promote therapeutic effects.
- Monitor laboratory values, when appropriate, to determine that the prescribed dose achieves a therapeutic drug level.

Minimizing Adverse Effects

Many of the nursing care strategies are directed at minimizing the adverse effects of drug therapy. Again, the strategies are specific to the drug, but some are common to all drug therapy:

- Before initiating drug therapy, verify that the patient is not allergic to the drug and that the drug is not contraindicated for this patient for some reason.
- Administer the drug in a manner consistent with standard safety protocols. For example, some drugs must be administered intravenously at a regular, steady rate, and the use of an IV infusion controller, or pump, is considered standard for these drugs.
- Monitor the patient and relevant laboratory findings closely for evidence of known adverse effects from drug therapy. Patients at high risk for developing a particular adverse effect should be monitored especially carefully.
- Discontinue or withhold a drug if the laboratory findings warrant doing so. Notify the prescriber of the findings and your actions.
- Report evidence of adverse effects to the prescriber as soon as possible.
- Modify administration techniques, when appropriate, to decrease the incidence of adverse effects. For example, if the drug causes the patient gastrointestinal distress on an empty stomach, administer the drug with food.
- Implement appropriate techniques for certain drugs to detect the onset of adverse effects. For example, monitor blood pressure before administering each dose of an antihypertensive drug to determine whether the blood pressure has decreased too much to administer the drug.

Intervention

The next phase of the nursing process is intervention: performing the plan. With intervention, the nurse integrates the devised strategies into the nursing plan of care for the patient receiving drug therapy. These strategies are relevant to the physical act of drug administration and to patient and family education about drug therapy, an essential part of implementing any therapeutic plan. The nurse integrates the recognized interactions of the core drug knowledge and the core patient variables into this patient and family education. Thus, the education is specific to the drug therapy and specific to the patient's needs.

Core Drug Knowledge

The nurse has a crucial role in educating patients and their families about drug therapy. The goal of patient education is for the individual patient to understand the drug and its effects well enough to self-medicate safely and effectively and to monitor the **drug response** (i.e., the anticipated therapeutic and adverse effects). Basic drug therapy education should include the name of the drug, the reason the drug was prescribed (pharmacotherapeutics), the intended effect of the drug (pharmacodynamics), and important adverse effects that may occur and should be reported to the nurse or health care provider. If the patient will be taking the drug at home, he or she also needs to know when, how frequently, and for how long to take it; how to store it; and what to do if a dose is missed. In addition, the patient must be aware of any special concerns regarding other drugs or foods taken (drug interactions) and trained in any special techniques needed for self-administration of the drug to maximize therapeutic or minimize adverse effects. This information is obtained from the prescription and from the core drug knowledge of pharmacokinetics and pharmacodynamics.

Core Patient Variables

Any or all of the core patient variables may have a bearing on the educational needs of the patient or the family. Patient variables may affect which educational materials should be provided and the format or method of presentation.

HEALTH STATUS

Education related to the core patient variable of health status includes information about those activities that must be performed while the patient receives the drug to maintain health or to detect early changes in health that are related to adverse effects of the drug. For example, there may be a need for periodic laboratory tests, such as monitoring levels of theophylline (a bronchodilator) or monitoring bleeding

time in a patient receiving an anticoagulant. Periodic examination or assessment by a health care provider may also be required, for example, to monitor blood pressure when the patient is receiving antihypertensives.

The current health status of the patient must also be considered. The following are questions a nurse considers when designing a patient education program for drug therapy:

- Has any current disease or condition impaired any organ or system functioning, leaving the patient at risk for certain adverse effects? If so, information on these adverse effects should be emphasized during educational sessions.
- Does the patient have impaired vision that may prohibit reading drug labels or contribute to making errors, such as misreading the number "3" as a "5" in the instruction, "Take 3 times a day"? A vision problem may also indicate that educational material cannot be presented in written form to this patient.
- Does the patient have a hearing loss that may interfere with the comprehension of oral teaching?
- Does the patient have difficulty with small motor movements, perhaps because of arthritis in the hands? If so, difficulty in opening drug bottles may be a problem.
- Does the patient remember spoken conversations well? If not, written education may be effective. If memory loss is severe, adherence to the prescribed drug regimen may be difficult to achieve, and devices or systems developed to help the patient remember to take the correct drugs at the correct time may be indicated.
- Does the patient have the mental capacity to understand the information presented on drug therapy? If not, another person may have to be responsible for administering the drug to the patient.

LIFE SPAN AND GENDER

The life span variable becomes important when a drug therapy has the potential to produce adverse effects on a developing fetus. Women of childbearing age need to be educated not to become pregnant while taking certain drugs. Age is also an important consideration when determining a patient education approach. For example, drug education for a preschooler will most likely be directed to the parents, whereas education for an adolescent is directed so that the adolescent becomes an active partner in the educational process.

LIFESTYLE, DIET, AND HABITS

When planning patient education, consider lifestyle and behavioral changes the patient may need to make during drug therapy because of the action or adverse effect of the drug. For example, a patient taking narcotics for pain will be drowsy because the drug depresses the central nervous system. This patient is cautioned not to drive a car or operate potentially hazardous machinery while taking the drug. A patient receiving an antihistamine for an allergic reaction may also experience drowsiness as an adverse drug effect and should be similarly cautioned. Other lifestyle changes may be indicated, such as avoiding alcohol or cigarettes because they may alter a drug's effect. For example, cimetidine is less effective in decreasing gastric acid production in a patient who smokes cigarettes while taking this drug.

The patient's lifestyle determines the value placed on patient education. The patient education information may be considered important by the nurse, but the patient may not share this view; thus, the educational process will not be very effective. The nurse needs to determine what the patient wants to know about the drug and what the patient believes has the most significance for him or her. Ideally, the educational process begins with the nurse giving answers to what the patient wants to know, even if the nurse believes that other, unasked questions may be more important. Meeting the needs of the patient will increase the effectiveness of the education and promote receptivity to additional teaching at a later time.

The nurse must consider the patient's learning style when selecting an approach to patient education. Some people are visual learners, and the use of videotapes may be a better teaching medium for them than printed information. Other people need to be physically involved in their learning, and role-playing or demonstration and return demonstration may be better educational techniques for them.

When using written educational materials, the nurse must take into consideration the patient's literacy level: Can the patient read and write in the language used in those materials? Written materials are appropriate for individuals who can read. However, they must be at the patient's reading level. If appropriate, standardized drug information sheets may be used. Many health care settings distribute these sheets for patient use. Additionally, some drug references are available that are designed to be photocopied and given to patients. If a standard information sheet is unavailable, the nurse can create one or simply write down instructions for taking the drugs along with a dosage schedule (Box 1.4).

BOX 1.4 Patient Education Guidelines

When preparing educational materials for patients receiving drug therapy, the nurse includes guidelines on the following:

- Drug name: generic and trade names
- Purpose of the drug
- Contraindication to taking the drug
- When to take the drug (time, frequency)
- Duration of treatment
- How to take the drug
- What to do if a dose is forgotten
- Special instructions related to lifestyle changes while on the drug
- Hazardous activities to avoid while on the drug
- Any dietary restrictions or additions
- Drug-food interactions
- Drug-drug interactions, including those that may result from over-the-counter drugs
- Adverse effects and instructions on what to do about them
- Special storage needs if applicable
- Special directions for drug disposal
- Therapeutic monitoring needed while taking the drug
- Periodic laboratory tests needed while taking the drug
- Precautions related to pregnancy or lactation
- Health care providers who should be notified about the drug therapy (e.g., dentist by patient taking an anticoagulant)
- Advisability of carrying or wearing a drug alert card or medical identification
- Period of time drug remains active after discontinuing therapy

ENVIRONMENT

Environment is an important consideration when educating a patient and family about drug therapy. The extent of teaching will vary, depending on the environment in which the patient receives the drug. Although some education is required regardless of the setting, more information is necessary if the patient will be taking the drug at home. These patients must know about all aspects of the drug so that its administration can be safely and effectively self-managed. If another person—family member or someone else—will be responsible for the patient's drug therapy at home, that person needs to be included in the educational process.

The physical properties of the home may also affect the patient education required; the home setup may increase the risk for injury or adverse effects from a drug. For example, if the home has scatter rugs, the patient needs to be educated about the increased risk for falls while receiving drug therapy that may cause an unsteady gait. General considerations for home- or community-based therapy are given in Box 1.5.

CULTURE AND INHERITED TRAITS

When educating the patient and family about drug therapy, the nurse needs to be sensitive to the patient's cultural frame of reference. A person's religious and ethnic background influences his or her beliefs about health, wellness, and the role of drug therapy in maintaining or restoring health. Cultural background may also influence communication patterns and determine the appropriate family member to be involved in educational sessions. Depending on the culture, this person may or may not be the patient. The patient's cultural background is neither right nor wrong. To provide effective education, the nurse must consider cultural issues and modify content or presentation accordingly. The nurse must adapt to meet the patient's needs. If it has been determined that the patient has a unique response to a particular drug therapy, the patient education must also be individualized.

BOX 1.5 General Considerations for Home- or Community-Based Drug Therapy

The nurse needs to explore considerations, such as those below, when assessing the ability of the patient or responsible others to self-manage drug therapy safely at home:

Patient Considerations

- Ability to see and read labels
- Ability to remember dosage schedule
- Ability to open medication containers
- Ability to perform any special techniques required for drug administration

Home Considerations

- Safe storage areas for keeping medications out of the reach of small children who may live in or visit the patient's home
- Adequate refrigeration if the medication needs to be chilled
- Convenient and safe storage areas for equipment, particularly the equipment needed to administer medication (e.g., intravenous (IV) pumps and controllers, nebulizers)
- Adequate and secure disposal containers for medication or equipment

Educational Considerations and Aids

- Thorough, clear, written instructions for medication administration
- Memory aids, such as a calendar, dosage chart, or a clock-faced picture with the appropriate medication doses identified at the correct times
- Organized, convenient system for accessing medication such as
  - Keeping all medication containers in a bowl, small box, or on a special shelf
  - Dispensing one day's medication in a pill box or commercially available organizer or the individual compartments of an empty egg carton
  - Numbering or color coding drug containers if the patient has a reading or language problem
- Organized, convenient system for drug delivery equipment (syringes, alcohol wipes, transdermal patches, drug pumps, IV tubing, and so forth), such as a box, a plastic storage container with a snap-on lid, or clean, dry glass jars with screw tops
- Impervious, puncture-proof containers with properly fitting lids, such as coffee cans or plastic milk jugs, for disposing of needles, syringes, and other equipment

Evaluation

Like the nursing process, nursing management in drug therapy ends with evaluation. At the end of the established time frame for achieving an expected outcome, the nurse measures the patient's progress. Was the outcome or goal achieved? Was the nursing management effective? These two measurements are not the same. An outcome can be achieved despite an ineffective plan. For example, a patient may not have adverse effects from drug therapy despite the nurse's not thoroughly identifying actions to minimize adverse effects. Or the management may have been appropriate, although the goal was not achieved. For example, the patient may experience an adverse drug effect even though the nurse appropriately identified and implemented strategies to minimize adverse effects. In evaluating the effectiveness of drug therapy, one of the most important aspects to consider is whether the drug achieved the desired effect. For example, an antihypertensive drug is given to lower blood pressure. Did the blood pressure drop to a safe and normal range? If so, then the evaluation shows that drug therapy was effective.

If the patient does not achieve the expected outcomes, the nurse must reassess to identify the barriers to success. Perhaps the nurse missed an important interaction between the core drug knowledge and the core patient variables. Perhaps the nurse did not identify a core patient variable. Perhaps the teaching strategies used were not effective for this patient, and a different approach should be attempted. Perhaps the identified outcome is not appropriate for this patient, or the outcome may be appropriate but the time frame inadequate. Evaluation is not merely determining whether the goals were achieved or the management was effective. The reason behind any treatment failure must be identified and steps taken to achieve desired results effectively.

CLINICAL PATHWAYS

Nursing management in drug therapy may be used in clinical pathways (also known as critical pathways). A clinical pathway is an interdisciplinary approach to care that establishes

common protocols for patients with the same medical diagnoses. These pathways specify the responsibilities, actions, and time frame required of each discipline (e.g., nursing, medicine, physical therapy, pharmacy, respiratory therapy) to meet the objectives required to complete the care plan.

Clinical pathways provide a standard of care for all patients with the same diagnosis. The pathway accounts for the drugs ordered as a treatment for or response to a specific condition. For example, the clinical pathway for a patient with deep vein thrombosis usually has drug therapy beginning with the anticoagulant heparin. After 3 to 4 days, the patient usually receives an oral anticoagulant, such as warfarin sodium. When the patient's blood tests indicate that the oral anticoagulant is at a therapeutic level, heparin therapy stops. If the patient meets the requirements of the pathway in the time specified, the therapy is evaluated as effective.

Nursing management in drug therapy still occurs with the use of the clinical pathway. Clinical pathways are not substitutes for nursing assessment and judgment. Assessing core drug knowledge and core patient variables, identifying their significant interactions, developing strategies to maximize therapeutic effects and minimize adverse effects, and providing patient and family education not only form the basis of astute nursing care but also contribute to early identification of a patient at risk for "falling off" the pathway. Early identification of the patient at risk alters plans of care, prevents complications, and minimizes additional inpatient days.

CHAPTER SUMMARY

- Core drug knowledge, which consists of basic pharmacologic facts about each drug, is composed of pharmacotherapeutics, pharmacokinetics, pharmacodynamics, contraindications and precautions, adverse effects, and drug interactions.
- Core patient variables are features that make a patient unique at any given time.
- The nurse determines which of the patient's core patient variables are relevant to a particular drug therapy. They include health status; life span and gender; lifestyle, diet, and habits; environment; and culture and inherited traits.
- The nurse determines which significant interactions will occur between the core drug knowledge and the core patient variables. The nurse then recommends strategies based on those interactions to maximize the therapeutic effect and minimize the adverse effects of drug therapy. The nurse integrates these strategies into a nursing plan of care. Patient and family education is also based on the interactions between core drug knowledge and core patient variables. This process is nursing management in drug therapy.
- A prototype drug is a drug that is representative of a class of drugs. Acquiring the core drug knowledge about the prototype provides the nurse with information about several other drugs in the same class as the prototype drug. Acquiring core drug knowledge organizes and simplifies learning about many different drugs.
- In providing nursing management of drug therapy, the steps of the nursing process are used. Nursing management of drug therapy occurs in all health care environments, including acute care, long-term care, and home and community settings.
- A thorough drug assessment provides the baseline information needed for effective nursing management of drug therapy. It includes the patient history, physical assessment, and examination of the medical record.
- Nursing diagnoses and outcomes are labels given to the identified interactions between core drug knowledge and core patient variables.
- Nursing diagnoses for patients receiving drug therapy reflect current or potential problems relevant to the therapy.
- Expected outcomes define the units of measure by which to gauge the effectiveness of drug therapy.
- Patient and family education is a crucial aspect of nursing management in drug therapy. Individualized education proceeds from the baseline core drug knowledge and core patient variables.
- Drug therapy is evaluated as effective if the desired effect of the drug occurs. The nurse also evaluates whether the management plan was effective. If conclusions drawn from the evaluation show that the drug effect or the management plan was not achieved, the nurse must determine why and then respond accordingly.
- An important goal of home-based drug therapy is for patients and caregivers to acquire the knowledge and skills needed to implement drug therapy safely and effectively. The nursing management of drug therapy must take the home setting into consideration. Education is structured so that patients and caregivers can assume maximal responsibility for administering and monitoring drug therapy safely and effectively.

QUESTIONS FOR STUDY AND REVIEW

1. How does the nurse assess core patient variables?
2. Why does the nurse need to assess the core drug knowledge of each drug a patient receives?
3. How does learning core drug knowledge about prototype drugs help the nurse?
4. How do the core patient variables affect the patient education that is provided?

? **Need More Help?**

Chapter 1 of the study guide for *Drug Therapy in Nursing* 2e contains NCLEX-style questions and other learning activities to reinforce your understanding of the concepts presented in this chapter. For additional information or to purchase the study guide, visit *http://connection.lww.com/go/aschenbrenner.*

REFERENCES AND BIBLIOGRAPHY

U.S. Pharmacopeia. (2004). [Online]. Available: *http://www.usp.org*.

Pharmaceuticals: Development, Safeguards, and Delivery

chapter 2

Learning Objectives

At the completion of this chapter the student will:

1. Identify key concepts relevant to nursing management in pharmacotherapy.
2. Name four main sources of drugs and biologic products.
3. Describe the differences in the ways that drugs are named.
4. Explain the significance of drug classifications.
5. Identify sources of drug information.
6. Describe the scope of nursing responsibilities related to pharmacology.
7. Discuss the application of the nursing process related to pharmacology.
8. Describe the intent, scope, and benefits of drug standards and legislation.
9. Identify several references and resources that list standards regulating drug development, distribution, and use.
10. Explain new drug development and the role of nurses in clinical trials.
11. Differentiate between over-the-counter and legend (prescription) drugs.
12. Discuss the significance of the 1970 Controlled Substance Act and its relationship to nursing practice.
13. Compare drug legislation in the United States with drug legislation in Canada.

KEY TERMS

Canadian Food and Drugs Act
chemical classification
chemical name
clinical trials
controlled substance
drug classification
Federal Food, Drug, and Cosmetics Act of 1938
generic name
genomics
legend drugs
National Formulary
physiologic classification
placebo response
Practitioners' Reporting Network
preclinical trials
Pure Food and Drug Act of 1906
therapeutic classification
trade name
United States Adopted Names Council
United States Pharmacopeia

FEATURED WEBLINK

http://www.fda.gov/cder/approval/index.htm
New drugs are approved by the FDA every month. Want to keep current? You can have up-to-date information automatically emailed to you.

CONNECTION WEBLINK

Additional Weblinks are found on Connection:
http://www.connection.lww.com/go/aschenbrenner.

What is a drug? By definition, a drug is any chemical that can affect living processes.

Virtually all chemicals can be considered drugs because when given in large enough amounts, all chemicals will have some effect on life.

Drugs have been used throughout the ages, even in prehistoric times. Drugs used today are essential in treating a variety of health problems ranging from hypertension and heart disease to cancer, pneumonia, and mental health disorders. Because pharmacotherapy is an integral piece of Western medicine, it is imperative that today's nurse understands the development, safeguards, and delivery of drugs.

HISTORICAL PERSPECTIVES OF DRUG DEVELOPMENT

Throughout history, humankind has been interested in the treatment and prevention of disease (Box 2.1). Early civilizations viewed disease with great superstition, and treatments were often directed toward driving away evil spirits and invoking religious and mystical powers. Pharmacologic knowledge up to the 19th century was derived from simple observation and practical experience. During the 19th century, however, pharmacology evolved into a highly specialized science, and the branch of pharmaceutical chemistry developed. The ability to isolate active components of drugs for study under controlled conditions facilitated the scientific method of inquiry; medicine based on systematic reasoning and rigorous testing of theory began to replace the more basic observational approach.

The emerging sciences of botany and physiology, quantitative chemistry, and systematic biology enabled modern pharmacology to emerge. Pharmacologists could study the action of pure drugs in the body and discover new active drugs in the plant world. Today, researchers examine rain forests and jungles for sources of new drugs to treat diseases. Scientists of the 21st century expect to develop new drugs through chemical synthesis, manipulation of enzymes and hormones, and genetic engineering, making pharmacology a complex science with a vast drug-manufacturing component. Highlights of advancements in pharmacology during the 20th century include the use of computer technology, which facilitates rational drug design and replaces some animal studies, and biotechnology, which permits the targeting of specific drug action and expands drug development procedures. One technique, receptor isolation, expands the potential for developing drugs with greater selectivity and reduced toxicity. Cell culture techniques permit the study of drug action at cellular and molecular levels. Immunochemistry leads to diagnosis that is more accurate and to the treatment of formerly untreatable diseases. The new drug classes that sometimes result from such advances in pharmacology provide novel means to treat and manage disease.

SOURCES OF DRUGS

As we have learned more about drugs and how they affect the human body, pharmaceutical companies have focused on four sources of current drug products: plants, animals, synthetic chemicals, and genetically engineered chemicals.

BOX 2.1 Pharmacology Across the Ages

- **Prehistory** (before written language). Archeological findings (some before 4000 B.C.) suggest tribal beliefs that evil spirits caused illness. Magical spells and potions of elemental substances (plants, animals, waters) used by tribal healers exorcised the evil spirits.
- **2700 B.C., China.** First pharmacology "textbook" documents medicinal use of natural substances (e.g., laxative properties of rhubarb and senna).
- **2100 B.C., Sumeria (Iraq).** Earliest prescriptions of medicinal mixtures are recorded.
- **2000 B.C., Babylon; North and South America.** Hammurabi's Code of Law provides protection from unskilled physicians (medical malpractice) and rewards for successful treatment of illness.
  - North American Iroquois Indians use herbs to stimulate taste.
  - South American Peruvian Incas use herbs as diuretics and respiratory stimulants.
- **1500 B.C., Egypt, Israel.** Early Egyptian scrolls record observations, diagnoses, remedies (e.g., aloe, castor oil, honey, opium, peppermint, vinegar), and medical data describing drug forms (gargles, poultices, powders); this is the beginning of polypharmacy.
  - Hebrew teacher-physicians use wine, fig poultices, and vinegar for medicine; Talmud records health practices and taboos.
  - The Mosaic Health Code records hygienic and sanitary practices.
- **400 B.C., Greece.** Writings of Hippocrates (father of medicine) identify more than 400 drugs and treatment methods (diet, exercise, lifestyle).
- **200 B.C., India.** Hindu priests record using colchicum, gentian, castor beans, and digitalis for medicinal purposes.
- **100 A.D., Greece.** Dioscorides writes *De Materia Medica,* a medical textbook, discussing drugs and their uses.
- **200 A.D., Greece.** Galen advocates medicinal use of vegetable preparations.
- **500–1500 A.D., Arab settlements; monastic gardeners of Europe.** Compendium of drugs (e.g., borax, ergot, cinnabar) and drug uses develops as Arabs practice pharmacy separately from medicine. The compilation systematizes the preparation of medicinal compounds and serves as the first set of drug standards.
  - Herbs such as clover, primrose, and belladonna were cultivated for medicinal purposes, although folk remedies and superstition still dominated pharmacology in Europe.
- **1500–1700 A.D., Europe and the Americas.** Interest in pharmacology and chemistry is renewed during the Renaissance. Spices are studied for medicinal properties.
  - In the Americas, Aztec and other Native American cultures record use of herbs and plants (e.g., balsam, chili, sarsaparilla, tobacco, cihuapatli [an oxytocic], and peyote [a hallucinogen]).
- **1700 A.D.–present, scientists worldwide.** Pharmacologic advances (e.g., antibiotics, enzymes, hormones, vaccines) are spurred by technology.

Plants

Drug sources from the plant world date to primitive times. Common drugs from plants include digitalis (purple foxglove), morphine (opium poppy), and vincristine (periwinkle). Drugs that come from plants are classified according to their physical and chemical properties:

- Alkaloids (alkaline substances) react with body acids to form a salt, which is readily soluble in body fluids.
- Glycosides contain a carbohydrate or sugar molecule.
- Gums are mucilaginous secretions—usually polysaccharides—with the ability to attract and hold water.

- Oils are insoluble in water and are classified as volatile or fixed. Volatile oils, which are derived strictly from plants, evaporate when exposed to air. Fixed oils, also known as fatty oils, are derived from both animals and plants; their consistency varies with temperature.
- Resins are solid or semisolid, water insoluble, organic substances of vegetable origin that are commonly used as laxative or caustic agents.

Animals

Traditionally, drugs from animal sources include agents such as insulin, pituitary hormones, some vitamins, antibiotics, and biologic agents (such as vaccines and immune serums). Today, genetically engineered hormones (including insulin, pituitary hormone, and erythropoietin) are rapidly replacing animal-based drugs. The advantage of genetically engineered drugs is their purity. Because no foreign proteins are involved, they do not induce antibody production.

Synthetic Chemicals

Most drugs used today are either partially or wholly synthetic chemical compounds that have been produced in a laboratory. A partially synthetic agent contains a derivative of a natural substance combined with a pure chemical. An example is penicillin V, known as Pen-Vee K. The penicillin molecule, which is unstable in gastric acid, is modified so that it can be given orally. An advantage of synthetic drugs is that they are pure chemicals and, unlike drugs from a natural source, are unaffected by pharmacodynamic changes—namely, deterioration in potency and stability. Another advantage of synthetic agents is that they are usually less expensive to produce than drugs from a natural source.

Genetically Engineered Chemicals

Genetically engineered drugs are also known as genomics-based drugs. **Genomics** is the study and identification of genes and gene function. Sequencing of the human genome has allowed scientists to discover more and more gene targets. This new knowledge has enabled researchers to manipulate the chemical formulas of drugs to produce more specifically targeted drugs with fewer adverse effects. Genomics has opened the door to the development of many drugs and treatments that had been only imagined in the past. The downside to genomics-based drugs is the high cost of development, which is reflected in the high cost of the drug to the consumer.

DRUG NOMENCLATURE

All drugs are known by at least three names: a **chemical name,** a **generic name** (sometimes called the official name), and a **trade name** (Figure 2.1).

The chemical name of a drug precisely describes the drug's atomic and molecular structure using exact chemical nomenclature (language) and terminology. The chemical name, which is usually long and complex, is not practical for everyday use but is useful to chemists and biochemists.

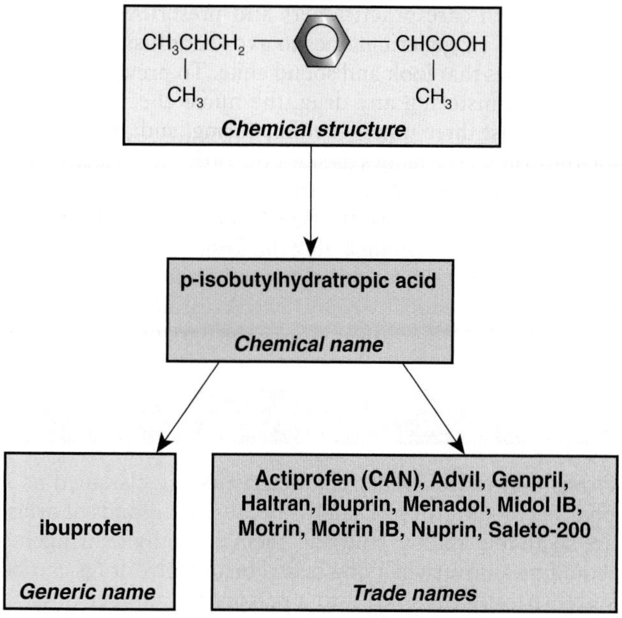

FIGURE 2.1 A drug called by another name may still be the same drug. Nomenclature is a core feature of pharmacology. The four configurations illustrate various names for the same drug.

The generic name of a drug is also known as its nonproprietary name. Each drug has only one generic name, which identifies the drug's active ingredient. As a general rule, generic names are less complicated than the chemical names from which they are derived, but they are more complicated than trade names. Generic names are easily recognizable because the first letter of the name is typically not capitalized. The **United States Adopted Names Council** assigns an official name to each drug, as mandated by the United States government in 1962. These names are published in the ***United States Pharmacopeia*** and the ***National Formulary.*** The official name for a drug is most often its generic name.

The trade name, also known as a brand or proprietary name, is given to a drug by its manufacturer. Trade names, which are usually easy to say and remember, are protected by trademark. The symbol ™ or ® after the trade name indicates that the drug molecule and name are registered by the drug manufacturer, and the use of the drug and its name are restricted to the drug's manufacturer. The manufacturer receives a 17-year patent on the drug, which provides an opportunity to recover part of the costs used in research, development, and testing of the drug. The trade name is easily recognizable because the first letter is capitalized and the ™ or ® symbol may be present. Unless governed by patent protection, any drug can be marketed in different formulations and by multiple drug companies. Consequently, the number of trade names a drug has can be extensive.

Implications for Nurses

Name recognition is important in drug therapy. The nurse has the responsibility of accurately transcribing drug orders, administering the drugs correctly, and documenting the patient's response. Usually, a drug is ordered by the generic name because numerous brand names may exist for the same

drug. Health care practitioners and prescribers typically order drugs by generic names to avoid confusion between brand names that look and sound alike. To prevent an error when administering any drug, the nurse checks the drug name at least three times—before, during, and after obtaining the drug. If the names used for the order and those on the drug label are different (e.g., trade name and generic equivalent), the nurse must verify that the two names refer to the same drug before administering the drug.

As a rule, generic formulations and trade name formulations are therapeutically equivalent. A distinct advantage of generic drugs is their lower cost to the patient.

DRUG CLASSIFICATIONS (FAMILIES)

Drugs that share similar characteristics are classified as a pharmacologic group or family. Because thousands of drugs are available today, studying them as individual agents would be an overwhelming task. Fortunately, drugs can be systematically classified into a reasonable number of drug groups known as **drug classifications** (or drug classes).

Drugs that share similar characteristics can be classified in several ways: by chemical composition, physiologic effect (on body systems), and therapeutic uses or actions (clinical indications). For example, the **chemical classification** of a drug such as morphine sulfate describes its chemical base of opium. Morphine sulfate, therefore, is classified as an opiate or opioid. The **physiologic classification** of morphine sulfate describes its effects on body systems; therefore, morphine sulfate is classified as a central nervous system depressant. The **therapeutic classification** of morphine sulfate describes the drug by its use in therapy; therefore, morphine sulfate is also known as an opioid narcotic analgesic. Thus, any one drug may belong to more than one drug class (family) depending on the classification system being used.

SOURCES OF DRUG INFORMATION

Because pharmacology is a dynamic science, new drugs are continually being developed, and new uses for existing drugs are frequently discovered. Nurses need reliable and up-to-date drug reference information. Awareness of reliable resources and the specific type of information provided in those resources enables the nurse to be efficiently and completely informed about safe drug administration and new therapeutic developments. Many drug-oriented publications help fill the need of nurses, health care providers, pharmacists, and others for current and detailed drug information. To be fully informed in a clinical situation, the nurse may have to consult several references (Table 2.1).

TABLE 2.1 Sources of Drug Information

Resource	Features	Evaluation and Commentary
Official Pharmacopeiae		
The United States Pharmacopeia (USP) and National Formulary (NF)	Drugs listed by official name Primary focus on sources, chemistry, physical properties of drugs; tests for identity, purity, and assay (measurement); and official storage requirements	• Federal Pure Food and Drug Act (1906) adopted USP and NF as official pharmacopeiae • Published every 5 y with periodic supplements • Formerly listed drugs deleted and replaced by newer or better drugs, or drug listing removed after high incidence of toxicity reported • More useful as a drug reference to the pharmaceutical industry than to the nursing profession
The British Pharmacopeia (BP)	Similar to USP and NF	• Adopted by Parliament (1968 Medical Act) for use in the United Kingdom • Published every 5 y
The International Pharmacopeia (2nd ed.)	Latin drug nomenclature	• Published by the United Nations • Used to encourage worldwide pharmacopeiae development and drug standardization • Official status conferred when adopted by individual nations • Published in English, French, and Spanish
Unofficial Compendia		
American Hospital Formulary Service (AHFS) Drug Information '02, '03, '04, etc.	Includes extensive drug information, particularly on drug classes Presents objective overviews of individual preparations of drugs available in the United States	• Published annually and updated with periodic supplements • Highly regarded drug reference
The British National Formulary (BNF)	Provides detailed descriptions of currently used preparations in medical practice	• Published by the British Medical Association and the Pharmaceutical Society of Great Britain

(continued)

TABLE 2.1 Sources of Drug Information (continued)

Resource	Features	Evaluation and Commentary
Facts and Comparisons	Provides concise but thorough monographs organized by drug class Begins each class section with a therapeutic overview followed by additional sections organized by chemical classifications Offers comparisons of drugs (including over-the-counter [OTC] products)	• Updated monthly with supplemental entries • Available in print or CD-ROM • Generally more usable than the Physician's Desk Reference (PDR) • Published by Facts and Comparisons, St. Louis, MO
Food and Drug Administration (FDA) Drug Bulletin	Offers recent FDA reviews of various drugs (usually common ones) and new clinical findings	• Free, quarterly newsletter • Includes a MedWatch form for reporting unusual clinical experiences with drugs to the FDA
USP Dispensing Information (USPDI)	Covers drug categories, prescribing precautions and considerations, side effects, drug actions, impact on lifestyle, dosage forms, and labeling data	• Written in nontechnical language • A major advantage is the presentation of side effect potential (rare to common) • Clearly identifies side effects to be reported to the health care provider • Highly valuable reference for nurses • Published annually and updated bimonthly
Pharmaceutical Package Inserts	Constitutes a concise compilation of specific drug information relative to clinical indications, safe dosage ranges, and unranked secondary (side) effects	• Manufacturer's leaflet enclosed with a drug product as it leaves the pharmaceutical distributor • Of limited value to the nursing process
Physician's Desk Reference (PDR)	Provides concise monograph of drug information similar to the manufacturer's package inserts	• Commonly consulted in clinical settings • Written by pharmaceutical company that manufactures the drug
PDR for Nonprescription Drugs	Besides concise monograph of OTC drug information, includes photographs of the drugs and a section on self-care of minor health problems	• Format similar to the PDR • First published in 1980 in response to the rapid growth and availability of OTC drugs and the general public's increasing health awareness and interest in managing self-care
Drug Interactions and Updates Quarterly	Presents drug interactions grouped together by drug class Rates drug-drug interactions according to clinical significance (e.g., minor, moderate, major)	• Fills needs emanating from constantly changing and increasing knowledge and experience with established and newly developed drugs • Covers changes in drug treatments and therapeutic regimens
Electronic Databases		
FDA web page, Medline, PharmInfoNet web page, Toxline, and others	Current drug-related information	• Available through the National Library of Medicine's on-line services
Cumulative Index to Nursing and Allied Health Literature (CINAHL)	Represents publications of major health care journals Abstracts available for many articles listed	• Available through private on-line services (e.g., Compuserve) • Libraries and schools have access through CD-ROM disks • Access through personal computers
Personal Digital Assistant Programs		
www.pdacortex.com	Offers up-to-date commentary on PDA practice Large selection of nursing-oriented programs Links to other PDA nursing-related sites	• User-friendly interface • Exceptional customer service • Many free programs developed by working nurses to assist in the clinical area • Access through personal computer
www.skyscape.com	Comprehensive selection of proprietary nursing programs	• Exceptional customer service • Access through personal computer
www.lexi.com	Comprehensive selection of proprietary nursing programs	• Exceptional customer service • Access through personal computer

SAFEGUARDS IN DRUG DEVELOPMENT, MANUFACTURE, AND DISTRIBUTION IN THE UNITED STATES

Most nurses administer drug therapy as part of their daily routine, and advanced practice nurses (such as nurse practitioners) may prescribe and dispense medications as well. Every state has its own Nurse Practice Act that fully describes nursing activities involving drug therapy. Nurses should be familiar with the Nurse Practice Act in their state because these acts define nurses' roles and responsibilities. Similarly, familiarity with governmental safeguards that promote drug safety, reliability, and uniformity help nurses administer drug therapy safely and appropriately. These regulations help to ensure that commercially available drugs are safe and effective.

New drugs are being developed at an unprecedented rate. Any new drug that comes to market undergoes years of testing to determine the drug's pharmacologic properties and its potential for toxicity.

Standards for Drug Purity and Content

Since 1820, the *United States Pharmacopeia* (USP) has been the source for standards of strength, quality, purity, and preparation of medicinal compounds. In 1888, the American Pharmaceutical Association began publishing another resource, the *National Formulary* (NF), which expanded this effort to set national standards for drug quality. Before that time, there was little need for standard resources because of the scarcity of effective drugs. In 1906, the Pure Food and Drug Act was passed, and the USP and NF compendiums became the official drug standards in the United States. Passage of the Pure Food and Drug Act in 1906 and the Food, Drug, and Cosmetic Act in 1938 protected the public from adulterated or mislabeled drugs and empowered the federal government to enforce these standards. The legislation required drug manufacturers to follow these standards to ensure that drugs were uniform, pure, and reliable. Later, amendments (1941–1945) to the Pure Food and Drug Act required that biologic products used as drugs (such as insulin and some antibiotics) be certified on a batch-by-batch basis by a government agency.

The USP is the current authoritative source for drug standards and is revised every 5 years by a group of experts in chemistry, microbiology, nursing, pharmaceutics, and pharmacology. Drugs are deleted when their clinical use shows unacceptably high toxicity or when newer, more effective agents are developed. Originally, the USP restricted its data to single drugs, and the NF was a reference for mixtures and formulas. Gradually, both reference books were expanded to include both single drugs and multiple-drug mixtures, and the two books have since been combined; the reference is now called the *United States Pharmacopeia–National Formulary.*

Legislation for Drug Safety and Efficacy

Federal legislation protects the public from drugs that are impure, toxic, ineffective, or not tested before marketing. The primary purpose of federal legislation is to ensure safety.

Pure Food and Drug Acts

The history of drug regulation reflects several medical and public health events. The **Pure Food and Drug Act of 1906** became law mostly because of revelations of unsanitary and unethical practices in the meatpacking industry and because of the many potent and dangerous drugs on the market. Although many of these drugs contained opioids (e.g., opium, morphine, or heroin), no law required the manufacturer to list the ingredients on the product label.

In addition, the Pure Food and Drug Act designated the USP and NF as the official standards and empowered the federal government to enforce those standards.

The **Federal Food, Drug, and Cosmetics Act of 1938** (FFDCA) was enacted largely in response to a considerable number of deaths (more than 100) caused by the marketing of a drug called elixir of sulfanilamide, which was not adequately tested for safety before marketing. Elixir of sulfanilamide contained the solvent diethylene glycol, which investigations later revealed to be nephrotoxic. The FFDCA established the Food and Drug Administration (FDA) as the agency for monitoring and controlling drug manufacturing and marketing, allowed the FDA to prohibit the marketing of any drug judged to be incompletely tested or dangerous, and stipulated that drugs must be labeled. According to the FFDCA, the drug label must contain the following:

- No false or misleading statements
- The suggested dose and frequency of use
- The name and business address of the manufacturer/packer or distributor
- The amount of all dependency-producing drugs in a product and the statement, "Warning: May Be Habit Forming"
- The kind, quantity, and percentage of certain specified ingredients that could be harmful (e.g., drugs containing alcohol, atropine, or digitalis)
- Complete, understandable directions for safe use and warnings against unsafe use by children, pregnant women, and people with contraindicating pathologic conditions

Kefauver-Harris Amendment

In the early 1960s, a drug-related tragedy altered drug-testing methods and expanded the scope of legislation regulating drugs. Based on results of animal testing, the sedative drug thalidomide was marketed across Europe as a nontoxic hypnotic. Hundreds of pregnant women who took the drug gave birth to infants with phocomelia, a condition characterized by severely shortened, deformed, or missing limbs. Thalidomide was not a widespread problem in the United States because the drug had been withheld by the FDA. Nonetheless, some babies with thalidomide-associated deformities were born in the United States to women who used the drug after obtaining it outside the country.

The thalidomide tragedy was one of the events that led to substantial changes in how drugs are regulated in the United States: requirements for more extensive testing of new drugs for teratogenic effects, stipulations that manufacturers prove both drug safety and efficacy, and passage of the 1962 Kefauver-Harris Amendment to the 1938 FFDCA. The Kefauver-Harris Amendment tightened controls on drug safety, especially experimental drugs, stating that adverse reactions and contraindications must be cited and included in the literature. Additionally, the amendment ordered evaluation of the testing methods used by manufacturers, specified

the process for withdrawal of approved drugs when safety and effectiveness were in doubt, and mandated the establishment of the clinical efficacy of new drugs before marketing. The law applied to both new and existing drugs. Furthermore, all drugs marketed between 1938 and 1962 were required to be tested for effectiveness to remain on the market. The Kefauver-Harris Amendment also authorized the FDA to establish official names for drugs, and in the early 1960s, the United States Adopted Names Council was established to ensure uniform drug nomenclature.

Procedure for Drug Development and Approval

The first step in the development of a new drug is in the discovery or synthesis of a potential new drug molecule. Years of research and millions of dollars go into the development of a new drug. When searching for new agents, a variety of methods may be used to identify potentially useful compounds. For example, manufacturers may start with known, active compounds and modify their chemical structure to alter pharmacokinetic or pharmacodynamic actions. Burgeoning technologic and scientific advances are expected to substantially increase the success of drug development efforts. As a result of these advances, pharmaceutical companies will be able to find much better compounds by being more selective (e.g., by screening out toxic compounds), which will ultimately decrease the average amount of time spent testing investigational drugs and getting them to market.

Once a potential new drug molecule is developed, it must be subjected to a battery of preclinical tests and **clinical trials** before it can be approved for use as a therapeutic agent. **Preclinical trials** are designed to provide basic safety, bioavailability, pharmacokinetic, and initial efficacy data about the drug and are carried out in animal subjects in the laboratory setting. Preclinical testing lasts approximately 3½ years. For every 1,000 compounds that enter laboratory testing, only one makes it to human testing.

Clinical Trials

At the conclusion of preclinical testing, the drug manufacturer submits the safety and effectiveness data from animal studies to the FDA in what is known as an investigational new drug (IND) application. The IND includes the following:

- All known information about the biologic, chemical, pharmacologic, and toxicologic properties of the new agent
- Precise details of how the drug is manufactured and storage requirements to preserve its stability
- The name and qualifications of each investigator who will participate in the clinical trial
- A signed affidavit by each investigator attesting that the study will be adequately supervised and that study volunteers have given informed consent
- Study protocols (guidelines) that clearly define how the drug is to be administered to study subjects (e.g., dose, route, duration) and what specific observations will be made during the clinical trial

If approved, the investigational new drug then undergoes clinical trials in humans. Clinical trials occur in four phases (I–IV) and may require from 5 to 9 years for completion (Figure 2.2). Phases I through III take place before a new drug is marketed. Phase IV testing is completed after marketing begins. Recently, the FDA has changed its policy to include women in early clinical trials (phases I and II), to determine whether differences in female physiology (e.g., menstrual cycle, menopause) influence pharmacotherapeutics, pharmacodynamics, and pharmacokinetics.

PHASE I

Twenty to 80 healthy human volunteers are given the drug, after which blood, urine, and other appropriate samples are taken to monitor drug metabolism. All pharmacologic and biologic effects of the drug are carefully noted. This information is useful in determining the potential of future testing. If the drug is expected to have significant toxicity, as is often the case in therapies for cancer and acquired immunodeficiency syndrome (AIDS), volunteers with the disease are used in phase I testing rather than healthy volunteers.

PHASE II

Assuming that no adverse effects are identified in the phase I trial, 100 to 300 patient volunteers are given various dosages of the test compound and studied in great detail. Dose response, toxicity, and pharmacotherapeutic effectiveness are carefully monitored, and dosage guidelines are usually determined in this phase. Results from the long-term animal studies are reviewed and compared with the human results—especially concerning the effects, if any, on fertility and reproduction.

PHASE III

If no serious problems are uncovered in phase II, the large-scale phase III trials can begin. Most of the risks associated with the new drug therapy are identified at this time. This widespread testing is also intended to uncover some infrequent or even rare adverse effects that sometimes affect only a small portion of the population. In this phase, 1,000 to 3,000 patient volunteers are enrolled in double-blind studies (studies in which neither the patient nor the researcher knows whether the drug or a placebo was given) and crossover design studies (studies comparing the study drug with an existing drug). These studies are monitored closely to evaluate the safety and effectiveness of the drug.

Nurses are generally most involved in this phase of clinical trials and may be responsible for administering investigational drugs to patients. Patients must be fully informed about the potential risks and benefits associated with the intended study. One of the nurse's roles is to address how patients feel about the clinical trial because these feelings may affect the quality and integrity of the investigation. Individual personal responses to an investigational drug may vary considerably. Some patients taking an investigational drug may believe that it is better than existing forms of therapy because it is new. These patients may have unrealistic expectations about the drug's usefulness or actions. Others may be more reluctant to participate in the study because they feel like "guinea pigs." Most patients tend to respond in a positive way to any therapeutic intervention by interested and caring health care personnel. This positive result is called the **placebo response** and may involve objective physiologic and biochemical changes as well as changes in subjective complaints (e.g., stomach upset, insomnia, sedation) associated with the disorder being treated. The placebo

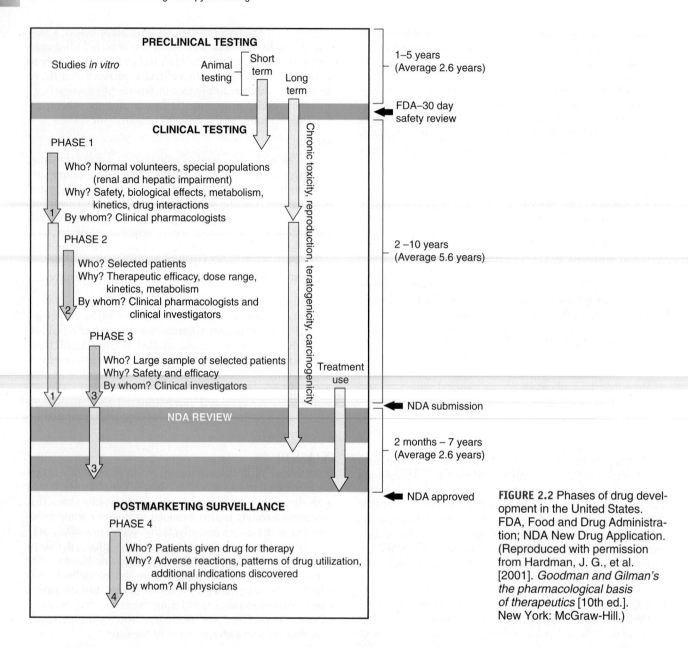

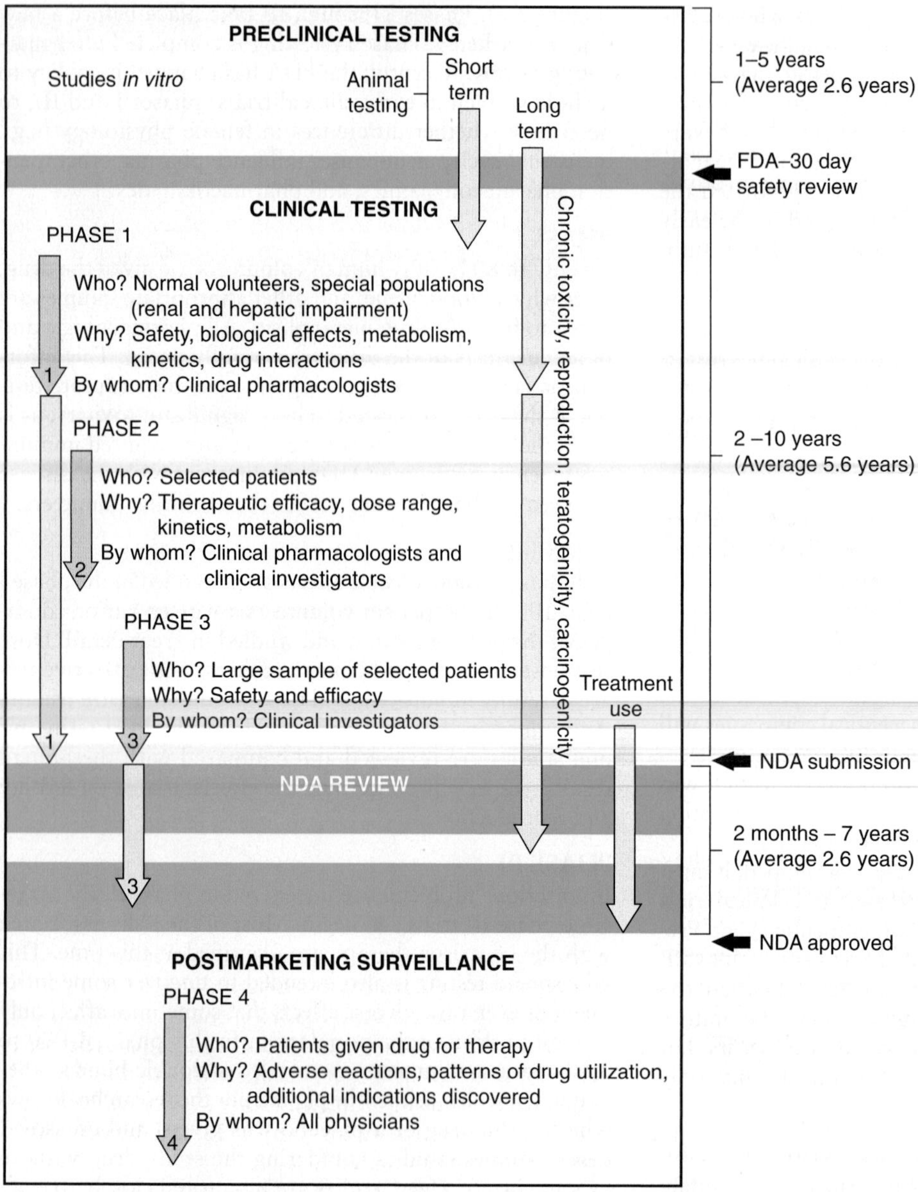

FIGURE 2.2 Phases of drug development in the United States. FDA, Food and Drug Administration; NDA New Drug Application. (Reproduced with permission from Hardman, J. G., et al. [2001]. *Goodman and Gilman's the pharmacological basis of therapeutics* [10th ed.]. New York: McGraw-Hill.)

response occurs relatively consistently in 20% to 40% of patients in almost all studies.

If the drug proves safe and effective through the first three phases of the clinical trial, the manufacturer may then apply for a new drug application (NDA). All clinical data, as well as the earlier preclinical data, are reviewed by the FDA. Approval of the NDA means that the drug may be marketed. The FDA now requires analysis by gender in almost all NDAs. Research has identified pharmacokinetic differences between men and women that may be harmful to women if dosages are not adjusted accordingly. Because the distribution patterns of fat differ in men and women, many dosing schedules have been found to be excessive, and even harmful, in women.

PHASE IV

Once a drug goes on the market, the FDA conducts postmarketing surveillance to monitor the drug for safety and any new developments while it is in widespread distribution. If safety problems appear, the agency limits the uses the drug is approved for or pulls the drug from the market. Another area of considerable interest in this phase is the effect of the drug on elderly patients and children because these groups are usually excluded from early clinical trials.

During phase IV, the pharmaceutical company that markets the drug keeps careful records on the results of therapy and must advise the FDA of any adverse effects and other effects on therapy. Occasionally, reports of toxicity occur with enough frequency that precautions for use are expanded and emphasized. For example, felbamate (Felbatol), a drug used to treat seizures, was found to cause aplastic anemia. Sometimes a drug is removed from the market because of serious side effects, as was the case with terfenadine (Seldane).

In recent years, the FDA and the USP have begun several programs to ensure adequate postmarketing surveillance of drugs. These programs rely heavily on health care practitioners, including nurses, pharmacists, and physicians, to

report problems or suspected problems with drug products to the FDA or USP. Examples of these programs include MedWatch and the Practitioners' Reporting Network.

MedWatch. The MedWatch program, sponsored by the FDA, encourages voluntary reporting from health professionals and consumers about adverse effects from drug products or medical devices directly to the FDA by mail, electronic mail (*www.fda.gov/medwatch*), or fax. Suspicion that a medical product may be related to a serious event is sufficient cause for a health professional to submit a MedWatch report. The goals of MedWatch are to increase awareness of serious reactions caused by drugs or medical devices, to facilitate the reporting of adverse reactions, and to provide the health care community with regular feedback about product safety issues.

Practitioners' Reporting Network. The **Practitioners' Reporting Network** sponsored by the USP involves four coordinated reporting programs:

- The USP Drug Product Problem Reporting Program specifically targets drug packaging and is dedicated to reporting problems with unclear labeling, defective packaging, poor product quality, suspected counterfeiting, or product tampering.
- The USP Drug Product Problem Reporting Program for Radiopharmaceuticals targets problems with adverse effects or quality of radioactive drugs.
- The Medication Errors Reporting Program looks for actual or potential medication errors that may involve labeling, packaging, miscalculations, or misinterpretation, as well as other problems in drug nomenclature, marketing, advertising, or use of abbreviations. To rank medication errors according to severity, the National Coordinating Council for Medication Error Reporting and Prevention developed the Medication Error Index to assist health care professionals in evaluating the extent of harm caused by an error (Box 2.2).
- The Medical Device and Laboratory Product Problem Reporting Program looks at quality, performance, and safety of medical devices.

The Approval Process

Only about 10% of new drugs that begin clinical trials prove safe and effective enough to win regulatory approval. Approving a drug for therapeutic use involves a long, complex, and expensive process. On average, it takes 12 years and $350 million for a new drug to be approved. The preclinical, clinical, and FDA review processes may be accelerated when an urgent need is perceived (e.g., with respect to AIDS or cancer therapy). In recent years, certain laws and protocols have been initiated to speed the drug approval process (Box 2.3).

Legislation to Promote Truth in Advertising

In 1912, Congress passed the Sherley Amendment to the 1906 Federal Pure Food and Drug Act, which prohibited drug manufacturers from making fraudulent therapeutic claims about their products. The FFDCA of 1938 bolstered this amendment by providing labeling requirements for the first time. Manufacturers were required to use standard drug

BOX 2.2 Medication Error Index

Category A	No error, although the circumstances or events may have resulted in an error.
Medication Errors Without Harm	
Category B	Error occurred but did not reach patient.
Category C	Error occurred and reached patient but did not cause harm.
Category D	Error occurred that reached patient, resulting in need for patient monitoring. No patient harm.
Medication Errors Causing Harm	
Category E	Error occurred, resulting in need for treatment or medical intervention. It caused temporary patient harm.
Category F	Error occurred, resulting in hospitalization (initial or prolonged). Caused temporary patient harm.
Category G	Error occurred, causing permanent patient harm.
Category H	Error occurred, causing a neardeath experience (anaphylaxis, cardiac or respiratory arrest, etc.).
Medication Error Resulting in Death	
Category I	Error resulted in patient death.

Developed by The National Coordinating Council for Medication Error Reporting and Prevention

nomenclature, and the presence and amount of certain potentially toxic drugs (including atropine, alcohol, or opiates) had to be disclosed. Directions for safe use and dosage had to be listed, and the manufacturer's or distributor's name had to be clearly marked. False or misleading statements were prohibited from appearing on the label.

Today, the Federal Trade Commission regulates the advertisement of medications aimed at the general public. The FDA regulates advertising of medications to medical personnel and relies on reports from practitioners and its own investigators to uncover abuses and fraud. Drug companies can be sanctioned for promoting the use of drugs in a manner that is not consistent with the agency-approved package insert.

The stated intent of the FDA is not to regulate medical practice but to guarantee the safety, purity, effectiveness, and reliability of drugs sold in the United States. However, the agency also aims to prevent manufacturers from promoting so-called off-label or unlabeled uses of drugs, in part to encourage the development of proper safety and efficacy data. Sanctions may also be imposed if a manufacturer advertises exaggerated claims of efficacy or reduced adverse effects in its product.

Legislation Regarding Controlled Substances

The Harrison Narcotic Law of 1914 legally defined the term *narcotic* and provided the first effective regulation regarding the manufacture and distribution of certain drugs known for their abuse potential, including cocaine, marijuana, and opium. The 1970 Comprehensive Drug Abuse Prevention and Control Act (also called the Controlled Substances Act, or CSA) established the Drug Enforcement Agency (DEA),

BOX 2.3 Streamlining the Drug Approval Process

Because of the high cost of research and development, many new and promising drugs never become available for consumers, primarily because of money: Manufacturers project that not enough revenue will be generated by drug sales to cover the cost of drug development.

Orphan Drugs

This is particularly true of drugs that have limited use, such as those used to treat rare or unusual diseases. These drugs are known as "orphans" because no pharmaceutical manufacturer is willing to assume the risk and expense of commercial development.

To meet the need of an individual who may benefit from an esoteric drug, the Orphan Drug Act of 1983 was enacted. The act provides certain tax benefits to companies that invest in drugs useful in the diagnosis, treatment, or prevention of rare diseases. Other legislation defined these rare diseases as those affecting fewer than 1 of every 200,000 people in the United States or diseases that may affect more than 1 of every 200,000 people but with no reasonable expectation that the company will recover development costs from sales within the United States.

Compassionate Use

Another recent development that helps to streamline the drug approval process is the compassionate use protocol, whereby certain drugs are made available to patients without complete Food and Drug Administration (FDA) approval. Since 1988, these protocols have enabled patients with life-threatening diseases to obtain investigational drugs without requiring them to enroll in a full clinical trial.

Expedited Process

All investigational new drugs (INDs) undergo the four phases of clinical evaluation; treatment INDs shorten this process, however. For example, acquired immunodeficiency syndrome (AIDS) poses a public health threat. Drug companies with AIDS drugs in phase II or III clinical trials may apply for FDA approval to use the drugs in patients who meet appropriate criteria.

The Prescription Drug User Free Act is legislation that Congress passed in 1992. Under pressure from both the pharmaceutical industry and AIDS activists, this Act, which allows the FDA to charge drug manufacturers for the FDA drug approval process, was passed. This influx of money allowed the FDA to hire additional reviewers, which accelerated the approval process.

formerly known as the Bureau of Narcotics and Dangerous Drugs (BNDD) of the United States Department of Justice, as the regulatory body responsible for the safe distribution and control of potentially addictive drugs. This act, which was designed to remedy the escalating problem of drug abuse, categorized and controlled drugs according to their abuse potential and medical usefulness on a scale of I to V, hence the term **controlled substance.** This act also defined the terms *drug dependency* and *drug addiction* and established education and treatment programs for drug abuse.

Under the CSA, five categories, known as schedules, were established, and controls were placed on prescribing, dispensing, and storing drugs in health care facilities according to the scheduled category (Table 2.2).

Drugs may be moved from one schedule category to another. For example, propoxyphene, which was originally assigned a C-V rank, was reassigned to the more restrictive C-IV category because of its popularity for misuse, abuse, and overdose. Tetrahydrocannabinol (THC, the active ingredient in marijuana)—ranked in the C-I category for many years—was moved to C-II because of its legitimate clinical use as a powerful antiemetic to relieve the adverse effects of cancer chemotherapy.

Nursing Management of Controlled Substances

The prescribing, dispensing, and storing of controlled substances is subject to considerably greater governmental control than the use of conventional prescription drugs. Procedures are precisely defined by law for virtually every step from manufacture to administration to wasting or discarding. Many hospitals use an automated system to electronically track the use of stock drugs, including controlled substances. In some health care environments, these automated systems are not used, and the nurse must document the administration of a narcotic on a narcotic log sheet. When using a narcotic log sheet, the nurse must document the following:

- Date and time of administration
- Drug name and dose
- Patient's name
- Prescriber's name
- Administering nurse's name

In a health care facility that does not use an automated system, stock supplies of narcotics must be kept in double-locked storage cabinets. Keys to the cabinet are restricted to licensed nurses, who are also responsible for the accurate accounting of all narcotics. The nurse finishing a shift and the nurse beginning a shift generally perform the narcotic count together to ensure an accurate account of all controlled substances.

The handling of controlled substances is a nursing responsibility that should never be taken lightly. Transfer of a C-II, C-III, or C-IV drug to anyone other than the person for whom it is prescribed is a crime. Violation of the CSA can result in a fine, imprisonment, or both. Any nurse who violates the CSA is also subject to loss of the nursing license and the right to practice nursing.

CRITICAL THINKING SCENARIO

Candidate for a new drug

Steve Smith has been diagnosed as having AIDS. He is being considered for treatment with a new drug during phase III clinical trials. Steve expresses concern about taking a new drug, especially in view of his declining health status and what he has heard about a shortened clinical evaluation process for AIDS drugs; he asks you, "What does the term 'new drug' mean?" What is your response?

Legislation Regarding Drug Distribution

The Durham-Humphrey amendments (1952) to the 1938 FFDCA separated drugs for the first time into two major classifications: nonprescription drugs and **legend** (prescription) **drugs.**

Prescription drugs must be identified by the legend (inscription) on the container: "Caution: Federal law prohibits dispensing without a prescription." Containers of controlled

TABLE 2.2 Schedule of Controlled Substances

Category	Abuse Potential	Dependence Liability	Examples	Rules Governing Prescription
C-I	High	Severe	Heroin, hashish, LSD, GHB	• No accepted medical use • Generally restricted to research
C-II	High	Severe	Amphetamines, some opioid narcotics (e.g., morphine, meperidine), dronabinol, short-acting barbiturates (e.g., pentobarbital, secobarbital)	• Prescription written in triplicate form (one copy forwarded to the DEA) • Refills require a new prescription.
C-III	Moderate	Moderate	Some opioid narcotics (e.g., codeine, hydrocodone), some CNS stimulants, anabolic steroids	• A written or telephone order is acceptable. • May be refilled 5 times within 6 months from the date of issue • Prescription must be rewritten after 6 months or 5 refills.
C-IV	Low	Limited	Benzodiazepine anxiolytics, anticonvulsants, muscle relaxants, and sedatives; nonbenzodiazepine hypnotics and intermediate-acting barbiturates. Opioid narcotics such as propoxyphene or pentazocine	• Same as C-III drugs
C-V	Limited	Lowest	Antidiarrheal preparations with diphenoxylate and loperamide; small amounts of narcotics such as codeine used as antitussives	• Many of these drugs may be obtained without a prescription.

substances must also display an additional warning label: "Caution: Federal law prohibits the transfer of this drug to any person other than the patient for whom it was prescribed." The Durham-Humphrey amendment further specifies procedures for the distribution of legend drugs. A prescription from a licensed practitioner is required before the drug can be dispensed, and refills are not permitted without authorization of the prescriber.

Labeling, according to the USP, is the written, printed, or graphic matter affixed to an immediate container, package, or wrapper in which the medication is enclosed. Informational sheets that are not attached (such as patient information/instruction sheets) are not considered part of the label. The prescription label remains a primary source of information to patients about the proper use of their medications. Cautions regarding use and storage are usually on auxiliary labels, and some medications require their use. The following are examples of auxiliary labels:

- Avoid prolonged or excessive exposure to sunlight or sunlamp while taking this medication.
- Avoid the use of grapefruit juice with this product.
- Avoid the use of laxatives with this product.
- Do not take this drug if you are pregnant or suspect that you may be pregnant.
- Do not take with dairy products or antacids, or ingest these products within 1 hour before or 2 hours after taking this medication.
- Do not use past the expiration date.
- May cause drowsiness. Alcohol may intensify this effect. Use care when operating a car or dangerous machinery.
- Must be refrigerated/do not freeze.
- Take all of this medication/complete the full course of therapy.
- Take on empty stomach, at least 1 hour before or 2 hours after meals.
- Take with full glass of water.

Online Pharmacies

Consumers are increasingly going online to meet their prescription drug needs. A combination of high-profile congressional hearings, sensational cases, anecdotal reporting by the media, and recently published scientific studies raises legitimate concerns about the potential for illegitimate Internet sites to put consumers' health at risk by selling prescription drugs without a valid physician–patient relationship. These sales are often from locations outside the United States. In 1999, Resolution 2763 (the Internet Pharmacy Consumer Protection Act) was introduced into the House of Representatives. This act would amend the FFDCA with respect to the sale of prescription drugs through the Internet and would require an Internet pharmacy page to provide:

- Name, address, and telephone number of the Internet pharmacy's principal place of business
- A listing of the states in which the Internet pharmacy is authorized by law to dispense prescription drugs
- Name of each individual who serves as a pharmacist for purposes of the site and each state in which the individual is authorized by law to dispense prescription drugs
- Names of all individuals (and their respective license numbers) who provide medical consultations through the site for purposes of providing prescriptions

Nongovernmental Institutional Controls

Health care institutions, such as hospitals and skilled nursing facilities, may adopt additional regulations to ensure safe drug therapy and drug distribution. The Joint Commission for Accreditation of Hospitals and Healthcare Organizations (JCAHO) is a watchdog group that provides the impetus for additional regulation. JCAHO sets the standards for quality of patient care and accreditation of health care institutions.

Generally, regulations to meet these standards of care for drug therapy vary greatly among institutions, but most guarantee that the therapy prescribed for any patient is continually reviewed for appropriateness, safety, and efficacy. Examples of these regulations include automatic discontinuation of antibiotic orders after 7 to 10 days of treatment or automatic discontinuation of narcotic or controlled substance orders after 48 to 72 hours. Institutional regulations exist to prevent prolonged, costly, and sometimes inappropriate administration of drugs. Development and implementation of such policies usually requires a collaborative effort among the nursing, pharmacy, and medical staffs.

SAFEGUARDS IN DRUG DEVELOPMENT, MANUFACTURE, AND DISTRIBUTION IN CANADA

Canadian drug laws are similar to those in the United States, and the Health Protection Branch of the Department of National Health and Welfare is responsible for maintaining quality and safety of drug development, manufacturing, and distribution. The Health Protection Branch is also responsible for administering and enforcing the **Canadian Food and Drugs Act,** the Canadian Narcotics Control Act, and the Proprietary or Patent Medicine Act. These acts are designed to protect the consumer from health hazards and fraud or deception in the sale and use of cosmetics, drugs, foods, and medical devices.

Canadian Food and Drugs Act

In 1953, the Canadian Food and Drugs Act established standards for labeling, packaging, manufacturing, quality, and advertising. The act is amended yearly (see *http://laws.justice.gc.ca/en/F-27/text.html*).

Schedule A of this act lists diseases such as alcoholism, arteriosclerosis, and cancer for which no cosmetic, drug, food, or device may be advertised or sold to the general public as a treatment, preventative, or cure.

Schedule B lists recognized compendiums such as the USP-NF, British Pharmacopoeia, Canadian Formulary, British Pharmaceutical Codex, and Compendium of Pharmaceuticals and Specialties. Section 10 of this act states that "Where a standard has not been prescribed for a drug, but a standard for the drug is contained in any publication referred to in Schedule B, no person shall label, package, sell or advertise any substance in such a manner that it is likely to be mistaken for that drug, unless the substance complies with the standard."

Drugs contained in Schedules C and D require inspection of the premises in which the drugs are manufactured. Section 12 of this act also states that the process and conditions of manufacture are suitable to ensure that the drugs are safe for human use.

Section 13 of this act states that the Ministry is responsible for ensuring that each batch of the drugs described in Schedule E is safe for use.

Schedule F contains drugs that are prohibited from sale to the general public in Canada. These are drugs that require assessment of the patient by a provider and authority to prescribe the drug in Canada.

Canadian Narcotics Control Act

In 1961, the Canadian Narcotics Control Act set forth regulations regarding the manufacture, sale, distribution, and possession of narcotics and other drugs of abuse. This act has been amended a number of times. The most recent Canadian drug legislation is the 1996 Narcotic Control Act. This law is similar in scope to the 1970 United States Comprehensive Drug Abuse Prevention and Control Act. Drugs are placed into categories depending on their potential for abuse (see Appendix A).

Canada, like the United States, has strict requirements for nurses, who must account for all narcotic drugs used within a health care institution or agency. Narcotics are dispensed only with a written prescription, and "N" must appear on the label.

EFFECT OF LEGAL AND INSTITUTIONAL CONTROLS ON NURSING MANAGEMENT OF DRUG THERAPY

Nurses need to be familiar not only with institutional protocols for safe and effective drug administration but also with official and professional regulations and laws. Drug laws and nurse practice acts vary from state to state, and these regulations define nursing responsibilities related to drug safety and effectiveness in patient care. Nurses must be familiar with the current regulations in their states and in their practice settings. Nurses can stay up to date by regularly consulting with representatives of regulatory bodies, arranging in-service training and information sessions, and understanding the policies of their own agencies.

In professional practice, nurses must adhere to and obey established drug control laws and protocols. They must avoid advising patients on the use of drugs, and they cannot provide drug therapy without proper authorization. Within the institution, nurses are responsible not only for drug security (to prevent unauthorized use or accidental loss) but also for the safe administration of drugs. Infraction of the laws and protocols that protect and promote patient safety may result in the loss of one's nursing license.

PATIENT EDUCATION AS A SAFEGUARD IN DRUG THERAPY

Educating patients is a key safeguard in drug therapy. Educating patients about drug therapy improves adherence to drug therapy and promotes therapeutic outcomes. In other

words, patients who understand the prescribed drug regimen have the best chance of achieving the maximum benefit from it.

Patient education requires a nurse to have skills in gathering data, individualizing instructions, prompting and supporting the patient, and assessing and evaluating the pharmacotherapeutic response for determining patient outcomes. An effective patient teaching program parallels the nursing process—the nurse assesses the patient's learning needs, formulates a diagnosis, identifies a desired outcome, develops and implements a teaching plan, and evaluates the teaching and learning that has occurred. Strategies for enhancing patient education are given in Box 2.4.

Patient Learning Needs

Learning needs for drug education vary among patients, as does each patient's adherence to the prescribed treatment regimen. Some variations result from clinical factors, such as the nurse–patient relationship. Others are related to the scope or complexity of drug therapy in relation to pharmacotherapeutic, pharmacokinetic, and pharmacodynamic parameters; contraindications, precautions, and adverse effects of therapy; and the potential for drug interactions with undesired effects. Variations may also relate to core patient variables: health status (Box 2.5); life span and gender; lifestyle, diet, and habits; environment; and culture and inherited traits.

Teaching Focus and Content

Because each patient processes information differently, the nurse attempts to individualize and communicate information so that the patient or the caregiver can understand it and act on it appropriately. If possible, the nurse prepares written or audiovisual materials for the patient to consult as needed (see Chapter 1, Box 1.4).

Evaluating and Documenting Educational Outcomes

Evaluation and documentation of patient education includes time of teaching, content of teaching, the patient's response to the teaching session, an evaluation of the patient's grasp of the subject matter, and an assessment of unmet or future learning needs. Like documentation of drug therapy and other nursing care, documentation of patient education activities becomes part of the clinical and legal record, serving as a reference for other health care professionals and helping guide future educational efforts.

BOX 2.4 Strategies for Enhancing Patient Education

- Avoid jargon; communicate in short words and sentences.
- Include written information using diagrams and illustrations.
- Promote understanding with repetition and reinforcement.
- Relate new information to the patient's existing knowledge and previous experiences.
- Highlight and recap important information. Ask the patient to repeat the instructions or demonstrate new techniques.

BOX 2.5 Assessment: Another Safeguard

To ensure the patient's safe adherence to drug therapy and to formulate an effective, relevant drug teaching plan, the nurse needs not only to assess the patient's learning needs, but also the patient's health history, asking about the following:

- Allergies or idiosyncratic reactions to drugs or foods
- Chronic conditions
- Drugs and other medications currently used (including vitamins, other supplements, and over-the-counter drugs)
- Pregnancy status now and future plans (for women of childbearing age)
- Use of alcohol, caffeine, nicotine, or illicit substances

Consumer Drug Information on the Internet

Patient education about drug therapy is particularly important in light of the explosive growth of the Internet, which has created countless opportunities for patients to access health-related information, products, and services. The Internet has forever changed the way many consumers obtain prescription drugs and health information. Opting for the convenience and privacy of the information-rich Internet, consumers have increasingly gone online for information on medications.

The quality of information provided on some Internet sites has become a concern for health care providers. Consumers may have difficulty recognizing the difference between accurate drug information and personal web pages that have biased opinions from nonmedical personnel. Because sites with the most accurate drug information frequently charge for their services, consumers may not be as likely to access these sites. Because information obtained from an Internet site may conflict with information provided by the health care provider, patients are counseled to discuss contradictory information they obtain from a website with the health care provider before changing a medication regimen.

IMPORTANCE OF NURSING MANAGEMENT OF DRUG THERAPY

The importance of pharmacotherapy in nursing practice continues to grow. Nurses are legally responsible for the drugs they administer and for safe drug administration. When caring for patients with acute health problems, the nurse is the health care provider who usually administers drugs. This function becomes substantially more demanding as more new drugs enter the marketplace, multiple-drug therapies grow more complex, and drug delivery systems become more sophisticated. Safe drug administration requires a thorough understanding of therapeutic drug actions and adverse drug reactions.

In some clinical settings, nurses are allowed to modify drug regimens according to specifically designed protocols, and almost all states now allow advanced practice nurses to prescribe drugs. Future nursing practice will likely involve the prescribing of selected drugs.

Application of the nursing process to the pharmacologic aspects of patient care is especially important because long-term use of drug therapy is frequently necessary to control chronic disease processes. Nursing management in drug therapy may be considered an applied science because it relies on knowledge and principles from many different disciplines, such as anatomy and physiology, anthropology, biochemistry, mathematics, microbiology, organic chemistry, psychology, and sociology.

CHAPTER SUMMARY

- Sources of drugs include plants, animals, minerals, and chemical substances.
- Each drug is identified by at least three names, including the chemical name; the generic (nonproprietary) name, which is a contraction or shortening of the chemical name; and the trade or brand (proprietary) name. In the United States, official names are assigned by the government and are usually the same as the generic name.
- Drugs that share similar characteristics are classified in several ways: by clinical indications, effects on body systems, or chemical composition.
- Drug classifications (also known as families) emphasize common characteristics of each grouping, usually identify a prototype drug, and facilitate the association of new drugs within an established family as new drugs become available.
- Sources of drug information include pharmacopeias, which are official sources; compendiums, which are unofficial sources; product-insert literature from pharmaceutical firms; published reports; and findings in journals and electronic databases.
- The development and delivery of drugs is guided by federal legislation that is continually being updated.
- The approval process for a new drug is lengthy and expensive. It involves four phases of clinical trials.
- The FDA program MedWatch takes reports from health professionals and consumers about adverse reactions and disseminates information about those reactions as well as information about labeling changes and other safety issues.
- Educating patients is a key safeguard in drug therapy. The nurse implements strategies that optimize patient learning.

QUESTIONS FOR STUDY AND REVIEW

1. What is the purpose of the USP and the NF?
2. Explain the ways in which drugs are named.
3. How are drugs classified? What is the purpose of placing drugs in classifications?
4. Discuss the purpose and intent of government regulations, such as the Food, Drug, and Cosmetics Act, the Durham-Humphrey amendments, or the Canadian Narcotics Control Act. What safeguards do these laws provide?
5. Explain the purpose and extent of clinical trials. Identify some advantages and disadvantages to clinical trials.
6. What are controlled substances? What are some nursing implications related to administering a controlled substance? What special precautions are required for handling controlled substances?
7. Identify some points about safe drug use that should be taught to all patients.
8. What kinds of information about drugs should be included in the patient teaching plan?

Need More Help?

Chapter 2 of the study guide for *Drug Therapy in Nursing* 2e contains NCLEX-style questions and other learning activities to reinforce your understanding of the concepts presented in this chapter. For additional information or to purchase the study guide, visit *http://www.connection.lww.com/go/aschenbrenner.*

REFERENCES AND BIBLIOGRAPHY

Food and Drug Administration. (2004). New drug approval process [Online]. Available: *http://www.fda.gov/cder/handbook/develop.htm.*

Food and Drug Administration. (2000). Drug prescription labels [Online]. Available: *http://www.fda.gov/cber/rules/labelreg.pdf.*

Fung, C. H., Woo, H. E., & Asch, S. M. (2004). Controversies and legal issues of prescribing and dispensing medications using the Internet. *Mayo Clinic Proceedings, 79*(2), 188–194.

Hardman, J. G. (2001). *Goodman & Gilman's the pharmacological basis of therapeutics* (10th ed.). New York: McGraw-Hill Health Professions Division.

Leake, C. D. (1975). *A historical account of pharmacology to the twentieth century.* Springfield, IL: Charles C. Thomas Press.

U.S. Department of Health and Human Services, Food and Drug Administration. (1999). *Task force report. Managing the risks from medical product use: Creating a risk management framework.* Washington, DC: U.S. Government Printing Office.

Drug Administration

chapter 3

Learning Objectives

At the completion of this chapter the student will:

1. Describe the three routes for administering drugs.
2. Differentiate systemic and local effects related to the various routes of drug administration.
3. Describe the variety of oral forms of enteral drugs.
4. Differentiate the three main methods of parenteral drug administration.
5. Describe the methods of topical administration.
6. Describe how the route of administration interacts with core drug knowledge.
7. Describe how the route of administration interacts with the core patient variables.
8. Describe nursing interventions to maximize therapeutic and minimize adverse effects based on drug administration route.

KEY TERMS

buccal
capsules
elixir
emulsion
enteral route
enteric coating
intra-arterial
intra-articular
intradermal
intramuscular
intrathecal
intravenous
intravenous piggyback
intravenous push
local effect
parenteral route
subcutaneous
sublingual
suspension
sustained release
syrup
systemic effect
tablet
topical route
troches

FEATURED WEBLINK

http://www.usp.org
Visit the United States Pharmacopeia site for information about patient safety in drug administration.

CONNECTION WEBLINK

Additional Weblinks are found on Connection:
http://www.connection.lww.com/go/aschenbrenner.

Drug therapy can be administered by several different routes or methods. These routes of administration require different preparations or forms of a drug. Most drugs are available from the drug manufacturer in multiple forms. The selection of the route and form is based on the interaction between core drug knowledge and core patient variables. In managing drug therapy, nurses use this information to assess patient needs, plan care, administer drugs, and evaluate the effectiveness of therapy. This chapter describes the different routes of drug administration, explains the different forms of drug preparations, and shows how the route and drug form interact with the core drug knowledge and the core patient variables.

DRUG ADMINISTRATION ROUTES: GENERAL CONSIDERATIONS

The three basic routes of drug administration are enteral, parenteral, and topical. (Some authorities place topical in the parenteral category.)

- The **enteral route** uses the gastrointestinal (GI) tract for the ingestion and absorption of drugs. The most common method of administering drugs through the enteral route is orally. The enteral route also includes drugs that are administered through a nasogastric (NG) or a gastrostomy (G) tube.
- The **parenteral route** avoids or circumvents the GI tract and is associated with all forms of injections: intramuscular (IM), subcutaneous (SC or SQ), and intravenous (IV). Less commonly used parenteral routes than IM, SC, and IV are intradermal (into the dermis), intrathecal (into the cerebrospinal fluid), intra-articular (into a joint), and intra-arterial (into an artery).
- The **topical route** is technically another parenteral route because it also bypasses the GI tract. Drugs administered topically are applied to the skin or mucous membranes, including those of the eyes, ears, nose, vagina, rectum, and lungs.

Drugs are administered for their local or systemic effects. For example, most drugs applied topically to the skin or mucous membranes exert their effect at that site, which is a **local effect.** An example is corticosteroid cream applied to relieve the itch from a rash. However, certain drugs given topically are absorbed by the skin and distributed throughout the body systems to produce a **systemic effect.** Drugs given for a systemic effect by any route must be capable of being transported into the blood and distributed through the body to a location distant from the administration site. An example is the narcotic used for pain relief, fentanyl, which is imbedded in a transdermal patch and applied to the skin.

Drugs administered by a route other than the enteral route have the advantage of avoiding the first-pass metabolism in the liver. Drugs administered enterally are absorbed from the stomach and small intestine. However, they first pass through the liver, the primary organ for drug metabolism, before being distributed throughout the body. Drugs administered parenterally and even some topical drugs are transported directly into the blood, thereby bypassing the liver. (See Chapter 4 for a complete discussion of the first-pass effect and the processes of pharmacokinetics.)

ENTERAL ROUTE AND FORMS

The enteral route involves using the GI tract for the administration and absorption of drugs. Enteral drugs, particularly oral drugs, are manufactured and prepared in a variety of forms, including solid tablets and capsules and liquid elixirs and syrups. Because the oral route of administration is the most common enteral route, oral dosage forms are the most common preparations. They are convenient, economical, and easy to use.

Some oral drugs, such as antacids and laxatives, are given for their local effect in the GI tract, but most are given to achieve a systemic effect. In most cases, patients can reliably self-medicate with oral drug forms.

Oral Drug Forms

Tablets

A **tablet** is a solid dosage form that is prepared by compressing or molding a drug into various sizes and shapes. In many cases, tablets are scored; that is, designed to be easily broken at a point so that one half or one quarter of the dose may be given. Unless a tablet is scored, it should never be broken because doing so could result in inaccurate dosage.

The active ingredients in tablets are commonly mixed with lactose or other sugars, binding agents, or other inert materials to facilitate manufacturing and ensure stability of the preparation. When the patient swallows the tablet, esophageal peristalsis propels it to the stomach, where it dissolves and releases the drug into the gastric contents.

Drugs that are appropriate for use in tablet form have some limitations. First, the drug must be stable in gastric contents. Because gastric juices may be highly acidic, drugs that rapidly degrade in acid environments may not be administered using conventional tablets. An additional consideration is flavor because the tablet will begin to dissolve as soon as it is placed in the mouth. Drugs determined by the pharmaceutical company to be bitter, irritating, or unpleasant tasting are not usually manufactured in conventional tablet form because they would be accepted poorly by patients. These limitations can be overcome by using a special coating on the tablet.

An **enteric coating** is a wax-like layer that is used on some tablets. This layer resists the acid environment of the stomach but dissolves in areas in which the local pH is neutral or slightly alkaline (e.g., the small intestine). Enteric coatings may be used to protect acid-labile drugs, to provide a sustained-release dose, or to guard against local adverse effects from a drug. Other types of commonly used coatings include film or sugar. Both of these coatings are used to protect the patient from bitter or unpleasant tasting drugs. These coatings do not impart any time-release characteristics.

Sustained-release (also called controlled-, timed-, extended-, or prolonged-release) tablets are formulated to release a drug slowly over an extended period, rather than

rapidly like conventional tablets. Sustained release occurs by several methods:

- Layers of enteric coatings may be applied, and the drug is released in response to changes in the surrounding pH of the GI fluid.
- The tablet may be formulated to release the drug in a steady, controlled manner.
- The tablet may be formulated to release the drug in a series of pulsations.
- In most cases, the total dose of drug in a sustained-release preparation is higher than that found in a regular tablet. The patient may safely take the higher dose because it is released in a controlled fashion, thereby preventing any adverse effects from overdosage.

Sublingual and Buccal Tablets

Sublingual and buccal preparations are tablet forms that are not used as often as oral tablets. These small, hard, compressed tablets are designed to dissolve rapidly in the vascular mucous membranes of the mouth. **Buccal** tablets are placed in the buccal pouch (between the cheek and gum), and **sublingual** tablets are placed under the tongue. Sublingual and buccal tablets must be relatively nonirritating, flavorless, and highly water soluble.

Because the buccal and sublingual areas are highly vascular, drugs are quickly absorbed into the bloodstream, and a rapid onset of drug effect occurs. At the same time, drugs administered in this way avoid the first-pass phenomenon because they are not ingested into the GI tract. Although these formulations typically are considered oral forms because they are placed in the mouth, most experts think of the sublingual and buccal forms as parenteral preparations because they are not absorbed in the GI tract. Others consider them a variation of the topical route.

Troches

Troches, also called pastilles or lozenges, are commonly used to achieve a local effect in the mouth or pharynx (throat). The drug is embedded in hard candy or another suitably flavored vehicle that the patient holds within the mouth, where it slowly dissolves. Antitussives, anti-infectives, local anesthetics, antihistamines, and analgesics are administered this way.

Capsules

Capsules are solid dosage forms in which the drug is usually encased in a shell of hard or soft gelatin. When the patient swallows the capsule, the drug is carried to the stomach, where the gelatin capsule quickly dissolves and releases the drug into the gastric contents. Because the active ingredients are enclosed in gelatin, foul-tasting drugs can be easily administered in capsules. Another advantage is that many patients find gelatin capsules easier to swallow than tablets. Unlike tablets, capsules cannot be easily divided or broken into equal pieces, so one disadvantage is that dosage may not be as flexible.

The most common capsules encase a powdered drug. Soft, elastic capsules are somewhat thicker and may be used to encase a drug paste, semiliquid, or liquid (provided the drug itself does not dissolve the capsule). In addition, the contents may be altered in one of several ways to produce a sustained-release dosage form as follows:

- Layers of enteric coatings may be applied to the drug particles, producing what is commonly known as microencapsulation. The drug is released in response to changes in the surrounding pH of the GI fluid. The rate of release is controlled by varying the thickness of the layers around the drug particles.
- The capsule may be formulated to release the drug in a steady, controlled manner from a matrix of drug encased in a slowly dissolving substance, such as wax.
- The drug is bound to ion-exchange resins, chemical compounds that form insoluble complexes within the capsule. Changes in the local environment, such as altered electrolyte content or pH, cause the drug to be released slowly from the resin matrix.

Like their tablet counterparts, sustained-release capsules may contain higher doses than those found in regular-release forms, but the patient may safely take the higher dose because the drug is released in a controlled fashion.

Syrups

A concentrated solution of sugar, such as sucrose, in water is known as a **syrup.** Most syrups that contain 65% or more sucrose are also resistant to mold, yeasts, and other microorganisms, and they have a reasonable shelf life with no need for refrigeration. Occasionally, sucrose may crystallize out of solution, clouding the syrup or giving it the appearance of particulate matter.

Elixirs

An **elixir** is a clear hydroalcoholic mixture that is usually sweetened or otherwise pleasantly flavored. Most elixirs contain ethanol and water, but glycerin, sorbitol, propylene glycol, flavoring agents, aspartase, and even syrups may also be found in elixirs. The alcohol content of elixirs varies greatly and can exceed 25%. Elixirs are stored at room temperature, and the alcohol content usually prevents the growth of any mold or other microorganisms. Elixirs should always be clear. Cloudiness indicates contamination.

Emulsions and Suspensions

Many drug preparations use mixtures of two chemically incompatible substances. These preparations may be administered orally. Rarely, they may be used topically.

An **emulsion** is created when two liquids that do not mix well are combined, and one liquid distributes uniformly through the other. Because these mixtures tend to separate rapidly, remember to shake the preparation well immediately before measuring a dose and to administer the dose soon after pouring and measuring. To enhance the stability of the mixture, an emulsifying agent is added. Most emulsions consist of a nonaqueous agent (oil or lipid phase) dispersed with an aqueous (water) agent. In general, nothing should be added to emulsions because additives may adversely affect the stability of the mixture.

A **suspension** is a drug preparation consisting of two agents: a finely divided solid dispersed within a liquid. The stability of the preparation depends on the ability of the dispersing medium to wet the solid particles. Surface-active agents may be used.

Nasogastric or Gastrostomy Tube Forms

Patients who cannot swallow but who have a functioning GI tract may have an NG (nasogastric) or G (gastrostomy) tube in place. An NG tube is a soft, flexible tube that is advanced through a nostril and into the stomach for administering food, fluids, and drugs, usually for a short time. An NG tube presents a risk for aspiration from gastric reflux because the tube prevents the gastroesophageal sphincter from closing. A G tube is surgically inserted into the stomach for administering food, fluids, and drugs to patients who need long-term care. Providing drugs and foods through a G tube is preferred over an NG tube because the G tube method leaves the gastroesophageal sphincter intact. Regurgitation is less likely with a G tube than with an NG tube.

Drugs administered through a tube should be either liquid or crushed and in a liquid vehicle. A liquid drug form is preferred because research has shown that this form causes less clotting of tubes than crushed and dissolved drugs. However, if a liquid form is not available, the tablet may be crushed as long as it is not an enteric-coated or sustained-release preparation. Sustained-release or enteric-coated tablets are never crushed.

NURSING MANAGEMENT IN ENTERAL DRUG ADMINISTRATION

Core Drug Knowledge

Although the oral method of drug delivery is most common, not all drugs can be administered orally. Gastric acids and enzymes destroy many drugs; others simply may not be absorbed.

Absorption may begin in the stomach, but most absorption of orally administered drugs occurs in the small intestine. Food may interfere with the dissolution and absorption of certain drugs, especially enteric-coated drugs, because of the considerable variation in individual gastric emptying times and therefore in the length of time a drug spends in the stomach.

Assessment of Relevant Core Patient Variables

Health Status

A primary consideration for administering an oral drug is the patient's condition. Can the patient tolerate an oral drug? Patients who are vomiting, uncooperative, or unconscious or whose condition requires that they receive nothing by mouth (i.e., no oral food or fluid) are not suited for oral drug therapy. Alternate routes should be used. If the patient cannot swallow at all but has a working GI system, the drug may be given through an NG or a G tube. If patients can take oral drugs but have difficulty swallowing tablets, pills, and capsules, the drugs may be crushed and mixed in a few milliliters of water or liquid or in a tablespoon of jelly, applesauce, or pudding. Large volumes of fluid or food are avoided because the patient must consume the full volume to receive the full drug dose. Alternately, a liquid drug form may be substituted. Sublingual drugs may be administered even to unconscious patients because these drug forms are so rapidly absorbed by the vasculature.

Life Span and Gender

The high sugar content of syrups can mask unpleasant drug flavors, making them useful vehicles for administering drugs orally to both adults and children. Because they usually contain little or no alcohol, syrups are especially good vehicles for drugs administered to children. Because of the potentially high alcohol content, elixirs are usually not used in children or in adults who should avoid ethanol.

Environment

Oral drug forms are easily self-administered by patients and can be used in home environments and acute or long-term care settings.

Planning and Intervention

Maximizing Therapeutic Effects

Capsules with sustained-release pellets in them can be opened and the pellets sprinkled on food or mixed with a liquid; the patient must eat or drink all the food or fluid.

Because emulsions and suspensions have a tendency to separate, they should be shaken well immediately before measuring a dose and then administered promptly.

Drugs administered through an NG or a G tube are instilled slowly without excessive force. Some may be allowed to flow in by gravity. The tube is flushed with 10 to 30 mL of water before and after drug administration to ensure that the patient receives the full dose and to maintain the patency of the tube.

Minimizing Adverse Effects

Drugs that have enteric coatings and drugs in sustained-release form should never be chewed, crushed, or broken. Doing so increases the risk for adverse effects, including toxicity, because a higher dosage of the drug is available all at once.

Repeated doses of sucrose-containing syrups may increase the risk for gingivitis or dental caries. Good oral hygiene should accompany the use of syrups. Also, patients with diabetes may need to monitor their glucose levels closely if they are receiving large doses of drugs in syrups.

Before administering drugs through an NG or G tube, the tube is assessed for proper placement. In addition, the head of the patient's bed is elevated to help prevent aspiration from reflux. If the patient is also receiving tube feedings, the nurse reviews information on the specific drug because some drugs are not absorbed well with tube-feeding formulas. When a tube-fed patient needs such a drug, the feeding must be shut off for a time both before and after drug administration.

To ensure safety, the nurse must closely follow the cardinal rules of drug administration (Box 3.1). Historically, these rules have been known as the Five Rights, but recently some authors have added a sixth right: documentation. To administer a drug at the "right time" using the "right route," the nurse must be able to read and interpret the

BOX 3.1 Six Rights of Drug Administration

In managing drug therapy safely and effectively, the nurse must heed the six rights of drug administration:

right	Patient
right	Drug
right	Time
right	Dose
right	Route
right	Documentation

medication order correctly. Standard abbreviations are frequently used in medication orders. The nurse must know these abbreviations (Table 3.1). To administer the "right dose," dosage calculation is often necessary. The most accurate method for doing dosage calculations is to use a calculator. Any drug dosage calculation book contains all of the necessary specific information. Many institutions require that all drug calculations be confirmed by two nurses before drug administration to prevent drug errors. Information about calculating pediatric doses is provided in Chapter 6. Occasionally, the nurse may need to convert the unit of measurement for the drug to another unit of measurement (Table 3.2).

TABLE 3.1 Abbreviations Related to Medication Administration

Abbreviation	Meaning
a.c.	before meals
p.c.	after meals
qd	every day
qod	every other day
qhs	every night at hour of sleep
qam	every morning
bid	twice a day
tid	three times a day (usually limited to hours awake)
qid	four times a day (usually limited to hours awake)
q4h	every four hours
q6h	every six hours
qh	every hour
prn	as needed
ad lib	as desired
IM	intramuscularly
IV	intravenously
SQ or SC	subcutaneous
PO	by mouth
SL	sublingual
OD	right eye
OS	left eye
OU	both eyes
STAT	immediately

TABLE 3.2 Measurement Equivalents

Metric	Household
1 milliliter or 1 cubic centimeter	
5 milliliters	1 teaspoon
15 milliliters	1 tablespoon
30 milliliters	2 tablespoons or 1 ounce
500 milliliters	1 pint
1,000 milliliters or 1 liter	1 quart or 2 pints
1 gram or 1,000 milligrams or 10,000 micrograms	
1 kilogram or 1,000 grams	2.2 pounds

PARENTERAL ROUTE

The parenteral route is associated with all forms of drugs administered by a syringe, needle, or catheter. The three most commonly used parenteral routes are intramuscular, subcutaneous, and intravenous.

Intramuscular Administration

The **intramuscular** technique involves injecting drugs into certain muscles. This method requires specific knowledge of anatomy and aseptic technique. Because muscles have a good blood supply, drugs that are injected into a muscle move directly into the bloodstream without having to be broken down and absorbed as oral drugs processed by the GI tract must be. Thus, the onset of action with intramuscular injections is faster. Muscles have more blood vessels than subcutaneous tissue; therefore, the onset of action after IM injection occurs more rapidly than after subcutaneous injection.

Drugs such as oils or irritating chemicals can be administered intramuscularly in solutions or suspensions. Many injectable drugs are dry powders and must be reconstituted before administration, possibly requiring a specific amount of diluent. Thin and watery solutions given intramuscularly move promptly into the blood vessels. Because suspensions or drugs with an oil base are thicker or more viscous than water-based solutions, they do not move as quickly into the blood vessels. A deposit of the drug is formed within the muscle that is slowly released into the bloodstream.

The most common sites for IM injection are the deltoid, dorsogluteal, ventrogluteal, rectus femoris, and vastus lateralis muscles (Figure 3.1). Injection in the dorsogluteal site carries a risk for damaging the sciatic nerve if the injection site is not located properly. Some experts and nursing fundamental texts no longer recommend using this site, and some state that it should be used only as a last resort. Consult your nursing practice textbooks for more information on the specific techniques used for administering intramuscular injections.

Subcutaneous Administration

Subcutaneous drugs are administered under the skin into fat and connective tissue. These drugs must be highly soluble, low volume (less than 2 mL in a good-sized adult), and non-

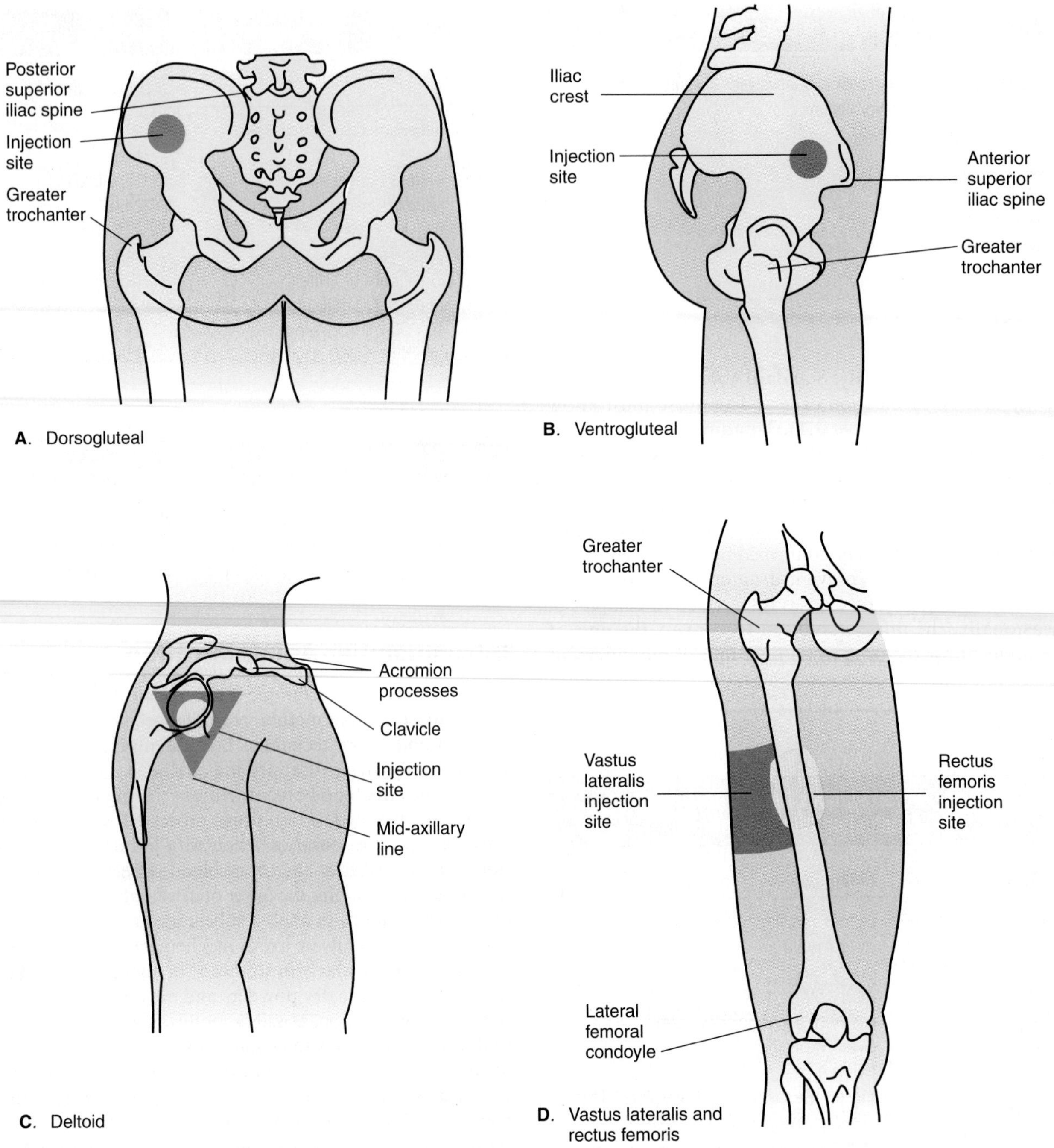

FIGURE 3.1 Anatomic landmarks and intramuscular (IM) injection sites: (**A**) dorsogluteal; (**B**) ventrogluteal; (**C**) deltoid; (**D**) vastus lateralis and rectus femoris.

irritating (to prevent tissue damage, tissue necrosis, and sterile abscess formation). Distribution of the drug is through the capillaries and is less rapid than by the IM route. Distribution slows if the patient has inadequate peripheral circulation or if the drug is administered into scar tissue, which is avascular; onset will therefore be delayed.

The SC route may be used for vaccines, insulin, heparin, and narcotics. The sites used for this route are the upper, lateral arm; anterior thigh; abdomen; and midback above the scapula (Figure 3.2). The size of the individual determines the angle of injection. Refer to nursing practice textbooks to review SC injection techniques.

Intravenous Administration

The **intravenous** technique administers a drug directly into the bloodstream, bypassing the need for absorption from the GI tract or transportation from other parts of the body, such as muscle or subcutaneous tissue. IV administration ensures prompt, sometimes immediate, onset of action and eliminates the uncertainty associated with varied absorption rates from other routes. Advantages of the IV route include the following:

- The IV route has immediate effect (e.g., nitroprusside for a patient in hypertensive crisis).

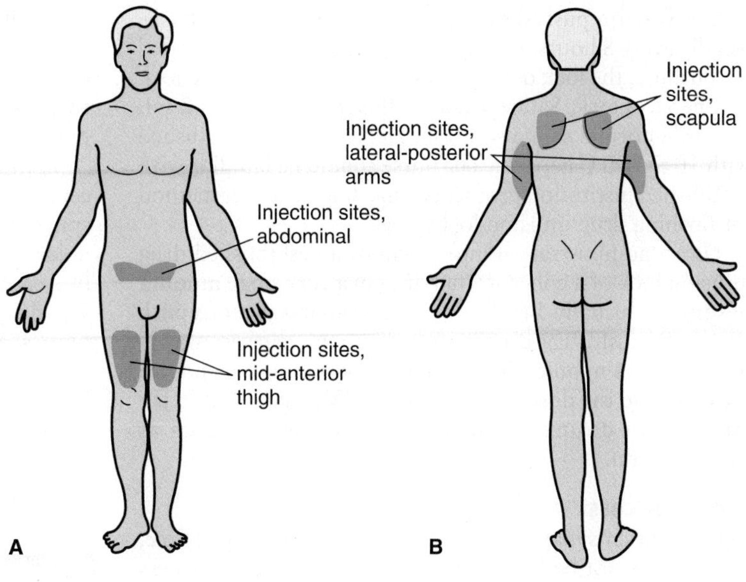

FIGURE 3.2 Subcutaneous (SC) injection sites: (**A**) anterior view: abdominal, mid-anterior thigh; (**B**) posterior view: scapula, lateral-posterior arms.

- The IV route allows administration of a large volume of drug (e.g., with certain antibiotics, such as cefoxitin).
- The IV route avoids tissue irritation or injury resulting from IM or SC administration (e.g., with chemotherapeutic drugs, vasopressors, such as norepinephrine [Levophed], or cardiac glycosides, such as digoxin [Lanoxin], because the blood buffers the drug).
- The IV route is acceptable when no other route is possible (e.g., in an unconscious patient).
- The IV route circumvents impaired circulation.
- The IV route has the potential for prolonged, continuous administration of solutions, such as lidocaine (Xylocaine) or aminophylline (Truphylline), which can be titrated (adjusted in small increments upward or downward) for the desired effect.

The IV route is also, however, one of the most dangerous routes. Once the drug is given, it cannot be retrieved, nor can its distribution through the body be slowed or stopped.

Peripheral Drug Delivery

A peripheral vascular access device, usually an angiocatheter or a butterfly set, is placed to give drugs intravenously. IV drug solutions may be run through tubing into the access device, either continually or intermittently.

Prescribed drugs may be given by continuous IV infusion to maintain a certain blood level of the drug. They are ordered either in volume (milliliters [mL]) per hour or strength (milligram [mg], micrograms [μg], or units [U]) per hour. Aminophylline, lidocaine, and heparin are examples of drugs that are given continuously to achieve maximum therapeutic effect.

IV drugs may also be given intermittently. When the patient receives continuous IV fluids and is also receiving intermittent IV drug therapy, the drug is given through a secondary IV tubing or through a volumetric dose chamber administration set, also called a metered-dose infusion set. When a secondary IV tubing is used to administer an IV drug, the tubing is added to the main line tubing, usually at a Y port. Adding secondary tubing is called "piggybacking" because the tubing with the drug rides on top of the primary fluid tubing.

Antibiotics are frequently given intermittently by **intravenous piggyback** (IV piggyback). Such drugs are diluted in a small volume of IV solution (usually 50 to 100 mL of sterile normal saline solution or 5% dextrose in water for an adult) and infused over 30 to 90 minutes (according to the specific drug). The main IV infusion then resumes at the original preset rate.

Volumetric-dose chamber administration sets connect to the main bag of IV fluid and are connected to IV tubing that in turn attaches to the peripheral venous access device. Volumetric-dose chamber administration sets can be used to run continuous infusions, in which fluid leaves the chamber and is replaced with fluid from the IV bag, or they can infuse only what is currently inside the chamber until manually refilled. When drugs are added to the chamber for infusion, the set is adjusted to infuse only what is in the chamber. When the drug is infused, the set may be returned to a continuous infusion, or refilled with only the main IV solution. These sets are primarily used when fluid restrictions are important, such as with pediatric, elderly, or critically ill patients.

Certain IV drugs, whether given by piggyback or through a metered-dose infusion set, may be incompatible with an existing continuous IV infusion. If this situation arises, the tubing should be flushed with 10 mL of an appropriate solution (usually sterile normal saline) before and after administration of the drug.

If intravenous drugs are prescribed intermittently, and other fluids are not running constantly, the access device is capped to prevent blood from coming out and bacteria from entering the body. This cap may be permanently attached to a small extension tubing set. This tubing is secured to the peripheral device. An access device equipped this way is called "locked," or the patient is said to have a "lock" in place.

Drug infusion locks are used for patients who require intermittent IV drugs but do not need continuous IV fluid administration. As with piggybacks, the drug is usually diluted in 50 to 100 mL of solution. When the drug infusion is complete, the tubing is disconnected from the lock, allowing the patient increased ease of movement. The lock is kept patent (open, without blood clotting occurring), with small volumes of either normal saline (0.9% sodium chloride) solu-

tion or heparin pushed through the lock on a routine basis, usually every 8 hours. Depending on the solution that is used for flushing, the lock device is commonly called a saline lock or a heparin lock. Saline locks are flushed with 0.5 to 2 mL of sterile normal saline solution. Heparin locks are flushed with 10 to 100 U heparin. The nurse should be familiar with established institution protocols regarding the exact method for flushing drug infusion locks.

Direct administration into a vein or an established drug infusion lock of a concentrated drug in a very small amount of solution (usually 1 to 2 mL) is called an **intravenous push** (IVP or IV push). The drug is pushed into the vein very slowly over at least 1 minute. The exact amount of time depends on the drug and the dose. Drugs given by IVP may be used for intermittent dosing or for treating emergencies, such as cardiac arrest.

Central Access

Certain patients may require IV access for a prolonged time, or they may not be able to have peripheral vascular access devices inserted. Devices used for these patients include single or multilumen central venous catheters and implantable venous access ports. A central venous catheter is inserted by the health care provider into a vein (jugular or subclavian) near the heart. The catheter may have as many as three lumens to allow the administration of various solutions and drugs. Peripherally inserted central lines (PICs) or peripherally inserted midlines can be inserted by nurses specifically skilled in the technique. These also may be multilumen lines, and drugs may be delivered continuously, intermittently, or by IVP.

An implantable vascular access port (VAP) is surgically implanted under the skin with the distal end inserted into a large central vein. A special needle (a Huber needle) is used to suffuse the drug into the port. These ports are used for intermittent infusions of, for example, antineoplastic drugs. Use of a VAP requires advanced skills and expertise on the part of the nurse.

Other Parenteral Delivery Routes

Other parenteral routes are the intradermal, intra-articular, intra-arterial, and intrathecal routes. These routes of parenteral administration are not as common as the IM, SC, and IV routes.

Intradermal injections are made into the dermis just below the epidermis. This technique is used primarily for local anesthesia and for sensitivity tests, such as allergy and tuberculin tests. A small needle (25- or 27-gauge) and small-volume syringes (less than 1 mL) are used for intradermal injections. The most common sites for intradermal injections are the medial forearm and the back over the scapula because the skin is thinner there.

An **intra-articular** injection is performed only by a skilled practitioner and involves injecting a drug into a joint. Corticosteroids are typically administered by intra-articular injection to relieve pain in an acutely inflamed joint. The effect is local. Nurses do not commonly administer medications by this route.

Intra-arterial drug administration requires a surgeon to insert a catheter into an artery leading directly to the targeted treatment area. The drug is delivered under positive pressure through the catheter. The positive pressure overcomes the pressure within the arterial system. For example, powerful undiluted chemotherapeutic agents can be delivered directly to a tumor by way of the artery that feeds it. Intra-arterial ports can also be implanted by a surgeon.

In **intrathecal** administration, a drug is delivered into the cerebrospinal fluid. It may be administered directly into the spinal subarachnoid space (a spinal) or outside the subarachnoid space (an epidural). Drugs are introduced into these areas by a catheter placed by specially trained health care providers. The drugs most commonly used are local anesthetics, antibiotics, and radiographic contrast media. This route is commonly used to deliver an anesthetic during labor and delivery. Pain relief can also be achieved with drugs given over this route by the nurse or by the patient using a patient-controlled analgesia device.

NURSING MANAGEMENT IN PARENTERAL DRUG ADMINISTRATION

Parenteral administration may be selected for a variety of reasons. This route allows drugs to be distributed directly to the vascular system without having to be absorbed by the GI tract and sent to the liver before circulating. The erratic absorption associated with the movement of the drug through the GI tract is avoided. Drugs that are highly metabolized by the first-pass mechanism can be given in smaller doses when given parenterally rather than orally because the parenteral route presents more drug to the vascular system initially than the enteral route does. Some drugs are almost completely metabolized during the first pass, so the parenteral route exclusively is chosen for these drugs. Moreover, drugs that are rapidly destroyed by GI secretions can be given parenterally to promote their effectiveness. Parenteral routes may also be necessary because of the GI irritant nature of the drug. Drugs administered by the parenteral routes have a faster onset of action than those administered orally or topically.

Assessment of Relevant Core Patient Variables

Health Status

A parenteral route may be chosen because the patient cannot tolerate oral drugs, cannot swallow, or has a condition that warrants resting the GI tract or keeping it empty. Muscle mass must be sufficient for the volume of a drug given intramuscularly. The gluteal muscle mass can deteriorate if the person does not walk (e.g., because of paralysis), and in such cases it should be avoided as a site for IM injections. The patient's veins must be able to accept a venous access device if drugs are to be given intravenously. When peripheral access devices cannot be inserted, central venous access devices may be used.

Life Span and Gender

Infants have small muscle mass. The largest muscle mass at birth is the vastus lateralis, which is the preferred site for IM injections in infants, although the rectus femoris may also be used. The deltoid is never used for IM injections in infants.

The gluteal muscles develop with walking and usually are not used for injections until the child has been walking for 1 year. Elderly people have decreased muscle mass overall and decreased tissue elasticity, which may result in drugs oozing from injection sites. Muscle mass must be determined before IM injections.

Lifestyle, Diet, and Habits

Parenteral forms of drugs are more expensive than oral forms. Parenteral administration requires specialized skills, equipment, and education. Placing IV access devices into peripheral veins may be difficult in patients who are IV substance abusers.

Environment

Patients, particularly diabetic patients who receive insulin, can be taught to give themselves SC injections at home. The techniques for IM injections can also be taught to patients and their families for home use, although this practice is not as common. IV administration of drugs is usually done in an acute or a long-term care setting; however, it can also be done in the home setting with a home health nurse administering the drug therapy.

Planning and Intervention

Maximizing Therapeutic Effects

Selecting the appropriate-sized syringe and needle is key to administering an IM or SC injection. Selection is based on the patient, the type of required injection, the administration site, and characteristics of the drug (how viscous, how irritating, and how much volume).

A continuous IV drug infusion should be monitored to ensure that therapeutic blood levels are achieved and that drug therapy is effective. After administration of an intermittent IV drug, the lock must be flushed to maintain patency. If heparin is used to keep the lock patent, flushing the lock is usually necessary before drug infusion with sterile normal saline solution, and then again after the infusion before flushing with the heparin. Flushing is necessary because many drugs are incompatible with heparin.

Minimizing Adverse Effects

To minimize adverse effects and drug errors, the nurse follows the six rights of drug administration when administering parenteral drug therapy. To prevent infections, the drug, all parts of the syringe that have come into contact with the drug, and the shaft of the needle that enters the patient's body must be sterile. Meticulous administration technique is necessary because most parenteral drugs enter the bloodstream readily, quickly spreading any organisms introduced with the injection.

Site selection is important because incorrect placement of the needle may damage blood vessels or nerves. Knowledge of the muscles, visible or palpable anatomic landmarks, and location of major nerves and blood vessels in the underlying tissue is an absolute necessity for safe administration.

The oils and irritating chemicals found in the solutions or suspensions of some parenteral drugs may be dangerous if given intravenously. Care must be taken by careful site selection and aspiration before injection to prevent inadvertently administering an IM drug into a blood vessel.

To prevent bacterial growth, reconstituted drugs usually require refrigeration if they are not completely used after dilution. The reconstituted drug container must be labeled with the patient's name, dilution date, and volume and type of diluent used.

When administering drugs that are very irritating to the tissues, the nurse may use an injection technique known as the Z-track method to prevent the drug from seeping up from the muscle into the subcutaneous tissue. Subcutaneous tissue is displaced to one side before inserting the needle into the muscle. The drug is then injected, the needle is withdrawn, and the subcutaneous tissue is allowed to go back into place. Consult your nursing practice texts for more detailed information.

Patients receiving drugs such as aminophylline, dopamine, and heparin by continuous IV infusion must be closely monitored. These drugs have powerful effects on the body, and their adverse effects can be serious or life threatening. The rate at which such drugs are administered should be regulated carefully by using an IV pump or controller. Because the drug enters the bloodstream directly, blood levels of the drug can rise above desired therapeutic levels quickly. Blood levels, therefore, should be closely monitored.

TOPICAL ROUTE AND FORMS

The topical route of drug administration involves applying drug preparations to the skin or mucous membranes, including the eyes, ears, nose, rectum, vagina, and lungs. The primary advantage is that topical drugs usually act locally, although some can have systemic effects. A disadvantage of topical drugs is that most are intended for only one specific site. For example, ophthalmic drugs are only used in the eyes, and dermatologic drugs are only used on the skin. Drugs that can be administered in topical forms include antibiotics, antiseptics, antifungals, anti-inflammatory agents, antipyretics, vasodilators, hormones, antismoking agents, analgesics, antiemetics, and débriding agents.

The most common and widely used topical agents are applied to the skin. Dermatologic preparations come in several forms: lotions, creams, liquids, ointments, and emol-

CRITICAL THINKING SCENARIO

Choosing the right drug administration site

Georgia Govans, 79 years old, is admitted with osteomyelitis of the hip, a severe infection, after a recent repair of a hip fracture. She has a temperature of 101°F (38.3°C) on admission and a history of severe peripheral vascular disease.

1. Which route will most likely be chosen to administer antibiotics to this patient?
2. Select and support a choice of drug delivery method based on the patient's history and her drug requirements.

lients. Emollients are applied liberally to dry skin. Most drugs applied to the intact skin have primarily local effects because little drug is absorbed through the outer epidermis. Absorption increases under the following circumstances:

- The skin is abraded or denuded.
- The drug is added to a specific solvent because only lipid-soluble substances are absorbed through the intact skin.
- The medicated skin is covered by an occlusive dressing (e.g., in treatment for psoriasis).

Most dermatologic drugs are applied in a thin layer or in a measured amount (topical nitroglycerin is applied in inches). Single-dose, adhesive-backed drug applications, called transcutaneous or transdermal drug delivery systems, are currently available. Some examples of the transdermal drug delivery route include nitroglycerin (Nitro-Dur) for patients with coronary artery disease, scopolamine (Transderm-Scop) for patients who suffer from motion sickness, and fentanyl (Duragesic) for patients with severe pain. Although this drug form can be expensive, its ability to avoid first-pass effects is an advantage. The transdermal system is convenient and usually requires less frequent application than other forms.

Drugs administered to the eye take the form of drops or ointments that are applied to the rim of the lower lid. Drugs administered in the ear are in the form of drops. Drugs administered through the rectum are either in suppositories (waxy, bullet-shaped systems that dissolve in the body from body heat) or ointments. Drugs administered into the vagina are in the form of suppositories, creams, foams, liquids, or tablets (moistened before insertion to promote dissolving inside the body).

Drugs given into the nose are either in liquid sprays, drops, or aerosol preparations. Inhalers, another form of aerosolized therapy, are used for respiratory conditions and have an effect on the lungs but are inhaled through mouth breathing. Patients should shake the inhaler well, exhale fully, and then inhale while pushing down on the inhaler to activate it. They should breathe in the puff of drug and hold the breath for several seconds before exhaling. The timing of this technique is difficult for many patients. The use of a spacer, which acts as a reservoir for the drug, is helpful for many patients. The patient activates the inhaler, and the drug enters the spacer. The patient then breathes in from the spacer. If multiple puffs of the inhaler are ordered, the patient should wait 1 to 2 minutes between puffs. The inhaler and the patient's mouth should be rinsed after drug administration.

NURSING MANAGEMENT IN TOPICAL DRUG ADMINISTRATION

Assessment of Relevant Core Patient Variables

For the most part, assessment involves inspecting the skin for integrity. If the skin is not intact, aseptic technique becomes an important factor in infection control.

Planning and Intervention

To maximize therapeutic effects and minimize adverse effects, the nurse should wear gloves or use an applicator when administering dermatologic drugs, to avoid infecting the patient and to protect his or her own skin from the drug. If the skin is broken, the nurse needs to use sterile technique when applying a dermatologic drug to prevent introducing bacteria and other organisms into the body. If an adverse effect occurs with drugs given by a transdermal system, removing the patch usually relieves the symptoms.

To ensure safety when administering all forms of topical drugs, the nurse must again observe the six rights of drug administration (see Box 3.1).

CHAPTER SUMMARY

- The three routes of drug administration are enteral, parenteral, and topical.
- The drug route may produce systemic effects, local effects, or both.
- Oral drugs may be available in sustained-release or enteric-coated form to delay onset of action of the drug.
- Food, fluids, and other drugs may alter the absorption of enteric drugs.
- The parenteral route avoids the GI tract and the irregularities of absorption, including the first-pass effect. The most common methods of parenteral drug administration are the IM, SC, and IV routes.
- Onset of drug action is more rapid with the parenteral than with the enteral route.
- Patient characteristics (age, weight, muscle mass) and drug characteristics (volume, viscosity, irritability) are considered when selecting a site for IM drug administration.
- Administration of IV drugs may be through continuous drip, intermittent infusion, or IVP methods into peripheral or central venous access devices.
- Topical drugs include those that are applied to the skin and mucous membranes of the eyes, ears, nose, rectum, and vagina.

QUESTIONS FOR STUDY AND REVIEW

1. Which route of drug administration is most frequently used?
2. What is the advantage of an enteric-coated tablet?
3. Why might a parenteral route of a drug be prescribed instead of an enteral route?
4. Which parenteral technique poses the greatest risk for rapid drug toxicity to a patient?

Need More Help?

Chapter 3 of the study guide for *Drug Therapy in Nursing* 2e contains NCLEX-style questions and other learning activities to reinforce your understanding of the concepts presented in this chapter. For additional information or to purchase the study guide, visit *http://connection.lww.com/go/aschenbrenner.*

■ REFERENCES AND BIBLIOGRAPHY

Anderson, R. P. (1998). Alternative routes of opioid administration in palliative care: Pharmacologic and clinical concerns. *Journal of Pharmaceutical Care in Pain & Symptom Control, 6*(1), 5–21.

Anonymous. (1997). Position statement. Insulin administration. *Diabetes Care, 20*(Suppl. 1), 546–549.

Basskin, L. E. (1999). New pharmacotherapy. Oral transmucosal fentanyl citrate: A new dosage form for breakthrough malignant pain. *American Journal of Pain Management, 9*(4), 129–138.

Belknap, D. C., Seifer, C. F., & Petermann, M. (1997). Administration of medications through enteral feeding catheters. *American Journal of Critical Care, 6*(5), 382–392.

Grond, S., Radbruch, L., & Lehmann, K. A. (2000). Clinical pharmacokinetics of transdermal opioids: focus on transdermal fentanyl. *Clinical Pharmacokinetics, 38*(1), 59–89.

McConnell, E. A. (1997). Clinical do's and don'ts. Using transdermal medication patches. *Nursing, 27*(7), 18.

Naysmith, M. R., & Nicholson, J. (1998) Nasogastric drug administration. *Professional Nurse, 13*(7), 424–427.

Roger, M. A., & King, L. (2000). Drawing up and administering intramuscular injections: A review of the literature. *Journal of Advanced Nursing, 31*(3), 574–582.

Sharar, S. R., Bratton, S. L., Carrougher, G. J., Edwards, W. T., Summer, G., Levy, F. H., & Cortiella, J. (1998). A comparison of oral transmucosal fentanyl citrate and oral hydromorphone for inpatient pediatric burn wound care analgesia. *Journal of Burn Care and Rehabilitation, 19*(6), 516–521.

Starr, C. (2000). Innovations in drug delivery. *Patient Care, 34*(1), 107–108, 113–114, 117–121.

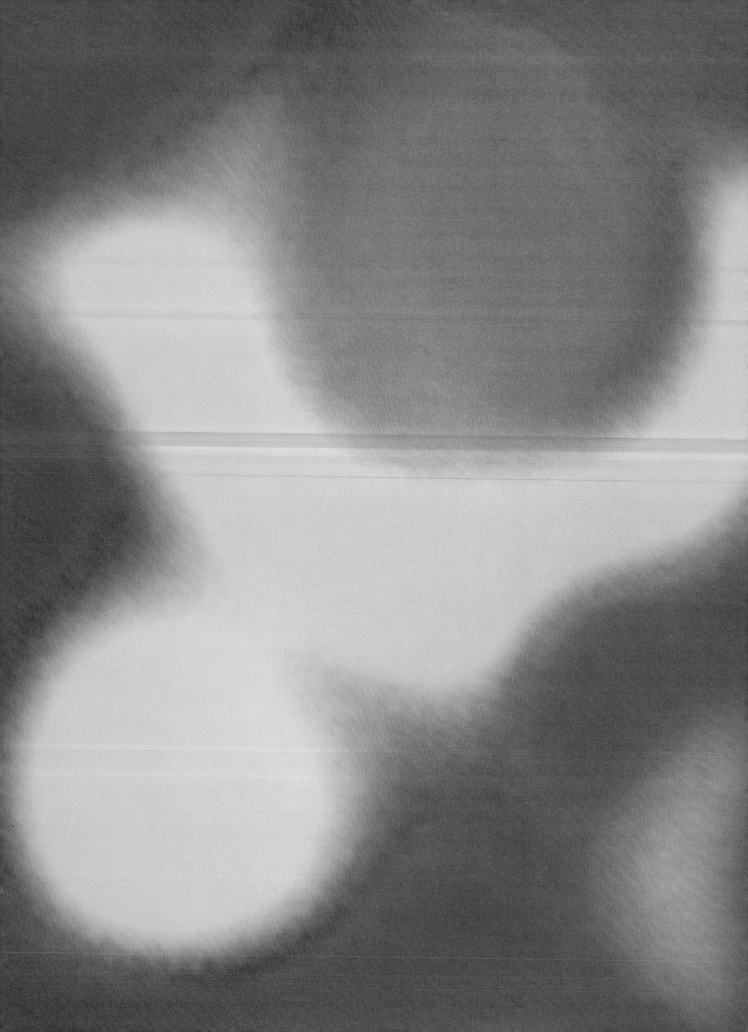

Core Drug Knowledge

unit 2

Pharmacotherapeutics, Pharmacokinetics, and Pharmacodynamics

chapter 4

Learning Objectives

At the completion of this chapter the student will:

1. Define pharmacotherapeutics, pharmacokinetics, and pharmacodynamics.
2. Describe the processes used as drugs move throughout the body.
3. Understand how the chemical makeup of a drug and the internal chemistry of the body affect a drug's ability to cross cell membranes.
4. Identify factors that affect absorption of drug molecules.
5. Describe factors that influence the distribution of drug molecules.
6. Discuss factors that may alter metabolism.
7. Identify how drug molecules are excreted from the body.
8. Identify the main mechanism drugs use to produce their effects on the body.
9. Describe the variables that influence the dose of a drug that is administered.

FEATURED WEBLINK

http://www.med.rug.nl/pharma/who-cc/ggp/ow-annx1.htm
For a good overview of essentials of pharmacology in daily practice, visit the World Health Organization's *Guide to Good Prescribing,* Annex 1.

CONNECTION WEBLINK

Additional Weblinks are found on Connection:
http://www.connection.lww.com/go/aschenbrenner.

KEY TERMS

absorption
affinity
agonist
antagonist
biotransformation
blocker
blood–brain barrier
clearance
distribution
efficacy
excretion
first-pass effect
half-life
intrinsic activity
loading dose
maintenance dose
metabolism
metabolites
P-450 system
pharmacokinetics
pharmacodynamics
pharmacotherapeutics
placebo
potency
prodrug
receptor
steady state
therapeutic index

Drug therapy in nursing involves more than passing the appropriately ordered drug to the right patient. The nurse must understand how drug therapy creates its effects in the body and be able to critically assess the patient's response to drug therapy. In order to do this, the nurse needs to know basic pharmacologic facts. These facts make up the Core Drug Knowledge related to a particular drug. As in all bodies of knowledge, there is a "language" of words that is specific to pharmacology and drug therapy. The nurse needs to understand this language and be able to correctly use the words in order to read and interpret written drug material and to clearly communicate with pharmacists, physicians, and other health professionals about drug therapy. This chapter examines the pharmacotherapeutics, pharmacokinetics, and the pharmacodynamics in Core Drug Knowledge.

PHARMACOTHERAPEUTICS

Pharmacotherapeutics is the achievement of the desired therapeutic goal from drug therapy. Essentially, it is the clinical purpose—the indication—for giving a drug. The terms *indications* and *therapeutics* are often substituted for the more formal term *pharmacotherapeutics*. For example, when a person has hypertension, we give drugs to lower the blood pressure to a normal level. In this way we treat, or manage, a chronic condition. The desired pharmacotherapeutics can also be used to induce a cure. For example, when a patient has a bacterial infection, we give an antibiotic that kills the infecting organism. The desired therapeutic effect of a drug can also be to prevent a problem. An example of this type of use is when a patient has had total joint replacement surgery. Because this procedure increases the patient's risk for developing a thrombus (blood clot), drug therapy with anticoagulants is used to prevent this undesirable outcome. Whatever the clinical or medical reason is for prescribing a drug, the pharmacotherapeutics is the desired outcome of administering that drug.

Labeled and Nonlabeled Uses

Generally, the pharmacotherapeutics of a drug is determined through clinical drug trials. Findings from these studies are submitted to the governmental agency that oversees approval of new drugs. In the United States, this agency is the Food and Drug Administration (FDA). If the clinical studies indicate that the effect a drug has on the desired outcomes of treatment is statistically significantly better than that achieved by a **placebo** (an inactive substance), the drug is approved for a particular indication or indications. This information is included when labeling the drug and in printed material about the drug.

After a drug is approved, however, it may be legally prescribed for a use that is not indicated on the label, if the prescriber believes it to be of benefit. Many "off-label" uses of drugs are based on the findings of additional research studies that are performed and reported in the professional literature. Case reports published in the literature may also support off-label uses of a drug. Off-label uses may become standard pharmacotherapeutic uses of a drug. The official drug label is modified only if the drug company goes back to the FDA with additional information and requests that a new pharmacotherapeutic indication be added. After an official review, the FDA may decide to alter the drug label. Because this process can be lengthy and expensive for the drug company, the company may not seek relabeling, even if the drug is commonly used in practice in this way. Nurses should not be overly concerned about off-label uses as long as the literature supports such use or the prescriber can explain why this drug is being used for a patient who does not have a condition for which the drug is indicated. Nurses do need to question all orders if the intended pharmacotherapeutics of a drug does not correlate with the patient's reason for receiving drug therapy. Such questions are necessary to help prevent medication errors in which the wrong drug has been prescribed. Nurses are also legally responsible for understanding the pharmacotherapeutics of all drugs that they administer.

PHARMACOKINETICS

Pharmacokinetics is the movement of the drug particles inside the body and the processes that occur during this movement. In general, pharmacokinetics is the effect of the body on the drug. Pharmacokinetics is made up of four phases: absorption, distribution, metabolism, and excretion. **Absorption** is the movement of the drug from the site of administration into the bloodstream. **Distribution** is movement of the drug through the bloodstream, into the tissues, and eventually into the cells. **Metabolism** is the conversion of the drug into another substance or substances. **Excretion** is the removal of the drug, or what the drug became after metabolism, from the body.

Drug molecules move during all phases of pharmacokinetics. To move throughout the body, the drug must cross membranes. Cells in most membranes are very close together, without much space between the cells. The membrane of the cell itself is mostly made up of lipid molecules. Drugs cross cell membranes in one of three ways. First, they can pass between the spaces or channels between the molecules in the membrane. Drug molecules can only cross a cell membrane this way if they are very small. Second, drugs can pass through the membrane with the help of a transport system. This method may or may not require the use of energy. Third, drugs can penetrate the membrane directly. To be able to penetrate the membrane, the drug must be lipophilic (soluble in lipids). Direct penetration is the method used by most drugs to cross the cell membrane.

The chemistry of the drug particles will also affect the movement of particles throughout the body. In some drug molecules, the positive charges (protons) and the negative charges (electrons) are grouped away from each other. These charged molecules are termed polar molecules. Although the charge in polar molecules is unevenly distributed, such molecules have an equal number of positive and negative charges, so that they have no net charge. Polar molecules are hydrophilic (soluble in water), not lipophilic. Therefore, polar drug molecules are not able to penetrate cell membranes. Nonpolar molecules are lipophilic; therefore, nonpolar molecules are able to penetrate cell membranes.

Ions are molecules that carry a net charge (either positive or negative). Very small ions move through the channels on

the cell membranes (the spaces between molecules). Other ions do not cross the cell membrane. Some molecules that normally do not carry a charge can be induced to carry a charge, depending on their environment. The process of inducing a molecule to carry a charge is called ionization because ions have a net charge. Acids give up a positive charge in a basic (alkaline) environment. Bases accept a positive charge in an acidic environment. Movement of molecules through a membrane occurs as long as the environment does not cause the molecule to ionize (i.e., become a charged molecule). If the environment promotes ionization, movement through the membrane stops. When the pH on either side of a membrane differs, drug molecules tend to move to the side where ionization will occur. This movement is termed ion trapping or pH portioning. Altering the pH on one side of a membrane thus alters the movement of the drug molecules.

Absorption

Several variables affect the completeness and rate of drug absorption. The completeness of absorption is the portion of the drug that is absorbed. Drugs given orally may not be completely absorbed because of other drugs or food that the patient is ingesting. The rate of absorption of a drug depends on the route of administration. The rate of absorption is also affected by the speed at which the drug dissolves, known as the rate of dissolution.

- Drugs that are administered orally generally take the longest to be absorbed because they must be broken down into small particles before they can move into the bloodstream. The presence of other drugs or food may also impair the rate of oral drug absorption.
- Drugs given parenterally are already dissolved and in a liquid form and therefore are absorbed more rapidly than drugs given orally.
- Drugs that are administered subcutaneously or intramuscularly are absorbed into the small capillaries fairly rapidly. Intramuscular absorption is somewhat more rapid than subcutaneous absorption.
- Drugs that are administered intravenously are placed directly into the bloodstream and are not technically absorbed, although some sources refer to intravenous drugs as being instantly absorbed.

Large surface areas increase the rate of absorption. Drugs administered orally are thus absorbed primarily in the small intestine, which has a larger surface area than the stomach, although some absorption occurs in the stomach. Blood flow also affects the rate of absorption—the greater the volume of blood flow, the faster the rate of absorption. Absorption speeds up with increased blood flow because increased flow carries more absorbed drug molecules away into the general circulation; in its place is blood without any particles of drug. Thus, the high concentration of drug moves into the blood where there is a low concentration of drug. Patients who have impaired circulatory systems (e.g., those with peripheral vascular disease) absorb drugs less rapidly than those with normally functioning systems. Lipid solubility also alters absorption. Drugs that are more lipid soluble usually are absorbed more rapidly than others because they can cross the lipid cell membranes easily. Finally, when pH differences between the site of administration and the plasma favor the drug molecules becoming ionized in the plasma, absorption is more rapid than when the molecules do not become ionized.

Finally, the physiologic condition of the patient affects drug absorption. Core patient variables that affect drug absorption are summarized in Box 4.1.

Distribution

The distribution of a drug throughout the body depends on three factors: blood flow to the tissues, the drug's ability to leave the blood, and the drug's ability to enter cells.

Once a drug is absorbed, it is transported to the tissues and cells through the circulatory system. In healthy individuals, all tissues are well perfused; thus, drug molecules can easily be distributed throughout the body. When there are pathophysiologic changes in the vascular system (such as narrowed, stiff, or occluded vessels), the distribution of drug molecules is impaired. This impairment may or may not affect distribution enough to decrease the therapeutic effect of the drug. For example, in a patient with peripheral vascular disease, circulation to the heart is not usually greatly impaired, although circulation to the legs and feet is. In this patient, a drug given for an altered cardiac rhythm may not be distributed well into the tissues in the legs, but plenty of drug molecules reach the heart, so that the drug is capable of achieving the desired pharmacotherapeutic effect. However, a drug given to treat cellulitis of the foot may not have adequate distribution to achieve the desired pharmacotherapeutic effect, because of the impaired circulation in the lower extremities.

Some tissues have little or no blood supply. Scar tissue is avascular, and adipose (fat) tissue has a poor blood supply. Two types of pathologic conditions—abscesses (pus-filled pockets surrounded by normal tissue) and solid tumors—have very limited blood supply, especially to their centers. Because drug therapy does not distribute well to these areas, it is difficult to treat problems that may develop (such as infections in the adipose tissue) or the pathology itself (i.e., the abscess or tumor) by drug therapy alone.

Once the drug has moved through the blood to the tissues, it must leave the bloodstream to enter the tissue itself. This transition is necessary because most drugs do not produce their effect while in the blood. The drug leaves the vascular space in the capillary bed. Because the cells of the capillary walls have fairly wide spaces between them, the drug molecules simply move between the cells to leave the capillaries and enter the tissues.

Protein Binding

Protein binding of drugs affects the distribution of a drug. Protein binding is an important concept to understand. Drug particles form reversible bonds with proteins in the blood, most specifically albumin. Because albumin is a large molecule, it cannot pass through capillary walls. Therefore, when the drug particle is attached to the albumin, the drug is prevented from passing through the capillary walls. Different drugs have different affinities, or attractions, to protein molecules. Some drugs are so attracted to protein that almost all of the drug will bind with protein if the protein is available.

BOX 4.1 Drug Absorption and Core Patient Variables

1. **Health status.** Any change in health status related to circulation, condition of the GI tract, or pH of body fluids (e.g., disease, trauma, strenuous physical exercise, or drug therapy) can reduce drug absorption. The condition of the gastric and intestinal surfaces affects oral drug absorption.
2. **Contact time, surface area of contact, and the condition of the absorptive surface** may increase or decrease the amount of drug absorbed. For example:
   - Large surfaces (e.g., pulmonary alveolar epithelium, intestinal mucosa) absorb drugs rapidly.
   - Decreased absorptive surface from damage (e.g., radiation), disease (e.g., inflammatory bowel disease) or surgery (e.g., surgically shortened intestine) lessens drug absorption.
3. Absorption from the GI tract depends on factors such as **gastric volume, GI pH, gastric emptying time, intestinal transit rate, gastric motility, and GI enzyme levels.**
   - Delayed transport from the stomach to the intestine (e.g., food in the stomach) will dilute the drug and increase the contact time by slowing gastric emptying.
   - Decreased GI motility (e.g., constipation) permits increased drug contact time with the GI mucosa, allowing extra time for absorption, which may lead to increased drug effects and toxicity.
   - Increased intestinal motility may enhance drug dissolution and absorption; a patient with increased intestinal motility (e.g., diarrhea), will move a drug very quickly through the GI tract, reducing the amount of time the drug remains in contact with the GI mucosa and impairing drug absorption.
4. **Life span and gender.** There are gender-related variations that alter absorption. For example:
   - Ingested solids versus liquids empty more slowly from women's stomachs, gastric acidity is lower in women, and women have lower gastric levels of alcohol dehydrogenase.
5. **Lifestyle, diet, and habits**
   - Diet may stimulate digestive enzymes and alter the gastric and intestinal mucosa. Generally, drugs ingested with food are slower absorbed than drugs taken on an empty stomach. Some drugs and food form complexes that cannot pass through the mucosal lining of the GI tract (e.g., tetracycline antimicrobials that bind with calcium, magnesium, iron, aluminum), and thus effective blood levels may not be reached. Some drugs are destroyed by the high acidity and peptic activity of gastric digestive enzymes.
   - The quality of blood flow to the site of absorption affects how much of the drug is absorbed. For example: Increased blood flow (e.g., application of heat or massage) enhances drug absorption because of the resulting increase in circulation. Similarly, absorption slows when blood flow decreases (e.g., shock or vasoconstriction). Some muscles normally have greater blood supply; for example, a drug injected into the deltoid muscle will be absorbed faster than one injected into the gluteus muscle because of the greater blood flow to the deltoid muscle.

These drugs are classified as highly protein bound. Other drugs have so little attraction that hardly any of the drug will bind with the available protein. Only drug molecules that are unattached to protein are capable of moving to their site of action (distribution) and achieving the desired therapeutic effect.

Another way of saying this is that only the free drug is active. Consider two drugs, A and B. Drug A is 95 % protein bound; Drug B is 25% protein bound. This means that for every 100 molecules of Drug A, 95 molecules will be bound with protein, and 5 molecules will be free and active. For every 100 molecules of Drug B, however, 25 will be bound to protein, and 75 will be free and active. Drug A may therefore require a larger dose than Drug B to achieve the same therapeutic effect because not as many of the molecules from each dose can distribute through the body and be active (Figure 4.1).

Protein binding can be compared with ninth-grade students at a school dance. If most of the students are interested in dancing, only a few of them are free to do as they please and to move about (and potentially cause trouble). If, however, most of the students are not that interested in dancing, then many are free to do as they please. The odds are increased that what they choose to do may be seen as troublesome to the teachers.

The bonds between the drug and protein molecules are not permanent. The bonds will dissolve in time, and the drug molecules will become free and active. Other drug molecules may then form a bond with the protein molecule.

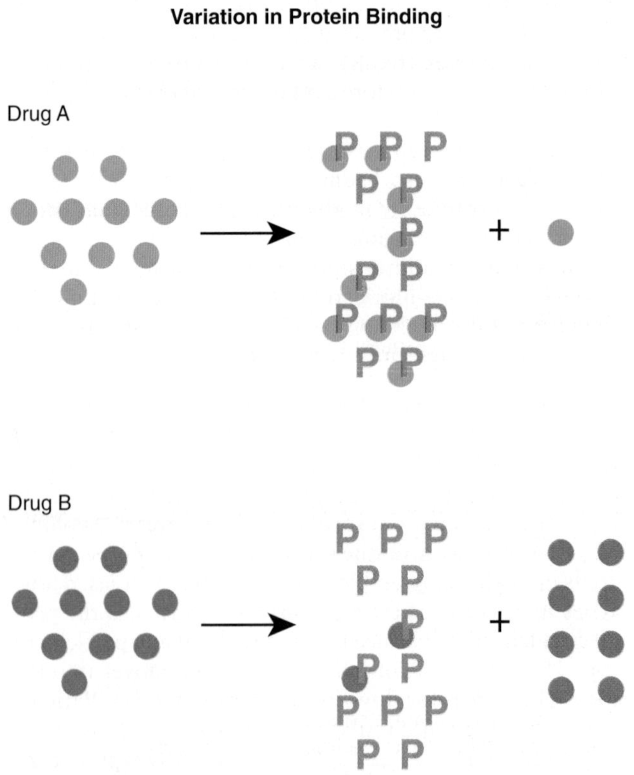

FIGURE 4.1 Drug A (●) is highly protein (P) bound. Little of the drug is free and active. Drug B (●) has low protein binding. A great deal of the drug is free and active.

The length of time the drug is bound varies, based on properties of the drug. In keeping with our analogy of a dance, students may dance with each other for quite some time, or for only one song. They then separate and choose new partners, or they may remain free.

Drug dosages are calculated based on the protein-binding characteristics of the drug. When the dose is determined, it is based on normal protein levels being available in the blood. When the patient has a lower-than-expected protein level (e.g., as a result of malnutrition, liver failure, or severe burns), the distribution of the drug is altered. Even if the drug normally has a high affinity for protein (i.e., it is highly protein bound), if protein is lacking, not as much drug can be bound. Less drug is bound because there is no place for the drug molecule to go. When less drug is bound, more drug is free and can be distributed to its site of action, thereby causing increased therapeutic, and possibly increased adverse, effects (Figure 4.2).

Because different drugs have different affinities for albumin, the administration of more than one drug simultaneously may also alter protein binding and consequently affect distribution of both drugs. For example, a particular drug is being administered. Part of that drug is bound to protein. Now, a second drug is also given, and it has a higher attraction to albumin than the first drug has. The second drug will bump or displace the first drug in order to bind with the protein (Figure 4.3). Displacement means that more of the first drug is free and active and will be distributed (as compared with distribution, when the first drug was the only drug being administered). The dosage of the first drug may have to be decreased to prevent excessive therapeutic or adverse effects.

In summary, protein binding plays an important role in distribution of active drug molecules. Changes in the expected protein-binding capabilities of a drug, either from pharmaceutical properties of other drugs or from patient-related variables, alter the effectiveness of drug therapy.

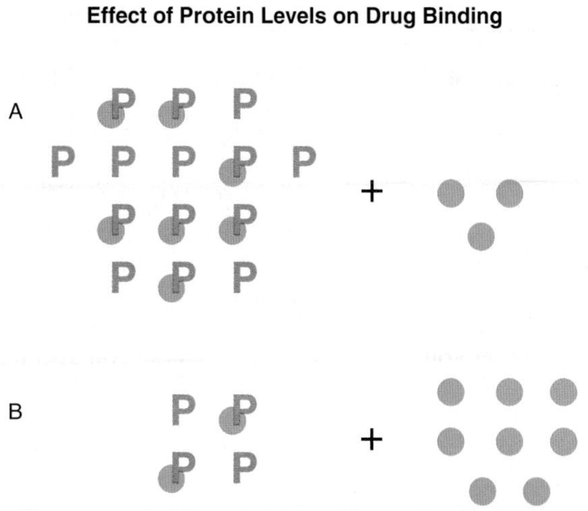

FIGURE 4.2 (**A**) High protein binding of a drug allows only a few drug molecules to be free and active. (**B**) When serum protein levels are below normal, the drug molecules have nowhere to bind. The number of drug molecules that are free is thus greater than would be normally expected. More therapeutic effects and adverse effects are likely to occur.

Blood–Brain Barrier

The capillary bed that services the brain is different from other capillary beds. Instead of wide spaces between the cells in the capillary walls, the cells are packed tightly together. This structure prevents drug molecules, and other foreign substances, from passing through and entering the brain. This system is called the **blood–brain barrier.** The purpose of the blood–brain barrier is to keep toxins and poisons from reaching the brain. This protective mechanism normally promotes health, but occasionally it prevents treatment of problems. For example, many antibiotics cannot cross the blood–brain barrier, making treatment of life-

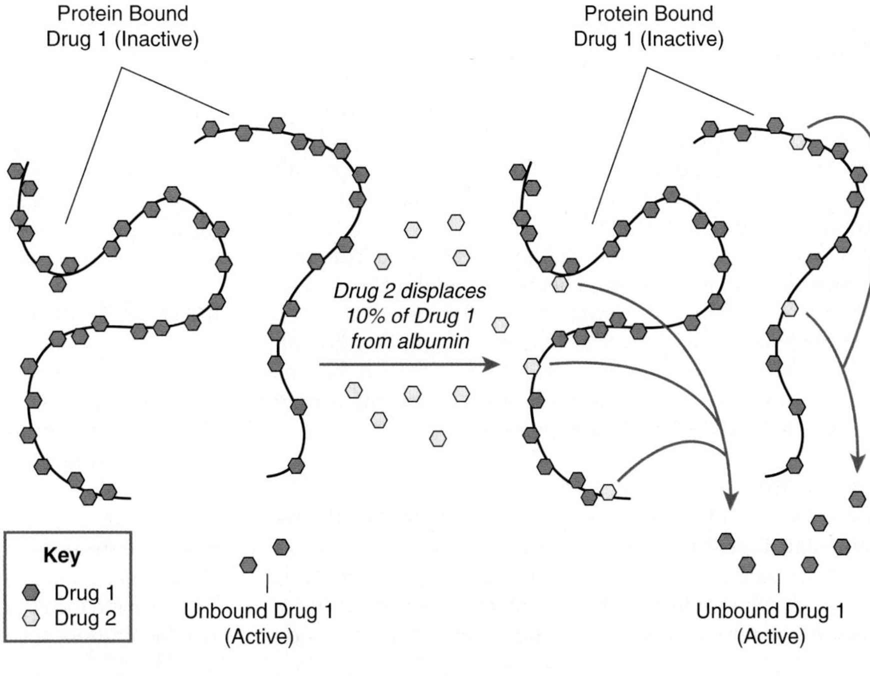

FIGURE 4.3 Consequence of drug displacement from albumin and other plasma proteins. Some drugs (e.g., "Drug 1") are greater than 90% bound to plasma proteins. The "free" (unbound) drug molecules, but not the bound molecules, are available to act at receptors. "Drug 2" displaces only five molecules of Drug 1, which more than triples the serum concentration of free (active) Drug 1. This increase could be fatal if Drug 1 has a narrow margin of safety. Displacement of drugs that are less highly protein bound is less significant. For example, if Drug 1 were 50% bound and 50% free, displacement of 10% of the bound fraction would increase the free fraction from 50% to 55%. This small increment is unlikely to be clinically relevant.

threatening infections of the brain, such as bacterial meningitis, difficult.

The way the blood–brain barrier works can be likened to a driver trying to exit a highway during rush hour. Imagine that you are driving in the far left lane of a three-lane highway. To exit the highway at one of the exit ramps, you must cross two lanes of traffic. If the traffic is light and there are great distances between the cars, exiting the highway can be accomplished easily. However, if the traffic is heavy and bumper to bumper, it is almost impossible to cross the other lanes to exit. In order to exit, you need to convince other drivers to let you pass through their lanes. You also might be able to move to the exit with the help of a police officer who is directing traffic.

In most tissues, the capillary walls have large spaces between the cells, like the times when the traffic is light and there are large spaces between the cars on the highway. In the brain, however, the cells that form the walls of the capillaries are packed together, like the cars on the highway during rush hour. Only drug molecules that are lipophilic (i.e., able to merge) or that have a transport system (i.e., a police officer directing traffic) can penetrate the barrier and get to the other side.

Placental Barrier

The placental membrane, which separates the maternal circulation from the fetal circulation, is not a barrier like the blood–brain barrier. Any drug that can pass through a membrane can pass through the placenta. In order to pass through the placenta, a drug must be lipophilic, not ionized, and not protein bound.

Core patient variables that influence drug distribution are summarized in Box 4.2.

BOX 4.2 Drug Distribution and Core Patient Variables

Health Status

1. Hepatic dysfunction alters the manufacture of albumin. For example, an alteration of health status (e.g., hepatic impairment), diet (e.g., malnutrition), and habits (e.g., ethanol consumption, smoking) directly affect the liver.
2. Conditions such as hypoalbuminemia, hepatic disease, and renal disease can decrease the extent of drug binding, particularly of acidic and neutral drugs. A diseased liver cannot synthesize the protein building blocks needed for albumin production. Thus, there is a greater concentration of free drug and a greater risk of increased drug response and toxicity.

Life Span and Gender

1. At birth, the blood–brain barrier is not fully developed; this causes an increased vulnerability of the infant to CNS poisons and greater sensitivity to drugs that act on the brain in comparison with older children and adults.
2. In pregnant women and fetuses, some drugs may be distributed to and bind with receptor sites in such a way that tissues may be adversely affected. For instance, bones and teeth, which contain calcium, can accumulate substances that bind with calcium (e.g., tetracycline antibiotics).
3. Blood albumins are not thought to possess a gender-dependent predilection, although levels of some globulin proteins (e.g., corticosteroid-binding and sex-hormone binding) are lower in women. Although the small differences in protein levels between the genders are unlikely to be clinically significant, lower blood albumin levels may increase the effect of drugs that are normally highly protein bound.

Metabolism

Metabolism of drugs occurs primarily in the liver. Some metabolism also occurs in other tissues, most notably the gastrointestinal (GI) tract, lungs, kidney, and skin. Recent research has shown that the intestinal mucosa is a major metabolic organ for some drugs and that intestinal metabolism greatly reduces the oral bioavailability of some drugs, such as nifedipine, a cardiovascular drug used to treat angina and hypertension (Doherty & Charman, 2002). Physiologic factors that impair the functioning of the liver, such as hepatitis and cirrhosis, decrease the ability of the liver to metabolize drugs. Other core patient variables that affect drug metabolism are given in Box 4.3.

When drugs are metabolized, they are changed from their original form to a new form. Therefore, metabolism is sometimes referred to as **biotransformation.** Drugs are generally metabolized from substances that are lipophilic into substances that are hydrophilic. The ability of a drug to become soluble in water is important because it allows the drug to be excreted through the renal system.

Metabolites

A product of metabolism is called a **metabolite.** Metabolism can create inactive metabolites; they will have no effect on the body as they travel throughout the body waiting to be excreted. Metabolism can also create active metabolites, which can achieve some independent effect on the body. Active metabolites may be beneficial. For example, after metabolism, codeine is changed to morphine, which is a stronger analgesic than codeine. Metabolism can convert a drug that has little or no therapeutic effect into the active, helpful form. Drugs that must be metabolized to be converted to an active form are called **prodrugs.** An example of a prodrug is primidone, used to control seizures. Primidone's primary anticonvulsant effect comes from the drug being metabolized into phenobarbital and PEMA, both strong anticonvulsants. Finally, an active metabolite may cause a different and potentially harmful effect from that of the original drug. An example of a prodrug with a harmful metabolite is meperidine, an analgesic, whose active metabolite is neurotoxic.

Rates of Metabolism and the First-Pass Effect

Metabolism occurs at different rates for different drugs. Some drugs are highly metabolized, meaning that every time drug molecules are circulated to the liver (about 25% of the cardiac output is sent to the liver), a large percentage of the drug molecules is metabolized. Other drugs are metabolized at slower rates, and a smaller percentage is metabolized each time the drug molecules circulate through the liver. Keep in mind that the percentage of drug that is metabolized each time the drug circulates, or passes, through the liver is the same, but the total number of drug molecules that are metabolized will be different (Figure 4.4). Highly metabolized drugs may

BOX 4.3 Drug Metabolism and Core Patient Variables

Life Span and Gender

1. Drug metabolism in patients whose enzymatic metabolic systems are either immature or functioning less efficiently (e.g., neonates, children, and older adults) is highly variable but is usually diminished. Decreased drug metabolism places the patient at increased risk of adverse effects from the drug.

Lifestyle, Diet, and Habits

1. Malnutrition may prolong drug effects as a result of poor hepatic microsomal metabolism.
2. In obese people, phase II transformations tend to occur more rapidly, thereby necessitating higher drug dosages. Obesity significantly influences distribution in drugs that are highly lipophilic (e.g., anesthetics, barbiturates).
3. Drug effects may be intensified if the specific drug places the person at nutritional risk by producing anorexia, increased appetite, nausea and vomiting, nutritional deficiencies, stomatitis, or toxic reactions, for example.
4. Diet may contribute to individual variations in drug metabolism. Charcoal-broiled foods and cruciferous vegetables induce one CYP isoenzyme, whereas grapefruit juice inhibits one.
5. Exposure to cigarette smoke and pesticides may cause a more rapid metabolism of some drugs because of enzyme induction.

Environment

1. Reduced partial pressure of oxygen at higher altitudes may affect enzymatic reduction systems.
2. Environmental pollutants may affect induction or inhibition of hepatic enzymes.
3. Light is a key modulator in the regulation of metabolic pathways and in specific settings may affect drug response (e.g., intensive care units that commonly remain constantly lit).

lose their therapeutic effectiveness quickly, especially drugs that are administered orally. After an oral drug is broken down and absorbed into the circulatory system, the first place the blood travels is to the liver, through the portal vein. Thus, drugs that are highly metabolized lose much of their effectiveness during this first pass through the liver, before they reach general circulation. This loss of effectiveness is called the **first-pass effect.** Drugs that experience a high first-pass effect may need higher oral doses to achieve a therapeutic level of circulating drug. To avoid the first-pass effect or the need for high oral doses of a drug, drugs that are highly metabolized are often given by another route that bypasses the liver initially. For example, the drug may be given intravenously. None of the drug given intravenously will initially go to the liver; all of it will return to the heart. From the heart, slightly more than 25% of the drug will be sent to the liver, where a percentage of it is metabolized.

P-450 System

Liver metabolism is predominantly achieved by specific liver enzymes. These microsomal enzymes are called the cytochrome P-450 system, or, more commonly, the **P-450 system.** This system is a combination of several types of cytochromes, called families. Of these, only three families—CYP1, CYP2, and CYP3—are involved in drug metabolism. The other enzymes in the P-450 group metabolize naturally occurring substances, such as fatty acids. Scientists have been able to identify specific members of each cytochrome family. These members are identified by a letter (representing the subgroup) and a number (representing the specific isoenzyme) after the family name (e.g., CYP1A2). This nomenclature is analogous to listing your name as follows: last name, middle name, first name. The enzyme CYP3A4 is the most common and is responsible for the metabolism of most drugs. Isoenzymes can also be found in other organs, such as those in the GI tract, and are responsible for the metabolism that occurs in these locations.

Some drugs either induce or inhibit the P-450 system, altering metabolism of other drugs. Usually, just one P-450 family is affected. Drugs that induce a hepatic enzyme increase the amount of that enzyme present in the liver. Induction is accomplished most frequently by stimulating enzyme synthesis. When a large quantity of one of these enzymes is present, more metabolism can occur through this pathway. Drugs that are metabolized by this pathway (also referred to as substrates of the enzyme) will therefore be metabolized more rapidly than drugs that are not. This increase in metabolism rapidly decreases the amount of circulating, active drug. Some drugs can induce the enzymes necessary for their own metabolism and thus can increase the rate of their own metabolism.

Number of Passes Through the Liver	Number of Drug Molecules Returning to the Liver Before Metabolism	Number of Drug Molecules Metabolized	Number of Drug Molecules Left After Liver Metabolism	Percent of Drug Metabolized
First	100	25	75	25%
Second	56.25	14.06	42.19	25%
Third	31.64	7.91	23.73	25%
Fourth	17.8	4.45	13.35	25%
Fifth	3.34	0.83	2.51	25%
Sixth	0.63	0.16	0.47	25%

FIGURE 4.4 For this hypothetical drug, 25% of the drug is metabolized every time the drug circulates to the liver for metabolism. Note that the percentage of drug metabolized stays the same each time but the total number of drug molecules metabolized varies. Why is there less drug returning to the liver than was left after the previous pass and metabolism? This is because only about 25% of any given cardiac output will be sent to the liver, the rest of the drug is sent elsewhere in the body from the heart.

Drugs that inhibit a particular hepatic enzyme slow the metabolism that occurs through this pathway, causing an increase in the amount of circulating, active drug. Metabolism returns to normal after the inducing or inhibiting drug is no longer administered, although it may take several days after an inducer is discontinued.

When two or more drugs are metabolized by the same hepatic enzymatic pathway, the drugs compete with each other for action from the enzyme. This competition results in at least one of the drugs having its metabolism impaired. To understand this concept entirely, consider the analogy of using the Internet through a dial-up connection. When there are few customers online, getting connected and using the online services is easy. However, when demand is very high, it may be difficult to get connected at all, and once connected, you may be abruptly disconnected, losing your ability to use the online services. Similarly, when the demand is high for the services of a particular hepatic enzyme, not every drug will receive attention immediately.

Drugs that affect the P-450 system are responsible for many drug interactions, as discussed in more detail in Chapter 5.

Excretion

Excretion is the process of removing a drug, or its metabolites, from the body. The most common route for drug excretion is through the urine. Other routes include bile in the GI tract, expired air from the lungs, breast milk, sweat from the skin, and saliva. Sweat and saliva are not therapeutically important routes of excretion, however.

Diseases and pathophysiologic changes in the kidney, such as renal failure, decrease the effectiveness of the kidney in drug excretion. Other patient variables that affect drug excretion are discussed in Box 4.4.

BOX 4.4 Drug Excretion and Core Patient Variables

Health Status

1. Renal impairment or renal failure decreases a drug's elimination from the body. If renal excretion is an important route of its elimination and the drug is given on a regular dosing schedule, its slowed removal from the body will produce a greater accumulation of drug in the body with an increased likelihood of additional therapeutic and adverse effects.
2. If cardiac output is decreased, the kidney may not be perfused adequately, decreasing the glomerular filtration rate as well as excretion of drugs.
3. Hepatic compromise or dysfunction will also decrease the elimination of drugs.
4. Drug therapy may produce nephrotoxicity as an adverse effect. Therefore, the renal elimination of all other drugs may be decreased.

Life Span and Gender

1. In elderly patients, the rate of drug clearance is reduced.
2. Some drugs have different rates of clearance depending on the sex of the patient.

Processes Involved in Renal Excretion

Three processes are involved in renal excretion of drugs. The first is glomerular filtration. Drugs come to the kidney through the capillaries surrounding Bowman's capsule. This capillary network is the glomerulus. Most drug particles pass easily through the spaces of the capillary walls into the urine in the proximal tubule. Only very large particles cannot pass. Proteins are examples of large molecules that are not filtered. Drug molecules bound to protein will therefore also not be filtered.

The second process is passive tubular reabsorption. Because a concentration gradient now exists, with more drug particles in the urinary tubule than in the bloodstream, the drug particles will try to move from the area of greater concentration to that of lesser concentration. Remember that for a drug to move through a membrane, it must be lipophilic. Therefore, for a drug to be able to move through the membranes separating the tubular and vascular structures, it must still be lipophilic. If it has been changed by metabolism into a form that is not lipid soluble (meaning that it is now an ion or a polar compound), passive tubular reabsorption cannot occur. Instead, the drug remains in the urine and is excreted.

The third process that affects excretion is active tubular secretion. Active transport systems in the renal tubule work to move some drugs from the blood and into the urine (Figure 4.5). There is one active transport system for organic acids and one for organic bases.

Factors That Affect Renal Excretion

Because ions cannot be passively reabsorbed from the tubule, drug excretion can be increased if the pH of the urine encourages the drug to become an ion. Remember that acids will ionize in basic environments and bases will ionize in acidic environments. Therefore, if another drug or some other agent is introduced that makes the urine more basic, acidic drugs will be ionized and not reabsorbed. Drug overdosage or ingestion of a poison is often treated in this way to promote excretion of the drug before it can harm the patient.

Overuse of the active transport system also affects excretion. Two drugs that rely on the active transport system for excretion will compete with each other for places on the transport system. As the transport system becomes overloaded, some of the drug particles will remain in the blood until they can be moved by the transport system. This residual portion will increase the circulating time of active drug in the body and slow the excretion of both drugs. This process is much like people waiting to ride a shuttle from the parking lot to a building. The shuttle bus has a limited number of seats and can only travel so fast between the two points. During the times when crowds are infrequent, everyone can find a seat on the shuttle without waiting. However, during rush hour, when crowds are large, not everyone can find a seat on the shuttle immediately. Some people will have to wait for their transportation to the building.

Two drugs can be given together to slow deliberately the rate of excretion of one or both of the drugs. A common example of this approach is giving probenecid, a drug used to treat gout, along with a penicillin or cephalosporin, antibiotics that are used to treat infections. In this situation, the probenecid is used not for its normal pharmacotherapeutic effect but solely to slow the rate of active transport and excretion of the antibiotic. This means that the antibiotic remains

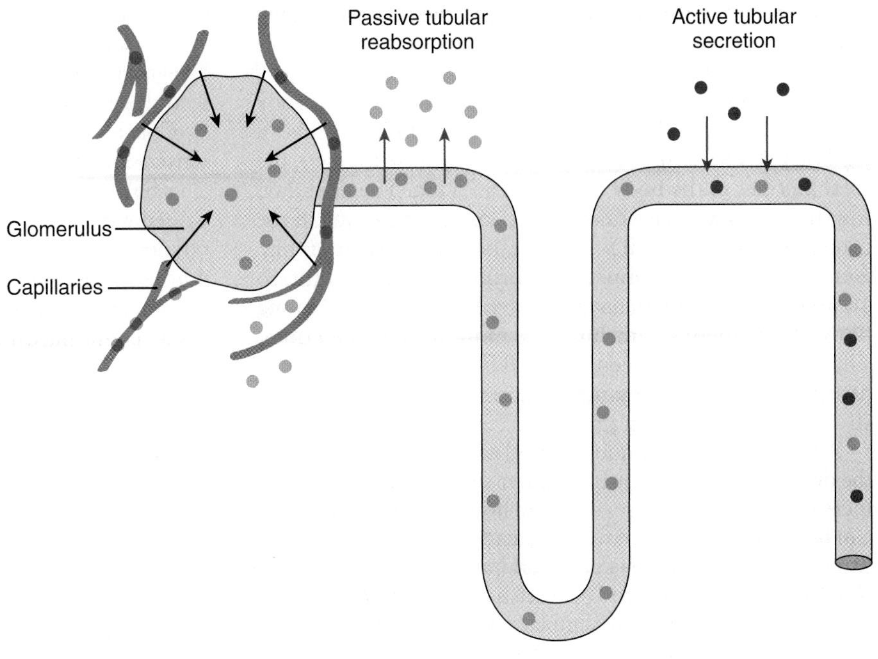

FIGURE 4.5 Renal excretion of drugs. Most drugs pass easily through the capillary walls and enter the tubules of the nephrons. Large molecules, such as proteins, cannot pass. Because of concentration gradients, some drug molecules will passively move back into the circulatory system (passive tubular reabsorption). Some drugs are actively moved into the tubule to be excreted.

in the blood and can continue to be active for a longer time than when given without the probenecid.

Factors That Affect Biliary Excretion

A factor that affects excretion of drugs through bile is enterohepatic recirculation. Some of the bile that leaves the liver and enters the intestine is reabsorbed back into the portal circulation and returned to the general circulation. Drug molecules that are in the bile are also reabsorbed. This process lengthens the time the drug is present in the bloodstream and can produce an effect.

Half-Life

The combined processes of metabolism and excretion are responsible for elimination of a drug from the body. The amount of time that is required to remove half (50%) of the blood concentration of a drug is called **half-life.** Drugs have various half-lives, based on their pharmacologic properties and rate of metabolism and excretion. Some drugs have half-lives measured in minutes; others have half-lives measured in days. It is important to understand that in one half-life, a set percentage of the drug molecules present in the blood will be eliminated, not an absolute set number of drug molecules. For example, if 1,000 drug molecules are present in the blood, 500 drug molecules will be left after one half-life. If there are 500 molecules, 250 will be left after one half-life. If there are only 10 drug molecules, 5 molecules will be left after one half-life. Each half-life removes 50% of the drug stored in the body; the number of molecules varies depending on the total load of drug in the body. See the Critical Thinking Scenario: Half-Life and Drug Dosing.

Steady State

There is a point at which the amount of drug being administered and the amount being eliminated balance off. Essentially, this balance means that what comes in equals what goes out. This balance creates a stable level of the drug in the blood. This stable level is called **steady state.** Technically, a 100% steady state cannot be achieved if a particular drug is given more than one time. However, the balance is almost even between the drug amount administered and that eliminated. At five half-lives, 97% of steady state will be achieved; therefore, steady state has been traditionally defined as five half-lives. However, most of steady state (94%) is achieved in four half-lives. In terms of clinical response from a given drug level, a drug at 94% of steady state will not achieve substantially less therapeutic effect than a drug at 97% of steady state. Because of this similarity in clinical response, it is now frequently stated that it takes four to five half-lives for steady state to be achieved.

When a particular dosage of one drug (i.e., a dose) is given at set repeated intervals (i.e., dosing intervals), it takes between four and five half-lives of the drug for the dose to equal the excretion rate of the drug. Imagine that the half-life of Drug A is 1 day and that 10 mg of Drug A is administered daily. On the second day, after one half-life, 5 mg of the drug is eliminated. An additional 10 mg dose is taken,

CRITICAL THINKING SCENARIO

Half-life and drug dosing

Gayle Herbert is 80 years old and has a history of renal insufficiency and congestive heart failure. She is receiving digoxin, a drug that strengthens the force of the heart's contraction, for congestive heart failure. Digoxin undergoes almost no metabolism but is primarily eliminated by renal excretion. The dose of the digoxin is to be increased, starting today. The half-life of digoxin is 30 to 40 hours.

1. If the new dose of digoxin were given orally once a day, how long would it take for the drug to reach steady state? Will Ms. Herbert's renal insufficiency affect the time to reach steady state?
2. Ms. Hawkins is also 80 years old and receives digoxin, but she does not have renal insufficiency. Would you expect Ms. Herbert's dose to be the same, less than, or greater than Ms. Hawkins' dose of digoxin? Why?

raising the total amount of the drug in the body to 15 mg (50% × 10 = 5; 5 + 10 = 15). The next day (after two half-lives), 7.5 mg of drug remains in the body. When that day's dose is administered, the total amount of drug in the body becomes 17.5 mg. The following day (after three half-lives), the body has 8.75 mg left. When the daily dose is given, the total amount in the body becomes 18.75 mg. The next day, four half-lives will have taken effect, leaving 9.375 mg of the drug in the body, which is 94% of the daily dose of 10 mg. Another dose is administered, bringing the amount to 19.375 mg. On the fifth day (after five half-lives), 9.6875 mg of the drug remains, which is 97% of the 10-mg daily dose. Thus, somewhere between four and five half-lives, the daily dosage is essentially the same as the amount left in the bloodstream after elimination (in = out) (Figure 4.6).

Although a larger amount (dose) of a given drug elevates the drug level found in the blood after steady state is achieved, increasing the dose has no effect on how *quickly* steady state can be achieved. Achievement of steady state is not based on drug dose. Steady state is achieved based on the amount of *time* required for four to five half-lives to occur, and half-life is related to the rate of elimination of the drug. Similarly, increasing the frequency of drug administration (i.e., dosing) *does not effect how quickly* the drug achieves steady state. Steady state is still achieved in the same amount of time, four to five half-lives.

The full pharmacotherapeutic response of a particular drug dose is measured when the drug has achieved steady state. Every time the dose is adjusted, it takes between four and five half-lives before the drug achieves steady state for that dose and for the full therapeutic effect to be assessed. This fact is important to remember when dose adjustments (up or down) are being considered in order to achieve a desired therapeutic effect. If the dose is modified before steady state is achieved, it is difficult to predict exactly what blood level will be achieved and, in turn, what therapeutic effect will be achieved from a drug dose. The result may be a blood level that is too low to be therapeutic or one that is too high, leading to adverse effects.

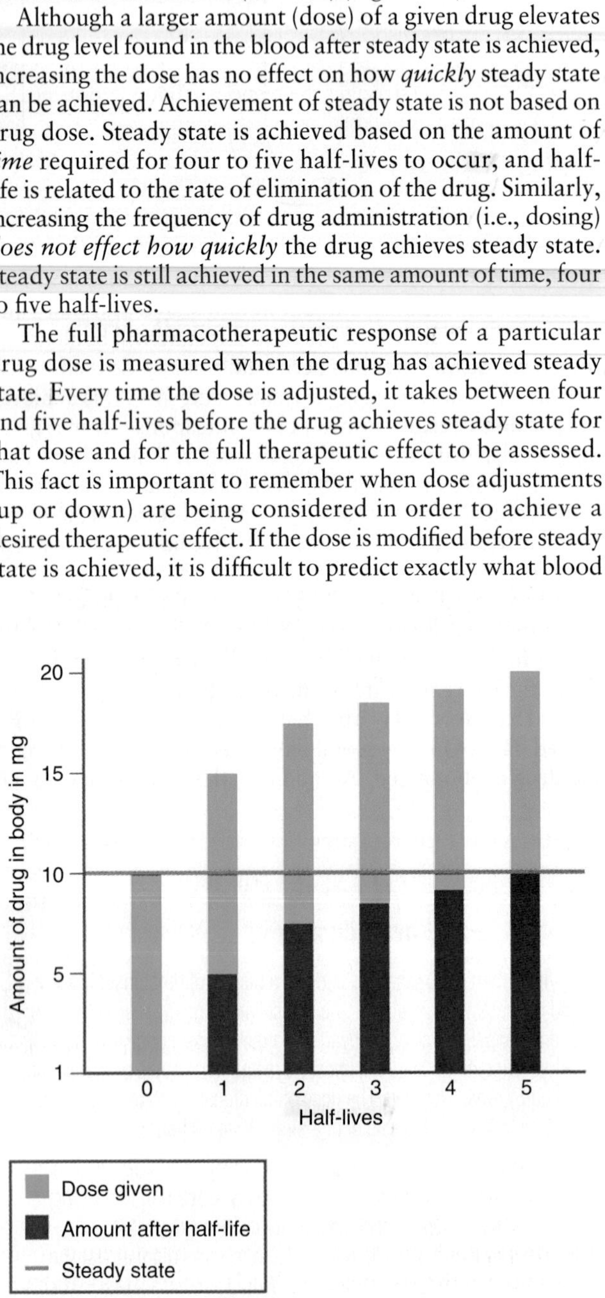

FIGURE 4.6 With each half-life, 50% of the drug in the body is eliminated. Note that steady state (in = out) is achieved in four to five half-lives.

Consider, for example, giving captopril to treat a hypertensive episode. The half-life of captopril is about 2 hours. This half-life means that in 10 hours, half of the drug administered will have been eliminated and the full effect of the initial dose of captopril will be evident. Let's say, however, that 4 hours after the drug is administered, the patient's blood pressure remains somewhat elevated. Two half-lives have occurred in this time. The physician orders a larger dose of captopril to be administered now. Twenty-five percent of the first dose remains in the patient's body after two half-lives. This residual drug is added to the new, larger dose. Later, the patient is found to be hypotensive, from too much effect of the medicine. In this particular case, not enough of the first dose had been eliminated before a second, but larger, dose was given. The combination created too high a blood level of the captopril. The drug did what it was intended to do: it lowered the blood pressure. But it lowered it too much. Had the dose been the same during the second administration of the drug, it is likely that the blood pressure would have dropped but stayed in the normal range. Decisions to alter the dose of a medication can most likely be made after four half-lives because this point is essentially steady state. Even after three half-lives, 90% of steady state has been achieved, which may be enough when making a clinical judgment to change the dose of the drug.

Clearance

Several pharmacokinetic factors work together to affect the rate at which drug molecules disappear from the circulatory system. This rate is called **clearance** or clearance rate of a drug. Renal excretion and hepatic metabolism are the major modes of clearance. Some drugs are primarily cleared by one mechanism rather than the other. For other drugs, the two mechanisms are both actively involved in clearance.

The gender of the patient can also alter the clearance of some drugs. Some drugs are cleared more rapidly in women (e.g., clozapine, erythromycin, and theophylline), whereas others are cleared more rapidly in men (e.g., lorazepam, acetaminophen, and digoxin). Slower clearance means that the drug particles stay in the circulation longer, increasing the half-life and the potential for increased therapeutic and adverse effects from the drug. It is important to recognize that even though a drug's clearance is shown to be statistically altered, this statistical difference does not necessarily create a clinical difference.

PHARMACODYNAMICS

Pharmacodynamics is the biological, chemical, and physiologic actions of a particular drug within the body and the study of how those actions occur. Essentially, it is how the drug affects the body. The pharmacodynamics of a drug can be affected by the age of the patient (Box 4.5).

Drugs cannot create new responses in the body; they can only turn on, turn off, promote, or block a response that the body is inherently capable of producing. Understanding the pharmacodynamics of a drug is critical to being able to

BOX 4.5 Pharmacodynamics: Age-Related Changes

- Increased myocardial sensitivity to anesthesia
- Increased analgesic effect from opioids (or other CNS depressants)
- Increased sedative effect from benzodiazepines (or other CNS depressants)
- Increased anticoagulant effect from anticoagulant therapy
- Exaggerated responses to cardiovascular drugs (normal homeostatic responsiveness is altered)

Note: When administering drug therapy to an elderly patient, the nurse should be alert to the possibility of moderate reductions in drug clearance and the potential for exaggerated pharmacodynamic responsiveness.

understand and critically assess a patient's response to drug therapy.

Drug–Receptor Interactions

Most drugs create their effects in the body by attaching to special sites, called **receptors,** on cells. At the receptor site, the drug is able to stimulate the cell to act in a way that the cell is designed to act. Drugs do this by attaching to the body's receptors for intrinsic elements such as hormones, neurotransmitters, or other internal methods of regulating cell function. Although each cell has many different receptor sites, the receptor sites do not all produce the same effects when stimulated. Each type of receptor is responsible for producing a particular effect in the cell. Drug molecules are able to attach only at certain receptors, and the receptors to which they attach determine the effect produced. Other drugs match up with different receptors, thus producing different effects.

When drug molecules attach to a receptor, they can stimulate the cell to act. Drugs that act in this way are described as **agonists,** meaning that they promote a function. Alternately, by attaching to a receptor, drug molecules can prevent something else from attaching and causing an effect. Drugs that act in this way are described as **antagonists** or **blockers.** Consider a busy parking garage at a mall. If other drivers have parked in all of the parking spaces before you get there, you are prevented from parking and going into the mall to shop. As you circle around waiting for a driver to leave a spot, you are in competition with all of the other drivers who are circling, looking for spots. At some point, a driver will vacate a parking space. If you are close by, you will be able to park and go in and shop. If other cars are closer, they will get the spot and again block you from parking. This scenario is similar to how drugs work on receptor sites.

A drug may latch onto a site to prevent a hormone or a neurotransmitter from attaching to the cell and turning on a function. If the drug is on the receptor, the other chemical cannot also be on the receptor. This fact is helpful when excessive internal stimulation of the cell causes the patient to experience pathologic changes. For example, in a patient with excessive stomach acid, the receptors in the stomach known as histamine-2 (H_2) receptors are overactivated, and the patient feels GI distress. When drugs called H_2 antagonists are given that attach to H_2 receptors and block the acid from attaching to the receptors, the person has a decrease in symptoms and feels better. The example of the parking garage also brings up an important point about drugs at receptor sites. The bonds that are formed are almost always temporary. When the drug molecule is no longer attached to the receptor, other drug particles may then attach, or the internal substance may then attach, to the receptor. Because there is competition for the receptor sites, the chemical that is present in the largest amount, either the drug or the internal regulator, is the most likely to be near an open receptor and attach to the receptor site. Most drugs that are antagonists are competitive; only a very few are not.

There are two theories about drug–receptor interactions: the single occupancy theory and the modified occupancy theory.

Single Occupancy Theory

The single occupancy theory has two aspects. First, the intensity of the body's response to the drug is directly related to the number of receptors occupied by the drug. The more receptors occupied, the stronger the response that is produced. Second, the maximum response occurs when all of the receptors have drug molecules attached. This theory does not explain, however, how two different drugs, each of which can attach to the same type of receptors, can produce different degrees of effect from stimulating the receptor. We know from common usage that different drugs need different doses to achieve their therapeutic effects. If you have two drugs that each relieve headaches, but the standard dose of Drug A is 20 mg and the standard dose of Drug B is 100 mg, there are obviously more drug molecules of Drug B than of Drug A. Thus, Drug B is attaching to and stimulating more receptors than Drug A, yet they both work to relieve a headache. Additionally, we know that, with some drugs, a ceiling effect occurs: at some point, no matter how much more drug you give, you cannot get any additional therapeutic response. Yet it would seem that all of the receptors are occupied, so that a maximal effect should be seen. The single occupancy theory, which assumes that all drugs have identical abilities to bind with receptors and that all drugs, once bound, have identical abilities to influence the functioning of the receptor, cannot be the only explanation for the way that drugs create an effect at receptor sites.

Modified Occupancy Theory

The modified occupancy theory is based on different assumptions about how drugs work at receptors. It states that different drugs have different strengths of attractions, or **affinity,** for receptor sites. Drugs with high affinity are strongly attracted to a receptor; drugs with low affinity are not very strongly attracted to a receptor. Drugs with strong affinity attach to a receptor even if not many drug particles are available. Drugs with low affinity attach only if large numbers of drug molecules are present. A comparison can be made with going to a movie. If you are very interested in seeing a particular movie, you'll make sure you go, even if you go alone or with only one friend. If you're not too interested in a movie, you'll go, but only if every one else is going, too. Thus, low doses of a drug with high affinity for a receptor will bind with that receptor and produce an effect.

Another assumption of the modified occupancy theory is that drugs, once attached to a receptor, have different abilities to stimulate the receptor. A drug's ability to stimulate its receptor is termed its **intrinsic activity.** Drugs with high intrinsic activity cause strong reactions from the receptor; drugs with low intrinsic activity cause low reactions from the recep-

tor. A drug with high affinity and high intrinsic activity is able to produce a strong effect from a small amount of drug.

Changes in Receptor Sensitivity

Receptors are not static; they can change or modify their response to a stimulus. Such change occurs when a receptor is continuously stimulated to act or continually inhibited from action. Receptor response can be modified either by changing the number of receptors on the cell or by changing the sensitivity of the current receptors.

Continual stimulation from an agonist usually makes the receptor desensitized to the drug and thus less active. Continual blockage from an antagonist usually makes the receptor become hypersensitive and much more likely to react.

Nonreceptor Responses

Although most drug effects are related to drug–receptor responses, some drugs exert their effect by reacting physically or chemically with other molecules in the body. For example, antacids create their effect by mixing with stomach contents to raise the pH, making it less acid. Another example is heparin, an anticoagulant. Heparin interferes with the conversion of prothrombin to thrombin (which is needed to form a stable clot) by inactivating factor X.

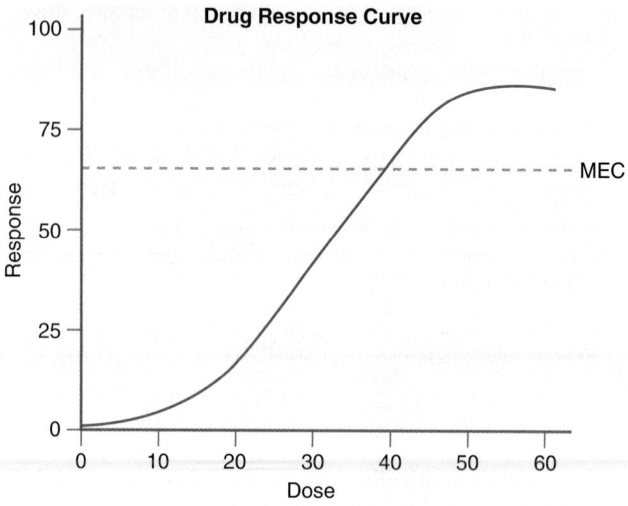

FIGURE 4.7 As the dose of a drug is increased, more response from the drug is achieved. Once the drug reaches the minimum effective concentration (MEC), a therapeutic effect can be observed. At a certain point, increasing the drug's dose fails to produce any greater response, and the curve flattens out. This point is the maximal efficacy of the drug.

VARIABLES THAT INFLUENCE THE DOSE OF A DRUG

Potency and Efficacy

From the drug–receptor theories, we see that the dose and characteristics of a drug have some relation to the pharmacotherapeutic effect achieved with drug therapy. A certain level of drug must be present in the body to produce an effect at all. This level is called the minimum effective concentration (MEC). After the MEC is reached, the strength of the response to a drug increases proportionately as more drug is given, until a plateau is reached and no additional therapeutic effect can be achieved, no matter the dose. When this relation between drug dose and response is plotted on a graph, it is referred to as a dose–response curve (Figure 4.7).

The amount of a drug that must be given in order to produce a particular response—its relative pharmacologic activity—is called the **potency** of a drug. A drug that is highly potent requires little of the drug to produce its effect. The affinity of a drug is related to its potency. Drugs with high affinity for a receptor need little drug to bind to the receptor and are thus highly potent drugs. How well a drug produces its desired effect is called **efficacy.** The efficacy of a drug is related to its intrinsic activity. Drugs with high intrinsic activity have greater efficacy.

Potency is not the same as efficacy. Two drugs may have different potencies but the same efficacy. For example, it might take 25 mg of Drug A to lower elevated blood pressure but 50 mg of Drug B to lower blood pressure by the same amount. Both drugs have equal efficacy, but Drug A is more potent than Drug B because fewer milligrams are needed to achieve the effect. Is the more potent drug the better drug? Not necessarily. Rarely is potency the most important consideration when selecting a drug. If the less potent drug, which is equal in efficacy, can be administered in a similarly sized pill as the more potent drug, patients and prescribers will view the drugs similarly. Other important considerations include the cost of each drug and the adverse effects from each one. If the less potent but equally effective drug is less expensive or is better tolerated by the patient, it will be the preferred drug. If the necessary route of administration is different, this consideration may also make one drug more desirable than the other. For example, if the more potent drug is administered only intravenously, but the less potent drug can be given orally, the less potent drug will usually be preferred when the patient is receiving drug therapy at home.

If drugs have similar potencies, but different efficacies, the drug that has better efficacy is usually preferred because this drug does a better job of achieving the desired therapeutic effect. However, if the largest effect that the drug can achieve (the maximal efficacy) is greater than the patient's clinical status warrants, a drug with a lower maximal efficacy may be chosen. For example, morphine has a higher maximal efficacy for relieving pain than acetaminophen. If the patient has postoperative pain at a surgical incision site, the morphine, with a higher maximal efficacy, is appropriate. If the patient has only a mild headache, the morphine is not appropriate, but the acetaminophen is.

ED_{50}, Maintenance, and Loading Doses

Because people are unique, how individuals respond to a drug dose varies. To determine what dose of a medicine should be given as the "usual dose," the distribution of doses needed to produce a response in a large and varied number of people is statistically calculated. The dose that is required to produce the therapeutic response in 50% of the population is called the effective dose 50% (ED_{50}). This dose is considered the standard or typical dose and is usually chosen as a starting dose. Once a dose is chosen and administered consistently

over time (e.g., every day), it is called the **maintenance dose.** Patients who are started on drug therapy using the standard maintenance dose arrive at steady state after four to five half-lives. The full therapeutic effect of any dose is achieved at steady state. For drugs that have long half-lives, achieving steady state may take days or weeks. The patient's medical condition may warrant immediate and full drug effect, however, in order to maintain health or life. When this is the case, a larger dose than usual is given initially. This initial large dose is called a **loading dose.** After one half-life, half of the administered dose is still available. The loading dose is computed so that after some of the drug is eliminated, the drug concentration in the body is still in the therapeutic range. The large initial loading dose is often divided into two or three portions, which are given more frequently than maintenance doses are administered. This dosing prevents the initial amount circulating in the patient from being so high that the patient experiences adverse effects.

Therapeutic Index

Just as people vary in the dose of a drug they need to achieve an effective therapeutic response, they vary as to the dose that will produce death. The lethal dose is computed in a laboratory setting and analyzed statistically. The point at which the dose would be fatal in 50% of the population receiving that dose is called lethal dose 50% (LD_{50}). To determine the safety of a drug, the ED_{50} is compared with the LD_{50}. The relation of ED_{50} to LD_{50} is called the **therapeutic index.** Therapeutic index can be explained by this equation, where TI represents the therapeutic index:

$$TI = \frac{ED_{50}}{LD_{50}}$$

If the amount of a drug required to be the ED_{50} is similar to the amount that is the LD_{50}, the mathematical ratio of the two values will equal a number close to one. For example, if the ED_{50} is 99 mg and the LD_{50} is 100 mg, the therapeutic index would be computed this way:

$$TI = \frac{99}{100}$$

$$TI = 0.99, \text{ which can be rounded to } 1.00$$

When the ED_{50} and the LD_{50} do not differ by much, the drug is considered to have a narrow therapeutic index. These drugs are not very safe and are therefore difficult to dose because the dose needed to be effective in half of the population will also kill half of the population. Drugs used in practice do not have a therapeutic index as narrow as in this example. However, the closer the two numbers are to each other, or the closer that the TI is to 1.00, the more difficult it is to use the drug to treat patients. For some types of conditions, however, the only appropriate drug is one that has a narrow therapeutic index. When patients receive these drugs, they must be closely monitored for adverse effects because adverse effects will become evident before death occurs. The current blood level of the drug is also monitored closely to make sure that the drug stays in the therapeutic range.

Thankfully, most drugs have a wide therapeutic index. A wide therapeutic index means that the amount required to be effective is very small, compared with the amount required to be lethal; for example:

$$TI = \frac{25}{1000}$$

$$TI = 0.025$$

In this example, the disparity between the ED_{50} and the LD_{50} is large. The therapeutic index is not close to 1.0. This drug is easy to dose; fatal effects are unlikely to occur because the LD_{50} is 40 times greater than the ED_{50}. Although this patient should be monitored for adverse effects, he or she is not at high risk for experiencing a problem, unlike the patient receiving a drug with a narrow therapeutic index.

Nurses should keep in mind that the therapeutic index is not something that they will need to compute. Furthermore, the numerical quotient of the comparison of the ED_{50} and the LD_{50} will not be published in the drug literature. Rather, what will be stated is that the drug has a narrow therapeutic index. If the drug does not have a narrow therapeutic index, usually no mention is made.

DRUG DOSAGE AND BLOOD CONCENTRATION

As previously stated, a minimum concentration of a drug is required to achieve the desired pharmacotherapeutic effect (the MEC). As drug levels within the body increase, the patient is more likely to experience adverse effects from drug therapy. For some drugs, these adverse effects may be very serious and potentially harmful to the patient. The goal of drug dosing is to give a dose that places the drug concentration above the MEC but below the level at which adverse effects occur. This range is called the therapeutic range.

To help determine whether a drug's dose is adequate to be in the therapeutic range, but not so high as to cause adverse effects, blood levels of the drug are often measured. Although most drugs do not achieve their therapeutic effect within the blood, blood samples are used because they are fairly easy to obtain. For many types of drugs, it would be too difficult to measure samples at the site of drug action. For example, drugs that alter cardiac function would require samples of tissue from the heart. Blood levels of a drug can be used, however, only if the relationship between the amount of drug circulating in the blood and the effects of the drug in the body are known. This information is not known for all drugs; therefore, blood samples are not drawn for every type of drug therapy. Acceptable target blood levels have been determined for most drugs that produce serious adverse effects.

Nurses need to monitor drug blood levels if samples are drawn and notify the physician or nurse practitioner if the level indicates that the patient is not in the therapeutic range or is greatly above the therapeutic range. Nurses should also seek orders for a blood level of a drug if a patient appears to be experiencing adverse effects. Because blood levels reflect the changes that have occurred from drug metabolism and excretion, it is important to note the exact time the last dose of the drug was administered on the drug blood level specimen slip. This record enables the laboratory to consider the pharmacokinetics of the drug during analysis.

The therapeutic range can only be considered an average, much like the temperature of 98.6°F is an average normal temperature. Some patients experience the therapeutic effects from a drug when their blood levels show that the drug is at "subtherapeutic" levels, whereas others experience adverse effects while the blood levels of the drug are in the "normal" range. The drug blood level is only one piece of data that must be considered when evaluating the patient's response to drug therapy. Changes to a drug's dose should be based on the total picture of the patient's response to therapy.

CHAPTER SUMMARY

- Pharmacotherapeutics is the clinical purpose or indication for giving a drug.
- Pharmacokinetics is the effect of the body on the drug. It is made up of four phases: absorption, distribution, metabolism, and excretion. Absorption is the movement of the drug from the site of administration into the bloodstream. Distribution is movement of the drug through the bloodstream and eventually into the cells. Metabolism refers to the changing of the drug into another substance or substances (i.e., metabolites). Excretion is the removal of the drug or its metabolites from the body.
- The blood–brain barrier is the body's natural defense to keep toxins and poisons from reaching the brain. It also may prevent the distribution of needed drug molecules from reaching their target.
- Drugs have different affinities for protein molecules, especially albumin, in the blood. Drugs that are highly protein bound have a lower proportion of their molecules available to produce the desired therapeutic effect. Only free drug is active.
- Metabolism of drugs occurs primarily in the liver. Liver metabolism is predominantly achieved by specific liver enzymes, known as the P-450 system. Some drugs can induce this system, increasing their own or other drugs' metabolism. When multiple drugs are metabolized by the same P-450 family, the metabolism of all the drugs is normally decreased. Anything that impairs liver functioning also decreases drug metabolism. Decreased metabolism leads to increased circulating levels of the drug, more therapeutic effect, and possibly more adverse effects.
- Drugs that are administered orally pass through the liver before going to the general circulation. If the drug is highly metabolized, a high first-pass effect occurs. This effect substantially decreases the amount of drug that is distributed to the body.
- The kidney is the primary organ responsible for drug excretion. There are three processes that affect the excretion of drugs in the urine: glomerular filtration, passive tubular reabsorption, and active tubular secretion. Anything that decreases kidney function decreases drug excretion, leading to increased circulating blood levels of the drug.
- Half-life of a drug is the amount of time needed to eliminate (by metabolism and excretion) half of the drug molecules currently in the body.
- Steady state is when the continuing dose of a drug is in balance with the elimination rate of the drug, that is, when the amount of drug entering the body equals the amount being removed. Steady state is achieved after four or five half-lives. Achievement of steady state is not related to the dosage of the drug or the frequency of drug administration.
- Most drugs create their effects in the body by attaching to special sites, called receptors, on cells. At the receptor site, the drug is able to stimulate the cell to act in a way that the cell is designed to act. Drugs that stimulate the cell to act are known as agonists. Drugs that attach to receptors to prevent other substances from attaching and "turning on" the cell are called antagonists or blockers.
- The single occupancy theory and the modified occupancy theory help to explain how drugs achieve their effects at receptors.
- Potency of a drug refers to how much of a drug is needed to create the desired therapeutic effect. Efficacy of a drug refers to how well the drug creates the desired therapeutic effect. Drugs may have different potencies but the same efficacy. Efficacy is a more important consideration than potency when selecting a particular drug.
- Loading doses are larger-than-normal doses used when therapy is initiated with drugs that have very long half-lives. The purpose of the loading dose is to achieve quickly a blood level of the drug that is in therapeutic range.
- Maintenance doses are the doses administered regularly throughout therapy.
- The therapeutic index is a measurement of the safety of the drug. Drugs that are described as having a narrow therapeutic index do not have much difference between the effective dose and the toxic or lethal dose. Patients receiving these drugs need to be monitored very closely for adverse effects. They also need to have their drug blood levels monitored closely.
- Drug dosages are adjusted to maintain a therapeutic level of the drug. Drug blood levels are one way of determining whether a dose needs to be either increased or decreased.

QUESTIONS FOR STUDY AND REVIEW

1. What is the difference between pharmacokinetics and pharmacodynamics?
2. What is the advantage of a drug being lipophilic during the distribution phase of pharmacokinetics?
3. Why are drugs metabolized to a hydrophilic form?
4. How do most drugs achieve their effect within the body?
5. Why would a drug that has a high first-pass effect be given by a route other than the oral route?
6. If a patient has renal insufficiency or poor hepatic functioning, how might the dose of a drug be adjusted? Why?
7. Your patient is receiving a drug that is known to be highly protein bound. The laboratory reports for this patient indicate that the albumin level is below normal. How might this affect the patient's risk for adverse effects of the drug therapy? Why?

Need More Help?

Chapter 4 of the study guide for *Drug Therapy in Nursing* 2e contains NCLEX-style questions and other learning activities to reinforce your understanding of the concepts presented in this chapter. For additional information or to purchase the study guide, visit *http://connection.lww.com/go/aschenbrenner.*

REFERENCES AND BIBLIOGRAPHY

Davis, M. W. (1998). Impact of gender on drug responses. *Drug Topics, 142*(9), 91–100.

Doherty, M. M., & Charman, W. N. (2002). The mucosa of the small intestine: How clinically relevant as an organ of drug metabolism? *Clinical Pharmacokinetics, 41*(4), 235–253.

Longo, D. L., Kasper, D. L., & Isselbacheter, K. J. (Eds.). (1999). *Harrison's online.* New York: McGraw-Hill.

Wetterberg, L. (1994). Light and biological rhythms. [Review]. *Journal of Internal Medicine, 235*(1), 5–19.

Adverse Effects and Drug Interactions

chapter 5

Learning Objectives

At the completion of this chapter the student will:

1. Identify the core drug knowledge of adverse effects and drug interactions.
2. Identify how adverse effects and drug interactions may alter the pharmacokinetics and pharmacodynamics of drug therapy.
3. Define the major toxicities that may occur as adverse effects.
4. Identify core patient variables related to adverse effects and drug interactions.
5. Relate the core drug knowledge of adverse effects and drug interactions to core patient variables.
6. Generate a nursing plan of care based on the interactions between core drug knowledge and core patient variables for adverse effects and drug interactions.
7. Describe nursing interventions to maximize therapeutic effects and minimize adverse effects and drug interactions in drug therapy.
8. Determine key points for patient and family education about adverse effects and drug interactions.

KEY TERMS

additive effect
adverse effect
allergic response
anaphylaxis
antagonistic drug interaction
cardiotoxicity
drug interaction
hepatotoxicity
idiosyncratic response
immunotoxicity
nephrotoxicity
neurotoxicity
ototoxicity
potentiation
synergistic effect

FEATURED WEBLINK

http://www.fda.gov/medwatch
The MedWatch program of the Food and Drug Administration (FDA) is a forum for reporting serious adverse drug effects.

CONNECTION WEBLINK

Additional Weblinks are found on Connection:
http://www.connection.lww.com/go/aschenbrenner.

In a perfect world, a perfect drug would produce only its desired therapeutic effect. Its effective dose would be easy to determine, it would be totally safe, and it would be so well tolerated that everyone who took it would adhere to and comply with the prescribed therapy. Alas, this is not a perfect world, and there is no perfect drug. All drugs can produce undesirable effects, some of them mild and annoying, others life threatening. Drugs can also produce altered effects because of interactions with other drugs, foods, or substances such as herbs and botanicals. These unexpected and nontherapeutic effects from drug therapy cause many patients to stop taking their prescribed drug therapy.

An **adverse effect** of drug therapy is a usually undesirable effect other than the intended therapeutic effect. It may occur even with normal drug dosing. An adverse effect may result from too much of a therapeutic effect (e.g., hypotension that may result from antihypertensive drug therapy) or from other pharmacodynamic effects of the drug (e.g., beta blockers are given for their effect on the heart, but they also have an effect on the bronchial tree). These effects are usually dose dependent and predictable. Adverse effects may also occur independently of the dose and be unpredictable. The term *adverse effect* encompasses all nontherapeutic responses to drug therapy and is used throughout this text.

A **drug interaction** occurs when two drugs or a drug and another element (such as food) have an effect on each other. This interaction may increase or decrease the therapeutic effect of one or both of the drugs, create a new effect, or increase the incidence of an adverse effect.

To maximize therapeutic effect, minimize adverse effects and drug interactions, and plan for appropriate patient and family education, nurses need to understand adverse effects and drug interactions and use this knowledge in their management of drug therapy. This chapter deals with these aspects of core drug knowledge.

ADVERSE EFFECTS

Every drug can produce adverse effects. Many adverse effects, such as nausea, are mild and bothersome perhaps only to the patient. Others, such as liver failure, are serious or even life threatening. Serious adverse effects lead to the withdrawal of a small number of drugs from the market every year. A drug is withdrawn not because it was approved without testing—clinical studies are done on all drugs under development, and all adverse effects in the study participants are identified. Sometimes, however, complete knowledge of adverse effects cannot be obtained until the drug has been used for a longer time than the length of the trial. Sometimes, adverse effects can be identified only when used extensively by patient populations that may not have been adequately represented in the study population, such as older adults, or patients with certain disease processes (e.g., renal disease).

It is important for nurses and other health care professionals to be alert for adverse effects from drug therapy. Sometimes, determining whether an adverse effect has occurred as a result of drug therapy is difficult. Adverse effects may be mistaken for changes associated with aging or disease pathology. For example, slight memory loss may be attributed to changes with aging, or hyperglycemia may be attributed to uncontrolled diabetes rather than to an adverse effect.

Serious adverse reactions to a drug, especially a newly approved drug, should be reported to a national database, such as the MedWatch reporting system sponsored by the FDA through its website (Figure 5.1). Reporting of serious adverse effects is necessary for corrective action to take place; examples of actions that may be taken to protect the public include revising the drug label, adding black box warnings for health care providers, creating patient Medication Guides, or withdrawing the drug from the market.

Adverse effects that are not predictable or dose related are caused by allergic or idiosyncratic responses. An **allergic response** is an immune system response. If the body interprets the drug as a foreign substance (antigen) and forms antibodies against the drug, the antigen–antibody response of the immune system is initiated when the drug is taken again. This response involves the release of histamine, which is responsible for many symptoms of allergy: redness, itching, swelling, rash, and hives. The allergic response may change over time, and symptoms may become more severe each time the drug is introduced into the body. The most serious allergic response is called **anaphylaxis.** During anaphylaxis, changes occur throughout the body, including constriction of bronchial smooth muscles (bronchospasms), vasodilation, and increased vascular permeability. The symptoms of anaphylaxis include acute respiratory distress, marked hypotension, edema (most importantly laryngeal edema), rash, tachycardia, cyanosis, and pale, cool skin. Convulsions may occur. If anaphylaxis is untreated, death is likely. Treatment includes the administration of vasopressor agents, bronchodilators (most often epinephrine, which is both a vasopressor and a bronchodilator), antihistamines (such as diphenhydramine), corticosteroids (to reduce swelling), oxygen therapy, and intravenous fluid administration. Endotracheal intubation and mechanical ventilation are often needed.

Idiosyncratic responses to a drug are another form of adverse effect. These responses are unusual and in fact may be the opposite of what is anticipated. They are sometimes called *paradoxical effects.* Idiosyncratic responses are related to an individual's unique response to a drug, rather than to the dose of a drug. They are considered to be genetically predetermined. The genetically inherited trait of responding to general anesthetics by developing malignant hyperthermia is an example of an idiosyncratic response to drug therapy.

Historically, different terms have been used to differentiate mild from serious nontherapeutic drug effects. The term *side effect* typically referred to a minor effect (such as nausea), whereas the term *toxic effect* referred to a more serious, potentially life-threatening effect (such as impaired renal function). In reality, the distinction between the terms is often blurry, and classification in one or the other category is somewhat arbitrary. For that reason, the newer term in pharmacologic literature is *adverse effect,* which is used to describe all undesired effects. Some practitioners use the term *side effect* as a synonym for *adverse effect.*

Specific patterns or groups of symptoms related to drug therapy that carry risk for permanent damage or death are called *toxicities.* The organ or system that is affected is used to name the toxicity (as in neurotoxicity, nephrotoxicity, cardiotoxicity). Drug toxicities are now listed as a type of adverse effect from a drug (e.g., nephrotoxicity is an adverse effect of aminoglycoside antibiotics). When two or more drugs taken by a patient can produce the same toxicity, the

U.S. Department of Health and Human Services

MEDWATCH

The FDA Safety Information and Adverse Event Reporting Program

For VOLUNTARY reporting of adverse events and product problems

Page ___ of ___

Form Approved: OMB No. 0910-0291, Expires: 03/31/05
See OMB statement on reverse.

FDA USE ONLY
Triage unit sequence #

PLEASE TYPE OR USE BLACK INK

A. PATIENT INFORMATION

1. Patient Identifier	2. Age at Time of Event:	3. Sex	4. Weight
In confidence	or ______ Date of Birth:	☐ Female ☐ Male	____ lbs or ____ kgs

B. ADVERSE EVENT OR PRODUCT PROBLEM

1. ☐ **Adverse Event** and/or ☐ **Product Problem** *(e.g., defects/malfunctions)*

2. **Outcomes Attributed to Adverse Event** *(Check all that apply)*
- ☐ Death: ______ *(mo/day/yr)*
- ☐ Life-threatening
- ☐ Hospitalization - initial or prolonged
- ☐ Disability
- ☐ Congenital Anomaly
- ☐ Required Intervention to Prevent Permanent Impairment/Damage
- ☐ Other: ______

3. **Date of Event** *(mo/day/year)*

4. **Date of This Report** *(mo/day/year)*

5. **Describe Event or Problem**

6. **Relevant Tests/Laboratory Data, Including Dates**

7. **Other Relevant History, Including Preexisting Medical Conditions** *(e.g., allergies, race, pregnancy, smoking and alcohol use, hepatic/renal dysfunction, etc.)*

Mail to: **MEDWATCH** 5600 Fishers Lane Rockville, MD 20852-9787 -or- FAX to: 1-800-FDA-0178

C. SUSPECT MEDICATION(S)

1. **Name** *(Give labeled strength & mfr/labeler, if known)*
#1
#2

2. **Dose, Frequency & Route Used**
#1
#2

3. **Therapy Dates** *(If unknown, give duration) from/to (or best estimate)*
#1
#2

4. **Diagnosis for Use** *(Indication)*
#1
#2

5. **Event Abated After Use Stopped or Dose Reduced?**
#1 ☐ Yes ☐ No ☐ Doesn't Apply
#2 ☐ Yes ☐ No ☐ Doesn't Apply

6. **Lot #** *(if known)*
#1
#2

7. **Exp. Date** *(if known)*
#1
#2

8. **Event Reappeared After Reintroduction?**
#1 ☐ Yes ☐ No ☐ Doesn't Apply
#2 ☐ Yes ☐ No ☐ Doesn't Apply

9. **NDC#** *(For product problems only)*
\- -

10. **Concomitant Medical Products and Therapy Dates** *(Exclude treatment of event)*

D. SUSPECT MEDICAL DEVICE

1. **Brand Name**

2. **Type of Device**

3. **Manufacturer Name, City and State**

4. **Model #** | **Lot #**
Catalog # | **Expiration Date** *(mo/day/yr)*
Serial # | **Other #**

5. **Operator of Device**
- ☐ Health Professional
- ☐ Lay User/Patient
- ☐ Other: ______

6. **If Implanted, Give Date** *(mo/day/yr)*

7. **If Explanted, Give Date** *(mo/day/yr)*

8. **Is this a Single-use Device that was Reprocessed and Reused on a Patient?**
☐ Yes ☐ No

9. **If Yes to Item No. 8, Enter Name and Address of Reprocessor**

10. **Device Available for Evaluation?** *(Do not send to FDA)*
☐ Yes ☐ No ☐ Returned to Manufacturer on: ______ *(mo/day/yr)*

11. **Concomitant Medical Products and Therapy Dates** *(Exclude treatment of event)*

E. REPORTER *(See confidentiality section on back)*

1. **Name and Address** | **Phone #**

2. **Health Professional?** ☐ Yes ☐ No

3. **Occupation**

4. **Also Reported to:**
- ☐ Manufacturer
- ☐ User Facility
- ☐ Distributor/Importer

5. **If you do NOT want your identity disclosed to the manufacturer, place an "X" in this box:** ☐

FORM FDA 3500 (12/03) **Submission of a report does not constitute an admission that medical personnel or the product caused or contributed to the event.**

FIGURE 5.1 Example of a MedWatch form for reporting an adverse event to the Food and Drug Administration (FDA). FDA authorities define a serious event as any occurrence that is fatal, life-threatening, permanently or significantly disabling, requires or prolongs hospitalization, results in a congenital anomaly, or requires intervention to prevent permanent impairment or damage.

risk that the patient will develop the drug toxicity increases. A description of the commonly referenced drug toxicities follows.

Neurotoxicity

Neurotoxicity, sometimes referred to as central nervous system (CNS) toxicity, is a drug's ability to harm or poison a nerve cell or nerve tissue. Signs and symptoms of neurotoxicity include drowsiness, auditory and visual disturbances, restlessness, nystagmus (involuntary cyclic movement of the eyeballs), and tonic-clonic (grand mal) seizures. Neurotoxicity can occur after exposure to drugs and other chemicals and gases (e.g., alcohol, solvents, insecticides, industrial vapors, and pollutants). Injury to the CNS is largely irreversible because the highly differentiated neurons of the brain cannot divide and regenerate. Immature nervous systems (e.g., fetal and neonatal nervous systems) can easily be damaged by drugs that produce neurotoxicity.

Hepatotoxicity

Hepatotoxicity is damage to the liver. Manifestations of hepatotoxicity include hepatitis, jaundice, elevated liver enzyme levels, and fatty infiltration of the liver. Hepatic anatomy and hepatic function both contribute greatly to the high susceptibility of the liver to toxicants. Blood draining from the stomach and small intestines is delivered directly to the liver by the hepatic portal vein. As a result, the liver is exposed to relatively large concentrations of ingested drugs or other potentially toxic substances. If the drug that was absorbed and is now present in the blood is hepatotoxic, liver damage will likely occur because of the large number of drug molecules presented to the liver. The liver is also responsible for metabolizing most drugs. If liver damage occurs, the drug will not be metabolized as efficiently, leaving more circulating drug to cause further liver damage.

Nephrotoxicity

Damage to the kidneys is called **nephrotoxicity.** Decreased urinary output, elevated blood urea nitrogen, increased serum creatinine, altered acid-base balance, and electrolyte imbalances can all occur with kidney damage. The renal system is similar to the hepatic system in that it is susceptible to poisoning because of its anatomy and function. The cells within the proximal tubule are frequently damaged by nephrotoxic drugs. These cells are responsible for filtering, concentrating, and eliminating toxic as well as nontoxic materials; as water is reabsorbed, instead of eliminated, the concentration of drug molecules in the tubule rises, thereby increasing the potential for damage.

Ototoxicity

Ototoxicity is damage to the eighth cranial nerve. Structures of the inner ear that may be affected include the cochlea (responsible for hearing) and the vestibule and semicircular canals (responsible for balance). Ototoxicity may or may not be reversible. Signs and symptoms of ototoxicity include tinnitus, which is a buzzing or ringing sound in the ear, and sensorineural hearing loss. Also called nerve deafness, sensorineural hearing loss usually begins with the loss of high-frequency sound and may worsen until low-frequency sound is also difficult to hear. Other signs and symptoms, particularly of vestibular toxicity, include light-headedness, vertigo, a spinning sensation from a seated position, and nausea and vomiting.

Cardiotoxicity

Irregularities in cardiac rhythms and conduction, heart failure, and even damage to the myocardium may result from an adverse effect known as **cardiotoxicity.** Exactly how some drugs produce cardiotoxicity is unknown. Older adults, who have less effective hearts than younger adults, and children younger than 2 years, whose hearts are still growing, are most susceptible to cardiotoxicity from drugs.

Immunotoxicity

When the immune system is significantly affected by drug therapy, the condition is called **immunotoxicity.** A wide variety of drugs can affect the immune system. Some may cause immunosuppression, whereas others may directly destroy immune system components. The effect of both kinds of immunotoxicity may be an increased incidence of bacterial, viral, and parasitic infections.

DRUG INTERACTIONS

Drug interactions occur when one drug (Drug A) is affected in some way by another drug (Drug B), a food, or some other substance that is taken concurrently. The effect may be to increase the therapeutic or adverse effects from Drug A or to decrease the therapeutic or adverse effects from Drug A. Rarely, a new and different effect may be induced.

Drug interactions may be beneficial (e.g., when the interaction increases the therapeutic effect of a drug or decreases its adverse effects). Sometimes, drugs are ordered specifically to bring about the desired drug interaction. For example, probenecid, a drug used to treat gout, is given to patients without gout to prevent the renal excretion of penicillin, thus allowing the penicillin to circulate longer and produce additional therapeutic effects.

Negative effects from drug interactions are those that decrease the therapeutic effect or increase the adverse effects of a drug. For example, consuming foods high in tyramine (such as smoked meats) while taking a monoamine oxidase inhibitor (MAOI) antidepressant can lead to pronounced elevation of blood pressure and may induce a hypertensive crisis. Drug interactions that alter the circulating level of one of the drugs are especially worrisome if the drug has a narrow therapeutic index. In this case, a slight elevation of the blood level of the drug may produce serious adverse effects, whereas a slight decrease in the blood level may cause the drug to become nontherapeutic.

Drug interactions may take place in any phase of pharmacokinetics—absorption, distribution, metabolism, or excretion. Drug interactions can also change the pharmacodynamics of a drug or the adverse effects of the drugs. When

two drugs can both independently cause the same adverse effect, there is an increased risk for that adverse effect when both drugs are taken. Drug interaction sites in the body are shown in Figure 5.2 and are discussed throughout the sections that follow.

Drug Interactions Affecting Pharmacokinetics

Drug Interactions Affecting Absorption

Drug absorption is often decreased because of drug interactions. If a drug binds with another substance in the gastrointestinal (GI) tract, less of the drug is available to be absorbed. For example, milk and antacids bind with the antibiotic tetracycline and prevent its absorption. This binding of a drug is termed *chelation.* Because drug absorption is related to how long the drug is present in the GI tract, changes in GI transit time alter drug absorption. Therefore, drugs such as laxatives, which hasten the transit time, can decrease the absorption of other drugs that are present in the GI tract at the same time. Finally, the mere presence of food in the GI tract can delay or reduce the absorption of many drugs.

Drug absorption may also be increased as a result of a drug interaction or the presence of food in the GI tract. For example, antacids increase the pH of the stomach contents. A less acidic environment decreases ionization of drugs that are basic, which promotes absorption of these drugs.

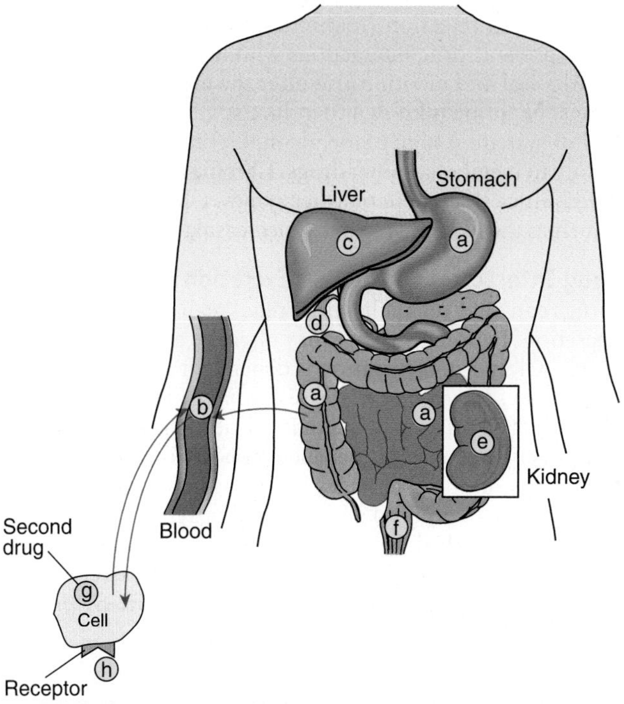

FIGURE 5.2 Drug interaction sites within the body. Drug interactions can occur in numerous body sites. Absorption can be enhanced or reduced in the gut (**a**); protein binding can be affected within the vasculature (**b**); metabolism can be affected in the liver (**c**); excretion can be affected either through bile (**d**); the kidney (**e**); or in feces (**f**); tissue binding of one drug can be affected by another (**g**); and finally, drugs may have an effect through action on specific receptors (**h**).

The exact extent of changes in drug absorption caused by drug interactions is often difficult to predict. The nurse needs to monitor for signs of decreased or less than anticipated drug effect to determine if there might be a drug interaction. Monitoring is warranted especially if the drug regimen changes (a new drug is added or one is stopped). Sometimes, separating the administration times of the two drugs by at least 2 hours is enough to prevent binding and loss of absorption and effectiveness. Other times, an increased dose of the affected drug may be indicated.

Drug Interactions Affecting Distribution

Distribution is affected by two types of drug interactions. The first is competitive protein binding. When two drugs compete for the same protein receptors, the drug that has a higher affinity for the site will displace the other drug. Thus, one of the drugs will have more free and active molecules to be distributed through the body than would normally be anticipated. (Protein binding is discussed in more detail in Chapter 4.)

The second way that drug distribution can be affected by drug interactions is when a drug alters the extracellular pH. A drug that increases the pH of the extracellular fluid (i.e., makes the extracellular fluid more basic) increases the ability of acidic drugs to ionize in the extracellular space. In this case, acidic drugs move from the low-pH environment found within the cells into the higher-pH environment in the extracellular space in order to be ionized. Thus, drug distribution is altered.

Drug Interactions Affecting Metabolism

Probably the most important and common drug interaction is one that alters the metabolism of a drug. As you recall from Chapter 4, metabolism of drugs is related to the cytochrome P-450 system. Some drugs either induce or inhibit the P-450 system, thus altering the metabolism of other drugs (Figure 5.3). Usually, just one P-450 family is affected.

Drugs that induce a hepatic enzyme increase the amount of that enzyme in the liver. Induction is accomplished most frequently by stimulating synthesis of the enzyme. When one of the hepatic enzymes is present in greater quantities than the others, more metabolism by this pathway can occur. Drugs that are metabolized by this pathway (also referred to as drugs that are substrates of the enzyme) are therefore metabolized more rapidly, which in turn rapidly decreases the amount of circulating, active drug. Some drugs can induce the enzymes necessary for their own metabolism and thus can increase the rate of their own metabolism. Drugs that inhibit a particular hepatic enzyme slow the metabolism that occurs through this pathway, causing an increase in the amount of circulating, active drug. Metabolism will return to normal after the inducing or inhibiting drug is no longer administered, although the return to normal may not occur until several days after an inducer is discontinued.

If two drugs that affect the cytochrome P-450 system must be administered to a patient together, the dose of one of the drugs may have to be adjusted. When two or more drugs are metabolized by the same hepatic enzyme pathway, they compete with each other for the action of the enzyme. This competition results in impaired metabolism of one or more of the drugs. Consider the analogy of using the Internet through a dial-up connection. When few customers are online, it is easy

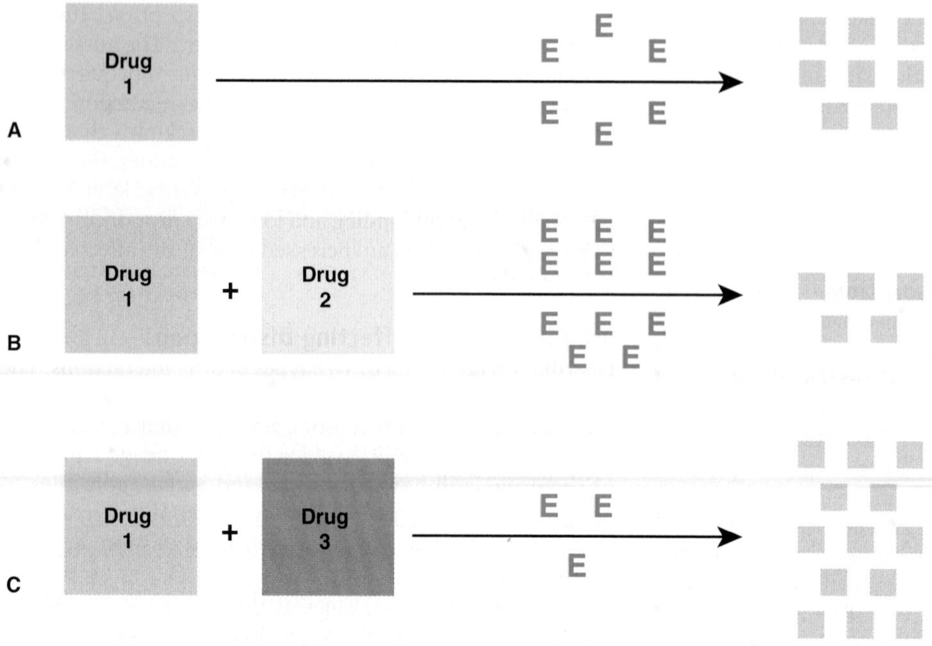

FIGURE 5.3 Drug interactions affecting P-450 metabolism. (**A**) Normal drug metabolism through the P-450 isoenzymes for Drug 1. (**B**) Drug 2 induces the P-450 system, increasing metabolism of Drug 1. Less Drug 1 than normal is left to circulate after this drug interaction. (**C**) Drug 3 inhibits the P-450 system; thus, metabolism is decreased for Drug 1. More Drug 1 than normal is left to circulate after this drug interaction.

to be connected and to use the online services. However, when there is very high demand, getting connected may be difficult, and once connected, you may be abruptly disconnected, losing the ability to use the online services. Similarly, when the demand is high for the services of a particular hepatic enzyme, not every drug will receive attention immediately.

In addition to drugs altering the metabolism of other drugs, grapefruit juice is also known to inhibit CYP3A4. Exactly how grapefruit juice inhibits this isoenzyme is not known. CYP3A4 is found in the liver and in the intestinal wall. Grapefruit juice primarily has an effect on CYP3A4 found in the intestinal wall. The inhibition of CYP3A4 decreases the GI metabolism of many drugs, which allows more of the drug to be absorbed, resulting in substantially higher blood levels than if grapefruit juice were not consumed. Because the amount of CYP3A4 in the intestine varies among individuals, the degree to which grapefruit juice alters drug metabolism also varies. In some people, the effect is great; in others, the effect is minimal. The more CYP3A4 that is present in the GI tract, the more drug metabolism can be increased (Lohezic-Le Devehat et al., 2002). The effect also appears to be dose dependent (i.e., the more grapefruit juice a person drinks, the more inhibition of CYP3A4 that occurs). If the patient regularly drinks grapefruit juice before drug therapy is started, the drug dosage can be adjusted to obtain a therapeutic level or therapeutic effect. In this case, the patient can safely continue to drink grapefruit juice. Problems arise, however, when a patient intermittently drinks grapefruit juice or starts to drink it after drug therapy has been started. In these situations, the grapefruit juice may alter drug levels unpredictably, and the potential exists for substantial elevations that may cause adverse effects. Patients who did not consume grapefruit juice before the initiation of drug therapy should avoid drinking it once drug therapy has begun. See Table 10-1 for a list of drugs that interact with grapefruit juice.

Some herbs and botanicals may also affect the CYP3A4 enzyme. St. John's wort, for example, contributes to the induction of CYP3A4 and enhances the metabolism of drugs that are substrates of this enzymatic pathway. Drugs that are substrates of the CYP3A4 enzymatic pathway include protease inhibitors (used to treat AIDS), oral contraceptives, tricyclic antidepressants, and the immunosuppressant cyclosporine. Coadministering St. John's wort with cyclosporine in patients who have received transplants has been known to cause organ rejection (Ioannides, 2002). Table 10-4 lists other possible drug interactions with herbs.

Alcohol and nicotine also alter the metabolism of some drugs. Nicotine is known to induce some isoenzymes in the P-450 system. A high blood alcohol level impairs the liver's ability to metabolize other drugs. Chronic use of alcohol may also induce some hepatic isoenzymes. Chronic alcoholism damages the liver permanently, decreasing drug metabolism.

Drug Interactions Affecting Excretion

Drugs can alter renal filtration, renal reabsorption, or renal secretion. In doing so, they may alter the excretion of other drugs. Glomerular filtration is dependent on blood flow to the kidney. Drugs that decrease cardiac output decrease the amount of circulating blood that is sent to the kidneys. Renal reabsorption of a drug is dependent on whether a drug is ionized. Drug-induced changes in urinary pH affect whether other drugs are ionized and excreted or remain nonionized and are reabsorbed. Renal secretion uses a transport system to move the drug molecules into the urine for excretion. If two drugs are dependent on the same transport system, the excretion rate of both is slowed.

Drug Interactions Affecting Pharmacodynamics

Drug interactions may affect the pharmacodynamics of one or both drugs administered. The overall effect may be positive or negative. Drug interactions can occur when both drugs act at the same receptor or at different receptors. Drugs that act at the same receptor compete to be attached to the receptor. The drug that has the weaker affinity for the receptor will

not be able to exert its therapeutic effect, as discussed in Chapter 4. Drugs that act in different ways, or at different receptors, can interact in several ways. They may create an additive effect, a synergistic effect, a potentiated effect, or an antagonistic effect.

Additive Effect

An **additive effect** occurs when two or more "like" drugs (in terms of therapeutic effect) are combined, and the result is the sum of the drugs' effects. If written as an equation, this concept would be expressed as: 1 (Drug A) + 1 (Drug B) = 2. An additive effect may be intentional or may unintentionally cause harm. Consider the following two examples:

- Codeine and acetaminophen work differently to reduce pain. When these two analgesic drugs are combined, the additive effect is better control of pain (compared with that resulting from the use of either drug alone).
- Alcohol and salicylates, such as aspirin, can both cause GI bleeding. When a salicylate and alcohol are consumed together, the risk for GI bleeding is greatly increased because each agent independently can cause GI bleeding.

Synergistic Effect

A **synergistic effect** occurs when two or more "unlike" drugs (in terms of therapeutic effect or mechanism of action) are used together to produce a combined effect, and the outcome is a drug effect greater than either drug's activity alone. As an equation, this concept would be expressed as: 1 (Drug A) + 1 (Drug B) = 3. Just like an additive interaction, a synergistic interaction may be intentional or may unintentionally cause harm. Consider the following examples:

- A beneficial synergistic effect occurs when two different types of antibiotics that work in very different ways are combined, such as penicillin G and an aminoglycoside antibiotic. This approach is commonly used in the treatment of subacute bacterial endocarditis.
- When three different types of antihypertensive drugs—an alpha-adrenergic blocker (a vasodilator), a beta-adrenergic blocker (a sympatholytic), and a diuretic—are combined, the antihypertensive effect is better than with any drug alone.
- A harmful synergistic effect is represented by the interaction between drugs that depress the CNS, such as morphine and alcohol; this interaction causes additional CNS depression that may be fatal.

Potentiated Effect

Potentiation best describes an interaction in which the effect of only one of the two drugs is increased. In other words, a drug that has a mild effect enhances the effect of a second drug. As an equation, this concept would be represented as ½ (Drug A) + 1 (Drug B) = 2. For example, when the antiemetic drug hydroxyzine, which has some CNS depressant effects and produces mild analgesic effects, is combined with a narcotic analgesic such as morphine, the pain-relieving ability of the morphine is increased without increasing the dose of the morphine.

Antagonistic Effect

An **antagonistic drug interaction** is the opposite of a synergistic effect. It results in a therapeutic effect that is less than the effect of either drug alone because the second drug either diminishes or cancels the effects of the first drug. As an equation, this concept would be expressed as: 1 (drug A) + 1 (drug B) = 0. For example, when the heparin antagonist protamine sulfate (a strong basic anticoagulant) is given as an antidote for heparin (a strong acidic anticoagulant) to halt heparin-induced bleeding, a stable salt forms, resulting in a loss of anticoagulant activity for both drugs. Antagonistic interactions can also occur at receptor sites when one drug is an agonist and the other drug is an antagonist for the same receptor, such as with morphine, a narcotic agonist, and naloxone, a narcotic antagonist used to correct narcotic overdosage.

DRUG INCOMPATIBILITIES

Drug incompatibilities are similar to drug–drug interactions in that a chemical inactivation or physical reaction occurs. This reaction may involve two or more drugs, inside the body or outside, before they are administered. While administering drugs parenterally (intravenously, intramuscularly, or subcutaneously), the nurse is especially alert to the possibility of drug incompatibilities and drug interactions. The most common kinds of incompatibilities are chemical and physical.

Chemical Incompatibilities

Chemical incompatibilities between drugs change both the drug's structure and its pharmacologic properties. The alteration may be beneficial. For example, heparin and protamine sulfate (a heparin antagonist) form an ionic bond that lacks any anticoagulant activity. Conversely, the chemical incompatibility may also be harmful; for example, combining multivitamins and antibiotics in the same intravenous (IV) solution changes the solution's pH and inactivates the antibiotic.

Physical Incompatibilities

Physical incompatibilities occur when two drugs are mixed together. The mixture results in the formation of a precipitate. Phenytoin and a diluent containing dextrose, for example, produce a cloudy, white precipitate. This kind of reaction usually interferes with the pharmacologic activity of one or both drugs. This is one of the reasons that manufacturers provide specific instructions for preparation, dilution, and addition of drugs to other solutions. These instructions should be followed carefully.

IMPLICATIONS FOR NURSING MANAGEMENT

When administering drug therapy, the nurse's main focus is on ensuring a beneficial outcome by maximizing therapeutic effects, minimizing adverse effects and drug interactions, and providing appropriate drug education for the patient and family. Beneficial outcomes are achieved by relating core drug knowledge to core patient variables throughout the nursing process. Understanding how core drug knowl-

edge and core patient variables interact to affect outcome is important because these interactions may predispose the patient to adverse effects from drug therapy.

Assessment of Core Patient Variables

Health Status

Concurrent medical conditions may increase the risk for adverse effects from drug therapy. For example, if a patient has diminished renal function and then takes a drug that may cause nephrotoxicity, the patient is more likely to develop adverse effects, even with a therapeutic dose. A patient's chronic health condition may also necessitate drug therapy that may interact with other drug therapy or promote adverse effects. For example, a patient with AIDS may be taking drug therapy that carries the risk for hepatotoxicity. If this patient develops tuberculosis, he or she will need to take additional drug therapy, which also may cause hepatotoxicity.

Life Span and Gender

A patient's age can greatly increase the risk for adverse effects from drug therapy. The liver and kidneys of both young children and older adults do not function as well as those of young adults. As a result, those populations are at increased risk for adverse effects and drug interactions. In addition, older adults are more likely to be receiving polypharmacy for multiple chronic illnesses and thus are more likely to experience drug interactions. Adverse effects from drug therapy taken by a pregnant woman may affect the unborn child. Many drugs can also be passed in breast milk, causing adverse effects in the infant. Life span issues are discussed in more detail in Chapters 6, 7, and 8.

Lifestyle, Diet, and Habits

What and when a patient eats and drinks and the patient's various habits and choices (e.g., the use of tobacco, alcohol, caffeine, street drugs, or over-the-counter herbs and botanicals) may influence the effects of drug therapy, either positively or negatively. For this reason, the nurse should remember to ask patients about diet and other habits when performing a drug history or when providing patient education on prescribed drug therapy. The nurse can then inform patients about possible interactions and describe how to maximize therapeutic effects or prevent or minimize adverse effects and drug interactions. (For more information on how lifestyle, diet, and habits influence drug therapy, see Chapters 9 and 10.)

Environment

The patient's environment may increase the likelihood that a certain adverse effect will occur. For instance, some antibiotics can cause the adverse effect of photosensitivity. Even brief exposure to sunlight or strong ultraviolet light can cause severe sunburn, hives, or a rash. Other drugs (e.g., anticholinergics, belladonna alkaloids) reduce the body's tolerance to heat or inhibit the body's ability to reduce temperature by perspiration. These types of drugs may make the patient vulnerable to heat stroke in hot weather or during exercise.

Environment can also play a role in the early detection of adverse effects. For example, a critically ill patient receives drug therapy under close supervision, which could lead to early detection of any adverse effects. However, a person who is receiving drug therapy in a community setting may be more at risk for adverse effects because the early signs of the adverse effect may not be identified as easily as they would be in a clinical setting. The relationship of environment to drug therapy is discussed in more detail in Chapter 11.

Culture and Inherited Traits

Researchers are beginning to study responses to drug therapy that are genetically determined in various ethnic and racial populations. These responses may place the patient at greater risk for adverse effects or drug interactions than the rest of the global population. Box 5.1 describes one study that focused on the metabolic activity of the P-450 system in two ethnic groups, Mexicans and European Americans. Culture and inherited traits and the ways that they influence drug therapy are discussed in more detail in Chapter 12.

Nursing Diagnoses and Outcomes

Nursing diagnoses are related to specific adverse effects of the ordered drug therapy and to drug interactions. Outcomes are directed at preventing or minimizing either occur-

FOCUS ON RESEARCH

Box 5.1 P-450 Similarities Between Ethnic Groups

Poland, R. A., Lin, K. M., Nuccio, C., et al. (2002). Cytochrome P450 2E1 and 3A activities do not differ between Mexican and European Americans. *Clinical Pharmacology and Therapeutics,* 72(3): 288–293.

The Study

In a very small study of 30 young, healthy Mexicans and 30 European Americans who were matched for age, sex, and weight, the metabolic activity of two of the P-450 enzymes, P-450 2E1 and P-450 3A4, was evaluated. Half of the patients received the drug chlorzoxazone, a drug that is metabolized by CYP2E1. Activation of CYP2E1 is believed to activate procarcinogens. The other half of the patients received the drug midazolam, which is metabolized by CYP3A4. No significant differences were found in the metabolism of the test drugs between the ethnic groups, which suggests that activation of the CYP2E1 enzyme carries an equal risk for precarcinogen activation in the Hispanic subgroup of Mexicans compared with European Americans. Thus, risk for adverse effects by this route is likely to be the same. The study also suggests that dosage for drugs that are metabolized by CYP3A4 can be the same for Mexicans and European Americans.

Nursing Implications

Because many drugs are metabolized by the P-450 pathway (with CYP3A4 the most frequently used pathway), it is important to know whether patients will respond differently to drug therapy based on inherent differences in drug metabolism. This limited study demonstrates that, for at least these two ethnic groups, the nurse most likely does not need to be concerned about differences in metabolism that could place certain patients at increased risk for adverse effects.

rence without harm to the patient. Some examples include the following:

- Risk for Infection related to drug-induced myelosuppression
  Desired outcome: *The patient will not develop infection while on drug therapy.*
- Altered Nutrition: Less Than Body Requirements related to drug-induced nausea, vomiting, anorexia, stomatitis
  Desired outcome: *Despite adverse effects, the patient will receive enough nourishment to meet physiologic needs.*
- Risk for Poisoning (Toxicity) related to use of drug with a narrow therapeutic index
  Desired outcome: *The patient will receive drug therapy without harmful or poisonous effects.*

Planning and Intervention

Maximizing Therapeutic Effects

When drug interactions are intentional and desirable, the nurse needs to give the drugs at the prescribed time intervals. They should be administered at the same time if necessary to achieve the interaction. When drug interactions are not desired but both drugs are needed for therapy, the doses must be administered at different times to promote the therapeutic effect of each drug.

Minimizing Adverse Effects

To help protect the patient from serious adverse effects and drug interactions, the nurse must obtain a drug history from the patient, beginning with a list of all drugs that the patient has taken. Drug references or databases may then be consulted for complete descriptions of known or suspected drug interactions.

If a patient is taking a drug that may interact with another drug in the current regimen, ideally the drugs should not be coadministered. The nurse can either stagger drug administration times, if that is sufficient to minimize an interaction, or contact the prescriber about changing one of the ordered drugs. If both drugs are required, additional monitoring of the patient or dose adjustment of one of the drugs may be warranted. If the interaction is potentially serious, the prescriber should be consulted before the nurse or patient begins administering the new drug. When a patient is receiving two or more drugs and either unexpected effects or no therapeutic effects occur, the nurse should suspect that a drug interaction may have occurred and investigate fully.

Throughout therapy, the patient is monitored for signs and symptoms of interactions and adverse effects and for alterations in health status that increase the risk for adverse effects. If a drug interaction is known to increase or decrease the circulating level of one of the drugs, serum drug levels are monitored to determine whether therapeutic levels are being maintained.

Providing Patient and Family Education

Before and throughout drug therapy, the nurse informs the patient and family about adverse effects and drug interactions. Initial instruction includes teaching the patient how to minimize the occurrence of these effects and how to cope with them. In addition, the nurse teaches the patient which effects to expect, which to report to the prescriber, and which require immediate medical attention.

Ongoing Assessment and Evaluation

During drug therapy, the nurse continues to monitor for adverse effects and drug interactions, including allergic responses. The nurse also considers the possibility of a drug interaction each time a new drug is added to the treatment plan. If none of these effects occurs and the therapeutic effect has been achieved, drug therapy is evaluated as successful.

CHAPTER SUMMARY

- Adverse effects are all unintended effects of drug therapy. All drugs have adverse effects. Adverse effects may be very mild and merely bothersome or serious and life threatening.
- Adverse effects are usually predictable or dose related. Adverse effects that are not predictable or dose related are attributable to allergic responses or idiosyncratic responses. The most serious allergic response is called anaphylaxis. Anaphylaxis can be fatal if not treated.
- Adverse effects that carry the risk for permanent damage or death and form specific patterns or groups of symptoms related to drug therapy are called toxicities. The major drug toxicities are hepatotoxicity, nephrotoxicity, neurotoxicity, cardiotoxicity, ototoxicity, and immunotoxicity.
- Drug interactions occur between two drugs or a drug and food or other substance, such as alcohol. Some drug interactions are beneficial, whereas others are harmful.
- Drug interactions may affect any aspect of pharmacokinetics: absorption, distribution, metabolism, or excretion.
- An important and common drug interaction is one that alters the metabolism of a drug by either inducing or inhibiting the P-450 system. Drug–drug interactions usually alter the P-450 system in the liver, whereas interactions between drugs and grapefruit juice primarily alter the P-450 enzymes in the GI tract.
- Drug interactions may also alter the pharmacodynamics of drug therapy. Two or more drugs may compete for the same receptor site, or they may work in different ways in the body with conflicting or cumulative results. Drugs that act in different ways, or at different recep-

CRITICAL THINKING SCENARIO

Suspected adverse effects

You are a nurse working in an emergency room of a community hospital. A patient with diabetes is brought in with complaints of nausea and abdominal pain. On physical assessment, she is found to have an enlarged, tender liver. Her liver enzymes are substantially elevated. During your assessment, you learn that the patient was started on a newly approved drug for her diabetes 3 months ago.

1. How would you determine whether her symptoms were known adverse effects from the drug therapy?
2. You determine that her symptoms are not listed as known adverse effects, but you still feel concerned that they may be related to her drug therapy. What action would be appropriate based on your suspicion?

When implementing pediatric drug therapy, the nurse must remember that children are different from adults in many ways. Although some drugs and administration routes are similar in adults and children, the nursing management of drug therapy varies greatly. For example, physiologic differences in children and the child's immature body systems, greater fluid composition, and smaller size all affect the core drug knowledge. These differences can exaggerate or diminish the pediatric patient's response to drug therapy, making some drug actions and outcomes less predictable in the child than in the adult.

Additionally, in children, core patient variables are different from those in adult patients and from child to child because of the differences across the developmental stages of childhood. The **pediatric patient** is usually defined as younger than 16 years and weighing less than 50 kilograms.

This chapter focuses on core drug knowledge that is relevant and unique to pediatric patients and on core patient variables that emphasize children's needs according to developmental changes. Special issues in managing pediatric drug therapy are explored, including maximizing therapeutic effects, minimizing adverse effects, and educating patients and families.

NURSING MANAGEMENT OF THE PEDIATRIC PATIENT

Core Drug Knowledge Related to Children

Pharmacotherapeutics

Therapeutic indications and effects of drug therapy are similar for children and adults. The major difference is in the drug dosage. Committing drug dosages to memory is difficult and unnecessary because child weights vary considerably. Unlike most adult drug dosages, almost all pediatric drug dosages are based on the weight of the child in kilograms. Dosage is usually specified in milligrams of drug per kilogram of body weight (mg/kg).

When a child dose is not specified, it can be determined from the adult dose based on the body surface area of the child. The **body surface area** is the external surface of the body expressed in square meters. The ratio of body surface area to weight is inversely proportional to length; therefore, the infant or young child who is shorter and weighs less than the adult has relatively greater surface area than would be expected from the weight. Body surface area is calculated using a standard formula found in Box 6.1.

Body surface area can also be determined by using a nomogram (Figure 6.1). A **nomogram** is a chart or a graph that shows relationships between numerical variables. A representative nomogram used to estimate body surface area in children may have several columns of calibrated measures representing height, surface area, and weight. Body surface area is calculated by drawing a line across the columns to connect the patient's height with the patient's weight. The point at which the line intersects the central surface area column is the patient's estimated body surface area.

Once body surface area is determined, the dosage can be computed using the formula in Box 6.1. A child's drug dosage may also be determined by comparing the child's weight to the recommended dose per kilograms of weight. Administering the correct drug dosage is crucial in pediatric drug therapy. The child's small and immature body systems make overdosages potentially lethal.

Pharmacodynamics

A drug's mechanism of action is the same in all individuals at all ages. However, what distinguishes individual responses is the ability of the organ systems to function fully and appropriately. In very young children, immature organ systems have less than optimal functioning, which may necessitate increasing or decreasing drug doses to prevent toxicity and to achieve a therapeutic drug level.

Pharmacokinetics

A child's age, growth, and maturation can affect how the body absorbs, distributes, metabolizes, and excretes a drug. By understanding how drugs affect pediatric patients differently from adult patients, the nurse can help maximize the therapeutic effects of a drug and minimize adverse effects. Dosages must often be lowered to account for immature or impaired body systems in neonates and infants.

Absorption

Absorption of a drug depends on various factors. In the pediatric patient, age, disease process, dosage form, route of administration, and foods and drugs present in the child's body have an effect on drug absorption.

The infant's gastrointestinal (GI) tract is less acidic and thus has a higher pH than that of an adult. Moreover, a premature infant's immature GI tract secretes less acid than the full-term newborn's or older child's. As the GI tract matures, the gastric pH decreases and the GI tract becomes more acidic, reaching adult values at approximately 1 year of age. These differences in pH affect drug absorption. For example, a drug such as digoxin is very well absorbed in an acidic environment. Therefore, less digoxin would be absorbed from the premature infant's GI tract than from the older child's or adult's GI tract.

Route of administration also affects absorption. Drugs administered intramuscularly (IM) or subcutaneously (SC) are affected by age. For example, the rate of absorption may be decreased in the infant or child because of erratic blood flow from the immature peripheral circulation. The neonate's blood flow is particularly slow and erratic. Conversely, increased absorption of topical drugs is common in pediatric patients, especially infants. Compared with adults, infants and children have a greater body surface area. The infant's skin exhibits greater permeability as well. An increased body surface area combined with increased permeability results in increased absorption of topical agents, which may result in adverse effects that usually do not occur in the adult patient.

Distribution

In a pediatric patient, drug distribution processes can differ from those in an adult because of differences in body water and fat, immature liver function, and an immature blood–brain barrier.

BOX 6.1 Calculating Pediatric Drug Dosages

Body Surface Area Method

Step 1. Determine the body surface area (BSA) of the child. It is measured in meters squared. A standard formula is used. Computations should be made with a calculator.

$$BSA = \sqrt{\frac{\text{Weight in kg} \times \text{Height in cm}}{3{,}600}}$$

Example: Child weighs 10 kg and is 45 cm tall

1. Multiply weight in kilograms by height in centimeters. $BSA = \frac{10 \times 45}{3{,}600}$
2. Divide product by 3,600. $= \frac{450}{3{,}600}$
3. Enter square root sign on calculator. $= \sqrt{0.125}$
4. Round the BSA to the nearest hundredth. $= 0.35\ m^2$

Step 2. Determine dose using the computed BSA and this formula:

$$\frac{\text{Child's BSA}}{1.7\ m^2 \text{ (average adult BSA)}} \times \text{Usual adult dose} = \text{Child's dose}$$

Example: Child's BSA = $0.35\ m^2$, and usual adult dose is 100 mg.

$$= \frac{0.35\ m^2}{1.7\ m^2} \times 100$$

= 20.588 (20.59) mg is child's dose.

Body Weight Method

Usual dose (in mg): 1 kg :: × dose (in mg): weight of child in kg

Example:

Usual dose is 10 mg/1 kg and child weighs 18 kg — 10 mg : 1 kg :: × mg : 18 kg × = 180 mg

Differences in Body Water and Fat. Compared with adults, children, especially infants, have a higher concentration of water in their bodies and a lower concentration of fat. Newborns have the greatest proportional water content, followed by infants, children, and then adults (Table 6.1). Because infants and children have a greater proportion of body water, water-soluble drugs are diluted to a greater degree, and for this reason, it is important to assess the amount of water in the body of an infant or child before administering water-soluble drugs. The drug moves to areas of water throughout the body, not just in the blood, resulting in lower concentrations of the drug in the blood. With drugs such as gentamicin, proportionately increased dosages may be required to achieve or maintain therapeutic levels.

To a lesser degree, fat-soluble drugs are affected by the proportionately lower fat in the infant and child. Fat distribution increases with age; thus, fat-soluble drugs are distributed to a greater degree in the adult. Because fat-soluble drugs are not widely distributed in the infant's or child's body, greater blood concentrations may result, leading to toxicity.

Immature Liver Function. In the infant and especially in the neonate, immature liver function affects drug distribution. The neonate's immature liver produces fewer plasma proteins, especially albumin; acidic drugs bind strongly to albumin. Pharmacologic effects of drugs result from unbound (i.e., free) drug. In the neonate and infant, more free drug is available because less drug is bound to plasma proteins. The result is increased blood levels of drugs, which in turn can cause greater adverse effects and toxicity in infants. Drug binding to serum proteins reaches adult levels by 6 months of age.

Multiple drugs administered to an infant may compete for the same binding sites, resulting in higher blood concentrations of both drugs or of the drug with less affinity for the binding site. Other naturally occurring substances in the body can also compete for fewer binding sites in the pediatric patient. For example, bilirubin, which may increase during the neonatal period, binds with plasma proteins. When sulfonamides are administered to the neonate who has an increased bilirubin level, it competes with bilirubin for binding sites, leaving more bilirubin free in the blood. Rarely, the bilirubin level can increase to a dangerous level, resulting in bilirubin accumulation in the central nervous system (CNS), a life-threatening condition called **kernicterus.**

Immature Blood–Brain Barrier. At birth, the blood–brain barrier is not fully developed. The blood–brain barrier prevents drugs in the general circulation from passing to the circulation of the brain, thereby protecting the brain from toxic substances. Therefore, newborns are particularly vulnerable to CNS toxicity. In the newborn, the effect of drugs that act on the CNS (e.g., phenobarbital and morphine) is intensified. In addition, infants experience exaggerated CNS responses to other drugs targeted for other body systems.

Metabolism

The liver metabolizes most drugs. However, the immaturity of the neonatal and infant liver results in decreased or incomplete metabolism of many drugs, which may necessitate lower drug dosages or an increased interval between

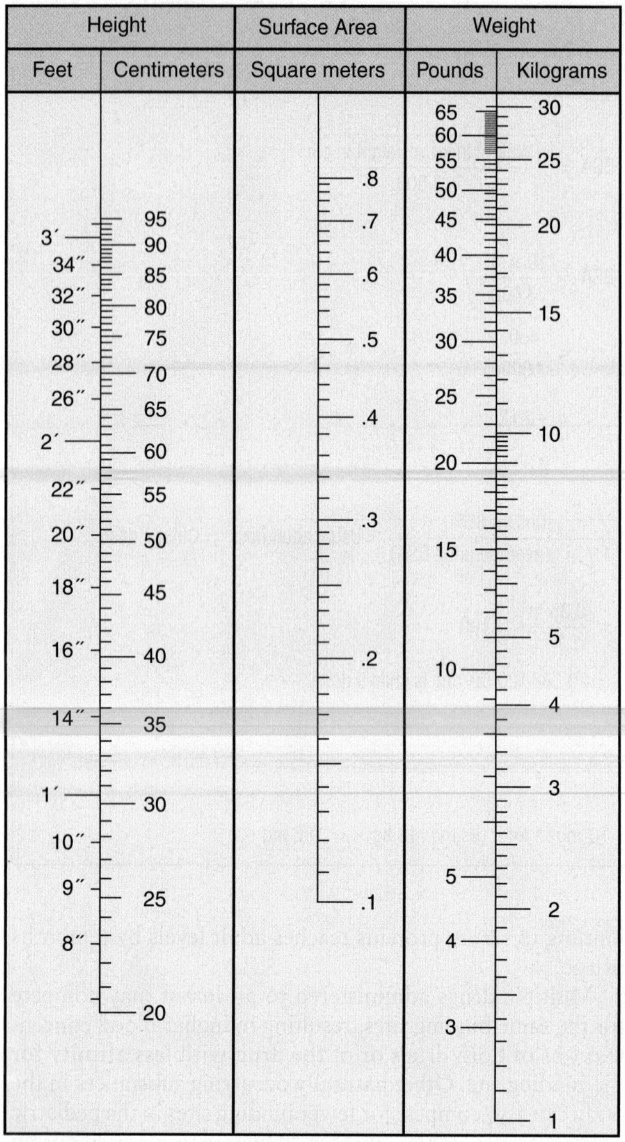

FIGURE 6.1 A pediatric nomogram is a device for estimating body surface area in children. To use it, draw a line from the child's height to the child's weight. The point at which this line intersects the surface area in the middle is the child's estimated body surface area.

TABLE 6.1 Proportional Water Content Across the Life Span

Age	Percentage of Body Water
Newborn	75%–85%
Infant	Approximately 85%
One year old	65%
Two years old	60%
Adult	50%–60%

doses to achieve appropriate blood levels. In children with liver disease, drug metabolism is further complicated by the liver's inability to detoxify drugs. A child with an immature liver or compromised liver function is at risk for drug toxicity.

Drugs requiring oxidation for metabolism are frequently more rapidly metabolized in children than in adults because children have a faster resting respiratory rate. These drugs include phenobarbital, phenytoin, and the methylxanthines (e.g., theophylline and caffeine). With these types of drugs, children may require higher dosages or more frequent administration schedules than adults do to maintain therapeutic blood levels.

Excretion

Most drugs are eliminated from the body through the urine. Drug elimination requires a functioning renal system, and its effectiveness depends on glomerular filtration rate, tubular reabsorption, and maturity of the renal system. In children with impaired renal function, drug dosages should be altered to achieve and maintain therapeutic drug levels.

The neonate, especially the preterm infant, has immature kidneys, and renal excretion of drugs is slow. Drug dosages and therapeutic drug levels must therefore be monitored closely to prevent toxicity. In addition, the reduced glomerular filtration rate and decreased tubular secretion and reabsorption during the first 6 months of life extend the half-life of many drugs (e.g., penicillins, sulfonamides, and cephalosporins). Drugs with a narrow margin between effective and toxic doses must be administered at longer dosage intervals to prevent toxicity. At about 3 months of age, the infant's kidneys can concentrate urine at the adult level, but urinary excretion remains low until the child is about 30 months old, when the kidneys become functionally mature.

A few drugs are excreted through the biliary tree into the intestinal tract. Biliary blood flow is decreased during the first few days of life, during which careful monitoring of drug levels and signs and symptoms of toxicity is imperative.

Contraindications and Precautions

Not all drugs that are safe for adults are safe for children, partly because not all drugs have been adequately tested in clinical trials on pediatric patients. Historically, it was considered unethical to enroll children in randomized, controlled drug studies. Because drugs in development were not tested on children, they were not labeled as approved for use in children. As a result, pediatricians have been forced to prescribe medications for off-label uses in children. At least 75% of drugs regularly prescribed to children in the United States are estimated to have never been labeled for use in any pediatric population. Additionally, the 10 most frequently prescribed drugs for outpatient use in children carry disclaimers on their labels about their use in children, or the labels lack adequate information about how to use the drug in children (with respect to correct dosing, or adverse effects) (Foundation for the National Institutes of Health website, 2003).

Compounding this problem was a lack of financial incentives for drug manufacturers to retest drugs already on the market to obtain approval for use in children. In recent years, the thinking has changed so that it is now considered *unethical* to exclude children from drug studies and not to

have child-specific prescribing information on drugs used in children. To meet this need, the United States Congress passed the Best Pharmaceuticals for Children Act in 2001. This act provides several avenues for drugs already on the market to be tested in clinical drug trials in children. Labeling changes will occur based on findings from these new studies. Until all drugs have been tested and labeled for use in children, nurses need to be aware that off-label use will occur. When a drug is prescribed off-label, the full therapeutic and adverse effects, as well as appropriate dosing, may be unknown. Off-label usage therefore requires cautious administration and careful, frequent assessments of the child. Some drugs are known to be dangerous in children and are labeled as such; these drugs are contraindicated. The core drug knowledge must be determined for each drug before the drug can be administered to a child.

Adverse Effects and Drug Interactions

Adverse effects of some drugs are more severe and more likely to occur in children because of the immature body systems of children. Newborns and young children may experience serious adverse effects from either direct administration of a drug or through their mother's use of a medication. In a review of adverse effects in infants and children younger than 2 years that were reported to the United States Food and Drug Administration (FDA) between 1997 and 2000, approximately 3.5% of the adverse effects accounted for half of the reported deaths in children. Of the total adverse effects reported, about one fourth of those were related to exposure from the mother during pregnancy, delivery, or lactation (Moore et al., 2002).

Other adverse effects on body systems occur only at specific phases of development. For example, tetracycline administered to a child between the ages of 4 months and 8 years will stain the permanent teeth. Glucocorticoids given to a child of any age will suppress growth if the child has not matured to full adult size. Drug receptor sensitivity varies with age; it may be increased or decreased for certain drugs. This variability may promote adverse effects and may necessitate lower or higher drug dosages than would normally be expected (see Chapter 5).

Drug interactions in children are similar to those occurring in adults.

Assessment of Core Patient Variables Related to Children

Health Status

A child's disease process can affect absorption of drugs from the GI tract. Diarrhea, for example, decreases intestinal transit time and therefore decreases the time available for drug absorption. Children with hepatic or renal disease cannot metabolize or excrete drugs as easily as other children and are more prone to adverse effects from drugs. As with adults, any chronic disease or condition may alter the effects of certain drugs and must be seriously considered in drug therapy.

Life Span

The nurse must always consider the developmental stage of the pediatric patient. In planning appropriate drug administration methods, the nurse needs to explain the treatment and enlist the child's cooperation. If doing so is not possible, the nurse must seek appropriate assistance to administer the drug therapy safely. Developmental considerations are especially important when the nurse communicates with the child. To elicit cooperation and obtain necessary information, the nurse must communicate at an appropriate level of understanding for the child. The following are age-appropriate considerations in administering drugs to infants and children. Box 6.2 provides more information regarding pediatric drug routes.

Infants (Birth to 12 Months)

Some infants with a well-developed sucking reflex may willingly swallow a pleasant-tasting liquid drug through a bottle nipple. Other babies may spit out oral medicine, making it difficult for the nurse to administer a full dose. Infant drops may be administered by gently squeezing the child's cheeks to open the mouth, and then placing the drops in the buccal pouch to ensure they will be swallowed. Drugs in rectal suppository form may be given to infants if necessary. However, to avoid expulsion of the suppository before the drug is absorbed, the nurse may need to hold the child's buttocks together for a short time.

If the IM route must be used, the nurse chooses the smallest gauge of needle appropriate for the drug. The preferred injection site for infants and children up to age 3 years is the vastus lateralis. This muscle is on the side of the thigh in the upper outer quadrant of the area between the greater trochanter and the knee. The vastus lateralis has few nerves and blood vessels and forms the largest muscle mass in this age group.

Normally, a $\frac{3}{8}$-inch needle is used for the vastus lateralis in infants; if one is not available, a needle no larger than $\frac{5}{8}$ inch should be used. With the longer needle, the angle of injection should be modified from the usual 90 degrees to 45 degrees toward the frontal plane of the knee. The 45-degree angle ensures that the needle does not traverse the blood vessel.

The rectus femoris is another possible injection site. This muscle is located near the vastus lateralis but is anterior midthigh; the needle should be injected at a 90-degree angle.

In infants, neither the deltoid nor the dorsogluteal muscle sites are used because the muscle masses are too small and undeveloped. The ventrogluteal muscle site, which is large at birth, is not recommended for use in infants because problems encountered in positioning the child make it difficult to locate the muscle site accurately.

Drugs may be administered intravenously to the infant through a peripheral site. These intravenous (IV) sites differ from those used for adults. Ideally, the nurse selects a site that is easy to access and that poses the least risk to the patient. In the neonate and infant, the scalp's many superficial veins

CRITICAL THINKING SCENARIO

Calling on core drug knowledge for children

You are caring for a premature newborn in the nursery. The newborn is receiving intravenous antibiotic therapy to treat an infection. Which specific aspects of core drug knowledge do you think will most help you anticipate any adverse effects of drug therapy?

BOX 6.2 Special Precautions for Pediatric Drug Routes

One way for nurses to promote a good outcome when administering drug therapy is to call on their knowledge of normal growth and development in children and their knowledge of safe administration techniques for specific routes.

Oral Route

- Drug volume should not exceed that which can be swallowed by a very small mouth. The drug dose should be mixed in a small amount of liquid so all of the dose is taken.
- Avoid adding a drug dose to formula. The infant may refuse future feedings because of the foul taste.
- Balance dosage schedules with feeding schedules. Consider whether the drug should be given with meals or on an empty stomach. Check for the possibility of a food-drug interaction.

Intramuscular Route

- Assess whether a less painful route is possible.
- If the IM route is unavoidable, apply a topical, local anesthetic, such as a lidocaine and prilocaine combination (EMLA cream), to numb the injection site.
- Locate anatomic landmarks and boundaries of injection sites.
- Evaluate muscle mass, skin condition, and potential complications related to the child's diagnosis.
- Rotate injection sites as needed, and use appropriate equipment and techniques.
- Seek help to hold the child still while administering the IM injection.

Intravenous Route

- Minimize initial pain on starting the IV by applying a topical anesthetic.
- Check the IV insertion site hourly for infiltration in infants and children.
- Monitor fluid status for signs of overload (risk is greatest in neonates and young infants because of their immature kidney function).
- Control the IV infusion rate by using volumetric pumps and microdrip calibrated chambers.
- Supply no more than 1 hour's worth of fluid when administering a continuous IV drip with an infusion pump (in case the pump malfunctions).
- Engage the lock feature on a volumetric pump to prevent unauthorized changes in the drop rate.

offer easy access. The superficial temporal vein just in front of the pinna of the ear and the metopic vein in the middle of the forehead are relatively easy to find and are less risky for patients (Figure 6.2). Other suitable IV sites for infants and older children include the vessels in the nondominant hand, forearm, upper arm, feet, and antecubital fossa. Distal IV sites are used first and are moved proximally as necessary. The feet provide good IV sites and are used in infants.

Toddlers (13 Months to 3 Years)

Toddlers can swallow liquid forms of drugs, and older toddlers can chew oral drugs. Because toddlers experience anxiety when separated from their parents, having a parent nearby usually helps the child's cooperation during drug therapy. The nurse attempts to elicit cooperation from the toddler but is prepared for the toddler to resist. A toddler's resistance may be associated with a past experience, such as unpleasantly flavored drugs or a painful injection.

Toddlers are also likely to be anxious or uncooperative during administration of rectal suppositories because of their experiences with toilet training and sphincter control. Toddlers have vivid imaginations but limited understanding of how the body works. A common fear is that important body contents will leak out from an injection site. As with infants, the vastus lateralis and rectus femoris remain the IM injection sites of choice for toddlers.

When IV drug therapy is necessary for toddlers, the scalp veins are still appropriate and can be used up to age 18 months. By this time, hair follicles mature and skin layers thicken, making IV access more difficult (Weinstein, 2000). Although the scalp provides excellent IV access, it is not the first choice because of the anxiety it causes parents. Parents feel uneasy because of the scalp's close proximity to the brain and because the area must be shaved at the IV site. If a scalp vein must be used and the site shaved, the nurse asks the parents whether they would like to save the hair and collect it for them if desired. Saving their child's hair makes the procedure less distressing to some parents. For toddlers, as for infants, other peripheral IV sites are also used. If possible, the nurse tries to avoid using the foot so as not to impede the toddler's mobility or cause undue frustration. The foot veins are used, however, in children who need to be immobile.

Preschoolers (3 to 5 Years)

Preschoolers are often uncooperative during drug administration. Strategies for enlisting cooperation include offering choices (e.g., between liquid medicines or chewable tablets) when feasible. Heightened awareness and the fear of punishment or body mutilation in this age group may influence the child's perception of and cooperation with drug therapy.

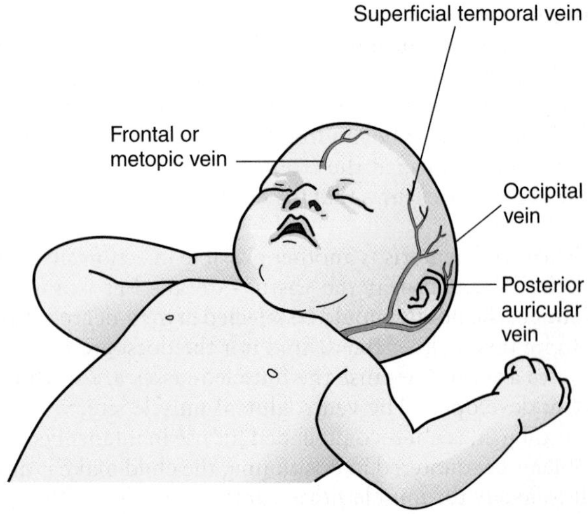

FIGURE 6.2 The scalp is an excellent site for intravenous (IV) therapy in the neonate and infant. The superficial temporal vein and the metopic vein in the central forehead are the preferred sites because they are easy to find and reasonably safe.

Nurses (and parents) should always reassure preschoolers that the drug is to help them feel better and keep them healthy.

When an IM injection must be given, the use of topical anesthetic creams (e.g., EMLA) to numb the site reduces pain in preschoolers during the injection (Cassidy et al., 2001). Several sites may be used for IM injections in preschoolers, most commonly the vastus lateralis, rectus femoris, and ventrogluteal sites. The ventrogluteal site is free of major nerves and blood vessels and is characterized by deep muscle mass. It is located above the greater trochanter between the anterior superior iliac spine and the posterior iliac crest. The drug is injected into the gluteus medius muscle, which is in the ventrogluteal site. Injection in the gluteus medius is less painful than injection in the vastus lateralis.

The dorsogluteal site can be used if necessary but only in children who have been walking for at least 1 year because the gluteus maximus muscle at this site is developed by walking. By 3 years (with the exception of developmentally delayed children), almost all preschoolers have been walking for at least 1 year. The dorsogluteal site is located by drawing an imaginary line from the head of the femur to the posterior superior iliac spine. The injection is then delivered into the gluteus maximus at the upper outer portion above the line. *The dorsogluteal site should be used only as a last resort because of potential damage to the sciatic nerve if the site is not chosen with precision.* Some authorities believe the site should be not used at all. When IV drug therapy is necessary, peripheral sites are selected for the preschooler. Scalp veins are no longer used.

School-aged Children (6 to 12 Years)

The school-aged child is often very cooperative. As with the preschooler, the nurse offers choices to help the school-aged patient exercise control. The school-aged child's greatest fears of drug therapy are usually related to negative past experiences. School-aged children can tolerate warning of drug therapy without becoming fearful and anxious. The school-aged child takes pride in accomplishments such as receiving an injection without incident.

Oral drugs may still be provided in liquid form or chewable tablets. Many school-aged children can also swallow pills. Generally, if rectal drug forms must be used, the school-aged child will feel embarrassment. School-aged and older children, like adults, must be ensured privacy at all times throughout the procedure.

The ventrogluteal site is recommended for an IM injection in the school-aged child, but the vastus lateralis and rectus femoris sites may also be used in this age group. The dorsogluteal site is again possible, *as a last resort.* Although it is not the preferred administration site, the deltoid muscle may also be used for small volumes of drugs (0.5 mL) or vaccines. This site is often considered less painful than the ventrogluteal site.

Adolescents (13 to 16 Years)

An adolescent's ability to cooperate is highly developed and much like an adult's. The nurse offers adolescents control whenever possible and lets them make choices. The nurse also offers support and encouragement without treating adolescents like children. Adolescents are more likely to cooperate and participate in drug therapy when they have a complete understanding of the treatment regimen. Adolescents are particularly sensitive about their bodies and their independence. Therefore, privacy and control are important issues to consider when administering drug therapy to this age group.

Routes of administration are similar to those for adults. Oral forms of drug therapy include tablets or pills. Suppositories can be used, but the adolescent is likely to be embarrassed. IM injection sites are usually the same as for adults unless the adolescent is particularly small. Careful examination is necessary to ensure that adequate muscle mass is available for IM injection. Site selection for IV therapy in adolescents is the same as for adults. The dorsogluteal site remains a last choice.

Lifestyle, Diet, and Habits

The infant's primary food intake is milk and formula. These substances decrease acidity and thus increase gastric pH. Drug absorption is usually affected by pH levels; therefore, food and drug interactions are a primary concern when administering oral drug therapy to infants.

In school-aged children and adolescents, the use and abuse of substances such as caffeine, alcohol, tobacco, and street drugs should be explored. During drug therapy, these substances cause the same complications in children as in adults. Adolescence is a time of experimentation, which includes experimentation with legal and illegal substances. Preadolescents may also experiment with these substances. Nurses must try to elicit this information from all school-aged or adolescent patients throughout drug therapy because potential adverse effects or interactions of these substances may cause serious complications. Regardless of the patient's age and appearance, the nurse never assumes that the child does or does not use or abuse certain substances. Questions regarding substance use are posed in the health assessment interview in a nonjudgmental, matter-of-fact manner.

The nurse questions the parent regarding the use of herbal therapy. Use of alternative therapies has become common, and its use is frequently not reported to the primary care provider. Patients and their families often do not consider these therapies "medications," or may not realize how they can interact with prescribed drug therapy. A recent study in a pediatric emergency department found that 45% of parents had administered an herbal therapy to their child. The most frequently reported herbal therapies were aloe plant/juice, echinacea, and sweet oil. Of the children who received herbal therapies, 27% had received three or more types within the last year. Most of the parents did not know if the herbal products had any adverse effects or if they could interact with prescribed medication. Less than half of the parents had discussed the use of herbs with their child's primary care provider (Lanski et al., 2003).

The economic circumstances of the patient and family are also considered. Are the parents concerned about paying for the child's drug therapy? Are insurance and other resources available?

Environment

Children may receive drug therapy in any setting, although some types of drugs may be administered primarily in one setting or another, just as in the adult population. Children receiving drug therapy at home need to have a parent or guardian responsible for ensuring that the child receives the prescribed therapy. General considerations about the

home need to be assessed just as they are assessed for adults. Does the home have electricity, a refrigerator, and indoor plumbing?

An important additional question that should be asked of the parent or caretaker is whether the home has a safe place to store prescription and nonprescription drugs away from children. Childhood ingestion of drugs is a serious concern because many drugs have serious adverse effects or may cause poisoning in children. Research has shown that unintentional ingestion of over-the-counter drugs is a serious problem and is related to several factors, such as absent or inadequate child-resistant packaging, lack of understanding by the parent or caregiver about the toxicity of the over-the-counter drug, and carelessness by parents or caregivers in the use and storage of the over-the-counter drug (Chien et al., 2003).

Culture and Inherited Traits

The beliefs of the family greatly affect a child's attitude and adherence to the therapeutic regimen. Questions to consider and assessment concerns include the following:

- Does the child's cultural background suggest suspicions about or taboos against drug therapy?
- Do health practices in the child's family rely on other forms of healing, such as using herbal or natural medicines, acupuncture, prayer, or mysticism?
- Do family religious beliefs directly conflict with the use of drug therapy?
- The child's cultural background and heritage must be considered quite seriously when planning drug therapy (see Chapter 12).

Nursing Diagnoses and Outcomes

Nursing diagnoses and outcomes related to specific drug therapy for children are much the same as they are for adults. However, many drug therapies are burdensome for families to maintain, present special concerns, or pose risks to a child's normal growth and development. Common nursing diagnoses and outcomes may include the following:

- Delayed Growth and Development
  Desired outcome: *The patient will achieve normal growth and development during drug therapy.*
- Ineffective Family Therapeutic Regimen Management
  Desired outcome: *Family members will master effective management strategies of the patient's drug regimen.*
- Caregiver Role Strain
  Desired outcome: *The patient and family will develop effective coping skills to avoid, reduce, or relieve stress on family caregivers.*

Planning and Intervention

Maximizing Therapeutic Effects

To administer drugs safely and effectively to children, the nurse must understand pediatric anatomy and physiology, the patient's developmental and cognitive levels, and the child's diagnosis and prognosis. The nurse uses this knowledge to select appropriate drug administration sites, equipment, and administration techniques.

Oral Drug Therapy

Although usually not painful, administration of oral medications can be traumatic, especially when the drug flavor is foul and the child protests. Many pediatric drugs come in liquid form and are drawn up into a syringe (without a needle) for accurate measurement. The drug can then be transferred to a medicine cup for older cooperative children who prefer this way of receiving the drug.

If the patient cannot swallow pills, some pills can be crushed and dissolved in a liquid or soft food (such as applesauce, gelatin, or ice cream) that masks the flavor of the drug. The nurse dilutes the drug in the smallest amount of liquid or food possible to ensure that the child receives the full dose and does not leave any in the residue. Another method of masking bad-tasting drugs for children is to offer a flavored ice pop or ice chips to help numb the taste buds and promote cooperation.

The nurse works carefully with the child to ensure that all of the drug is taken. If the child drools or spits out some of the drug, the nurse calculates the amount of drug lost. If the total is considerable, the nurse reports the estimated amount lost to the prescriber and obtain an order for a replacement dose. For drugs that pose a high risk for toxicity, another dose is unlikely to be ordered. For example, when digoxin (which slows the heart) is given to children with congestive heart failure, an overdose can be lethal.

Parenteral Drug Therapy

To ensure accurate parenteral drug delivery, the nurse must choose age-appropriate equipment. For example, the length and gauge of a needle must be suited to the child's age and growth level. A needle that is too long for the child's size delivers a drug into the muscle rather than into the subcutaneous tissue, thereby speeding the rate of absorption.

When offering a child choices for the sake of gaining his or her cooperation during drug administration, the nurse presents only those choices that truly exist. For example, the nurse does not ask a preschooler if he or she would like to take medicine now if the child does not really have the choice to refuse. Instead, the nurse asks which drug the child wants to take first or how many bandages the child would like to apply after an injection.

Rectal Drug Therapy

The nurse always gives a full explanation to the patient and family regarding the need to administer a drug rectally and asks the child to attempt to retain the drug for as long as possible. As always, the developmental level of the child is taken into consideration with the rectal administration of drugs. To allow time for the drug to be absorbed, young children are dissuaded from going to the bathroom and encouraged to participate in a quiet activity. Older children and adolescents need to have their privacy maintained during the administration of rectal suppositories.

Minimizing Adverse Effects

Calculating Drug Dosages Accurately

When determining a drug dosage, the nurse must remember that muscle mass, body water, fat content, gastric pH levels, and liver function vary greatly from the child to the adult. These variations affect the rate of absorption, making

it vital that dosage calculations be correct. Overdosage of many drugs can cause serious or even fatal effects in children. Because pediatric dosages are small in volume, even a small error may produce serious adverse effects. The nurse must remember that the pediatric drug dosage is not merely a reduced adult dosage; rather, it is calculated by specific equations adjusted to the child's weight and body surface area (see Box 6.1).

Although many nursing drug references give dosage ranges for children, they do not include dosages specific to preterm and full-term neonates. Nurses administering drugs to these patients use a pediatric drug guide that gives ranges of pediatric dosages in mg/kg of body weight or by dose for all children.

The nurse is responsible for ensuring the accuracy of a prescribed drug dose before it is administered. To prevent mathematical errors, drug dosage calculations, even when previously computed by the physician, pharmacist, or both, are always double-checked by the nurse before administering any dose to a child. Research has shown that when equations or math calculations are required to determine the correct dose, 10-fold dose-prescribing errors are more likely to occur in children than in adults (Lesar, 2002; Box 6.3).

Reducing Psychological Stress and Anxiety

Some adverse effects in pediatric drug therapy involve psychological distress of the child or parent. The nurse who understands age-related emotional needs can use appropriate communication techniques to help allay anxiety and negative, stress-provoking feelings regarding drug therapy. For school-aged children and adolescents, feelings are addressed and questions discussed and answered as simply and honestly as possible.

Although infants do not converse, they do communicate nonverbally. Parents are helpful in providing a history of the infant's experiences, behaviors, and schedule, and they can also provide an interpretation of the infant's nonverbal cues. Infants are very much in tune with their parents and can sense their feelings. If the parents are anxious, the infant is likely to be anxious as well. Therefore, parents are offered reassurance and full explanations regarding procedures and rationales. During therapy, the parents may comfort the infant by maintaining eye contact, gently stroking the head, or talking in soothing tones. Parents are not asked to restrain the infant but should be at hand to comfort the child. After drug therapy is administered, they should cuddle and comfort the child.

Because toddlers need to view drug therapy as positively as possible, they should be comforted and praised after receiving a drug regardless of whether they were cooperative or uncooperative. Whatever their behavior, they should never be referred to as a "bad boy" or "bad girl." Toddlers take pride in their accomplishments, and positive feedback and praise enhance their sense of self-esteem.

Play therapy is useful for reducing a child's anxiety and promoting understanding of drug therapy. To familiarize the child with an administration procedure, the nurse encourages role-playing with dolls and appropriate medical equipment. During role-playing, the nurse can further encourage the child to express any feelings of anxiety or anger.

For preschoolers and school-aged children, care is taken to explore the child's experiences with the health care system. These experiences strongly influence the behavior of these children, which, like the behavior of toddlers, are accepted without value judgments. Similarly, the nurse takes advantage of opportunities to provide positive feedback and avoid negativity.

Providing Patient and Family Education

A crucial step in administering pediatric drug therapy is educating the child, the parents, and other family members or caregivers. Providing honest and detailed explanations and rationales helps reassure those caring for the child. Patient and family education is especially important if drug therapy continues when the child returns home. It is important to include the child in drug education. Children have a right to appropriate information regarding any medicine they take. The nurse provides age-appropriate explanations. Including children in drug education, starting at an early age, helps them to grow into the role of informed consumers. The position paper *Ten Guiding Principles for Teaching Children and Adolescents About Medicines* issued by the United States Pharmacopeia encourages educating children about drug therapy. Additional resources for teaching children about medications, including guidelines for creating age-appropriate teaching materials, are also available from the United States Pharmacopeia.

For toddlers, the rationale for drug therapy and type of administration is fully explained to the parents in private, away from the toddler. Toddlers are given a very brief, straightforward, honest explanation before they receive drug therapy and especially before an invasive procedure. Otherwise, their fears and anxiety will escalate.

FOCUS ON RESEARCH

Box 6.3 Medication Administration Errors

Lesar, T. S. (2002). Tenfold medication dose prescribing errors. *Annals of Pharmacotherapy, 36*(12):1833–1839.

The Study

An analysis was done of 200 consecutive tenfold prescribing errors made in a tertiary-care teaching hospital. The prescribing errors had occurred in pediatric and adult patients, with approximately 20% of the errors in pediatric patients. About half of the errors overall were rated as potentially serious or severe. Factors that were associated with the errors included multiple zeros in the dose, the use of equations or calculations to determine the dose, a dose amount of less than one full dose, and conversion of the unit of measure. Of all the errors studied, those involving an equation or a calculation to determine the appropriate dose occurred overwhelmingly (more than 90% of the time) in pediatric patients. A misplaced decimal point was the most frequent cause of a tenfold error (43.5% of the errors), followed by adding an extra zero (in about one third of the cases), and omitting a zero (in about one fourth of the cases).

Nursing Implications

Nurses need to be able to calculate drug dosages accurately. Accuracy is especially important for pediatric drug doses. The nurse provides the final check, after the physician and pharmacist, for the accuracy of the calculated dose. Every drug dose should be checked before it is administered to prevent medication errors and maximize patient safety.

Preschoolers require simple explanations. They often understand more than they can articulate. The information on the drug therapy should be accurate but brief. Giving preschoolers a simple description of the medication administration procedure and calmly informing them—for example, telling them that they might feel a momentary "pinch" or "stick"—is generally sufficient to prepare them. The information is supplied just before a procedure so that little time is left for their fears and anxiety to escalate. Parents or primary caregivers are usually permitted to be with the child during the procedure.

The school-aged child can understand somewhat more in-depth explanations and will ask many specific questions regarding drug therapy. Answers and explanations are honest and as detailed as necessary for the patient and parents. Information is provided on what the child wants to know, not just what the health care provider believes the child should know.

Adolescents are treated like adults with regard to full explanations and rationale for drug therapy. The nurse invites adolescents to be involved in these discussions and encourages them to ask questions and express their feelings. Nurses stress the importance of therapeutic adherence because adolescents are at the age when they assume more responsibility for their own health and well-being. Many adolescents take responsibility for scheduling and administering their own drug therapy.

At a minimum, initial education for school-aged children, adolescents, and parents include the following:

- Generic and trade names of drugs
- Rationale for drug therapy
- Description of the intended therapeutic drug effect
- Route by which drug will be administered
- Schedule and duration of administration
- Potential adverse effects
- Special drug-related precautions or restrictions (e.g., relating to exercise or diet)

In addition, the nurse educates as many family members or other caregivers as possible. Doing so promotes accurate and safe drug administration to the child at home and ensures that sources of information about the child's drug history are easily found, especially in an emergency.

School-aged children and adolescents typically require instruction in proper techniques for self-administering drug therapy. For example, children with diabetes need to learn how to select injection sites and administer injections. Children with asthma need instruction in using respiratory inhalers. Other patients may need instruction in how to mix, shake, or otherwise prepare drugs before measuring the dose.

Parents and pediatric patients are given as much opportunity to practice drug administration techniques as possible while the nurse observes and offers feedback. For example, techniques are reevaluated frequently during admissions to the hospital or at scheduled medical visits because problems related to poor technique frequently arise. Providing parents with a dosing spoon or syringe with a line marked at the correct dose and asking them to again demonstrate how they measure the dose is an effective technique for teaching how to measure a dose properly. Spoken instructions on administering the drug are much less effective.

The importance of administering a drug at the appropriate times and continuing therapy for the full course of treatment must be emphasized to parents and children. Sometimes, parents stop administering a drug once the child no longer exhibits signs or symptoms of an illness, which is especially true if the child protests or has difficulty taking the drug. Nurses stress that interrupting drug therapy before treatment is completed may cause problems such as recurrence of an infection or development of a drug-resistant infection.

The importance of education and health promotion in pediatric drug therapy cannot be overemphasized. Preventing illness and injury helps eliminate the need for many types of drug therapy and the subsequent risk for adverse effects (Box 6.4).

Ongoing Assessment and Evaluation

Nursing management of drug therapy in children is considered effective when the developmental needs of the patient have been met, the care has involved the family, and the drug has achieved its therapeutic effect without adverse effect to the child. Children who are receiving drug therapy for chronic conditions need to be reassessed frequently and evaluated during regular yearly pediatric checkups to ensure that they are safely adhering to prescribed drug therapy, self-administering drug therapy as indicated, and growing and developing normally while undergoing drug therapy.

COMMUNITY-BASED CONCERNS

Box 6.4 Health Education to Minimize Drug Therapy Use and Adverse Effects in Children

- Involve the child in education about drug therapy at an age-appropriate level.
- Explain the role of childhood immunizations in maintaining health, the need to follow the recommended schedule of immunizations, the importance of receiving all recommended immunizations, and the potential adverse effects that may follow the immunization.
- Show the family and child how to perform frequent, thorough hand washing. Explain how this practice prevents the spread of infections, including cold and influenza viruses.
- Teach families the importance of the regular use of sunscreen with children to prevent sunburn resulting from drug-induced photosensitivity and to protect the child against skin cancer later in life.
- Caution families to avoid accidental overdosage and poisonings by keeping all drugs (prescription and over-the-counter products) out of the reach of children, insisting on childproof caps for drug containers, and installing child-resistant latches on cupboards where drugs and other dangerous products are stored. Instruct family members never to describe drugs as "candy."
- Help patients and families develop hygienic practices that will prevent or minimize transmitting parasitic infections by fecal–oral contamination (from not washing hands after using the toilet or touching soiled diapers) or by sharing hairbrushes or hats contaminated by lice.
- Demonstrate how to use car seats appropriately for children of different ages and sizes to prevent injury in car accidents.

CHAPTER SUMMARY

- Children are different from adults both physically and emotionally, and these differences seriously affect the planning of safe and effective drug therapy.
- A child's age, growth, and development are crucial considerations in relating core drug knowledge with core patient variables in drug therapy.
- A child's age, weight, body surface area, water content, and fat content must be considered when determining the proper dose of a drug. Drug dosage is calculated for each child using mathematical formulas.
- Pediatric dosages must be accurate because even small errors can cause adverse effects, toxicity, or death. The nurse verifies all dosage calculations made by other health care providers.
- To maximize the therapeutic effect of any drug, the nurse must ensure that all of the appropriate dose is administered by the desired route.
- Many of the adverse effects of drug therapy can be avoided or minimized by ensuring that the child receives the appropriate drug dosage calculated specifically for him or her. Nurses should have access to a pediatric drug reference or guide that gives the pediatric ranges for drug doses, including those for preterm and full-term neonates.
- One of the adverse effects in pediatric drug administration is psychological distress in the child or parent. The nurse who uses knowledge of age-related emotional needs and communication techniques can greatly help relieve this emotional distress and enhance compliance with drug therapy.
- Patient and family education regarding drug therapy should include information needed to help the child take the drug safely and effectively. Teaching involves giving honest and straightforward explanations about drug therapy, answering questions and allaying patient and family anxiety, and emphasizing the importance of drug compliance.

QUESTIONS FOR STUDY AND REVIEW

1. How does the neonate's and infant's liver function affect drug distribution?
2. What is body surface area?
3. What dose adjustment might be expected when a water-soluble drug is given to an infant?
4. Are all drugs that are safe for adults also safe for children?
5. What is the appropriate site of an IM injection for an infant?
6. Why is it important to assess the preschooler's or school-aged child's past experience with health care providers and drug therapy? Why is patient and family education important with pediatric patients?

Need More Help?

Chapter 6 of the study guide for *Drug Therapy in Nursing* 2e contains NCLEX-style questions and other learning activities to reinforce your understanding of the concepts presented in this chapter. For additional information or to purchase the study guide, visit http://connection.lww.com/go/aschenbrenner.

REFERENCES AND BIBLIOGRAPHY

Cassidy, K. L., Reid, G. J., McGrath, P. J., et al. (2001). A randomized double-blind, placebo-controlled trial of the EMLA patch for the reduction of pain associated with intramuscular injection in four- to six-year-old children. *Acta Paediatricia, 90*(11), 1329–1336.

Chien, C., Marriott, J. L., Ashby, K., et al. (2003). Unintentional ingestion of over the counter medications in children less than 5 years old. *Journal of Paediatrics and Child Health, 39*(4), 264–269.

Foundation for the National Institutes of Health. (2003). The best pharmaceuticals for children fund [Online]. Available: *http://www.fnih.org/programs/translational_research/best_pharmaceuticals.shtml.*

Lanski, S. L., Greenwald, M., Perkins, A., et al. (2003). Herbal therapy use in a pediatric emergency department population: expect the unexpected. *Pediatrics, 111*(5 Pt 1), 981–985.

Lesar, T. S. (2002). Tenfold medication dose prescribing errors. *Annals of Pharmacotherapy, 36*(12), 1833–1839.

Moore, T. J., Weiss, S. R., Kaplan, S., et al. (2002). Reported adverse drug events in infants and children under 2 years of age. *Pediatrics, 110*(5), e53.

United States Food and Drug Administration. (2001). The best pharmaceuticals for children act [On-line]. Available: *http://www.fda.gov/opacom/laws/pharmkids/pharmkids.html.*

United States Pharmacopeia. (1999). Position statement. Ten guiding principles for teaching children and adolescents about medicines [On-line]. Available: *http://www.usp.org/drugInformation/children/principles.html.*

Weinstein, S. (2000). *Plummer's principles and practice of intravenous therapy* (7th ed.). Philadelphia: Lippincott Williams & Wilkins.

Life Span: Pregnant or Breast-Feeding Women

chapter 7

KEY TERMS

eclampsia

fetal alcohol syndrome

fetal hydantoin syndrome

gestational diabetes

hyperemesis gravidarum

lactation

organogenesis

preeclampsia

teratogenic

Learning Objectives

At the completion of this chapter the student will:

1. Identify how core drug knowledge of drug therapy in pregnant or breast-feeding patients may vary from core drug knowledge in other life-span groups.
2. Identify how normal physiologic changes with pregnancy alter the pharmacokinetics of drug therapy.
3. Define teratogenic effect and its relevance in managing drug therapy in the pregnant patient.
4. Differentiate the classifications of drugs for use in pregnancy.
5. Describe why adverse effects of drug therapy may be overlooked in pregnant patients.
6. Identify how the pregnant or breast-feeding patient's core patient variables in drug therapy may vary from the core patient variables of other life-span groups.
7. Relate the core drug knowledge to core patient variables when providing drug therapy in pregnant or breast-feeding patients.
8. Generate a nursing plan of care from the interactions between core drug knowledge and core patient variables for drug therapy in pregnant or breast-feeding patients.
9. Describe nursing interventions to maximize therapeutic effects and minimize adverse effects in drug therapy in pregnant or breast-feeding patients.
10. Determine key points for patient and family education in drug therapy for pregnant or breast-feeding patients.

FEATURED WEBLINK

http://www.perinatology.com/exposures/druglist.htm
This website provides listings of known effects of drugs on pregnant and breast-feeding women.

CONNECTION WEBLINK

Additional Weblinks are found on Connection:
http://www.connection.lww.com/go/aschenbrenner.

Although the prevalence varies, drug therapy during pregnancy is common. Nursing management of drug therapy for pregnant women is challenging for several reasons. The main issue is that nursing care is needed for both the patient and the fetus because most drugs pass through the placental membrane to the fetus (usually by diffusion) or through breast milk to the infant.

Drug therapy in pregnant women is used primarily for two reasons: to treat a preexisting medical condition or to treat complications that arise during pregnancy. Although drug therapy may be indicated during pregnancy or during **lactation** (the secretion of breast milk), nursing management must focus on both the therapeutic effects on the patient and the potential adverse effects on the developing fetus or infant being breast-fed.

The nurse must know about the physiologic changes that occur during pregnancy and how they may alter the patient's response to a drug. The nurse must also understand the adverse effects of certain drugs on the developing fetus. Although adverse effects of drug therapy to the breast-fed infant are generally less severe than those to the fetus during pregnancy, the nurse must also be familiar with the potential adverse effects from drug therapy during lactation.

This chapter presents core drug knowledge and core patient variables that pertain to pregnancy and lactation. In addition, some general guidelines are presented for maximizing therapeutic effects, minimizing adverse effects, and providing patient and family education for any drug therapy.

NURSING MANAGEMENT OF THE PREGNANT OR BREAST-FEEDING PATIENT

Core Drug Knowledge

Pharmacotherapeutics

Pharmacotherapeutics are no different in a pregnant woman than in a woman who is not pregnant. The important consideration in drug therapy for pregnant women is the potential adverse effects on the developing fetus. A clear clinical indication for drug therapy must exist before a drug is prescribed or self-administered. Although the range for most drug dosages remains the same for the pregnant patient, the nurse must always consider the risk for fetal effects. The lowest therapeutic dose of a drug should be administered to the pregnant woman to help minimize fetal effects.

Some health problems occur secondarily to pregnancy and require drug therapy. These problems include **preeclampsia** (a serious hypertensive condition that can develop during pregnancy) or **eclampsia** (a life-threatening condition resulting from uncontrolled preeclampsia, involving cerebral edema and convulsions). **Gestational diabetes,** a form of diabetes that develops during pregnancy, may also occur. Occasionally, if the fetus has a health problem, drugs are administered to the pregnant woman with the intent of treating the fetus as the drug passes through the placenta. For example, digoxin is administered to the mother to treat fetal tachycardia and congestive heart failure.

Pharmacokinetics

Several physiologic and anatomic changes occur during pregnancy. They can alter the pharmacokinetics of drugs and involve the endocrine, gastrointestinal (GI), cardiovascular, circulatory, and renal systems.

Absorption

Changes in the GI system are influenced by pregnancy hormones and mechanical pressure from the growing uterus. Progesterone decreases gastric tone and motility and prolongs stomach emptying time, which may alter the pharmacokinetics of orally administered drugs. Progesterone also promotes functional respiratory system changes during pregnancy. Tidal volume increases 30% to 40%, with a 50% increase in minute volume by term. These increases, along with the pulmonary vasodilation that occurs during pregnancy, enhance the absorption of drugs that are inhaled.

Distribution and Metabolism

Hemodynamic changes in the cardiovascular system alter heart rate, cardiac output, venous and arterial blood pressures, blood volume, circulation, and coagulation. The heart rate increases about 10 to 15 bpm above baseline as a result of a 40% increase in blood volume. A 50% increase in plasma volume causes a hemodilution of plasma albumin, which potentiates changes in drug distribution. Plasma lipid levels increase throughout pregnancy as a result of the more complete absorption and decreased elimination of fats during pregnancy. These changes in lipid levels may alter drug transport mechanisms and drug distribution. Drugs are distributed by the circulatory system to the fetus by passing through the placenta, usually by diffusion. Drugs may compete with the hormones of pregnancy for albumin-binding sites, which may result in a larger amount of unbound (or free) drug in circulation, leaving the drug available to cross the placental membrane and enter the fetal circulation. Drugs that are lipophilic (fat soluble) and not bound to protein pass easily through the placenta's lipid membrane.

Drugs are also distributed into breast milk. Drugs that are widely distributed throughout the mother's body are usually minimally passed into breast milk, producing low drug concentrations in breast milk. Other drugs, such as those with increased lipid solubility and low protein binding (e.g., central nervous system [CNS] agents), pass more easily and may produce high drug concentrations in breast milk. Lipophilic drugs pass easily because breast milk contains a high percentage of fat. Drugs that are not highly protein bound have more active, free drug molecules in the bloodstream, which can then diffuse into breast milk. Other drugs that are more likely to diffuse into breast milk include drugs with lower molecular weights and those with organic bases; these drugs may become "trapped" in breast milk because of its low pH, producing high drug concentrations.

Not all drugs present in breast milk are well absorbed by the neonate. Drug levels in breast milk are not equivalent to drug levels in the mother's blood, and so drugs with poor bioavailability usually do not achieve high concentrations in the neonate's circulation. A breast-feeding infant usually ingests less than 2% of the mother's total dose.

Drug metabolism is not altered by pregnancy or breast-feeding.

Excretion

Changes in renal function during pregnancy result from changes in renal plasma flow, glomerular filtration rates, and renal tubular reabsorption. By the third trimester, the renal blood flow has increased 40% to 50% from the prepregnancy level. Increases in renal plasma flow cause greater capillary pressures, requiring an increase in filtration through the glomerulus. The glomerular filtration rate increases by approximately 50% and contributes to increased excretion rates. Therefore, drug excretion rates may be increased during pregnancy.

Pharmacodynamics

Two dramatic physical changes occur in the mother during pregnancy: by 32 weeks' gestation, cardiac output is increased by 50%; and from the second trimester on, arterial blood pressure is decreased. These conditions necessitate careful evaluation of a drug's pharmacodynamics.

Contraindications and Precautions

Some drugs and vaccines are contraindicated during pregnancy, and others should be given with caution if they pose a threat to the developing fetus by passing through the placenta (Box 7.1). Some drugs and vaccines can cause **teratogenic** effects (physical defects) in the developing fetus. For example, the most commonly prescribed anticonvulsant, phenytoin (Dilantin), a hydantoin, has been found to cause **fetal hydantoin syndrome.** This syndrome is characterized by craniofacial abnormalities, limb defects, growth deficiency, and mental deficiency (Hansen & Smith, 1975). These abnormalities are believed to occur because phenytoin competes for folic acid–binding sites.

The precise effects of drug therapy on the fetus are mostly undetermined. A recent review of all drugs approved in the United States between 1980 and 2000 found that the teratogenic risk in human pregnancy was still undetermined for more than 90% of those drugs. The longer the drug had been on the market, the more likely it was that the exact teratogenic risk was unknown (Lo & Friedman, 2002).

The identification of a drug as a teratogen is traditionally based on the findings of animal teratology studies. This method is problematic because animal models are frequently poor predictors of whether a drug is a human teratogen. Nonhuman primates are good predictors of human teratogenicity because they are the most genetically similar to humans; however, nonhuman primates are rarely used in experiments because of the expense involved. Rodents are used most frequently in teratology studies, but unfortunately they are very dissimilar to humans in terms of their physiology, metabolism, and ontogenetic development. Although animal studies do not provide all of the information in determining teratogenicity of a drug, they currently are the most-used tool to screen drugs for their potential to cause human birth defects. Clinical studies in pregnant women have not been done because of ethical concerns about experimentation on the fetus.

The ultimate assessment of drug safety during pregnancy, unfortunately, comes from the use of the drugs in humans. To address the need for more information about how drugs affect a pregnancy, the United States Food and Drug Administration (FDA) has established Pregnancy Registries (U.S. FDA, Office of Women's Health, 2004). Women who take medication during pregnancy for a chronic or acute condition may elect to join one of these registries. The information regarding their experience is added to a national database, whose purpose is to provide more definitive information about the teratogenic affects of various drug therapies.

COMMUNITY-BASED CONCERNS

Box 7.1 Smallpox Vaccine

In collaboration with the Food and Drug Administration (FDA) and the Department of Defense in the United States, the Centers for Disease Control and Prevention (CDC) established the National Smallpox Vaccine in Pregnancy Registry. The registry includes women found to be pregnant when vaccinated, those who became pregnant within 28 days of vaccination, and those who, while pregnant, were in close contact with a person who had received the smallpox vaccine within the past 28 days. Women who are reported to this registry will be monitored throughout the pregnancy and at the conclusion of the pregnancy to document pregnancy outcomes.

Women who are pregnant or might become pregnant within 4 weeks after vaccination should not be vaccinated against smallpox unless there is active circulating disease because of the risk for fetal vaccinia, which is a rare but serious infection of the fetus. Fetal vaccinia is manifested by skin lesions and internal organ involvement and can result in fetal or neonatal death or premature birth. Smallpox vaccine has not been clearly shown to cause other teratogenic effects or other adverse effects in the fetus or newborn. People who have close personal contact with a pregnant woman should also not be vaccinated.

The CDC has recommended that screening for pregnancy before vaccination is paramount to preventing exposures in pregnant women. The screenings that have occurred as part of the current immunization campaign against smallpox appear to have been effective in minimizing exposure of pregnant women to the vaccine.

Source: Centers for Disease Control. (2003). *Women with smallpox vaccine exposure during pregnancy reported to the national smallpox vaccine in pregnancy registry—United States, 2003* [Electronic version]. *MMWR, 52* (17), 386–388. Available: *http://www.cdc.gov/mmwr/preview/mmwrhtml/mm5217a3.htm.*

Pregnancy Categories

In 1980, the FDA developed a categorical ranking based on research findings to help classify drugs by the risks posed to the fetus, weighed against the potential benefits to the pregnant woman. The categories are A, B, C, D, and X (Box 7.2). Categories A and B (and to some extent, C) are generally based on increasing risk. Categories D and X (and to some extent, C) are based on risk versus potential benefit.

To inform health care providers making decisions about drug administration, drug manufacturers are required by law to state these pregnancy categories in all printed drug reference materials and package inserts. Recently, several concerns have been voiced about the categorical ranking system currently in use, including the following:

- The categories do not supply enough information for providers and consumers to make informed decisions about drug therapy.

BOX 7.2 FDA Pregnancy Categories

Category A: Controlled human studies in pregnant women fail to demonstrate a risk to the fetus.
Category B: Animal studies fail to demonstrate fetal risk, but there are no controlled human studies in pregnant women; or animal studies demonstrate fetal risk that was not confirmed in controlled human studies in pregnant women.
Category C: Animal studies demonstrate fetal risk, and there are no controlled human studies in pregnant women to rule out fetal risk, or there are no animal or human studies. Drugs are given if the benefit justifies risk.
Category D: Controlled human studies demonstrate positive evidence of fetal risk. In life-threatening situations, the benefit may be acceptable despite the risk.
Category X: Controlled human studies demonstrate fetal risk. The fetal risk outweighs any possible benefit. Use in pregnant or potentially pregnant women is contraindicated.

- The FDA, in trying to keep the categories simple, has grouped together drugs that do not have identical risks.
- The alphabetical progression leads people to believe that the seriousness of the risk increases with each letter, which is not correct.

Based on these concerns, the FDA Pregnancy Labeling Task Force has been revising the current pregnancy labeling system. One recommendation is to replace the current letter categories and text description with a more informative narrative. Another major goal of the task force is to determine how animal teratogenicity contributes to knowledge about human teratogenicity, with special emphasis on reevaluating category C. Many drugs are grouped into category C because human studies of those drugs do not exist and animal studies indicate adverse effects on the fetus. This categorization may falsely elevate the number of drugs that actually pose a threat to human pregnancies because animal studies do not always closely predict human responses to drug therapy. The information gained from the Pregnancy Registries should help clarify how drugs must be labeled relative to their actual risk to the fetus (U.S. FDA, Center for Drug Evaluation and Research, 2001).

Lactation Categories

In 2001, the American Academy of Pediatrics Committee on Drugs published its updated recommendations on drugs and breast-feeding (American Academy of Pediatrics, 2001). The report identified several categories of drugs and their potential to cause problems with breast-feeding, which are as follows:

- Cytotoxic drugs that may interfere with cellular metabolism of the nursing infant
- Drugs of abuse for which adverse effects on the infant during breast-feeding have been reported
- Radioactive compounds that require temporary cessation of breast-feeding
- Drugs for which the effect on nursing infants is unknown but may be of concern
- Drugs that have been associated with significant effects on some nursing infants and should be given to nursing mothers with caution
- Maternal medication usually compatible with breast-feeding
- Food and environmental agents: effects on breast-feeding

All contraindicated drugs have been reported to cause signs and symptoms in the infant or produce an adverse effect with lactation. The American Academy of Pediatrics states that this list is not complete and recommends that all drugs of abuse should be avoided by lactating women, even though reports of neonatal adverse effects are not found in the literature for all substances. If a breast-feeding woman is receiving any radioactive compounds, such as those used for treating malignant tumors or an overactive thyroid gland, the patient should pump her breasts during the time that breast milk is radioactive and discard that milk in a biohazard container designed for radioactive materials. Breast-feeding can resume when the drug is stopped and the breast milk contains no radioactivity.

Drugs with unknown effects on the neonate that may be of concern include psychotropic drugs (antianxiety drugs, antidepressants, and neuroleptic drugs). These drugs appear in low concentrations in breast milk after maternal ingestion. However, these drugs have long half-lives, and because of immature hepatic and renal function in newborns, the drugs or some of their metabolites may reach measurable amounts in nursing babies' plasma and tissues and in organs such as the brain. Nursing mothers should be informed that if they take one of these drugs, the infant will be exposed to it. These drugs affect neurotransmitter function in the developing CNS, and the long-term neurodevelopmental effects that can occur from newborn exposure are unknown.

Other drugs with unknown effects on the neonate that may be of concern are several anti-infectives, including chloramphenicol (Chloromycetin), metoclopramide (Reglan), and metronidazole (Flagyl).

Drugs that are associated with significant neonatal effects after breast-feeding and that should be used with caution include aspirin, clemastine (Tavist), 5-aminosalicylic acid (Paser Granules), phenobarbital, primidone (Mysoline), and sulfasalazine (Azulfidine). Most reported effects for these drugs include sedation and diarrhea.

Often, drugs identified as being compatible with breast-feeding are not part of large research studies. Rather, information is obtained from single case reports or a small series of reports. However, most drugs that are taken by the mother for treatment are believed to pose no harm to the breast-fed newborn.

Adverse Effects

The two major considerations when evaluating adverse effects of drug therapy in pregnant women are common side effects of pregnancy and the adverse effect that maternal drug therapy can have on the fetus. Symptoms such as nausea and vomiting, light-headedness or hypotension, constipation, heartburn, urinary frequency, heart palpitations, and fatigue may mask the adverse effects of drug therapy in pregnant patients, making adverse effects more difficult to assess. When considering the effects of drugs on the fetus, several factors are important, including dose and duration of drug

therapy, the type of adverse effect that may appear, and when during pregnancy the drug is taken. The timing of drug exposure is critical because of the vulnerability of the fetus during constant changes in development. Before implantation, the fertilized ovum may not be affected by maternal drug use, although some drugs, such as alcohol, produce a hostile intrauterine environment that can prevent implantation and cause a spontaneous abortion. The time from conception to implantation is theorized as the "protected period"; that is, without a vascular interface between the mother and the conceptus, drugs in the mother's circulation are believed to be unable to pass to the conceptus and have an effect on it.

The critical period of **organogenesis,** during which the major fetal organs form, is from implantation up to approximately day 58 to 60 after conception. If drugs that cause teratogenic effects are administered during this period, major malformations of fetal organ systems may result (Table 7.1). Malformations that are lethal to the embryo will result in spontaneous abortion. If possible, drug therapy should be delayed until after this time. Unfortunately, most women do not realize they are pregnant or do not seek prenatal care until after this early period, so that accidental exposure to teratogens may occur.

After 60 days, the embryonic phase is complete, and the fetal phase begins. This phase continues through the remainder of the pregnancy, during which fetal exposure to drugs continues to have the potential for harm. The fetal effects that may occur are of four primary types:

- Damage to structures or organs that were formed normally during organogenesis
- Damage to systems undergoing tissue development
- Growth retardation
- Fetal death or stillbirth

Combinations of these effects may also occur. Damage to the fetus may be caused by teratogens but may also be caused by agents that have no apparent potential to produce abnormal development. An example is coumarin derivatives used as anticoagulants, which may produce eye and brain defects from hemorrhagic accidents in the fetus. Growth retardation is the most common fetal effect. However, it is difficult to determine whether this effect is caused by the drug therapy or the primary condition for which the drug therapy is prescribed. For example, the antihypertensive drug propranolol is associated with fetal growth retardation, but untreated hypertension is also associated with this condition.

Additionally, some drugs create adverse neonatal effects (Table 7.2). These agents do not normally cause teratogenic effects but instead create a situation that makes it difficult for the neonate to adapt to life outside the uterus. Examples are floppy infant syndrome from the use of benzodiazepines (antianxiety agents, sedatives) near the time of delivery and premature closing of the ductus arteriosus from the use of prostaglandin synthetase inhibitors (i.e., nonsteroidal anti-inflammatory drugs such as aspirin or indomethacin [Indocin]).

The risk for adverse effects of drug therapy on the breast-feeding infant are not as great as those relating to drug therapy during pregnancy because the breast-feeding infant usually ingests less than 2% of the total dose of the drug given to the mother. However, because the risk for adverse effects still exists, breast-feeding is contraindicated with many drug therapies and is strongly discouraged with others. Again, knowledge is limited because of the dearth of controlled clinical studies of drugs' effects on a breast-fed child. Breast-feeding confers many advantages to the baby and is being encouraged more and more by health professionals and public health officials. As this trend continues, nurses need to know more about whether the administration of a particular drug poses a risk to the breast-feeding infant.

TABLE 7.1 Examples of Teratogenic Drugs

Teratogenic Drug or Drug Class	Indication
aminopterin, methylaminopter, busulfan, cyclophosphamide, thalidomide*	Antineoplastic
androgenic hormones, diethylstilbestrol	Hormone replacement
coumarin	Anticoagulant
etretinate	Psoriasis
isotretinoin	Recalcitrant cystic acne
lithium	Antimanic
methimazole	Antithyroid
penicillamine	Cystinuria and rheumatoid arthritis
phenytoin, trimethadione, valproic acid	Anticonvulsant
tetracycline	Antibiotic

*Originally used as a tranquilizer and sedative; also currently used as an anti-infective for leprosy.

TABLE 7.2 Selected Nonteratogenic Drugs with Adverse Fetal Effects

Nonteratogenic Drug	Adverse Fetal Effects
acetaminophen	Renal failure
adrenocortical hormones	Adrenocortical suppression, electrolyte imbalance
amphetamines	Withdrawal
cocaine	Vascular disruption, withdrawal, intrauterine growth retardation
meperidine	Neonatal depression
phenobarbital (excess)	Neonatal bleeding, death
cigarette smoking	Premature births, intra-uterine growth retardation
thiazide diuretics	Thrombocytopenia, salt and water depletion, possible neonatal death

Drug Interactions

Drug interactions are unchanged during pregnancy and breast-feeding.

Assessment of Core Patient Variables Relevant to Pregnancy and Breast-Feeding

Health Status

Several considerations must be taken into account when assessing health status during pregnancy. First, if the patient has a preexisting condition that requires drug therapy, the health care providers must consider whether the prescribed drug therapy will have adverse effects on the fetus. Second, any adverse effects the pregnancy may have on the mother's health must be identified because they may require changes in drug therapy. Third, if the pregnancy does induce changes in health status that require new drug therapy, any adverse effects of this drug therapy on the fetus will have to be determined.

Pregnant women, especially those being treated with drug therapy, must be assessed for preexisting conditions. Special attention should be given to any cardiovascular problems because the cardiovascular system undergoes many changes and stresses during pregnancy. The pregnancy may necessitate changes in drug selection or dosage. The also assesses the woman's use of over-the-counter drugs, which may also pose risks to the fetus.

Seizure disorder is important to consider during pregnancy. A woman with a seizure disorder who is planning a pregnancy must first seriously consider how anticonvulsant drug therapy might affect the fetus. Many traditional, established anticonvulsants have well-known teratogenic potential because of their mechanism of action. However, stopping all drug therapy for the pregnant woman with epilepsy is not necessarily advisable because seizures and status epilepticus, which can occur when drug therapy is stopped, are responsible for most excess maternal deaths in women with epilepsy (i.e., beyond what would be expected to occur statistically). Controversy exists regarding what harm maternal seizures can cause the fetus (Barrett & Richens, 2003). Some clinical experts have hypothesized that seizures in a pregnant woman may cause fetal hypoxia, leading to CNS damage. This "between a rock and a hard place" reality demonstrates the difficulty of making drug therapy decisions that are in the best interest of both the mother and the baby.

If anticonvulsants must be continued during pregnancy, drug selection is important. Within the last few years, new types of anticonvulsants have been developed that prevent seizures in different ways and therefore do not pose the same risks to the developing fetus. These drugs do not appear to be teratogenic in animals, although as stated earlier, animal teratology studies may not be reliable predictors of human teratology (Palmieri & Canger, 2002). Certain anticonvulsants (e.g., trimethadione [Tridione] and valproic acid [Depakote]) should still be avoided. However, only drugs of pregnancy class X are strictly contraindicated. The decision whether to maintain therapy with drugs having a class D or even a class C rating must be made based on the ratio of risk to benefit. It is important to remember that these contraindications are relative and that there is no clear definition of the precise risks and benefits. Anticonvulsants may be discontinued for select patients upon medical consultation.

Another health condition that may warrant assessment is depression. With the increased use of antidepressants, concerns have arisen about the effects these drugs might have during pregnancy, but there is little information on this subject to date. However, one study examined the effect of three different drugs in one class of antidepressants, the selective serotonin reuptake inhibitors. These drugs did not appear to cause increased risk for neonatal complications or congenital anomalies. High doses of one of the drugs, fluoxetine (Prozac), may be associated with a risk for low birth weight (Hendrick et al., 2003); further study is needed.

Diabetes, whether preexisting or developed during pregnancy, is another important condition to consider. Between 1% and 5% of women have diabetes before pregnancy. Another 2% to 3% of pregnant women develop gestational diabetes, in which the secretion of placental hormones (human placental lactogen, cortisol, progesterone, and catecholamines) causes the pregnant woman to develop insulin resistance as the pregnancy progresses. In either case, hyperglycemia may result, which requires either an increase in insulin therapy for those women already receiving it or initiation of insulin therapy for those with gestational diabetes. Because hyperglycemia is believed to increase the incidence of congenital anomalies (particularly during the first trimester), the primary goal for the pregnant patient is to maintain normal blood glucose levels. Insulin is the drug of choice for controlling blood glucose levels because, unlike oral hypoglycemic drugs, it does not cross the placenta. After the neonate is delivered, maternal insulin needs should return to baseline levels, and insulin therapy is usually no longer necessary for women who did not need it before becoming pregnant.

Another change in health status that may occur during pregnancy is **hyperemesis gravidarum,** commonly called pernicious vomiting of pregnancy. When hyperemesis gravidarum is severe, antiemetic drug therapy is needed to control the vomiting. Currently, antiemetic drug therapy consists of drugs from the piperazine class (e.g., meclizine [Antivert] and cyclizine [Marezine]) and the phenothiazine class (e.g., chlorpromazine [Thorazine], prochlorperazine [Compazine], and promethazine [Phenergan]). The piperazines are not known to be teratogenic. The phenothiazines are generally considered safe with low and infrequent usage, although some studies show that animal or human infant malformations can occur. Therefore, when using antiemetics, especially during the first trimester, the risk for adverse fetal effects must be considered.

Preeclampsia is another serious condition that can develop and require drug therapy during pregnancy. This hypertensive condition of pregnancy typically develops after the 24th gestational week. Preeclampsia is characterized by a triad of symptoms—hypertension, edema, and proteinuria. Uncontrolled preeclampsia may lead to eclampsia, a condition characterized by cerebral edema and convulsions. The primary goal of preeclampsia treatment is to prevent eclampsia and stabilize the patient until the fetus reaches maturity. Treatment for preeclampsia is aimed at decreasing CNS irritability and reducing maternal blood pressure to enhance placental and maternal circulation to the organs. Drug therapy for preeclampsia includes magnesium sulfate, which is

the drug of choice for preventing convulsions (see Chapter 55), and hydralazine, a drug used to treat hypertension (see Chapter 27). Other drugs used in treating hypertension in preeclampsia include diazoxide (Hyperstat IV), nifedipine (Procardia), and labetalol (Trandate).

Another condition that may occur secondary to pregnancy is thrombus formation. The decreased venous return and increased levels of clotting factors and fibrinogen that are characteristic in pregnancy produce a state of hypercoagulation, which increases the risk for clot formation. Pregnant women who develop thrombosis are treated with heparin.

Lifespan and Gender

Teenage pregnancy continues to be a problem in the United States. A recent study suggests that the pregnancies of teenage girls may be at additional risk for teratogenic drug effects because of sharing of prescription medication and the unplanned nature of these pregnancies. More than 20% of the girls surveyed reported borrowing or sharing their medications with others. The reasons they gave for this behavior were: having the same prescription, getting medication from a family member, having the same type of problem as the person who had the medication, or wanting something strong for pimples or oily skin (Daniel, Honein, & Moore, 2003). Nurses assess for this risky behavior.

Lifestyle, Diet, and Habits

The lifestyle, diet, and habits of pregnant or breast-feeding women can have a serious impact on the course of the pregnancy and the development of the fetus or infant. For example, alcohol is a known human teratogen. **Fetal alcohol syndrome** is a serious pattern of teratogenic effects seen in infants born to women who may have consumed alcohol chronically during pregnancy. Fetal alcohol syndrome is marked by specific physical malformations at birth and severe growth retardation, mental retardation, and microcephaly. Cocaine abuse is also known to cause adverse fetal effects and is suspected to be a human teratogen. Opiate abuse does not appear to significantly increase the risk for congenital anomalies, but other adverse outcomes are associated with the use of opiates, including abruptio placentae, neonatal withdrawal, preterm birth, and fetal growth retardation. Smoking tobacco also has adverse fetal effects, most notably fetal growth retardation. A recent study showed that cigarette smoking before and during pregnancy was associated with smaller and lighter newborns. A higher incidence of cesarean birth was also found among women who smoked (Kirchengast & Hartmann, 2003). Box 7.3 further explores the effects of substance abuse in pregnancy.

Environment

Although some changes in health status that occur in pregnancy require drug therapy administered in the hospital setting, such as magnesium sulfate for preeclampsia, most drug therapy given during pregnancy or breast-feeding is administered in the patient's home.

Culture and Inherited Traits

Cultural beliefs may affect whether a woman accepts certain drug therapies while she is pregnant or breast-feeding. Assess for these beliefs when managing drug therapy in the pregnant or breast-feeding woman. For more about the effects of culture on pharmacotherapeutics, see Chapter 12.

FOCUS ON RESEARCH

Box 7.3 Pregnancy and Substance Abuse

Ebrahim, S. H., & Gfroerer, J. (2003). Pregnancy-related substance use in the United States during 1996-1998. *Obstetrics and Gynecology, 101*(2), 374–379.

The Study

To determine the national prevalence of illicit drug use during pregnancy, data from the National Household Survey on Drug Abuse were analyzed. These data were collected between 1996 and 1998 and are considered a representative sample of noninstitutionalized women aged 18 to 44 years. Of the 22,303 women surveyed, 1,249 were pregnant. Of the pregnant women, 2.8% reported that they used illegal drugs, compared with 6.4% of nonpregnant women. Three fourths of the drug-abusing women used marijuana, and one tenth of them used cocaine. Knowledge of pregnancy promoted abstinence from illegal drug use; 28% of pregnant women abstained during the first trimester, and 93% abstained by the third trimester. However, there was considerable relapse in drug use after delivery, with only 24% of the women remaining drug free after delivery. More than half of the pregnant drug-abusing women also reported that they smoked cigarettes and drank alcohol, compared with two thirds of the nonpregnant women. The highest rate of substance abuse in pregnant women was found in those who were younger than 30 years of age, were unmarried, and had less than a high school education. Age and marital status were related to drug use in nonpregnant women, but not education.

Nursing Implications

Substance abuse poses a significant risk to developing fetuses. During any 4-week period, an estimated 6 pregnancies per 1,000 women of childbearing age occur in the United States. Pregnancy is often not detected until at least one menstrual period is missed. Drug use and abuse during this interval poses special risks because it is also the time of organ development. Nurses need to recognize that a sizable number of childbearing women abuse illegal substances, in addition to using cigarettes and alcohol—all of which are risks for adverse fetal effects. Education about the effects of both illegal and legal substances on child development is important to promoting healthy pregnancies. Therefore, this kind of education should be included as part of routine health care to women of childbearing age who may use these substances.

Nursing Diagnoses and Outcomes

Nursing diagnoses formulated for the pregnant or breast-feeding patient receiving drug therapy are similar to diagnoses made for patients with other concerns relating to life span. The main difference is that for the pregnant or breast-feeding woman, the nursing diagnosis must address the needs of both the patient and her child. Relevant nursing diagnoses may include the following:

- Risk for Injury to the fetus related to adverse effects of maternal drug therapy
  Desired outcome: *The patient will demonstrate therapeutic drug effects with minimal adverse effect to the fetus or infant by avoiding unnecessary drugs throughout pregnancy and lactation and by using nonpharmacologic measures to relieve common discomforts of pregnancy.*

- Anxiety related to perceived danger of drug therapy to fetus or infant
  Desired outcome: The patient's anxiety will be minimal during drug therapy.
- Risk for Injury to the patient related to failure to receive needed drug therapy because of its potential adverse effects on the fetus or infant
  Desired outcome: The patient will not sustain an injury from choices made about receiving drug therapy.

Planning and Intervention

The nurse and other health care providers have a responsibility to the pregnant patient to consider the risk-to-benefit ratio of drug therapy, to educate the childbearing patient regarding possible teratogenic effects, and to support the patient's decision to accept or refuse drug therapy.

Maximizing Therapeutic Effects

If a prescribed drug therapy does not have adverse effects for the developing fetus or the child of the breast-feeding woman, this absence of known risk should be emphasized when teaching patients. Women may be reluctant to take needed drug therapy if they believe it may be harmful to the fetus.

Minimizing Adverse Effects

Limiting drug use in pregnancy decreases maternal and fetal adverse effects. No drug can be considered absolutely safe when administered during pregnancy, although general guidelines can assist the health care provider with decisions relating to drug therapy. Women of childbearing age should always be assessed for pregnancy before any drug therapy is initiated. During pregnancy, nonpharmacologic alternatives to drug therapy should be used if possible, especially for common discomforts of pregnancy, such as nausea and vomiting, light-headedness or hypotension, constipation, heartburn, urinary frequency, heart palpitations, and fatigue. If drug therapy is required, the nurse first checks the drug's FDA pregnancy category to determine safety. An evaluation of the risks versus the benefits shows whether administering a drug is justified. When a drug is to be administered, the nurse consults with the prescriber so that the minimum therapeutic dose is used for as short a time as possible. If possible, drug therapy is delayed until after the first trimester of pregnancy, during which all major fetal organ systems are forming, especially if the drug has the potential for causing teratogenic effects.

The pregnant woman and the fetus are monitored for both therapeutic and adverse effects of drug therapy. If prolonged drug use is necessary and poses risk to the woman or fetus, serum levels of the drug are monitored to detect elevations that may lead to adverse effects. Dosage adjustments or discontinuation of the drug may be needed to reverse adverse effects or prevent toxicity. To reduce the risk for adverse effects, only drugs that are absolutely necessary are administered when complications of pregnancy occur. To help relieve typical discomforts of pregnancy, the nurse teaches the patient how to use nonpharmacologic strategies, such as eating dry crackers first thing in the morning to prevent nausea.

When evaluating a patient, the nurse must be careful to distinguish discomforts of pregnancy (e.g., nausea, vomiting, heartburn, light-headedness, urinary frequency, heart palpitations) from possible adverse drug effects. In addition, the pediatrician should be informed about maternal drug therapy. Knowledge of fetal exposure to drugs assists the pediatrician in making appropriate health care decisions regarding the neonate.

When questions and concerns arise regarding drug therapy and breast-feeding, similar strategies are used to prevent adverse effects. The various approaches include using nonpharmacologic remedies, determining the safest drug possible based on the amount of the drug that is transferred to breast milk and the possible neonatal effects, and assessing blood concentrations of the drug in the breast-feeding infant. Each drug administered to the lactating patient is evaluated for its potential adverse effects on the neonate, and the nurse also assesses the infant for adverse effects of the drug. Other methods used to reduce neonatal drug exposure include scheduling drug therapy just after breast-feeding or before the infant is going to sleep for a long time. Some drugs, such as antineoplastic drugs and drugs of abuse, are contraindicated during lactation, and breast-feeding is discontinued if the patient is taking any of these drugs. Agents such as general anesthetics, sedatives, and radioactive compounds required for a short-term diagnostic test should be cleared from the patient's circulation before she resumes breast-feeding. The nurse must know the drug's half-life and duration of action to be able to determine when breast-feeding can begin again. The risks to the neonate must be balanced against the advantages of the drug to the woman.

Providing Patient and Family Education

The nurse's role in counseling about pregnancy and fetal drug effects ideally begins before pregnancy. This counseling helps women make informed choices about drug therapy and helps minimize the risk for accidental exposure to teratogens in the early stages of pregnancy (from conception to day 60). Informing women of childbearing age about fetal drug effects can help them make decisions about planning pregnancy and about what to do when they become pregnant.

Patient and family education during pregnancy and breast-feeding is primarily focused on adverse effects to the fetus and infant. If the woman has used a drug before learning that she is pregnant, she will need information regarding what degree of risk the fetus has been exposed to, if any. Each pregnant patient should be given information on a drug's effects, both therapeutic and adverse, and should be permitted to make an informed decision about whether to receive the drug therapy.

The pregnant patient should also be taught how to anticipate adverse effects of drug therapy and distinguish them from normal pregnancy-related problems. The nurse instructs the patient to notify the health care provider if adverse drug

CRITICAL THINKING SCENARIO

Ensuring drug safety during lactation

Your patient, a breast-feeding mother, tells you that she frequently gets stress headaches and takes aspirin for them. She would like the aspirin to have as little effect on the baby as possible. What advice can you offer her?

effects occur. The woman who is lactating also is informed of possible adverse effects of drug therapy on the infant and is instructed to report those findings immediately to the health care provider.

Ongoing Assessment and Evaluation

Nursing management of drug therapy during pregnancy and lactation is considered effective when maternal therapeutic needs have been met without harm to the fetus or the breast-feeding infant. Other measures of effective drug therapy include successful patient- and family-oriented drug education and assessment findings indicating that the mother and child are not experiencing adverse drug effects.

CHAPTER SUMMARY

- Drug therapy may be indicated for pregnant or lactating women to manage preexisting or newly developed conditions. Although therapeutic effects may be achieved in the woman, drug therapy may adversely affect the fetus or infant.
- The physiologic changes that occur during pregnancy may alter drug absorption, distribution, and elimination.
- Some drugs are contraindicated in pregnancy, and caution is advised for using others because drugs may pass through the placenta to the fetus and cause teratogenic effects. The potential fetal risks must be compared with maternal benefits when drug therapy is required.
- The effects of most approved drugs on a developing human fetus are not known. Voluntary enrollment by pregnant women in Pregnancy Registries for different drug therapies is one new mechanism for gaining knowledge about drugs and their effects on the developing fetus.
- Drugs may be excreted into breast milk, although the total received by the infant is a small percentage of the maternal dose. The nurse should be familiar with the prescribed drugs and the substances of abuse that are contraindicated during breast-feeding.
- Symptoms of pregnancy may mask adverse effects of drug therapy in the mother. Discomforts commonly associated with pregnancy, such as nausea and vomiting, light-headedness or hypotension, constipation, heartburn, urinary frequency, heart palpitations, and fatigue, are also frequent adverse drug effects.
- Limiting drug use during pregnancy and lactation decreases maternal and fetal adverse effects. Nonpharmacologic alternatives to drug therapy should be used if possible, particularly when treating the common discomforts of pregnancy.
- Substances of abuse are contraindicated during pregnancy and lactation because they can cause serious teratogenic effects, such as fetal alcohol syndrome, or harm the breast-feeding infant.
- The minimum therapeutic dose should be used for as short a time as possible during pregnancy. If possible, drug therapy should be delayed until after the first trimester of pregnancy, during which the fetal organ systems are forming.
- Both the pregnant patient and the fetus should be monitored for therapeutic and adverse effects of drug therapy, and that practice should continue for the lactating patient and breast-feeding infant.

QUESTIONS FOR STUDY AND REVIEW

1. Which FDA pregnancy category rating includes the criterion, "The fetal risk outweighs any possible benefit," and what does that mean?
2. Explain what types of drugs are most easily transferred across the placenta to the fetus.
3. Explain why gestational weeks 3 through 8 are considered critical when drug administration is considered during pregnancy.
4. Describe the physiologic changes in the renal system that increase drug excretion rates.
5. Why are lipophilic drugs more likely to enter breast milk than nonlipophilic drugs?

? Need More Help?

Chapter 7 of the study guide for *Drug Therapy in Nursing* 2e contains NCLEX-style questions and other learning activities to reinforce your understanding of the concepts presented in this chapter. For additional information or to purchase the study guide, visit *http://connection.lww.com/go/aschenbrenner.*

REFERENCES AND BIBLIOGRAPHY

American Academy of Pediatrics. (2001). Policy statement. The transfer of drugs and other chemicals into human milk [Online.] Available: *http://www.aap.org/policy/0063.html.*

Barrett, C., & Richens, A. (2003). Epilepsy and pregnancy: Report of an epilepsy research foundation workshop. *Epilepsy Research, 52*(3), 147–187.

Daniel, K., Honein, M. A., & Moore, C. A. (2003). Sharing prescription medication among teenage girls: Potential danger to unplanned/undiagnosed pregnancies. *Pediatrics, 111*(5 Part 2), 1167–1170.

Hansen, J. W., & Smith, D. W. (1975). The fetal hydantoin syndrome. *Journal of Pediatrics, 87*(2), 285–290.

Hendrick, V., Smith, L. M., Suri, R., et al. (2003). Birth outcomes after prenatal exposure to antidepressant medication. *American Journal of Obstetrics and Gynecology, 188*(3), 812–815.

Kirchengast, S., & Hartmann, B. (2003). Nicotine consumption before and during pregnancy affects not only newborn size but also birth modus. *Journal of Biosocial Science, 35*(2), 175–188.

Lo, W. Y., & Friedman, J. M. (2002). Teratogenicity of recently introduced medications in human pregnancy. *Obstetrics and Gynecology, 100*(3), 465–473.

Palmieri, C., & Canger, R. (2002). Teratogenic potential of the newer antiepileptic drugs: what is known and how should this influence prescribing? *CNS Drugs, 16*(11), 755–764.

U.S. Food and Drug Administration, Office of Women's Health. (2004). Promoting healthy pregnancies [Online]. Available: *http://www.fda.gov/womens/registries/default.htm.*

U.S. Food and Drug Administration, Center for Drug Evaluation and Research. (2001). CDER Women's Health Subcommittee [Online]. Available: *http://www.fda.gov/cder/audiences/women/subcommittee_new.htm.*

Life Span: Older Adults

chapter 8

Learning Objectives

At the completion of this chapter the student will:

1. Identify how core drug knowledge of drug therapy in older adults may vary from core drug knowledge in younger adults.
2. Identify how normal physiologic changes with aging alter pharmacokinetics of drug therapy.
3. Define polypharmacy and its relevance in managing drug therapy in the older adult.
4. Describe why adverse effects of drug therapy may be overlooked in older adults.
5. Identify how the older adult's core patient variables in drug therapy may vary from the younger adult's core patient variables.
6. Relate the interaction of core drug knowledge to core patient variables when providing drug therapy in older adults.
7. Generate a nursing plan of care based on the interactions between core drug knowledge and core patient variables for drug therapy in older adults.
8. Describe nursing interventions to maximize therapeutic and minimize adverse effects in drug therapy in older adults.
9. Determine key points for patient and family education in drug therapy for older adults.

KEY TERMS

benefit:risk ratio

frail elderly

geriatric patient

nonadherence

older adult

paradoxical excitement

polypharmacy

FEATURED WEBLINK

http://www.guideline.gov/summary/summary.aspx?ss=15&doc_id=3513&nmbr=2739
At this site, you'll find the most current clinical guideline related to medication administration for hospitalized, older adults. The guideline emphasizes assessment and interventions to prevent adverse events.

CONNECTION WEBLINK

Additional Weblinks are found on Connection:
http://www.connection.lww.com/go/aschenbrenner.

Many physiologic changes occur with normal aging, which is accompanied by a decline in general organ and system function. In general, aging organs and body systems are less responsive than young ones to a drug's effect. Age-related changes affect the patient's response to drug therapy because both the therapeutic and the adverse effects are altered. This state creates specific risks and needs for the older adult receiving drug therapy. To manage drug therapy safely and effectively in the older adult, the nurse must be aware of these changes. The nurse also needs to be aware that many older adults take multiple prescribed and over-the-counter (OTC) drugs. Taking several drugs simultaneously is called **polypharmacy.**

The **older adult** (or **geriatric patient**) is defined as a person who is 65 years or older. This population is divided into three subgroups: the young-old (65 to 74 years), the middle-old (75 to 84 years), and the old-old (85 years and older). Of these, the old-old group is the fastest growing and most medically needy and will generate the greatest consumption of societal resources for the next half century.

Many older adults are independent and in generally good health. They may receive drug therapy for chronic conditions (many of them related to normal aging changes), but their physiologic conditions are well controlled, and they do not consider themselves "sick." Some older adults, however, are not independent and are in poor or compromised health. These are the **frail elderly,** a term that describes all individuals older than 65 years who have one or more debilitating conditions. Being frail and elderly places a person at higher risk for developing serious adverse drug effects.

This chapter presents the ways that core drug knowledge and core patient variables may be altered because of age. This chapter also presents general guidelines for maximizing therapeutic effects, minimizing adverse effects, and providing patient and family education for the older adult.

NURSING MANAGEMENT OF OLDER ADULTS

Core Drug Knowledge

Pharmacotherapeutics

The pharmacotherapeutics of drug therapy for older adults is similar to that for younger adults. Some drug therapies are more frequently used than others in older adults because their therapeutic effects offset the decreased functioning of body organs and systems that occurs with normal aging. Older adults are prone to certain disease processes or pathologic conditions, such as congestive heart failure, chronic renal disease, and hypertension; certain drug therapies used to treat these conditions are used frequently in older adult patients.

Pharmacokinetics

The processes of drug absorption, distribution, metabolism, and excretion may be affected or impaired by the normal physiologic changes of aging. Changes in the gastrointestinal (GI), cardiovascular, and circulatory systems; reduced body mass; and disturbances in liver and kidney function can alter the pharmacokinetics of drug therapy. Box 8.1 identifies these age-related physiologic changes in the older patient. These changes ultimately affect the extent and duration of systemic availability of a drug and the possibility and probability of adverse drug effects.

BOX 8.1 Pharmacokinetic Changes in Older Adults

Physiologic Changes Related to Normal Aging

Absorption
- Increased gastric pH
- Decreased absorptive surface
- Decreased blood flow
- Decreased gastrointestinal motility

Distribution
- Decreased cardiac output
- Decreased total body water
- Decreased lean body mass
- Decreased serum albumin
- Increased alpha1-acid glycoprotein
- Increased body fat

Metabolism
- Decreased hepatic mass
- Decreased hepatic blood flow

Excretion
- Decreased renal blood flow
- Decreased glomerular function
- Decreased tubular secretion

Absorption

Although absorption seems to be the least affected pharmacokinetic process during aging, several physiologic changes related to absorption affect drug therapy. In the older adult, increased gastric pH levels, decreased rate of blood flow, decreased GI motility, and reduced body surface area may influence the rate of absorption. However, the degree to which these factors affect absorption is unclear. Disease processes are more likely than age-related changes to alter an older adult's absorption patterns.

With age, the GI tract undergoes several changes that can alter oral drug absorption or affect bioavailability. For example, the stomach's response to food decreases, typified by reduced gastric acidity. Drugs that require an acidic environment to dissolve may take longer to disintegrate and be absorbed by the body; this delay may ultimately decrease systemic availability of a drug.

Circulation problems (e.g., reduced blood flow to organs) and reduced surface area of the GI tract are common in older adults. Drug absorption from the GI tract is highly dependent on both blood flow to the GI tract and the surface area of the GI tract; consequently, the extent or rate of drug absorption may be decreased in older adults. Additionally, decreased blood flow to tissues and muscles can alter the absorption of drugs administered subcutaneously or intramuscularly in older adults. Altered absorption can be further complicated by disease processes, such as peripheral vascular disease. Therefore, an intramuscular (IM) drug injection in the older adult may produce erratic blood concentrations because

of changes in tissue perfusion and reduced muscle mass (another common age-related change).

Because GI motility decreases in older adults, substances take longer to move through the GI tract. Because of the extended GI transit time, a drug is in contact with the GI membranes for a longer time; therefore, the extent of drug absorption increases. For many drugs, the effects of increased contact time with the GI membranes are balanced by the effect from the decreased surface area.

The overall effects of aging on the GI tract result in a slowed drug absorption rate yet allow for the extent of drug absorption to be almost as complete as that in younger adults. However, this slowing in the rate of absorption not only results in slower onset of action but also alters the intensity of peak response because peak serum drug concentrations are blunted by the slowed absorption. Such an effect on the rate and extent of drug absorption may or may not have immediate clinical consequences, but the patient may require an increase in drug dosage if therapeutic effects decrease substantially below desired levels.

Distribution

Several physiologic factors affect the distribution of a drug in older adults, including decreased body mass, reduced levels of plasma albumin, and a less effective blood–brain barrier. Other age-related factors that may affect drug distribution include declining cardiac output, extreme changes in body weight, poor nutrition, dehydration, inactivity, and extended bed rest.

The body mass of an individual decreases with age. In the older adult, the proportion of body fat increases as the percentage of lean muscle mass decreases. Consequently, body water decreases in proportion to the total body weight. The higher proportion of body fat to lean muscle mass and decreased body water can substantially alter the distribution patterns of most drugs, depending on whether they are fat soluble or water soluble. In older adults, a highly fat-soluble drug (e.g., diazepam [Valium]) exhibits an increased volume of distribution; this increase will result in a prolonged distribution phase, a prolonged half-life, and an increased duration of action. The increased volume of distribution for a given drug dose means that concentrations are lower in the blood but higher in the tissues. Therefore, when diazepam is given to older patients, one can anticipate a greater response to the drug and a greater likelihood of adverse effects than in a young adult.

In contrast to fat-soluble drugs, highly water-soluble drugs (e.g., gentamicin) exhibit a decreased volume of distribution because of the decrease in total body water in the older patient. Even at standard doses, more of these drugs will circulate in the blood, making toxic blood levels a potential hazard.

Plasma levels of the protein albumin, which is produced by the liver, are also reduced in the elderly, often by as much as 13%. The reduced plasma albumin level reflects declining metabolic activity in the liver. Plasma albumin is responsible for binding, transporting, and distributing many drugs throughout the body, particularly acid-based drugs. In contrast, amounts of plasma alpha-1 acid glycoproteins, which principally bind and transport alkaline-based drugs, are not depressed in older adults. Hence, the acid or alkaline base of drugs can cause significant alterations in the older patient's response to drugs. In addition, when plasma albumin levels decline in the older adult, fewer binding sites are available for drugs. This scarcity of binding sites results in higher concentrations of unbound forms of a drug, which increases target organ exposure, pharmacologic activity, and the risk for adverse effects. Although higher concentrations of free drug also increase the amount of the drug available for metabolism and renal excretion, normal age-related decreases in liver and kidney function offset any increase in these pharmacokinetic processes. Overall, low plasma protein levels place older adults at increased risk for adverse effects from drug therapy. This risk is especially high when the drug is normally highly protein bound. An example would be the anticonvulsant phenytoin (Dilantin), a highly protein-bound drug. Polypharmacy further complicates the effects of decreased albumin levels in older adults. Recall that highly protein-bound drugs compete for protein-binding sites even in younger patients. When fewer sites are available to start with, and several drugs must compete for fewer sites, the drugs may be unable to locate a protein-binding site. Ultimately, the effects of drug therapy will increase because more free or unbound drug is available to be active.

Age-related changes in the central nervous system (CNS) can alter drug distribution. Normally, the blood–brain barrier prevents drugs from affecting the brain, but with advancing age, the efficiency of the blood–brain barrier declines. This decline permits higher levels of drug than normal to penetrate the brain.

Metabolism

The liver's efficiency at metabolizing substances gradually declines throughout the aging process. In the older adult, three major physiologic changes greatly affect the efficiency of the liver. First, the size of the liver changes, and the number of metabolically active hepatocytes may decrease as much as 50%. Most change occurs when adults are in their 60s or 70s. Second, because cardiac output declines with age, blood flow to the liver declines as well. With less blood-borne oxygen available, the liver's capacity to remove many metabolic by-products is reduced. Third, the overall ability of the liver to metabolize drugs and other chemicals is reduced.

Normal hepatic metabolism of substances occurs in two major phases. Phase I metabolic reactions include oxidation, reduction, and hydrolysis of drug molecules. During phase I, the liver creates metabolites that may retain some degree of pharmacologic activity. Phase II reactions combine the drug or other metabolites produced in phase I with highly water-soluble forms of acetate, glucuronic acid, sulfate, or an amino acid. These reactions produce an inactive metabolized form of the drug that is excreted in the urine or feces. Ultimately, most phase I and II reactions make drugs more water soluble, which restricts their access to the tissues, promotes removal from the body, and thereby terminates pharmacologic activity.

Aging affects the efficiency of both phases of metabolic activity but tends to alter phase I more than it alters phase II reactions. Because drug metabolism is slowed by reduced oxidation in phase I, drug blood levels are higher and drug half-lives are extended in older adults. This effect usually alters the appropriate dose and dosing interval and the duration of adverse effects. For example, when elderly adults receive a benzodiazepine (e.g., to relieve anxiety or promote

sleep), they may experience associated cognitive impairments, such as sedation, confusion, and decreased mental alertness, for a longer time than normal after drug therapy ceases. Often, standard half-life parameters are inaccurate for the elderly patient. Nurses obtain age-related drug half-life information to evaluate drug responses accurately in older patients. Nurses who are unfamiliar with age-related differences may mistakenly interpret an older patient's altered cognitive function as a normal sign of aging rather than as a residual drug effect.

Excretion

Efficient renal function is a crucial factor in ensuring drug clearance from the blood and excretion from the body, and in terminating drug action. Aging can substantially decrease renal efficiency by altering the two main processes by which the kidneys remove drugs from the blood: glomerular filtration and renal tubular secretion. Both of these processes decline in efficiency with age and ultimately result in slower drug excretion and altered drug half-life.

One of the standard markers for renal function is the serum creatinine concentration, which reflects creatinine clearance from the blood by way of glomerular filtration. Despite the decline in the efficiency of glomerular filtration in the older patient, serum creatinine levels often remain in the normal range (Table 8.1). The normal range is maintained because creatinine production declines in the older patient as muscle mass decreases; therefore, less creatinine overall exists in the older adult to be filtered. These so-called normal creatinine levels can be misleading and should not be interpreted as an indication of normal renal function in elderly patients.

Pharmacodynamics

Decreased organ efficiency in the older adult alters pharmacodynamic responses. Because absorption is prolonged in the older adult, response to single doses of drugs is commonly delayed substantially. For example, the older adult taking aspirin for intermittent joint pain usually experiences a longer onset of action than normal. This delayed onset is not experienced for drugs that the older adult takes on a regular basis because doses taken at regular intervals maintain steady blood levels.

Most drug responses are based on the drug–receptor interaction. A patient's response to a particular drug depends on how efficiently that drug's receptor system operates or on the number of available receptors for that drug. An example of this interrelationship is the elderly patient and the beta-adrenergic receptor system. As a result of aging, the beta-adrenergic receptor system seems to operate less efficiently and possibly with fewer receptors. This decline in efficiency explains why the older adult is typically less responsive to beta-adrenergic agonists (stimulants), such as isoproterenol (Isuprel). Age-related changes affect the parasympathetic muscarinic-receptor system as well. Generally, the older adult has an increased response to anticholinergic drugs, such as atropine, and to the anticholinergic effects of drugs such as the tricyclic antidepressants.

Decreases in the number of receptors are also associated with decreases in the respective neurotransmitters themselves. Older patients, for example, have decreased amounts of the neurotransmitters dopamine and acetylcholine.

Contraindications and Precautions

Drug contraindications are generally similar for older adults and younger adults. Some diseases or conditions that may contraindicate certain drug therapies are more likely to occur in older adults. Moreover, because of the older adult's decreased renal function and possibly metabolic function, many drugs should be used with caution. Some drugs or drug classes cause substantially more adverse effects in older adults than in other age populations. These drugs are generally considered inappropriate for older adults; however, with proper clinical management, monitoring, and dose limitations, these drugs may be used. Use of inappropriate drugs may be a substantial problem in the current health care system. The nurse needs to work closely with physicians, nurse practitioners, and pharmacists to minimize the use of drugs that are generally contraindicated in older adults, by seeking safer alternative drug therapy. Simultaneously, the nurse must realize that there will be occasions when an "inappropriate" drug will be used because it is the best therapy to treat the older adult. During these occasions, the nurse will need to work closely with the rest of the health care team, providing clinical care to minimize potential adverse outcomes to the patient.

Adverse Effects

Although the same adverse effects from any given drug therapy will occur in older adults as in other age groups, physiologic changes in older adults place them at greater risk for certain adverse effects. Adverse drug effects are an important cause of hospital admissions in older adults (Wu & Pantaleo, 2003). Adverse drug effects are also a serious concern for older adults who receive medication in ambulatory care settings. Research has found that the more serious adverse effects are frequently preventable (Box 8.2) (Gurwitz et al., 2003).

Because of the less effective blood–brain barrier, older adults may be more vulnerable to CNS side effects, such as increased depressant or sedative activity of drugs. In addition, decreased dopamine concentrations in the brain of older adults render them more susceptible to parkinsonian effects

TABLE 8.1 Age-Related Differences in Creatinine in Men

Age (Yr)	Creatinine Clearance Levels*	Serum Creatinine
17–24	140	0.808
25–34	140	0.808
35–44	133	0.813
45–54	127	0.829
55–64	119	0.837
65–74	109	0.825
75–84	96	0.843

*Ccl_{cr} = (140 – age) (weight)/(72) (serum creatinine)

NOTE: Women also demonstrate a similar decline in Ccl_{cr} with age. Ccl_{cr} for women is about 85% of values in men.

FOCUS ON RESEARCH

Box 8.2 Can Adverse Drug Effects Be Prevented?

Gurwitz, J. H., Field, T. S., Harrold, L. R., et al. (2003). Incidence and preventability of adverse drug events among older persons in the ambulatory setting. *Journal of the American Medical Association, 289*(9), 1107–1116.

The Study

All Medicare enrollees cared for by a multispecialty group practice in an ambulatory setting were assessed over a 1-year period to determine whether they had incurred adverse drug effects. The medical records and all relevant institutional records of the patients were reviewed. The overall rate of adverse drug events was found to be 50.1 per 1,000 person-years; more than one fourth of events were identified as preventable. The adverse drug effects that were considered to be serious, life-threatening, or fatal composed 38% of the total adverse effects. The more serious adverse effects were more likely to be preventable than the less serious adverse effects. Preventable adverse effects were associated with errors in prescribing and monitoring as well as older patient errors in self-administration of medications. The drug classes most frequently associated with preventable adverse drug effects were cardiovascular agents, diuretics, nonopioid analgesics, hypoglycemics, and anticoagulants.

Nursing Implications

Adverse effects from drug therapy cause substantial morbidity and mortality in older adults. Although many adverse effects cannot be prevented, nurses should be vigilant to help protect patients from those that are preventable. Nurses should question any medication order in which the wrong drug or dose appears to have been ordered for the patient. Nurses also need to recognize the importance of patient education concerning proper administration of prescribed drug therapy. Multiple teaching sessions and the use of various teaching techniques, including written information, role play, and return demonstration, should be used when providing the older adult with drug information. Special attention should be given when the patient is prescribed one of the drug classes highly associated with preventable adverse effects.

of dopamine antagonists, such as the phenothiazine antipsychotics and metoclopramide (see Chapter 18 for details). Some research has shown that hospitalized older adults who currently have depression are more at risk than others for developing adverse drug effects. The exact cause is unknown, and further research is warranted (Onder et al., 2003).

Older adults are also more responsive to anticholinergic drugs and drugs with anticholinergic adverse effects (see Chapter 14).

Depending on the severity of these adverse responses, drug dosages may be limited or contraindicated for a particular patient.

Drug-induced behavioral changes often affect the older adult. Sometimes, they occur unexpectedly. For example, when beginning drug therapy with a sedative or a benzodiazepine to treat anxiety, the older patient may experience an effect that is the opposite of the intended effect. This effect is known as **paradoxical excitement,** whereby the patient is wide awake and hyperactive rather than calm and relaxed.

Determining whether an older patient is experiencing an adverse effect or a normal age-related health problem is difficult. Age-related health problems often mimic the adverse effects of drug therapy. For example, hearing loss can be a sign of aging, or it can be a serious adverse effect of some antimicrobial drugs (e.g., gentamicin). Loss of balance and unsteadiness while walking are often experienced by older patients and may be confused with the adverse effects of some drugs that cause dizziness or light-headedness. Clearly, the nurse needs to distinguish between these two conditions.

Drug Interactions

Drug interactions are the same for older adults as for other populations, but because older adults tend to take more drugs, they are at higher risk for interactions. It is not uncommon for older adults to be taking between 8 and 12 prescribed and OTC drugs to treat a variety of diseases. Often, the combination of so many different drugs causes serious drug interactions. For example, a patient who is taking a total of 10 different prescriptions and OTC drugs risks 45 different two-drug combinations that could interact to produce an adverse effect. Research has shown that drug interactions can decrease the effectiveness of one or both of the drugs or increase the risk for adverse effects. Drug interactions are common in older adults (Bjorkman et al., 2002).

Assessment of Relevant Core Patient Variables Related to Older Adults

Health Status

Aging is associated with a decline in normal bodily maintenance and function. The major organ systems (cardiovascular, respiratory, GI, genitourinary, endocrine, and others) all become much less efficient with advancing age and cause a multitude of health problems that often require drug therapy. When assessing the older patient's health status, the nurse assesses for polypharmacy, which has the potential for causing serious drug interactions and adverse effects. The compromised health status of the older adult can further alter the pharmacokinetics of certain drugs and is of equal concern. In such cases, the nurse assesses the functional ability of the older adult's body systems and determines whether the patient has any diseases that may affect prescribed drug therapy. Particular attention is given to cardiovascular, renal, and circulatory problems because these problems can greatly alter the patient's responses to drug therapy.

When assessing the older patient's renal function status, nurses must remember that normal laboratory value ranges may be deceptive. As discussed, the older patient with compromised renal function may have serum creatinine levels or

CRITICAL THINKING SCENARIO

Thinking about age-related core patient variables

Antonio Mendez, a 70-year-old man with insulin-dependent diabetes, has been admitted to your unit for the second time in a month with diabetic ketoacidosis. His blood glucose level on admission is elevated at 600 mg/dL. The prescriber writes an order for 15 U of NPH insulin mixed with 5 U of regular insulin every morning. As the patient's nurse, you are assessing why this patient continues to have elevated blood glucose levels. What relevant core patient variables should you investigate with this patient?

blood urea nitrogen (BUN) levels in the normal range. Hence, normal serum creatinine or BUN levels are not a true indicator of the older patient's renal status.

Assessment should always include a thorough inventory of all the drugs the patient is currently taking, dosage, and dosing schedule. This inventory will help alert the nurse to any possible drug interactions. If possible, the nurse confirms this information with the patient's medical record or primary care provider. A recent study of older adults seen in an emergency department showed that less than half of them could correctly identify all of their prescription medications. About one third of them could name the correct dosage for each medication. They were better able to name the correct interval for taking their medications (more than half could do so correctly) and to state all of the correct indications for their drug therapy (two thirds of them were able to do so) (Chung & Bartfield, 2002). Gaps in the knowledge of older adult patients indicate that teaching about drug therapy is needed.

The nurse also assesses whether the older adult patient is taking the medication as prescribed. Research indicates that when a medication regimen is followed at home, older adults may take the medication more often than indicated or less often than indicated. Low adherence with therapy was associated with a high number of daily prescribed medications and impaired cognitive ability among older patients (Gray et al., 2001). Information from the assessment also indicates what information the nurse needs to emphasize in patient education.

The older adult patient must be asked about all OTC drugs because many patients do not consider these medicines "drugs" and may not mention them unless specifically asked. For example, many older adults take laxatives to relieve constipation, a common problem associated with age-related slowing of GI motility. Most older patients are unaware that laxatives can interact with and complicate prescribed drug therapy by decreasing absorption of some drugs. Unless the nurse specifically asks about laxative use, the patient may not volunteer the information. The nurse also assesses the ability of the older adult to open drug bottles and read drug labels if he or she will be self-administering drugs at home.

Lifestyle, Diet, and Habits

Because lifestyle, diet, and habits of the older adult affect the pharmacokinetics and pharmacodynamics of drug therapy, the nurse assesses several basic areas of daily living, such as how active the patient is and what his or her daily routine includes. Moderate, regular exercise promotes circulation, absorption of drugs given intramuscularly or subcutaneously, and distribution of drugs through the GI tract.

Dietary patterns and habits are also important. If older adults have difficulty swallowing solid food and eat only soft or chopped foods, they may need to have oral drugs (such as pills or tablets) crushed and mixed with a diluent for swallowing or have the drugs prescribed in a liquid form.

The use of alternative medications, such as herbs and botanicals, has increased with older adults as it has with the general population. Because older adults tend to take more prescribed medications than other age groups, they are at higher risk for drug interactions if they take alternative medications. The nurse asks the older patient if he or she takes any alternative medications and then documents the findings. Documentation is important to help all health care providers identify any potential drug–herb interactions. One study showed that although 64% of the older adult patients queried used alternative medications, only one third of these complementary therapies were documented in the patient record (Cohen et al., 2002).

Another important assessment is how drug therapy and the related adverse effects have altered the older adult's lifestyle or impaired the quality of life. How have the activities of daily living been impaired? How have adverse effects interfered with the patient's involvement in community or family events? Some drugs place the older adult at risk for injury and therefore can greatly limit the quality of life. For example, drugs that cause dizziness or light-headedness when standing put the older patient at great risk for falls and broken bones. Drugs that cause postural hypotension, such as many antihypertensives, have been associated with falls and hip fractures.

The mental status of older patients is extremely important to their quality of life. Many older patients are depressed because they are lonely or have limited ability to function and participate in life's enjoyments. Sometimes, drug therapy can further decrease the older patient's quality of life because of adverse drug effects. Depression, delirium, dementia, and low self-esteem are commonly cited adverse effects of drug therapy.

Habits regarding drug therapy should be considered when planning drug administration in the hospital. The nurse assesses whether the older adult patient has a preferred schedule for taking drug therapy at home because it may be more therapeutic to maintain the patient's established routine and dosage schedule than to readjust them to fit hospital routines. Maintaining the same drug schedule not only promotes similar drug actions and reactions but also helps reduce stress and anxiety in older patients who may have difficulty adjusting to changes in routine.

Because older adults typically have fixed incomes, the nurse questions patients to determine whether their health insurance includes payment or partial payment for drug therapy. Coverage may influence whether the older patient can afford the prescribed drug therapy. As mentioned, many older patients take several drugs for various health problems, and drug therapy may be extremely costly.

Environment

Assessing the older patient's environment is another important element when considering drug therapy. The nurse needs to determine whether the patient lives alone or with other family members or caregivers who can help obtain and administer drug therapy if needed. Other considerations are as follows:

- Is the pharmacy accessible to the older adult?
- Can the patient drive or take a bus to the pharmacy, or is someone available to go for him or her?
- Does the pharmacy make deliveries?

If ready access is not available, the nurse may need to make referrals to other sources for drug therapy, such as mail-order pharmacies.

Culture and Inherited Traits

Whenever assessing older adults, the nurse must be sensitive to beliefs and cultural values that may have an effect on drug therapy. Some ethnic or cultural groups still practice folk medicine, preferring home remedies or herbal treatments to traditional drug therapy. These patients may be skeptical or afraid of new or unfamiliar methods of drug therapy. Moreover, they may not understand the drug regimen. Among cultural groups that may practice folk medicine are Eastern Europeans, Hispanic Americans, Native Americans, Asians, some African Americans, and some patients from remote or rural areas of the United States, such as Appalachia, the Ozark Mountains, or Alaska.

Nursing Diagnoses and Outcomes

Nursing diagnoses specific to drug therapy in older adults are similar to those for patients in other age groups. However, because of age-related health problems of older patients, decreased organ functioning, and polypharmacy, some diagnoses more commonly apply. They include the following:

- Risk for Injury related to adverse effects of drug therapy stemming from polypharmacy and drug interactions secondary to increased therapeutic effect, delayed elimination, and prolonged drug half-life
  Desired outcome: *The older adult patient will not sustain an injury while on drug therapy.*
- Ineffective Therapeutic Regimen Management because of impaired memory
  Desired outcome: *The patient will effectively manage the therapeutic regimen with the help of memory aids.*

Planning and Intervention

Maximizing Therapeutic Effects

For any drug therapy to be therapeutic, the appropriate dose must be taken at the appropriate times. The more complicated the overall therapeutic regimen, the greater the likelihood of poor adherence to the drug therapy. **Nonadherence** does not always mean that the patient directly refuses to follow the recommended drug therapy schedule. It may indicate that the patient cannot adhere to the prescribed drug course for various reasons. Older adults who have multiple drug therapies are at increased risk for nonadherence. They may have difficulty remembering to take all of their different drugs, or they may have difficulty remembering which drug to take for which health problem and when. The expense of multiple drug therapies may also cause the older adult to be nonadherent to the treatment plan. The nurse needs to determine the true cause of nonadherence in order to make an appropriate plan of care.

Nurses and prescribers can improve adherence by making drug regimens as easy to follow and as uncomplicated as possible. For example, some drugs are available in sustained-release forms that can be taken once or twice a day, rather than four or more times a day. Some combination drug forms are available that incorporate two drugs, allowing the patient to take only one preparation instead of two. The health care provider should be consulted for appropriate orders if such options are available for the patient's specific drug therapy.

When new drug therapy begins, a new drug schedule should be planned to coincide with other prescribed schedules whenever possible. If the patient already takes a drug three times a day with meals, and the new drug must be taken once a day, the patient should take the new drug with breakfast when other drugs are taken. In this way, the patient need not remember another time to take a drug. This kind of planning promotes therapeutic adherence.

After simplifying drug therapy as much as possible, the nurse verifies that the patient can remember to take the drug. If the patient is having trouble remembering which drug should be taken at which time, the nurse assists the older adult by creating memory aids. Pill boxes are available with compartments labeled by the hours of the day or by meal times (B, L, D), as are pill boxes labeled with days of the week. The patient places each drug in its appropriate slot at the beginning of the day and can then easily check whether each dose was taken on schedule. An inexpensive adaptation of the commercial pill box is an egg carton with hand-labeled hours of the day on each egg compartment.

When recommending types of drug preparations for each patient, the nurse considers which form can be self-administered easily. A chewable tablet or a liquid may be easier to take if the patient has difficulty swallowing pills. If a choice of dosage forms is possible, the prescriber can be consulted about selecting the form that is most easily used. To improve the ability to self-administer drug therapy correctly, the patient is advised of options that can be requested from the dispensing pharmacy. For example, containers with easy-to-remove, nonchildproof caps and large-print labels promote therapeutic adherence for patients with arthritis or vision impairments. The nurse also verifies whether the patient can obtain prescriptions and refills from the pharmacy independently or with assistance.

Older adults must be monitored diligently for initial and continuing therapeutic drug effects. To detect improvements or deterioration in the patient's condition, the nurse performs periodic comparative assessments of current and previous status and identifies changes in therapeutic effectiveness that may necessitate a dosage adjustment.

Minimizing Adverse Effects

Whenever possible, alternatives to drug therapy should be considered as the initial treatment for problems. For example, if the older adult complains of difficulty sleeping, encouraging some mild exercise during the day (e.g., walking) or suggesting minor dietary changes (e.g., avoiding large meals near bedtime) may be enough to promote sleep. Sedatives and other drug therapy should only be used if absolutely necessary. Reducing the number of prescribed medications decreases the risk for adverse drug effects and drug interactions (Schafer, 2001).

Drugs should be used with great caution in older adults because these patients exhibit a narrow **benefit:risk ratio** compared with younger adults. A benefit:risk ratio is the margin between desired therapeutic effects and adverse consequences of drug therapy. Obviously, the beneficial therapeutic outcomes must be considered in relation to the associated physical risk factors.

Because the renal and metabolic systems of most older adults do not function as efficiently as those of younger patients in metabolizing and eliminating drugs from the body,

older adults are at increased risk for drug overdose or toxicity. Because of diminished renal function in older patients, the nurse closely monitors for signs and symptoms of possible drug toxicity when the patient is taking drugs (e.g., digoxin) that do not undergo significant metabolism. When potentially nephrotoxic drugs (e.g., gentamicin, certain cephalosporin antibiotics, and nonsteroidal anti-inflammatory drugs) are used, the nurse is particularly careful because the older adult patient is particularly prone to rapid onset of action and severe nephrotoxicity. Serum blood levels are monitored to detect whether toxic drug levels are developing.

Additionally, the nurse distinguishes carefully between the normal signs and symptoms of aging and the onset of adverse effects from drug therapy. Some adverse effects—impaired cognition, memory, or alterations in mood—mimic signs of aging. For example, the patient who falls repeatedly may be experiencing drug-induced light-headedness or drowsiness from benzodiazepines. Those with difficulty communicating may be experiencing aphasia as a result of antipsychotic drug therapy. The nurse consults with the pharmacist for assistance in determining whether behaviors or symptoms exhibited by the older adult stem from adverse drug reactions or drug interactions.

Many older patients demonstrate atypical adverse effects that mimic signs of aging and paradoxical effects. If drug-induced symptoms are misinterpreted by the nurse, proper interventions may be neglected, and the older adult may unnecessarily suffer long-term effects. Unless the nurse knows the patient's history, health status, and potential adverse effects of the drugs the patient is taking, he or she will not be able to distinguish between drug-induced symptoms or excessive therapeutic effect and age-related problems.

The nurse obtains a current drug profile and an accurate history of the patient's usual abilities and changes in abilities or health status. By establishing this baseline information, the nurse is alert to any new signs and symptoms in the patient that could be drug related. Older adults are asked if they believe they are having adverse effects from drug therapy because they are frequently correct in recognizing such effects. If the older adult patient has any communication impairments, the nurse talks with family members or others who know the older adult patient well to determine the patient's baseline behaviors.

The nurse also becomes familiar with the core drug knowledge regarding possible adverse effects and drug interactions of the patient's specific drug therapy. The older patient is monitored carefully for development of adverse effects caused by physiologic changes or polypharmacy. If the older adult shows any signs of adverse effects, the nurse seeks appropriate changes in the drug therapy. Box 8.3 discusses the identification and management of polypharmacy problems.

The nurse helps devise a drug schedule that will minimize the risks of adverse effects. For example, if the patient is to take a drug that causes sedation, the dose may be given at bedtime, if possible, to avoid daytime drowsiness and to lessen the risk of falling. In general, the prescriber may start the older adult's therapy with a low dose and increase the dose gradually as needed to reach a therapeutic level. Once the desired therapeutic effects occur, the dosage can be stabilized at that level. Using the minimal therapeutic dosage minimizes the risk for adverse effects.

COMMUNITY-BASED CONCERNS

Box 8.3 Identification and Management of Polypharmacy Problems

- Question the patient about any and all drug therapy that he or she is taking or has taken in the past. Remember to ask about any non-prescribed, over-the-counter (OTC) preparations.
- Ask to see the drug bottles to verify the physician's or nurse practitioner's orders and evaluate the patient's knowledge about the drugs. Frequently, patients will pull out plastic bags or boxes full of drugs.
- Read the labels carefully. Attempt to identify drugs unknown to the patient or unclear prescriptions. If the prescriptions have changed frequently, or the patient has a long history of chronic health problems, the drug labels may be worn, faded, or difficult to read.
- Determine which drug prescriptions and OTC preparations are for current use. Some patients keep drugs for problems they no longer have.
- Determine whether therapy can be simplified. Consult with the physician or nurse practitioner as indicated.
- Assist the patient in creating a time schedule to take all prescribed drugs appropriately but in accordance with the patient's lifestyle. Use memory aids as needed.

Providing Patient and Family Education

The nurse can educate patients about drug therapy in various ways. Written instructions regarding drug use and times of administration may be developed and emphasized to help prevent confusion. This education is especially important when patients are receiving several drugs.

Patients and families are also taught about expected or possible adverse effects and how to differentiate between them and normal signs of aging. Also, patients need to understand which adverse effects should be reported immediately to the health care provider or nurse practitioner. Patients and families can be taught methods to assist with accurate dosage and administration of drugs.

Ongoing Assessment and Evaluation

Because the physiologic changes associated with aging often greatly alter the pharmacologic properties of drug therapy, the nurse assesses the older patient continually for therapeutic and adverse effects of drug therapy. In many situations, the nurse also assesses the home environment and family support to determine the older patient's ability to adhere to drug therapy. Consistent and regular monitoring of the older patient is extremely important because of polypharmacy, which is common in older patients and puts them at high risk for drug interactions, decreased therapeutic effects, and nonadherence. Drug therapy is effective in the older adult when therapeutic effects are achieved without serious adverse effects that diminish quality of life.

CHAPTER SUMMARY

- Older adults share common age-related changes and risk factors that alter drug administration, dosage, and expected response to drug therapy.
- Aging alters all of the pharmacokinetic processes, placing older adults at increased risk for adverse drug effects.

- Serum creatinine levels often remain in the normal range despite impaired kidney function.
- Pharmacodynamics of drug therapy may be decreased in older adults because of changes in the receptor systems. Older adults also have decreased amounts of the neurotransmitters dopamine and acetylcholine.
- Some drugs or drug classes produce more adverse effects in the older adult, partly related to decreased organ functioning. Dose modifications and close clinical monitoring are necessary if these drugs must be used in older adults.
- Many signs and symptoms of health problems in older adults result from the normal aging-related decline in organ or system function. These symptoms often mimic the adverse effects of drug therapy. The nurse must be careful to distinguish between the normal signs and symptoms of aging and the onset of adverse effects from drug therapy.
- Polypharmacy is an important concern in older adults because it greatly increases the risk for drug interactions and adverse effects.
- Lifestyles of older adults may affect the pharmacokinetics of drug therapy. Nurses need to assess patients' circumstances and cultural preferences or barriers to determine whether patients have the means and ability to obtain and comply with prescribed treatments, dietary recommendations, daily routine, and activity levels that can affect drug therapy.
- Nurses can promote older patients' adherence to prescribed drug therapy by minimizing the use of drug therapy when possible, simplifying the therapeutic regimen as much as possible, titrating doses upward gradually as prescribed to minimize adverse effects, helping with drug administration scheduling, assisting with memory aids if needed, and providing teaching and instructions in writing.

▲ QUESTIONS FOR STUDY AND REVIEW

1. Describe the effects of aging on the liver and its functioning.
2. How do normal changes in the renal system place the older adult at risk for adverse effects from drug therapy?
3. What is polypharmacy? Why is it an important issue for the nurse to consider in older adult patients?
4. Why are adverse drug effects often overlooked in older adults?
5. Why is it important to consider the core patient variables of lifestyle, diet, and habits with older adults receiving drug therapy?

? Need More Help?

Chapter 8 of the study guide for *Drug Therapy in Nursing* 2e contains NCLEX-style questions and other learning activities to reinforce your understanding of the concepts presented in this chapter. For additional information or to purchase the study guide, visit *http://connection.lww.com/go/aschenbrenner.*

■ REFERENCES AND BIBLIOGRAPHY

Bjorkman, I. K., Fastbom, J., Schmidt, I. K., et al., for the Pharmaceutical Care of the Elderly in Europe Research (PEER) Group. (2002). Drug-drug interactions in the elderly. *Annals of Pharmacotherapy, 36*(11), 1675–1681.

Chung, M. K., & Bartfield, J. M. (2002). Knowledge of prescription medications among elderly emergency department patients. *Annals of Emergency Medicine, 39*(6), 605–608.

Cohen, R. J., Ek, K., & Pan, C. X. (2002). Complementary and alternative medicine (CAM) use by older adults: A comparison of self-report and physician chart documentation. *Journal of Gerontology. Series A, Biological Sciences and Medical Sciences, 574,* M223–227.

Gray, S. L., Mahoney, J. E., & Blough, D. K. (2001). Medication adherence in elderly patients receiving home health services following hospital discharge. *Annals of Pharmacotherapeutics, 35*(5), 539–545.

Gurwitz, J. H., Field, T. S., Harrold, L. R., et al. (2003). Incidence and preventability of adverse drug events among older persons in the ambulatory setting. *Journal of the American Medical Association, 289*(9), 1107–1116.

Onder, G., Penninx, B. W., Landi, F., et al., the Investigators of the Gruppo Italiano di Farmacoepidemiologia nell'Anziano Study. (2003). Depression and adverse drug reactions among hospitalized older adults. *Archives of Internal Medicine, 163*(3), 301–305.

Schafer, S. L. (2001). Prescribing for seniors: It's a balancing act. *Journal of the American Academy of Nurse Practitioners, 13*(3), 108–112.

Wu, W. K., & Pantaleo, N. (2003). Evaluation of outpatient adverse drug reactions leading to hospitalization. *American Journal of Health-System Pharmacy, 60*(3), 253–259.

Lifestyle: Substance Abuse

chapter 9

Learning Objectives

At the completion of this chapter the student will:

1 Describe the scope of substance abuse in the United States.
2 Identify etiologic factors associated with substance abuse.
3 Identify frequently abused drugs and list common medical problems associated with abuse of these drugs.
4 Describe the pharmacologic basis for physical and psychological drug dependence, tolerance, and addiction.
5 Explain the adverse effects associated with chronic abuse of alcohol, cocaine, marijuana, and opioids.
6 Discuss the nursing management of patients who abuse substances, including alcohol, cocaine, marijuana, hallucinogenics, and opioids.

KEY TERMS

abstinence syndrome
addiction
cross-dependence
cross-tolerance
habituation
physical dependence
psychedelic
psychoactive
psychological dependence
substance abuse
tolerance
withdrawal syndrome

FEATURED WEBLINK

http://www.drugabusestatistics.samhsa.gov/
Drug abuse is an enormous problem in the United States. For current statistical information log on to this site.

CONNECTION WEBLINK

Additional Weblinks are found on Connection:
http://www.connection.lww.com/go/aschenbrenner.

Lifestyle, diet, and habits is a core patient variable that exerts one of the most important effects on a patient's response to drug therapy. The use of substances such as alcohol, tobacco products, and illicit or "street" drugs can seriously complicate drug therapy as well as the patient's general condition. Box 9.1 summarizes highlights from a national survey concerning the use of alcohol, tobacco, and illicit drugs in the United States.

Substance abuse is the inappropriate and usually excessive self-administration of a drug substance for nonmedical purposes. Drugs with a high abuse potential have the ability to stimulate compulsive drug-seeking behavior. Contemporary substance abuse has pervasive economic, legal, medical, moral, psychological, religious, and social implications. Substance abuse occurs throughout the life span and cuts across all racial, socioeconomic, ethnic, and cultural groups. Furthermore, factors in the patient's environment, family, or community can influence susceptibility to substance abuse and lead to drug addiction.

Drug **addiction** is a complex process involving interactions among the drug (availability, cost, pharmacology, toxicology); the user (personal resources, psychiatric profile, temperament); and society (family and peer influences, positive and negative advertising, and social attitudes). Broadly speaking, drug addiction alters the patient's life in a harmful way; for example, drug-related activity may result in a jail sentence.

Substance use and abuse interact with drug therapy in several ways:

- Drug therapy may become drug abuse.
- Chronic abuse may create health problems that require treatment with drug therapy.
- Treating or preventing symptoms of withdrawal from a substance may require drug therapy.
- Concurrent use of a substance may interact with drug therapy prescribed for a physiologic problem.

This chapter discusses various factors involved in substance abuse, several commonly abused drug categories and how they affect the body, and nursing management of substance-abusing patients.

CAUSES OF SUBSTANCE ABUSE

Dopamine Hypothesis

Scientists are becoming increasingly convinced that a link exists between the neurotransmitter dopamine and drugs of abuse and that dopamine plays a key role in a wide range of addictions. Dopamine is associated with feelings of pleasure and elation. Dopamine levels can be elevated by a hug or kiss, a word of praise, a winning poker hand, or the effects of a drug. Cocaine use stimulates a surge of dopamine in an

COMMUNITY-BASED CONCERNS

Box 9.1 How Many Substance Abusers?

Substance Abuse and Mental Health Services Administration (SAMHSA) National Survey on Drug Use & Health [formerly called the National Household Survey on Drug Abuse (NHSDA)] is the primary source of information on the prevalence, patterns, and consequences of alcohol, tobacco, and illegal drug use and abuse in the general U.S. civilian non-institutionalized population, aged 12 years and older. The following information is highlighted in the 2002 report:

- In 2002, an estimated 19.5 million Americans, or 8.3% of the population aged 12 years or older, were current illicit drug users. Current drug use means use of an illicit drug during the month preceding the survey interview.
- In 2002, an estimated 2.0 million persons (0.9%) were current cocaine users, 567,000 of whom used crack. Hallucinogens were used by 1.2 million persons, including 676,000 users of Ecstasy. There were an estimated 166,000 current heroin users.
- Among youths aged 12 to 17 years, 11.6% were current illicit drug users. The rate of use was highest among young adults (18 to 25 years) at 20.2%. Among adults aged 26 years or older, 5.8% reported current illicit drug use.
- Among pregnant women aged 15 to 44 years, 3.3% reported using illicit drugs in the month before their interview. This rate was significantly lower than the rate among women aged 15 to 44 who were not pregnant (10.3%).
- In 2002, an estimated 11.0 million persons reported driving under the influence of an illicit drug during the past year. This number represents 4.7% of the population aged 12 or older. The rate was 10% or greater for each age from 17 to 25 years, with 21-year-olds reporting the highest rate of any age (18.0%). Among adults aged 26 years or older, the rate was 3.0%.
- An estimated 120 million Americans aged 12 years or older reported being current drinkers of alcohol in the 2002 survey (51.0%). About 54 million (22.9%) participated in binge drinking at least once in the 30 days preceding the survey, and 15.9 million (6.7%) were heavy drinkers.
- An estimated 71.5 million Americans (30.4% of the population aged 12 years or older) reported current use (past month use) of a tobacco product in 2002. About 61.1 million (26.0%) smoked cigarettes, 12.8 million (5.4%) smoked cigars, 7.8 million (3.3%) used smokeless tobacco, and 1.8 million (0.8%) smoked tobacco in pipes.
- The percentage of youths aged 12 to 17 years who had ever used marijuana declined slightly from 2001 to 2002 (21.9% to 20.6%). Among young adults aged 18 to 25 years, the rate increased slightly from 53.0% in 2001 to 53.8% in 2002.
- The percentage of youths aged 12 to 17 years who had ever used cocaine increased slightly from 2001 to 2002 (2.3% to 2.7%). Among young adults aged 18 to 25 years, the rate increased slightly from 14.9% in 2001 to 15.4% in 2002.
- The rate of lifetime daily cigarette use among youths aged 12 to 17 years declined from 10.6% in 2001 to 8.2% in 2002. There also was a small decline in lifetime prevalence among young adults (37.7% to 37.1%) from 2001 to 2002.

addict's brain, which essentially triggers the cocaine high. Research studies have demonstrated that in dopamine-rich areas of the brain, nicotine behaves in a manner remarkably similar to that of cocaine. Brain imaging technology can track increases in dopamine and link them to feelings of euphoria. This dopamine hypothesis—although controversial and incomplete—gives rise to the recognition that there may be a clear biologic basis for drug dependence; addiction may be a disorder of the brain no different from other forms of mental illness.

The major drugs of abuse mimic the structures of neurotransmitters. Neurotransmitters serve as a basis for every thought and emotion, for memory, and for learning; they carry the signals between all the neurons in the brain. At a purely chemical level, every enjoyable experience amounts to an explosion of dopamine in the brain.

Several other factors, including physiologic, genetic, developmental, and environmental factors, play a role in determining why some people abuse substances. Box 9.2 explores factors that may place individuals at risk for substance abuse.

Physiology

The physiologic effects of drugs with a high potential for abuse involve the body's adaptation to the toxic effects of the drugs at the biochemical and cellular level. Several physiologic changes characterize this process: tolerance, physical dependence, and psychological dependence. It is important to note that tolerance or physical dependence alone does not imply addiction.

Tolerance

With drug use over time, tolerance develops. **Tolerance** occurs when the body develops a natural resistance to the drug's physical or euphoric effects, making it necessary to take increasing doses more frequently to achieve the desired effect. Actual changes occur in liver cells as a result of drug use, which help the body to metabolize drugs more rapidly. When a patient becomes tolerant to a class of drugs, **cross-tolerance** may also occur, meaning that tolerance to a drug in a particular class may be transferred to other drugs in the same class. For example, tolerance to clonazepam (Klonopin) may result in tolerance to diazepam (Valium). Cross-tolerance does not extend to drugs in another class. For example, tolerance to clonazepam, a benzodiazepine, would not induce tolerance to meperidine (Demerol), an opiate drug.

Physical Dependence

Physical dependence occurs when actual changes in body cells, secondary to tolerance, cause the body to "need" the drug for homeostasis. Abstinence will result in a withdrawal syndrome. Physical dependence is related to the amount and duration of drug abuse. The higher the dose and the longer the duration, the more physically dependent the patient becomes. Drugs associated with a high degree of physical dependence include heroin, morphine, alcohol, benzodiazepines, barbiturates, nicotine, and caffeine.

Physical dependence alone does not define addiction. A patient may be physically dependent on a drug without showing behavior patterns associated with addiction. For instance, a patient with chronic pain syndrome may be dependent on opioid drugs. However, this dependence on opioid drugs does not constitute an addiction. In reality, taking these drugs enhances the patient's quality of life.

Patients may also experience **cross-dependence.** When a patient is dependent on a specific drug in one drug class, they may also be dependent on a similar drug in the same class. For example, if a patient who is dependent on clonazepam does not have access to that drug but is able to obtain diazepam, the patient will not experience a withdrawal syndrome.

Abstinence syndrome, or **withdrawal syndrome,** develops when dependent drug use is stopped or interrupted. This interruption results in physical signs and symptoms of withdrawal as the body tries to return to "normal." Signs and symptoms of withdrawal syndrome are specific to the class of drug abused and are generally the opposite effects of the drug action. The severity of withdrawal syndrome is directly correlated with the degree of physiologic dependence.

Psychological Dependence

Psychological dependence, thought by some experts to be the most important factor in addiction, involves the compulsive use of, and craving for, a drug. It results from the direct influence of drugs on brain chemistry. The drug causes an altered state of consciousness and distorted perceptions that are pleasurable and satisfying to the user. The recollection of these pleasurable feelings, along with the physiologic changes caused by tolerance and the fear of withdrawal symptoms, reinforce continued use of the drug. Thus, patients with a psychological addiction are motivated by the feelings the drug provides, rather than the body's need for the drug.

Genetics

Genetic factors also play an important role in drug dependence, and this genetic vulnerability varies. For example, certain genes may predispose an individual to, or protect the person from, alcoholism.

Several studies emphasize the effects of heredity and maintain that the disease of addiction—a chronic, progressive, recurrent, incurable, and potentially fatal condition—is a consequence of genetic deficiencies in brain tissues or neurotransmitters. For example, a vast body of evidence from studies of alcoholism suggests that genetic factors are more influential than environmental factors, and that alcoholism is a multifactorial disorder in which biologic and genetic factors

BOX 9.2 Who's at Risk for Substance Abuse?

- Individuals with chronic pain (e.g., back, joint, musculoskeletal disorders) who may occasionally misuse or abuse their prescribed drugs (Longo, et al., 1999)
- Teenagers—especially if they are dealing with self-esteem issues
- The socioeconomically disadvantaged—they may be desperate to "escape their world" selling and using drugs to survive
- Health care professionals (e.g., physicians, nurses, pharmacists) who have easy access to drugs and may begin using drugs or substances to promote sleep or arousal, decrease physical discomfort, and manage stress and anxiety
- Individuals with a family history of substance abuse, including alcoholism
- Individuals with a history of child abuse or sexual assault

interact. These conclusions are supported by animal research (breeding of "alcoholic" rats), studies of twins (alcohol metabolism, alcohol drinking patterns, each twin's response to alcohol), and studies of adoptees whose biologic parents suffered from alcoholism.

Development and Environment

Developmental and environmental influences can trigger changes in brain hormones. For example, chronic stress can decrease brain levels of neurotransmitters, such as metenkephalin, dopamine, norepinephrine, and serotonin. Many sociologic studies suggest that physical or emotional stress caused by abuse, anger, peer pressure, and other environmental stressors can cause individuals to seek and sustain use of mind-altering drugs, leading to drug dependence. Several kinds of developmental and environmental factors may influence a person's substance abuse, including personality traits, mood disorders, availability of drugs, cultural attitudes, and socioeconomic circumstances.

Personality Traits

No absolute addictive personality has been identified, and the ability to respond to stress and peer pressure varies among individuals. However, substance abusers are frequently described as having a low tolerance for frustration, being impulsive and manipulative, and experiencing fears of failure. Feelings of inadequacy, resentment, hostility, and anger are other common characteristics thought to predispose a person to substance abuse. People with one or several of these personality traits may use substances to escape from reality or to relieve emotional discomfort.

Mood Disorders

The literature and clinical findings provide evidence that mood disorders have a major effect on health status, quality of life, and likelihood of substance abuse. About 32% of all patients with mood disorders (e.g., depression and anxiety, dependent personality, antisocial personality) are substance dependent or substance abusers at some time in their lives.

Patients who have depression or anxiety and who cannot cope with life's daily pressures and problems may try to escape from a mental or physical environment perceived as anxiety ridden, bleak, and joyless. People with a dependency disorder are unable to face everyday experiences independently. Instead, they use drugs to help them feel powerful and secure. Often, this behavior pattern becomes a vicious cycle. Larger or stronger amounts of drug may be needed to resolve the discomfort. People who have an antisocial personality may initially use substances to help them relate socially and to relieve their loneliness. The effects of alcohol and drugs may provide the courage to be social and have fun.

Availability of Drugs and Drug Diversion

Availability of a drug is an important factor in developing and maintaining abuse. Drugs are readily available in hospitals and clinics, which helps explain, in part, the potential for drug abuse among health care providers, nurses, and pharmacists. Although diversion of prescription drugs is a relatively small aspect of the overall drug abuse problem, drug diversion is estimated to cost employers and insurance companies $25 billion annually.

The most commonly diverted prescription medications are scheduled controlled substances, including stimulants (e.g., methylphenidate), narcotic analgesics (e.g., hydrocodone), and central nervous system (CNS) depressants, especially benzodiazepines. The most abused, nonscheduled drug in the United States is carisoprodol (Soma), a centrally acting muscle relaxant. Carisoprodol is metabolized to meprobamate—a C-IV antianxiety agent. Illicit uses of carisoprodol include taking it with diphenhydramine, hydrocodone, or methadone; the combination of these drugs produces a heroin-type high.

Socioeconomic Circumstances

Economic circumstances have made drug abuse a major problem in many cities and towns across the United States. Some individuals may use or traffic drugs to escape harsh surroundings of poverty and illiteracy and change their perceptions of reality. Those who are not economically disadvantaged may use psychoactive drugs as a form of recreation and relaxation or for a variety of other reasons. Common reasons for using drugs include altering mood, exploring feelings, promoting social interaction, escaping boredom, stimulating creativity, improving physical performance, or enhancing the senses.

SUBSTANCE ABUSE AND THE CENTRAL NERVOUS SYSTEM

Virtually all abused drugs have some effect on the CNS and, with continued use, result in a physiologic or a psychological dependence, otherwise known as **habituation** and addiction. However, used with medical supervision, many drugs that affect the CNS have a therapeutic influence. These drugs are invaluable therapeutically because of the very specific physiologic and behavioral changes that result. Drugs that selectively affect the CNS may be used for analgesic, anticonvulsant, antipyretic, antiemetic, or anorectic purposes or to suppress movement disorders. These drugs can also be used without altering consciousness to treat mood and thought disorders.

The excessive use of these drugs, however, can have adverse effects when their use leads to dependence. In combination with alcohol, additive pharmacologic effects may occur after administration of all antihistamines, anxiolytics, CNS depressants, and narcotics. Commonly abused drugs that affect the CNS are classified into five main categories:

1. CNS depressants
2. CNS stimulants (**psychoactive** drugs)

CRITICAL THINKING SCENARIO

Considering substance abuse among professionals

As a nursing student, you may become aware of health care professionals who jeopardize their careers and their patients' safety by using drugs inappropriately. Propose some reasons why you think that a colleague might misuse drugs.

3. Hallucinogens (**psychedelic** drugs)
4. Cannabis
5. Miscellaneous drugs

A miscellaneous category of abused substances includes inhalants such as airplane or model glue, gasoline, or nitrous oxide; designer drugs such as analogues of fentanyl; antipsychotic drugs such as lithium; anabolic or androgenic steroids such as testosterone analogues; and over-the-counter (OTC) drugs, such as diet pills and antihistamines that contain caffeine and phenylpropanolamine. Figure 9.1 depicts selected drugs of abuse.

Central Nervous System Stimulants

The most commonly abused CNS stimulants include cocaine and the amphetamines. These CNS stimulants initially increase heart rate and blood pressure. The more potent stimulants energize muscles, decrease appetite, cause some degree of mental and physical alertness, produce feelings of self-confidence, and induce some degree of euphoria. Psychoactive drugs, particularly cocaine and methamphetamine, affect nerve impulses by disrupting the normal functioning of stimulatory neurotransmitters—dopamine, norepinephrine, and serotonin. The body responds to more frequent and higher doses of the drug by releasing smaller quantities of these neurotransmitters. Excess amounts can cause insomnia, hypertension, and cardiovascular problems—especially if the individual has a sensitivity to the drug. Intoxication with amphetamines, cocaine, hallucinogens, and marijuana may cause panic attacks. Prolonged use may lead to anxiety, confusion, dependency, depression, exhaustion, anhedonia (inability to experience normal pleasure), irritability, paranoia, and violence as the body's own neurotransmitters are depleted. Synthesis of the depleted neurotransmitters may take months to occur after chronic, heavy use.

The CNS stimulants have a wide range of effects that increase their potential for abuse. Caffeine, nicotine, amphetamines, and cocaine increase alertness and energy, lessen drowsiness and fatigue, increase concentration and thinking, alleviate moodiness, and impart a "high" or happy feeling. All stimulant drugs pose a risk for both physical and psychological dependence.

Caffeine is categorized as a mild CNS stimulant. It is found in coffee, tea, cocoa, colas and other soft drinks, and chocolate. It is also found in many OTC products, such as analgesics and weight-control products.

Nicotine is a highly addictive drug found in tobacco products such as cigarettes, cigars, pipe tobacco, and snuff. Tobacco use is the principal cause of preventable morbidity, disability, and premature death in the United States. Nicotine gum and transdermal patches are available by prescription or OTC to facilitate withdrawal.

Amphetamines are anorexiants used medically in short-term use for treating obesity, narcolepsy (a chronic disorder characterized by recurrent attacks of drowsiness and sleep during daytime), and attention deficit hyperactivity disorder (ADHD). Drug abusers typically take large oral doses or inject amphetamine—known as "speed"—for an intense "rush" that lasts only a short time. Studies have demonstrated that abnormal brain chemistry associated with methamphetamine abuse is evident months after the drug abuse has stopped.

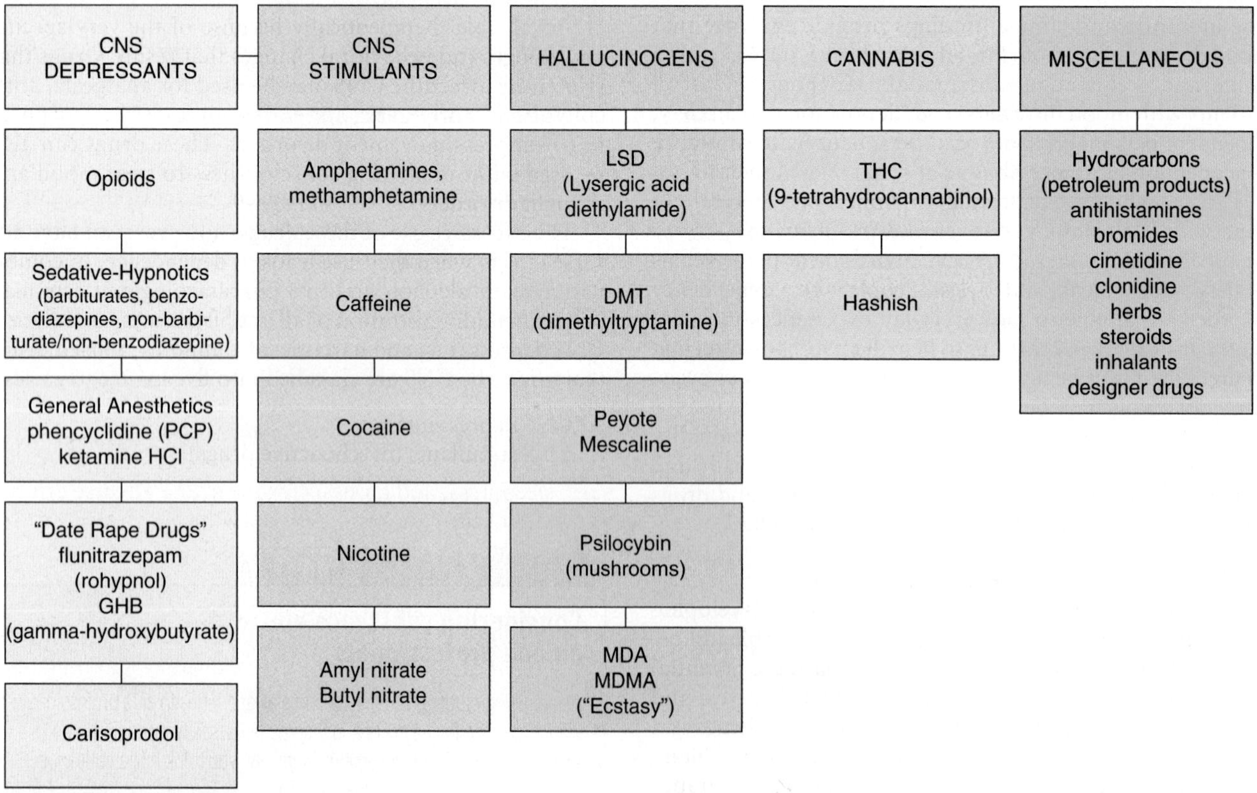

FIGURE 9.1 Selected drugs of abuse.

Brain scans have demonstrated reduced *N*-acetyl-aspartate compounds in the basal ganglia. Although no direct correlation is known, these reduced *N*-acetyl-aspartate levels are associated with a variety of diseases, including dementias, epilepsy, multiple sclerosis, brain tumors, and cerebral infarction.

Cocaine, another popular drug of abuse, produces a powerful but short-acting effect. Cocaine is not only psychologically addicting, it is also physically addicting because of its effect on neurotransmitters. The life-controlling effect of cocaine can lead an addict to exclude everything from his or her life except the pursuit of cocaine. A cocaine habit can cost an addict thousands of dollars a week to maintain.

As a general rule, intoxication with stimulant drugs is more dangerous than withdrawal. Acute intoxication may cause severe and prolonged seizure activity; withdrawal symptoms include nausea, sleep disorders, cravings, depression, irritability, agitation, and fatigue. Withdrawal symptoms occur within 24 hours and can last as long as 1 week or more.

Central Nervous System Depressants

Small doses of CNS depressants decrease heart rate, respiration, and reaction time, although initially they induce some euphoria. They relax the muscles, suppress physical and mental pain, diminish inhibitions, and promote sedation. CNS depressants, such as the opioids, can also decrease muscular coordination and energy and cause constipation, depression, nausea, vomiting, physical dependence, and withdrawal symptoms if used to excess.

Commonly abused CNS depressants include sedative-hypnotics, the most common of which are alcohol, barbiturates, and benzodiazepines. Sedative-hypnotic drugs can cause physical and psychological dependence. Regular use of these drugs over a long period leads to drug tolerance and a need for larger and larger doses to achieve the desired effect.

Alcoholism is the number one drug problem in America. Because of its complex nature, alcoholism is difficult to define. Generally, people are considered alcoholics if their lifestyle is dominated by acquiring and consuming alcoholic beverages and if this behavior interferes with personal, professional, social, or family responsibilities and relationships.

Barbiturates, once the mainstay of sedative-hypnotic drugs, are also used as anesthetics and anticonvulsants. Many barbiturates are short-acting drugs, which helps explain the problem with abuse; that is, the person needs to use more drug to sustain the desired effect. Examples of barbiturates habitually used include pentobarbital, secobarbital, and amobarbital. Methaqualone has been withdrawn from the market and is no longer legally manufactured.

Benzodiazepines, which were initially developed as an alternative to the highly dependency-producing barbiturates, are longer-acting drugs. However, they still cause physical and psychological dependence if taken regularly over a prolonged period. Benzodiazepines, which are used primarily to relieve anxiety and to provide a hypnotic, or sedative, effect, are widely prescribed and therefore readily available. Some common benzodiazepines habitually used are diazepam, alprazolam, clorazepate, clonazepam, and lorazepam.

Abrupt withdrawal from long-term use of sedative-hypnotic drugs should never be attempted because withdrawal symptoms are serious and potentially fatal. Withdrawal symptoms include agitation, dysphoria, insomnia, vomiting, diarrhea, ataxia, hallucinations, acute psychosis, muscle and abdominal cramps, anorexia, and seizures. These symptoms may occur 12 to 72 hours after the last use of the drug and may last up to 14 days.

Opioids

Opioids (also known as narcotic analgesics) are commonly prescribed to relieve pain, suppress coughing, enhance anesthetic effect for surgery, and relieve severe diarrhea. These narcotic drugs have a high potential for abuse and are extremely addicting both physically and psychologically. Frequently used and abused opioids include heroin, opium (paregoric), morphine, meperidine (Demerol), codeine, pentazocine (Talwin), and propoxyphene (Darvon). Administered orally, heroin and morphine undergo first-pass metabolism and have only one third to one sixth the effect of heroin or morphine administered parenterally. Therefore, abusers of these drugs usually administer them by injection or inhalation.

All opioids affect the CNS and cause cerebral changes, mood changes, confusion, euphoria, and analgesia. Regular use of narcotics over several weeks usually results in tolerance to the drug's effects. Withdrawal effects from narcotics induce muscle pain, nausea and vomiting, abdominal cramps, and diarrhea. Although these symptoms can be severe, they are not generally lethal. However, death may occur if the patient becomes severely dehydrated and experiences profound electrolyte imbalances. Withdrawal symptoms occur within 8 to 12 hours and can persist for up to 10 days.

Tranquilizers

Certain tranquilizing drugs, known as "date rape" drugs, have made headlines. They are Rohypnol and gamma-hydroxybutyrate (GHB). Rohypnol is the trade name for flunitrazepam—a sedative-hypnotic benzodiazepine that produces muscle relaxation and amnesia. Outside the United States, Rohypnol is legally manufactured and is prescribed for the short-term treatment of severe sleep disorders. It is widely available in Europe, Mexico, and Colombia, but is neither manufactured nor approved for sale in the United States. Rohypnol is 10 times more potent than diazepam (Valium). Initially, Rohypnol was a tasteless and odorless drug that dissolved clear in liquids, making it difficult to detect. In 1999, the manufacturers of Rohypnol reformulated the drug so that it turns blue in liquids. Unfortunately, many mixed drinks and punches are themselves dark in color, making these drinks ideal vehicles for administering the drug to unsuspecting victims. Rohypnol induces slowing of psychomotor performance, muscle relaxation, decreased blood pressure, sleepiness, and amnesia. Some of the adverse effects associated with use are drowsiness, headaches, memory impairment, dizziness, nightmares, confusion, and tremors. Although classified as a depressant, Rohypnol can induce aggression, excitability, and even death.

Gamma-hydroxybutyrate (GHB) is a powerful, rapidly acting CNS depressant initially developed as an anesthetic agent in the 1960s. GHB is produced naturally by the body in small amounts, but its physiologic function is unclear. GHB was sold in health food stores as a performance-enhancing additive in bodybuilding formulas until the United States Food and Drug Administration (FDA) banned it in 1990.

GHB is currently marketed in some European countries as an adjunct to anesthesia. GHB, which became a Schedule I Controlled Substance in March 2000, is abused for its ability to produce euphoric and hallucinogenic states and for its alleged function as a growth hormone, which releases agents to stimulate muscle growth. The popularity of GHB stems from its ease of manufacture—home chemistry kits and instructions can be found on the Internet. Like Rohypnol, GHB is a colorless, tasteless, and odorless drug that dissolves in liquids. Effects occur in 15 to 30 minutes and last for 3 to 6 hours. Adverse effects associated with GHB include nausea, vomiting, delusions, depression, vertigo, hallucinations, seizures, respiratory distress, loss of consciousness, slowed heart rate, lowered blood pressure, amnesia, and coma. The margin between GHB's anesthetic dose and its lethal dose is very narrow. In 1994, there were 54 documented GHB-related emergency room visits. In 2001, an estimated 3340 emergency room visits were attributed to the use of GHB. Since January 2000, the United States Drug Enforcement Administration (DEA) has documented more than 60 deaths relating to GHB.

Because of concern about Rohypnol, GHB, and other similarly abused sedative-hypnotics, Congress passed the Drug-Induced Rape Prevention and Punishment Act of 1996 in October 1996. This legislation increased federal penalties for using any controlled substance to aid in sexual assault.

Hallucinogens

Hallucinogenic drugs have pronounced mental and emotional effects because they distort the way the brain interprets sensory information. They can also mimic certain mental illnesses such as schizophrenia. Included in this category are the naturally occurring substances (marijuana, mescaline, and psilocybin) and the synthetic substances (lysergic acid diethylamide [LSD], dimethyltryptamine [DMT], and phencyclidine hydrochloride [PCP]). Psychedelic drugs are, with the exception of marijuana, not used medically. Psychedelics do not cause physical dependence, and only marijuana has been shown to produce psychological dependence.

Relatively new amphetamine-derivative drugs with special stimulatory effects on the brain are termed hallucinogenic amphetamines (e.g., 3,4-methylenedioxymethamphetamine [MDMA], "Ecstasy"). These drugs can be inhaled, injected, or swallowed. They cause a long-lasting reduction in the brain's supply of serotonin and produce powerful psychic changes.

Another drug, ketamine, an anesthetic used in animals, is used frequently for conscious sedation in humans. It produces some emergent hallucinogenic effects (hallucinations and sensory distortion) that immobilize the user and detach him or her from reality. Ketamine does not depress the circulatory or respiratory systems. Its effects are equivalent to those of being severely inebriated.

Inhalants

The term "inhalants" refers to products that can be abused by inhaling them through the nose or mouth to achieve an intoxicating effect (Box 9.3). Because they are easily accessible, inexpensive, and easy to conceal, inhalants are some of the first substances abused. These substances can be inhaled in various ways. Common methods include inhaling directly from containers (products such as rubber cement or correction fluid), sniffing fumes from plastic bags held over the mouth and nose, or sniffing a cloth saturated with the substance.

BOX 9.3 Commonly Abused Commercial Products

Adhesives: Model airplane glue, rubber cement, household glue
Aerosols: Spray paint, hair spray, air freshener, deodorant, fabric protector
Anesthetics: Nitrous oxide, ether, chloroform
Cleaning agents: Dry cleaning fluid, spot remover, degreaser
Food products: Vegetable cooking spray, whipped cream, and other products in aerosol containers (nitrous oxide "whippets")
Gases: Butane, propane, helium
Solvents: Nail polish remover, paint thinner, typing correction fluid and thinner, toxic markers, pure toluene, toluol, cigarette lighter fluid, gasoline

Effects of inhalant use resemble alcohol inebriation. As the user inhales, the body becomes starved of oxygen. As a compensatory effect, the heart rate increases in an attempt to increase blood flow to the brain. The user initially experiences stimulation, a loss of inhibition, and a distorted perception of reality and spatial relations. After a few minutes, the senses become depressed, and a sense of lethargy arises as the body attempts to stabilize blood flow to the brain, usually referred to as a "head rush." Users can become intoxicated several times over a few hours because of these chemicals' short-acting, rapid-onset effect. Many users also experience headaches, nausea, vomiting, slurred speech, loss of coordination, and wheezing.

The nurse should suspect inhalant abuse when observing paint or stains on the body or clothing, spots or sores around the mouth, red or runny eyes and nose, chemical odor on the breath, a drunken or dazed appearance, loss of appetite, excitability, and irritability.

Tolerance and physical dependence may occur with heavy or long-term use. Withdrawal symptoms may include sweating, rapid pulse, hand tremors, insomnia, nausea, vomiting, physical agitation, anxiety, hallucinations, and grand mal seizures.

Designer Drugs

These drugs are similar in chemical structure to existing drugs and are developed with relative ease in illegal laboratories. They are extremely potent, and when used recreationally, they have addictive capabilities greater than those of existing drugs. For example, alpha-3-methyl fentanyl (the street version of fentanyl), which may be represented as "China white" (heroin), is 35 times more potent than heroin. Fentanyl, a narcotic analgesic legitimately used during and after surgery, is an example of an existing drug "designed" into another form. These analogues of existing substances, which offer similar psychoactive properties, are primarily designed to bypass federal regulation and control by means of their chemical formulations, which differ from those of existing drugs and are thus not covered by existing laws. Two meperidine analogues that have appeared on the street include MPPP (1-methyl-4-phenyl-4-propionoxypiperidine) and PEPAP (1-[2-phenylethyl]-4-acetyloxypiperidine). They are often marketed as "new heroin." MPPP is popular among drug

abusers because when it is injected, it produces a euphoria similar to that produced by heroin. An impurity formed during the illicit manufacture of MPPP, called MPTP (1-methyl-4-phenyl-1,2,3,6-tetrahydro-pyridine), destroys brain cells and much of voluntary muscular movement. MPTP produces a crippling condition that closely resembles Parkinson disease.

Anabolic Androgenic Steroids

Anabolic androgenic steroids are synthetic formulations of the male hormone testosterone. The abuse of these drugs in men and women to increase strength and enhance athletic performance is widespread. Anabolic androgenic steroids also have a dramatic effect on emotions and make the user feel more confident and aggressive. Continued use of anabolic androgenic steroids may lead to emotional instability, rage, depression, or psychosis. Serious health problems are associated with both short- and long-term use of anabolic androgenic steroids. These problems include sex hormone imbalances (including amenorrhea or erectile dysfunction), changes in secondary sexual characteristics (e.g., gynecomastia, hypomastia, testicular atrophy, and ovarian atrophy), permanent sterility, hepatic cancer, and myocardial infarction. In light of the risks associated with these substances, many athletic organizations have banned their use.

COMMONLY ABUSED DRUGS

Of the most commonly abused drugs, alcohol, cocaine, heroin, and marijuana appear to receive the most publicity and are involved in some of the most dramatic abuse situations encountered in clinical practice.

The drugs discussed in this chapter are commonly abused drugs that have little, if any, therapeutic medicinal use. These substances are not legal, with the exception of alcohol, and in some instances, marijuana.

NURSING MANAGEMENT IN COMMONLY ABUSED DRUGS

The nurse's role in substance abuse involves having core knowledge related to specific drugs and to abuse prevention, assessing potential or actual abuse, and formulating nursing diagnoses related to the assessment findings. Once the nurse has gathered the data and developed nursing diagnoses, outcome criteria can be identified, and interventions can be implemented. Finally, the nurse evaluates whether the outcome criteria have been met and what further patient care is needed.

Core Drug Knowledge in Alcohol Abuse

Pharmacokinetics

Alcohol, known clinically as ethanol (ETOH), does not require digestion before absorption. It is completely absorbed by the stomach and small intestine within 2 hours of ingestion. However, food in the stomach decreases the effects of alcohol, delays gastric emptying time, and retards absorption from the small intestine. Once in the systemic circulation, alcohol is immediately distributed to the rest of the body at a rate proportional to blood flow and water content. Consequently, high concentrations in the brain, liver, lung, and kidney develop rapidly. Once absorption is complete, brain and blood alcohol levels are very similar.

The liver metabolizes alcohol by two different pathways—using the enzyme alcohol dehydrogenase and the microsomal ethanol-oxidizing system (MEOS). In the average adult, 90% to 98% of an ingested dose of alcohol is converted to acetaldehyde by alcohol dehydrogenase. The acetaldehyde is then oxidized to acetate by aldehyde dehydrogenase. The acetate is finally oxidized in the liver to carbon dioxide and water. These actions primarily take place in the cytoplasm and mitochondria of the hepatocyte. The remaining 2% to 10% is excreted unchanged in the urine and expired air. The average rate of metabolism of alcohol by nontolerant individuals is 100 mg/kg of body weight per hour (or 7 g per hour in a person who weighs 70 kg).

People with chronic alcoholism metabolize alcohol by way of the MEOS, which occurs primarily in the endoplasmic reticulum. Metabolism of ethanol by this pathway produces an end product of acetaldehyde and free radicals, both of which damage liver cells. Metabolism by this pathway is also dangerous because cytochrome P-450, an enzyme that is integral to the pathway, is required by the liver to transform toxins, drugs, and excess fat-soluble vitamins. If P-450 is being used to metabolize alcohol, it cannot perform its other tasks. The result is susceptibility to organ damage from other toxins, drugs, and vitamins. Alcohol is excreted in urine by the kidneys, in the breath by the respiratory system, and in sweat by the skin.

Pharmacodynamics

Alcohol affects many body systems (Box 9.4). Alcohol is thought to interfere with the transmission of nerve impulses at synaptic junctions, although this exact mechanism is unclear. It is similar in action to that of general anesthetics and probably exerts its action on the brain by dissolving in neuronal plasma membranes rather than by acting on a specific receptor.

BOX 9.4 Health Problems Related to Alcohol Abuse

- Cardiac arrhythmias and cardiomyopathy
- Cancers of the upper GI tract, liver
- Cirrhosis of the liver
- Gastritis and GI bleeding
- Hepatic dysfunction and hepatitis
- Hypertension
- Impotence
- Malnutrition and vitamin deficiencies
- Increased incidence of peptic ulcer disease
- Pancreatitis
- Peripheral neuritis
- Pregnancy complications and neonatal drug dependency
- Seizures
- Wernicke-Korsakoff syndrome

Like the general anesthetics, alcohol sequentially depresses the CNS (i.e., the cerebrum, cerebellum, spinal cord, medulla). However, the excitatory stage of alcohol is longer, and the anesthetic stage is equivalent to toxicity. The margin between alcohol's anesthetic dose and its lethal dose is very narrow.

Adverse Effects

Alcohol depresses the CNS. However, the depressant effects may appear to be stimulatory because alcohol depresses the higher centers of the brain, causing individuals to shed behavioral and social inhibitions. The degree of depression produced is directly proportional to the quantity of alcohol consumed. Table 9.1 presents blood alcohol levels and stages of intoxication.

Awareness of these two effects may depend on the excitability of the CNS at the time of drug administration, which is influenced by the environmental setting in which the drug is used and the personality of the user. For example, in a quiet, nonsocial environment, the excitatory influence may be impaired, and the drug's CNS depressant effects of sedation and drowsiness may dominate. In a social setting, where sensory input is increased, the effects of low doses of alcohol may be perceived as stimulation because the drinker may demonstrate talkativeness, increased self-confidence, and a release of usual inhibitions.

Alcohol impairs muscular coordination. It increases the heart rate and dilates the blood vessels, causing body heat loss and, in low doses, lowers the blood pressure, which is thought to reduce the risk for myocardial infarction in patients with high levels of high-density lipoproteins. With large doses of alcohol, however, dangerous levels of cardiovascular depression can occur. Prolonged alcohol use causes hypertension and cardiovascular damage such as alcoholic cardiomyopathy.

TABLE 9.1 Blood Alcohol Levels and Stages of Intoxication

Blood Alcohol Level (mg/dL)	Physical and Behavioral Effects
<50	Body sway, euphoria, excitement, impaired judgment, incoordination, increased sociability, loss of inhibitions
50–100	Disturbed gait, impaired ability to operate machinery (e.g., motor vehicles), increased reaction time, increasingly impaired judgment, distractibility, slurred speech
100–140	Ataxia, increasingly impaired mental and motor skills, impaired short-term memory
140–200	Inability to operate a motor vehicle, staggering gait
200–300	Blackouts; in combination with other CNS depressants, death secondary to additive effects
>300	Severe respiratory and cardiovascular depression, coma, death

Alcohol irritates the gastrointestinal (GI) tract by causing an increase in digestive enzymes. Ulceration of the gastric mucosa is a serious complication of excessive alcohol consumption. Alcohol also causes altered bowel function, inducing either constipation or diarrhea. The risk for developing alcoholic liver disease is related to the quantity and duration of alcohol consumption. Excessive alcohol consumption creates fatty deposits in the liver. These deposits can damage and scar the liver and lead to complications, such as cirrhosis, ascites, esophageal varices, and portal hypertension. Excess alcohol consumption inhibits antidiuretic hormone and therefore increases urine production. Finally, alcohol disrupts endocrine functions, causing alterations and fluctuations in blood glucose, catecholamine, and aldosterone levels. Alcoholics are frequently immunologically compromised, with an increased risk for mortality resulting from cancers of the upper GI tract and liver. Additionally, patients with alcohol abuse behaviors are frequently malnourished, resulting in hypoalbuminemia. Patients with hypoalbuminemia have altered protein-binding ability. Thus, the potential for adverse effects and drug toxicity during any type of drug therapy is increased.

Drug Interactions

Alcohol has no nutritional value, and it interferes with the absorption of vitamins and minerals. Alcohol can affect iron absorption, folate activities, and platelets. These harmful effects can result in a variety of anemias. Table 9.2 gives more information about drug interactions with alcohol.

Core Drug Knowledge in Cocaine Abuse

Cocaine is derived from the leaves of *Erythroxylon coca.* It is available in two forms: crystalline cocaine hydrochloride and highly purified cocaine alkaloid. Cocaine hydrochloride is usually administered orally, intravenously, or by nasal insufflation because it is water soluble and unstable when exposed to heat. The alkaloid form of cocaine—called "crack" because of the popping sound it makes when the crystals are heated—is stable on exposure to heat but is water insoluble; therefore, it is usually administered by inhalation. On the street, pure cocaine is diluted or "cut" with other substances to increase its quantity and thereby increase profits to the sellers.

Freebasing consists of converting the cocaine alkaloid to a freebase rock form using a solvent such as diethyl ether. This rock is then heated, and the fumes are inhaled. This practice is potentially dangerous because the fumes are potent and diethyl ether is flammable; in addition to the risk for burns, many users report being addicted after only one use. Treatment for cocaine addiction is difficult because of the extreme physical and psychological dependence associated with its use.

Pharmacokinetics

Cocaine is rapidly absorbed into the bloodstream, regardless of whether it is snorted, inhaled, or injected. Cocaine has a 1- to 2-minute onset of action and a 30-minute duration of action after smoking or intravenous (IV) injection; peak effects after inhaling cocaine occur in 30 to 60 minutes, with a duration of action of several hours. Cocaine is only 30% to 40% bioavailable after oral administration, and GI absorp-

TABLE 9.2 Agents That Interact With Alcohol

Interactants	Effect and Significance	Nursing Management
Analgesics (e.g., aspirin)	Combination may cause severe stomach irritation	Monitor for upper or lower GI bleeding.
Anesthetics*	Potentiation of the anesthetic effect	Observe during patient's recovery from anesthetic effects. Recovery may be prolonged.
Anticoagulants	Potentiation of the anticoagulant effect, leading to possible hemorrhage	Observe for signs of bleeding: bruising, black tarry stools.
Anticonvulsants	Accelerated anticonvulsant drug metabolism	Monitor for poor seizure control. Also monitor for seizures and provide for patient safety.
Antidiabetics, hypoglycemics	Unpredictable; rise or fall of blood glucose level	Monitor blood glucose levels regularly.
Antihistamines	Additive sedative effects; increased incidence of accidents due to drowsiness and increased response time	Caution patient that drinking and driving do not mix.
Antihypertensives	Additive hypotensive effects	Monitor blood pressure. Explain strategies for coping with orthostatic hypotension.
Antipsychotics* (e.g., phenothiazines)	Significant respiratory depression	Monitor breathing. Provide respiratory assistance if needed.
Barbiturates	Significant synergistic effects with alcohol	Monitor for severe respiratory depression.
Diuretics	Significant increased hypotensive effects due to antidiuretic hormone and diuresis	Monitor fluid and electrolyte levels. Caution patient about orthostatic hypotension.
Narcotics*	Synergistic, intensified CNS depressant effects	Provide respiratory support if significant respiratory depression occurs.
Sedative-hypnotics*	Additive effects; adverse effects on alertness and performance	Caution patient that sedative drugs and alcohol should not be consumed together.
Vitamins	Continuous alcohol use interferes with vitamin absorption and synthesis	Monitor for nutritional deficiencies (thiamine, folate, B_{12}) and paresthesias.

*These are potentially hazardous when ingested by a heavy drinker, patient with long-term alcoholism, or patient recovering from alcoholism.

tion may continue for several hours. Orally administered cocaine has a slower onset of action, approximately 1 hour.

Cocaine is extensively metabolized in the liver and the blood. Metabolites may be detected in the urine for 2 or more days. Because cocaine is so rapidly metabolized in the liver, the user must inhale, inject, or smoke the drug approximately every 30 minutes to maintain the high. Cocaine is characterized by tachyphylaxis (a rapidly decreasing response to the drug following administration of the initial doses). Therefore, its psychoactive effects diminish rapidly, despite its continued presence in the plasma.

The elimination half-life for cocaine is similar for all forms of administration—about 50 minutes for the oral route, 80 minutes for the intranasal route, and 60 minutes for the IV route.

Pharmacodynamics

Cocaine has pronounced effects on the central and peripheral nervous systems. It impairs the uptake of norepinephrine and epinephrine by presynaptic nerve endings, thus activating the adrenergic systems and causing hypertension, tachycardia, and vasoconstriction. Cocaine interferes with serotonin uptake, causing dramatic alterations in the sleep–wake cycle and evoking feelings of intense energy. It also impairs dopamine reuptake, thus activating the dopaminergic system and causing euphoria, thereby strongly reinforcing use. With long-term use, dopamine becomes progressively depleted from nerve endings, causing the dysphoria that is so prominent during withdrawal. Dopamine depletion and dysphoria frequently lead to drug craving, causing a very high rate of relapse. Cocaine also interferes with sodium ion activity in peripheral nerves, causing local anesthetic actions.

Adverse Effects

Adverse reactions to cocaine include:

- CNS stimulation, including severe agitation, anxiety, excitement, paranoid psychosis, and seizures
- Cardiovascular effects, including atrioventricular arrhythmias, severe hypertension, cardiomyopathy, coronary and peripheral vasoconstriction, myocardial infarction, and intestinal or renal ischemia
- Pulmonary complications, including pneumothorax, pulmonary edema, and respiratory arrest
- Metabolic complications, including disseminated intravascular coagulation, hepatotoxicity, hyperthermia, renal failure, and rhabdomyolysis
- Complications of nasal inhalation, including anosmia, nasal mucosal atrophy, nasal septal necrosis, and rhinorrhea

High doses of pure cocaine in freebase form (crack) can overtax the cardiovascular system and cause sudden death from acute myocardial infarction or rupture of the aorta. Cocaine sensitizes cardiac cells and causes an increase in contractility. Corresponding high levels of epinephrine secondary

to excitement from cocaine cause the individual to be particularly susceptible to cardiac arrest.

Core Drug Knowledge in Opioid Abuse

Heroin, the most abused opioid in the United States, is a synthetically manufactured drug that possesses morphine-like pharmacologic activity. It has a poor oral availability; therefore, abusers often begin by smoking the drug. As the abuser becomes tolerant to the drug, he or she begins to use the drug by IV injection. When abusers can no longer find a site for IV injection, they will start subcutaneous administration, also known as "skin-popping." Pure heroin is very expensive and dangerously powerful. For these reasons, street heroin is usually mixed with fillers, such as sugars, starches, or quinine, resulting in a mixed substance that contains only 1% to 10% heroin.

Pharmacokinetics

The rate of heroin's absorption by the bloodstream depends on the method of administration. Absorption rate increases from oral use to IV injection. Typically, effects are felt within about 30 minutes after oral administration and with a range of 5 to 15 minutes after smoking or injecting. Depending on the dose, the effects of injected heroin persist approximately 4 to 6 hours. Most heroin is converted to morphine and excreted by the kidneys. Insignificant quantities of unconverted heroin may be found in urine and feces.

Pharmacodynamics

Heroin acts on the body in a manner similar to that of other opioids. An intense rush follows IV administration of heroin. This rush subsides in a few minutes, and the effects resemble those following oral dosing. The abuser feels relaxed, carefree, somewhat dreamy, but able to carry on with many normal activities. Taking daily doses of heroin (at least 24 mg) usually results in a clinically significant dependence in a few weeks.

Adverse Effects

The pathophysiologic effects of heroin are also similar to those of the other opioids (see Chapter 23); however, the degree of some effects is greater. An overdose of heroin may result in severe respiratory depression, pulmonary edema, coma, and possibly death. Some pathophysiologic effects specific to IV heroin use include infection with human immunodeficiency virus (HIV) or hepatitis from contaminated needles, toxic reactions to contaminants injected along with the heroin, vasculitis, and thromboembolic complications.

Core Drug Knowledge in Marijuana Abuse

The most commonly abused psychedelic drug is marijuana, which is derived from the hemp species, *Cannabis sativa*. Marijuana refers to the entire plant chopped and dried; the more potent hashish is the dried resinous exudate of the flowering tops.

The major ingredient of marijuana is 9-tetrahydrocannabinol (THC). The THC concentration in the average marijuana cigarette has increased substantially during the past 3 decades. A typical marijuana cigarette delivers a dose of THC ranging from 2.5 mg to 5 mg.

Pharmacotherapeutics

An oral form of marijuana, dronabinol (Marinol), is now used in the United States to treat anorexia in patients with acquired immunodeficiency syndrome (AIDS) and for reducing nausea and vomiting in patients with cancer who are undergoing chemotherapy. Studies are ongoing related to its effectiveness in reducing intraocular pressure associated with glaucoma.

Pharmacokinetics

The systemic availability of THC after smoking is about 25%, with a peak plasma concentration occurring after 10 to 30 minutes. The duration of the entire effect is about 2 to 3 hours. The effectiveness of THC after oral ingestion is less than after smoking it: systemic availability is less (6% to 20%), onset of CNS effects is 30 to 60 minutes, peak plasma concentrations are reached within 2 to 3 hours, and the duration of effect is about 4 to 6 hours for psychoactive effects and more than 24 hours for appetite stimulant effects.

THC is converted quite rapidly to a pharmacologically active metabolite, 11-hydroxy-9-THC. Further metabolism yields an inactive metabolite (11-nor-9-carboxy-9-THC), which is excreted in the urine. The plasma half-life of THC is approximately 13 days, and the urinary elimination half-life for 11-nor-9-carboxy-9-THC is approximately 10 days. The concentrations of these metabolites, however, do not correlate well with THC's clinical effects and are poor predictors of behavioral impairment or intoxication. The slow urinary elimination provides an ideal marker for detecting marijuana use in drug testing.

Pharmacodynamics

The mechanism of action of THC is unknown; however, antiemetic and other pharmacologic effects occur within minutes of use. THC produces minor cognitive effects, such as an altered sense of time, a period of euphoria followed by sedation, less discriminate hearing, and enhanced visual stimuli.

Adverse Effects

Some of the adverse effects of THC include decreased myocardial oxygen supply, a dose-related increase in heart rate (20 to 50 bpm after one or two marijuana cigarettes), and impaired fertility. Cannabinoid receptors are concentrated most heavily in the cerebellum, the part of the brain that controls motor coordination, and in the hippocampus, which governs learning and memory. Large numbers are also found in the cerebral cortex, the seat of higher thinking, and lesser numbers are scattered in the immune system. They are largely absent from the brainstem regions that govern heartbeat and respiration. At high levels of intake, a cannabis psychosis may occur, and regular heavy cannabis users may suffer repeated psychotic episodes and personality changes. Chronic use of THC appears to cause permanent brain damage, as evidenced by loss of short-term memory, decreased motivation, impaired performance of simple and complex motor tasks, development of acute anxiety that may reach panic proportions, and severe psychological dependence.

Although smoking marijuana is often thought to be relatively safe compared with smoking tobacco, the smoke is virtually identical in both cases. Smoking marijuana involves inhaling larger volumes of smoke and holding the breath as much as four times longer than with tobacco, which ultimately makes smoking three to four marijuana joints a day equivalent to smoking 1 pack of tobacco cigarettes a day and a "possible causal role for marijuana in the pathogenesis of . . . bullous emphysema" (Johnson, 2000).

Tolerance to the effects of marijuana develops quite slowly. Evidence that marijuana is addictive has been obscured partly because THC is readily stored in body fat, and marijuana users who quit are often "weaned" off the drug slowly as small amounts continue to filter into the bloodstream. Several studies, however, have shown that a "flulike" syndrome occurs during withdrawal from marijuana. The National Institute of Drug Abuse (which funds most of the marijuana research in the United States) estimates that 100,000 people seek treatment every year for marijuana dependency.

Core Drug Knowledge in Hallucinogen Abuse

Although often associated with the 1960s, LSD and PCP are still used. LSD is taken orally, and PCP can be taken orally, smoked, or injected. Tolerance develops with continued use of these drugs. However, psychological dependence is rare, and physical dependence does not occur. In addition, no specific withdrawal syndrome is associated with these drugs. LSD and PCP have no accepted medical use and are classified as Schedule I drugs.

Pharmacokinetics

The effects of LSD and PCP usually occur 30 to 90 minutes after ingestion or inhalation and can last between 8 and 12 hours. The effects depend on the amount taken, the user's personality, the user's mood and expectations, and the setting in which the drug is used.

PCP is rapidly metabolized in the liver to inactive metabolites. Large doses of PCP may result in accumulation of large amounts of nonmetabolized PCP in the urine. PCP has a half-life of 30 minutes to 1 hour in small amounts and of 1 to 4 days in large doses.

Pharmacodynamics

The mechanism of action is unclear, although some experts think serotonin-antagonistic activity within the brain is responsible for its hallucinogenic properties. Alterations in sensory perception, distortions of size, body image distortions, and surreal feelings of separation of body parts are prominent features of LSD intoxication. Sensory input is also enhanced, which creates vivid visual illusions, hallucinations, and intensely colored visual images.

Adverse Effects

Subjective effects and mood changes are quite variable with LSD. A dream-like state with feelings of good humor, euphoria, relaxation, and a sense of wonderment may predominate. Conversely, "bad trips" may occur. These consist of dysphoria, nervousness, anxiety, disorientation, hallucinations, panic attacks, and severe psychotic attacks. LSD produces adrenergic effects, most notably hypertension, hyperpnea, tachycardia, hyperthermia, pupillary dilation, and hyperreflexia. Diaphoresis, salivation, lacrimation, nausea, and vomiting may also occur.

Dopaminergic and anticholinergic effects on the body occur with PCP use. In addition, this drug shares some of the dysphoric properties of the opioids. After low doses, the user has a sense of thinking and acting swiftly. Moods may range from euphoria and a sense of "bouncing" to depression. Larger doses cause changes in mood, which are quite unpredictable and labile. A sense of unreality predominates. Under the influence of PCP, an individual may experience a bad trip and become irrational, extremely combative, and violent. The lack of pain secondary to its anesthetic effect seems to exaggerate the individual's perception of his or her own strength. In some cases, PCP can cause severe psychoses, seizures, respiratory depression, intracerebral hemorrhage, hyperpyrexia, and death.

Flashbacks—hallucinatory episodes that occur days to years after taking the drug—occur with LSD and PCP use. Prolonged psychotic episodes (lasting several days to several months) with visual hallucinations have been precipitated by LSD and PCP.

Core Drug Knowledge in Inhalant Abuse

Inhalants, another type of psychedelic drug, are volatile chemicals and gases that produce behavioral effects and are subject to abuse. Commonly abused inhalants include model glue, spray paint and hair spray propellants, cleaning solvents, gasoline, and kerosene. Nonmedical nitrous oxide is another popular inhalant.

These substances are generally sniffed from rags, paper or plastic bags, gauze, or ampules. Long-term inhalant abuse can cause permanent CNS, hepatic, renal, and bone marrow damage and greatly reduced mental and physical abilities.

Pharmacokinetics

Inhalants are rapid-acting substances. Their effects are almost immediate. The duration of the effect depends on the substance used. For example, the effects of glue, paint, or gasoline usually last several or more hours, whereas the effects of nitrous oxide typically last less than 5 minutes. The effects of amyl nitrate (or butyl nitrate) last from a few seconds to several minutes.

Pharmacodynamics

Inhaling volatile chemicals and gases produces a short-lived, mild intoxication that typifies the early stages of anesthesia. These agents produce a sense of exhilaration and lightheadedness. Judgment, vision, memory, and perception of reality are impaired. These substances are slightly hallucinogenic and cause CNS depression because of the hypoxia they induce. Abusive, violent behavior has also been known to occur in people who abuse inhalants.

Adverse Effects

Psychological dependence can develop, but physical dependence is rare. Tolerance to the substance can develop over time, and more of the substance is needed over time to produce the same effect.

Toxicities depend on the properties of the individual solvents. The consequences of inhaling these substances can be severe. Abuse of inhalants has been implicated in severe brain damage, cancer, neuropathies, kidney failure, liver damage, respiratory failure, and cardiac arrest.

Assessment of Core Patient Variables in Substance Abuse

Health Status

When the nurse suspects that a patient may be abusing substances, a physical, psychological, and functional health assessment is performed. The assessment focuses on the physical, psychological, emotional, and functional status of the patient.

Substance abuse screening may be easily incorporated into a health habits survey, with questions moving from legal and less stigmatized substances, such as caffeine, nicotine, and alcohol, to inquiries about street drugs. Questions about drug use or abuse should cover lifetime experience because recovering users remain at risk for relapse. In addition, a complete health and drug history is taken. During this time, the nurse tries to obtain as much information about legal and illegal drug use as possible. When providing this information, the patient may use street names to refer to particular drugs or drug classes. Therefore, the nurse must be familiar with commonly used street names for legal and illicit drugs. Table 9.3 provides a list of street names of commonly abused drugs.

At this time, the nurse also asks the patient about any family history of substance abuse. During the physical assessment, the nurse conveys a nonjudgmental attitude, which may encourage the patient to communicate. A person is more likely to open up to someone who appears open and nonjudgmental. The nurse also should not assume someone is or is not a drug user. There is no stereotypical drug user. People who abuse drugs are from all socioeconomic and cultural backgrounds. Table 9.4 describes characteristics of drug abuse.

Life Span and Gender

Substance abuse throughout the life span poses serious problems for patients, families, and the community.

Effects in Pregnancy

An estimated 10% of infants are exposed to illicit drugs during the gestational period. When alcohol, caffeine, and nicotine are considered, some researchers report as many as 33% of all pregnant women have used a psychoactive drug during pregnancy.

Alcohol use during pregnancy increases the risks for spontaneous abortions, fetal demise, problematic pregnancies, lower birth rate, and neonates who are slower to grow postnatally. Specific toxic effects of alcohol on the developing fetus are known as fetal alcohol syndrome (FAS). The incidence of FAS in some parts of the United States is estimated to be as high as 1 in 300 births. It is a common cause of preventable birth defects. FAS causes growth deficiency, CNS dysfunction, craniofacial abnormalities, microcephaly, and other major organ defects. No amount of alcohol has been established as safe during pregnancy or lactation, nor has any time during pregnancy been determined as safe for drinking it. Alcohol is teratogenic, but unlike other teratogens, alcohol does not uniformly affect all fetuses exposed to it.

Fetal physiology differs from neonatal and adult physiology. These differences suggest that maternal ingestion of psychoactive substances may produce a more dramatic effect in the fetus.

Fetal nourishment occurs through the placenta. To reach the fetus, drugs in the maternal environment must cross over the continuous lipid membrane of the placenta. Substances with a molecular weight of less than 600 (such as alcohol and cocaine) cross over easily. Drug effects may persist for a greater length of time in the fetal environment because fetal blood is moderately acidotic and contains fewer protein-binding sites, and undeveloped hepatic function decreases the fetus' ability to metabolize and excrete the substance. Although excretion occurs through the placenta, the drug may be recirculated throughout the amniotic fluid before it is excreted.

The effects of opioid abuse during pregnancy include preterm birth, intrauterine growth retardation, and low birth weight. Cocaine use during pregnancy has disastrous effects on the fetus; it causes potent vasoconstriction that reduces placental blood flow by about 50%. This reduction results in fetal hypoxia and alters the maternal–fetal nutrient exchange. Fetal effects of maternal cocaine and methamphetamine use include abruptio placentae, preterm labor and delivery, intrauterine growth retardation, microcephaly, low birth weight, and cerebral infarction. Fetal exposure can be recognized in a neonate who exhibits a withdrawal syndrome characterized by tremor, poor feeding, increased muscle tone, abnormal sleep patterns, and high-pitched crying.

Women who use these drugs should be counseled to avoid breast-feeding because these drugs are concentrated in breast milk.

Effects in Infancy

Opioid-exposed infants experience several common complications: hypoglycemia, septicemia, and hyperbilirubinemia. In addition to metabolic problems, term infants are at risk for pneumonia and meconium aspiration. Preterm and full-term infants alike experience withdrawal symptoms. Narcotic abstinence syndrome, which contributes substantially to neonatal morbidity, is characterized by CNS hyperirritability, GI dysfunction, increased muscle tone, respiratory distress, tremor, and vague autonomic symptoms such as fever, skin mottling, sneezing, and yawning. Initially, some infants may require drug therapy and treatment in the neonatal intensive care unit. Some symptoms may persist for 3 or 4 months or more.

Effects in Childhood

Children of people with alcoholism face a broad range of problems that vary in severity and are associated with all phases of the life span. They are at risk for a range of cognitive deficits, especially those related to verbal ability, ADHD, antisocial personality disorder, anxiety, and depression. The prevalence of alcoholism is higher than normal in all first-degree relatives of patients with alcoholism, and on average, children of people with alcoholism are three to five times more likely to develop alcoholism than children of people who do not have alcoholism. Many children of alcoholics develop intensely resilient personalities.

TABLE 9.3 Identifying Drug Street Names

Drug	Selected Street Names
CNS depressants	
Barbiturates	Downers, reds, red devils, RDs, yellows, blues, rainbows, Christmas trees
Benzodiazepines (general)	Coral, idiot pills, M&Ms, tranq, Uncle Milty, ups & downs
Chlordiazepoxide (Librium)	Green and whites, libs, roaches
Diazepam (Valium)	V, vals
Flunitrazepam (Rohypnol)	Circles, forget me drug, forget me pill, getting roached, La Rocha, lunch money drug, Mexican Valium, pingus, R-2, reynolds, rib roach-2, roapies, robutal, roofies, rope, rophies, row-shay, ruffles, wolfies
Nonbenzodiazepines (general)	Ludes, Qs, 714s, vitamin Q
GHB	Cherry meth, liquid X, fantasy, organic quaalude, GBH, salty water, Georgia home boy, scoop, great hormones at bedtime, sleep-500, grievous bodily harm, soap, liquid E, somatomaz, liquid ecstasy, Vita-G, max, goop
Ketamine	Special K, super K, super acid, vitamin K, cat Valium, jet, K
Opioids	
Fentanyl	China white, king ivory, dance fever, jackpot
Heroin	Al Capone, antifreeze, ballot, Bart Simpson, big bag, big, H, brown sugar, capital H, cheese, chip, crank, dead on arrival, dirt, Dr. Feelgood, ferry dust, George, smack, golden girl, good horse, hard candy, hazel, hero, hombre, horse, HRN, isda, jee gee, joy, junk, lemonade, Mexican brown, nice and easy, noise, ogoy, old Steve, orange line, P-dope, pangonadalot, peg, perfect high, poison, pure, rawhide, ready rock, salt, sweet dreams, train, white boy, zoquete, downtown
Hydromorphone	Drug stores
Methadone	Dolls, dollies
Morphine	Miss Emma, Mort, M
CNS stimulants	
Amphetamines	Uppers, whites, minibennies, hearts, dexies, black beauties
Cocaine	Snow, flake, blow, rock, whiff, cola, oca, toot, nose candy, girl, crack, uptown
Methamphetamine	Blue mollies, chalk, crank, crystal, glass, go-fast, ice, LA glass, meth, methlies, quick, Mexican crack, shabu, quartz, sketch, speed, stove-top, West Coast
Inhalants	
General	Air blast, bagging, discorama, glading, gluey, kick, Medusa, moon gas, Oz, poor man's pot, snorting
Amyl nitrite	Ames, amys, boppers, pearls, poppers
Isobutyl nitrite	Aroma of men, bolt, climax, quicksilver, rush, snappers, thrust, whiteout
Nitrous oxide	Buzz bomb, laughing gas, shoot the breeze, whippets
Cannabis	Pot, grass, weed, Colombian, Jamaican red, Mexican commercial, sinsemilla, kona gold, joint, roach, honey, reefer, ganja, mota
Hallucinogens	
LSD	Acid, L, microdots, sunshine, windowpane, paper acid, blotter acid
MDA (Ecstasy)	Speed for lovers, X Adam, B-bombs, cristal, disco biscuit, Eve, iboga, pollutants, sweeties, Bens, love drug, scooby snacks, wheels, clarity, dex, essence, hug drug, morning shot, speed for decadence, E, go
Peyote	Button, mesc, mescal, cactus
Psilocybin	Shrooms, magic mushrooms
PCP	Angel dust, peace pill, elephant tranquilizer, rocket fuel, shermans, kools, zombie, tictac

TABLE 9.4 **Characteristics of Substance Abuse**

Drug	Intoxication Effects	Symptoms of Overdose	Health Consequences
Alcohol	Bloodshot and watery eyes, alcohol breath, motor incoordination, slurred speech, elevated blood pressure, nystagmus, mood swings and irritability, sedation	Severe vomiting or vomiting while "sleeping" or passed out and not waking up after vomiting; not responding to verbal or tactile stimulation; ataxic gait; slow, labored breathing; cold, clammy skin; rapid pulse; respiratory depression or arrest	Hypertension, GI bleeding, liver dysfunction, pancreatitis, gastric cancer
Anabolic steroids	None	None	Hypertension; changes in cholesterol/blood clotting, acne, hostility/aggression, suicide, cancer, or liver and kidney disease Adolescents: inhibition of growth Males: prostate cancer, reduced sperm production, shrunken testicles, breast enlargement Females: menstrual irregularities, facial hair, masculine characteristics
Barbiturates	Reduced pain or anxiety, feeling of well-being, lowered inhibitions, sedation/drowsiness, slowed pulse and breathing, decreased blood pressure, poor concentration	Respiratory depression and arrest, cardiovascular collapse, death	Confusion, dizziness, slurred speech, excitement, irritability, depression, fatigue, fever, addiction, impaired coordination/memory/judgment
Benzodiazepines	Same as barbiturates	Same as barbiturates	Confusion, dizziness, impaired coordination/memory/judgment, fatigue, addiction
Cannabis	Euphoria, slowed thinking/reaction time, confusion, impaired balance/coordination	Fatigue, paranoia, acute psychosis	Impaired memory/learning, anxiety, panic attacks, cough, frequent respiratory infection, increased heart rate, addiction
Cocaine	Increased heart rate/blood pressure/temperature, mental alertness, feelings of exhilaration, energy, pupil dilation, motor agitation	Agitation, paranoia, acute psychosis, seizures, respiratory failure, stroke, death	Reduced appetite, nausea, headaches, rapid/irregular heartbeat, chest pain, heart failure
Flunitrazepam (Rohypnol)	Reduced pain/anxiety, feelings of well-being, lowered inhibitions, slowed pulse/breathing, decreased blood pressure, poor concentration	Respiratory depression and arrest, death	Confusion, fatigue, memory loss for time under the drug's effects, impaired coordination/memory/judgment, visual/gastrointestinal disturbances, urinary retention
Methylphenidate	Increased or decreased blood pressure/heart rate, mental alertness, energy, feelings of exhilaration	Vomiting, agitation, tremors, hyperreflexia, muscle twitching, convulsions (may be followed by coma), euphoria, confusion, hallucinations, delirium, sweating, flushing, headache, hyperpyrexia, tachycardia, palpitations, cardiac arrhythmias, hypertension, mydriasis, dryness of mucous membranes	Reduced appetite, digestive problems, rapid/irregular heartbeat, heart failure

(continued)

TABLE 9.4 Characteristics of Substance Abuse (continued)

Drug	Intoxication Effects	Symptoms of Overdose	Health Consequences
Nicotine	Increased heart rate/blood pressure, mental alertness, energy, feelings of exhilaration	Agitation, anxiety, seizures	Reduced appetite, rapid/irregular heartbeat, adverse pregnancy outcomes, chronic lung disease, cardiovascular disease, stroke, cancer, addiction
Opioids	Apathy, euphoria, staggering gait, pinpoint pupils, sedation	Unconsciousness, respiratory depression and arrest, death	Nausea, constipation, confusion, sedation, addiction
PCP and analogues	Increased or decreased heart rate and blood pressure, impaired motor function, numbness	Violent behavior, paranoia, seizures, acute psychosis, heart failure, death	Memory loss, nausea or vomiting, loss of appetite, depression, panic, aggression, violence
Hallucinogens	Altered perception and feelings, tremor, numbness, insomnia, loss of appetite, weakness	Acute psychosis, death (frequently from trauma)	Chronic mental disorders, flashbacks

Effects in Adolescence

The greatest physical and emotional changes occur during adolescence. The struggle toward independence is a time of great conflict, and rebellion is common during this period. Common forms of rebellion include style of dress and appearance, although rebellion can take destructive forms, such as illicit drug use and excessive alcohol drinking.

Several risk factors have been identified for adolescent substance abuse:

- Family constitution and stressful family events
- Poor parent–child relationships
- Low self-esteem
- Psychological disturbances, such as depression
- Low academic motivation
- Other problem behaviors
- Absence of religion
- High level of thrill-seeking behavior
- High family and peer substance use
- Early tobacco use

Effects in Older Adults

In the United States, adults who are 65 years and older are the fastest-growing segment of the population. Retirement often brings changes in the older person's societal role as well as a decrease in social and financial status. Declining health, financial problems, and illness and death of family and friends are common losses of aging. Depressive symptoms related to these losses are common in older people. For some, alcohol or drug use becomes a way of coping with age-related changes, which normally cause physiologic changes. These changes have an important effect on how the body metabolizes drugs. Reductions in blood flow with age may result in an inability of the liver and kidneys to process drugs as efficiently as in youth; benzodiazepines, for example, are metabolized at about half the rate seen in a younger individual, making these drugs more difficult to use in the older population.

Alcohol- and drug-related medical problems may not be recognized because multiple medical problems are common in the elderly, and they may be mistaken for age-related problems. Confusion, depression, falls and other accidents, idiosyncratic reaction to prescribed drugs, inattention to self-care, incontinence, labile moods, and malnutrition are all conditions that can be related to either normal age-related changes or to the use of alcohol or drugs.

Environment

As with other chronic drug use, heavy and chronic use of cocaine and methamphetamine is especially accompanied by dysphoria and anhedonia. Former substance abusers are at risk for relapse because the perceived cure for the dysphoria is more drug use. Recurrence of symptoms and intense drug craving may occur even after long abstinence. Environmental triggers may produce intense desire for the drug even after years of recovery.

Culture and Inherited Traits

Some populations, most notably East Asians and American Indians, exhibit an unusual response of facial flushing, vasodilation, and tachycardia after consuming ethanol. These individuals have a genetic deficiency in the enzyme aldehyde dehydrogenase, which leads to an accumulation of acetaldehyde even after consuming relatively small amounts of ethanol.

Nursing Diagnoses and Outcomes

A comprehensive nursing assessment yields subjective and objective data helpful in formulating nursing diagnoses and desired outcomes relevant to short- or long-term drug history and actual or potential health problems related to substance abuse. Nursing diagnoses may vary according to which substances are used and what symptoms appear. In addition to Deficient Knowledge, Disturbed Sensory Perception (Visual and Auditory), and Risk for Poisoning, additional

typical nursing diagnoses and outcomes may include the following:

- Ineffective Denial related to impaired ability to accept consequences of behavior
  Desired outcome: *The patient will acknowledge an alcohol or substance abuse problem; explain the psychological and physiologic effects of alcohol or drug use; abstain from alcohol and drug use; state recognition of the need for continued treatment; express a sense of hope; use alternative coping mechanisms to cope with stress; and have a plan for high-risk situations for relapse.*
- Risk for Other-Directed Violence related to drug or alcohol abuse
  Desired outcome: *The patient will demonstrate control of behavior with assistance from others; have a decreased number of violent responses; and describe causation and possible preventive measures.*
- Ineffective Health Maintenance related to substance abuse
  Desired outcome: *The patient will identify barriers to health maintenance and will engage in (or verbalize an intent to engage in) health maintenance behaviors, including abstinence and sobriety.*
- Self-concept Disturbance related to self-destructive behavior (substance abuse)
  Desired outcome: *The patient will appraise self-situations in a realistic manner without distortions; verbalize and demonstrate increased positive feelings; and demonstrate healthy adaptation and coping skills.*

Planning and Intervention

In general, nursing interventions involve maximizing the therapeutic effects of the treatment plan, minimizing factors that may contribute to resumption of substance abuse, and providing patient education to help the patient cope with denial and recognize the importance of his or her substance abuse problem.

Maximizing Recovery

Initial nursing interventions in acutely intoxicated patients are generally directed toward preventing life-threatening or debilitating effects from the substance itself or its withdrawal. These nursing interventions evolve from the specific physiologic and psychological effects of the particular substance. For example, if the patient is experiencing hallucinogen and CNS-stimulant intoxication or withdrawal, the nurse monitors vital signs and mental status and provides a quiet, dim, nonstimulating, nonthreatening environment. Additional monitoring focuses on emotional status and possible seizure activity.

Because physical or psychological withdrawal symptoms may follow abrupt cessation of a substance, the first intervention is medical detoxification if the person entering treatment is currently under the influence of drugs. Physiologic symptoms associated with drug withdrawal may be treated with various pharmacotherapies. For example, diazepam or lorazepam is used to modify the symptoms of alcohol withdrawal and prevent the seizures it can precipitate. Clonidine (Catapres) is frequently used to manage the symptoms of opioid and cocaine withdrawal.

Minimizing Relapse

For alcohol, cocaine, or narcotic abusers, treatment is lifelong, and relapses do occur. However, several therapies may promote motivation to remain substance free and increase the patient's chances for success. They include psychotherapy and support groups and administration of withdrawal and anticraving drugs. Nursing management strategies in alcoholism are summarized in Box 9.5.

Some patients who have withdrawn from alcohol and who desire to achieve continued sobriety may elect to take the drug disulfiram (Antabuse). Its effects rely on a drug interaction (between ethanol and disulfiram) to produce unpleasant and undesirable symptoms as a deterrent to alcohol ingestion. The very unpleasant symptoms of a disulfiram–ethanol reaction include facial flushing, throbbing headache, hyperventilation, tachycardia, palpitations, nausea and copious vomiting (within 60 minutes after alcohol ingestion), hypotension, shortness of breath, vertigo, syncope, confusion, and profuse diaphoresis. In very severe reactions, myocardial infarction, cardiovascular collapse, unconsciousness, convulsions, and even death may occur.

Patients withdrawing from cocaine addiction may be treated with amantadine (Symmetrel), bromocriptine (Parlodel), buprenorphine (Buprenex), carbamazepine (Tegretol), desipramine (Norpramin), and lithium. These drugs have been used clinically with varying degrees of success.

Treatment for heroin addicts is possible. However, the process is slow, and some methods used are somewhat

BOX 9.5 Nursing Management Strategies in Alcoholism

Nursing interventions are modified according to the problems and complications encountered in patients with alcoholism. Some general interventions follow.

Acute Alcohol Intoxication

- Maintain an open and adequate airway.
- Support respiration and blood pressure.
- Alleviate hypoglycemia, ketoacidosis, dehydration, and neurologic deficit by administering glucose and IV fluids containing potassium, magnesium, phosphate, and vitamins (thiamine, pyridoxine, and folic acid).

Alcohol Withdrawal Syndrome

- Administer drug therapy as prescribed (e.g., primarily benzodiazepines chlordiazepoxide or lorazepam) to suppress the withdrawal syndrome.

Chronic Alcoholism

- Inform the patient of the necessity for complete abstinence from alcohol use, including alcohol in "benign" products such as cough syrups and food flavoring (vanilla extract).
- Refer the patient and family to social and environmental support groups, such as Alcoholics Anonymous, Alateen, Al-Anon.
- Teach about preventive medical and pharmacologic treatments, such as aversion therapy with disulfiram (Antabuse), hypnotherapy, psychotherapy, and treatment programs in private or public clinics outside of a hospital setting.

BOX 9.6 Treating Heroin Addiction

For many substance abusers, overcoming heroin or other opioid addiction is a long and difficult process. Over the years, many treatment interventions have been proposed and used with varying degrees of success, failure, and controversy.

Methadone (Dolophine, Methadose)

Oral methadone is substituted for heroin at a dose sufficient to suppress opioid withdrawal and then, theoretically, reduced by 50% every other day. This treatment effectively suppresses withdrawal symptoms and has a long duration of action (24 hours). About 1 mg of methadone is equivalent to 1.5 mg heroin.

Methadone treatment is controversial for several reasons: some practitioners argue that methadone therapy simply substitutes one addicting substance for another. Although the goal is to be drug free, many patients continue to take methadone rather than be tapered from the drug. Additionally, illicit methadone markets have developed because of the widespread use of methadone programs and the fact that patients are allowed to take larger quantities home and make fewer clinic visits.

Clonidine (Catapres)

Clonidine, an adrenergic agonist and antihypertensive drug, is useful in treating mild heroin dependence and withdrawal. It suppresses the sensory nervous system and the hyperactivity that accompanies withdrawal. Clonidine facilitates withdrawal in two ways: it may be substituted for methadone (after methadone facilitates withdrawal) and then withdrawn, or it may be used with the long-acting opioid antagonist naltrexone (Trexan) as a substitute for methadone. Ultimately, the clonidine is withdrawn, leaving the patient solely on naltrexone.

Naltrexone (Trexan, ReVia)

A recent treatment option for heroin addiction is long-term naltrexone. Naltrexone is a long-acting narcotic antagonist. An oral dose of 50 mg effectively blocks the receptors for 24 hours so that heroin has no effect and the patient experiences no real pleasure from taking the drug. The decision to "do drugs" must be made a day in advance.

Buprenorphine (Buprenex, Suboxone, Subutex)

Buprenorphine, a semisynthetic mixed opiate agonist-antagonist, is the first therapy approved for in-office prescribing for opioid dependence under the federal Drug Addiction Treatment Act of 2000. In supervised drug rehabilitation programs, it is administered as a sub-lingual tablet. In unsupervised programs, buprenorphine is given as an oral drug combined with naloxone (an opioid antagonist). If the buprenorphine tablet is dissolved in water and injected, the full antagonistic effect of naloxone occurs. This effect does not occur when the drug is taken orally. In contrast to methadone, buprenorphine is given three times per week.

Psychiatric Treatment and Support Programs

Traditional psychiatric treatment has been relatively ineffective for heroin and other opioid addicts. Therapeutic communities led by health care professionals and ex-addicts appear to be somewhat more effective in treating recently detoxified users. These organizations help restructure the addict's lifestyle and orientation through leadership, group help, and self-help.

controversial. Box 9.6 discusses the treatment of heroin addiction.

Treatment for marijuana abuse consists mainly of nonpharmacologic interventions combined with an exercise program to help deal with withdrawal symptoms and cravings for the drug.

Because no addiction results from LSD or PCP use, no withdrawal syndrome results, and no treatment is required. Treatment for LSD and PCP is necessary only when the user experiences a bad trip. Box 9.7 provides guidelines for intervening on a bad trip.

Treatment for acute inhalant intoxication is similar to that for CNS depressant overdosage. Patients need oxygen and other respiratory assistance. They should not receive any vasopressor therapy, such as injected epinephrine, because the interaction between a vasopressor and an inhalant may trigger serious arrhythmias.

Providing Patient and Family Education

After identifying a substance abuse problem, the nurse intervenes by assisting the patient and family to develop ways to prevent substance abuse, such as communicating and reinforcing healthy coping strategies and stress-reduction behaviors; recognizing the patient's values, beliefs, and support systems; and identifying and encouraging contact with self-help groups, community resources, rehabilitative organizations, and support groups.

BOX 9.7 Intervening on a "Bad Trip"

Nursing interventions for managing the terrifying perceptions and hallucinations or "bad trips" resulting from LSD or PCP use rely on decreasing sensory stimuli and providing comfort and support. Some guidelines follow:

LSD

- Place the patient in a quiet room to decrease sensory stimuli.
- Remain with the patient, and help the patient to calm down by talking to him or her while panic and agitation is at a peak. This approach will help to alleviate fear and anxiety.
- Administer tranquilizers, barbiturates or benzodiazepines, or nicotinic acid as prescribed to counteract the chemical effects of LSD. Do not administer phenothiazines. They may induce hypotension, confusion, and an increased panic reaction because of their influence on the anticholinergic-like effects of LSD.

Ketamine (or PCP)

- Put the patient in a dark, quiet room, and closely observe him or her.
- Avoid verbal communication because any sensory stimuli may cause further reaction and agitation.
- If pharmacologic therapy is prescribed (e.g., benzodiazepines), administer as directed. As with bad LSD trips, phenothiazines should be avoided because of their addictive anticholinergic effects.

The nurse can help family members identify their feelings and responses to the substance abuse problem and cope with these feelings. Family members can be referred to counseling services and emotional support groups. Entry into substance abuse treatment programs is frequently through an evaluation and referral center. This is also an opportune time for the nurse to teach the family more about the hazards of substance abuse. The nurse can also explain that relapses may occur and that support groups (e.g., Alcoholics Anonymous, Alateen, Narcotics Anonymous) exist for helping the patient and family members to deal with relapses and to work through new problems related to recovery and altered relationships. The goal of treatment—longer and longer periods of abstinence and sobriety—is emphasized. Relapse prevention includes teaching patients to identify and manage feelings, recognize high-risk situations, and develop effective coping strategies.

Ongoing Assessment and Evaluation

Health consequences of substance abuse are usually manifested by changes in physiologic and behavioral functioning; therefore, evaluative guidelines related to detoxification, withdrawal, and rehabilitation will correspond to signs that the patient has returned to normal physiologic and psychological functioning.

Nurses and other health care professionals have a community responsibility to provide information about substance abuse. Meeting this responsibility may involve providing information and counseling or referring patients, friends, and neighbors to treatment resources. The nurse should be familiar with the community resources and keep up-to-date on common drug abuse problems and their treatment.

Recovery is lifelong and requires total abstinence from the abused substance. The recovering person can never return to controlled use without rekindling the addiction.

CHAPTER SUMMARY

- Substance abuse is a substantial problem nationwide and worldwide.
- Strong evidence supports a dopamine hypothesis of drug abuse and addiction and a biologically inherited tendency toward alcoholism.
- Drug abuse is a complex biopsychosocial problem that does not lend itself to simple solutions.
- Characteristics of drug abuse include tolerance, physical dependence, and psychological dependence.
- Drugs of abuse are categorized as CNS stimulants, CNS depressants, hallucinogens, cannabis, and miscellaneous drugs.
- The most commonly abused drugs are alcohol, cocaine, heroin, marijuana, caffeine, and nicotine.
- The nurse's role in substance abuse involves understanding core drug knowledge related to specific drugs, preventing abuse, assessing potential or actual abuse, and formulating nursing diagnoses related to the assessment findings.
- The nurse is pivotal in maximizing recovery, minimizing relapse, and providing patient and family education.

QUESTIONS FOR STUDY AND REVIEW

1. What adverse effects can occur if alcohol is taken concurrently with barbiturates, benzodiazepines, or other CNS depressants?
2. Define the following: drug abuse, drug misuse, addiction, physical dependence, and psychological dependence.
3. Explain the use of disulfiram (Antabuse).
4. What factors place an individual at high risk for substance abuse?
5. Methadone maintenance for opioid addiction is controversial. Why is this so?
6. Describe nursing interventions for an individual experiencing a hallucinogenic "bad trip."
7. Name several drugs that are frequently associated with abuse, and propose some reasons that they are abused.

Need More Help?

Chapter 9 of the study guide for *Drug Therapy in Nursing* 2e contains NCLEX-style questions and other learning activities to reinforce your understanding of the concepts presented in this chapter. For additional information or to purchase the study guide, visit *http://connection.lww.com/go/aschenbrenner.*

REFERENCES AND BIBLIOGRAPHY

Ahmadi, J., Toobaee, S., Kharras, M., et al. (2003). Psychiatric disorders in opioid dependents. *Journal of Social Psychiatry, 49*(3), 185–191.

American Academy of Child and Adolescent Psychiatry. (1999). Children of alcoholics [Online]. Available: *http://www.aacap.org/publications/factsfam/alcoholc.htm.*

Anderson, C. E., & Loomis, G. A. (2003). Recognition and prevention of inhalant abuse. *American Family Physician, 68*(5), 869–874.

Conners, N. A., Bradley, R. H., Mansell, L. W., et al. (2003). Children of mothers with serious substance abuse problems: An accumulation of risks. *American Journal of Drug and Alcohol Abuse, 29*(4), 743–758.

Jacob, T., Waterman, B., Heath, A., et al. (2003). Genetic and environmental effects on offspring alcoholism: New insights using an offspring-of-twins design. *Archives of General Psychiatry, 60*(12), 1265–1272.

Johnson, M. K., Smith, R. P., Morrison, D., et al. (2000). Large lung bullae in marijuana smokers. *Thorax, 55*(44), 340–342.

Langbehn, D. R., Cadoret, R. J., Caspers, K., et al. (2003). Genetic and environmental risk factors for the onset of drug use and problems in adoptees. *Drug and Alcohol Dependence, 69*(2), 151–167.

Longo, D. L., Kasper, D. L., & Isselbacheter, K. J. (Eds.). (1999). Harrison's online. New York: McGraw-Hill.

Monahan, G. (2003). Drug use/misuse among health professionals. *Substance Use and Misuse, 38*(11–13), 1877–1881.

National Association for Children of Alcoholics. (1998). Children of alcoholics: Important facts [Online]. Available: *http://www.nacoa.net/impfacts.htm.*

Rudgley, R. (1998). The encyclopedia of psychoactive drugs. New York: St. Martin's Press.

Trull, T. J., Waudby, C. J., & Sher, K. J. (2004). Alcohol, tobacco, and drug use disorders and personality disorder symptoms. *Experimental and Clinical Psychopharmacology, 12*(1), 65–75.

United States Drug Enforcement Administration. (2003). Drug descriptions [Online]. Available: *http://www.usdoj.gov/dea/concern/concern.htm.*

Lifestyle, Diet, and Habits: Nutrition and Complementary Medications

chapter 10

Learning Objectives

At the completion of this chapter the student will:

1. Discuss the role of nutrition in health maintenance.
2. Identify common nutritional factors affecting drug efficacy.
3. Identify common ways that drug therapy may alter nutritional status.
4. Differentiate prescribed uses of vitamins and herbal and botanical preparations from nonprescribed uses.
5. Identify core patient variables that increase the risk for the occurrence of drug–nutrient interactions.
6. Identify key aspects of nursing management to maximize therapeutic effect and minimize adverse effects from drug interactions with diet, diet supplements, and herbal and botanical preparations.

KEY TERMS

alternative therapy
botanical preparations
complementary therapy
herbal preparations
mineral cations
phytomedicinals
trace elements
vitamins

FEATURED WEBLINK

http://www.eatright.org/Public/
Staying healthy requires good nutrition. The website of the American Dietetic Association provides comprehensive nutrition information.

CONNECTION WEBLINK

Additional Weblinks are found on Connection:
http://www.connection.lww.com/go/aschenbrenner.

The core patient variable of lifestyle, diet, and habits represents the way a person lives his or her life and the choices he or she makes to accept or reject behaviors that influence health. In drug therapy, this variable is assessed according to how these factors interact with the prescribed drug therapy. Chapter 9 examined an unhealthy lifestyle choice (the use and abuse of substances) and its relation to drug therapy. This chapter focuses on normal dietary habits, including the use of herbal, botanical, and nutritional supplements.

The core patient variable of diet interacts with the patient's health in several ways. First, a well-balanced diet may prevent chronic illness and therefore indirectly decrease the need for drug therapy. Additionally, a well-balanced diet influences the pharmacokinetics of many drugs. Second, the nutritional status of a patient can be altered by a chronic disease or as an adverse effect of drug therapy. Nutritional supplements and herbal or botanical preparations may also be taken to increase wellness or to meet normal nutritional needs. Lastly, certain foods, beverages, dietary supplements, and herbal or botanical preparations can affect the absorption and effectiveness of some drugs or produce an adverse effect. These points are discussed in this chapter.

DIETARY FACTORS AFFECTING DRUG EFFICACY

Health status in general has a nutritional base. A proper well-balanced diet provides a healthy person with an adequate supply of nutrients. Predicted drug response in the body is based on the ideal of a body that has the normal balance of elements, including dietary factors. When dietary factors are altered, drug therapy may produce different effects in the body than would normally occur.

Several factors related to malnutrition are believed to alter drug disposition. Box 10.1 describes various pharmacokinetic and nutrient interactions. Protein levels are one important factor. Diminished protein status results in lower amounts of plasma proteins and can substantially increase the concentration of free drug available. Because only free drug is active, this increase in free drug increases the drug's pharmacologic effect and the risk for adverse effects. Adequate protein levels are especially important for drugs that are normally highly protein bound. As explained in Chapter 4, albumin is the most important protein, in terms of drug action, because most protein binding by drugs occurs with albumin molecules. Drug binding to albumin is also affected by high-fat meals and fasting. Both of these situations lead to high serum levels of free fatty acids that compete with the drug for albumin-binding sites. Additionally, a diet poor in proteins may inhibit the biotransformation of drugs because protein deficiency may make drug-metabolizing systems less effective.

Malnourished individuals exhibit decreased oxidative metabolism and reduced glomerular filtration rate, potentially increasing blood concentrations of the drug or an active metabolite. This nutritional state increases the effect of the drug and the potential for adverse effects.

Dietary factors that promote obesity have an indirect effect on drug therapy. Body composition is an important consideration in determining drug response. For example, distribution of fat-soluble drugs is increased in obese and the elderly people because of the increased proportion of adipose tissue to lean body mass.

Excessive intake of vitamins may also adversely affect the action of some drugs. For example, increased pyridoxine intake may adversely affect the therapeutic effect of levodopa by increasing its metabolism. Increased or decreased intake of some elements may alter the absorption or reabsorption of a drug. For example, changes in the dietary intake of sodium will alter the reabsorption of lithium in the renal tubule. Sig-

BOX 10.1 Pharmacokinetic and Nutrient Interactions

Absorption

- Changing the acidity of the digestive tract e.g., rapid-acting carbohydrates, (such as candy, causing sustained- or timed-release medication to dissolve too quickly)
- Stimulating secretion of digestive enzymes (e.g., griseofulvin is absorbed better when taken with foods—especially fat—that stimulate the release of digestive enzymes)
- Altering the rate of absorption (e.g., acidic foods and beverages interfere with nicotine absorption from nicotine gum used for smoking cessation; aspirin is more slowly absorbed when taken with food)
- Binding to drugs (e.g., calcium binds to tetracycline, limiting drug absorption)
- Competing for absorption sites in the intestines (e.g., dietary amino acids interfere with levodopa absorption)

Distribution

- Changing binding of drug allows more free drug in bloodstream (low protein)

Metabolism

- Acting as structural analogues (e.g., anticoagulants and vitamin K)
- Competition for metabolic enzyme systems (e.g., phenobarbital and folate)
- Altering enzyme activity and contributing pharmacologically active substances (e.g., monoamine-oxidase inhibitors and tyramine)

Excretion

- Changing the acidity of the urine (e.g., vitamin C can alter urinary pH and limit the excretion of aspirin)

CRITICAL THINKING SCENARIO

Malnutrition and drug action

Larry Willis, a 35-year-old homeless man, is brought to the emergency department by the police, who found him collapsed and having a seizure on the street. He is malnourished. He is admitted to the hospital and started on a standard dose of phenytoin, a drug used to prevent seizures in epilepsy, which is a highly protein-bound drug. He is showing signs of adverse effects from the phenytoin.

Use your knowledge of the effect of diet on drug actions to determine why this man is having adverse effects.

nificant decreases in dietary sodium will result in extra lithium being reabsorbed, higher circulating levels of lithium, and potential drug toxicity from elevated lithium levels.

Food and nutrient intake can affect drug excretion by changing the urinary pH. For example, acidic drugs are more rapidly excreted in alkaline urine. A diet rich in meat or in vegetables may also influence the urine pH—either acidic or basic—and in this way the renal excretion of drugs may be changed considerably because drugs are generally either weak organic acid or bases. Conversely, drugs may also interfere with the availability and use of certain nutrients (e.g., vitamins, electrolytes, or trace elements); this interaction may occur with the long-term administration of certain drugs (e.g., antibiotics, oral contraceptives, anticonvulsants, laxatives) or the chronic consumption of alcohol. Deficiency of certain nutritional factors or even diseases may be the consequence of such interactions.

A particular food, or the manner in which food is prepared, can also affect drug disposition. For example, grapefruit juice is a potent inhibitor of the intestinal cytochrome P-450 3A4 system (specifically, CYP3A4-mediated drug metabolism), which is responsible for the first-pass metabolism of many medications. This interaction can lead to increases in bioavailability and corresponding increases in serum drug levels. Table 10.1 describes drugs that interact with grapefruit or its juices. Cruciferous vegetables (broccoli, brussel sprouts,

TABLE 10.1 Drugs That Interact With Grapefruit or Its Juices

Class	Interaction
Antihistamines	
Terfenadine	Potential for fatal cardiac dysrhythmias
Fexofenadine	Decreased efficacy of fexofenadine
Antianxiety drugs	Increased serum concentration; sedation
Alprazolam	
Buspirone	
Diazepam	
Midazolam (oral)	
Triazolam	
Antihypertensive drugs	
Eplerenone	Decreased metabolism
Calcium-channel blocking agents	Increased bioavailability Tachycardia Profound hypotension
Anti-infective drugs	
Albendazole	Increased bioavailability
Halofantrine	Decreased metabolism
Praziquantel	Increased serum concentration
Voriconazole	Increased serum concentration
Antiretroviral drugs	Increased serum concentration
Amprenavir	
Atazanavir	
Indinavir	
Fosamprenavir	
Saquinavir	
Antiseizure drugs	
Carbamazepine	Increased serum concentration
Zonisamide	Decreased metabolism
Cardiac drugs	
Amiodarone	Potential drug accumulation
Dofetilide	Decreased metabolism
Quinidine	Inhibits conversion to major metabolite
Cholesterol-lowering drugs	Increased risk for myopathy and rhabdomyolysis
Atorvastatin	
Cerivastatin	
Lovastatin	
Simvastatin	
Corticosteroids	
Budesonide	Increased bioavailability
Methylprednisolone	Increased effects

(continued)

TABLE 10.1 Drugs That Interact With Grapefruit or Its Juices (continued)

Class	Interaction
Erectile dysfunction drugs	Decreased metabolism
Sildenafil	
Tadalafil	
Vardenafil	
Ergotamine derivatives	Decreased metabolism
Estrogens	Decreased metabolism
Immunosuppressants	Increased bioavailability
Cyclosporine	Risk for toxicity
Sirolimus	
Tacrolimus	
Opiates	
Buprenorphine	Decreased metabolism
Methadone	Increased serum concentration
Psychiatric drugs	
Escitalopram	Increased serum concentration
Pimozide	Increased risk for toxicity
Sertraline	Decreased metabolism
Miscellaneous	Decreased acetaminophen-induced hepatotoxicity
Acetaminophen	
Dextromethorphan	Increased bioavailability
Caffeine	Increased clinical effects and duration
Cilostazol	Unknown
Cinacalcet	Increased serum concentration
Modafinial	Decreased metabolism
Sibutramine	Unknown
Tolterodine	Decreased metabolism

cabbage, cauliflower, rutabaga, turnips, kohlrabi, and kale as well as greens such as mustard and collards) markedly induce chemical oxidations when added to the diet and increase drug metabolism. The polycyclic hydrocarbons—similar to those found in cigarette smoke—generated from charcoal broiling of foods may increase drug metabolism. As you remember, inducing drug metabolism results in a lower serum concentration (or a subtherapeutic level) of the drug.

Finally, the time that food and beverages are consumed, in relation to the time drug therapy is taken, may alter the effectiveness of the drug therapy. Some drugs must be taken on an empty stomach to promote absorption; some drugs bind with certain types of foods, which prevents drug absorption; and some drugs must be taken with food for best results.

DRUG THERAPY AND NUTRITIONAL STATUS

Drugs potentially affect the status of almost every nutrient. Particularly important to consider are vitamin A and the B vitamins folate and pyridoxine because intake of these vitamins is often marginal and many commonly used drugs affect them. Some drugs affect nutrient metabolism and excretion by an "antivitamin" process. They inhibit the synthesis of specific enzymes by competing for the vitamins or vitamin metabolites necessary to their structure. For example, the antineoplastic drug methotrexate is a folic acid antagonist. Without folic acid, synthesis of deoxyribonucleic acid (DNA) is inhibited, cell replication ceases, and cell death results. A drug may also form a complex with a nutrient, thereby making it unavailable for use by the body. For example, the antituberculosis drug isoniazid forms a complex with pyridoxine, interfering with its metabolism and resulting in vitamin B_6 deficiency.

Other "antivitamin" drugs include hydralazine and L-dopa (which affect levels of vitamin B_6) and the coumarin anticoagulants (which block the action of vitamin K to prolong bleeding time).

Some commonly used drugs have nutrition-related actions. For example, chronic phenytoin therapy is associated with folate deficiency and megaloblastic anemia. Folic acid and phenytoin are structurally similar and are thought to compete with each other for the same surface receptors. Diuretic drugs increase the excretion of nutrients by interfering with reabsorption in the renal tubules. Chronic use may result in depletion of potassium, magnesium, and zinc because renal excretion of these minerals is increased.

COMPLEMENTARY NUTRITIONAL THERAPIES

The use of nutritional supplements and herbal and botanical preparations is often considered an **alternative therapy** for health. Although these choices have been traditional in

some non-Western cultures, they are now being used more frequently in Western cultures, where they have come to be viewed less as alternative practices to Western medicine and more as augmentations or supplements to health care. The term **complementary therapy** is now often used for these choices. Complementary nutritional therapies include supplements of basic food elements, vitamins, and minerals, as well as the use of herbs and botanicals.

Nutritional Supplements

If patients do not have enough of a nutrient, oral supplements of that nutrient may be prescribed as adjuncts to drug therapy.

Protein

Protein, which provides 4 kcal/g, is one of the most important and abundant substrates in the body. The body may draw on dietary or tissue protein to obtain needed energy when the supply from carbohydrates and fats is inadequate. Proteins are polymers of essential amino acids, nonessential amino acids, or both. Although animal proteins generally contain sufficient essential amino acids, many plant proteins do not, and vegetarians may not eat a wide enough variety of plants to ensure an adequate supply. Quality protein should provide approximately 15% to 20% of a healthy person's well-balanced diet.

Individuals wishing to build muscle mass may take amino acid supplements and eat excess protein in the belief that increased protein intake facilitates the deposition of protein into muscles. Ingested amounts exceeding those needed to replace body losses, however, are simply converted into fat and stored. Some amino acids (e.g., L-carnitine) have gained popularity as preventive or therapeutic agents and are taken as dietary supplements. Their use may be hazardous in that there may be competition for transport with other amino acids into cells or the central nervous system (CNS). The research supporting their use is nonexistent or considered marginal by many nutritional experts. Supplements containing the essential amino acids lysine and arginine, promoted as regulators of body composition and muscle growth because these amino acids stimulate growth hormone secretion, have been proved clinically to lack these effects. Tryptophan has been used to enhance brain serotonin concentrations as a sleep inducer and in conjunction with weight-loss regimens.

Carbohydrates

Carbohydrates—especially sugars and starches—are the most common dietary component; they provide 4 kcal/g and constitute the body's primary source of fuel for heat and energy. A well-balanced diet for a healthy person supplies approximately 50% to 60% of the total kilocalories from carbohydrates. Simple sugars (e.g., fructose, sucrose), refined sugars used primarily in soft drinks and baked goods, may cause an increase in serum insulin and triglyceride concentrations because they are absorbed rapidly. Conversely, starches are complex carbohydrates that must be digested; thus, absorption of glucose is slower, and serum levels of glucose, insulin, and triglycerides remain more stable. Complex carbohydrates are useful adjuncts to drug therapy for patients with diabetes mellitus (both types 1 and type 2) and for patients with atherosclerotic vascular disease or hyperlipidemia.

Fat

Dietary fats from animal and plant sources provide the body's alternate or storage form of heat and energy. Fat—a more concentrated fuel—supplies 9 kcal/g. Fat should supply no more than 25% to 30% of the total intake of a well-balanced diet in a healthy person. Triglycerides are the predominant dietary lipids. Other important natural and dietary lipids include cholesterol and its esters and phospholipids. Cholesterol is an important component of cell membranes and a precursor of steroid hormones. Phospholipids, like cholesterol, are important components of cellular membranes and intracellular organelles. Although the body is able to synthesize adequate amounts of phospholipids, phospholipid compounds are marketed over the counter as health aids (e.g., lecithin) for treating or preventing aging, cancer, heart disease, obesity, and other conditions. Data to support these claims are limited or nonexistent.

Essential fatty acids—linolenic acids (omega-3; derived from corn, peanuts, soybeans) and linoleic acids (omega-6; derived from halibut, salmon)—must be supplied in the diet. Patients who are receiving all of their nutrition parenterally need to have fats administered to meet all their nutritional needs.

Dietary Fiber

Dietary fiber—a group of plant substances resistant to human digestion—is categorized by the food industry as soluble (dissolves in neutral or acid detergent) or insoluble (does not dissolve). Important characteristics of fiber are its water retention ability, cation exchange properties, and antioxidant actions. Fiber added to the diet may be recommended to treat or prevent constipation, which can be an adverse effect of some drug therapies. If the patient cannot consume sufficient oral dietary fiber, drug therapies of bulk-producing laxatives, such as psyllium, may be prescribed.

Vitamins

Vitamins are a chemically diverse group of organic compounds needed by the body to maintain health by regulating metabolism and assisting in the biochemistry of food digestion as cofactors for enzymes. Small quantities of each necessary vitamin must be obtained exogenously, either because the vitamin cannot be synthesized in humans or because its rate of synthesis is too slow to produce sufficient quantities. The Food and Drug Administration considers nearly all vitamin products to be dietary supplements, and they are controlled by the Dietary Health and Supplement Education Act. Vitamins are generally classified as water soluble or lipid soluble. There are 13 vitamins—A, D, E, K (lipid soluble), vitamin C, and 8 B-complex vitamins (water soluble). Water-soluble vitamins are stored in the body only to a limited extent, and frequent consumption of these compounds is needed to maintain adequate body levels. Conversely, lipid-soluble vitamins are maintained in the body much longer, do not require such frequent ingestion, and have a greater potential for toxicity if taken in excess.

Recommended dietary allowances (RDAs), established by the federal government, were designed to serve as dietary guidelines based on the idea that people would obtain essential and nonessential nutrients from a variety of foodstuffs. However, the eating habits of people vary widely. Therefore, a major industry supplying vitamin and mineral products

has developed, which focuses on these "missing" nutrients. Vitamins may be prescribed when general nutritional status is poor, oral intake is insufficient, or the body has additional demands for a vitamin, such as vitamin C to promote wound healing. Vitamin supplements may also be prescribed to correct for general malnutrition to achieve optimal health or to maximize the therapeutic effects and minimize the adverse effects from drug therapy. When vitamins and minerals are taken in excess, potential adverse effects may occur. At the same time, many drugs can contribute to the deficiency of many vitamins. Table 10.2 presents selected vitamins and possible drug interactions.

Minerals

MAJOR MINERAL CATIONS

Major **mineral cations** include calcium, magnesium, potassium, and sodium. Their movement across cell membranes is highly regulated; they function in energy metabolism, membrane transport, and maintenance of membrane potential.

Potassium is the principal intracellular cation in body tissues. It has an important role in many physiologic processes, including transmission of nerve impulses; contraction of cardiac, skeletal, and smooth muscle; acid-base balance; and maintenance of normal renal function. Sodium functions to maintain the body's balance of calcium and potassium. It has an important effect in cardiac function, regulating osmotic pressure in the cells and fluids, acting as an ion balance in the tissues, producing a buffering action in the blood, and guarding against excessive loss of water from the tissues. No RDA for potassium and sodium has been established. Calcium is a critical component of the skeleton and is vital to neuromuscular transmission, cellular signaling, and blood clotting. The adult RDA is 800 mg. Menopausal women especially at risk for osteoporosis are recommended to consume 1,500 mg daily. Magnesium is involved in a great number of enzymatic reactions. Deficiency produces osteomalacia, neuromuscular disorders, seizures, and cardiac dysrhythmias. The adult RDA is 280 to 350 mg daily. Excess magnesium may cause CNS changes, hypotension, and cardiac toxicity including cardiac arrest.

If a patient is severely deficient in one or more of these electrolytes, intravenous (IV) replacement is used to prevent serious complications, and oral replacements may be ordered to treat less severe deficits. Electrolyte imbalances may increase the risk for adverse effects from some drug therapies. They may also occur as an adverse effect resulting from some drug therapies. Supplements are often used as adjuncts to

TABLE 10.2 Selected Vitamins and Possible Drug Interactions

Vitamin	Possible Drug Interaction
Vitamin B_1 (thiamin)	Aspirin, antibiotics, antacids, caffeine, diuretics, estrogens, and sulfa drugs contribute to vitamin B_1 deficiency.
Vitamin B_2 (riboflavin)	Antibiotics, antidepressants and oral contraceptives contribute to vitamin B_2 deficiency.
Vitamin B_3 (niacin)	Increased niacin may exacerbate symptoms in patients with peptic ulcers, gout, glaucoma, diabetes mellitus, and liver dysfunction. Aspirin, oral contraceptives, estrogens and sleeping medications contribute to vitamin B_3 deficiency.
Vitamin B_5 (pantothenic acid)	Aspirin, diuretics, antibiotics, antacids, and sleeping medications contribute to vitamin B_5 deficiency.
Vitamin B_6 (pyridoxine)	Pyridoxine accelerates the peripheral conversion of levodopa into dopamine, thus decreasing the amount of levodopa that is available to cross into the CNS. Antidepressants, antacids, amphetamines, oral contraceptives, estrogens, diuretics, and some antibiotics contribute to vitamin B_6 deficiency.
Vitamin B_7 (biotin)	Antibiotics and sulfa drugs may inhibit the bacteria responsible for the formation of vitamin B_7.
Vitamin B_{12} (cobalamin)	Laxatives, antacids or proton pump inhibitors, aminoglycoside antibiotics, sulfonylureas, oral contraceptives, and colchicine contribute to vitamin B_{12} deficiency.
Vitamin M (folic acid)	Increased folic acid changes the function of anticonvulsants. Oral contraceptives, aspirin, PSIs, sulfa antibiotics, sulfonylureas, and anticonvulsants contribute to folic acid deficiency.
Vitamin C (ascorbic acid)	Antacids, alcohol, antidepressants, oral contraceptives, PSIs, and steroids contribute to ascorbic acid deficiency.
Vitamin A (palmitate)	Chronic use of lubricant laxatives or bile acid sequestrants may cause vitamin A deficiency.
Vitamin D (calciferol)	Laxatives, bile acid sequestrants, antituberculosis agents, and use of sun-blocking agents contribute to vitamin D deficiency.
Vitamin E (tocopherol)	Bile acid sequestrants, oral contraceptives, antituberculosis agents, and estrogens contribute to vitamin E deficiency.
Vitamin K (menadione)	Increased vitamin K levels decrease the anticoagulant effect of warfarin. Chronic antibiotic use decreases vitamin K by interfering with the bacteria that produces it. Bile acid sequestrants may contribute to vitamin K deficiency.

PSI, prostaglandin synthetase inhibitor.

drug therapy for these reasons. Table 10.3 describes potential drug interactions with electrolytes and minerals.

Trace Elements

There are a number of essential **trace elements,** also known as microminerals. The most important of these include chromium, copper, iron, selenium, and zinc. Trace elements are present in minute amounts in body tissues and are essential to optimal growth, health, and development. Seafood is usually rich in nearly all micronutrients except manganese, which is readily available from plant sources.

Chromium improves insulin action, and a deficiency may cause elevated levels of blood sugar, cholesterol, and triglycerides. Copper is used in making blood cells and is active in the metabolism of iron. Copper-containing enzymes are involved in immune functions. Severe illness, high-dose zinc supplementation, and antacids can reduce absorption of copper. Supplementation may be necessary with zidovudine treatment (because zidovudine reduces copper levels) and with total parenteral nutrition.

Iron is an essential nutrient. It is needed to make red blood cells; deficiency results in anemia. Iron participates in oxidation and reduction reactions. It must be tightly bound to serum proteins to prevent potentially destructive oxidant effects. Bound to serum proteins, it is first stored and then distributed throughout the body.

Selenium is an especially important antioxidant. Its levels correlate with immune function—specifically, albumin levels, lean body mass, and total lymphocyte count. Deficiency occurs in infection and increased metabolic rates. Deficiency is also associated with heart disease and anemia. Zinc is absorbed in the small intestine; high-fiber diets limit its absorption. Zinc promotes wound healing and functions in antibody production. Deficiency impairs protein metabolism and the immune response.

The trace minerals may be administered if dietary intake is low or the patient is malnourished. They are usually included in a multivitamin formula. Correction of generalized malnourishment is often an adjunct to drug therapy to achieve maximum therapeutic effect from the drug or to prevent adverse effects from drug therapy.

Herbal and Botanical Preparations

Herbal preparations and **botanical preparations** are those substances derived from a plant source and used as a dietary supplement or as a medication. Although herbal and botanical preparations have been traditional in some non-Western cultures, they are now being used more frequently in Western cultures as augmentations or supplements to health care. To illustrate this point, recent Gallup surveys report more than 28 million Americans taking one or more herbal supplements. This revival of interest in herbal, botanical, and dietary supplements in the United States during the past two decades can be attributed to an aging population with a large number of chronic diseases. Many of these diseases have no satisfactory conventional medical treatments, or the conventional treatment for them involves severely limiting adverse effects. Interest can also be attributed to a pervasive "back to nature" movement in a society increasingly attracted to good nutrition, exercise, and preventive health care as a means of remaining young and active.

Plants have historically been used for medicinal purposes. Many drugs used today are derived from plants. Therapeutic agents derived from plants or the preparations made from them are called **phytomedicinals.** Aspirin, for example, comes from the bark of the willow tree, and digoxin is derived from digitalis or purple foxglove. Today, many herbs and other plant substances are being sold over the counter. Many of the most popular herbal, botanical, and dietary preparations are marketed as a means of preventing aging-associated disorders, providing energy enhancement and a feeling of well-being, and assisting with weight loss; they are also sold for more traditional therapeutic uses. Regulation of these products may be limited because they are considered food sources rather than drug therapies. The bioavailability, or activity, of a preparation may vary widely between manufacturers. Consumers tend to think of these substances as harmless because

TABLE 10.3 Potential Drug Interactions With Electrolytes and Minerals

Drug	Electrolytes and Minerals
Antacids	Potassium, calcium, copper, iron, magnesium, zinc
Antigout; colchicine	Sodium
ACE inhibitors	Potassium, zinc
Antibiotics	
Aminoglycoside antibiotics	Iron, magnesium, nitrogen, potassium, sodium
Tetracycline	Calcium, magnesium, zinc
Antituberculosis agent: isoniazid	Calcium
Anti-inflammatory agents: ASA, PSIs	Iron, zinc
Antisecretory agent: omeprazole	Calcium, magnesium
Beta-adrenergic blocking agents	Potassium, calcium, magnesium
Corticosteroids	Calcium, potassium, selenium, zinc
Diuretics	Potassium, sodium, magnesium, zinc
Thyroid replacement	Calcium

ACE, angiotensin-converting enzyme; ASA, acetylsalicylic acid; PSI, prostaglandin synthetase inhibitor.

they are sold over the counter. In actuality, they, like prescription drugs, can cause substantial adverse effects. Box 10.2 describes some of these adverse effects. Furthermore, herbs may interact with prescribed drugs in ways that affect their therapeutic response. Table 10.4 presents selected herbs and possible drug interactions.

Because of the increased over-the-counter use of herbs and botanicals, Western medicine has recently examined many of these substances in clinical studies. Some findings support using these substances to treat or manage disease or altered physiology. For example, a health care provider may prescribe an herb such as St. John's wort for depression or saw palmetto for benign prostatic hypertrophy.

NURSING MANAGEMENT OF THE PATIENT WITH DIETARY CONSIDERATIONS

Assessment of Relevant Core Patient Variables

Abnormal dietary intake and the use of herbs and nutritional supplements may have a bearing on drug therapy; therefore, the nurse questions the patient during an initial drug assessment to uncover relevant information. If the

BOX 10.2 Herbal and Botanical Preparations and Potential Adverse Effects

Borage: possible hepatotoxicity from toxic alkaloids
Calamus: nephrotoxicity and seizures
Chaparral: acute hepatitis, hepatic failure, and renal failure
Coltsfoot: hepatotoxicity, photosensitivity, and possible carcinogenicity
Comfrey: hepatotoxicity, possible carcinogenicity
Ephedra/ephedrine (*ma huang*): arrhythmias, cerebrovascular accident, heart failure, hypertension, myocardial infarction, nephrolithiasis, psychosis, and seizures
Germander: hepatitis and hepatic cell necrosis
Hemlock: seizures and respiratory failure
Kava: oculogyric crisis and exacerbation of Parkinson disease
Life root: venoocclusive disease
Lily of the valley: digitalis-like toxicity
Pennyroyal: abortifacient and hepatic failure
Sassafras: hallucinations, hepatotoxicity, and possible carcinogenic activity
Senna: syncope, loss of bowel function and death from cardiac dysrhythmias
Willowbark: Reye syndrome

TABLE 10.4 Selected Herbs and Possible Drug Interactions

Herb	Possible Drug Interactions
Bromelain	Increases the risk for bleeding with anticoagulants
	Increases the effects of antibiotics
Chamomile	Increases the risk for bleeding with anticoagulants
Cranberry	Decreases the elimination of many renally excreted drugs
Echinacea	May interfere with or counteract immunosuppressant therapy
Ephedrine (ma huang)	May increase CNS stimulation and adverse effects from caffeine, decongestants, sympathomimetics, bronchodilators, and CNS stimulants
Evening primrose	May interact with antipsychotic agents
	Increases the risk for temporal lobe epilepsy
Garlic	May interfere with hypoglycemic therapy
	May potentiate the antithrombotic effects of anti-inflammatory drugs
	May increase bleeding times with antiplatelet or anticoagulant therapy
Ginger root	High doses may interfere with cardiac, antidiabetic, or anticoagulant therapy
Ginseng	May increase the effect of monoamine oxidase inhibitors, antihypertensives, and hypoglycemics
	May interfere with the action of steroids
	Red ginseng may increase the CNS stimulant effects of coffee or tea
Hawthorn	Can potentiate the cardiac glycoside actions of digitalis
Kava	May intensify the effect of barbiturates and alcohol
Saw palmetto	May change the effects of hormones in oral contraceptives, patches, or hormone replacement therapy
St. John's wort (hypericum)	Serotonin syndrome may occur when used with other serotonergic drugs such as SSRIs, trazodone, tricyclic antidepressants, or amphetamines
	May produce increased drug effects when given with other antidepressants
Valerian	May potentiate CNS depression from sedatives

SSRI, selective serotonin reuptake inhibitor.

assessment reveals an abnormal dietary intake, such as low protein or malnutrition, the deficiency must be corrected in some way. The nurse determines why the patient is malnourished. Does the patient make poor choices as to what to eat, or is there a lack of money to buy food? Is there insufficient knowledge about what types of food should be in a balanced diet? Is the patient unable to feed himself because of muscle weakness? Is impaired cognition causing the patient to forget to eat? Does the patient have nausea or loss of appetite either from a disease process or as an adverse effect of drug therapy?

To assess the use of herbs and nutritional supplements, the nurse focuses data collection on what substances the patient takes (e.g., drugs, nutritional supplements, herbs, and other preparations); why the patient takes them; which brands are used; and who recommended their use. This information is important and will help the nurse determine whether the desired effect of self-administered drug therapy is based on fact, fad, or tradition.

The nurse also documents the patient's age and life span status because many of these therapies are not recommended for use with children, during pregnancy, or during lactation. The nurse carefully assesses older adults, those who are chronically ill, those with a history of marginal or inadequate nutritional intake, and anyone receiving multidrug therapy over an extended period because such patients are likely to have drug-induced nutritional deficiencies. Because the effects of drug therapy can be altered by specific foods, the time that a patient normally consumes food and beverages before self-administering drug therapy at home should be determined.

Nursing Diagnoses and Outcomes

Nursing diagnoses and outcomes related to nutritional considerations will vary depending on the dietary factor and the drug therapy that the patient is receiving. Some potential general diagnoses include:

- Risk for Injury related to low protein levels and malnutrition
  Desired outcome: *Protein levels and malnutrition will be corrected to prevent adverse effects from drug therapy.*
- Risk for Injury related to adverse effects from excessive use of vitamins or herbs
  Desired outcome: *The patient will not develop any adverse effects while using nutritional supplements.*
- Risk for Injury related to drug interactions of vitamins, herbs, or food intake with prescribed drug therapy
  Desired outcome: *Drug interactions will be prevented while the patient is on drug therapy.*
- Deficient Knowledge related to interactions of vitamins or herbs with drug therapy
  Desired outcome: *The patient will obtain sufficient knowledge to make knowledgeable choices about the use of vitamins and herbs while on drug therapy.*
- Health-Seeking Behaviors related to the use of nutritional supplements
  Desired outcome: *The patient will effectively use nutritional supplements to complement drug therapy to increase health.*

Planning and Intervention

Maximizing Therapeutic Effects and Minimizing Adverse Effects

If the patient has been determined to have low protein levels, the nurse consults with the physician or nurse practitioner about protein replacement. Oral protein supplements or a high-protein diet may be ordered. If levels are substantially below normal, intravenous infusions of albumin may be indicated. If the patient is generally malnourished but eating, a well-balanced diet should be encouraged. The nurse verifies that the patient is capable of feeding himself and offer appropriate assistance if needed. The nurse works with the physician or nurse practitioner to alleviate nausea, vomiting, or loss of appetite related to disease process or drug therapy that prevents sufficient oral intake.

If the patient cannot take in enough food orally, vitamins or other nutritional supplements may be ordered. In some cases, enteral nutrition (i.e., tube feedings) or total parenteral nutrition may be necessary to correct the imbalances.

If the assessment reveals that the patient is at risk for an interaction among a prescribed drug and foods, nutrients, herbs or nutritional supplements, the nurse can discuss with the patient the many ways that these interactions affect nutritional status and drug therapy effectiveness. The nurse may also need to discuss these findings with the prescriber of drug therapy.

Many of the nurse's actions to maximize the therapeutic effect or minimize the adverse effect of drug therapy, in relation to dietary factors, are centered around patient education.

Providing Patient and Family Education

- Teach the patient about the potential interactions of food, nutrients, and complementary nutritional therapies with prescribed drug therapy.
- Emphasize to the patient and family the importance of being well nourished while receiving prescribed drug therapy.
- Teach the patient when to take the prescribed drug in relation to meals if timing is relevant for the particular drug (e.g., should the drug be taken on an empty stomach to promote absorption?).
- Encourage the patient to inform all of his or her health care providers about all dietary supplements used.
- Teach the patient that botanical supplements should be used as treatment for serious health conditions only with the advice and supervision of a qualified health practitioner.
- Instruct the parents of children and pregnant women or breast-feeding mothers not to use botanical products unless advised to do so by a qualified health practitioner, particularly if using these products is associated with toxicity or drug and food interactions.
- Counsel the patient about the variable quality of nutritional products.
- Advise the patient to watch for any unusual reactions to any medication and to report them to the health care provider.

Ongoing Assessment and Evaluation

The nurse assesses for potential drug interactions when a patient is taking any dietary supplement or herbal preparation in addition to prescribed drug therapy. These interactions may reduce the therapeutic effect of the prescribed drug, or cause adverse effects from either the prescribed drug or the supplemental therapy. Drug therapy can be evaluated as effective if dietary factors have not impaired drug action or produced adverse effects. Dietary treatments may be evaluated as effective if they return the patient to a normal physiologic status, or if they work efficiently as adjuncts to drug therapy.

CHAPTER SUMMARY

- Numerous medications and nutrients interact, which can lead to imbalances or interfere with drug effectiveness.
- Supplementary use of vitamins, herbals, and botanicals may be prescribed by a health care provider to meet normal nutritional needs or to treat diseases or pathologies. The use of these nutritional supplements may also be self-prescribed by the patient.
- Foods and nutrients can alter the absorption, distribution, metabolism, and excretion of medications.
- Adverse drug–nutrient interactions are most likely to occur with medications taken for chronic conditions, if several medications are taken, or if nutrition status is poor or deteriorating.
- When assessing for the extent of drug–nutrient interactions, it is important for the nurse to consider the patient's age, drug dose, and duration of therapy with medications known to have an adverse effect on nutrients.
- Patients may not recognize the importance of mentioning their use of dietary supplements or their normal dietary patterns during a drug history. Nurses need to be aware of this lack of awareness and routinely ask patients about this information.

QUESTIONS FOR STUDY AND REVIEW

1. What factors in a patient's drug history suggest a likelihood of drug–nutrient interactions?
2. Describe how drugs and nutrients can interact and alter metabolism.
3. Describe how foods can alter drug absorption.
4. Why is it important for the nurse to routinely assess patients for their use of dietary supplements or herbal preparations?

Need More Help?

Chapter 10 of the study guide for *Drug Therapy in Nursing* 2e contains NCLEX-style questions and other learning activities to reinforce your understanding of the concepts presented in this chapter. For additional information or to purchase the study guide, visit *http://connection.lww.com/go/aschenbrenner.*

REFERENCES AND BIBLIOGRAPHY

Clinical Pharmacology website. Available: *http://cp.gsm.com.*

Gallup Organization website. Available: *http://www.gallup.com.*

Gottesman, M. M. (2003). Healthy eating and activity together (HEAT): Weapons against obesity. *Journal of Pediatric Care, 17*(4), 210–215.

Huang, S. M., Hall, S. D., Watkins, P., et al. (2004). Drug interactions with herbal products and grapefruit juice: A conference report. *Clinical Pharmacology and Therapeutics, 75*(1), 1–12.

Hurst, J. W. (2002). Can fish save us? *Medscape Cardiology, 6*(2). [Online]. Available: *http://www.medscape.com/viewarticle/441945.*

John, J. H., et al. (2002). Effects of fruit and vegetable consumption on plasma antioxidant concentrations and blood pressure: A randomised controlled trial. *Lancet, 359*(9322), 1969–1974.

Physicians Desk Reference. (2002). *The PDR family guide to nutritional supplements: An authoritative A-Z resource on the 100 most popular therapies and nutraceuticals.* New York: Random House.

Willett, W. C. (2002). *Eat, drink, and be healthy: The Harvard Medical School guide to healthy eating.* New York: Simon and Schuster.

Wolinsky, I., & Williams, L. (2003). *Nutrition in pharmacy practice.* Washington, DC: APHA Publications.

Environment: Influences on Drug Therapy

chapter 11

Learning Objectives

At the completion of this chapter the student will:

1. Identify environmental settings appropriate for pharmacotherapy.
2. Identify limitations for drug therapy for each specific environmental setting.
3. Discuss environmental influences on drug stability and effectiveness.
4. Discuss environmental influences on adverse effects of drug therapy.
5. Identify the relationship between environment and occupation.
6. Identify the role of the nurse regarding environmental influences on drug therapy.

KEY TERMS

environment

hepatic drug-metabolizing enzymes

industrial chemicals

pollutants

FEATURED WEBLINK

http://www.hc-sc.gc.ca/english/protection/environment.html
Environment and health have an important relationship with pharmacotherapy. For fact sheets and more information, visit this Weblink.

CONNECTION WEBLINK

Additional Weblinks are found on Connection:
http://www.connection.lww.com/go/aschenbrenner.

The core patient variable of **environment** also is relevant to drug therapy. Three aspects of environment relate to drug administration. The first aspect of environment is the physical setting in which the drug is administered. The second aspect of environment is environmental influences that may affect the stability or efficacy of certain drugs or drug classes. The third aspect of environment is the factors that may increase the risk for adverse effects, injury, or toxicity from drug therapy (Figure 11.1).

These interactions of environment are discussed in this chapter, as is the nurse's role regarding environment and pharmacotherapy.

PHYSICAL SETTINGS FOR DRUG THERAPY

Drug therapy may be administered in a variety of settings. These settings include acute care hospitals, acute rehabilitative units, transitional care units, outpatient units, long-term care facilities, and the home or community environment. Many factors influence whether a particular drug or class of drugs may be administered safely in a specific physical setting.

Acute Care Hospitals

Although most types of drugs are administered in acute care hospitals, certain drugs or drug classes are given in specific areas of these hospitals. For instance, the patient receiving intravenous digoxin (Lanoxin) requires continuous heart monitoring. This requirement necessitates that the drug be administered in a critical care unit, step-down unit, or other specialized area that has both a specially trained nurse and the appropriate equipment to monitor the patient safely.

Surgical patients receive inhaled anesthetics such as tubocurarine (Tubarine) only in the surgical suite where the anesthesiologist or nurse anesthetist monitors the patient. Patients in active labor or immediately after delivery receive drugs such as oxytocin (Pitocin) in the delivery suite or postpartum unit. Alternately, in an emergency, oxytocin may also be administered in the emergency department. Although these drugs are used for totally different medical problems, the common theme is that they require specialized nurses to administer them in a specialized unit of the acute care hospital.

Although most oncology drugs, such as 5-fluorouracil (5-FU), may be given on any medical unit, the administration of these agents is restricted to specially trained nurses. These nurses must understand specifics about handling chemotherapeutic drugs, recognizing and administering rapid

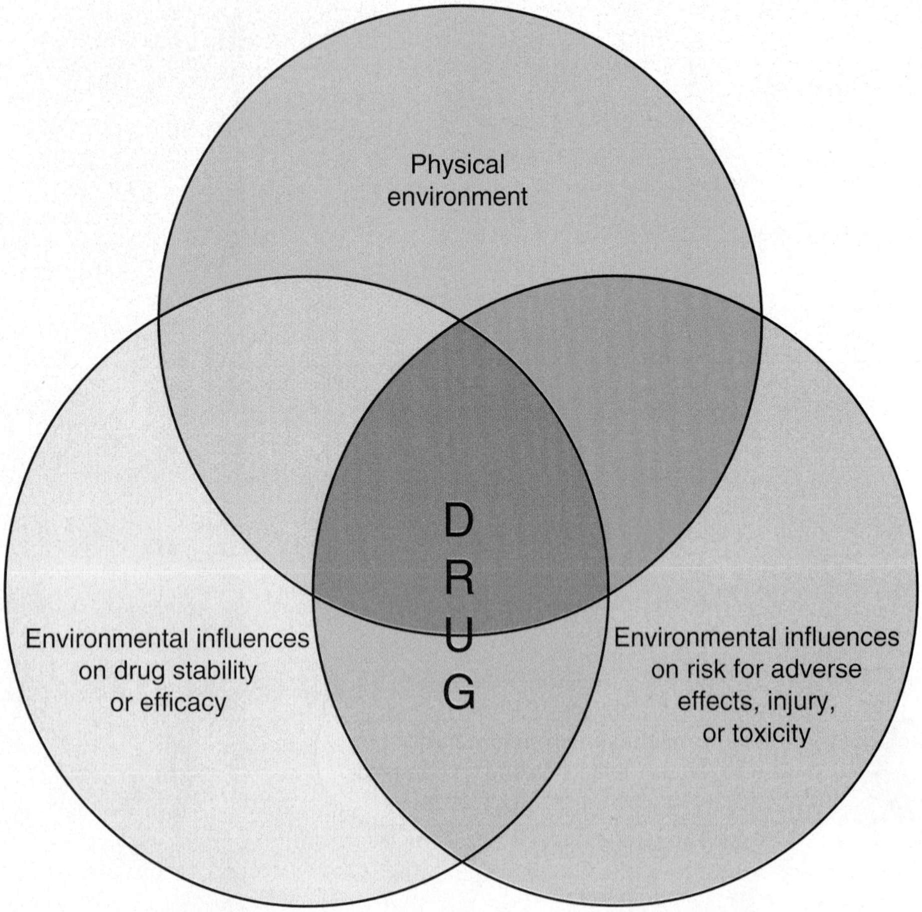

FIGURE 11.1 The physical environment, environmental influences on drug stability or efficacy, and environmental influences that increase the patient's risk for adverse effects, injury, or toxicity intersect to affect the action of the drug.

treatment of severe adverse effects, and properly disposing of oncologic drugs (see Chapter 35).

Acute Rehabilitative Units

Acute rehabilitative units (ARUs) may be located in a portion of the acute care facility or another site off the main campus of the hospital. Although drugs given by most routes, including intravenous (IV) drugs, can be administered on these units, the units are developed to focus on the physical rehabilitation of the patient. Therefore, if the patient needs medication that requires close monitoring, or equipment such as heart monitors, the patient is generally moved back into the acute care hospital.

Transitional Care Units

Transitional care units (TCUs) have been developed to continue care of patients who are well enough to be discharged from the acute care facility but may not be eligible for a long-term facility because they need IV drug therapy or intense physical therapy. Like an ARU, these units may be in a portion of the acute care facility or in a totally different location. Because the patient-to-nurse ratio is higher in the TCU, drug therapy that requires close monitoring or equipment such as heart monitors limits the type of pharmacotherapy administered in this type of unit.

Outpatient Units

In the acute care facility, the term *outpatient* refers to the patient who arrives in the morning for a procedure with the expectation of returning home after the procedure is completed. Occasionally, the patient has a complication that requires that she or he be admitted to the acute care facility after the procedure.

In the community, *outpatient* refers to a patient who receives health care in an environment other than the acute care setting. These environments may include urgent care centers, doctor offices, mental health clinics, or outpatient surgical suites.

Most pharmacotherapy may be administered in outpatient units as long as the individual site has the ability to monitor the patient closely and has life-saving equipment and drugs readily available. In some cases, on-site laboratory testing may also be required. For instance, before administering intramuscular gold salts, a complete blood count and urinalysis must be performed.

Outpatient chemotherapy is done routinely. The limitation in the acute care setting—the need for specialized personnel—is also pertinent in the outpatient setting. Additionally, disposal of chemotherapeutic agents must be addressed carefully in this setting.

Long-Term Care Facilities

Long-term care facilities generally admit patients who do not require intense observation. These patients range from trauma patients to elderly people who will live out the remainder of their lives in the facility. Long-term care facilities may have a very limited scope of care or a much broader scope, depending on the philosophy of the institution. Most facilities are capable of administering IV medications but do not do so if the particular medication also requires special monitoring equipment. Some facilities provide acute long-term care, including the use of ventilators. Medication administration depends on the scope of the individual facility and its ability to monitor patients closely. Additionally, certain drugs also require the ability to intervene with life-saving equipment and drugs.

Home Environment

Most drug routes are safe for administering medication in the home environment. Limiting factors include the need to monitor the patient closely and the need for special monitoring equipment. Although some patients receive pharmacotherapy from a home health nurse, many other patients are taught to self-administer medications, or family members and friends are taught to deliver the drugs safely.

The decision to teach the patient or family to administer drugs is made after a careful evaluation of the home environment by the home health nurse. Assessing the patient's environment may give important clues to its potential influence on therapeutic effectiveness, the patient's adherence to the drug regimen, and the potential risks from drug therapy itself. For example, if a patient is receiving a drug that causes dizziness as an adverse effect, stairs in the home may pose a risk for falls or injury.

General factors to consider in the home include cleanliness; lighting; adequate heat, water, and refrigeration; and walkways in and around the house that are unobstructed and in good repair. The nurse also needs to determine whether the patient lives alone or with other family members or caregivers who can help with the responsibilities of health care and assist with obtaining and administering drug therapy if needed.

The nurse must assess whether the patient has the required financial resources, transportation, and knowledge to obtain the drugs. Additionally, the nurse must assess for the correct equipment for measuring dosages and administration of the drug. Finally, the nurse must assess the patient's ability to monitor therapeutic effects and recognize any adverse drug effects.

ENVIRONMENTAL INFLUENCES ON DRUG STABILITY AND EFFECTS

Many drugs are sensitive to the physical environment. For example, excess heat, light, or moisture or sudden temperature changes can affect the stability of a drug, and many drugs lose their potency when exposed to these elements. Interactions between drugs and the environment may involve storage of the drug or the effect of the environment on the drug's pharmacokinetic and pharmacodynamic processes. The nurse determines where and how the patient's drugs are stored because some individuals do not leave their drugs in the original containers.

The environment can also modify drug effects. For example, temperature affects drug activity. Heat relaxes peripheral vessels, accelerates the circulation, and thus intensifies the actions of some drugs such as vasodilators; cold has the opposite effect—it retards drug action by constricting the blood vessels and slowing circulation. High altitude puts the body under stress, and relative oxygen deprivation at high altitudes

may make some drugs ineffective, whereas it will increase the sensitivity to others, such as alcohol and central nervous system depressants.

In some cases, environmental influences can actually abate the action of certain drugs. For instance, nitroglycerin, a drug used for acute anginal pain, is affected by air, light, and moisture. Because of these environmental interactions, the drug needs to remain in its original container and to be replaced frequently.

Environmental influences can affect pharmacotherapy in any environmental setting, not just the home environment. For instance, some intravenous drugs that are administered in the acute hospital setting, such as nitroprusside and amphotericin-B, must be covered in aluminum foil or with a brown bag during administration to avoid light sensitivity.

ENVIRONMENTAL INFLUENCES ON ADVERSE EFFECTS AND INJURY

Environmental chemicals are increasingly being recognized as agents that cause substantial drug interactions in some individuals. For example, polychlorinated biphenyls (found in industrial solvents or used as flame retardant), polycyclic aromatic hydrocarbons (caused by incomplete combustion of organic materials and found in cigarette smoke), chlorinated hydrocarbons (found in pesticides), and consumption of ethanol are active inducers of **hepatic drug-metabolizing enzymes.** People chronically exposed to these chemicals metabolize some drugs (e.g., cimetidine, theophylline) more rapidly than normal.

A patient's environment may also influence the relationship between physiologic function, drug effects, and adverse effects or injury. Alcohol, tobacco, or pesticides may alter the pharmacokinetics of certain drugs and increase the patient's risk for adverse drug effects. For example, benzodiazepines such as lorazepam (Ativan), in combination with alcohol, may increase the adverse effect of respiratory depression to such an extent that death may occur. Another example is heat and antihypertensive drugs. Almost all of the antihypertensive drugs may cause the adverse effect of orthostatic hypotension. Combine pharmacotherapy for hypertension with a patient who enjoys soaking in a spa or hot tub and the outcome may be syncope. Photosensitivity is another potentially adverse effect that is associated with many different types of drugs. When a patient is taking a drug that causes photosensitivity, the nurse assesses the patient's environment for potential exposure to sunlight and emphasizes ways to minimize this potential adverse effect. Appendix I lists common drugs that may induce photosensitivity.

The role of the home health nurse, described in more detail above, is to assess the physical environment of the patient to determine the limitations for home pharmacotherapy. That assessment should also extend to finding ways to decrease the potential for injury related to pharmacotherapy. For example, many patients receive narcotic analgesics to control pain when they return home. Some of the most frequent adverse effects to narcotic analgesics are sedation and dizziness. The home health nurse identifies potential hazards in the home environment, such as stairs and loose rugs, to teach the patient to avoid these potential hazards when feeling sedated or dizzy.

Simple daily activities may also be affected by environmental influences of pharmacotherapy. For instance, the patient who is a stay-at-home mother may not recognize that the heat of her home can increase the adverse effects of sedation and weakness when taking certain drugs. When she attempts to make dinner, a simple task such as cutting up vegetables may become hazardous.

In the broad context of environmental influences, the patient's occupation must also be considered. Certain types of adverse effects, such as sedation and dizziness, are enhanced by environmental influences and can lead to serious or deadly harm to patients with certain occupations. For instance, sedation or dizziness in a patient who works as a taxicab driver may lead to accident and injury to the patient as well as others in his or her cab. Drugs that cause photosensitivity may actually cause partial-thickness burns to a patient who works as a lifeguard. Before the patient is discharged from the hospital, the nurse evaluates the patient's risk for adverse events based on his or her occupation.

Patients who work in an environment that exposes them to **industrial chemicals** and pesticides have the highest risk for adverse effects and drug toxicity because these environmental **pollutants** affect drug biotransformation. These factors are thought to be responsible for decreased efficacy, prolonged pharmacologic effects, and increased toxicity.

A large number of drugs and chemicals, environmental pollutants, and endogenous substances are extensively metabolized in the liver before being excreted from the body. The environment can influence the metabolism of these substances. A variety of factors in the environment can influence the metabolism of chemicals by CYP450-dependent enzymes. These include concurrent drug treatment, cigarette smoking, and exposure to occupational and environmental pollutants.

THE NURSE'S ROLE

The nurse's role is extending more frequently beyond inpatient hospital settings to homes, schools, and industry. The nurse's role now includes the expanded range of health care concerns of health education, home health care, hospice, and public health because individuals are now being discharged from health care institutions at increasingly early stages in their treatment. Nurses monitor drug response and provide patient education about medication in a variety of patient care environments.

NURSING MANAGEMENT OF THE PATIENT WITH ENVIRONMENTAL CONSIDERATIONS

Assessment

Drug action is not exclusively a biologic phenomenon. Environment is an important determinant of drug response. A number of components of the institutional environment are under the control of nursing. In the hospital, the nurse assesses factors that influence drug outcome, such as a new or strange environment; unfamiliar people, noises, and equipment or procedures; and lack of physical activity. All of these factors may increase the need for some medications, such as analgesics, laxatives, and sedative-hypnotics. For example, providing a quiet, cool environment and reducing

external stimuli to decrease tension and stimulation will enhance the anxiolytic effects of sedative drugs.

Controlling the environment after discharge is a much more difficult task for the nurse. The nurse must determine the environment in which the drug will be administered because drug therapies may occur in multiple environments. For example, patients may start chemotherapy or antidiabetic therapy in one environment, such as the acute care hospital, and continue therapy in the home environment.

Individuals may not realize that environmental factors may affect their prescribed drug therapy. With that possibility in mind and to safeguard the patient, the nurse needs to conduct a complete drug assessment focusing on environmental and occupational influences.

Nursing Diagnoses and Outcomes

- Risk for Injury related to environmental hazards such as falls from stairs or loose rugs
  Desired outcome: *The patient will remain without a fall.*
- Risk for Injury related to decreased drug stability stemming from environmental factors
  Desired outcome: *The patient will store drugs as directed.*
- Impaired Skin Integrity related to environmental exposure to sunlight
  Desired outcome: *The patient will take measures to control the amount of direct sunlight to exposed skin and use sunscreen at all times.*

Planning and Intervention

The planning and intervention phases of the nursing process contain short- and long-term goals. Often, these goals are modified as therapy proceeds. When working with patients to blend the element of environment into a regimen that promotes health maintenance and disease prevention, the nurse's role may be broad and include elements of advocacy, education, referral, consultation, clinical care, management, organization, research, and evaluation. At this stage of the nursing process, however, the nurse's primary role usually focuses on patient education.

The rapport established early in the nurse–patient relationship provides the basis for the trust that is needed as the nurse continues to collaborate with the patient. To maximize the benefits of drug therapy as it is affected or changed by environment, the nurse teaches the patient about safe therapy and promotes collaboration among health care providers and the patient. It may be necessary for the nurse to teach patients how to evaluate their personal and occupational environments for hazardous chemicals and, if appropriate, suggest wearing or using protective equipment. Another aspect of patient education is teaching the patient about the proper way to discard medications. Therapeutic drugs can contaminate the environment through metabolic excretion, improper disposal, or industrial waste.

The extent of teaching will vary, depending on the environment in which the patient will receive the drug (e.g., home, clinic, group home, hospice). Although some education is required whatever the setting, more information is necessary if the patient will be taking the drug at home than if the patient receives the drug in a rehabilitation center or other facility. The patient must be knowledgeable about all aspects of the drug regimen so that it can be self-administered safely and effectively. If another person—a family member or someone else—will be responsible for the patient's drug therapy at home, that person needs to be included in the educational process.

Ongoing Assessment and Evaluation

The nurse evaluates the patient for increased or decreased drug effectiveness related to environmental stimuli. The nurse assesses the patient for signs of adverse effects that may have been induced by environmental factors. The nurse reviews measures to control environmental factors with the patient at each clinic visit.

CHAPTER SUMMARY

- Environmental settings include acute care hospitals, acute rehabilitative units, transitional care units, outpatient units, home, and community.
- Limitations of pharmacotherapy for any setting include need for close monitoring of the patient, need for specialized equipment, need for life-saving equipment and drugs, and need for specialized personnel.
- Environmental influences can affect the stability of a drug.
- Environmental influences can affect the effectiveness of a drug.
- Environmental influences can increase the risk for adverse effects, toxicity, and patient injury.
- Environmental influences can increase the risk for injury in specific occupations.
- The nurse's role is to identify possible environmental influences on pharmacotherapy and institute appropriate patient education.

QUESTIONS FOR STUDY AND REVIEW

1. Identify elements of the environment essential for the nurse to assess regarding drug therapy.
2. How can smoking, alcohol, or environmental chemical exposures influence a patient's drug response?
3. What is the nurse's role in managing the patient with environmental considerations?

? Need More Help?

Chapter 11 of the study guide for *Drug Therapy in Nursing* 2e contains NCLEX-style questions and other learning activities to reinforce your understanding of the concepts presented in this chapter. For additional information or to purchase the study guide, visit *http://connection.lww.com/go/aschenbrenner.*

REFERENCES AND BIBLIOGRAPHY

Hardman, J. G. (2001). *Goodman and Gilman's the pharmacological basis of therapeutics* (10th ed.). New York: McGraw-Hill Health Professions Division.

Katzung, B. C. (2001). *Basic and clinical pharmacology* (8th ed.). New York: McGraw-Hill.

Levine, R. R., Walsh, C. T., & Schwartz-Bloom, R. D. (2004). *Pharmacology: Drug actions and reactions* (7th ed.). New York: Pantheon Publishing Group.

Culture and Inherited Traits: Considerations in Drug Therapy

chapter 12

Learning Objectives

At the completion of this chapter the student will:

1. Identify the influences that culture and ethnicity have on health and illness.
2. Recognize similarities and differences among the five major ethnic groups in the United States.
3. Describe why it is important to assess a patient's culture and inherited traits when managing his or her drug therapy.
4. Describe techniques that can be used in nursing management in drug therapy when working with patients and families of different cultures and ethnicities.
5. Describe how an individual's genetic makeup can alter the pharmacokinetics of a drug.

KEY TERMS

biocultural ecology
cultural blindness
cultural competence
culture
ethnicity
ethnocentrism
pharmacogenetics
pharmacogenomics
stereotyping

FEATURED WEBLINK

http://www.nigms.nih.gov/pharmacogenetics/
This National Institute of Health site has information about clinical research in pharmacogenetics and links to educational literature about genetics and medication selection and genetic causes of diseases.

CONNECTION WEBLINK

Additional Weblinks are found on Connection:
http://www.connection.lww.com/go/aschenbrenner.

North America has been called a "melting pot." A better term of description might be "cultural mosaic," because this term signifies that individuals who emigrate to North America blend into society while retaining their individuality in terms of their culture. **Culture** is the shared customs and traditions, norms and values, institutions, arts, history, and folklore of a group. Similarly, **ethnicity** refers to a group that shares a common cultural heritage and that is linked by race, nationality, or language. An ethnic group is part of a larger social group.

The United States is becoming an increasingly multicultural society. In terms of nursing management and drug therapy, this diversity means that a patient's basic beliefs about health and disease may vary based on his or her cultural heritage. American society is primarily composed of five major ethnic population subgroups: white Americans, black Americans, Asian–Pacific Islander Americans, Hispanic Americans, and Native Americans. Each native and immigrant group has specific cultural attitudes about health, illness, and health care practices. Within each group, cultural attitudes, customs, and values may also vary widely (i.e., not all members of a culture have identical beliefs and practices). Members of minority cultures also tend to assume some or all of the practices and beliefs of the majority. Some aspects of minority cultures also become assimilated into the practices of the majority, producing a blend of cultural beliefs and attitudes.

Nurses today are being challenged to learn more about how cultural differences affect health, influence health-seeking behaviors, influence a patient's adherence or nonadherence to treatment regimens, and alter their responses to drug therapy. Nurses already know that language and economics continue to be the main barriers to appropriate health care for many culturally diverse populations.

As patient populations become more culturally diverse, cultural competence becomes another feature of skillful nursing. **Cultural competence** requires maintaining awareness of one's own values and beliefs without letting them have undue influence on those of other backgrounds, demonstrating knowledge and understanding of another's culture, accepting and respecting cultural differences, and considering a patient's culture carefully.

Nurses must be aware that patients with various cultural and ethnic backgrounds may have beliefs and practices that differ from their own. These beliefs and practices are not wrong or inferior, merely different. Regardless of the patient's ethnicity or cultural background, nurses must be mindful of patients' beliefs and practices and consider them respectfully when managing drug therapy.

Ethnic groups share similarities in biologic and cultural characteristics. The term **biocultural ecology** (Purnell & Paulanka, 2003) refers to specific inherited physical, biologic, and psychological variations in ethnic and racial groups. These variations include skin color; physical body differences; genetic, endemic, and topographic diseases; individual psychological makeup; and biologic differences that affect the ways drugs are metabolized.

Recent pharmaceutical research has revealed that drug metabolism, dosing requirements, therapeutic response, and adverse effects differ among racial and ethnic groups. Additionally, research has found genetic variations within apparently homogeneous populations. For the purposes of this text, the core patient variable of culture and inherited traits is to be interpreted extremely broadly. In this text, the term *culture* refers to religious practices and beliefs, the use of medical or other health practices, and ethnicity—all of which may influence a patient's behavior in health and in illness. *Inherited traits,* or genetic variations, are also part of this core patient variable.

WORLD VIEW

Culture represents a way of perceiving, behaving in, and evaluating the world. A person's cultural identify influences his or her perception of the environment. Beliefs about the causes and effects of illness, health practices, and health-seeking behaviors are all influenced by a person's or group's perception of the environment—their world view. Three kinds of world-view health beliefs have been identified. These perspectives are known as biomedical health beliefs, magicoreligious health beliefs, and holistic health beliefs.

Biomedical Health Beliefs

In general, North Americans describe health from the scientific point of view. Scientific thinking underlies the biomedical view of health, in which life and life processes are controlled by physical and biochemical processes that can be manipulated by humans. For example, specific causes (bacteria, viruses) for an illness can be identified, and a specific treatment (drug therapy, surgery) can be developed to effect a cure.

Magicoreligious Health Beliefs

Predominant themes of magicoreligious health beliefs among some cultural groups focus on the concept of supernatural forces controlling health and illness and on the idea that illnesses are the result of "being bad" or "opposing God's will." Those who subscribe to these views perceive health as a gift from God and illness as an opportunity to realign with God. Prayer to God is used to cope with disease and to seek intervention for healing. Some cultures (e.g., West Indian) believe that magic, voodoo, or a hex or spell by a sorcerer or witch can cause illness. Some Mexican-American and other Latin-American groups believe that illness results from selection by the evil eye, or *mal ojo*. In these cases, the person will seek treatment from a traditional or folk healer, perhaps in addition to scientific therapies. The person's subscription to magicoreligious health beliefs influences his or her approach to health care.

Holistic Health Beliefs

A harmonious balance of the forces of nature is the basis of holistic health beliefs. According to this view, everything in the universe has a place and a function to perform according to natural laws that maintain order. Disturbing these laws creates imbalance, chaos, and disease. Four facets of the individual's nature—physical, mental, emotional, and spiritual—must be in balance and harmony for the individual to be healthy.

Traditional Native-American and Chinese-American cultures have a holistic belief system. Disease occurs when an imbalance exists in the individual's nature. An example of holistic health beliefs among Chinese-American groups is the yin and yang theory of health and illness; among Mexican-American and other Hispanic groups, it is the hot and cold theory of illness. Therapies that may be used to restore a state of balance may include exercise, herbal remedies, meditation, and nutritional or dietary changes.

For example, within the biomedical world view of health, tuberculosis is clearly defined as an infection caused by *Mycobacteria*. According to a holistic world view, however, in which disease results from multiple environmental "hot" interactions, tuberculosis is caused by the interrelationships of poverty, malnutrition, overcrowding, and mycobacteria.

EFFECT OF CULTURAL DIVERSITY ON HEALTH CARE

Purnell's Model for Cultural Competence

To understand any culture thoroughly, examining it with the use of a conceptual framework is helpful. Purnell and Paulanka's evolving model for cultural competence (Purnell & Paulanka, 2003) is an example of a conceptual framework that is geared specifically to health care providers. This model identifies 12 aspects (or domains) of every culture that health care providers should consider. The domains are:

1. Overview (heritage and residence)
2. Communication
3. Family roles and organization
4. Workforce issues
5. Biocultural ecology
6. High-risk health behaviors
7. Nutrition
8. Pregnancy and childbearing practices
9. Death rituals
10. Spirituality
11. Health care practices
12. Health care practitioners

This text does not present comprehensive descriptions of every culture in the United States, nor does it provide instructions for performing a comprehensive cultural assessment. The intention of this text is to provide general knowledge of cultural concerns relevant to nursing management in drug therapy, using a brief description of those factors in the five most common cultures in the United States. Although Purnell and Paulanka's model is evolving, certain domains are easily applicable to nursing management in drug therapy. These aspects are overview (heritage and residence), communication, family roles and organization, spirituality, health care practices, and biocultural ecology.

According to Purnell and Paulanka's model, heritage describes where the people come from, and residence describes where they currently live. Heritage and residence are important factors to consider because they provide clues about potential illnesses or conditions that may be present in the patient and require drug therapy. For example, new immigrants to the United States who have lived in areas where malaria is prevalent (e.g., Egypt, Italy, Turkey, Vietnam) may need to be screened for malaria, and if they test positive, to receive drug treatment. Another example is patients who currently live in crowded, poor urban areas who may need to be screened for tuberculosis.

Communication is an important part of culture for the nurse to assess. Communication includes verbal language (including dominant language; dialects; contextual use of words; and paralanguage variations, such as voice volume, tone, and inflection) and nonverbal language (e.g., eye contact, facial expression, use of touch, and temporality of world view). Temporal relationships are defined according to whether a culture is oriented to the past, present, or future (Purnell & Paulanka, 2003). Past-oriented cultures (e.g., German) may value the importance of providing historical background before presenting new information. Present-oriented cultures (e.g., Chinese) place more importance on the "here and now" than on the past or future. Future-oriented cultures (e.g., white American, European) believe it is important to prepare for what lies ahead. Punctuality is also part of temporal relationships; some cultures see promptness as important for all aspects of life, whereas others may be more relaxed about time, especially in social situations. The nurse needs to be mindful of all of these issues when working with patients. The ability to communicate effectively with a patient will have a major effect on assessment, teaching, and the entire nurse–patient relationship.

The domain of family roles and organization defines the relationships among those inside and outside the family. Family roles and organization include head of household and gender roles; family goals and priorities; developmental tasks of children and adolescents; roles of the aged and extended family; social status; and acceptance or nonacceptance of nontraditional lifestyles (e.g., divorce, single parenting, same-sex relationships). This information is important for the nurse to consider when providing teaching to the patient and family. For example, some Middle Eastern men may feel that the health care provider does not respect them as the head of the family if patient education is directed toward a female family member (even if the woman is the patient).

Spirituality includes all formal religious beliefs and the use of prayer. It also includes all behaviors that provide meaning to life and strength to the individual. Spirituality may influence nutrition, health care practices, and the other cultural domains. Identifying sources of strength and comfort for patients is important because these resources assist in promoting health and high-level wellness. The nurse considers spirituality to treat the patient holistically.

Health care practices include the focus of typical care (acute or preventive); the basis for health care (traditional, magicoreligious, or biomedical); beliefs about individual responsibility for health; self-medicating practices; views about mental illness, chronic illness, rehabilitation, organ donation, and transplantation; and responses to pain and the sick role. These practices influence not only how a patient responds to health and illness but also his or her acceptance of drug therapy. Drug interactions may occur from self-medication or the use of alternative therapies (e.g., herbs). The knowledge of health care practices not only assists the nurse in assessing the patient but also provides a basis for appropriate patient education.

Biocultural ecology identifies specific physical, biologic, and physiologic variations that stem from ethnic and racial background. Some diseases have a genetic predisposition, placing certain ethnic groups at increased risk. These diseases may require drug therapy. For example, blacks are slightly more than 1.5 times more likely to develop hypertension than are whites. Most important for nurses managing drug therapy, some racial and ethnic variations alter drug metabolism. Active pharmacokinetic processes (e.g., protein binding and metabolism) are more likely to be affected by ethnic differences than passive pharmacokinetic processes (e.g., absorption).

Although data in this field are limited, more studies are being done to examine drug therapy for interracial variations.

Pharmacogenetics and Drug Therapy

Pharmacogenetics is the study of inherited differences in response to clinical drug therapy. People with some genetically carried traits have been observed to metabolize drugs at rates that differ from the norm, placing them at risk for developing adverse effects or clinical failure from drug therapy. These genetic factors therefore alter the dose necessary to be therapeutic but avoid toxicity. This link between genetic makeup and drug response may be related to race or ethnicity; however, research increasingly is showing individual variation within population groups that is not related to race or ethnicity. Understanding how different people will respond to a particular drug and adjusting the drug dose to meet each individual's unique needs is essentially the concept of "one drug for many people."

Pharmacogenomics is the "... study of patterns of human genome variations that are in or near genes known to influence drug action" (Prows & Prows, 2004). The genome of an organism contains all of its genetic information. Pharmacogenomics entails the use of databases to identify disease-relevant drug targets in the human genome at the molecular level and to target drugs to clinical populations that share unique genetic profiles. This approach is essentially the concept of "many drugs for many people" (Norbert & Roses, 2003). Pharmacogenomics, although still in its infancy, may become an important tool in developing new drugs in the future.

The observation that people metabolize drugs in different ways was the initial impetus for the study of pharmacogenetics. New knowledge is showing that genetic variations also occur in drug receptors or drug target systems, such as transport proteins or cell membrane enzymes. Genetic variations that have a low incidence in the population (<1%) are termed *mutations*. Genetic variations that have an incidence in the population of 1% or greater are called *polymorphisms*. Polymorphisms may be the result of variations in the DNA sequence—that is, changing one nucleotide (the most common cause), inserting or deleting one or several hundred DNA bases, or inserting or deleting DNA repeating sequences (Siest et al., 2003).

Although many diseases are carried genetically, individual variation can still occur in a person's genetic makeup. Genotype is a person's specific gene composition; this composition reflects any variations unique to that individual. Phenotype is the observable or measurable expression of a genotype (Prows & Prows, 2004). All people with a similar phenotype will experience a particular disease or disorder, but they will not necessarily have the identical genotype. These variations in genotype account for different responses to drug therapy. For example, a chromosomal variation known as the Philadelphia chromosome is present in most, but not all, patients with chronic myeloid leukemia. Chronic myeloid leukemia is a type of cancer in which large numbers of mature myeloid cells are found in the peripheral blood and in the bone marrow. The variation in genotype expressed as the Philadelphia chromosome produces a certain abnormal protein. Cells with this abnormal protein do not respond to drug therapy but continue to reproduce. Research that explained how this particular protein malfunctioned enabled creation of a specific drug, imatinib (Gleevec), with a mode of action aimed specifically at the dysfunctional protein. This drug is much more successful than others in treating chronic myeloid leukemia, but only if the genotype variation of the Philadelphia chromosome is present (Prows & Prows, 2004).

Because drug metabolism through the P-450 hepatic enzymes has been studied the longest, some conclusions about genetic variations in the enzymes responsible for drug metabolism are known. Some of these data show variation among races, although great individual variation exists within any population group (i.e., specific race). For example, the isoenzyme CYP2D6 is known to be active in metabolism of some drugs. Between 7% and 10% of white individuals lack an active CYP2D6 enzyme and therefore metabolize drugs poorly through this pathway. A small percentage of whites have a phenotype in which the CYP2D6 gene is duplicated, so that they have two active genes, making them ultrarapid metabolizers. Interethnic variability has been shown with Asian and black African/African-American populations having reduced CYP2D6 activity compared with whites (Oscarson, 2003). A good bit of data support individual genetic variation in CYP3A4 and CYP2C9 and the effects these variations have on drug interactions, drug metabolism, and drug dosing (Daly & King, 2003; Siest et al., 2003; Schmitz & Drobnik, 2003). (See also Chapters 4 and 5 for more information.) Genetic testing for some CYP alterations is available and is increasingly used at many clinical sites. Laboratories that perform this procedure are testing for only the most common gene variations that produce either poor or ultrarapid metabolism. Because the patient may have other genetic variations that will go undetected by these tests, he or she may still experience changes in drug metabolism (Prows & Prows, 2004).

Two other mechanisms of drug metabolism are enzymes: *N*-acetyltransferases (NATs) and thiopurine methyltransferase (TPMT). NATs speed up the rate of the chemical reaction in which an acetyl group is transferred to a particular drug, increasing its water solubility and promoting renal excretion. Mutations or polymorphisms of NAT genes are responsible for slowing the metabolism of drugs such as isoniazid (an antitubercular agent) and some cardiovascular drugs, among others. Patients with genetic variations that affect these enzymes are at risk for higher circulating levels of drug and adverse effects. Tests to predict these variations are not currently part of routine clinical practice.

TPMT is necessary for the metabolism of certain types of drugs, known as thiopurine drugs. This chemical class of drugs is used for a variety of purposes, such as treating rheumatoid arthritis, preventing rejection of transplanted

organs, treating pediatric acute lymphoblastic leukemia, and treating steroid-resistant inflammatory bowel disease. These drugs are highly toxic and have a narrow therapeutic index; thus, finding the proper dose for a patient is crucial to prevent adverse effects and injury. In some clinical areas, lab analysis for TPMT—rather than the conventional method of using the patient's weight—is considered the current standard for determining the proper dose of a thiopurine drug. Patients with an alteration in one TPMT gene begin therapy at 65% of the usual standard dose, whereas patients with an alteration in both TPMT genes begin therapy at 6% to 10% of the standard dose (Prows & Prows, 2004).

Currently, pharmacogenetics is still a relatively new area of study; pharmacogenomics is even more in its infancy. As more information is learned and technology develops to identify genetic variations easily and accurately, drug therapy will be individualized to meet each patient's needs optimally while minimizing risks for adverse effects.

Cultural Differences Among Major Ethnic Groups

The following sections describe some of the differences in the five predominant ethnic groups in the United States, using the parameters described in Purnell and Paulanka's model. Every culture includes variations; therefore, these are general characteristics. Any statement that describes a general characteristic of a culture risks being considered stereotypical. Therefore, these descriptions must not be considered applicable to every person in any given culture. Indeed, many aspects of the dominant culture are usually also present in the nondominant cultures of our society. Every patient needs to be assessed individually for beliefs and practices.

White Americans

The most prevalent culture in the United States is that of whites. The people in this cultural group trace their ancestors to various European countries. Although they exhibit differences, white Americans have many common cultural traits.

White Americans speak English; a few may also speak a second language. White Americans tend to be future oriented and encourage work and sacrifice today as an investment for the future. People in this cultural group expect to delay the purchase of nonessential items to provide for drug therapy, medical treatment, and other health care needs, in the belief that doing so will help ensure a healthier future. White Americans have a linear sense of time (e.g., this action or event happens at this time followed by another action or event at a particular time). Time is highly valued, and people in this cultural group tend to be punctual for meetings, appointments, and social gatherings (Purnell & Paulanka, 2003).

Married white Americans generally live in traditional nuclear families of a man and woman and their children. However, nontraditional, nonnuclear families are becoming more common. Although historically the man worked and the woman stayed at home to care for the children, this division of labor now occurs less frequently, and more households have two working spouses.

The predominant religious belief is Christianity, with multiple denominations represented (e.g., Protestant, Roman Catholic). However, some white Americans are Jewish. Some religious beliefs may affect a patient's acceptance of certain drug therapies. For example, Roman Catholicism does not support the use of birth control. This doctrine could alter a woman's acceptance of oral contraceptives, even when given for medical management of irregular menstrual periods.

Most white Americans share a bioscientific view of disease and health management, although nontraditional health care practices are becoming more accepted and common. Some white Americans hold strong religious views and rely on prayer to regain health. Many white Americans hold a combined belief in the abilities of science and prayer or faith to restore health. Health care practices are based primarily on traditional Western medicine, although alternative therapies are also used to some extent.

White Americans have been found to have more acid glycoproteins than other ethnic groups. Therefore, when they take drugs that bind to these proteins, they have lower amounts of free (or active) drug than when the same dose is given to someone of another ethnic group (Johnson, 2000). Most clinical drug studies have been done on white men; therefore, the pharmacokinetic information from the study may or may not be applicable to white women or to other ethnic groups. More studies are now being done that include white women.

Black Americans

The largest group of black Americans is African American. This group will be discussed as illustrative of black Americans, although some differences exist among African-American and non–African-American blacks. African Americans trace their ancestors to Africans who were brought to North America as slaves. African Americans speak English and may also speak a black dialect of English. Generally, African Americans tend to be more present oriented than past or future oriented. Having a circular view of time, rather than a linear view, they are more relaxed about time than whites. It may be more important for some African Americans to have made an appointment than to be punctual. Many African Americans, however, share the dominant culture's belief in linear time (Purnell & Paulanka, 2003).

African Americans may have extended families, with the grandmother having an important role. Historically, the families tend to be matriarchal, although patriarchal families are not uncommon now.

African Americans tend to be very spiritual and actively practice their religions. Most African Americans are practicing Christians, with Baptist and Methodist being the most common denominations. However, several other Christian denominations are represented in African-American culture, as are the Nation of Islam and other Islamic sects. Islamic lifestyle is strictly regulated, and important parts of this lifestyle include cleanliness pertaining to specific religious beliefs. During times of crisis (e.g., critical illness, imminent death), these patients and their families turn to religion. Because they believe that life is precious, they perceive almost any medical treatment (e.g., transfusion) needed to support survival as acceptable, unless it is contradicted by their religious beliefs.

Historically, access to traditional health care for African Americans was uncertain. As a result, folk medicine became a necessity for treating illness. Even today, some African Americans may turn to folk medicines and practices much as their ancestors did, viewing health as a state of harmony

of body, mind, and spirit and illness as a state of disharmony resulting from natural causes, evil spirits, or divine punishment. Health-related folk practices are intended to restore harmony. The art of healing stems from a fundamental belief that healing power is a gift from God. Prayer, rituals, or the laying on of hands often accompanies the use of home remedies. Certain people within the community may be identified as having this power to cure. The traditional healers of the African-American community are usually women, who are proficient in using home remedies. Some African Americans may also seek advice from a voodoo practitioner. Additionally, African Americans use bioscientific medicine to treat disease and illness. Traditional or folk medicines may be used before, or concurrently, with Western medicine.

In general, African Americans respond to some drugs differently than whites. For example, they are less responsive to beta blockers (e.g., propranolol) and more responsive to monotherapy for hypertension than whites. The pathology of hypertension, a substantial health problem in this group, is caused by volume expansion, decreased levels of renin, and increased intracellular concentration of sodium and calcium. Because African Americans usually have dark eyes, their eyes dilate less than the eyes of people with light eyes in response to mydriatic drugs used during ophthalmologic procedures. Other biomedical differences include a higher incidence of extrapyramidal effects from tricyclic antidepressants and the antipsychotic haloperidol and greater susceptibility to tricyclic antidepressant delirium and other adverse effects of psychotropic drugs. These differences are based on pharmacogenetic differences in drug metabolism.

Asian and Pacific Islander Americans

Asian and Pacific Islander Americans have their ancestral origins in China, Japan, Korea, Vietnam, Cambodia, and other Asian countries and in the various Pacific Islands. Cultural differences among Asian–Pacific Islander Americans are many, owing to their diverse backgrounds. Because the Chinese-American population is the largest, however, it is discussed separately here.

Generally, Chinese Americans speak English. Older Chinese Americans may speak a Chinese dialect as their first language and may or may not speak English. Younger Chinese Americans speak predominantly English and may or may not also speak some Chinese.

The Chinese concept of time is related to the natural cycles of birth, life, and death. Therefore, time is to be integrated into life, rather than mastered (as whites attempt to do). Some Chinese Americans see little value in punctuality; whereas others, who view tardiness as a sign of disrespect and therefore as unharmonious, are prompt and expect the same promptness from others.

Traditional Chinese Americans place great significance on family and family roles. They emphasize the male relatives: fathers, sons, and uncles. Usually, the established head of the household—a man—has great authority and assumes all major responsibilities for the family.

Many Chinese Americans consider formal religion to be superstition, whereas others practice Buddhism, Roman Catholicism, Protestantism, Taoism, or Islam. Religion is considered a personal expression, prayer is a source of comfort, and formal group services are minimal.

Chinese Americans believe that harmony with nature is essential for physical and spiritual well-being and that harmony comes from a balance among the cycles and elements of nature (fire, water, wood, earth, and metal) and the cycles of life. Traditional Chinese Americans view the body and spirit as a gift given to them by their parents and ancestors. Therefore, the body and spirit must be cared for and well maintained. Care and maintenance are accomplished through the powers that govern the universe: yin and yang. Although these forces are in opposition to one another, they function in unison. A person whose yin is flourishing and whose yang is steadily active or energized is considered to be healthy.

Yang represents the positive male energy that produces light, warmth, and fullness or satisfaction. Matters that are ascending, brilliant, dynamic, and external belong to yang. Yin, in contrast, represents the negative female energy of darkness, cold, and emptiness. Things that are descending, dull, internal, regressive, and static belong to yin. For example, the surface of the body and the back are yang; the inside of the body and the front are yin.

Yin also represents the five viscera of the five solid organs (heart, kidney, liver, lungs, and spleen; referred to as *ts'ang*), which collect and store secretions. Diseases of winter and spring are thought to be yin. Yang represents five hollow organs (bladder, gallbladder, large intestine, small intestine, and stomach), referred to as *fu,* and the diseases associated with the warmer seasons of summer and fall.

The pulses are controlled by both yin and yang. For example, if yin is too strong, the individual is nervous, apprehensive, and catches colds easily. Disease is caused by an upset in the balance of yin and yang, and weather has an effect on the body's balance (e.g., heat is injurious to the heart; cold is injurious to the lungs). According to this culture, improper balance of yin and yang will shorten an individual's life span.

Chinese-American health care practices vary. Younger Chinese Americans usually seek Western medical care first and traditional Chinese treatment as a follow-up. Older Chinese Americans may seek health care in the reverse order. Traditional Chinese health care is based on the concept of harmonious yin and yang.

Herbal medicines and Western foods and drugs may affect some Chinese Americans in important ways. Chinese Americans are also more likely than most other Americans to have certain inherited conditions. For example, alpha thalassemia, an inherited disorder of hemoglobin metabolism, affects Chinese Americans with greater frequency than it affects other cultural groups (except those of Mediterranean origin), placing them at greater risk for anemia. In addition, a sex-linked genetic disease—a deficiency of glucose-6-phosphate dehydrogenase (G6PD)—is common in the Chinese American (Gaspard, 2002). This disease is characterized by a lack of the G6PD enzyme and results in anemia. Chinese-American populations also have a relatively high incidence of lactose intolerance, which leads to gastric symptoms, such as diarrhea, when milk or other dairy products are consumed. Certain drugs are metabolized differently and have different effects in Chinese Americans. Among these drugs are mephenytoin (Mesantoin); diazepam (Valium; poorly metabolized in 15% to 20% of Chinese Americans); beta blockers, atropine (Sal-Tropin), and alcohol (increased sensitivity); antidepressants and neuroleptics (increased responses at lower doses); and analgesics (decreased sensitivity, but increased

gastrointestinal [GI] adverse effects). Specific variations of drug metabolism among Chinese Americans are difficult to determine because most clinical drug studies have not differentiated them from other Asians.

Some variation of drug response among Chinese Americans is unrelated to differences in drug metabolism. Lithium carbonate (Eskalith), used in managing bipolar disorder, is a drug that is not metabolized, but it has a different effect in Chinese Americans than in Europeans and whites. Chinese Americans require lower levels of lithium to achieve a therapeutic response. Part of the explanation for the differences in drug response lies in the number and type of drug receptors present. Just as different drugs can be metabolized only by specific liver enzymes, receptors are custom designed to accept only certain drug configurations. As with enzymes, the number and type of receptors are influenced by genetics. Chinese Americans, and other Chinese people, appear to have a greater number of lithium-activated receptors than other groups.

Hispanic Americans

Hispanic Americans are a large minority in the United States because of birth rates and immigration. Members of the Hispanic-American community have their origins primarily in Puerto Rico, and in Mexico, Cuba, and other Latin American countries. The culture of Mexican Americans is described here.

Mexican Americans may speak either Spanish or English as their primary language. They may also be bilingual. Historically, Mexican Americans have been more present oriented than future oriented. Because time is viewed as relative, punctuality is relaxed, especially in social situations, although in modern society, the trend is toward greater punctuality. Mexican-American families tend to be patriarchal, with the male head of the household as the primary decision maker. These roles too are changing, with greater responsibility being shared with female family members.

Although some Mexican Americans tend to view life as chance, believing that health is purely the result of good luck (if one's luck changes, so does one's health), others have a dominant fatalism and hold the opinion that God is responsible for delivering health or illness, and that good health should not be taken for granted. Still others are deeply involved in formal religions, primarily Catholicism, but some worship with the Church of Jesus Christ of Latter Day Saints (LDS), Jehovah's Witnesses, Seventh Day Adventists, Presbyterians, and Baptists. In this context, appropriate ways of preventing ill health involve using herbs and spices, praying and wearing religious artifacts, and maintaining a balanced diet and physical activity. Socioeconomic and educational backgrounds influence the beliefs held by the individual Mexican American.

Individuals are expected to maintain equilibrium by eating and working properly. Good health exists when the biologic, psychosocial, and spiritual natures are holistically balanced in relation to the environment. The more serious physical and mental-emotional illnesses are brought to the male *curandero* or female *curandera,* who is a holistic healer in the community. The use of herbs (commonly in the form of teas and poultices) is a popular treatment offered by folk healers. Western medicine is also used.

As with other cultural groups, Mexican Americans believe that disease occurs when there is an imbalance between opposing life forces. For Mexican Americans, these forces are perceived as hot, cold, wet, and dry. The body is composed of four kinds of fluids (also known as humors), which may vary in temperature and moisture content. They are blood (hot and wet), yellow bile (hot and dry), phlegm (cold and wet), and black bile (cold and dry). Imbalances may exist among these fluids, and these imbalances are manifested as illness. Maintaining a balance between these fluids is important to promote wellness. When the four humors are balanced, the body is healthy.

These concepts provide a way of determining the remedy for a particular illness. Illness is thought to be caused by prolonged exposure to hot or cold; to cure the illness, the opposite quality of the etiologic agent is applied to absorb the hot or cold. For example, a cold substance is used to treat a hot illness. Hot conditions include constipation, diarrhea, fever, infections, kidney problems, liver problems, rashes, skin ailments, sore throat, and ulcers. Cold foods include barley water, chicken, fish, dairy products, fresh vegetables, goat meat, honey, raisins, and tropical fruits. Cold herbs and medicines include linden, milk of magnesia, orange-flower water, sage, and sodium bicarbonate.

Conversely, hot substances are used to treat cold conditions. Cold conditions include cancer, colds, dysmenorrhea, earache, headache, joint pains, malaria, paralysis, pneumonia, rheumatism, stomach cramps, teething pain, and tuberculosis. Hot foods include aromatic beverages, beef, cheese, chili peppers, chocolate, eggs, pork, liquor, goat milk, onions, peas, temperate-zone fruits, and whole grains (except barley). Hot herbs and medicines include anise, aspirin, cinnamon, castor oil, cod-liver oil, iron preparations, garlic, ginger, penicillin, tobacco, and vitamin preparations.

Hot and cold do not refer to temperature but are descriptive of the nature of a particular substance. Food, beverages, animals, and people possess the characteristics of hot and cold in varying degrees. Other Hispanic groups also consider items as hot or cold, but different substances are classified into these categories.

Few clinical drug studies have separated Mexican Americans from other Hispanic groups, so that information about variations in drug metabolism must be generalized from findings in Hispanic groups. Some studies have shown that Hispanics may metabolize some drugs differently from other cultural groups. For example, studies indicate that Hispanics need lower doses of antidepressants than do other groups and experience greater adverse effects from these drugs. Further complicating the issue is the fact that many Mexican Americans have mixed heritage. Therefore, generalizations may not be accurate for all Mexican Americans.

Native Americans and Alaska Natives

The Native American and Alaska Native population in the United States consists of more than 500 tribes that are recognized by the federal government; many others that are not. Native Americans (or American Indians) and Alaska Natives are the original inhabitants of North America, and each tribal community is unique in its cultural beliefs. The Navajo Indians are the largest tribe. A person must have at least one-quarter Navajo blood to be considered part of the tribe. The Navajo Indians are presented as the example of Native Americans and Alaska Natives.

CRITICAL THINKING SCENARIO

Diversity, drug therapy, and implications for teaching

Forty-nine-year-old Maria Alvarez is a bilingual Mexican American. She is newly diagnosed with type 2 diabetes with prescribed "diabetic teaching" related to insulin administration. The nurse reviews cultural phenomena affecting health and health care among Mexican Americans and adult teaching-learning principles before working with Mrs. Alvarez.

1. What are some of the most significant considerations for the nurse to explore prior to teaching Mrs. Alvarez?
2. During one of the teaching sessions, the nurse plans to use pamphlets to teach Mrs. Alvarez about insulin. What may be a limitation of printed material?

The Navajo tribe lives in a large reservation that consists of portions of Arizona, Utah, and New Mexico. In New Mexico, the Navajo tribe is scattered and lives with Zuñi Indians and settlers from the LDS church. A nomadic people, the Navajo tribe will travel great distances searching for adequate grazing grounds for their sheep. Navajo Indians speak Navajo, which until the 1970s was only a spoken language. A few older Navajo people speak some English or Spanish; younger Navajo people are usually bilingual and speak Navajo and English. The Navajo and Apache have similar languages, but their dialects are different. Minor variations in the pronunciation of Navajo words may change the meaning of the word or phrase spoken. Navajo Indians believe that silence is an appropriate way to communicate nonverbally and feel comfortable even during long silences. Navajos, especially older people, take their time to respond carefully and thoughtfully to what is said to them.

In contrast to whites, who view time in a present–future–past sequence, Navajo Indians view time in a present–past–future sequence. This outlook means that Native Americans attach little value to planning for the future, often considering it foolish. Time has little meaning or importance. Activities begin when people or members of a group gather.

The Navajo, like most other Native Americans, are matrilineal. Men are important, but grandmothers and mothers are the center of society. No decisions are made unless the appropriate older woman is present.

Native American religion predominates among the Navajo, although some have been converted to Christian religions, such as the LDS church, Jehovah's Witnesses, and some evangelical groups. The Navajo view spirituality as being in a state of harmony with one's surroundings. Prayer is important. Spirituality cannot be separated from healing and is important in healing ceremonies. Illnesses result from not being in harmony with nature; from the spirits of an evil person, such as a witch; or from violating tribal taboos. Healing ceremonies restore mental, physical, and spiritual balance. The Navajo may use Western medicine in addition to healing from tribal ceremonies.

Type 2 diabetes is very common among Navajo people, as it is among all Native Americans and Alaska Natives. Other health problems common to the Navajo people are severe combined immunodeficiency syndrome (failure of antibody response and cell-mediated immunity, not related to acquired immunodeficiency syndrome [AIDS]), Navajo neuropathy (an inherited condition in which myelinated fibers are completely absent, and death occurs before the age of 24 years), albinism, and genetic blindness. Although little research has been conducted on variation in drug metabolism in Navajos, or other Native Americans and Alaska Natives, it is known that Navajo people can have increased adverse effects to some medications. For example, adverse reactions to lidocaine (Xylocaine), an anesthetic and antiarrhythmic, occur in 29% of Navajos but only in 11% to 15% of whites.

NURSING MANAGEMENT OF CULTURALLY DIVERSE GROUPS

In administering drug therapy to culturally diverse patient populations, the nurse respects each patient's cultural heritage, beliefs, and practices. A health care provider not fully aware of a patient's background may be unable to understand many of the patient's health beliefs and practices. Lack of knowledge or misunderstanding may unintentionally turn what should be a therapeutic experience into a degrading and humiliating experience for patients of other cultures. If possible, every effort should be made to accommodate the patient's traditional practices with standard drug therapy while providing nursing care to maximize therapeutic effects, minimize adverse effects, and promote health and safety for the patient and the family.

When caring for patients, the nurse must be conscious of ethnocentrism, stereotyping, and cultural blindness. Because culture influences individuals so strongly in the way they feel, think, act, and judge the world, individuals often subconsciously restrict their view of the world to the point of being unable to accept other cultures. This inability is called **ethnocentrism.** Ethnocentrism inhibits acceptance of others and may lead to a clash of values and poor communication. Health care providers exhibit ethnocentricity when they act from the mistaken belief that only their own cultural and ethnic beliefs are normal, superior, or right. **Stereotyping** means making the assumption that all patients of a particular culture or ethnic group will have the same response. Health care providers may exhibit **cultural blindness** if they proceed as if differences do not exist. Because the American health care system is based on the dominant pattern of Western scientific health beliefs and practices, it is not uncommon for health care providers to dismiss any deviations from the established pattern. The implication of all this is clear—throughout care, nurses must remember to be nonjudgmental and to convey respect.

Nursing Diagnoses and Outcomes

When developing nursing diagnoses, the nurse needs to be aware of cultural beliefs, values, and behaviors that may influence the patient's situation. Although all nursing diagnoses may have related cultural factors, some can be specifically identified as having strong cultural implications. Box 12.1 presents nursing diagnoses and outcomes related to drug therapy and cultural diversity.

BOX 12.1 Nursing Diagnoses and Outcomes Related to Drug Therapy and Cultural Diversity

Impaired Verbal Communication
Desired outcome: Effective communication about drug therapy will be established among the patient, patient's family, and health care providers, despite possible language differences.
Anxiety related to new drug treatment
Desired outcome: Patient will recognize and express feelings of anxiety and will identify potential and actual sources of anxiety when health care practices during drug therapy interfere with cultural habits and health practices.
Fear of Health-Seeking Behaviors related to barriers to health care (e.g., caregiver's judgments of nonadherence or deviant behaviors) or fear of being criticized for traditional practices and inability to communicate these needs effectively in the English language
Desired outcome: Patient will recognize and express feelings of spiritual distress when health care practices, such as drug therapy, interfere with spiritual beliefs.
Ineffective Health Maintenance
Desired outcome: Patient (and family) will verbalize an understanding of beneficial, neutral, and harmful cultural health practices as they relate to drug therapy.
Ineffective Coping or Disabled Family Coping
Desired outcome: Individual (or family) will more effectively deal with stress after talking with a health care provider who explains the reason for, or expected outcome of, planned drug therapy as it relates to cultural beliefs and practices.
Spiritual Distress
Desired outcome: Patient will recognize feelings of spiritual distress when health care practices, such as drug therapy, interfere with traditional beliefs and habits.

Planning and Intervention

After the beliefs of the patient and family about health and disease, drugs and drug therapy, personal health habits, and chronic illness are assessed, planning and implementation may proceed.

Maximizing Therapeutic Effects

When drug therapy is recommended, the nurse makes an effort to determine whether prescribed therapies are consistent with the patients' physical needs, cultural backgrounds, religious preferences, dietary preferences, and self-care practices. The nurse can then incorporate these aspects into nursing practice whenever possible and when not contraindicated for health reasons.

Minimizing Adverse Effects

Nurses and patients need to be aware that certain cultural practices (e.g., using herbal preparations in addition to conventional drug therapy) may create drug toxicity or herb–drug interactions. Conventional prescribed drugs may have similar or antagonistic actions to an herb or herbal product. For example, overmedication may result when ginseng (a tonic stimulant and an antihypertensive) is taken in combination with antihypertensive drugs. Some foods may also interact with some drug therapies; normal dietary patterns must be assessed to help prevent food–drug interactions (see Chapter 10).

Providing Patient and Family Education

The communication style of the patient should be considered when preparing to provide patient education. The reasons for a treatment plan must be shared with patients and families and explained in language and at levels they can understand. When planning educational materials for patients whose primary language is not English, the nurse makes every effort to obtain interpreters or translations of written materials. Interpreters are preferred to translators because an interpreter will make sure that the meaning behind the message is the same; translators merely change the words from one language to another. Box 12.2 provides guidelines for communicating with patients who speak another language. Pictures that reinforce the content of the verbal and written instructions are also helpful. Many computer systems are available that can automatically translate instructions into other languages (e.g., Spanish). Computer programs can also alter the level of language to make it appropriate for the patient's educational background. The nurse compiles and maintains a listing of community resources that are available to assist patients of different cultures.

If the patient is present oriented, his or her understanding of acute and chronic illness may be affected by the perception of time. In such cases, the nurse teaching a patient about drugs for a chronic disease (e.g., hypertension) may be more successful emphasizing short-term problems (e.g., what may happen if the drug is not taken on time) than long-term problems, such as stroke and myocardial infarction.

The nurse also considers gender roles and the importance of various family relationships to the patient when teaching about drug therapy. The nurse ascertains that the appropriate person is present before beginning. For example, this person might be the grandmother of a Navajo Indian patient or the husband of a Mexican-American woman.

BOX 12.2 Communicating With Patients Who Speak Another Language

Use an interpreter (preferably) or a translator. Use dialect-specific interpreters (if possible) trained in health care. If possible, use an interpreter of the same age and same gender as the patient.

- Look at the patient when you speak, not at the interpreter.
- Speak slowly.
- Do not raise your voice or exaggerate your mouth movements.
- Provide time for interpretation or translation.
- Allow time for the patient to think before he or she responds.
- Avoid using relatives and children as interpreters; they may not be objective and the patient or relative may be embarrassed by the content of the discussion.
- Listen attentively.

If an interpreter or translator is not available:

- Remember that patients often understand more language than they can speak.
- Limit the number of words you use, and include as many words of the patient's language as possible.
- Speak slowly, but not loudly.
- Use nonverbal language.

Ongoing Assessment and Evaluation

To evaluate the effectiveness of nursing care for a patient of another culture, the nurse determines the extent to which the goals have been met by comparing the patient's current status with the identified outcome criteria.

CHAPTER SUMMARY

- Pharmacogenetics, which may or may not be related to ethnicity or race, accounts for individual variation in the response to drug therapy. This is a new field, and the knowledge about genetic variations affecting drug therapy is rapidly growing, although it is still somewhat limited today.
- Many cultural groups in North America embrace both their original culture and the dominant North American culture.
- Although generalizations may be made about the beliefs of different cultural groups, these statements cannot be applied to all individuals sharing a cultural background. Every individual must be assessed to determine his or her unique beliefs.
- Individual health-seeking behaviors and health practices exist and differ, sometimes markedly, among the major cultural groups in the United States.
- Medicinal plants and symbolic rituals play important roles in the health practices of many cultural groups.
- Patients should be advised of the potential for chemical interactions between folk medicine or herbal remedies and traditional (Western) drug therapy.
- Factors related to communication, time, and environmental control influence the relationship between the nurse and the patient whose backgrounds are culturally different.
- Individual variation in response to the effects of drugs and pharmacokinetic drug differences may occur because of biologic and genetic differences among individuals. For example, some patients may metabolize certain drugs more slowly because of a genetically induced enzyme deficiency.
- Nursing management emphasizes a thorough assessment of a patient's health beliefs, traditional practices, and cultural influences, so that the nurse and other health care providers may implement interventions that complement the patient's values. Therapeutic regimens that accommodate a patient's cultural values (and traditional rituals) are more likely to foster adherence to drug therapy and discourage alienation from the health care system.
- Cultural, ethnic, and environmental influences add complex issues to pharmacotherapy.

QUESTIONS FOR STUDY AND REVIEW

1. How does culture differ from ethnic group?
2. How is an awareness of cultural differences helpful when providing nursing management in drug therapy?
3. Describe strategies that can be used when your patient does not speak the same language as you.
4. Explain how an individual's concept of time will influence patient teaching about drug therapy.
5. Why are clinical drug studies that describe a drug's altered pharmacokinetic process in Hispanics not always applicable to Mexican Americans?

Need More Help?

Chapter 12 of the study guide for *Drug Therapy in Nursing* 2e contains NCLEX-style questions and other learning activities to reinforce your understanding of the concepts presented in this chapter. For additional information or to purchase the study guide, visit *http://connection.lww.com/go/aschenbrenner.*

REFERENCES AND BIBLIOGRAPHY

Daly, A. K., & King, B. P. (2003). Pharmacogenetics of oral anticoagulants. *Pharmacogenetics, 13*(5), 247–252.

Gaspard, K. J. (2002). The red blood cell and alterations in oxygen transport. In C. M. Porth (Ed.). *Pathophysiology: Concepts of altered health states* (6th ed., pp. 271–289). Philadelphia: Lippincott Williams & Wilkins.

Johnson, J. A. (2000). Predictability of the effects of race or ethnicity on pharmacokinetics of drugs. *International Journal of Clinical Pharmacology and Therapeutics, 38*(2), 53–60.

Norbert, P. W., & Roses, A. D. (2003). Pharmacogenetics and pharmacogenomics: Recent developments, their clinical relevance and some ethical, social, and legal implications. *Journal of Molecular Medicine, 81*(3), 135–140.

Oscarson, M. (2003). Pharmacogenetics of drug metabolizing enzymes: Importance for personalized medicine. *Clinical Chemistry and Laboratory Medicine, 41*(4), 573–580.

Prows, C. A., & Prows, D. R. (2004). Medication selection by genotype: How genetics is changing drug prescribing and efficacy. *American Journal of Nursing, 104*(5), 60–70.

Purnell, L. D., & Paulanka, B. J. (2003). *Transcultural health care.* Philadelphia: F. A. Davis.

Schmitz, G., & Drobnik, W. (2003). Pharmacogenomics and pharmacogenetics of cholesterol-lowering therapy. *Clinical Chemistry and Laboratory Medicine, 41*(4), 581–589.

Siest, G., Ferrari, L., Accaoui, M. J., et al. (2003). Pharmacogenomics of drugs affecting the cardiovascular system. *Clinical Chemistry and Laboratory Medicine, 41*(4), 590–599.

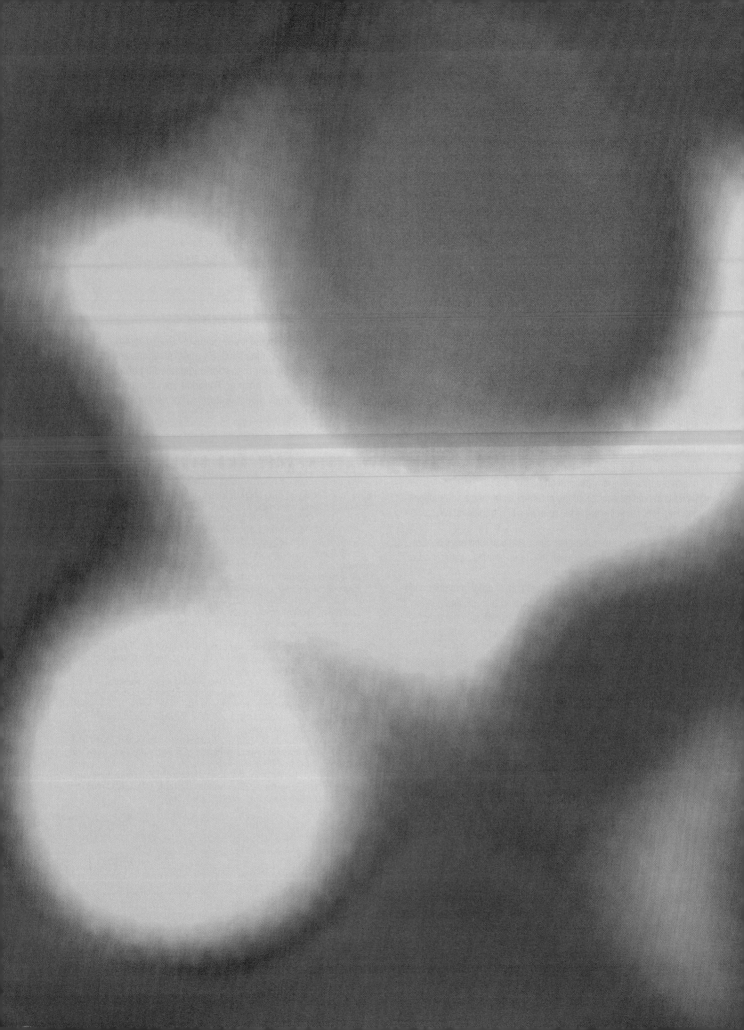

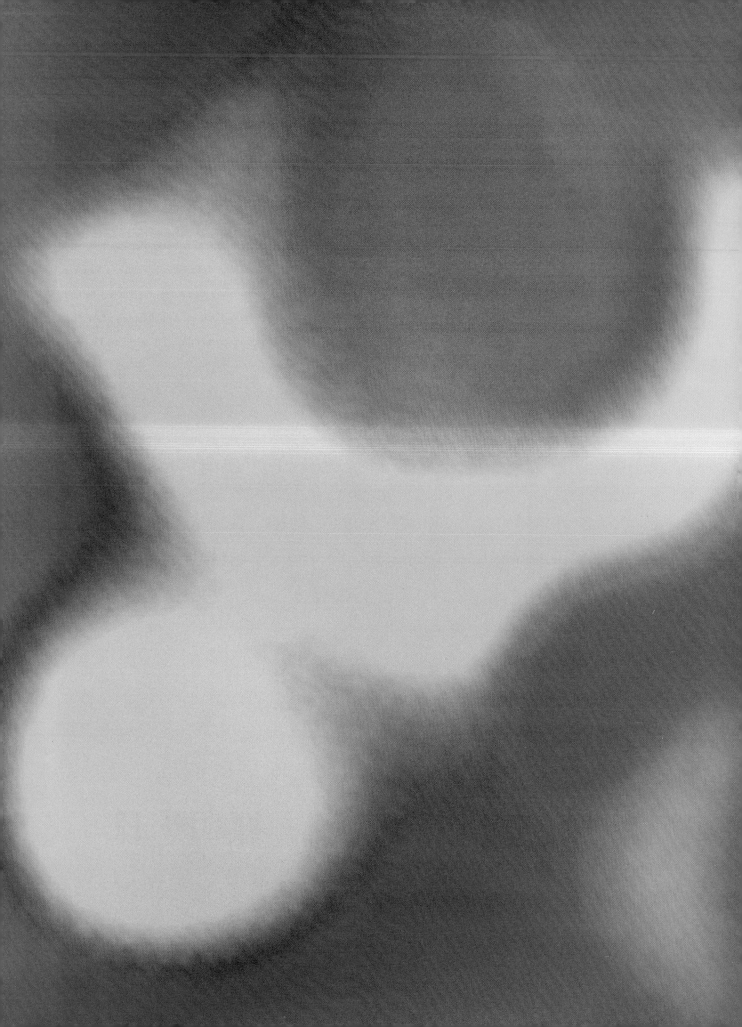

2. If you administered a cholinergic drug, why would you assess your patient for flushing of the skin, a headache, a sudden drop of blood pressure, and decreased pulse rate?
3. How would you respond to and manage a cholinergic crisis?
4. You may have encountered a way of remembering anticholinergic poisoning through the terms "mad as a hatter, blind as a bat, red as a beet, and dry as a bone." How does "dry as a bone" relate to adverse anticholinergic effects?

Need More Help?

Chapter 14 of the study guide for *Drug Therapy in Nursing* 2e contains NCLEX-style questions and other learning activities to reinforce your understanding of the concepts presented in this chapter. For additional information or to purchase the study guide, visit *http://connection.lww.com/go/aschenbrenner.*

REFERENCES AND BIBLIOGRAPHY

Clinical Pharmacology [Online]. Available: *http://cp.gsm.com.*

Diokno, A. C. (2004). Medical management of urinary incontinence. *Gastroenterology, 126*(1 Suppl 1), S77–81.

Facts and Comparisons. (2004). *Drug facts and comparisons.* Philadelphia: Lippincott Williams & Wilkins.

Fox, R. I. (2003). Sjögren's syndrome: Evolving therapies. *Expert Opinion Investigational Drugs, 12*(2), 247–254.

Gill, S. S., Mamdani, M., & Rochon, P. A. (2004). Management of overactive bladder. *New England Journal of Medicine, 350*(21), 2213.

Hardman, J. G. (2001). *Goodman & Gilman's the pharmacological basis of therapeutics* (10th ed.). New York: McGraw-Hill Health Professions Division.

Katzung, B. (2004). *Basic and clinical pharmacology* (9th ed.). New York: McGraw-Hill/Appleton & Lange.

Lehne, R. A. (2004). *Pharmacology for nursing care* (5th ed.). St. Louis: W. B. Saunders

Micromedex Healthcare Series [Online]. Available: *http://healthcare.micromedex.com.*

Tatro, D. S. (2004). *Drug interaction facts.* Philadelphia: Lippincott Williams & Wilkins.

and tridihexethyl chloride (Pathilon). All are oral agents; however, glycopyrrolate may also be given parenterally. Since the advent of histamine-2 blockers and proton pump inhibitors, these antisecretory anticholinergics have fallen out of favor because they induce a myriad of adverse effects. However, for patients unresponsive to histamine-2 blockers or proton pump inhibitors, these drugs may be effective.

Benztropine

Benztropine (Cogentin) is a centrally acting oral and parenteral synthetic muscarinic receptor antagonist that is structurally similar to atropine and can be given both orally and parenterally. It is used adjunctively with other agents to treat all types of parkinsonian syndromes including antipsychotic-induced extrapyramidal symptoms. It produces less CNS stimulation than does trihexyphenidyl, another commonly used anticholinergic drug used in the management of Parkinson disease. The drug may be helpful in geriatric patients who cannot tolerate cerebral-stimulating agents. Onset of therapeutic effect may take 2 to 3 days. Adverse effects are similar to atropine.

Hyoscyamine

Hyoscyamine (Cystospaz) relaxes smooth muscle spasm resulting from parasympathetic stimulation. It inhibits gastrointestinal propulsive motility and decreases gastric acid secretion. It also controls excessive pharyngeal, tracheal, and bronchial secretions. It requires only half the dose of atropine; therefore, it has a lower potential to induce adverse effects.

Ipratropium

Ipratropium bromide (Atrovent) is a synthetic anticholinergic agent that is structurally very similar to atropine. It may be administered by oral or nasal inhalation. The actions of ipratropium parallel those of atropine on bronchial smooth muscle, salivary glands, the gastrointestinal tract, and the heart when administered intravenously. However, when administered by oral inhalation, ipratropium exhibits greater antimuscarinic activity on the bronchial smooth muscle, and systemic effects are minimal. Compared with atropine, ipratropium is roughly twice as potent as a bronchodilator, and it affects bronchodilation more than it inhibits salivary secretion.

Intranasal administration of ipratropium produces a localized parasympatholytic effect. This action reduces watery hypersecretion from mucosal glands of the nose, thereby relieving rhinorrhea associated with the common cold or allergic or nonallergic perennial rhinitis.

Although ipratropium may be used for the management of asthma, it is more commonly used for cholinergic-mediated bronchospasm associated with chronic obstructive pulmonary disease.

Scopolamine

Scopolamine (Isopto Hyoscine) is a naturally occurring anticholinergic agent found in belladonna leaf. Compared with atropine, scopolamine is more potent in its anticholinergic effects on the iris, ciliary body, and the salivary, bronchial, and sweat glands. It is less potent than atropine on the heart and on bronchial and gastrointestinal smooth muscle. In contrast to atropine, scopolamine at therapeutic doses produces CNS depression characterized by drowsiness, euphoria, amnesia, fatigue, and dreamless sleep resulting from decreased periods of rapid eye movement. Paradoxical CNS excitation manifested as restlessness, hallucinations, or delirium can occur, especially when the patient is experiencing severe pain. Scopolamine is very effective for the prevention of motion sickness, and this indication represents the most common clinical use. Other uses for scopolamine include treatment of iritis, uveitis, and Parkinson disease.

Trihexyphenidyl

Trihexyphenidyl (Artane) is a centrally acting anticholinergic used adjunctively to treat all types of parkinsonian syndromes including antipsychotic-induced extrapyramidal symptoms. This drug is frequently used in combination with other antiparkinsonian agents, and it is effective in 50% to 75% of patients. In general, anticholinergic agents can help control tremor but are less effective for treating bradykinesia or rigidity. Additionally, trihexyphenidyl can block dopamine reuptake, thereby prolonging dopamine's effects. Tolerance to the effects of trihexyphenidyl can occur with prolonged use.

Urinary Relaxants

Cholinergic antagonists such as tolterodine (Detrol), oxybutynin (Ditropan) and flavoxate hydrochloride (Urispas) are used in patients with urinary incontinence. Urge incontinence is generally caused by involuntary contraction of the detrusor muscle of the bladder. Relaxation of this muscle results in bladder control.

CHAPTER SUMMARY

- Parasympathetic or cholinergic drugs can be stimulating or blocking in their action. The cholinergic stimulating drugs are known as cholinergic agonists, and the cholinergic blocking agents are known as cholinergic antagonists or anticholinergics.
- Drugs that interfere with acetylcholinesterase's breakdown of acetylcholine are known as anticholinesterase agents.
- In the parasympathetic system, the transmitter is acetylcholine, and the receptors may be muscarinic or nicotinic.
- Therapeutic uses of cholinergic drugs are varied and related to providing extra cholinergic stimulation or blockage to normal autonomic nervous system functioning.
- A prototype of a direct-acting muscarinic agonist is pilocarpine, which is used for simple and acute glaucoma, preoperative and postoperative intraocular tension, and mydriasis.
- A prototype direct-acting nicotinic agonist is nicotine, which is used as an adjunct to smoking cessation programs.
- A prototype indirect-acting cholinergic receptor stimulant is neostigmine, which is used to control the symptoms of myasthenia gravis. As with any of the cholinergic drugs, adverse effects involve many of the major organ systems.
- Atropine is the prototype of the antimuscarinic anticholinergic drugs. It is most commonly used preoperatively to dry postoperative secretions.

QUESTIONS FOR STUDY AND REVIEW

1. After abdominal surgery, a common postoperative drug order is for bethanechol. Why is this ordered, and how would you know whether it has been effective? If the patient became short of breath after a few doses of bethanechol, what would you do?

- Constipation related to adverse effects of drug
  Desired outcome: *The patient will continue baseline elimination pattern.*
- Risk for Injury related to drug-induced drowsiness and blurred vision
  Desired outcome: *The patient will understand adverse effects and develop a repertoire of strategies for their management.*
- Ineffective Sexuality Patterns or Sexual Dysfunction related to anticholinergic impact on erection and ejaculation in men and on vaginal secretions in women
  Desired outcome: *The patient and partner will adjust sexual functioning and develop a repertoire of strategies to maintain satisfaction.*

Planning and Intervention

Maximizing Therapeutic Effects

Two factors should be considered for the person receiving atropine because they arise directly from the interactions between core drug knowledge and core patient variables. First, patients taking atropine for peptic ulcer disease should adhere to dietary restrictions established to prevent exacerbations of the disease, thereby allowing the therapeutic potential of the atropine to be achieved. The nurse may suggest administering the larger dose at bedtime to decrease sleep-disturbing pain. Second, patients need to be encouraged to take their atropine exactly as prescribed and at the required dosage frequency to enhance therapeutic potential.

Minimizing Adverse Effects

Because a prominent anticholinergic effect is dry mouth, good oral hygiene is important. Dryness may be relieved with hard candies, chewing gum, or lip gloss. Blurred vision and mydriasis can be hazardous for drivers, particularly at night; therefore, driving is best avoided. Bright lights and photophobia may be counteracted with sunglasses. For patients with a complaint of dry eyes, artificial tears should be administered.

Atropine alters the body's ability to regulate temperature; therefore, extremes of heat and strenuous exercise are minimized, and the patient is adequately and deliberately hydrated. Constipation is a troubling adverse effect that may be managed by adding fiber to the diet, promoting hydration, and exercising moderately.

In longer-term therapy, the nurse stresses the importance of mouth care and monitors the need for urinary catheterization or measures to relieve constipation and abdominal distention. A distressing adverse effect for many patients relates to their preferred modes of sexual expression, which may be dramatically changed with anticholinergic drugs. If appropriate, supportive counseling or directive teaching about alternatives to intercourse may be useful, although many of these issues are better managed by a sex therapist.

Providing Patient and Family Education

Important aspects of patient and family teaching include recognizing and managing adverse effects:

- Older men are informed of the need to report any changes in urinary stream because it may be a prodromal symptom of prostatic hypertrophy.
- Aids to elimination are suggested, including adequate exercise, added dietary fiber, and increased fluid intake.
- It is particularly important to stress the hazards associated with driving, especially at night, because night vision may be altered significantly by atropine.
- The nurse reminds the patient to avoid all OTC and herbal medications without the direct approval of the health care provider. As previously mentioned, these medications frequently contain atropine-like ingredients.

Ongoing Assessment and Evaluation

Assessment of goal attainment is relatively straightforward for patients receiving anticholinergic therapy with atropine. Ongoing assessment includes data about elimination patterns, sexual functioning and adjustment, and recognition and management of side effects. The ongoing assessments may be tailored to the clinical indications for which atropine or other anticholinergics are prescribed, but they should include any concurrent drug therapy to rule out the possibility of drug interactions. Vital signs measured at onset of therapy are compared with vital signs throughout therapy and used to monitor and detect adverse effects.

Bowel and bladder function are assessed on an ongoing basis because of the profound impact that drug therapy may have on elimination. Because of the potential for confusion, anyone at risk for adverse CNS effects should have a mental status assessment.

Drugs Closely Related to [P] Atropine

Antisecretory Anticholinergics

There are many anticholinergic drugs used to decrease the secretion of gastric acids. These include anisotropine (Valpin), clidinium (Quarzan), glycopyrrolate (Robinul), hexocyclium (Tral Filmtabs), isopropamide (Darbid), mepenzolate (Cantil), methantheline (Banthine), methscopolamine (Pamine), oxyphencyclimine (Daricon), propantheline (Pro-Banthine),

MEMORY CHIP

[P] Atropine

- An antimuscarinic drug that is commonly given preoperatively to reduce postoperative secretions; the drug of choice for cholinergic crisis
- Major contraindications: hypersensitivity to sulfites, myasthenia gravis, acute myocardial infarction
- Most common adverse effects: blurred vision, constipation, dry mouth, urinary retention
- Most serious adverse effect: severe bradycardia
- Maximizing therapeutic effects: Take the medication exactly as prescribed and the required dosage.
- Minimizing adverse effects: good oral hygiene, fluid replacement
- Most important patient education: safety issues for blurred vision, avoid OTC and herbal medications without the direct approval of the health care provider

myasthenia gravis because the drug competes with the small amount of acetylcholine that has potential to act in the body. Atropine is relatively contraindicated in acute myocardial infarction because the drug can potentiate arrhythmias. In addition, the increase in heart rate caused by atropine increases the oxygen demand on the heart and can exacerbate myocardial ischemia. Precautions should be observed with patients who drive or perform hazardous tasks for a living (because of the adverse effects of drowsiness and blurred vision). Precautions are also needed for the elderly as well as those with glaucoma, severe forms of hepatic disease, ulcerative colitis, renal disease, prostatic hypertrophy, coronary artery disease, congestive heart failure, arrhythmias, tachycardia, hypertension, asthma, and allergies. Finally, precautions are needed for anyone with increased sensitivity (e.g., infants and small children) and for patients with brain damage, hyperthyroidism, and hyperthermia. All of these circumstances may be exacerbated with atropine and other anticholinergics.

Adverse Effects

The most common adverse effects of atropine are blurred vision, dry mouth, constipation, and urinary retention. The most serious potential adverse effect is an anticholinergic overdose. This is characterized by the hallmarks of "mad as a hatter (CNS psychotic effect), dry as a bone (salivary), red as a beet (peripheral vasodilation), and blind as a bat (mydriasis)."

In the CNS, the predominant effect is drowsiness, sometimes with confusion, especially in the elderly. Other potential adverse effects include elevation of intraocular pressure, decreased ability to sweat, and tachycardia. Although anticholinergic drugs are used in the management of asthma, the drying of respiratory secretions may result in mucus plugs that may actually induce bronchospasm and asthma attacks.

Atropine is an FDA pregnancy category C drug and should be avoided by pregnant and lactating women.

Drug Interactions

Atropine interacts with phenothiazine antipsychotics and with haloperidol (Table 14.7). Cardiac status, as measured by electrocardiography (ECG), may be affected by atropine. Atropine may interfere with ECG measurements through its cardiovascular effects and result in spurious cardiac findings. The ECG interpretation should note the atropine therapy.

Assessment of Relevant Core Patient Variables

Health Status

Because atropine has many actions on the body, the nurse carefully assesses the patient for contraindications or precautions to its use before administering the drug. It is important to determine whether the patient has acute angle-closure glaucoma, obstructive disease of the gastrointestinal tract, paralytic ileus, obstructive uropathy, intestinal atony (particularly in elderly or debilitated patients), megacolon complicating ulcerative colitis, unstable cardiovascular status in acute hemorrhage, tachycardia secondary to cardiac insufficiency of thyrotoxicosis, myasthenia gravis, toxemia of pregnancy, or previous exposure to high temperatures.

Positive findings are communicated to the health care provider. The nurse also determines whether the patient has chronic obstructive lung disease, severe heart disease, hypertension, ulcerative colitis, ileus, chronic lung disease, hyperthyroidism, autonomic neuropathy, hepatic or renal disease, prostatic hypertrophy, esophageal reflux, or hiatal hernia. Because these conditions may be exacerbated with atropine therapy, the nurse provides close monitoring of these patients. The nurse also assesses the patient's use of OTC or herbal medications. These drugs frequently contain atropine-like ingredients that may induce severe adverse effects.

Life Span and Gender

The nurse documents the age of the patient. Atropine must be used carefully with infants, young children, and anyone older than 40 years because the adverse effects may be more pronounced in these age groups.

Environment

The nurse documents the patient's occupation and daily activities. People treated with atropine may experience mydriasis and hence difficulties adjusting to changing light intensities. These effects may have considerable impact on people working in transportation (airline flight crew, drivers) and those working at night (because of photophobia and temporary blindness in response to bright lights).

Nursing Diagnoses and Outcomes

- Urinary Retention related to adverse effects of drug
  Desired outcome: *The patient will eliminate without difficulty.*

TABLE 14.7 Agents That Interact With P Atropine

Interactants	Effect and Significance	Nursing Management
phenothiazines	Decreased antipsychotic efficacy of phenothiazines	Adjust phenothiazine dosage.
haloperidol	Decreased serum haloperidol levels, worsening of symptoms, onset of tardive dyskinesia	Avoid concurrent atropine or lower haloperidol dosage; monitor carefully.

TABLE 14.6 Summary of Selected (C) Cholinergic Antagonists (continued)

Drug (Trade) Name	Selected Indications	Route and Dosage Range	Pharmacokinetics
hyoscyamine (Cystospaz)	Abdominal cramps, anticholinesterase poisoning, biliary disorders, colic, diverticulitis, dysentery, enterocolitis, GI disorders, irritable bowel syndrome, neurogenic bowel disturbances, Parkinson disease, peptic ulcer, pylorospasm, spastic colon, splenic flexure syndrome, pancreatitis, rhinitis	*Adult:* PO, 0.125–0.25 mg q4h, PO (sustained-release product), 375–0.75 mg q12h; SC, IM, IV push, 0.25–0.5 mg	*Onset:* PO, 5–20 min; IV, 2 min *Duration:* 4–12 h $t_{1/2}$: Not applicable
ipratropium (Atrovent; *Canadian:* Alti-Ipratropium)	Asthma, chronic bronchitis, chronic obstructive lung disease, rhinorrhea	*Adult:* inhaler, 36 μg qid	*Onset:* 15 min *Duration:* 3–4 h $t_{1/2}$: 1.6 h
oxybutynin (Ditropan)	Urinary incontinence	*Adult:* PO, 5 mg bid–tid, ER tabs, 5 mg qd syrup, 1 tsp bid–tid *Children > 5 y:* PO, 5 mg bid syrup, 1 tsp bid	*Onset:* 30–60 min *Duration:* 6–10 h $t_{1/2}$: Unknown
pralidoxime (Protopam)	Anticholinesterase or organophosphate poisoning	*Adult:* IV initially, 1–2 g/100 mL in normal saline solution over 30 min, then PO, 1–3 g repeated in 5 h	*Onset:* IV, rapid *Duration:* Not applicable $t_{1/2}$: 0.8–2.7 h
propantheline (Pro-Banthine, Propantheline Bromide; *Canadian:* Propanthel)	Duodenal ulcer, GI spasmolytic, hyperhidrosis, sialorrhea, urinary incontinence	*Adult:* PO, 15–30 mg 30 min before meals and 30 mg at bedtime or 15–30 mg q4–6h	*Onset:* 30–60 min *Duration:* 6 h $t_{1/2}$: 3–4 h
scopolamine (Scopolamine Hydrobromide, Hyoscine Hydrobromide)	Motion sickness Preanesthetic premedication, obstetric amnesia, antidelirium Glaucoma, ophthalmology, uveitis	*Adult:* PO or transdermal patch, 0.6–1.0 mg *Adult:* PO, 1 mg 1–4 h before anesthesia; IM, 0.4–0.6 mg 45–60 min before anesthesia *Adult:* topical, 1–2 drops of 0.25% solution in eye 1 h before refraction; 1–2 drops up to four times daily for uveitis	*Onset:* PO/IM, 30 min *Duration:* 4–6 h $t_{1/2}$: 8 h
tolterodine (Detrol)	Urinary incontinence	*Adult:* PO, 2 mg bid or 4 mg qd	*Onset:* 1–2 h *Duration:* 6–8 h $t_{1/2}$: 1.9–3.7 h

(see Table 14.6). Topical administration to the eyes may take 30 to 40 minutes to produce cycloplegia (paralysis of ciliary muscles), whereas intravenous (IV) administration produces rapid effects. Atropine is partially metabolized in the liver with about 60% of a dose eliminated unchanged through the kidneys.

Pharmacodynamics

Atropine is a competitive inhibitor at autonomic postganglionic cholinergic receptors. These receptors are found in gastrointestinal and pulmonary smooth muscle, exocrine glands, the heart, and the eye. The principal actions of atropine are a reduction in salivary, bronchial, and sweat gland secretions; mydriasis; cycloplegia; changes in heart rate; contraction of the bladder detrusor muscle and of the gastrointestinal smooth muscle; decreased gastric secretion; and decreased gastrointestinal motility.

The action of atropine on the heart rate is dose dependent. In doses of 0.4 to 0.6 mg, atropine causes a slight sinus bradycardia through vagal stimulation. In larger doses (1 to 2 mg), it causes sinus tachycardia secondary to inhibition of vagal control of the sinoatrial node in the heart.

Contraindications and Precautions

Contraindications to atropine use include hypersensitivity to anticholinergics or sulfites. Atropine is contraindicated in

doxime is not effective in reversing overdose of reversible anticholinesterase drugs. It works best when given immediately after the exposure. It does not cross the blood–brain barrier and, therefore, is ineffective in reversing anticholinesterase in the CNS.

C CHOLINERGIC ANTAGONISTS

The cholinergic antagonists are drugs that antagonize, or block, muscarinic or nicotinic receptors directly. They may be clustered into three categories: antimuscarinic drugs (the largest group), antinicotinic drugs (with two subcategories: ganglionic blockers and neuromuscular blockers), and cholinesterase regenerators.

The ganglionic blockers include mecamylamine (Inversine) and trimethaphan (Arfonad). Their clinical importance is in decreasing blood pressure in critical situations; accordingly, they are covered in Chapter 27. The neuromuscular blockers, which are covered in Chapter 15, include succinylcholine and the curare derivatives. The antimuscarinic drugs of clinical significance include atropine, benztropine, scopolamine, ipratropium, and hyoscyamine. Table 14.6 summarizes selected cholinergic antagonists. Atropine is the ideal prototype for the antimuscarinic group of cholinergic antagonists.

NURSING MANAGEMENT OF THE PATIENT RECEIVING P ATROPINE

Core Drug Knowledge

Pharmacotherapeutics

Atropine has a multitude of therapeutic uses. It is used in emergency situations, such as symptomatic bradycardia, pulseless electrical activity, ventricular asystole, or cardiopulmonary resuscitation. Preoperatively, it is used to decrease respiratory secretions, and during surgery, it is used to block cardiovagal reflexes and succinylcholine-induced arrhythmias. Other uses include reversal of organophosphate insecticide toxicity or neuromuscular blockade, induction of mydriasis or cycloplegia, treatment of iritis or uveitis, and management of traveler's diarrhea. It is also used as an adjunctive treatment of gastrointestinal disorders, such as duodenal ulcer, irritable bowel syndrome, and gastrointestinal hypermotility caused by cholinergic stimulation.

Pharmacokinetics

Following intramuscular administration, onset of effect is usually rapid, peaking at 30 minutes and lasting up to 5 hours

TABLE 14.6 Summary of Selected C Cholinergic Antagonists

Drug (Trade) Name	Selected Indications	Route and Dosage Range	Pharmacokinetics
P atropine (Atropine Sulfate; *Canadian:* Apo-Benztropine)	Anesthesia induction, premedication for surgery Bradycardia Biliary spasm, GI radiography, irritable bowel syndrome, peptic ulcers, urinary incontinence, asthma, bronchitis, reversal of bronchospasm, hiccups, organophosphate poisoning, arrhythmias (e.g., angiography induced, postmyocardial infarction, succinylcholine induced), myelodysplasia, neuromuscular blockade reversal, hyperhidrosis, hypothermia, rhinorrhea, tetanus asystole, dental procedures	*Adult:* SC, IM, or IV, 0.3–0.6 mg 60 min before inducing anesthesia *Adult:* IV, 0.5–2.0 mg *Adult:* 0.3–1.2 mg q4–6h any route for GI or anticholinergic uses	*Onset:* SC, varies; IM, 10–15 min; IV, immediate *Duration:* 4 h $t_{1/2}$: 2.5 h
benztropine (Benztropine Mesylate, Cogentin)	Drug-induced extrapyramidal symptoms, akathisia, dystonic reactions, haloperidol-induced acute dystonic reaction, parkinsonism, drooling, myoclonus, priapism	*Adult:* PO, IM, IV, 1–4 mg daily or bid	*Onset:* PO, 1 h; IM, IV, 15 min *Duration:* PO, IM, IV 6–10 h $t_{1/2}$: 4–8 h
flavoxate (Urispas)	Urinary incontinence	*Adult:* PO, 100–200 mg tid–qid *Children:* Safety not demonstrated	*Onset:* Rapid *Duration:* 24 h $t_{1/2}$: 6 h

(continued)

MEMORY CHIP

[P] Neostigmine

- An indirect-acting cholinoceptor stimulant used in the management of myasthenia gravis
- Major contraindications: GI obstruction or ileus, urinary tract obstruction, peritonitis
- Most common adverse effects: nausea or vomiting, diarrhea, abdominal pain, miosis, salivation, diaphoresis, sinus bradycardia
- Most serious adverse effects: cholinergic crisis, cardiac arrest
- Maximizing therapeutic effects: Administer at regular intervals throughout the day to ensure adequate blood levels.
- Minimizing adverse effects: availability of atropine, the antidote for cholinergic crisis
- Most significant nursing responsibility: Differentiate between cholinergic crisis and myasthenic crisis.
- Most important patient education: symptoms of cholinergic crisis and need for immediate medical attention

Drugs Closely Related to [P] Neostigmine

Ambenonium Chloride

Ambenonium chloride (Mytelase) is an oral, slowly reversible anticholinesterase agent. It is indicated for use in patients with myasthenia gravis to improve muscle strength. Ambenonium chloride has actions similar to those of the oral cholinesterase inhibitor pyridostigmine, but it tends to produce more muscarinic side effects. Contraindications, adverse effects, and drug interactions are similar to those of neostigmine.

Demecarium

Demecarium (Humorsol) is a long-acting cholinesterase inhibitor and potent miotic. Because of its potential toxicity, it is reserved for use in patients with open-angle glaucoma or other chronic glaucoma not satisfactorily controlled with the short-acting miotics or other agents. Demecarium decreases intraocular pressure by lowering the resistance to the outflow of the aqueous humor.

Demecarium is contraindicated in patients with hypersensitivity and in women who are pregnant or breast-feeding. Because miotics may aggravate inflammation, demecarium should not be used in active uveal inflammation.

Demecarium may cause local or systemic adverse effects. Local effects include burning, redness, stinging, or other irritation of the eyes. More serious local effects include eye pain and retinal detachment. Adverse effects related to systemic absorption include bradycardia, bronchospasm, hypotension, increased sweating, loss of bladder control, muscle weakness, and gastrointestinal distress. Systemic effects are infrequent when demecarium is instilled carefully. Compression of the lacrimal duct for several seconds immediately following instillation minimizes drainage into the nasal chamber where extensive absorption may occur.

Edrophonium

Edrophonium (Tensilon) is a rapid-acting, short-duration, parenteral cholinesterase inhibitor. It is the drug of choice for diagnosing myasthenia gravis because of its rapid onset of action and reversibility. Other uses include assessing cholinesterase inhibitor therapy, differentiating cholinergic and myasthenic crises, and reversing the effects of nondepolarizing neuromuscular blockers after surgery.

Physostigmine

Physostigmine (Antilirium) is a parenteral and ophthalmic cholinesterase inhibitor. The difference between physostigmine and neostigmine is that physostigmine is a tertiary amine, whereas neostigmine is a quaternary amine. This difference accounts for the increased activity of physostigmine in the CNS. Physostigmine is most commonly used as an ophthalmic agent in the treatment of open-angle glaucoma. It is also used to counteract toxic anticholinergic effects (both central and peripheral) of other drugs, particularly in overdose situations. In the past it was used to treat tricyclic antidepressant overdose, but this use has lost favor because of physostigmine's own potentially harmful effects. It has also been used to treat Alzheimer disease and hereditary ataxias.

Pyridostigmine

Pyridostigmine (Mestinon) is an oral cholinesterase inhibitor. It is somewhat longer acting than neostigmine and also possesses fewer muscarinic effects. Pyridostigmine is marketed in both regular and sustained-release tablets and is the most commonly used agent of the group for oral treatment of myasthenia gravis. It is also used to reverse the actions of nondepolarizing neuromuscular blockers after surgery.

Tacrine

Tacrine hydrochloride (Cognex) is another oral cholinesterase inhibitor. It is the first drug approved for improving cognitive symptoms, such as problems with memory, attention, reason, language, and the ability to perform simple tasks associated with Alzheimer disease. Elevated levels of acetylcholine in the cerebral cortex are believed to be responsible for improvement in cognition. This mechanism requires that intact cholinergic neurons are present. As dementia progresses, fewer intact cholinergic neurons remain, and tacrine becomes less effective. There is no evidence that tacrine alters the underlying pathologic processes of dementia.

Drugs Significantly Different From [P] Neostigmine

Most of the irreversible cholinesterase inhibitors are in the organophosphate category. Because of the phosphate element of these drugs, they are highly lipid soluble and are easily absorbed from any administration site. Their ease of absorption, coupled with their potential toxicity, is the basis for their use as insecticides and chemical warfare agents.

There are a few therapeutically useful irreversible inhibitors, such as echothiophate and isoflurophate (Floropryl), which are used for glaucoma that is refractory to the usual miotics.

Overdose or accidental overexposure to irreversible anticholinesterase drugs is characterized by cholinergic crisis. The antidote of choice is pralidoxime (Protopam, PAM). Prali-

Life Span and Gender

The nurse documents the age and gender of the patient. Because they have lower body mass than other adults and decreased renal functioning, elderly patients may be more prone to the psychotogenic effects of cholinergic overdose, including restlessness, anxiety, and agitation. The nurse also determines whether the patient is pregnant or breast-feeding because these patients should avoid neostigmine.

Lifestyle, Diet, and Habits

The nurse documents the patient's occupation, daily activities, and rest and exercise patterns. Patients taking neostigmine for myasthenia gravis may need to pace their daily activities to allow the peak and duration effects of neostigmine dosing to support their muscular and respiratory work.

Environment

The nurse is aware of the environment in which the drug will be administered and assesses the home or living environment, if appropriate. Neostigmine in its oral form may be administered in any setting by health care providers, nurses, the patient, or family members.

Nursing Diagnoses and Outcomes

- Impaired Gas Exchange related to drug-induced bronchospasm, increased secretions, or respiratory paralysis
  Desired outcome: *The patient will maintain effective gas exchange.*
- Ineffective Airway Clearance
  Desired outcome: *The patient will maintain effective airway clearance.*
- Ineffective Breathing Pattern related to drug dosage
  Desired outcome: *The patient will maintain effective breathing patterns.*
- Self-Care Deficit (Feeding, Bathing/Hygiene, Dressing/Grooming, Toileting) related to the impact of neuromuscular weakness secondary to overdose
  Desired outcome: *The patient will seek assistance in carrying out self-care as needed.*

Planning and Intervention

Maximizing Therapeutic Effects

Neostigmine is administered at regular intervals throughout the day to ensure effective blood levels. If the patient has difficulty swallowing or breathing, the parenteral form of neostigmine should be administered until oral therapy can be tolerated.

Minimizing Adverse Effects

As with other cholinergic stimulants, the use of neostigmine requires the availability of an antidote in case of systemic overdose or cholinergic crisis. Atropine is the usual antidote. For patients with known allergies or suspected hypersensitivity, life-support measures must be available in case of bronchial spasm or hypersensitivity reactions. Because adverse systemic effects include stimulation of sphincters, patients may need access to a bedpan or urinal in case of rapid responses.

If the patient has a history of allergies or asthma or chronic obstructive lung disease, careful monitoring of the first few doses of neostigmine is required to ensure that respiratory difficulties do not occur.

Providing Patient and Family Education

The key considerations for patient and family education include managing serious adverse effects and recognizing crisis states that may require prompt and expert intervention:

- Exploring aspects of long-term therapy that sometimes escape the attention or resources of acute care staff, such as decreased libido, is usually productive.
- Patients and their families may need assistance in understanding how to recognize myasthenic crisis (undermedication) and distinguish it from cholinergic crisis (overmedication), and in knowing how to respond to either situation. In myasthenic crisis caused by undermedication, muscle weakness becomes pronounced and may cause quadriparesis, quadriplegia, shortness of breath, respiratory insufficiency, and difficulty swallowing. Conversely, in a cholinergic crisis caused by overmedication, there is an increase in gastrointestinal motility with diarrhea and cramping, bradycardia, muscle fasciculation, pupillary constriction, and increased salivation and sweating. The nurse advises the patient and family to seek immediate care should any of these symptoms occur.

Ongoing Assessment and Evaluation

The nurse is familiar with procedures for detecting and managing myasthenic or cholinergic crises. The achievement of therapeutic goals relates to detailed therapeutic monitoring of neuromuscular functioning, vital signs, respiratory rate and capacity, mobility, self-care levels, and self-esteem.

An important component of the ongoing assessment is the patient's neuromuscular status. The focus is on vital capacity (respiratory status), presence of ptosis, presence of diplopia, ability to chew and swallow, strength of hand grip bilaterally, and quality of gait if the patient is ambulatory. Acute care settings often provide a detailed assessment sheet designed specifically for the person with myasthenia gravis. Other data should include baseline and ongoing measurements of blood pressure and pulse and respiratory rates.

CRITICAL THINKING SCENARIO

Neostigmine therapy

Amy Rose, a 27-year-old legal assistant, has been admitted to your unit with a diagnosis of myasthenia gravis. She has been started on neostigmine therapy, and you are wondering how to differentiate between undermedication with the possibility of a myasthenic crisis, and overmedication with the possibility of a cholinergic crisis.

1. Explain the key differences between the two situations, and propose a nursing management strategy that you could use for either situation.
2. Discuss the implications of a health care provider–ordered edrophonium test. Why do you think this test would be ordered?

Contraindications and Precautions

Neostigmine is absolutely contraindicated in patients with gastrointestinal obstruction or ileus and urinary tract obstruction because it increases contractions of smooth muscle. It should not be used in patients with peritonitis because it increases gastrointestinal motility, which would exacerbate the disorder. Neostigmine should be used with caution in patients with peptic ulcer disease because it stimulates gastric acid secretion, again inducing an exacerbation of the disorder. The CNS stimulation induced by neostigmine may exacerbate hyperthyroidism or seizure disorders.

Neostigmine should be used cautiously in patients with hypotension and bradycardia because it can further decrease blood pressure and heart rate by increasing vagal tone. Neostigmine also has direct stimulatory effects on the myocardium, which can increase oxygen demand. This state can be dangerous for patients with cardiac disease, particularly coronary artery disease alone or in association with cardiac arrhythmias. In the respiratory system, neostigmine may induce bronchoconstriction; therefore, it should be used cautiously in patients with asthma, chronic bronchitis, or chronic airway limitation.

Adverse Effects

The most serious adverse effects result in a cholinergic crisis, which may be life threatening. Symptoms include nausea and vomiting, diarrhea, salivation, sweating, peripheral vasodilation, bronchial constriction, and respiratory arrest. In patients with myasthenia gravis, it is sometimes necessary to distinguish between a cholinergic crisis and a myasthenic crisis. In the case of a cholinergic crisis, it is likely that too much anticholinesterase has been given, whereas a myasthenic crisis may be the result of inadequate dosages failing to control myasthenic symptoms. A challenge dose of edrophonium (Tensilon) will differentiate the two states. If there is no relief or if an increase in muscle weakness follows, then the patient is receiving too much anticholinesterase. If there is an improvement with edrophonium, then an increase in cholinesterase inhibitor dosage is indicated.

The most common unwanted effects of neostigmine's cholinergic stimulation of end organs are nausea and vomiting, diarrhea, abdominal pain, miosis, salivation, diaphoresis, sinus bradycardia, bronchospasm, and increased bronchial secretions.

Drug Interactions

Neostigmine and the anticholinesterase drugs in general interact with steroids, aminoglycoside antibiotics, depolarizing muscle relaxants, local anesthetics and some general anesthetics, and magnesium, all of which have an influence on the neuromuscular junction (Table 14.5). Steroids may decrease the anticholinesterase effects of neostigmine, with a resulting worsening of the myasthenic condition. This exacerbation may require an increased dose of neostigmine or alternate dosing of each class of agent. Some of the aminoglycosides cause a mild neuromuscular blockade, which may antagonize the effects of neostigmine. For the depolarizing muscle relaxants, such as succinylcholine, neostigmine may increase the time of neuromuscular blockade; thus, concurrent usage in people with myasthenia is contraindicated.

Assessment of Relevant Core Patient Variables

Health Status

Before administering the drug, the nurse performs a baseline physical assessment to document the current status of the patient, especially respiratory status and muscle strength. Myasthenia affects the muscles of respiration and other muscle groups; therefore, respiratory function may be further compromised in the presence of upper respiratory tract infections or allergies. Undertreatment or overtreatment is of particular concern because it can lead to life-threatening crises.

The nurse also assesses for a history of diseases or disorders that contraindicate the use of neostigmine. Positive findings are communicated to the health care provider before neostigmine is administered.

TABLE 14.5 Agents That Interact With P Neostigmine

Interactants	Effect and Significance	Nursing Management
aminoglycoside antibiotics (neomycin, streptomycin, kanamycin)	Mild nondepolarizing blocking action	Monitor for increased neuromuscular blockade.
corticosteroids	Decreases effect of anticholinesterase therapy in myasthenia gravis	Ensure respiratory support if needed.
depolarizing muscle relaxants (succinylcholine) and mivacurium	Increased, prolonged neuromuscular blockade	Avoid use if possible. If not, administer these drugs only as directed and only if indicated. Provide emergency respiratory support.
magnesium	Antagonizes and counteracts beneficial effects of neostigmine	Avoid magnesium-containing drugs and foods.
anticholinesterase drugs	Excessive GI stimulation and symptoms of cholinergic crisis or underdosage in patients with myasthenia gravis	Have antidote (atropine or belladonna) available to treat overdosage.

to minimize skin reactions. Upper respiratory tract effects may be counteracted with a room humidifier. Adverse effects that cannot be managed and that may be specific to the delivery system warrant a change to a different system on a trial basis.

Providing Patient and Family Education

- The nurse cautions patients receiving nicotine replacement therapy about adverse effects and the possibility of overdosing with concomitant use of tobacco smoking during therapy.
- The nurse watches the patient demonstrate the correct use of sprays or transdermal patches to ensure safe, optimal self-dosing.
- The nurse instructs the patient on how to manage adverse effects and encourages the patient to contact the health care provider if self-management is ineffective or if serious or persistent adverse effects continue.
- If toxicity or overdosing is suspected, the therapy must be discontinued until the effects abate and then a decreased dosage or frequency of dosing can be reintroduced.
- The nurse encourages the patient to avoid other stimulants during nicotine therapy, including caffeine-containing beverages, because they may lead to exaggerated CNS stimulation experienced as irritability and nervousness.
- The nurse cautions the patient and family to keep nicotine out of the reach of children.
- The nurse incorporates all other smoking cessation program measures in the educational effort because replacement therapy is only a short-term adjunct measure.

Ongoing Assessment and Evaluation

During therapy, symptoms of tobacco craving should gradually subside. Throughout therapy, the nurse remains alert for signs and symptoms of overdosing, which indicate that the patient is "cheating" and smoking tobacco while taking the nicotine replacement. Dizziness, nausea, and headaches may result and promote nonadherence to the therapeutic use of nicotine. Other evaluative measures include assessing the quantitative decrease of adverse effects and promoting therapeutic adherence.

MEMORY CHIP

P Nicotine

- A direct-acting nicotinic agonist used as an adjunct to smoking cessation programs
- Major contraindications: immediately post MI, life-threatening dysrhythmias, severe angina
- Most common adverse effects: erythema, pruritus, burning, headache, insomnia
- Most serious adverse effect: vasculitis
- Maximizing therapeutic effects: adherence to the recommended dosing
- Minimizing adverse effects: Limit timing of last dose to promote rest and sleep.
- Most important patient education: correct use of multiple administration routes, avoidance of other stimulants

C Indirect-Acting Cholinergic Agonists

Synaptic transmission of neurotransmitters was discussed in Chapter 13. To review, the final step of synaptic transmission is termination. After the neurotransmitter crosses the synaptic gap and binds to a receptor, the neurotransmitter is cleared from the synaptic gap by either enzymatic degradation, reuptake, or diffusion. Acetylcholine, the neurotransmitter of the cholinergic nervous system, is cleared from the synaptic gap by acetylcholinesterase, also known as cholinesterase. Any drug that inhibits cholinesterase will be the functional equivalent of a cholinergic receptor stimulant—or agonist—because of its ability to prolong the activity of acetylcholine at the synapse. For this reason, some indirect-acting cholinergic agonists are also known as *cholinesterase inhibitors* or *anticholinesterase agents.* It is important to remember that acetylcholine stimulates both nicotinic and muscarinic receptor sites; therefore, cholinesterase inhibitors prolong the action of acetylcholine throughout the body.

The two major groups of indirect-acting cholinergic receptor stimulants are the reversible and "irreversible" cholinesterase inhibitors. Neostigmine (Prostigmin) is the prototype for reversible cholinesterase inhibitors.

NURSING MANAGEMENT OF THE PATIENT RECEIVING P NEOSTIGMINE

Core Drug Knowledge

Pharmacotherapeutics

The most significant indication for neostigmine therapy is myasthenia gravis. In this disease, the neuromuscular junction is affected by an autoimmune process that diminishes the number of functional nicotinic receptors at the junction. The result is the characteristic weakness and fatigue that accompany exercise in people with this disease. The use of neostigmine effectively increases the amount of acetylcholine available at the myoneural junction, resulting in enhanced strength of muscle contraction.

Other clinical indications include urinary retention and paralytic ileus. Neostigmine is also used as an antidote for nondepolarizing neuromuscular blocking agents.

Pharmacokinetics

Neostigmine is administered both orally and parenterally. It is poorly absorbed when given orally. Onset of action occurs within 2 to 4 hours when taken orally, and within 10 to 30 minutes when given parenterally. The drug is metabolized by microsomal liver enzymes and hydrolyzed by cholinesterases. Duration of effect varies considerably among patients. Approximately 80% of neostigmine is excreted in the urine within 24 hours as unaltered drug and metabolites (see Table 14.2).

Pharmacodynamics

Neostigmine is a reversible inhibitor of postsynaptic cholinesterase and therefore acts as a cholinergic agent by increasing the synaptic presence of acetylcholine.

TABLE 14.4 Agents That Interact With P Nicotine

Interactants	Effect and Significance	Nursing Management
adenosine	Enhanced cardiovascular effects of adenosine	Advise patients undergoing stress tests to avoid chewing nicotine gum or reduce adenosine dosage to avoid angina.
lithium	Potentiates effects of nicotine	Monitor for increased effect.

Assessment of Relevant Core Patient Variables

Health Status

A careful history and physical examination will identify contraindications and precautions pertaining to the person beginning nicotine replacement therapy. The patient's desire to cease smoking or the requirement not to smoke usually prompts nicotine replacement therapy. Before therapy begins, the nurse ensures that the patient has had neither a recent myocardial infarction nor symptoms of significant cardiovascular disease (e.g., arrhythmias and angina pectoris) because these conditions are contraindications to therapy. Before application of transdermal nicotine patches, skin test results should be reviewed to determine sensitivity to the drug.

Life Span and Gender

The nurse documents the age and gender of the patient and assess women of childbearing age for pregnancy and lactation. If the patient is pregnant, nicotine therapy should be used only if necessary—for example, in cases in which the benefits of smoking cessation are important. If the patient is breast-feeding, the infant should be monitored for respiratory or CNS stimulation. If such stimulation occurs, the timing of breast-feeding or the administration of the nicotine may need to be staggered to minimize adverse effects. Older adults undergoing nicotine therapy may be at increased risk for dizziness and sleep disturbances resulting from CNS stimulation.

Lifestyle, Diet, and Habits

The nurse documents the patient's occupation and daily activities. Patients are advised not to smoke during nicotine therapy to avoid overdosage and adverse effects. Patients whose jobs require shift work should be aware that sleep disturbances may disrupt their rest. In addition, the nurse inspects the patient's oral cavity for dentures and other significant dental work. Nicotine gum is heavier and stickier than regular gum and may affect artificial teeth or other dental work.

Environment

The nurse is aware of the environment in which the drug will be administered. Nicotine in any of its dosage forms may be administered in any setting by health care providers, nurses, or patients themselves. In institutional or other smoke-free settings, nicotine replacement therapy may be almost obligatory.

Culture and Inherited Traits

The nurse explores the patient's underlying cultural beliefs and values regarding smoking. In many cultural groups, such as Japanese American, Austrian, Polish immigrant, and highly acculturated Latino, smoking tobacco is popular and widely accepted. It is important to recognize that some patients may have more difficulty giving up smoking than others because of cultural influences.

Nursing Diagnoses and Outcomes

- Risk for Injury to mouth, teeth, or dental work related to gum viscosity, and sore throat or mouth related to use of the intranasal spray
  Desired outcome: *The patient will remain free of injury or problems related to adverse effects of therapy.*
- Disturbed Sleep Pattern related to drug-induced insomnia
  Desired outcome: *The patient will experience undisturbed sleep.*

Planning and Intervention

Maximizing Therapeutic Effects

The following interventions by the nurse may help to maximize the beneficial effects of nicotine therapy:

- The patient is encouraged to adhere to the recommended dosage schedule because it is the one most likely to reduce craving.
- Because nicotine replacement therapy is an adjunctive measure in smoking cessation programs, all other program measures are promoted and encouraged.
- Because craving is substantially increased when patients are exposed to others who smoke (promoting effects from secondary smoke inhalation, reinforcing old habits, and prompting recollection of pleasurable sociocultural influences), the nurse encourages the patient to minimize exposure to these influences initially.

Minimizing Adverse Effects

Overstimulation of the CNS may be counteracted by promoting good sleep hygiene and adjusting the dosage and timing of the last nicotine dose of the day. Other adverse effects may require the episodic use of analgesics for headaches.

Avoiding gastrointestinal effects requires good mouth care (particularly for the patient using nicotine gum) and possibly the use of antiemetics (for nausea) or antidiarrheals, as needed. For patients using the transdermal nicotine patches, good skin care and rotation of patch sites will help

secretions; hence, patients with asthma, chronic bronchitis, or chronic obstructive pulmonary disease should be closely monitored.

Methacholine

Methacholine (Provocholine) is a parasympathomimetic inhalation agent used to help diagnose bronchial airway hyperreactivity in patients who do not have clinically apparent asthma. Methacholine induces bronchoconstriction in asthmatic patients more readily than in nonasthmatic patients.

Contraindications and precautions include hypersensitivity to parasympathomimetic agents, concurrent beta-antagonist therapy, epilepsy, cardiovascular disease characterized by bradycardia, peptic ulcer disease, thyroid disease, urinary tract obstruction, and clinically apparent asthma, wheezing, or very low baseline pulmonary function test results.

Women of childbearing age should be given this diagnostic test within 10 days of the first day of their menses or within 2 weeks following a negative pregnancy test result. Methacholine should not be administered to women who breast-feed because it is unknown whether the drug is excreted in breast milk. When given to patients receiving beta blockers, the effects of methacholine can be exaggerated or prolonged. Common adverse effects include headache, throat irritation, light-headedness, and pruritus. Because acute respiratory distress may occur, emergency equipment and medications should be at the bedside during this diagnostic test.

(C) Direct-Acting Nicotinic Agonists

The direct-acting nicotinic agonists are also called ganglionic stimulating agents. These drugs stimulate nicotinic receptors directly. The two significant classes of nicotinic stimulants are the ganglionic stimulants (e.g., nicotine) and the neuromuscular nicotinic stimulants that are discussed in Chapter 15.

Nicotine is an important drug, although its selection as a prototype may be considered controversial by some. However, because of its great abuse potential in smoking and chewing tobacco and its therapeutic uses in smoking cessation, it is presented as the prototype for direct-acting nicotinic agonists.

NURSING MANAGEMENT OF THE PATIENT RECEIVING [P] NICOTINE

Core Drug Knowledge

Pharmacotherapeutics

Nicotine replacement is used as an adjunct to smoking cessation programs. Various formulations are available, such as gum, transdermal patches, and nasal spray. The nicotine gum and transdermal patches are available over the counter (OTC) in the United States. The patches are preferred for maintenance therapy during smoking cessation programs, unless the patient is allergic to the patches. Gum or nasal spray may be useful for episodic or bolus effects of nicotine and in institutional settings in which smoking is not allowed (see Table 14.2).

Pharmacokinetics

When delivered as a chewing gum, nicotine is readily absorbed through the buccal mucosa when the gum is chewed. However, the amount of nicotine absorbed depends on how long the saliva remains in the mouth. Very little nicotine is absorbed from the gastrointestinal tract because of extensive first-pass metabolism through the liver. Regular use of the gum provides steady-state blood levels of nicotine similar to those achieved by smokers. However, peak plasma levels occur much more slowly than when tobacco smoke is inhaled. Nicotine levels reach the brain within 7 seconds of a single puff on a cigarette, but peak concentrations of the gum can take 14 to 20 minutes; the transdermal patch can require as long as 4 hours to reach peak concentrations.

Nicotine is widely distributed in the body tissues, particularly the CNS. It crosses the placenta and is secreted in milk. The concentrations of nicotine in amniotic fluid and fetal serum exceed those in maternal serum. Detectable amounts also appear in the serum and urine of infants of nursing mothers who smoke.

Nicotine is metabolized in the liver by oxidation and excreted by the kidneys as unchanged nicotine and metabolites.

Pharmacodynamics

Nicotine is a potent ganglionic and CNS stimulant, with actions that are mediated through specific nicotine receptors. In small doses, all autonomic ganglia are stimulated; in larger doses, initial stimulation is followed by blockade. The dependency potential of nicotine is based mostly on its CNS stimulant effects.

Contraindications and Precautions

Nicotine in any dosage form should not be used in patients immediately after myocardial infarction, or in those with life-threatening arrhythmias or severe or worsening angina pectoris. It should not be used in patients who have allergies to any of the components of the delivery system, including gum, nasal spray, and transdermal patches. Smoking should be avoided during nicotine therapy because of the potential for overdose and toxicity (with manifestations including dizziness, nausea, and headache).

Adverse Effects

The adverse effects of nicotine in the cardiovascular system include peripheral vasoconstriction and tachycardia. In the CNS, the effects may include headache, paresthesias, fatigue, insomnia, nervousness, nausea, hot flashes, and nightmares. Diarrhea, dry mouth, nausea, and dyspepsia are adverse effects on the gastrointestinal system. Use of Nicotrol spray may cause nasal irritation, lacrimation, throat irritation, sneezing, and coughing. The transdermal patches may cause erythema, pruritus, edema, or rash at the site of administration.

The nicotine transdermal system and nasal spray are classified as FDA pregnancy category D, although the benefits of nicotine replacement therapy during pregnancy appear to outweigh the risks of continued smoking during pregnancy.

Drug Interactions

Adenosine and lithium carbonate interact with nicotine (Table 14.4).

Oral pilocarpine is administered at regular intervals throughout the day.

Minimizing Adverse Effects

As with all cholinergic agonists, the use of pilocarpine requires the availability of an antidote in case of systemic overdose or cholinergic crisis. Atropine is the usual agent for this purpose. For patients with known allergies or suspected hypersensitivity, life support measures must be available in case of bronchial spasm or allergic reactions. Systemic side effects include stimulation of sphincters, so that patients may need access to a bedpan or urinal.

Contact lenses should be removed before ophthalmic treatment. If pilocarpine drops are applied to the eyes when soft contact lenses are in place, the lenses can deteriorate or absorb the drug. It also is possible that hard contact lenses can cause corneal abrasion or roughening of the corneal surface. Corneal abrasion can increase systemic absorption, possibly causing toxicity.

Providing Patient and Family Education

- Patients are cautioned about blurred vision and its hazards.
- Patients are taught to recognize systemic adverse effects and how to manage them.
- Patients using the Ocusert system need instruction on inserting and removing the ocular device safely and antiseptically.

Ongoing Assessment and Evaluation

During therapy, monitoring of therapeutic effects should reveal the decrease in frequency or severity of target symptoms or the resumption of the problem for which pilocarpine was prescribed. Nurses familiar with ophthalmic surgery and conditions are adept at continuous assessment and evaluation of changes in intraocular pressure. Moreover, they can use a tonometer to gauge substantial changes in intraocular pressure. Other evaluations include whether adverse side effects are effectively minimized.

MEMORY CHIP

P Pilocarpine

- A direct-acting muscarinic agonist used for simple and acute glaucoma, preoperative and postoperative intraocular tension, mydriasis, and xerostomia
- Major contraindications (ophthalmic): hypersensitivity, history of retinal detachment, and acute iritis
- Major contraindications (oral): hypersensitivity, severe respiratory diseases
- Most common adverse effects: blurred vision, myopia
- Most serious adverse effects: cholinergic crisis, bronchospasm
- Maximizing therapeutic effects: Administer ophthalmic solution into the conjunctival cul-de-sac.
- Minimizing adverse effects: availability of antidote, aseptic technique for ophthalmic administration
- Most important patient education: symptoms of cholinergic crisis and need for immediate medical attention

Drugs Closely Related to P Pilocarpine

Acetylcholine

As a drug, acetylcholine (Miochol) is limited to use in the management of ophthalmologic surgery. It produces complete miosis in cataract surgery, keratoplasty, iridectomy, and other anterior segment surgery in which rapid miosis is required. Because it is given topically, systemic adverse effects rarely occur. However, it may cause problems for patients with acute cardiac failure, bronchial asthma, peptic ulcer, hyperthyroidism, gastrointestinal spasms (cramps), urinary tract obstruction, or Parkinson disease. It is contraindicated for use in patients with acute iritis and acute inflammatory disease of the anterior chamber of the eye.

Bethanechol

Bethanechol (Urecholine) is a synthetic muscarinic stimulant with primary effects on the urinary and gastrointestinal tracts. Its effect on the bladder results from stimulation of muscarinic receptors in the detrusor muscle. As the detrusor contracts, the bladder capacity decreases, resulting in micturition. Bethanechol also stimulates ureteral peristalsis and relaxes the trigone and external sphincter. Because bethanechol is a direct-acting agonist, spinal cord injury does not compromise its actions. Stimulation of muscarinic receptors in the gastrointestinal tract restores peristalsis, increases motility, and increases the resting lower esophageal sphincter pressure. Bethanechol also stimulates the lower gastrointestinal tract, resulting in defecation. It is the preferred drug in the treatment of postpartum and postoperative nonobstructive urinary retention. It is also used in the management of urinary retention related to phenothiazine or tricyclic antidepressant therapy.

As an oral agent, bethanechol may induce systemic adverse effects similar to those of pilocarpine. As with pilocarpine, drug interactions include other cholinergic or anticholinergic drugs. In addition, bethanechol in conjunction with ganglionic blocking agents may result in a critical decrease in blood pressure.

Carbachol

Carbachol (Isopto Carbachol) is used in the management of glaucoma. It is administered as an ophthalmologic solution up to three times daily. Like pilocarpine, it works by direct stimulation of the muscarinic cholinergic receptors in the eye. Contraindications and adverse effects are similar to pilocarpine.

Cevimeline

Cevimeline (Evoxac) is a cholinergic agonist that is indicated for the treatment of symptoms of dry mouth in patients with Sjögren syndrome. It binds with muscarinic receptors and increases secretion of exocrine glands such as salivary and sweat glands. Cevimeline is contraindicated in patients with known hypersensitivity, uncontrolled asthma, acute iritis, or narrow-angle (angle-closure) glaucoma. It is used with caution in patients with cardiovascular or pulmonary diseases. Cevimeline can alter cardiac conduction or heart rate; therefore, patients with significant cardiovascular disease may be unable to compensate for transient changes in hemodynamics or rhythm. Also, cevimeline can increase airway resistance, bronchial smooth muscle tone, and bronchial

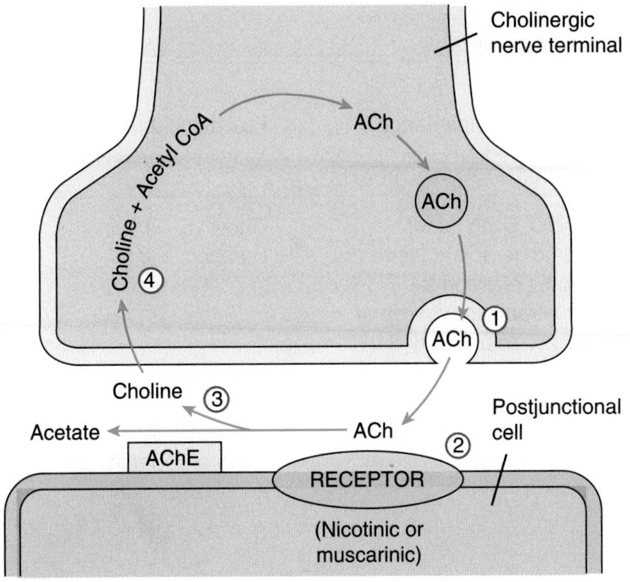

FIGURE 14.2 Activation and degradation of acetylcholine. (1) ACh release, (2) binding to cholinergic receptor, (3) degradation of ACh, and (4) reuptake.

TABLE 14.1 Cholinergic Receptor Subtypes' Location and Action

Location	Response to Stimulation
Nicotinic$_N$	
All autonomic nervous system ganglia	Stimulation of sympathetic and parasympathetic *postganglionic* transmission
Adrenal medulla	Release of epinephrine
Nicotinic$_M$	
Neuromuscular junction	Contraction of skeletal muscle
Muscarinic	
Eye	Miosis (pupillary constriction) Contraction of the ciliary muscle
Heart	Decreased rate
Lung	Bronchoconstriction Increased bronchial secretions
Blood vessels	Vasodilation Hypotension
GU system	Micturition
GI tract	Increased salivation Increased intestinal tone and motility Increased gastric secretions Defecation
Sweat glands	Increased sweating
Sex organs	Erection

Nicotinic$_M$ receptors are located on skeletal muscle. Stimulation of nicotinic$_M$ receptors results in skeletal muscle contraction.

Muscarinic Receptors

Muscarinic receptors respond to acetylcholine and also bind muscarine, an alkaloid substance isolated from mushrooms. They are located on postsynaptic cells, muscles, and glands. Of interest is the presence of muscarinic receptors on blood vessels; however, these receptors are not associated with the nervous system. Although their physiologic activation is unclear, their pharmacologic response is vasodilation, resulting in decreased blood pressure.

PATHOPHYSIOLOGY

The tissues and organs that are innervated by the ANS are diverse, and few discrete disorders are directly related to compromise of the parasympathetic nervous system. Instead, the therapeutic uses of parasympathetic drugs are related to providing extra cholinergic stimulation or blockade of normal ANS functioning. Disorders of the bronchi, cardiovascular system, gastrointestinal or genitourinary tract, skeletal muscle, eyes, and various glands may respond to cholinergic stimulation through their muscarinic and nicotinic receptors.

Ⓒ CHOLINERGIC AGONISTS

Cholinergic agonists include direct-acting muscarinic agonists, direct-acting nicotinic agonists, and indirect-acting cholinergic agonists (Table 14.2).

Ⓒ Direct-Acting Muscarinic Agonists

Direct-acting muscarinic agonists are drugs that bind to the muscarinic receptors located in various tissues and organs throughout the body. Their activation elicits a response that resembles the action of the parasympathetic nervous system; therefore, they are also called parasympathomimetic agents. The muscarinic drugs are the choline esters, such as acetylcholine (Miochol), bethanechol (Urecholine), carbachol (Isopto Carbachol), cevimeline (Evoxac), methacholine (Provocholine), and the alkaloid pilocarpine (Akarpine). Although pilocarpine has limited therapeutic scope, it is the ideal prototype for the direct-acting muscarinic agonists.

NURSING MANAGEMENT OF THE PATIENT RECEIVING P PILOCARPINE

Core Drug Knowledge

Pharmacotherapeutics

Pilocarpine is a direct-acting cholinergic agonist with ophthalmic uses. The major indications for pilocarpine are open-angle glaucoma, acute treatment of angle-closure glaucoma,

TABLE 14.2 Summary of Selected (C) Cholinergic Agonists

Drug (Trade) Name	Selected Indications	Route and Dosage Range	Pharmacokinetics
(C) Direct-Acting Muscarinic Agonists			
[P] pilocarpine (Akarpine)	Dry mouth from chemotherapy	*Adult:* PO, 5 mg tid for chemotherapy-induced dry mouth (xerostomia)	*Onset:* 10–30 min *Duration:* 4–8 h $t_{1/2}$: 3/4–1-1/2 h
	Open-angle glaucoma, changes in intraocular pressure, reversal of mydriasis	*Adult:* intraocular, 1 drop of 1%–2% solution q6–8 h or 20–40 mg/h by intraocular delivery device (Ocusert)	
acetylcholine (Miochol)	Cataract extraction, iridectomy, iris incarceration, keratoplasties, ophthalmic surgery, peripheral iridectomy, parotitis, renal failure, respiratory distress syndrome	*Adult:* intraocular, 5–20 mg intraocular as 0.5–2.0 mL solution	*Onset:* 10–30 min *Duration:* 10 min $t_{1/2}$: Minutes
bethanechol (Bethanechol Chloride; *Canadian:* Duvoid)	Decompensated bladder, lower motor neuron lesions, neurogenic bladder, postpartum urinary retention, urinary retention, postoperative urinary retention, atonies, sexual dysfunction, bladder dysfunction, parotitis, motion sickness	*Adult:* PO, 10–50 mg tid or qid	*Onset:* 30–90 min *Duration:* 1–6 h $t_{1/2}$: Variable
carbachol (Isopto Carbachol)	Glaucoma	*Adult:* topical, 2 drops of 0.75%–3.0% solution tid for glaucoma	*Onset:* 10–20 min *Duration:* 8 h $t_{1/2}$: Minutes
cevimeline (Evoxac)	Xerostomia associated with Sjögren's syndrome	*Adult:* PO, 30 mg	*Onset:* 60–90 min *Duration:* Unknown $t_{1/2}$: 5 h
methacholine (Provocholine)	Diagnosis of bronchial airway hyperactivity	Individualized	*Onset:* Rapid *Duration:* 15–75 m $t_{1/2}$: Unknown
(C) Direct-Acting Nicotinic Agonists			
[P] nicotine (Nicotrol, Prostep)	Smoking cessation	*Adult:* PO, 2 mg chewing gum prn; transdermal, 5–22 mg daily depending on number of weeks without cigarettes	*Onset:* Transdermal 1–2 h *Duration:* 2–24 h $t_{1/2}$: 3–4 h
(C) Indirect-Acting Cholinergic Agonists			
[P] neostigmine (Neostigmine Methylsulfate, Prostigmin; *Canadian:* PMS Neostigmine Methylsulfate)	Myasthenia gravis (MG) Neuromuscular blockade reversal Paralytic ileus and urinary retention	*Adult:* PO, 150 mg/d *Adult:* SC/IM, 0.5 mg *Adult:* 0.5 mg, then 0.5 mg q3h up to five times	*Onset:* PO, 2–4; SC/IM, 20–30 min; IV, 60 s *Duration:* PO, 2.5–4 h; IV 1–2 h $t_{1/2}$: 50–90 min
ambenonium (Mytelase)	MG, parotitis	*Adult:* PO, 5–25 mg tid or qid	*Onset:* 20–30 min *Duration:* 3–8 h $t_{1/2}$: Unknown
demecarium (Humorsol *Canadian:* Phospholine iodide)	Glaucoma	*Adult:* 1-2 gtt 1–2 x d *Child:* 1 gtt daily	*Onset:* ≤ h *Duration:* 1 m $t_{1/2}$: Unknown

(continued)

TABLE 14.2 Summary of Selected C Cholinergic Agonists (continued)

Drug (Trade) Name	Selected Indications	Route and Dosage Range	Pharmacokinetics
edrophonium (Tensilon)	Diagnosis of MG, differentiation between cholinergic and myasthenic crises, antagonism of neuromuscular blockade, parotitis, supraventricular tachycardia, Eaton-Lambert syndrome	*Adult:* IV, 1–10 mg depending on the indication	*Onset:* IV, 30–60 s *Duration:* IV 5–10 min $t_{1/2}$: 5–10 min
physostigmine (Antilirium, Isopto Eserine, prazosin hydrochloride)	Alzheimer's disease	*Adult:* PO 6–18 mg in four to nine divided doses daily	*Onset:* IV, 3–5 min *Duration:* 30–60 min $t_{1/2}$: 15–40 min
	Antidote for anticholinergic overdose	*Adult:* IV, 2 mg slow push over 2 min or more	
	Glaucoma, parotitis, acute myelogenous leukemia, chronic pain	*Adult:* 0.25% or 0.5%, 1 drop up to four times daily or 1 cm 0.25% ointment one to three times daily	
pyridostigmine (Mestinon, Regonol)	Motion sickness	*Adult:* PO, 30 mg tid	*Onset:* PO, 35–45 min; IV, 5 min *Duration:* 3–6 h $t_{1/2}$: 1.9–3.7 h
	MG	*Adult:* PO, 600 mg paced throughout the day	
	Reversal of nondepolarizing neuromuscular blockade	*Adult:* IV, 0.1–0.25 mg/kg	
tacrine (Cognex)	Alzheimer disease, AIDS dementia, tardive dyskinesia, anticholinergic overdose	*Adult:* PO, 10 mg qid increasing by 40 mg/d every 6 wk; IV slow push, 0.25–0.5 mg/kg	*Onset:* Varies *Duration:* Unknown $t_{1/2}$: 2–4 h

induction of **miosis** (pupillary constriction) to counteract mydriatic effects of sympathomimetics used in surgery, and miosis induction following ophthalmoscopy to counteract the effects of cycloplegics and mydriatics. Oral pilocarpine is used to treat xerostomia (dry mouth) caused by hypofunction of the salivary gland arising from radiotherapy for cancer of the head or neck.

Pharmacokinetics

Pilocarpine may be applied topically by solution or in an ocular system that allows sustained release over 7 days. With topical administration, miosis occurs within 10 to 30 minutes, and a maximal decrease in intraocular pressure occurs within 2 to 4 hours (see Table 14.2). When pilocarpine is given as an oral agent, peak effects are achieved in about 1 hour. Peak effects may take longer if the drug is taken with food. The mechanism for inactivation of pilocarpine is not clear but is thought to occur at the neuronal synapses and in plasma. Pilocarpine and its degradation products are excreted in the urine.

Pharmacodynamics

Pilocarpine directly stimulates cholinergic receptors. It produces miosis by contracting the iris sphincter. In open-angle glaucoma, pilocarpine contracts the ciliary muscle, increasing the outflow of aqueous humor, which reduces intraocular pressure. In closed-angle glaucoma, pilocarpine-induced miosis opens the angle of the anterior chamber of the eye, allowing the aqueous humor to exit. Pilocarpine also counteracts the mydriatic effects of sympathomimetic agents used in ophthalmologic examinations. When administered orally, pilocarpine stimulates secretions of the exocrine glands. All secretory glands may be affected, with results including an increase in salivary flow.

Contraindications and Precautions

Some contraindications may not be applicable to ophthalmic use, and others are not applicable to oral use. Hypersensitivity is a contraindication regardless of the formulation utilized.

Ophthalmic pilocarpine is contraindicated for use in patients with a history of retinal detachment. Miotics can precipitate detachment of the retina, resulting in a sudden drop in intraocular pressure. Ophthalmic pilocarpine is also contraindicated for use in patients with acute iritis or other conditions that would be exacerbated by pupillary constriction.

Because of its systemic effects, oral pilocarpine has more contraindications and precautions. These contraindications and precautions occur because of pilocarpine's ability to mimic the effects of the parasympathetic nervous system. For example, patients with asthma, chronic bronchitis, or chronic airway limitation may have exacerbations of these conditions because pilocarpine stimulates the mucous cells of the respiratory tract and increases bronchial smooth muscle tone and airway resistance. Pilocarpine causes contractions of the gallbladder or biliary smooth muscle, possibly resulting in biliary obstruction, cholangitis, or cholecystitis. Patients with cardiac disease may not be able to compensate for the transient changes in heart rhythm or hemodynamics caused by oral pilocarpine. Pilocarpine increases ureteral smooth muscle tone and may precipitate renal colic, especially in patients with

nephrolithiasis. Oral pilocarpine may induce dose-related central nervous system (CNS) effects that could exacerbate conditions of psychiatric disturbances or cognitive disturbances.

Pilocarpine is classified as a pregnancy category C drug. The oral dosage form should only be used if the benefits outweigh the risks to the fetus.

Finally, patients using ophthalmic or oral preparations of pilocarpine should be cautioned about nighttime driving, particularly the elderly and those with opaque lenses. Loss of visual acuity and accommodation is greater in poor light.

Adverse Effects

The ophthalmic adverse effects of pilocarpine include transient stinging and burning, tearing, and ciliary spasm. The ocular system (Ocusert) may cause conjunctival irritation. Systemic adverse effects include hypertension, tachycardia, bronchiolar spasm, pulmonary edema, salivation and sweating, and nausea and vomiting. When systemic effects occur with other cholinergic agonists, a **cholinergic crisis** may arise. Cholinergic crisis must be recognized quickly and managed effectively. It is caused by cholinergic toxicity and results in medullary paralysis (central respiratory paralysis), peripheral respiratory paralysis, excessive tracheobronchial and salivary secretions, bronchospasm, and laryngospasm. These effects may cause respiratory failure, which can be reversed with the maintenance of a patent airway. Muscle twitching, fasciculations, and paralysis may also occur. All symptoms of cholinergic crisis may be reversed with atropine, an anticholinergic drug.

Drug Interactions

There are no known important interactions between pilocarpine and other drugs, although other cholinergic agonists or blockers may enhance or antagonize its effects (Table 14.3).

Assessment of Relevant Core Patient Variables

Health Status

Cholinergic agonists such as pilocarpine do not have a wide range of therapeutic uses, but when they are used, they may cause systemic side effects and interact with preexisting disorders in life-threatening ways. A careful history and physical assessment will identify contraindications and precautions necessary for the person taking pilocarpine.

The nurse determines whether the patient has uncontrolled asthma or acute iritis, which are contraindications to pilocarpine therapy. Patients are assessed for significant cardiovascular disease because they may be unable to compensate for transient changes in hemodynamics or rhythm induced by pilocarpine. Pilocarpine should be used cautiously in patients with chronic bronchitis or chronic airway limitation because it may increase airway resistance, bronchial smooth muscle tone, and bronchial secretions. Patients with a history of biliary disease or nephrolithiasis are also closely monitored.

Life Span and Gender

The nurse documents the age and gender of the patient and assesses women of childbearing age for pregnancy and lactation. If the patient is pregnant, this drug should be used only if necessary because it is not known whether pilocarpine causes fetal abnormalities. If the patient is breast-feeding, the infant is monitored for cholinergic stimulation; if such stimulation occurs, the drug may need to be discontinued. Elderly patients may be at higher risk for injury because of blurred vision.

Lifestyle, Diet, and Habits

The nurse documents the patient's occupation and daily activities. Patients are advised to exercise caution when driving or operating machinery at night or in low light because miosis compromises dark adaptation.

Environment

The nurse is aware of the environment in which the drug will be administered and assesses the home or living environment if appropriate. Pilocarpine may be administered in any setting by a health care provider, nurse, or the patient.

Nursing Diagnoses and Outcomes

- Risk for Injury related to blurred vision
  Desired outcome: The patient will remain free of injury.
- Disturbed Sensory Perception (Visual) secondary to instillation of topical miotic.
  Desired outcome: The patient will adapt to blurring and adapt activity accordingly.
- Acute Pain related to local corneal irritation by miotic instillate
  Desired outcome: The patient will remain free from irritation.

Planning and Intervention

Maximizing Therapeutic Effects

Because pilocarpine is usually instilled, the nurse demonstrates how to instill drops into the conjunctival sac. To obtain the optimal intraocular hypotensive effect using the Ocusert system, the nurse must also demonstrate the placement and insertion of the system into the inferior conjunctival sac.

If both the solution and gel are used, the solution is applied first, and the gel is applied 5 minutes later. Following administration of the solution, finger pressure is applied on the lacrimal sac for 1 to 2 minutes.

TABLE 14.3 Agents That Interact With P Pilocarpine

Interactants	Effect and Significance	Nursing Management
cholinergic drugs	Enhanced cholinergic effect	Monitor increased and prolonged cholinergic stimulation.
anticholinergic drugs	Decreased cholinergic effect	Keep in mind that a dosage adjustment may be needed.

As described in Chapter 13, the **autonomic nervous system** (ANS) is divided into the sympathetic (adrenergic) and parasympathetic (cholinergic) nervous systems. These systems work in combination or opposition to maintain homeostasis within the body. This chapter identifies drugs used to treat the major disorders that are affected by deficiencies or excesses in cholinergic neurotransmission. It also discusses the wide range of therapeutic uses of cholinergic drugs. This chapter presents the cholinergic drugs that are categorized into cholinergic stimulants, called **cholinergic agonists,** cholinergics, or parasympathomimetics, and cholinergic blockers, known as **cholinergic antagonists,** anticholinergics, or parasympatholytics.

The cholinergic drugs are also categorized by the type of cholinergic receptor they affect. For example, pilocarpine (Akarpine) is the prototype direct-acting muscarinic agonist, whereas nicotine (Nicotrol, ProStep) is the prototype direct-acting nicotinic agonist. Neostigmine (Prostigmin) is the prototype indirect-acting cholinergic agonist, also known as an anticholinesterase or cholinesterase inhibitor. The prototype representing the cholinergic antagonists is atropine (Atropine Sulfate).

PHYSIOLOGY

Function of the Autonomic Nervous System

As mentioned in Chapter 13, the autonomic nervous system is an involuntary system responsible for the control of smooth muscle, cardiac muscle, and exocrine glands. These regulatory functions of the body are monitored by both the **sympathetic nervous system** and the **parasympathetic nervous system.** The sympathetic and parasympathetic nervous systems work either as complementary or oppositional systems to maintain the involuntary functions of the body. Chapter 13 includes a discussion of synaptic transmission and regulation of physiologic processes.

Cholinergic Neurotransmitters

Cholinergic drugs act on the parasympathetic nervous system, one of the subdivisions of the ANS. Acetylcholine (ACh) is the presynaptic and postsynaptic neurotransmitter in the parasympathetic nervous system (Figure 14.1). The precursors to ACh are choline and acetyl-coenzyme A. After formation and storage, ACh is released in response to an action potential and binds to cholinergic receptors on the target organs or tissues. After dissociation, ACh is degraded into two inactive products, acetate and choline, by acetylcholinesterase (AchE) (Figure 14.2).

Cholinergic Receptors

There are three types of cholinergic receptors: nicotinic$_N$, nicotinic$_M$, and muscarinic (Table 14.1).

Nicotinic Receptors

The **nicotinic receptors** (nicotinic$_N$ and nicotinic$_M$) are called *nicotinic* because they are stimulated primarily by nicotine, a plant alkaloid, but they will also respond to acetylcholine. They have a very low affinity for muscarine. Nicotinic$_N$ receptors are located on the cell bodies of all postganglionic neurons in both the sympathetic and parasympathetic nervous systems and in the adrenal medulla. Activation of nicotinic$_N$ receptors in the adrenal medulla results in the release of epinephrine.

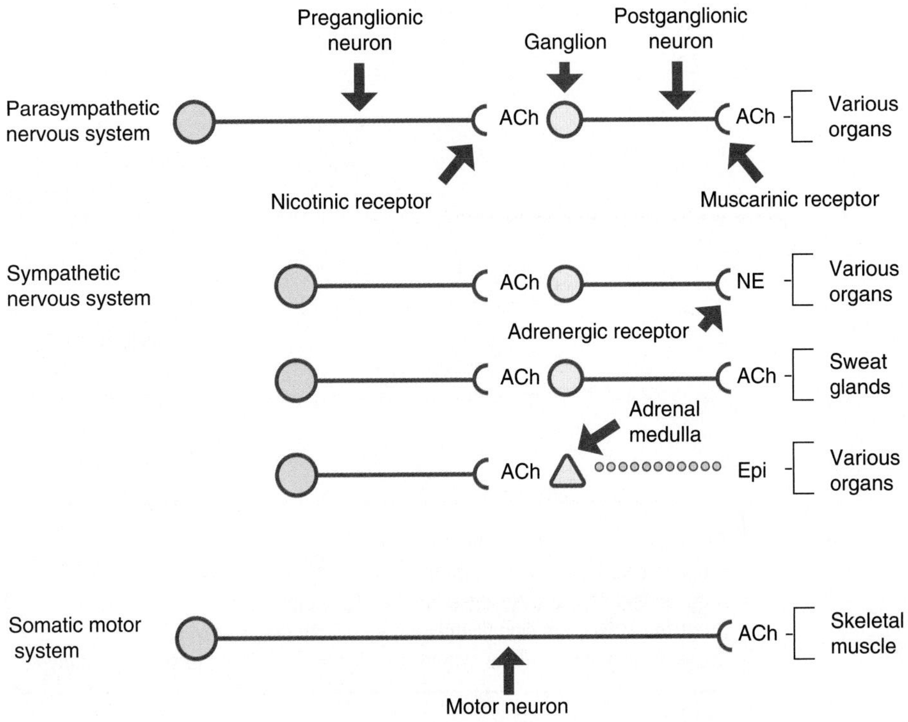

FIGURE 14.1 Neurotransmitters.
Acetylcholine
- All preganglionic neurons
- Postganglionic neurons to sweat glands in ANS
- Postganglionic neurons in PSNS
- Motor neurons in somatic motor system

Norepinephrine
- Postganglionic neurons to most organs in SNS

Epinephrine
- Released by adrenal medulla

Drugs That Affect Cholinergic Function

Ⓒ Cholinergic agonists

Ⓒ Direct-acting muscarinic agonists

- **P pilocarpine**
- acetylcholine
- bethanechol
- carbachol
- cevimeline
- methacholine

Ⓒ Direct-acting nicotine agonists

- **P nicotine**

Ⓒ Indirect-acting cholinergic agonists

- **P neostigmine**
- ambenonium chloride
- demecarium
- edrophonium
- physostigmine
- pyridostigmine
- tacrine
- irreversible cholinesterase inhibitors

Ⓒ Cholinergic antagonists

- **P atropine**
- antisecretory anticholinergics
- benztropine
- hyoscyamine
- ipratropium
- scopolamine
- trihexyphenidyl
- urinary tract relaxants

The symbol Ⓒ indicates the **drug class.**
Drugs in **bold type** marked with the symbol **P** are prototypes.
Drugs in blue type are closely related to the prototype.
Drugs in red type are significantly different from the prototype.
Drugs in black type with no symbol are also used in drug therapy; no prototype

Drugs Affecting Cholinergic Function

chapter 14

Learning Objectives

At the completion of this chapter the student will:

1. Describe the anatomy and physiology of the cholinergic nervous system.
2. Describe synaptic transmission.
3. Describe the role of cholinergic agonists and antagonists in a variety of therapeutic uses.
4. Identify core drug knowledge about drugs that act as cholinergic agonists or antagonists.
5. Identify core patient variables relevant to drugs that act as agonists or cholinergic antagonists.
6. Relate the interaction of core drug knowledge to core patient variables for drugs that act as cholinergic agonists or antagonists.
7. Generate a nursing plan of care from the interactions between core drug knowledge and core patient variables for drugs that act as cholinergic agonists or antagonists.
8. Describe nursing interventions to maximize therapeutic and minimize adverse affects for drugs that act as cholinergic agonists or antagonists.
9. Determine key points for patient and family education for drugs that act as cholinergic agonists or antagonists.

KEY TERMS

autonomic nervous system

cholinergic agonists

cholinergic antagonists

cholinergic crisis

miosis

muscarinic receptor

nicotinic receptor

parasympathetic nervous system

sympathetic nervous system

FEATURED WEBLINK

http://www.healthatoz.com/healthatoz/Atoz/ency/cholinergic_drugs.html.
Cholinergic agonists are used in a variety of diseases and disorders. For more information, log on to this website.

CONNECTION WEBLINK

Additional Weblinks are found on Connection:
http://www.connection.lww.com/go/aschenbrenner.

Sotalol

Sotalol (Betapace) is an oral, nonselective beta-adrenergic blocking agent. Unlike other beta blockers, sotalol has no sympathomimetic activity or membrane-stabilizing effects but does possess class III antiarrhythmic properties similar to those of amiodarone. As a result, sotalol is used as an antiarrhythmic. It is primarily used in the management of ventricular arrhythmias and angina.

CHAPTER SUMMARY

- Regulation of physiologic processes in the autonomic nervous system (ANS) is managed by oppositional or complementary stimulation by the adrenergic and cholinergic nervous systems.
- To effect an action, a neurotransmitter needs to bind with an appropriate receptor site on the effector organ or tissue.
- Alpha-1 adrenergic agonists, such as phenylephrine, stimulate alpha-1 receptors directly. They are most commonly used as nasal decongestants and in ophthalmology to achieve mydriasis. They may also be used as vasopressors to treat vascular failure and related shock.
- Nonselective adrenergic agonists, such as epinephrine, are used to treat anaphylactic shock, asthma, hemorrhage, and ventricular fibrillation. The nonselective activity stimulates all four adrenergic subtypes.
- Dopamine, a vasopressor, is used to correct the hemodynamic imbalances present in shock. Dopamine is a naturally occurring catecholamine and a precursor to norepinephrine. It stimulates alpha-1 and beta-1 receptors directly and indirectly (by releasing the stored epinephrine). It has either no effect or only minimal effect on beta-2 receptors. It also has dopaminergic effects including increased renal perfusion, increased cardiac output, increased or decreased peripheral resistance (depending on the dose), and increased blood pressure.
- Fenoldopam, a dopamine-1 agonist, is used in the management of acute hypertension for rapid reduction of blood pressure. It is also indicated for renal high-risk patients before contrast dye diagnostics.
- Alpha-adrenergic antagonists, such as prazosin, are used to treat hypertension and benign prostatic hypertrophy (BPH).
- Beta-adrenergic antagonists, such as propranolol, are used to treat hypertension, angina, and cardiac arrhythmias.
- Alpha- and beta-adrenergic antagonists, such as labetalol, are used to treat hypertension and heart failure.

QUESTIONS FOR STUDY AND REVIEW

1. You have been assigned to a cardiac care unit and are particularly interested in patients with angina. Which parameters are key to your predrug therapy assessments for a patient about to receive beta blockers?
2. When working with patients who have angina, which factors are most important to you during therapeutic monitoring?
3. How will you recognize impending toxicity in a patient receiving propranolol?
4. What will you do if it appears that the patient is showing cardiotoxic effects from propranolol?
5. Why is dopamine dosage determined by urinary output and cardiovascular response?
6. What is the purpose of administering fenoldopam to patients who are having a diagnostic test using radiocontrast dye?
7. What precautions are taken before the first-dose administration of prazosin? Why?

> **? Need More Help?**
>
> Chapter 13 of the study guide for *Drug Therapy in Nursing* 2e contains NCLEX-style questions and other learning activities to reinforce your understanding of the concepts presented in this chapter. For additional information or to purchase the study guide, visit *http://connection.lww.com/go/aschenbrenner.*

REFERENCES AND BIBLIOGRAPHY

Brown, G. A., & Sussman, D. O. (2004). A current review of medical therapy for benign prostatic hyperplasia. *Journal of the American Osteopathic Association, 104*(2 Suppl 2), S11–16.

Clinical Pharmacology [Online]. Available: *http://cp.gsm.com.*

de Reijke, T. M., & Klarskov, P. (2004). Comparative efficacy of two alpha-adrenoreceptor antagonists, doxazosin and alfuzosin, in patients with lower urinary tract symptoms from benign prostatic enlargement. *British Journal of Urology International, 93*(6), 757–762.

Facts and Comparisons. (2004). *Drug facts and comparisons.* Philadelphia: Lippincott Williams & Wilkins.

Hardman, J. G. (2001). *Goodman and Gillman's the pharmacological basis of therapeutics* (10th ed.). New York: McGraw-Hill Health Professions Division.

Katzung, B. (2004). *Basic and clinical pharmacology* (9th ed.). New York: McGraw-Hill/Appleton & Lange.

Lehne, R. A. (2004). *Pharmacology for nursing care* (5th ed.). St. Louis: W. B. Saunders.

Micromedex Healthcare Series [Online]. Available: *http://healthcare.micromedex.com.*

Moser, M., & Setaro, J. (2004). Continued importance of diuretics and beta-adrenergic blockers in the management of hypertension. *Medical Clinics of North America, 88*(1), 167–187.

Patel, M. R., & Gattis, W. (2003). Which beta-blocker for heart failure? *American Heart Journal, 147*(2), 238.

Tabrizchi, R. (2003). Should beta-blockers form the cornerstone for the treatment of congestive heart failure? *Expert Review of Cardiovascular Therapeutics, 1*(2), 157–160.

Tatro, D. S. (2004). *Drug interaction facts.* Philadelphia: Lippincott Williams & Wilkins.

MEMORY CHIP

[P] Propranolol

- Beta blocker
- Treats hypertension, angina, cardiac arrhythmias, migraine
- Decreases heart rate and contractility, slows conduction, suppresses automaticity
- Major contraindications: bradycardia, complete heart block, cardiogenic shock, uncompensated cardiac failure, reactive airway diseases, and Raynaud disease
- Most common adverse effects: postural hypotension, bronchospasm
- Most serious adverse effect: myocardial infarction
- Maximizing therapeutic effects: Take the medication exactly as prescribed, never double a dose.
- Minimizing adverse effects: Minimize situational and environmental stressors, stress safety issues.
- Most important patient education: self-monitoring techniques for pulse rate and heartbeat, safe mobility related to postural hypotension, and never abruptly stop taking the medication

Drugs Closely Related to [P] Propranolol

Atenolol

Atenolol (Tenormin) is a competitive, beta-1 selective adrenergic antagonist similar to metoprolol. It may be administered orally or parenterally. Atenolol has a longer plasma half-life than metoprolol, reducing the frequency of administration. As with all selective beta blockers, high doses result in attenuated or lost selectivity for the beta-1 receptor. Atenolol does not possess membrane-stabilizing activity, as do pindolol and propranolol. In addition, atenolol has the lowest lipid solubility within the class, which affects its route of elimination and, theoretically, its potential for causing CNS side effects.

Metoprolol

Metoprolol (Lopressor) is a competitive, beta-1 selective adrenergic antagonist similar to atenolol. It is only administered orally. Metoprolol does not have intrinsic sympathomimetic activity and does not exhibit membrane-stabilizing activities. Metoprolol is more lipid soluble than atenolol, but less so than propranolol. Metoprolol has one of the shortest plasma half-lives of the orally administered cardioselective beta blockers.

Pindolol

Pindolol (Visken) is an oral, nonselective beta-receptor antagonist. It has intrinsic sympathomimetic activity (ISA), which means that it has partial agonist activity. Pindolol is the beta blocker with the highest degree of ISA and nonselective antagonist qualities. The effect of ISA, as with beta blockade in general, can be selective or nonselective in nature. The partial agonist potential of pindolol is greater for beta-2 than for beta-1 receptors, resulting in the ability to be partially vasodilatory.

Nadolol

Nadolol (Corgard) is an oral, nonselective beta-adrenergic receptor antagonist similar to propranolol. Nadolol does not demonstrate appreciable intrinsic sympathomimetic or membrane-stabilizing activities. Unlike propranolol, nadolol possesses a low degree of lipid solubility. It also has the longest plasma half-life of all the beta-adrenergic blocking agents.

Timolol

Timolol (Blocadren) is a nonselective beta-adrenergic receptor antagonist similar to propranolol and nadolol. Timolol does not demonstrate appreciable intrinsic sympathomimetic or membrane-stabilizing activities. Like propranolol, timolol possesses a relatively high degree of lipid solubility and is subject to first-pass metabolism by the liver. Timolol is available for oral ophthalmic use.

Drugs Significantly Different From [P] Propranolol

Carvedilol

Carvedilol (Coreg) is a combined alpha selective and nonselective beta blocker. Although it has some pharmacologic similarities to labetalol, the ratio of beta-1 to alpha-1 effects is much greater for carvedilol than for labetalol. Carvedilol also possesses antioxidant properties (an effect not shared by other beta blockers). Carvedilol has multiple actions that make it a useful cardiovascular drug. Similarly to labetalol, carvedilol antagonizes both alpha-1 and beta receptors. However, the ratio of beta blockade to alpha-1 blockade for carvedilol is in the range of 10:1 to 100:1. The ratio for labetalol is 1.5:1. Carvedilol is indicated for the management of hypertension, heart failure, and stable angina and as post-myocardial infarction prophylaxis. It is frequently administered with other antihypertensive agents to gain additive therapeutic effects.

When initiating carvedilol therapy, the patient should have a standing blood pressure measurement 1 hour after dosing. An initial dose of 6.25 mg should be maintained for 7 to 14 days; then, the patient should be evaluated for the effectiveness of the dose. If further control of diastolic blood pressure is needed, the dosage may be increased to 12.5 mg orally twice daily for an additional 7 to 14 days. If needed, the dosage may be further increased to the maximum recommended dosage of 25 mg orally twice daily if tolerated. If the pulse rate drops below 55 bpm, the dosage of carvedilol should be reduced. Doses should be taken with food to slow the rate of absorption and reduce the risk for orthostatic hypotension.

Labetalol

Labetalol (Normodyne) is a competitive nonselective beta-adrenergic and selective postsynaptic alpha-1 adrenergic receptor blocker that can be given orally and parenterally. Labetalol blocks beta-1 receptors in the heart, beta-2 receptors in bronchial and vascular smooth muscle, and alpha-1 receptors in vascular smooth muscle. The beta-blocking activity is 3 to 7 times as potent as the alpha-blocking ability. The result of labetalol's actions at alpha and beta receptors leads to vasodilation and decreased total peripheral resistance, which results in decreased blood pressure without a substantial decrease in resting heart rate, cardiac output, or stroke volume.

Desired outcome: The patient will sleep normally and awaken rested.

- Activity Intolerance related to lethargy and weakness secondary to beta blockade
  Desired outcome: *The patient will maintain a satisfactory activity level.*
- Risk for Deficient Fluid Volume related to drug-induced diarrhea
  Desired outcome: *The patient will remain adequately hydrated and nourished despite adverse GI effects. The patient will report any intolerable GI effects.*

Planning and Intervention

Maximizing Therapeutic Effects

The nurse instructs the patient to take propranolol exactly as prescribed and at the required dosage frequency to enhance the therapeutic potential. Patients taking propranolol in sustained-release form are advised to swallow the whole drug and not to chew, crush, or break it. Patients may also take the drug with food to increase the drug's bioavailability and to avoid possible GI upset (e.g., diarrhea).

Patients are informed about what to do if they miss a dose. If the next dose is more than 4 hours away (8 hours for sustained-release forms), the patient is advised to take the missed dose as soon as possible. If the next dose is scheduled to occur within the next 4 hours (8 hours for sustained-release forms), the patient should skip the missed dose and return to the regular schedule.

Minimizing Adverse Effects

Some standards of care relating to beta-adrenergic antagonists such as propranolol are concerned with safety and require the nurse to perform certain interventions:

- The nurse checks the apical and peripheral pulses before giving propranolol. If the pulse is irregular or if there is bradycardia, the drug is withheld and the prescriber notified because signs may be early indications of adverse or cardiotoxic effects.
- The nurse monitors blood pressure, pulmonary wedge pressure, and cardiac rhythm and conduction (by ECG), particularly when adrenergic antagonists such as propranolol are administered intravenously, because bronchoconstriction and altered cardiac output may result from adrenergic blockade.
- In patients with angina, the nurse monitors the frequency of anginal pain episodes and tolerance of activity.
- In patients with hypertension, the nurse assesses drug effectiveness by monitoring blood pressure and comparing the findings with baseline measurements.
- In patients with impaired renal or hepatic function, the nurse monitors for signs of drug accumulation and potential toxicity.

Providing Patient and Family Education

- Sympatholytic drugs interfere with compensatory and homeostatic mechanisms regulated by the normal functioning of the SNS, particularly in response to stress. Therefore, it is crucial to identify and monitor environmental stressors for patients receiving adrenergic antagonists, such as propranolol.
- Careful teaching about adverse effects is important. This includes teaching patients how to take their own pulses and detect irregular rhythms or bradycardias.
- Therapeutic adherence is promoted by reminding patients and their family members that drug therapy is meant to control certain life-threatening or debilitating conditions and should be continued even when the patient is feeling well and has no symptoms.
- If drug therapy is being discontinued, it is important to stress tapering or gradual withdrawal to prevent rebound symptoms and to adjust the activity levels to suit the reduced blockade.
- As another safety factor, the patient is taught to change position slowly to reduce dizziness and light-headedness and to avoid operating machinery or driving until full adaptation to side effects has occurred. Factors known to enhance postural hypotension (e.g., heat, exercise, and alcohol consumption) should be avoided.

CRITICAL THINKING SCENARIO

Thinking critically about beta-blocker therapy

Mr. DiGiovanni is a 65-year-old man with hypertension and angina. His health care provider recently increased his propranolol dosage from 40 mg qid to 60 mg qid. He complains to you that he is experiencing erectile dysfunction.

1. Discuss what you know about the effects of propranolol on sexual performance.
2. Choose elements related to propranolol therapy to include in a teaching plan for Mr. DiGiovanni, and provide rationale for your choices.
3. What other health care professionals may work with the nurse to provide the best care for Mr. DiGiovanni?

Ongoing Assessment and Evaluation

The same assessment focus is used for adrenergic antagonists as for the adrenergic agonists. All patients with cardiovascular disorders are considered worthy of extra attention when taking an adrenergic antagonist such as propranolol. When evaluating the success of nursing management in propranolol therapy, the nurse anticipates the absence of signs and symptoms for the condition being treated, as well as minimal adverse effects.

If propranolol is being given for angina or hypertension, blood pressure should be within normal limits, the frequency of anginal attacks should be reduced, and there should be tolerance to reasonable activity. For antiarrhythmic indications, no arrhythmias should be evident on ECG findings. Moreover, the patient should be free from injury resulting from postural hypotension or dizziness. The patient may report sexual adjustment. Ideally, the patient and family can understand, recognize, and cope with adverse effects.

TABLE 13.9 Agents That Interact With P Propranolol

Interactants	Effect and Significance	Nursing Management
clonidine	Life-threatening increases in blood pressure after discontinuation of clonidine therapy	When clonidine is to be withdrawn from concomitant therapy with a beta blocker, discontinue the beta blocker first, and monitor blood pressure carefully. Consult with prescriber: Labetalol (alpha/beta blocker) or alpha blockers (e.g., prazosin, doxazosin) may prevent rebound hypertension.
epinephrine	Initial hypertension followed by bradycardia	Monitor blood pressure carefully for serious hypotension.
verapamil	Increased hypotensive effects of both drugs	Monitor for signs and symptoms of theophylline toxicity.
aminophylline	Reduced elimination of theophylline	Monitor for increased blood pressure.
barbiturates	Decreased propranolol levels resulting from barbiturate induction	Monitor respiration. Administer concomitant therapy with caution.
phenothiazines	Increased levels of both drugs; phenothiazines inhibit first-pass metabolism of propranolol	Monitor phenothiazine level, and decrease dosage if prescribed.
cimetidine	May increase propranolol level twofold	Monitor cardiac function carefully (i.e., blood pressure, heart rate), and lower dosage of propranolol as prescribed.
ergot derivatives	Peripheral ischemia and cold extremities	If used together, monitor for peripheral ischemic effects (i.e., cold extremities), and substitute a selective beta blocker (e.g., atenolol) if ischemia occurs.
hydralazine	Increased levels of both drugs	If concurrent therapy is required, administer with food or switch to a sustained-release beta blocker. Monitor blood pressure carefully.
nonsteroidal anti-inflammatory drugs	Decreased propranolol level	Monitor blood pressure.
insulin	Prolonged hypoglycemia with masking of symptoms	Monitor blood glucose level regularly. Anticipate adjustment in drug dosages. Consult prescriber about lowering propranolol dosage, and monitor impact on blood glucose level.
lidocaine	Increased, potentially toxic lidocaine level	Consult prescriber about lower lidocaine dosage. Monitor for enhanced inotropic effect of propranolol.
prazosin	Increased postural hypotension from prazosin	Monitor blood pressure. Caution patient to rise slowly from seated position and use hand railings, particularly on stairs.
quinidine	Moderate increase in drug levels	Use caution with concomitant administration. Monitor for hypotension, bradycardia, arrhythmias, and heart failure.
alcohol	Decreased absorption and increased elimination of propranolol, resulting in tachycardia and possible increase in hypertension	Advise patient to avoid ethanol. Monitor blood pressure and heart rhythm.
rifampin	Rifampin-induced enzymes that decrease beta blocker levels by increasing metabolism and clearance	If concurrent therapy is required, monitor blood pressure carefully. A higher dose of propranolol may be required in patients receiving rifampin for longer than 1 to 2 wk. Or the prescriber may substitute atenolol or nadolol for propranolol.

Nursing Diagnoses and Outcomes

- Sexual Dysfunction related to decreased libido or erectile dysfunction secondary to beta blockade
  Desired outcome: *The patient will adapt to altered sexual functioning and understand that decreased libido or erectile dysfunction will be reversible on cessation of therapy.*
- Risk for Injury related to dizziness secondary to beta blockade
  Desired outcome: *The patient will not sustain injury and will learn safe methods for dealing with dizziness and postural hypotension.*
- Disturbed Sleep Pattern, Insomnia and Drowsiness, secondary to beta blockade

release formulation). With IV dosing, half-life is shorter (see Table 13.8).

Pharmacodynamics

Propranolol is a nonselective beta-blocking drug that has similar effects on beta-1 (cardiac) and beta-2 (bronchial, vascular smooth muscle) receptors. Beta-1 blockade decreases heart rate and myocardial contractility during periods of high sympathetic activity (such as during physical exercise), which results in decreased cardiac output. As cardiac output decreases, so does blood pressure. In cardiac conduction tissue, beta blockade results in slowing of atrioventricular conduction and suppression of automaticity. These actions result in decreased oxygen demand, thus suggesting its use as an antianginal agent. Propranolol also blocks beta-1 receptors in the kidneys. This action decreases the release of renin, which results in decreased blood pressure. Many of the adverse effects of propranolol are attributable to its overlapping beta-2 blockade. These include bronchospasm, hypoglycemia, and peripheral vasoconstriction. Although its role in reducing hypertension is complex, propranolol is an effective antihypertensive.

Contraindications and Precautions

The main contraindications for propranolol include severe bradycardia, complete heart block, cardiogenic shock, uncompensated cardiac failure, airway diseases, Raynaud syndrome, and concomitant use of antidepressant drugs. The action of propranolol depresses conduction through the atrioventricular node and decreases contractility. These actions can exacerbate cardiac disorders. Beta blockade results in bronchoconstriction, which exacerbates symptoms of chronic airway disorders. In Raynaud disease, symptoms can be exacerbated secondary to a reduced cardiac output and a relative increased alpha stimulation. Propranolol has been associated with major depression, although the mechanism is unclear. Abrupt discontinuation of propranolol in patients with hyperthyroidism may induce a thyroid storm.

Caution is used in patients with pheochromocytoma and vasospastic angina because unopposed alpha stimulation may result in hypertension. Propranolol is used cautiously in patients with diabetes because beta blockade can mask the signs of hypoglycemia, especially palpitations, tachycardia, and tremors. Patients receiving propranolol during surgery are monitored closely because of the cardiodepressant effects of general anesthetics. Patients with renal and hepatic diseases also require close monitoring to ensure clearance of the drug from the body. Other conditions that may be exacerbated by propranolol therapy include myasthenia gravis and psoriasis. Propranolol is secreted in breast milk; therefore, women who are breast-feeding should not take this drug.

Adverse Effects

If propranolol or a similar beta blocker is withdrawn abruptly, myocardial ischemia, infarction, ventricular arrhythmias, severe hypertension, or angina may occur. In the CNS, propranolol may cause cognitive dysfunction or depression. Hallucinations and psychosis have been reported with high doses of the drug. These CNS effects are seen more frequently in elderly patients and resolve after discontinuation. The drug predisposes patients with type 1 diabetes to hypoglycemia and may trigger hyperthyroidism in susceptible individuals. In the GI system, diarrhea is common and may be severe enough to require discontinuation of the drug. With long-term therapy, weight gain is common.

Drug Interactions

Beta antagonists have many interactions with other drugs. Some of the more significant interactions include those with clonidine, epinephrine, verapamil, aminophylline, barbiturates, phenothiazines, cimetidine, ergot derivatives, hydralazine, NSAIDs, insulin, lidocaine, prazosin, quinidine, and rifampin (Table 13.9).

Elevated bilirubin levels may occur in patients who have chronic renal failure and who are taking propranolol because its metabolites interfere with the bilirubin analysis. In addition, food enhances the bioavailability of propranolol, which may account for slight fluctuations in beta blockade or adverse effects (depending on dose scheduling).

Assessment of Relevant Core Patient Variables

Health Status

The nurse assesses for conditions for which the drug is contraindicated or for which special precautions might be necessary (e.g., uncontrolled asthma or chronic obstructive lung disease, severe sinus bradycardia, right ventricular hypertrophy or failure secondary to pulmonary hypertension, second- or third-degree atrioventricular block, cardiac failure, or cardiogenic shock). It is also important to determine whether any other drugs are being taken concurrently to identify significant potential drug interactions.

Because propranolol is used mainly to treat angina, cardiac arrhythmias, migraine headaches, hypertension, and tremors, the physical assessment includes blood pressure, cardiovascular status, genitourinary function, and mental and neurologic status. Heart and lung sounds are auscultated as well.

Life Span and Gender

The nurse documents the age and gender of the patient and assesses women of childbearing age for pregnancy and lactation. If the patient is pregnant, propranolol is administered only if necessary. This drug is classified as FDA pregnancy risk category C, and the possibility of inducing fetal abnormalities is not established. If the patient is breast-feeding, the infant is monitored for adrenergic blockade. If it occurs, the administration may need to be discontinued. Elderly patients may be at risk for injury resulting from blurred vision related to propranolol use.

Lifestyle, Diet, and Habits

The nurse documents the patient's occupation and daily activities. Patients, particularly those in hazardous occupations, are advised to exercise caution when driving or operating machinery at night or in bright light conditions. Mydriasis may cause temporary night blindness, which may prove perilous.

Environment

The nurse is aware of the environment in which the drug will be administered and assesses the home or living environment, if appropriate. Propranolol may be administered in any setting by health care providers, nurses, or patients themselves.

and only 10% of the drug is excreted unchanged by the kidneys. As with alfuzosin, its pharmacokinetics are altered in patients with severe renal or hepatic dysfunction.

Contraindications, precautions, adverse effects, and drug–drug interactions are similar to alfuzosin. Although tamsulosin is a pregnancy category B drug, it is only used in the management of BPH and so is not indicated for use in women.

The nurse teaches the patient not to open, crush, or chew the capsule to maintain its prolonged action.

Terazosin

Like prazosin and doxazosin, terazosin (Hytrin) is an alpha-adrenergic blocking agent used in the treatment of hypertension and BPH. The duration of action of terazosin is longer than that of prazosin but shorter than that of doxazosin. In a head-to-head comparison with finasteride (Proscar), terazosin achieved superior results in the management of BPH. In addition to its alpha-1 blockade, terazosin also alters lipid metabolism, decreasing the levels of total cholesterol, low-density lipoprotein (LDL) cholesterol, and very low-density lipoprotein (VLDL) cholesterol.

Antihypertensive effects are seen within 15 minutes, and peak plasma levels are observed approximately 1 hour after administration. The plasma half-life is about 12 hours. Excretion of terazosin occurs as both unchanged drug and metabolites in the urine and in the feces. Only 10% of the terazosin dose is excreted renally as unchanged drug; therefore, impaired renal function has no significant effect on the elimination of terazosin.

Contraindications, precautions, drug interactions, and adverse effects are almost identical to those of prazosin.

Drugs Significantly Different From [P] Prazosin

Phentolamine

Unlike prazosin, phentolamine (Regitine) blocks both alpha-1 and alpha-2 receptors. It is used in the management of tissue necrosis caused by extravasation of parenterally administered drugs and in the management of symptoms from a pheochromocytoma, an adrenaline-secreting tumor. It may induce adverse effects similar to those of prazosin, but it is more likely to cause reflex tachycardia because of its ability to block alpha-2.

Phentolamine is contraindicated in patients with a known hypersensitivity. It is also contraindicated for use in patients with a history of acute myocardial infarction or any evidence of coronary artery disease because of its cardiac-stimulating effects and resultant increase in myocardial oxygen demand. Also, reflex tachycardia can exacerbate angina. Phentolamine is used with caution in patients with gastric and duodenal ulcers because the drug has a histamine-like effect. Phentolamine can stimulate secretion of gastric acid and pepsin in the stomach, which can aggravate peptic ulcer disease.

Phentolamine should not be used in conjunction with epinephrine. Phentolamine can antagonize epinephrine's alpha receptor–mediated actions and exaggerate its beta-adrenergic responses, resulting in hypotension, vasodilation, and tachycardia. Potential adverse reactions are similar to those of prazosin.

Phenoxybenzamine

Like phentolamine, phenoxybenzamine (Dibenzyline) blocks both alpha-1 and alpha-2 receptors. It is useful in the treatment of sweating and hypertension associated with pheochromocytoma, urinary symptoms of BPH, and symptoms of certain peripheral vasospastic conditions such as acrocyanosis, Raynaud phenomenon, and frostbite. The effects of phenoxybenzamine are similar to those of phentolamine. Phenoxybenzamine has a slower onset of action and a longer duration of action than phentolamine—its effects begin several hours after administration, and the effects of a single dose may last 3 to 4 days.

(C) Beta-Adrenergic Antagonists

Beta-adrenergic antagonists are frequently and more commonly called beta blockers. They comprise a significant group of drugs that can be grouped according to their specificity of action at the beta-1 and beta-2 receptors. If the predominant actions of stimulation of each of the two groups of beta-adrenergic receptors are considered, it follows that sometimes a therapeutic effect will require stimulation of beta-1 only (tachycardia, increased lipolysis, inotropy) or sometimes of both beta-1 and beta-2 receptors (vasodilation, decreased peripheral resistance, bronchodilation).

Beta-1 blockade is effected by atenolol, acebutolol, alprenolol, metoprolol, betaxolol, and esmolol; beta-2 blockade has only one specific drug that triggers vasodilation, bronchodilation, and peripheral vascular resistance—namely butoxamine, which has no significant clinical application. The nonselective beta blockers include propranolol, metipranolol, nadolol, penbutolol, pindolol, timolol, carteolol, and sotalol. Propranolol is the prototype nonselective beta blocker.

NURSING MANAGEMENT OF THE PATIENT RECEIVING [P] PROPRANOLOL

Core Drug Knowledge

Pharmacotherapeutics

Propranolol is used in the treatment of hypertension, angina, irregular cardiac rhythms, paroxysmal atrial tachycardias, ventricular tachycardias, digitalis intoxication, myocardial infarction, pheochromocytoma, migraine, hypertrophic subaortic stenosis, and essential tremor. It has been used to treat a wide variety of other disorders, including situational anxiety and substance withdrawal.

Pharmacokinetics

Propranolol is well absorbed following oral administration, and peak serum levels are observed within 2 to 6 hours of ingestion; however, hypotensive stability may not occur for 2 to 3 weeks. Beta blockade may occur within 1 to 2 hours. Parenteral dosing speeds the onset and lowers the duration. Much of an ingested dose is subjected to first-pass metabolism in the liver. Metabolites are excreted through urine. Propranolol crosses the placenta and is excreted into breast milk. It has a half-life of 3 to 5 hours (longer with the sustained-

Desired outcome: The patient will receive adequate nourishment by practicing appropriate dietary management.

- Risk for Injury related to orthostatic hypotension
  Desired outcome: The patient will remain free of injury.

Planning and Intervention

Maximizing Therapeutic Effects

The nurse emphasizes the importance of taking the prescribed dose on a daily basis exactly as instructed. The nurse explains the importance of refraining from OTC drug use because many OTC drugs contain ingredients that decrease the effectiveness of prazosin.

Minimizing Adverse Effects

Nursing strategies to minimize adverse effects include having the patient take the first dose just before bedtime, having the patient lie down if syncope occurs, monitoring the patient's weight, and checking for edema. The nurse explains the importance of changing position slowly to avoid orthostatic hypotension.

Providing Patient and Family Education

- Patients are advised to take the drug as prescribed and to avoid operating machinery or driving for about 4 hours after the first dose.
- The nurse teaches the patient about additional adverse effects, such as dizziness and weakness (after changing position rapidly, in hot weather, after exercising, and after drinking alcohol). To avoid injury from these effects, the patient may need to avoid driving or engaging in tasks that require alertness until the body adjusts to the drug, to change positions slowly, to use caution when climbing stairs, to cool down when exercising, and to avoid consuming alcoholic beverages.
- The nurse highlights the symptoms that should be reported to the provider if they occur. These symptoms include blurred vision, difficulty breathing, fainting spells, lightheadedness, irregular heartbeat, palpitations or chest pain, mental depression, swelling of the legs and ankles, protracted vomiting, and prolonged, painful erections.

Ongoing Assessment and Evaluation

Monitoring of blood pressure, heart and lung sounds, and edema is important. To identify significant potential drug interactions, the nurse also determines whether any other drugs are being taken concurrently with prazosin.

MEMORY CHIP

P Prazosin

- Vasodilator
- Treats refractory CHF, hypertension, Raynaud vasospasm, prostatic obstruction
- Major contraindication: hypersensitivity
- Most common adverse effects: lightheadedness, dizziness, headache, drowsiness, weakness, lethargy, nausea, and palpitations
- Most serious adverse effect: "first dose syncope"
- Maximizing therapeutic effects: Refrain from administering any OTC drug in combination with prazosin.
- Minimizing adverse effects: Stress safety issues regarding CNS effects.
- Most important patient education: safe ways to cope with postural hypotension

Drugs Closely Related to P Prazosin

Alfuzosin

Alfuzosin (UroXatral) is another alpha-1 antagonist drug that is more specific to alpha-1a receptor sites than prazosin is. Because approximately 70% of the alpha-receptor sites in the prostate are alpha-1a subtypes, alfuzosin is indicated for the management of benign prostatic hypertrophy (BPH). Blockade of these receptors causes smooth muscles in the bladder neck and prostate to relax, which reduces pressure on the urethra. As a result, the urine flow rate improves, and the symptoms of BPH decrease.

Alfuzosin is an oral sustained-release tablet. It is metabolized in the liver by the P-450 3A4 (CYP3A4) pathway. It is excreted in feces and by the kidneys. Pharmacokinetics is greatly altered in patients with renal and liver dysfunction.

Contraindications, precautions, and adverse effects are similar to those for prazosin. Like prazosin, alfuzosin may interact with other antihypertensive agents and drugs for erectile dysfunction. In addition, because it is a P-450–metabolized drug, it may interact with cimetidine, diltiazem, azole antifungal agents, macrolide antibiotics, and protease inhibitors.

Because alfuzosin is used only in the management of BPH, it is not indicated for use in women, although it has been classified as pregnancy category B.

Doxazosin

Like prazosin, doxazosin (Cardura) is an oral alpha-adrenergic blocking agent used in the treatment of hypertension and benign prostatic hyperplasia. It is pharmacologically similar to prazosin and terazosin but has the longest duration of action of agents in the group. Because of its duration, it may be dosed once daily.

Doxazosin is highly metabolized in the liver, and an oral dose is mostly eliminated in feces, suggesting enterohepatic recycling. The remainder is excreted in urine. Neither advanced age nor renal failure significantly alters the elimination half-life.

Doxazosin interacts with more drugs than prazosin does but has minimal adverse reactions. Drug interactions include other antihypertensive agents, dopamine, epinephrine, estrogens, metaraminol, methoxamine, nonsteroidal anti-inflammatory agents (NSAIDs), and phenylephrine.

Tamsulosin

Tamsulosin (Flomax) is another alpha-1 antagonist drug with specificity to alpha-1a subtype receptors. Like alfuzosin, it is indicated for use in the management of BPH. Tamsulosin causes less hypotension than other alpha blockers and may be given concurrently with other antihypertensive agents.

Tamsulosin is a once-a-day oral capsule that should be taken with a meal. It undergoes extensive hepatic metabolism,

TABLE 13.2 Adrenergic Receptor Subtypes' Location and Action

Location	Response to Stimuli
Alpha-1	
Arteries and veins	Constriction
Bladder neck	Contraction
Eyes	Mydriasis (dilation) of the pupil
Male sex organs	Ejaculation
Prostatic capsule	Contraction
Alpha-2	
Central nervous system	Inhibits release of norepinephrine
Beta-1	
Heart	Increased rate Positive inotropic action Increased atrioventricular conduction
Kidney	Release of renin
Beta-2	
Arterioles	Dilation
Bronchi	Dilation
Liver	Glycogenolysis
Skeletal muscle	Contraction, glycogenolysis
Uterus	Relaxation
Dopamine-1 (DA-1)	
Vessels	Peripheral vasodilation
Proximal tubule	Maintain or increase GFR
Renal tubules	Natriuresis Diuresis
Dopamine-2 (DA-2)	
Vessels	Peripheral vasodilation
Glomerulus	Deceased renal blood flow
Renal nerves	Decreased GFR
Adrenal cortex	Decreased Na and H_2O excretion Decreased aldosterone

GFR, glomerular filtration rate.

Adapted from Lehne, R. A. (2004). *Pharmacology for nursing care* (5th ed., p. 107). St. Louis: Saunders.

duration of action, may be given orally, and do cross the blood–brain barrier.

Adrenergic agonists are also classified according to their selectivity. Agents that stimulate multiple adrenergic subtype receptors are called **nonselective-acting drugs.** Nonselective adrenergic agonists stimulate both alpha and beta receptors. Agents that target a specific subtype receptor are called **selective-acting drugs.** To maximize therapeutic effects and minimize adverse effects, selective-acting drugs are used more frequently than nonselective drugs. It is important to remember that selectivity is not exclusive. Although a selective-acting drug is preferential to a given subtype receptor, given in higher doses it may also stimulate other subtype receptors.

C Nonselective Adrenergic Agonists

Nonselective adrenergic agonists stimulate most receptors; therefore, they have a multitude of uses. It is important to remember that these drugs stimulate all of the subtypes, regardless of which subtype would be most helpful for a specific pathology.

The prototype for nonselective adrenergic agonists is epinephrine. This drug stimulates alpha-1, alpha-2, beta-1, and beta-2 receptors. The only adrenergic receptor subtype it does not stimulate is the dopamine receptor. A summary of selected adrenergic agonists is provided in Table 13.3.

TABLE 13.3 Summary of Selected (C) Adrenergic Agonists

Drug (Trade) Name	Selected Indications	Route and Dosage Range	Pharmacokinetics
(C) Nonselective Adrenergic Agonists			
P epinephrine (Adrenalin, Epinephrine)	Anaphylactic shock, asthma, cardiopulmonary resuscitation, glaucoma, adjunct in topical anesthesia, ventricular fibrillation, cataracts, chloroquine poisoning, cluster headaches, croup, gastrointestinal hemorrhage, herpes simplex, hyperkalemia, hypothermia, mastocytosis, obstetric analgesia, open heart surgery, priapism, septic shock, wheezing in infants	*Adult:* IV, 1–4 mg/min of 4 mg/mL [15–60 mL/h]; other special dosages for ICU use *Child:* SC (asthma), 0.01 mL/kg/dose (1:1000), with maximum of 0.4–0.5 mL, repeated every 15–20 min for three to four doses or q4h if needed; IM/SC (anaphylaxis), 0.01 mL/kg, with maximum 0.3 mL of 1:1,000 solution; if response inadequate, IV 0.1 mL/kg of 1:10,000 solution every 5–10 min; inhalation, 0.05 mL/kg to a max of 0.5 mL/dose of 2.25% solution	*Onset:* IV, instant; SC > 1 h *Duration:* 20–30 min; SC, 4 h $t_{1/2}$: NA
ephedrine (*Canadian:* Omni-Tuss)	Asthma, enuresis, nasal congestion, rhinorrhea, sinusitis Hypotension	*Adult:* PO, 25–50 mg q3–4h *Adult:* IM, 25–50 mg; IV, 10–25 mg IV slow push	*Onset:* PO, 15–60 min; IM, 10–20 min; IV, instant *Duration:* PO, 3–5 h; IM/IV, 1 h $t_{1/2}$: 3–6 h
norepinephrine (Levophed)	Hypotension, shock, GI bleeding, glaucoma, hypothermia, ventricular fibrillation	*Adult:* IV, 8–12 mg/min at 2–3 mL/min	*Onset:* 1–2 min *Duration:* 1–2 min $t_{1/2}$: 7–18 h
(C) Alpha-1 Adrenergic Agonists			
P phenylephrine (Dristan, Dimetapp, Neo-Synephrine, others); *Canadian:* Dionephrine	Nasal congestion, common cold, glaucoma, shock, hypotensive crisis, anesthetic adjunct, PSVT	*Adult:* Topical, 1–2 sprays of 0.25%–1% solution q3–4h; IM, 2–5 mg; IV, 0.2– 0.5 mg (IM/IV adjusted for indication)	*Onset:* IM, 10–15 min; IV, immediate *Duration:* IM 30–120 min; IV, 15–20 min $t_{1/2}$: 2–3 h
methoxamine (Vasoxyl)	Hypotension, blood pressure maintenance during anesthesia, shock, SVT	*Adult:* IM, 10–15 mg; IV, 3–10 mg by slow push depending on condition	*Onset:* 30–120 s *Duration:* 60 min $t_{1/2}$: NA
(C) Alpha-2 Adrenergic Agonists			
P clonidine (Catapres; Canadian: Apo-Clonidine) (see Chapter 26)	Cancer pain (epidural), antihypertensive, alcohol withdrawal, diabetic diarrhea, menopausal flushing, opiate detoxification, herpetic neuralgia, ulcerative colitis	*Adult:* PO, 100–300 μg bid; IM/IV, 150 μg; epidural, 75–150 μg	*Onset:* 30–60 min *Duration:* 24 h $t_{1/2}$: 12–16 h
P dopamine (Intropin; *Canadian:* Revimine)	Hemodynamic imbalances	*Adult:* IV, 2–5 μg/kg/min *Seriously Ill Adult:* IV, 5 μg/kg/min up to a rate of 20–50 μg/kg/min *Child:* Safety and efficacy not established	*Onset:* IV, 1–2 min *Duration:* IV, length of infusion $t_{1/2}$: 2 min
dobutamine (Dobutrex)	Cardiac decompensation due to decreased contractility	*Adult:* IV infusion, 2.5–10 μg/kg/min	*Onset:* 1–2 min *Duration:* Unknown $t_{1/2}$: 2 min

(continued)

TABLE 13.3 Summary of Selected C Adrenergic Agonists (continued)

Drug (Trade) Name	Selected Indications	Route and Dosage Range	Pharmacokinetics
P isoproterenol (Isuprel)	Asthma, CPR, COLD, MI, cerebral vasospasm, status asthmaticus, torsades de pointes, hypothermia, poisoning, AV block, bradycardia	*Adult:* SL, 10–20 mg up to tid for asthma; IM, 0.2 mg followed by 0.02–1.0 mg contingent on response; IV, 2–10 μg/min until response	*Onset:* Rapid *Duration:* 2 h $t_{1/2}$: Unknown
mephentermine (Wyamine)	Hypotension attendant to spinal anesthesia Hypotension following spinal anesthesia Shock following hemorrhage	*Adult:* IM, 30–45 mg 10–20 min prior to procedure *Adult:* IV, 30–45 mg as a single injection *Adult:* IV, 0.1% solution in 5% dextrose in water just until blood replacement achieved	*Onset:* IM, 10–15 min; IV, immediate *Duration:* IM, 1–2 h $t_{1/2}$: 15–20 min
metaraminol (Aramine)	Prevention and/or treatment of acute hypotensive state	*Adult:* Prevention, IM or SC 2–10 mg; treatment, IV infusion, 15–100 mg	*Onset:* IM, 10 min; SC 5–20 min; IV, 1–2 min *Duration:* IM, SC; 20–60 min $t_{1/2}$: Unknown
C Dopamine Agonists			
P fenoldopam (Corlopam)	Severe hypertension, renal vasodilation	*Adult:* IV, 0.01–1.6 μg/kg/min	*Onset:* 50% of maximal effect within 15 min *Duration:* 50% of effect lost within 15 min $t_{1/2}$: 5 min

NURSING MANAGEMENT OF THE PATIENT RECEIVING P EPINEPHRINE

Core Drug Knowledge

Pharmacotherapeutics

Epinephrine has a wide variety of indications, including anaphylactic shock, asthma, cardiopulmonary resuscitation, simple glaucoma, ventricular fibrillation, cataracts, chloroquine poisoning, cluster headaches, croup, GI hemorrhage, herpes simplex infection, hyperkalemia, hypothermia, mastocytosis, obstetric analgesia, priapism, septic shock, and wheezing in infants. It is also used in open heart surgery and as an adjunct in topical anesthesia.

Pharmacokinetics

Epinephrine may be administered parenterally, topically, or by inhalation. Depending on the administration method, epinephrine exerts its effects very quickly and is metabolized rapidly. It is well absorbed after intramuscular (IM) or subcutaneous (SC) injection, and its duration of action ranges between 1 and 4 hours. It is metabolized in the liver and excreted through the kidneys.

Pharmacodynamics

Epinephrine is a potent sympathomimetic drug with profound effects on a variety of organ systems. It stimulates all adrenergic receptors and causes the greatest adverse effects in the cardiovascular system and CNS. It acts directly on the postsynaptic adrenergic receptors.

After activation of the receptor, epinephrine is terminated by reuptake into adrenergic nerves or inactivated by the enzymes COMT and MAO. Depending on the location and distribution of receptors, epinephrine exerts a variety of responses in different effector organs and tissues. In the cardiovascular system, epinephrine exerts positive inotropic and chronotropic effects on the myocardium by stimulating beta-1 adrenergic receptors. In the skin and viscera, epinephrine stimulates alpha-adrenergic receptors, causing vasoconstriction and vasodilation in skeletal muscle vessels. The overall effect is to increase systolic pressure and slightly decrease diastolic pressure. In the respiratory system, epinephrine causes bronchodilation by stimulation of beta-2 adrenergic receptors and is used in this way to treat patients with asthma or to manage anaphylactic shock.

Contraindications and Precautions

Absolute contraindications to epinephrine include hypersensitivity, sulfite sensitivity, closed-angle glaucoma, and its use during labor. It is also absolutely contraindicated in patients with severe organic cardiac disease, in shock states other than anaphylactic shock, and in patients receiving cyclopropane, chloroform, or trichloroethylene general anesthesia. The action of epinephrine can exacerbate the symptoms of closed-angle glaucoma. As a beta-2 agonist, epinephrine administered during labor can delay progression to the second

stage. The cardiovascular effects of epinephrine, such as increased myocardial oxygen demand, increased heart rate, vasoactivity, and potential to induce arrhythmias, may be detrimental to patients with severe cardiac disorders. These same cardiovascular effects may worsen shock states, although epinephrine is used to manage anaphylactic shock and ventricular fibrillation. In patients receiving general anesthetic agents, epinephrine may induce myocardial sensitization to catecholamines, resulting in cardiac irritability.

Relative contraindications include cerebrovascular disease, such as cerebral arteriosclerosis or organic brain syndrome. The alpha effects of epinephrine have the potential to induce cerebrovascular hemorrhage with these disease states, especially when epinephrine is administered intravenously. Another relative contraindication is hypertension because the vascular effects of epinephrine can worsen this condition. Patients with hyperthyroidism may become more sensitive to catecholamines, resulting in cardiotoxic symptoms. Epinephrine also increases glycogenolysis in the liver. Patients with diabetes mellitus are monitored for hyperglycemia.

Adverse Effects

Adverse effects are frequent because of epinephrine's ability to stimulate the four major adrenergic subtypes. Potential severe adverse effects include hypertensive crisis, angina, cerebral hemorrhage, and cardiac arrhythmias. If extravasation occurs during parenteral administration, necrosis may result because of epinephrine's potent vasoconstrictive properties.

Patients with hyperthyroidism or hypertension are more susceptible to headaches, anxiety, fear, and palpitations after taking epinephrine. In others, the main adverse effects are tremor, weakness, dizziness, anxiety, pallor, palpitations, apprehensiveness, sweating, nausea, and vomiting. Because of the breakdown of glycogen that is stimulated in response to epinephrine's effect on beta-2 receptors in the liver and in skeletal muscle, epinephrine may increase blood glucose levels in patients with diabetes.

Drug Interactions

Epinephrine interacts with a variety of different classes of compounds, including tricyclic antidepressants, oxytocics, halogenated anesthetics, beta blockers, and blood glucose measurements (Table 13.4). Because epinephrine increases blood glucose levels and promotes hepatic glycogenolysis, it may interfere with blood glucose determinations.

Assessment of Relevant Core Patient Variables

Health Status

The nurse documents preadministration vital signs. If Epi is being given for respiratory distress, the nurse auscultates and documents the patient's lung sounds. In patients with diabetes, the nurse obtains a baseline glucose level.

Before administering epinephrine in a nonemergency situation, the nurse evaluates for diseases, disorders, or medications that contraindicate the safe use of epinephrine or require special monitoring. If possible, the nurse assesses the patient for a history of sulfite sensitivity because some epinephrine formulations contain sulfites that may induce a reaction (Box 13.1). It is also important to evaluate the use of over-the-counter (OTC) or herbal medications because these agents may contain sympathomimetic ingredients. However, when epinephrine is administered during an emergency, the potential benefits always outweigh the risks associated with it.

Life Span and Gender

The nurse documents the age and gender of the patient and assesses women of childbearing age for pregnancy and lactation. Epinephrine is in the U.S. Food and Drug Administration (FDA) pregnancy risk category C, and its use should be avoided in pregnant or lactating women. It must be administered carefully to infants, small children, and very old patients because adverse drug effects may be more pronounced in these age groups. In children with asthma, epinephrine may produce hypotension and syncope.

Lifestyle, Diet, and Habits

The nurse documents the patient's occupation and daily activities. Patients treated for glaucoma with epinephrine may develop corneal pigmentation, which may impair their vision. This condition may have a significant impact on people working in transportation (e.g., airline flight crew, truck drivers) and those working at night in low-light conditions.

Patients with diabetes who receive epinephrine for chronic conditions (e.g., asthma) should monitor blood glucose closely. Insulin dosages may need to be adjusted.

TABLE 13.4 Agents That Interact With P Epinephrine

Interactants	Effect and Significance	Nursing Management
tricyclic antidepressants	Potentiation of epinephrine's vasopressor effect	Consult prescriber about adjusting epinephrine dosage.
oxytocic drugs used in labor and delivery	Synergistic vasoconstriction, resulting in hypertension (when epinephrine is administered to correct hypotension)	Monitor patient's blood pressure and vital signs carefully.
beta blockers	Hypertension resulting from beta-agonist action of epinephrine	Monitor blood pressure; avoid concurrent use if possible.
halogenated anesthetics	Arrhythmias resulting from sensitization of the myocardium to catecholamines	Monitor patient's cardiovascular status and ECG carefully during and after anesthesia.

BOX 13.1 Sulfite Sensitivity

Although rare in the general population, sulfite sensitivity may be seen in asthmatics or nonasthmatics with atopic diseases. Many of the drugs affecting the adrenergic nervous system have formulations that contain sulfites. These drugs include epinephrine, norepinephrine, phenylephrine, methoxamine, dopamine, dobutamine, metaraminol, and fenoldopam. Symptoms of sulfite sensitivity include:

- **Central nervous system symptoms:** dizziness, loss of consciousness
- **Cardiovascular symptoms:** hypotension, syncope
- **Integumentary symptoms:** clammy or flushed skin, pruritus, urticaria, cyanosis
- **Respiratory symptoms:** bronchospasm, wheezing, shortness of breath, laryngeal edema or respiratory arrest

Environment

The nurse is aware of the environment in which the drug will be administered and assesses the home or other relevant setting if appropriate. When epinephrine is administered intravenously, it is given in a hospital setting or possibly by trained emergency personnel in the community. It may be administered by other routes in any setting.

Nursing Diagnoses and Outcomes

- Imbalanced Nutrition: Less Than Body Requirements related to drug-induced anorexia or nausea
  Desired outcome: *The patient will maintain adequate nutrition by learning how to cope with adverse effects or use an antiemetic agent if recommended.*
- Disturbed Sleep Pattern, Insomnia, related to CNS excitation secondary to adrenergic drug therapy
  Desired outcome: *The patient will learn about and practice sleep hygiene or take bedtime sedatives as prescribed so that normal sleep patterns will be maintained.*
- Disturbed Sensory Perception related to impaired vision
  Desired outcome: *The patient will notify the provider if vision changes occur.*
- Ineffective Tissue Perfusion (Cardiopulmonary) related to cardiovascular effects of epinephrine
  Desired outcome: *The patient will notify the provider if tachycardia, chest pain, or palpitations occur.*

Planning and Intervention

Maximizing Therapeutic Effects

In addition to therapeutic monitoring, administering adrenergic agonists requires close monitoring of vital signs and careful monitoring for adverse effects. Physical measures to treat a stopped heart, such as chest compressions, are used before epinephrine. The IV route is preferred for treatment of cardiac arrest, although intramyocardial injection or insertion through an endotracheal tube may be done by trained personnel if IV access cannot be established. For treatment of respiratory problems, the SC or IV routes may be used. Patients who receive epinephrine for other (nonemergency) uses need to be encouraged to take the epinephrine exactly as prescribed and at the required dosage frequency to enhance therapeutic potential.

Minimizing Adverse Effects

When epinephrine is given to treat anaphylactic shock or cardiac arrest, monitor the patient's blood pressure carefully for hypertension. Monitor the patient's pulse and electrocardiogram (ECG) for changes in rhythm. If given intravenously, check the site frequently for patency to prevent extravasation. Should extravasation occur, infiltrate the region with phentolamine to minimize injury.

Patients receiving epinephrine for its cardiovascular effects are closely monitored. The nurse is prepared to intervene if adverse effects to epinephrine occur during therapy. For symptoms such as angina, tachycardia, or cardiac arrhythmias, the nurse is prepared to administer beta-adrenergic blocking agents. For hypertension, the nurse is prepared to administer alpha-adrenergic blocking agents.

Nursing strategies to minimize adverse effects include providing the patient with light, comfortable bedding, soothing baths, and optimal skin care. Patients receiving epinephrine for bronchodilation may experience restlessness and sweating. If the patient tires easily, the nurse may need to help with self-care activities to minimize fatigue. In addition, promotion of sleep hygiene is important so that the patient can overcome the CNS stimulation that may occur with epinephrine.

Assisting the patient with menu planning may help to promote appetite and counteract the anorectic influence of epinephrine. Monitor the patient for signs of sulfite sensitivity (see Box 13.1). Finally, key interventions for patients with cardiovascular problems include monitoring for anginal pain and arrhythmias, whereas interventions for asthma patients include regular auscultation of lung sounds and assessment of respiratory functioning.

Epinephrine may be used for its vasoconstrictive properties in conjunction with local anesthetic agents to decrease bleeding during laceration repair. The nurse reads the label carefully to avoid administering epinephrine to an area of the body where vasoconstriction may cause damage, such as the fingers, toes, nose, ears, or male genitalia.

Providing Patient and Family Education

- Many patients who take epinephrine are acutely ill; therefore, it is inappropriate to provide complex instructions. Teaching should be brief, simple, and supportive. Once the acute illness resolves, the patient and family members may realize a greater benefit from instruction, particularly if the patient will be discharged on epinephrine or a similar adrenergic drug.
- For patients taking epinephrine for bronchodilation, the nurse explains the proper use and care of a nebulizer or a metered-dose inhaler and advises patients and families about common adverse effects. Emphasize the timing of doses to prevent disrupting sleep.
- For patients taking epinephrine in ophthalmic form, the nurse can teach how to instill topical eye drugs properly.
- Other teaching concerns include the importance of avoiding OTC drugs containing sympathomimetic ingredients, which may potentiate the effects of epinephrine.
- It is important for the nurse to remind patients with diabetes to monitor their blood glucose levels carefully.

Ongoing Assessment and Evaluation

The patient is assessed for resolution of the presenting problem. For example, when epinephrine is administered for the management of bronchoconstriction, the effect of treatment is a decrease in wheezing. Regardless of the presenting problem, the patient is constantly monitored for adverse effects related to the action of epinephrine. It is important to remember that epinephrine is a nonselective adrenergic agonist. Therefore, all receptor subtypes (alpha-1, alpha-2, beta-1, and beta-2) are stimulated, and the potential for adverse reactions is high.

Drugs Closely Related to P Epinephrine

Ephedrine

Like epinephrine, ephedrine stimulates alpha-1, alpha-2, beta-1, and beta-2 receptors. Unlike epinephrine, it is not a catecholamine. Ephedrine, also known as ma huang, is derived from plants of the genus *Ephedra* and has been used in Chinese medicine for more than 5,000 years. Ephedrine is metabolized to norephedrine, which is responsible for the stimulating effects of the drug on the CNS.

In Western medicine, ephedrine is primarily used intravenously to prevent or treat hypotension associated with spinal anesthesia and topically for the treatment of sinus congestion. Ephedrine is used extensively in OTC medications because of its ability to stimulate multiple adrenergic receptors. It is a frequent ingredient in OTC bronchodilators as well as in many drugs used for colds and flu. Oral ephedrine has been misused as an agent for weight loss and is often included in herbal products and dietary supplements that supposedly increase strength, decrease weight, and produce an "herbal high." One of its more recent uses is as a substrate for the illegal synthesis of amphetamine and methamphetamine. When used inappropriately, potential severe adverse effects of ephedrine include heart attack, stroke, paranoid psychosis, vomiting, fever, palpitations, convulsions, and coma.

MEMORY CHIP

P Epinephrine

- Stimulates all adrenergic receptors, particularly those of the cardiovascular and central nervous systems
- Treats shock (supplied on crash cart), cardiac emergencies, asthma, glaucoma, and other problems
- Major contraindications: hypersensitivity, during active labor, closed angle glaucoma, general anesthesia, severe organic cardiac disease, and shock states other than anaphylaxis
- Most common adverse effects: fatigue, sleep disturbances, tremor, weakness, dizziness
- Most serious adverse effect: cardiovascular stimulation
- Maximizing therapeutic effects: Monitor cardiovascular status closely.
- Minimizing adverse effects: Schedule doses to minimize sleep disruption and allow appetite and meal times to coincide.
- Most important patient education: use of inhalers and nebulizers

Norepinephrine

Norepinephrine (Levophed) is very similar to epinephrine. Its major difference is that NE does not stimulate beta-2 receptors. Like epinephrine, NE is a catecholamine and may not be administered orally. Adverse effects and drug interactions are identical to those of epinephrine with the exception that NE does not promote hyperglycemia. Clinically, NE is used in the management of hypotension and cardiac arrest.

C Alpha-1 Adrenergic Agonists

The alpha-1 adrenergic agonists are drugs that stimulate the alpha-1 receptor directly. These drugs include phenylephrine and methoxamine. Phenylephrine (Allerest) is an ideal prototype for the alpha-1 adrenergic agonists.

NURSING MANAGEMENT OF THE PATIENT RECEIVING P PHENYLEPHRINE

Core Drug Knowledge

Pharmacotherapeutics

Phenylephrine may be used parenterally for treatment of vascular failure in shock, shock-like states, or drug-induced hypotension. Other parenteral uses include overcoming paroxysmal supraventricular tachycardia, prolonging spinal anesthesia, maintaining blood pressure during spinal and inhalation anesthesia, and vasoconstriction in regional anesthesia. Although approved for these uses, phenylephrine is generally not the drug of choice for management of these conditions. More commonly, phenylephrine is used topically for relief of nasal and nasopharyngeal mucosal congestion and to produce mydriasis for ophthalmologic procedures.

Pharmacokinetics

Phenylephrine is poorly absorbed orally and is usually given parenterally or topically. Following IM administration, a vasopressor effect is apparent within 15 to 20 minutes and lasts for 1 to 2 hours (see Table 13.3). The drug is metabolized in the liver and excreted mainly in urine. It has an elimination half-life of 2 to 3 hours. Even if phenylephrine got into breast milk, it would probably be destroyed in the infant's intestines before absorption.

Pharmacodynamics

Phenylephrine is structurally similar to epinephrine and is a powerful alpha-1 adrenergic agonist with very little activity at beta-adrenergic receptors. The predominant actions of phenylephrine are in the vascular system, where it acts as a vasopressor by stimulating alpha-1 vascular receptors and thus causes vasoconstriction. As a result, renal perfusion and cardiac output are decreased, and blood pressure is increased by the increase in peripheral resistance.

Contraindications and Precautions

The main contraindications to phenylephrine are drug hypersensitivity, sulfite sensitivity, severe hypertension, ventricular tachycardia, and closed-angle glaucoma. Precautions need

to be observed for hyperthyroid states and pregnancy and in patients who are elderly or have diabetes, myocardial disease, arteriosclerosis, uncorrected hypovolemia, or asthma.

Adverse Effects

The main adverse effects of phenylephrine are headache, restlessness, excitability, and reflex bradycardia following an increase in blood pressure. Restlessness and excitability are experienced by many people who take OTC nasal decongestants containing sympathomimetics, with effects similar to those of phenylephrine.

Drug Interactions

Phenylephrine interacts with monoamine oxidase inhibitors (MAOIs), tricyclic antidepressants, and oxytocics used in labor and delivery (Table 13.5).

Assessment of Relevant Core Patient Variables

Health Status

The nurse assesses for medical disorders such as diabetes, hyperthyroidism, heart disease, cerebral arteriosclerosis, bronchial asthma, idiopathic orthostatic hypotension, chronic bronchitis, and chronic obstructive pulmonary disease. Phenylephrine may increase airway resistance and bronchial smooth muscle tone and therefore should be given only if absolutely necessary. The nurse also assesses for a history of sulfite sensitivity because some formulations of phenylephrine contain sulfites that may induce a reaction (see Box 13.1). Finally, the nurse also assesses for recent use of prescription drugs (e.g., tricyclic antidepressants and MAOIs). Positive findings are communicated to the health care provider in nonemergency situations before phenylephrine is administered.

The nurse obtains pretreatment vital signs to establish a baseline for therapeutic monitoring and detection of potential adverse effects. During therapy, the nurse needs to monitor therapeutic effects to evaluate the decrease in frequency or severity of target symptoms or the resumption of functions that were previously changed.

Life Span and Gender

The nurse documents the age and gender of the patient. The nurse assesses women of childbearing age for pregnancy and lactation. During pregnancy, phenylephrine is used only if absolutely necessary because it is not known whether phenylephrine causes fetal abnormalities. If the patient is breast-feeding, the infant is monitored for adrenergic stimulation. If such stimulation occurs, the drug may have to be discontinued.

Elderly patients may be at increased risk for blurring of vision from mydriasis. The topical 10% ophthalmic phenylephrine solution is avoided in infants and used cautiously with the elderly because there is an increased risk for systemic absorption.

Lifestyle, Diet, and Habits

The nurse documents the patient's occupation and activities of daily living. It is important to advise the patient to exercise caution when driving or operating machinery at night or under very bright light because mydriasis may cause temporary blindness. Additionally, the nurse asks the patient about his or her use of OTC cough, cold, or herbal remedies containing sympathomimetic ingredients, which intensify the effects of phenylephrine.

Environment

The nurse knows where the drug will be administered and assesses the home or living environment, if appropriate. Phenylephrine is administered in the hospital for treatment of hypotension and shock. For other uses, it may be self-administered by the patient in any environment.

Nursing Diagnoses and Outcomes

- Impaired Gas Exchange related to bronchoconstriction or bronchospasm
  Desired outcome: Gas exchange will remain unimpaired by coughing or drug-induced bronchoconstriction.
- Imbalanced Nutrition: Less Than Body Requirements related to anorexia or nausea secondary to use of an adrenergic drug

TABLE 13.5 Agents That Interact With P Phenylephrine

Interactants	Effect and Significance	Nursing Management
monoamine oxidase inhibitors	Increased amount of norepinephrine available for release, resulting in headache, hypertension, hyperpyrexia, and possibly in hypertensive crisis	Avoid concurrent use if possible.
tricyclic antidepressants	Inhibition of reuptake of norepinephrine in the neuron and diminished pressor effect of phenylephrine	Anticipate dosage adjustment of phenylephrine. Monitor patient carefully for hypertension and cardiac arrhythmias.
oxytocics	Synergistic vasoconstriction, resulting in hypertension (when epinephrine is administered to correct hypotension)	Monitor patient's blood pressure and vital signs carefully.

Desired outcome: The patient will take sufficient nourishment, manage diet adequately, and use antiemetics if necessary.

- Disturbed Sleep Pattern, Insomnia, related to CNS excitation secondary to phenylephrine use
  Desired outcome: *The patient will maintain normal sleep patterns by practicing sleep hygiene measures and using a sedative at bedtime if necessary.*

Planning and Intervention

Maximizing Therapeutic Effects

Blood loss or volume deficits are corrected before IV phenylephrine is used to treat hypotension. Phenylephrine may be used concurrently with replacement therapy if necessary to prevent cerebral or coronary artery ischemia. For topical use, the following factors are considered:

- To produce optimal mydriasis, the nurse must be careful to instill the ophthalmic form of phenylephrine into the conjunctival cul-de-sac.
- If the phenylephrine is in the form of a nasal spray, the nurse demonstrates the proper way to administer the spray. The patient can then perform a repeat demonstration.
- The patient is encouraged to use phenylephrine exactly as prescribed and at the required dosage frequency to enhance therapeutic effects.

Minimizing Adverse Effects

When given to treat hypotension, IV phenylephrine is administered through a large vein, preferably in the antecubital space. This method will help prevent extravasation, which may cause necrosis as a result of vasoconstriction. The IV site is checked frequently for patency. If extravasation does occur, the antidote is the potent alpha blocker phentolamine (Regitine), which is injected subcutaneously into the affected tissue with a fine-gauge needle. The nurse also monitors for signs of sulfite sensitivity.

The following are strategies to teach the patient to minimize adverse effects during topical drug therapy:

- Avoid driving at night because blurred vision can be hazardous. Wearing sunglasses, however, may relieve the glare of bright lights and reduce photophobia.
- Time doses to prevent disrupting sleep, and use effective sleep hygiene measures (dimmed lights, reduced noise, soothing music).
- Avoid OTC drugs that contain sympathomimetic ingredients that potentiate the effect of phenylephrine.

Providing Patient and Family Education

- The nurse stresses the hazards associated with driving and operating heavy or dangerous machinery until the effects of the drug on the individual are known.
- The nurse teaches the patient about drug interactions and advised not to use phenylephrine if they are taking MAOIs, tricyclic antidepressants, or drugs that treat glaucoma.
- The nurse teaches the patient to recognize and report signs and symptoms of adverse effects requiring medical attention, such as a fast, pounding, or irregular heartbeat; chest pain that lasts longer than 5 minutes; trouble breathing; or tingling in the hands or feet.

Ongoing Assessment and Evaluation

Determining whether therapy is successful for patients taking phenylephrine and other adrenergic drugs is relatively straightforward. Because the contraindications and precautions for phenylephrine are many, it is important to assess lifestyle and occupation and be able to recognize and manage adverse effects. Completing a detailed and thorough history and physical examination on any patient anticipating long-term adrenergic drug therapy is essential.

Drugs Closely Related to P Phenylephrine

Methoxamine (Vasoxyl) is a parenteral vasopressor agent used for blood pressure support during surgery and for terminating some supraventricular tachycardias. It increases blood pressure by increasing peripheral resistance through the alpha receptors.

Methoxamine is contraindicated for use in patients with sulfite sensitivity, severe hypertension, hyperthyroidism, bradycardia, partial atrioventricular block, myocardial disease, severe arteriosclerosis, or sulfite hypersensitivity.

Like phenylephrine, methoxamine may interact with MAOIs, tricyclic antidepressants, and oxytocics. In addition, methoxamine may interact with bretylium, which results in arrhythmias. It may partially or fully reverse the antihypertensive effects of guanethidine. Lastly, use with halogenated hydrocarbon anesthetics can sensitize the myocardium to the effects of catecholamines.

Potential adverse effects include hypertension, ventricular ectopic beats, nausea and vomiting, headache, anxiety, sweating, pilomotor response, uterine hypertonus, fetal bradycardia, and urinary urgency.

MEMORY CHIP

P Phenylephrine

- Alpha-adrenergic agonist and vasopressor (constricts blood vessels, raises blood pressure)
- Treats hypotension, shock related to vascular failure, nasal congestion; also used during anesthesia
- Major contraindications: hypersensitivity, severe hypertension, ventricular tachycardia, and closed angle glaucoma
- Most common adverse effects: hypertension, headache, sleep disturbances
- Most serious adverse effect: reflex bradycardia
- Important drug–drug interaction: possible life-threatening interaction with monoamine oxidase inhibitors
- Maximizing therapeutic effects: Instill eye drops in conjunctival cul-de-sac.
- Minimizing adverse effects: Avoid situations that increase blurred vision.
- Most important patient education: Stress safety related to blurred vision.

Ⓒ Alpha-2 Adrenergic Agonists

Stimulation of alpha-2 receptors at the presynaptic nerve terminal results in minimal clinical response. However, stimulation of alpha-2 receptors in the CNS decreases sympathetic outflow by inhibiting the release of norepinephrine. The prototype alpha-2 adrenergic agonist is clonidine (Catapres), which has a narrow range of specific clinical indications. Because clonidine is used primarily as an antihypertensive agent, it is covered in depth in Chapter 27. See Table 13.3 for a brief summary of the drug.

Ⓒ Beta-Adrenergic Agonists

Beta-adrenergic agonists also mimic the action of the SNS; therefore, they are also known as sympathomimetic agents. They exert their effects by stimulation of one or both beta-adrenergic receptors. Like the alpha-adrenergic drugs, they are classified as either a catecholamine or noncatecholamine.

Beta-adrenergic agonists are also labeled according to their selectivity. Drugs that stimulate both beta-1 and beta-2 receptors are nonselective. Those that target either beta-1 or beta-2 are selective. To maximize therapeutic effects and minimize adverse effects, selective drugs are used most frequently. Again, as with alpha-adrenergic drugs, selectivity is preferential but not exclusive. The prototypical beta-adrenergic agonist is dopamine.

NURSING MANAGEMENT OF THE PATIENT RECEIVING P DOPAMINE

Core Drug Knowledge

Pharmacotherapeutics

Dopamine (Intropin) is used to correct the hemodynamic imbalances present in shock due to myocardial infarction, trauma, endotoxic septicemia, open heart surgery, renal failure, and chronic cardiac decompensation (i.e., congestive heart failure) (see Table 13.3). For the treatment to be most effective, the patient should not be experiencing severe disruptions in urine production, myocardial function, and blood pressure. In other words, the earlier the signs of shock are recognized and treatment is started with fluids and dopamine, the more successful the therapy will be.

Pharmacokinetics

The onset of dopamine's action is within 5 minutes. Duration of action is less than 10 minutes. The drug is distributed widely in the body but does not cross the blood–brain barrier. Dopamine is metabolized in the liver, kidneys, and plasma by MAO and COMT to inactive compounds. About one fourth of it is taken up into adrenergic nerve terminals that are specialized neurosecretory vesicles. There, through hydroxylation, it becomes norepinephrine. Dopamine is excreted mainly by the kidneys.

Pharmacodynamics

Dopamine is a naturally occurring catecholamine and a precursor to norepinephrine. It stimulates alpha-1 and beta-1 receptors through direct methods and indirectly through the release of stored epinephrine. It also has dopaminergic effects. Beta-1 stimulation produces increased cardiac output by increasing the force of contraction and heart rate. Although dopamine causes the oxygen needs of the myocardium to increase, this effect is less pronounced than when isoproterenol is administered. Tachyarrhythmias usually do not occur. Systolic blood pressure increases, whereas if any increases in diastolic pressure occur, they are usually minimal. Total peripheral resistance (from alpha effects) is not changed substantially if dopamine is given at low or intermediate levels. Although blood flow to the peripheral beds may decrease, blood flow to the mesenteric beds increases. Dopamine dilates renal and mesenteric vasculature as well as the cerebral and cardiac beds. This dilation, which is believed to arise from stimulation of dopaminergic receptors, produces an increase in renal blood flow, glomerular filtration rate, and urinary output. The dopaminergic zero effect in the peripheral resistance is lost as the dose becomes high because the alpha stimulation takes precedence. The alpha stimulation produces increased peripheral resistance, raising blood pressure as the dose of dopamine increases. The drug's dosage is titrated upward until adequate perfusion of vital organs is achieved.

Contraindications and Precautions

Dopamine is contraindicated in pheochromocytoma, uncorrected tachyarrhythmias, and ventricular fibrillation. Any underlying hypovolemia is corrected before therapy begins. Acidosis decreases the effectiveness of dopamine and other vasopressors. It is important to correct acidosis before starting therapy or as soon as it occurs. Dopamine must be administered in an environment where blood pressure, cardiac output, urinary flow, and pulmonary wedge pressure can be monitored closely.

Adverse Effects

The most frequent adverse effects from dopamine are ectopic beats, nausea and vomiting, tachycardia, angina, palpitation, dyspnea, headache, hypotension, and vasoconstriction. Infrequent effects are abnormal conduction, bradycardia, widened QRS complex, and piloerection. High doses may cause ventricular arrhythmias and dilated pupils. High doses given over a long time have caused gangrene. Gangrene has also occurred in patients receiving low doses who had occlusive vascular disease.

Overdosage is evidenced by excessive hypertension. If overdosage occurs, reduce the rate or stop the infusion until the patient is stabilized.

Drug Interactions

A few drugs are known to interact with dopamine (Table 13.6).

Assessment of Relevant Core Patient Variables

Health Status

The absence of pheochromocytoma, uncorrected tachyarrhythmias, and ventricular fibrillation must be confirmed because these conditions are contraindications to the use of dopamine. The nurse verifies that existing volume deficits have been corrected. The nurse also assesses for drug use

TABLE 13.6 Agents That Interact With P Dopamine

Interactants	Effect and Significance	Nursing Management
guanethidine	Partial or total reversal of the antihypertensive effects of guanethidine. This may be desirable if hypotension from shock is present.	Monitor blood pressure.
halogenated hydrocarbon anesthetics	May sensitize the myocardium to the effects from a catecholamine. This may cause a serious arrhythmia	Use a cardiac monitor and assess cardiac function carefully. Use extreme caution.
monoamine oxidase inhibitors; furazolidone (antimicrobial with MAOI action)	Increase the pressor effect of dopamine 6- to 20-fold as dopamine metabolism is inhibited	Avoid this combination. If given by mistake, administer phentolamine.
oxytocic drugs	Severe persistent hypertension	Avoid combination if possible. Monitor BP closely if must be given.
phenytoin	Simultaneous infusion has led to seizures, severe hypotension, and bradycardia	Discontinue phenytoin and provide supportive measures.
tricyclic antidepressants	The pressor response of dopamine may be decreased, causing it to be less effective	Increase dosage of dopamine if necessary

known to cause interaction, especially MAOIs. It is important to determine whether the patient has a history of occlusive vascular disease (such as arteriosclerosis, arterial embolism, Raynaud disease, or frostbite) because these patients may be more likely to develop necrosis from vasoconstriction with dopamine. If possible, the nurse assesses for a history of sulfite sensitivity because some dopamine formulations contain sulfites (see Box 13.1).

Life Span and Gender

The nurse assesses for pregnancy because dopamine is a category C drug. Whether dopamine is excreted into breast milk is unknown. The nurse also notes the patient's age before administering dopamine. Dopamine's effect and safety in children has not been established, although it has been used in a limited number of pediatric cases.

Environment

Because dopamine is an IV drug, the nurse knows that it is administered only in acute care settings where continuous monitoring of the patient's cardiovascular status can occur.

Nursing Diagnoses and Outcomes

- Risk for Ineffective Tissue Perfusion to Vital Organs related to drug effect
  Desired outcome: *The patient will maintain sufficient perfusion of vital organs to prevent serious damage.*
- Risk for Injury related to adverse effects of drug therapy
  Desired outcome: *Adverse effects of drug therapy will not occur or will be minimized to prevent injury.*

Planning and Intervention

Maximizing Therapeutic Effects

The nurse administers IV dopamine using an infusion pump to regulate flow. It is important to start at low doses and titrate up until the desired renal or hemodynamic response is attained. Oxidizing agents, iron salts, or alkaline solutions such as 5% sodium bicarbonate are not added because these substances deactivate dopamine.

Minimizing Adverse Effects

If the drug is not prediluted, the nurse must follow the manufacturer's instructions for dilution because dopamine is a potent drug that may cause extravasation. It is imperative to use an infusion pump. Before treatment, hypovolemia must be corrected with whole blood or plasma as indicated. The nurse monitors the blood pressure, urinary flow, cardiac output, and pulmonary wedge pressure closely throughout therapy.

The nurse assesses for a disproportionate rise in diastolic blood pressure, which may indicate predominant vasoconstriction. Patients with a history of occlusive vascular disease are monitored closely for changes in temperature or color of skin or extremities. If these changes occur, the nurse consults with the physician to determine the benefits of dopamine compared with the risk for developing necrosis.

The nurse monitors the insertion site for patency, free flow, and signs of extravasation. Using a large vein such as the antecubital fossa decreases the potential for extravasation. Should extravasation occur, the nurse injects the affected area with phentolamine in the subcutaneous space to minimize the potential for necrosis or sloughing of tissues.

When discontinuing dopamine, the nurse gradually decreases the dose and then monitors the resulting effects. Sudden discontinuation of dopamine may induce hypotension.

Providing Patient and Family Education

- Dopamine is administered during an acute medical crisis. Patient education is therefore limited at that time.
- If the patient is awake and alert, the nurse informs the patient that his or her blood pressure is low and that the medication will raise blood pressure to a normal level.
- It is important to reassure the patient and family that the patient will be monitored closely during administration of the drug.

Ongoing Assessment and Evaluation

Dopamine therapy is effective if blood pressure stabilizes, urinary output returns to normal, cardiac output returns to normal, and the patient does not have serious adverse effects from the drug.

Drugs Closely Related to [P] Dopamine

Dobutamine (Dobutrex)

Dobutamine is chemically similar to dopamine. Like dopamine, its primary influence is on beta-1 receptors, with similar effects on the force of contraction. Dobutamine is somewhat less effective than dopamine at increasing the rate at the sinoatrial (SA) node. Also like dopamine, dobutamine's beta-2 effects on vasodilation are minimal. Unlike dopamine, dobutamine has almost no effect on alpha receptors to cause vasoconstriction. Although cardiac output and blood pressure are similarly increased with both drugs, dobutamine does not produce the increased renal output that dopamine does. Furthermore, dobutamine always increases peripheral resistance, whereas dopamine may increase or decrease peripheral resistance. Dobutamine does not cause the release of endogenous norepinephrine that dopamine causes.

The pharmacotherapeutic uses of dobutamine differ from those of dopamine. Dobutamine is indicated in the short-term treatment and support of patients experiencing cardiac decompression because of depressed contractility. The decreased contractility may be secondary to either organic heart disease or cardiac surgery. Patients with atrial fibrillation and a rapid ventricular rate are treated with digoxin before dobutamine treatment to protect the ventricles.

MEMORY CHIP

[P] Dopamine

- Used to treat the hypotension resulting from shock because it stimulates alpha and beta receptors to increase cardiac output, blood pressure, and renal perfusion
- Correct hypovolemia before administering
- Major contraindications: pheochromocytoma, uncorrected tachyarrhythmias, and ventricular fibrillation
- Most common adverse effects: ectopic beats, nausea and vomiting, tachycardia, angina, palpitations, dyspnea, headache, hypotension, and vasoconstriction
- Most serious adverse effect: ventricular arrhythmias
- Important drug–drug interaction: monoamine oxidase inhibitors
- Maximizing therapeutic effects: Use infusion pump, titrate drug until desired effect is obtained.
- Minimizing adverse effects: Monitor blood pressure, urinary output, cardiac output, and pulmonary wedge pressure throughout therapy.
- Most important patient education: Reassure patient that close monitoring will be maintained.

Dobutamine is metabolized by two methods: methylation of the catechol and conjugation. Byproducts are excreted in the urine. Onset of action is 1 to 2 minutes, but up to 10 minutes may be needed for the peak effect to occur. A contraindication unique to dobutamine is the presence of idiopathic hypertrophic subaortic stenosis. Although elevated pulse usually does not occur when using dobutamine, tachycardia can occur. Accompanying the tachycardia is a rapid and substantial increase in blood pressure, with the systolic pressure rising 50% or more. These adverse effects are usually dose related, and reducing the dose promptly corrects the problem. Interestingly, dobutamine also can cause significant hypotension if given in excessive amounts; again, decreasing the dose usually corrects the problem. Dobutamine may cause or exacerbate ventricular ectopic beats, although ventricular tachycardia is rare. Other rare adverse effects include nausea, headache, anginal pain, nonspecific chest pain, palpitations, and shortness of breath. Phlebitis and local inflammation at the IV site may occur; a large vein is chosen to minimize the patient's risk for developing these complications.

As with dopamine, patients receiving dobutamine require continuous cardiac monitoring while receiving the drug. Blood pressure is checked frequently. Pulmonary wedge pressure and cardiac output are checked whenever possible.

Isoproterenol (Isuprel)

Like dopamine, isoproterenol has a strong effect on beta-1 receptor and produces similar increases in contractility. However, isoproterenol's effects on heart rate and vasodilation are much greater than those of dopamine. Isoproterenol does not stimulate the alpha receptors for vasoconstriction. Like dopamine, isoproterenol increases cardiac output. Renal perfusion is also affected, although unlike dopamine, isoproterenol can either increase or decrease it. Peripheral resistance always is decreased, but blood pressure may go up or down from isoproterenol. Although isoproterenol may be used to treat shock, the practice is uncommon because of the tachycardia that may occur. Isoproterenol is used in respiratory drugs used to manage asthma, bronchitis, and emphysema.

Mephentermine (Wyamine)

Mephentermine has a weaker effect than dopamine on the beta-1 receptors, causing less increase in contractility and heart rate. However, it has a stronger effect on the beta-2 receptors, producing moderate vasodilation. It has only a weak effect on alpha-1 receptors, causing a small increase in vasoconstriction. Its pharmacodynamics, when compared with those of dopamine, are in some ways similar. It increases cardiac output and blood pressure. It may have no effect on peripheral resistance or it may increase it, and renal perfusion may increase or decrease. Mephentermine is used to treat hypotension from ganglionic blockade or spinal anesthesia. It can be used on an emergency basis to maintain blood pressure during hypovolemic shock, but only until blood or blood substitutes become available.

Metaraminol (Aramine)

Metaraminol is similar to mephentermine in that it has only minor effects on beta-1 receptors, creating mild increases in contractility and heart rate. It has more effect on vasoconstriction from alpha-1 stimulation than mephentermine, but less than dopamine has. It has no effect on vasodilation

from beta-2 stimulation. It primarily increases blood pressure by increasing peripheral resistance. Unlike dopamine, it lowers cardiac output and renal perfusion. Although it stimulates the sinoatrial node somewhat (which theoretically should increase the heart rate), the net effect on the heart is bradycardia, resulting from a strong reflexive response to the significant vasoconstriction. Metaraminol is used in the prevention and treatment of acute hypotensive states occurring with spinal anesthesia. It is an adjunct treatment for hypotension due to hypovolemia, reactions to drug therapy, surgical complications, and shock associated with brain damage due to trauma or tumor. Unlike dopamine, it can be given by IM or SC injection, in addition to being given as an IV infusion.

Respiratory Beta Agonists

Many drugs are used in the management of chronic airway limitation (CAL) diseases. They may be given orally, parenterally, by nebulizer, or by metered-dose inhalers. These drugs may be nonselective or selective of beta-2 receptors. To minimize adverse effects, use of beta-2 selective drugs has become the community standard. Beta-2 respiratory agonists differ from each other in the way they are delivered as well as in their onset and duration of action. These drugs are discussed in Chapter 47.

Drugs Significantly Different From [P] Dopamine

Midodrine raises blood pressure, but it is not used as a vasopressor in shock. Instead, it is used in the symptomatic treatment of orthostatic hypotension in patients whose lives are impaired significantly despite standard clinical treatment. An unlabeled use is in the treatment of urinary incontinence. It is administered orally. Midodrine is a prodrug that becomes active when it changes into the metabolite desglymidodrine. The metabolite is an alpha-1 agonist that increases the tone of the arteriolar and venous vasculature, increasing peripheral resistance. It results in increased standing, sitting, and lying blood pressures in orthostatic hypotension. Because it increases supine blood pressure, midodrine is not given less than 4 hours before bedtime. Suggested dosing times are shortly before or just after rising in the morning, midday, and late afternoon. This dosing schedule helps the patient maintain his or her normal daytime activities and prevent supine hypertension during the night. If supine hypertension does occur, it may be controlled by preventing the patient from lying completely flat (e.g., by lying with the head of the bed elevated).

(C) DOPAMINERGIC AGONISTS

Although there are five types of dopamine receptors, only dopamine-1 (DA1) and dopamine-2 (DA2) receptors mediate responses in the adrenergic nervous system. Stimulation of DA1 and DA2 receptors results in peripheral vasodilation; however, stimulating both receptors may have either complementary or opposing effects. Fenoldopam (Corlopam) is a DA1 agonist and the prototype for dopaminergic agonist drugs.

NURSING MANAGEMENT FOR THE PATIENT RECEIVING [P] FENOLDOPAM

Core Drug Knowledge

Pharmacotherapeutics

Fenoldopam is used for in-hospital, short-term (up to 48 hours) management of severe hypertension when rapid and selective but quickly reversible emergency reduction of blood pressure combined with renal vasodilation is necessary. Although it is not an FDA-approved indication, administration of fenoldopam with contrast agents decreases the risk for radiocontrast dye–induced renal impairment in high-risk patients, including those with acute renal failure.

Pharmacokinetics

Fenoldopam is administered as a constant infusion. Steady-state concentrations are achieved within 20 minutes. There is a predictable relationship between the dose and the plasma concentration of fenoldopam. Metabolism of fenoldopam is by conjugation and does not involve cytochrome P-450 enzymes. Ninety percent of infused fenoldopam is eliminated in urine, 10% in feces.

Pharmacodynamics

Fenoldopam is a selective peripheral DA1 agonist. Unlike dopamine, it does not bind with DA2, alpha, or beta receptors. It provides rapid vasodilation to the coronary, renal, mesenteric, and peripheral arteries. The pharmacokinetics of fenoldopam is not influenced by age, gender, or race in hypertensive emergency patients (see Table 13.3).

Contraindications and Precautions

Fenoldopam is contraindicated in patients with known hypersensitivity to sulfites. Patients with a history of glaucoma or intraocular hypertension are monitored closely because fenoldopam may increase intraocular pressure during infusion. Patients with hypokalemia also require close monitoring because fenoldopam may reduce serum potassium when administered for more than 6 hours. Fenoldopam is given cautiously to patients with acute cerebral infarction or hemorrhage because it may cause hypotension.

Adverse Effects

Fenoldopam may induce symptomatic hypotension; therefore, close monitoring of blood pressure is essential. Fenoldopam may also cause dose-related tachycardia, especially with infusion rates greater than 0.1 μg/kg/min. Tachycardia diminishes over time but remains elevated with higher doses. Patients may also experience flushing of the face, neck, or upper chest; headache; nausea; and vomiting. Less common adverse effects include abdominal or back pain, GI effects, sweating, and CNS effects such as insomnia, dizziness, nervousness, or anxiety.

Drug Interactions

No formal drug–drug interaction studies have been done with fenoldopam. Fenoldopam should be avoided with beta

blockers and diuretics (Table 13.7). Theoretically, the potential exists for drug–drug interactions with the concomitant administration of antihypertensive agents such as alpha blockers, calcium-channel blockers, or angiotensin-converting enzyme (ACE) inhibitors.

Assessment of Relevant Core Patient Variables

Health Status

The nurse assesses for a history of sulfite sensitivity because fenoldopam contains sulfites that may induce a reaction (see Box 13.1). The nurse also assesses for a history of glaucoma or intraocular hypertension and determines whether antihypertensive medications were used recently. The nurse documents preinfusion baseline vital signs, especially the blood pressure and heart rate. In a nonemergent situation, the nurse obtains a baseline serum potassium level.

Life Span and Gender

Fenoldopam is a pregnancy category B drug; however, because animal reproduction studies are not always predictive of human response, fenoldopam is used during pregnancy only if clearly needed. Whether fenoldopam is excreted in breast milk is unclear. Its safety and efficacy in pediatric use have not been established.

Environment

Fenoldopam is administered only in the acute care hospital setting. When used for antihypertensive emergent therapy, the drug is administered in a critical care environment. Fenoldopam for renal vasodilation before diagnostic testing with contrast media may be administered in any unit within the acute care hospital.

Nursing Diagnoses and Outcomes

- Risk for Ineffective Tissue Perfusion related to hypotension, tachycardia, or increased intraocular pressure
  Desired Outcome: *The patient will maintain adequate tissue perfusion throughout therapy.*
- Risk for Injury related to hypokalemia
  Desired Outcome: *The patient will maintain a serum potassium level within normal limits throughout therapy.*

Planning and Intervention

Maximizing Therapeutic Effects

The nurse dilutes the fenoldopam ampule concentrate with 0.9% sodium chloride or 5% dextrose. The drug is administered using an infusion pump to regulate flow. Fenoldopam is never administered as an IV push. The initial dose is titrated upward or downward, no more frequently than every 15 minutes and less frequently as goal blood pressure is approached. The recommended increments for titration are 0.05 to 0.1 μg/kg/min.

For patients receiving fenoldopam as a protective agent before radiocontrast dye diagnostics, the nurse starts the infusion 2 hours before the procedure at a rate of 0.1 μg/kg/min. The infusion continues at a rate of 0.5 μg/kg/min during the procedure and for up to 4 hours after the administration of the IV contrast medium.

Minimizing Adverse Effects

The nurse visually inspects the drug ampule. If particulate matter or cloudiness is observed, the nurse discards the medication. The nurse starts at low doses and titrates up to avoid reflex tachycardia. The nurse monitors the heart rate and blood pressure continuously throughout the infusion. Fenoldopam may be abruptly discontinued in the presence of hypotension. In patients receiving fenoldopam for more than 6 hours, the nurse obtains baseline and periodic electrolyte levels, especially for potassium. The nurse discards diluted solution that is not used within 24 hours of preparation.

Providing Patient and Family Education

- The nurse explains to the patient and family the rationale for the use of fenoldopam.
- The nurse explains the importance of reporting adverse effects during the infusion.
- The nurse explains the necessity of frequent heart rate and blood pressure measurement.
- The nurse reassures the patient that close monitoring will be maintained.

Ongoing Assessment and Evaluation

It is important for the nurse to monitor vital signs throughout fenoldopam infusion. In the hypertensive patient, the nurse evaluates the efficacy of fenoldopam by monitoring the reduction in blood pressure. In the patient receiving fenoldopam before contrast dye diagnostics, the nurse monitors urinary output.

TABLE 13.7 Agents That Interact With P Fenoldopam

Interactants	Effect and Significance	Nursing Management
Beta-adrenergic blocking agents	Potential inhibition of reflex tachycardia resulting in decreased cardiac output	Advise provider if patient has been on recent beta-blocker therapy. Avoid concomitant use.
Diuretics	The natriuretic and diuretic properties of fenoldopam could lead to worsening volume depletion.	Advise provider if patient has been on recent diuretic therapy. Avoid concomitant use.

MEMORY CHIP

P Fenoldopam

- Used to treat hypertension by stimulating dopamine-1 receptors, resulting in peripheral vasodilation
- Also used for renal protection in patients receiving contrast dye diagnostics
- Major contraindications: sulfite hypersensitivity
- Most common adverse effects: hypotension, tachycardia
- Most serious adverse effect: hypotension
- Important drug–drug interaction: beta-blocking agents and diuretics
- Maximizing therapeutic effects: Titrate the drug slowly.
- Minimizing adverse effects: Continuously monitor heart rate and blood pressure.
- Most important patient education: Reassure the patient that close monitoring will be maintained.

C ADRENERGIC ANTAGONISTS

C Alpha-Adrenergic Antagonists

Alpha-adrenergic antagonists block the stimulation of alpha receptors. Alpha-1 receptors have three distinct subtypes: alpha-1a, alpha-1b, and alpha-1d. Alpha-1a receptors mediate human prostatic smooth muscle contraction, whereas alpha-1b and alpha-1d receptors are involved in vascular smooth muscle contraction. Clinically relevant drugs in current use block alpha-1 receptors in the vasculature and the prostate. There are no therapeutic agents approved by the FDA for alpha-1 blockade receptors located in the eye or for alpha-2 blockade. The prototype for alpha-adrenergic antagonists is prazosin (Minipress).

NURSING MANAGEMENT OF THE PATIENT RECEIVING P PRAZOSIN

Core Drug Knowledge

Pharmacotherapeutics

Prazosin is used in the management of refractory congestive heart failure, Raynaud vasospasm, and treatment of prostatic outflow obstruction. It is frequently used in treating hypertension, alone or in combination with other drugs.

Pharmacokinetics

Prazosin is given orally and is metabolized in the liver and excreted in the bile, feces, and urine. It crosses the placenta and may enter breast milk. A single oral dose has a 10-hour duration of action and a half-life of 2 to 4 hours (Table 13.8).

Pharmacodynamics

Prazosin selectively blocks postsynaptic alpha-1 adrenergic receptors, decreasing sympathetic tone of the vasculature, dilating arterioles and veins, and lowering supine and standing blood pressure.

Contraindications and Precautions

The main contraindication to prazosin use is hypersensitivity. Prazosin is used cautiously in patients with angina pectoris because severe hypotension may cause or worsen angina. Prazosin is also used cautiously in patients who are pregnant or who have congestive heart failure or renal failure.

Adverse Effects

The most common adverse effects of prazosin are light-headedness, dizziness, headache, drowsiness, weakness, lethargy, nausea, and palpitations. These effects may spontaneously resolve or be alleviated with a decreased dosage. Other common adverse effects include reflex tachycardia, orthostatic hypotension, nasal congestion, and inhibition of ejaculation.

Prazosin is well known for causing "first-dose syncope." This may be avoided by administering a lower first dose with food. Prazosin-induced syncope is unpredictable and does not correlate with serum prazosin levels. Syncope may be preceded by tachycardia (120 to 160 bpm) and occurs more frequently with dosage increases alone or when increases are combined with the adjunctive use of other antihypertensive agents.

Prazosin may cause adverse effects in practically any body system. Adverse effects include edema, dyspnea, and angina. Prazosin therapy may also induce rash, pruritus, priapism, urinary frequency, incontinence, blurred vision, dry mouth, pancreatitis, liver function test abnormalities, diaphoresis, fever, arthralgia, positive ANA titer, and mental depression.

Drug Interactions

Prazosin may interact with other antihypertensive medications, especially other alpha- or beta-blocking agents. It may also interact with drugs for erectile dysfunction.

Assessment of Relevant Core Patient Variables

Health Status

The nurse assesses the patient's history for diseases or disorders that may contraindicate the use of prazosin. Positive findings are communicated to the provider before the drug is given. Before and throughout therapy, the nurse closely monitors the patient's heart rate and blood pressure and assists the patient with position changes and ambulation.

Life Span and Gender

The nurse documents the age and gender of the patient. The nurse assesses women of childbearing age for pregnancy and lactation. If the patient is pregnant, prazosin must be used cautiously if at all because it is in FDA pregnancy risk category C. Safety and efficacy have not been established in pediatric patients. Elderly patients are more likely than other adults to be affected by postural hypotension and syncope.

Lifestyle, Diet, and Habits

The nurse documents the patient's occupation and daily activities. Patients should be cautious when operating

TABLE 13.8 Summary of Selected Ⓒ Adrenergic Antagonists

Drug (Trade) Name	Selected Indications	Route and Dosage Range	Pharmacokinetics
Ⓒ Alpha-Adrenergic Antagonists			
P prazosin (Minipress; *Canadian;* Alti-Prozosin)	Hypertension, angina, CHF, BPH, Raynaud vasospasm	*Adult:* PO 3–20 mg daily in divided doses (initial dose 0.5–1 mg to minimize hypotension syncope)	*Onset:* Varies *Duration:* 10 h $t_{1/2}$: 2–3 h
doxazosin (Cardura)	Hypertension, BPH	*Adult:* PO 1–16 mg daily according to individual response	*Onset:* 2 h *Duration:* 24 h $t_{1/2}$: 22 h
alfuzosin (Uroxatral)	BPH	*Adult:* PO, 10 mg daily	*Onset:* Unknown *Duration:* Unknown $t_{1/2}$: 5 hrs
tamsulosin (Flomax)	BPH	*Adult:* PO, 0.4 mg 30 min following a meal	*Onset:* Unknown *Duration:* Unknown $t_{1/2}$: 14–15 hr
terazosin (Hytrin; *Canadian:* Alti-Terazosin)	Hypertension BPH	*Adult:* PO 1–5 mg per day PO 10–20 mg per day	*Onset:* 1–2 h *Duration:* Unknown $t_{1/2}$: 12 h
phentolamine (Regitine; *Canadian:* Rogitine)	Drug infiltration	Infiltrate area with small amount of solution made by diluting 5–10 mg in 10-mL 0.9% sodium chloride	*Onset:* 15–20 min IV immediate *Duration:* IM; 30–45 min; 15–30 min $t_{1/2}$: 19 min
	Pheochromocytoma-induced hypertension (HTN) and sweating, micturitional disorders, Raynaud vasospasm, impotence	*Adult:* 2.5–5 mg IV *Child:* 0.05–0.1 mg/kg IV	
phenoxybenzamine (Dibenzyline)	Pheochromocytoma-induced HTN and sweating, micturitional disorders, Raynaud vasospasm, impotence	*Adult:* PO 20–30 mg bid; can be given IV, but not IM or SC, because drug is an irritant	*Onset:* 2 h *Duration:* 3–4 d $t_{1/2}$: 24 h
Ⓒ Beta-Adrenergic Antagonists			
P propranolol (Inderal; *Canadian:* Apo-Propanolol)	Cardiac arrhythmias, MI, hypertrophic asubaortic stenosis, HTN, pheochromocytoma, prophylaxis of migraine, angina, essential tremor	*Adult:* PO, 80–320 mg/d in divided doses; IV, 1–3 mg at 1 mg/min with monitoring	*Onset:* PO, 20–30 min, IV, immediate *Duration:* PO, 6–12 h; IV, 4–6h $t_{1/2}$: 3–5 h
atenolol (Tenormin; *Canadian:* Tenolin)	Angina, HTN, post-MI, arrhythmias, CHF, anxiety, irritable bowel syndrome, alcohol withdrawal	*Adult:* PO, 50–100 mg daily	*Onset:* PO, varies *Duration:* 24 h $t_{1/2}$: 6–7 h
acebutolol (Sectral; *Canadian:* Apo-Acebutolol)	Ventricular arrhythmias, angina, HTN	*Adult:* PO, 200 mg bid *Adult:* PO, 400–800 mg/d using graded dosages until blood pressure is controlled	*Onset:* Varies *Duration:* 6–8 h $t_{1/2}$: 3–4 h
metoprolol (Betaloc, Lopressor, Toprol XL; *Canadian:* Apo-Metoprolol)	Angina, HTN, post-MI	*Adult:* PO, 12.5–400 mg/d depending on patient's condition and response; IV, 2–20 mg titrated to response	*Onset:* PO, 15 min; IV, immediate *Duration:* 15–19 h $t_{1/2}$: 3–4 h
pindolol (Visken; *Canadian:* Apo-Pindolol)	HTN	*Adult:* PO, 5 mg bid	*Onset:* Varies *Duration:* Unknown $t_{1/2}$: 3–4 h
	Angina	*Adult:* PO, 2.5–5.0 mg/d up to 40 mg/d	*Onset:* Varies *Duration:* Unknown $t_{1/2}$: 3–4 h

(continued)

TABLE 13.8 Summary of Selected Ⓒ Adrenergic Antagonists (continued)

Drug (Trade) Name	Selected Indications	Route and Dosage Range	Pharmacokinetics
penbutolol (Levatol)	HTN	*Adult:* PO, 10–40 mg/d	*Onset:* Varies *Duration:* 20 h $t_{1/2}$: 5 h
betaxolol (Betopic, Kerlone)	HTN, cardiovascular disorders	*Adult:* PO, 10–40 mg/d	*Onset:* 30–60 min *Duration:* 12–15 h $t_{1/2}$: 14–22 h
	Glaucoma	*Adult:* topical, 1 drop 0.5% solution in affected eye(s) bid	*Onset:* Unknown *Duration:* Unknown $t_{1/2}$: 14–22 h
metipranolol (OptiPranolol)	Glaucoma	*Adult:* topical, 1 drop 0.3% solution in affected eye(s) bid	*Onset:* 0.5–3 h *Duration:* <24 h $t_{1/2}$: 3 h
	Ocular HTN	*Adult:* PO, 10–40 mg bid	
sotalol (Betapace; *Canadian:* Alti-Sotalol)	Ventricular arrhythmias, angina, HTN	*Adult:* PO, 80–320 mg daily in divided doses; IV, 0.2–1.5 mg/kg over 5 min with monitoring	*Onset:* 2–3 h *Duration:* 24 h $t_{1/2}$: 7–18 h
nadolol (Corgard; *Canadian:* Apo-Nadol)	Angina, HTN, cardiovascular disorders	*Adult:* PO, 40–160 mg daily; IV, 0.01–0.05 mg/kg at 1 mg/min to 10 mg maximum	*Onset:* Varies *Duration:* 17–24 h $t_{1/2}$: 20–24 h
timolol (Blocadren; *Canadian:* Gen-Timolol)	HTN, angina, arrhythmias, post-MI, prophylaxis of migraine	*Adult:* PO, 10–60 mg daily or bid in divided doses; IV, 0.5 followed by oral dosing	*Onset:* 0.5–3 h *Duration:* NA $t_{1/2}$: NA
	Glaucoma	*Adult:* topical, 1 drop of 0.25% solution in affected eyes bid	*Onset:* 15–20 min *Duration:* NA $t_{1/2}$: NA
Ⓒ Alpha/beta Adrenergic Antagonists			
labetalol (Normodyne)	HTN	*Adult:* 100 mg bid; maintenance, 200–400 mg qd *Child:* 4 mg/kg d in two divided doses	*Onset:* PO, 20 min; IV, 2–5 min *Duration:* PO, 8–24 h; IV, 2–4 h $t_{1/2}$: 2.5–8 h
carvedilol (Coreg)	HTN	*Adult:* 6.25 mg PO bid 7–10 d, then increase to 12.5 mg PO bid, maximum 25 mg PO bid *Child:* Not approved	*Onset:* 1–2 h *Duration:* Unknown $t_{1/2}$: 7–10 h
	heart failure	*Adult:* 3.125 mg PO bid × 2 wk; then 6.25 mg PO bid; maximum 25 mg PO bid *Child:* Not approved.	
	Static angina	*Adult:* 25–50 mg PO bid	
	Post-MI	*Adult:* 2.5 mg IV followed by 12.5–25 mg/PO bid × 6 mo.	

machinery, exercising, driving, changing positions, or climbing stairs.

Environment

The nurse is aware of the environment in which the drug will be administered and assess the home or living environment, if appropriate. Prazosin may be administered in any setting, by health care providers, nurses, or the patients themselves.

Nursing Diagnoses and Outcomes

- Ineffective Tissue Perfusion related to prazosin-induced hypotension
  Desired outcome: *The patient will maintain adequate tissue perfusion.*
- Imbalanced Nutrition: Less Than Body Requirements related to nausea secondary to prazosin use

TABLE 13.1 Receptor Activation of Selective Adrenergic Agonists

	Alpha-1	Alpha-2	Beta-1	Beta-2	Dopamine
Catecholamines					
Dobutamine			—		
Dopamine	—		—		—
Epinephrine	—	—	—	—	
Isoproterenol			—	—	
Norepinephrine	—	—	—		
Noncatecholamines					
Clonidine		—			
Ephedrine	—	—	—	—	
Fenoldopam		—			—
Mephentermine			—	—	
Metaraminol	—		—		
Phenylephrine	—				
Respiratory drugs			—	—	

are related to providing extra-adrenergic stimulation or blockade of normal ANS functioning. Because adrenergic receptors are distributed throughout the body and because adrenergically innervated organs and tissues show a predominance of one type of receptor over another, it is important to examine the major effects mediated by the different types of receptors to understand the implications of drug treatment in differing pathologic states (Table 13.2).

One of the most frequent indications for adrenergic agonist drugs is **shock.** Shock is the result of inadequate tissue perfusion, leaving the cells without the oxygen and nutrients they need to function normally and survive. When cell dysfunction is widespread, the patient can die. Shock has multiple causes. Hypovolemic shock results from a decrease in circulating blood volume from bleeding or hemorrhage. It occurs when intravascular volume decreases more than 15% and as much as 25%. Cardiogenic shock is the result of the heart's inability to pump enough blood to adequately perfuse the vital organs. This type of shock may be caused by myocardial infarction, ventricular arrhythmias, severe cardiomyopathy, or congestive heart failure. Septic shock occurs when a severe infection brings about circulatory insufficiency. Obstructive shock is caused by a massive blockage in blood flow that results in inadequate tissue perfusion. Obstructive shock can originate with a large pulmonary embolus, cardiac tamponade, restrictive pericarditis, or severe cardiac valve dysfunction. Neurogenic shock is uncommon. It occurs because of a blockade of neurohormonal outflow that may be induced by drugs (e.g., spinal anesthesia) or trauma to the spinal cord.

Shock has two phases—early (compensated) and late (noncompensated). In early shock, the body tries to compensate for the decreased perfusion. The heart and respiratory rates increase, and blood pressure is generally maintained, or it may be low-normal. The body begins to shunt some blood flow away from the skin, although the skin is still perfused. Urine output decreases slightly as renal blood flow is reduced. Emotionally, the patient may be anxious or confused. When the body is no longer able to make up for changes brought on by shock, the patient develops late, or uncompensated, shock. Tachycardia persists, but the blood pressure falls dramatically, and the rate of respiration falls. Venous constriction occurs, and with the circulation shut off, the skin becomes cold and clammy. Urine output declines dramatically and may cease when the kidneys are no longer perfused. The patient becomes nonresponsive and unconscious.

C ADRENERGIC AGONISTS

Adrenergic agonists are drugs that mimic the action of the SNS; thus, they are also known as sympathomimetic agents. They exert their effects by direct or indirect stimulation of adrenergic receptors. Indirect mechanisms include increasing the transmission of NE, inhibiting NE reuptake, and inhibiting MAO or COMT. Inhibiting the reuptake of NE or inhibiting MAO or COMT is related to the dissociation and termination of NE binding to adrenergic receptors, which results in the continuation of the effects of NE.

These drugs are generally divided into two groups: catecholamines and noncatecholamines. Catecholamines are so named because of a chemical structure they have in common. Because of this chemical similarity, they also possess three similar characteristics. First, they have a short duration of action, resulting in their need to be administered in a continuous fashion (i.e., by intravenous [IV] infusion). Second, they cannot be given orally. As oral agents, they cannot be given continuously, and certain substances in the body (MAO and COMT) would degrade them before they reached systemic circulation. Third, because of their chemical structure, they do not cross the blood–brain barrier. Noncatecholamines have directly opposite characteristics. They have a longer

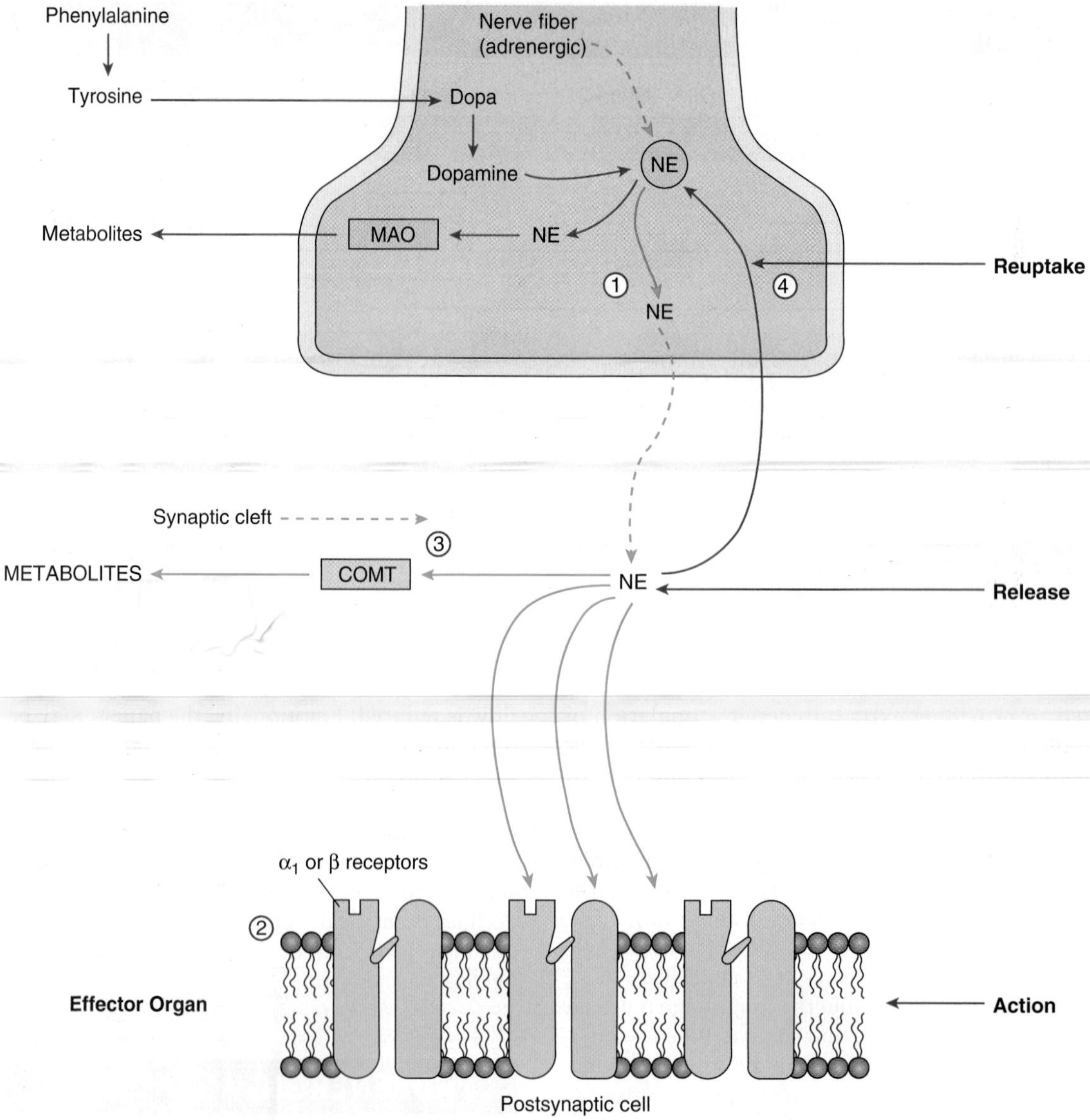

FIGURE 13.3 Norepinephrine release and degradation. (1) Norepinephrine release, (2) binding to receptor, (3) degradation of norepinephrine, and (4) reuptake.

Adrenergic Receptors

Receptors are either adrenergic or cholinergic. In the SNS, there are several types of adrenergic receptors, including alpha-adrenergic and beta-adrenergic receptors. Another type of receptor, the dopaminergic receptor, is related to adrenergic receptors in that dopamine is the precursor to NE. As such, it can activate both alpha- and beta-adrenergic receptors. Dopaminergic receptors are known to exist as subtypes, and at least five have been identified. Dopaminergic receptors in the periphery are located primarily in the kidney.

There are also subtypes of alpha- and beta-adrenergic receptors. The current significant adrenergic subtypes are alpha-1, alpha-2, beta-1, and beta-2 receptors. Alpha-1 receptors are located in the eyes, blood vessels, bladder, male sex organs, and prostatic capsule. Alpha-2 receptors are located in presynaptic nerve terminals. Beta-1 receptors are found primarily in the heart but also in the kidney. Beta-2 receptors are located in the arterioles of the heart, lung, and skeletal muscles as well as in the bronchi, uterus, liver, and skeletal muscle.

The subtypes respond to stimulation by one or more neurotransmitters. Alpha-1 and beta-1 receptors respond to all three sympathetic neurotransmitters (Epi, NE, and dopamine). Alpha-2 receptors respond to epinephrine and NE, whereas beta-2 receptors respond only to epinephrine. In addition to alpha-1 and beta-1 receptors, dopamine also affects dopaminergic receptors. The relative selectivity of various adrenergic agonists can be used to therapeutic benefit in determining which effector organs or tissues should be targeted (Table 13.1).

PATHOPHYSIOLOGY

Diverse tissues and organs are innervated by the ANS, and few discrete disorders are directly related to compromise of the SNS. Instead, the therapeutic uses of sympathetic drugs

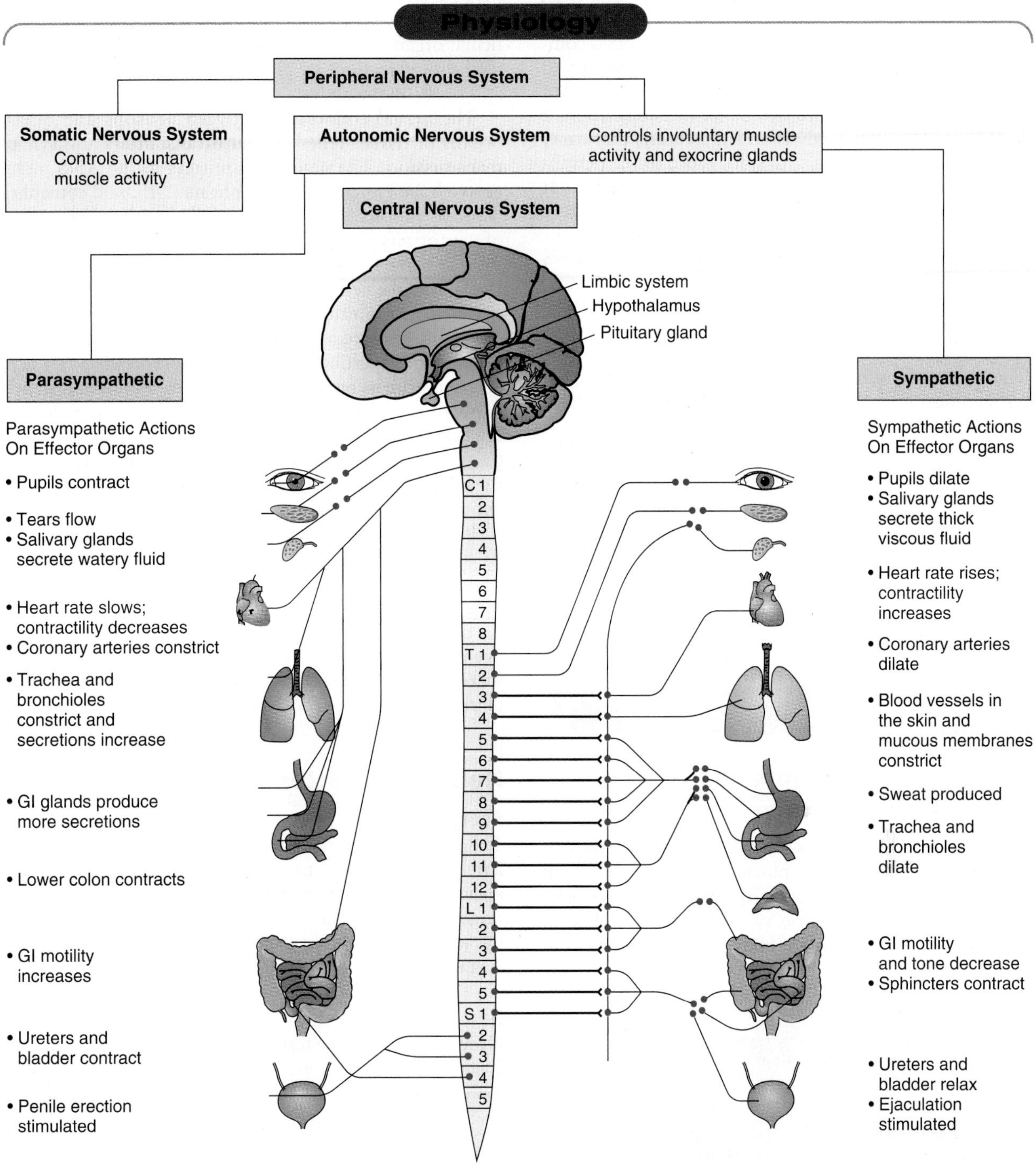

FIGURE 13.2 Actions of the nervous system. Whereas the brain and spinal cord make up the central nervous system (CNS), the neurons found outside the CNS make up the peripheral nervous system, which carries nerve impulses to and from the CNS over afferent (to the brain and spinal cord) and efferent (from the brain and spinal cord) pathways. The efferent pathways, which make up the autonomic nervous system, regulate voluntary and involuntary activities of the smooth muscles and glands. The autonomic nervous system is in charge of the parasympathetic and sympathetic nervous systems. The parasympathetic nerves govern craniosacral impulses, whereas the sympathetic nerves govern impulses associated with the thoracolumbar region. The parasympathetic nervous system is associated with decreased exocrine gland activity (tearing and salivation) and increased gastrointestinal activity (motility, secretion, and contraction). Drugs that affect parasympathetic function are known as cholinergic drugs. Those that stimulate parasympathetic activity are called cholinergic agonists; those that inhibit or block parasympathetic activity are called cholinergic antagonists or anticholinergic drugs. Drugs that affect sympathetic function are known as adrenergic or sympathetic drugs. Those that stimulate sympathetic activity are called adrenergic agonists or sympathomimetic agents. Those that inhibit or block sympathetic activity are called sympathetic or adrenergic antagonists.

The nervous system is divided into two main branches, the **central nervous system** (CNS) and the **peripheral nervous system** (PNS) (Figure 13.1). The CNS is composed of the brain and spinal cord. The PNS consists of all neurons that are found outside the brain and spinal cord and is further subdivided into two major divisions: efferent and afferent. The efferent division has neurons that carry signals away from the brain and spinal cord to the periphery, whereas the afferent division contains neurons that carry impulses from the periphery to the CNS. The efferent division may be further subdivided into the somatic nervous system and the **autonomic nervous system** (ANS). The ANS is in turn subdivided into the **sympathetic nervous system** (SNS), also known as the **adrenergic nervous system,** and the **parasympathetic nervous system** (PSNS), also known as the cholinergic nervous system.

This chapter focuses on drugs that affect the SNS. These drugs include adrenergic and dopaminergic **agonists** (stimulators) and adrenergic **antagonists** (blockers). The prototype nonselective adrenergic agonist is epinephrine. The prototype alpha-1 adrenergic agonist is phenylephrine, and the prototype alpha-2 adrenergic agonist is clonidine. The prototype beta-adrenergic agonist is dopamine. The prototype dopaminergic agonist is fenoldopam.

The adrenergic antagonists are categorized similarly. Prazosin is the prototype alpha antagonist, whereas the prototype beta-adrenergic antagonist (more commonly referred to as a beta-adrenergic blocker) is propranolol.

PHYSIOLOGY

Function of the Autonomic Nervous System

The ANS has been identified as an involuntary system responsible for the control of smooth muscle (e.g., in bronchi, blood vessels, and the gastrointestinal [GI] tract), cardiac muscle, and exocrine glands (e.g., gastric, sweat, and salivary glands). These regulatory functions of the body are monitored by both the SNS and PSNS. Some organs and tissues are regulated by both systems. When both the SNS and PSNS stimulate a particular organ or tissue, the action may be oppositional or complementary. Figure 13.2 presents the major effects of the SNS and PSNS on the body.

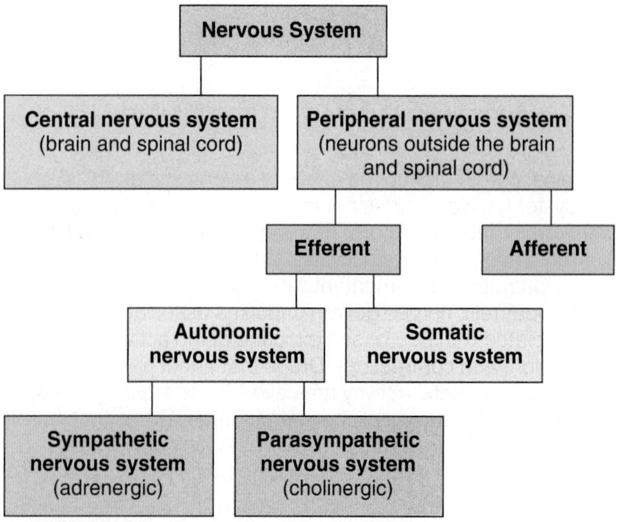

FIGURE 13.1 The human nervous system.

The actual connection between neurons and effector organs or tissues relies on **neurotransmitters** and **synaptic transmission.** The neurotransmitters in the ANS include acetylcholine (ACh), norepinephrine (NE), and epinephrine (Epi). Synaptic transmission initially involves the synthesis of neurotransmitters in the nerve terminal with subsequent storage of the neurotransmitter awaiting an action potential that allows the neurotransmitter to be released. After release, the neurotransmitter diffuses across the synaptic gap and reversibly binds to a receptor on the postsynaptic cell. After binding and exerting an effect, the neurotransmitter is dissociated from its binding site by a variety of mechanisms that allow the neurotransmitter to be degraded or to undergo reuptake for reuse (Figure 13.3). To effect an action, the neurotransmitter needs to bind with an appropriate receptor site on the effector organ or tissue. This simple statement reflects the entire concept of neuropharmacologic drug therapy.

In the SNS, preganglionic transmission is mediated by ACh, whereas postganglionic transmission is mediated by NE. ACh also stimulates the adrenal medulla to release Epi. Once the postganglionic neurons transmit their impulse to the effector organs or tissues through their neurotransmitters, several events may occur. For example, beta-1 stimulation by NE increases the heart rate, while at the same time beta-2 stimulation induces bronchodilation.

Neurotransmitters

Acetylcholine

The precursors to ACh are choline and acetyl coenzyme A. After formation and storage, ACh is released in response to an action potential, then binds to cholinergic receptors on the target organs or tissues. After dissociation, ACh is degraded by acetylcholinesterase (AchE) into two inactive products, acetate and choline.

Norepinephrine

Norepinephrine is the terminal neurotransmitter in the SNS. The precursors to NE include phenylalanine, tyrosine, dopa, and, as the final step, dopamine. NE is produced and stored in the presynaptic nerve terminals of the SNS. As with ACh, it responds to an action potential. NE may bind to presynaptic alpha-2 receptors or postsynaptic alpha-1 and beta-adrenergic receptors. Transmission is terminated by reuptake of NE back to the nerve terminal where it can be restored for further use or degraded by monoamine oxidase (MAO) in the nerve ending or catechol-O-methyltransferase (COMT) within the synaptic cleft (see Figure 13.3).

Epinephrine

Epinephrine is actually a hormone that is converted enzymatically from NE in the adrenal medulla. It is stored in the adrenal medulla and, like neurotransmitters, responds to an action potential. It then travels through the bloodstream throughout the body to target organs. Its termination occurs through hepatic metabolism.

Ⓒ Adrenergic Agonists

Ⓒ Nonselective adrenergic agonists
- P **epinephrine**
- ephedrine
- norepinephrine

Ⓒ Alpha-1 adrenergic agonists
- P **phenylephrine**
- methoxamine

Ⓒ Alpha-2 adrenergic agonist
- P **clonidine**

Ⓒ Beta adrenergic agonists
- P **dopamine**
- dobutamine
- isoproterenol
- mephentermine
- metaraminol
- respiratory beta agonists
- midodrine

Ⓒ Dopaminergic agonist
- P **fenoldopam**

Ⓒ Adrenergic Antagonists

Ⓒ Alpha-adrenergic antagonists
- P **prazosin**
- alfuzosin
- doxazosin
- tamsulosin
- terazosin
- phentolamine
- phenoxybenzamine

Ⓒ Beta-adrenergic antagonists
- P **propranolol**
- atenolol
- metoprolol
- pindolol
- nadolol
- timolol
- carvedilol
- labetalol
- sotalol

The symbol Ⓒ indicates the **drug class.**
Drugs in **bold type** marked with the symbol P are prototypes.
Drugs in blue type are closely related to the prototype.
Drugs in red type are significantly different from the prototype.
Drugs in black type with no symbol are also used in drug therapy; no prototype

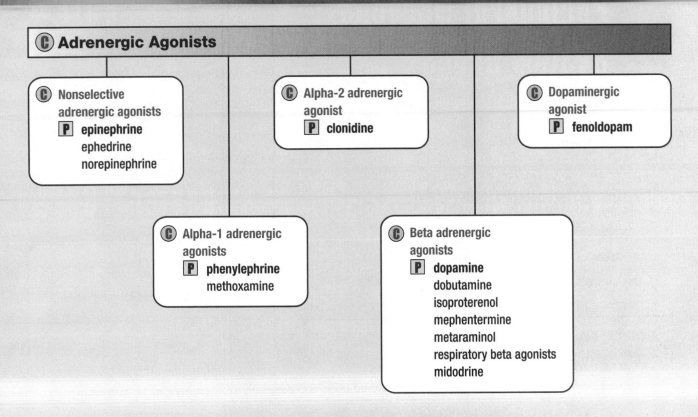

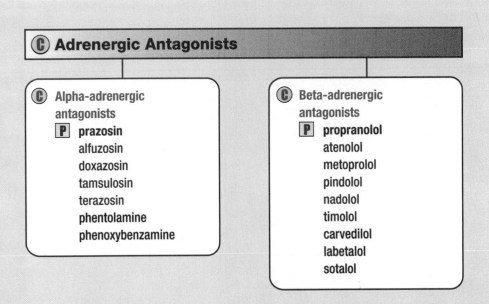

Peripheral Nervous System Drugs

unit 4

Drugs Affecting Adrenergic Function

chapter 13

Learning Objectives

At the completion of this chapter the student will:

1. Describe the anatomy and physiology of the adrenergic nervous system.
2. Describe synaptic transmission.
3. Describe the role of adrenergic agonists and antagonists in a variety of therapeutic uses.
4. Identify core drug knowledge about drugs that act as adrenergic agonists or antagonists.
5. Identify core patient variables relevant to drugs that act as adrenergic agonists or antagonists.
6. Relate the interaction of core drug knowledge to core patient variables for drugs that act as adrenergic agonists or antagonists.
7. Generate a nursing plan of care from the interactions between core drug knowledge and core patient variables for drugs that act as adrenergic agonists or antagonists.
8. Describe nursing interventions to maximize therapeutic effects and minimize adverse affects for drugs that act as adrenergic agonists or antagonists.
9. Determine key points for patient and family education for drugs that act as adrenergic agonists or antagonists.

FEATURED WEBLINK

http://www.healthcentral.com/mhc/top/000185.htm
Adrenergic agents are used for many diseases and disorders. For information on using adrenergic agents for shock, visit the Health Central website.

CONNECTION WEBLINK

Additional Weblinks are found on Connection:
http://www.connection.lww.com/go/aschenbrenner.

KEY TERMS

adrenergic nervous system
agonists
antagonists
autonomic nervous system
central nervous system
neurotransmitters
nonselective-acting drugs
parasympathetic nervous system
peripheral nervous system
shock
selective-acting drugs
sympathetic nervous system
synaptic transmission

Central Nervous System Drugs

unit 5

Drugs Producing Anesthesia and Neuromuscular Blocking

chapter 15

Learning Objectives

At the completion of this chapter the student will:

1 Describe the physiology of the central nervous system as it relates to anesthesia and neuromuscular blocking.
2 Identify observable changes in stages of anesthesia and neuromuscular blockade.
3 Identify risk and disease factors that may influence a patient's response to anesthetics and neuromuscular blocking agents.
4 Identify core drug knowledge about anesthetic and neuromuscular blocking agents.
5 Identify core patient variables related to anesthetic and neuromuscular blocking agents.
6 Relate the interaction of core drug knowledge and core patient variables for anesthetic and neuromuscular blocking agents.
7 Generate a nursing plan of care based on the interactions between core drug knowledge and core patient variables for anesthetic and neuromuscular blocking agents.
8 Describe nursing interventions to maximize therapeutic effects and minimize adverse effects for anesthetic and neuromuscular blocking agents.
9 Determine key points for patient and family education about anesthetic and neuromuscular blocking agents.

KEY TERMS

anesthesia
balanced anesthesia
depolarizing drugs
dissociative anesthesia
end plate
general anesthesia
local anesthesia
narcoanalysis
neuroleptanesthesia
nondepolarizing drugs
paralysis

FEATURED WEBLINK

http://health.discovery.com/diseasesandcond/encyclopedia/2947.html
General anesthetics are used during surgical procedures. Never had surgery? Visit this website for an overview of surgical procedures.

CONNECTION WEBLINK

Additional Weblinks are found on Connection:
http://www.connection.lww.com/go/aschenbrenner.

Drugs Producing Anesthesia and Neuromuscular Blocking

(C) General Anesthetic Agents

(C) Inhalent agents

- [P] **isoflurane**
- desflurane
- enflurane
- haloflurane
- sevoflurane
- nitrous oxide

(C) Parenteral agents

- [P] **propofol**
- thiopental
- etomidate
- ketamine
- fentanyl
- benzodiazepines

(C) Local Anesthetic Agents

- [P] **lidocaine**
- bupivacaine
- etidocaine
- mepivacaine
- prilocaine
- procaine
- topical anesthetics

(C) Neuromuscular Blocking Agents

(C) Nondepolarizing agents

- [P] **tubocurarine**
- atracurium
- cisatracurium
- doxacurium
- mivacurium
- pancuronium
- pipecuronium
- rocuronium
- vecuronium

(C) Depolarizing agents

- [P] **succinylcholine**

The symbol (C) indicates the **drug class.**
Drugs in **bold type** marked with the symbol [P] are prototypes.
Drugs in blue type are closely related to the prototype.
Drugs in red type are significantly different from the prototype.
Drugs in black type with no symbol are also used in drug therapy; no prototype

Anesthesia produces a loss of feeling or sensation. It is used to avoid sensations (especially pain) and memories associated with surgery and diagnostic procedures. Anesthetics are classified as general or local agents. **General anesthesia** is characterized by a state of unconsciousness, analgesia, and amnesia, with skeletal muscle relaxation and loss of reflexes. General anesthetic drugs are subdivided into inhaled agents and parenteral agents. **Local anesthesia** occurs when sensory transmission from a specific area of the body to the central nervous system (CNS) is blocked. These drugs are used to perform minor surgical procedures for a conscious patient. Neuromuscular blocking agents are used to cause **paralysis** (loss of motor function) for surgical procedures or to facilitate mechanical ventilation. These agents are subdivided into **nondepolarizing drugs** (which induce paralysis by muscle flaccidity) and **depolarizing drugs** (which excite muscles and promote contraction, ultimately leading to muscle paralysis after repeated excitation).

This chapter discusses drugs used to induce anesthesia and skeletal muscle paralysis. Inhaled anesthetics are represented by the prototype drug isoflurane (Forane). Parenteral anesthetics are represented by the prototype drug propofol (Diprivan). Local anesthetics are represented by the prototype drug lidocaine (Xylocaine). Nondepolarizing neuromuscular junction (NMJ) blockers are represented by the prototype drug tubocurarine (Tubarine). Depolarizing NMJ blockers are represented by the prototype drug succinylcholine (Anectine).

PHYSIOLOGY

Central Nervous System Anesthesia

The CNS is responsible for providing control systems and surveillance for many vegetative and conscious functions, including appetite, satiety, attention, arousal, and movement. Various sleep and arousal mechanisms are linked to the brain, particularly the raphe nuclei and locus ceruleus in the pons and other parts of the reticular activating system (RAS). Sensations of pain may disrupt the usually smooth regulation of arousal, and activity may result.

At the synaptic level in the CNS, normal arousal mechanisms are affected through presynaptic release of neurotransmitters, such as norepinephrine, serotonin, and dopamine. As described in Chapter 13, these transmitters diffuse across the synaptic cleft to the postsynaptic effector membrane, which is usually another neuron. The postsynaptic membrane contains receptors for the transmitters. The transient combination of the transmitter with the receptor causes membrane changes, leading to propagation of the action potential. An action potential is the brief reversal of electrical polarization of a nerve or muscle cell membrane. In the neuron, the action potential constitutes the nerve impulse. The transmitter can be metabolized by postsynaptic enzymes (such as monoamine oxidase) or removed from further activity through reuptake into the presynaptic storage vesicles. Anesthetics may provoke a decreased release of neurotransmitters or an increased reuptake and inhibition of the postsynaptic enzymes. The result is a diminished postsynaptic response, leading to decreased arousal, decreased sensation (including pain), and loss of consciousness.

Local Anesthesia

Nerve impulses depend on the flow of ion currents through channels in the cell's membrane. Nerve cells are negatively polarized at rest, a state that is maintained by active Na^+/K^+ exchange. When a cell is stimulated, it becomes depolarized, and an action potential occurs. Local anesthetics reversibly block all nerve impulses by disrupting membrane permeability to sodium during an action potential.

Neuromuscular Blockade

Muscle relaxation and paralysis can take place at a variety of sites, including the CNS, somatic nerves, motor nerve terminals, acetylcholine receptor sites, the motor **end plate** (the terminal branch of a motor nerve, which forms part of the NMJ), the muscle membrane, or the internal contractile units of muscle. Normal muscle function involves the arrival of a nerve impulse at the motor nerve terminal followed by the release of the neurotransmitter acetylcholine into the synaptic cleft. Neuromuscular blockade occurs at acetylcholine receptor sites where acetylcholine reacts with the muscle cell membrane, causing depolarization and subsequent muscle relaxation.

Nondepolarizing drugs prevent neural communication by depolarizing the muscle, so that the muscle remains in a relaxed state. Depolarizing drugs cause muscle depolarization and prevent repolarization; that is, the muscle experiences rapid contractions followed by flaccid paralysis, at which point it is unable to receive further neural communication.

PATHOPHYSIOLOGY

Anesthetics are called functional drugs because they are not used to treat a pathologic disease or disorder. However, patients have a variety of conditions that require anesthesia. General anesthetics are used to induce and maintain anesthesia during surgery, **narcoanalysis** (the use of sedating drugs to help uncover unconscious material during psychoanalysis), electroconvulsive therapy, **dissociative anesthesia** (which causes a loss of perception of certain stimuli, while that of others remains intact), and **neuroleptanesthesia** (also called conscious sedation).

Neuromuscular blocking agents are used in conjunction with inhalation or parenteral anesthetics during surgical procedures or to facilitate induction and maintenance of mechanical ventilation.

Ⓒ GENERAL ANESTHETIC AGENTS

The action of general anesthetics produces a state of unconsciousness and whole-body anesthesia. After administration of a general anesthetic, loss of consciousness and sensation usually follows increasing levels, or stages, of CNS depression. Slower-acting anesthetics allow some differentiation of these stages, whereas faster-acting anesthetics do not show precise delineation. Classic studies with early anesthetics indicate the presence of four stages, which are differentiated through increasing influence on reflex activity, muscle tone, and respiration. Stages I and II constitute anesthetic induction;

keeping the patient at stage III is anesthetic maintenance. Reversal of the stages to the conscious state is the process of recovery. The four stages of anesthesia are as follows:

- Stage I, analgesia: the patient remains conscious, may be able to converse, and experiences some analgesia as the anesthetic reduces sensory transmission in the spinothalamic tract.
- Stage II, excitement: systolic pressure rises, and the patient may experience excitation and restlessness along with an increased respiratory rate. In addition, the patient may experience delirium. Stage II is usually circumvented by intravenously administering a short-acting barbiturate beforehand.
- Stage III, surgical anesthesia: stage III may have four planes, or levels, characterized by differential responses of the ocular muscles, eye reflexes, and pupils. It begins in plane I with the resumption of regular respiration and the beginning of muscle relaxation. By plane IV, spontaneous respiration ceases. Most surgery occurs when the patient is in planes II and III.
- Stage IV, medullary depression: the respiratory and vasomotor centers are depressed, and spontaneous respiration has ceased. Unless rapid intervention and support occur, coma and death follow.

It is not always desirable to produce general anesthesia with a single agent because too deep a level of unconsciousness may ensue. To avoid this possibility, a process called **balanced anesthesia** is used. Balanced anesthesia relies on a combination of drugs to produce loss of consciousness, analgesia, and muscle relaxation, while producing and maintaining a lighter stage of anesthesia. Drugs used in balanced anesthesia include inhaled or parenteral anesthetics, ultrashort-acting barbiturates, neuromuscular blocking agents, benzodiazepines, and opioid analgesics. The minute-to-minute maintenance of anesthesia is sensitively adjusted with the inhaled anesthetic.

As previously mentioned, general anesthetics are subdivided into inhaled and parenteral agents.

(C) Inhaled Anesthetic Agents

Inhaled anesthetic agents include isoflurane (Forane), desflurane (Suprane), enflurane (Ethrane), haloflurane, sevoflurane (Ultane), and nitrous oxide. The inhalant anesthetics are typified by isoflurane (Forane), a halogenated ether that is the prototype for this group. A drug significantly different from isoflurane is nitrous oxide.

NURSING MANAGEMENT OF THE PATIENT RECEIVING [P] ISOFLURANE

Core Drug Knowledge

Pharmacotherapeutics

Isoflurane is used to induce and maintain anesthesia and is typically part of balanced anesthesia. It is used in intensive care units for sedation, in obstetrics for analgesia, and in ocular surgical procedures (such as cataract removal, lens implantation, and reconstructions) because it lowers intraocular pressure.

Pharmacokinetics

Isoflurane produces surgical anesthesia within 7 to 10 minutes and is usually administered with 50% to 70% nitrous oxide. It is administered slowly because its pungent odor would otherwise tend to cause breath holding or coughing. It is absorbed through the alveoli and is minimally biotransformed. A tiny fraction of the inhaled dose is transformed in the liver into trifluoroacetic acid and excreted in the urine as fluoride ion. Most isoflurane is excreted unchanged through expired air. Table 15.1 provides a comparison of the pharmacokinetic properties of halogenated general anesthetic agents.

Pharmacodynamics

The exact mechanism of action of isoflurane—and for the inhaled anesthetics altogether—is unknown. Several theories have been postulated (Figure 15.1). It is likely that the effects are mediated through physicochemical properties of the gases, rather than through specific binding with receptors or through potentiation or inhibition of specific neurotransmitters.

The minimum alveolar concentration (MAC) is a measure of potency. It is the concentration of anesthetic gas required to eliminate movement in 50% of patients challenged by a standardized skin incision. The smaller the MAC, the more potent the agent is. The MAC of isoflurane is 1.15% for adults when it is administered alone, but it decreases to 0.5% when administered with 70% nitrous oxide.

Contraindications and Precautions

The main contraindications to isoflurane are hypersensitivity to halogenated compounds and predisposition to malignant hyperthermia, which is often determined from the individual or family history. In patients with increased intracranial pressure (ICP), isoflurane will increase cerebral blood flow, which can further exacerbate the ICP.

Isoflurane may cause intraoperative hyperglycemia and leukocytosis, which may be of concern for patients with diabetes. Isoflurane is assigned to pregnancy category C and should be used in pregnant women only when the benefits outweigh the risks. Use of isoflurane in patients with myasthenia gravis can cause an increase in muscular weakness because of the neuromuscular blocking effects of anesthetics.

Adverse Effects

With many anesthetics, blood pressure drops during induction and returns following surgical stimulation. Prolonged hypotension may occur with isoflurane, but otherwise, the myocardium appears stable with this agent. Malignant hyperthermia, characterized by a sudden temperature spike, is a possibility with this agent, although the reported incidence is low. Like other anesthetics, isoflurane depresses renal function. However, it is not generally nephrotoxic, and it has a higher cardiovascular and respiratory margin of safety than halothane, desflurane, or enflurane. Respiratory depression occurs with all inhaled anesthetics, resulting in the need for mechanical ventilation throughout surgery. Rarely, postanesthesia respiratory depression may occur, especially in

TABLE 15.1 Summary of Selected (C) Inhalant Anesthetic Agents

Drug (Trade) Name	Selected Indications	Route and Dosage Range	Pharmacokinetics
P isoflurane (Forane)	Anesthesia: induction, maintenance	*Adult:* 1.5%–3% in oxygen or in oxygen/nitrous oxide for induction, 1%–2.5% for maintenance	*Onset:* 7–10 min *Duration:* 7–19 min $t_{1/2}$: minimal biotransformation
desflurane (Suprane)	Anesthesia: induction, maintenance	*Adult:* 3%–11% in oxygen or in oxygen/nitrous oxide (monitored anesthesia care 2.8%–7.5%)	*Onset:* 2–2.6 min *Duration:* 5–7 min $t_{1/2}$: 2.5 min
enflurane (Ethrane)	Anesthesia, patient-controlled obstetric analgesia	*Adult:* 2%–4.5% in oxygen or in oxygen/nitrous oxide for induction, 0.5–3% for maintenance	*Onset:* 2.3 min *Duration:* 5 min $t_{1/2}$: 2–3 min
sevoflurane (Ultane)	Anesthesia: induction, maintenance	*Adult:* 1.8%–5% in oxygen or in oxygen/nitrous oxide for induction, 0.75%–3% for maintenance	*Onset:* 1–2 min *Duration:* 4–14 min $t_{1/2}$: 2–3 min

obese patients. Tremor and shivering may occur in response to a decreased body temperature, but these adverse effects are generally self-limiting. Nausea and vomiting may also occur. During surgery, the airway is protected by the endotracheal tube. If vomiting occurs after surgery, aspiration is another potential adverse effect. During labor and obstetric delivery, isoflurane can produce uterine relaxation, which can delay delivery and increase postpartum hemorrhage.

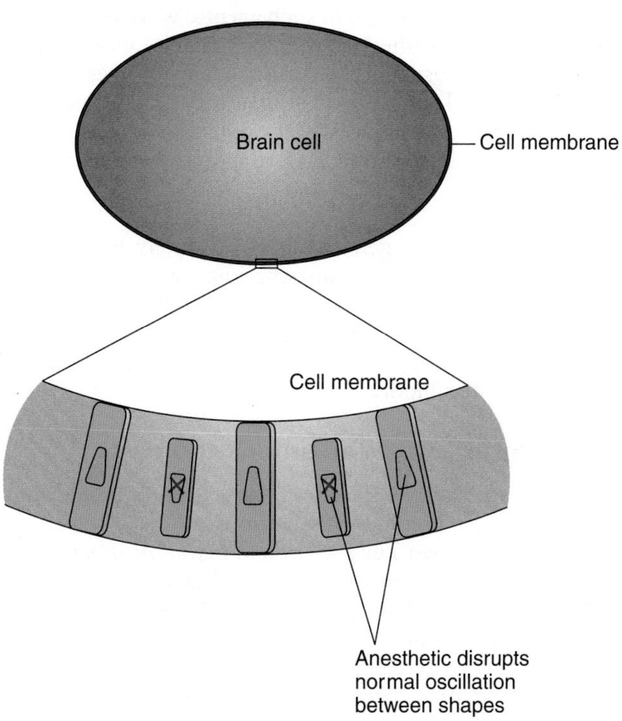

FIGURE 15.1 New theories of the mechanism of anesthesia. Older theories of anesthetic mechanisms of action suggest that anesthetics bind to or dissolve in the lipid layers of cell membranes, causing swelling, disruption, and loss of feeling. A newer theory suggests that multiple mechanisms may be at play. These mechanisms involve the cell membrane proteins, which are thought to oscillate between two shapes. Now it is thought that anesthetics disrupt this oscillation.

Chronic accidental exposure, which can occur in operating room personnel, may increase the incidence of spontaneous abortions, birth defects, and stillbirths. Isoflurane has been observed to react with carbon dioxide dry adsorbents in anesthetic circle systems to form carbon monoxide and cause carboxyhemoglobinemia. To avoid this adverse effect, carbon dioxide adsorbents are changed frequently.

Drug Interactions

If isoflurane is administered to a patient receiving labetalol, a synergistic hypotensive effect occurs. Combined use of these drugs increases the time to the resumption of spontaneous respirations. Extra caution is needed when caring for these patients during postanesthesia recovery. Additional interactions are identified in Table 15.2.

Assessment of Relevant Core Patient Variables

Health Status

Take a careful health history. Many factors influence the process of anesthetic induction, maintenance, and recovery, including lung conditions, cardiovascular status, obesity, previous drug history, and comorbidity. Inhalation anesthetics are administered through the lungs and absorbed across alveolar surfaces. Therefore, a lung condition may have a profound impact on the efficacy and nature of anesthesia. Patients with chronic obstructive lung disease, asthma, or a history of cigarette smoking present potential problems in anesthesia based on changes in lung compliance, bronchoconstriction, and ventilation-to-perfusion ratios. Patients with compromised pulmonary function have a substantially increased rate of postoperative complications. Similar issues arise for patients with cardiovascular compromise or disease because absorption, distribution, metabolism, and excretion

TABLE 15.2 Agents That Interact With P Isoflurane

Interactants	Effect and Significance	Nursing Management
nondepolarizing muscle relaxants, such as atracurium, doxacurium, gallamine, metocurine, mivacurium, pancuronium, pipecuronium, tubocurarine, vecuronium	Potentiates effects of neuromuscular blockers and prolongs blockade	Monitor respiratory function (dosage may need to be reduced). Prepare to provide ventilatory support.
alfentanil	Prolongs respiratory depression and increases incidence of bradycardia	Monitor respiratory and cardiac function. Provide ventilatory support.
labetalol	Additive hypotensive effects and decreased cardiac output	Monitor cardiac function. Use extra caution if interaction is anticipated.
herbal drugs • St. John's wort • *Hypericum perforatum*	Herbal drugs may intensify or prolong the effects of isoflurane.	Advise patient to stop herbal medications 2–3 weeks before surgery.
hepatic inducers • alcohol • barbiturates • carbamazepine • INH • phenytoin • rifampin	Chronic use of agents that induce hepatic enzymes can increase isoflurane metabolism, thus increasing the risk for hepatic injury.	Document the use of these agents in the medical record. Advise anesthesiologist of the use of these drugs.

of inhalant anesthetics are all affected by blood flow through the lungs and the rest of the body.

Life Span and Gender

Document the age of the patient. Challenges with isoflurane administration differ by age group. Isoflurane is not used for infants and children because it causes respiratory irritation. Additionally, in neonates and infants, the size of the airway and larynx may contribute to difficulties with intubation.

In older adults, especially those with failing organ systems, difficulties may occur in detoxification and excretion of administered anesthetic agents, which may lead to increased intensity and duration of drug effects, including toxic effects.

Assess women of childbearing age for pregnancy. Isoflurane has a low pregnancy safety rating (pregnancy category C). In animal studies, isoflurane showed the potential for fetotoxicity; however, no human studies have been performed. Its use during pregnancy is determined by the balance between potential benefit and harm to both the woman and the fetus.

Lifestyle, Diet, and Habits

Measure the patient's height and weight. The patient with morbid obesity who requires anesthesia may experience problems with isoflurane administration. The obese patient may be particularly prone to longer recovery times and a greater incidence of adverse effects with fat-soluble anesthetics such as isoflurane and methoxyflurane. Compounding these difficulties, obese patients often present with other comorbid conditions, such as hypertension, cardiac insufficiency, respiratory difficulties, and diabetes, all of which can generate their own special anesthetic challenges.

One other important category of anesthetic challenge is drug abusers; drug abuse often coexists with disease states that require special attention during anesthesia. For example, alcohol abuse is often associated with an elevated level of hepatic enzymes, which may increase the requirement for anesthetic drugs. In addition, liver dysfunction may lead to changes in the metabolism of such agents. With drug dependency, the postanesthetic period may require more careful monitoring than usual in case abstinence syndromes develop (see Chapter 9). Take a careful drug history to reveal previous use or abuse of drugs that have the potential to cause severe interactions with isoflurane and other anesthetic agents.

Environment

Isoflurane and other general anesthetics may be administered in special settings by anesthesiologists (a type of specialist physician) and nurse anesthetists (advanced practice nurses trained in anesthesiology). Administration usually occurs only in settings that allow for postanesthetic recovery and full life support.

Nursing Diagnoses and Outcomes

- Ineffective Airway Clearance related to suppressed cough reflex and the presence of secretions
  Desired outcome: *The patient will maintain effective airway clearance by being suctioned as necessary and by performing deep breathing and coughing exercises.*
- Ineffective Breathing Pattern related to respiratory depression secondary to drugs used during anesthesia
  Desired outcome: *The patient will maintain effective breathing despite respiratory depression by administration of oxygen as appropriate.*
- Risk for Aspiration related to drug-induced nausea and vomiting, gastrointestinal (GI) distention, hypoxia, and stimulation of the vomiting center
  Desired outcome: *The patient's nausea and vomiting will be minimized by preanesthetic administration with antiemetics to reduce the risk for aspiration and nausea.*

- Ineffective Thermoregulation related to CNS depression secondary to drugs used during anesthesia
  Desired outcome: *The patient will be warmed as necessary during the postanesthetic disturbance of thermoregulation.*
- Disturbed Sensory Perception, varied, related to CNS depression secondary to drugs used during anesthesia
  Desired outcome: *The patient will remain free of sensory or perceptual alterations through careful reorientation, repeated as necessary.*

Planning and Intervention

Maximizing Therapeutic Effects

Preinduction and induction should be carried out in a place where environmental stimulus, particularly noise, is kept to a minimum. Inform the patient about induction procedures and describe measures that are useful for promoting uncomplicated recovery. Also, give preoperative support and reasonable reassurance to concerns voiced by the patient. In addition, advise patients scheduled for surgery to avoid stressors and to aim for a good night's sleep before surgery, whether the patient is at home or already in the hospital.

Minimizing Adverse Effects

After anesthesia, monitor blood pressure and temperature to detect residual hypotension and the possibility of malignant hyperthermia. Because gaseous or volatile inhalational agents (such as isoflurane) are expired quickly through the lungs, the recovery phase is often short. Shivering and tremors, which are common following surgery, can be managed with blankets. Until normal respiration resumes, adequate respiratory support must be maintained, by taking steps such as administering oxygen and asking the patient to cough, perform deep-breathing exercises, or change position. After the patient awakens, assess the need for postoperative analgesia.

Recovering patients need to be in a room in which the air supply is continually replaced and exhaled gases are carried out through exhaust vents. You can prevent aspiration by helping the patient into a side-lying position and by administering antiemetic drugs. Monitor vital signs frequently to prevent complications such as shock. When the patient returns to the room or unit from the postanesthesia care unit (PACU), continue monitoring vital signs, bowel sounds, and urine output because these signs are directly affected by isoflurane.

Providing Patient and Family Education

Family and patient education falls into preoperative and postoperative categories:

- Provide preoperative teaching to help the patient anticipate the surgery and anesthesia without excessive fear and assimilate routines that will aid postoperative recovery.
- Postoperatively, instruct the patient to avoid nonprescribed CNS depressants or herbal agents unless approved by the prescriber.
- For outpatient surgery, discharge the patient into the care of a responsible adult and instruct the patient not to drive or engage in any hazardous activities requiring full alertness or coordination.

Ongoing Assessment and Evaluation

The evaluation of progress in the recovery phase is often carried out in two stages. Initially, the unconscious patient may be transferred to a postanesthesia recovery area. The patient should regain consciousness, orientation, some stability of vital signs, and an ability to cooperate with instructions during this stage. After the immediate postsurgery, postanesthesia goals have been reached in the PACU, the patient can be transferred back to a room or unit, and a less stringent postoperative protocol may be followed. Other assessments specifically related to the procedure or surgery are distinct from those required for the postanesthesia state. When the patient returns to the room or unit, continue to monitor vital signs, bowel sounds, and urine output, as was done in the PACU.

Drugs Closely Related to [P] Isoflurane

Desflurane

Desflurane (Suprane) is an inhaled volatile liquid general anesthetic with a MAC of 7.0. It is used for induction or maintenance of anesthesia during surgery for adults. It is not recommended for use in children because of a high incidence of associated cough and laryngospasm. Desflurane is also contraindicated for use in patients with coronary artery disease, increased heart rate, or hypertension.

Enflurane

Enflurane (Ethrane) is a halogenated inhaled anesthetic used for general anesthesia with a MAC of 1.70. Both onset of action and recovery from anesthesia are rapid. As with most inhaled anesthetics, enflurane is typically used with adjunctive medications such as narcotics and nitrous oxide, and it can be given in low doses to provide analgesia for procedures not requiring loss of consciousness. Enflurane is an excellent muscle relaxant, providing enough relaxation for intra-abdominal surgery. Contraindications, precautions, and adverse effects are similar to those for isoflurane.

Haloflurane

Haloflurane is used less often than other inhaled anesthetics in North America because of the availability of agents

MEMORY CHIP

[P] Isoflurane

- A potent inhalation anesthetic
- Major contraindications: hypersensitivity to halogenated compounds, predisposition to malignant hyperthermia
- Most common adverse effects: hypotension, hypothermia, nausea, or vomiting
- Most serious adverse effect: respiratory depression
- Maximizing therapeutic effects: low-stimulus environment, preoperative teaching regarding anesthetic induction
- Minimizing adverse effects: Monitor need for respiratory support.
- Most important patient education: preoperative teaching regarding anesthesia and surgical procedures

with less severe adverse effects. Hepatotoxicity occurs in 1:10,000 adults but is rare in children; hence, halothane is used mainly for pediatric anesthesia. Haloflurane has a MAC of 0.78.

Sevoflurane

Although expensive, a newer inhaled agent, sevoflurane (Ultane), appears to offer advantages above and beyond others in its class. Adjusting the depth of anesthesia is easier with sevoflurane than with enflurane, halothane, or isoflurane. Induction of and recovery from anesthesia are rapid, and cardiorespiratory depression is minimal, which makes sevoflurane generally safe in patients with coronary artery disease. Additionally, because of its low tissue solubility and nonirritating odor, sevoflurane is an appropriate agent for pediatric patients.

The disadvantages of sevoflurane include metabolism to inorganic fluoride and degradation in soda lime to potentially toxic metabolites. Additionally, no well-designed clinical trials have documented clinically important advantages of sevoflurane over isoflurane.

Drug Significantly Different From P Isoflurane

Nitrous oxide is a colorless, odorless, tasteless, nonflammable, nonirritating, inorganic gas rather than a halogenated ether. It is used commonly as an adjunct in balanced anesthesia to decrease the MAC of halogenated agents. It is a powerful analgesic but a relatively weak inhaled anesthetic. Nitrous oxide is also used in low doses to provide analgesia in obstetrics and during procedures that do not require unconsciousness, as well as in dental procedures.

Nitrous oxide is readily absorbed into the blood through the pulmonary capillary system. It has a relatively low solubility in blood and a MAC of 100%. Nitrous oxide is rapidly eliminated in the expired breath, essentially unchanged, with minimal diffusion through the skin.

The benefits must outweigh the risks of use of nitrous oxide during pregnancy because animal studies show that it can cause fetal death, growth retardation, and skeletal anomalies. Prolonged administration of nitrous oxide can cause inactivation of methionine synthase, a vitamin B_{12}–dependent enzyme, resulting in leukopenia and anemia. This effect does not occur within the time frame of clinical surgery, but it poses a potential problem for providers who are chronically exposed to nitrous oxide.

C Parenteral Anesthetic Agents

Parenteral anesthetics are also known as induction agents. Several classes of drugs are used as parenteral anesthetics in balanced anesthesia, including barbiturates, benzodiazepines, opioid analgesics, and nonbarbiturate hypnotic agents. Parenteral anesthetics that will be discussed include propofol (Diprivan), thiopental (Pentothal), etomidate (Amidate), ketamine (Ketalar), fentanyl (Sublimaze), and the benzodiazepines.

Propofol (Diprivan), a nonbarbiturate hypnotic agent, is the prototype for parenteral anesthetics (Table 15.3). Propofol appears as a milky white solution because it is formulated in a solution with soybean oil, glycerol, and egg phospholipids—accordingly, it has been given the nickname "the milk of anesthesia." Drugs significantly different from propofol are ketamine, fentanyl, and the benzodiazepines.

NURSING MANAGEMENT OF THE PATIENT RECEIVING P PROPOFOL

Core Drug Knowledge

Pharmacotherapeutics

Propofol is used for induction and maintenance of general anesthesia and maintenance of sedation in the intensive care unit (ICU). It may also be used to treat refractory status epilepticus; however, it has a higher risk profile than benzodiazepines.

Pharmacokinetics

Propofol is administered intravenously and is rapidly distributed to all tissues in the body. Loss of consciousness usually occurs within 40 seconds. The duration of a bolus injection is 3 to 5 minutes.

Propofol crosses the placenta and is distributed into breast milk. Propofol is metabolized in the liver but also through extrahepatic routes. Recovery from anesthesia is rapid and is associated with minimal psychomotor impairment. The kinetics of propofol do not appear to be affected by chronic hepatic or renal disease.

Pharmacodynamics

The cellular mechanism of action of propofol is unknown, but it is thought to mediate activity of the gamma-aminobutyric acid (GABA) receptors. However, the clinical response is clear: anesthesia is immediate and short-lived. Cardiorespiratory depression occurs, as well as decreased cerebral blood flow and intraocular pressure. Apnea and substantial hypotension may occur and may be dose related. Propofol is a weak analgesic agent; therefore, it is generally administered with other analgesics. However, concomitant use of opiates may intensify cardiorespiratory depression.

Contraindications and Precautions

Propofol is contraindicated for patients with a hypersensitivity to propofol or any of the ingredients of its emulsion vehicle. It is also contraindicated during pregnancy and lactation. Propofol is relatively contraindicated in patients with a seizure disorder because they are at an increased risk for developing convulsions during the recovery phase. Propofol should be used with caution in patients with cardiac or peripheral vascular disease because the cardiovascular depressive and hypotensive effects of propofol can aggravate these conditions.

Propofol should be used cautiously in patients with cerebrovascular disease, impaired cerebral blood flow, or increased ICP because it can cause a substantial reduction in mean arterial pressure and cerebral perfusion. Propofol is used with caution in patients who are hypotensive, hypovolemic, or hemodynamically unstable because of its hypotensive effects. Because disorders of lipid metabolism can be aggravated by the emulsion vehicle in which propofol is deliv-

TABLE 15.3 Summary of Selected (C) Parenteral Anesthetic Agents

Drug (Trade) Name	Selected Indications	Route and Dosage Range	Pharmacokinetics
P propofol (Diprivan)	Anesthesia induction and maintenance, monitored anesthesia care (MAC), sedation for diagnostic and surgical procedures, continuous sedation in intensive care unit.	*Adult:* IV, 5 mg/kg/min for 5 min for sedation, 2–2.5 mg/kg for induction, 6–12 mg/kg/h for maintenance, 0.5 mg/kg over 3–5 min for MAC initiation, 1.5–4.5 mg/kg/h for maintenance	*Onset:* 30 sec *Duration:* 3–10 min $t_{1/2}$: biphasic initial: 40 min; terminal: 1–3 d
droperidol (inapsine, innovar)	Tranquilization and antinauseant/antiemetic in surgical and diagnostic procedures; premedication; induction and adjunct in general and regional anesthesia; neuroleptanalgesia	*Adult:* IM, 2.5–10 mg 30–60 min preop	*Onset:* 3–10 min *Duration:* 2–4 h $t_{1/2}$: 2.2 h
etomidate (Amidate)	Anesthetic induction or adjunct, cardioversion, status epilepticus, head injury	*Adult:* 0.3 mg/kg IV over 15–60 s or 10–20 μg/kg/min for maintenance	*Onset:* 20 s *Duration:* 4–10 min $t_{1/2}$: 1.5–4 min (serum); 2.6 h (elimination)
ketamine (Ketalar)	Anesthesia for short surgical or diagnostic procedures not requiring skeletal muscle relaxation	*Adult:* IM, 5–10 mg/kg for induction, 2–4 mg/kg for sedation; IV, 1–2 mg/kg over 60 s for induction and 0.1–0.5 mg/min for maintenance	*Onset:* IM, 3–4 min; IV, 30 s *Duration:* IM, IV, 5–10 min $t_{1/2}$: 10–15 min (initially), 2.5 h
midazolam (Versed)	Anesthesia induction, cardiac catheterization, conscious sedation, endoscopy, gastroscopy, premedication	IM, IV, titrated	*Onset:* IM, 15 min; IV, 3–5 min *Duration:* 30–60 min $t_{1/2}$: 1.2–12.3 h

ered, patients with diabetic hyperlipidemia, pancreatitis, or primary hyperlipoproteinemia should be monitored closely.

Adverse Effects

The most common adverse effects of propofol are nausea and vomiting. Another frequent adverse effect is involuntary muscle movement. Propofol may produce a dose-related degree of hypotension or decrease in systemic vascular resistance. Apnea occurs in 50% to 84% of patients. Anaphylaxis may also occur. High-dose or long-term propofol use in the critical care setting can induce the production of bright-green urine.

Local adverse effects include pain on injection, transient muscle twitching, and tremor. The solution in which propofol is prepared can support bacterial growth because it contains soybean oil, glycerol, and egg phosphatide.

Drug Interactions

Propofol may interact with benzodiazepines, droperidol, CNS depressants, and theophylline (Table 15.4).

Assessment of Relevant Core Patient Variables

Health Status

Assess the patient for a history of hypersensitivity to propofol, soybean oil, glycerol, or egg phospholipids. Also, assess the patient for diseases or disorders that contraindicate the use of propofol and for concomitant use of drugs that may interact with propofol, such as theophylline in the case of asthma or emphysema and benzodiazepines or phenothiazines in the case of patients with mental health issues. Positive responses should be communicated to the anesthesiologist or nurse anesthetist before surgery.

When propofol is used for sedation in an ICU, obtain serum triglyceride levels before administering propofol and every 3 to 7 days of therapy.

Life Span and Gender

Document the age of the patient. Elderly, debilitated, and dehydrated patients are typically more sensitive to the effects of propofol than younger patients are. In addition, elderly patients typically have reduced total-body clearance of propofol and should be given lower induction doses and slower infusion rates for anesthesia maintenance.

Environment

Propofol must be given in a controlled environment, such as an operating room, recovery room, or ICU. A cardiac monitor, blood pressure monitor, and ventilator generally are required during administration.

Nursing Diagnoses and Outcomes

- Ineffective Breathing Pattern related to respiratory depression secondary to drugs used during anesthesia

TABLE 15.4 Agents That Interact With P Propofol

Interactants	Effect and Significance	Nursing Management
CNS depressants • Alcohol • Anesthetics • Benzodiazepines • Barbiturates • Histamine-1 blockers • Opioids • Phenothiazines • Tricyclic antidepressants	The pharmacologic effects of propofol may be enhanced, resulting in increased sedation and respiratory depression.	Provide continuous patient assessment. Monitor sedation. Monitor respiratory status. Provide supportive therapy as needed.
carbidopa-levodopa	When levodopa is abruptly withdrawn, a symptom complex resembling neuroleptic malignant syndrome may occur.	Administer levodopa as soon as patient is able to resume PO medications. Monitor for muscular rigidity, hyperthermia, mental changes, increased creatine phosphokinase concentration, diaphoresis, and tachycardia.
catecholamines	Propofol and catecholamines may drive each other in a progressively myocardial depressive loop, which could lead to cardiac arrhythmias or cardiac failure.	Monitor cardiovascular status. Follow standing protocols for titrating these drugs.
droperidol	Coadministration may increase frequency of postoperative nausea and vomiting.	Avoid coadministration.
herbal medications • St. John's wort • *Hypericum perforatum*	Coadministration of propofol with herbal medications may intensify or prolong the effects of propofol.	Advise the patient to discontinue herbal medication 2–3 weeks before surgery.
warfarin	Propofol is emulsified with soybean oil 10%, which contains vitamin K.	Monitor efficacy of anticoagulation.

Desired outcome: *The patient will maintain effective breathing despite respiratory depression by administration of oxygen as appropriate.*

- Risk for Aspiration related to drug-induced nausea and vomiting, GI distention, hypoxia, and stimulation of the vomiting center

  Desired outcome: *The patient's nausea and vomiting will be minimized by premedication with antiemetic agents.*
- Disturbed Sensory Perception, varied, related to CNS depression secondary to drugs used during anesthesia

  Desired outcome: *The patient will remain free from sensory or perceptual alterations through careful reorientation, repeated as necessary.*

Planning and Intervention

Maximizing Therapeutic Effects

For the surgical patient, preinduction and induction should be done in a low-stimulus environment, as with isoflurane. Preoperative patient education is imperative to minimize the patient's anxiety, which, in turn, helps maximize the therapeutic effects of propofol.

In the critical care setting, a low-stimulus environment is also important. To avoid overstimulation, interact with the patient only when necessary. Evaluate the depth of analgesia and adjust the infusion of propofol according to the health facility's standing orders.

Minimizing Adverse Effects

Visually inspect the propofol preparation for particulate matter and discoloration before administration. If the emulsion appears to be separated, do not use it. Because the propofol emulsion does not contain preservatives, it is important to limit its duration of administration to avoid bacterial growth. When used for critical care sedation, propofol should be discarded after 12 hours if administered directly from the container provided from the pharmacy or within 6 hours if transferred to a syringe or other container.

Providing Patient and Family Education

- Provide preoperative patient education about the induction process to minimize fears of anesthesia.
- In the critical care unit, explain the purpose of the light anesthesia state and reassure patients that they are being constantly monitored.
- For outpatient surgery, discharge the patient to the care of a responsible adult and instruct the patient not to drive or engage in any activity that requires full alertness or coordination.

Ongoing Assessment and Evaluation

Patients receiving propofol as an induction agent for balanced anesthesia should be monitored in the postanesthesia recovery room until they are awake and have stable vital signs.

In the critical care unit, when propofol is used to maintain light anesthesia, continuously monitor blood pressure,

cardiac output, and pulmonary capillary wedge pressure. Assess the patient's lung sounds frequently for respiratory depression. Because the patient remains motionless, turn the patient every 2 hours and assess for skin breakdown. Constantly monitor the level of sedation and titrate propofol to maximize sedation. As previously mentioned, serum triglycerides should be monitored every 3 to 7 days.

Drugs Closely Related to P Propofol

Thiopental

Thiopental (Pentothal) is a barbiturate anesthetic agent. Its rapid onset and short duration of action are ideal for an induction agent. Its onset of action after intravenous (IV) administration is less than 1 minute, and the hypnotic action lasts only a few minutes. Metabolism of thiopental takes place in the liver slowly, and the drug accumulates to a toxic level in the tissues after repeated administrations. Thiopental differs from propofol in that it is not used for the duration of anesthesia by continuous infusion. It does not provide any analgesia.

Etomidate

Etomidate (Amidate) is a nonbarbiturate, nonanalgesic anesthetic used primarily for induction, but it can be used for IV anesthesia when supplemented by a narcotic analgesic. Induction is rapid, and recovery from a single dose takes only a few minutes because of rapid redistribution of drug to other tissues. Etomidate is metabolized by the liver and has a much shorter elimination time than propofol does. There appears to be less respiratory and cardiovascular depression than with barbiturates and propofol. Additionally, etomidate does not release histamine.

The popularity of etomidate has diminished because of its adverse effects, including involuntary movements during induction, a high incidence of nausea and vomiting during recovery, and adrenocortical suppression.

Drugs Significantly Different From P Propofol

Ketamine

Both chemically and pharmacologically, Ketamine (Ketalar) closely resembles phencyclidine, which is a street drug with a pronounced effect on sensory perception. Thus, ketamine produces pharmacologic actions distinctly different from other IV anesthetics. It produces dissociative anesthesia, resulting in catatonia, amnesia, and analgesia. The patient may appear awake and reactive but does not respond to sensory stimuli. Ketamine is used for short procedures not requiring muscle relaxation, including diagnostic tests and surgery. It can be used as a general anesthetic agent for children. Because of the high incidence of postoperative psychological phenomena (sensory and perceptual illusions and vivid dreams) associated with its use, ketamine is not commonly used in adult patients. However, it is considered useful for high-risk geriatric patients and patients in shock, because of its cardiostimulatory properties.

After IV administration, ketamine has an initial half-life of 10 to 15 minutes, which subsequently changes to a longer half-life of 2.5 hours, corresponding with redistribution from the CNS and hepatic biotransformation. The metabolites of ketamine are excreted in the urine. Cardiovascular and respiratory stimulation occurs shortly after injection, peaks after a few minutes, and subsides within 15 minutes.

No muscle relaxation is associated with ketamine use, and laryngeal and pharyngeal reflexes stay intact. Under ketamine anesthesia, the higher centers of the brain do not perceive auditory, visual, or painful stimuli. This effect is thought to occur through ketamine action at opioid and nonopioid receptors, including muscarinic receptors. It may be that different receptors are involved in analgesia and loss of consciousness.

Ketamine is contraindicated in patients for whom a substantial increase in blood pressure would be hazardous. It is not used for patients with psychiatric disorders, because of the potential for a reaction during emergence from anesthesia, which may include hallucinations and agitation. It also should be avoided in cases of known hypersensitivity. Caution is advised using ketamine in cases involving mild to moderate hypertension, pregnancy or lactation, alcohol abuse, acute intermittent porphyria, elevated intraocular pressure or ICP, and hyperthyroidism.

Hypertension and tachycardia are common cardiovascular effects of ketamine that are probably mediated through sympathetic stimulation. Nausea and vomiting are also common. In addition, ketamine may enhance the actions of the nondepolarizing neuromuscular blockers (discussed later in this chapter) and prolong respiratory depression. Theophylline should not be coadministered with ketamine because the two interact and may cause unpredictable seizures. Patients on thyroid enhancement therapy may experience hypertension and tachycardia when taking ketamine.

Nursing care of the patient under ketamine anesthesia is largely protective because of the dissociative state that it causes and the likelihood of emergence reactions. Take vital signs and a brief mental status examination as a pretreatment assessment.

The expected outcomes for ketamine anesthesia are effective and safe anesthesia, adequate airway maintenance, and minimal emergence reaction. Emergence reactions may be avoided or diminished if you are careful to reduce external stimuli during the recovery phase and allow the patient to wake up spontaneously. Frightening emergence symptoms can be stopped with diazepam. Because emergence reactions may occur up to 24 hours after anesthesia, instruct the patient

MEMORY CHIP

P Propofol

- A parenteral anesthetic used in the management of general anesthesia, sedation induction or maintenance, and status epilepticus
- Major contraindications: hypersensitivity to soybean oil, glycerol, or egg phosphatide
- Most common adverse effects: nausea, vomiting, involuntary movements
- Most serious adverse effects: apnea and anaphylaxis
- Maximizing therapeutic effects: low-stimulus environment
- Minimizing adverse effects: Time the administration to avoid potential bacterial growth.
- Most important patient education: Reassure the patient that he or she is being constantly monitored.

to avoid hazardous activities, including driving, for at least that long. Ambulatory patients must be discharged into the care of a responsible adult. Instruct the patient to avoid alcohol and other CNS depressants for 24 hours. The nurse in the PACU and the nurse in charge of the patient on his or her return to the unit should evaluate outcomes achieved and compare them with what would be expected under normal conditions.

Fentanyl

Fentanyl (Sublimaze) is a narcotic agent used with a neuroleptic drug, such as droperidol, to produce a state of consciousness called neuroleptanesthesia. Fentanyl and droperidol are manufactured as the combination drug Innovar. To induce neuroleptanesthesia, fentanyl and droperidol are administered intravenously in combination with nitrous oxide and oxygen. This type of anesthesia is useful for procedures such as bronchoscopy that require freedom from pain but the patient's ability to cooperate. The most important adverse effect of neuroleptanesthesia is respiratory depression or arrest. Chapter 23 discusses narcotic agents in depth.

Benzodiazepines

Benzodiazepines (e.g., diazepam, lorazepam, midazolam) have been used as parenteral agents in balanced anesthesia. Midazolam is water soluble at low pH and has been reported to cause less pain on injection and a lower incidence of venous thrombosis than diazepam does. Additionally, midazolam can be administered intramuscularly. Chapter 16 discusses benzodiazepines in depth.

C LOCAL ANESTHETIC AGENTS

Local anesthetic agents are divided into esters and amides. Important practical differences exist between these two groups. Esters are relatively unstable in solution and are rapidly hydrolyzed in the body by plasma cholinesterase and other esterases. One of the main breakdown products is para-aminobenzoic acid (PABA), which is associated with allergic phenomena and hypersensitivity reactions. In contrast, amides are relatively stable in solution and are slowly metabolized by hepatic amidases; hypersensitivity reactions to amide local anesthetics are extremely rare. In current clinical practice, the esters have largely been superseded by the amides.

Local anesthetics produce local or regional anesthesia by blocking nerve conduction and abolishing sensations in a limited and well-defined area of the body without loss of consciousness (Figure 15.2). The blockade affects all nerve fibers sequentially: autonomic, then sensory, then motor, with effects diminishing in reverse order. Clinically, the loss of nerve function affects temperature first; then pain, touch, proprioception, and finally, skeletal muscle tone.

Local anesthetics share the same mechanism of action, but they differ in their potency, onset of action, and duration (Table 15.5). Examples of local anesthetic agents include lidocaine (Xylocaine), bupivacaine (Marcaine), etidocaine (Duranest), and procaine (Novocain). The prototype discussed in this chapter is lidocaine (Xylocaine), an amide local anesthetic agent.

NURSING MANAGEMENT OF THE PATIENT RECEIVING P LIDOCAINE

Core Drug Knowledge

Pharmacotherapeutics

Lidocaine is used as a local anesthetic in a variety of situations, including regional blocks, nerve blocks, ophthalmic anesthesia, obstetric anesthesia, dental anesthesia, and infiltration anesthesia to repair full-thickness skin lacerations. It can be applied topically for dental pain, postherpetic neuralgia, neuropathic pain, and stomatitis. When administered intranasally, it is also effective for migraine headaches.

In addition to its uses as a local anesthetic, lidocaine is also used intravenously for ventricular tachycardia and ventricular fibrillation. See Chapter 26 for a discussion of lidocaine as an antiarrhythmic agent.

Pharmacokinetics

Lidocaine may be administered topically, orally, subcutaneously, intradermally, submucosally, and intravenously. Only minimal amounts of lidocaine enter the circulation

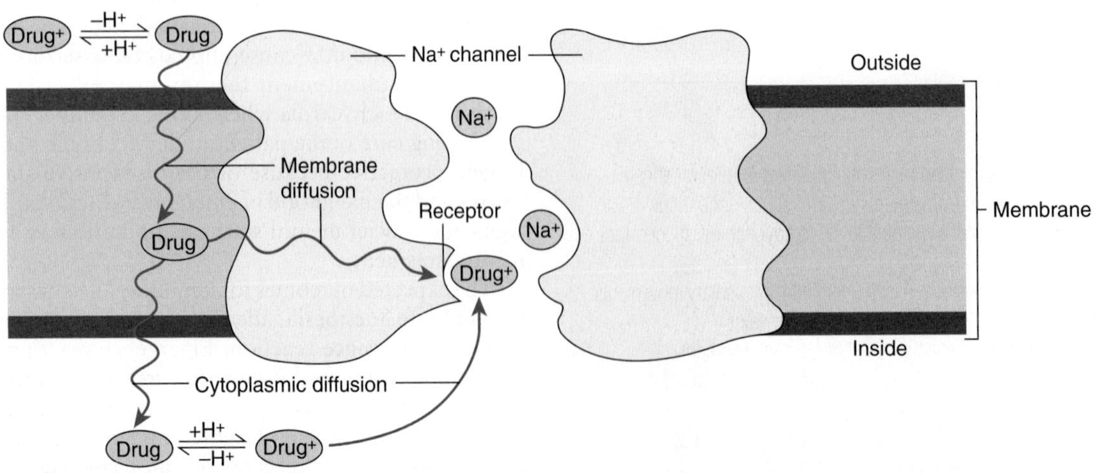

FIGURE 15.2 Local anesthetics' mechanism of action.

TABLE 15.5 Summary of Selected (C) Local Anesthetic Agents

Drug (Trade) Name	Selected Indications	Route and Dosage Range	Pharmacokinetics
[P] lidocaine (Xylocaine)	Infiltration anesthesia Topical anesthesia Peripheral nerve blocks IV regional nerve blocks Epidural and spinal blocks	*Adult and child:* maximum, 3 mg/kg; with adrenalin: maximum: 7 mg/kg	*Onset:* Rapid *Duration:* 1–3 h $t_{1/2}$: 7–30 min
bupivacaine (Marcaine)	Infiltration anesthesia Peripheral nerve blocks Epidural and spinal blocks	*Adult and child:* maximum: 2 mg/kg; with adrenalin, maximum: 2 mg/kg	*Onset:* 1–10 min *Duration:* 3–9 h $t_{1/2}$: neonates: 8.1 h $t_{1/2}$: adults: 3.5 h
etidocaine (Duranest)	Infiltration anesthesia Peripheral nerve block Extradural blocks	*Adult:* maximum: 4 mg/kg *Child:* maximum dose not established	*Onset:* 2–8 min *Duration:* 4.5–13 h $t_{1/2}$: neonates: 4–8 h $t_{1/2}$: adults: 2.7 h
mepivacaine (Carbocaine, Polocaine)	Infiltration anesthesia Peripheral nerve blocks	*Adult:* 400 mg as a single regional dose not to exceed 1000 mg/24 h *Child:* 5–6 mg/kg	*Onset:* 5–4 min *Duration:* 1–2 h $t_{1/2}$: neonates: 8.7–9 h $t_{1/2}$: adults: 1.9–3.2 h
prilocaine (Citanest)	Infiltration anesthesia Peripheral nerve blocks IV regional nerve blocks	*Adult and child:* 6 mg/kg; with adrenalin, 9 mg/kg	*Onset:* <2 min *Duration:* 1–2 h $t_{1/2}$: 1.25 h
procaine (Novocain)	Dental anesthesia Infiltration Anesthesia Local anesthesia Peripheral nerve block Regional anesthesia Severe pain Spinal anesthesia Sympathetic nerve block	*Adult:* single dose of 350–600 mg *Child:* 15 mg/kg	*Onset:* 2–5 min *Duration:* 1 h $t_{1/2}$: 7.7 min

following subcutaneous injection. The duration of action of subcutaneously administered lidocaine is 1 to 3 hours, depending on the strength of the lidocaine preparation used. Adding epinephrine to lidocaine in proportions of 1:200,000 to 1:100,000 slows the vascular absorption of lidocaine and prolongs its effects.

Lidocaine is nearly completely absorbed following oral administration but undergoes extensive first-pass metabolism in the liver, resulting in a systemic bioavailability of only 35%. Some systemic absorption is possible when using oral viscous solutions.

Transdermal absorption of lidocaine is related to the duration of application and the surface area over which the patch is applied. When the lidocaine patch is used as directed, very little systemic absorption occurs. After topical administration of viscous solutions or jelly to mucous membranes, the duration of action is 30 to 60 minutes, with peak effects occurring within 2 to 5 minutes.

Local dental anesthesia starts to occur within 2.5 minutes of applying the DentiPatch to intact mucous membranes and continues for approximately 30 to 40 minutes.

Pharmacodynamics

Lidocaine produces its analgesic effects through a reversible nerve conduction blockade, which diminishes the nerve membrane's permeability to sodium. This action decreases the rate of membrane depolarization, thereby increasing the threshold for electrical excitability. Direct penetration of the nerve membrane is necessary for effective anesthesia, which is achieved by applying the anesthetic topically or injecting it subcutaneously, intradermally, or submucosally around the nerve trunks or ganglia supplying the area to be anesthetized.

Contraindications and Precautions

Lidocaine is contraindicated in patients with hypersensitivity to amide local anesthetics and in patients with hypersensitivity to sulfites or the preservative methylparaben. To avoid systemic absorption of lidocaine, its administration as a nerve block or as epidural, local, or spinal anesthesia is contraindicated in patients with infection or inflammation at the injection site.

Applying lidocaine preparations to severely traumatized mucosa (large skin abrasions, eczema, burns) can increase its absorption, which in turn increases the risk for systemic toxicity. Application to the oral mucosa can interfere with swallowing and increase the risk for aspiration. Lumbar and caudal epidural anesthesia should be used with extreme caution in patients with existing neurologic disease, spinal deformities, sepsis, and severe hypertension, because the risk for adverse effects increases.

Adverse Effects

Allergic reactions such as urticaria, angioedema, bronchospasm, and anaphylactic shock may occur with lidocaine administration. Some preparations contain sulfites and methylparaben, which can cause severe allergic reactions, including status asthmaticus, in susceptible patients.

Local anesthetic agents are relatively free from adverse effects if they are administered in an appropriate dosage and in the correct anatomic location. However, systemic and localized toxic reactions may occur, usually from accidental intravascular or intrathecal injection, or from an excessive dose of the local anesthetic agent. Systemic reactions to local anesthetics primarily involve the CNS and the cardiovascular system.

Transoral or transdermal application of lidocaine is unlikely to cause systemic adverse reactions because of the small amount of lidocaine absorbed. Potential local reactions include erythema, edema, and dysesthesia (abnormal sensations including numbness, tingling, prickling, or burning). These reactions are usually mild and transient, resolving within a few minutes to a few hours.

Drug Interactions

Drug interactions occur most frequently with IV administration of lidocaine. Subcutaneous administration rarely causes drug interactions unless lidocaine is inadvertently administered into an artery or vein.

Local anesthetics can interact with antihypertensive agents, cholinesterase inhibitors, monoamine oxidase inhibitors, and opiate agonists (Table 15.6). These interacting drugs will be discussed in more detail in subsequent chapters.

Assessment of Relevant Core Patient Variables

Health Status

Assess for hypersensitivity to lidocaine or any other drug with "caine" in the name. Positive findings should be communicated to the provider before lidocaine is administered.

Before using topical anesthesia, inspect the area. Topical anesthesia should not be applied to abraded or denuded skin. For viscous lidocaine, assess for the patient's ability to swallow before using the drug.

Life Span and Gender

Lidocaine should be used with caution in patients who are pregnant or breast-feeding. Although lidocaine is a pregnancy category B drug, local anesthetics can cross the placenta rapidly when administered for epidural, paracervical, pudendal, or caudal block anesthesia, resulting in fetal bradycardia. The frequency and extent of toxicity are dependent on the procedure performed. Maternal hypotension can result from regional anesthesia, and elevating the feet and positioning the patient on her left side can alleviate this problem. When lidocaine is used as epidural anesthesia during labor and delivery, it may prolong the second stage of labor. Monitor for cardiovascular and CNS depression in the fetus or neonate.

Lifestyle, Diet, and Habits

Viscous lidocaine may be provided for patients with stomatitis or chronic ulceration in the mouth. It is important that the patient assess his or her ability to swallow before eating or drinking to avoid biting the interior of the mouth or aspirating foods or fluids.

Environment

Lidocaine is used in a variety of settings, including hospitals, outpatient surgical settings, clinics, private doctor's offices, and dental offices. Topical or viscous lidocaine may be administered in the home environment.

Nursing Diagnoses and Outcomes

- Fear related to traumatic injury and concern about pain during the surgical procedure
  Desired outcome: *The patient will be assured that pain will not occur during the procedure.*

TABLE 15.6 Agents That Interact With [P] Lidocaine

Interactants	Effect and Significance	Nursing Management
antihypertensive agents	Epidural administration of local anesthetics with antihypertensive agents may result in additive hypotensive effects due to loss of sympathetic tone.	Monitor vital signs.
cholinesterase inhibitors	Local anesthetics can antagonize the effects of cholinesterase inhibitors by inhibiting neuronal transmission in skeletal muscle.	Dosage adjustment of the cholinesterase inhibitor may be necessary to control the symptoms of myasthenia gravis.
monoamine oxidase inhibitors (MAOIs)	Concomitant administration of MAOIs and local anesthetics increases the risk of hypotension.	MAOIs should be discontinued 10 days before surgery requiring a regional block.
opiate agonists alfentanil fentanyl morphine sufentanil	Concomitant use of low-dose local anesthetics with opiate agonists may increase analgesia and decrease opiate dosage requirements.	Monitor for analgesic efficacy. Monitor CNS depression.

- Risk for Peripheral Neurovascular Dysfunction related to action of drug
  Desired outcome: The patient will refrain from activities that may induce injury while area is numb.
- Impaired Swallowing related to administration of viscous lidocaine
  Desired outcome: The patient will refrain from eating or drinking for 1 hour after swallowing viscous lidocaine.

Planning and Intervention

Maximizing Therapeutic Effects

Assist with the administration of lidocaine after the patient is informed about the process. Use a calm, reassuring approach and allow the patient to voice concerns before the procedure begins.

Minimizing Adverse Effects

Read the drug label carefully before helping the provider to administer lidocaine. Preparations containing preservatives should not be used for spinal or epidural anesthesia. Preparations with adrenaline should not be administered in areas such as fingers, toes, nose, or penis because prolonged vasoconstriction may damage these areas of the body. Restrict food and fluids for 1 hour after viscous lidocaine is swallowed.

Providing Patient and Family Education

- Tell the patient and family how local anesthetics such as lidocaine work. Assure the patient that the area will be numb before the procedure begins. Encourage the patient to verbalize any discomfort during the procedure.
- Advise the patient receiving topical anesthesia at home first to place the anesthetic on the dressing and then to place the dressing on the site. Remind patients receiving viscous lidocaine that it causes numbness of the tongue, cheeks, and throat. The patient should not eat or drink for 1 hour to keep from biting the cheeks or tongue and to avoid aspiration.
- Advise the patient of the expected duration of lidocaine's effects. The patient should contact the provider if sensation does not return.

Ongoing Assessment and Evaluation

Evaluate for the lack of sensation before starting a procedure and remind the patient to assess for sensation before resuming food or fluid intake.

Drugs Closely Related to P Lidocaine

Bupivacaine

Bupivacaine (Marcaine) is a long-acting local amide anesthetic recommended for local or regional anesthesia. It has the ability to separate sensory and motor blockade because its effect on motor function varies with concentration. With bupivacaine administration, analgesia persists longer than anesthesia, which postpones the need for postoperative narcotics. Bupivacaine is also used in epidural patient-controlled analgesia (PCA) in combination with narcotics.

MEMORY CHIP

P Lidocaine

- Used for infiltration anesthesia, regional blocks, nerve blocks, ophthalmic anesthesia, obstetric anesthesia, or dental anesthesia
- Major contraindications: hypersensitivity to amide local anesthetics, sulfites, or methyl paraben; infection or inflammation at the site of administration
- Most common adverse effects: minimal adverse reactions unless accidental intravascular or intrathecal injection occurs
- Most serious adverse effect: allergic reactions
- Maximizing therapeutic effects: calm reassurance by staff
- Minimizing adverse effects: Read labels carefully. Be sure to use the right preparation for the right procedure.
- Most important patient education: safety due to lack of sensation

Etidocaine

Etidocaine (Duranest) is a long-acting local anesthetic of the amide type. It is used for epidural, local, and retrobulbar anesthesia in surgical and dental procedures. Like lidocaine, etidocaine has a rapid onset of sensory and motor blockade, but the duration of analgesia is 1.5 to 2 times longer than it is with lidocaine. Its profound motor blockade may last up to 9 hours when given peridurally.

Mepivacaine

Mepivacaine (Carbocaine, Polocaine) is a local amide anesthetic with an intermediate duration of action. Compared with lidocaine, it produces less vasodilation and has a more rapid onset and longer duration of action. Mepivacaine is indicated for infiltration (administration of a local anesthetic into the area to be numbed) and transtracheal anesthesia and for peripheral, sympathetic, regional, and epidural nerve blocks in surgical and dental procedures.

Prilocaine

Prilocaine (Citanest) is another local anesthetic of the amide class used primarily for dental anesthesia. It has an intermediate duration of action and is longer acting than lidocaine. Prilocaine causes the least systemic toxicity of the amides but at high doses may cause methemoglobinemia, a condition marked by high levels of a hemoglobin compound that does not carry oxygen.

Procaine

Procaine hydrochloride (Novocain) is a short-acting local anesthetic of the ester type used for local or regional anesthesia and dental applications. It has no topical anesthetic activity. Procaine is more likely to cause a hypersensitivity reaction and vasodilation than amide-type local anesthetics.

Topical Anesthetics

Local anesthetics may be applied to the skin, the eyes, the ears, the nose, and the mouth, as well as to other mucous membranes. In general, cocaine, lidocaine, and prilocaine are the most useful and effective local anesthetics for topical administration, and when used for that purpose, they usually have a rapid onset of action (5 to 10 minutes) and a moderate duration of action (30 to 60 minutes). In

addition to its use as a topical anesthetic, cocaine is a potent vasoconstrictor.

Absorption of local anesthetics through intact skin is usually slow and unreliable, and high concentrations are required. EMLA cream is a mixture of local anesthetics (lidocaine and prilocaine in an emulsion) that may be used to provide surface anesthesia of the skin, particularly for children. Cutaneous contact (usually under an occlusive dressing) should be maintained for at least 60 minutes before venipuncture.

C NEUROMUSCULAR BLOCKING AGENTS

Neuromuscular blocking agents are divided into two categories: nondepolarizing drugs, which prevent neural communication from depolarizing the muscle (keeping the muscle in a relaxed state); and depolarizing drugs, which cause muscle depolarization and prevent repolarization (so that the muscle contracts and is unable to go into a relaxed state to receive further neural communication). Neuromuscular blockers are not mediated by the CNS. Rather, they work by directly interfering with transmission at the end plate, which is the site of communication between a nerve and a muscle (Figure 15.3). Box 15.1 summarizes the potential effects of the NMJ blocking agents discussed in this chapter.

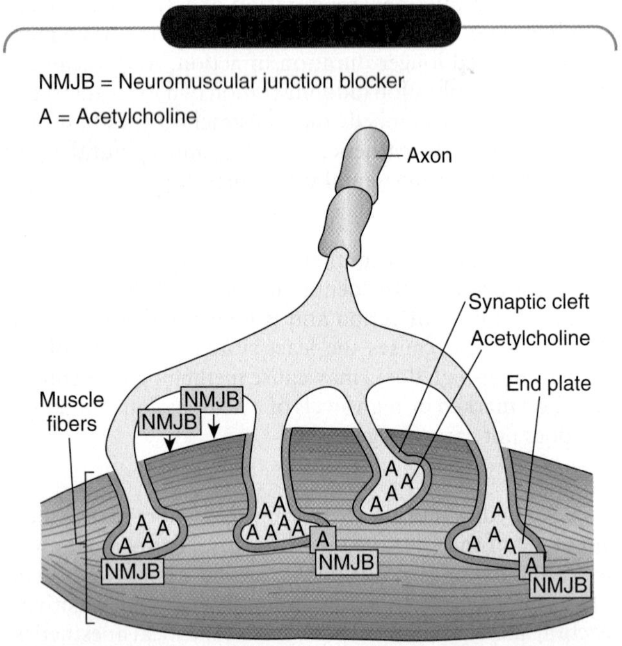

FIGURE 15.3 How neuromuscular blockers work. Motor end plates are the terminal branches of motor nerves. They are found within muscle fibers, but they are separated from the muscle itself by a synaptic cleft. Normally, the neurotransmitter acetylcholine is found in the axon of the motor nerve. However, when the nerve is stimulated, the acetylcholine is released and moves to receptor sites on surface of the muscle cell. Neuromuscular blockers inhibit the action of acetylcholine (muscle contraction) by competing for these receptor sites.

BOX 15.1 Potential Effects of Neuromuscular Junction Blocking Agents

Histamine Release
tubocurarine
atracurium
mivacurium
succinylcholine

Vagolytic Activity
pancuronium

Sympathetic Stimulation
pancuronium

Ganglionic Blockade
tubocurarine

Vagal Stimulation
succinylcholine

C Nondepolarizing Neuromuscular Blocking Agents

Nondepolarizing neuromuscular blocking agents include tubocurarine (Tubarine, Tubocurarine), pancuronium bromide (Pavulon), pipecuronium (Arduan), and vecuronium (Norcuron) (Table 15.7). The prototype drug of this class is tubocurarine.

NURSING MANAGEMENT OF THE PATIENT RECEIVING P TUBOCURARINE

Core Drug Knowledge

Pharmacotherapeutics

Tubocurarine is a skeletal muscle relaxant used as an adjunct to general anesthetics in facilitating endotracheal intubation and mechanical ventilation. In the ICU or cardiac intensive care setting, tubocurarine is used to minimize a patient's movement to conserve energy or to reduce agitation that may increase ICP. It is also used to prevent trauma during electroconvulsive therapy and to diagnose myasthenia gravis.

Pharmacokinetics

Tubocurarine is available only for IV use. The onset of muscle paralysis occurs within 2 minutes after administration and peaks at 3 to 5 minutes. Muscle paralysis starts to subside within 20 to 30 minutes but may be prolonged to 90 minutes or more. Up to 75% of tubocurarine is excreted unchanged by the kidneys in the first 24 hours. Another 11% may undergo biliary excretion. Only a negligible amount of the drug is metabolized. Tubocurarine crosses the placenta; whether it enters breast milk is unknown.

TABLE 15.7 Summary of Selected (C) Neuromuscular Blocking Agents

Drug (Trade) Name	Selected Indications	Route and Dosage Range	Pharmacokinetics
Nondepolarizing Neuromuscular Junction Blockers			
[P] tubocurarine (Tubarine, Tubocurarine)	Adjunct to general anesthesia and neuromuscular blockade	*Adult:* IV, 6–9 mg followed by 3–4.5 mg in 3–5 min if necessary *Child:* IV, 0.2–0.5 mg/kg followed by 0.04–0.1 mg/kg prn to maintain paralysis *Neonate <1 mo:* IV, 0.3 mg/kg followed by 0.1 mg/kg to maintain paralysis	*Onset:* 2 min *Duration:* 20–90 min $t_{1/2}$: 170–270 min
	Electroconvulsive therapy	*Adult:* IV, 0.165 mg/kg administered slowly	
	Myasthenia gravis diagnosis	*Adult:* IV, 0.004–0.033 mg/kg	
atracurium (Tracrium)	Endotracheal intubation, neuromuscular blockade	*Adult and child >2 y:* IV, 0.4–0.5 mg/kg followed by 0.08–0.1 mg/kg 20–45 min after the first dose as needed; reduce doses if used with general anesthetics *Child 1 mo–2 y:* IV, 0.3–0.4 mg/kg	*Onset:* 2–3 min *Duration:* 20–40 min $t_{1/2}$: 2–3 min
	Mechanical ventilation	*Adult:* IV, 5–9 μg/kg/min by continuous infusion	
cisatracurium (Nimbex)	Endotracheal intubation, neuromuscular blockade	*Adult:* IV, 0.15–0.20 mg/kg followed by 0.03 mg/kg every 20 min *Child >2 y:* IV, 0.1 mg/kg followed by 1–2 μg as needed	*Onset:* 2–3 min *Duration:* 30–40 min $t_{1/2}$: 22 min
	Mechanical ventilation	*Adult:* IV, 0.5–10.2 μg/kg/min	
doxacurium (Nuromax)	Endotracheal intubation	*Adult:* IV, 0.05 mg/kg over 5–10 sec *Child 2–12 y:* IV, 0.03–0.05 mg/kg	*Onset:* 5–6 min *Duration:* 12–54 min $t_{1/2}$: Unknown
	Neuromuscular blockade maintenance	*Adult and child:* IV, 0.0005–0.1 mg/kg every 60–100 min over 5–10 sec (Child may need more frequent dosing)	
mivacurium (Mivacron)	Endotracheal intubation	*Adult:* IV, 0.15 mg/kg over 5–15 sec (over 60 sec in patients with cardiovascular disease) *Child 2–12 y:* IV, 0.9–0.2 mg/kg	*Onset:* 1.5–3 min *Duration:* 15–20 min $t_{1/2}$: 2 min
	Neuromuscular blockade maintenance	*Adult and child:* IV, 0.1 mg/kg every 15 min	
	Continuous infusion	*Adult:* IV, Initial 9–10 μg/kg/min then reduce to 4 μg/kg/min *Child:* IV, 10–15 μg/kg/min	
pancuronium (Pavulon)	Neuromuscular blockade, agitation	*Adult and child:* IV, 0.04–0.1 mg/kg initial dose; may give additional doses of 0.01 mg/kg at 30- to 60-min intervals	*Onset:* 2–3 min *Duration:* 40–60 min $t_{1/2}$: 110 min

(continued)

TABLE 15.7 Summary of Selected (C) Neuromuscular Blocking Agents (continued)

Drug (Trade) Name	Selected Indications	Route and Dosage Range	Pharmacokinetics
pipecuronium (Arduan)	Endotracheal intubation	*Adult and child:* IV, 85–100 μg/kg, ideal body weight, given as rapid bolus over 5–10 sec	*Onset:* 2–3 min *Duration:* 120–150 min $t_{1/2}$: 1.7 h
	Neuromuscular blockade maintenance	*Adult and child:* IV, 5–25 μg/kg as needed for long procedures	
rocuronium (Zemuron)	Rapid-sequence intubation	*Adult:* IV, 0.6–1.2 mg/kg	*Onset:* 1–2 min *Duration:* 30 min $t_{1/2}$: 1–2 min
	Endotracheal intubation	*Adult:* IV, 0.6 mg/kg *Child >3 mo:* IV, 0.6 mg/kg	
	Neuromuscular blockade continuous infusion	*Adult:* IV, 0.01–0.012 mg/kg/min *Child >3 mo:* IV, 0.012 mg/kg/min	
vecuronium (Norcuron)	Endotracheal intubation	*Adult and child >10 y:* IV, 80–100 μg/kg *Child 1–10 y:* IV, Individualized; may need slightly more than adult dose *Infant 7 wk–12 mo:* Individualized *Neonate:* Safe dose not established.	*Onset:* 2–3 min *Duration:* 45–60 min $t_{1/2}$: 4 min
	Neuromuscular blockade as adjunct to general anesthesia with enflurane or isoflurane	*Adult and child >10 y:* IV, 60–85 μg/kg IV; then 10–15 μg/kg after 25–40 min; then readminister every 12–15 min *Child 1–10 y:* IV, Individualized; may need slightly more than adult dose *Infant 7 wk–12 mo:* 0.08–0.1 mg/kg followed by 0.05–0.1 mg/kg every hour as needed *Neonate:* IV, 0.1 mg/kg followed by 0.03–0.15 mg/kg every 1–2 h	
	Neuromuscular blockade as adjunct to general anesthesia with succinylcholine	*Adult and child >10 y:* IV, 40–60 μg/kg under inhalation anesthesia, or 50–60 μg/kg under balanced anesthesia *Child 1–10 y:* IV, Individualized; may need slightly more than adult dose *Infant 7 wk–12 mo:* Individualized *Neonate:* Safe and effective dose not established.	

(continued)

TABLE 15.7 Summary of Selected C Neuromuscular Blocking Agents (continued)

Drug (Trade) Name	Selected Indications	Route and Dosage Range	Pharmacokinetics
Depolarizing Neuromuscular Junction Blockers			
P succinylcholine (Anectine, Quelicin)	Endotracheal intubation	*Adult:* IV, 0.3–1.1 mg/kg; IM, 3–4 mg/kg *Adolescent and older child:* IV, 1 mg/kg; IM, 3–4 mg/kg *Small child and infant:* IV, 2 mg/kg; IM, 3–4 mg/kg	*Onset IV:* 30–60 sec *Onset IM:* 2–3 min *Duration IV:* 4–6 min *Duration IM:* 10–20 min $t_{1/2}$: *Unknown*
	Neuromuscular blockade (short procedures)	*Adult:* IV, 0.3–1.1 mg/kg over 10–30 sec *Adult, child, and infant:* IM, 3–4 mg/kg	
	Neuromuscular blockade (long procedures)	*Adult:* IV, 0.3–1.1 mg/kg followed by 0.04–0.07 mg/kg as needed *Child and infant:* Not recommended	
	Electroconvulsive therapy	*Adult:* IV, 10–30 mg 1 min before ECT: IM, 3–4 mg/kg, not to exceed 150 mg	

Pharmacodynamics

Tubocurarine is found in certain plants in the Amazon rain forest. It is a component of the paralytic agent curare, which is extracted from these plants. Tubocurarine and other NMJ blockers are antagonists of acetylcholine; they compete with the neurotransmitter for the cholinergic receptor sites at the motor end plate. This antagonism causes a decrease in the response of the muscle to acetylcholine, resulting in a flaccid or relaxed paralysis. Tubocurarine does not cross the blood–brain barrier and has no action on the CNS. For this reason, anesthesia is induced before neuromuscular blockade is started; otherwise, the unanesthetized patient would have the frightening experience of paralysis and the inability to breathe.

It is also important to remember that NMJ blockers do not affect consciousness or alter sensation; therefore, benzodiazepines and analgesics are administered concurrently to manage fear, anxiety, and pain, especially when NMJ blockers are used to facilitate mechanical ventilation in the ICU or other critical care units.

The neuromuscular blocking actions of tubocurarine may be reversed with anticholinesterases such as neostigmine, pyridostigmine, and edrophonium. These drugs block the normal breakdown of acetylcholine at the motor end plate, causing the neurotransmitter to accumulate and returning muscle stimulation.

Contraindications and Precautions

Tubocurarine is contraindicated in patients who have ever shown hypersensitivity to the drug or to any other nondepolarizing blocker. It is classified as a pregnancy category C drug, and it is contraindicated for use in early pregnancy because it can cause congenital fetal fractures.

Tubocurarine is used with caution in patients who have pre-existing pulmonary disease or lung cancer. Neuromuscular blockade may be enhanced in these patients. Patients with asthma, bronchospasm, hypotension, and cardiac disease may be affected by the histamine release and vasodilation effects of tubocurarine, which may exacerbate these conditions. Tubocurarine is also used with caution in patients with dehydration, electrolyte imbalance, or an acid-base imbalance because these disorders may alter its affects. In patients with hypothermia, the action or duration of tubocurarine may be decreased.

Tubocurarine should be used with extreme caution in patients with decreased renal function because the drug is excreted unchanged primarily by the kidneys. Tubocurarine should be used with caution in patients with myasthenia gravis, unless it is being used as a diagnostic aid.

Adverse Effects

The principal adverse effects of tubocurarine result from its blockade of neuromuscular activity at all neuromuscular end plates. Prolonged paralysis can cause immobility that leads to pressure sores (decubitus ulcer formation). Prolonged apnea can result from the paralysis of the respiratory muscles. Therefore, assisted ventilation is needed until the drug's effects resolve or anticholinesterase administration is successful.

Neuromuscular blockade of the GI tract can result in decreased GI tone and mobility and may render the patient more prone to regurgitation, vomiting, and aspiration. Relaxation of arterial muscles results in vasodilation, which can promote flushing, hypotension, slow or rapid heart rate, or worsening of pre-existing heart problems.

Histamine release associated with the NMJ blockers may result in respiratory difficulty, including wheezing and bronchospasm. Additionally, the release of histamine

causes dilation of peripheral vessels, increased secretions, and anticoagulation that may in turn cause hypotension. Occasionally, patients may respond to their first exposure to tubocurarine or other NMJ blockers with an extreme hypersensitivity reaction or even malignant hyperthermia, which is characterized by massive muscle contraction, sharply elevated body temperature, severe acidosis, and if the reaction is uncontrolled, death.

Drug Interactions

Drugs that may decrease the effectiveness of tubocurarine include carbamazepine and the hydantoins and theophyllines. Drugs that potentiate the action of tubocurarine include antibiotics, inhalation anesthetics, ketamine, magnesium salts, quinine derivatives, thiopurines, trimethaphan, and verapamil. Table 15.8 discusses these potential drug interactions.

Assessment of Relevant Core Patient Variables

Health Status

Evaluate the patient for a history of hypersensitivity to any NMJ blocker or for any renal, hepatic, cardiovascular, or respiratory diseases. Place a note on the chart and the drug administration record (Kardex) identifying the need to monitor patients with a history of any of these disorders closely.

Before administration, perform a physical assessment. The physical examination should include body weight, temperature, state of hydration (skin turgor, pulses), reflexes and muscle tone, pulse, blood pressure, respiratory rate, and adventitious breath sounds. Assess laboratory tests to establish baseline electrolyte values and renal and hepatic status.

TABLE 15.8 Agents That Interact With P Tubocurarine

Interactants	Effect and Significance	Nursing Management
antibiotics aminoglycosides lincosamide polypeptides tetracycline	Potentiate the action of tubocurarine, resulting in profound and severe respiratory depression	Avoid combination. Provide life support as needed. Provide anticholinesterases as indicated.
anticonvulsants carbamazepine hydantoins	In combination, may decrease the duration or efficacy of tubocurarine	Monitor for decreased muscle relaxant effectiveness. Titrate drug as necessary.
inhalation anesthetics	Potentiate the actions of tubocurarine	Monitor respiratory function. Titrate drug as necessary. Provide life support as needed.
ketamine	May enhance the actions of tubocurarine, resulting in profound and severe respiratory depression	Monitor respiratory function. Titrate drug as necessary. Provide life support as needed.
magnesium salts	May enhance the actions of tubocurarine, resulting in profound and severe respiratory depression	Monitor respiratory function. Titrate drug as necessary. Provide life support as needed.
opioids	May enhance hypotensive effects of tubocurarine	Monitor BP. Titrate as necessary. Provide life support as needed.
quinine derivatives	Have a synergistic action with tubocurarine, resulting in profound and severe respiratory depression	Monitor neuromuscular function. Titrate drug as necessary. Provide life support as needed.
theophyllines	May antagonize the activity of tubocurarine	Monitor for efficacy of tubocurarine. Increase dose of tubocurarine if needed.
thiopurines	May inhibit phosphodiesterase, resulting in an anticurare action; may decrease the activity of tubocurarine	Monitor for efficacy of tubocurarine. Increase dose of tubocurarine if needed.
trimethaphan	Augments the neuromuscular blockade of tubocurarine, resulting in prolonged apnea	Avoid combination if possible. Monitor respiratory function. Titrate drug as necessary. Provide life support as needed.
verapamil	May enhance the action of tubocurarine because of its blockage of calcium channels in skeletal muscle	Avoid combination if possible. Monitor respiratory function. Titrate drug as necessary. Provide life support as needed.

Life Span and Gender

Assess women of childbearing age for pregnancy. Tubocurarine is contraindicated in early pregnancy because of its potential for teratogenic effects. However, it can be used safely as an adjunct to anesthesia in cesarean deliveries. After birth, closely observe the infant for any signs of respiratory depression because the drug crosses the placenta.

Environment

Be aware of the environment in which the drug will be administered. Like all neuromuscular blocking agents, tubocurarine causes respiratory impairment and paralysis. It should be administered only by a person skilled in administering NMJ blockers. Necessary equipment for intubation, controlled ventilation, and administration of oxygen must be immediately available.

Nursing Diagnoses and Outcomes

- Impaired Spontaneous Ventilation related to respiratory paralysis
  Desired outcome: *The patient will be maintained with artificial ventilation until the ability to sustain spontaneous respirations returns.*
- Impaired Skin Integrity related to paralysis
  Desired outcome: *The patient will remain free of skin breakdown.*
- Fear related to paralysis and helplessness
  Desired outcome: *The patient will be reassured and comforted to prevent fear and sympathetic effects of fear during paralysis.*

Planning and Intervention

Maximizing Therapeutic Effects

You can maximize the therapeutic effects of tubocurarine by helping patients understand the reason for the therapy and by helping to decrease their fear and anxiety. Monitor the patient carefully for pain or distress; responses of the pupils, blood pressure, and heart rate, although not foolproof, are probably the most reliable guide to the patient's condition. Also, frequently reassure the patient that the staff is aware of the patient's feeling of helplessness. The hearing of these patients is not impaired; therefore, procedures and interventions should be explained.

Minimizing Adverse Effects

Have resuscitation equipment and drugs at the bedside throughout therapy. Evaluate the depth of paralysis by use of a stimulator and use cholinesterase inhibitors to overcome excessive or prolonged neuromuscular blockade.

If paralysis is prolonged, change the patient's position frequently to prevent venous stasis or decubitus ulcer formation and provide frequent skin care to prevent skin breakdown.

Providing Patient and Family Education

- Before administration, explain to the patient and family that the drug will paralyze muscles and the patient will be unable to speak, move, or breathe unassisted. It is important to explain that these effects should subside a short time after the drug is discontinued.
- Advise the patient that adverse effects may occur after administration. These effects include sore muscles, constipation, difficulty voiding, and dizziness on arising. Explain to the patient the importance of reporting these symptoms to avoid potential injury.

Ongoing Assessment and Evaluation

Monitor the respiratory and cardiac status of the patient every 15 minutes while tubocurarine is administered. For patients with prolonged paralysis, monitor skin status frequently. Conscious patients should be monitored for any sign of distress, which is especially important because they are unable to talk or move. Keep in mind, however, that patients can still hear. For patients with prolonged paralysis, turn the patient every 2 hours and monitor for skin breakdown. Provide protection to the corneas by taping eye pads in place and by using artificial tears. Continue use of benzodiazepines and analgesic agents to provide a calm environment for these patients.

Drugs Closely Related to [P] Tubocurarine

Atracurium Besylate

Atracurium (Tracrium) is an intermediate-acting NMJ blocking agent used as an aid to tracheal intubation and as an adjunct to general anesthesia during surgery or mechanical ventilation to provide skeletal muscle relaxation. Atracurium is metabolized in plasma by ester hydrolysis and by a chemical reaction called Hofmann elimination. It is used frequently in patients with multisystem failure because its metabolism is independent of hepatic or renal function. Atracurium produces less histamine release than tubocurarine does, and recovery is more rapid with atracurium than with tubocurarine or pancuronium. Histamine release may occur if doses exceed 0.6 mg/kg or if atracurium precipitates in the syringe or vein. Precipitation can occur if atracurium is injected immediately after thiopentone. Atracurium is used with caution in patients with respiratory diseases because of its potential for histamine release. Although it is a pregnancy category

MEMORY CHIP

[P] Tubocurarine

- A nondepolarizing neuromuscular junction blocking agent used to facilitate endotracheal intubation and mechanical ventilation
- Used in critical care patients to conserve energy and prevent agitation
- Major contraindications: hypersensitivity, early pregnancy
- Most common adverse effects: flushing, hypotension
- Most serious adverse effects: prolonged paralysis, apnea, malignant hyperthermia
- Maximizing therapeutic effects: Decrease anxiety and fear.
- Minimizing adverse effects: Have resuscitation equipment and cholinesterase inhibitor antidote at the bedside.
- Most important patient education: Reassure the patient that he or she is being constantly monitored.

C drug, it is widely used in obstetrics because placental transfer is minimal. Drug–drug interactions are similar to those for tubocurarine.

Cisatracurium Besylate

Cisatracurium (Nimbex) is another intermediate-acting NMJ blocking agent. It is one of several isomers of atracurium and is three times as potent as atracurium. Its metabolism is similar to that of atracurium; thus, it is useful in patients with multisystem failure. Unlike atracurium, cisatracurium does not cause dose-related increases in histamine release. For this reason, cisatracurium can be used safely in patients with cardiovascular disease. Clinical uses include skeletal muscle relaxation, facilitation of tracheal intubation in combination with general anesthesia, and skeletal muscle relaxation in ICU patients who require mechanical ventilation. Cisatracurium interacts with lactated Ringer's solution, propofol, and ketorolac injection.

Doxacurium

Doxacurium (Nuromax) is a long-acting NMJ blocking agent used to cause skeletal muscle relaxation as an adjunct in general anesthesia, endotracheal intubation, or in facilitating mechanical ventilation. Doxacurium is 2.5 to 3 times more potent than pancuronium, another long-acting nondepolarizing agent. Doxacurium lacks substantial histamine-releasing properties and is not metabolized by plasma cholinesterase. It is frequently used for long surgical procedures, especially in patients with cardiovascular disorders, because of its extended duration of action and minimal cardiovascular effects. Doxacurium is a pregnancy category C drug and may be used in children older than 2 years.

Mivacurium

Mivacurium (Mivacron) is a short-acting, nondepolarizing NMJ blocking agent used to cause skeletal muscle relaxation as an adjunct to general anesthesia or for endotracheal intubation. Its onset of action is similar to that of atracurium, but it has a shorter duration of action. Like succinylcholine, mivacurium is metabolized by plasma cholinesterase; therefore, patients with pseudocholinesterase deficiency may experience a prolonged duration of action. (Succinylcholine, the prototype depolarizing blocker, is discussed in the next section.) Unlike tubocurarine or pancuronium, it does not affect cardiac muscarinic receptors, which minimizes the risk for tachycardia and hypotension. However, mivacurium does have the potential for substantial histamine release with its attendant risk for hypotension and bronchospasm. At recommended doses, mivacurium has no clinically important hemodynamic effects. Drug–drug interactions are similar to those for tubocurarine.

Pancuronium Bromide

Pancuronium bromide (Pavulon) is another IV nondepolarizing NMJ blocking agent. Although similar to tubocurarine, it is five times as potent. Pancuronium is used to induce relaxation of the skeletal muscles during surgery, to facilitate pulmonary compliance during mechanical ventilation, and to treat agitation in patients in intensive care.

Pancuronium is contraindicated for use in neonates. Some preparations of pancuronium contain benzyl alcohol as a preservative, which has been associated with "gasping syndrome," a fatal toxic reaction. One major difference between pancuronium and tubocurarine is that pancuronium produces little histamine release and no ganglionic blockade. For this reason, hypotension and bronchospasm are not associated with its use.

Pipecuronium

Pipecuronium (Arduan) is a parenteral, long-acting, nondepolarizing neuromuscular blocker. Like other NMJ blockers, it is used as an adjunct to general anesthesia or for endotracheal intubation. Because of its long action, it should be used only for procedures expected to last more than 90 minutes.

Rocuronium

Rocuronium (Zemuron) is a short-acting NMJ blocking agent that was developed out of a need for an agent with rapid onset, short duration of action, and low risk for side effects. Its onset of action is comparable to that of succinylcholine, but its duration of action is considerably longer. Because of its rapid onset, rocuronium may be a useful alternative to succinylcholine for rapid-sequence induction. In addition to its therapeutic actions, rocuronium can cause an increase in heart rate, but this side effect is minimal at normal doses. Rocuronium produces little histamine release and no ganglionic blockade; thus, hypotension and bronchospasm are not associated with its use. Children generally require larger doses per kilogram than adults do to achieve muscle relaxation.

Vecuronium

Vecuronium bromide (Norcuron) is a short-acting, IV, nondepolarizing neuromuscular blocking agent. Vecuronium is more potent than pancuronium, but the blockade produced is short-lived in comparison with other NMJ blockers. The advantage of vecuronium is that it is the least active histamine releaser of the NMJ blockers and has minimal effect on cardiovascular function.

(C) Depolarizing Neuromuscular Junction Blockers

Depolarizing NMJ blockers work by causing the muscle cell membrane to depolarize or become excited, which causes muscle contraction. This action leads to paralysis of the muscle after repeated excitation. This mechanism differs from that of nondepolarizing NMJ blockers, which prevent excitation. Succinylcholine (Anectine) is the prototype depolarizing NMJ blocker.

NURSING MANAGEMENT OF THE PATIENT RECEIVING [P] SUCCINYLCHOLINE

Core Drug Knowledge

Pharmacotherapeutics

Succinylcholine is used primarily for rapid endotracheal intubation and endoscopic procedures. It is also of value in modifying muscle contractions and preventing fractures during electroconvulsive therapy because it produces a complete neuromuscular blockade within 1 minute that lasts for a few minutes, allowing sufficient time to complete the ther-

apy. The use of succinylcholine as an adjunct to anesthesia or to facilitate prolonged mechanical ventilation has been largely replaced by the use of more effective and less toxic NMJ blockers.

Pharmacokinetics

Succinylcholine is administered intravenously and intramuscularly. It has a rapid onset and a short duration of action. Following IV administration, complete muscle relaxation occurs in 30 seconds to 1 minute, lasts for 2 to 3 minutes, and then dissipates within 10 minutes. After IM injection, muscle relaxation occurs in 2 to 3 minutes and lasts 10 to 30 minutes.

Succinylcholine is distributed in the extracellular fluid but does not readily cross the placental barrier. Succinylcholine has a complex excretion pattern. Approximately 10% of the dose is excreted unchanged in the urine. Succinylcholine is mostly hydrolyzed by plasma pseudocholinesterase to metabolites. One of the metabolites, succinylmonocholine, has nondepolarizing muscle relaxation properties. It, in turn, is excreted partly in urine, and the remainder is broken down into inactive metabolites. Succinylmonocholine is hydrolyzed slowly. If accumulation occurs, as it does with hepatic dysfunction, prolonged muscle relaxation may cause apnea.

Pharmacodynamics

Succinylcholine acts as an agonist at the cholinergic nicotinic receptors of the motor end plate. Like the usual neurotransmitter acetylcholine, it depolarizes the postsynaptic membrane, producing repetitive excitation of the motor end plate. Muscular fasciculations (rapid contractions) result, followed by flaccid paralysis. Because of this effect, patients often experience postoperative muscle pain. The ensuing paralysis is short lived because the succinylcholine is hydrolyzed by plasma pseudocholinesterase.

Contraindications and Precautions

Succinylcholine is contraindicated in any patient with a known hypersensitivity to the drug. Because it can induce malignant hyperthermia, it is also contraindicated in anyone with a personal or family history of the disorder. Because succinylcholine may interact with acetylcholine to produce prolonged apnea, it is contraindicated in patients with familial plasma pseudocholinesterase disorders. Succinylcholine is also contraindicated in patients with an open eye injury or acute narrow-angle glaucoma because it causes a transient elevation in intraocular pressure immediately after injection.

Succinylcholine should be used with caution in patients prone to low pseudocholinesterase levels. Decreased concentrations of serum pseudocholinesterase, the major enzyme that degrades succinylcholine, can lead to very high levels of the drug and prolonged action.

Succinylcholine should also be used with caution in patients who have or are at risk for hyperkalemia. Intense muscle contraction and potassium release from succinylcholine may induce hyperkalemia and provoke complications of hyperkalemia, such as cardiac arrhythmias. Caution is advised especially with children and adults who have compromised cardiac function, degenerative or dystrophic neuromuscular disease, or paraplegia. These patients tend to become severely hyperkalemic when succinylcholine is administered.

Adverse Effects

The principal adverse effects of succinylcholine are associated with muscle paralysis caused by the drug. Prolonged apnea can result from the paralysis of the respiratory muscles, and assisted ventilation is needed until the drug's effects are known. Increased intraocular pressure can aggravate or precipitate glaucoma, and the immobility caused by prolonged paralysis can result in the formation of decubitus ulcers.

A mild histamine release associated with succinylcholine may result in respiratory difficulty, including wheezing and bronchospasm, cardiac arrhythmias, hypotension, and even cardiac arrest in susceptible patients. Malignant hyperthermia has been reported infrequently. Other metabolic effects include hyperkalemia, with its resultant muscular and cardiac effects, and myoglobinemia and myoglobinuria, which are associated with extreme muscle contraction. Patients may complain of intense muscle pain that may persist for several days after they have received the drug.

Drug Interactions

Succinylcholine interacts with aminoglycosides, anticholinesterases, procaine, and trimethaphan (Table 15.9). It also interacts with drugs that decrease plasma cholinesterase, such as cyclophosphamide, echothiophate, lidocaine infusion, metoclopramide, and quinine derivatives.

Assessment of Relevant Core Patient Variables

Health Status

Assess the patient's personal or family history for low pseudocholinesterase levels. Patients at risk for low pseudocholinesterase levels include those with severe burns, malnutrition, dehydration, severe hepatic disease, cancer, severe anemia, or myxedema. Also, assess for a history of slow recovery from anesthesia or difficulty during anesthesia.

Before administering succinylcholine, perform a physical assessment. The physical examination should include body weight and temperature, state of hydration (skin turgor, pulses), reflexes and muscle tone, pulse rate, blood pressure, respiratory rate, and adventitious breath sounds.

Life Span and Gender

Document the age and gender of the patient and assesses women of childbearing age for pregnancy. Succinylcholine is used cautiously in children because it can cause severe bradycardia or cardiac arrest. The drug is in pregnancy category C. Although it is uncertain whether it causes fetal harm, it should be used cautiously during pregnancy because the drug places the patient at risk for increased drug effects, such as prolonged apnea. Succinylcholine is commonly used during cesarean section. If repeated dosing is required during delivery, the neonate should be monitored closely for apnea and flaccidity.

Environment

Be aware of the environment in which the drug will be administered. Like tubocurarine, succinylcholine causes respiratory impairment and paralysis. It should be administered

TABLE 15.9 Agents That Interact With P Succinylcholine

Interactants	Effect and Significance	Nursing Management
aminoglycosides	Potentiate neuromuscular effects of succinylcholine	Use combination with caution. Delay administration of aminoglycosides as long as possible after recovery of spontaneous respirations. Monitor for respiratory depression. Have mechanical ventilation available.
anticholinesterases	Inhibition of plasma cholinesterase by anticholinesterases may delay hydrolysis of succinylcholine	Use this combination with caution. Monitor patients' spontaneous muscle activity, which must continue for 5 minutes before longer acting agents are administered.
plasma cholinesterase inhibitors cyclophosphamide echothiophate lidocaine infusion metoclopramide quinine derivatives oral contraceptives	Plasma cholinesterase (pseudocholinesterase) necessary to hydrolyze succinylcholine; decreased plasma cholinesterase interferes with the inactivation of succinylcholine, may prolong neuromuscular blockade	Measure serum cholinesterase levels for patients who have been receiving drugs that inhibit plasma cholinesterase. Reduce succinylcholine dosage if plasma cholinesterase levels are decreased. Monitor for respiratory depression. Have mechanical ventilation available.
procaine	Procaine and succinylcholine both hydrolyzed by plasma cholinesterase; competition for the enzyme possibly resulting in prolonged effects of succinylcholine	Monitor for respiratory depression. Have mechanical ventilation available.
trimethaphan	Potent noncompetitive inhibitor of plasma cholinesterase; directly decreases the sensitivity of the respiratory center, increasing risk for respiratory depression	Avoid this combination. Substitute nitroprusside for trimethaphan.

only by a qualified clinician. Necessary equipment for intubation, controlled ventilation, and administration of oxygen must be immediately available.

Nursing Diagnoses and Outcomes

- Impaired Spontaneous Ventilation related to respiratory paralysis
  Desired outcome: *The patient's breathing will be maintained with artificial ventilation until the ability to sustain spontaneous respiration returns.*
- Impaired Physical Mobility related to drug-induced paralysis
  Desired outcome: *The patient will remain free from disorders related to immobility, such as skin breakdown.*
- Fear related to paralysis and helplessness
  Desired outcome: *The patient will be reassured and comforted to prevent fear and sympathetic effects of fear during paralysis.*

Planning and Intervention

Maximizing Therapeutic Effects

You can maximize the therapeutic effects of succinylcholine by helping the patient understand the rationale for the therapy and by helping to decrease fear and anxiety.

Minimizing Adverse Effects

To decrease muscle fasciculations, the patient should receive a small dose of a nondepolarizing NMJ blocker before succinylcholine is given. This step is especially important when succinylcholine is used in children.

Providing Patient and Family Education

- Before administration, explain to the patient and family that the drug will paralyze muscles and the patient will be unable to speak, move, or breathe unassisted. It is important to explain that these effects should subside soon after the drug is discontinued.
- Because this drug may be used in an emergency situation, explain the effects of the drug to the patient even if he or she appears to be unconscious.

Ongoing Assessment and Evaluation

Monitor for symptoms of malignant hyperthermia, such as muscle rigidity (especially the jaw), tachycardia, tachypnea, and elevated body temperature. Dantrolene should be on standby in case malignant hyperthermia occurs. Also, monitor the cardiac and respiratory status of the patient while succinylcholine is being administered.

MEMORY CHIP

P Succinylcholine

- A depolarizing neuromuscular junction blocking agent used to facilitate endotracheal intubation and short procedures such as endoscopy or electroconvulsive therapy
- Major contraindications: hypersensitivity, history of malignant hyperthermia, familial plasma pseudocholinesterase disorders, and narrow-angle glaucoma
- Most common adverse effects: increased ocular pressure, histamine release, muscle pain
- Most serious adverse effects: prolonged paralysis and apnea
- Maximizing therapeutic effects: Decrease anxiety and fear.
- Minimizing adverse effects: Have resuscitation equipment at the bedside.
- Most important patient education: Reassure the patient that he or she is being constantly monitored.

CHAPTER SUMMARY

- Anesthesia is a loss of feeling or sensation.
- Balanced anesthesia is a combination of anesthetic agents used to decrease the depth of anesthesia and keep the patient safe.
- Anesthetic agents are divided into inhaled and intravenous agents.
- Isoflurane (Forane) is a halogenated inhaled anesthetic. Nursing management of patients recovering from isoflurane anesthesia includes carefully monitoring residual CNS depression, manifested as respiratory depression.
- Nitrous oxide is an inflammable gas used to increase the effectiveness of halogenated agents without severely depressing the depth of coma.
- Propofol (Diprivan) is the prototype intravenous anesthetic. It has a quick onset and short duration of action.
- Neuroleptic drugs, such as propofol and narcotic opiates, are used in combination with nitrous oxide to effect a state of consciousness called neuroleptanesthesia.
- Ketamine (Ketalar) causes dissociative anesthesia. It is generally not used in adults because of its psychological adverse effects.
- Local anesthetics such as lidocaine produce local or regional anesthesia by blocking nerve conduction. They are used to facilitate various types of procedures.
- Nondepolarizing NMJ blockers, such as tubocurarine, prevent nerve impulses from exciting muscle; paralysis ensues because the muscle is unable to respond.
- Depolarizing NMJ blockers, such as succinylcholine, cause muscle paralysis by overexcitement (depolarization) and subsequent exhaustion of the muscle.
- The NMJ blockers are primarily used as adjuncts to general anesthesia, to facilitate endotracheal intubation, or to facilitate mechanical ventilation.

QUESTIONS FOR STUDY AND REVIEW

1. What is balanced anesthesia?
2. What environmental safeguards are needed for patients receiving anesthesia?
3. Propofol is administered in a special emulsion vehicle. What problems does this vehicle pose?
4. What unusual adverse effect may occur with high-dose or long-term propofol administration?
5. Describe the potential systemic adverse effects of locally administered lidocaine (Xylocaine).
6. What is the difference in the mechanism of action between non-depolarizing NMJ blockers and depolarizing NMJ blockers?
7. Mrs. Smith has just returned to the intensive care unit after surgery. She is being maintained on pancuronium bromide. The charge nurse comes into the room and starts to discuss Mrs. Smith's prognosis. What should you do?
8. Your patient is scheduled to receive succinylcholine for a surgical procedure. What teaching points would you need to include in a plan for this patient to prepare him or her for the postoperative experience?

Need More Help?

Chapter 15 of the study guide for *Drug Therapy in Nursing* 2e contains NCLEX-style questions and other learning activities to reinforce your understanding of the concepts presented in this chapter. For additional information or to purchase the study guide, visit *http://connection.lww.com/go/aschenbrenner.*

REFERENCES AND BIBLIOGRAPHY

Clinical Pharmacology [Online]. Available: *http://cp.gsm.com*. Accessed August 2004.

Facts and Comparisons. (2004). *Drug facts and comparisons.* Philadelphia: Lippincott Williams & Wilkins.

Elcock, D. H., & Sweeney, B. P. (2002). Sevoflurane vs. isoflurane: A clinical comparison in day surgery. *Anaesthesia, 57*(1), 52–56.

Gupta A., Stierer, T., Zuckerman, R., et al. (2004). Comparison of recovery profile after ambulatory anesthesia with propofol, isoflurane, sevoflurane and desflurane: A systematic review. *Anesthesia and Analgesia, 98*(3), 632–641.

Hardman, J. G. (2001). *Goodman & Gilman's the pharmacological basis of therapeutics* (10th ed.). New York: McGraw-Hill Health Professions Division.

Hogarth, D. K., & Hall, J. (2004). Management of sedation in mechanically ventilated patients. *Current Opinion in Critical Care, 10*(1), 40–46.

Katzung, B. (2004). *Basic and clinical pharmacology* (9th ed.). New York: McGraw-Hill/Appleton & Lange.

Micromedex Healthcare Series [Online]. Available: *http://healthcare.micromedex.com*. Accessed August 2004.

Meistelman, C. (2003). Effect sites of neuromuscular blocking agents and the monitoring of clinical muscle relaxation. *Advanced Experiments in Medical Biology, 523,* 227–238.

Niermeijer, J. M., Uiterwaal, C. S., & Van Donselaar, C. A. (2003). Propofol in status epilepticus: Little evidence, many dangers? *Journal of Neurology, 250*(10), 1237–1240.

Tatro, D. S. (2004). *Drug interaction facts.* Philadelphia: Lippincott Williams & Wilkins.

Drugs Relieving Anxiety and Producing Sleep

chapter 16

Learning Objectives

At the completion of this chapter the student will:

1. Describe the varied therapeutic uses of benzodiazepines.
2. Identify core drug knowledge about drugs that relieve anxiety and promote sleep.
3. Identify core patient variables related to drugs that relieve anxiety and promote sleep.
4. Relate the interaction of core drug knowledge to core patient variables for drugs that relieve anxiety and promote sleep.
5. Generate a nursing plan of care from the interactions between core drug knowledge and core patient variables for drugs that relieve anxiety and promote sleep.
6. Describe nursing interventions to maximize therapeutic and minimize adverse effects for drugs that relieve anxiety and promote sleep.
7. Determine key points for patient and family education for drugs that relieve anxiety and promote sleep.

KEY TERMS

anxiety

anxiolytics

GABA

insomnia

NREM

REM

FEATURED WEBLINK

http://www.nimh.nih.gov/publicat/anxiety.cfm

The National Institute of Mental Health (NIMH) Anxiety Disorders website provides information about the various anxiety disorders, the role of research in understanding and treating anxiety disorders, various treatments for anxiety disorders, how to get help for an anxiety disorder, strategies to make treatment more effective, and information about relevant clinical trials. For more information, check the home page of the NIMH website.

CONNECTION WEBLINK

Additional Weblinks are found on Connection:
http://www.connection.lww.com/go/aschenbrenner.

Drugs Relieving Anxiety and Producing Sleep

RELIEVING ANXIETY

(C) Benzodiazepines

(P) lorazepam

Benzodiazepines for anxiety
- alprazolam
- chlordiazepoxide
- clorazepate
- diazepam
- halazepam
- oxazepam

Nonbenzodiazepines for anxiety
- buspirone
- hydroxyzine
- meprobamate
- selective serotonin reuptake inhibitors
- tricyclic antidepressants

PRODUCING SLEEP

(C) Benzodiazepines

(P) lorazepam

Benzodiazepines for sleep
- estazolam
- flurazepam
- quazepam
- temazepam
- triazolam

Nonbenzodiazepines for sleep
- barbiturates
- chloral hydrate
- paraldehyde
- zolpidem

The symbol (C) indicates the **drug class.**
Drugs in **bold type** marked with the symbol (P) are prototypes.
Drugs in blue type are closely related to the prototype.
Drugs in red type are significantly different from the prototype.
Drugs in black type with no symbol are also used in drug therapy; no prototype

Depression of the central nervous system (CNS) can cause a variety of effects. Sometimes, depression of the CNS system is thought of as a continuum of effects ranging from relieving anxiety and producing relaxation to producing anesthesia and loss of consciousness. Some drugs that depress the CNS, such as the benzodiazepines, can produce multiple effects depending on the dose and the route of administration. Two of those effects, relieving anxiety and promoting sleep, are discussed in this chapter. Benzodiazepines used in seizure disorders are presented in Chapter 19, and those used as muscle relaxants are mentioned in Chapter 20.

The prototype benzodiazepine for this chapter is lorazepam (Ativan). Lorazepam is primarily used to treat anxiety, although it may also be used to promote sleep and rest. Other benzodiazepines in the class that are primarily used for anxiety include alprazolam (Xanax), chlordiazepoxide (Librium), clorazepate (Tranxene), diazepam (Valium), halazepam (Paxipam), and oxazepam (Serax). Benzodiazepines represented by the prototype but primarily used to treat insomnia are estazolam (ProSom), flurazepam (Dalmane), temazepam (Restoril), triazolam (Halcion), and quazepam (Doral).

This chapter also discusses drugs outside the benzodiazepine class that are used to relieve anxiety or induce sleep. Drugs significantly different from the prototype that are used to treat anxiety are the selective serotonin reuptake inhibitors, the tricyclic antidepressants, and the drugs buspirone (BuSpar), hydroxyzine (Vistaril), and meprobamate (Equanil). Nonbenzodiazepine drugs used to treat insomnia are zolpidem (Ambien), chloral hydrate, paraldehyde, and barbiturates.

PHYSIOLOGY

Emotions and Neurotransmitters

Human emotions, although universal, are not well understood. The limbic system in the brain is known to be primarily responsible for emotions, but why a particular situation might create a severe emotional response in one individual but not in another individual is still unknown. Much of the research that has been done on the emotions of fear and anxiety has centered on the amygdala, an almond-shaped structure, and on the hippocampus, both located within the brain. The amygdala receives incoming sensory signals and then communicates with the frontal lobes of the brain where information is interpreted. The amygdala can signal the brain that a threat is present and set off a fear response or anxiety. When a stimulus is interpreted as highly threatening, the amygdala floods the brain with danger messages, demanding immediate action and not allowing time for the rest of the brain to process the information with rational and systematic thought.

For example, if your eyes saw that you were in the pathway of a falling tree, your cerebral cortex of the brain would interpret the sight, compare it to known past experiences, determine that the tree will hit you if you do not move out of the way, and send messages to various body systems to respond. In this case, the heart will beat faster to provide more blood supply to the muscles, and the muscles will contract to run. However, the amygdala determines that the tree is extremely dangerous to the body's well-being and demands that the body respond and *run now,* think later.

Another part of the brain, the hippocampus, is responsible for processing threatening or traumatic stimuli. The hippocampus helps encode information into memories. To continue with the above example, the next time you encounter a stimulus similar to the falling tree (such as the cracking noise the tree made before it began to fall), the hippocampus will remember this traumatic stimulus and send the message to the amygdala, which will then sense immediate danger and flood the brain with messages to flee for safety.

The brain sends its messages to the body by way of the nervous system. Various neurotransmitters assist in moving messages along the nervous system. Some of those neurotransmitters stimulate the nerve to respond and some of them inhibit response from the nervous system. One of those inhibitory neurotransmitters is gamma-aminobutyric acid, better known as **GABA.** The inhibitory action of GABA works in opposition to the excitatory neurotransmitter glutamate. GABA is released into the synapse, crosses the synapse, and then attaches to a postsynaptic receptor site. Once it is attached, an influx of negatively charged chloride ions enters the postsynaptic neuron. Hyperpolarization of the cell occurs and prevents the cell from functioning.

Figure 16.1 depicts the action of GABA on the cell's receptors.

Sleep

Sleep is a time of bodily rest, although the brain remains active. Sleep usually occurs once every 24 hours, on a circadian rhythm, and lasts several hours. Throughout the remaining 24 hours, the person is awake. However, many people have a long period of sleep at night and a short nap in the afternoon. While the eyes are closed during sleep, periodic rapid eye movements can be observed. Sleep, therefore, has two stages; the first has no rapid eye movements (**NREM**), and the second has rapid eye movements (**REM**). NREM sleep is divided into four stages:

- Stage 1—light sleep; muscles relax; brain waves are irregular and rapid.
- Stage 2—brain waves are larger than in stage 1 with bursts of electrical activity.
- Stages 3 and 4—deep sleep occurs, with even larger, slower brain waves called delta waves; this stage is often referred to as slow-wave sleep.

After stage 4 sleep, the body begins REM sleep. During REM sleep, brain waves are almost the same as they are during waking hours. Dreaming occurs during REM sleep. The body becomes essentially paralyzed during REM sleep, so that it cannot act out the dreams. After a period of REM sleep, the person will cycle through the NREM stages before again returning to REM sleep. The pattern is repeated about four to five times during the night. Arousal from sleep is fairly easy when in REM, but can be difficult from NREM. A person awakened from NREM sleep may be confused and disoriented until completely awake, a process that can take up to 5 minutes. Approximately 75% of sleep time is non-REM sleep, and 25% is REM sleep. REM periods generally become longer and more frequent during the later part of the sleep cycle.

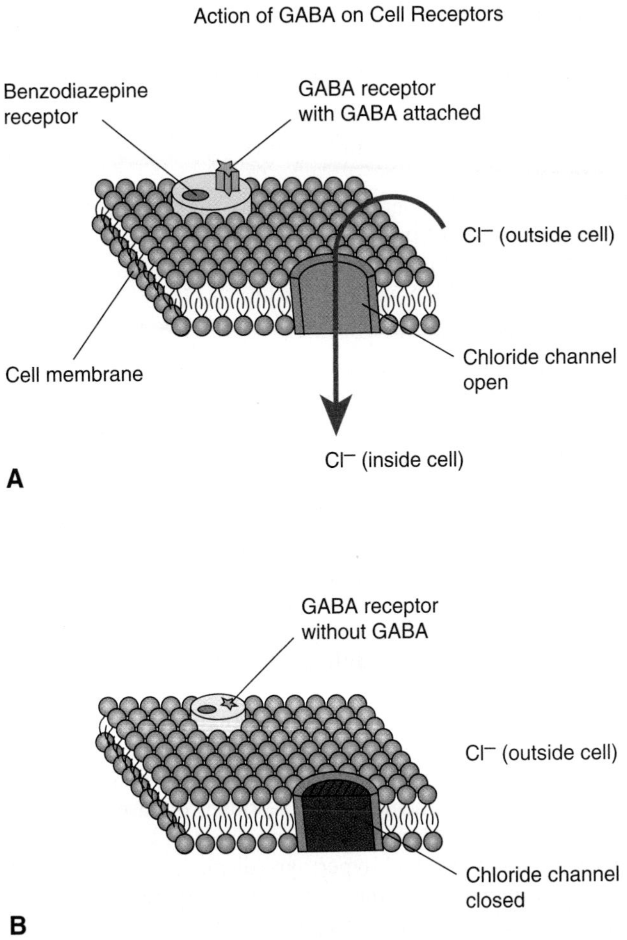

FIGURE 16.1 (**A**) When GABA attaches to the cell's receptors, it causes the chloride channel to open. The rush of chloride ions gives the inside of the cell a highly negative charge, which decreases the cell's ability to fire. GABA has an inhibitory action on the nervous system and has receptor sites on the cells. Benzodiazepines can occupy these receptor sites. When the receptor is occupied, it keeps the chloride channel open longer, thereby potentiating GABA's inhibitory effect. (**B**) When GABA is not attached to a receptor, the chloride channel closes. As the interior of the cell becomes more positive, it can fire.

A number of physiologic changes occur during sleep. The low point of the 24-hour cycle for temperature occurs at night during sleep, although sleep does not cause the decrease. Urine secretion falls during sleep. The heart rate and respirations are slower and more regular during NREM sleep and then more rapid and less regular during REM sleep. Blood flow to the brain is increased during REM sleep. Autonomic nervous functions tend to be active during REM, with irregular breathing, variable pulse rate and blood pressure levels, and an increased metabolic rate. Penile erections can occur during sleep and are more frequent during REM sleep. Hormone levels can fluctuate during sleep. Secretion of growth hormone increases during the first 2 hours, and surges of adrenocorticotropic hormone (ACTH) and cortisone secretion occur in the second half of the sleep period. Luteinizing hormone secretion is increased for both boys and girls during puberty, and prolactin is secreted at an increased rate in both men and women, especially immediately after the onset of sleep.

The amount of sleep needed by an individual varies throughout the life span, with infants requiring the most sleep and adults requiring the least. The time in each phase of the sleep cycle will also vary throughout the life span. Additionally, sleep requirements among individuals vary greatly.

PATHOPHYSIOLOGY

Anxiety

Anxiety is a feeling of unease that something bad or undesirable may happen. Some anxiety is normal; it is a protective mechanism that has evolved to help people recognize danger and take action for self-preservation. Anxiety becomes pathologic, however, when it is severe and chronic and interferes with an individual's ability to function in normal life.

Anxiety is actually several related disorders. Each anxiety disorder has its own distinct features, but they all share characteristics of excessive and irrational fear and dread. Anxiety is a serious illness that affects approximately 19 million American adults (National Institute of Mental Health, 2003). Anxiety disorders can become progressively worse if they are untreated. Treatment includes counseling ("talk therapy") and drug therapy.

The following disorders are types of anxiety disorders:

- Panic disorder—sudden feelings of terror that come on suddenly and repeatedly without warning. Panic disorder is often comorbid with depression, drug abuse, or alcoholism. People with panic disorder may avoid places or situations where a previous attack occurred; some people may be so affected that they do not leave the house.
- Obsessive-compulsive disorder—anxious, recurrent, unwelcome thoughts or rituals that cannot be controlled. For example, a patient may be filled with doubts and repeatedly check situations that cause concern. The recurring thoughts demonstrate obsessions; the behaviors that deal with those thoughts are compulsions.
- Post-traumatic stress disorder (PTSD)—a debilitating condition that can develop following a terrifying event. A person experiences persistent frightening thoughts and memories of the ordeal, which may come during the day or at night. People with PTSD may feel emotionally numb and have difficulty relating to people they were once close to.
- Social phobia (also called social anxiety disorder)—overwhelming anxiety and excessive self-consciousness in everyday social situations. People with this phobia have persistent, intense, and chronic fears of being watched and judged by others and fear being embarrassed by their own actions. This disorder often occurs with other anxiety disorders or depression.
- Specific phobias—an intense fear of a particular thing or situation that poses little or no actual danger. Common examples are fear of heights, elevators or enclosed spaces, or flying.
- Generalized anxiety disorder—chronic anxiety that lasts more than 6 months and causes the person to have exaggerated worry and tension every day. In this disorder, the person always anticipates disaster and worries excessively

over issues such as health, money, work, and family. Severe generalized anxiety disorder can make it difficult to partake in ordinary daily activities. Women have a higher prevalence of generalized anxiety disorder than men, although the course of the illness and the prognosis for both sexes is not measurably different.

Emotional memories stored in the amygdala are believed to play a role in disorders involving very distinct fears, such as phobias. Other parts of the brain may be involved with other types of anxiety. The hippocampus, for example, shrinks in people who have experienced severe stress because of child abuse or military combat, which may explain why people with PTSD have flashbacks, deficits in explicit memory, and fragmented memory of details of the traumatic event. Other research indicates that the basal ganglia and striatum in the brain are involved in obsessive-compulsive disorder (National Institute of Mental Health, 2003).

Studies of twins and families indicate that both genes and experience influence the development of anxiety disorders. Studying the interaction of these two factors might lead to ways to prevent or treat anxiety (National Institute of Mental Health, 2003).

Neurotransmitters are known to play a role in anxiety, although exactly how they do so is not known. GABA has long been known to have a role in diminishing anxiety, and antianxiety drugs (**anxiolytics**) enhance the action of GABA. Serotonin and norepinephrine have also recently been discovered to function in anxiety, and other neurotransmitter systems, such as corticotropin-releasing factors and substance P, appear to be abnormally regulated in patients who have anxiety. More research is needed to determine whether drugs that are antagonists to these systems might be helpful in treating anxiety. Also, because GABA works to counteract glutamate, decreasing glutamate or diminishing its activity might decrease anxiety (Gorman et al., 2003).

Sleep Disorders

At least 40 million Americans have a sleep disorder. Sixty percent of adults report that they have sleep problems at least a few nights a week; 40% of adults report that at least a few days every month they have daytime sleepiness severe enough to interfere with daily activity (National Sleep Foundation, 2003, citation 1).

Sleep disorders are many and varied. They include the following problems:

- Narcolepsy—sudden irresistible sleep attacks of unknown origin lasting from seconds to minutes, two to six times a day
- Sleep apnea—a group of disorders characterized by cessation of breathing during sleep, lasting 10 seconds or longer and occurring 30 or more times during a night's sleep
- Sleepwalking—getting up and walking about while still asleep, although the eyes are open; usually occurs in children
- Night terrors—occur only in children, with periods of fright, crying, moaning, or screaming after a brief time asleep; episodes usually do not last long and are not generally remembered in the morning
- Excessive daytime sedation
- Insomnia

Of these disorders, **insomnia** occurs most frequently. Insomnia is the perception or complaint of inadequate or poor-quality sleep. It has many presentations, which include:

- Difficulty falling asleep or staying asleep
- Waking up too early in the morning without being able to return to sleep
- Waking up frequently during the night with difficulty returning to sleep
- Not sleeping long enough
- Feeling that sleep was not restful
- Sleeping poorly

Because individuals vary greatly in their need for sleep and their satisfaction with sleep, insomnia cannot be defined merely by the number of hours a person sleeps or by how long it takes to fall asleep. Insomnia is instead classified by frequency of occurrence: transient (occurring a single night to a few weeks), intermittent (occurring from time to time), or chronic (occurring most nights and lasting a month or more). Insomnia has many causes. Transient and intermittent insomnia are often related to stress, environmental noise, extreme temperatures, change in the surrounding environment, sleep–wake schedule problems such as jet lag, or adverse effects of drug therapy. Chronic insomnia is more complex and often results from more than one cause, including underlying physical or mental disorders. One of the most common causes of chronic insomnia is depression. Other underlying causes include arthritis, kidney disease, heart failure, asthma, sleep apnea, narcolepsy, restless legs syndrome, Parkinson disease, and hyperthyroidism. Chronic insomnia may also be related to the core patient variable of life span, diet, and habits. The following behaviors are associated with chronic insomnia: overuse of caffeine, misuse of alcohol or other substances, disrupted sleep–wake cycles such as from shift work, and chronic stress. Some people also have insomnia related to smoking cigarettes just before bedtime, excessive napping in the afternoon or evening, and expecting or worrying about sleep difficulties.

Insomnia can be found in all age groups, although older adults seem to have more difficulty sleeping than other age groups. It is unclear whether older adults actually have problems with insomnia or if they simply require less sleep as they get older (National Sleep Foundation, 2003, citations 2 and 3). Women tend to have insomnia more often than men, especially after they reach menopause.

Although lifestyle changes can prevent insomnia in most people with transient or intermittent insomnia, some patients need short-term drug therapy to help them sleep. Chronic insomnia can be treated by diagnosing and treating any underlying medical or psychological problems. Stopping behaviors that contribute to insomnia is also helpful. Patients may also need to apply behavioral techniques such as relaxation therapy, sleep restriction therapy, and reconditioning in order to overcome chronic insomnia. Relaxation techniques such as progressive relaxation and rhythmic breathing allow the muscles to relax and the mind to stop "racing," thereby allowing natural sleep to occur. Sleep restriction may be used when people spend too much time in bed trying to fall asleep. These patients are allowed only a few hours in bed at night for a while, and then the time in bed is gradually increased until a more normal night's sleep occurs. Reconditioning helps people reconnect being in bed and bedtime with sleeping. They

need to avoid using their beds for any activity besides sleeping or sex. If they are unable to sleep, they are instructed to get out of bed and return to bed only once they are sleepy, so that eventually the body will associate the bed with sleeping. They are also coached to avoid naps and to continue going to bed and getting up in the morning at the same time every day. The use of drug therapy to treat chronic insomnia is very controversial. Generally, drug therapy is considered best if used for the shortest duration possible.

DRUGS TO RELIEVE ANXIETY

(C) Benzodiazepines

Benzodiazepines are used for a number of therapeutic effects, including anxiety relief, sleep promotion, anticonvulsant effects, muscle relaxation, treatment of acute alcohol withdrawal, induction of general anesthesia, preoperative sedation, and conscious sedation. Some of these drugs have other specific uses, many of them off label. As a class, benzodiazepines appear to potentiate the effects of GABA. Because GABA is an inhibitory neurotransmitter, this benzodiazepine-mediated intensification of the effects of GABA leads to more CNS depression than would normally be found.

Benzodiazepines bind to specific receptor sites to produce their effects. At least two types of these receptors are believed to exist, BZ_1 and BZ_2. Sleep mechanisms are thought to be related to BZ_1, and memory, motor, sensory, and cognitive functions related to BZ_2. Activity of the benzodiazepines may involve the following sites: spinal cord (muscle relaxation), brainstem (anticonvulsant activity), cerebellum (ataxia effects), and the limbic and cortical areas (emotional behavior). The antianxiety effects of benzodiazepines are separate from those that nonspecifically depress the CNS (leading to sedation and motor impairment). Much larger doses of benzodiazepines are required to produce the effects of ataxia and sedation than to produce antianxiety effects.

As a drug class, benzodiazepines have a high margin of safety (i.e., a wide therapeutic index) and are therefore the drug class of first choice to treat anxiety. All of the benzodiazepines have similar efficacy; they differ by pharmacokinetics and cost. Lorazepam is the prototype benzodiazepine used to treat anxiety. Other drugs in this class represented by the prototype are alprazolam (Xanax), clorazepate (Tranxene), chlordiazepoxide (Librium), diazepam (Valium), halazepam (Paxipam), and oxazepam (Serax).

NURSING MANAGEMENT OF THE PATIENT RECEIVING [P] LORAZEPAM

Core Drug Knowledge

Pharmacotherapeutics

Lorazepam (Ativan) is used in treating anxiety disorders and for short-term relief of anxiety that occurs with depression. Day-to-day stress and anxiety should not be treated with antianxiety drugs. Lorazepam, when given intramuscularly or intravenously preoperatively and before anesthesia, produces sedation, relieves anxiety, and decreases the patient's ability to recall events surrounding surgery. Unlabeled uses of lorazepam include treating status epilepticus, chemotherapy-induced nausea and vomiting, the symptoms of acute alcohol withdrawal, and psychogenic catatonia. Oral lorazepam is also used to treat chronic insomnia.

Pharmacokinetics

Lorazepam, like other benzodiazepines, is readily absorbed from the gastrointestinal (GI) tract. Unlike some of the other benzodiazepines, lorazepam is readily absorbed when it is given intramuscularly. Because of its high lipid solubility, lorazepam is widely distributed in the body tissues, and it is also highly protein bound (85%). Compared to other benzodiazepines, lorazepam has an intermediate speed of onset when taken orally. Lorazepam is hepatically metabolized to an inactive substance, making it—along with oxazepam (Serax)—unusual among the drugs in the class, which are otherwise metabolized to active compounds. This easy inactivation is an advantage for patients with liver disease and for older adults. Lorazepam is eliminated through the urine.

Intravenous lorazepam is distributed quickly to the brain, which makes it effective in treating status epilepticus (discussed further in Chapter 19). Unlike diazepam, another benzodiazepine given for status epilepticus, lorazepam redistributes out of the brain slowly, providing prolonged protection against further seizures. Although the half-life of lorazepam in the blood is rather short, its effectiveness in controlling seizures is related to how long it is at the site of action—the brain, not the bloodstream. Table 16.1 provides a summary of selected benzodiazepines and a comparison of their pharmacokinetic properties.

Pharmacodynamics

Like all benzodiazepines, lorazepam increases the effects of GABA, which has an inhibitory effect on the CNS. However, none of the benzodiazepines act like GABA or increase the amount of GABA present. The intrinsic amount of GABA is limited; hence, the effects from benzodiazepines are also limited. Tolerance to lorazepam and the other benzodiazepines can occur if they are used long term, requiring larger doses to achieve a therapeutic effect.

Contraindications and Precautions

The contraindications to the use of lorazepam, which apply to all the benzodiazepines, are hypersensitivity, psychoses, acute narrow-angle glaucoma, intra-arterial use, and use in children younger than 6 months. Prolonged administration of lorazepam or any other benzodiazepine produces physical dependence, and withdrawal symptoms will occur if the drug is stopped suddenly. Like most other benzodiazepines, lorazepam is a pregnancy category D drug. These drugs have been found in maternal and cord blood, indicating transfer to the baby; therefore, they should not be used for obstetric uses during labor and delivery.

Paradoxical reactions have been reported with lorazepam and other benzodiazepines, evidenced by excitement,

TABLE 16.1 Summary of Selected (C) Benzodiazepines

Drug (Trade) Name	Selected Indications	Route and Dosage Range	Pharmacokinetics
(P) lorazepam (Ativan; *Canadian:* Novo-Lorazepam)	Anxiety, anesthetic premedication, status epilepticus, alcohol withdrawal, chronic insomnia	*Adult:* PO, 2–6 mg/d; IM, 0.05 mg/kg; IV, 2 mg *Child:* Not recommended; IV/IM, oral dose not established	*Onset:* PO, 1–3 h; IM, 15–30 min; IV, 1–5 min *Duration:* 12–24 h $t_{1/2}$: 10–20 h
alprazolam (Xanax; *Canadian:* Nu-Alpraz)	Anxiety, panic disorder, agoraphobia	*Adult:* PO, 0.25–1.0 mg tid *Child:* Not established	*Onset:* 30 min *Duration:* 4–6 h $t_{1/2}$: 6.3–26.9 h
chlordiazepoxide (Librium; *Canadian:* Corax)	Anxiety, alcohol withdrawal, anesthetic premedication	*Adult:* PO, 5–10 mg tid–qid (50–100 mg for alcohol withdrawal); IM/IV, 50–100 mg *Child >6 y:* PO, 5 mg bid–qid; IM/IV, 25–50 mg; not recommended under 6 y	*Onset:* PO, varies; IM, 10–15 min *Duration:* 48–72 h $t_{1/2}$: 5–30 h
diazepam (Valium; *Canadian:* Diazemuls)	Anxiety, status epilepticus, skeletal muscle relaxant	*Adult:* PO, IM, 2–10 mg/bid–qid; rectal, 0.2 mg/kg qd–bid; IV, 5–10 mg prn *Reduced dosage in geriatric or debilitated patients* *Child >2 y:* PO, 1–2.5 mg tid–qid; IM and IV, up to 0.25 mg/kg; Rectal, 0.5 mg/kg	*Onset:* PO, 30–60 min; IM, 15–30 min; rectal, rapid; IV, 1–5 min *Duration:* 3 h (1 h IV) $t_{1/2}$: 20–50 h
flurazepam (Dalmane; Canadian: Somnal)	Insomnia	*Adult:* 15–30 mg at bedtime *Child:* Not for use <15 y	*Onset:* 15–30 min *Duration:* 7–8 h $t_{1/2}$: 2–3 h; 47–100 h (active metabolite)
midazolam (Versed)	Preoperative sedation, anxiolysis, amnesia Sedation Anesthesia	*Adult:* IM, IV: 1–5 mg *Child:* 0.025–0.15 mg/kg *Dose individualized/reduced in patients >60 years of age, debilitated, or chronically ill.*	*Onset:* IM, *Adult:* 15 min; *Child:* 5 min; IV, 1–3 min *Duration:* 6 h $t_{1/2}$: 1.8–6.4 h
(C) Benzodiazepine Antagonist			
flumazenil (Romazicon; *Canadian:* Anexate)	Benzodiazepine antagonist	*Adult:* IV, 0.2 mg q 60 seconds up to 1 mg (reversal of conscious sedation); 0.2 mg, then 0.3 mg q 30 seconds up to 3 mg (management of benzodiazepine overdose).	*Onset:* 20–30 sec *Duration:* 72 h $t_{1/2}$: 7–15 min; 41–79 min (repeated doses)

stimulation, and acute rage. These effects have been noted mostly in patients with psychiatric disorders and in hyperactive, aggressive children. Other symptoms that may occur are acute hyperexcited states, anxiety, hallucinations, increased muscle spasticity, insomnia, and sleep disturbances. These effects usually occur within the first 2 weeks of therapy.

Adverse Effects

Lorazepam, like other benzodiazepines, is generally well tolerated, with few adverse effects. Mild drowsiness is common but transient, occurring in the first few days of therapy and then dissipating. Ataxia and confusion may also occur, especially in older adults and in debilitated patients. Dose adjustments should be made if these effects persist. Respiratory disturbances and partial airway obstruction may occur if excessive lorazepam is given intravenously before a procedure. A number of other adverse effects are possible, although they are rare. Many relate to the CNS depression that occurs with the drug therapy. These adverse effects are as follows:

- *Cardiovascular:* bradycardia, tachycardia, cardiovascular collapse, hypertension, hypotension, decreased systolic blood pressure, palpitations, edema, and phlebitis and thrombosis at intravenous (IV) sites
- *CNS:* problems with arousal and energy (sedation, sleepiness, depression, lethargy, apathy, fatigue, hypoactivity,

restlessness, stupor, coma); balance and movement (lightheadedness, syncope, rigidity, tremor, dystonia, vertigo, dizziness, unsteadiness, ataxia, impaired coordination, weakness, akathisia, hemiparesis, hypotonia, psychomotor retardation, seizures); mood and emotions (crying, sobbing, euphoria, nervousness, irritability, agitation); cognitive (memory impairment, disorientation, delirium, anterograde amnesia, confusion, difficulty in concentration, inability to perform complex mental functions); speech (slurred speech, aphonia, dysarthria); other (vivid dreams, "glassy eyed" appearance, headache, extrapyramidal symptoms, paradoxical reactions)

- *Dermatologic:* urticaria, pruritus, rash, dermatitis, hair loss, hirsutism, ankle and facial edema
- *GI:* constipation, diarrhea, dry mouth, coated tongue, sore gums, nausea, anorexia, change in appetite, vomiting, difficulty swallowing, increased salivation, gastritis
- *GU:* incontinence, changes in libido, urinary retention, menstrual irregularities
- *Ophthalmic:* visual disturbances, diplopia, nystagmus
- *Psychiatric:* behavioral problems, hysteria, psychosis, suicidal tendencies
- *Hematologic:* elevated liver enzymes, leukopenia, blood dyscrasias, anemia, thrombocytopenia, eosinophilia
- *Miscellaneous:* decreased hearing, nasal congestion, auditory disturbances, hiccups, fever, diaphoresis, gynecomastia, changes in weight, dehydration, lymphedema, joint pain, and burning or pain at the IM injection site

Drug Interactions

Several drug interactions are possible with lorazepam, the most important of which occur when lorazepam is coadministered with other drugs or substances that also depress the CNS. When lorazepam or other benzodiazepines are administered with alcohol, narcotics, barbiturates, or other CNS depressants, the effect on the CNS is additive. These combinations may depress respiratory drive, create severe hypotension or bradycardia, and substantially alter level of consciousness. Although lorazepam and other benzodiazepines are very safe when taken by themselves, when combined with other CNS depressants, especially in large quantities, the effects can be deadly. Table 16.2 presents agents that interact with lorazepam.

Assessment of Relevant Core Patient Variables

Health Status

Assess the patient for any contraindications to using lorazepam before initiating therapy. Assess for renal and hepatic impairment, which may alter the circulating levels of the

TABLE 16.2 Agents That Interact With P Lorazepam

Interactants	Effect and Significance	Nursing Management
alcohol, CNS depressants (opioid narcotics, barbiturates)	Increased CNS effects of lorazepam	Evaluate patient for additive CNS-depressant effects. Monitor serum levels (if appropriate) for therapeutic levels. Avoid concomitant administration if possible.
antacids	Altered rate of absorption of lorazepam, but generally not the extent of absorption	Administer antacid 1 hour before or 2 hours after lorazepam.
digoxin	Increased serum concentration of digoxin and possible toxicity	Assess serum digoxin levels closely. Monitor the patient's cardiac status frequently for changes.
levodopa	Decreased control of parkinsonian symptoms	Administer lorazepam cautiously to patients receiving levodopa for Parkinson disease. Assess patient for increasing muscle rigidity, tremors, and drooling.
oral contraceptives	Increased clearance of lorazepam may affect symptom management	Change in lorazepam dosage may be needed.
phenytoin	Increased serum concentration of phenytoin leading to possible toxicity	Monitor serum phenytoin levels closely.
probenecid	Interference with hepatic conjugation leading to more rapid onset or prolonged effect of lorazepam	Assess patient for continued sedative effects. Assess for dosage change as indicated.
rifampin	Increased hepatic microsomal enzyme metabolism of lorazepam leading to decreased effectiveness of lorazepam	Assess for dosage change of lorazepam as indicated. Assess patient for changes in seizure control or decrease in sedative effect.
scopolamine	Increased sedation when administered with parenteral form of lorazepam	Institute safety measures. Assess patient for signs of increased drowsiness, dizziness, and ataxia.
theophylline	Possible antagonism of sedative effects of lorazepam	Assess for lorazepam dosage adjustment.

drug. In patients who have depression along with anxiety, assess for risk for suicide. Obtaining a baseline level of hepatic enzymes and a complete blood count will provide a reference for comparison when these levels are checked throughout long-term therapy.

Life Span and Gender

Assess the patient's age. Intravenous lorazepam is not recommended in children younger than 18 years of age because data regarding its effects are minimal. Similarly, the efficacy and safety of oral lorazepam have not been established for children younger than 12 years of age. When it is used in children, the initial dose should be small, and it should be increased in very small increments. Lorazepam is contraindicated in children younger than 6 months.

Data suggest that women metabolize all benzodiazepines differently from men and that the desired and adverse effects of the drug may also be different for men and women. The exact nature of these differences is not known at this time (Howell et al., 2001). Assess whether the woman is pregnant because lorazepam is a pregnancy category D drug and should generally be avoided during pregnancy. It is not known whether lorazepam enters breast milk, although other benzodiazepines do. The age of the adult should be assessed when starting lorazepam therapy. Lorazepam may cause excessive ataxia or lethargy in older adults; in these patients, the drug should be started at a small dose and increased slowly. Older adults receiving lorazepam, or other benzodiazepines, may also be at increased risk for urinary incontinence. Box 16.1 presents research on this topic.

Lifestyle, Diet, and Habits

Assess the patient for the use of alcohol, narcotics, and other CNS depressants, which have an additive effect with lorazepam. The patient who has a history of alcohol or substance abuse may be a poor candidate for lorazepam because he or she may be more likely to develop dependence on the drug. Determine whether the patient regularly drives, operates heavy machinery, or participates in other activities that require mental alertness. These activities may be dangerous during the initial period of drug use, because of drowsiness caused by the drug.

Environment

Oral lorazepam may be administered in any environment. IV infusions of lorazepam require that the patient be in a monitored environment. Equipment to maintain a patent airway should be at the bedside.

Culture and Inherited Traits

Studies have shown that some benzodiazepines have a longer half-life in Asians than in whites. These results suggest that Asians should receive lower doses of the drug than whites, although no specific studies with lorazepam in Asians have been done.

Nursing Diagnoses and Outcomes

- Risk for Injury related to drowsiness and other adverse effects
  Desired outcome: *The patient will not sustain an injury while on lorazepam.*
- Anxiety related to disease process
  Desired outcome: *The patient will achieve symptom control.*
- Deficient Knowledge related to newly prescribed drug therapy
  Desired outcome: *The patient will learn the actions and adverse effects of lorazepam and how to safely self-administer the drug.*

FOCUS ON RESEARCH

Box 16.1 Benzodiazepines and Frail Older Persons

Landi F, Cesari M, Russo A, et al., for the Italia Silver Network Home Care Study Group. (2002). Benzodiazepines and the risk of urinary incontinence in frail older persons living in the community. Clinical Pharmacological Therapeutics, *72*(6), 729–734.

The Study

Data from 4,583 frail older adult patients who were admitted to home care programs and enrolled in a large collaborative observational study group (the Italia Silver Network Home Care Project) were analyzed to determine whether there was a relationship between urinary incontinence and the use of benzodiazepines. A total of 1,475 individuals (21% of whom were 60 to 74 years of age and 38% of whom were 75 years of age or older) reported urinary incontinence. Those who were taking benzodiazepines had a 45% greater risk for urinary incontinence than those not taking benzodiazepines. Benzodiazepines with the longest half-lives produced the most problems.

Nursing Implications

Why benzodiazepines increase the risk for urinary incontinence is not clear from this study. Also, the type of incontinence is not specified (such as stress or urge incontinence), which is an important consideration. However, increased risk for urinary incontinence may be related to increased drowsiness and sedation, which would impair the patient's ability to reach a toilet before being incontinent (perhaps most relevant in urge incontinence). Additionally, it can be hypothesized that CNS depression decreases the patient's ability to consciously maintain control over the external sphincter, which may be most important in stress incontinence. What the study does point out is the need to assess the older adult on benzodiazepine therapy for onset of urinary incontinence. If noted, drug therapy may have to be decreased or stopped and another drug class substituted if possible.

Planning and Intervention

Maximizing Therapeutic Effects

Lorazepam has a fairly short duration of action; therefore, the daily dosage for treating anxiety is split into two or three doses, administered throughout the day to achieve continued therapeutic effect. If one of the symptoms of anxiety experienced is difficulty sleeping, the largest dose of the day should be administered at bedtime to promote sleep. If the drug is given solely as a sleep aid, the entire dose is given at bedtime. IV solutions of lorazepam should be protected from light and stored in the refrigerator to prevent loss of potency.

To help the patient learn coping skills and further decrease anxiety on a more permanent basis, talk therapy or counseling should accompany drug therapy with lorazepam.

Minimizing Adverse Effects

If GI distress occurs, lorazepam may be taken with food. Monitor for paradoxical reactions and stop the drug if they occur. Hepatic function and blood cell counts should be assessed periodically during therapy to determine whether any adverse effects have occurred. To prevent undue adverse effects, older adults and children should be started on small doses of lorazepam, and the dose should then be increased slowly as necessary. Coadministration of lorazepam with other CNS depressants should be avoided if possible. If it is necessary to coadminister these agents, assess the patient carefully for signs of significant CNS depression. If paradoxical effects occur, the drug should be discontinued.

Dilute injectable lorazepam with an equal volume of compatible solution, such as sterile water for injection, sodium chloride for injection, or 5% dextrose solution, and inject at a rate not to exceed 2 mg/minute. Give IV lorazepam only in a monitored environment with equipment to maintain a patent airway at the bedside. Monitor patient closely during administration.

Patients with depression and anxiety should be assessed carefully for suicidal tendencies. The number of pills dispensed to the patient should be the least amount feasible.

To prevent withdrawal symptoms when lorazepam is to be discontinued, the drug should be slowly tapered off if the patient has been on the drug for a long time or if a high dose of the drug was being taken.

Providing Patient and Family Education

- To prevent additive CNS depression, teach the patient to avoid taking alcohol and other CNS depressants while on lorazepam.
- Warn the patient that drowsiness, sedation, and ataxia may occur when the drug is first started, but that these effects should disappear once the patient accommodates to the drug. Until the effects of the drug on the patient are known, the patient should avoid driving, operating machinery, or any other tasks that require mental alertness and concentration.
- If the patient experiences GI distress from lorazepam, instruct him or her to take the drug with food.
- Warn women of childbearing age to avoid becoming pregnant while on lorazepam because it is a pregnancy category D drug. Women should not breast-feed while on lorazepam because it is not known whether the drug distributes into breast milk, although other benzodiazepines do.
- Inform the patient of the importance of returning for follow-up blood work if lorazepam therapy is to continue for an extended period.
- Teach the patient and family what the paradoxical effects of lorazepam are and explain that if they occur, the patient should stop taking the drug and immediately contact the prescriber.

Box 16.2 provides teaching guidelines for the patient who is prescribed benzodiazepines to be taken at home.

Ongoing Assessment and Evaluation

Lorazepam therapy is effective if the patient reports a reduction in feelings of anxiety and begins to develop other, more positive coping mechanisms for life problems. For lorazepam therapy to be effective, adverse effects either should not occur or should be tolerable and manageable so that the patient does not need to stop therapy. Throughout therapy, assess for therapeutic response and onset of adverse effects.

MEMORY CHIP

[P] Lorazepam

- Used to treat anxiety disorders
- Works by increasing the inhibitory effects of GABA
- Major contraindications: psychoses and acute narrow-angle glaucoma
- Most common adverse effects: mild drowsiness, ataxia, confusion
- Most serious adverse effects: paradoxical reactions
- **Life span alert: contraindicated in children under 6 months; pregnancy category D; older adults more likely to develop ataxia and confusion**
- Maximizing therapeutic effects: Daily dose should be split into two or three doses to give sustained daily therapeutic effect; counseling ("talk therapy") should be given while on drug therapy.
- Minimizing adverse effects: Assess for suicidal tendencies; discontinue long-term treatment by tapering dose slowly.
- Most important patient education: Avoid taking alcohol and other CNS depressants while on lorazepam to prevent additive CNS depression.

COMMUNITY-BASED CONCERNS

Box 16.2 Teaching for Patients Prescribed Home Benzodiazepine Therapy

Patients are often prescribed benzodiazepines, such as lorazepam, to be taken at home. In addition to the initial drowsiness that the drug can cause, CNS depression may also impair cognition and processing of information and may slow response time, all of which place these patients at considerable risk for having an accident while driving. This risk increases with the additive CNS depression that can occur if benzodiazepines are taken with alcohol and other CNS depressants, including prescription medications. Patients may forget about additive effects from alcohol use once they adapt to lorazepam therapy or if they do not experience drowsiness in the first place. Ensure that patients who are to start on lorazepam understand the following precautions:

- They should avoid driving until the effects of the drug on them are known.
- They should avoid drinking alcohol.
- If they ingest alcohol, they should have someone else (who has not been drinking) drive.
- If it is necessary to start another CNS depressant medication, they should again use extra caution driving until the combined effects of the drugs are known.

CRITICAL THINKING SCENARIO

Lorazepam and anxiety

Lena Hawthorne, 24 years old, was started on lorazepam for anxiety 3 days ago. She calls the clinic and tells you that the dosage must not be large enough because her symptoms of anxiety have increased. She complains of feeling so anxious that she feels she "might jump out of her skin." She also complains of having insomnia since she started on lorazepam.

1. What is your assessment of her problem?
2. What interventions would you carry out or suggest at this time?

Drugs Significantly Different From [P] Lorazepam

Selective Serotonin Reuptake Inhibitors

Some people do not respond to the antianxiety effects of benzodiazepines. Low serotonin levels are known to be present in severe stress and in many mood and anxiety-related disorders. Research on generalized anxiety disorder has indicated that dysfunction of the serotonin and norepinephrine systems is a neurobiological link between depression and generalized anxiety disorders (Gorman et al., 2002). Research has also shown that deletion of serotonin receptors in mice produces increased anxiety and causes changes in their GABA receptors, making them less responsive to benzodiazepine therapy (Sibille et al., 2000). Based on the knowledge of the link between low serotonin and anxiety, it has been determined that a class of antidepressant drugs that increase the availability of serotonin at the receptor site (known as the selective serotonin reuptake inhibitors, or SSRIs) is effective in decreasing anxiety, even if depression is not also present.

The SSRIs tend to be well tolerated and do not cause substantial adverse effects in most people. Unlike the benzodiazepines, they do not cause diminished alertness or ataxia. SSRIs can produce some nausea or jitteriness when first started, but these adverse effects usually go away with continued use. These medications can also cause sexual dysfunction. Unlike the benzodiazepines, which can reduce anxiety from one dose, the SSRIs must be taken for several weeks for their full anxiety-relieving effect to be evident. SSRIs that are prescribed for anxiety include citalopram (Celexa), fluvoxamine (Luvox), paroxetine (Paxil), fluoxetine (Prozac), and sertraline (Zoloft). They are used in panic disorder, obsessive-compulsive disorder, social anxiety disorder, PTSD, and generalized anxiety disorder. Venlafaxine, a drug closely related to the SSRIs, is also used in treating generalized anxiety disorder. The SSRIs are discussed in more depth in Chapter 17.

Tricyclic Antidepressants

Tricyclic antidepressants work by affecting the regulation of serotonin or norepinephrine in the brain. They act similarly to the SSRIs, which is most likely why they are effective in treating anxiety disorders. Tricyclic antidepressants are as effective as the SSRIs in treating anxiety, but they produce more adverse effects and are therefore not used as often. Adverse effects include dizziness, drowsiness, dry mouth, and weight gain. As with the SSRIs, several weeks of therapy on tricyclics are necessary before anxiety begins to diminish. The tricyclics that are used for anxiety are doxepin (Adapin), nortriptyline (Aventyl), amitriptyline (Elavil), imipramine (Tofranil), maprotiline (Ludiomil), desipramine (Norpramin), trimipramine (Surmontil), and protriptyline (Vivactil). They are used to treat panic disorder and PTSD. Clomipramine (Anafranil) is used to treat obsessive-compulsive disorder. The tricyclics are discussed in more depth in Chapter 17.

Buspirone

Buspirone (BuSpar) is an azaspirodecanedione that is not chemically or pharmacologically related to the benzodiazepines or any other sedative or anxiolytic drug. It is used to treat symptoms of anxiety, although exactly how it works is unknown. In laboratory studies, it shows a high affinity for serotonin receptors, but it has no effect on GABA receptors. Buspirone also has moderate affinity for one type of brain dopamine receptor; it may act as a presynaptic dopamine agonist. It also increases norepinephrine metabolism in the locus ceruleus.

Optimum relief of anxiety usually occurs after 3 to 4 weeks of treatment, although some improvement is often seen within 7 to 10 days of starting therapy. Although buspirone is intended for short-term therapy, patients who have been treated with buspirone for up to 1 year have not required a dosage increase to maintain therapeutic effect, and withdrawal symptoms did not occur if the drug was stopped suddenly. Buspirone produces much less sedation than lorazepam and does not produce substantial functional impairment. It can, however, cause dizziness, nausea, headache, nervousness, lightheadedness, or excitement as adverse effects. Because it is difficult to predict what effects any particular patient will experience, patients should be cautioned to avoid driving or operating machinery until the effects of the drug on them are known.

Hydroxyzine

Hydroxyzine (Vistaril) is a miscellaneous antianxiety drug that exerts CNS depressant activity in subcortical areas. It rapidly produces a feeling of calm and relieves anxiety without impairing mental alertness. Hydroxyzine also has bronchodilatory, antihistamine, analgesic, antispasmodic, and antiemetic effects. It can be administered intramuscularly or orally. It may be coadministered with a narcotic to control pain while minimizing the nausea that may be an adverse effect from the narcotic. Adverse effects of hydroxyzine include dry mouth, drowsiness (usually transient in continuous therapy), and involuntary motor activity (which usually occurs at higher-than-recommended doses).

Meprobamate

Meprobamate (Equanil) is also used for short-term management of anxiety symptoms. Meprobamate has selective effects at multiple sites within the CNS, including the thalamus and the limbic system. It may also inhibit multineuronal spinal reflexes. It has mild tranquilizing properties and some anticonvulsant and muscle-relaxant properties.

Meprobamate can produce several CNS adverse effects, such as drowsiness, ataxia, dizziness, slurred speech, headache, vertigo, weakness, impaired visual accommodation, euphoria, overstimulation, paradoxical excitement, and fast electroencephalographic (EEG) activity. Cardiovascular adverse effects include tachycardia, arrhythmias and palpitations, transient electrocardiographic (ECG) changes, syncope, and hypotensive crisis. Nausea, vomiting, and diarrhea are possible, as are potentially severe allergic responses.

Meprobamate is a pregnancy category D drug that is associated with congenital malformations if taken in the first trimester. It is also excreted into breast milk at levels two to four times that found in the maternal plasma. It should therefore be avoided in pregnant women, women who might become pregnant, and breast-feeding women.

DRUGS TO PROMOTE SLEEP

Benzodiazepines

In addition to their use in treating anxiety, benzodiazepines are used to treat insomnia or in situations in which a restful sleep is desired, such as the night before surgery. The benzodiazepine receptor subtype BZ_1 is thought to be associated with sleep mechanisms; BZ_1 receptors are specific GABA receptors located in the limbic, neocortical, and mesencephalic reticular systems in the brain. All of the benzodiazepines decrease the number of times the person awakens during the night. Stage 2 sleep is lengthened by all benzodiazepines. Most benzodiazepines shorten stages 3 and 4 (slow-wave sleep). Almost all benzodiazepines decrease the amount of time spent in REM sleep.

Five of the benzodiazepines have been approved for use as sleep aids (hypnotics). These are estazolam (ProSom), flurazepam (Dalmane), quazepam (Doral), temazepam (Restoril), and triazolam (Halcion). The major difference among these drugs is their half-life. Triazolam has the shortest half-life, at 1.5 to 5.5 hours, whereas quazepam has the longest half-life, at 41 hours. Table 16.3 presents the indications and half-lives for selected benzodiazepines. The drugs with shorter half-lives cause fewer problems with daytime sedation, although they may produce more early-morning insomnia.

The use of benzodiazepines as sleep aids should be short term. If benzodiazepines are used for as long as 3 or 4 weeks and then discontinued, REM rebound may occur (i.e., the REM sleep will occur more than usual in the sleep cycle). Abruptly discontinuing triazolam may produce rebound sleep disorder, in which the insomnia is worse than it was before treatment. The rebound effect is less likely to occur with estazolam, flurazepam, or quazepam, which have longer half-lives. Anterograde amnesia (inability to remember events that occur after the drug is taken) is more likely to occur with high doses of triazolam, but it may also occur with lower doses of triazolam or with the other benzodiazepines. Unlike lorazepam, these benzodiazepines are classified as pregnancy category X. These drugs are teratogenic when used during the first trimester, and if they are given to the mother during the last weeks of pregnancy, their distribution through the placenta results in neonatal CNS depression. Other adverse effects and characteristics of benzodiazepines are similar to those for lorazepam.

The use of benzodiazepines in older adults to treat insomnia is somewhat controversial because the daytime sedation that can occur places the older adult at increased risk for falls and other accidents. The impaired cognitive function that can come with continuous use of these drugs also places older adults at increased risk for injury (Petrovic et al., 2003).

Zolpidem

Zolpidem (Ambien) is used for short-term treatment of insomnia—generally not for more than 7 to 10 days. Although it is not chemically related to the benzodiazepines, zolpidem does interact with the GABA-BZ receptor complex and shares some pharmacologic properties with the benzodiazepines. Zolpidem generally preserves all of the

TABLE 16.3 Labeled Therapeutic Indications and Half-Lives of Benzodiazepines

Name	$t_{1/2}$ (h)	Anxiety	Insomnia	Seizures	Muscle Spasms	Alcohol Withdrawal	Anesthesia Induction
alprazolam	6.3–26.9	✓					
chlordiazepoxide	5–30	✓				✓	
clonazepam	18–50			✓			
clorazepate	40–50	✓		✓		✓	
diazepam	20–80	✓		✓	✓	✓	✓
estazolam	8–28		✓				
flurazepam	2–3 (47–100 metabolites)		✓				
halazepam	14	✓					
lorazepam	10–20	✓		✓		✓	✓
midazolam	1.8–6.4						✓
oxazepam	5–20	✓				✓	
quazepam	41 (47–100 metabolites)		✓				
temazepam	3.5–18.4 (9–15 metabolites)		✓				
triazolam	1.5–5.5		✓				

sleep stages and has only minor effects on REM sleep. Zolpidem is rapidly absorbed from the GI tract and has a short half-life. Hepatic dysfunction prolongs its half-life, but renal failure does not seem to increase the circulating level of zolpidem. Zolpidem does not seem to produce residual effects the next morning or cause a rebound effect when the drug is discontinued. However, withdrawal symptoms can be seen if the drug is stopped abruptly. Zolpidem induces sleep rapidly and should be taken immediately before going to bed. Zolpidem causes CNS depression, and as with all other CNS depressants, an additive effect will be seen if zolpidem is combined with alcohol or other CNS depressant drugs. Impaired motor or cognitive performance may occur in older adults after taking zolpidem; thus, initial doses should be small. Zolpidem is a pregnancy category B drug. The most common adverse effects from zolpidem are drowsiness, dizziness, and diarrhea. Caution patients that the drug may produce drowsiness and that he or she should take precautions until the effects of the drug are known.

Chloral Hydrate

Chloral hydrate is a nonbarbiturate hypnotic used to induce sleep and to cause preoperative sedation in order to lessen anxiety. It can be used as an adjunct to opiates and analgesics in pain control; it can also suppress or prevent alcohol withdrawal symptoms when given by rectal suppository. It is for short-term use only because it loses much of its effectiveness in producing and maintaining sleep after 2 weeks of use. Its exact mechanism of action is not known, although it is known to produce mild cerebral depression and quiet, deep sleep. In therapeutic doses, chloral hydrate has little effect on respirations, blood pressure, or reflexes. It does produce numerous adverse effects in the CNS, including disorientation, incoherence, paranoid behavior, excitement, delirium, nightmares, and confusion, among others. Prolonged use may result in psychological and physical dependency and tolerance. Sudden withdrawal may cause CNS excitation with tremor, anxiety, hallucinations, or even delirium, and may be fatal. Chloral hydrate has largely been replaced by other drugs that promote sleep in a safer and more effective manner.

Paraldehyde

Paraldehyde (Paral), a polymer of acetaldehyde, produces nonspecific, reversible depression of the CNS. With typical therapeutic doses, it produces little effect on respiration and blood pressure, but large doses may cause respiratory depression and hypotension. It is a liquid that tastes sharply of acetic acid; therefore, it must be mixed in milk or iced fruit juice to mask the taste and odor. Paraldehyde has generally been replaced by other drugs.

Barbiturates

Barbiturates such as phenobarbital (Bellatal), secobarbital (Seconal), and pentobarbital (Nembutal) were used to treat insomnia before the availability of the benzodiazepines. Although they are effective for short-term treatment of insomnia, they are also highly habit forming. Patients can develop tolerance and physical and psychological dependence on the drugs. Withdrawal symptoms can be severe and can lead to death. Patients who develop tolerance to a barbiturate are likely to overdose in an attempt to self-medicate and obtain therapeutic response. Overdosage results in severe respiratory depression as well as general CNS depression, likely followed by death. Because of these problems, barbiturates are not generally used to treat insomnia.

Phenobarbital is sometimes used as an adjunct for seizure disorders (see Chapter 19). Phenobarbital, as well as other barbiturates such as pentobarbital and secobarbital, is used parenterally as an adjunct to anesthesia.

CHAPTER SUMMARY

- Benzodiazepines, such as lorazepam, are used frequently to treat anxiety and sleep disorders. They work by intensifying the effects of GABA at specific receptors. They have fewer adverse effects and are generally better tolerated than older drug classes used for these conditions. They are generally very safe to use because they have a large therapeutic index.
- Benzodiazepines can also be used in treating seizures and muscle spasms, as adjuncts to anesthesia, and in managing acute alcohol withdrawal. Specific benzodiazepines are approved for different uses.
- Benzodiazepines differ mainly by their onset of action and half-life. They are generally recommended for short-term use in anxiety and insomnia, although their use in practice may vary.
- Other drug classes used to treat anxiety are the selective serotonin reuptake inhibitors (SSRIs) and the tricyclics, both classes of antidepressants. Their effectiveness in anxiety treatment, irrespective of whether the patient has depression, is believed to be attributable to their effect on serotonin levels.
- The use of barbiturates and chloral hydrate as treatments for insomnia is now limited because other drugs depress the CNS more safely and effectively.

QUESTIONS FOR STUDY AND REVIEW

1. How does lorazepam, a benzodiazepine, decrease anxiety?
2. What is an advantage of lorazepam over the SSRIs in treating patients with anxiety?
3. Why might lorazepam be the benzodiazepine of choice for a patient with anxiety and decreased liver function?
4. Why might an older adult be more at risk for falls than a younger adult when taking lorazepam at home?
5. Explain why triazolam, used to treat patients who have difficulty falling asleep, may also cause the adverse effect of early-morning insomnia.

? Need More Help?

Chapter 16 of the study guide for *Drug Therapy in Nursing* 2e contains NCLEX-style questions and other learning activities to reinforce your understanding of the concepts presented in this chapter. For additional information or to purchase the study guide, visit *http://connection.lww.com/go/aschenbrenner.*

REFERENCES AND BIBLIOGRAPHY

Gorman, J. M., Hirschfeld, R. M., & Ninan, P. T. (2002). New developments in the neurobiological basis of anxiety disorders. *Psychopharmacology Bulletin, 36*(Suppl 2), 49–67.

Howell, H. B., Brawman-Mintzer, O., Monnier, J., et al. (2001). Generalized anxiety disorders in women. *Psychiatric Clinics of North America, 24*(1), 165–178.

National Institute of Mental Health. (2003). Anxiety disorders [Online]. Available: *http://www.nimh.nih.gov/publicat/anxiety.cfm.* Accessed August 2004.

National Sleep Foundation. (2004). The importance of sleep [Online]. Available: *http://www.sleepfoundation.org/about.cfm#sleepl.* Accessed August 2004.

National Sleep Foundation. (2003). Sleep in America. Poll: Comparing sleep of older and young adults [Online]. Available: *http://www.sleepfoundation.org/NSAW/2003presskit/pk_compare.html.* Accessed August 2004.

National Sleep Foundation. (2003). Sleep, health and aging: The experts speak [Online]. Available: *http://www.sleepfoundation.org/NSAW/2003presskit/pk_experts.html.* Accessed August 2004.

Petrovic, M., Mariman, A., Warie, H., et al. (2003). Is there a rationale for prescription of benzodiazepines in the elderly? Review of the literature. *Acta Clinica Belgica, 58*(1), 27–36.

Sibille, E., Pavlides C., Benke D., et al. (2000). Genetic inactivation of the serotonin (1A) receptor in mice results in downregulation of major $GABA_A$ receptor alpha subunits, reduction of $GABA_A$ receptor binding, and benzodiazepine-resistant anxiety. *Journal of Neuroscience, 20,* 2758–2765.

Drugs Treating Mood Disorders

chapter 17

Learning Objectives

At the completion of this chapter the student will:

1. Identify risk factors for the development of depression.
2. Identify the symptoms of major depression.
3. Identify the symptoms of bipolar disorder.
4. Identify the core drug knowledge of drugs used to treat mood disorders.
5. Relate the interaction of core drug knowledge to core patient variables for drugs used to treat mood disorders.
6. Generate a nursing plan of care from the interactions between core drug knowledge and the core patient variables for drugs used to treat mood disorders.
7. Describe nursing interventions to maximize therapeutic and minimize adverse effects for drugs that affect mood.
8. Determine key points for patient and family education for drugs that affect mood disorders.

KEY TERMS

antidepressants

bipolar disorder

depression

dysregulation

mania

mood

mood stabilizers

neurotransmitters

psychotropic

serotonin reuptake inhibitor withdrawal syndrome

serotonin syndrome

FEATURED WEBLINK

http://www.acnp.org

Want to find out about the latest research pertaining to neuropsychopharmacology? The American College of Neuropsychopharmacology maintains a website that is an excellent source of information. Content is presented in newsletter, journal, and electronic book forms.

CONNECTION WEBLINK

Additional Weblinks are found on Connection:
http://www.connection.lww.com/go/aschenbrenner.

Drugs Treating Mood Disorders

(C) Antidepressants

(C) Selective serotonin reuptake inhibitors

- [P] **sertraline**
- citalopram
- fluoxetine
- fluvoxamine
- paroxetine
- bupropion
- trazodone
- venlafaxine

(C) Tricyclic antidepressants

- [P] **nortriptyline**
- amitriptyline
- amoxapine
- clomipramine
- doxepin
- imipramine
- maprotiline
- mirtazapine
- protriptyline
- trimipramine

(C) Monoamine oxidase inhibitors

- [P] **phenelzine**
- isocarboxazid
- trancyclopromine
- **selegiline**
  (see Chapter 21)

(C) Mood Stabilizers

- [P] **lithium**
- carbamazepine
- gabapentin
- valproic acid

The symbol (C) indicates the **drug class**.
Drugs in **bold type** marked with the symbol [P] are prototypes.
Drugs in blue type are closely related to the prototype.
Drugs in red type are significantly different from the prototype.
Drugs in black type with no symbol are also used in drug therapy; no prototype

"I'm depressed." We've all heard people say that or maybe even said it ourselves. These statements are often made without any formal diagnosis by a physician. And no one who says such a thing would ever think of saying "I have diabetes," . . . "I have liver failure," or even, "I have heart disease" in the absence of a formal diagnosis by a physician. So when people say, "I'm depressed," what do they actually mean? What are they trying to tell us? Most likely what they're trying to explain is that they are experiencing a decline in their mood.

A **mood,** as defined by the American Psychiatric Association, is "a pervasive and sustained emotion that colors the perception of the world." The prevalence of the term depression in our everyday language merely confirms what the experts have long known: Depression is the oldest and most common psychiatric illness. A landmark epidemiologic study of the 48 contiguous United States found the lifetime prevalence of major depression to be 16.2% (Kessler et al., 2003). The World Health Organization–supported Global Burden of Disease study predicts that major depression will become second only to ischemic heart disease as the leading cause of disability worldwide by 2020 (Murray & Lopez, 1997). Among U.S. workers alone, lost productive work time is estimated at $31 billion per year for workers with depression (Stewart et al., 2003). These statistics are only a few of those available to illustrate how important it is for you to be familiar with mood disorders and the medications used to treat them.

People with mood disorders no longer are solely psychiatric inpatients being cared for by psychiatric nurses. Mood disorders include depression and bipolar disorder, which is characterized by periods of depression and periods of mania. People who have mood disorders and take medicine to treat these illnesses can be found in all nursing practice settings. Furthermore, associations are increasingly being recognized between some mood disorders and physical illness, as described in Box 17.1. For these reasons, you must be ready to provide safe and competent care by having adequate knowledge about mood disorders and their treatment with medications.

The medications used to treat mood disorders can be broadly grouped as either **antidepressants** or **mood stabilizers.** The antidepressants can be further divided into several classes of medications. Among the antidepressants, the most widely prescribed drug class is the selective serotonin reuptake inhibitors (SSRIs). Sertraline (Zoloft) is the prototype SSRI that will be discussed in this chapter. Drugs significantly different from the prototype include bupropion (Wellbutrin), trazodone (Desyrel), and venlafaxine (Effexor).

Another class of medications is the tricyclic antidepressants. The prototype tricyclic antidepressant for this chapter is nortriptyline (Pamelor). Monoamine oxidase inhibitors (MAOIs), represented by the prototype phenelzine (Nardil), are another class of antidepressant. Drugs closely related to phenelzine are isocarboxazid (Marplan) and tranylcypromine (Parnate).

The mood stabilizers include the prototype lithium (Eskalith). Drugs significantly different from lithium are carbamazepine (Tegretol), valproic acid (Depakene), divalproex sodium (Depakote), and gabapentin (Neurontin).

FOCUS ON RESEARCH

Box 17.1 Depression Affects the Heart in More Ways Than One

Todaro, J. F., Shen, B. J., Niaura, R., et al. (2003). Effect of negative emotions on frequency of coronary heart disease (the Normative Aging Study). *American Journal of Cardiology, 92*(8), 901–906.

Tiemeier, H., Breteler, M. M., van Popele, N. M., et al. (2003). Late-life depression is associated with arterial stiffness: A population-based study. *Journal of the American Geriatric Society, 51*(8), 1105–1110.

The Study

The "baby boomer" generation is now reaching the age at which chronic diseases become increasingly apparent. These studies look at two of these illnesses, coronary heart disease (CHD) and depression. Todaro and colleagues examined the relation between negative emotions and the development of CHD in 498 elderly men over a period of 3 years. Not only were symptoms of anxiety and depression significantly associated with development of CHD, but men with the highest symptom scores were the most likely to develop CHD. The researchers concluded that people experiencing negative emotions have a significantly higher risk for developing CHD than other people do. Tiemeier and colleagues screened 3,704 elderly people for depression and arterial stiffness. Their analysis shows an association between arterial stiffness and depression in the elderly that further supports the proposed relationship between depression and vascular disease.

Nursing Implications

These are just two of many studies that support the belief that a definite connection exists between disorders of the mind and body. Psychoneuroimmunology is the growing field in which scientists focus on this very connection. However, increasing evidence within many of the other specialties supports the existence of this connection as well. It is important, therefore, for you to recognize that if you are caring for a patient in a medical or coronary care unit with the primary presentation of coronary artery disease, this patient may also have undiagnosed depression or already be receiving antidepressant therapy. It is equally important when caring for a depressed patient on a psychiatric unit to recognize that the patient may have undiagnosed coronary artery disease or be receiving medications for this illness.

PHYSIOLOGY

The brain contains billions of specialized cells called neurons. For these neurons to function as a cohesive system, they must communicate with one another. The communication from one neuron to another is called neurotransmission, and it takes place in the space between two neurons (a synapse). The axon of one neuron and the dendrite of another neuron communicate at the synapse. For neurotransmission to take place between two neurons at the synapse, chemicals called **neurotransmitters** must be present. Several neurotransmitters exist, each of which travels to a specific neuroreceptor site. Neurotransmission plays a role in both normal and abnormal brain function. (For a further discussion of neurotransmitters and receptors, see Chapter 13).

What seems obvious, but is often forgotten, is that the mind and the brain are the same organ. Certain activities are often thought of as belonging to either the mind or the brain.

In practical terms, critical thinking, emotions, and control of behavior are thought of as occurring in the mind, whereas activities such as controlling muscles of the body and regulating breathing, digestion, and body temperature are thought of as occurring in the brain. Conceptualizing the information in this way makes it easier to understand how illnesses in the brain can affect not only the emotions that a person experiences but also bodily functions such as movement and digestion.

PATHOPHYSIOLOGY

The 1990s were identified as the decade of the brain by the National Institutes of Health. During this time, unprecedented research about the brain and how it works improved the lives of people suffering with mood disorders. Improved techniques of brain imaging have brought about greater understanding of neural circuits and neurotransmitters. Genetic studies have identified a specific gene that predisposes some people to develop depression when exposed to emotional stressors (Caspi et al., 2003).

Specific neurotransmitters are believed to affect mood. Illnesses resulting in mood disorder are associated with an imbalance or **dysregulation** of neurotransmitters. Much remains to be discovered about the exact etiology and treatment of mood disorders.

Major Depressive Disorder

Everyone has some sense of what it's like to be sad and have a low mood. Being depressed or having major **depression** is more than just having a low mood. Specific criteria to describe and diagnose depressive disorders are outlined by the American Psychiatric Association in the *Diagnostic and Statistical Manual for Mental Disorders,* fourth edition, text revision (DSM-IV-TR), which helps health care providers diagnose psychiatric illnesses.

Diagnosing major depression is partly a process of elimination. A patient's symptoms cannot be the result of a general medical condition such as cancer or hypothyroidism, nor can they be the result of drug abuse or an adverse effect of medication, although some drug classes are associated with depression. Box 17.2 lists these drug classes.

A pattern of other signs and symptoms must be present to complete an accurate diagnosis of major depression. Within a 2-week period, a person must manifest a depressed, even tearful mood or report or demonstrate to others a diminished interest or lack of pleasure in all activities most of the day. The symptoms must cause impairment at work or other social functions. Additionally, four other symptoms must be present from the following: changes of appetite, weight, sleep, or energy; a decrease in concentration; recurring death wishes; or thoughts of suicide. Thus, in addition to mood, major depression affects a person's body and ability to think.

According to epidemiologic studies, 16.2% of people in the United States will experience these symptoms within their lifetimes (Kessler, 2003). Risk factors for depression include:

- Having previously been depressed
- Having a first-degree relative diagnosed with depression
- Being a woman, an adolescent, or a young adult

Approximately half of the people diagnosed with major depression will experience an additional episode at some point in their lives (Solomon et al., 2000). Elderly patients may have an even greater risk for experiencing an additional episode of depression (Mueller et al., 2004). Because only one third of depressed people seek help, are accurately diagnosed, or obtain the appropriate treatment, 15% of severely depressed patients will commit suicide. However, antidepressant treatment can result in a 50% reduction of symptoms in 70% of patients, according to one study (Tamminga et al., 2002). Furthermore, another study demonstrated that no greater financial burden was incurred in the United States by providing treatment for more patients with major depression between 1990 and 2000 (Greenberg et al., 2003). This information suggests that increased diagnosis and treatment of major depression will not only improve the health status of the affected individual but also does not negatively affect the economy of the United States. In fact, the economy may be slightly improved because treated workers do not lose productivity through the absenteeism that a depressive disorder can cause.

BOX 17.2 Drug Classes Associated With Depression

Alcohol	H_2 antagonists
Anticonvulsants	Narcotic analgesics
Antihypertensive agents	Oral contraceptives
Antiparkinsonian agents	Psychotropic agents
Antituberculosis agents	Steroids

Bipolar Disorder

Bipolar disorder is diagnosed when a person experiences symptoms of depression at some times and symptoms of mania at others. To better understand this disorder, one must first know the diagnostic criteria for mania. **Mania** is diagnosed when a person has an elevated or irritable mood lasting at least one week (or less if hospitalization is necessary) and at the same time has three or more of the following symptoms:

- Grandiosity
- Distractibility
- Decreased sleep
- More goal-directed activities or psychomotor agitation
- Belief that there is pressure to keep talking
- Subjective expression of racing thoughts
- Excessive involvement in pleasurable activities that have a high potential for painful consequences (American Psychiatric Association, 2000)

Throughout their lifetimes, approximately 0.5% to 2% of the general population is at risk for developing bipolar disorder. Unlike risk for major depression, with which women are diagnosed more frequently than men, the risk

for bipolar disorder is even among men and women. Most diagnoses are made in early adulthood. Current research continues to support a genetic predisposition to bipolar disorder (Chen et al., 2003). In 60% to 70% of cases, people with bipolar disorder experience a manic episode immediately before or after a major depressive episode. Throughout his or her lifetime, each person will establish a particular pattern of illness. However, with treatment, 70% to 80% of individuals experience an ability to live meaningful, productive lives.

C ANTIDEPRESSANTS

Imagine going to the doctor and explaining that you are experiencing a particular pain. The doctor responds that he or she knows exactly what you are experiencing. The best part of all is that a medicine is available to treat this pain. However, it will take about 1 to 2 weeks before the pain is gone. For patients experiencing emotional pain, such as depression, this is their very experience.

Most antidepressant drugs have a lag period of 10 days to 4 weeks before a therapeutic response is noted. Increasing the dose will not shorten this period but rather increase the incidence of adverse reactions. Although antidepressants can bring about an immediate change at neuroreceptor sites, it is unclear why a corresponding immediate relief of depressive symptoms does not occur. A current hypothesis about depression is that the postsynaptic receptors, which participate in nerve impulse neurotransmission, may have as important a role as the presynaptic receptors where regulation of neurotransmitter release and reuptake occur. It is possible that long-term antidepressant drug therapy produces changes in both presynaptic and postsynaptic neuroreceptors, increasing the sensitivity at the postsynaptic sites while decreasing sensitivity at the presynaptic sites. This activity corrects an abnormal receptor–neurotransmitter relationship. As the dysregulation is corrected, the clinical symptoms of depression cease. For the patient with an acute depressive disorder, this delay is difficult to accept. By the time a person seeks treatment for these illnesses, he or she wants immediate relief from pain. It's important not to minimize the pain and distress experienced by patients with mood disorders.

There are three main categories or types of antidepressants: the selective serotonin reuptake inhibitors (SSRIs), tricyclic antidepressants (TCAs), and monoamine oxidase inhibitors (MAOIs). There are also several miscellaneous agents that are used as antidepressants. Each type of antidepressant works a little differently, but they all change the brain chemistry to improve neurotransmission. Table 17.1 presents a summary of selected drugs used to treat depression and other mood disorders.

Although all types of antidepressants are similarly effective in treating depression, each type has unique adverse effects. The goal in antidepressant therapy is to bring about the greatest relief of symptoms while minimizing any unpleasant adverse effects as much as possible (DePaulo & Horvitz, 2002). Table 17.2 compares the adverse effects of selected antidepressant drugs; Table 17.3 describes methods of managing these adverse effects.

C Selective Serotonin Reuptake Inhibitors

Currently, the selective serotonin reuptake inhibitors (SSRIs) are the first choice for treating depression. They are preferred over the TCAs and the MAOIs because they can be less damaging to the heart and have minimal anticholinergic and hypotensive effects.

In 1987, fluoxetine (Prozac) became the first SSRI approved by the Food and Drug Administration (FDA) for use as an antidepressant in the United States. It immediately became popular because of its ease in dosing and few adverse effects. Its effectiveness, combined with the increasing social acceptance of antidepressant use, led many patients to ask their doctors for Prozac. Its great marketing success is thought to have stimulated widespread research and subsequent introduction of other newer antidepressants. Prozac has been around long enough that its patent has now expired, resulting in generic availability of this drug. But in the United States, the cultural impact is such that most people still think of Prozac when they think of antidepressants.

Currently, sertraline (Zoloft) is the most widely prescribed SSRI in the United States. Although its use in treating children and adolescents is currently under review, some studies have demonstrated that sertraline is safe and effective for treating major depressive disorder in this population (Wagner et al., 2003). At this time, however, sertraline is not approved by the FDA for use in children. Because of its widespread use, sertraline has been chosen as the prototype SSRI. Other SSRIs include citalopram (Celexa), fluoxetine (Prozac), fluvoxamine (Luvox), and paroxetine (Paxil).

NURSING MANAGEMENT OF THE PATIENT RECEIVING P SERTRALINE

Core Drug Knowledge

Pharmacotherapeutics

Sertraline (Zoloft) was approved by the FDA in 1991 for treating depression in the United States. Treating acute depressive disorder requires several months or longer of drug therapy with sertraline, as well as other antidepressants. Additional approved uses for sertraline include: obsessive-compulsive disorder, panic disorder, and post-traumatic stress disorder. It is also used off-label to treat pediatric depression and generalized social phobia.

Pharmacokinetics

Sertraline is well absorbed following oral administration, with peak plasma levels occurring within 4.5 to 8.4 hours. It has a 26- to 104-hour elimination half-life (with metabolites) and reaches a steady state within 7 days. SSRIs like sertraline are extensively metabolized by the liver and should be used with caution in patients with severe liver impairment. Food does not appear to affect systemic bioavailability of sertraline, although it may delay absorption.

TABLE 17.1 Summary of Selected (C) Drugs for Treating Mood Disorders

Drug (Trade) Name	Selected Indications	Route and Dosage Range	Pharmacokinetics
(C) Selective Serotonin Reuptake Inhibitors (SSRIs)			
P sertraline (Zoloft)	Major depression, obsessive-compulsive disorder	*Adult:* PO, 50–200 mg/d *Child:* OCD use, 25–200 mg/d	*Onset:* 4.5–8.4 h *Duration:* 12–20 h $t_{1/2}$: 26 h (104 h for active metabolite)
citalopram (Celexa)	Major depression	*Adult:* 20–40 mg/d *Child:* Safety and efficacy have not been established for <18 y	*Onset:* Slow *Duration:* Unknown $t_{1/2}$: 35 h
fluoxetine (Prozac; *Canadian:* Gen-Fluoxetine)	Major depression, obsessive-compulsive disorder, panic disorder, posttraumatic stress disorder, bulimia nervosa	*Adult:* PO, 20–60 mg/d not to exceed 80 mg/d *Child:* PO, 10–20 mg/d	*Onset:* Slow *Duration;* 10–12 h $t_{1/2}$: 1–3 d (7 to 9 d for S-norfluoxetine, active metabolite)
fluvoxamine (Luvox)	Obsessive-compulsive disorder	*Adult:* PO, 50–300 mg/d *Child:* Safety and efficacy have not been established for <18 y	*Onset:* Rapid *Duration:* 4–16 h $t_{1/2}$: 13.5–15.6 h
paroxetine (Paxil)	Major depression, obsessive-compulsive disorder, panic disorder	*Adult:* PO, 20–50 mg/d *Child:* Safety and efficacy have not been established for <18 y	*Onset:* 5.2 h *Duration:* 12–16 h $t_{1/2}$: 21 h
(C) Tricyclic Antidepressants			
P nortriptyline (Pamelor; *Canadian:* Norventyl)	Major depression	*Adult:* PO, 75–150 mg/d *Child:* Use not recommended	*Onset:* Varies *Duration:* 2–4 wk $t_{1/2}$: 18–44 hr
amitriptyline (Elavil; *Canadian:* Apo-Amitriptyline)	Major depression	*Adult:* 75–150 mg/d; IM, 20–30 mg qid *Child:* Not recommended for <12 y	*Onset:* Varies *Duration:* >20 h $t_{1/2}$: 31–46 h
amoxapine (Asendin)	Major depression	*Adult:* PO, 200–300 mg/d *Child:* Not recommended for <16 y	*Onset:* Varies *Duration:* 2–4 wk $t_{1/2}$: 8–30 h
clomipramine (Anafranil; *Canadian:* Gen-Clomipramine)	Obsessive-compulsive disorder	*Adult:* PO, 25–100 mg/d *Child:* PO, 25 mg/d with gradual increases to a maximum of 3 mg/kg/d or 100 mg/d	*Onset:* Slow *Duration*: 1–6 wk $t_{1/2}$: 19–37 h
desipramine (Norpramin; *Canadian:* Alti-Desipramine)	Major depression	*Adult:* PO, 100–200 mg/d *Child:* Not recommended for <12 y	*Onset:* Varies *Duration:* 3–4 d $t_{1/2}$: 12–24 h
doxepin (Sinequan; *Canadian:* Novo-Doxepin)	Major depression Depression, associated anxiety	*Adult:* PO, 75–150 mg/d *Child:* not recommended for <12 y	*Onset:* Varies *Duration:* Unknown $t_{1/2}$: 8–24 h
imipramine (Tofranil; *Canadian:* Apo-Imipramine)	Major depression	*Adult:* PO, 75–150 mg/d; IM, 100 mg/d *Child:* PO, 1.5 mg/kg/d	*Onset:* Varies *Duration:* Unknown $t_{1/2}$: 11–25 h
protriptyline (Vivactil)	Major depression	*Adult:* PO, 15–40 mg/d divided into 3 or 4 doses *Child:* Use not recommended	*Onset:* Slow *Duration:* Unknown $t_{1/2}$: 67–89 h

(continued)

TABLE 17.1 Summary of Selected (C) Drugs for Treating Mood Disorders (continued)

Drug (Trade) Name	Selected Indications	Route and Dosage Range	Pharmacokinetics
maprotiline (Ludiomil)	Major depression, bipolar disorder	*Adult:* PO, 75–225 mg/d *Child:* Use not recommended; safety and efficacy have not been established	*Onset:* Slow *Duration:* 2–3 wk $t_{1/2}$: 61 h
mirtazapine (Remeron)	Major depression	*Adult:* PO, 15–45 mg/d single dose at bedtime *Child:* Safety and efficacy have not been established	*Onset:* Slow *Duration:* 2–4 wk $t_{1/2}$: 20–40 h
trimipramine (Surmontil; *Canadian:* Nu-Trimipramine)	Major depression	*Adult:* PO, 75–150 mg/d *Child:* Use not recommended	*Onset:* Varies *Duration:* Unknown $t_{1/2}$: 7–30 h
(C) Monoamine Oxidase Inhibitors (MAOIs)			
P phenelzine (Nardil)	Major depression	*Adult:* PO, 15 mg tid, increasing to 60 mg/d; maximum 90 mg/d	*Onset:* Approximately 4 wk *Duration:* 48–96 h $t_{1/2}$: Unknown
trancyclopromine (Parnate)	Major depression	*Adult:* PO, 30 mg/d maximum dose 60mg/d in divided doses	*Onset:* 7–10 d *Duration:* Unknown $t_{1/2}$: 2.5 h
(C) Mood Stabilizers			
P lithium (Eskalith; *Canadian:* Lithizine)	Mania of bipolar disorder	*Adult:* 1800 mg/d (slow release) for acute mania; 900–1200 g/d for maintenance *Child:* Safety and efficacy have not been established for <12 y	*Onset:* 5–7 d *Duration:* Unknown $t_{1/2}$: 10–50 h
(C) Other Antidepressants			
trazodone (Desyrel; *Canadian:* Trazorel)	Major depression	*Adult:* PO, 150–600 mg/d *Child:* Safety and efficacy have not been established	*Onset:* Varies *Duration:* Varies $t_{1/2}$: 4–9 h

Pharmacodynamics

Sertraline is a potent and selective inhibitor of neuronal serotonin (5-HT) reuptake and has a weak effect on norepinephrine (NE) and dopamine (DA) neuronal reuptake. Because the SSRIs do not have a high affinity for muscarinic (Ach), histaminergic (H_1), and alpha-adrenergic receptors, their capacity for causing anticholinergic, sedative, cardiac, and orthostatic hypotensive effects is considerably less than that of the TCAs. Achieving antidepressant effects from sertraline, as with other antidepressants, can take anywhere from 10 days to 4 weeks. Some symptoms of depression, such as loss of energy, may be corrected before the mood is fully elevated.

Contraindications and Precautions

Sertraline should be administered with caution in patients with compromised liver function. Adjustments such as a lower or less-frequent dosing schedule may be made for these patients. Although no studies have been conducted specifically in patients with seizure disorders, the incidence of seizures in patients taking sertraline is 0.2%, which is similar to other antidepressant and placebo studies. A history of seizures therefore requires cautious use of sertraline.

Some concern exists that SSRI antidepressants such as sertraline may increase the risk for suicide in some pediatric patients. At this time, it is unclear whether sertraline and other SSRIs actually induce suicidal ideation, or whether the drugs' ability to restore energy levels before elevating mood provides depressed patients with the ability to act on their depressed mood. Box 17.3 explores some of these questions. Although using sertraline to treat depression in children is a nonlabeled use, the FDA has asked manufacturers of this and other antidepressant drugs to revise their warning labels to indicate that both adults and children taking sertraline, as well as other SSRIs, should be closely monitored for worsening of depression and the emergence of suicidal

TABLE 17.2 Adverse Effects of Selected Antidepressant Drugs

	Anticholinergic*	Agitation, Insomnia	Drowsiness	Cardiac Arrhythmia	Orthostatic Hypotension	Gastrointestinal Distress	Weight Gain
SSRIs							
sertraline	0	2	0	0	0	3	0
citalopram	1	3	0	0	0	3	0
fluoxetine	0	2	0	0	0	3	0
fluvoxamine	0	2	0	0	0	3	0
paroxetine	0	2	0	0	0	3	0
Tricyclics							
nortriptyline	1	0	1	2	2	0	1
amitriptyline	4	0	4	3	4	0	4
clomipramine	4	1	4	3	1	1	3
doxepin	3	0	4	2	2	0	3
imipramine	3	1	3	3	4	1	3
trimipramine	1	0	4	2	2	0	3
amoxapine	2	2	2	3	2	0	1
desipramine	1	1	1	2	2	0	1
protriptyline	2	1	1	2	2	0	0
maprotilene	2	0	4	1	0	0	2
mirtazapine	1	1	4	0	2	1	2
Other							
nefazodone	1	1	3	0	2	3	0
bupropion	0	2	0	1	0	1	0
trazodone	0	2	0	1	0	1	0
venlafaxine	0	0	4	1	1	1	1
MAOIs							
phenelzine	1	2	1	0	2	1	1
trancyclopromine	1	2	1	0	2	1	1

*Dry mouth, blurred vision, urinary hesitancy, and constipation.
0, absent or rare to 4, common.

thoughts and tendencies (Food and Drug Administration, 2004). As this book goes to press, the issue is still under debate; for the most recent information, visit the FDA website: *http://www.fda.gov.*

Adverse Effects

Compared with the tricyclics (TCAs), sertraline and other SSRIs have fewer adverse anticholinergic and cardiovascular effects and usually do not cause weight gain. Adverse effects, which are mild and brief, include gastrointestinal distress (anorexia, nausea, vomiting, and diarrhea), headache, fatigue, insomnia, and sexual function disturbances (delayed ejaculation, inability to achieve orgasm). Some of these adverse effects are transient, subsiding within the first 1 to 2 weeks of therapy. Other adverse effects may include hematologic problems, such as blood dyscrasias, leukopenia, and altered platelet function. For some patients, the most limiting adverse effects of SSRIs are disturbances of sexual function. This effect may not be a concern to the depressed patient beginning therapy, but it may become a greater concern as the patient regains interest in sexual activity. The presence of this adverse effect is a frequent reason that patients consider stopping drug therapy. In clinical trials, only 10% to 15% of patients required discontinuation of treatment because of an adverse event. As noted earlier, sertraline and other SSRIs may increase the risk for suicide, although the incidence of suicide is extremely small. Suicidal thoughts or attempts that occur early in the course of therapy may be related to the drug beginning to work; remember that the energy level of the patient will increase before the depression is fully relieved.

Drug Interactions

Sertraline is highly bound (98%) to plasma protein. If it is administered with another drug that is highly protein bound, increased free concentrations of either drug may result. The activity of isoenzyme cytochrome P-450 2D6 may be substantially inhibited by sertraline. Any drug that is metabolized by this isoenzyme should therefore be administered with caution because expected plasma levels will be altered. Consuming caffeinated beverages can increase the stimulant

TABLE 17.3 Management of Adverse Effects of Antidepressants

Symptoms	Strategies for Management
Gastrointestinal	
Nausea, anorexia	Administer with food (or antacids) if drug absorption is unaffected.
Diarrhea	Use antidiarrheal medication (if not contraindicated).
Constipation	Diet change (increase fiber and fluids), exercise, stool softener (avoid laxatives); wait for tolerance to drug effects.
Sexual dysfunction	Discuss methods available for satisfactory sexual expression.
Anorgasmia	Encourage talk with health care provider regarding dosage reduction or drug holiday.
Erectile dysfunction	
Impaired ejaculation	
Orthostatic hypotension	Use calf exercises, wear support hose, increase fluid intake.
Anticholinergic effects (dry eyes and mouth)	Use artificial tears, frequent dental hygiene, sugar-free chewing gum; wait to develop tolerance to drug effects.
Tremor/"jitteriness"	Slow gradual titration of increasing dosages; encourage discussion with health care provider regarding dosage reduction or drug holiday.
Insomnia	Take medication in the morning (exception is trazodone).
Sedation	Caffeine (if not contraindicated), take medication at bedtime (exception is bupropion in afternoon).
Headache	Evaluate diet, stress, other drugs used; suggest dosage reduction to health care provider.
Weight gain	Decrease carbohydrate intake; consume low-fat diet; exercise.

sensation experienced by the patient taking sertraline and other SSRIs. Nicotine intake from cigarette smoking may cause an increase in the metabolism of the sertraline and other SSRIs. The combined intake of an SSRI and another drug that enhances serotonergic neurotransmission, such as an MAOI, can cause a rare, life-threatening event called **serotonin syndrome.** This syndrome is believed to result from overactivation of the central serotonin receptors that leads to symptoms such as sweating, fever, increased blood pressure, tachycardia, abdominal pain, diarrhea, muscle spasm, increased motor activity, irritability, hostility, and altered mental state. In its most severe presentation, cardiovascular shock or even death may result. Table 17.4 summarizes potential drug interactions with sertraline.

Assessment of Relevant Core Patient Variables

Health Status

Review the patient's drug history for current drugs used, health history for any illnesses that may complicate therapy, and mental status. Assess for a history of seizures because SSRIs such as sertraline are used with caution in patients with such a history. The drug should be discontinued if seizures occur. Additionally, because anxiety, nervousness, and insomnia occur in 2% to 22% of patients treated with SSRIs, careful consideration should be given to the use of these antidepressants in patients who already exhibit one or more of these symptoms. SSRIs, such as sertraline, may not be the antidepressant drug class of choice for the extremely underweight depressed patient because approximately 3% to 9% of patients treated with SSRIs experience substantial weight loss. However, only rarely has weight loss required patients to discontinue therapy. Also, assess for the presence of suicidal ideation before starting therapy and closely monitor the patient for evidence of worsening depression or onset of suicidal ideation while receiving sertraline or other SSRIs. The most critical time to closely monitor the patient for behavioral changes is during the first few weeks of drug therapy.

Life Span and Gender

Consider the patient's age. Although some research indicates that this drug has been proved safe and effective for use in children (for some indications), this drug is not approved for use in children. When it is used in children, the pediatric dose is usually half that for adults because of children's smaller body size. Concern exists that sertraline may increase depression and risk for suicide in children. Again, whether the increased risk for suicide is related to the drug itself or to an increase in energy that enables action on suicidal thought is still under debate. Recommendations regarding the use of sertraline and other SSRIs in children may change. The risk for suicide is also present in adults.

The adverse effect profile in the elderly patient is similar to that in younger healthy adults. However, because of decreased clearance of the drug in the older patient, smaller doses and slower increases should be made when prescribing sertraline or other SSRIs.

Ask female patients of childbearing age whether they are pregnant, intend to become pregnant, or are breast-feeding. The FDA classifies sertraline in pregnancy risk category C. Use caution when prescribing SSRIs to women who are breast-feeding because some of the SSRIs are excreted into breast milk. A few infants have developed adverse effects while being breast-fed by women taking SSRIs. All of the adverse effects cleared easily, however, after the infants stopped receiving the breast milk.

Lifestyle, Diet, and Habits

The SSRIs can affect sexual functioning. Men may report delayed ejaculation or ejaculatory failure, whereas women may report the inability to achieve orgasm. However, sexual

COMMUNITY-BASED CONCERNS

Box 17.3 SSRI Use in Adolescents

Warnings were recently added to SSRI labels that an increased risk of suicidality may occur in all age groups receiving SSRI therapy for depression. This warning was the outcome of an FDA review of all SSRI clinical trials. The review was prompted by case reports of suicidality and suicide in adolescents receiving SSRIs. The adolescents in the anecdotal reports were not enrolled in any clinical trial nor were they hospitalized; they were treated in the community.

The American College of Neuropsychopharmacology, in its preliminary report of the task force on SSRIs and suicidal behavior in youth, stated several points. Existing research proving the safety and efficacy of SSRIs in treating children and adolescents with depression far outweighs the dangers suggested by the anecdotal reports. No other antidepressants have been shown to be safe for this population. The TCAs, particularly, have even been found to be harmful. Untreated depression presents a greater risk for suicide and suicidal ideation than treatment does.

The current debate is reminiscent of the one that arose when SSRIs were first used to treat depressed adults 10 years ago. At that time, similar reports emerged of adults in the community who received Prozac, the first SSRI, for depression and who subsequently became suicidal. Now, after years of adult use, SSRIs are considered the standard drug in combination with "talk therapy" (psychotherapy) for treating depression. A recent multisite study, involving a large number of adolescents who received Prozac and talk therapy for depression, further supports the safety of SSRIs and the effectiveness of this combination. There were no deaths, and the number of suicide attempts was too small to analyze statistically (March et al., 2004).

Any nurse involved with treating depressed adolescents and children in the community will reach one clear conclusion: **Safe and successful treatment of a depressed patient depends on much more than merely giving the correct dosage of an antidepressant.** Because most antidepressant drugs, but particularly SSRIs, are physically activating, the newly energized but still depressed patient must be kept safe. To achieve this outcome in the community, you must make two critical interventions: First, develop a trusting therapeutic relationship with the patient, to facilitate honest communication and education. This bond will encourage the patient to take active responsibility for his or her own safety. Second, involve the family or care providers in teaching about depression and antidepressant therapy, so that they too will be prepared to play an integral role in providing a safe environment for the patient. Although the increased risk of suicide is slight, it cannot be dismissed. All precautions must be taken to maintain the safety of the patient. There is much more to treating depressed patients in the community than suggesting that they just take a pill a day and be on their way.

functioning can also be adversely affected by the very depression that the SSRI is prescribed to treat. Therefore, a baseline assessment of sexual functioning should be performed before starting treatment with sertraline. Assess the normal use of caffeine in patients who will be starting sertraline because caffeine interacts with sertraline. Also, assess for alcohol use and determine whether or not the patient smokes cigarettes because these agents also interact with sertraline.

Culture and Inherited Traits

Consider the patient's cultural background. Some individuals with a polymorphism in the P-450 isoenzyme 2D6 may lack this enzyme and would therefore be poor drug metabolizers, have higher circulating drug doses, and could possibly experience adverse effects from the SSRIs, even at low doses. Research conducted by Lin and Poland (1995) identifies a range of differences found globally among various ethnic groups. Their finding suggests that poor metabolizing is least common in East Asians, followed by African Americans, then in Hispanics, with whites exhibiting this condition most frequently. For this reason, an East Asian patient may respond less than an African American patient, a Hispanic patient, or even a white patient, even if they all receive the same dose of an SSRI. More research is necessary, however, to confirm these findings. Also, Native Americans must be included in further studies because very few data exist for this group.

Nursing Diagnoses and Outcomes

- Risk for Suicide related to increased energy from sertraline without relief of suicidal ideations or low mood
  Desired outcome: *The patient will identify alternative coping mechanisms.*
- Restlessness related to psychomotor agitation secondary to sertraline use
  Desired outcome: *The patient will identify appropriate interventions to promote relaxation.*
- Sleep Pattern Disturbance: Less than Body Requirements related to psychomotor agitation secondary to sertraline use
  Desired outcome: *The patient will identify appropriate interventions to promote sleep.*
- Nausea, Abdominal Pain, or both related to abnormal peristalsis secondary to sertraline use
  Desired outcome: *The patient will report a decrease of nausea.*
- Diarrhea and Loose Stools related to adverse effects of medication secondary to sertraline use
  Desired outcome: *The patient will re-establish and maintain normal pattern of bowel functioning.*
- Sexual Dysfunction related to disrupted sexual response pattern, such as impotence or anorgasmia, secondary to sertraline use
  Desired outcome: *The patient will identify satisfying and acceptable sexual practices and some alternative ways of dealing with sexual expression.*

Planning and Intervention

Maximizing Therapeutic Effects

By the time patients begin drug therapy, they may be at their most hopeless state. This state sometimes can even be compounded by their initial response to the medication. Equally important to remember is that the patient does not experience the maximum therapeutic effect for several weeks. To maximize the therapeutic effect of antidepressant therapy, establish a therapeutic, trusting relationship with the patient by offering the hopeless patient hope for the future by being candid about the therapeutic effects and adverse effects of the medication. Properly administering the medication at regular times, without missing doses, is important as well.

Minimizing Adverse Effects

Remember that any possible adverse effects of sertraline often occur immediately or early in the treatment course.

TABLE 17.4 Agents That Interact With Sertraline

Interactants	Effect and Significance	Nursing Management
alcohol	Additive CNS depression may occur.	Monitor for adverse effects.
benzodiazepines	Decreased metabolism of benzodiazepines through hepatic oxidation route. Significance not known.	Monitor for adverse effects of benzodiazepines.
cimetidine	Increases half-life, AUC, and C_{max} of sertraline, but clinical significance is unknown.	Adjust sertraline doses as necessary.
clozapine	May elevate clozapine levels.	Monitor for adverse effects of clozapine.
cyproheptadine	May decrease or reverse pharmacologic effects of SSRIs.	Monitor for reduced efficacy of sertraline.
drugs metabolized by P-450 2D6	Sertraline or other SSRIs may substantially inhibit the activity of P-450 2D6 (especially during the beginning of therapy); metabolism of these other drugs may be reduced, potentially resulting in adverse effects.	Monitor for adverse effects. Lower doses of sertraline may be needed.
drugs that are highly protein bound	Because sertraline and other SSRIs are highly protein bound, sertraline may displace the other drug from the protein, causing increased circulating levels of the other drug and possibly adverse effects. If other drugs are started while the patient is on sertraline, the sertraline may be displaced from the protein, resulting in higher circulating levels of sertraline, and possibly adverse effects.	Monitor for adverse effects.
hydantoin	Sertraline may increase hydantoin levels.	Monitor for increased hydantoin levels.
MAOIs	Serotonin syndrome, with serious, sometimes fatal, reactions such as hyperthermia, rigidity, vital sign changes, mental status changes, and autonomic nervous system instability.	Avoid sertraline and other SSRIs when MAOIs are used and within 14 days of stopping an MAOI.
phenytoin	May increase phenytoin levels.	Monitor for adverse effects of phenytoin. Check blood phenytoin levels when starting therapy or changing dose of sertraline.
sumatriptan	Concurrent use increases serotonin levels, potentially leading to serotonin syndrome.	Avoid concurrent use.
sympathomimetic drugs	Increases sensitivity to the effects of sympathomimetics. Serotonin syndrome is more likely to occur.	Monitor for adverse effects.
tolbutamide	Coadministration has been shown to decrease the clearance of tolbutamide. Clinical significance unknown.	Monitor tolbutamide levels.
TCAs	May increase serum TCA levels.	Monitor for adverse effects. Monitor TCA blood levels. TCA dose may have to be reduced.
tryptophan	Concurrent use increases serotonin levels, potentially leading to serotonin syndrome.	Avoid concurrent use.
warfarin	Increases prothrombin time and may cause bleeding.	Monitor prothrombin time.

AUC, area under the curve; C_{max}, maximum concentration.

Restlessness or even insomnia may be reported by patients at the beginning of therapy. To minimize these effects, give the medication early in the day, when the patient will be most active and least likely to be bothered by such effects. The adverse effects of nausea and diarrhea can be minimized as well, by giving the medication with food or even by dividing the daily dose into more frequent, smaller doses. Carefully assess the patient on drug therapy for worsening of depression or signs of suicidal ideation. *Close monitoring of all patients, but especially children, is imperative to minimize the risk for suicide.* Closest monitoring needs to be done during the beginning of therapy and at each dose change. To further guard against suicide, sertraline and other SSRIs should be administered only in addition to counseling and therapy, not in its place.

To help the patient minimize any sexually related adverse effects, demonstrate a willingness to discuss these matters with the patient in an open and honest manner. Inquire about

any changes in sexual functioning because changes associated with medication use may lead to nonadherence to drug therapy. Patients should always be discouraged from consuming alcohol while undergoing sertraline therapy because increased central nervous system (CNS) depression may result. It is also important to protect the patient from ultraviolet light until his or her individual photosensitivity response is known. When a patient decides to stop use, the sertraline dose should be tapered rather than stopped abruptly. Consider the length of time the patient has been taking the medicine, the dosage, and the half-life of the drug to decrease any risk for **serotonin reuptake inhibitor withdrawal syndrome.** The symptoms of this syndrome can be remembered by using the mnemonic FLUSH (Preskorn, 1999):

Flu-like (e.g., fatigue, myalgia, loose stools, nausea)
Lightheadedness, dizziness, or both
Uneasiness, restlessness, or both
Sleep and sensory disturbances
Headache

Symptoms of sertraline toxicity or overdose are dilated pupils, tachycardia, electrocardiographic (ECG) changes, anxiousness with decreased level of consciousness, and vomiting. No deaths have been reported by overdose involving sertraline alone. However, a few fatalities have occurred when sertraline was mixed with alcohol or other drugs in a deliberate overdose. Management of overdose should include treating presenting symptoms. There are no specific antidotes. Activated charcoal may be as effective as emesis or lavage.

Providing Patient and Family Education

- Educate the patient and family about realistic expectations for antidepressant therapy. Include information about the delay in relief of symptoms and the necessity of continuing with the medication even after relief of symptoms is achieved.
- Educate the patient and family about potential suicidal ideation. The family needs special help to learn how to recognize behavioral changes that may indicate suicidal ideation because the patient may not recognize it in himself or herself.
- Emphasize the risk for SSRI withdrawal syndrome if the patient abruptly stops taking his or her medication.
- Inform the patient about possible adverse effects (such as nausea, restlessness, insomnia, sexual dysfunction) and advise the patient on how to minimize disruption to his or her lifestyle. Emphasize that adverse effects may occur before therapeutic effects and that many of them are transient.
- Discuss the increased stimulant effect that results when sertraline and caffeine are combined and advise the patient to modify the diet accordingly.
- Teach the patient to avoid alcohol and other CNS depressant drugs to avoid any cumulative depressant effect.
- Caution the patient about using heavy machinery or driving until individual response to the drug is known.

Ongoing Assessment and Evaluation

Continue to assess the patient's mood and observe any increase in anxiety, nervousness, restlessness, or insomnia. If the patient becomes physically energized yet experiences little improvement in mood, assess the patient especially closely for suicidal thoughts because he or she is at greater risk for acting on these thoughts under these conditions. Periodically monitor laboratory tests that assess liver function and measure total blood cholesterol and triglycerides to assess the patient for any possible changes. As sertraline therapy continues, expect patients to report an increased interest in their surroundings and more energy to participate in daily activities. Sertraline therapy is considered effective when depression is relieved and no serious adverse effects occur.

Drugs Significantly Different From [P] Sertraline

Bupropion

Bupropion (Wellbutrin) is a weak blocker of neuronal uptake of NE and 5-HT. It also inhibits, to some extent, neuronal reuptake of DA. Bupropion has the benefit of being somewhat energizing for patients with major depression. It also may be coadministered with other SSRIs to decrease the effect of the primary medication when sexual functioning is adversely affected. Although the usual dose is 300 mg/day, the risk for seizure may be four times greater when bupropion is given at doses between 300 and 450 mg/day. This risk further increases to almost 10 times greater when given at doses between 450 and 600 mg/day. Bupropion should be administered with caution to any patient who has an increased seizure risk. Missed doses should never be doubled; seizure may result.

Trazodone

Trazodone (Desyrel) is a weak serotonin transport inhibitor as well as a serotonin receptor ($5\text{-}HT_2$) blocker. This combination diminishes some troubling adverse effects associated with 5-HT transporter inhibitors, such as insomnia,

MEMORY CHIP

[P] Sertraline

- Selective serotonin reuptake inhibitor used to treat depression, obsessive-compulsive disorder, panic disorder, and post-traumatic stress disorder
- Major contraindications: Cautious use in patients with decreased liver or kidney function (lower the initial dose)
- Most common adverse effects: gastrointestinal distress, headache, sleep disturbance, and abnormal ejaculation
- Most serious adverse effect: may possibly increase the risk for suicide, especially in pediatric populations
- **Life span alert: pregnancy category C**
- Maximizing therapeutic effects: Encourage patient to continue medicine, even though immediate response does not occur, and continue medication well after an improvement is experienced.
- Minimizing adverse effects: Give with food; avoid ultraviolet light.
- Most important patient education: Teach that a lag time occurs between beginning therapy and relief of symptoms; avoid alcohol and drugs.

jitteriness, and sexual dysfunction. Trazodone is also an adrenergic receptor blocker that affects both alpha-1 and alpha-2 receptors, so it can cause dizziness and orthostatic changes. It is not recommended for use by patients during the initial recovery phase of a heart attack. Patients with preexisting cardiac disease should also be monitored closely, particularly for cardiac arrhythmias. Administered orally, the drug is well absorbed; food enhances its absorption. Therapeutic response usually occurs within 2 weeks. Metabolism in the liver is extensive; none of its metabolites is believed to be pharmacologically active. Trazodone may cause priapism, a prolonged and often painful penile erection rarely associated with sexual arousal.

Venlafaxine

Venlafaxine (Effexor) is a mixed NE and 5-HT reuptake inhibitor. It has no significant affinity for adrenergic receptor blockade (alpha-1 or alpha-2), H_1, or Ach receptors. Its pharmacologic effects are dose related, and it exhibits triphasic pharmacologic effects within its dosage range. At the lowest effective dose, venlafaxine primarily affects 5-HT reuptake. Its effects on NE and DA occur at higher concentrations (dosages of more than 300 mg/day). It may cause constipation, diaphoresis, dizziness, hypertension, nausea, nervousness, somnolence, and disturbance in sexual function. When increasing the dosage, gradual titration is important to maximize venlafaxine's therapeutic effect. Minimizing adverse effects may be accomplished by giving an extended-release formulation of venlafaxine (Effexor XR), which provides more stable plasma and CNS drug levels than the rapidly absorbed and rapidly eliminated immediate-release drug formulation.

(C) Tricyclic Antidepressants

The TCAs were named for their molecular structure, which features a three-ring nucleus. They are generally categorized as secondary or tertiary amines. Most secondary amines (e.g., desipramine, nortriptyline, and protriptyline) are better tolerated than tertiary amines (e.g., amitriptyline, clomipramine, doxepin, imipramine, and trimipramine). Although they are similar in treating depression, they differ in potency and selectivity. Patients taking tertiary amines generally experience an increased incidence of anticholinergic effects, cardiovascular adverse effects, and impaired memory and cognition. The tertiary amines have a very narrow therapeutic index; even a moderate overdose, such as a dose greater than 1 g, is toxic and can be fatal. These are a few of the reasons secondary amine tricyclics are preferred over the tertiary amine tricyclics.

All TCAs enhance the activity of NE and 5-HT by blocking neuronal reuptake of these neurotransmitters. Their lack of specificity affects other receptor systems and is associated with anticholinergic, neurologic, and cardiovascular adverse effects.

The prototype TCA is nortriptyline, a secondary amine. Although secondary amines do not have as many of the adverse effects of the tertiary amines, they do share the same potential for cardiovascular toxicity. It is because of this risk that the TCAs are not considered a first-choice treatment for depression.

NURSING MANAGEMENT OF THE PATIENT RECEIVING [P] NORTRIPTYLINE

Core Drug Knowledge

Pharmacotherapeutics

Nortriptyline (Pamelor) is used to relieve the symptoms of depression. It is also used off-label at dosages of 75 to 300 mg/day as adjunctive analgesia for phantom limb pain and chronic pain (such as in migraine, chronic tension headache, diabetic neuropathy, trigeminal neuralgia, cancer pain, painful peripheral neuropathy, postherpetic neuralgia, and arthritic pain) and for cocaine withdrawal, panic disorder, bulimia nervosa, and premenstrual syndrome.

Pharmacokinetics

Nortriptyline is well absorbed from the gastrointestinal tract, achieving peak plasma concentrations in 2 to 4 hours. It undergoes a substantial first-pass effect and is highly bound (more than 90%) to plasma proteins, lipid soluble, and widely distributed in tissues, including the CNS. Wide individual variation occurs in steady-state plasma levels at a given dosage, primarily because of differences in the rate of metabolism or first-pass effect. Effective dosage levels vary greatly and must be individualized. Metabolism of nortriptyline and the other TCAs occurs in the liver, through the P-450 enzyme system.

Pharmacodynamics

Nortriptyline specifically blocks reuptake of NE into nerve terminals, thereby allowing increased concentration at postsynaptic effector sites. The chemical structure and pharmacologic activity of nortriptyline resemble those of the phenothiazine antipsychotics (see Chapter 18). Three major pharmacologic actions of nortriptyline are blocking of the amine pump, sedation, and peripheral and central anticholinergic action. Other pharmacologic and clinical effects include inhibition of histamine, sedation, and mild peripheral vasodilator effects.

Contraindications and Precautions

Nortriptyline should be used with extreme caution in patients with cardiovascular disorders because of the possibility of conduction defects, arrhythmias, congestive heart failure, sinus tachycardia, myocardial infarction, stroke, and tachycardia. These patients require cardiac surveillance at all dosage levels of the drug. In high doses, nortriptyline may produce arrhythmias, sinus tachycardia conduction defects, and prolonged conduction time. Elderly patients and patients with a history of cardiac disease are at special risk for developing cardiac abnormalities. Patients with hyperthyroidism or those receiving thyroid medications require close supervision because of the possibility of cardiovascular toxicity, including arrhythmias.

Nortriptyline can slow cardiac conduction and cause arrhythmias. It is possible that a patient will be sensitive to any of the TCAs once he or she has developed sensitivity to one of them.

Because nortriptyline, like other TCAs, lowers the seizure threshold, it should be used with caution in patients with a history of seizures or other predisposing factors (e.g., brain damage of varying etiology, alcoholism, concomitant drugs known to lower the seizure threshold). However, seizures have also occurred following administration of TCAs to patients with no history of seizure disorders. Because of its anticholinergic effects, nortriptyline should be used with caution in patients with a history of urinary retention, glaucoma, or increased intraocular pressure because even an average dose may precipitate a recurrence. Human fetal risk has been demonstrated during clinical trials and postmarketing surveillance, which puts nortriptyline in pregnancy category D. With other TCAs such as amitriptyline and imipramine, there have been clinical reports of congenital malformations and limb-reduction anomalies.

Adverse Effects

Adverse effects are related to nortriptyline's effects on neurotransmitters. In comparison to drugs in this class that are tertiary amines, nortriptyline and other secondary-amine TCAs have less effect on the histamine, cholinergic, and alpha-1 adrenergic receptor sites. At usual therapeutic concentrations, they block NE reuptake. Patients report sedation and anticholinergic effects most frequently, although they usually develop tolerance to these effects. Other adverse effects include disturbed concentration and confusion (especially in older adults), headache, tremors, nausea, vomiting, bone marrow depression, urinary retention, sexual function disturbances, skin rash, nasal congestion, and weight gain. In agitated patients, increased anxiety or agitation may occur. Schizophrenic or paranoid patients may exhibit a worsening of their psychoses. Because photosensitivity may occur, patients receiving nortriptyline should avoid sun exposure or use protective measures to prevent skin reactions.

Nortriptyline can cause skin rashes or "drug fever" in susceptible individuals. These allergic reactions are rarely severe. They are most likely during the first few days of treatment but may also occur later. The drug should be discontinued if the patient develops rash or fever.

At the upper limit of the therapeutic range, serious and potentially life-threatening cardiac and CNS effects may begin to develop. Overdosage produces symptoms that are primarily an extension of the common adverse reactions. Cardiac irregularities, especially tachycardia and conduction disturbances, are common and create the most serious hazards. Fatal arrhythmias may occur as late as 56 hours after overdose. Other problems include metabolic acidosis, respiratory depression, seizures, and extremely high fever (McEvoy et al., 2002). Box 17.4 describes emergency measures for TCA overdose.

Drug Interactions

Nortriptyline is associated with multiple drug interactions because it, like other TCAs, is metabolized through the P-450 liver enzyme system. Drugs with potential for interaction with nortriptyline include sedative-hypnotics, alcohol, antihypertensives, antiarrhythmics, and anticholinergics. Nortriptyline and other highly protein-bound substances, such as aspirin, phenytoin, and phenothiazines, may compete for binding sites. Other drugs, such as methylphenidate, oral contraceptives, and antipsychotics, may interfere with the metabolism of nortriptyline. Nortriptyline may prevent the antihypertensive action of some drugs by their primary and secondary effects at the NE synapses. Administering nortriptyline with an MAOI may result in severe CNS toxicity. Nortriptyline potentiates the sedative effects of alcohol. Table 17.5 summarizes interactions that can occur with nortriptyline.

BOX 17.4 Emergency Measures for TCA Overdose

- Provide symptomatic and supportive care.
- Monitor cardiac changes continually.
- Administer phenytoin, lidocaine, or propranolol as prescribed for life-threatening cardiac arrhythmias.
- Avoid giving drugs such as quinidine, procainamide, and disopyramide. These agents depress myocardial conductivity and contractility.
- Reserve administration of the cholinergic agonist physostigmine for life-threatening, refractory anticholinergic symptoms.

Assessment of Relevant Core Patient Variables

Health Status

Assess patients for pre-existing cardiovascular disease because these patients are especially sensitive to the potential cardiotoxicity of nortriptyline. Patients should be carefully assessed for a history of seizure activity or organic brain disease because nortriptyline lowers the seizure threshold.

Life Span and Gender

Consider age-related factors associated with nortriptyline therapy. Lower dosages are recommended for adolescents and older adults. The dosage should be increased slowly depending on the clinical response and any evidence of intolerance.

Children are especially susceptible to the cardiotoxic and seizure-inducing effects of high doses of nortriptyline. Because of these safety issues and the uncertain benefit to children and adolescents, other types of antidepressants should be considered before nortriptyline or other TCAs (Geller et al., 1999). Elderly patients may be especially sensitive to the anticholinergic adverse effects of nortriptyline, and this sensitivity can result in confusion, disorientation, delusions, and hallucinations. The combination of these symptoms can continue to worsen, to the extent that the patient even becomes delirious. Older adults may be at an increased risk for falls during drug therapy with nortriptyline.

Assess the woman of childbearing age for pregnancy or intention to become pregnant because the safety of nortriptyline during pregnancy has not been established. Therefore, it should be used only when potential benefits to the mother outweigh potential hazards to the fetus. Also, ask if a female patient is breast-feeding because TCAs are excreted into breast milk in low concentrations.

Lifestyle, Diet, and Habits

Adverse effects of nortriptyline can be very similar to the symptoms of depression. For this reason, it is important evaluate the patient's symptoms within the context of his or her lifestyle before starting nortriptyline therapy.

TABLE 17.5 Agents That Interact With P Nortriptyline

Interactants	Effect and Significance	Nursing Management
alcohol	Increased sedative effects	Avoid coadministration
anticholinergic agents	Increased anticholinergic effects	Assess patient for increasing tachycardia, dry mouth, blurred vision, constipation, and urinary retention. Coadminister with caution.
barbiturates	Decreased serum concentration of nortriptyline Potential additive CNS depression	Anticipate need for increase in nortriptyline dosage. Institute safety measures. Monitor neurologic status closely.
cimetidine, haloperidol, SSRIs	Increased plasma concentration of nortriptyline	Monitor serum levels as appropriate. Assess for signs of nortriptyline toxicity.
clonidine	Increased risk for hypertension and hypertensive crisis	Monitor blood pressure closely. Avoid coadministration.
dicumarol	Increased anticoagulant effects	Assess for signs and symptoms of bleeding. Anticipate need for decreased dosage of dicumarol. Avoid coadministration.
guanethidine	Antagonism of guanethidine action	Monitor blood pressure closely.
disulfiram	Increased risk for organic brain syndrome Increased effect of nortriptyline	Avoid coadministration.
levodopa	Delayed levodopa absorption and decreased bioavailability	Assess for therapeutic effects of both drugs.
MAOIs	Hyperpyrexia, sweating, confusion, seizures, tachycardia, tachypnea, hypotension, coma, DIC, and death	Avoid coadministration. Discontinue MAOIs 7–10 days before starting nortriptyline.
oral contraceptives, phenothiazines	Inhibition of hepatic enzyme system metabolism of nortriptyline leading to increased plasma levels	Monitor for signs and symptoms of nortriptyline toxicity.

Ask the patient whether he or she performs activities that require mental alertness, manual dexterity, or motor coordination. Nortriptyline may impair concentration and coordination; hence, the patient receiving nortriptyline should perform such activities with caution until actual drug effects on the individual are known.

Photosensitivity may also develop as a result of nortriptyline therapy. Patients whose lifestyles expose them to the outdoors need to protect themselves from overexposure to sunlight.

Culture and Inherited Traits

Keep in mind inherited traits relevant to therapy with nortriptyline. Very little published information exists concerning differences in antidepressant pharmacology among African Americans, Hispanic Americans, and white Americans of European descent (Wood & Zhou, 1991); however, some studies have suggested that ethnicity influences the pharmacokinetics, pharmacotherapeutics, and pharmacodynamics of **psychotropic** drugs (agents that affect the mind, emotions, or behavior). For example, results of one study showed that plasma nortriptyline levels were 50% higher in African American patients than in white Americans. Another reported that Hispanic American patients have greater sensitivity than others to the anticholinergic effects of tricyclics and therefore require a lower dosage. Collected survey data from multiple Asian countries indicated that imipramine and amitriptyline dosages were much lower than those customary in the United States, suggesting that Asians achieve significantly higher plasma concentrations of tricyclics and have lower clearance rates than whites. Although these studies have been criticized for improper control of independent variables, such as dosage for body weight or smoking and even diet or alcohol consumption, it is prudent to give some consideration to a patient's ethnic background until more conclusive studies prove otherwise (Wood & Zhou, 1991).

Nursing Diagnoses and Outcomes

Several nursing diagnoses may apply to the depressed patient receiving nortriptyline therapy. Examples include:

- Constipation or Diarrhea related to medication use
  Desired outcome: *The patient will establish normal bowel habits.*
- Disturbed Sleep Pattern related to medication-induced somnolence or insomnia
  Desired outcome: *The patient will report a satisfactory balance of rest and activity.*

In addition to these, selected nursing diagnoses for treatment with nortriptyline include the following:

- Risk for Poisoning related to TCA toxicity
  Desired outcome: *The patient will identify factors that increase the risk for and verbalize practices to prevent poisoning.*

- Risk for Injury related to adverse effects (e.g., blurred vision, drowsiness, and hypotension) secondary to nortriptyline use
  Desired outcome: *The patient will identify factors that increase the risk for and relate intent to practice safety measures to prevent injury.*
- Imbalanced Nutrition: More than Body Requirements related to adverse effects of nortriptyline
  Desired outcome: *The patient will verbalize reasons for a risk for weight gain, identify normal nutritional needs, and discuss methods to control weight.*
- Disturbed Sensory Perception related to chemical alterations secondary to nortriptyline therapy
  Desired outcome: *The patient will experience normal sensory perception.*

Planning and Intervention

Maximizing Therapeutic Effects

A single daily dose of nortriptyline may be used for maintenance therapy. A single daily dose at bedtime, if convenient, will minimize the daytime adverse effect of sedation. The sedative effect at bedtime may be beneficial in patients with concomitant sleep disorders.

Use therapeutic drug monitoring to monitor effective plasma drug levels to achieve the greatest likelihood of antidepressant response and the smallest risk for adverse effects. Optimal serum concentrations for nortriptyline are 50 to 150 ng/mL.

Following remission, the patient may require maintenance medication for a longer time at the lowest dose that will maintain remission. Maintenance therapy should continue for at least 3 months to decrease the possibility of relapse.

Minimizing Adverse Effects

Although the half-life of nortriptyline is long enough to permit single daily dosing, adverse reactions may require divided dosing schedules. Because older adults have an increased risk for experiencing adverse effects, they should receive initial doses equivalent to one half to one third of the dose administered to younger adults. Ultimately, elderly patients may benefit by receiving nortriptyline in split doses because they may be unable to tolerate single daily doses. Regular ECG monitoring of cardiac rhythm is essential for any individual taking nortriptyline. Therapy may induce neutropenia; clinical indicators such as fever or sore throat may signal serious neutrophil depression, and therapy should be discontinued if such evidence of pathologic neutropenia occurs. In addition to serum levels of the drug, blood studies, including a complete blood count with differential, serum glucose level, and renal and hepatic function should be monitored periodically. Monitoring helps detect adverse effects so that intervention can occur before interrupted drug therapy or nonadherence compromises the therapeutic effect. Patients with glaucoma are closely monitored during drug therapy because nortriptyline may precipitate an acute episode of angle-closure glaucoma. As with all antidepressant therapy, continue assessing the patient for low mood and suicidal thoughts. When a patient is most depressed, he or she may have thoughts of suicide but at the same time may not have enough energy or concentration to plan and follow through on these thoughts. However, the risk for suicide increases if the suicidal thoughts remain while the patient's concentration and energy improve to the point at which he or she can act on the suicidal thoughts. This fact is particularly important with the patient taking TCAs because the very drug taken to treat the depression can also be taken in a lethal dose to commit suicide. The patient's safety can be increased by closely monitoring the number of pills that are accessible to him or her.

Providing Patient and Family Education

- Teach the patient and family that the therapeutic response will not be immediate. Several weeks may pass before any measurable clinical effect is noted. The symptoms of depression may come and go during the earliest stages of treatment. If this possibility is not discussed, patients may become even more hopeless, thinking that they will never be symptom free. Also, discuss the ongoing risk for suicide with the patient and the patient's family.
- It is also important to teach the patient about the need to continue with nortriptyline therapy even after initial relief of depressive symptoms. Inform the patient that stopping the medication at this time will most likely result in a relapse of the depressive symptoms.
- Stress the importance of taking the drug exactly as prescribed and of not stopping the drug abruptly or without consulting with the health care provider. Abrupt discontinuation may cause nausea, headache, and malaise.
- Help the patient stay motivated to continue treatment. To promote adherence to the therapeutic regimen, educate the patient and family about the medication effects—both therapeutic and adverse. Advise the patient about adverse effects that, if unexplained, may contribute to nonadherence. These effects include sweating, weight gain, and sexual dysfunction.
- Warn the patient of the possibility of photosensitivity reactions. Advise the patient to avoid prolonged exposure to sunlight or bright artificial light, to apply sunscreen before exposure, and to wear protective clothing.
- Emphasize the importance of keeping the drug safely stored and away from curious children. Children are very susceptible to nortriptyline-induced cardiotoxicity.
- Caution the patient to avoid operating machinery, driving a vehicle, or engaging in activities that require focus and concentration until the patient is aware of his or her own individual response to the medication. Most antidepressants cause some degree of sedation and may impair mental alertness and physical coordination. Because certain drug combinations produce an additive CNS depressant effect, patients should not use antidepressants concurrently with alcohol or sleep-inducing drugs such as sedative-hypnotics.
- Advise the patient to wear or carry medical identification, such as a Medic Alert tag, regarding antidepressant therapy because nortriptyline can interact with many other drugs.

Ongoing Assessment and Evaluation

Continually assess depressed patients for suicidal thoughts during nortriptyline therapy. As with all antidepressant therapy, the depressed patient with suicidal thoughts is at greatest risk for self-harm once he or she has become sufficiently energized to act on the thoughts. Because of the potential for

drug-related toxicity to the heart, all patients, particularly those receiving higher than usual dosages of nortriptyline or other TCAs, should have periodic ECG examinations regardless of normal cardiac functioning before treatment. Patients with pre-existing cardiovascular disease should be closely monitored, with ECG tracings performed routinely.

Patients on multidrug therapies should be monitored for other effects as well because other drugs, such as antihypertensives, alcohol, and therapeutic hormones, may cause depression.

Obtain baseline and periodic laboratory blood tests to monitor leukocyte counts, differential blood cell counts, and liver function studies. Also, monitor drug serum levels to ensure that therapeutic levels are maintained. Nortriptyline therapy is considered effective when depression is relieved and adverse effects either do not occur or are minimal.

Ⓒ Monoamine Oxidase Inhibitors

The monoamine oxidase enzyme system is widely distributed throughout the body. This system is responsible for metabolizing amines such as DA, epinephrine, NE, and 5-HT. Drugs described as MAOIs inhibit monoamine oxidase enzymes, thereby increasing the concentration of those amines.

There are two subtypes of monoamine oxidase. Monoamine oxidase A, found primarily in the GI tract, liver, and peripheral adrenergic nerves, predominantly metabolizes NE, 5-HT, and tyramine. Monoamine oxidase B, found in the brain, primarily metabolizes DA. Although the precise antidepressant mechanism of MAOIs is unclear, it is thought that the increases in NE and 5-HT or changes in other amine concentrations in the CNS are responsible.

MAOIs were initially used to manage tuberculosis. It was observed that patients taking these drugs often experienced an elevation in their mood and hypotension. Although they are effective as antidepressants and antihypertensives, their use is limited by their potential to cause intense adverse effects and potentially fatal interactions, such as hypertensive crisis. Potentially fatal pharmacodynamic drug–drug interactions can occur with MAOIs when they are combined with a variety of drugs that are NE or 5-HT agonists or with foods rich in tyramine, such as cured or fermented foods, aged cheeses, red wine (especially Chianti), coffee, and soy sauce. Generally, any high-protein food that is aged should be avoided. Because MAOIs are irreversible inhibitors of monoamine oxidase, up to 2 weeks may be required for normal amine metabolism to be restored once the drug is discontinued.

In general, nonselective MAOIs are indicated for patients who are unresponsive to other antidepressant pharmacotherapy. They are rarely first-choice drugs. The prototype MAOI is phenelzine (Nardil).

MEMORY CHIP

[P] Nortriptyline

- Tricyclic secondary amine antidepressant used to treat symptoms of depression
- Major contraindications: cautious use in patients with pre-existing cardiovascular disease
- Most common adverse effect: drowsiness, dry mouth, constipation, hypotension
- Most serious adverse effect: arrhythmias caused by changes in atrioventricular conduction
- **Life span alert: not recommended for children; decrease or divide the dosage for elderly patients**
- Maximizing therapeutic effects: Maintain a therapeutic serum plasma level; continue therapy at least 3 months to prevent relapse.
- Minimizing adverse effects: Give entire dose at bedtime to decrease drowsiness.
- Most important patient education: Symptom relief is not immediate and may take several weeks; when symptoms are relieved, medication must be continued.

NURSING MANAGEMENT OF THE PATIENT RECEIVING [P] PHENELZINE

Core Drug Knowledge

Pharmacotherapeutics

Phenelzine is used mainly to treat depression that is unresponsive to other drug therapy or treatments. Patients may have mixed anxiety and depression with phobic or hypochondriacal features. In some cases, phenelzine is used to treat bulimia, cocaine addiction, and panic disorder associated with agoraphobia.

Pharmacokinetics

Phenelzine appears to be well absorbed following oral administration, and peak levels of phenelzine are reached in 2 to 4 hours. However, maximum inhibition of phenelzine does not occur for 5 to 10 days. Antidepressant action can take from 7 days to 8 weeks. Phenelzine is excreted in the urine, mostly as metabolites.

Half-life is fairly short and unrelated to the length of enzyme inhibition, which is prolonged: The clinical effects of phenelzine may continue for up to 2 weeks after therapy is discontinued.

Pharmacodynamics

Phenelzine increases the concentrations of DA, NE, and serotonin within the neuronal synapse because it inhibits the enzyme monoamine oxidase. Phenelzine, a hydrazine derivative, irreversibly inhibits both monoamine oxidase A and monoamine oxidase B.

Contraindications and Precautions

Poor liver function is a contraindication for using phenelzine because hydrazine compounds damage the functional tissues of the liver. Phenelzine is also contraindicated in patients with congestive heart failure. Cautious use is advised in patients with ischemic heart disease or a history of stroke or myocardial infarction because phenelzine may produce cardiovascular depressing effects, such as orthostatic hypotension, bradycardia, and decreased contractility of the heart muscle.

Adverse Effects

Toxic drug levels, which may damage the liver, can occur and appear to be unrelated to phenelzine dosage or treatment duration. Other adverse effects are anticholinergic, including blurred vision, constipation, and dry mouth. These effects are more pronounced at dosages above 45 mg/day. CNS-related adverse effects include akathisia, ataxia, dizziness, drowsiness, headache, insomnia, and nystagmus. Adverse effects related to other systems include agranulocytosis, anemia, leukopenia, thrombocytopenia, sexual function disturbances, and urinary retention.

The most serious adverse reactions involve changes in blood pressure and hypertensive crisis. Use of these drugs in elderly or debilitated patients or in patients with hypertension, cardiovascular problems, or cerebrovascular disease is inadvisable.

Drug Interactions

Pseudoephedrine and phenylpropanolamine, which are examples of mixed-acting sympathomimetics, are common ingredients in over-the-counter (OTC) decongestants, appetite suppressants, and weight-loss products. They release NE from adrenergic nerve endings. The indirect-acting sympathomimetics also trigger NE release. Acute, severe, and potentially fatal hypertensive crises are possible when combining phenelzine with drugs from either of these classes, tyramine, or tryptophan. Table 17.6 lists drugs that can interact with phenelzine.

TABLE 17.6 Agents That Interact With P Phenelzine

Interactants	Effect and Significance	Nursing Management
anesthetics	Adverse cardiovascular effects from sympathetic stimulation	Monitor heart rate, rhythm, and blood pressure for adverse effect from sympathetic stimulation.
antihypertensives (e.g., guanethidine, methyldopa)	Loss of antihypertensive effects	Monitor blood pressure for degree of control.
beta-adrenergic blockers	Bradycardia possible during concurrent use of MAOIs and beta adrenergic blockers	Monitor heart rate, rhythm, and cardiac output for adverse effect from bradycardia.
dextromethorphan	Hyperpyrexia, hypotension, and death associated with this combination*	Caution patients taking MAOIs to avoid OTC cold and cough preparations.
levodopa	Hypertensive reactions with combinations of levodopa and MAOIs	Avoid concurrent administration. Monitor cardiovascular status for adverse effect.
L-tryptophan	Coadministration resulting in hyperreflexia, confusion, disorientation, amnesia, ataxia, and Babinski signs	Caution the patient taking MAOIs to avoid food supplements, herbal/homeopathic, or home remedies without approval from the health care provider.
meperidine	Coadministration may result in agitation, seizures, fever, apnea, and death with possible adverse reactions weeks after MAOI withdrawal	Avoid concomitant administration of MAOIs and meperidine. For analgesia, administer other narcotic analgesics with caution.
SSRI, TCA, or venlafaxine antidepressants	Potential serious (occasionally fatal) reactions, including hyperthermia, rigidity, autonomic instability with labile blood pressure, myoclonus, and extreme agitation	Monitor neurologic and cardiovascular status for adverse effect.
sulfonamide compounds	Coadministration may cause either sulfonamide or MAOI toxicity	Avoid concurrent administration.
sulfonylurea antidiabetic agents	Possible potentiation of hypoglycemic response and delayed recovery from hypoglycemia	Monitor patients with diabetes for level of control and incidence of hypoglycemic episodes.
sumatriptan	Coadministration may cause sumatriptan toxicity	Avoid concurrent administration.
sympathomimetics (mixed acting or indirect acting, including anorexiants)	MAOI potentiation of sympathomimetic substances may cause severe headache, hypertension, hyperpyrexia possibly resulting in hypertensive crisis	Avoid concurrent administration.†
thiazide diuretics	Exaggerated hypotensive effects may result from concurrent use	Avoid concurrent administration. Monitor cardiovascular status and blood pressure for degree of control.

*Interaction inconclusive due to lack of adequate patient data.

†Direct-acting agents appear to interact minimally (if at all).

These drug–drug or drug–food interactions occur because phenelzine and the other agents act in peripheral adrenergic nerve endings to increase the buildup of NE, although they prevent the release of NE in response to normal nerve activity. When phenelzine is combined with the mixed-acting and indirect-acting sympathomimetics, however, NE release is not inhibited. The result is an intense adrenergic response because of the extra supply of NE. Ingesting a tyramine-containing food or a sympathomimetic drug may precipitate a hypertensive crisis. Normally, monoamine oxidase enzymes in the liver metabolize these substances rapidly. However, when monoamine oxidase enzymes are inhibited, tyramine metabolism decreases and triggers the release of accumulated NE, triggering a hypertensive episode. The earliest symptom may be a severe headache. The necessity of avoiding these substances to prevent a life-threatening hypertensive crisis is the major limitation of MAOIs. Box 17.5 lists the tyramine-rich foods that should be avoided by patients taking MAOIs.

BOX 17.5 The MAOI Diet

General Guidelines

- Eat fresh, freshly cooked, or canned foods.
- Avoid foods and beverages that are aged, salted, smoked, pickled, or fermented and those that are stored for a long time.

High-Tyramine Foods

Do not consume.

Alcohol: ales, beers, Burgundy or Chianti wine, sherry, vermouth
Bread: homemade, high-yeast, or made with aged cheeses, meats, or yeast extracts
Dairy products: aged or processed cheeses, such as cheddars, Swiss cheese, blue cheeses, Camembert, and cheese spreads
Fruit: banana peels; overripe or spoiled fruits
Meat and other proteins: aged, dried, cured meats, including jerkies; dried or pickled fish; leftovers that may be partly fermented; liver; meat extracts; salami or other dry sausages; game; any salted, smoked, or pickled meat or fish
Vegetables: fava bean pods, Italian or broad green beans, kim chee (fermented cabbage), lentils, lima beans, sauerkraut
Other: brewer's yeast, bouillon or broth with yeast, commercially prepared gravies, crackers made with cheese, Marmite and other yeast spreads, miso (fermented soybean paste) and soy sauce, yeast extracts

Moderate-Tyramine Foods

Consume no more than ¼ to ½ cup total each day.

Beverages: bouillon, distilled liquors; red (other than Burgundy or Chianti), white, and port wines
Breads: commercial breads without, or low in, yeast
Dairy products: cultured products such as buttermilk, sour cream, yogurt; unpasteurized milk products
Fruits: avocados, raspberries, red plums
Meat and other proteins: fish roe and caviar, meat pâtés, peanuts
Vegetables: Chinese pea pods, spinach
Other: limit intake of coffee, tea, colas (no more than 2 cups total per day); chocolate products (1 small serving per day); monosodium glutamate (MSG); teriyaki sauce (2–4 Tbsp per day)

Assessment of Relevant Core Patient Variables

Health Status

Perform a baseline cardiovascular assessment and complete blood count and liver function tests for the patient taking phenelzine. Assess the patient's orientation, mood, and affect because phenelzine may cause memory and emotional changes, irritability, and nervousness.

Life Span and Gender

Consider the patient's age and its relation to phenelzine therapy. Phenelzine is not recommended for patients younger than 16 years. Because patients older than 60 years may be more prone to adverse drug effects, their dosages (<60 mg/day) should be increased gradually and adjusted accordingly.

Ask the woman of childbearing age if she is pregnant, intends to become pregnant, or is breast-feeding. Phenelzine is in FDA pregnancy category C. It crosses the placenta and enters breast milk.

Lifestyle, Diet, and Habits

Assess the patient's lifestyle to determine whether he or she performs activities requiring alertness, physical coordination, or manual dexterity. Because of possible associated adverse effects such as ataxia, drowsiness, and blurred vision, patients need to exercise caution when driving or operating machinery. Also, evaluate the patient's nutritional status. Pyridoxine deficiency, frequently observed as numbness and swelling, is associated with phenelzine use. For this reason, the patient may need a pyridoxine (vitamin B_6) supplement. Ask the patient about his or her participation in outdoor activity because phenelzine may cause photosensitivity. The patient should wear sunscreen and protective clothing in prolonged outdoor exposure, such as recreational or occupational pursuits. Assess the patient for willingness to adhere to the dietary restrictions required with phenelzine therapy. Assess for use of herbal preparations such as St. John's wort, L-tryptophan, and ginseng because they can interact with phenelzine.

Environment

Consider the environment in which phenelzine will be administered. The drug should be kept in a tightly closed container away from light and heat.

Culture and Inherited Traits

Consider the patient's ethnic background when beginning drug therapy with phenelzine. Acetylation inactivates phenelzine and its metabolites. About one half of Americans and Europeans (and more in Asia) are slow acetylators of hydrazine-type drugs, including phenelzine. This fact may contribute to the exaggerated effects observed in some patients who receive standard doses of phenelzine (Hardman, 2001).

Nursing Diagnoses and Outcomes

- Risk for Injury related to drug–nutrient, drug–drug, or drug–environment interactions or hypertensive crisis secondary to phenelzine antidepressant therapy

Desired outcome: The patient will remain safe and injury free during drug therapy.

- Ineffective Therapeutic Regimen Management related to MAOI-required dietary restrictions
  Desired outcome: *The patient will acknowledge an understanding of the need to follow a low-tyramine diet and demonstrate appropriate dietary choices.*
- Imbalanced Nutrition: More than Body Requirements related to adverse effect of phenelzine
  Desired outcome: *The patient will understand and acknowledge the risk for weight gain, identify normal nutritional needs, and discuss methods to control weight.*

Planning and Intervention

Maximizing Therapeutic Effects

Before phenelzine therapy is initiated, platelet monoamine oxidase enzyme activity (mostly B subtype) is usually measured. After therapy is underway, an inhibition of more than 85% is associated with therapeutic response (Hardman, 2001). Platelet enzyme inhibition exceeding 95%, however, increases the risk for serious drug and food interactions.

Minimizing Adverse Effects

The primary difficulties with phenelzine are the numerous dietary and medication restrictions that the patient must obey to avoid drug–food and drug–drug interactions. Taking phenelzine with foods high in tyramine or with certain drugs (e.g., ephedrine, dextromethorphan, cocaine, decongestants, appetite suppressants) increases the potential for a hypertensive crisis. The symptoms of hypertensive crisis include severe occipital headache, stiff neck, nausea, vomiting, diaphoresis, and extremely elevated systolic and diastolic blood pressure.

Advise the patient to avoid herbal preparations such as St. John's wort, L-tryptophan, and ginseng because they can interact with MAOIs. Encourage the patient to consult with the prescriber of the medication before using any OTC products. Alcohol (especially beer, ale, sherry, and Chianti wine), stimulants, and illicit drugs should never be used because they increase the likelihood of adverse effects or hypertensive crisis. Dosages exceeding 30 mg/day may result in postural hypotension, leading to syncope. If dosage increases are necessary, they should be made gradually. Other measures to minimize adverse effects include maintaining a tyramine-restricted diet during and for at least 2 weeks after phenelzine therapy and giving the drug with food or milk if gastrointestinal discomfort is problematic. If the patient has been on fluoxetine therapy, at least 6 weeks should elapse before phenelzine therapy begins.

Providing Patient and Family Education

- Warn all patients taking phenelzine against eating foods with high tyramine content or consuming alcohol during and for 2 weeks following phenelzine treatment. Ensure that the patient taking phenelzine understands and follows the special required dietary guidelines. Any high-protein food that is aged has the potential to produce a hypertensive crisis in patients taking phenelzine.
- Caution patients against self-medication with certain proprietary agents such as cold, hay fever, or weight-reduction preparations containing sympathomimetic amines while undergoing phenelzine therapy.
- Instruct patients not to consume excessive amounts of caffeine in any form.
- Stress the importance of not discontinuing the medication, adjusting dosage, or ingesting any other medication, even OTC preparations, except on the advice of the prescriber. Alert the patient that phenelzine may cause drowsiness or blurred vision and warn him or her to exercise caution when driving or performing other tasks that require alertness, coordination, or physical dexterity until effects of the drug are known.
- Alert the patient to the possibility of dizziness, weakness, or fainting when arising from a sitting position.
- Emphasize to the patient and family that antidepressant effects may be delayed a few weeks. Caution them to notify the health care provider if the patient develops severe headache, palpitation, tachycardia, a sense of constriction in the throat or chest, sweating, dizziness, neck stiffness, nausea, vomiting, or other unusual symptoms.

Ongoing Assessment and Evaluation

Observation of the patient is necessary to identify the therapeutic effects of phenelzine. These effects may occur within 7 days after therapy begins, although in some patients, a therapeutic response may not occur for up to 6 to 8 weeks. Effectiveness of phenelzine is demonstrated by improved mood and increased social activity in depressed patients. The patient's appetite, energy, and sleep pattern will improve as well.

During therapy, blood pressure should be monitored frequently to detect any abnormal response. Periodic liver function tests, such as aspartate transaminase, alanine transaminase, and bilirubin, should be performed. Phenelzine should be discontinued at the first sign of liver failure. Therapy should be discontinued immediately if the patient reports palpitations or frequent headaches because these signs may signal a hypertensive crisis. Drug therapy with phenelzine is considered effective if depression is alleviated and serious adverse effects are avoided.

MEMORY CHIP

P Phenelzine

- Monoamine oxidase inhibitor used to treat depression unresponsive to other treatments or drug therapy
- Major contraindications: congestive heart failure, impaired liver or kidney function
- Most common adverse effects: restlessness, orthostatic hypotension, blurred vision
- Most serious adverse effects: hypertensive crisis
- **Life span alert: Avoid giving to children 16 and younger; reduce dosage for older adults.**
- Maximizing therapeutic effects: Platelet monoamine oxidase inhibition activity should be monitored to achieve a goal between 85% and 95%.
- Minimizing adverse effects: Avoid tyramine-rich foods and over-the-counter cold remedies with dextromethorphan.
- Most important patient education: Adhere strictly to a tyramine-free diet (MAOI diet) during and 2 weeks after medication is stopped; antidepressant effect may take several weeks, take only as prescribed and do not stop abruptly.

MOOD STABILIZERS

When a person has been diagnosed with bipolar disorder and is experiencing a manic episode, he or she will be treated with drugs that are categorized as mood stabilizers. Treatment with these drugs decreases the extreme range of mood experienced by the patient. In addition to mood, a manic episode also increases energy and disorganizes cognition.

Lithium carbonate (Eskalith), usually simply called lithium, is the prototype mood stabilizing or antimanic drug. Other drugs used to treat bipolar disorder and stabilize mood include carbamazepine, gabapentin, and valproic acid. These drugs may be combined with lithium for a greater therapeutic effect.

NURSING MANAGEMENT OF THE PATIENT RECEIVING [P] LITHIUM

Core Drug Knowledge

Pharmacotherapeutics

Lithium is called a mood stabilizer because its primary action is to prevent extreme mood swings. The drug also has several unlabeled uses. It increases the neutrophil count in patients with cancer chemotherapy-induced neutropenia and in patients with acquired immunodeficiency syndrome (AIDS) who receive zidovudine therapy. It also is useful in preventing cluster headache and in treating bulimia, alcoholism, and postpartum-affective and corticosteroid-induced psychoses. The therapeutic range for lithium is 0.5 to 1.2 mEq/L.

Pharmacokinetics

The intestinal tract provides nearly complete absorption of lithium within 6 hours. Food does not substantially slow absorption. Peak plasma levels occur in 0.5 to 3 hours, and plasma half-life is about 20 hours. Onset of action is slow (5–7 days, with full therapeutic effects established in 10–21 days). Lithium is not protein bound or biotransformed into metabolites. Excretion occurs almost entirely in the urine (95%) and varies with pregnancy, age, and renal status. Lithium and sodium compete for resorption in the proximal renal tubule, where 80% of lithium is reabsorbed. Many factors, such as sodium imbalance, dehydration, or diuretic use, can affect lithium clearance because of the competition between lithium and sodium for resorption. Dose-related adverse effects are not usually serious if serum levels are maintained below 1.5 mEq/L.

Distribution approximates total body water and is complete within 6 to 10 hours. Higher concentrations occur in the bones, thyroid gland, and portions of the brain than in the serum. Although distribution across the blood–brain barrier is slow, the cerebrospinal fluid level is 40% of the plasma concentration. Elimination half-life is 24 hours, with a range between 10 and 50 hours. A steady state is reached after 5 to 7 days without dose changes.

Pharmacodynamics

Lithium competes with calcium, magnesium, potassium, and sodium in body tissues and at binding sites. It alters sodium transport in nerve and muscle cells. It also affects the synthesis, storage, release, and reuptake of central monoamine neurotransmitters, including acetylcholine, DA, gamma-aminobutyric acid, NE, and 5-HT. Although the contributions of these effects are uncertain, its antimanic effects are thought to result from increases in NE reuptake and increased serotonin receptor sensitivity. Lithium has a very narrow therapeutic index.

Contraindications and Precautions

Lithium is contraindicated in patients with severe cardiovascular or renal disease and in patients who are pregnant or breast-feeding.

Adverse Effects

The adverse effects of lithium can be classified as acute, chronic, and toxic. Acute effects include increased thirst, nausea, increased urination, and a fine hand tremor. Chronic adverse effects include increased urination, weight gain, hair loss, acne, and cognitive impairment. Low thyroid function and lack of kidney response to antidiuretic hormones may also occur in patients receiving long-term lithium therapy. However, discontinuing lithium treatment reverses these effects. Long-term lithium therapy (exceeding 10 years) commonly impairs the ability of the kidneys to concentrate urine, although this effect is not associated with a reduced glomerular filtration rate or with renal insufficiency. Lithium toxicity is dose related; the higher the circulating blood level of lithium, the more likely the patient will experience adverse effects and toxicity. The most serious effects occur when serum concentrations exceed 2 mEq/L, although some patients may experience toxicity even if their serum drug measurements are considered to be in the normal range. Early symptoms include a coarse hand tremor, severe gastrointestinal upset (vomiting and diarrhea), blurred vision, drowsiness, mental dullness, slurred speech, confusion, muscle twitching, and a dizzy or spinning sensation. Serious, later symptoms include seizures, coma, arrhythmias, and permanent neurologic impairment. A serious lithium overdose can be life threatening.

CRITICAL THINKING SCENARIO

Bug or drug?

Your patient is a 55-year-old man with a diagnosis of bipolar disorder whose manic symptoms have recently been stabilized using lithium, 600 mg PO once in the morning and once in the evening, and haloperidol, 10 mg PO once in the evening. He comes to you asking for medicine to treat his diarrhea, stating that he has been experiencing this symptom for 2 days now, and it must be something going around or something he ate.

1. As his nurse, what are your concerns?
2. What further assessments and interventions should you take?

Drug Interactions

Lithium interacts substantially with other drugs that deplete sodium. Examples of such drugs include thiazide diuretics and angiotensin-converting enzyme inhibitors. This interaction may lead to toxicity secondary to decreased renal elimination of lithium. Table 17.7 lists agents that can interact with lithium.

Assessment of Relevant Core Patient Variables

Health Status

Take a complete health history that includes a complete physical assessment and a complete drug history. Lithium's interaction with many other drugs makes this thoroughness essential. Health conditions that increase sodium resorption, such as congestive heart failure or cirrhosis of the liver, may also increase lithium resorption and lead to lithium toxicity. It is essential that patients who are taking lithium inform all health care providers, including dentists, that they are using this drug.

Life Span and Gender

Consider the patient's age, keeping in mind that lithium clearance in the kidneys decreases as a person ages. Elderly patients should use lithium cautiously because older adults experience more profound or toxic CNS effects. Older adults also are more likely to develop clinical hypothyroidism, lithium-induced goiter, and nephrogenic diabetes insipidus. Ask the woman of childbearing age whether she is pregnant, intends to become pregnant, or is breast-feeding. Lithium is

TABLE 17.7 Agents That Interact With P Lithium Carbonate

Interactants	Effect and Significance	Nursing Management
alkalinizing agents: potassium acetate, potassium citrate, sodium bicarbonate, sodium citrate, sodium lactate, tromethamine	Increased renal clearance of lithium	Anticipate possible dosage adjustment.
caffeine	Reduced serum lithium concentrations	Counsel patients about possibly decreased effectiveness of therapy, and identify sources of caffeine (coffee, tea, chocolate, carbonated colas, and other beverages).
verapamil	Possible lithium toxicity	Avoid concurrent use.
diuretics	Increased or decreased lithium levels depending of diuretic: enhanced lithium reabsorption with diuretics that act in distal tubule (thiazides, spironolactone, triamterene) or enhanced renal clearance with diuretics that act at the proximal tubule (osmotic diuretics, carbonic anhydrase inhibitors)	Monitor lithium levels carefully; anticipate dosage adjustments accordingly.
methyldopa	Possible lithium toxicity	Coadminister cautiously.
NSAIDs	Elevated lithium serum concentration from reduced excretion	Monitor lithium levels carefully; observe for signs of toxicity.
phenothiazines, haloperidol, carbamazepine	Neurotoxicity (delirium, seizures, encephalopathy, hyperpyrexia, EPS)	Monitor lithium levels carefully; observe for signs of toxicity.
acetazolamide, theophylline	Increased excretion of lithium	Monitor lithium levels closely. Anticipate dosage adjustment.
TCAs	Increased pharmacologic effect of TCAs	Monitor patient carefully for signs and symptoms of TCA toxicity. Anticipate dosage adjustment for TCAs.
neuromuscular blocking agents	Increased neuromuscular blocking effect with severe respiratory depression	Assess respiratory and neurologic status closely. Anticipate dosage reduction of neuromuscular blocking agent. Coadminister with caution.
fluoxetine	Increased lithium levels	Monitor lithium levels closely. Assess for signs and symptoms of lithium toxicity.

classified in pregnancy risk category D. It crosses the placenta, and serum concentration is equal in the mother and fetus. Lithium may cause fetal harm when given to a pregnant woman. Data from lithium birth registries suggest an increase in cardiac and other anomalies.

Lifestyle, Diet, and Habits

Review the patient's diet because sudden changes in sodium intake may alter lithium resorption, changing the amount of drug that is available in the bloodstream. Assess the patient's use of alcohol and other drugs, including caffeine. Concurrent drug or alcohol abuse reduces responsiveness to drug therapy. Alcohol and caffeine-containing foods and beverages, such as coffee, tea, and some sodas, increase lithium excretion. Consider the patient's daily activities. Lithium therapy causes drowsiness and may impair activities that require alertness or physical coordination.

Environment

Be aware of the environments in which lithium may be administered. Lithium can be administered safely in acute care, chronic care, and home care settings.

Culture and Inherited Traits

Consider the patient's ethnic heritage. For example, in Japan, lower lithium doses result in the same serum blood lithium levels. This fact would support lower dosing of patients with Japanese heritage here as well.

Nursing Diagnoses and Outcomes

- Ineffective Therapeutic Regimen Management related to questions about the benefits of the regime (a patient experiencing a manic episode may not want to take medicine that will interfere with his or her feelings of grandiosity or boundless energy)
  Desired outcome: *The patient will adhere to taking lithium as prescribed to maintain a therapeutic serum lithium level.*
- Excess Fluid Volume related to water retention secondary to lithium therapy
  Desired outcome: *The patient will adopt strategies to restore and maintain proper fluid balance.*
- Risk for Poisoning related to effects of lithium toxicity
  Desired outcome: *The patient will comply with regular monitoring of blood lithium levels to maintain a therapeutic serum level.*

Planning and Intervention

Maximizing Therapeutic Effects

You play an important role in helping patients with bipolar disorder remain in remission. Instruct the patient about early warning signs of a relapse, ways to manage psychosocial problems, and the importance of health-conscious behaviors. Patients may miss the highs of mania, considering life very flat while on lithium therapy. Offer emotional support to patients who feel this way and encourage them to continue with lithium therapy. If the patient cannot abstain from alcohol, advise moderate intake. Help the patient to arrange a work schedule that provides regular eating and sleeping schedules to minimize stress.

Minimizing Adverse Effects

Monitor the patient's blood level of lithium carefully when first starting therapy or whenever the dose is increased, to prevent toxicity from occurring. Serum lithium levels are monitored once or twice weekly during initiation of therapy and monthly thereafter, to ensure dosage is within therapeutic ranges. Blood specimens are obtained 8 to 12 hours after drug administration. Obtain a drug blood level at the first symptom of toxicity. Consuming lithium with food or dividing the dose minimizes gastrointestinal distress. Lithium is best taken with, or shortly after, meals. Administration should be accompanied by 10 to 12 glasses of water (8 oz) each day to prevent possible dehydration. In order to maintain a therapeutic lithium level, patients should be encouraged not to make any major changes in their consumption of water or salt. Hemodialysis is effective in removing lithium from the body and may be indicated in cases of severe overdose or toxicity.

Providing Patient and Family Education

- Teach the symptoms of lithium toxicity and emphasize that the patient must report any such symptoms to the prescriber at once.
- Stress the importance of adhering to a schedule of follow-up laboratory and medical appointments.
- Caution the patient to avoid OTC products containing nonsteroidal anti-inflammatory drugs (NSAIDs), except for aspirin, because these products decrease renal clearance. Patients should not use NSAIDs without first consulting the health care provider.
- Caution the patient against changing sodium intake, starting new drug therapy, or even using OTC drugs without first consulting the prescriber. Changes such as these may result in the patient reaching toxic lithium levels. In addition, explain the relationship between lithium activity and dietary sodium and teach the patient how to maintain a constant level of sodium and fluid intake to avoid fluctuations in lithium level.
- Teach strategies to prevent dehydration during lithium therapy.

Ongoing Assessment and Evaluation

Monitor serum lithium levels throughout therapy as described above. Observe the patient's neurologic and psychiatric functioning and assess neuromuscular, gastrointestinal, cardiovascular, kidney, and thyroid function routinely. To evaluate emotional stability, contrast pretreatment behaviors and patient's report of mood state with current observations and patient report. It is equally important to observe the patient's adherence to the therapeutic regimen. Lithium therapy is considered effective when the bipolar disorder is controlled and the patient does not experience serious adverse effects.

Drugs Significantly Different From [P] Lithium

Selective anticonvulsant agents, such as carbamazepine, valproic acid, and gabapentin, demonstrate antimanic effectiveness in patients who do not respond or are intolerant of

MEMORY CHIP

P Lithium Carbonate

- Mood stabilizer for treating bipolar affective disorder, particularly manic episodes
- Changes in sodium or fluid intake will alter blood levels of lithium.
- Major contraindications: severe cardiovascular or kidney disease, pregnancy or lactation, sodium imbalance
- Most common adverse effects: increased thirst or urge to drink, frequent urination, nausea, fine hand tremor
- Most serious adverse effects: lithium toxicity (slurred speech, unsteady gait, weakness, drowsiness, diarrhea, vomiting, confusion, and irregular heartbeat, possibly even seizure)
- **Life span alert: Older adults are at greater risk for hypothyroidism, drug-induced goiter, and nephrogenic diabetes insipidus.**
- Maximizing therapeutic effects: Promote a healthy lifestyle (balanced diet and activity level); encourage adherence.
- Minimizing adverse effects: Monitor serum levels regularly.
- Most important patient education: Have serum lithium levels monitored, avoid major changes in sodium and fluid intake, consult with the prescriber before using any other drugs, even over-the-counter products (especially nonsteroidal anti-inflammatory drugs).

lithium (although these are unlabeled uses). The anticonvulsants are discussed in more depth in Chapter 19.

Carbamazepine

Carbamazepine is an alternative to lithium for managing acute mania and for maintenance therapy. It is thought to reduce the sensitization of the brain to repeated episodes of mood swing. Mood-stabilizing use of carbamazepine does not appear to cause the blood dyscrasias that complicate its use as an anticonvulsant.

Gabapentin

Gabapentin appears effective in most patients who have bipolar disorder but have not responded to lithium or other mood stabilizers. Moreover, gabapentin may have substantially more sedative and calming potency than either carbamazepine or valproic acid.

Valproates

Valproic acid and divalproex sodium appear as effective as lithium in treating mania but are less effective in managing the depressive component of the disorder. This weak effect on depression may very well be the reason that Goodwin and colleagues (2003) found that the risk for suicide was also greater in bipolar patients being treated with divalproex than in those treated with lithium. Long-term therapy appears to reduce the frequency and severity of bipolar episodes.

CHAPTER SUMMARY

- Illnesses resulting in mood disorder are associated with an imbalance or dysregulation of neurotransmitters.
- Antidepressant therapy is used to treat depressive disorders. The three major classes of antidepressants are selective serotonin reuptake inhibitors (SSRIs), tricyclic antidepressants (TCAs), and monoamine oxidase inhibitors (MAOIs). Several miscellaneous agents are also used as antidepressants.
- Antidepressants appear to relieve depression by creating changes in both presynaptic and postsynaptic neuroreceptors, correcting the neurotransmitter imbalance. The neuroreceptors affected by antidepressant therapy are the serotonin, norepinephrine, dopamine, acetylcholine, histamine, and alpha-1 adrenergic receptors. Antidepressants stimulate these receptors differently, depending on the drug class. The effects at serotonin, norepinephrine, and dopamine receptors are generally responsible for the therapeutic effects, whereas effects at the other receptor sites are generally responsible for adverse effects.
- All antidepressant therapy requires sustained use of the drug to achieve a therapeutic effect, sometime between 10 days and 4 weeks of therapy. Energy levels may return before the depressed mood is elevated, placing patients at great risk for suicide during this time, because they still have the mindset for suicide, but now they have the physical ability to act on their mood.
- No ideal antidepressant exists because all produce adverse effects. Some adverse effects are mild and transient, whereas others may be serious. Important functions that you fulfill are teaching the patient and family safe and effective use of these agents, offering strategies to minimize adverse effects, and offering hope to patients that drug therapy will help to lift their mood.
- Sertraline is the prototype SSRI; it is the most frequently prescribed antidepressant and is generally well tolerated by patients. Nortriptyline is the prototype TCA. Its adverse effect profile includes difficulty concentrating, cardiac irregularities, and seizures. Older adults are particularly prone to these adverse effects. Phenelzine is the prototype MAOI. It is the least used of the antidepressants because of its adverse effects. Hypertensive crisis is the most serious toxic effect of phenelzine and other MAOIs. It may occur after ingesting certain foods containing high amounts of tyramine or with concomitant use with several other drugs.
- Bipolar disorder is characterized by mood shifts that include mania and depression. The mood stabilizer lithium is considered the drug of choice for bipolar disorder.
- Lithium ions are managed in the body the same way that sodium ions are managed. Changes in either sodium or fluid intake therefore can affect how much lithium the kidney reabsorbs and changes the circulating level of lithium in the bloodstream.
- Lithium has a narrow therapeutic index. Serum drug levels of lithium must be monitored closely throughout therapy to prevent lithium toxicity.

QUESTIONS FOR STUDY AND REVIEW

1. Identify the three main classifications of antidepressant drugs.
2. What is an additional assessment that you must make, in addition to medication efficacy, once the depressed patient has begun antidepressant therapy?
3. Identify an important point that you must teach the patient and his or her family to enhance adherence to antidepressant therapy.
4. What teaching can you give to a patient who complains of gastrointestinal distress associated with sertraline therapy?
5. What are common adverse effects produced by nortriptyline?
6. What are some dietary restrictions during phenelzine treatment?
7. What are the symptoms of an MAOI hypertensive crisis?
8. Identify the pharmacologic agents used to treat bipolar disorder.
9. What is the therapeutic range or level for lithium therapy?
10. What are the symptoms of lithium toxicity?

Need More Help?

Chapter 17 of the study guide for *Drug Therapy in Nursing 2e* contains NCLEX-style questions and other learning activities to reinforce your understanding of the concepts presented in this chapter. For additional information or to purchase the study guide, visit *http://connection.lww.com/go/aschenbrenner.*

REFERENCES AND BIBLIOGRAPHY

American Psychiatric Association. (2000). *Diagnostic and statistical manual of mental disorders* (4th ed., text revision). Washington, DC: Author.

Caspi, A., Sugden, K., Moffitt, T. E., et al. (2003). Influence of life stress on depression: Moderation by a polymorphism in the 5-HTT gene. *Science, 301*(5631), 386–389.

Chen, Y. S., Akula, N., Detera-Wadleigh, S. D., et al. (2003). Findings in an independent sample support an association between bipolar affective disorder and the G72/G30 locus on chromosome 13q33. *Molecular Psychiatry, 9*(1), 87–92.

DePaulo, J. R., & Horvitz, L. A. (2002). *Understanding depression: What we know and what you can do about it.* New York: John Wiley & Sons.

Food and Drug Administration. FDA Talk Paper. (March 22, 2004). *FDA issues public health advisory on cautions for use of antidepressants in adults and children* [Online]. Available: *http://www.fda.gov/bbs/topics/ANSWERS/2004/ANS01283.html.*

Geller, B., Reising, D., Leonard, H. L., et al. (1999). Critical review of tricyclic antidepressant use in children and adolescents. *Journal of the American Academy of Child and Adolescent Psychiatry, 38*(5), 513–516.

Goodwin, F. K., Fireman, B., Simon, G. E., et al. (2003). Suicide risk in bipolar disorder during treatment with lithium and divalproex. *Journal of the American Medical Association, 290*(11), 1467–1473.

Greenberg, P. E., Kessler, R. C., Birnbaum, H. G., et al. (2003). The economic burden of depression in the United States: How did it change between 1990 and 2000? *Journal of Clinical Psychiatry, 64*(12), 1465–1475.

Hardman, J. G. (2001). *Goodman & Gilman's the pharmacological basis of therapeutics* (10th ed.). New York: McGraw-Hill Health Professions Division.

Kessler, R. C., Berglund, O., Demier, O., et al. (2003). The epidemiology of major depressive disorder: Results from the National Comorbidity Survey Replication (NCS-R). *Journal of the American Medical Association, 289*(23), 3095–3105.

Lin, K. M., & Poland, R. E. (1995). Ethnicity, culture, and psychopharmacology. In F. E. Bloom & D. I. Kupfer (Eds.). *Psychopharmacology: The fourth generation of progress.* New York: Raven Press.

March, J., Silva, S., Petrycki, S., et al., for the Treatment for Adolescents With Depression Study (TADS) Team. (2004). Fluoxetine, cognitive-behavioral therapy, and their combination for adolescents with depression: Treatment for Adolescents with Depression Study (TADS) randomized controlled trial. *Journal of the American Medical Association, 292*(7), 807–820.

McEvoy, G. K., Litvak, K., & Welsh Jr., O. H. (Eds.). (2002). *Drug information.* Bethesda, MD: American Hospital Formulary Service.

Mueller, T. I., Kohn, R., Leventhal, N., et al. (2004). The course of depression in elderly patients. *American Journal of Geriatric Psychiatry, 12*(1), 22–29.

Murray, C. J. L., & Lopez, A. D. (1997). Alternative projections of mortality and disability by cause, 1990–2020: Global Burden of Disease Study. *Lancet,* 349, 1498–1504.

Preskorn, S. H. (1999). *Outpatient management of depression: A guide for the primary-care practitioner* (2nd ed.). Caddo, OK: Professional Communications.

Solomon, D. A., Keller, M. B., Leon, A. C., et al. (2000). Multiple recurrences of major depressive disorder. *American Journal of Psychiatry, 157*(2), 229–233.

Stewart, W. F., Ricci, J. A., Chee E., et al. (2003). Cost of lost productive work time among US workers with depression. *Journal of the American Medical Association, 289*(16), 3135–3144.

Stuart, G. W., & Laraia, M. T. (2000). *Principles and practice of psychiatric nursing.* Charleston, SC: Harcourt Health Sciences, Medical University of South Carolina.

Tamminga, C. A., Nemeroff, C. B., Blakely, R. D., et al. (2002). Developing novel treatments for mood disorders accelerating discovery. *Biological Psychiatry, 52*(6), 589–609.

U.S. Department of Health and Human Services, Public Health Service, Agency for Health Care Policy and Research. (1993). *Depression Guideline Panel: Depression in primary care, Vol.2, Treatment of major depression.* Clinical practice guideline, No. 5 (AHCPR publication no. 93-0551), Rockville, MD: USDHHS.

Wagner, K. D., Ambrosini, O., Rynn, M., et al. (2003). Efficacy of sertraline in the treatment of children and adolescents with major depressive disorder. *Journal of the American Medical Association, 290*(8), 1033–1041.

Wood, A. J., & Zhou, H. H. (1991). Ethnic difference in drug disposition and responsiveness. *Clinical Pharmacokinetics, 20,* 350–373.

Drugs Treating Psychotic Disorders and Dementia

chapter 18

Learning Objectives

At the completion of this chapter the student will:

1. Identify diseases and disease processes in which psychotic disorders or dementia are present.
2. Identify the symptoms of psychotic disorders or dementia.
3. Identify the "positive and negative symptoms" of schizophrenia.
4. Identify core drug knowledge of drugs used to treat psychotic disorders or dementia.
5. Name the types of drugs that are used to treat psychotic disorders or dementia.
6. Identify core patient variables relevant to drugs that affect psychotic disorders or dementia.
7. Relate the interaction of core drug knowledge to core patient variables for drugs to treat psychotic disorders or dementia.
8. Generate a nursing plan of care from the interaction between core drug knowledge and the core patient variables for drugs to treat psychotic disorders or dementia.
9. Describe nursing interventions to maximize therapeutic and minimize adverse effects for drugs that affect psychotic disorders or dementia.
10. Identify the signs and symptoms of neuroleptic malignant syndrome.
11. Determine key points for patient and family education for drugs that affect psychotic disorders or dementia.

KEY TERMS

Alzheimer disease

delirium

dementia

extrapyramidal symptoms

neuroleptic malignant syndrome

psychosis

schizophrenia

tardive dyskinesia

vascular dementia

FEATURED WEBLINK

http://www.nami.org

The website of the National Alliance for the Mentally Ill—a not-for-profit, grassroots, self-help organization—offers information, discussion groups, and resources for people with mental illness.

CONNECTION WEBLINK

Additional Weblinks are found on Connection: **http://www.connection.lww.com/go/aschenbrenner.**

Drugs Treating Psychotic Disorders and Dementia

Ⓒ Antipsychotics

Ⓒ Typical antipsychotics

- **[P] haloperidol**
- fluphenazine
- loxapine
- molindone
- perphenazine
- pimozide
- thiothixene
- trifluoperazine
- triflupromazine
- chlorpromazine
- mesoridazine
- thioridazine

Ⓒ Atypical antipsychotics

- **[P] olanzapine**
- quetiapine
- risperidone
- ziprasidone

Drugs for Alzheimer-Type Dementia

Ⓒ Acetylcholinesterase enzyme inhibitors

- **[P] rivastigmine**
- donepezil
- tacrine
- galantamine hydrobromide

The symbol Ⓒ indicates the **drug class.**
Drugs in **bold type** marked with the symbol [P] are prototypes.
Drugs in blue type are closely related to the prototype.
Drugs in red type are significantly different from the prototype.
Drugs in black type with no symbol are also used in drug therapy; no prototype

Although it is impossible to read a person's mind, much less to know precisely whether his or her thoughts are ordered or disordered, a person's thoughts influence his or her perception of reality, interpretation of the environment, speech, and behavior. **Psychosis** is the inability to perceive and interpret reality accurately, think clearly, respond correctly, and function in a socially appropriate manner. Disordered thoughts can produce speech and behavior patterns that are confusing and even frightening to the individual and those around him. The presence of these symptoms is used to make a diagnosis of a psychotic disorder, such as schizophrenia. Historically, treating psychotic disorders involved containing the sick person and protecting society from what that person might do. The setting more closely resembled a jail than a hospital. The first drug therapy was aimed at sedating the patient in order to control behavior. It was not until the mid-1950s that drug therapy to control symptoms was devised. These drugs were very effective and constituted a major breakthrough in patient care. Unfortunately, these early drug therapies had many undesirable adverse effects, many of which were chronic, and some even permanent. The goal in creating new therapies has not necessarily been to create a more effective drug, but rather to create one with fewer adverse effects. Indeed, the original drugs are still considered the gold standard for effective symptom control. As brain imaging techniques advanced in the 1990s, it became possible to learn more about the sophisticated functioning of the brain; this new understanding enabled the development of drug therapies that worked at specific neuroreceptor sites in the brain and central nervous system (CNS). This targeted drug therapy not only was effective in relieving symptoms of psychotic disorders, such as delusions and hallucinations, but also minimized adverse effects by limiting the number of receptors that were stimulated by the drug. Recent research suggests that targeted therapy may improve adherence (Box 18.1).

Drugs that relieve symptoms of psychotic disorders are generally referred to as antipsychotics. They are also called neuroleptics, to reflect the fact that the drugs work in the nervous system at neuroreceptor sites. Both terms are currently used and are interchangeable. Table 18.1 presents a summary of selected antipsychotic drugs.

Antipsychotic agents are further divided into typical and atypical antipsychotics. The prototype typical antipsychotic is haloperidol. It is considered a high-potency typical antipsychotic. Drugs in this class represented by the prototype are molindone, perphenazine, loxapine, trifluoperazine, fluphenazine, thiothixene, and pimozide. Drugs closely related to the prototype that are considered low-potency typical antipsychotics are chlorpromazine, thioridazine, and mesoridazine. The prototype atypical antipsychotic is olanzapine. Drugs in this class represented by the prototype include risperidone, ziprasidone, aripiprazole, clozapine, and quetiapine.

Drugs used in the treatment of dementia and Alzheimer disease are also discussed in this chapter. The prototype Alzheimer drug is rivastigmine (Exelon). Drugs represented by the prototype include donepezil and tacrine.

FOCUS ON RESEARCH

Box 18.1 Comfort is the Key to Adherence

Lieberman, J. A., Tollefson, G., Tohen, M., et al., for the HGDH Study Group. (2003). Comparative efficacy and safety of atypical and conventional antipsychotic drugs in first-episode psychosis: A randomized, double-blind trial of olanzapine versus haloperidol. *American Journal of Psychiatry, 160*(8), 1396–1404.

The Study

This double-blind study, which compared the effects of haloperidol and olanzapine in 263 patients during a 12-week period, found that these drugs were equally effective in reducing acute psychotic symptoms. However, the patients receiving olanzapine participated in the study for longer than patients receiving haloperidol, and fewer of the olanzapine recipients dropped out of the study because of adverse events.

These results suggest that patients receiving an atypical antipsychotic such as olanzapine probably experience benefits other than merely reduced psychotic symptoms. In this study, the patients were more likely to adhere to treatment with an atypical antipsychotic, presumably because fewer adverse effects with this agent meant that therapy was more comfortable for them.

Nursing Implications

When caring for any patient receiving an antipsychotic, you should continually assess not only for absence of symptoms, but also for absence of adverse effects. You must not merely wait for the patient to complain of adverse effects, but rather elicit from the patient information that will confirm that he or she is comfortable with the prescribed regimen and will therefore adhere to treatment.

PHYSIOLOGY

The cerebrum, the highest functional area of the brain, is concerned with activities such as creative thought, judgment, memory, and reason, and it is divided into two hemispheres. The frontal lobes control voluntary body movement, expression of feelings, perceptual interpretation of information, and thinking. The temporal lobes also play a role in the expression of emotions. Other major CNS functional systems include the extrapyramidal system responsible for muscle coordination; the limbic system responsible for the emotions of anger, anxiety, fear, pleasure, sorrow, learning, and memory; and the reticular activating system responsible for consciousness, filtering, and stimulus alert.

Within the nervous system, communication between neurons depends on neurotransmission. The movements of electrical impulses cause neurotransmitters to be released from the presynaptic cell (axon) into the synapse, where they are received by the postsynaptic cell (dendrite) of the next cell. The axons are insulated by a coating called myelin. The myelin sheath can be compared to the coating on an extension cord. It protects the internal wires from damage and prevents the electrical impulses from escaping into the surrounding area.

Thought, like mood, is controlled by neurotransmitters that stimulate neuroreceptors in the brain. The brain has unique receptors, unlike receptors elsewhere in the body. These receptors activate thought processes, and other unique receptors in the brain activate mood response. A combination of neurotransmitters is thought to play a role in the workings of the brain. The primary neurotransmitter related to thought processing is believed to be dopamine. Dopamine is secreted by neurons originating in the midbrain that function in coordination, emotion, and voluntary decision making.

TABLE 18.1 Summary of Selected Ⓒ Antipsychotics

Drug (Trade) Name	Selected Indications	Route and Dosage Range	Pharmacokinetics
Ⓒ Typical Antipsychotics			
High Potency			
[P] haloperidol (Haldol; *Canadian:* Peridol)	Psychotic disorders, hyperexcitability in children	*Adult:* PO, 0.5–2 mg bid to tid; IM, 5–30 mg/d *Child:* PO, 0.05–0.15 mg/d	*Onset:* PO, varies, IM, 15–30 min *Duration:* PO, 24–72 h; IM, 4–8 h $t_{1/2}$: 21–14 h
acetophenazine (Tindal)	Psychotic disorders	*Adult:* PO, 20–80 mg/d in divided doses *Child:* Not recommended	*Onset:* 2–3 h *Duration:* 36–48 h $t_{1/2}$: 10–20 h
fluphenazine enanthate (Prolixin; *Canadian:* Apo-Fluphenazine)	Psychotic disorders	*Adult:* IM/SC, 12.5–25 mg *Child:* Not recommended	*Onset:* 24–72 h *Duration:* 1–3 wk $t_{1/2}$: 3.7 d
perphenazine (Trilafon; *Canadian:* Apo-Perphenazine)	Psychotic disorders	*Adult:* PO, 4–8 mg tid to qid; IM, 5–15 mg/d	*Onset:* Varies *Duration:* 6–12 h $t_{1/2}$: Unknown
thiothixene (Navane)	Psychotic disorders	*Adult:* PO, 2–30 mg/d; IM, 4–30 mg/d	*Onset:* 1–6 h *Duration:* 12–24 h $t_{1/2}$: 34 h
Low Potency			
chlorpromazine (Thorazine; *Canadian:* Chlorprom)	Psychotic disorders, such as schizophrenia	*Adult:* PO, 10–25 mg, bid, tid, or qid to maximum of 2,000 mg/d; IM 25–50 mg repeated in 4 h if needed *Child:* 5–12 y, 23–46 kg, 75 mg/d; 6 mo–5 y (up to 23 kg), 40 mg/d; IM, 0.55 mg/kg q6–8h	*Onset:* PO, 30–60 min; IM, 10–15 min *Duration:* 4–6 h $t_{1/2}$: 23–37 h
loxapine (Loxitane; *Canadian:* Loxapac)	Psychotic disorders	*Adult:* PO, 10–100 mg/d; IM, 12.5–50 mg/d	*Onset:* PO, 30 min; IM, rapid *Duration:* 12 h $t_{1/2}$: 19 h
mesoridazine (Serentil)	Schizophrenia, alcohol withdrawal, acute/chronic alcoholism	*Adult:* PO, 50–400 mg/d (lower dosage for alcohol withdrawal)	*Onset:* Varies *Duration:* 4–8 h $t_{1/2}$: 24–48 h
molindone (Moban)	Psychotic disorders	*Adult:* PO, 50–225 mg/d in divided doses	*Onset:* Varies *Duration:* 24–36 h $t_{1/2}$: 1.5 h
pimozide (Orap)	Tourette syndrome	*Adult:* PO, 1–10 mg/d in divided doses	*Onset:* Varies *Duration:* Unknown $t_{1/2}$: 55–154 h
thioridazine (Mellaril; *Canadian:* Apo-Thioridazine)	Psychotic disorders; agitation, depression, sleep disturbance, and fear in geriatric patients; hyperactivity and related symptoms in children	*Adult:* PO, 50–800 mg/d *Child 2–12 y:* PO, 0.5–3.0 mg/kg/d	*Onset:* Varies *Duration:* 8–12 h $t_{1/2}$: 10–12 h
Ⓒ Atypical Antipsychotics			
[P] olanzapine (Zyprexa)	Pyschotic disorders	*Adult:* PO, 5–15 mg/d	*Onset:* Unknown *Duration:* Unknown $t_{1/2}$: 21–54 h, average 30 h
clozapine (Clozaril)	Schizophrenia unresponsive to other antipsychotic drugs	*Adult:* PO, 25–450 mg/d	*Onset:* Varies *Duration:* 4–12 h $t_{1/2}$: 8–12 h
Benzisoxazoles			
risperidone (Risperdal)	Psychotic disorders	*Adult:* PO, 1 mg bid to 16 mg/d	*Onset:* Varies *Duration:* Unknown $t_{1/2}$: 20 h

Many areas of the brain secrete acetylcholine; reductions in the amount of this neurotransmitter cause cognitive changes. Acetylcholine has a number of functions, including arousal, coordination of movement, memory acquisition, and memory retention. Research is also being conducted on the extent to which norepinephrine and serotonin might be involved in thought processes. For a complete discussion of the physiology of brain and nervous function, see Chapter 17.

PSYCHOTIC DISORDERS

In psychiatry, psychotic disorders are described by different diagnoses. Each diagnosis has its own etiology, symptoms, and treatments, although a given drug may be useful in more than one diagnosis.

Schizophrenia

Schizophrenia is a particular kind of psychosis that is characterized mainly by a clear sensorium but a marked disturbance in thinking. Schizophrenia is a complex illness with uncertain etiology. Schizophrenia interferes with a person's ability to think clearly, manage emotions, make decisions, and relate to others. Schizophrenia affects approximately 1% to 2% of all populations worldwide, including approximately 2.2 million American adults. That is, approximately 1.1 percent of the population aged 18 and older in a given year has schizophrenia.

Schizophrenia often appears earlier in men, usually in the late teens or early 20s, than it does in women, who are generally affected in the 20s or early 30s. Current research implies that schizophrenia has a strong genetic component; however, the illness is still considered to have multiple causes. With a genetic predisposition, the various stressors that may occur in a person's life can trigger the disorder's symptoms. This effect could be compared to what can happen to a bridge made of wooden planks. The structure is strong enough to accommodate light loads safely, but if a heavy truck drove over the bridge, it would be likely to collapse.

Other hypotheses exist for the pathogenesis of schizophrenia, especially with regard to changes in brain chemistry, because schizophrenia is associated with an unusual imbalance of neurotransmitters. The dopamine hypothesis is the most fully developed of these hypotheses. It is based on the unexpected discovery that agents that diminish dopaminergic activity have beneficial effects in reducing the acute symptoms and signs of psychosis, specifically agitation, anxiety, and hallucinations. These agents reduce delusions and social withdrawal less dramatically, however. Imaging studies have lent credence to the belief that excessive dopamine activity is involved in schizophrenia, particularly on the left side, where the most recognizable "positive" symptoms occur. This imbalance appears to arise not from overproduction of dopamine, but rather from an increase in specific chemical receptors that attract dopamine. Moreover, there appears to be low activity of a subset of dopamine (D_1) receptors in the prefrontal cortex of the brain where so-called negative symptoms originate. (Positive and negative symptoms are explained later.)

The term schizophrenia is derived from the Greek words that indicate a broken or shattered personality, separating the cognitive and emotional aspects of the personality. Many people mistakenly believe that schizophrenia involves multiple personalities. People with schizophrenia do not have multiple personalities. Another common misconception is that affected individuals are prone to violence. Although patients with schizophrenia may sometimes become violent, they are far more likely to withdraw from society. In fact, these people are more often the victims rather than the perpetrators of violence. Fears and misperceptions persist, however, and integrating patients with psychotic symptoms into society remains challenging (Box 18.2).

Schizophrenia is characterized by symptoms described as positive, negative, and disorganized. The positive symptoms of schizophrenia, and the most recognizable symptoms, include delusions (e.g., paranoia or distorted perceptions of other people's intentions) and hallucinations. For example, individuals with schizophrenia may have beliefs or thoughts that are fixed and false; these beliefs or thoughts are a type of delusion. Hallucinations, on the other hand, can affect any one of the five senses. Auditory hallucinations are the most common type of hallucination; a person with auditory hallucinations might hear voices talking to or about him or her. A person experiencing a visual hallucination may see persons or objects that are not there. Hallucinations are considered positive symptoms because they add a layer of something new to the person. They are an excess or a distortion of normal brain function.

The negative symptoms of schizophrenia include flat or blunted emotions, lack of pleasure or interest in things (anhedonia), and limited speech. These symptoms take away from the person's personality and are thus considered "negative." They also represent a loss or diminishing of normal brain function. For example, individuals with schizophrenia may have difficulty understanding their feelings or expressing their emotions clearly. Furthermore, they view the world and society as uninteresting and not worth participating in, and they often may not say much or speak

COMMUNITY-BASED CONCERNS

Box 18.2 Easing Fears About Mental Illness

It is an unfortunate reality that what little attention mental illness receives in the media mostly focuses on episodes of sensational violence, committed by people who are clearly psychotic. However, the overall number of people suffering from mental illnesses, particularly illnesses involving psychosis, is far greater than the number of those who behave violently. Psychotic people most often are the victims, rather than the perpetrators, of injury. Despite this reality, sensational stories of mental illness persist, and prisons fill with untreated mentally ill patients.

All nurses have a responsibility to continue to educate patients, their families, and all members of the community about the symptoms of various mental illnesses and about any resources available for treatment. Rallying the support of the community is crucial to increase the resources that will help patients receive appropriate treatment. More drugs for treating specific symptoms of mental illness are available today than ever before. These advances also mean that there is less need to fear the psychotic patient and more reason than ever before for the patient to be integrated as a functioning member of the community.

unless spoken to. Consequently, the individual may have trouble relating to others, which in turn can lead to periods of intense withdrawal and profound isolation.

Symptoms of disorganized thinking and speech may cause the following problems for schizophrenic individuals:

- Trouble thinking clearly and understanding what other people say
- Using words in a way that make no sense to anyone else
- Inability to plan ahead
- Inability to solve relatively small problems

The disorganized behavior may make the individual do things that do not make sense, such as repeated, rhythmic gestures or ritualistic movements.

Some symptoms of schizophrenia differ between men and women. For example, the negative symptoms are more often present in men; mood symptoms, especially depression, are more commonly seen in women. Additionally, delusions in women appear less bizarre, with more somatic and romantic preoccupation. Men are more concerned with political conspiracy and undercover activities and have more grandiose delusions of power, royalty, and divinity. Many individuals with schizophrenia have a combination of these symptoms.

Other Psychotic Disorders

Compared with schizophrenia, which is a permanent illness, other psychotic disorders may be short lived. As defined earlier, a psychotic episode is one in which the person loses touch with reality. In addition to being present in schizophrenia, psychosis can also be present in states of depression or mania. The causes of psychosis are varied and can include electrolyte imbalances, metabolic imbalances (e.g., diabetic ketoacidosis), drug abuse (either from drug intoxication or withdrawal), adverse effects from prescribed drug therapy, or hormonal shifts, such as those that occur during the postpartum period.

COGNITIVE DISORDERS

Dementia

Dementia is a clinical syndrome of progressive, degenerative loss of memory and of one or more of these abilities:

- Language skills
- Higher-level skills such as judgment, comprehension, and problem solving
- Ability to recognize or identify objects despite intact sensory function
- Ability to perform motor skills (American Psychiatric Association, 2000)

Mood and behavior may also be affected in dementia. Agitation or withdrawal, hallucinations, delusions, insomnia, emotional apathy, and loss of inhibitions are also common.

There are many types of dementia, including Alzheimer-type dementia, vascular dementia, and other dementia caused by diseases such as acquired immunodeficiency syndrome (AIDS). Dementia can also be a result of brain damage from substance abuse, such as alcoholism or inhalant use, or from exposure to environmental chemicals. In all of these circumstances, symptoms of dementia develop gradually, and although the deterioration is not necessarily diffuse or "global," it often affects some areas of intellectual functioning while sparing others. Early in the disease, the patient may be aware of changes in intellectual ability and become depressed or anxious and attempt to compensate by writing down information, attempting to structure routines, and simplifying responsibilities. These coping mechanisms may give patients the appearance of intact cognitive abilities for a while, even though they are actually in decline.

Alzheimer Disease

Alzheimer disease (AD) is one form of progressive dementia. Alzheimer disease, the most common cause of dementia among people 65 years of age and older, affects an estimated 4 million Americans. The duration of illness, from onset of symptoms to death, averages 8 to 10 years.

At this time, there is no cure or way to prevent Alzheimer disease. As more and more Americans live longer, the number affected by Alzheimer disease will continue to grow, unless a cure or effective prevention is discovered. Alzheimer disease causes a gross, diffuse atrophy of the cerebral cortex. It is associated with extracellular plaques with beta-amyloid protein deposits and neurofibrillary tangles in the cortical neurons, with eventual loss of neurons. The earliest loss of neurons occurs in the nucleus basalis and the entorhinal cortex, where cholinergic neurons are preferentially affected. As the illness progresses, up to 90% of cholinergic neurons in the nucleus basalis baseline may be lost. Cholinergic deficiency in Alzheimer disease is most prominent at the more advanced stages.

Typically, Alzheimer disease begins insidiously with short-term memory loss, whereas long-term memory is initially spared. Eventually, long-term memory is also lost as the disease progresses. In addition to memory loss, other cognitive deficits also impair activities of daily living. Individuals with Alzheimer disease frequently repeat questions, forget phone messages and appointments, do not pay bills, and get lost driving. Individuals with Alzheimer disease may lose weight because they no longer shop for food, cook, or eat. Furthermore, the cognitive deficits are relentlessly progressive; affective, behavioral, and motor signs become more common as the disease advances.

In addition to the cognitive deficits, behavioral and psychiatric symptoms (e.g., abnormal sleep, delusions, depression, hallucinations, mania, and wandering) tend to occur at some point in most patients with Alzheimer-type dementia.

Vascular Dementia

Vascular dementia results from damage to brain tissue, caused by cerebrovascular events such as transient ischemic attacks. The areas that experience infarcts are associated with specific neurologic functions, so that an infarct in the cerebellum, for example, can produce problems with motor coordination or balance. Although vascular dementia and Alzheimer dementia differ in cause, many of the symptoms are similar (Groves et al., 2000).

Other Dementia

Dementia can also be caused by a variety of medical conditions. The primary mechanism of this diagnosis is the presence of or a noted history of a disease, such as AIDS,

Parkinson disease, Huntington chorea, hypothyroidism, normal pressure hydrocephalus, brain tumor, or vitamin B_{12} deficiency. The symptoms caused by these conditions are also similar to those described earlier for Alzheimer disease. Box 18.3 presents risks for and causes of dementia, both irreversible and potentially reversible.

Delirium

Delirium is a sudden disruption in cognitive functioning, most often caused by a physical change in the body, rather than by changes within the brain. This physical change prevents the brain from receiving some critical element (e.g., blood or oxygen) that it needs to function effectively. This event can be conceptualized as "brain failure," just as any other organ will experience failure from physical impairment. A hallmark symptom of this "brain failure" is a disturbance in the level of consciousness that comes and goes throughout the day or days when delirium is present. This pattern is called waxing and waning. Another symptom of delirium, as with dementia, is that psychotic-like symptoms can occur in which the person loses touch with reality. Thus, the patient may experience hallucinations and delusions. Some causes of delirium include substance withdrawal, infection (e.g., septicemia and urinary tract infections), sensory deprivation, metabolic disturbances (arising from renal failure, diabetic ketoacidosis, hypoxia, and fluid or electrolyte imbalance), and adverse effects from some medications. One major difference between delirium and dementia is its onset. Unlike that of dementia, which is slow and gradual, the onset of delirium is rapid. To treat delirium effectively, the underlying cause must first be identified. *Untreated delirium can be fatal because the underlying condition is not diagnosed and treated.* Use of an antipsychotic or sedative will calm the patient but not resolve the cause of the delirium.

BOX 18.3 Risk Factors and Possible Causes of Dementia

Irreversible Risk Factors/Causes

- Age over 65 years
- Cerebral infarction or ischemia
- Diseases such as cardiovascular disorders, type 1 diabetes, degenerative (e.g., Parkinson disease), neoplasms
- Male gender
- Genetic factors such as apolipoprotein E gene on chromosome 19 and chromosome 10

Potentially Reversible Risk Factors/Causes

- Depression
- Diseases such as type 2 diabetes, hyperlipidemia, hypertension, infections
- Drugs with iatrogenic/idiosyncratic effect or polypharmacy
- Lifestyle habits such as excessive alcohol consumption, smoking, illicit drug use, among others
- Metabolic disorders
- Nutritional disorders
- Toxins
- Trauma

C ANTIPSYCHOTICS

C Typical Antipsychotics

The typical antipsychotics were the first antipsychotic drugs created. They are sometimes referred to as the conventional antipsychotics. Use of the original drug in this class, chlorpromazine (Thorazine), has become limited because of its substantial adverse effect profile. Haloperidol (Haldol) is a commonly used typical antipsychotic and is the prototype for the class.

NURSING MANAGEMENT OF THE PATIENT RECEIVING P HALOPERIDOL

Core Drug Knowledge

Pharmacotherapeutics

Haloperidol is used to treat psychotic disorders such as schizophrenia. It is also used to treat Tourette disorder and in pediatric patients with hyperactivity or severe behavioral problems. Off-label, it is used to treat nausea, vomiting, intractable hiccups, psychosis, and agitation in dementia and in PCP-induced psychosis. Haloperidol can be administered orally, intramuscularly, and intravenously.

Pharmacokinetics

Haloperidol is fairly well absorbed. Its bioavailability from oral doses is 60% to 65%. It is highly protein bound at 92%. Its exact mechanism of metabolism is unknown, although almost all of it is eliminated by metabolism; about 1% is eliminated in the urine and stool. Ethnicity has been found to influence the pharmacokinetics of haloperidol. Asians were found to achieve a 50% higher plasma concentration of haloperidol than whites who received the same dose. It is hypothesized that this difference is attributable to inherent differences in metabolism, but the precise reason is not known (Lin & Poland, 2000).

Pharmacodynamics

Haloperidol can take several days to reach its full therapeutic effect. The exact cause of this delay is unknown. The delay is frequently more frustrating to the nursing staff than to the patient. Haloperidol produces its effects by blocking dopamine (specifically D_2), alpha, serotonin, and histamine receptors. It has minimal blocking effects at cholinergic receptors.

Blockade of dopaminergic receptors produces a decrease in movement disorders, relief of hallucinations and delusions, relief of psychosis, worsening of negative symptoms, and release of prolactin. Dopamine blockade also quiets the chemoreceptive trigger zone in the brain that produces nausea and vomiting, thereby relieving these symptoms.

Blockade of alpha receptors produces many of the cardiac adverse effects of haloperidol treatment. Other adverse effects, related to alterations in mood, are caused by the blockade of serotonin receptors. Blockade of histamine receptors produces adverse effects such as sedation.

Anticholinergic effects from haloperidol are modest but explain the adverse effects such as dry mouth. Blockade of dopamine receptors actually creates the net effect of too much cholinergic stimulation because the delicate balance between these two systems is altered. Many of the adverse effects from haloperidol are related to this relative imbalance between dopamine and cholinergic neurotransmitters.

Haloperidol may also decrease the seizure threshold in patients with seizure disorder. Haloperidol controls the positive symptoms of schizophrenia but has no effect on the negative symptoms. Occasionally, the negative symptoms may worsen with haloperidol therapy.

Contraindications and Precautions

Haloperidol is contraindicated if the patient has hypersensitivity to any of the drug's components. It is also contraindicated in Parkinson's disease because cholinergic stimulation in that disorder is already excessive.

Haloperidol should be administered with caution to patients who:

- Have been exposed to extreme heat or phosphorous insecticides
- Use atropine or other anticholinergic drugs
- Are currently withdrawing from alcohol
- Have any disorder of the skin (dermatosis) or other allergic reactions to phenothiazine derivatives (because of the risk for cross-sensitivity)
- Have experienced an idiosyncratic response to other centrally acting drugs
- Are pregnant, because it is a pregnancy category C drug

Adverse Effects

Adverse effects, which can be perceived as a substantial nuisance or a source of embarrassment to the patient, are the primary reason that patients stop taking the haloperidol. Although many adverse effects can be managed or minimized pharmacologically, some patients will need to accept that they will experience some adverse effects in order to have their psychotic symptoms controlled.

The major risk to the patient receiving haloperidol comes from a group of symptoms called **extrapyramidal symptoms** (EPS). The cause of these symptoms is the relative lack of dopamine stimulation and relative excess of cholinergic stimulation. EPS symptoms are the most common adverse effects of haloperidol. The risk for EPS increases if drug therapy is repeatedly and abruptly stopped and then restarted.

There are four major presentations of EPS. The first is Parkinson-like effects (also known as pseudoparkinsonianism). With this adverse effect, the patient demonstrates symptoms that are typically seen in Parkinson disease, such as cog-wheeling muscle rigidity, fine tremor, slow motor responses, and a flat affect (a mask-like facial expression). It is important to distinguish this flat affect from the primary symptom of schizophrenia, which is flat affect without the mask-like features, combined with social withdrawal.

The second presentation of EPS is akathisia, a constant feeling of restlessness that the patient cannot control or explain. This presentation must be distinguished from signs of anxiety related to an identifiable source of worry. The third presentation of EPS is acute dystonia, which is prolonged muscular contractions and spasms. The spasms may present as arching and twisting of the neck, arching of the back, rolling of the eyes up toward the back of the head, or spasms of the laryngeal-pharyngeal muscles (which may occlude the airway, if the spasms are severe, and can be life-threatening). These symptoms cannot be controlled, occur suddenly, and may be frightening and painful.

The remaining way that EPS can present is called **tardive dyskinesia.** Tardive dyskinesia generally occurs late in haloperidol therapy and usually is irreversible. It is most commonly related to high doses and long-term use. Approximately 1 in 25 patients treated for a period of 1 year develops tardive dyskinesia. Risk factors for developing this adverse effect are listed in Box 18.4. However, after treatment for 7 years, the incidence increases to one in four patients. Symptoms of tardive dyskinesia include involuntary lip smacking, chewing, mouth movements, tongue protrusion, blinking, grimacing, and involuntary muscle twitching of the limbs.

Other adverse effects of haloperidol that are fairly common include drowsiness, sedation, somnolence, lethargy, and dysphoria (a decline in mood). It has been hypothesized that the complaints of drowsiness and sedation may actually be signs of drug-induced depression that have been misinterpreted by the patient and the clinician. More research is needed to help devise antipsychotic drugs that do not produce these adverse effects, so that the quality of life can be improved for patients requiring long-term therapy (Voruganti & Awad, 2004).

Use of antipsychotics puts the patient at risk for developing a relatively rare, although potentially fatal, adverse effect called **neuroleptic malignant syndrome** (NMS). This syndrome is characterized by fever, sweating, tachycardia, muscle rigidity, tremor, incontinence, stupor, leukocytosis, elevated creatinine phosphokinase (CPK) levels, and renal failure. Patients are more likely to develop neuroleptic malignant syndrome if they are dehydrated or taking large doses of haloperidol. Neuroleptic malignant syndrome can occur with use of any of the typical antipsychotics. In addition to having an underlying psychotic illness, the patient now also becomes delirious.

Another potentially fatal, although extremely rare, adverse effect that patients can develop is agranulocytosis. Although this adverse effect is possible with haloperidol, it is more common with the atypical antipsychotics.

BOX 18.4 Risk Factors for Tardive Dyskinesia (TD)

If the patient is receiving treatment with "typical" antipsychotics, additional factors that place the patient at risk for TD include:

- 6 months of antipsychotic therapy
- Increased length of antipsychotic therapy
- Antipsychotic dosage change—either increased or decreased
- Diagnosis of organic mental disorder or mood disorder
- Increased age
- Diabetes
- Genetic predisposition
- Race (African Americans may be twice as likely to develop TD than whites)

A variety of other adverse effects can possibly occur from use of haloperidol. They are categorized as:

- Cardiovascular (electrocardiographic [ECG] changes, hypertension, hypotension, QT-interval prolongation, tachycardia)
- CNS (agitation, anxiety, catatonia-like state, confusion, convulsions, depression, euphoria, hallucinations, headache, insomnia, libido increases, transient dyskinetic signs, vertigo)
- Dermatologic (acne, alopecia, maculopapular skin reactions, photosensitivity)
- Gastrointestinal (anorexia, constipation, diarrhea, dry mouth, dyspepsia, nausea, salivation, vomiting)
- Genitourinary (breast engorgement, galactorrhea, gynecomastia, impotence, breast pain, menstrual irregularities, priapism (prolonged erection), urinary retention)
- Hematologic and lymphatic (anemia, hyperglycemia, hypoglycemia, hyponatremia, leukocytosis, leukopenia, elevated blood ammonia levels, lymphomonocytosis)
- Hepatic (jaundice, impaired liver function)
- Musculoskeletal (severe spasms causing arching of the body from head to toe)
- Respiratory (bronchospasms, laryngospasm, increased depth of respiration)
- Special senses (cataracts, blurred vision, visual disturbances, retinopathy)
- Miscellaneous (sudden death, withdrawal syndrome, heat stroke, local tissue reactions from injection)

Drug Interactions

A few drug interactions are known to occur with haloperidol. Cigarette smoking has been linked with lower serum levels of haloperidol. Table 18.2 lists agents that interact with haloperidol.

Assessment of Relevant Core Patient Variables

Health Status

Assess the patient to determine whether he or she has an illness that is treated suitably with antipsychotics. Ensure that the patient does not have Parkinson disease, which is a contraindication for use of haloperidol. Also, assess for other conditions that require precautions for haloperidol use. Assess for a history of seizure disorder because haloperidol decreases the seizure threshold. Dehydration places patients at greater risk for developing neuroleptic malignant syndrome.

Life Span and Gender

Assess the patient's age. Determine whether the patient is pregnant or could become pregnant because haloperidol is a pregnancy category C drug. Safety and efficacy in children has not been assessed. Infants should not be breast-fed if the mother is receiving haloperidol. Oral haloperidol should not be used in children younger than 3 years. Young adult males, especially young black males, have the highest risk for the various dystonias. Older adult women have the highest risk for tardive dyskinesia.

Lifestyle, Diet, and Habits

Assess the patient's typical daily fluid intake to determine whether the patient is sufficiently hydrated. Determine whether the patient smokes cigarettes because smoking may decrease the effectiveness of haloperidol. Alcohol may have additive CNS effects with haloperidol, leading to profound CNS depression.

Environment

Assess the environment where the drug will be given. Intravenous (IV) administration is restricted to an inpatient setting. Intramuscular (IM) doses may be administered in an outpatient setting. Some formulations act as drug depots and slowly release the drug over several weeks. Other times, IM doses may be administered as an emergency treatment until the person can be admitted to an inpatient setting, or the acute symptoms are controlled. Oral haloperidol can be administered in any environmental setting. Because photosensitivity is a possible adverse effect, assess whether or not the person is outside frequently.

Culture and Inherited Traits

Assess the patient's ethnicity because Asians have a 50% higher serum level of haloperidol than whites do. This difference may affect the dose required to be effective.

Nursing Diagnoses and Outcome

- Risk for Injury related to EPS from haloperidol
  Desired outcome: *The patient will remain injury free from haloperidol as EPS are prevented or minimized.*

TABLE 18.2 Agents That Interact With P Haloperidol

Interactants	Effect and Significance	Nursing Management
anticholinergic agents	Decreased haloperidol serum concentrations	Coadminister with caution
azole antifungal agents	May elevate haloperidol serum concentrations	Adjust dose as needed
carbamazepine	Therapeutic effects of haloperidol may be decreased	Adjust dose as needed
charcoal	Charcoal can decrease absorption	Do not give together
lithium	Alterations in consciousness, encephalopathy, EPS, fever	Discontinue either drug if interaction is suspected
Maalox	Impairs absorption of typical (and possibly atypical) antipsychotics	Do not take within 1 hour of taking haloperidol
rifamycins	May decrease haloperidol serum concentrations	Adjust dose as needed

- Altered Thought Processes related to hallucinations and delusion
  Desired outcome: The patient's hallucinations and delusions will be controlled by haloperidol therapy.
- Risk for Ineffective Management of Therapeutic Regimen, Individual, related to adverse effects of drug therapy or poor understanding of the need for drug therapy
  Desired outcome: The patient will take haloperidol therapy as directed.

Planning and Intervention

Maximizing Therapeutic Effects

Encourage the patient to take the drug routinely. Ensure that the patient has swallowed the medication when it is administered and that the patient has not kept the medication in his or her cheek (a practice referred to as "cheeking") in order to spit it out and avoid taking the medication.

Minimizing Adverse Effects

Adverse effects are common and dose related. The goal of therapy is to find a dose that effectively controls the psychotic symptoms but produces minimal adverse effects.

Some of the adverse effects (e.g., sedation and drowsiness) are transient, and patients need to be encouraged to be patient and see whether the adverse effects dissipate with continued use of the drug. If adverse effects are distressing to the patient, modify the treatment plan to make the therapy more acceptable to the patient. For example, instead of giving two equal-sized doses daily to a patient, the larger dose or the entire daily dose could be given at bedtime if daytime sedation is a major problem. Additionally, the patient might be encouraged to be as active as possible during the daytime hours to help ward off sedation.

Many of the adverse effects that are not transient can be minimized to some extent. For example, you should encourage the patient with akathisia to walk when he or she feels restless. Because many of the adverse effects are related to a relative excess of cholinergic stimulation, anticholinergic drugs—most commonly diphenhydramine, benztropine, or trihexyphenidyl—may be administered to treat or minimize these effects. The choice of drug and the route of drug administration are dependent on the severity of the extrapyramidal symptoms present and the degree of patient distress. If the patient is experiencing acute dystonic symptoms, diphenhydramine (Benadryl) or benztropine may be used either intramuscularly or intravenously. Diphenhydramine works rapidly to alleviate acute dystonia, especially those forms that could be life threatening. Once a patient experiences acute EPS, the likelihood increases that acute EPS will recur. To prevent recurrence, benztropine or trihexyphenidyl is added to existing drug therapy on a continuing basis. Sometimes, these drugs are started prophylactically to prevent extrapyramidal symptoms. However, remember that these drugs carry their own adverse effects (see Chapter 21 for more information).

Extrapyramidal symptoms are more likely to occur if the patient repeatedly stops and restarts therapy; thus, the patient should be encouraged to stay on drug therapy once started. Akathisia is sometimes difficult to differentiate from anxiety. If this difficulty arises, the prescriber may treat for one or the other, assess the effectiveness of therapy, and change the drugs if the patient does not respond positively to drug therapy.

Another adverse effect of neuroleptics, and one that is life-threatening, is neuromalignant syndrome. If the patient develops neuromalignant syndrome, stop the antipsychotic immediately. Notify the prescriber that the medication has been stopped for this reason. The patient is then treated symptomatically. Large volumes of normal saline are normally infused as quickly as the patient can tolerate, which not only rehydrates the patient but also flushes the drug from the person's body. Antipyretics may also be given. Because of the delirium that can occur with neuromalignant syndrome, safety precautions may have to be implemented. These precautions may include staying with the patient continuously, decreasing environmental stimuli, or applying physical restraints (although restraints are usually used only as a last resort).

Providing Patient and Family Education

- Teach the patient and family about realistic expectations of antipsychotic therapy. Include information about the delay before relief of symptoms and the necessity of continuing with the medication even after symptom relief is achieved.
- Inform patients and families about possible adverse effects. Patients and families need to understand that some adverse effects will have to be managed because it may not be possible to eliminate them completely.
- Encourage the patient to report adverse effects so that these effects can be managed appropriately.
- Teach the patient to avoid using alcohol and other CNS depressant drugs in order to avoid any additive effects that will produce CNS depression.
- Encourage patients to wear protective covering and sunscreen if they are outside a great deal. Advise them to balance the need to wear clothing to protect from photosensitivity with the need to choose clothing that is cool enough to prevent overheating and heat stroke. Remind patients to drink extra fluids when they are out in the heat in order to prevent dehydration that could lead to neuromalignant syndrome.
- Caution the patient about use of heavy machinery or driving until individual response to the drug is known.

Ongoing Assessment and Evaluation

Treatment with haloperidol is considered effective if the psychotic symptoms are controlled or reduced and the patient does not develop serious adverse effects.

CRITICAL THINKING SCENARIO

What's wrong with this patient?

Your patient, Mr. Jones, has schizophrenia and a history of heart disease. He has been receiving haloperidol, 10 mg twice a day; benztropine, 2 mg twice a day; and verapamil, 80 mg three times a day. This morning, as you approach him to administer his medicine, you notice sweat on his forehead. Upon being questioned, he also complains of discomfort in his arms. You observed that, whereas his gait was previously steady, it now has a slight shuffle.

1. As this patient's nurse, what do you think is happening to Mr. Jones?
2. As this patient's nurse, what initial action should you take?

MEMORY CHIP

[P] Haloperidol

- Typical antipsychotic used to treat schizophrenia and other psychotic illnesses
- Creates its effects by blocking dopamine (specifically D_2), alpha, serotonin, and histamine receptors; minimal blocking effects at cholinergic receptors
- Major contraindication: Parkinson disease
- Most common adverse effect: extrapyramidal symptoms (EPS) such as pseudoparkinsonism, akathisia, acute dystonia, and tardive dyskinesia
- EPS adverse effects are caused by relative lack of dopamine stimulation.
- Most serious adverse effect: neuromalignant syndrome
- **Life span alert: Young adult males, especially young black males, have the highest risk for dystonias. Older adult women have the highest risk for tardive dyskinesia.**
- Maximizing therapeutic effects: Encourage patient to take therapy; check that patient has swallowed drug.
- Minimizing adverse effects: Keep dose as low as possible; avoid going on and off the drug therapy because this behavior increases risk for EPS; administer anticholinergic drugs to treat or prevent EPS adverse effects.
- Most important patient education: importance of continued therapy; how to cope with transient adverse effects and minimize impact of chronic adverse effects

Drugs Significantly Different From [P] Haloperidol

Chlorpromazine (Thorazine), thioridazine (Mellaril), and mesoridazine (Serentil) are all considered low-potency antipsychotics compared with haloperidol, which is a high-potency antipsychotic. This distinction means that a higher dosage of the low-potency drug is necessary to achieve the same antipsychotic effect that is achieved with haloperidol. There is no difference in efficacy between the high-potency and low-potency antipsychotics in treating psychotic symptoms. Recall that the definition of potency is how many milligrams of drug are needed to achieve an effect, and that efficacy refers to how effective the drug is in achieving the therapeutic goal. See Chapter 4 for a complete discussion of these terms. These antipsychotic drugs differ distinctly, however, in their adverse effect profiles. High-potency antipsychotics such as haloperidol cause little sedation or anticholinergic adverse effects such as blurry vision, constipation, dry mouth, urinary hesitation, and delirium, whereas they have a very high likelihood of causing extrapyramidal symptoms such as dystonias, akathisia, and Parkinson-like adverse effects. Low-potency antipsychotics such as chlorpromazine, on the other hand, tend to produce sedation and frequent anticholinergic adverse effects, while presenting a low probability of EPS. Table 18.3 presents a comparison of the risks for various adverse effects with high- and low-potency antipsychotic agents.

Because the high-potency and low-potency antipsychotics alleviate psychotic symptoms to a similar degree, most prescribers consider which type has the least desirable adverse effect profile for each patient. A patient may also express a particular preference for one drug over another. The prescriber chooses the antipsychotic agent accordingly. For example, because an older adult is more sensitive to the anticholinergic effects on the body, a drug that produces little anticholinergic effect, such as haloperidol, may be used. Another example would be a patient who has previously experienced an EPS such as akathisia from taking haloperidol, who may agree to try thioridazine, which, although more sedating, has much less likelihood of causing EPS.

[C] Atypical Antipsychotics

Atypical antipsychotics differ from the typical antipsychotics in that they target specific dopamine receptors, instead of all of them. This specificity creates a much lower adverse effect

TABLE 18.3 Risk for Adverse Effects With High- and Low-Potency Typical Antipsychotics

	Risk of Adverse Effects		
Drug Name	Anticholinergic	Extrapyramidal	Sedating
High Potency			
fluphenazine haloperidol loxapine molindone perphenazine pimozide thiothixene trifluoperazine triflupromazine	Low	High	Low
Low Potency			
chlorpromazine mesoridazine thioridazine	High	Low	High

profile. Another major advantage of the atypical antipsychotics is that they treat both the negative and positive symptoms of schizophrenia. The first atypical antipsychotic was clozapine. This drug causes a serious adverse effect, agranulocytosis, and for this reason is not often used in the United States. When clozapine is used, strict guidelines must be followed. Box 18.5 outlines these guidelines. Olanzapine (Zyprexa), which does not carry a risk for agranulocytosis, is the prototype atypical antipsychotic.

NURSING MANAGEMENT OF THE PATIENT RECEIVING [P] OLANZAPINE

Core Drug Knowledge

Pharmacotherapeutics

Olanzapine is used to treat psychotic symptoms in schizophrenia and for short-term treatment of bipolar mania. Recent research has shown that it can be effectively used off-label, especially if combined with an SSRI antidepressant, for chronic management of bipolar disorder (Tohen et al., 2002; 2003). Other unlabeled uses include agitation, Alzheimer-type dementia, other dementias, and obsessive-compulsive disorder that does not respond to selective serotonin reuptake inhibitors.

Pharmacokinetics

Olanzapine is moderately absorbed and achieves a bioavailability of 60%. The drug is highly protein bound at 93%. It is metabolized by gluconidation and oxidation through the cytochrome P-450 system, particularly CYP1A2 and CYP2D6. Elimination is through the urine and the feces, with about twice as much being eliminated in the urine as in the stool. Half-life is between 21 and 54 hours. This long half-life allows the drug to be dosed once a day.

Pharmacodynamics

Olanzapine works by blocking several neuroreceptor sites, including serotonin, dopamine, muscarinic, histamine-1 (H_1), and alpha-1. Olanzapine has high affinity for these sites but lower affinity for gamma-aminobutyric acid (GABA), benzodiazepine, and beta receptor sites, although blockade at these receptor sites also occurs. Olanzapine, like other atypical antipsychotics, affects the negative symptoms as well as the positive symptoms of schizophrenia. (Typical antipsychotics, such as haloperidol, affect only the positive symptoms.) Olanzapine, as well as other atypical antipsychotics, may elevate blood glucose levels, sometimes to extremely high levels, through an unknown mechanism.

Contraindications and Precautions

There are no labeled contraindications for olanzapine. Precautions should be taken if the patient has diabetes because all use of atypical antipsychotics is associated with substantially elevated blood glucose levels.

Adverse Effects

In general, atypical antipsychotics are well tolerated and produce few adverse effects. In patients who do experience adverse effects, the most common are related to the CNS: drowsiness and sedation, insomnia, agitation, nervousness, hostility, and dizziness. The most important adverse effects with olanzapine are tardive dyskinesia and neuroleptic malignant syndrome, although these effects occur very rarely. Hyperglycemia for diabetic patients may be pronounced enough to require insulin adjustments; patients without diabetes are unlikely to have problems from increases in blood glucose. A wide variety of other adverse effects can potentially occur, including:

- CV (hypotension, tachycardia, hypertension, bradycardia, cardiac arrest, cerebrovascular accident, congestive heart failure, palpitation, vasodilation, pulmonary embolus, and premature atrial fibrillation)
- CNS (asthenia, abnormal gate, akathisia, akinesia, tremor, amnesia, ataxia, delirium, dysarthria, hypesthesia, hypokinesia, incoordination, increased libido, vertigo, intense or abnormal dreams, euphoria, paresthesia, suicidal thoughts, neuroleptic malignant syndrome, and pseudoparkinsonism)
- Dermatologic (rash)
- GI (constipation, abdominal pain, weight gain, increased appetite, and dry mouth)
- Genitourinary (premenstrual syndrome)
- Musculoskeletal (arthralgia, neck rigidity, twitching, hypertonia, and tremor)
- Ocular (dimmed vision)
- Respiratory (rhinitis, cough, and pharyngitis)

Drug Interactions

The risks of using olanzapine in combination with other drugs have not been extensively evaluated. Caution should be used when olanzapine is taken in combination with other centrally acting drugs or alcohol. Coadministering either

BOX 18.5 Clozaril Treatment/Patient Management System

Results of early clinical studies with clozapine indicated that it was associated with 1% to 2% incidence of potentially lethal agranulocytosis. To minimize this risk, clozapine is available only through treatment systems that ensure a weekly or biweekly WBC testing prior to delivery of the next supply of medication. During the 5 years of WBC monitoring with the "Clozaril National Registry," the risk for agranulocytosis was reduced to approximately 0.38%. Guidelines for the Clozaril treatment/patient management system include:

- Treatment systems may include facilities with on-site pharmacies, facilities without on-site pharmacies, and individual treating physicians.
- Patients taking clozapine are enrolled in the "Clozaril National Registry."
- Clozaril is only available through weekly or biweekly distribution systems.
- WBC evaluation is required prior to initiation of therapy, weekly or biweekly during therapy, and for 4 weeks after discontinuation.
- All WBC evaluations (normal and abnormal results) must be promptly reported to the "Clozaril National Registry" within 7 days of collection.
- The "Clozaril National Registry" must be promptly notified of all patients who discontinue.

ethanol or diazepam with olanzapine potentiated the orthostatic hypotension observed with olanzapine. Because of its potential for inducing hypotension, olanzapine may enhance the effects of certain antihypertensive agents. Olanzapine also may antagonize the effects of levodopa and dopamine agonists.

Agents that induce CYP1A2 or glucuronyl transferase enzymes, such as omeprazole and rifampin, may increase olanzapine clearance. Inhibitors of CYP1A2 could potentially inhibit olanzapine clearance. Although olanzapine is metabolized by multiple enzyme systems, induction or inhibition of a single enzyme may appreciably alter olanzapine clearance. Therefore, a dosage increase (for induction) or a dosage decrease (for inhibition) may have to be considered with specific drugs.

Carbamazepine therapy (200 mg twice daily) increases the clearance of olanzapine by approximately 50%, likely because carbamazepine is a potent inducer of CYP1A2 activity. Higher daily doses of carbamazepine may cause an even greater increase in olanzapine clearance. Fluvoxamine, a CYP1A2 inhibitor, decreases the clearance of olanzapine, resulting in a mean increase in olanzapine maximum concentration (C_{max}) following fluvoxamine of 54% in female nonsmokers and 77% in male smokers. Mean increases in olanzapine area under the curve (AUC) are 52% and 108%, respectively. Lower doses of olanzapine should be considered in patients receiving concomitant treatment with fluvoxamine. Table 18.4 lists potential drug interactions with olanzapine.

Assessment of Relevant Core Patient Variables

Health Status

Obtain the patient's baseline vital signs and other measurements, such as weight, serum glucose, triglyceride levels, and complete blood count, before olanzapine therapy begins. It is critical that a patient's serum glucose levels be monitored before and throughout any atypical antipsychotic therapy. Also, assess for various individual factors that can alter drug response, such as liver function and gastric absorption.

Life Span and Gender

Document the age and gender of the patient. Explore the sexual patterns and reproductive goals of the patient because reproductive effects such as changes in libido, amenorrhea, irregular menses, impotence, and ejaculatory failure may occur. The elderly patient receiving atypical antipsychotics should be considered at higher risk for adverse effects.

Lifestyle, Diet, and Habits

Evaluate the patient's caffeine intake and diet because the efficacy of olanzapine may be affected by fluctuations in caffeine intake. Also assess for use of dong quai and St. John's wort (because these herbal medicines may cause photosensitization) and for the use of kava kava, gotu kola, valerian, St. John's wort, and ethanol (because these agents may increase CNS effects).

Document the patient's occupational and recreational activities because orthostatic hypotension, drug-related dizziness, and blurred vision may impair coordination and dexterity, and hypotension may occur with hot tubs, hot showers, or tub baths.

Environment

Document the climate in which the drug will be administered because drug-related heatstroke may occur in hot weather.

Nursing Diagnoses and Outcomes

Several nursing diagnoses may apply to the patient receiving atypical antipsychotics. Examples include:

- Imbalanced Nutrition: More than Body Requirements related to increased appetite and secondary to olanzapine use
  Desired outcome: *The patient will state that there is a risk for weight gain and will identify the effects of a low-fat diet and exercise on weight control.*
- Risk for Injury related to drug-induced dizziness, blurred vision, and orthostatic hypotension
  Desired outcome: *The patient will identify factors that increase the risk for injury and will relate intent to use safety measures and practices to prevent injury.*
- Risk for Fluid and Electrolyte Imbalance and Hyperglycemia related to adverse effects of medication
  Desired outcome: *The patient will maintain appropriate fluid and electrolyte balance while receiving medication.*
- Risk for Sedation related to adverse effects of the medication

TABLE 18.4 Agents That Interact With P Olanzapine

Interactants	Effect and Significance	Nursing Management
carbamazepine	Therapeutic effects of olanzapine may be decreased	Adjust dose as needed
charcoal	Charcoal can decrease absorption	Do not give together
CYP1A2 inducers (e.g., carbamazepine, omeprazole, rifampin)	May decrease olanzapine serum concentrations	May need to increase olanzapine dose
CYP1A2 inhibitors (e.g., fluvoxamine)	May increase olanzapine serum concentrations	May need to decrease dose
fluoxetine	Coadministration resulted in a small (16%) decrease in olanzapine clearance	May need to decrease olanzapine dose

Desired outcome: The patient will maintain appropriate level of wakefulness while receiving medication.

Planning and Intervention

Maximizing Therapeutic Effects

Maintaining adherence to any medication regimen once a patient experiences relief of symptoms is an ongoing challenge for all health care providers. With patients experiencing disturbances of their thoughts and perceptions, it is essential that you focus, from the very start, on developing a trusting therapeutic relationship. This trust that develops between you and the patient frequently will be what enables the patient to develop the insight necessary to continue taking medication. This same trust can also form the basis on which you and the patient candidly discuss the many benefits of continuing with the medication, even if adverse effects occur. By focusing on the patient's own hopes and aspirations for the quality of life he or she wishes to have, adherence to the medication regimen will be enhanced.

Minimizing Adverse Effects

Assess fasting blood sugar before drug therapy is initiated. Fasting blood sugar must be monitored throughout therapy in some patients, especially if the patient has diabetes. To minimize daytime drowsiness, you can give the entire daily dose at night.

Providing Patient and Family Education

- Teach the signs of hyperglycemia; patients with diabetes may need to be taught to monitor blood sugar more frequently than before olanzapine therapy.
- Teach the patient and family that the therapeutic response will not be immediate.
- Stress the importance of continuing drug therapy even in the absence of psychotic symptoms.
- Help the patient to stay motivated to continue treatment. To promote adherence to the therapeutic regimen, educate the patient and family about the effects of medication—both therapeutic and adverse. Advise the patient about adverse effects that, if unidentified, may contribute to nonadherence. An example of this kind of effect is sedation.
- Ensure that the patient understands the importance of keeping the drug safely stored and away from curious children.

Ongoing Assessment and Evaluation

Treatment with an atypical antipsychotic such as olanzapine requires ongoing assessment and evaluation, because of the ongoing, chronic nature of most illnesses in which they are used. For this reason, you must continue to assess the patient for the originally presenting symptoms for which the drug therapy was initiated. You also will evaluate the patient's ability to meet the therapeutic goals identified by the entire treatment team. Throughout this process, you must continue monitoring for any adverse effects that the patient may develop.

MEMORY CHIP

P Olanzapine

- Atypical antipsychotic used to treat schizophrenia and bipolar mania
- Olanzapine works by blocking serotonin, dopamine, muscarinic, H_1, and alpha-1 receptor sites
- Most common adverse effects: normally well tolerated; if adverse effects occur, CNS effects such as drowsiness, sedation, dizziness
- Most serious adverse effects: tardive dyskinesia and neuroleptic malignant syndrome (both rare)
- **Life span alert: Older adults are more at risk for adverse effects.**
- Maximizing therapeutic effects: Encourage patient to take medication regularly.
- Minimizing adverse effects: Give daily dose at bedtime to decrease daytime sedation.
- Most important patient education: Full therapeutic effect will take time to achieve; patient may need to tolerate some adverse effects until they pass.

DRUGS FOR ALZHEIMER-TYPE DEMENTIA

C Acetylcholinesterase Enzyme Inhibitors

Acetylcholine is a neurotransmitter for several CNS circuits that are located in the basal forebrain, the hippocampus, and parts of the cerebral cortex. Agents that augment this system have been under investigation to treat Alzheimer disease for more than 20 years, and numerous types of drugs that augment levels of acetylcholine to compensate for losses of cholinergic function in the brain have been used in these patients. These drugs have included acetylcholine precursors, muscarinic agonists, nicotinic agonists, and acetylcholinesterase inhibitors. The only FDA-approved drugs to treat the symptoms of Alzheimer disease are the acetylcholinesterase inhibitors. Acetylcholinesterase (AChE) is the enzyme that breaks down acetylcholine. By inhibiting the action of AChE, acetylcholinesterase inhibitors (AChEIs) prolong the activity of acetylcholine on cortical cholinergic receptors and in the synapse. The mechanism of action of the three AChEIs—tacrine, donepezil, and rivastigmine—is essentially the same. These agents increase concentrations of the memory-regulating and cognition-regulating neurotransmitter acetylcholine by reversibly inhibiting the enzyme cholinesterase. Although these drugs have not been shown to alter the course of the dementing process, it is anticipated that disease effects will lessen as the disease process advances and fewer cholinergic neurons remain intact.

Drugs used to treat dementia and Alzheimer disease include donepezil, rivastigmine, and tacrine. Rivastigmine (Exelon) is the prototype Alzheimer drug. Table 18.5 summarizes selected Alzheimer drugs.

TABLE 18.5 Summary of Selected Drugs for Alzheimer Disease

Drug (Trade) Name	Selected Indications	Route and Dosage Range	Pharmacokinetics
P rivastigmine (Exelon)	Mild to moderate Alzheimer type dementia	*Adult:* PO, 3 to 6 mg bid to a maximum of 12 mg/d *Child:* Not currently indicated	*Onset:* Intermediate *Duration:* 10 h $t_{1/2}$: 1.5 h
donepezil (Aricept)	Mild to moderate Alzheimer type dementia	*Adult:* 5–10 mg/d *Child:* Safety and efficacy not established	*Onset:* Unknown *Duration:* Unknown $t_{1/2}$: 70 h
tacrine (Cognex)	Mild to moderate Alzheimer type dementia	*Adult:* 10 mg qid *Child:* Safety and efficacy not established	*Onset:* Unknown *Duration:* 6 h $t_{1/2}$: 2–4 h

NURSING MANAGEMENT OF THE PATIENT RECEIVING P RIVASTIGMINE

Core Drug Knowledge

Pharmacotherapeutics

Rivastigmine is indicated for treating mild to moderate dementia of the Alzheimer type. In clinical studies, it has been shown to enhance cognition (memory, language, orientation) and improve the ability to perform activities of daily living among patients with mild to moderate Alzheimer disease.

Pharmacokinetics

Rivastigmine is rapidly and completely absorbed, with peak plasma concentrations reached in 1 hour. Administering rivastigmine with food delays (by about 1.5 hours), but does not impair, drug absorption. Rivastigmine may be taken with food if gastrointestinal adverse effects are problematic.

Rivastigmine is widely distributed throughout the body. It penetrates the blood–brain barrier, reaching peak concentrations in cerebrospinal fluid in 1.4 to 2.6 hours. Rivastigmine is 40% bound to plasma proteins.

Rivastigmine is rapidly and extensively metabolized by acetylcholinesterase; minimal metabolism occurs by the major CYP450 isozymes. Thus, no CYP450 drug interactions have been observed. It is about equally metabolized through the hepatic cytochrome P-450 enzyme system and excreted as unchanged drug in the urine. The elimination half-life is 1.5 hours, with most elimination as metabolites excreted from the kidneys. The oral solution and capsules may be interchanged at equal doses.

Pharmacodynamics

Rivastigmine is a carbamate derivative that is believed to exert its therapeutic effect by enhancing cholinergic function. This enhancement occurs by increasing the concentration of acetylcholine through reversible inhibition of acetylcholinesterase. Rivastigmine does not alter the course of the underlying dementing process.

Contraindications and Precautions

Rivastigmine is contraindicated in patients with hypersensitivity to carbamate derivatives. No adequate or well-controlled studies have been performed in children or in pregnant or lactating women; therefore, rivastigmine should be used cautiously in these patients. Rivastigmine is in FDA pregnancy category B. It is not known whether rivastigmine is excreted in breast milk. Like other drugs that increase cholinergic activity, rivastigmine should be used with care in patients with a history of asthma or obstructive pulmonary disease.

Adverse Effects

Rivastigmine is associated with substantial gastrointestinal adverse reactions, including nausea and vomiting, anorexia, and weight loss. Other adverse effects include dizziness, headache, chest pain, peripheral edema, vertigo, joint pain, agitation, nervousness, delusion, paranoid reaction, coughing, generalized rash, and urinary incontinence. Rivastigmine may have vagotonic effects on heart rates (resulting in bradycardia) because the drug increases cholinergic activity. These vagotonic effects may be particularly important in patients with "sick sinus syndrome" or other supraventricular cardiac conduction conditions. Because it increases cholinergic activity, rivastigmine may cause urinary obstruction and may have some potential for causing seizures, although seizure activity also may be a manifestation of Alzheimer disease.

Drug Interactions

Pharmacokinetic drug interactions are not believed to occur with rivastigmine because only minimal metabolism of the drug occurs through the major CYP450 isozymes.

Synergistic effects can be expected when acetylcholinesterase inhibitors are given with succinylcholine, similar neuromuscular blocking agents, or cholinergic agonists, such as bethanechol. Because of their mechanism of action, AChEIs have the potential to interfere with the activity of anticholinergic medications.

Assessment of Relevant Core Patient Variables

Health Status

Assess body systems thoroughly. The patient's cardiac status may be adversely affected by AChEIs because these drugs

increase cholinergic activity and may cause bradycardia from vagal effects on heart rate. The cholinergic activity of the AChEIs may cause urinary retention or obstruction; men with benign prostatic hypertrophy may be especially at risk.

Evaluate the patient's renal and hepatic function. Dosage adjustments may be necessary in patients with renal or hepatic function impairment. Review the patient's respiratory function because respiratory depression may occur. Carefully assess the patient's gastrointestinal status because AChEIs such as rivastigmine may increase gastric acid secretion, cause gastritis, and exacerbate peptic ulcer disease. Assess and closely monitor individuals with a history of ulcer disease or those receiving nonsteroidal anti-inflammatory drugs for symptoms of active or occult gastrointestinal bleeding.

Life Span and Gender

Document the age of the patient. The mean oral clearance of rivastigmine is 30% lower in elderly individuals taking rivastigmine. Assess women of childbearing age for pregnancy and lactation. If appropriate, explore potential benefits of rivastigmine therapy compared with potential risks to the fetus or child.

Lifestyle, Diet, and Habits

Assess the patient for tobacco use because nicotine use moderately increases the oral clearance of rivastigmine (by 23%).

Environment

Be aware of the environment in which the drug will be administered. If appropriate, assess the patient's home or living environment. Secure all medication to avoid accidental inappropriate ingestion by the patient.

Nursing Diagnoses and Outcomes

- Imbalanced Nutrition: Less than Body Requirements related to decreased desire to eat secondary to nausea and vomiting from drug therapy
  Desired outcome: *The patient will ingest daily nutritional requirements in relation to activity level and metabolic needs.*
- Risk for Injury related to adverse effect of sedation
  Desired outcome: *The patient will establish appropriate sleep and rest patterns, participate in activities, and establish priorities for daily and weekly activities.*

Planning and Intervention

Maximizing Therapeutic Effects

It is important to detect and correct any treatable factors that can cause or contribute to cognitive impairment. Be aware that any cognitive impairment may be exacerbated by hearing or visual deficits, depression, delirium arising from a urinary tract infection, heart failure, electrolyte imbalance, or anemia.

Minimizing Adverse Effects

Offer small frequent meals or give the drug with food to offset GI effects of nausea and vomiting. Monitor weight throughout therapy. If weight loss occurs, encourage intake of nutrient- and calorie-rich foods that are acceptable to patient, such as Ensure or Boost beverages, milkshakes, or puddings.

Providing Patient and Family Education

The irreversible nature of Alzheimer disease and its progressive, deteriorating course have devastating effects on affected individuals, their caregivers, and their families. Although drug therapy is directed toward enhancing cognitive and functional abilities, or at least slowing the cognitive decline, teaching considerations reflect more issues regarding the disease process and its progressive nature as well as the burdens facing the caregiver.

- Advise the patient and family that nausea and vomiting are likely with rivastigmine use and that anorexia and weight loss may result. Encourage them to monitor for these adverse events and to inform the prescriber if they occur.
- To increase the likelihood that the patient will accept the medication from caregivers willingly, teach helpful communication techniques, such as using concrete language, maintaining social greetings and rituals, using a soft tone of voice, and simplifying and repeating instructions frequently.

Ongoing Assessment and Evaluation

Rivastigmine, as with other AChEIs, produces modest improvement in some measures of cognitive functioning and in other areas of functioning in the patient with mild to moderate Alzheimer disease, apparently slowing the progression of the disease. However, you must advise patients and their families to maintain realistic expectations regarding what the drug can do.

CHAPTER SUMMARY

- Thought, like mood, is controlled by combinations of neurotransmitters that stimulate neuroreceptors in the brain. The primary neurotransmitter related to thought processing is believed to be dopamine.
- Another important neurotransmitter is acetylcholine. Many areas of the brain secrete acetylcholine; reduction in the amount of this neu-

MEMORY CHIP

P Rivastigmine

- Used in Alzheimer dementia
- Works by inhibiting acetylcholinesterase (the enzyme that breaks down acetylcholine), thus increasing the amount of active acetylcholine
- Major contraindication: hypersensitivity to carbamate derivatives
- Most common adverse effects: gastrointestinal
- Most serious adverse effects: vagotonic effects in patients with "sick sinus syndrome" or other supraventricular cardiac conduction conditions
- Maximizing therapeutic effect: Assess for and correct any treatable factors that may impair cognition.
- Minimizing adverse effects: Offer small, frequent meals; monitor weight; offer nutritional supplements.
- Most important patient and family education: that drug therapy will not cure Alzheimer disease but will minimize symptoms; importance of monitoring weight; and techniques to gain patient acceptance of medication

Drugs Treating Seizure Disorders

chapter 19

Learning Objectives

At the completion of this chapter the student will:

1. Identify the three basic mechanisms of action of the antiepileptic drugs.
2. Identify common core drug knowledge about prototype drugs belonging to the major antiepileptic drug (AED) classifications.
3. Identify core patient variables of concern related to the major AEDs.
4. Generate a nursing plan of care based on the interactions between core drug knowledge and core patient variables for the major AEDs.
5. Describe nursing interventions to maximize therapeutic effects and minimize adverse effects for the major AEDs.
6. Relate key points for patient and family education for major AEDs.

KEY TERMS

absence seizure
convulsions
epilepsy
GABA
generalized seizure
glutamate
partial seizure
postictal
seizure
status epilepticus
tonic-clonic seizure

FEATURED WEBLINK

http://www.ninds.nih.gov
From the National Institute of Neurological Disorders and Stroke home page, click on the link for disorders. General information about epilepsy and other neurologic disorders is available. The site also provides links to current clinical research trials and published research on epilepsy.

CONNECTIONS WEBLINK:

http://www.connection.lww.com/go/aschenbrenner.

rotransmitter causes cognitive changes. Acetylcholine has a number of functions including arousal, coordination of movement, memory acquisition, and memory retention. Norepinephrine and serotonin are other neurotransmitters that are believed to be important to normal thought, but their exact mechanisms are not known yet.

- Schizophrenia, a psychotic disorder, has components termed positive and negative symptoms. The term "positive symptom" does not mean that the changes are beneficial to the patient. The positive symptoms of hallucinations and delusions add a layer of something new to the person. They are in excess of or are a distortion of normal brain function. The "negative symptoms" take away from the person's personality and represent a loss or a diminishing of normal brain function. Negative symptoms include flat or blunted emotions, lack of pleasure or interest in things (anhedonia), and limited speech.
- Haloperidol (Haldol) is the prototype typical antipsychotic. It is used to treat psychotic disorders, such as schizophrenia, and relieves primarily positive symptoms. The full therapeutic effect from haloperidol can require several days to develop. Haloperidol creates its effects by blocking dopamine (specifically D_2), alpha, serotonin, and histamine receptors. It has minimal blocking effects on cholinergic receptors.
- Haloperidol's blockade of dopaminergic receptors produces decreased symptoms of movement disorders, relief of hallucinations and delusions, relief of psychosis, worsened negative symptoms, a release of prolactin, and a quieting of the chemoreceptive trigger zone in the brain. Its blockade of alpha, serotonin, histamine, and cholinergic receptors produces many of its adverse effects.
- The most common reason patients stop taking antipsychotic medications like haloperidol is the occurrence of adverse effects. The higher the dose of haloperidol, the more likely the patient will experience adverse effects. Stopping and starting therapy also increases the likelihood of developing extrapyramidal symptoms (EPS). Encourage the patient to stay with therapy because some of the adverse effects are transient and can be managed.
- Chlorpromazine (Thorazine), thioridazine (Mellaril), and mesoridazine (Serentil) are all considered low-potency typical antipsychotics, compared with haloperidol, which is a high-potency antipsychotic. A higher dosage of these drugs is necessary to achieve the same antipsychotic affect as those achieved with haloperidol. Both types of typical antipsychotics have the same effectiveness, although they have different adverse effects. High-potency typical antipsychotics, such as haloperidol, have a very high likelihood of causing EPS (e.g., dystonias, akathisia, and Parkinson-like adverse effects). Low-potency typical antipsychotics are more likely to produce sedation and anticholinergic adverse effects but are unlikely to produce EPS.
- Atypical antipsychotics differ from the typical antipsychotics in that they target specific dopamine receptors instead of all of them and that they treat both the negative and positive symptoms of psychotic disorders.
- In general, atypical antipsychotics such as olanzapine are well tolerated and produce few adverse effects, although some patients experience sedation and dizziness. Elevated blood glucose levels can also be problematic, especially for patients with diabetes.
- Drugs that augment levels of acetylcholine, by preventing its breakdown by acetylcholinesterase, compensate for losses of cholinergic function in the brain and are used to treat Alzheimer-type dementia. Rivastigmine (Exelon) is the prototype acetylcholinesterase inhibitor (AChEI).
- Rivastigmine produces modest improvement in some measures of cognitive functioning and in other areas of functioning in the patient with mild to moderate Alzheimer disease, apparently slowing the progression of the disease. The most common adverse effects are gastrointestinal.

▲ QUESTIONS FOR STUDY AND REVIEW

1. What are the major differences between high-potency and low-potency typical antipsychotic drugs?
2. Define EPS.
3. What are the differences between typical antipsychotics such as haloperidol and atypical antipsychotics such as olanzapine?
4. Why can acute dystonias be a medical emergency?
5. Describe some of the suggestions that you could offer to a patient to help him or her cope with sedation and drowsiness when haloperidol therapy is first initiated.
6. Describe how rivastigmine produces therapeutic effects in Alzheimer-type dementia.

? Need More Help?

Chapter 18 of the study guide for *Drug Therapy in Nursing* 2e contains NCLEX-style questions and other learning activities to reinforce your understanding of the concepts presented in this chapter. For additional information or to purchase the study guide, visit *http://connection.lww.com/go/aschenbrenner.*

■ REFERENCES AND BIBLIOGRAPHY

American Psychiatric Association. (2000). *Diagnostic and statistical manual of mental disorders* (4th ed., text revision). Washington, DC: Author.

Groves, W. C., Brandt, J., Steinberg, M., et al. (2000). Vascular dementia and Alzheimer disease: Is there a difference? A comparison of symptoms by disease duration. *Journal of Neuropsychiatry and Clinical Neuroscience, 12*(3), 305–315.

Executive summary of mental health: Culture, race, ethnicity [Online]. Available: *http://www.surgeongeneral.gov/library/mentalhealth/cre/execsummary-1.html.* Accessed August 2004.

Lieberman, J. A., Tollefson, G., Tohen, M., et al., for the HGDH Study Group. (2003). Comparative efficacy and safety of atypical and conventional antipsychotic drugs in first-episode psychosis: A randomized, double-blind trial of olanzapine versus haloperidol. *American Journal of Psychiatry, 160*(8), 1396–1404.

Lin, K. M., Poland, R. E., Lau, J. K., et al. (1988). Haloperidol and prolactin concentrations in Asians and Caucasians. *Journal of Clinical Psychopharmacology, 8*(3), 195–201.

Lin, K. M., & Poland, R. E. (2000). Ethnicity, culture, and psychopharmacy. American College of Neuropsychopharmacology. [Online]. Available: *http://www.acnp.org-g4-GN401000184/CH180.html.*

Pelegrin, G. M. (2003). Poor compliance [Online]. *Pharmacy Times.* Available: *http://www.pharmacytimes.com/article.cfm?ID=563.*

Tohen, M., Baker, R. W., Altshuler, L. L., et al. (2002). Olanzapine versus divalproex in the treatment of acute mania. *American Journal of Psychiatry, 159*(6), 1011–1017.

Tohen, M., Vieta, E., Calabrese, J., et al. (2003). Efficacy of olanzapine and olanzapine-fluoxetine combination in the treatment of bipolar I depression. *Archives of General Psychiatry, 60*(11), 1079–1088.

Voruganti, L. I. V., & Awad, A. G. (2004). Neuroleptic dysphoria: Towards a new synthesis. *Psychopharmacology, 171,*121–132.

Drugs Treating Seizure Disorders

(C) Antiepileptics

Antiepileptic drugs that decrease sodium influx

- [P] **phenytoin**
- ethotoin
- fosphenytoin
- mephyenytoin
- carbamazepine
- felbamate
- lamotrigine
- levetiracetam
- oxcarbazepine
- topiramate
- valproic acid

Antiepileptic drugs that decrease calcium influx

- [P] **ethosuximide**
- methsuximide
- phensuximide
- zonisamide

Antiepileptic drugs that increase the effects of GABA

- (C) **benzodiazepines**
- clonazepam
- clorazepate
- diazepam
- [P] **lorazepam** (see also Chapter 16)

Antiepileptic drugs significantly different from benzodiazepines

- gabapentin
- phenobarbital
- primidone
- tiagabine
- vigabatrin

Antiepileptic drugs used in seizures related to pre-eclampsia and eclampsia

- **lorazepam** (see also Chapter 55)

The symbol (C) indicates the **drug class.**
Drugs in **bold type** marked with the symbol [P] are prototypes.
Drugs in blue type are closely related to the prototype.
Drugs in red type are significantly different from the prototype.
Drugs in black type with no symbol are also used in drug therapy; no prototype

Epilepsy, a brain disorder, is not a single entity, but rather a group of neurologic disorders in which CNS neurons display hyperexcitability. This excessive neurologic activity produces a wide variety of effects, from loss of consciousness with generalized muscle twitching to mild alterations in consciousness such as confusion or a blank stare with repetitive blinking. All of these effects from altered neurologic activity are termed **seizures.** More than 2 million people in the United States have experienced an unprovoked seizure or have been diagnosed with epilepsy (National Institutes of Health, 2004). Patients with patterns of seizures who are diagnosed with epilepsy are treated with antiepileptic drugs (AEDs). Many of the AEDs, especially the newer drugs, are not chemically related to each other and do not fit into a drug class with other drugs. The three main ways that AEDs work are by decreasing the rate at which sodium flows into the cell, inhibiting calcium flow rate into the cell through specific channels, and increasing the effect of the neuroinhibitor gamma-aminobutyric acid (GABA). Some drugs work in more than one way. Three main classes of drugs used to treat seizures are discussed in this chapter: drugs that decrease sodium influx, represented by the prototype phenytoin (Dilantin); drugs that decrease calcium influx, represented by the prototype ethosuximide (Zarontin); and drugs that increase the effectiveness of GABA, represented by the benzodiazepines. The prototype benzodiazepine, lorazepam, is discussed at length in Chapter 16.

Drugs in the same class and represented by the prototype of phenytoin are ethotoin (Peganone), fosphenytoin (Cerebyx), and mephenytoin (Mesantoin). Drugs that also inhibit the influx of sodium but that are significantly different from phenytoin are carbamazepine (Tegretol), valproic acid (Depakote), topiramate (Topamax), lamotrigine (Lamictal), oxcarbazepine (Trileptal), levetiracetam (Keppra), and felbamate (Felbatol).

Drugs that are in the same class and represented by the prototype ethosuximide are methsuximide (Celontin) and phensuximide (Milontin). A drug significantly different from the prototype that also decreases calcium influx is zonisamide (Zonegran).

The use of benzodiazepines to treat seizures is covered in this chapter. Drugs that are significantly different from the benzodiazepines but that also increase the effectiveness of GABA are gabapentin (Neurontin), phenobarbital, primidone (Mysoline), tiagabine (Gabitril), and vigabatrin (Sabril).

A drug used specifically to treat seizures associated with pre-eclampsia and eclampsia that is significantly different from all of the prototypes is magnesium sulfate.

PHYSIOLOGY

Action potentials within neurons are initiated by an influx of sodium into the cell through special sodium channels in the cell membrane. For sodium to enter through the cell membrane, the channels have to be open and in an active state. As soon as sodium enters, the channels close and return to an inactive state. When the voltage-dependent channel is inactive, sodium cannot enter through the cell membrane. Influx of calcium through specialized voltage-dependent channels also plays a role in creating an action potential. Usually, this has a limited effect, except in the neurons of the hypothalamus. The movement of these two ions into the cell is controlled by special mechanisms to maintain homeostasis and prevent excessive formation of action potentials. Neurons normally fire at about 80 times a second.

When the cell fires and the action potential spreads across the presynaptic terminal, release of neurotransmitters into the synaptic cleft occurs. Some of these neurotransmitters, such as **glutamate,** produce excitation, and others, such as GABA, inhibit the nervous system. **GABA** normally acts as a counterbalance to glutamate, preventing hyperexcitation, and works at specialized receptors; it is present throughout the brain. After GABA is released into the synapse, it is taken back up by the nerve cell to be either degraded or re-released. Some GABA is taken up by glial cells, which are nonnerve cells in the supporting tissue around the brain and spinal column. GABA in glial cells is metabolized into the amino acid glutamine, which is used by nerve cells to create more GABA or glutamate (Figure 19.1).

PATHOPHYSIOLOGY

When a group of neurons exhibits coordinated, high-frequency discharge, it is termed a focus. The causes of a focus include head trauma, tumor growth, hypoxia, and inherited birth defects. When the activity from a focus spreads to other areas of the brain causing other neurons to join in the hyperactivity, seizures result. These patients may have either high levels of glutamate or low levels of GABA, which allow the focus to take over in the brain. In epilepsy, the neurons may fire as many as 500 times a second, in great excess of the normal range. The classifications of seizures are based on how widespread the neural hyperactivity is within the brain. The two basic types of seizures are partial (also known as focal) and generalized. Subtypes are found within each of the two types. Figure 19.2 presents the classifications of seizures. **Partial seizures** occur when focus activity is limited to an area of the brain, within one hemisphere. The hyperactive neurons are in the cerebral cortex, and the effect on the adjacent cortical areas is limited. When the focus activity has spread to both hemispheres, **generalized seizure** symptoms will occur. The spread of focus activity can be compared to teenagers at a party. Although a few partygoers might get hyperactive and a little out of control, the parents in the house inhibit the spread of such behavior, and the party should stay on track. If no parents are present, no direct inhibition on the partygoers' actions occurs, and the hyperactive and wild behavior will spread to more and more people at the party, possibly resulting in a melee.

Partial seizures can be further divided into two main subgroups, simple and complex. The defining difference between them is that the level of consciousness is altered in some way in complex partial seizures. Simple partial seizures may manifest as twitching in a particular muscle grouping, for example, in the right leg; no loss of consciousness occurs. Complex partial seizures likely have some involuntary muscle twitching or movement also, but the patient seems confused or exhibits odd behavior, both of which are evidence of an impaired level of consciousness.

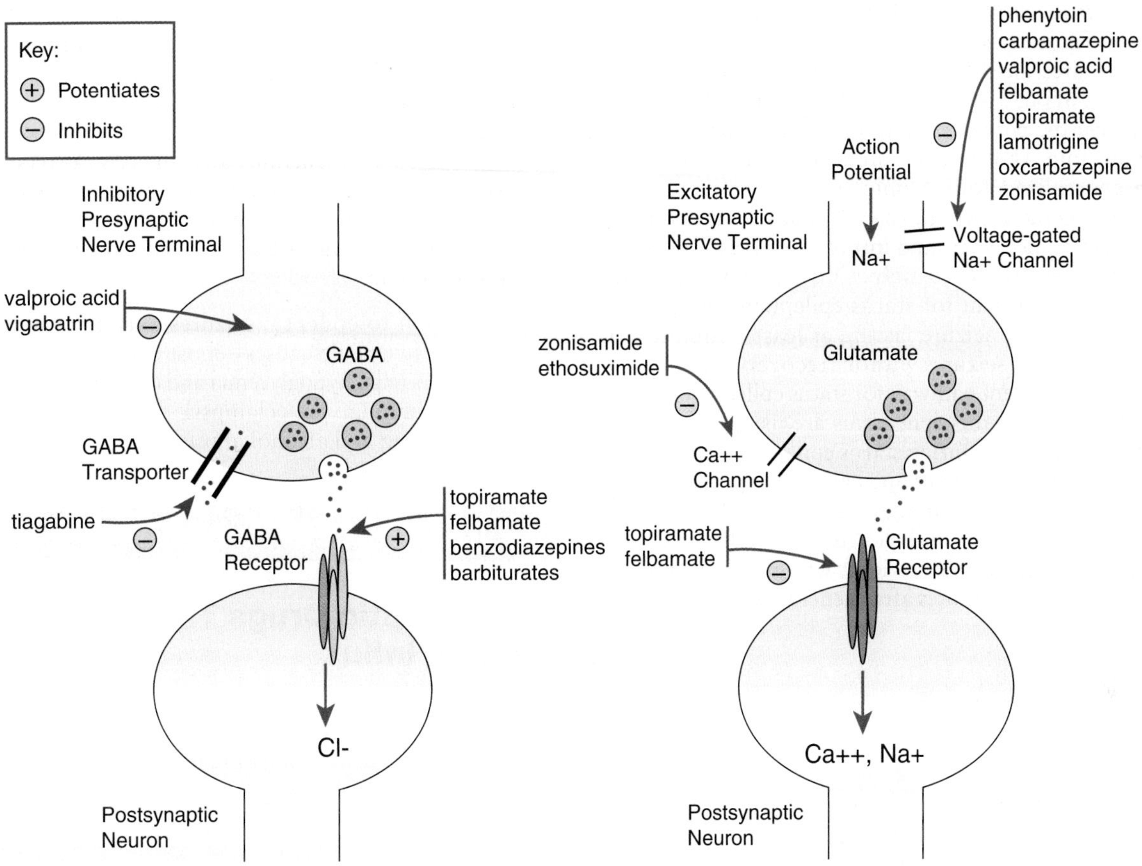

FIGURE 19.1 Mechanisms of antiepileptic drugs. Reprinted with permission from Drug Topics, Medical Economics Company, July 3, 2000.

Generalized seizures are broken into several subtypes: tonic-clonic (also referred to as grand mal), absence (also referred to as petit mal), atonic, myoclonic, status epilepticus, and febrile. A brief description of these generalized seizures follows:

- **Tonic-clonic seizure** (grand mal)—the entire cerebral cortex is altered by hyperexcited neurons. Initially, the person experiences stiffness and rigidity (tonic phase) and falls to the ground. The person loses consciousness, and no movement follows for several seconds. Then, massive muscle spasms (**convulsions**) occur, with the muscles alternating between contracting and relaxing (clonic phase). Urinary or bowel incontinence and biting the tongue can occur during this phase. Premonitions or auras may occur before the onset of tonic-clonic seizures. Following the convulsions, the person will gradually regain consciousness. The patient does not remember the events of the seizures and may not fully recover for up to several days. This period is referred to as the **postictal** state.
- **Absence seizure** (petit mal)—very brief loss of consciousness, lasting several seconds but less than 1 minute, is characteristic. Some mild symmetric motor activity, such as eye blinking, often occurs. A blank stare and loss of attention may also be observed. Many times, the seizures are so brief that others do not notice them when they happen. These seizures usually occur in children. More than 100 absence seizures may occur in one day.
- Atonic seizure—a sudden loss of muscle tone occurs. If the muscles affected are just in the neck, "head drop" will be observed. If the loss of tone is more widespread, the patient will fall suddenly to the ground in a "drop attack."
- Myoclonic seizure—sudden rapid muscle contractions occur. The contractions can be limited to a body region, such as one limb, or can be generalized throughout the body.
- **Status epilepticus**—when one seizure follows another without recovery of consciousness between events, or the seizure lasts longer than 10 minutes. All types of seizures in which consciousness is lost can progress to status epilepticus (Alldredge, 2002). The most common causes of status

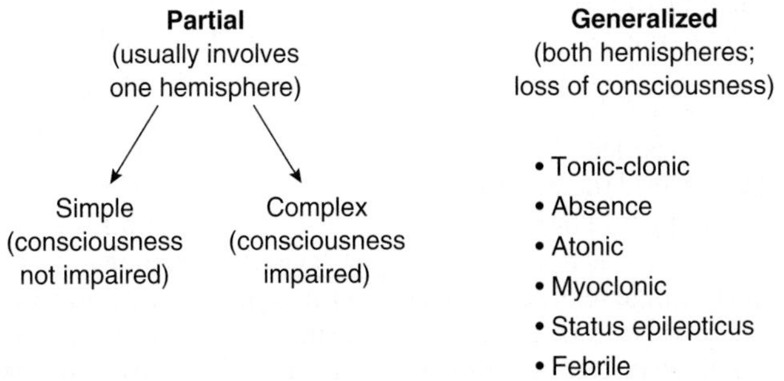

FIGURE 19.2 Classification of seizures.

epilepticus are stopping AED therapy and alcohol withdrawal. The death rate from status epilepticus in the United States has been estimated to be about 25% in adults and about 3% in children (DeLorenzo et al., 1996). The longer the period of status epilepticus, the higher the mortality rate. The most life-threatening condition results from generalized tonic-clonic seizures, referred to as generalized convulsive status epilepticus. This condition is a medical emergency, and intravenous (IV) drug intervention is needed immediately. Current clinical practice is to begin treatment for status epilepticus when a patient has a single seizure lasting at least 5 minutes, or has two or more seizures without recovery. Figure 19.3 presents a treatment pathway for status epilepticus. Treatment failures in status epilepticus are usually related to insufficient dosing. During status epilepticus, the patient may not maintain a patent open airway, the cardiac function may be altered, and high fever (hyperthermia) can occur. Lactic acidosis and elevated blood levels of carbon dioxide may follow. Patients who remain comatose for more than 30 minutes after generalized clonic status epilepticus is controlled may be experiencing subtle status epilepticus. Generalized tonic-clonic motor activity is not associated with subtle status epilepticus; diagnosis is based on electroencephalogram (EEG) readings showing persistent ictal discharges.

- Febrile seizures—generalized seizures can also occur as a result of high fevers in infants and young children and are termed febrile generalized seizures. These types of seizures do not increase the risk for developing epilepsy as the child grows up.

In addition to epilepsy, seizures may also occur from known and reversible causes—most commonly, metabolic abnormalities (e.g., hypoglycemia and electrolyte imbalance), meningitis, uremia, pre-eclampsia and toxemia of pregnancy, and drug and alcohol abuse.

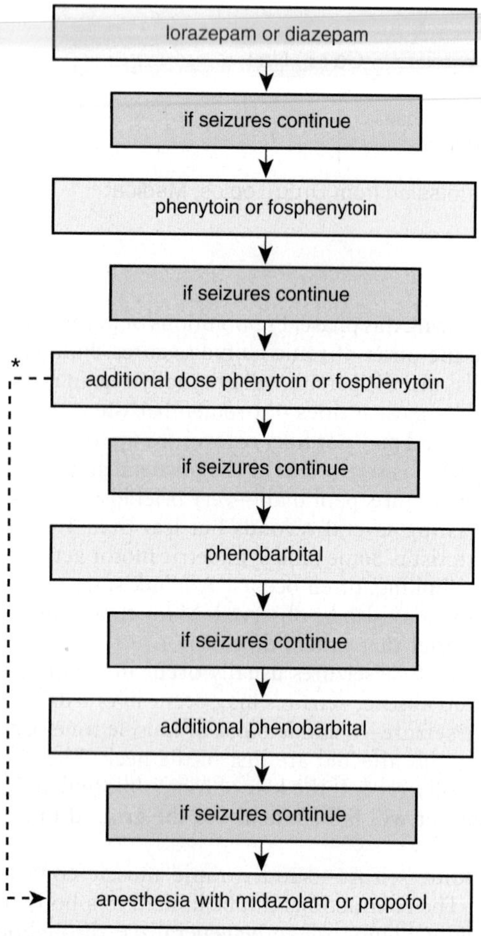

* If patient not controlled after benzodiazepine and two rounds of phenytoin treatment, go directly to anesthesia under these conditions:
- patient in ICU setting and
- has severe systemic effects (e.g., extreme hyperthermia) or
- seizing for more than 60 to 90 minutes

FIGURE 19.3 Treatment pathway for status epilepticus.

C ANTIEPILEPTIC DRUGS

Antiepileptic Drugs That Decrease Sodium Influx

Phenytoin is the prototype drug that controls seizures by decreasing sodium influx into the cells. It is also representative of a class of drugs called the hydantoins.

NURSING MANAGEMENT OF THE PATIENT RECEIVING P PHENYTOIN

Core Drug Knowledge

Pharmacotherapeutics

Phenytoin is used to control generalized (grand mal) and other psychomotor seizures. It is also used to prevent and treat seizures that occur either during or following neurosurgery. Parenterally, it is used to treat status epilepticus after a benzodiazepine. A Veterans Affairs study (Treiman et al., 1998) showed that lorazepam was greatly superior to phenytoin in treating status epilepticus. Unlabeled uses of phenytoin include its common use as an antiarrhythmic drug, especially when the arrhythmia is induced by cardiac glycoside drugs, such as digoxin. Another unlabeled use of phenytoin is as an alternative to magnesium sulfate for treating severe pre-eclampsia during pregnancy. Other uses of phenytoin include treatment of trigeminal neuralgia (also called tic douloureux).

Therapeutic effects of phenytoin are closely related to the serum level of the drug. The therapeutic blood level of phenytoin is between 10 and 20 μg/mL. However, it is possible for patients to achieve therapeutic effects at levels below the standard therapeutic range because great variability exists among people in how phenytoin is processed and how the body responds to the drug. Slight deviations from the therapeutic range may produce nontherapeutic effects or adverse effects related to the unique pharmacokinetics of phenytoin as well. Determining an accurate and effective dose is therefore somewhat difficult. Adjustments to the initial dose

will most likely be needed when therapy is started. Be aware that dosing of phenytoin should be individualized to the patient's needs and that achieving the therapeutic range should be considered a guide, but not an absolute rule.

Pharmacokinetics

Phenytoin is slowly absorbed when given orally. The rate and extent of absorption and bioavailability of phenytoin vary among individuals and also depend on the product formulation. Oral phenytoin reaches peak serum levels in 1.5 hours to 3 hours for prompt-onset preparations and within 12 hours for extended-release products. Intramuscularly administered phenytoin is very slowly and erratically absorbed because the drug will precipitate at the injection site within the muscle. Absorption from the site may occur for 5 days or longer. Serum levels reached by intramuscular injection never equal those reached by oral dosing. Phenytoin is highly protein bound (about 90%). Phenytoin is metabolized in the liver to inactive metabolites, which can be excreted in the urine by tubular excretion. However, the biotransformation of phenytoin to the metabolite has a limit at any given time. In lower doses of phenytoin, complete metabolism occurs fairly easily. However, as the dose increases, not all of the drug can be metabolized at once, and the half-life of phenytoin will increase as the dose increases. At low dosage levels, which are frequently subtherapeutic, the half-life is 6 to 24 hours; as the dose is increased to achieve the therapeutic range, the half-life increases to between 20 and 60 hours. Because of these pharmacokinetics, small changes in the dose of phenytoin may produce larger than expected changes in the serum concentration of phenytoin. This variability in the metabolism rate makes phenytoin different from most other drugs. To further complicate the process of metabolism, the rate of metabolism varies greatly among individuals. This limitation on rate of metabolism is an inherited trait. Table 19.1 summarizes the actions of selected antiepileptic drugs.

Pharmacodynamics

The primary site of action of phenytoin, and of other hydantoins, is believed to be the motor cortex. Phenytoin reversibly binds to sodium channels while they are in the inactive state. This binding delays the return of the channel to an active state. Because sodium can only enter the cell to initiate an action potential when the channels are active, the time between action potentials is greatly lengthened, the neurons cannot fire at an excessive rate, and excessive muscle contractions that occur in grand mal–type seizures are prevented. Phenytoin selectively binds to sites with hyperactive neurons; it does not alter the sodium movement into neurons that fire normally. This ability to selectively work at neurons that are firing abnormally explains why phenytoin is also effective in treating cardiac arrhythmias from ectopic foci.

Contraindications and Precautions

Because of its effects on ventricular automaticity, phenytoin is contraindicated in patients with sinus bradycardia, sinoatrial block, second- and third-degree atrioventricular (AV) block, or Adams-Stokes syndrome. Phenytoin is also contraindicated if the patient is hypersensitive to hydantoins; phenytoin hypersensitive reactions are not typical.

Because phenytoin may cause blood dyscrasias, it should not be administered with other drugs that also have this effect, if at all possible. If such drugs must be used, the patient should be monitored closely for blood dyscrasias.

Other precautions include patients with acute intermittent porphyria (rare inherited metabolic disorder characterized by excessive excretion of porphyrins, acute abdominal pain, and neurological disturbances) because phenytoin may precipitate a crisis. Use caution in diabetic patients because phenytoin may elevate blood glucose levels.

Phenytoin should not be abruptly stopped because doing so can precipitate status epilepticus. Phenytoin use has been associated with osteomalacia, a softening and flexibility of the bones in adults. Phenytoin is a pregnancy category D drug. The use of phenytoin during pregnancy is somewhat complicated and confusing. On the one hand, phenytoin, as well as other antiepileptic drugs, has been associated with an increased incidence of birth defects in infants whose mothers used the drug. These congenital malformations include cleft lip, cleft palate, and heart malformations. A fetal hydantoin syndrome has been identified that includes prenatal growth deficiency, microcephaly, and mental deficiency. However, these features of intrauterine growth retardation have all been associated with other causes as well as hydantoin use; therefore, phenytoin use may or may not be solely responsible for their onset. Most women taking phenytoin, however, deliver normal, healthy babies. There have also been reports that maternal ingestion of phenytoin can produce bleeding in the newborn, usually within 24 hours of birth. The defect is characterized by low levels of vitamin K–dependent clotting factors and by prolonged prothrombin times, partial thromboplastin times, or both. On the other hand, stopping the use of phenytoin and other AEDs during pregnancy is likely to induce seizures, including status epilepticus, which places the fetus at risk for being without sufficient oxygen. Even minor seizures may pose a risk to the well-being of the developing fetus, although the exact effects are not known. No easy answer exists to the question of whether to use phenytoin during pregnancy. In general, it is now thought that phenytoin should not be discontinued if the nature, frequency, and severity of the seizures pose a serious threat to either the patient or the fetus. In other words, benefits should outweigh risks. Box 19.1 discusses anticonvulsants and pregnancy.

Adverse Effects

The most frequent adverse effects of phenytoin occur in the central nervous system (CNS) and include nystagmus, ataxia, dysarthria, slurred speech, mental confusion, dizziness, insomnia, transient nervousness, numbness, tremor, and headache. Reducing the dose is often effective in eliminating these adverse effects. Other common adverse effects of phenytoin are nausea and gingival hyperplasia (overgrowth of the gums).

Rare but potentially life-threatening adverse effects of phenytoin are dermatologic reactions (Stevens-Johnson syndrome, lupus erythematosus syndrome, and bullous, exfoliative, or purpuric dermatitis), liver damage, and hematopoietic effects (blood dyscrasias). When given intravenously, phenytoin may cause cardiovascular collapse (hypotension, cardiac arrhythmias) if it is administered too rapidly.

TABLE 19.1 Summary of Selected (C) Antiepileptic Drugs

Drug (Trade) Name	Selected Indications	Route and Dosage Range	Pharmacokinetics
Drugs That Decrease Sodium Influx			
P phenytoin (Dilantin; *Canadian:* Diphenylan)	Tonic-clonic seizures, psychomotor seizures, status epilepticus	*Adult:* PO, use to serum levels of 5–20 µg/mL	*Onset:* Slow *Duration:* 6–12 h $t_{1/2}$: 6–24 h
carbamazepine (Tegretol; *Canadian:* Carbamaz)	Tonic-clonic seizures, mixed seizures, psychomotor seizures	*Adult:* PO, 400–1,000 mg/d *Child 6–12 y:* PO, 200–1,000 mg/d	*Onset:* Slow *Duration:* 4–5 h $t_{1/2}$: 25–65 h initially, 12–17 h with multiple dosing
felbamate (Felbatol)	Adjunctive or monotherapy of partial seizures in adults; adjunctive therapy in children with Lennox-Gastaut syndrome	*Adult (>14 y):* 1,200–3,600 mg/d *Child 2–14 y:* PO, 15 mg/kg/d	*Onset:* Rapid *Duration:* Dose proportional $t_{1/2}$: 20–23 h
fosphenytoin (Cerebyx)	Status epilepticus	*Adult:* IV, dilute in D_5W or 0.9% NaCl to a concentration of 1.5–25 mg phenytoin equivalent (PE)*/mL; administer at rate of ≤150 mg PE/mL	*Onset:* Rapid *Duration:* 1–2 h $t_{1/2}$: 6–24 h
oxcarbazepine (Trileptal)	Adjunctive treatment of partial seizures	*Adult:* PO, 1,200 mg/d as adjunctive therapy; 2,400 mg/d as monotherapy. *Child 4–16 y:* PO, 30–46 mg/kg/d as adjunctive therapy	*Onset:* 1 h *Duration:* 3–13 h $t_{1/2}$: 2*–9**
valproic acid (Depakene; *Canadian:* Deproic)	Sole or adjunctive treatment for simple or complex absence seizures	*Adult:* PO, 10–60 mg/kg/d	*Onset:* Varies depending on dosage form *Duration:* 1–4 h $t_{1/2}$: 5–20 h (average, 10.6 h)
Drugs That Increase Effectiveness of GABA			
clonazepam (Klonopin; Canadian: Rivotril)	Myoclonic seizures, absence seizures, akinetic seizures, variant absence seizures (Lennox-Gastaut)	*Adult:* PO, 1.5–20 mg/d *Child:* PO, 0.01–0.05 mg/kg/d	*Onset:* 20–60 min *Duration:* 6–12 h $t_{1/2}$: 18–60 h
clorazepate (Tranxene; *Canadian:* Apo-Clorazepate)	Partial seizures	*Adult:* PO, 7.5 mg tid *Child:* PO, 7.5 mg bid	*Onset:* 15–45 min *Duration:* 7–8 h $t_{1/2}$: 30–100 h
diazepam (Valium, *Canadian:* Vivol)	Adjunct in convulsant seizures, status epilepticus	*Adult:* PO, 2–10 mg bid or tid *Adult:* IV (initial), 10–15 mg/kg *Child:* IV (initial), 5–10 mg/kg	*Onset:* PO, 30–60 min; IV, 1–5 min *Duration:* PO, 3 h, IV, 15–66 min $t_{1/2}$: 20–80 h, PO
gabapentin (Neurontin)	Partial seizures in adults with and without secondary generalization	*Adult:* PO, 900–1,800 mg/d	*Onset:* Rapid *Duration:* 6–8 h $t_{1/2}$: 5–7 h
phenobarbital (*Canadian:* Barbita)	Status epilepticus, cortical local, tonic-clonic seizures	*Adult:* PO, 60–100 mg/d to serum level of 10–40 µg/mL; IM/IV, 200–320 q6h *Child:* PO, 3–6 mg/kg/d; IM/IV, 10–15 mg/kg/d	*Onset:* PO, 30–60 min; IM, 10–30 min; IV, 5 min *Duration:* 8–15 h $t_{1/2}$: 53–140 h

(continued)

TABLE 19.1 Summary of Selected (C) Antiepileptic Drugs (continued)

Drug (Trade) Name	Selected Indications	Route and Dosage Range	Pharmacokinetics
tiagabine (Gabitril)	Adjunctive treatment of partial seizures	Dosage ranges not established	*Onset:* Rapid *Duration:* 6–12 h $t_{1/2}$: Varies (4.5–13.4 h)
Drugs That Decrease Calcium Influx			
(P) ethosuximide (Zarontin)	Absence seizures	*Adult:* PO, 500 mg/d to serum level of 40–100 μg/mL *Child:* PO, 250 mg/d (3–6 y) or 500 mg/d (6 y or older)	*Onset:* Varies *Duration:* 3–7 h $t_{1/2}$: 40–60 h in adults; 30 h in children 7–9 y
zonisamide (zonegran)	Adjunctive treatment of partial seizures	*Adult:* PO, 100–400 mg/d	*Onset:* 2–6 h *Duration:* More than 105 h $t_{1/2}$: 63 h

*Parent drug.

**Active metabolite.

A number of other adverse effects are possible but not common; these include:

- *Dermatologic:* rash, hirsutism, alopecia
- *Endocrine:* diabetes insipidus, hyperglycemia
- *Gastrointestinal (GI):* vomiting, diarrhea, constipation
- *Hepatic:* hepatitis, jaundice
- *Respiratory:* pneumonia, pharyngitis, sinusitis, hyperventilation, rhinitis, apnea, aspiration pneumonia, asthma, dyspnea, atelectasis, increased cough, epistaxis, hypoxia, pneumothorax, hemoptysis, bronchitis, chest pain, pulmonary fibrosis
- *Senses:* tinnitus, diplopia, taste perversion, amblyopia, deafness, visual-field defect, eye pain, conjunctivitis, photophobia, hyperacusis, mydriasis, parosmia, ear pain, taste loss
- *Miscellaneous:* polyarthropathy, weight gain, chest pain, edema, immunoglobulin A (IgA) depression, fever, photophobia, conjunctivitis, gynecomastia, periarteritis nodosa, pulmonary fibrosis, soft tissue injury at the injection site, lymph node hyperplasia (may represent a hypersensitivity reaction)

Drug Interactions

Numerous drugs interact with phenytoin. Be certain to check for drug interactions when patients are receiving phenytoin and any other drug. These interactions occur because of phenytoin-inducing effects on hepatic microsomal enzyme systems (also referred to as P-450). Pharmacologic induction of these enzymes enhances the metabolism of both endogenous and exogenous substances, including other AEDs.

Drug interactions may increase or decrease the effect of phenytoin or the other drug (Table 19.2). Several enteral feeding preparations (tube feedings) may decrease phenytoin

BOX 19.1 Anticonvulsants and Pregnancy

Teratogenic Effects
- Possible with all AEDs
- Risk increases with first-trimester exposure and multidrug therapy
- Little data on new AEDs because no studies; do not appear to cause malformation in monotherapy
- Innate ability to metabolize and eliminate AEDs increases risk
- Metabolism of hormonal contraceptives is increased by AEDs, decreasing their effectiveness, increasing risk for unplanned pregnancy

Competitive Inhibitors of Vitamin K
- Neonatal hemorrhage possible
- Phenytoin, carbamazepine, ethosuximide, phenobarbital, and primidone have high mortality from hemorrhage
- Transferred in breast milk

Loss of Seizure Control
- Concentration of AEDs decreases during pregnancy (even with steady or increasing dose)
- Concentration decreases differently for different AEDs
- One fourth to one third of pregnant women will have increased incidence of seizures related to decreased drug concentration

CRITICAL THINKING SCENARIO

What happens when antiepileptic therapy stops abruptly?

Rudy Hernandez, 26 years old, is brought to the emergency room by ambulance, accompanied by his wife. He is currently unconscious, is having tonic-clonic convulsions, and has been incontinent of urine. He had two seizures at home without regaining consciousness before the ambulance arrived. His wife states that he was on phenytoin and valproic acid for seizure prevention and that he has been on medication since he was a teenager. She also reports he stopped his medication last week because he didn't like the adverse effects.

1. What type of seizure is Mr. Hernandez exhibiting? What is the likely cause of this seizure?
2. What nursing actions are indicted upon his arrival in the emergency room?
3. What drug therapy or therapies do you expect that he will receive?

TABLE 19.2 Agents That Interact With P Phenytoin

Interactants	Effect and Significance	Nursing Management
allopurinol, amiodarone, benzodiazepines, cimetidine, clonazepam, disulfiram, ethanol, fluconazole, ibuprofen, isoniazid, metronidazole, miconazole, omeprazole, phenothiazines, salicylates, succinimides, sulfonamides, tricyclic antidepressants, trimethoprim, valproic acid	Increased pharmacologic effects of phenytoin from inhibition of its metabolism	Monitor patient for changes in seizure control. Monitor serum phenytoin levels. Assess for signs of phenytoin toxicity.
barbiturates, ethanol (chronic ingestion), rifampin, theophylline	Decreased pharmacologic effects of phenytoin due to its increased metabolism	Assess patient for increased seizure frequency and changed seizure control. Monitor serum phenytoin levels at regular intervals.
antacids, charcoal, sucralfate	Decreased phenytoin effects due to decreased absorption	Assess patient for increased seizure frequency and changed seizure control. Monitor serum phenytoin levels at regular intervals.
acetaminophen, carbamazepine, cardiac glycosides, corticosteroids, disopyramide, doxycycline, estrogens (and oral contraceptives), haloperidol, methadone, mexiletine, quinidine, theophylline	Decreased pharmacologic effects of interactants from increased metabolism by phenytoin Analgesic effects of acetaminophen may be reduced by concomitant phenytoin use; the potential hepatotoxicity of acetaminophen may be increased Corticosteroid use may mask systemic manifestations of phenytoin hypersensitivity reactions	Evaluate patient for changed seizure control. Assess patient for evidence of therapeutic effects of interacting drugs. Monitor patient for therapeutic serum levels (if applicable) of interacting drugs.

levels either by impairing absorption or through some other mechanism. Phenytoin may interfere with results of diagnostic endocrine tests that use dexamethasone.

Assessment of Relevant Core Patient Variables

Health Status

Determine whether the patient is hypersensitive to phenytoin or if he or she has any of the cardiac conditions that are contraindications for the use of the drug. Because phenytoin is highly protein bound, assess whether the patient has chronic conditions, such as liver failure, that alter the level of albumin protein. Check ordered blood work to determine whether albumin levels are abnormal.

Before starting therapy, also confirm that the patient has either grand mal or other psychomotor seizures that respond to phenytoin.

Life Span and Gender

Before phenytoin therapy begins, assess whether the patient is pregnant. The use of AEDs such as phenytoin poses some risk to the developing fetus and, if possible, should not be started during a pregnancy. Women of childbearing age should use birth control to prevent pregnancy, although AEDs may make doing so more difficult because of their effects on contraceptives (Food and Drug Administration, 2000). Exposure during the first trimester of pregnancy increases the risk for malformations in the child; taking multiple AEDs increases the risk even more. Teratogenicity may be related to an individual woman's genetic makeup, which influences how well she metabolizes and eliminates AEDs. When metabolism and elimination are slower than would normally be predicted, the risk for teratogenic effects on the infant increases. Phenytoin, like other AEDs, is a competitive inhibitor of vitamin K; this action increases the risk for neonatal hemorrhage in the first 24 hours after birth. Phenytoin is associated with a high mortality rate in neonatal hemorrhage. Suddenly stopping phenytoin during pregnancy carries the risk for inducing seizures, as previously mentioned. If possible, the woman should be weaned off phenytoin before becoming pregnant. Phenytoin is passed in breast milk, and so is the competitive inhibition of vitamin K; women taking phenytoin should not breast-feed.

Drug therapy with phenytoin, as with other AEDs, need not be lifelong. Box 19.2 presents some guidelines for using and discontinuing AEDs.

Older adults are more likely to experience hypotension and cardiac arrhythmias when phenytoin is given intravenously.

Lifestyle, Diet, and Habits

Assess for conditions that may make the patient more likely to have decreased blood protein levels. Does the patient have

COMMUNITY-BASED CONCERNS

Box 19.2 Starting and Stopping AED Therapy

Although AED therapy has often been considered lifelong, many patients can be successfully weaned off of therapy. AEDs all contain possible adverse effects; about 1 in 30,000 patients taking an AED will experience a serious adverse effect, and 15% will need to have the drug discontinued because of adverse effects. Some of those adverse effects become more prevalent the longer the drug therapy is taken. In many patients, the risks from drug therapy may outweigh the risk for occasional seizure activity. Almost 70% of patients will achieve long-term remission once AEDs are withdrawn. What follows are some current guidelines regarding the use and discontinuation of AEDs.

Starting Therapy: Adults

- After first seizure: if abnormal EEG, structural lesions related to stroke or tumor, general tonic-clonic seizures, status epilepticus, or substantial occupational risk
- After two seizures: almost all patients (those with simple, partial, or widely spaced seizures may not be treated)

Starting Therapy: Children

- After first seizure: almost never (possible exception—first seizure is status epilepticus and child younger than 3 years)
- After two seizures: depends on type, duration, frequency, psychosocial issues, parent/child preference
- After three seizures: usually

Stopping Therapy: Adults

Still somewhat unknown. Generally:

- Seizure free at least 2 years
- On single drug therapy

Less likely to relapse if:

- Short duration of treatment
- Less severe EEG changes
- Less than 100 seizures before control
- Not complex partial seizures with secondary generalization, or generalized seizures

Stopping Therapy: Children

- Seizure free for 2 years; may start to taper before 2-year anniversary
- If possible, do before they reach driving age

alcoholism? Is the patient malnourished? Is the patient's dietary protein intake severely limited? These conditions put the patient at greater risk for having greater amounts of free, active drug in the blood because less protein albumin is available for binding than would normally be expected. Therefore, the patient is more at risk for having adverse effects from the phenytoin. Chronic ingestion of alcohol also increases the metabolism of phenytoin and therefore alters blood drug levels.

Environment

Oral phenytoin can be administered in any setting. IV phenytoin should be given in a hospital setting, ideally with the patient in a monitored bed.

Nursing Diagnoses and Outcomes

- Disturbed Sensory Perception related to adverse effects of drowsiness and sedation
  Desired outcome: *The patient will not experience adverse effects to the degree that sensory perception is altered enough to impair quality of life.*
- Risk for Injury related to the adverse effects of drowsiness and sedation
  Desired outcome: *The patient will not sustain any injury while taking phenytoin.*
- Altered Oral Mucous Membrane related to the adverse effect of gingival hyperplasia
  Desired outcome: *The patient will demonstrate knowledge of optimal oral hygiene and experience no deterioration in dental health.*
- Risk for Injury related to adverse effects of blood dyscrasias
  Desired outcome: *The patient will return for follow-up blood work while taking phenytoin and will have no life-threatening blood disorders.*

Planning and Intervention

Maximizing Therapeutic Effects

Therapeutic effect of phenytoin is normally related to achieving a therapeutic blood level of the drug. Monitor blood levels to determine whether they are therapeutic. If the blood level is not therapeutic, and the patient is still having seizures, notify the physician or other prescriber to inquire about increasing the dose. Remember that some patients achieve therapeutic results even when their blood levels of phenytoin are not in the ideal therapeutic range. The drug should be adjusted in very small increments because of the unusual pharmacokinetics of phenytoin. The risk is that a dosage change will move the blood phenytoin level from just marginally therapeutic to toxic. Titrating the dose upward gradually will help to minimize this risk.

Phenytoin absorption is compromised when administered with enteral tube feedings. Check gastric residuals and refrain from administering the drug for 1 to 2 hours if the residual is greater than 100 mL. Continuous tube feedings should be held for 1 hour before and after administering the phenytoin.

Minimizing Adverse Effects

Adverse effects from phenytoin are frequently related to excessively high blood drug levels. It is important to monitor the patient's blood levels of phenytoin as well as the patient's physical response to drug therapy. Drug levels should be monitored most closely at the initiation of therapy or after every increase in the dose. If the patient is demonstrating adverse effects, the drug dosage may need to be decreased. Dosage changes downward should also be done in small increments to avoid decreasing the blood level so much that it is below the therapeutic level. It is important to analyze the patient's mental and neurologic function and behavior regularly for changes from baseline behavior to determine whether CNS adverse effects are present. If the patient is having difficulty with dizziness, safety measures should be instituted to prevent falls and injury. Administer the drug with meals if the patient is experiencing nausea and GI distress; however, antacids should be avoided because they may impair absorption. Diabetic patients may experience

elevated glucose levels; their glucose levels should be measured more frequently until the effects of phenytoin on them are determined.

Administer IV push phenytoin no faster than 50 mg/minute in adults or 1 to 3 mg/kg/minute in neonates because fast administration is associated with cardiovascular collapse. Careful monitoring of the pulse and blood pressure is essential during IV administration. Follow the administration of phenytoin with sterile saline through the same IV catheter to avoid local venous irritation from the alkalinity of the phenytoin. Phenytoin is not given as a continuous IV infusion. Intramuscular (IM) administration should be avoided because of irregular and delayed absorption.

Evaluate blood counts, bleeding tendencies, and white blood cell counts regularly to determine whether any hematologic adverse effects have occurred. Notify the prescriber if any abnormalities are detected to prevent serious adverse effects. Vitamin D and calcium supplements are recommended for patients showing symptoms of osteomalacia and also for those at high risk for developing osteomalacia. Report any signs and symptoms of skin rash. Although a rash is usually not serious, phenytoin may need to be discontinued to minimize the risk for severe reactions such as Stevens-Johnson syndrome.

To minimize the risk for neonatal hemorrhage, pregnant women taking phenytoin should receive 10 mg per day of vitamin K during the last week of pregnancy.

Providing Patient and Family Education

Much of the patient and family education regarding phenytoin is common to any AED that is prescribed. Box 19.3 contains guidelines for patient and family education common to AEDs. Some educational points specific for phenytoin are:

- Teach the importance of shaking suspension forms of phenytoin thoroughly before pouring and measuring the dose.
- Teach the patient and family the importance of good dental hygiene to prevent gingival hyperplasia and gum softening. Encourage the patient to brush the teeth at least twice daily with a soft toothbrush and to floss daily.
- Suggest that patients take phenytoin with food to minimize GI distress.
- Teach the diabetic patient to frequently check capillary blood glucose.
- You might suggest bleaching or electrolysis if hirsutism is a problem for female patients because shaving or depilatories often leave stubble.
- Teach the patient to notify the physician if he or she experiences skin rash, severe nausea or vomiting, swollen glands, bleeding, swollen or tender gums, yellowish discoloration of the skin or eyes, joint pain, unexplained fever, sore throat, unusual bleeding or bruising, persistent headache, malaise, and any indication of an infection or bleeding tendency, which are signs of serious adverse effects. Female patients should also notify the physician if they become pregnant.
- Teach women who have delivered a baby about the risks involved in breast-feeding.

Ongoing Assessment and Evaluation

Ongoing assessments include monitoring patients closely for therapeutic responses, seizure control, and adverse effects to

BOX 19.3 Patient and Family Education Common to AEDs

AEDs require that much of the same information be shared with patient and family. The nurse providing education for the epileptic patient should include the following information.

- AED therapy does not cure the seizure disorder; it suppresses seizure activity.
- The condition in which seizures recur so frequently that consciousness or normal function cannot be regained in the interval between seizures is known as status epilepticus; this is a medical emergency.
- Sudden withdrawal of the AED may cause epileptic control to be lost and the patient may experience seizures or status epilepticus.
- Double dosing of an AED should be avoided. If a dose is missed, instruct the patient to take the dose as soon as it is remembered unless it is close to the time for the next dose.
- Follow-up appointments with the health care provider and periodic laboratory testing are important because they provide an ongoing record of response (both positive and negative) to AED therapy.
- A "seizure record" should be kept. This record can provide information about changes in the type or frequency of seizures over time, the effect of different medications on seizure control, adverse effects of medications, and seizure-provoking factors. This record should include the date and time, as well as the type, of seizure. If a precipitating factor is suspected (e.g., lack of sleep, missed medication, stress, menstrual period), the patient should write it down. For women, it may be helpful to keep track of the relationship between seizures and the menstrual cycles. It is also helpful to record the medication, dosage, and blood drug levels (if known). Recommend that the patient and family (or caregiver) show this record to the health care provider during follow-up visits.
- A form of medical identification (e.g., MedicAlert) indicating the medical condition and the drugs prescribed for it, including dosage in case of an emergency, should be carried or worn by the patient.
- Use of OTC preparations, herbal preparations, and dietary supplements should be avoided unless approved by the physician or nurse practitioner.
- Transient mild drowsiness and dizziness are common in the first few days of therapy until the patient becomes accustomed to the drug therapy. Observe caution while driving, operating machinery or performing other tasks requiring mental alertness and motor coordination until effects of the drug are known.
- Alcohol consumption should be avoided because it may increase the CNS-depressant effect of the AED as well as precipitate incidence of seizures.
- Environmental factors (e.g., flashing lights, alcohol) and physiologic factors (e.g., hypoglycemia, fatigue, stress) may increase the frequency of seizures. If stress aggravates seizure activity, teach the patient to develop effective stress management techniques.
- AEDs can have significant effects on hormonal homeostasis, although epilepsy itself may play a role in causing these problems. Men may experience reduced libido and sexual potency; women may experience sexual arousal disorders. Seizure frequency may increase during menses because of the increase in sex hormones that alter the excitability of cortical neurons.
- The risk of having a child with a congenital defect may be 2–3 times greater in epileptic women who received AEDs in the early stages of pregnancy. Most AEDs are not recommended during pregnancy and lactation. Many women receiving AEDs, however, deliver healthy infants.

drug therapy. Blood levels of the drug should be monitored whenever the dose is changed, or if the patient is having seizures. Because phenytoin interacts with so many drugs through its effect on the enzymes of hepatic metabolism, also determine the likelihood of drug interactions between phenytoin and other newly ordered drugs or newly discontinued drugs. Phenytoin therapy is effective if seizures can be controlled and the patient experiences no serious adverse effects.

Drugs Significantly Different From P Phenytoin

Carbamazepine

Carbamazepine is used to treat partial seizures with complex symptoms. It can also be used in treating generalized tonic-clonic seizures, mixed seizure patterns, or other partial or generalized seizures. Although effective in all of these types of seizures, carbamazepine seems to produce the most effect in treating partial seizures with complex symptoms. Carbamazepine is also used to treat trigeminal neuralgia. Nonlabeled uses for carbamazepine include its common use in treating several psychiatric disorders (bipolar disorder, depression, schizoaffective illness, schizophrenia resistant to other drug therapies, dyscontrol syndrome associated with limbic system dysfunction, intermittent explosion disorder, post-traumatic stress disorder, and atypical psychosis). Other nonlabeled uses are management of alcohol, cocaine, and benzodiazepine withdrawal; restless legs syndrome; non-neuritic pain syndromes, painful neuromas, or phantom limb pain; neurogenic or central diabetes insipidus; and hereditary or nonhereditary chorea in children. Therapeutic blood level for controlling seizures is 2 to 4 µg/mL.

Carbamazepine is chemically related to the tricyclic antidepressants. Its mode of action is similar to that of phenytoin; it is believed to suppress the inflow of sodium into the cell, thereby decreasing frequency of action potentials and controlling seizures. It is generally well absorbed. Bioavailability of the drug is essentially the same for conventional tablets, extended-release tablets, and oral suspension. Peak times differ among these routes, however, with the quickest peak (about 1.5 hours) from the suspension and the slowest peak (3–12 hours) from the extended-release format. Therapeutic blood level for the drug ranges from 4 to 12 µg/mL for an adult. Carbamazepine is less protein bound than phenytoin, at 76%. Although carbamazepine is metabolized through the liver, like phenytoin, the characteristics of metabolism are different. The metabolite formed also has anticonvulsant activity; its half-life is shorter than that of carbamazepine. The half-life of carbamazepine is initially 25 to 65 hours, with repeated doses of the drug the half-life decreases to 12 to 17 hours. Excretion of the drug and metabolite are primarily through the urine, but some is also excreted through the feces.

Like phenytoin, carbamazepine is a pregnancy category D drug; and the same concerns exist about its use in pregnancy and sudden discontinuation of the drug during pregnancy.

The most common adverse effects from carbamazepine are similar to those from phenytoin: dizziness, drowsiness, unsteadiness, nausea, and vomiting. A major difference in the adverse effects of these two drugs is the black box warning carried by carbamazepine in regard to its potential to cause three fatal blood dyscrasias. These are aplastic anemia (lack of red blood cells caused by disorders of bone marrow), thrombocytopenia (lack of platelets), and agranulocytosis (complete lack of white blood cells). Carbamazepine has been found to increase the risk for developing these fatal disorders; patients taking the drug are between five and eight times more likely to develop these hematologic problems than the general population not taking the drug. Still, even with this increased risk, the likelihood that aplastic anemia, thrombocytopenia, or agranulocytosis will develop is very low. Many patients have transient or persistent decreased red blood cell, platelet, or white blood cell counts and do not go on to develop the more serious conditions. Patients receiving carbamazepine need to be monitored for these conditions; the patient should be monitored more carefully if any changes occur in the blood cell counts. Drug therapy should be discontinued if considerable depression of bone marrow function is apparent. Patients who have hematologic abnormalities should not receive carbamazepine.

Valproic Acid

Valproic acid, also called valproate, is a broad-spectrum AED that is effective against all seizure types. It is the most widely prescribed AED worldwide (Perucca, 2002). In the United States, the only FDA approved use is for absence seizures, although in practice it is used for tonic-clonic, atonic, myoclonic, and partial seizures. Additionally, valproic acid is approved to treat mania and migraine headaches. Although

MEMORY CHIP

P Phenytoin

- Used to treat generalized tonic-clonic (grand mal) and other psychomotor seizures; status epilepticus
- Binds to receptors on sodium channels, keeping the channels in a closed position longer, preventing influx of sodium ions and excessive firing of the cell
- Major contraindications: sinus bradycardia, sinoatrial block, second- and third-degree AV block, and Adams-Stokes syndrome
- Most common adverse effects: CNS (dizziness, ataxia, blurred vision), nausea, and gingival hyperplasia
- Most serious adverse effects: life-threatening dermatologic reactions, liver damage, and blood dyscrasias; cardiovascular collapse if given too rapidly by IV push
- **Life span alert: can cause fetal hydantoin syndrome, infant death from neonatal hemorrhage, and decreased effectiveness of hormonal contraceptives; circulating level will decrease during pregnancy, increasing risk for seizures**
- Maximizing therapeutic effect: Monitor for therapeutic blood level, avoid coadministration with enteral tube feedings
- Minimizing adverse effects: Change dose upward or downward in small increments; monitor blood levels when dosage is changed or if symptomatic of adverse effects; give IV push very slowly during status epilepticus; vitamin K before date of delivery
- Most important patient education: Be careful driving or operating machinery until effects of drug are known; potential risks to fetus if patient becomes pregnant

no controlled trials have been conducted, some open-label trials with valproic acid indicate that it is effective in treating status epilepticus (Alldredge, 2002). The therapeutic blood level for seizure control is 50 to 150 µg/mL.

Valproic acid works through a number of different mechanisms. Like phenytoin, it blocks the voltage-gated sodium channels. Unlike phenytoin, it also increases GABA transmission and modulates the transmission of dopamine and serotonin (Perucca, 2002).

Oral absorption of valproic acid is rapid, and all oral formulations have almost 100% bioavailability. Like phenytoin, valproic acid is highly protein bound, although as the dosage of valproic acid increases, the percentage of drug that is bound decreases. Valproic acid is metabolized through the liver; however, unlike phenytoin, it does not induce hepatic enzymes, although it can potentially inhibit the drug metabolism of some drugs. The half-life of valproic acid is between 9 and 18 hours, shorter half-lives of 5 to 12 hours can occur in patients also being medicated with enzyme-inducing agents such as phenytoin, carbamazepine, or barbiturates.

The most common adverse effects of valproic acid are GI problems, tremor, and weight gain. Adverse effects, which are not common but very serious and potentially lethal, are elevated blood ammonia levels (hyperammonemia), possibly with encephalopathy symptoms; platelet disorders; pancreatitis (life threatening); and liver toxicity (including liver failure and death). Liver toxicity appears to be more of a risk in children younger than 2 years who are on multiple-AED therapy. Other adverse effects that can occur include CNS effects (sedation, ataxia, confusion); dermatologic effects (transient hair loss, skin rash, photosensitivity, Stevens-Johnson syndrome); endocrine effects (irregular menses, breast enlargement); psychiatric effects (depression, psychosis, aggression); and miscellaneous effects (weakness, fever, hearing loss, otitis media).

Valproic acid is a pregnancy category D drug. Case reports in the literature indicate an increased risk for neural tube defects (such as spina bifida) when the drug is used during pregnancy, with about 1% to 2% of births having neural tube defects. This adverse effect is usually associated with the use of higher doses. However, no controlled studies exist to substantiate this association.

Valproic acid may cause falsely elevated urine ketone tests, when used in diabetic patients, and altered thyroid tests.

Topiramate

Topiramate is used to treat partial-onset seizures and tonic-clonic seizures; unlabeled uses include cluster headaches, infantile spasms, and Lennox-Gastaut syndrome. Like phenytoin, topiramate has an effect on the sodium influx into cells, blocking formation of action potentials. Unlike phenytoin, topiramate has two other methods of action. Topiramate enhances the effectiveness of GABA, increasing the inhibitory effects of the neurotransmitter. Topiramate also blocks the receptors for glutamate, a stimulating neurotransmitter. Therapeutic serum levels have not been determined.

Topiramate is easily absorbed when taken orally. Bioavailability of tablets is about 80%; it is not altered by food intake. Peak levels occur in about 2 hours. The half-life of topiramate is 18.7 to 23 hours. Steady state is reached in about 4 days in patients with normal renal function. Unlike phenytoin, topiramate has low protein binding, about 13% to 17%. Also unlike phenytoin, topiramate is mostly excreted unchanged in the urine. Only a small percentage of the drug is metabolized.

Topiramate is a weak carbonic anhydrase inhibitor and, like other carbonic anhydrase inhibitors (e.g., acetazolamide and dichlorphenamide), it promotes kidney stone formation by reducing urinary citrate excretion and increasing the urinary pH. The concurrent use of topiramate and other carbonic anhydrase inhibitors increases the risk for kidney stone formation.

Topiramate carries a warning that oligohidrosis (decreased sweating) and hyperthermia, with potentially serious sequelae, may occur. These adverse effects have infrequently required hospitalization. This warning is based on postmarketing reports that have been received. Most cases have been associated with high environmental temperatures or vigorous exercise. Caution needs to be used if topiramate is prescribed with other drugs that can predispose the patient to heat-related disorders, such as other carbonic anhydrase inhibitors or drugs with anticholinergic effects. Topiramate is ranked as a pregnancy category C drug. Animal studies have found that teratogenic effects can occur if given during the time of organ development. No studies have been done with humans.

The adverse effects that are most common are the CNS effects (psychomotor slowing; difficulty with concentration; speech or language problems, especially word-finding difficulties; somnolence and fatigue). Other CNS effects are also possible, but not as common. Generally, however, the drug is well tolerated.

Topiramate is available in tablets and in sprinkle capsules. Tablets should be swallowed whole because they have a bitter taste if broken. Instruct patients to open the sprinkle capsules and to sprinkle the entire contents onto a teaspoon of soft food, such as applesauce, and swallowed immediately, not chewed. Follow with water to guarantee that all the drug is swallowed.

Teach all patients, especially parents of children prescribed topiramate, to monitor for decreased sweating and elevated temperature and to seek medical help if these occur. Proper hydration in hot weather, especially before and during exercise or activity, is helpful to decrease the effects from oligohidrosis and hyperthermia.

Lamotrigine

Lamotrigine is approved as an adjunct therapy for treating partial seizures in adults and generalized seizures of Lennox-Gastaut syndrome (the most severe form of childhood epilepsy, characterized by very frequent seizures of several different types; it is usually nonresponsive to other AED therapy) in pediatric and adult patients. Lamotrigine has been found to be effective in clinical studies as add-on therapy or as monotherapy. In many cases, the patient can be converted from add-on therapy to monotherapy successfully (Jozwiak & Terczynski, 2000).

Lamotrigine is not chemically related to other AEDs. It appears to act by decreasing the sodium influx into the cells. A standardized serum blood level has not been determined.

Lamotrigine is easily absorbed from the GI tract and has about 98% bioavailability, which is not affected by food. Peak serum levels are reached in 1.4 hours to 4.8 hours. Lamotrigine is much less protein bound than phenytoin at

about 55%. Lamotrigine will not displace other protein-bound AEDs. An unusual feature of lamotrigine is its ability to bind in melanin-containing skin (e.g., in eyes and pigmented skin). Lamotrigine is metabolized by hepatic enzymes and is capable of inducing its own metabolism with repeated administration. When it is administered with other AEDs that induce hepatic enzymes, its elimination is increased. The exception to this effect is when lamotrigine is administered along with valproic acid. Valproic acid more than doubles the half-life of lamotrigine, requiring dose adjustments of lamotrigine.

The most common adverse effects of lamotrigine are CNS effects (dizziness, double vision, ataxia, blurred vision, somnolence, and headache), GI effects (nausea and vomiting, which are dose related), and rash. Although rashes can be common, serious life-threatening rashes, including Stevens-Johnson syndrome, can occur. Life-threatening rashes are more common in children treated with lamotrigine. For this reason, children younger than 16 years should not be treated with lamotrigine unless they have Lennox-Gastaut syndrome resistant to other drug therapies. Administering lamotrigine with valproic acid also appears to increase the incidence of rash. Because it is not possible to distinguish which rashes will become serious, drug therapy should be stopped at the first sign of a rash. Unfortunately, even stopping drug therapy immediately may not prevent a rash from becoming life-threatening or permanently disfiguring.

Lamotrigine is a pregnancy category C drug. Animal studies have shown maternal and fetal toxicity, but teratogenic effects have not been determined, although lamotrigine is known to decrease the fetal folate concentrations in animals.

Oxcarbazepine

Oxcarbazepine is chemically similar to the metabolite of carbamazepine; it was designed to mimic efficacy, while minimizing adverse effects and risks for drug interactions. Oxcarbazepine is used as either monotherapy or adjunctive therapy in adults with partial seizures and as adjunctive therapy for children 4 to 16 years old with partial seizures. Although the precise mechanism of action for oxcarbazepine is not known, it is believed to block voltage-sensitive sodium channels, similar to phenytoin. Its effects on increasing potassium conduction and suppressing high-voltage calcium channels may also contribute to the anticonvulsant properties of oxcarbazepine. The drug is rapidly absorbed. It has moderate low protein binding at 40%. The drug is rapidly converted to its active metabolism; all of the drug's effects are achieved through the metabolite. The metabolites are excreted through the urine.

There seems to be some cross-hypersensitivity between oxcarbazepine and carbamazepine. Between 25% and 30% of patients who have exhibited hypersensitivity to carbamazepine will also have hypersensitivity to oxcarbazepine. Oxcarbazepine is a pregnancy category C drug. Although no human studies exist to confirm the drug's teratogenicity in humans, its similar chemical structure to carbamazepine, a known teratogen, makes it likely that oxcarbazepine also causes human teratogenic effects.

The most common adverse effects of oxcarbazepine are related to the CNS (dizziness, somnolence, diplopia, abnormal vision, fatigue, ataxia, abnormal gait, and tremor) and the GI system (nausea, vomiting, abdominal pain, and dyspepsia). Hyponatremia can also occur with oxcarbazepine use; clinically important hyponatremia generally occurs within the first 3 months of treatment.

Oxcarbazepine is a CYP3A4/5 inducer and can cause substantial drug interactions with some other AED drugs that are also inducers of this pathway. The circulating levels of oxcarbazepine decrease when it is given with carbamazepine, phenytoin, valproic acid, or phenobarbital. Coadministering these drugs causes only phenytoin and phenobarbital levels to rise. Verapamil, a calcium-channel blocker used in several cardiac conditions, causes oxcarbazepine levels to decrease substantially. Oxcarbazepine causes the circulating levels of oral contraceptives to decrease by up to half.

Nursing management unique to oxcarbazepine includes the need for routine assessment of sodium levels and teaching women taking oral contraceptives that they need to use an additional form of birth control.

Levetiracetam

Levetiracetam is an adjunct AED used to treat partial-onset seizures in adults. It is chemically unrelated to other AEDs. Unlike phenytoin, its exact mechanism of action is not known, although it does *not* inhibit seizures by any mechanism related to inhibitory or excitatory neurohormones. Levetiracetam may prevent hypersynchronization of epileptiform burst firings and propagation of seizure activity from the hippocampus.

Levetiracetam is rapidly absorbed, and food does not affect the extent of absorption. Two thirds of the drug is renally excreted unchanged. The one third that is metabolized is not metabolized through any of the P-450 isoenzymes. Dosing needs to be decreased if renal impairment develops.

Two frequent adverse effects of levetiracetam that may have serious effects on the daily life of patients are somnolence and asthenia (weakness). Both can occur in about 15% of patients taking levetiracetam, although somnolence can occur in close to half of the patients if the dose is not slowly increased upward to the desired dose. Other adverse effects that are fairly common are dizziness and infections. Levetiracetam does not have any known drug interactions, unlike phenytoin and other AEDs. It is a pregnancy category C drug.

Felbamate

Felbamate is not a first-line AED. It is approved to treat partial seizures, either with or without generalization in adults, and Lennox-Gastaut syndrome in children, but it is only used if other therapies have not been effective and the epilepsy is considered severe. This restriction is attributable to the fact that felbamate greatly increases the risk for aplastic anemia (lack of red blood cells from bone marrow damage). The incidence of aplastic anemia among those who are taking felbamate may be more than 100 times the incidence found in the general population of those not receiving the drug. Death occurs in 20% to 70% of the patients who develop aplastic anemia, depending on the severity of the disorder. Aplastic anemia usually occurs as a full-blown syndrome; thus, there are no clinical warning signs or indications, and lab work does not indicate early signs of problems.

Monitoring lab work will, however, provide indication of full-blown aplastic anemia. Felbamate also greatly increases the risk for liver failure. Liver function tests must be monitored during therapy. Because of these serious consequences, felbamate is only used if other therapies have failed and the benefit to the patient outweighs these considerable risks. Therapeutic blood levels have not been determined.

The exact manner in which felbamate decreases seizure activity is unknown, which is a significant difference from phenytoin.

Felbamate is well absorbed from the GI tract. About half of the drug is metabolized to several metabolites, and the other half is excreted in the urine unchanged. Terminal half-life of felbamate is 20 to 23 hours.

In addition to the serious adverse effects listed previously, felbamate can produce photosensitivity as well as many other adverse effects, all of which are not common. Felbamate is a pregnancy category C drug.

Antiepileptic Drugs That Decrease Calcium Influx

The prototype antiepileptic drug that inhibits influx of calcium is ethosuximide.

NURSING MANAGEMENT OF THE PATIENT RECEIVING [P] ETHOSUXIMIDE

Core Drug Knowledge

Pharmacotherapeutics

Ethosuximide is used to treat absence (petit mal) seizures. A therapeutic serum level is 40 to 100 µg/mL.

Pharmacokinetics

Readily absorbed from the GI tract, ethosuximide can reach a peak serum level in 3 to 7 hours. Ethosuximide is extensively metabolized to inactive metabolites, and 20% is excreted unchanged by the kidneys. The plasma half-life is 30 hours in children and 60 hours in adults.

Pharmacodynamics

Ethosuximide, one of the succinimides, works by inhibiting the influx of calcium ions when they travel through a special set of channels, known as T-type calcium channels. Although an electric current will be generated when the calcium moves through the T-type channels, in most neurons, this current has only a minimal role in creating an action potential. However, in the hypothalamus neurons, this electric current does play an important role in creating an action potential. Because hypothalamic neurons are responsible for absence seizures, control of action potentials in this location reduces the incidence of absence seizures.

Contraindications and Precautions

Hypersensitivity to succinimides is the only contraindication for ethosuximide. Caution should be used if ethosuximide is used as monotherapy in mixed types of epilepsy because it may increase the frequency of tonic-clonic (grand mal) seizures in some patients. Caution should be used if the patient has pre-existing renal or liver disease. Ethosuximide is a pregnancy class D drug.

Adverse Effects

Common adverse effects of ethosuximide are drowsiness, dizziness, and lethargy. The patient usually accommodates to these adverse effects. Nausea and vomiting are also common. Other CNS and GI effects are possible but not common. Serious adverse effects include blood dyscrasias, with and without bone marrow suppression. Some of the cases of blood dyscrasias have been fatal. Another serious adverse effect is the development of systemic lupus erythematosus. Liver or renal function may also be impaired.

Adverse effects, which are uncommon, include:

- *Dermatologic:* pruritus, urticaria, Stevens-Johnson syndrome, pruritic erythematous rashes, skin eruptions, erythema multiforme, alopecia, hirsutism
- *Genitourinary:* urinary frequency, renal damage, vaginal bleeding, microscopic hematuria
- *Psychiatric:* confusion, instability, mental slowness, depression, hypochondriacal behavior, sleep disturbances, night terrors, aggressiveness, inability to concentrate (these are most often in patients who have previously had psychological disorders)
- *Miscellaneous:* periorbital edema, hyperemia, muscle weakness, swollen tongue, gum hypertrophy

Drug Interactions

Ethosuximide is known to interact with some of the other AEDs. Table 19.3 describes these interactions, effects and significance, and nursing management.

Assessment of Relevant Core Patient Variables

Health Status

Patients should have absence seizures in order to receive ethosuximide. Confirm that the patient does not have a hypersensitivity to the drug before starting therapy. Determine whether the patient has pre-existing renal or hepatic disease, both of which indicate caution with ethosuximide use.

Life Span and Gender

Like all AEDs, ethosuximide may cause teratogenic effects if given during pregnancy. However, as with other AEDs, suddenly discontinuing ethosuximide may cause an increase in seizures. Women of childbearing age should be aware of the risks related to pregnancy. Assess whether a woman is pregnant before starting drug therapy.

Environment

Ethosuximide can be administered in all environmental settings.

Nursing Diagnoses and Outcomes

- Imbalanced Nutrition: Less than Body Requirements related to adverse GI drug effects of anorexia, abdominal complaints, nausea, and vomiting

TABLE 19.3 Agents That Interact With P Ethosuximide

Interactants	Effect and Significance	Nursing Management
valproic acid	Increased pharmacologic effects of ethosuximide Both increases and decreases in ethosuximide levels have occurred	Monitor patient for changes in seizure control. Assess patient for evidence of therapeutic effects of interacting drugs.
phenytoin	Serum hydantoin levels may increase	Evaluate patient for changed seizure control. Assess patient for evidence of therapeutic effects of interacting drugs. Check for therapeutic serum levels of interacting drugs.
primidone	Lower primidone and phenobarbital levels may occur	Evaluate patient for changed seizure control. Assess patient for evidence of therapeutic effects of interacting drugs. Check for therapeutic serum levels of interacting drugs.

Desired outcome: The patient will not experience major nutritional imbalances while receiving ethosuximide.

- Risk for Injury from falls related to CNS adverse effects of ethosuximide
  Desired outcome: *The patient will not sustain an injury while receiving ethosuximide.*
- Risk for Injury from blood dyscrasias related to adverse effects of ethosuximide
  Desired outcome: *The patient will not experience major changes in his or her complete blood cell counts.*

Planning and Intervention

Maximizing Therapeutic Effects

When initiating therapy or changing a dose, monitor the drug serum level to determine whether a therapeutic range has been obtained.

Minimizing Adverse Effects

Assess complete blood counts regularly to determine whether any low blood cell counts are present. If patients develop signs of infection (sore throat, fever), the blood cell counts should also be checked at that time. Periodic urinalysis and liver function studies will help to identify early any complications that might be from ethosuximide therapy. Like all AEDs, taper the dose gradually if it is necessary to discontinue the drug to minimize the risk for seizures, including absence status.

Providing Patient and Family Education

Much of the teaching for ethosuximide is similar to that for phenytoin and other AEDs. Specific teaching includes the following:

- Teach the patient to take the drug with milk or food if GI upset occurs.
- Teach the patient to notify the physician if any of the following occurs: skin rash, joint pain, unexplained fever, sore throat, unusual bleeding or bruising, severe drowsiness, severe dizziness, blurred vision, or pregnancy.
- Teach women of childbearing age to use birth control because drug therapy carries some risks if they become pregnant. Women who wish to become pregnant while taking this drug need to be counseled about the importance of discussing their options with their physicians first.

Ongoing Assessment and Evaluation

Ongoing assessments include monitoring patients closely for therapeutic responses, seizure control, and adverse effects of drug therapy. Blood levels of the drug should be monitored whenever the dose is changed or if the patient is having seizures. Ethosuximide therapy is effective if seizures can be controlled and the patient experiences no serious adverse effects.

Drugs Significantly Different From P Ethosuximide

Zonisamide is used as an adjunct drug in treating partial seizures in adults. It is a sulfonamide drug. Therapeutic level has not been determined. Although the exact mechanism of action is not known, it is believed to block calcium flow through T-type calcium channels, like ethosuximide. Additionally, zonisamide appears to alter sodium influx.

MEMORY CHIP

P Ethosuximide

- Used to treat absence (petit mal) seizures
- Works by inhibiting the influx of calcium ions through T-type calcium channels
- Most common adverse effects: drowsiness, dizziness, lethargy, nausea and vomiting
- Most serious adverse effects: blood dyscrasias, systemic lupus erythematosus
- Maximizing therapeutic effect: Monitor serum levels.
- Minimizing adverse effects: Monitor serum levels and complete blood counts.
- Most important patient education: Notify the physician of skin rash, joint pain, signs of infection, unusual bleeding or bruising, or pregnancy.

Zonisamide also facilitates dopamine and serotonin transmission. It has *not* been shown to increase the effectiveness of GABA.

Absorption is fairly slow with oral administration, and peak time is within 2 to 6 hours. If food is present when the drug is administered, peak will not occur until 4 to 6 hours; however, the bioavailability is not changed with the presence of food. Zonisamide has fairly low protein binding at 40%. Zonisamide binds extensively in erythrocytes as opposed to the plasma. Eight times as much zonisamide is in red blood cells compared with the plasma. The half-life of zonisamide varies; it is 63 hours from the plasma and 105 hours from the red blood cells. A steady state will occur in 14 days. Metabolism occurs in the liver, but most of the drug is eliminated in the urine unchanged. If taken with other drugs that induce hepatic enzymes, the rate of metabolism will be increased.

Hypersensitivity to the drug or to sulfonamides is a contraindication. Death can occur, although rarely, related to a hypersensitivity reaction to sulfonamides. Zonisamide is a pregnancy category C drug.

Common adverse effects include dizziness, somnolence, fatigue, ataxia, decreased mental functioning, nausea, headache, irritability, and renal calculi. Serious adverse effects include Stevens-Johnson syndrome, aplastic anemia, and agranulocytosis. Lack of sweating and elevated temperatures in children were noted during clinical testing. The drug is not approved for use in children.

Zonisamide is known to increase the levels of the following lab tests: serum creatinine, blood urea nitrogen, and serum alkaline phosphatase.

Antiepileptic Drugs That Increase the Effects of GABA

Benzodiazepines

Benzodiazepines produce their many effects by potentiating the effects of the neurotransmitter, GABA, which is an inhibitory neurotransmitter. Certain benzodiazepines are approved for different therapeutic uses, although all of the drugs in the class share many similarities. The prototype benzodiazepine is lorazepam and is discussed in Chapter 16. This chapter highlights diazepam, clonazepam, and clorazepate for their use as AEDs. Benzodiazepines are the drugs of first choice in treating status epilepticus.

Diazepam

Diazepam is used as an adjunct to other AED therapy in convulsive disorders. It has historically been the drug of first choice to treat status epilepticus, although lorazepam is now often used and has some advantages over diazepam. Diazepam is also used to treat anxiety, as a muscle relaxant, in the treatment of acute alcohol withdrawal, and as a preoperative medication to reduce anxiety, tension, and recall of events. An unlabeled use is for treating panic attacks. The therapeutic blood level of diazepam has not been determined. Diazepam works like all benzodiazepines by increasing the effectiveness of GABA.

Onset of action when taken orally is very rapid for diazepam, and peak plasma levels are reached in 30 minutes to 2 hours. The drug is very highly protein bound, higher than lorazepam, at 98%. Like lorazepam, diazepam is metabolized through the liver; unlike lorazepam, it is metabolized to an active metabolite. Elimination half-life is 20 to 80 hours; this time is lengthened in obese patients. Like other benzodiazepines, diazepam is excreted in the urine.

Unique pharmacokinetic differences exist between diazepam and lorazepam, which are relevant when the drugs are used to treat status epilepticus. Although both drugs achieve therapeutic effects within a few minutes of IV administration, the anticonvulsant effect of diazepam is short lived, and seizures often reoccur 30 to 60 minutes after disruption of status epilepticus. This phenomenon occurs because diazepam is distributed quickly to the brain, where it creates its effect, but then is rapidly redistributed out of the brain to other body tissues (Alldredge, 2002; Brown, 1990). Lorazepam, on the other hand, has a much slower redistribution out of the brain and therefore a longer duration of action in status epilepticus—that is, more than 12 hours (see Chapter 16 for more information).

Diazepam is similar to lorazepam and other benzodiazepines in contraindications, precautions, adverse effects, and drug interactions. Because diazepam is used as an adjunct therapy and coadministered with other AEDs, additional CNS depression may occur, and patients need to be cautioned when the drug is added to their therapy.

Diazepam is administered intravenously during status epilepticus; the small veins in the dorsum of the hand or the wrist should be avoided. It should be injected very slowly, no faster than 5 mg in 1 minute. Diazepam should not be mixed or diluted with other solutions or drugs, either in the syringe or in IV bags of fluid. Diazepam interacts with plastic containers and administration sets, substantially decreasing availability of drug delivered. If it is not possible to give diazepam directly into the vein, it can be administered through the IV infusion tubing as close to the insertion site into the vein as possible. Although a deep intramuscular route could be used if absolutely necessary, IM injections produce low or erratic plasma levels and may not control status epilepticus easily. For this reason, the IM route is normally avoided. IV diazepam, as well as lorazepam, has been found to be safe and effective in controlling status epilepticus when administered by emergency medical technicians in patients' homes (Alldredge et al., 2001).

Clonazepam

Clonazepam is used alone or as adjunctive treatment for Lennox-Gastaut syndrome (absence variety) and akinetic and myoclonic seizures. It may be useful to patients with absence seizures who have failed to respond to succinimides, such as ethosuximide. Unlabeled uses include periodic leg movements during sleep, parkinsonian (hypokinetic) dysarthria, acute manic episodes of bipolar disorders, multifocal tic disorders, adjunct treatment for schizophrenia, and neuralgias. Therapeutic serum levels are 20 to 80 mg/mL.

Like other benzodiazepines, clonazepam increases the effectiveness of GABA. Clonazepam suppresses the spike and wave discharge that occurs with absence seizures and decreases the frequency, amplitude, duration, and spread of neuronal discharge in motor seizures. The onset of action of clonazepam is intermediate, with peak plasma level being reached in 1 to 2 hours. Clonazepam is highly protein bound at 97%. It is metabolized through the liver to five metabolites. The elimination half-life is 18 to 50 hours.

Tolerance to the antiseizure effects of clonazepam can occur within months. Abrupt withdrawal of the drug will induce seizures, including status epilepticus.

Clonazepam can produce an increase in salivation as an adverse effect. It should be used with caution in patients for whom increased salivation causes respiratory difficulty. Like diazepam, when given with other AED therapy, clonazepam will cause additive CNS depression.

Other adverse effects, precautions, and drug interactions are similar to the prototype, lorazepam.

Clorazepate

Clorazepate is used as adjunctive treatment for partial seizures; it is also used to treat anxiety disorders and for symptom management in acute alcohol withdrawal. The therapeutic blood level for clorazepate has not been determined. It has a fast onset of action, reaches peak in 1 to 2 hours, and has an elimination half-life of 40 to 50 hours. It is highly protein bound at 97% to 98%. It is metabolized in the liver by the same pathway as diazepam. Like all benzodiazepines, it achieves its effects by enhancing the effects of GABA. Additional core drug knowledge about clorazepate is similar to the prototype, lorazepam.

Drugs Significantly Different From the Benzodiazepines

Gabapentin

Gabapentin is an adjunct AED used in treating partial seizures, with or without secondary generalization, in patients older than 12 years. It is also used in treating partial seizures in children 3 to 12 years of age. Nonlabeled uses include multiple sclerosis, amyotrophic lateral sclerosis, neuropathic pain, bipolar disorder, and prophylaxis for migraine headaches. A therapeutic blood level of gabapentin has not been established.

Gabapentin is structurally related to the neurotransmitter GABA, but it does not interact at GABA receptors. It is believed to promote the release of GABA. It is absorbed through the GI tract, and food does not affect its absorption. It is almost entirely free from protein binding, with only 3% bound. Gabapentin is excreted renally, without undergoing metabolism. Elimination half-life is 5 to 7 hours. Patients with renal failure or renal disease may have additional risks for adverse effects from the drug.

Gabapentin is a pregnancy category C drug. It is secreted into breast milk and should generally be avoided during nursing because the safety and efficacy in children younger than 3 years is not known. The most common adverse effects of gabapentin for patients older than 12 years are CNS effects: somnolence, dizziness, ataxia, fatigue, and nystagmus. In children between the ages of 3 and 12 years, the most common adverse effects of gabapentin are viral infection, fever, nausea and vomiting, somnolence, and hostility. Children younger than 12 years could have other neuropsychiatric adverse effects such as behavior problems, aggressive behavior, thought disorders with trouble concentrating or changes in school performance, restlessness, and hyperactivity. Usually, the occurrence of these effects is mild to moderate in intensity.

Because gabapentin does not affect hepatic enzymes responsible for metabolism of other drugs, it is very free of drug interactions. This advantage makes it ideal to combine with other AEDs for seizure treatment. The only important drug interaction is with antacids. Antacids will reduce the bioavailability or gabapentin by 20%; to avoid this interaction, gabapentin should be administered at least 2 hours after administering antacids.

Older adults should have the dose increased gradually because they may have age-related kidney function deterioration. As for all AEDs, gabapentin should be withdrawn slowly and gradually to prevent the onset of seizures.

Phenobarbital

Phenobarbital is used to treat generalized tonic-clonic and cortical focal seizures. Phenobarbital is also used to treat acute convulsive episodes that require emergency intervention (e.g., status epilepticus, eclampsia, cholera, meningitis, tetanus, and toxic reactions to strychnine or local anesthetics), as a preanesthetic, and to induce sleep (see Chapter 16). Phenobarbital is a general CNS depressant that suppresses the sensory cortex, decreases motor activity, alters cerebellar function, and produces drowsiness, sedation, and hypnosis. Phenobarbital's anticonvulsant activities are relatively nonselective. It stimulates GABA receptors, thereby elevating the seizure threshold and limiting the spread of seizure activity by affecting the CNS neuronal pathway neurotransmitters. Tolerance does not occur to the anticonvulsant effects of phenobarbital, as it does to the sedative effects. The therapeutic blood level of phenobarbital is 15 to 40 µg/mL.

Phenobarbital is absorbed through the GI tract; time to reach a peak plasma level varies from 30 minutes to more than 1 hour. It is only moderately protein bound at 40% to 60%. It is metabolized in the liver and induces the hepatic enzyme system. It can induce its own metabolism. Its half-life is long, 53 to 143 hours. One fourth of phenobarbital is excreted in the urine unchanged.

Phenobarbital is classified as FDA pregnancy category D, and fetal abnormalities are possible if used during pregnancy.

Adverse effects are related to CNS depression, and respiratory depression is the most serious. The degree of respiratory depression is dose dependent. The dosage used to control seizures is rarely involved with substantial respiratory depression. Drowsiness occurs commonly with phenobarbital use in the treatment of seizures; tolerance to this effect, however, develops with chronic use. Other CNS effects may occur. In some instances, phenobarbital will produce CNS effects that are the opposite of what would normally be expected. Therefore, agitation, hyperactivity, insomnia, irritability, and CNS stimulation may occur. Children and older adults are particularly prone to these paradoxical effects. Adverse cognitive effects in children may also include impaired short-term memory and deficits on neuropsychologic tests and memory concentration tasks. Fever may occur with chronic use. Like other AEDs, status epilepticus may occur if phenobarbital is stopped suddenly after chronic use. Like other AEDs, additive CNS depression will occur if phenobarbital is taken with other CNS depressants. Because it induces the hepatic enzyme system and alters the metabolism of a large number of other drugs, phenobarbital is characterized by many drug–drug interactions. Because of its many adverse effects and drug interactions, phenobarbital use has greatly decreased since the creation of the newer AEDs.

When given for emergency use, phenobarbital is administered intravenously and may require at least 15 minutes before peak concentration is reached in the brain to control

the seizure. Because of phenobarbital's long half-life, if it is administered continuously until the seizure activity ceases, severe barbiturate-induced CNS depression, including respiratory depression and excessive hypotension, can occur. Because of the length of time needed to reach a therapeutic effect and control status epilepticus, more rapidly acting drugs, such as diazepam or lorazepam, are normally used to treat status epilepticus initially. Phenobarbital is used as a third-line drug after interventions with a benzodiazepine and phenytoin have failed.

Primidone

Primidone is used to control grand mal, psychomotor, or focal epileptic seizures, either alone or used in combination with other AED therapy. An unlabeled use of primidone is benign familial tremor. Although primidone is actually considered to be an adjuvant AED, one of the active metabolites of primidone is phenobarbital. The other active metabolite is phenylethylmalonamide (PEMA). Although primidone has anticonvulsant properties of its own, much of its effect comes from the anticonvulsant properties of phenobarbital and PEMA. Animal studies have shown that PEMA also potentiates the effects of phenobarbital. Phenobarbital accounts for between 15% and 25% of the metabolites formed by primidone.

Primidone has a half-life of 5 to 15 hours. PEMA and phenobarbital have longer half-lives (10–18 hours and 53–140 hours, respectively) and accumulate with chronic use. About 40% of primidone is excreted unchanged in the urine. The remainder of the drug is excreted as unconjugated PEMA and as phenobarbital and its metabolites.

The therapeutic effects and adverse effects of primidone are similar to those of phenobarbital and other AEDs. Nursing management of the patient is also similar.

Tiagabine

Tiagabine is used as an adjunct therapy in treating partial seizures. Like the benzodiazepines, it is believed to enhance the effectiveness of GABA. Unlike the benzodiazepines, tiagabine binds to the sites associated with GABA reuptake. By binding to these sites, it inhibits GABA reuptake, and the neurotransmitter can further stimulate the receptors on the postsynaptic cells. Tiagabine is sometimes referred to as a GABAergic drug.

Tiagabine is absorbed rapidly and almost completely from the GI tract and peaks in about 45 minutes if taken on an empty stomach; a high-fat meal will slow the rate but not the extent of absorption. Tiagabine is highly protein bound at 96%. Metabolism of tiagabine is in the liver through hepatic enzymatic pathways, mostly CYP3A, although other isoenzymes may also be involved. Although half-life is 7 to 9 hours in healthy adults, it can be decreased considerably (up to 65%) if taken with other AEDs that induce hepatic isoenzymes, such as phenytoin, carbamazepine, primidone, or phenobarbital. An unusual feature of the pharmacokinetics of tiagabine is that it exhibits a diurnal effect; steady-state values are 15% lower after the evening dose than after the morning dose. A therapeutic drug level for tiagabine has not been established.

Like all other AEDs, tiagabine is not recommended to be used during pregnancy or breast-feeding. It is classified as a pregnancy category C drug because animal studies have indicated teratogenic effects. However, no related controlled studies have been done in women. Tiagabine is excreted in breast milk.

Although tiagabine is usually well tolerated, the most common adverse effects are related to the CNS system. These include dizziness, muscle weakness, somnolence, nervousness, tremor, insomnia, difficulty with concentration or attention, ataxia, and confusion. GI problems of nausea, diarrhea, or vomiting are also common.

Nursing management for tiagabine is similar to that for other AEDs. Although animal studies indicate a risk for visual-field impairment from tiagabine, clinical research has not borne this potential out (Box 19.4).

Vigabatrin

Vigabatrin is used to treat resistant partial epilepsy in cases in which other drug therapy has failed to control seizures. Vigabatrin is a GABAergic drug, like tiagabine. Unlike tiagabine, vigabatrin has been found to significantly increase the risk for visual-field impairment (see Box 19.4). About one third of the patients treated with vigabatrin develop visual-field defects characterized by a bilateral, absolute concentric constriction of the visual field; the severity of the impairment can be mild or severe. Sometimes, the damage to the retina is permanent. Adults seem to be at higher risk for developing the adverse effect (although more research is needed with pediatric pop-

FOCUS ON RESEARCH

Box 19.4 Same Mode of Action, Different Adverse Effects

Krauss, G. L., Johnson, M. A., Sheth, S., et al. (2003). A controlled study comparing visual function in patients treated with vigabatrin and tiagabine. *Journal of Neurology, Neurosurgery, and Psychiatry, 74*(3), 339–343.
Hosking, S. L., Roff Hilton, E. J., Embleton, S. J., et al. (2003). Epilepsy patients treated with vigabatrin exhibit reduced ocular blood flow. *British Journal of Ophthalmology, 87*(1):96–100.

The Study

An analysis of patients who received either tiagabine or vigabatrin, both of which raise GABA levels, and other AEDs was performed. Patients who received other AEDs were considered the control. The vision in these groups was compared for visual acuity, color vision, static and kinetic perimetry, and electroretinograms. Only patients treated with vigabatrin had marked visual-field constrictions in kinetic perimetry and abnormal electroretinography results; both those treated with tiagabine and those treated with the control drugs displayed normal responses. This disparity showed that the visual-field impairment was unique to vigabatrin. The cause of this difference is still somewhat hypothetical. Vigabatrin is known to achieve higher retinal concentrations than tiagabine can achieve. Additionally, another small study showed that vigabatrin reduced ocular perfusion more than other AEDs. Either of these factors, alone or in combination, or some other unknown factor, may explain why vigabatrin produces such a high incidence of visual-field impairment.

Nursing Implications

These studies have broad and very important implications for nurses. You need to understand that although drugs may share many similar characteristics, including mode of action or assigned drug class, all actions and effects of the drug are not necessarily identical. Although learning about a prototype teaches you a good bit about drugs in that class, when administering drug therapy or teaching patients about their drug therapies, it is important to look up each individual drug to check for unique adverse effects or drug interactions.

ulations), and men have about twice the risk of women for developing these problems. Data suggest that the incidence increases during the first 2 years of treatment and with initiating therapy when the daily dose is up to 2 kg. Risk for visual-field impairment stabilizes at 3 years and after the total daily dose reaches 3 kg (Kalviainen & Nousiainen, 2001). Because of these serious adverse effects, patients should be started on vigabatrin only if all other combinations of AED therapy have been tried and were unsuccessful. Patients receiving vigabatrin should regularly have their vision tested. Vigabatrin is not currently approved for use in the United States, but it is available in Canada and other parts of the world.

DRUGS USED IN SEIZURES RELATED TO PRE-ECLAMPSIA AND ECLAMPSIA

Magnesium sulfate is a drug that is completely different from all of the other AEDs. Magnesium sulfate is used in treating seizures related to severe pre-eclampsia or eclampsia in pregnant women. It is also used to control preterm labor. Magnesium has a depressive effect on the CNS. It prevents or controls seizures by blocking the neuromuscular transmission of acetylcholine and decreasing the amount of this neurotransmitter liberated at the end plate by motor nerve impulses. This drug is discussed in more detail in Chapter 55.

CHAPTER SUMMARY

- Antiepileptic drugs work by inhibiting influx of sodium ions through sodium channels into the cell, inhibiting calcium ion influx into special calcium channels, or altering the effectiveness of GABA.
- All AEDs carry risks for teratogenicity. Stopping drug therapy also carries the risk for inducing seizures, which is risky to the mother and the fetus. Most babies born to epileptic mothers on drug therapy are normal.
- Status epilepticus is a medical emergency and requires IV drug therapy. The first line of treatment is a benzodiazepine, either diazepam or lorazepam. Phenytoin is used next. Phenobarbital is a third-line drug used if neither the benzodiazepine nor the phenytoin is effective.
- AED therapy can be successfully discontinued in about 70% of people once they are seizure free for 2 years.
- Nursing management procedures for the AEDs are similar in many respects. Patients need to understand the disease process, how the disease and drug therapy may affect their lives, and possible adverse effects of drug therapy.

QUESTIONS FOR STUDY AND REVIEW

1. What is the difference between a seizure and a convulsion?
2. Why is phenytoin useful in treating both seizures and some cardiac arrhythmias?
3. What is the first-line drug of choice in treating status epilepticus?
4. Why should dosage changes of phenytoin be made in small increments?
5. Why would patients with low serum albumin levels be more at risk for adverse effects from phenytoin?
6. How does ethosuximide reduce absence seizures?
7. How do benzodiazepines suppress seizure activity?

Need More Help?

Chapter 19 of the study guide for *Drug Therapy in Nursing* 2e contains NCLEX-style questions and other learning activities to reinforce your understanding of the concepts presented in this chapter. For additional information or to purchase the study guide, visit *http://connection.lww.com/go/aschenbrenner.*

REFERENCES AND BIBLIOGRAPHY

Alldredge, B. K. (2002). Issues in the initiation of treatment for status epilepticus. *Profiles in seizure management: Pharmacy series* [Online]. Princeton Media. Available: *http://www.princetoncme.com/public/2002-31-1/report89.html.*

Alldredge, B. K., Gelb, A. M., Isaacs, S. M., et al. (2001). A comparison of lorazepam, diazepam, and placebo for the treatment of out-of-hospital status epilepticus. *New England Journal of Medicine, 345*(9), 631–637.

Brown, T. R. (1990). The pharmacokinetics of agents used to treat status epilepticus. *Neurology, 40*(Suppl. 2), 28–32.

DeLorenzo, R. J., Hauser, W. A., Towne, A. R., et al. (1996). A prospective, population-based epidemiologic study of status epilepticus in Richmond, Virginia. *Neurology, 46*(4), 1029–1035.

Food and Drug Administration. (2000). Complications with the use of anticonvulsants in pregnancy [Online]. Slide presentation by M. Yerby. Available: *http://www.fda.gov/cder/present/clinpharm 2000/Yerby/sld001.htm.*

Jozwiak, S., & Terczynski, A. (2000). Open study evaluating lamotrigine efficacy and safety in add-on treatment and consecutive monotherapy in adult patients with epilepsy resistant carbamazepine and valproate. *Seizure, 9*(7), 486–492.

Kalviainen, R., & Nousiainen, I. (2001). Visual field defects with vigabatrin: Epidemiology and therapeutic implications. *CNS Drugs, 15*(3), 217–230.

National Institutes of Health. National Institute of Neurological Disorders and Stroke. (2004). Seizures and epilepsy: Hope through research [Online]. Available: *http://www.ninds.nih.gov/health_and_medical/pubs/seizures_and_epilepsy_htr.htm#Epilepsy.* Accessed August 13, 2004.

Perucca, E. (2002). Pharmacological and therapeutic properties of valproate: A summary after 35 years of clinical experience. *CNS Drugs, 16*(10), 695–714.

Reports from the 54th Annual Meeting of the American Academy of Neurology. (2002). Practical seizure management: Starting and stopping AEDs [Online]. Available: *http://www.neurologyreviews.com/oct02/nr_oct02_seizure.html.*

Treiman, D. M., Meyers, P. D., Walton, N. Y., et al. (1998). A comparison of four treatments for generalized convulsive status epilepticus. Veterans Affairs Status Epilepticus Cooperative Study Group. *New England Journal of Medicine, 339*(12), 792–798.

Drugs Affecting Muscle Spasm and Spasticity

chapter 20

KEY TERMS

centrally acting

clonic

peripherally acting

spasm

spasmolytics

spasticity

tonic

Learning Objectives

At the completion of this chapter the student will:

1. Correlate the pathophysiology of muscle spasm and spasticity with appropriate pharmacotherapy.
2. Identify core drug knowledge about pharmacologic therapies that affect muscle spasm and spasticity.
3. Identify core patient variables related to drugs that affect muscle spasm and spasticity.
4. Relate the interaction of core drug knowledge with core patient variables for pharmacologic therapies that affect muscle spasm and spasticity.
5. Generate a nursing plan of care from the interactions between core drug knowledge and core patient variables for pharmacologic therapies that affect muscle spasm and spasticity.
6. Describe nursing interventions to maximize therapeutic effects and minimize adverse effects for drugs that affect muscle spasm and spasticity.
7. Determine key points for patient and family education about drugs that affect muscle spasm and spasticity.

FEATURED WEBLINKS

http://www.msif.org/en
http://www.spinalcord.org

Spasmolytic agents are frequently used for managing multiple sclerosis (MS) and spinal cord injury. To enhance your knowledge of MS, visit the first site listed above. For more information regarding spinal cord injury, visit the second site.

CONNECTION WEBLINK

Additional Weblinks are found on Connection:
http://www.connection.lww.com/go/aschenbrenner.

Drugs Affecting Muscle Spasm and Spasticity

Ⓒ Centrally Acting Muscle Relaxants

- [P] **cyclobenzaprine**
- carisoprodol
- chlorzoxazone
- metaxalone
- methocarbamol
- orphenadrine
- diazepam

Ⓒ Spasmolytics

Ⓒ Centrally acting

- [P] **baclofen**
- tizanidine
- gabapentin

Ⓒ Peripherally acting

- [P] **dantrolene**
- botulinum toxin type A

The symbol Ⓒ indicates the **drug class.**
Drugs in **bold type** marked with the symbol [P] are prototypes.
Drugs in blue type are closely related to the prototype.
Drugs in red type are significantly different from the prototype.
Drugs in black type with no symbol are also used in drug therapy; no prototype

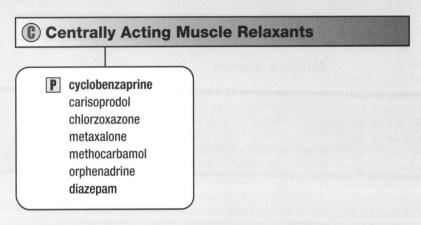

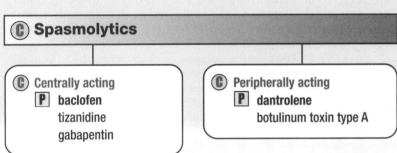

Drugs used to manage muscle spasm and spasticity can be divided into two major therapeutic groups: skeletal muscle relaxants and **spasmolytics.** Muscle spasms are treated with a combination of physical therapy, centrally acting muscle relaxants, and anti-inflammatory agents (see Chapter 24). Spasticity is treated with physical therapy and drugs called spasmolytics. Spasmolytics are categorized as **centrally acting** or **peripherally acting.** As their names imply, these agents act in the brain or in the peripheral muscles.

This chapter discusses the centrally acting muscle relaxant cyclobenzaprine (Flexeril), the centrally acting spasmolytic baclofen (Lioresal), and the peripherally acting spasmolytic dantrolene sodium (Dantrium). Table 20.1 presents a summary of these drugs. In addition, this chapter addresses core drug knowledge, core patient variables, nursing management practices, potential nursing diagnoses, and patient education guidelines related to the use of these drugs. For discussion of physical methods for managing spasm and spasticity, refer to an appropriate medical-surgical textbook.

PHYSIOLOGY

The human body contains approximately 600 skeletal muscles. Skeletal muscle is voluntary, meaning a person can contract it at will. Seen under a microscope, skeletal muscle fibers show a pattern of cross-banding, which gives rise to its other name: striated muscle. The striations are caused by the alignment of bands, the most prominent of which are the A bands, I bands, and Z lines. The unit between two Z lines is called the sarcomere (Figure 20.1).

Striated muscle is composed of two contractile proteins: actin and myosin. The thin filaments are made of actin, which is attached to the Z lines and is found in both A bands and I bands. The thick filaments, found in A bands, are made of myosin. In the process set forth in the sliding filament theory, the sarcomere shortens, and the Z lines move closer together when muscle contracts. The filaments slide together because myosin attaches to, and pulls on, actin. The myosin head attaches to the actin filament, forming a crossbridge. After formation of the crossbridge, the myosin head bends, pulling on the actin filaments and causing them to slide. The result is that the Z lines move closer together, the I band becomes shorter, and the A band stays the same (see Figure 20.1). Muscle contraction is like climbing a rope. The crossbridge cycle is one of grabbing, pulling, and releasing, repeated over and over.

Muscle contraction is triggered by a sudden inflow of calcium ion (Ca^{2+}). In the resting state, the protein tropomyosin winds around actin and covers the myosin-binding sites. The Ca^{2+} binds to a second protein, troponin; this action causes the tropomyosin to be pulled to the side, exposing the myosin-binding sites. With the sites exposed, muscle will contract in the presence of adenosine triphosphate (ATP). Muscle contraction stops when Ca^{2+} is removed from the immediate environment of the myofilaments.

PATHOPHYSIOLOGY

Muscle Spasm

A muscle **spasm** is a sudden violent involuntary contraction of a muscle or group of muscles. Spasm is usually related to a localized skeletal muscle injury from acute trauma. Spasms may also stem from disorders such as hypocalcemia, hypokalemia or hyperkalemia, chronic pain syndromes, or epilepsy. Pain and interference with function attend muscle spasm, producing involuntary movement and distortion. When a muscle goes into spasm, it freezes in contraction and becomes a hard knotty mass, rather than normally contracting and relaxing in quick succession. During spasm, the blood vessels that normally feed the muscles and supply oxygen constrict, further compounding the problem.

Tonic spasm, or cramp, is characterized by an unusually prolonged and strong muscular contraction, with relaxation occurring slowly. In the other form of spasm, called **clonic** spasm, contractions of the affected muscles occur repeatedly, forcibly, and in quick succession, with equally sudden and frequent relaxations.

Spasticity

Spasticity is a condition in which certain muscles are continuously contracted. This contraction causes stiffness or tightness of the muscles and may interfere with gait, movement, or speech. Damage to the portion of the brain or spinal cord that controls voluntary movement usually causes spasticity. Spasticity may be associated with spinal cord injury, multiple sclerosis (MS), cerebral palsy, anoxic brain damage, brain trauma, severe head injury, and some metabolic diseases, such as adrenoleukodystrophy and phenylketonuria. Symptoms may include hypertonicity (increased muscle tone), clonus (a series of rapid muscle contractions), exaggerated deep tendon reflexes, muscle spasms, scissoring (involuntary crossing of the legs), and fixed joints. The degree of spasticity varies from mild muscle stiffness to severe, painful, and uncontrollable muscle spasms. The condition can interfere with daily activities and with rehabilitation in patients with certain disorders.

C CENTRALLY ACTING MUSCLE RELAXANTS

The centrally acting muscle relaxants are a group of drugs with similar pharmacologic properties. They act in the central nervous system (CNS). The prototype for centrally acting muscle relaxants is cyclobenzaprine. Other drugs in this class include carisoprodol, chlorphenesin, chlorzoxazone, metaxalone, methocarbamol, and orphenadrine.

Diazepam (Valium), a benzodiazepine, is also mentioned in this chapter because it is used in managing both muscle spasms and spasticity. Its pharmacodynamics make it significantly different from centrally acting muscle relaxants.

TABLE 20.1 Summary of Selected Drugs That Affect Muscle Spasm and Spasticity

Drug (Trade) Name	Selected Indications	Route and Dosage Range	Pharmacokinetics
C Centrally Acting Muscle Relaxants			
P cyclobenzaprine (Flexeril, *Novo-Cycloprine*)	Muscle spasms Muscle relaxation	*Adult:* PO 10 mg tid; maximum 60 mg qid *Child <15 y:* not recommended	*Onset:* 1 h *Duration:* 12–24 h $t_{1/2}$: 8 h
carisoprodol (Soma)	Muscle spasms Muscle relaxation	*Adult:* PO 350 mg qid *Child:* not recommended	*Onset:* 3–5 d *Duration:* 4–6 h $t_{1/2}$: 1–3 d
chlorzoxazone (Paraflex)	Muscle spasms Muscle relaxation	*Adult:* PO 250–500 mg tid/qid *Child:* PO 20 mg/kg/d in divided doses	*Onset:* 30–60 min *Duration:* 3–4 h $t_{1/2}$: 60 min
metaxalone (Skelaxin)	Muscle spasms Muscle relaxation	*Adult and child >12 y:* PO 800 mg tid–qid	*Onset:* 1 h *Duration:* 4–6 h $t_{1/2}$: 2–3 h
methocarbamol (Robaxin)	Muscle spasms Muscle relaxation	*Adult:* 1,500 mg qid; 1,000 mg qid for maintenance *Child:* not recommended	*Onset:* 30 min *Duration:* 8 h $t_{1/2}$: 1–2 h
	Tetanus	*Adult:* IV 2–4 g up to 3 g/d *Child:* not recommended	*Onset:* rapid *Duration:* unknown $t_{1/2}$: 1–2 h
orphenadrine (Norflex, *Orfenace*)	Muscle spasms Muscle relaxation	*Adult and child >12 y:* PO 200–250 mg/d in divided doses; IV 60 mg q 12 h *Child <12 y:* not recommended	*Onset:* 1–2 h *Duration:* 4–6 h $t_{1/2}$: 14–16 h
C Centrally Acting Spasmolytics			
P baclofen (Lioresal; *Canadian:* Apo-Baclofen)	Spasticity	*Adult:* PO 5–20 mg tid; Intrathecal 5–25 µg *Child:* not recommended	*Onset:* 3–4 d *Duration:* 24–48 h $T_{1/2}$: 3–4 h
tizanidine (Zanaflex)	Spasticity MS Muscle relaxation	*Adult:* 2–4 mg tid; maximum dose 36 mg/d *Child:* not recommended	*Onset:* 1 h *Duration:* 3–6 h $T_{1/2}$: 2.5 h
gabapentin (Neurontin)	Spasticity	*Adult:* PO, 600–1200 mg/d in divided doses *Child:* not recommended	*Onset:* 30 min *Duration:* 8 h $T_{1/2}$: 5–7 h
C Peripherally Acting Spasmolytics			
P dantrolene (Dantrium)	Athetosis cerebral palsy, MS, hemiplegia, paraplegia, Parkinson disease, spasticity, CVA, spinal cord injury	*Adult:* PO 25–100 mg 2–4 times qid *Child <5y:* not approved *Child >5y:* 0.5 mg/kg bid, maximum 100 mg qid	*Onset:* 4–7 d *Duration:* dose related $T_{1/2}$: 7–9 h
	Prevention of malignant hyperthermia	IV: 2.5 mg/kg 1 h before surgery PO: 4–8 mg/kg in divided doses 1–2 d before surgery with last dose 3–4 h after surgery	
	Malignant hyperthermia (adult and child)	IV: 1 mg/kg	
	Postcrisis follow-up	PO: 4–8 mg/kg in four divided doses for 1–3 d	
botulinum toxin type A (Botox)	Chronic spasticity	*Adult:* 1 m; extremely individualized	*Onset:* 3 d–2 wk *Duration:* 3 mo $T_{1/2}$: 10 h

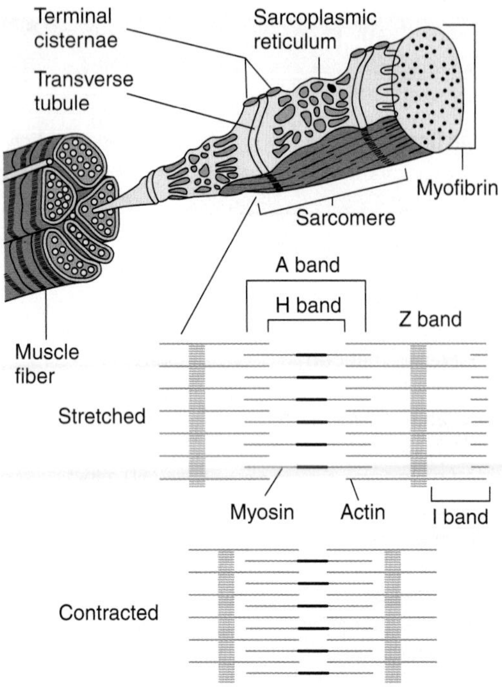

FIGURE 20.1 When stimulation stops, calcium ions are actively transported back into the sarcoplasmic reticulum, resulting in decreased calcium ions in the sarcoplasm. The removal of calcium ions restores the inhibitory action of troponin-tropomyosin; crossbridge action is impossible in this state.

NURSING MANAGEMENT OF THE PATIENT RECEIVING P CYCLOBENZAPRINE

Core Drug Knowledge

Pharmacotherapeutics

Cyclobenzaprine is used to manage muscle spasms associated with acute musculoskeletal disorders, such as low back strain. It is also used as supportive therapy in patients with tetanus or fibromyalgia.

Pharmacokinetics

Cyclobenzaprine is administered orally. It is well absorbed from the gastrointestinal (GI) tract and probably undergoes first-pass metabolism because plasma levels vary considerably among patients. Onset of skeletal muscle relaxation occurs in about 1 hour, and duration of action ranges from 12 to 24 hours. Optimal effects may take 1 to 2 days to fully develop. Cyclobenzaprine undergoes extensive metabolism and is excreted mainly as conjugated inactive metabolites in the urine and as unchanged drug through bile in the feces. Its half-life ranges from 1 to 3 days.

Pharmacodynamics

Cyclobenzaprine relieves muscle spasms through a central action, possibly at the level of the brain stem, with no direct action on the neuromuscular junction or the muscle involved. It reduces pain and tenderness and improves mobility. Because of its structural similarity to the tricyclic antidepressants (TCAs), cyclobenzaprine may reduce tonic somatic motor activity by influencing both alpha and gamma motor neurons. Cyclobenzaprine is ineffective for treating spasticity associated with cerebral or spinal cord disease or in children with cerebral palsy.

Contraindications and Precautions

Cyclobenzaprine is contraindicated for patients with hyperthyroidism because of a possible increased risk for developing arrhythmias or an exacerbation of tachycardia. Because of its similarity to the TCAs, cyclobenzaprine is also contraindicated for use within 14 days of administration of monoamine oxidase inhibitors (MAOIs).

In overdoses, TCAs cause conduction disturbances and have been associated with torsades de pointes (an atypical tachycardia) and death. Because it is closely related to the TCA amitriptyline, cyclobenzaprine should be used cautiously in patients with heart failure, cardiac arrhythmias, or atrioventricular (AV) block or other conduction disturbances, or in those who are in the acute recovery phase following myocardial infarction (MI).

Cyclobenzaprine possesses anticholinergic activity. Patients with increased intraocular pressure, angle-closure glaucoma, or urinary retention require careful monitoring. Cyclobenzaprine should be used with caution in pregnant or breast-feeding women. Studies for determining safe use during pregnancy have not been performed.

Adverse Effects

The common adverse effects of cyclobenzaprine are related to its CNS depression and anticholinergic activity. The most common adverse effects are drowsiness, dizziness, and dry mouth. Other frequent adverse effects include fatigue, asthenia (loss of strength and energy), nausea and vomiting, constipation, dyspepsia, dysgeusia, blurred vision, headache, nervousness, and confusion. Serious adverse effects, including arrhythmias, seizures, and MIs, can occur because of cyclobenzaprine's similarity to the TCAs.

Drug Interactions

Interactions between cyclobenzaprine and CNS depressants or antimuscarinic drugs may be extensive. Cyclobenzaprine may also interact with tramadol, guanethidine, MAOIs, histamine-1 blocking agents, and various herbal remedies. These interactions are highlighted in Table 20.2.

Assessment of Relevant Core Patient Variables

Health Status

Assess the patient for a history of cyclobenzaprine hypersensitivity or pre-existing diseases such as hyperthyroidism, cardiac dysfunction, recent MI, and glaucoma. Also, assess for use of medications that may interact with cyclobenzaprine, such as MAOIs. Communicate positive findings to the prescriber before administering the drug. Also, assess for over-the-counter (OTC) drugs used for allergies or hay fever because these drugs usually have an anticholinergic effect,

TABLE 20.2 Agents That Interact With P Cyclobenzaprine

Interactants	Effect and Significance	Nursing Management
CNS depressants • sedatives • tranquilizers • alcohol • opioids	Cyclobenzaprine, in combination with other CNS depressants, may induce additive effects, resulting in increased CNS depression.	Avoid this combination. Monitor for sedation and dizziness. Provide ambulatory assistance. Ensure patient's safety.
Tramadol	Cyclobenzaprine may react with tramadol, resulting in seizure activity.	Use of tramadol with cyclobenzaprine is not recommended. Monitor for seizure activity.
Guanethidine	Cyclobenzaprine may react with guanethidine, decreasing guanethidine's antihypertensive effect.	Use of guanethidine with cyclobenzaprine is not recommended. Monitor blood pressure. Discuss possible increased dosage of guanethidine with health care provider.
MAOIs	Although the mechanism of action is unknown, it is likely that concurrent administration of cyclobenzaprine and MAOIs enhances adrenergic activity, increasing the likelihood of oretic (hydrochlorothiazide) crisis, severe seizures, and death.	A minimum of 14 days should elapse between the discontinuance of MAOIs and the initiation of cyclobenzaprine therapy.
H_1-blocking agents	H_1 drugs and cyclobenzaprine have antimuscarinic properties. When used in combination, anticholinergic side effects can be additive.	Monitor for paralytic ileus.
Phytomedicinal herbs • Valerian • *Valeriana officinalis* • Kava kava • *Piper methysticum*	Combination therapy can cause additive effects of sedation and dizziness, which can impair the patient's ability to undertake tasks that require mental alertness.	Monitor for sedation and dizziness. Provide ambulatory assistance. Ensure patient's safety. Dosage adjustments of either or both medications may be necessary.

and additive effects occur when anticholinergic drugs are given concurrently with cyclobenzaprine.

Life Span and Gender

In working with older adult patients, assess them for the anticholinergic and CNS depressant effects of cyclobenzaprine because increased age makes a patient more susceptible to them. Evaluation of the female patient's pregnancy and lactation status is important. Safety during pregnancy has not been documented, although cyclobenzaprine is a pregnancy category B drug. Distribution of the drug into breast milk has not been established, but TCAs are found in breast milk. Because of its structural similarity to the TCAs, cyclobenzaprine may also distribute into breast milk.

Lifestyle, Diet, and Habits

Assess for use of alcohol or any other CNS depressant, which will increase the sedating effects of cyclobenzaprine. Advise the patient to assess the depth of sedation related to cyclobenzaprine use before driving a vehicle or attempting activities that require mental alertness or motor coordination. Long-term use of cyclobenzaprine may result in physical dependence. Assess for potential abuse of this drug.

Environment

Cyclobenzaprine may be administered in any environment, but it is most often given on an outpatient basis. Because it can cause sedation, discuss with the patient possible hazards in the home environment.

Nursing Diagnosis and Outcome

- Risk for Injury related to CNS depressant effects and potential cardiovascular effects.
  Desired outcome: *The patient will remain free from injury throughout therapy.*

Planning and Intervention

Maximizing Therapeutic Effects

The patient should take cyclobenzaprine with a full glass of water at evenly spaced intervals. Coordinate physical modalities such as physical therapy, whirlpool, and cold or hot compresses to the affected area.

Minimizing Adverse Effects

While the patient is hospitalized, ensure the patient's safety by keeping the bed in the lowest position. Accompany the patient during ambulation until the degree of sedation is ascertained. Also, caution the patient about the potential for orthostatic hypotension resulting in dizziness and teach the patient to change positions slowly. Finally, remind the patient of the potential for synergistic effects when cyclobenzaprine is taken with other CNS depressants, especially alcohol. Because cyclobenzaprine can cause physical dependence,

slowly withdrawing the drug over 1 to 2 weeks is important to prevent abstinence syndrome (see Chapter 9).

Providing Patient and Family Education

- Instruct patients to take cyclobenzaprine exactly as prescribed. If patients miss a dose, they should take it as soon as they remember but should never double the dose.
- Explain that adverse effects such as mild drowsiness, dizziness, or clumsiness may accompany cyclobenzaprine therapy. Although these symptoms will often improve with time, patients must refrain from driving or performing hazardous tasks until their level of sedation is ascertained. Advise patients to contact the prescriber if sedation persists or is bothersome. Also, emphasize the need to refrain from alcohol, which may exacerbate these adverse effects.
- Advise patients to contact the prescriber immediately if they experience severe headache, confusion, hallucinations, or sudden or increased weakness. Female patients should contact the prescriber immediately if they suspect they may be pregnant.
- Instruct patients to avoid using any OTC or prescription drugs without first consulting the prescriber. Many of these drugs can cause dangerous adverse effects when taken with cyclobenzaprine.
- Finally, instruct patients never to abruptly cease cyclobenzaprine if therapy has been with high doses or over a prolonged period; rather, they should decrease the dosage gradually over 2 weeks.

Ongoing Assessment and Evaluation

Constantly evaluate the patient's safety. Monitor the level of sedation and report to the prescriber if it is severe. In addition to CNS symptoms, monitor for GI symptoms, such as gastric distress or constipation. Provide analgesics for headache, offer small and frequent meals to decrease GI upset, and establish a bowel program if constipation becomes a problem. Successful cyclobenzaprine therapy is marked by decreased muscle spasms and no injury to the patient related to adverse effects.

MEMORY CHIP

P Cyclobenzaprine

- Centrally acting spasmolytic is used for muscle spasms; ineffective for spasticity
- Most common adverse effect: sedation; safety is a nursing priority
- Most serious adverse effects: occur with abrupt withdrawal and include agitation, auditory or visual hallucinations, seizures, or psychotic symptoms
- **Life span alert: Older adult patients are more prone to sedation and anticholinergic effects.**
- Maximizing therapeutic effects: Take medication exactly as prescribed.
- Minimizing adverse effects: Avoid use of other CNS depressants.
- Most important patient education: Never abruptly stop medication; withdraw medication over a 2-week period.

Drugs Closely Related to P Cyclobenzaprine

Carisoprodol

Carisoprodol (Soma) is an oral skeletal-muscle relaxant used in treating musculoskeletal injuries. Although carisoprodol is itself a nonscheduled drug, it can be very addictive; it is metabolized into meprobamate; a Schedule IV controlled substance. Its ability to produce dependence and the availability of newer agents has diminished its use.

Carisoprodol works by depressing the CNS, resulting in sedation and alteration of pain perception. It has no direct action on skeletal muscle. It is widely distributed in the body, crosses the placenta, and enters breast milk. It is hepatically metabolized and renally excreted. Therefore, carisoprodol should be given cautiously to patients with impaired hepatic or renal function.

Adverse effects of carisoprodol are similar to those of cyclobenzaprine. Symptoms of overdose include stupor, shock, and respiratory depression. Abrupt withdrawal may induce seizures. Treatment of overdose is supportive, following attempts to enhance drug elimination.

Chlorzoxazone

Chlorzoxazone (Paraflex, Parafon Forte) is another centrally acting muscle relaxant. Although its exact mechanism of action is unknown, its effects are thought to be related to its depression of the CNS, which results in reduced skeletal muscle spasms. Pain relief is thought to result from alterations in the perception of pain. Chlorzoxazone has been used for many years. It is widely distributed throughout the body, metabolized by the liver, and excreted by the kidneys.

Because chlorzoxazone is metabolized in the liver, it should be used with caution in patients with hepatic disease. A metabolite of chlorzoxazone is rapidly excreted in the urine; therefore, it should be used with caution in patients with renal impairment because it may alter excretion and possibly cause toxicity. Chlorzoxazone has not been evaluated for safe use during pregnancy, and thus its effects on the fetus are unknown. It should be used only when the benefits to the pregnant woman outweigh the risks to the fetus. Whether chlorzoxazone is distributed into breast milk is unknown. Finally, chlorzoxazone is not recommended for use in older adults because of the potential for anticholinergic side effects, sedation, and weakness.

Adverse effects are sedation, dizziness, and hepatotoxicity. Hepatotoxicity ranges from a mild elevation in hepatic enzymes to hepatic necrosis.

Metaxalone

Metaxalone (Skelaxin), like other centrally acting muscle relaxants, has no direct effect on the contractile mechanism of striated muscle, the motor end plate, or the nerve fiber. Its mode of action may be related to its sedative properties. Administration is oral, metabolism is hepatic, and excretion is renal.

Metaxalone is contraindicated in patients with severe renal impairment. The drug is also contraindicated in patients with a history of drug-induced hemolytic anemia or other anemias. Because metaxalone is metabolized in the liver, it should be used with caution in patients with hepatic disease. Metaxalone is contraindicated in patients with severe hepatic impairment. The safety and effectiveness of metaxalone have

not been established in children 12 years of age or younger. Metaxalone is not recommended for use in older adults because of the potential for anticholinergic side effects, sedation, and weakness. Metaxalone should be used during pregnancy only if the potential benefits to the pregnant woman outweigh the possible risks to the fetus. Distribution of metaxalone into breast milk is not known; therefore, it should be used with caution in breast-feeding women.

Adverse effects of metaxalone include elevated hepatic enzymes, such as increased serum concentrations of aspartate transaminase (AST), alanine transaminase (ALT), and alkaline phosphatase, and increased levels of bilirubin. Liver function tests should be performed periodically on patients receiving metaxalone. The most frequent reactions to metaxalone include nausea and vomiting, GI upset, drowsiness, dizziness, headache, anxiety, and irritability. Rare but serious adverse effects include leukopenia, hemolytic anemia, and jaundice.

Methocarbamol

Methocarbamol (Robaxin) is a centrally acting agent that may be administered by oral, intramuscular (IM), and intravenous (IV) routes. In addition to its use for muscle spasm, methocarbamol is used in managing tetanus. As with other centrally acting agents, its exact mechanism of action is not understood but is thought to be its CNS depressant properties. Its short duration of action limits methocarbamol therapy.

Methocarbamol is widely distributed throughout the body, crosses the placental barrier, and is concentrated in the liver and kidneys. It is extensively metabolized in the liver and renally excreted. Its distribution into breast milk is unknown.

Contraindications for methocarbamol include hepatic or renal disorders, age younger than 12 years or older than 60 years, and pregnancy. It is used with caution in patients with seizure disorders because it may exacerbate seizure activity.

When methocarbamol is given intravenously, the rate should not exceed 300 mg/min (3 mL of 10% injection). Because the solution is hypertonic, extravasation may occur, resulting in thrombophlebitis, sloughing, and pain at the injection site.

The most common adverse effects of methocarbamol are related to its CNS depressant effects. Diplopia, dyspepsia, flushing, hypotension, metallic taste, mild muscular incoordination, nystagmus, sinus bradycardia, syncope, and vertigo have followed IM or IV administration of methocarbamol. IV injections occasionally have been associated with hemolysis, resulting in hematuria.

Orphenadrine

Orphenadrine (Norflex) is the last centrally acting muscle relaxant. Administration is oral or parenteral. Orphenadrine is used as adjunct therapy for acute, painful musculoskeletal conditions and in managing quinine-resistant leg cramps. It has also been used adjunctly in treating arteriosclerotic, idiopathic, or postencephalic parkinsonism. Like other centrally acting agents, orphenadrine does not directly affect muscles, but works by its depression of the CNS. It also possesses anticholinergic effects and some antihistaminic and local anesthetic capability. Orphenadrine is distributed throughout the body and may cross the placenta. Its distribution into breast milk is unknown.

Orphenadrine should be used with caution in conditions that are affected by its anticholinergic and antihistaminic effects, which include bladder obstruction, prostatic hypertrophy, GI obstruction, peptic ulcer disease, gastroesophageal reflux disease (GERD), asthma, glaucoma, and myasthenia gravis (MG). Orphenadrine should also be used with caution in older patients who do not tolerate anticholinergics well. Additionally, caution should be taken when administering to patients with cardiac insufficiency or thyrotoxicosis. The safety of orphenadrine in children or pregnant or breast-feeding women has not been established.

Orphenadrine interacts with haloperidol, worsening schizophrenic symptoms and possibly contributing to the development of tardive dyskinesia. It also interacts with amantadine, with resultant additive anticholinergic effects. Orphenadrine decreases the action of phenothiazines when given concurrently. In addition to having CNS effects similar to those of other centrally acting skeletal muscle relaxants, orphenadrine may induce aplastic anemia or anaphylactic reaction. The most common adverse effects to orphenadrine result from its anticholinergic and antihistaminic effects, including dry mouth, agitation, blurred vision, constipation, dizziness, drowsiness, gastric irritation, hallucinations, and headache. Additionally, the peripheral anticholinergic effects of orphenadrine may decrease or inhibit salivary flow, thereby contributing to the development of caries, periodontal disease, oral candidiasis, or oral discomfort.

Drug Significantly Different From P Cyclobenzaprine

Diazepam (Valium) is a benzodiazepine that can produce any level of CNS depression required, including sedation, hypnosis, skeletal muscle relaxation, anticonvulsant activity, or coma. Diazepam and baclofen are the only two centrally acting drugs that are used for spasticity as well as muscle spasm. Although diazepam is an extremely effective muscle relaxant, its use as a maintenance drug for spasms is limited because of its potential for physical and psychological dependence. Additionally, withdrawing diazepam abruptly may induce seizure activity. For further information on benzodiazepines, see Chapter 16.

C CENTRALLY ACTING SPASMOLYTICS

The centrally acting spasmolytics work in the CNS to reduce excessive reflex activity and to allow muscle relaxation. This class includes baclofen and tizanidine. The prototype for the centrally acting spasmolytics is baclofen (Lioresal).

NURSING MANAGEMENT OF THE PATIENT RECEIVING P BACLOFEN

Core Drug Knowledge

Pharmacotherapeutics

Baclofen relieves some components of spinal spasticity—involuntary flexor and extensor spasms and resistance to passive movements. It is useful in MS and traumatic lesions

of the spinal cord that result in paralysis. Baclofen is not useful in treating spasms that follow a cerebrovascular accident (CVA, or stroke) or those that occur in Parkinson disease or Huntington chorea (see Table 20.1).

Baclofen has been used in patients with focal dystonic movements, including torticollis (wry neck). It has been used with some success in Meige syndrome (blepharospasm-oromandibular dystonia) and stiff-man syndrome, also known as Moersch-Woltmann syndrome. Stiff-man syndrome occurs primarily in men. It is characterized by muscular rigidity accompanied by paroxysmal painful spasms precipitated by physical or emotional stimuli.

Baclofen has been effective in treating intractable hiccups. It may also be used to manage trigeminal neuralgia and various types of neuropathic pain, including migraine headaches.

Surgically implanted pumps are used to deliver intrathecal baclofen to patients who have long-term needs or poor control with oral medications. Among these patients are those with MS or traumatic spinal cord lesions.

Pharmacokinetics

Baclofen is rapidly absorbed orally and peaks in 2 to 3 hours. It is distributed throughout the body and crosses the blood–brain barrier. Baclofen also crosses the placenta and passes into breast milk. The half-life ranges from 2 to 4 hours. The kidneys excrete 70% to 85% of a dose as unchanged drug and active and inactive metabolites. The liver metabolizes the remainder, which is excreted through the feces.

Pharmacodynamics

Baclofen is a derivative of the neurotransmitter gamma-aminobutyric acid (GABA) and acts specifically at the spinal end of the upper motor neurons at $GABA_B$ receptors to cause hyperpolarization. This action reduces excessive reflex activity underlying muscle hypertonia, spasms, and spasticity and allows muscle relaxation. The mechanism of action explains why baclofen is not used for spasticity resulting from CVA or Parkinson disease because these disorders involve lesional or functional impairment of basal ganglia coordination, in an area of the CNS above the spinal motor neurons.

Contraindications and Precautions

Baclofen is contraindicated in anyone who has demonstrated previous hypersensitivity to it. It is also contraindicated for spasticity of cerebral origin (e.g., in cerebral palsy or CVA) or for reducing the rigidity of parkinsonism or Huntington chorea because it is ineffective in these disorders.

Baclofen is classified as a pregnancy category C drug and should be used during pregnancy only when the benefits to the pregnant woman outweigh the risks to the fetus. Baclofen appears in small amounts in breast milk; therefore, caution should be used in administering it to breast-feeding women. Baclofen has not been approved for use in children younger than 12 years.

Baclofen should be used with caution in patients who have any pre-existing muscle weakness. Pre-existing weakness may be exacerbated when decreased spasticity diminishes support for the legs. Extreme caution must be used when spasticity is necessary to maintain posture, balance in locomotion, or function.

Baclofen is used with caution in patients who have seizure disorders. It has caused deterioration in seizure control and electroencephalographic changes in patients with epilepsy. When given to patients with CNS disorders, such as cerebral hemorrhage or a prior CVA, baclofen may increase the risk for developing CNS, respiratory, or cardiovascular depression and ataxia. Baclofen can increase blood glucose concentrations and should therefore be used cautiously in patients with diabetes mellitus. Patients with pre-existing psychiatric disorders are more likely to develop baclofen-induced psychiatric disturbances. Baclofen should also be used with caution in patients who have renal impairment because most of the drug is excreted unchanged in the urine.

Adverse Effects

The most common adverse effects of baclofen therapy include drowsiness, weakness, dizziness and lightheadedness, headache, nausea and vomiting, hypotension, constipation, lethargy and fatigue, confusion, insomnia, and increased urinary frequency. Other effects in the CNS include euphoria, excitement, depression, and hallucinations. Baclofen may also cause paresthesias, myalgias, or tinnitus. The patient may experience difficulty with coordination, tremors, rigidity, or ataxia. The patient may also experience vision disturbances such as nystagmus, strabismus, miosis, mydriasis, or diplopia. Adverse effects in the GI system include xerostomia, anorexia, dysgeusia, abdominal pain, and diarrhea. Cardiovascular adverse effects, such as palpitations, angina, excessive diaphoresis, and syncope, are possible. Genitourinary (GU) effects may include urinary incontinence or retention, dysuria, erectile dysfunction, ejaculation dysfunction, and nocturia. Integumentary adverse effects may include rash and pruritus.

Drug Interactions

Baclofen has the potential to cause clinically important interactions with other CNS depressants or TCAs. Baclofen has also been reported to cause false-positive results on tests for occult blood in the stool. Additionally, baclofen may induce elevations in levels of AST, alkaline phosphatase, or serum glucose (Table 20.3).

Assessment of Relevant Core Patient Variables

Health Status

Assess for a history of baclofen hypersensitivity or pre-existing disorders that contraindicate the use of baclofen. Also assess for muscle spasms and their causes. Baclofen therapy will not affect skeletal muscle spasms resulting from CVA, cerebral palsy, or parkinsonism.

Perform a physical examination that includes baseline assessments of neurologic function, cardiac function, kidney function, and muscle strength and spasticity. Laboratory assessments should include baseline liver and kidney function values and blood glucose level.

Life Span and Gender

Older patients are more susceptible to baclofen-induced sedation and psychiatric disturbances, including hallucinations, excitation, and confusion. Therefore, continually assess older patients taking baclofen for such adverse effects. Evaluate the patient for pregnancy. Baclofen may be used during pregnancy when the benefits to the pregnant woman outweigh the risks to the fetus. Baclofen should not be used in children younger than 12 years.

TABLE 20.3 Agents That Interact With P Baclofen

Interactants	Effect and Significance	Nursing Management
CNS depressants • alcohol • benzodiazepines • barbiturates • opioids	In combination with dantrolene, CNS depressant drugs may have additive effects, increasing CNS depression.	Monitor for increased sedation. Institute safety measures, especially with ambulation.
Nonsteroidal anti-inflammatory agents	Baclofen may decrease the clearance of NSAIDs and increase the potential for renal toxicity.	Monitor fluid intake and output.
Phytomedicinals • *Valeriana officinalis* • kava kava • *Piper methysticum*	In combination with dantrolene, phytomedicinals may have additive effects, increasing CNS depression.	Monitor for increased sedation. Institute safety measures, especially with ambulation.
Tricyclic antidepressants	Baclofen and TCAs can potentiate muscle relaxation and enhance anticholinergic effects. This combination may result in severe weakness, memory loss, and loss of muscle tone.	Monitor for adverse effects. Provide ambulatory assistance. Increase fluids or consume sugarless candies for dry mouth. Monitor for urinary retention or constipation.

Lifestyle, Diet, and Habits

Caution the patient about the concurrent use of alcohol and baclofen. Alcohol may increase the risk for CNS depression and other CNS adverse effects. Also, caution patients to assess their level of alertness (which may be affected by CNS depression) before attempting to drive, use machinery, or perform activities that require concentration.

Environment

Oral baclofen can be given in any environment and is generally self-administered in the home. Intrathecal baclofen administration requires a surgical procedure to implant the device. The prescriber refills the reservoir every 4 to 12 weeks, depending on the daily dose.

Nursing Diagnoses and Outcomes

- Acute Pain related to headache, muscle pain, GI disturbances, or rash
  Desired outcome: *The patient will be provided with measures to decrease the discomfort of drug therapy and the possibility of nonadherence.*
- Risk for Disturbed Sensory Perception related to visual changes, vestibular dysfunction, and somatosensory changes
  Desired outcome: *The patient will be protected from injury if dizziness, weakness, visual changes, or perceptual changes occur.*

Planning and Intervention

Maximizing Therapeutic Effects

The patient should take baclofen with a full glass of water at evenly spaced intervals.

Minimizing Adverse Effects

Ensure the patient's safety by keeping the bed in the lowest position with the side rails up. Assist ambulatory patients with locomotion because sedation and muscle weakness may increase. Advise the patient to change positions slowly to prevent dizziness.

Withdrawing baclofen abruptly may result in agitation, auditory and visual hallucinations, seizures, psychotic symptoms, or, most commonly, acute exacerbations of spasticity. Ensure gradual reduction of the baclofen dosage over 1 to 2 weeks. For patients with GI distress, coordinate small, frequent meals.

Providing Patient and Family Education

- Education for patients receiving baclofen is similar to that for patients receiving cyclobenzaprine. As with cyclobenzaprine, caution patients to avoid sudden cessation of the drug; instead, patients should taper doses of the drug over 2 weeks.
- Another major point is to remind patients to refrain from alcohol or any other CNS depressant agents. Advise patients that it may take them up to 1 month to experience the full benefit of baclofen therapy.
- Advise patients of the importance of contacting the prescriber should they experience severe headaches, confusion, hallucinations, or sudden or increased weakness. Advise all female patients to contact the prescriber immediately if they become pregnant.
- Additionally, instruct patients with diabetes to use capillary blood glucose monitoring because baclofen may cause blood and urine glucose levels to rise. These patients should notify their prescribers if serum glucose level elevations persist.

Ongoing Assessment and Evaluation

To ensure safety, assess the patient for the CNS effects of baclofen throughout therapy. Monitor for the emergence of hallucinations or psychotic episodes and consult with the prescriber immediately about the possibility of reducing the

dose or discontinuing the drug. Also, monitor the patient for integumentary, GI, or GU system complaints. Suggest approaches for dealing with minor symptoms, such as analgesics for headache or small, frequent meals for GI upset. Help establish a bowel program if constipation occurs. For GU effects such as erectile dysfunction, refer the patient to the prescriber and ensure that the patient does not abruptly stop the medication. Box 20.1 provides guidelines for ensuring successful baclofen therapy in the home.

COMMUNITY-BASED CONCERNS

Box 20.1 Ensuring Successful Baclofen Therapy in the Home

Surgically implanted drug delivery pumps are frequently used to deliver intrathecal infusions of baclofen in long-term treatment of patients with spasms that are not adequately controlled by oral baclofen. These patients (particularly those with MS and traumatic spinal cord lesions) are being managed more frequently in the community setting, primarily because the cost of institutionalization for drug therapy is formidable. As a result, the community health system is facing an increasingly complex management issue.

Patients with neuromuscular diseases present a wide variety of management challenges—from feeding and providing for daily activities to promoting locomotion and the highest level of attainable function. Frequently, patients with painful, contracting muscle spasms related to MS or spinal cord injury can benefit from continual intrathecal baclofen infusion. This therapy is accomplished with an indwelling catheter and a portable infusion pump.

Issues facing the community health nurse charged with supervising this therapy are the risk for infection introduced through the catheter and the need to maintain a continual infusion. The community health nurse must ensure that the infusion equipment remains patent and in good operating condition and that the patient receives effective nursing care.

When managing a patient receiving IV baclofen therapy at home, typical interventions include the following:

- Assess the home environment for designated "clean" areas needed for storing supplies, dressing, and so forth.
- Include at least one, and ideally more, of the patient's family members or friends in all instructions about mixing drug solution, storage and care of the drug, and use and maintenance of the infusion pump and IV catheter insertion site.
- Identify community resources for ensuring that the patient does not run out of the drug and that the pump, whether battery operated or electrical, can be adequately and continually charged. Frequently, the power company in an area has provisions for maintaining power to the pump in case of emergency.
- Prepare and post a list of phone numbers of emergency and support systems in the patient's home, preferably near a telephone.
- Discuss the mechanics of baclofen therapy with other caregivers who may be working with this patient, so that the entire health care team is aware of the associated needs and potential problems.
- Post a list of warning signs. Include signs of infection at the catheter insertion site, adverse drug effects, and increasing weakness. List telephone numbers of appropriate people to call for help.
- Consult the health resources in the area for support groups or respite services for the patient and for family members or others involved in the patient's care.

Therapeutic monitoring during baclofen therapy will show improvement in symptoms of spasticity and a decrease in resistance to passive movement of limb joints.

Drug Closely Related to P Baclofen

Tizanidine (Zanaflex) is an oral agent used to treat spasticity related to spinal cord pathology and MS. It is structurally and pharmacologically similar to clonidine, an alpha-2 adrenergic agonist. The efficacy of tizanidine in treating spasticity is equivalent to that of baclofen.

Tizanidine is used cautiously in patients with hypotension, hepatic disease, psychosis, or renal impairment. An important interaction with tizanidine occurs with oral contraceptives. When the two are given concurrently, the clearance of tizanidine may be 50% lower, resulting in toxicity. Tizanidine also has additive effects when given with other antihypertensive agents, alpha-2 agonists, or ethanol. Adverse effects parallel those of other alpha-2 adrenergic agonists, including dry mouth, drowsiness, dizziness, GI disturbances, and liver function abnormalities. Because of its adrenergic action, hypotension and orthostatic hypotension may also occur. Tizanidine produces greater drowsiness and sedation than baclofen does. Slow upward titration of the dose can minimize adverse effects.

Drug Significantly Different From P Baclofen

Gabapentin (Neurontin) is a miscellaneous anticonvulsant drug that has demonstrated efficacy in the management of neuropathic pain and spasticity. It is useful in managing spasticity associated with MS, although that is an off-label indication. Although its exact mechanism of action is not known, it is thought to interact with voltage-gated calcium channels to decrease pain and spasticity. Gabapentin is orally administered and rapidly absorbed. It is highly lipid soluble, crosses the blood–brain barrier, and is widely distributed in the CNS. Gabapentin is not metabolized and is excreted unchanged in the urine; therefore, monitoring renal function is important.

MEMORY CHIP

P Baclofen

- Centrally acting spasmolytic is used for muscle spasms or spasticity
- Major contraindication: patients who use spasticity to maintain posture or balance
- Most common adverse effect: sedation; safety is a nursing priority
- Most serious adverse effects: occur with abrupt withdrawal and include agitation, auditory or visual hallucinations, seizures, or psychotic symptoms
- **Life span alert: Older patients are more prone to sedation and other effects on the central nervous system.**
- Maximizing therapeutic effects: Administer at evenly spaced intervals.
- Minimizing adverse effects: Assist in changing positions slowly; withdraw medication over a 2-week period.
- Most important patient education: Never abruptly stop medication.

Gabapentin is unusual in that it does not interact with other drugs. Common adverse effects include drowsiness, somnolence, nausea, and fatigue. For additional information regarding gabapentin, see Chapter 19.

C PERIPHERALLY ACTING SPASMOLYTICS

Peripherally acting spasmolytics relax muscles through direct action on the skeletal muscle fibers. They do not interfere with neuromuscular communication, nor do they have CNS effects. Peripherally acting spasmolytics include dantrolene, botulinum toxin, and ibuprofen. Dantrolene (Dantrium) is the most frequently used peripheral agent and the prototype for the peripherally acting spasmolytics.

NURSING MANAGEMENT OF THE PATIENT RECEIVING P DANTROLENE

Core Drug Knowledge

Pharmacotherapeutics

IV dantrolene is the drug of choice, when accompanied by supportive measures, for acute treatment of malignant hyperthermia. Preoperatively, it can be used orally or intravenously to prevent malignant hyperthermia in patients considered at risk.

Dantrolene has several other pharmacotherapeutic uses. It has been effective in treating upper motor neuron disorders, such as hereditary spastic paraplegia. It has also been used to treat heatstroke and to prevent and treat the rigors associated with amphotericin B. It is useful in managing spasticity resulting from spinal cord and cerebral injuries, MS, cerebral palsy, and possibly CVA. Dantrolene is not effective in treating acute muscle weakness of local origin or muscle weakness resulting from rheumatoid spondylitis, arthritis, or bursitis.

Pharmacokinetics

Approximately 35% of an oral dose of dantrolene is absorbed; peak plasma concentrations are reached in approximately 5 hours. The liver metabolizes dantrolene to weakly active metabolites, which are excreted in the urine. The elimination half-life is reported to be about 9 hours in healthy adults and 7.3 hours in children. Therapeutic effects in patients being treated for upper motor neuron disorders may not appear for 1 week or more. Dantrolene crosses the placenta and enters breast milk.

Pharmacodynamics

Dantrolene reduces the force of contraction of skeletal muscle through a direct effect on muscle cells. It reduces the amount of Ca^{2+} released from the sarcoplasmic reticulum, thereby uncoupling (relaxing) muscle contraction from excitation. Interference with the release of Ca^{2+} from the sarcoplasmic reticulum may prevent the increase in intracellular Ca^{2+}, which activates the acute catabolic events of malignant hyperthermia. Dantrolene has little or no effect on contraction of cardiac or intestinal smooth muscle. It may decrease hyperreflexia, muscle stiffness, and spasticity in patients with upper motor neuron disorders.

Contraindications and Precautions

Dantrolene is contraindicated in patients who rely on spasticity to maintain an upright posture and balance, such as patients with cerebral palsy. It is also contraindicated in patients with active liver disease because of its associated liver toxicity. No contraindications apply to IV administration of dantrolene to prevent or acutely treat malignant hyperthermia crisis.

Dantrolene should be used with caution in patients with pre-existing myopathy or neuromuscular disease with respiratory depression. The risk for perioperative complications is increased in patients with these conditions who receive dantrolene for prevention of malignant hyperthermia.

Dantrolene should also be used with caution in patients with cardiac disease and pulmonary dysfunction, particularly chronic obstructive pulmonary disease (COPD). For patients with cardiac disease, dantrolene can precipitate pleural effusions or pericarditis. In patients with pulmonary dysfunction, dantrolene can precipitate respiratory depression.

Dantrolene is classified as a pregnancy category C drug; therefore, pregnant or lactating women should avoid its use.

Adverse Effects

The most common adverse effect of dantrolene therapy is muscle weakness. Manifestations of such muscle weakness may include drooling, slurred speech, drowsiness, dizziness, malaise, and fatigue. Serious adverse effects seen with dantrolene therapy include potentially fatal hepatitis, seizures, and pleural effusion with pericarditis.

In the GI system, symptoms include diarrhea, constipation, GI bleeding, anorexia, difficulty swallowing, abdominal cramps, and nausea and vomiting. Diarrhea is usually transient, but in some cases it can be severe, and the drug may have to be withheld. Hematologic adverse reactions with dantrolene therapy include aplastic anemia, leukopenia, and lymphocytic lymphoma.

Rash, acne, abnormal hair growth, and photosensitivity are possible integumentary effects. IV dantrolene may cause edema and thrombophlebitis. Rarely, IV administration may cause erythema and urticaria.

Drug Interactions

Drugs that interact with dantrolene include clofibrate, estrogens, verapamil, and warfarin. Table 20.4 discusses these potential interactions.

Assessment of Relevant Core Patient Variables

Health Status

Elicit a comprehensive health history, including any history of active hepatitis, estrogen use in women older than 35 years, impaired cardiac or pulmonary function, any liver disease, or spasticity used to sustain upright posture and balance in locomotion or to obtain or maintain increased function. Communicate positive findings for any of these factors to the prescriber.

TABLE 20.4 Agents That Interact With P Dantrolene

Interactants	Effect and Significance	Nursing Management
Calcium channel blockers • diltiazem • verapamil	In combination with dantrolene, calcium channel blockers may increase hyperkalemia and myocardial depression.	Avoid coadministration, if possible. Monitor cardiac function. Monitor potassium levels.
Clindamycin	In combination with dantrolene, clindamycin may increase neuromuscular blockade.	Monitor for increased effects of dantrolene.
Clofibrate	Clofibrate may decrease plasma protein binding of dantrolene, resulting in decreased effects of dantrolene.	Monitor for efficacy of dantrolene therapy.
CNS depressant drugs • alcohol • benzodiazepines • barbiturates • opioids	In combination with dantrolene, CNS depressant drugs may have additive effects, increasing CNS depression.	Monitor for increased sedation. Institute safety measures, especially with ambulation.
Estrogens	Mechanism of interaction is unknown; women older than 35 years are at risk for hepatotoxicity when estrogens and dantrolene are coadministered.	Monitor for signs of hepatotoxicity. Coordinate periodic liver function tests for long-term therapy.
Phytomedicinals • *Valeriana officinalis* • kava kava • *Piper methysticum*	In combination with dantrolene, phytomedicinals may have additive effects, increasing CNS depression.	Monitor for increased sedation. Institute safety measures, especially with ambulation.
Psychotropic drugs • MAOIs • phenothiazines	In combination with dantrolene, psychotropic drugs may increase neuromuscular blockade.	Monitor for increased effects of dantrolene.
warfarin	Warfarin may decrease plasma protein binding of dantrolene, resulting in decreased effects of dantrolene.	Monitor for efficacy of dantrolene therapy.

Perform a physical examination before initiating therapy. Assessment of the musculoskeletal system should include the patient's posture, ability to walk, reflexes, and muscle tone. Document the amount and location of spasticity. Other assessments should include the CNS and GI systems. Laboratory tests should include a complete blood count (CBC), and AST, ALT, alkaline phosphatase, and total bilirubin levels.

Life Span and Gender

Consider the patient's age relative to dantrolene therapy. Liver damage occurs most commonly in patients older than 30 years, especially women older than 35 years who are taking estrogens. Children younger than 5 years should not receive dantrolene. Older patients are more vulnerable to the adverse effects of dantrolene. Before giving dantrolene, assess the patient for pregnancy and breast-feeding because the safety of dantrolene therapy has not been established for pregnant or lactating women.

Lifestyle, Diet, and Habits

Dantrolene capsules contain lactulose. Therefore, assess the patient for lactose intolerance before the drug is given.

Environment

Caution the patient about the potential for photosensitivity. Patients should wear appropriate clothing and sunscreen whenever they are in direct sunlight. Because dantrolene causes muscle weakness, also discuss with the patient any barriers in the home (such as stairs) that may affect dantrolene therapy. In addition, caution the patient to assess the drug's effects before attempting to ambulate without assistance.

Nursing Diagnoses and Outcomes

- Risk for Injury related to muscular weakness
  Desired outcome: *The patient will be injury free despite muscular weakness.*
- Diarrhea or Constipation related to drug effects
  Desired outcome: *The patient will maintain baseline bowel habits.*
- Risk for Disturbed Sensory Perception: Kinesthetic related to dizziness, malaise, and fatigue
  Desired outcome: *The patient will remain free of injury from adverse effects.*
- Disturbed Body Image related to drug-related dermatologic effects
  Desired outcome: *Any adverse effects will be resolved by the end of therapy.*

Planning and Intervention

Maximizing Therapeutic Effects

Administer dantrolene with food or milk to avoid gastric distress. For patients with difficulty swallowing, mix the contents of the capsule with fruit juice and administer immedi-

ately. If extended-release capsules or tablets are prescribed, they should not be opened or crushed.

Minimizing Adverse Effects

To avoid injury, supervise the transfer or ambulation of patients taking dantrolene. Also, provide frequent skin care and hygiene measures to prevent skin breakdown and request treatment for acne if appropriate. Protecting the patient from exposure to ultraviolet light is important, as is providing sunscreen if exposure is inevitable.

Therapy is initiated at low doses and gradually increased to minimize dose-related side effects. This practice also determines the minimum effective dose and allows a smooth induction of antispastic effects.

Providing Patient and Family Education

- Before the drug is given, explain to patients and family that the drug is being used to relieve spasticity and that muscle weakness may occur. Family members should be instructed to assist patients with ambulation and ensure safety precautions.
- Inform patients that one of the most dangerous adverse effects of dantrolene therapy is hepatitis. Write down a list of symptoms for patients to report to the prescriber immediately, including loss of appetite, nausea, vomiting, yellowed skin or eyes, and changes in color of urine or stool. Also, explain that regular follow-up medical care, including blood tests, is necessary to monitor the effects of the drug on the body.
- Advise patients that other adverse effects may occur, such as drowsiness, dizziness, GI upset, diarrhea or constipation, or rash. Discuss self-care measures to alleviate common symptoms and urge patients to contact the prescriber if the symptoms do not abate. To avoid photosensitivity, advise patients to wear appropriate clothing and use sunscreen when in direct sunlight.

Ongoing Assessment and Evaluation

Monitor for improvement in symptoms of spasticity and decrease in resistance to passive movement of the limb joint. Beneficial effects in spasticity may take 1 week or more to appear. Assist ambulatory patients with locomotion, because muscle weakness may increase.

Monitor for signs of adverse effects, especially hepatitis and hematologic effects. Coordinate periodic laboratory tests to evaluate liver function and the CBC. Withhold dantrolene and contact the prescriber if clinical signs of hepatitis appear.

Drug Closely Related to P Dantrolene

Botulinum toxin type A (Botox) is a neurotoxin used for its muscle-relaxing properties. It is a protein that is produced by the anaerobic bacterium *Clostridium botulinum*. As many as seven serotypes of botulinum neurotoxin exist, but only types A and B are in clinical use at this time. Botulinum toxin type B (Myobloc) is less potent and shorter-acting than botulinum toxin type A.

MEMORY CHIP

P Dantrolene

- Peripherally acting spasmolytic is used for muscle spasms or spasticity.
- Drug of choice for preventing or treating malignant hyperthermia
- Major contraindications: patients who use spasticity to maintain posture or balance (such as patients with cerebral palsy) or who have active hepatic disorders
- Most common adverse effect: muscle weakness; safety is a nursing priority
- Most serious adverse effect: fatal hepatitis, especially in women older than 35 years who are taking estrogens
- Maximizing therapeutic effects: Give with food or milk to decrease GI distress.
- Minimizing adverse effects: Assist with ambulation.
- Most important patient education: Advise patients of symptoms of hepatitis and the importance of notifying the prescriber should any occur.

Botulinum toxin type A is produced under controlled laboratory conditions and is given in extremely small therapeutic doses (0.05–0.1 mL per injection site). It blocks neuromuscular conduction by binding to receptor sites on motor nerve terminals, entering nerve terminals, and inhibiting the release of acetylcholine. Conditions that are treated with botulinum toxin injections include muscle contraction headaches, chronic muscle spasms in the neck and back, torticollis (severe neck muscle spasms), myofascial pain syndrome, and spasticity from multiple sclerosis or stroke. Botulinum toxin type A is given as an IM injection. Gradual relaxation of muscle spasm develops 1 to 2 weeks after the injection. The reduction of muscle spasm lasts for 3 to 4 months, and pain relief can last even longer. Potential adverse effects from the injection may include temporary increase in pain, weakness in the muscles injected, body aches, dry mouth, hoarseness, and flu-like symptoms.

CHAPTER SUMMARY

- Drugs used to manage muscle spasm and spasticity are divided into muscle relaxants and spasmolytics. Muscle spasm is a sudden, violent, involuntary contraction of a muscle or group of muscles.

CRITICAL THINKING SCENARIO

Adjusting to Dantrolene Therapy

J.J. was born with cerebral palsy, which has been successfully managed medically for 18 years. He recently finished high school and enrolled in a community college. During his second week at college, he began having uncontrollable muscle spasms that were painful and embarrassing to him. The college health service recommended treating the spasms with dantrolene.

1. Prioritize the assessment factors that the college health service nurse must consider before and during therapy.
2. Suggest steps that may need to be taken at J.J.'s school as a result of the drug therapy.

Drugs for Treating Parkinson Disease and Other Movement Disorders

Ⓒ Antiparkinson Drugs

- **P carbidopa-levodopa**
- amantadine
- bromocriptine
- pergolide
- pramipexole
- ropinirole
- selegiline
- entacapone
- tolcapone

Ⓒ Anti-ALS Drugs

- **P riluzole**
- creatine

Ⓒ Anti-MS Drugs

- **P glatiramer**
- interferon beta-1a
- interferon beta-1b

Drugs for Other Movement Disorders

Myasthenia gravis
- neostigmine
- pyridostigmine

Huntington disease
- haloperidol
- phenothiazines

Tourette syndrome
- clonidine
- fluphenazine
- haloperidol
- pimozide

The symbol Ⓒ indicates the **drug class**.
Drugs in **bold type** marked with the symbol **P** are prototypes.
Drugs in blue type are closely related to the prototype.
Drugs in red type are significantly different from the prototype.
Drugs in black type with no symbol are also used in drug therapy; no prototype

Movement disorders can be chronic, severe, and debilitating. These disorders are incurable, and patients with them have various responses to treatment. As a result of a disorder's progression, patients may become socially isolated and depressed. As patients become increasingly disabled and the drugs become minimally effective, your primary role shifts from one of medical intervention to psychosocial and functional care, with the aim of helping the patient maximize remaining capacities. This chapter limits the discussion to the nurse's pharmacologic role. Information on the nonpharmacologic role of the nurse can be found in a medical-surgical textbook or subject-specific website.

This chapter discusses three major movement disorders—Parkinson disease, amyotrophic lateral sclerosis (ALS), and multiple sclerosis (MS)—focusing on drugs used to inhibit the symptoms associated with these diseases. In addition, it discusses core drug knowledge, core patient variables, nursing management, potential nursing diagnoses, and patient education related to the use of these drugs. Table 21.1 summarizes selected drugs used to manage movement disorders.

PHYSIOLOGY

The extrapyramidal system is responsible for coarse control of voluntary muscles. This "system" is composed of basal ganglia, cortical areas of the brain that project to the basal ganglia, cerebellar areas of the brain that project to the basal ganglia, and parts of the reticular formation and thalamic nuclei that connect to the basal ganglia. Motor activity requires integration of the actions of the cerebral cortex, basal ganglia, and cerebellum.

The **basal ganglia** are a group of functionally related nuclei located in paired groups in each cerebral hemisphere. Two primary nuclei are the **corpus striatum,** located deep within the cerebrum, and the **substantia nigra,** a group of darkly pigmented cells located in the midbrain. When the basal ganglia are stimulated, muscle tone in the body is inhibited, and voluntary movements are refined.

The regulatory neurotransmitter dopamine is produced in the substantia nigra and adrenal glands, and then transmitted to the basal ganglia along a neural pathway for secretion when needed. Recently, five dopamine receptors have been identified in the brain. Three of these receptors (dopamine-1, dopamine-2, and dopamine-3—usually called D_1, D_2, and D_3, respectively) appear to play important roles in properly balancing the stimulation of the basal ganglia involved in normal motor function. Acetylcholine, an excitatory neurotransmitter, is produced by the basal ganglia and in the nerve endings in the periphery of the body. When the body wants to make a movement (e.g., walking or picking up a cup of coffee), the striatum releases dopamine and acetylcholine through the nervous system to the appropriate muscles, which enables initiation, modulation, and completion of smooth, coordinated movement within a fraction of a second.

PATHOPHYSIOLOGY

Parkinson Disease

Parkinson disease is also called idiopathic parkinsonism or **paralysis agitans.** This disease is naturally occurring in that an external stimulus, such as a virus or trauma, does not trigger it. Parkinson disease generally afflicts patients aged 50 years and older and progresses slowly. In Parkinson disease, unexplained loss of dopamine-containing neurons occurs in the substantia nigra, resulting in reduced dopamine in the nerve terminals of the nigrostriatal tract. Consequently, an imbalance exists between dopamine inhibition and acetylcholine excitation (Figure 21.1).

Additionally, unopposed acetylcholine stimulates the release of gamma-aminobutyric acid (GABA). The combination of excessive acetylcholine and GABA is the basis for most symptoms of Parkinson disease, such as muscle rigidity, tremor at rest, **akinesia** (loss of voluntary movement) or **bradykinesia** (abnormal slowness of movement), and postural instability. As the disease progresses, patients may also experience depression, emotional changes, and sleep problems. Memory loss and slow thinking may develop, although the ability to reason remains intact. Whether people actually suffer intellectual loss (also known as dementia) from Parkinson disease is a controversial issue that is still being studied.

Parkinsonism is a syndrome with characteristics similar to Parkinson disease that are secondary to other conditions that structurally damage the dopaminergic pathway or interfere with dopamine's action within the basal ganglia. Well-known precipitants of parkinsonism are drugs such as the phenothiazines, metoclopramide, and reserpine. Drug-induced parkinsonism is usually reversible when the drugs are discontinued. Parkinsonism may also result from trauma, encephalitis, or heavy-metal poisoning.

Amyotrophic Lateral Sclerosis

ALS is a progressive neurologic disorder that affects motor function. It is also known as Lou Gehrig disease after the famous baseball player who succumbed to the disorder. The etiology of ALS is unknown. It presents in adulthood, usually between ages 40 and 70 years, and affects men two to three times more often than women. ALS affects both the upper motor neurons in the cerebral cortex and the lower motor neurons in the brain stem and spinal cord. Although this disorder is neurologic, one of its classic features is that it spares the entire sensory system and the intellect. Additionally, it also spares the cranial nerves that innervate movement of the eye (cranial nerves III, IV, and VI).

The disease begins in the distal neurons and then progresses in a centripetal but asymmetric fashion. The loss of upper motor neurons results in spastic paralysis and hyperreflexia. The loss of lower motor neurons results in decreased muscle tone and reflexes and flaccid paralysis. Ultimately, neuronal cell death leads to muscular weakness, muscle atrophy and fasciculations, spasticity, dysarthria, dysphagia, and respiratory compromise. Although periods of remission may occur, ALS typically progresses rapidly, and death occurs within 5 years for 50% of patients diagnosed with the disease.

Multiple Sclerosis

MS is a major cause of neurologic disability among young and middle-aged adults. Some patients experience exacerbations and remissions, whereas others have a steadily progressive pattern. MS is characterized by more than one area of inflammation and scarring of the myelin in the brain and spinal cord. When myelin is damaged, messages between the brain and other parts of the body are affected. The most common characteristics of MS include fatigue, weakness, spasticity, balance problems, bladder and bowel problems,

TABLE 21.1 Summary of Selected Drugs for the Management of Movement Disorders

Drug (Trade) Name	Selected Indications	Route and Dosage Range	Pharmacokinetics
(C) Antiparkinson Agents			
(C) Dopaminergics			
(P) carbidopa-levodopa (Sinemet)	Parkinson disease	*Adult:* PO 25/100 bid–qid to a maximum of 200/2,000 mg/d *Child:* Not recommended	*Onset:* Rapid *Duration:* 6–12 h $t_{1/2}$: 1–2 h
amantadine (Symmetrel; *Canadian:* Endantadine)	Parkinson disease Antiviral agent	*Adult:* PO 100–400 mg/d as needed *Adult and child >9 y:* PO 100 mg bid *Child 1–9 y:* 2–4 mg/lb	*Onset:* 36–48 h *Duration:* Unknown $t_{1/2}$: 15–24 h
levodopa (Dopar, Larodopa)	Parkinson disease	*Adult:* PO 500–1,000 mg/d in divided doses every 6–12 h maximum 8,000 mg/d *Child:* PO 0.5 g/m²	*Onset:* Variable *Duration:* 6–12 h $t_{1/2}$: 1.2–2.3 h
selegiline (Eldepryl)	Parkinson disease	*Adult:* PO 5 mg taken at breakfast and lunch *Child:* Not recommended	*Onset:* 1 h *Duration:* 24–72 h $t_{1/2}$: 9 min; 20.5 h for active metabolites
Dopamine Agonists			
bromocriptine (Parlodel; *Canadian:* Apo-Bromocriptine)	Parkinson disease Acromegaly Hyperprolactinemia	*Adult:* PO 5–50 mg bid *Adult:* PO 30–30 mg/d *Adult:* PO 5–7.5 mg/d *Child:* Not recommended	*Onset:* 1 h *Duration:* 14 h $t_{1/2}$: biphasic Initial 6–8 h Terminal 50 h
pergolide (Permax)	Parkinson disease	*Adult:* PO 1 mg tid *Child:* Not recommended	*Onset:* Varies *Duration:* Unknown $t_{1/2}$: 27 h
pramipexole (Mirapex)	Parkinson disease	*Adult:* PO 1.5–4.5 mg/d *Child:* Not recommended	*Onset:* Rapid *Duration:* Unknown $t_{1/2}$: 8–12 h
ropinirole (Requip)	Parkinson disease	*Adult:* PO 1 mg tid *Child:* Not recommended	*Onset:* 30–40 min *Duration:* 16 h $t_{1/2}$: 6 h
COMT Inhibitors			
tolcapone (Tasmar)	Parkinson disease	*Adult:* PO 100–200 mg tid *Child:* Not recommended	*Onset:* 1 h *Duration:* Unknown $t_{1/2}$: 2–3 h
entacapone (Comtan)	Parkinson disease	*Adult:* PO 200 g with each dose of carbidopa-levodopa not to exceed 1,600 g qd *Child:* Not recommended	*Onset:* 1 h *Duration:* Unknown $t_{1/2}$: 1–2 h
entacapone, carbodopa, levodopa (Stalevo)	Parkinson disease		Same as for individual agents
Anticholinergics			
benztropine (Cogentin; *Canadian:* Apo-Benztropine)	Parkinson disease	*Adult:* PO/IM/IV, 0.5–6 mg/d *Child:* Not recommended	*Onset:* PO, 1 h; IM/IV, 15 min *Duration:* Unknown $t_{1/2}$: 6–10 h
diphenhydramine (Benadryl; *Canadian:* Allerdyl)	Parkinson disease	*Adult:* PO, 25–100 mg/d; IM/IV, 10–50 mg *Child:* PO > 10 kg 12.5–25 g 3–4 times daily, max 300 g qid; IV 5 mg/kg/d	*Onset:* PO, 15–30 min; IM 20–30 min; IV, rapid *Duration:* 4–8 h $t_{1/2}$: 2.5–7 h
trihexyphenidyl (Artane; *Canadian:* Apo-Trihex)	Parkinson disease	*Adult:* PO, 1–15 mg in divided doses *Child:* Safety and efficacy not established	*Onset:* Varies *Duration:* Unknown $t_{1/2}$: 5–10 h

(continued)

TABLE 21.1 Summary of Selected Drugs for the Management of Movement Disorders (continued)

Drug (Trade) Name	Selected Indications	Route and Dosage Range	Pharmacokinetics
C Anti-ALS Agents			
P riluzole (Rilutek)	ALS	*Adult:* PO 50 mg q 12 h *Child:* Not recommended	*Onset:* Rapid *Duration:* Unknown $t_{1/2}$: 2–3 h
creatine	ALS	*Adult:* PO, 1 packet dissolved 1 fruit juice qd	*Onset:* Rapid *Duration:* Unknown $t_{1/2}$: Unknown
C Anti-MS Agents			
P glatiramer (Copoxone)	MS	*Adult:* SC, 20 mg/mL qd	*Onset:* Unknown *Duration:* Unknown $t_{1/2}$: Unknown
interferon beta-1a (Avonex, Rebif)	MS	*Adult:* Avonex: 30 µg IM every week Rebif: 44 µg SC 3× week	*Onset:* Rapid *Duration:* $t_{1/2}$: Avonex, 8.6–10 h $t_{1/2}$: Rebif, 69 h
interferon beta-1b (Betaseron)	MS	*Adult:* SC, 0.25 mg every other day	*Onset:* Rapid *Duration:* Rapidly degraded $t_{1/2}$: 8 min–4.3 h
natalizumab (Tysabri)	MS	*Adult:* IV, 3 mg/kg every 4 weeks	*Onset:* 1 mo *Duration:* 8 wk $t_{1/2}$: 90–170 h

numbness, vision loss, tremor, and vertigo. The signs and symptoms reflect the location of the lesions; therefore, not every patient experiences every symptom of MS.

C ANTIPARKINSON DRUGS

The relative lack of dopamine combined with the relative excess of excitatory acetylcholine cause the symptoms of Parkinson disease. The goal of therapy is to restore the balance between dopamine and acetylcholine, which can be accomplished by increasing the activity of dopamine or blocking the action of acetylcholine (Figure 21.2).

Drugs that promote activation of dopamine receptors or slow the loss of dopamine are called **dopaminergics;** drugs that prevent the activation of cholinergic receptors are called anticholinergics. Both types of drugs are used to treat Parkinson disease at different stages. Dopaminergics are dis-

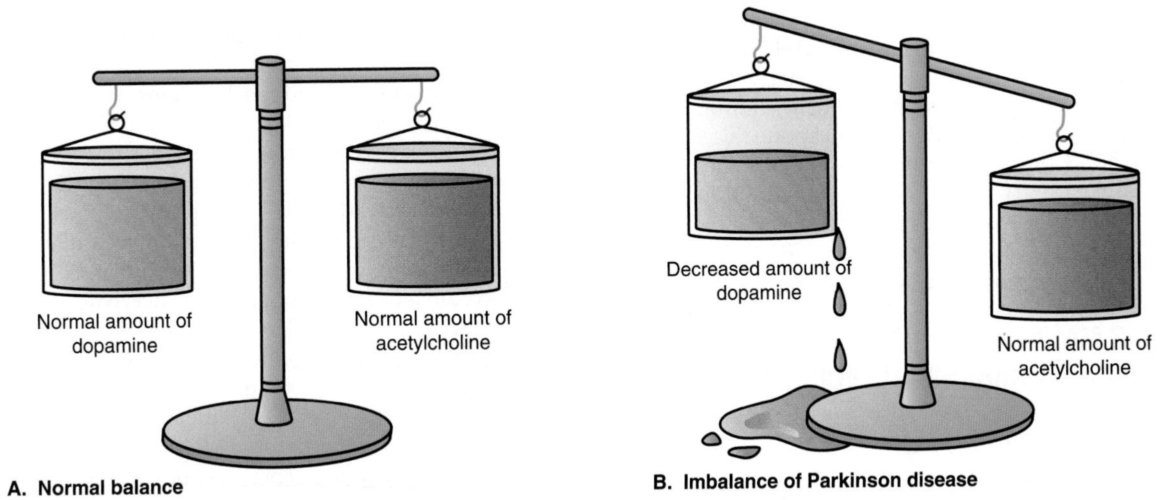

FIGURE 21.1 (**A**) Normal balance. This figure depicts the body at rest when the dopamine and acetylcholine systems are balanced. When the body moves, the brain understands the movement the body wants to make and it sends out a balance of dopamine and acetylcholine messages to keep that movement smooth. (**B**) Imbalance in Parkinson disease. This figure represents Parkinson disease, in which the normal levels of acetylcholine and dopamine are imbalanced and abnormal movement affects the body until chemical balance can be restored, to a degree.

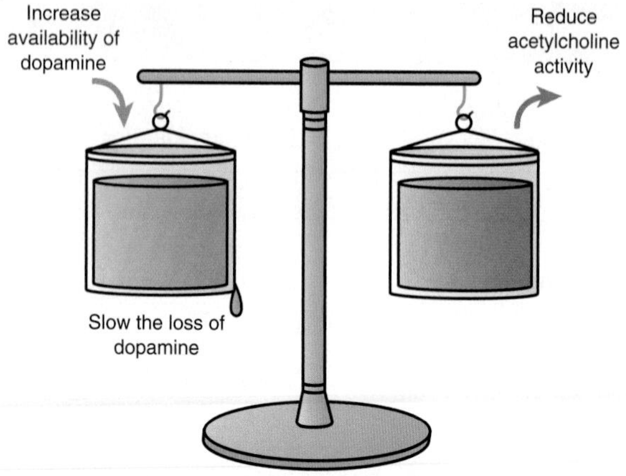

FIGURE 21.2 The goal of pharmacologic treatment for Parkinson disease is to restore the homeostatic balance between acetylcholine and dopamine, which can be accomplished by increasing the amount or availability of dopamine, slowing the loss of dopamine, or blocking the activity of acetylcholine.

cussed fully in this chapter; anticholinergics are only briefly summarized here but are discussed in depth in Chapter 14.

(C) Dopaminergics

The combination drug carbidopa-levodopa (Sinemet, Parcopa) is the prototype for the dopaminergics.

The logical solution to the imbalance in Parkinson disease is to administer dopamine to the patient; however, dopamine does not cross the blood–brain barrier. Levodopa, the precursor to dopamine, is occasionally used alone in treating Parkinson disease; however, it is largely deactivated in the periphery of the body. When levodopa is administered as a single drug, approximately 2% actually crosses the blood–brain barrier. To increase the amount of levodopa available to cross the blood–brain barrier, it is combined with the drug carbidopa. Carbidopa does not cross the blood–brain barrier, but it decreases peripheral destruction of levodopa.

In addition to carbidopa-levodopa and levodopa alone, other dopaminergics are used in treating Parkinson disease. Dopamine agonists include pramipexole (Mirapex), ropinirole (Requip), bromocriptine (Parlodel), and pergolide (Permax). Amantadine (Symmetrel) is an oral antiviral drug that also has dopaminergic activity. Selegiline (Eldepryl), another dopaminergic agent, inhibits monoamine oxidase type B (MAO-B). Tolcapone (Tasmar) and entacapone (Comtan) inhibit the enzyme catechol-O-methyltransferase (COMT), which degrades dopamine in the periphery of the body.

NURSING MANAGEMENT OF THE PATIENT RECEIVING [P] CARBIDOPA-LEVODOPA

Core Drug Knowledge

Pharmacotherapeutics

Carbidopa-levodopa (Sinemet, Parcopa) is a combination drug used in treating Parkinson disease. It is also used to treat restless-leg syndrome.

Pharmacokinetics

With oral administration, carbidopa-levodopa may begin to take effect after 2 to 3 weeks, although some patients require up to 6 months of therapy before noting an effect. The plasma half-life of both carbidopa-levodopa and carbidopa alone is roughly 1 to 2 hours, and the duration of action of a dose is 5 hours. Most carbidopa-levodopa is metabolized into dopamine in the periphery of the body, whereas carbidopa itself is minimally metabolized. Carbidopa-levodopa is eliminated renally as dopamine metabolites and in small amounts as unchanged drug. In addition, carbidopa-levodopa crosses the placenta and is present in breast milk. Table 21.1 summarizes selected drugs used to manage movement disorders.

Pharmacodynamics

Carbidopa-levodopa diffuses levodopa into the central nervous system (CNS), where it is converted to dopamine. The resulting change in dopamine–acetylcholine balance is believed to improve nerve impulse control and to form the basis of the drug's antiparkinsonian activity. Carbidopa does not cross the blood–brain barrier.

When carbidopa is administered in combination with levodopa, it inhibits the conversion of levodopa to dopamine in the periphery of the body, thereby increasing the amount of levodopa available to diffuse into the CNS. Because the bioavailability of dopamine increases in the CNS, the dosage of levodopa can be reduced. This reduction minimizes the potential for adverse reactions from levodopa. The carbidopa-levodopa combination also enables more rapid and even titration of effect.

Contraindications and Precautions

Patients with hypersensitivity to carbidopa-levodopa should not take the drug. Carbidopa-levodopa, marketed as Dopar, contains tartrazine. Therefore, patients with tartrazine sensitivity should avoid carbidopa-levodopa if Dopar is the only formulation available. Carbidopa-levodopa can worsen malignant melanoma; thus, the drug is contraindicated in patients with undiagnosed pigmented lesions or a history of melanoma. Although carbidopa-levodopa may not be used in patients with closed-angle glaucoma, it may be used in patients with open-angle glaucoma if intraocular pressure is closely monitored and controlled. Simultaneous administration of carbidopa-levodopa with monoamine oxidase inhibitors (MAOIs) can result in hypertensive crisis. Therefore, MAOIs should be discontinued 2 to 4 weeks before therapy with carbidopa-levodopa begins.

Precautions to carbidopa-levodopa therapy include cardiac disease (especially arrhythmias or past myocardial infarction [MI]), pulmonary disease, peptic ulcer disease, and diabetes mellitus. Carbidopa-levodopa may exacerbate symptoms in patients with these disorders.

Additionally, carbidopa-levodopa may cause mental status changes and should be used with caution in patients with a history of psychosis. All patients receiving carbidopa-levodopa should be monitored closely for signs of mental disturbances, including depression or suicidal thoughts.

Adverse Effects

Adverse gastrointestinal (GI) effects are common in patients receiving carbidopa-levodopa and include nausea

and vomiting, anorexia, and weight loss. Another common adverse effect to carbidopa-levodopa therapy is orthostatic hypotension.

Of the more serious adverse effects of carbidopa-levodopa therapy, abnormal movements are the most common. These abnormal movements result from the increased dopamine in the brain. They include choreiform, dystonic reactions and dyskinetic movements. Other involuntary movements that may develop include the following:

- **Bruxism** (clenching the teeth, associated with forceful lateral or protrusive jaw movements, resulting in rubbing, gritting, or grinding the teeth)
- Protrusion of the tongue
- Opening and closing of the mouth
- Bobbing of the head
- Rhythmic movements of the feet or hands
- Quick movements of the shoulder
- **Ballismus** (jerking, flinging movements of an extremity)

Abnormal movements are usually dose related and may resolve with a reduction in dose. Unfortunately, with a dose reduction, the symptoms of Parkinson disease may recur.

Psychiatric disturbances may develop with the administration of carbidopa-levodopa. Symptoms include memory loss, anxiety, nervousness, agitation, restlessness, confusion, insomnia, nightmares, daytime somnolence, euphoria, malaise, and fatigue. Patients taking carbidopa-levodopa are also at risk for developing severe mental depression, suicidal tendencies, dementia, hallucinations, paranoid delusion, psychoses, and hypomania.

Cardiac arrhythmias can occur during carbidopa-levodopa therapy but are relatively infrequent. Other cardiovascular symptoms include flushing and hypertension. For patients taking carbidopa-levodopa for a prolonged period, **bradykinetic episodes,** also known as the **"on–off effect,"** may occur. Characteristics of this syndrome include akinesia, a sudden return of the effectiveness of the drug, and akinesia paradoxica (an abrupt hypotonic reaction in which the patient usually falls as he or she begins to walk). The akinetic episode can last from 1 minute to 1 hour. A sudden return of effectiveness may follow, and the cycle can recur many times each day. Recently, the Food and Drug Administration (FDA) approved a new drug to treat these episodes in patients with Parkinson disease (Box 21.1).

Neuroleptic malignant syndrome (NMS, also called parkinsonian crisis) is characterized by an abrupt onset of marked rigidity, akinesia, tremor, and hyperpyrexia. It can follow abrupt discontinuation of carbidopa-levodopa therapy, and it occurs most frequently in patients who are also receiving antipsychotic drugs.

Other adverse effects associated with carbidopa-levodopa include episodic hyperventilation, bizarre breathing patterns, hoarseness, and increased nasal secretions. Urinary retention, polyuria, and urinary incontinence may also occur. Rarely, leukopenia may occur, necessitating discontinuing the drug temporarily.

Drug Interactions

Carbidopa-levodopa can interact substantially with hydantoins, MAOIs, pyridoxine, phenothiazines, or tricyclic antidepressants (TCAs). Table 21.2 presents a list of agents that interact with carbidopa-levodopa. Carbidopa-levodopa may also cause elevated serum and urinary pH levels, false-positive reactions for urinary glucose and ketones, and false elevations of urinary catecholamines.

COMMUNITY-BASED CONCERNS

Box 21.1 Treating Hypomobility in Parkinson Disease

Patients with advanced Parkinson disease who are taking levodopa may experience bradykinetic episodes, also known as "on–off syndrome." These episodes are characterized by a shift from the ability to be mobile (on) to an unpredictable period of immobility (off). The intensity, duration, and frequency of "off" periods vary from patient to patient. Intensity ranges from partial loss of movement to total immobility. On–off syndrome is thought to be related to an increased sensitivity in the brain to small changes in serum levels of dopamine.

Apomorphine hydrochloride (Apokyn) has been approved by the FDA as an orphan drug for treating acute, intermittent episodes of hypomobility. Apomorphine hydrochloride helps the patient walk, talk, or move more easily, but it does not prevent hypomobility, nor does it replace the patient's drugs for Parkinson disease.

Apomorphine hydrochloride is given as a subcutaneous injection. Symptoms improve within 15 minutes; the effect lasts for approximately 2 hours. The drug must be given with an antiemetic, because it can induce nausea and vomiting. It should not be given concurrently with antiemetic agents classified as 5-HT_3 antagonists because this type of antiemetic drug can induce hypotension or loss of consciousness. Examples of these drugs include ondansetron, granisetron, dolasetron, palonosetron, and alosetron. Common adverse effects associated with apomorphine hydrochloride include yawning, dyskinesias, nausea and vomiting, sedation or sleepiness, dizziness, runny nose, hallucinations, edema, chest pain, increased sweating, flushing, and pallor. Apomorphine hydrochloride is a pregnancy category C drug. It is unknown whether it enters breast milk.

When educating patients about apomorphine hydrochloride, you must emphasize the importance of continuing all drugs prescribed for Parkinson disease, despite symptom relief with apomorphine hydrochloride. You must also emphasize the importance of taking the drug with an antiemetic drug. Monitor the first injection to evaluate the patient or caregiver's ability to administer a subcutaneous injection correctly; emphasize the importance of aspirating before injecting to avoid intravenous administration.

Assessment of Relevant Core Patient Variables

Health Status

Assess the patient for tartrazine allergy, melanoma, and closed-angle glaucoma. Assess also for a history of psychiatric disorders that necessitate administration of MAOIs. If the patient has any of these disorders, notify the prescriber before administering carbidopa-levodopa.

Assess for previous levodopa or carbidopa-levodopa therapy. After 2 to 5 years of continuous therapy, these drugs lose their overall effectiveness in controlling symptoms of Parkinson disease. Administering a higher dose may affect symptoms but will also increase the patient's risk for adverse effects.

TABLE 21.2 Agents That Interact With P Carbidopa-Levodopa

Interactants	Effect and Significance	Nursing Management
hydantoins	Mechanism of action unknown, but decrease effectiveness of carbidopa-levodopa	Monitor for decreased therapeutic effects. Consider alternative anticonvulsant therapy.
MAOIs	Inhibit peripheral metabolism of carbidopa-levodopa, resulting in increased levels of dopamine; may result in hypertensive crisis	Do not coadminister these drugs. If accidental administration occurs, phentolamine is the antidote.
pyridoxine	Increases the peripheral metabolism of carbidopa-levodopa, resulting in decreased dopamine levels	This effect is more pronounced in patients receiving levodopa as a single agent. Monitor for decreased therapeutic effects.
phenothiazines	May inhibit dopamine receptors in the CNS	Monitor for decreased therapeutic effects.
tricyclic antidepressants	Delay the absorption of carbidopa-levodopa and may decrease its bioavailability	Monitor for decreased therapeutic effects.

Perform a complete physical examination, including mental status. Carbidopa-levodopa can exacerbate diseases or disorders in every body system; therefore, evaluate baseline functioning. Appropriate laboratory or diagnostic tests are determined in part by the patient's pre-existing conditions. Patients with cardiovascular disorders require a baseline electrocardiogram. Patients with pulmonary disorders should have baseline pulmonary function tests. Patients with glaucoma should have intraocular pressure measured at baseline. For patients with diabetes, a glycosylated hemoglobin (HbA_{1C}) level should be obtained. Baseline hepatic function or renal function tests are included for patients with disorders in those body systems.

Throughout the physical examination, document the signs and symptoms of Parkinson disease, such as abnormal posture and gait, muscle rigidity, and tremors. This baseline information will be used to assess the efficacy of carbidopa-levodopa therapy and progression of the disease.

Some patients receiving carbidopa-levodopa have experienced postoperative bleeding episodes; therefore, hematologic studies are recommended for all patients who undergo surgery while receiving the drug.

Life Span and Gender

Carbidopa-levodopa is a pregnancy category C drug and therefore should be used with caution during pregnancy. It should not be given to breast-feeding women because carbidopa-levodopa enters breast milk and may inhibit lactation. Therefore, assess all female patients for pregnancy or breast-feeding. In addition, carbidopa-levodopa should not be administered to children younger than 18 years of age, so confirm that the patient is 18 years or older.

Lifestyle, Diet, and Habits

Coordinate a consultation with a nutritionist for patients taking carbidopa-levodopa. Patients should attempt weight control because increased body weight increases the work of the body, especially the muscles. A high-protein diet can slow or prevent absorption of carbidopa-levodopa. Therefore, moderate amounts of protein should be divided equally for consumption throughout the entire day. Pyridoxine (vitamin B_6) increases the action of decarboxylases that destroy levodopa in the periphery of the body, resulting in reduced effects of carbidopa-levodopa. Accordingly, patients should avoid foods containing large amounts of pyridoxine, such as avocados, bananas, beef liver, oatmeal, halibut, chicken, pork, mashed potatoes, wheat germ, and sunflower seeds. Patients should also increase dietary fiber and fluids to offset the potential for constipation.

Environment

Carbidopa-levodopa is usually administered in the home environment. Assess patients for their ability to understand the prescriber's directions and to physically self-administer drugs. A new formulation of the combination drug, which dissolves rapidly on the tongue, may improve patients' ability to self-medicate. Home care referrals are necessary for patients who cannot self-medicate. Because carbidopa-levodopa does not affect the progression of the disease, coordinate counseling and physical and occupational therapies for the patient to optimize therapeutic outcome.

Culture and Inherited Traits

In decarboxylation, carbidopa-levodopa is metabolized by COMT, which antagonizes the therapeutic effects of carbidopa-levodopa. COMT activity destroys levodopa in the periphery of the body and is found in higher amounts in people of Chinese, Filipino, or Thai descent. Therefore, ask patients about their ethnic heritage as part of the assessment.

Nursing Diagnoses and Outcomes

- Disturbed Thought Processes related to adverse CNS effects
  Desired outcome: *The patient will remain oriented and communicate effectively.*
- Disturbed Sleep Pattern related to drug therapy
  Desired outcome: *The patient will report alterations in sleep patterns affecting activities of daily living.*
- Impaired Physical Mobility related to on–off effect
  Desired outcome: *The patient will immediately report incidents of the on–off effect to the prescriber.*
- Risk for Injury related to drug-induced orthostatic hypotension
  Desired outcome: *The patient will learn to change position slowly, carefully, and safely to minimize effects of orthostatic hypotension.*

Planning and Intervention

Maximizing Therapeutic Effects

Carbidopa-levodopa should be taken on an empty stomach to facilitate absorption of the drug. If the patient has trouble swallowing pills, the rapid-dissolving formulation should be used. Monitor the patient's diet to limit foods high in protein and pyridoxine. If the drug causes severe nausea, give the patient a small amount of food 15 to 30 minutes after administering drug therapy.

Minimizing Adverse Effects

Carbidopa-levodopa should be administered at evenly spaced intervals; the dose should always be titrated. The dose is slowly increased to prevent nausea, vomiting, or orthostatic hypotension and is slowly decreased to prevent NMS (parkinsonian crisis).

Providing Patient and Family Education

- Advise patients that carbidopa-levodopa therapy is palliative and will not cure the disease. Patients must understand that it takes weeks to months to notice benefits from therapy. Caution patients not to change the drug dosage in an attempt to hasten the therapeutic benefits, nor to discontinue the drug abruptly because they think treatment has failed.
- Advise patients to notify the prescriber about any of the following adverse reactions: uncontrollable movements of the face, eyelids, mouth, tongue, neck, arms, hands, or legs; mood or mental changes; irregular heartbeat or palpitations; difficult urination; severe or persistent nausea or vomiting; appetite loss; difficulty swallowing; or distorted taste.
- Demonstrate how to change positions slowly to avoid dizziness or fainting. Advise patients to assess how the drug affects them before driving, using machinery, or performing tasks that require mental alertness.
- Discuss the potential for "on–off effect" described under the section on Adverse Reactions. Ensure that patients understand that they are at risk for injury from falls during the off periods. Convey the importance of contacting the prescriber immediately if patients experience an akinetic episode.
- Include necessary dietary changes in patient education. Patients should avoid vitamins or foods high in pyridoxine, high-protein foods when the drug is ingested, and alcohol.
- Caution patients with pre-existing disorders such as arrhythmias, pulmonary diseases, or peptic ulcer disease that carbidopa-levodopa may exacerbate their condition. Patients must contact their prescriber if their symptoms increase in frequency or intensity. Caution patients with diabetes to monitor their glucose by capillary blood testing because carbidopa-levodopa may induce false-positive urinary glucose results. Finally, carbidopa-levodopa sometimes darkens urine and sweat. Assure patients that this effect is no cause for concern.

Ongoing Assessment and Evaluation

Monitor for improvement in the patient's ability to perform daily activities and for decreased muscle rigidity and tremors. During periods of dose adjustment, monitor blood pressure every 4 hours. When dose adjustment is done in the home, teach a family member how to monitor blood pressure.

Monitor for signs of adverse effects from carbidopa-levodopa therapy. Dosage changes may increase adverse effects; thus, notifying the prescriber if these signs occur is important. Monitor for signs of personality, behavioral, or mental changes. Eliciting information regarding these potential changes from the family and patient is important. Patients should also receive a periodic eye examination because carbidopa-levodopa may affect intraocular pressure.

Monitor for signs or symptoms of NMS. If signs or symptoms of NMS develop, assess for adherence to drug therapy to ensure proper dosing. Report any signs of NMS to the prescriber immediately, and instruct the patient and family members that they should report any signs of NMS to the prescriber immediately.

With successful therapy, you should observe decreased muscular rigidity and tremors and improved mobility. The patient should be able to verbalize an understanding of the importance of contacting the prescriber immediately if any adverse reactions occur and of the need for periodic reevaluation by the prescriber.

Drugs Closely Related to P Carbidopa-Levodopa

Dopaminergics

AMANTADINE

Amantadine (Symmetrel) is a dopaminergic agent that is not a dopamine agonist. Amantadine is an oral antiviral drug that is also effective in treating Parkinson disease. Little is known about its precise mechanism of action in the brain. It has traditionally been considered a dopaminergic drug, but recent studies suggest that it may affect other neurochemical pathways containing the chemical messengers glutamate or acetylcholine. Amantadine's efficacy diminishes within a short time. Its effects may decrease within as little as 3 to 6 months.

MEMORY CHIP

P Carbidopa-Levodopa

- Dopaminergic drug used in managing Parkinson disease
- Major contraindications: known hypersensitivity, allergy to tartrazine, melanoma, closed-angle glaucoma, and breast-feeding
- Most common adverse effects: abnormal movements, orthostatic hypotension, and GI effects
- Most serious adverse effects: neuroleptic malignant syndrome, which may occur with abrupt cessation of the drug; precautions necessary with cardiac disease, pulmonary disease, peptic ulcer disease, diabetes mellitus, psychosis, and pregnancy
- Maximizing therapeutic effects: Take drug on an empty stomach and reduce protein and pyridoxine in the diet.
- Minimizing adverse effects: Titrate the drug upward to avoid GI effects; titrate the drug downward to avoid neuroleptic malignant syndrome.
- Most important patient education: Caution about hypotension and "on–off effect."

Amantadine tends to cause insomnia as well as daytime fatigue. Other adverse effects can include swollen feet, anxiety, dizziness, urinary retention, and hallucinations. The patient may also experience effects similar to those of anticholinergic drugs, such as blurred vision, constipation, urinary retention, and xerostomia (dry mouth). These effects may be enhanced when amantadine is given concurrently with other drugs that have anticholinergic effects.

An adverse effect specific to amantadine is "livedo reticularis," a reddish-blue netlike mottling of the skin. Fortunately, this condition is benign and disappears when amantadine therapy is stopped.

SELEGILINE

Selegiline (Eldepryl) is another dopaminergic agent that is not a dopamine agonist. It is an oral selective inhibitor of MAO-B, the chemical that breaks down dopamine. It should not be confused with the MAOIs used to treat depression. Selegiline decreases the destruction of dopamine, whether the dopamine is extrinsic, such as the dopamine produced from carbidopa-levodopa, or intrinsic. It is thought to slow the progression of Parkinson disease. Selegiline delays the need for carbidopa-levodopa and effectively prolongs the efficacy of pharmacotherapy. As with amantadine, its action diminishes rapidly; the therapy is viable for only 12 to 24 months.

Selegiline is metabolized in the liver into two metabolites: amphetamine and methamphetamine. These metabolites may be responsible for the most common adverse effect of selegiline, which is insomnia. Concurrent administration of selegiline with carbidopa-levodopa may enhance adverse effects such as orthostatic hypotension, dyskinesias, nausea, and psychological disturbances.

Dopamine Agonists

BROMOCRIPTINE

The pharmacologic action of a dopamine agonist differs from that of carbidopa-levodopa. Bromocriptine (Parlodel), a dopamine agonist, is an oral synthetic agent that has been used to treat Parkinson disease for many years. Its other indications include acromegaly, amenorrhea, galactorrhea, infertility, and prolactin-secreting pituitary adenomas. It is being investigated for use in treating insulin resistance in patients with type 2 diabetes mellitus.

Bromocriptine works by stimulating D_2 receptors and antagonizing D_1 receptors in the hypothalamus and striatum. For treating Parkinson disease, the effect is to increase the availability of dopamine. Additionally, bromocriptine suppresses prolactin secretion from the anterior pituitary gland, enabling ovulation and ovarian function in amenorrheic patients and suppressing lactation in women with normal ovarian activity.

The adverse effects of bromocriptine therapy limit its use. Symptoms such as psychiatric disturbances, nausea, and orthostatic hypotension are very common. Bromocriptine exacerbates pre-existing conditions such as psychiatric illness, peripheral vascular disease, and peptic ulcer disease. In addition, bromocriptine may cause patients with a history of MI to experience serious cardiac problems.

Bromocriptine should not be administered with drugs that antagonize its actions. Such drugs include those that increase the concentration of prolactin, such as haloperidol (Haldol), loxapine (Loxitane), molindone (Moban), MAOIs, imipramine (Tofranil), amitriptyline (Elavil), methyldopa (Aldomet), phenothiazines, and reserpine (Serpalan). Estrogens or progestins can produce amenorrhea or galactorrhea and should not be given concurrently.

PERGOLIDE

Pergolide (Permax), the second dopamine agonist, is an oral agent similar in action to bromocriptine, with 10 times the potency of bromocriptine at the D_2 receptors. Unlike bromocriptine, pergolide stimulates D_1 receptors as well. Pergolide directly activates dopamine receptors in the striatum, inhibits the secretion of prolactin, and decreases luteinizing hormone. The effects on prolactin secretion persist much longer than the antiparkinsonian action.

Because pergolide is a potent dopamine receptor agonist, it should not be administered with dopamine receptor antagonists (i.e., neuroleptics such as phenothiazines, haloperidol, and thiothixene). Dopamine receptor antagonists can antagonize the effects of pergolide.

Adverse effects of pergolide are nausea, vomiting, confusion, hallucinations, lightheadedness, and fainting. A rare side effect known as fibrosis (thickening or scarring of the membrane lining of body organs) has also been reported.

PRAMIPEXOLE

Pramipexole (Mirapex) is the third dopamine agonist used to treat Parkinson disease. Carbidopa-levodopa is converted in the brain into dopamine. In contrast, dopamine agonists such as pramipexole help alleviate the symptoms of Parkinson disease by acting directly on dopamine receptors in the brain. Pramipexole is a selective agonist at D_2 and D_3 receptors in the brain. It is more selective for these receptors than either bromocriptine or pergolide.

Pramipexole has been approved for treating both early and late stages of Parkinson disease. With early-stage monotherapy, pramipexole (like selegiline) will delay the need for carbidopa-levodopa, thus extending the pharmacotherapeutic benefits of carbidopa-levodopa when it is used to treat more advanced stages of Parkinson disease. Additionally, in later stages of Parkinson disease, coadministering pramipexole and carbidopa-levodopa can decrease the dosage of carbidopa-levodopa by 25%. This reduction decreases the potential for carbidopa-levodopa's adverse effects.

In the early stages of Parkinson disease, the most frequent adverse effects of pramipexole are nausea, dizziness, drowsiness, insomnia, and postural hypotension. In advanced stages of Parkinson disease, additional adverse effects include dyskinesias, extrapyramidal syndromes, and hallucinations. Inform all patients that postural hypotension may occur more frequently during initial treatment and that hallucinations can occur at any time during the course of treatment.

ROPINIROLE

Ropinirole (Requip), the last dopamine agonist, is similar to pramipexole. Like pramipexole, ropinirole may be used in early Parkinson disease or in later stages in conjunction with carbidopa-levodopa. With ropinirole, the dose of carbidopa-levodopa may be reduced, which may in turn help decrease the on–off fluctuations that affect some patients who have been on carbidopa-levodopa for many years.

Administering ropinirole as monotherapy can induce adverse effects in every system of the body. In the autonomic

nervous system, the most common adverse effects include diaphoresis, flushing, and dry mouth. In the overall body, the most common adverse effects include asthenia, chest pain, dependent edema, fatigue, malaise, pain, and peripheral edema. Cardiovascular adverse reactions include atrial fibrillation, extrasystoles, hypertension, hypotension, orthostatic hypotension, palpitations, sinus tachycardia, and syncope (sometimes with sinus bradycardia). Most cases of syncope occurring with ropinirole therapy are reported more than 4 weeks after initiation and are usually associated with a recent increase in dosage. In the GI system, common adverse effects include abdominal pain, anorexia, dyspepsia, flatulence, and nausea and vomiting. The most common adverse reactions affecting the CNS and peripheral nervous system include dizziness, hyperesthesia, restlessness, and vertigo. The metabolic and nutritional adverse effect is weight loss, whereas respiratory adverse effects include bronchitis, dyspnea, pharyngitis, rhinitis, sinusitis, visual impairment, and xerophthalmia (conjunctival dryness).

Psychiatric adverse reactions include amnesia, impaired concentration, confusion, hallucinations, drowsiness, and yawning. There have been many reports of patients who have fallen asleep while driving or performing other normal daytime activities while taking ropinirole. The episodes have occurred as late as 1 year after initiating treatment. Some patients have reported feeling completely alert before these events. It is not clear whether the medication, the sleep status of the patient, or the Parkinson disease itself contributed to these episodes.

In addition to the above adverse effects, ropinirole in combination with carbidopa-levodopa may induce additional effects, including dyskinesia, falls, headache, hypokinesia, paresis, paresthesias, tremor, constipation, diarrhea, dysphagia, flatulence, hypersalivation, anemia, upper respiratory infections, pyuria, urinary incontinence, and diplopia. Additionally, anxiety, abnormal dreaming, hallucinations, nervousness, and somnolence (drowsiness) may also occur. The potential advantage of ropinirole over carbidopa-levodopa is a lower incidence of dyskinesia and lower propensity to induce adverse psychiatric effects.

Drugs Significantly Different From P Carbidopa-Levodopa

Tolcapone

Tolcapone (Tasmar) is a new adjunct to carbidopa-levodopa therapy. It inhibits the enzyme COMT, which degrades dopamine in the periphery of the body. The higher and more sustained plasma concentrations of levodopa that result translate into more constant dopaminergic stimulation in the brain, which in turn leads to greater effects on the signs and symptoms of Parkinson disease. The decreased destruction of levodopa allows a decrease in the daily dosage of carbidopa-levodopa. Tolcapone is indicated for treating Parkinson disease in patients who are experiencing fluctuations in symptoms and are not responding to or are not appropriate candidates for other adjunctive therapies.

COMT also metabolizes medications other than levodopa, including dopamine, dobutamine, epinephrine, norepinephrine, isoproterenol, methyldopa, and bitolterol. The dosage of these agents may have to be reduced in patients who are treated with tolcapone.

Because COMT and MAO are the two major enzyme systems involved in the metabolism of catecholamines, the possibility exists that the combined use of tolcapone and a nonselective MAOI such as phenelzine or tranylcypromine would inhibit most pathways involved in normal catecholamine metabolism. Therefore, the concurrent use of these agents should be avoided. Tolcapone can, however, be used with the selective MAO-B inhibitor selegiline, and these agents have been used together in antiparkinsonian regimens without difficulty.

The most frequent adverse effects of tolcapone are dyskinesia, nausea, increased daytime sleepiness, dystonia, orthostatic hypotension, diarrhea, dizziness, and hallucinations. Tolcapone may elevate liver transaminase concentrations in the blood. Because of reports of fatal liver injury, the manufacturers of tolcapone advise that its use should be reserved for patients who do not respond to or are not appropriate candidates for other available treatments. Extensive liver function testing is required for all patients before and during therapy.

Entacapone

Entacapone (Comtan) is the second COMT inhibitor to be approved and is indicated as an adjunct to carbidopa-levodopa in treating patients with idiopathic Parkinson disease who experience the signs and symptoms of end-of-dose "wearing-off." This agent has no antiparkinsonian effect of its own, and it must be administered with carbidopa-levodopa. Like tolcapone, adding entacapone to a carbidopa-levodopa regimen increases the bioavailability of levodopa. Entacapone is also available as a fixed-dose combination pill with carbidopa-levodopa (Stalevo).

Entacapone has the same adverse effect profile as tolcapone, with the exception that entacapone is not associated with hepatotoxicity or clinically important elevations of liver enzymes. This exception represents an important advantage over tolcapone. Potential drug–drug interactions with entacapone are similar to those for tolcapone.

Centrally Acting Anticholinergic Drugs

The centrally acting anticholinergic drugs work by blocking the access of acetylcholine to cholinergic receptors in the striatum. Centrally acting anticholinergic drugs are less effective than carbidopa-levodopa. They can be used as monotherapy in early Parkinson disease or in combination with dopaminergic drugs in later stages. They are used with caution in older patients because of the potential for severe CNS effects. The anticholinergics used most frequently in treating Parkinson disease are benztropine (Cogentin), diphenhydramine (Benadryl), and trihexyphenidyl (Artane). For additional information concerning anticholinergic drugs, see Chapter 14.

C ANTI-AMYOTROPHIC LATERAL SCLEROSIS DRUGS

Historically, there has not been specific pharmacotherapy for treating ALS. In December 1995, the FDA approved riluzole (Rilutek), the first drug for treatment of ALS. Riluzole,

the prototype anti-ALS drug, does not cure ALS. Rather, it is used to delay the need for tracheostomy or mechanical ventilation in patients who have ALS. Research for additional ALS medications is ongoing.

NURSING MANAGEMENT OF THE PATIENT RECEIVING P RILUZOLE

Core Drug Knowledge

Pharmacotherapeutics

Riluzole is indicated for treating ALS because it slows down the disease's progression by delaying for several months the loss of muscle strength and limb function. The drug is given to extend survival time before tracheostomy is necessary, but it is not a cure.

Pharmacokinetics

Riluzole is administered orally in 50-mg doses every 12 hours. Its onset of action is slow, and its duration of action is 3 to 5 days. Well absorbed from the GI tract, riluzole has a half-life of 12 hours. Hepatic metabolism of riluzole is extensive, producing six major and several minor metabolites. The cytochrome P-450 enzyme system is involved in hydroxylation and glucuronidation. The main isozyme involved in hydroxylation is CYP1A2. Riluzole crosses the placenta and enters breast milk.

Excretion of riluzole is mainly renal and 5% fecal. Riluzole is largely excreted as metabolites, with about 2% excreted as unchanged drug. Renal clearance of riluzole is individualized, possibly because of the variability of CYP1A2 (see Table 21.1).

Pharmacodynamics

The etiology of ALS is unknown. One of the leading theories of its pathogenesis is that glutamate injures motor neurons. Although the mode of action of riluzole in treating ALS is also unknown, it may work by inhibiting glutamate release, inactivating voltage-dependent sodium channels, or interfering with intracellular events that follow transmitter binding at excitatory amino acid receptors.

Contraindications and Precautions

The only contraindication to riluzole therapy is a hypersensitivity to any of its components. Many precautions, however, are issued.

Riluzole has affected fetal development and viability in animal studies; however, adequate studies on human pregnancy have not been completed. It is assigned to pregnancy category C and should be administered only when the benefits to the mother outweigh the risks to the fetus throughout pregnancy.

Hepatic disease, renal disease, or renal impairment can affect the clearance of riluzole, which is extensively metabolized in the liver and excreted in the urine. Patients with pre-existing hepatic or renal disease should be given riluzole with caution.

Adverse Effects

Evaluating adverse effects caused by riluzole can be difficult because ALS has several manifestations that may be mistaken for adverse effects. In reviewing the adverse effects for patients taking riluzole, consider natural disease progression.

Potential side effects are fatigue, nausea, dizziness, diarrhea, anorexia, vertigo, and somnolence. When these symptoms become troublesome, treatment should be discontinued. Riluzole increases levels of hepatic enzymes in 50% of patients. This increase occurs in patients with no history of hepatic injury. Rarely, jaundice may also occur.

Many potentially adverse reactions have been reported with riluzole therapy, involving every system of the body. These adverse reactions, however, have occurred in less than 1% of patients receiving riluzole. One of the most serious potential adverse effects is neutropenia. Although such reactions are rare, a complete blood count (CBC) should be monitored for the patient's safety.

Drug Interactions

As previously mentioned, riluzole may cause hepatic injury. The potential exists for increased risk for hepatic injury when riluzole is used concurrently with potentially hepatotoxic drugs. Additionally, drugs that induce the hepatic enzyme system may also increase the risk for hepatic injury.

The principal isoenzyme involved in the metabolism of riluzole is CYP1A2. Inhibitors or inducers of this enzyme may change plasma concentrations, resulting in toxic or subtherapeutic concentrations of the drug. Table 21.3 presents agents that may interact with riluzole.

Assessment of Relevant Core Patient Variables

Health Status

Elicit a careful history, including any pre-existing hepatic or renal dysfunction. Assess also for a history of cigarette smoking. Communicate any positive findings to the prescriber.

Completing a physical examination of the patient before initiating therapy is important. Riluzole can induce adverse effects in every body system. With the exception of hepatic injury, the chance of these adverse reactions is less than 1%. Baseline data are helpful should any of the reactions occur. All patients should have baseline CBC and renal and hepatic function tests documented.

Life Span and Gender

Older patients are more likely to have age-related changes in hepatic or renal function. No specific recommendations for dosage in older adults have been made, but closely monitor older patients for adverse effects.

The metabolism of riluzole depends largely on the activity of a specific isozyme, CYP1A2. This isozyme reportedly is more active in men than women. Higher blood concentrations of riluzole and its metabolites may be present in women, which may increase the risk for adverse effects in women. Continually assess female patients for these effects.

Lifestyle, Diet, and Habits

Evaluate the patient's diet for high fat content, use of caffeine products, and high intake of charcoal-broiled foods, and determine whether the patient is a smoker. The absorption of riluzole may be diminished by up to 20% in patients who consume a high-fat diet. Caffeine products can inhibit

TABLE 21.3 Agents That Interact With P Riluzole

Interactants	Effect and Significance	Nursing Management
CYP1A2 inhibitors • amitriptyline • caffeine • quinolones • theophylline	Administering riluzole with drugs that inhibit CYP1A2 has the potential to increase plasma concentrations of riluzole by decreasing the rate of clearance.	Monitor for toxicity. Monitor serum plasma levels.
CYP1A2 inducers • cigarette smoke • charcoal-broiled foods • omeprazole • rifampin	Administering riluzole with substances that induce CYP1A2 has the potential to increase plasma concentrations of riluzole by increasing the rate of clearance.	Monitor for efficacy of riluzole therapy. Monitor serum plasma levels.
hepatic enzyme inhibitors • barbiturates • carbamazepine	Administering riluzole with hepatic enzyme inducers has the potential to increase the risk for hepatotoxicity.	Monitor liver function tests. Monitor for signs of hepatic dysfunction.
hepatotoxic drugs • allopurinol • aminoglycosides • leflunomide • methyldopa • methotrexate • sulfasalazine	Administering riluzole with other drugs known for their hepatotoxic effects has the potential to increase the risk for hepatotoxicity.	Monitor liver function tests. Monitor for signs of hepatic dysfunction.

CYP1A2, resulting in increased serum concentration of riluzole. Conversely, charcoal-broiled foods and tobacco smoking can induce CYP1A2, which may increase the elimination of riluzole from the body.

Environment

Riluzole is usually administered in the home environment. Assess patients for their ability to understand the prescriber's directions and to physically self-administer drugs. Appropriate home care referrals are necessary for patients unable to self-medicate. Riluzole is extremely expensive. Evaluate patients' financial circumstances and refer patients and families for social services as appropriate.

Culture and Inherited Traits

Determine whether the patient is of Japanese descent. Riluzole clearance in ethnic Japanese patients is 50% less efficient than in whites. It is uncertain whether this effect is related to a difference in metabolic function in ethnic Japanese or to environmental factors such as smoking, alcohol or coffee intake, or diet.

Nursing Diagnoses and Outcomes

- Risk for Injury related to hepatic dysfunction, anemia, and CNS and cardiovascular effects of riluzole therapy
  Desired outcome: *The patient will immediately report any signs of hepatic dysfunction (fatigue, rash, jaundice), anemia (fatigue, sore throat, easy bruising), or CNS or cardiovascular effects to the prescriber.*
- Disturbed Thought Processes related to adverse CNS effects
  Desired outcome: *The patient will remain oriented and able to communicate effectively.*

Planning and Intervention

Maximizing Therapeutic Effects

Administer riluzole with a full glass of water. It is best for riluzole to be taken on an empty stomach, at least 1 hour before or 2 hours after meals. For patients who will be self-medicating, explain the importance of correct administration.

Minimizing Adverse Effects

At the beginning of therapy, riluzole may cause dizziness or sedation. Caution the patient to refrain from driving, using machinery, or performing tasks that require mental alertness until the effects of riluzole have been established.

Providing Patient and Family Education

- The most important patient and family education is explaining that riluzole will not change the course of the disorder. At best, riluzole will delay the need for tracheostomy and mechanical ventilation. Patients must understand what the eventual sequelae of ALS are and have a legal document in place if they choose to refuse life-sustaining measures.
- Advise patients to take riluzole on an empty stomach at 12-hour intervals. Present dietary concerns, such as the case for a low-protein diet. Also, advise patients to refrain from caffeine, alcohol, and charcoal-broiled foods.
- Advise patients of the potential adverse effects of riluzole. Because progression of the disease may mimic common adverse effects, patients should always contact the prescriber should any symptoms occur.
- Advise patients about the importance of regular follow-up and the need for periodic blood testing. Present symptoms of hepatic dysfunction and emphasize the importance of contacting the prescriber if any appear.

Ongoing Assessment and Evaluation

Coordinate regular follow-up evaluations of the patient. At each visit, evaluate the patient for the onset of adverse effects and complete a physical examination. CBC and alanine transaminase (ALT) levels should be taken monthly during the first 3 months of treatment, then every 3 months for the remainder of the first year. After the first year, ALT levels should be monitored periodically. Patients with elevated ALT levels require more frequent monitoring. Discontinuation of riluzole therapy should be considered when ALT levels become five times the normal range. Reinforce the necessity dietary and smoking restrictions during each encounter with the patient.

Effective therapy should delay deterioration of the respiratory muscles. The patient should acknowledge the importance of contacting the prescriber immediately if any adverse reactions occur. The patient should also acknowledge the importance of periodic re-evaluation by the prescriber.

Drugs Significantly Different From P Riluzole

Creatine

Creatine monophosphate is a dietary supplement granted FDA orphan drug status for use in patients with ALS. It is similar to the natural compound creatine phosphate, which is an essential component of the energy-converting system in muscle cells. Creatine's primary function is to maintain adenosine triphosphate (ATP) levels within muscle. Muscles use the energy supplied by ATP during anaerobic activity, such as lifting weights. Creatine also promotes an anabolic environment in the muscle, which promotes protein synthesis that is important for muscle growth and repair. Studies have shown that increasing the amount of creatine in the muscle increases ATP production and therefore improves high-power activity and muscle growth, which is important for ALS patients because retained muscle strength leads to a better prognosis and quality of life. Creatine may also be combined with the antibiotic minocycline for managing ALS.

Creatine should be used cautiously in people with preexisting renal disease that produces renal impairment or renal failure. Creatine generates an increased amount of creatinine that must be eliminated by the kidneys. Studies have not been done to show the safety of creatine in children or during pregnancy.

MEMORY CHIP

P Riluzole

- Used in managing ALS to delay need for mechanical ventilation
- Major contraindication: hypersensitivity to any components of riluzole
- Most serious adverse effect: neutropenia; adverse effects possible in every body system but may simply indicate progression of disease
- Maximizing therapeutic effects: Recommend dietary decreases in protein and avoidance of caffeine, charcoal-broiled foods, tobacco, and alcohol.
- Minimizing adverse effects: Refrain from tasks that require concentration until the effects of riluzole are known.
- Most important patient education: Have CBC and ALT monitored monthly for first 3 months, then every 3 months thereafter.

CRITICAL THINKING SCENARIO

Riluzole and reality

Mrs. Baxter has been diagnosed with ALS. She has moderate weakness in her extremities and uses a walker to ambulate. During your home visit, Mr. Baxter tells you, "I'm so glad they have started my wife on riluzole. I was thinking of having our attorney come over and do all that paperwork about the will because I was so scared. Now I don't have to."

1. How would you respond to Mr. Baxter?
2. What specific topics would you cover with him?

Drugs for Symptom Abatement

Patients with ALS are affected by diverse symptoms, including spasticity, muscle cramping, depression, gastric reflux, excessive salivation, viscous phlegm, pain, constipation, urinary urgency, and in the final stages of the disease, breathing difficulty. Drugs used to decrease spasticity include baclofen, tizanidine, and diazepam (see Chapter 20). For muscle cramps, patients may be prescribed quinine, baclofen, or clonazepam (see Chapters 17 and 20). Gastric reflux is managed with use of histamine-2 blocking agents or proton pump inhibitors (see Chapter 48). For excessive salivation, patients are prescribed anticholinergics or antihistamines (see Chapter 14). Viscous phlegm can be decreased with guaifenesin (see Chapter 46). Pain is managed initially with acetaminophen or prostaglandin synthetase inhibitors such as ibuprofen (see Chapter 24). As the disease progresses, pain management may require narcotic administration (see Chapter 23).

Constipation is a major problem and may be treated with laxatives, prune juice, enemas, or a bowel program (see Chapter 49). Urinary urgency is controlled with tolterodine (see Chapter 28). Because many of these drugs can be purchased over the counter, educate the patient to consult with the prescriber before using these drugs in an effort to avoid drug–drug interactions.

C ANTI-MULTIPLE SCLEROSIS DRUGS

Pharmacotherapy for MS uses a multilayered approach. Drugs used to affect the progress of the disease are called "ABC therapy." These drugs are interferon beta-1a (Avonex), interferon beta-1b (Betaseron), and glatiramer (Copaxone). The interferons are also used in managing hepatitis C and other viral illnesses and are discussed in Chapter 43. Glatiramer is the prototype drug for managing MS.

NURSING MANAGEMENT OF THE PATIENT RECEIVING P GLATIRAMER

Core Drug Knowledge

Pharmacotherapeutics

Glatiramer is used to reduce the frequency of attacks in patients with relapsing-remitting multiple sclerosis.

Pharmacokinetics

The pharmacokinetics of glatiramer in humans has not been studied, and no direct and sensitive analytical method exists for measuring glatiramer in serum. In animal studies, it is readily absorbed after subcutaneous injection, and no evidence exists of any tissue accumulation of glatiramer (see Table 21.1).

Pharmacodynamics

Glatiramer acetate is a synthetic chemical that is similar in structure to myelin basic protein. Its action is unclear; however, the drug is thought to modify immune processes that cause MS by acting as a decoy to locally generated autoantibodies. This effect results in decreased tissue destruction.

Contraindications and Precautions

Absolute contraindications include intravenous (IV) administration and hypersensitivity to mannitol. It should be used with caution in already immunocompromised patients and in patients receiving vaccinations because the action of glatiramer is to modulate the immune response.

Adverse Effects

Glatiramer may induce chest pain or tightness, breathing difficulties, hives or severe rash, pounding heartbeat, and unusual muscle weakness or tiredness. These symptoms should be reported to the provider immediately.

The most common adverse effects include lumps, pain, and redness at the site of injection. Other common adverse effects include anxiety, bleeding, inflammation, itching, dizziness, flushing, joint aches, muscle stiffness, nausea or vomiting, tremor, and weakness. These symptoms may become quite bothersome, and the patient should contact the provider if they do not subside.

Drug Interactions

Although no known drug–drug interactions occur, glatiramer can alter the results of a Papanicolaou test (Pap smear); therefore, women should tell their obstetrician-gynecologist if they are taking glatiramer.

Assessment of Relevant Core Patient Variables

Health Status

Elicit a patient history, especially questioning hypersensitivity to mannitol or pre-existing immunocompromise. Document patient limitations related to MS to serve as a baseline for evaluating the effectiveness of glatiramer therapy.

Life Span and Gender

Glatiramer is a pregnancy category B drug. It is not known whether glatiramer is excreted into breast milk. Glatiramer has not been studied in patients younger than 18 years.

Lifestyle, Diet, and Habits

Glatiramer has no known interactions with lifestyle, diet, or habits. Much literature has been published on the appropriate diet for a patient with MS, but diet does not affect the use of glatiramer.

Environment

Glatiramer may be used in any environment and is most frequently self-administered at home. It should be kept in the refrigerator before use and should not be exposed to high temperature or intense light. Emphasize the need to place used syringes in a puncture-resistant container and then return the container to the prescriber for proper disposal.

Nursing Diagnoses and Outcomes

- Weakness related to glatiramer injection
  Desired outcome: *The patient will recognize weakness and take measures to decrease its impact on activities of daily living.*
- Skin Integrity, Impaired, related to injection site reactions
  Desired outcome: *The patient will employ strategies to minimize injection site reactions.*
- Disturbed Sensory Perception related to anxiety and dizziness
  Desired outcome: *The patient will notify the provider if these adverse effects occur.*

Planning and Intervention

Maximizing Therapeutic Effects

Explain that glatiramer should be kept in the refrigerator until it is used. Teach the patient and family how to transfer sterile water into the glatiramer using aseptic technique, gently swirl the vial, and then allow the mixture to stand at room temperature until all of the powder is dissolved. Advise the patient and family using glatiramer from prefilled glass syringes to allow the syringe to sit at room temperature approximately 20 minutes before injection.

Minimizing Adverse Effects

Teach the patient and family to administer the subcutaneous injection correctly. It is important to deliver the medication into the subcutaneous tissues and avoid either intradermal or intravenous administration. Explain the importance of rotating the injection site so that no one spot is used more than once a week.

Providing Patient and Family Education

- Review the potential adverse effects of glatiramer, focusing on how common adverse differ from serious effects that should be reported to the provider.
- Review appropriate subcutaneous injection sites. Appropriate sites include the thigh, back of the hip, stomach, and upper arm.
- Review proper reconstitution of glatiramer powder.
- Review aseptic technique for subcutaneous administration.
- Review appropriate disposal of syringes.

Ongoing Assessment and Evaluation

Elicit a history from the patient at each subsequent visit, focusing on improvement of baseline symptoms or acquisition of new symptoms. Question the patient about adverse effects and document them in the medical record.

Effective therapy should decrease the intensity of baseline symptoms and prolong the intervals between acute exacerbations of MS. The patient should recognize important adverse effects that require contact with the provider.

MEMORY CHIP

P Glatiramer

- Used in managing MS to delay the progression of the disease
- Major contraindication: IV administration, hypersensitivity
- Most serious adverse effect: chest pain or tightness, breathing difficulties, hives or severe rash
- Maximizing therapeutic effects: Keep medication refrigerated; reconstitute medication correctly.
- Minimizing adverse effects: Correct procedure to subcutaneous administration.
- Most important patient education: Avoid accidental IV administration.

Drugs Significantly Different From P Glatiramer

Interferons

Interferon beta is also used in treating MS. Interferon beta is available as interferon beta-1a (Avonex, Rebif) and interferon beta-1b (Betaseron). Interferon beta works by decreasing interferon gamma and other proinflammatory cytokines. Interferon gamma is believed to be one of the major factors responsible for triggering the autoimmune reaction resulting in MS. In MS, T cells migrate across the blood-brain barrier in response to interferon gamma and attack antigens on nervous system tissues. By reducing interferon gamma, T-cell migration is reduced, resulting in less tissue damage. Another action of interferon beta is an increased production of nerve growth factor (NGF), which may have a favorable effect of remyelination.

A recombinant process produces both drugs, but in other respects, they differ greatly. In therapy, 1-mg interferon beta-1a represents 200 million units of activity, whereas 1 mg of interferon beta-1b represents 32 million units of activity. Interferon beta-1a shows a reduction in relapse rate and slows disease progression. Interferon beta-1b shows a very substantial clinical benefit in decreasing relapse but has not been shown to slow disease progression. Interferon beta-1a as Avonex is administered by intramuscular injection, whereas interferon beta-1b is administered by subcutaneous injection. Interferon beta-1a has not been associated with injection-site necrosis, whereas roughly 85% of patients receiving interferon beta-1b experienced an injection-site reaction.

Interferon beta should not be administered to patients with hypersensitivity to interferon beta or albumin. It is a pregnancy category C drug and should be avoided during pregnancy because of the risk for spontaneous abortion. It should also be avoided during breast-feeding because serious adverse reactions may occur in the infant. Interferon beta is also used with caution in patients who have a history of cardiac arrhythmias, heart failure, or myocardial infarction. Suicidal ideation has occurred in patients on interferon beta therapy. It is unclear whether this ideation is related to the drug or to the disease process of MS.

Biologic Response Modifiers

Natalizumab (Tysabri), a monoclonal antibody, is an alpha-4 integrin antagonist in a class known as selective adhesion molecule inhibitors. It is FDA approved to treat patients with relapsing forms of MS to reduce the frequency of symptom flare-ups or exacerbations of the disease. During its clinical trials, it reduced the rate of clinical relapses by up to 66% and reduced the development of new or newly enlarging MRI-detected brain lesions (Miller et al., 2003). It is still under investigation for the treatment of Crohn's disease (Ghosh et al., 2003) and may be effective for other types of inflammatory diseases.

Natalizumab works by blocking the ability of $\alpha_4\beta_1$ integrin and $\alpha_4\beta_7$ integrin to bind to their receptive vascular-cell adhesion molecules. Binding to adhesion molecules is an important step in white cells crossing arterial blood vessels and entering into the brain to attack myelin in MS. Because of its different mechanism of action, natalizumab is expected to be an important therapeutic option in the management of MS.

Natalizumab is given intravenously every 4 weeks in the health care provider's office. It is given cautiously in patients with pre-existing hepatic insufficiency. Common adverse effects include headache, fatigue, urinary tract infection, depression, lower respiratory tract infection, joint pain, and abdominal discomfort. It is expected that the drug may cost at much as $20,000 per year.

Drugs for Symptom Abatement

As in ALS, many other classes of drugs are used to manage the symptoms that accompany MS. Pharmacotherapy for symptoms of MS may include glucocorticoids to shorten the duration of an acute attack or delay the progression of optic neuritis. Other drugs useful in managing symptoms include tolterodine for bladder incontinence; carbamazepine or gabapentin for shooting sensory pain; baclofen, carisoprodol, or benzodiazepines for muscle spasticity; and tizanidine for low back pain.

OTHER MOVEMENT DISORDERS AND RELATED DRUG THERAPY

The following disorders and the drugs used to treat them are important to include in any discussion of drugs used to treat movement disorders. The drugs commonly used to treat these disorders are covered in depth in other chapters in this textbook. Therefore, the disorders and drugs commonly used to treat them are discussed briefly in this chapter. For more detailed information about the specific drugs, refer to the appropriate chapter in this textbook.

Myasthenia Gravis

Myasthenia gravis (MG) is an autoimmune disorder that impairs the receptors for acetylcholine at the myoneural junction. In this disease, immunoglobulin G (IgG) antibodies to acetylcholine receptors are formed, then block, and ultimately destroy the receptors so that the muscle cannot be stimulated. The patient experiences skeletal muscle weakness and rapid fatigue of the affected muscles.

The first symptoms of MG are usually weakness of the eye muscles and ptosis, and the disease progresses from ocular weakness to generalized weakness. The proximal limbs are weaker than the distal limbs. Symptoms are generally worse in the afternoon or as environmental temperature rises.

Diagnosis of MG is based on the edrophonium (Tensilon) test. In this test, the patient is induced into weakness by being required to maintain a position. Edrophonium, a short-acting acetylcholinesterase inhibitor, is administered intravenously. Patients with MG will have a dramatic transitory improvement in muscle function.

As with other movement disorders, MG has no cure. The treatments of choice are neostigmine (Prostigmin) or pyridostigmine (Mestinon). Both are presented in Chapter 14.

Huntington Disease

Huntington disease (chorea) is an inherited disorder that remains undiagnosed until midlife when symptoms first occur. The two main symptoms of the disease are progressive mental status changes leading to dementia and choreiform (rapid, jerky) movements. The inhibitory neurotransmitter GABA is depleted in the basal nuclei and substantia nigra. Levels of acetylcholine in the brain also appear to be reduced. Dopamine, however, is unaffected.

The first symptoms of Huntington disease are restlessness and choreiform movements of the arms and face. Symptoms in early disease include intellectual impairment such as loss of problem-solving skills, poor judgment, inability to concentrate, and memory lapses. As the disease progresses, personality changes, moodiness, and behavior disturbances occur. The dementia, which accompanies progressive disease, may be related to excessive amounts of dopamine. As atrophy of the brain continues, rigidity and akinesia develop.

No effective treatment exists for Huntington disease. Treatment of choreiform movements includes antipsychotic drugs such as haloperidol (Haldol) or phenothiazines, which block dopamine receptors. These drugs are discussed in depth in Chapter 18. Research to find other agents that will be useful in treating this disorder is ongoing (Box 21.2).

FOCUS ON RESEARCH

Box 21.2 Coenzyme Q_{10} (Ubiquinone) and Its Use in the Treatment of Neurodegenerative Diseases

The Huntington Study Group. (2001). A randomized, placebo-controlled trial of coenzyme Q10 and remacemide in Huntington's disease. *Neurology, 57*(3), 397–404.

Shults, C. W., et al. (2002). Effects of coenzyme Q10 in early Parkinson disease: Evidence of slowing of the functional decline. *Archives of Neurology, 59*(10), 1541–1550.

The Study

Coenzyme Q_{10} (CoQ_{10}) is a nonprescription dietary supplement, or nutriceutical. It is an endogenously synthesized provitamin, which is involved in a variety of cellular processes and plays a vital role in ATP production. It has also been noted to have antioxidant properties, such as free radical scavenging. Researchers at Massachusetts General Hospital conducted a study that investigated whether CoQ_{10} can exert neuroprotective effects in Huntington's disease. They were able to demonstrate very small decreases in the rate of decline on the total functional capacity (TFC) scale as well as the HD Independence Scale.

An additional study was done at the University of California for patients with Parkinson disease (PD). In that study, CoQ_{10} appeared to slow the progressive deterioration of function in PD. Researchers in both studies felt the results needed to be confirmed in larger studies.

Nursing Implications

Because CoQ_{10} can be purchased over the counter, you may encounter patients who are taking the supplement. The recommended daily dose of CoQ_{10} is between 50 mg and 300 mg per day, usually in divided doses, depending on the condition for which it is taken. To enhance absorption, CoQ_{10} should be taken with food. Side effects may include insomnia, nausea, loss of appetite, diarrhea, rash, irritability, headache, and increased levels of hepatic enzymes, but these events are rare. Potential drug interactions include those with warfarin, oral hypoglycemics, and cholesterol-lowering medications.

Gilles de la Tourette Disease

Gilles de la Tourette disease (Tourette syndrome, TS) is an autosomal dominant inherited tic disorder appearing in childhood and characterized by multiple motor or vocal tics lasting more than 1 year. Patients may also have obsessive-compulsive behavior, attention deficit hyperactivity disorder, or other psychiatric disorders. Coprolalia (involuntary utterances of vulgar or obscene words) and echolalia (involuntary parrot-like repetition of a word or sentence just spoken by another person) can occur but are rare.

Motor and vocal tics from this disease may respond to haloperidol (Haldol) and similar D_2 receptor blockers (see Chapter 18). Up to 80% of patients with TS initially benefit from haloperidol, sometimes dramatically; however, only approximately 20% of patients continue haloperidol for an extended period. Patients often discontinue the drug because of the emergence of side effects such as excessive fatigue, weight gain, dysphoria, parkinsonian symptoms, intellectual dulling, memory problems, personality changes, feeling "zombie-like," akathisia, school or social phobias, loss of libido, sexual dysfunction, and, especially after chronic use of high doses, tardive dyskinesia.

Pimozide (Orap) is another drug used for TS. It is chemically distinctive from haloperidol and phenothiazines, with potent dopamine-blocking properties. Its side effects are similar to those of haloperidol but may be less severe and appear in fewer patients. Routine electrocardiographic studies before and periodically during treatment are advised because of potential cardiotoxicity.

Other phenothiazines, particularly fluphenazine (Prolixin), may be effective alternatives to haloperidol and pimozide. Fluphenazine's side effects are the same as those associated with haloperidol but are better tolerated by some patients. Other neuroleptics that have been reported to be effective in a few patients include thiothixene (Navane), chlorpromazine (Thorazine), and trifluoperazine (Stelazine). These drugs are also discussed in Chapter 18.

Another drug useful in treating TS is clonidine (Catapres), an imidazoline compound with alpha-adrenergic agonist activity. In low doses, clonidine decreases the release of central norepinephrine, resulting in decreased motor tics. In addition to reducing the simple motor and phonic symptoms in TS, clonidine seems especially useful in ameliorating complex motor and phonic symptoms and improving attention problems. It has a low incidence of associated side effects. Perhaps its greatest importance is that it does not have the potential to cause tardive dyskinesia. Clonidine is covered in depth in Chapter 27.

CHAPTER SUMMARY

- Movement disorders are chronic, severe, and debilitating.
- Parkinson disease is a naturally occurring disorder characterized by rigidity, rest tremor, bradykinesia or akinesia, and postural instability.
- Parkinsonism is a syndrome of symptoms resembling Parkinson disease but caused by trauma, drugs, or infection.
- Amyotrophic lateral sclerosis (ALS) is a neuromuscular degenerative disease that progresses quickly until the patient experiences respiratory compromise and ultimately death.
- Drugs used to treat movement disorders are not curative.
- Dopaminergic drugs are used to treat Parkinson disease by increasing the action of dopamine in the CNS. The prototype dopaminergic drug is carbidopa-levodopa (Sinemet, Parcopa).
- Drugs that decrease the action of acetylcholine (anticholinergic drugs) are also used to treat Parkinson disease.
- The only FDA-approved anti-ALS drug is the prototype riluzole (Rilutek).
- Riluzole delays the need for tracheostomy and mechanical ventilation.
- Multiple classes of medications are used to manage the symptoms of ALS.
- Multiple sclerosis is generally treated with the "ABC" approach. This term is derived from the names of the drugs interferon beta-1a (Avonex), interferon beta-1b (Betaseron), and glatiramer (Copaxone).
- Other movement disorders and the drugs used to treat them include myasthenia gravis (MG), neostigmine; Huntington disease (chorea), haloperidol or phenothiazines; Tourette syndrome, haloperidol, clonidine, and fluphenazine.

QUESTIONS FOR STUDY AND REVIEW

1. How do dopaminergic and anticholinergic drugs work to decrease the symptoms of Parkinson disease?
2. Why is carbidopa-levodopa considered more efficient than levodopa alone?
3. What is neuroleptic malignant syndrome? When is it most likely to occur?
4. What is a bradykinetic episode?
5. What diet restrictions should be discussed when a patient starts carbidopa-levodopa therapy?
6. What assessments should you make throughout carbidopa-levodopa therapy?
7. What is the goal of riluzole therapy?
8. For patients taking riluzole, why is assessing adverse effects difficult?
9. What dietary restrictions should you discuss with the patient starting riluzole therapy?
10. How does glatiramer differ from the interferons in managing MS?
11. What pharmacodynamic similarities of glatiramer and interferon beta may affect patient adherence to therapy?

? Need More Help?

Chapter 21 of the study guide for *Drug Therapy in Nursing* 2e contains NCLEX-style questions and other learning activities to reinforce your understanding of the concepts presented in this chapter. For additional information or to purchase the study guide, visit *http://connection.lww.com/go/aschenbrenner.*

REFERENCES AND BIBLIOGRAPHY

Anonymous. (2004). Stalevo for Parkinson's disease. *The Medical Letter on Drugs and Therapeutics, 46*(1182), 39–40.

Biglan, K. M., & Holloway, R. G. (2002). A review of pramipexole and its clinical utility in Parkinson's disease. *Expert Opinions in Pharmacotherapeutics, 3*(2), 197–210.

Bonuccelli, U. (2003). Comparing dopamine agonists in Parkinson's disease. *Current Opinions in Neurology, 16*(Suppl. 1), S13–19.

Clinical Pharmacology [Online]. Available: *http://cp.gsm.com.*

Facts and Comparisons. (2004). *Drug facts and comparisons.* Philadelphia: Lippincott Williams & Wilkins.

Ghosh, S., Goldin, E., Gordon, F. H., et al. (2003). Natalizumab for active Crohn's disease. *New England Journal of Medicine, 348*(1), 24–32.

Hardman, J. G. (2001). *Goodman and Gilman's the pharmacological basis of therapeutics* (10th ed.). New York: McGraw-Hill Health Professions Division.

Hauser, R. A. (2004). Levodopa/carbidopa/entacapone (Stalevo). *Neurology, 62*(1 Suppl. 1), S64–S71.

The Huntington Study Group. (2001). A randomized, placebo-controlled trial of coenzyme Q_{10} and remacemide in Huntington's disease. *Neurology, 57*(3), 397–404.

Katzung, B. (2004). *Basic and clinical pharmacology* (9th ed.). New York: McGraw-Hill/Appleton & Lange.

Micromedex Healthcare Series [Online]. Available: *http://healthcare.micromedex.com.*

Miller, D. H., Khan, O. A., Sheremata, W. A., et al. (2003). A controlled trial of natalizumab for relapsing multiple sclerosis. *New England Journal of Medicine, 348*(1), 15–23.

Montgomery, E. B. (2002). Two advances in the management of Parkinson disease. *Cleveland Clinic Journal of Medicine, 69*(8), 639–643.

Shoulson, I. (2002). Experimental neurotherapeutics: Leaps and bounds. *Archives of Neurology, 59*(5), 689–691.

Shults, C. W., Oakes, D., Kieburtz, K., et al. (2002). Effects of coenzyme Q_{10} in early Parkinson disease: Evidence of slowing of the functional decline. *Archives of Neurology, 59*(10), 1541–1550.

Tatro, D. S. (2004). *Drug interaction facts.* Philadelphia: Lippincott Williams & Wilkins.

Traynor, B. J., Alexander, M., Corr, B., et al. (2003). An outcome study of riluzole in amyotrophic lateral sclerosis—a population-based study in Ireland, 1996–2000. *Journal of Neurology, 250*(4), 473–479.

Drugs Stimulating the Central Nervous System

chapter 22

Learning Objectives

At the completion of this chapter the student will:

1. Describe the physiology of the central nervous system (CNS) as related to arousal and stimulation.
2. Describe the various therapeutic uses of CNS stimulants.
3. Identify core drug knowledge about pharmacotherapies that stimulate the CNS.
4. Identify core patient variables relevant to drugs that stimulate the CNS.
5. Relate the interaction of core drug knowledge to core patient variables for therapies that stimulate the CNS.
6. Generate a nursing plan of care from the interactions between core drug knowledge and core patient variables for therapies that stimulate the CNS.
7. Describe nursing interventions to maximize therapeutic and minimize adverse effects for drugs that stimulate the CNS.
8. Determine key points for patient and family education for drugs that stimulate the CNS.

KEY TERMS

analeptics

anorectic

attention deficit hyperactivity disorder

cataplexy

hypercapnia

hypnagogic hallucinations

narcolepsy

obesity

overweight

sleep paralysis

FEATURED WEBLINKS

http://www.obesity.org

http://www.surgeongeneral.gov/topics/obesity

Need more information regarding obesity? Two great sites are given above.

CONNECTION WEBLINK

Additional Weblinks are found on Connection: **http://www.connection.lww.com/go/aschenbrenner.**

Drugs Stimulating the Central Nervous System

Ⓒ Centrally Acting Stimulants

- P **dextroamphetamine**
- amphetamine salts
- dexmethylphenidate
- methylphenidate
- pemoline
- cocaine
- atomoxetine
- antihypertensive agents
- antidepressants
- khat

Ⓒ Anorectic Agents

- P **sibutramine**
- phentermine
- adrenergic drugs
- serotonergic drugs
- orlistat

Ⓒ Respiratory Stimulants

- P **caffeine**
- doxapram

The symbol Ⓒ indicates the **drug class.**
Drugs in **bold type** marked with the symbol P are prototypes.
Drugs in blue type are closely related to the prototype.
Drugs in red type are significantly different from the prototype.
Drugs in black type with no symbol are also used in drug therapy; no prototype

Many substances are used to stimulate the central nervous system (CNS). These substances, sometimes called **analeptics,** include drugs that are used for therapeutic effects and nontherapeutic effects, both legal and illegal. Substances with therapeutic effects are categorized as central, anorectic, or respiratory stimulants. Central and respiratory stimulants are generally used to stimulate the CNS, whereas **anorectic** agents depress the appetite. The central stimulants are used to treat narcolepsy and as adjuncts in treating attention deficit hyperactivity disorder (ADHD). The anorectic agents suppress appetite or the sensation of hunger, mainly through serotonergic activity or central sympathomimetic effects. They are used as adjuncts to diet and exercise in the short-term management of moderate to severe obesity. The respiratory stimulants are rarely used, but as analeptics, they are representative of drugs that affect the brain stem and respiratory centers.

This chapter presents dextroamphetamine (Dexedrine), the prototype for centrally acting CNS stimulant drugs; sibutramine (Meridia), the prototype anorectic agent; and caffeine, the prototype respiratory stimulant. In addition, this chapter discusses core drug knowledge, core patient variables, nursing management, potential nursing diagnoses, and patient education related to the use of these drugs.

PHYSIOLOGY

The CNS is responsible for providing control systems and surveillance for many vegetative and conscious functions, including appetite, satiety, attention, arousal, activity, and respiration. The hypothalamus mediates appetite and satiety. Various sleep and arousal mechanisms are linked to the raphe nuclei and locus ceruleus in the pons and other parts of the reticular activating system (RAS).

The control of respiration occurs in the pons and medulla. Functional, structural, or lesional disorders may lead to disruptions in the usually smooth regulation of appetite, arousal, and activity. Figure 22.1 is a schema of the brain that shows the location of some regulatory centers involved in appetite, arousal, activity, and respiration.

At a synaptic level in the CNS, normal arousal mechanisms are affected through presynaptic release of neurotransmitters, such as norepinephrine, serotonin, and dopamine (Figure 22.2). These transmitters diffuse across the synaptic cleft to the postsynaptic effector cell, which is usually another neuron. The postsynaptic membrane contains receptors for the transmitters. In normal arousal, the transient combination of the transmitter with the receptor causes membrane changes that lead to propagation of the action potential. The transmitter can be metabolized by postsynaptic enzymes such as monoamine oxidase (MAO) or removed from further activity through reuptake into the presynaptic storage vesicles. CNS stimulants may provoke an increased release of neurotransmitters, a decreased reuptake of neurotransmitters, or inhibition of postsynaptic enzymes. The result is a heightened postsynaptic response, leading to increased arousal. Similar mechanisms occur in the sympathetic nervous system, where drugs such as the amphetamines act as indirect adrenergic agonists.

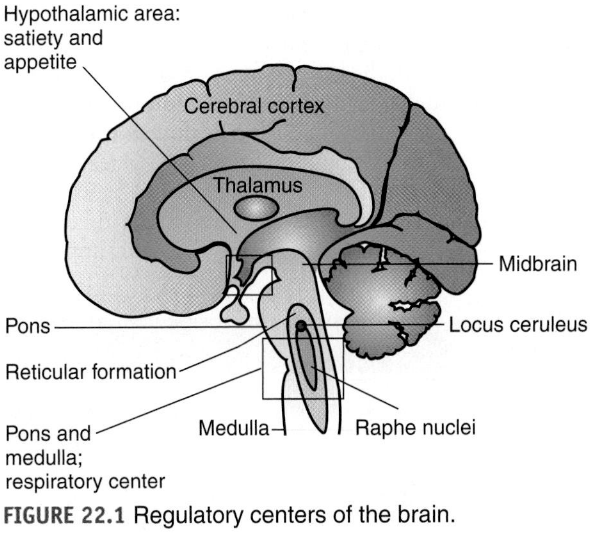

FIGURE 22.1 Regulatory centers of the brain.

PATHOPHYSIOLOGY

The CNS stimulants are indicated in various disorders and conditions, including narcolepsy, ADHD, obesity, and respiratory stimulation.

Narcolepsy

Narcolepsy, a neurologic condition that affects approximately 1 of every 1000 people, is characterized by irresistible bouts of rapid-eye-movement (REM) sleep during nonsleep cycles. Associated features include disturbed nocturnal sleep and REM sleep disturbances such as cataplexy, sleep paralysis, hypnagogic hallucinations, and abnormal sleep-onset REM periods. **Cataplexy** is a brief, sudden loss of motor control. In the person with narcolepsy, cataplexy usually manifests itself as a postural collapse to the ground, even though the individual maintains full consciousness. **Sleep paralysis** usually precedes the onset of sleep and involves being unable to speak or move, even though awareness of external events remains intact. The elapsed time is usually brief but may seem inordinately long to the person who experiences it.

Hypnagogic hallucinations are auditory, visual, or kinesthetic sensations without stimuli, appearing in the transition period between wakefulness and sleep. For example, the waking person may sense another person in the room but when fully awake recognizes that he or she is alone. Most people notice such hypnagogic hallucinations occasionally; however, they occur with greater intensity and frequency in patients with narcolepsy. Restoration of more normal physiologic arousal leads to the return of more normal sleep-activity cycles and forms the basis of CNS stimulant pharmacotherapy for narcolepsy.

Attention Deficit Hyperactivity Disorder

Attention deficit hyperactivity disorder (ADHD) is characterized by a persistent pattern of inattention or hyperactivity-impulsivity that is more frequent and severe than typically observed in individuals of a comparable developmental level.

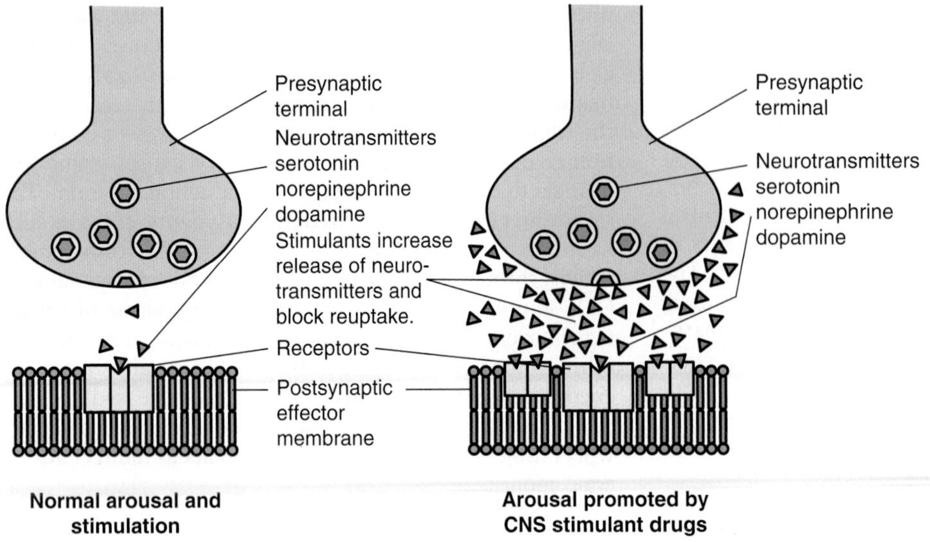

FIGURE 22.2 CNS arousal.

It afflicts between 3% and 5% of children and may persist into adult life at prevalence rates of 1% to 2%. Symptoms of ADHD include low frustration tolerance, short attention span, impulsivity, distractibility, and usually hyperactivity. These symptoms may result in poor school performance and difficulty with peer or parental relationships. Some studies suggest that the etiology of ADHD involves a dopamine deficiency because the three most effective stimulants for this disorder—dextroamphetamine, pemoline, and methylphenidate—all enhance dopamine concentrations. The management of the disorder may be complex but usually involves pharmacotherapy with one or more of the CNS stimulants. In people with ADHD, the stimulants act paradoxically and cause a quieting response, allowing for increased concentration and attention and decreased impulsivity and purposeless activity.

Overweight and Obesity

The United States Department of Health and Human Services monitors the health status of Americans. The department developed the National Health and Nutrition Examination Survey (NHANES) in 1971 and has periodically updated the data. The data from NHANES III, released in 1998, indicate that obesity in the United States is epidemic. The most alarming measurement is the increase in the number of Americans who are classified as obese rather than overweight (Table 22.1).

Overweight refers to an excess of body weight compared to set standards. The excess weight may come from muscle, bone, fat, or body water. **Obesity** refers specifically to having an abnormally high proportion of body fat. One can be overweight without being obese, as in the example of a bodybuilder or other athlete who has a lot of muscle. However, many people who are overweight are also obese.

To determine obesity, the measurement of choice for researchers and health care providers is body mass index (BMI). BMI is a direct calculation based on height and weight and is not gender specific. To determine BMI, divide a person's weight in kilograms by height in meters squared [weight (kg)/height squared (m^2)]. Although BMI does not directly measure percentage of body fat, it provides a more accurate measure of overweight and obesity than weight alone. Box 22.1 lists BMI index categories.

In addition to BMI, health professionals may also rely on a person's waist measurement to determine the location of excess body fat and the corresponding health risks. Health risks increase as waist circumference increases. A woman whose waist measures more than 35 inches and a man whose waist measures more than 40 inches may be at particular risk for developing health problems. An increased percentage of abdominal or upper-body fat is related to the risk for developing heart disease, diabetes, high blood pressure, gallbladder disease, stroke, and certain cancers. Body fat concentrated in the lower body (e.g., around the hips) may be less harmful in terms of mortality and morbidity with the exception of varicose veins and orthopedic problems.

Weight regulation is multifactorial. Key endocrine systems involved in weight regulation include the hypothalamic–pituitary axis (HPA), the leptin system, insulin, neuropeptide Y, leptin-regulated hormones, and the autonomic nervous system. Although major endocrine dysfunction may cause obesity, by far the most common causes are overeating and a sedentary lifestyle.

Treating obesity involves a combination of different methods, including modifying eating behavior, implement-

TABLE 22.1 Prevalence of Obesity in the United States

	NHANES II (1976–1980)	NHANES III (1988–1994)	NHANES (1999–2000)
Overweight or obese (BMI ≥25.0)	47%	56%	64%
Obese (BMI ≥30.0)	15%	23%	31%

BOX 22.1 Body Mass Index (BMI) Categories

- Underweight = <18.5
- Normal weight = 18.5–24.9
- Overweight = 25–29.9
- Obese = ≥30

ing and maintaining an exercise program, and using adjunctive pharmacologic therapy to reduce appetite. Drugs used to manage appetite include 5HT and norepinephrine reuptake inhibitors such as sibutramine, stimulants such as methylphenidate, lipase inhibitors such as orlistat, selective serotonin reuptake inhibitors (SSRIs) such as fluoxetine, and serotonin agonists such as phentermine. In morbidly obese patients, surgical intervention called "bariatric" surgery, has been found to be most effective for long-term weight loss.

Respiratory Stimulation

In patients at risk for postoperative pulmonary complications, respiratory depression may be a complication arising from chronic obstructive lung disease and frequent hypercapnia. **Hypercapnia** is a buildup of carbon dioxide levels that may result from pulmonary compromise, frank lung disease, or changes in ventilatory efficacy. The increased levels of carbon dioxide depress the CNS, including the respiratory center, and further compound the problem.

Preterm infants may experience hypercapnia because of their immature respiratory systems. They are prone to postoperative respiratory depression and apnea severe enough to warrant pharmacologic respiratory stimulation. Pharmacologic management of respiratory depression includes administering CNS stimulants such as caffeine and doxapram that act directly on the respiratory center to stimulate effective ventilation and reverse hypercapnia.

C CENTRALLY ACTING CNS STIMULANTS

The centrally acting CNS stimulants are drugs that stimulate the CNS directly or indirectly. This group of drugs includes the amphetamines, methylphenidate, pemoline, and cocaine. Khat and betel are two naturally occurring CNS stimulants. The ideal and most widely used CNS stimulant is dextroamphetamine (Dexedrine, Dextrostat), an amphetamine. This drug is the prototype for the purposes of discussing the central CNS stimulants. Table 22.2 presents a summary of selected CNS stimulants.

NURSING MANAGEMENT OF THE PATIENT RECEIVING P DEXTROAMPHETAMINE

Core Drug Knowledge

Pharmacotherapeutics

The major therapeutic uses of dextroamphetamine include treatment of narcolepsy and ADHD and anorectic adjunct therapy in obesity. Dextroamphetamine is occasionally used to treat refractory depression, which is an unlabeled use. As a stimulant, dextroamphetamine is classified as a Schedule II drug, which means its use is tightly controlled.

Pharmacokinetics

Following oral ingestion, dextroamphetamine has an onset of 20 to 60 minutes and a duration of 5 hours. The sustained-release form of the drug has an onset of 60 to 90 minutes and lasts 6 to 10 hours. The half-life ranges between 10 and 30 hours. Dextroamphetamine is metabolized by the liver and is excreted, partly unchanged and partly in the form of inactive metabolites, in the urine. This process peaks at 12 to 24 hours.

Pharmacodynamics

The exact mechanism of action of dextroamphetamine is unknown, although it is likely that indirect alpha- and beta-adrenergic activity mediates both central and peripheral effects. Dextroamphetamine causes the release of norepinephrine and, in higher doses, dopamine in adrenergic nerve terminals. It also interferes with the reuptake of dopamine. The sites of action in the CNS are the cerebral cortex and the RAS. The drug's anorectic effects are likely secondary to CNS stimulation in the hypothalamic satiety-feeding center.

Contraindications and Precautions

Dextroamphetamine is contraindicated in patients with advanced arteriosclerosis, symptomatic cardiovascular disease, moderate to severe hypertension, hyperthyroidism, known hypersensitivity or idiosyncratic reactions to other sympathomimetic drugs, glaucoma, or a history of drug abuse. Dextroamphetamine use in patients with these disorders places them at risk for hypertension, increased intraocular pressure, or abuse of the drug. Because of its pressor effects, dextroamphetamine is contraindicated during the first 14 days after discontinuing monoamine oxidase inhibitor (MAOI) therapy, because MAOI therapy itself may predispose the patient toward elevated blood pressure. Therefore, this 14-day washout period for MAOIs must be observed to prevent hypertensive crisis. Stimulant drugs should not be used in children with ADHD and concomitant Tourette syndrome or tics because stimulants will exacerbate these motor disorders.

Caution is warranted in older adult patients with even mild hypertension because the adrenergic stimulation of the amphetamines increases blood pressure. Monitoring the growth and development of children who take amphetamines is important because amphetamines have been associated with increased growth hormone secretion. Growth suppression is also common in children, although the two phenomena may be distinct. Dextroamphetamine is assigned to pregnancy category C, and women should not use it during the first trimester of pregnancy or during lactation. If its use is required during such periods, the prescriber should monitor treatment carefully to prevent fetal growth abnormalities or irritability in the breast-fed infant.

Some formulations of dextroamphetamine contain yellow dye No. 5 (tartrazine), which may cause allergic-type reactions (including bronchial asthma) in certain susceptible individuals. This sensitivity is rare, although it is frequently seen in patients who also have aspirin hypersensitivity.

TABLE 22.2 Summary of Selected (C) CNS Stimulants

Drug (Trade) Name	Selected Indications	Route and Dosage Range	Pharmacokinetics
Stimulants			
(P) dextro-amphetamine (Dexedrine, Dextrostat, Dexedrine Spansules)	ADHD, narcolepsy	Dexedrine, Dextrostat *Adult:* PO, initially, 5 mg bid to a maximum of 60 mg/d in divided doses q4–5h *Child:* PO, 2.5–10 mg/d in single dose up to maximum of 40 mg/d	*Onset:* 20–60 min *Duration:* 5 h $t_{1/2}$: 10–30 h
	Exogenous obesity	*Adult:* PO, 5–30 mg/d in divided doses of 5–10 mg, 30–60 min before meals or 10–15 mg in the morning (long-acting form) *Child:* Not recommended for children <12 y	
	ADHD, narcolepsy	Dexedrine Spansules *Adult:* PO, 10 mg qd	*Onset:* 60–90 min *Duration:* 6–10 h $t_{1/2}$: 10–30 h
amphetamine salts (Adderall, Adderall XR)	ADHD	Adderall *Adult and adolescent:* PO, initially, 5 mg 1–2 times/d; maximum dose: 60 mg/d *Child 6–12 y:* initially, 5 mg, 1–2 times/d; maximum dose: 40 mg/d *Child 3–5 y:* PO, initially, 2.5 mg PO once daily; maximum: 0.1–0.5 mg/kg/d *Child <3 y:* safety and efficacy not established.	*Onset:* 30–60 min *Duration:* 4–6 h $t_{1/2}$: 10–13 h
	Narcolepsy	*Adult and adolescent:* PO, 5–60 mg PO per day in divided doses; initially, 10 mg once daily *Child 6–12 y:* PO, 5–60 mg PO per day in divided doses; initially, 5 mg once daily *Child <6 y:* safety and efficacy not established.	
	ADHD	Adderall XR *Adult, adolescent, and child >6 y:* PO, initially, 10 mg once daily; maximum: 30 mg/d *Child <6 y:* safety and efficacy not established.	*Onset:* 30–60 min *Duration:* 9 h $t_{1/2}$: 10–13 h
dexmethylphenidate (Focalin)	ADHD	*Adult and child ≥6 y:* PO, initially, 2.5 mg twice daily; may adjust dose at weekly intervals in 2.5–5 mg increments; maximum: 20 mg/d (10 mg PO twice daily) *Child <6 y:* safety and efficacy have not been established.	*Onset:* Rapid *Duration:* 2–5 h $t_{1/2}$: 2.2 h
methylphenidate (Ritalin, Ritalin SR, Ritalin LA)	ADHD, narcolepsy	Ritalin *Adult:* PO, initially, 5 mg bid to a maximum of 10–60 mg/d in 2–3 divided doses, 30–45 min before meals *Child ≥6 y:* PO, 0.3–2 mg/kg/day; Maximum dosage: 60 mg/day *Child <6 y (weight ≥25 kg):* PO, 2.5–5 mg twice daily before breakfast and lunch; maximum dose: 20 mg tid *Child <6 y (weight <25 kg):* PO, 2.5 mg twice daily before breakfast and lunch; maximum dose: 15 mg tid	*Onset:* 15–30 min *Duration:* 2.5–4 h $t_{1/2}$: 1.5–2.5 h
		Ritalin SR *Adult, adolescent, and child ≥6 y:* PO, 20 mg qd to a maximum of 60 mg/d *Child <6 y:* safety and efficacy not established.	*Onset:* 15–30 min *Duration:* 6–8 h $t_{1/2}$: 4 h
		Ritalin LA *Adult, adolescent, and child ≥6 y:* PO, 20 mg once daily in the morning; maximum of 60 mg/d *Child <6 y:* safety and efficacy not established.	*Onset:* 15–30 min *Duration:* 8 h $t_{1/2}$: 2–7 h

(continued)

TABLE 22.2 Summary of Selected (C) CNS Stimulants (continued)

Drug (Trade) Name	Selected Indications	Route and Dosage Range	Pharmacokinetics
methylphenidate (Metadate CD, Metadate ER)	ADHD, narcolepsy	Metadate CD *Adult, adolescent, and child* ≥*6 y:* PO, 20 mg once daily in the morning; maximum: 60 mg/d PO. *Child <6 y:* safety and efficacy not established Metadate ER *Adult, adolescent, and child* ≥*6 y:* PO, 20 mg tid *Child <6 y:* safety and efficacy not established.	*Onset:* 15–30 min *Duration:* 8 h $t_{1/2}$: 6.8 h *Onset:* 15–30 min *Duration:* 8 h $t_{1/2}$: 3–4 h
methylphenidate (Concerta)	ADHD	*Adult, adolescent, and child* ≥*6 y:* PO, initially, 18 mg qd; maximum, 54 mg/d *Child <6 y:* safety and efficacy not established.	*Onset:* 1 h *Duration:* 12 h $t_{1/2}$: 3.5 h
methylphenidate (Methylin, Methylin Chewable, Methylin ER)	ADHD Narcolepsy	Methylin; Methylin Chewable *Adult:* PO, 20–30 mg in divided doses preferably before meals; maximum dose: 60 mg/d *Child >6 y:* 5 mg bid before breakfast and lunch; maximum dose: 60 mg/d Methylin ER *Adult:* PO, 20 mg bid maximum, 60 mg/d	*Onset:* Rapid *Duration:* 4–6 h $t_{1/2}$: 3 h *Onset:* 15–30 min *Duration:* 6 h $t_{1/2}$: 3–4 h
pemoline (Cylert, Cylert chewable)	ADHD	*Adult and child >6 y:* PO, 37.5–112.5 mg/d	*Onset:* 30–45 min *Duration:* 8–12 h $t_{1/2}$: 11–13 h
	Narcolepsy; excessive day-time sleepiness	*Adult:* PO, 50–200 mg/d in divided doses	
Nonstimulants			
atomoxetine (Straterra)	ADHD	*Adult and child* ≥*6 y and weight* ≥*70 kg:* PO, 40 mg/d in 1 or 2 divided doses; titrate slowly to maximum dose of 100 mg/d in 1 or 2 divided doses; maximum: of 80 mg/d if administered with other cytochrome P-450 enzyme (CYP) 2D6 inhibitor *Adolescent and child* ≥*6 y and weight <70 kg:* PO, 0.5 mg/kg/d in 1 or 2 divided doses; titrate slowly to a maximum dose of 1.2 mg/kg/d in 1 or 2 divided doses *Child <6 y:* safety and efficacy not established.	*Onset:* Rapid *Duration:* Unknown $t_{1/2}$: 4–5.2 h

Dextroamphetamine should be used with caution to avoid overdose or dependence. The least amount feasible should be prescribed or dispensed at any one time to minimize the possibility of overdosage. Patients should be advised not to discontinue therapy abruptly because rebound symptoms may occur. As tolerance develops, particularly to the anorectic effects of the drug, the recommended dose should not be exceeded in an attempt to increase the effect. Instead, the drug should be discontinued. Patients who have recently ceased smoking cigarettes or using other products that contain nicotine may show a hypertensive sensitivity to dextroamphetamine, partly because of the absence of the vasoconstrictive toning effects of nicotine.

Adverse Effects

Dextroamphetamine may produce the prototypical effects of all CNS stimulants: decreased appetite, rebound irritability and depression, headache, jittery feeling, GI upset, sleep difficulties, anxiety, and increased blood pressure or heart rate. Blood glucose may also elevate; therefore, diabetic patients need to monitor their blood glucose closely. Increased ocular irritation, resulting from decreased lacrimation, and mydriasis are two visual adverse effects that may interfere with activities such as driving. Occasionally, those with allergic tendencies may experience urticaria when taking dextroamphetamine. Finally, the pronounced sympathomimetic action of dextroamphetamine may lead to an inability to ejaculate and either increased or decreased libido.

Drug Interactions

Considerable care must be exercised when administering dextroamphetamine with many other classes of drugs. One noteworthy feature of anorectic drugs is their ability to cause rapid change in nutritional status, which may lead to cachexia and hypoproteinemia and thus possibly alter the pharmacokinetics of other drugs. CNS depressants, if

administered with CNS stimulants, will counteract each other and leave only residual adverse effects. Table 22.3 lists agents that interact with dextroamphetamine.

Dextroamphetamine may cause elevations in plasma corticosteroid levels beyond normal diurnal variations, which may interfere with serum or urinary steroid determinations. Dextroamphetamine use in children with ADHD has been associated with increased levels of growth hormone and with hyperkalemia from rhabdomyolysis caused by the drug.

Maximal absorption of dextroamphetamine occurs in the alkaline environment of the small intestine. Therefore, acidic juices and fruits may impair GI absorption. In addition, foods that acidify urine increase the renal clearance of dextroamphetamine and may lower serum levels. This effect is seen with the anorectic influence of dextroamphetamine, which prompts a form of fasting ketoacidosis and leads to enhanced excretion.

Assessment of Relevant Core Patient Variables

Health Status

Evaluate the patient for pre-existing medical or mental health problems that may exacerbate the symptoms of ADHD. Checking the patient's history is important for ruling out any contraindications to the pharmacotherapy, including other drug therapies and drug and alcohol abuse. Question the patient regarding the use of nonprescription drugs, particularly those with sympathomimetic effects, because patients often do not report the occasional use of over-the-counter (OTC) drugs unless questioned.

Evaluate the patient for advanced arteriosclerosis, symptomatic cardiovascular disease, moderate to severe hypertension, hyperthyroidism, glaucoma, agitated states, a history of drug abuse, a recent history of MAOI use, or known hypersensitivity or idiosyncrasy to the sympathomimetic amines, all of which are contraindications for the use of dextroamphetamine.

Document baseline physical assessment data including height, weight, and vital signs. In addition, an electrocardiogram (ECG) is important for ruling out any cardiovascular abnormalities that CNS stimulants might exacerbate.

Life Span and Gender

Ask whether the patient is pregnant. If the patient is pregnant, dextroamphetamine should be used only if absolutely necessary because it is not known whether dextroamphetamine causes fetal abnormalities (pregnancy category C). If the patient is breast-feeding, monitoring the infant for CNS stimulation is important. In the event of CNS stimulation in the infant, the mother may need to discontinue the drug. Very young and very old patients may be at higher risk for injury because of CNS adverse effects of agitation and restlessness. Monitoring children's growth is important because dextroamphetamine may cause growth retardation.

Lifestyle, Diet, and Habits

Ask the patient about his or her regular consumption of caffeine-containing drinks such as tea, coffee, and cola because they may increase the adverse effects associated with dextroamphetamine.

Support adherence to the drug regimen to enhance the patient's quality of life. People involved in shift work need

TABLE 22.3 Agents That Interact With P Dextroamphetamine

Interactants	Effect and Significance	Nursing Management
acidifying agents, GI acidifying agents (guanethidine, reserpine, glutamic acid HCl, ascorbic acid, fruit juices)	Decreased absorption of dextroamphetamine Lowered blood levels of dextroamphetamine	Instruct patient to avoid acidic foods. Inform patient of possibly reduced effect of medication (especially of the antihypertensive guanethidine).
Urinary acidifying agents (ammonium chloride, sodium acid phosphate)	Increased urinary excretion and lowered blood levels of dextroamphetamine	Drug may be of therapeutic use in overdose.
alkalinizing agents, GI alkalinizing agents (sodium bicarbonate)	Increased absorption of dextroamphetamine Higher blood levels of dextroamphetamine	Avoid administering alkaline agents or increase dosing interval.
urinary alkalinizing agents (sodium bicarbonate)	Prolonged effects of dextroamphetamine	Avoid administering alkaline agents or increase dosing interval.
tricyclic antidepressants	Enhanced dextroamphetamine effects	Avoid administering dextroamphetamine to a patient taking a tricyclic antidepressant, if possible. Otherwise, monitor patient closely for seizures, hypertension.
MAO inhibitors	Exacerbation of dextroamphetamine effects, hypertensive crisis, cerebral bleeding	Avoid; allow proper MAOI washout period.
furazolidone	Increased sensitivity to anorexiants	Monitor for signs and symptoms of amphetamine toxicity; reduce dose as prescribed.
phenothiazines	Diminished effects of dextroamphetamine; may increase psychosis	Avoid; may be of therapeutic use in overdose.

to adjust the timing of their doses to avoid sleep disturbances and allow for normal appetite. Be mindful of the high abuse potential for dextroamphetamine and assess patients carefully for a history of drug or alcohol abuse.

Environment

Dextroamphetamine may be administered in any setting by physicians, nurses, or patients. Therefore, assess the safety of the patient's environment. When the patient is a child, it is advisable for parents to store and monitor the drugs.

Culture and Inherited Traits

In some immigrant populations, alternative therapies and drug use are a part of religious or cultural practice. Therefore, it is important to determine the nature and type of alternative therapy or ritual drug use to avoid drug–drug interactions and to maximize the therapeutic effects of dextroamphetamine.

Nursing Diagnoses and Outcomes

- Disturbed Sleep Pattern related to drug effects or caffeine use
  Desired outcome: *The patient maintains normal sleep patterns through proper use of sleep hygiene measures and bedtime (hour of sleep [HS]) sedation.*
- Delayed Growth and Development related to drug effects
  Desired outcome: *The patient maintains a normal growth and development profile.*
- Disturbed Sensory Perception related to drug response
  Desired outcome: *The patient remains free from sensory and perceptual disturbances.*
- Imbalanced Nutrition: Less than Body Requirements related to amphetamine abuse and anorexia
  Desired outcome: *The patient maintains adequate nutrition.*
- Nonadherence to Therapeutic Regimen related to lack of motivation, poor self-image, or negative effects of prescribed drug
  Desired outcome: *The patient adheres to the drug regimen.*

Planning and Intervention

Maximizing Therapeutic Effects

It is important to administer dextroamphetamine with food in the morning and no fewer than 6 hours before bedtime, preferably longer for the sustained-release formulations. Inform patients and family members that improvements may not be seen until several weeks after the treatment is initiated. A great deal of emotional and psychological support is necessary during this interval, particularly because families often feel guilty about the disorders being treated. It is important to explain to the obese individual that anorectic agents are used only to supplement a combined program of calorie reduction, nutritional counseling and adjustment, and systematic exercise of large muscle blocks. Enhance support by encouraging the individual to attend self-support groups and psychotherapy. Explain that individuals suffering from narcolepsy, ADHD, or obesity will usually benefit from programs designed to foster and enhance self-esteem.

Minimizing Adverse Effects

Monitor for adverse effects of dextroamphetamine and intervene if they occur. In patients experiencing decreased appetite, administer the morning dose of medication before or with breakfast to ensure a good caloric intake at the beginning of the day. Monitor for rebound irritability and depression as the stimulant wears off. Consult with the prescriber to change the time or frequency of dosing if these symptoms are intolerable. Monitor also for headache. Intermittent headaches may be treated with acetaminophen; however, if frequent headaches occur, contact the prescriber to decrease the dose of stimulant or possibly change to a different formulation. To minimize gastrointestinal (GI) distress, administer the medication with meals.

In the event of toxicity or overdose, it is necessary to monitor vital signs and anticipate use of anticonvulsants and antipsychotics. Patients who are experiencing drug toxicity or overdose are vulnerable, and they must be placed in a nonstimulating yet supportive environment where they are protected from hurting themselves and kept from injuring others. Reassure the patient with drug toxicity or overdose, particularly because profound depression of systems initially stimulated by the drug may occur.

Providing Patient and Family Education

An important component of health promotion is the encouragement and support of patients taking dextroamphetamine and their families. Ensure that patient and family education includes explaining the importance of adhering to dosing instructions and dosage scheduling, and understanding recommendations regarding possible adverse effects, other drugs to avoid, drug storage, missed doses, abuse potential, and monitoring the effects of therapy.

- Cautioning all patients treated with dextroamphetamine therapy about adverse effects and the possibility of overdosing is important. Advise patients and their families about managing adverse effects and about when to consult with their caregivers if self-management is ineffective or if serious and persistent adverse effects continue. If toxicity or overdosing is suspected, it is important to decrease frequency of dosing.
- Encourage patients to avoid other stimulants during dextroamphetamine therapy, including caffeinated beverages, because these may lead to exaggerated CNS stimulation, irritability, and nervousness.
- Alert patients and parents or caregivers to keep dextroamphetamine in safe storage, out of children's reach.

CRITICAL THINKING SCENARIO

Pharmacotherapy and attention deficit hyperactivity disorder

A family friend has a child who has been diagnosed with ADHD. The friend asks you what you think about treating this disorder with drugs. Instead of giving an opinion, construct a patient teaching plan to help this person understand how to maximize the effects of pharmacotherapy. Present three topics for discussion with the family, and explain how you would prioritize these topics.

- Advise patients to take dextroamphetamine early in the day, unless otherwise instructed, to avoid nighttime insomnia. If the tablets are sustained release or long acting, advise patients not to crush or chew them. Tell patients to notify their prescriber if they experience nervousness, restlessness, insomnia, dizziness, dry mouth, diarrhea, constipation, or an unpleasant taste; a dosage adjustment may be necessary. It is also important to tell patients to avoid all other drugs (including OTC drugs) while taking dextroamphetamine unless the prescriber recommends them.
- Tell patients and family members what to do if they miss a dose of dextroamphetamine. When the patient misses one dose, it is important for him or her to take that dose as soon as possible to prevent trouble sleeping. However, the dose should be taken no later than 6 hours before bedtime for the short-acting form, and no later than 10 to 14 hours before bedtime for the long-acting form. If the patient does not remember the missed dose until the next day, he or she should skip the missed dose and return to the normal dosing schedule. The patient must never take double doses of the drug.
- Advise patients that dextroamphetamine may impair their ability to engage in potentially hazardous activities, such as operating machinery or driving vehicles, particularly if the effects of drug therapy on the patient are not yet known.

Ongoing Assessment and Evaluation

Monitor periodic growth and development data for children throughout therapy. Monitor for adverse effects such as anorexia, irritability, depression, headache, GI distress, anxiety, cardiovascular changes, and sleep deprivation. Review the patient's diet periodically and remind the patient to abstain from caffeine-rich products.

It is important to monitor patients for responses to therapy, including improvements in mental and behavioral symptoms in children, decreased baseline rate of motor activity, weight loss, and decreased frequency of narcoleptic attacks.

The patient should show a reduction in symptoms or symptom severity. Patients receiving dextroamphetamines for ADHD should show improved attention span or decreased impulsivity. Patients receiving dextroamphetamines for obesity should show documented weight loss. Patients receiving dextroamphetamines for narcolepsy should have fewer or less severe episodes. The patient and family should show an increased understanding of how to recognize and manage adverse effects and explain how to store and administer drug therapy safely.

MEMORY CHIP

P Dextroamphetamine

- Releases dopamine and norepinephrine in adrenergic nerve terminals and interferes with the reuptake of dopamine; sites of action in the CNS are the cerebral cortex and the reticular activating system
- Most common adverse effects: restlessness, insomnia, dizziness, overstimulation, palpitations, tachycardia, hypertension, dry mouth, unpleasant taste, and diarrhea
- Maximizing therapeutic effects: Take with food in the morning and not less than 6 hours before bedtime.
- Minimizing adverse effects: Obtain a baseline nursing history and physical assessment to compare with treatment outcomes; important assessment items include sleep disturbances, nervousness, complete diet history (including use of caffeine), height, weight, ECG, and drug or alcohol abuse.
- Most important patient education: importance of adhering to dosing instructions, dosage scheduling, possible adverse effects, other drugs to avoid, drug storage, missed doses, abuse potential, and monitoring the effects of therapy

Drugs Closely Related to P Dextroamphetamine

Amphetamine Salts

Amphetamine salts (Adderall, Adderall XR) are a combination of amphetamine and dextroamphetamine. Adderall was formerly marketed as Obetrol, a product used primarily for adjunctive short-term treatment of exogenous obesity. The current formula consists of mixed salts of amphetamine aspartate, amphetamine sulfate, dextroamphetamine saccharate, and dextroamphetamine sulfate. It is approved to treat ADHD or narcolepsy. Like dextroamphetamine, the mechanism of action of Adderall on mental and behavioral conditions is unclear. However, its ability to improve symptoms in ADHD is well documented. These include improved attention span, decreased distractibility, increased ability to follow directions or complete tasks, and decreased impulsivity and aggression. The contraindications and the adverse effect profile of Adderall are similar to those for dextroamphetamine. The benefit of Adderall is its once-daily dosing and its longer duration of action than that of dextroamphetamine. For patients with difficulty swallowing, the Adderall XR capsule may be opened and the beads sprinkled in applesauce.

Methylphenidate

Methylphenidate (Ritalin, Ritalin SR, Ritalin LA, Metadate-ER, Metadate-CD, Concerta) is an orally administered CNS stimulant that is chemically and pharmacologically similar to the amphetamines. It is clinically used to treat ADHD and narcolepsy. The CNS actions of methylphenidate are milder than those of the amphetamines and have more noticeable effects on mental activities than on motor activities. Methylphenidate shares the abuse potential of the amphetamines and is a Drug Enforcement Administration (DEA) Schedule II controlled substance.

Methylphenidate comes in many formulations. Although the active ingredient is the same, these drugs have different pharmacokinetics because of their structure or method of delivery. Ritalin is the oldest available medication for ADHD and is considered the drug of choice by many prescribers. Its quick onset and short duration make it possible to individualize dosing. Ritalin SR is an extended release form of methylphenidate with an approximate duration of 8 hours. Ritalin SR tablets must be swallowed whole. Ritalin LA is a long-acting formulation of methylphenidate that provides all-day treatment with one morning dose. This dosing regimen eliminates the social stigma felt by children who have to bring

medication to school and decreases the possibility of medication misuse. Advantages include once-daily dosing and the potential for sprinkle administration, if needed.

Methylin is another trade name of methylphenidate. It has three formulations: Methylin and Methylin Chewable tablets, which are comparable to Ritalin; and Methylin-ER, which is comparable to Ritalin SR and Metadate-ER. Methylin Chewable tablets should be taken with 8 ounces of water to minimize the risk for choking. Methylin is also available as a transdermal patch; however, at this time, the patch is not approved by the FDA for use in the United States.

Metadate-ER is another extended-release form that uses a two-phase process to deliver an initial rapid release of methylphenidate followed by a second continuous-release phase. Metadate-CD has a controlled delivery system that uses a multiparticulate bead system, with each bead acting as a drug reservoir. The individual beads are coated with different polymers that dissolve and release at different times. Metadate-CD capsules contain immediate-release and extended-release beads in a ratio of 30:70. It is similar to Concerta in its duration of action; however, serum drug levels of Metadate-CD are higher than Concerta for the initial 4 hours of activity. Advantages of Metadate-CD include once-daily dosing, which is especially important for school-aged children, and the ability for sprinkle administration, if necessary. Disadvantages include cost and the fixed ratio of immediate-release to extended-release beads.

Concerta is a once-a-day formulation of methylphenidate that is targeted at patients with moderate ADHD. There is a dose-related size problem with the capsules. Many patients have difficulty swallowing the larger-dose capsules. Patients with severe ADHD frequently need a larger dose of methylphenidate than can be offered in the Concerta formulation. The size of the capsule is related to its unique delivery system. The outside of the capsule dissolves and releases the initial methylphenidate within an hour. The inner core has a push layer and a drug layer.

Once in the GI tract, water enters the osmotic system and dissolves or suspends the drug in the tablet's core. The drug is then released by osmotic pressure at a controlled rate through a laser-drilled hole in the membrane. The capsule itself is excreted in the feces. Because of its delivery system, Concerta cannot be crushed, chewed, or opened in any way. Its major advantage is the long duration of action. Its major disadvantage is the size of the capsules.

Yet another variation on methylphenidate dosing, achieved with drug holidays, is the subject of ongoing research (Box 22.2).

Dexmethylphenidate

Dexmethylphenidate (Focalin) is a CNS stimulant that is chemically similar to the amphetamines and is an isomer of methylphenidate. It is used in managing ADHD. Dexmethylphenidate is thought to block the reuptake of norepinephrine and dopamine into the presynaptic neuron and increase the release of these monoamines into the extraneuronal space. This activity results in improved attention spans, decreased distractibility, increased ability to follow directions or complete tasks, and decreased impulsivity and aggression in patients with ADHD. Although dexmethylphenidate does not produce a physical dependence, it may induce tolerance or psychic dependence. The adverse effects of dexmethylphenidate are similar to those of other stimulant drugs. They occur relatively frequently but are usually mild at normally prescribed dosages. They may be more frequent or severe during the initial days of therapy, but most adverse effects disappear within a few weeks of continued use.

FOCUS ON RESEARCH

Box 22.2 Methylphenidate and Drug Holidays

Martins, S., Tramontina, S., Polanczyk, G., et al. (2004). Weekend holidays during methylphenidate use in ADHD children: A randomized clinical trial. *Journal of Child and Adolescent Psychopharmacology, 14*(2), 195–206.

The Study

In this double-blind, 28-day study, the researchers assessed whether weekend drug "holidays" (brief cessation of drug therapy) during methylphenidate treatment would alter the efficacy and tolerability of methylphenidate in 40 children with attention deficit hyperactivity disorder (ADHD). The children (all male) were randomized into two groups: the first group received methylphenidate twice daily for 7 days; the second group received methylphenidate twice daily on weekdays and placebo on the weekends. Parents completed the Conners' Abbreviated Rating Scale (ABRS) to assess ADHD symptoms and the Barkley's Side Effect Rating Scale (SERS) to assess adverse effects on weekends. Additionally, teachers completed the ABRS on each Monday. Overall, ABRS scores decreased significantly in both groups, indicating a reduction in symptoms during methylphenidate therapy. The difference in ABRS scores between the two groups was not significantly different, either on weekends or on weekdays. However, the group that took drug holidays had significantly less severe insomnia and somewhat less interference with appetite. The researchers concluded that weekend holidays during methylphenidate therapy reduce the adverse effects of insomnia and appetite suppression without increasing the symptoms of ADHD, either on weekends or upon return to the classroom.

Nursing Implications

Drug holidays during treatment of ADHD is a controversial topic. The American Academy of Pediatrics (AAP) recommends that the treating clinician, the parents, and the child, in collaboration with school personnel, should identify specific target outcomes to guide management. They recommend use of stimulants along with appropriate behavior therapy, using the target outcomes to guide changes in medication or behavior therapy. Teach the patient and family the goals of therapy and caution parents to consult with the child's clinician before initiating a drug holiday.

Pemoline

Pemoline (Cylert) is an oral CNS stimulant with pharmacologic actions similar to those of the amphetamines and methylphenidate; however, its sympathomimetic effects are minimal. Benefits to pemoline therapy include once-a-day dosing because of its long half-life and its classification as a DEA Schedule IV controlled substance.

Pemoline is indicated for use in ADHD. Pemoline has been used off-label to fight fatigue in patients with multiple sclerosis (MS), as an alternative treatment for narcolepsy, and to fight fatigue associated with sustained military operations. Pemoline has caused hepatic dysfunction, including autoimmune hepatitis, jaundice, and elevated hepatic enzymes and hepatic failure resulting in death. If no noticeable symptomatic improvement occurs within 3 weeks, pemoline should be discontinued because of its risk for hepatic failure.

Periodic liver function tests should be obtained for patients on long-term therapy.

Cocaine

Cocaine is used therapeutically as a local anesthetic. Its widest use, however, is as an illicit stimulant, which represents a substantial abuse problem.

Drugs Significantly Different From P Dextroamphetamine

Atomoxetine

Atomoxetine (Straterra) is a selective norepinephrine reuptake inhibitor initially evaluated for use as an antidepressant. Although it failed to demonstrate efficacy as an antidepressant, further research showed it to be highly effective for ADHD. Atomoxetine is the first ADHD medication that is not a stimulant. Although its true mechanism of action is unknown, it is thought involve the selective inhibition of the presynaptic norepinephrine transporter. Atomoxetine is metabolized by the cytochrome P-450 2D6 isoenzyme. Concurrent use of drugs that inhibit this pathway, such as SSRIs, increases the serum concentration of atomoxetine and extend its half-life substantially. The only contraindication to the use of atomoxetine is concurrent use of MAOIs. In patients who have been exposed to both drug classes, a 2-week washout period should take place after discontinuing either drug or before starting either drug. Atomoxetine appears to have a substantial and dose-related effect on growth. Patients may lose weight and gain height while on atomoxetine. It may also increase blood pressure and heart rate and can cause additive cardiovascular effects with albuterol and pressor agents. Atomoxetine is generally well tolerated, with the most common adverse effects listed in pediatric patients being dyspepsia, nausea, vomiting, fatigue, appetite suppression, dizziness, and mood swings. The most common adverse effects listed in adult patients are constipation, dry mouth, nausea, appetite suppression, dizziness, insomnia, sexual dysfunction, urinary dysfunction (hesitation or retention), and dysmenorrhea. The major advantage of atomoxetine is that, because it is not a stimulant, it is not a Schedule II drug—samples can be provided to physicians, prescriptions can be refilled, and the drug does not have be securely stored.

Antihypertensive Agents

Antihypertensive agents such as clonidine (Catapres) and guanfacine (Tenex) may be prescribed with a stimulant to manage the symptoms of ADHD. These drugs help with impulsivity, sleep problems, frustration tolerance, and activity. They do not have any known effect on inattention. Common adverse effects include drowsiness, dry mouth, and constipation. In-depth information regarding these antihypertensive agents is located in Chapter 27.

Antidepressants

Antidepressants may be used in managing ADHD, especially if comorbid diagnoses are suspected. Tricyclic antidepressants (TCAs), such as such as amitriptyline (Elavil), desipramine (Norpramin), nortriptyline (Pamelor), and imipramine (Tofranil), improve concentration, mood, and hyperactivity and help regulate emotional ups and downs. It is important to monitor cardiac activity, especially in children, when patients are taking these drugs. SSRIs, such as fluvoxamine (Luvox), paroxetine (Paxil), and fluoxetine (Prozac), are used primarily when mood or anxiety disorders are thought to coexist. SSRIs may increase impulsivity. Venlafaxine (Effexor) is thought to provide the benefits of both TCAs and SSRIs. It is not generally used in children. Common adverse effects with antidepressant drugs include headache, insomnia, weight loss, nervousness, and either constipation or diarrhea. Many of these adverse effects abate after continued use of the drug. For more information regarding antidepressant drugs, see Chapter 17.

Khat

Khat (pronounced "cot") is a natural CNS sympathomimetic stimulant from the *Catha edulis* plant, also known as qat, kat, chat, kus-es-salahin, mirra, tohai, tschat, catha, quat, Abyssinian tea, African tea, and African salad. In the United States, khat usage is usually seen among East African and Middle Eastern immigrants, particularly in large cities that have large representative subpopulations of these immigrants.

The active ingredients in khat are cathinone and cathine, both of which are structurally similar to dextroamphetamine. Fresh leaves contain both ingredients, whereas older leaves contain only cathine. The user typically chews a mouthful of fresh leaves, leaving the wad inside the mouth so that intermittent chewing will release further active components. Users report a mild euphoria similar to that experienced with amphetamine or cocaine but without the "rush" sensation. In addition to the euphoria, users report that khat sharpens and clarifies thinking and lifts the spirits; however, after the effects wear off, the user usually experiences a mild let-down or depressive mood.

Khat is used traditionally for religious and recreational purposes and is not considered a drug of abuse. Because khat is a sympathomimetic, users sometimes present with precipitated cardiovascular complaints or with psychiatric symptoms from excessive use. Under these circumstances, complete a culturally sensitive assessment and ask about religious and recreational rituals.

Khat is freely available in shops and restaurants that cater to the ethnic and national groups of Yemen, Somalia, and Ethiopia, even though one of its ingredients, cathinone, is classified as a Schedule I narcotic. Cathine, the ingredient that remains in khat after 48 hours, is classified as a Schedule IV substance. Illegal drug trade laboratories have generated a synthetic variant of cathinone, known as methcathinone or "cat," which has the same effects and uses.

C ANORECTIC AGENTS

Obesity is a complex problem that is very difficult to treat. Current views concerning the cause of obesity favor a disturbance in the hypothalamic set-point, which mediates caloric intake and use and energy expenditure. Although drug therapy is helpful, drugs alone cannot manage weight loss. Diet and exercise are equally important. Common agents used as anorectics include sibutramine, phentermine, adrenergic drugs, serotonergic drugs, and orlistat. This section focuses on sibutramine (Meridia), the prototype anorectic drug. Table 22.4 presents a summary of selected anorectic and respiratory CNS stimulants.

TABLE 22.4 Summary of Selected (C) Anorectic and (C) Respiratory CNS Stimulants

Drug (Trade) Name	Selected Indications	Route and Dosage Range	Pharmacokinetics
(C) Anorectic Stimulants			
[P] sibutramine (Meridia)	Adjunct in obesity	*Adult:* 10 mg qd titrate to a maximum of 15 mg qd *Child <16 y:* not approved	*Onset:* Rapid *Duration:* Unknown $T_{1/2}$: 1.1 hr
benzphetamine (Didrex)	Adjunct in obesity	*Adult:* PO, 25–50 mg once daily *Child:* Not recommended for children younger than 12 y	*Onset:* NA *Duration:* NA $t_{1/2}$: NA
diethylpropion (Tenuate, Dospan, Tepanil)	Adjunct in obesity	*Adult:* PO, 25 mg tid 1 h before meals or 75 mg controlled release at midmorning	*Onset:* Within 1 wk *Duration:* 4–12 h $t_{1/2}$: 8 h
mazindol (Mazanor, Sanorex)	Adjunct in obesity Narcolepsy	*Adult:* PO, 1 mg tid 1 h before meals *Adult:* PO, 3–8 mg/d in single or divided doses	*Onset:* Within 2 wk *Duration:* NA $t_{1/2}$: 30–50 h
phendimetrazine (Adipost, Bontril)	Adjunct in obesity	*Adult:* PO, 35 mg tid; sustained release, 105 mg qid in AM	*Onset:* NA *Duration:* NA $t_{1/2}$: 2–4 h
phentermine (Adipex, Fastin, Zantryl, Obe-Nix)	Adjunct in obesity	*Adult:* PO, 24–30 mg/d 2 h after breakfast or 8 mg tid 30 min before meal *Child:* 12 y, PO, 5–15 mg/d	*Onset:* 1–2 wk *Duration:* Multiple dose, 12 wk $t_{1/2}$: 20 h
phenylpropanolamine (Dexatrim)	Adjunct in obesity	*Adult:* PO, 25 mg q4h or 50 mg q8h or 75 mg SR q12h, not to exceed 150 mg/d	*Onset:* rapid *Duration:* 24 hr $t_{1/2}$: 6 h
Orlistat (Xenical)	Adjunct in obesity	*Adult:* 120 mg TID with meals	*Onset:* 24–48 h *Duration:* Unknown $T_{1/2}$: 1–2 h
(C) Respiratory Stimulants			
[P] caffeine (OTC: Caffedrine, Tirend, NoDoz; prescription: caffeine and sodium benzoate)	Adjunct for analgesia (eg, headache), stimulant effects Postdural puncture headache Neonatal apnea	*Adult:* PO, 100–200 mg q3–4 h *Adult:* IV, 500 mg in 1 to 2 doses; PO, 300–400 as single dose (for postdural headache only) *Child:* IV/PO, 20 mg/kg as a loading dose, then 5–10 mg/kg maintenance dose	*Onset:* PO, 15–45 min *Duration:* NA $t_{1/2}$: 3–5 h
doxapram (Dopram)	Postanesthetic respiratory depression or postanesthetic shivering Drug-induced CNS depression Chronic airway limitation	*Adult:* IV, single injection of 0.5–1 mg/kg, not to exceed 1.5 mg/kg as single dose or 2 mg/kg as multiple doses at 5-min intervals *Adult:* IV, inject priming dose of 2 mg/kg, repeat in 5 min and every 1–2 h until patient awakens *Adult:* IV, mix 400 mg in 180 mL of IV infusion at 1–2 mg/min; do not use longer than 2 h *Child:* Do not give to children younger than 12 y	*Onset:* 20–40 s *Duration:* 5–12 min $t_{1/2}$: 3.4 h

NURSING MANAGEMENT OF THE PATIENT RECEIVING [P] SIBUTRAMINE

Core Drug Knowledge

Pharmacotherapeutics

Sibutramine is a Schedule IV drug used to manage obesity by promoting weight loss and its maintenance. It is indicated for patients with an initial BMI greater than or equal to 30 kg/m^2, or greater than or equal to 27 kg/m^2 with other risk factors such as diabetes mellitus, dyslipidemia, or hypertension.

Pharmacokinetics

Following oral administration, sibutramine is rapidly absorbed from the GI tract and undergoes extensive first-pass metabolism into two pharmacologically active metabolites: M1 and M2. Sibutramine is rapidly and extensively

distributed into tissues. It has a relatively low transfer rate to the fetus during pregnancy.

Sibutramine is metabolized primarily in the liver by the cytochrome P-450 3A4 (CYP3A4) isoenzyme to the active metabolites M1 and M2. These active metabolites are further metabolized into pharmacologically inactive metabolites, M5 and M6. The primary route of excretion for M1 and M2 is hepatic metabolism; for M5 and M6, the primary route is renal excretion.

Pharmacodynamics

Sibutramine inhibits the central reuptake of dopamine, norepinephrine, and serotonin. Unlike other anorectic drugs, it does not release these neurotransmitters. Sibutramine's action on dopamine reuptake is less dramatic than its effects on norepinephrine and serotonin. It is thought that the serotonin mechanism enhances satiety, whereas the norepinephrine mechanism raises the metabolic rate. Sibutramine has no anticholinergic or antihistaminic activity.

Contraindications and Precautions

Because sibutramine is an appetite suppressant, it is contraindicated in patients who are taking other centrally acting appetite suppressant drugs and in patients who have anorexia nervosa. Sibutramine is also contraindicated for use in patients with untreated or poorly controlled hypertension. Because sibutramine undergoes hepatic metabolism and renal excretion, it should not be used in patients with severe hepatic disease or severe renal impairment. Before prescribing sibutramine, the prescriber should exclude organic causes of obesity.

The concomitant use of sibutramine and MAOIs is contraindicated. Because sibutramine substantially increases blood pressure and heart rate in some patients, it should be used cautiously in patients with a history of hypertension, coronary artery disease (CAD), congestive heart failure (CHF), cardiac dysrhythmias, or stroke.

Sibutramine can cause mydriasis and therefore should be used cautiously in patients with closed-angle glaucoma. It should also be used cautiously in patients with a history of seizures. It should be discontinued in any patient who develops seizures while receiving the drug.

Sibutramine should be used cautiously in patients with pre-existing cholelithiasis because weight loss can precipitate or exacerbate gallstone formation.

Adverse Effects

Sibutramine is well tolerated. The most common adverse reactions are anorexia, constipation, insomnia, headache, and dry mouth.

CNS adverse effects include dizziness, nervousness, emotional liability, and CNS stimulation. Cardiovascular adverse effects include tachycardia, vasodilation, hypertension, palpitations, and chest pain. In the GI tract, sibutramine may induce dyspepsia, dysgeusia, abdominal pain, and paradoxical increased appetite.

Because of its effects on serotonin uptake, sibutramine may have an effect on platelet function, resulting in ecchymosis. Rarely, sibutramine may induce seizures.

Drug Interactions

Drug interactions with sibutramine may result in "serotonin syndrome," characterized by CNS irritability, motor weakness, shivering, myoclonus, and altered consciousness. This syndrome may occur when sibutramine is used in conjunction with dextromethorphan, ergot alkaloids, lithium, MAOIs, meperidine, 5-HT receptor agonists, and SSRIs. Drugs that are mediated by CYP3A4 may also interact with sibutramine. Table 22.5 presents these drug interactions.

Assessment of Relevant Core Patient Variables

Health Status

Assess for disorders that contraindicate or require precautions with sibutramine therapy. Assess also for current or recent use of medications that may interact with sibutramine, especially MAOIs. Communicate positive findings to the prescriber before starting sibutramine therapy.

Perform a physical examination that includes calculating the BMI. Sibutramine is indicated for use only with morbidly obese patients. Obtain baseline blood pressure and heart rate parameters because sibutramine may increase both. Weight loss should occur slowly; accordingly, the patient will receive this medication for a prolonged duration. Because of the prolonged duration of sibutramine therapy, it is important to obtain baseline results for laboratory tests, including complete blood count (CBC), liver function, and renal function tests.

Life Span and Gender

Assess female patients for pregnancy or the intention to become pregnant. Sibutramine is classified as pregnancy category C drug because adequate, well-controlled studies with sibutramine have not been conducted in pregnant women. Women of childbearing potential should use adequate contraception while taking sibutramine. Advise patients to notify their physician if they become or intend to become pregnant during sibutramine therapy. Additionally, it is unknown whether sibutramine or its metabolites are excreted in breast milk; therefore, sibutramine is not recommended for breastfeeding mothers. Accordingly, assess female patients for lactation.

Assess for age-related considerations. In older adults, peak plasma concentrations are similar to those in young adults; however, dosing in older adults should be done cautiously, because of a greater likelihood of decreased hepatic, renal, or cardiac function. Safety and effectiveness for patients younger than age 16 years has not been established.

Lifestyle, Diet, and Habits

Assess the patient's diet and make modifications to optimize therapy. Ingesting sibutramine with food delays peak concentration but does not alter efficacy of therapy. Sibutramine is most effective when combined with a low-calorie diet and behavior modification counseling.

Environment

Sibutramine may be administered in any setting by physicians, nurses, or patients. Assess the patient's environment to ensure safety.

Nursing Diagnoses and Outcomes

- Imbalanced Nutrition: Less than Body Requirements, related to anorexia

TABLE 22.5 Agents That Interact With P Sibutramine

Interactants	Effect and Significance	Nursing Management
dextromethorphan	Serotonergic effects of these agents may be additive.	Concurrent use is not recommended. If concurrent use is unavoidable, monitor patient for symptoms of serotonin syndrome.
ergot alkaloids • dihydroergotamine • ergotamine • methysergide	Serotonergic effects of these agents may be additive.	Concurrent use is not recommended. If unavoidable, monitor patient for symptoms of serotonin syndrome.
• lithium	Serotonergic effects of these agents may be additive.	Concurrent use is not recommended. If unavoidable, monitor patient for symptoms of serotonin syndrome.
MAOIs • isocarboxazid • phenelzine • tranylcypromine	Serotonergic effects of these agents may be additive.	Concurrent use is contraindicated. Allow 2 weeks after stopping MAOIs before starting treatment with sibutramine. Allow 2 weeks after stopping sibutramine before starting treatment with MAOIs.
meperidine	Serotonergic effects of these agents may be additive.	Concurrent use is not recommended. If unavoidable, monitor patient for symptoms of serotonin syndrome.
SSRIs • fluoxetine • fluvoxamine • nefazodone • paroxetine • sertraline • venlafaxine	Serotonergic effects of these agents may be additive.	Concurrent use is not recommended. If unavoidable, monitor patient for symptoms of serotonin syndrome.
5-HT receptor agonists • naratriptan • risatriptan • sumatriptan • solmitriptan	Serotonergic effects of these agents may be additive.	Concurrent use is not recommended. If unavoidable, monitor patient for symptoms of serotonin syndrome.
cytochrome P-450 3A4 drugs • erythromycin • clarithromycin • danazol • azole antifungal agents • cimetidine • quinidine • diltiazem • verapamil • loratadine • niacin • propoxyphene	Concurrent use of drugs metabolized by cytochrome P-450 3A4 may inhibit the metabolism of sibutramine, resulting in toxicity.	Monitor blood pressure and heart rate. Monitor for adverse effects.

Desired outcome: *The patient maintains adequate nutrition.*

- Nonadherence to Therapeutic Regimen related to lack of motivation, poor self-image, or negative effects of prescribed drug

  Desired outcome: *The patient adheres to drug regimen.*

Planning and Intervention

Maximizing Therapeutic Effects

Patients should take sibutramine on an empty stomach to maximize peak concentration levels. They should take it only once a day. It is important to remember that sibutramine should be used in conjunction with a low-calorie diet and daily exercise routine for maximum results. Some patients benefit from writing a food journal to assess the amount of food intake and the types of foods consumed.

Minimizing Adverse Effects

Adverse effects are minimized by adhering to the contraindications and precautions for this medication. Refraining from using drugs that may induce serotonin syndrome or elevate the blood pressure and heart rate is especially important. At least 2 weeks should elapse between discontinuing MAOI therapy and initiating sibutramine therapy. Similarly, at least 2 weeks should elapse after stopping sibutramine

therapy and starting MAOI therapy. It is also important for female patients to take precautions to avoid pregnancy and to contact the prescriber immediately if pregnancy occurs.

Providing Patient and Family Education

- An important component of health promotion is encouragement and support of the patient's commitment to weight loss. Remind the patient that sibutramine is only one component in the recipe for weight loss. Behavior modification and exercise are equally important in reaching the patient's goal.
- Educate the patient and family about drugs that may interact with sibutramine and encourage the patient to contact the prescriber before adding any daily medications, even OTC drugs.
- Instruct the patient regarding possible adverse effects of sibutramine therapy, especially the potential for hypertension. When possible, teach the patient and family how to take blood pressure and pulse.
- When working with women, discuss contraception and the importance of notifying the prescriber if the patient becomes pregnant. Discuss also the need to refrain from sibutramine therapy if the patient is breast-feeding.

Ongoing Assessment and Evaluation

Calculate BMI at each follow-up visit in addition to obtaining gross weight measurement. Assessing vital signs is equally important, with a focus on blood pressure and heart rate. When possible, review the patient's food journal and assess the progress of the patient's behavior modification. Reinforce the need for daily exercise to complement sibutramine therapy. Finally, arrange for serial laboratory tests, including CBC, liver function, and renal function tests.

Evaluating the patient routinely is important for assessing progress. With sibutramine therapy, an adequate diet, and regular exercise, the patient should lose between 8 and 10 pounds per month. The patient should not remain on sibutramine therapy if weight loss does not occur. The time frame will depend on the individual's specific variables.

Drugs Closely Related to P Sibutramine

Phentermine

Phentermine is a Schedule IV drug classified as an indirect sympathomimetic. It is used as an adjunct in treating exogenous obesity. Phentermine is available as the hydrochloride salt (Fastin, Zantryl, Adipex-P, Obe-Nix, and others) or as the resin complex (Ionamin). Because phentermine is structurally and chemically related to the amphetamines, the pharmacologic effects are also similar. Appetite suppression is believed to occur through direct stimulation of the satiety center in the hypothalamic and limbic regions. Tolerance to the anorectic effects of phentermine usually develops within a few weeks of starting therapy; therefore, it is indicated for short-term therapy. When tolerance develops to the anorectic effects, it is generally recommended that phentermine be discontinued rather than increased.

Phentermine is contraindicated in patients with advanced arteriosclerosis, agitated states, moderate to severe hypertension, glaucoma, or symptomatic cardiovascular disease including cardiac arrhythmias. Phentermine is not recommended for use in patients with cardiac disease including valvular heart disease. Phentermine should not be combined with any other drug class used to decrease weight.

Adverse effects can affect several body systems. CNS effects include dizziness, dyskinesia, dysphoria, euphoria, headache, insomnia, overstimulation, restlessness, and tremor. Potential ocular effects include blurred vision, mydriasis, and ocular irritation. Cardiovascular effects include hypertension, palpitations, and sinus tachycardia. GI effects include constipation, diarrhea, dysgeusia, nausea and vomiting, and dry mouth. Other adverse reactions include impotence, libido increase, libido decrease, and urticaria.

Adrenergic Drugs

The adrenergic drugs are primarily phenethylamines—drugs similar to amphetamines. These drugs were created by altering the side chain and ring structure of amphetamines to produce drugs that have appetite-suppressing effects with markedly decreased risks for CNS stimulation and abuse. Their mechanism of action is not fully known, but they are thought to directly stimulate the satiety center in the hypothalamus. These drugs include benzphetamine (Didrex), diethylpropion (Tenuate), mazindol (Mazanor, Sanorex), and phendimetrazine (Adipost, Bontril).

Serotonergic Drugs

Anorectic drugs that affect the serotonergic receptors in the brain include SSRIs, which are approved only as antidepressants. They do, however, induce weight loss in the short term. Fluoxetine (Prozac) is the SSRI known best for its ability to induce anorexia. Other SSRI drugs in this class that cause anorexia are venlafaxine (Effexor) and sertraline (Zoloft). These drugs are discussed in depth in Chapter 17.

MEMORY CHIP

P Sibutramine

- Used only for patients with a body mass index diagnostic for morbid obesity
- Inhibits dopamine, norepinephrine, and serotonin
- Major contraindications: uncontrolled hypertension
- Most serious adverse effects: "serotonin syndrome" and hypertension
- Most important patient education: Drug must be used in conjunction with a low-calorie diet and exercise plan.

Drug Significantly Different From P Sibutramine

Orlistat is a GI lipase inhibitor indicated for weight loss and subsequent weight maintenance in morbidly obese patients. As with sibutramine, orlistat is used in conjunction with a reduced-calorie diet and physical activity. Orlistat works nonsystemically to block the absorption of dietary fat by approximately 30%. A thorough discussion of orlistat appears in Chapter 48.

C RESPIRATORY STIMULANTS

Respiratory stimulants are used to manage postsurgical respiratory depression and apnea in preterm neonates. The primary respiratory stimulants are caffeine and doxapram. Caffeine is the prototype respiratory stimulant. It is used to manage postsurgical respiratory depression and apnea in preterm neonates. Because of its CNS stimulation, it is also used to maintain alertness and decrease fatigue. Caffeine is also used nontherapeutically in foods such as cocoa and chocolate and in beverages such as coffee, tea, and colas. It is chemically related to theophylline and possesses some bronchodilatory effects. (Table 22.6 presents potential drug interactions with caffeine.)

NURSING MANAGEMENT OF THE PATIENT RECEIVING P CAFFEINE

Core Drug Knowledge

Pharmacotherapeutics

Caffeine is used in managing neonatal apnea, asthma, drowsiness, and fatigue. It is used in combination with many other drugs such as aspirin, acetaminophen, propoxyphene, and butalbital for treating migraine and other types of headache. Caffeine is also sold without a prescription in products marketed to treat drowsiness or mild water-weight gain.

Pharmacokinetics

Caffeine may be administered orally and intravenously. Orally administered caffeine in an adult is well absorbed from the GI tract, reaching peak plasma concentrations within 50 to 75 minutes. In neonates, oral administration results in peak concentrations in 30 to 120 minutes. Formula feedings do not affect the time to maximum concentrations after oral dosing. Caffeine is distributed rapidly to all body tissues and readily crosses the blood–brain and placental barriers. It is distributed into breast milk.

In adults, caffeine is partially metabolized in the liver. Caffeine metabolism in neonates is limited because of their immature hepatic enzyme systems. Unchanged caffeine and its metabolites are excreted in the urine (see Table 22.5).

Pharmacodynamics

Caffeine is a mild, direct stimulant at all levels of the CNS, which also stimulates the cardiovascular system. Caffeine also stimulates the medullary respiratory center and relaxes bronchial smooth muscle. Caffeine stimulates voluntary muscle and gastric acid secretion, increases renal blood flow, and is a mild diuretic. Caffeine is preferred over theophylline in neonates because of the ease of once-daily administration, reliable oral absorption, and a wide therapeutic window. The cellular mechanism of action is unclear.

Contraindications and Precautions

Caffeine should be used cautiously in patients with anxiety disorders, panic disorder, or both because as a CNS stimu-

TABLE 22.6 Agents That Interact With P Caffeine

Interactants	Effect and Significance	Nursing Management
oral contraceptives	Serum concentrations of caffeine may be increased during concurrent administration with oral contraceptives.	Monitor for nausea or tremors. Limit caffeine intake with oral contraceptives.
fluoroquinolone antibiotics • ciprofloxacin • levofloxacin • norfloxacin • enoxacin	Fluoroquinolone antibiotics decrease the clearance of caffeine, resulting in the potential for caffeine toxicity.	Avoid concomitant use of caffeine with fluoroquinolone antibiotics if possible. Monitor for caffeine toxicity.
• lithium	Caffeine reduces serum lithium concentration.	Monitor serum lithium levels. Counsel patients taking lithium regarding caffeine intake.
MAOIs	Dangerous cardiac arrhythmias or severe hypertension may occur because of potentiation of sympathomimetic effects.	Do not administer caffeine within 2 weeks of MAOI therapy. Counsel patient taking MAOIs of potential adverse effect with caffeine.
phenylpropanolamine	A combination of caffeine and phenylpropanolamine has resulted in cerebrovascular accident.	Do not combine these agents.
psychostimulants • dextroamphetamine • methylphenidate • modafinil • nicotine • pemoline • pseudoephedrine • sympathomimetic agents	When combined with any of these medications, an additive effect may occur resulting in nervousness, irritability, insomnia, or cardiac arrhythmias.	Avoid these combinations when possible. Monitor blood pressure and heart rate. Monitor for adverse effects.

lant, it can aggravate these conditions. Caffeine is contraindicated for patients suffering from insomnia because insomnia is one of its most frequent adverse effects. In overdoses, caffeine has been associated with seizures; therefore, it should be prescribed cautiously to any patient with a seizure disorder.

Caffeine may stimulate the force of contraction and increase heart rate and blood pressure. It may also increase left ventricular output and stroke volume. Patients who have cardiac disease, angina, hypertension, or a history of cardiac dysrhythmias should be given caffeine cautiously. Patients should not take caffeine within 14 days of a myocardial infarction (MI).

Patients with chronic disorders such as diabetes mellitus, hyperthyroidism, and peptic ulcer disease should not receive or should minimize their intake of caffeine. In patients with diabetes, caffeine can either increase or decrease blood sugar. In neonates, both hypoglycemia and hyperglycemia have been observed with the use of caffeine. In patients with hyperthyroidism, the stimulatory effects of caffeine can be augmented. Because caffeine can stimulate gastric secretions, it may also aggravate stomach ulcerations.

Caffeine should be used cautiously in patients with hepatic disease or hepatic impairment. Caffeine clearance may be delayed, leading to toxicity. Using caffeine cautiously is especially important in neonates because their hepatic metabolism is underdeveloped. Additionally, renal impairment in premature neonates may delay caffeine clearance because caffeine elimination depends more on renal clearance in neonates than in older infants or adults.

Adverse Effects

Many adverse reactions to caffeine are an extension of caffeine's pharmacologic actions. Caffeine can cause tremor, sinus tachycardia, and heightened attentiveness. Other adverse reactions include diarrhea, excitement, irritability, insomnia, headache, muscle twitches, and palpitations. Because caffeine is a mild diuretic, polyuria is a possibility.

Cardiac arrhythmias, seizures, and delirium are possible after deliberate overdoses. In neonates, intolerance or overdose of caffeine may manifest as tachypnea, hyperglycemia, azotemia, fever, or seizures.

High caffeine intake has been reported to inhibit spermatogenesis in male animals. Adverse effects may also occur when a patient abruptly discontinues use of caffeine. Caffeine withdrawal syndrome is characterized by lethargy, anxiety, dizziness, or headache.

Drug Interactions

Caffeine has many potential drug–drug interactions, including with oral contraceptives, psychostimulants, sympathomimetic agents, fluoroquinolone antibiotics, lithium, and MAOIs. Caffeine may also interact with grapefruit juice. Table 22.6 presents these potential drug interactions.

Assessment of Relevant Core Patient Variables

Health Status

Assess for disorders that contraindicate or require precautions with caffeine therapy. Assess for current or recent use of medications that may interact with caffeine, especially MAOIs and sympathomimetic drugs. Assessing for the use of OTC drugs is important because many of them have sympathomimetic ingredients. Communicate positive findings to the prescriber before starting caffeine therapy.

Obtain baseline vital signs. When caffeine is used for respiratory depression or neonatal apnea, appropriate monitoring equipment should be used.

Life Span and Gender

Ask the female patient whether she is pregnant or would like to become pregnant. Couples who are pursuing pregnancy should probably limit excessive intake of caffeine. Caffeine drug products are generally classified in FDA pregnancy category B; however, injectable forms are classified in FDA pregnancy risk category C because caffeine easily crosses the placenta. It is generally recommended that pregnant women avoid the intake of caffeine-containing beverages (e.g., coffee, teas, colas) or limit their use to no more than one or two caffeine-containing beverages per day. Likewise, pregnant women should use caffeine-containing medications only when absolutely necessary.

The American Academy of Pediatrics generally considers the casual use of caffeinated beverages to be compatible with lactation. Lactating women should use caffeine-containing drug products cautiously. When breast-fed infants are prescribed caffeine for apnea, their mothers should avoid the use of caffeine.

In neonates, there is a possible association between the use of methylxanthines like caffeine and the development of necrotizing enterocolitis. All preterm neonates treated with caffeine should be monitored for the development of gastric adverse effects such as abdominal distension, vomiting, bloody stools, and lethargy. In addition, monitoring serum caffeine levels is recommended. Neonates should receive caffeine without sodium benzoate.

The benzoate may displace bilirubin and induce kernicterus. In addition, elevated serum concentrations of benzoate have been associated with neurologic disturbances such as hypotension, gasping respiration, and metabolic acidosis.

Lifestyle, Diet, and Habits

Caffeine is found in many foods and beverages. To avoid toxicity, patients should limit their intake of these foods while taking drugs that contain caffeine. To avoid caffeine withdrawal syndrome, patients should decrease their intake of caffeine daily rather than stop caffeine ingestion abruptly. Patients should never take caffeine tablets with grapefruit juice, which increases the effects of caffeine.

Environment

Oral preparations of caffeine may be administered in any setting by physicians, nurses, or patients. When used for respiratory depression or neonatal apnea, injectable caffeine must be administered in a monitored setting with appropriate life-sustaining equipment available.

Nursing Diagnoses and Outcomes

- Disturbed Sleep Pattern related to insomnia
  Desired outcome: *The patient will maintain adequate sleep and rest cycles.*

- Anxiety related to stimulatory effects of caffeine
  Desired outcome: The patient will remain calm throughout therapy.
- Deficient Fluid Volume related to diuretic effect of caffeine and potential diarrhea
  Desired outcome: The patient will remain well hydrated.

Planning and Intervention

Maximizing Therapeutic Effects

Ensure that the patient takes the caffeine tablets or caplets as directed. It is very important that the patient does not take more than prescribed. If administering an extended-release form of caffeine, advise the patient to swallow the tablet whole, not to crush or chew it. If administering chewable tablets, advise the patient to chew well and then swallow. Consistent intake of caffeine results in tolerance to its effects. Patients obtain maximum therapeutic effects when they use caffeine intermittently.

Minimizing Adverse Effects

Adverse effects are minimized when patients adhere to the contraindications and precautions for caffeine therapy. Patients taking caffeine for its therapeutic effects should limit their ingestion of caffeine from food and beverage sources. The patient should also refrain from taking OTC products that contain caffeine, especially cold and cough medications that also have a sympathomimetic effect.

Providing Patient and Family Education

- The general public typically does not view caffeine as a drug. Convey to the patient that caffeine is a drug and as such may create serious adverse effects. Review the contraindications and precautions of caffeine therapy with the patient and family before initiating therapy. Review potential drug–drug interactions and explain the importance of refraining from OTC drug use without prescriber's knowledge.
- Instruct the patient regarding the potential adverse effects of caffeine and ways to minimize their potential. Tell the patient to contact the prescriber if symptoms such as anxiety or panic reactions, confusion, dizziness, lightheadedness or fainting spells, fast or irregular breathing or heartbeat (palpitations), muscle twitching, nausea and vomiting, seizures, or trembling occur.
- Alert women of childbearing age to the potential difficulty of becoming pregnant when they ingest large amounts (more than 500 mg/day) of caffeine daily. Inform men of the potential for inhibiting spermatogenesis.
- Review dietary sources of caffeine and explain the importance of limiting caffeine from these sources while taking therapeutic caffeine. Discuss the interaction between caffeine and grapefruit juice to avoid caffeine toxicity.

Ongoing Assessment and Evaluation

Caffeine is indicated for short-term or intermittent therapy. When used for respiratory depression or neonatal apnea, monitor the patient's vital signs carefully. When administering for migraine or other types of headaches, monitor for potential adverse effects, especially CNS and cardiovascular stimulation. Conversely, also monitor for signs of caffeine withdrawal.

Drug Closely Related to P Caffeine

Doxapram (Dopram), a parenteral analeptic agent, is used to stimulate postanesthesia respiratory depression or drug-induced CNS depression and to treat chronic pulmonary disease associated with acute hypercapnia. It has an unlabeled use for neonatal apnea. Doxapram works by activating the peripheral carotid chemoreceptors, thereby increasing respiratory rate. It is not usually the drug of choice because of its narrow margin of safety. Adverse effects include hypertension, sinus tachycardia, arrhythmias, skeletal muscle hyperactivity, dyspnea, headache, dizziness, apprehension, disorientation, pupil dilation, convulsions, cough, tachypnea, laryngospasm, bronchospasm, nausea and vomiting, diarrhea, and urinary retention.

CHAPTER SUMMARY

- The CNS acts as a system of control and surveillance for many unconscious and conscious functions. Normal arousal mechanisms are affected through presynaptic release of neurotransmitters, such as norepinephrine, serotonin, and dopamine.
- The CNS stimulants are used therapeutically to treat several pathologic conditions, including narcolepsy, ADHD, obesity, and respiratory depression. CNS stimulants can be divided into three drug classes according to the specific effects they have on the body: central CNS stimulants, anorectic CNS stimulants, and respiratory CNS stimulants.
- The central CNS stimulants stimulate the CNS directly or indirectly, and drugs in this class include those that are used therapeutically and nontherapeutically. Those that are used therapeutically include dextroamphetamine, amphetamine salts, methylphenidate, pemoline, and cocaine. Those used nontherapeutically include amphetamines, cocaine, strychnine, nicotine, caffeine, and khat.
- The prototype centrally acting CNS stimulant is dextroamphetamine. It is used to treat ADHD, narcolepsy, and obesity. Nursing management concerns regarding dextroamphetamine relate to preventing abuse,

MEMORY CHIP

P Caffeine

- Used therapeutically for neonatal apnea, asthma, drowsiness, and fatigue
- Ingested nontherapeutically in cocoa, chocolate, coffee, tea, and cola
- Stimulates medullary respiratory center, CNS, and cardiovascular systems
- Most common adverse effects: usually an extension of its pharmacologic actions; caffeine withdrawal syndrome occurs with abrupt cessation after long-term or high intake of caffeine

promoting adherence to the therapeutic regimen, and recognizing and managing adverse effects.

- Other classes of drugs used in the management of ADHD include nonstimulants such as atomoxetine, antihypertensive medications, and antidepressant medications.
- The anorectic CNS stimulants may directly stimulate the satiety center in the hypothalamus. These drugs include sibutramine, benzphetamine, diethylpropion, mazindol, phendimetrazine, phentermine, and phenylpropanolamine. Their mechanisms of action relate to adrenergic or serotonergic inhibition of the hypothalamic satiety center.
- Anorectic drug use is controversial and not effective as monotherapy. These drugs should be used as part of an overall strategy to control obesity.
- All anorectic drugs except phenylpropanolamine are available by prescription only. They all exhibit a wide range of adverse effects.
- Nursing management for anorectic drugs should focus on careful pretreatment assessment, adequate therapeutic monitoring, and proper patient and family education.
- The respiratory CNS stimulants directly affect the brain stem and respiratory centers. Respiratory CNS stimulants include caffeine and doxapram.

▲ QUESTIONS FOR STUDY AND REVIEW

1. Many stimulants are used in the management of ADHD. Develop a learning tool to differentiate between short-acting, intermediate-acting, and long-acting stimulants.
2. You are working in an outpatient setting that specializes in the management of ADHD in children. Develop a series of questions that you would ask parents during follow-up visits. Develop a list of observations that you should document after each visit.
3. You have been telephoned by the daughter of your discharged patient, Mrs. Christo. Mrs. Christo was sent home last week with a diagnosis of narcolepsy and was taking dextroamphetamine, 30 mg/day. Her daughter wants to know how effective this drug is. What questions would you ask her to be able to answer her question properly?
4. You are talking with a colleague who tells you, "I must be allergic to my home. Every weekend I have a terrible headache. I feel tired, dizzy, and lethargic. I never feel this way at work. What could be wrong with me?"
5. Your patient has morbid obesity. She is prescribed sibutramine. What are the most important teaching points for this patient?
6. How do sibutramine and orlistat differ in their mechanisms of action?

? Need More Help?

Chapter 22 of the study guide for *Drug Therapy in Nursing* 2e contains NCLEX-style questions and other learning activities to reinforce your understanding of the concepts presented in this chapter. For additional information or to purchase the study guide, visit *http://connection.lww.com/go/aschenbrenner.*

■ REFERENCES AND BIBLIOGRAPHY

Anonymous. (2004). An update on attention deficit disorder. *Harvard Mental Health Letter, 20*(11), 4–7.

Biederman, J., Spencer, T., & Wilens, T. (2004). Evidence-based pharmacotherapy for attention-deficit hyperactivity disorder. *International Journal of Neuropsychopharmacology, 7*(1), 77–97.

Clinical Pharmacology [Online]. Available: *http://cp.gsm.com.*

Facts and Comparisons. (2004). *Drug facts and comparisons.* Philadelphia: Lippincott Williams & Wilkins.

Finer, N. (2002). Sibutramine: Its mode of action and efficacy. *International Journal of Obesity and Related Metabolic Disorders, 26*(Suppl. 4), S29–S33.

Hardman, J. G. (2001) *Goodman and Gilman's the pharmacological basis of therapeutics* (10th ed.). New York: McGraw-Hill Health Professions Division.

Katzung, B. (2004). *Basic and clinical pharmacology* (9th ed.). New York: McGraw-Hill/Appleton & Lange.

Kociancic, T., Reed, M. D., & Findling, R. L. (2004). Evaluation of risks associated with short- and long-term psychostimulant therapy for treatment of ADHD in children. *Expert Opinions on Drug Safety, 3*(2), 93–100.

Leonard, B. E., McCartan, D., White, J., et al. (2004). Methylphenidate: A review of its neuropharmacological, neuropsychological and adverse clinical effects. *Human Psychopharmacology, 19*(3), 151–180.

Leung, W. Y., et al. (2003). Weight management and current options in pharmacotherapy: Orlistat and sibutramine. *Clinical Therapeutics, 25*(1), 58–80.

Micromedex Healthcare Series [Online]. Available: *http://healthcare.micromedex.com.*

NHANES study [Online]. Available: *http://www.cdc.gov/nchs/products/pubs/pubd/hestats/obese/obse99.htm.*

Poston, W. S., & Foreyt, J. P. (2004). Sibutramine and the management of obesity. *Expert Opinions in Pharmacotherapy, 5*(3), 633–642.

Reeves, G., & Schweitzer, J. (2004). Pharmacological management of attention-deficit hyperactivity disorder, *Expert Opinions in Pharmacotherapy, 5*(6), 1313–1320.

Spencer, J. T. (2004). ADHD treatment across the life cycle. *Journal of Clinical Psychiatry, 65*(Suppl. 3), 22–26.

Tatro, D. S. (2004). *Drug interaction facts.* Philadelphia: Lippincott Williams & Wilkins.

Wilens, T. E., Spencer, T. J., & Biederman, J. (2002). A review of the pharmacotherapy of adults with attention-deficit/hyperactivity disorder. *Journal of Attention Disorders, 5*(4), 189–202.

Analgesic and Anti-inflammatory Drugs

unit 6

Drugs Treating Severe Pain

chapter 23

Learning Objectives

At the completion of this chapter the student will:

1 Define pain.
2 Describe the physiology of the central nervous system (CNS) as it relates to pain.
3 Differentiate the types of pain.
4 Differentiate the various methods used in pain management.
5 Be able to assess pain.
6 Describe the effects of agonist stimulation and antagonist stimulation at the opiate receptors.
7 Identify core drug knowledge about narcotic drugs.
8 Identify core patient variables related to narcotic drugs.
9 Relate the interaction of core drug knowledge to core patient variables for narcotic drugs that relieve pain.
10 Generate a nursing plan of care from the interactions between core drug knowledge and core patient variables for narcotic drugs used to control pain.
11 Describe nursing interventions that maximize therapeutic effects and minimize adverse effects when narcotics are given for pain management.
12 Describe the key points for patient and family education when narcotics are used in pain management.

KEY TERMS

acute pain
addiction
adjunct analgesics
analgesics
breakthrough pain
chronic pain
dependence
narcotic
neuropathic pain
nociceptic pain
opioid
pain
rescue dose
tolerance

FEATURED WEBLINK

http://www.jcaho.org/news+room/health+care+issues/pain+mono_npc.pdf

Would you like to learn more about assessing and managing pain? Download the complete 2001 position paper from the National Pharmaceutical Council (NPC) and Joint Commission on Accreditation of Healthcare Organizations (JCAHO). It provides general information about pain, pain assessment, and pain management, and gives specific drug information.

CONNECTION WEBLINK

Additional Weblinks are found on Connection:
http://www.connection.lww.com/go/aschenbrenner.

Drugs Treating Severe Pain

Ⓒ Narcotic Analgesics

Ⓒ Strong narcotic agonists

- [P] **morphine**
- alfentanil
- fentanyl
- hydromorphone
- levorphanol
- meperidine
- methadone
- oxycodone
- oxymorphone
- remifentanil
- sufentanil
- naloxone

Ⓒ Mild narcotic agonists

- [P] **codeine**
- hydrocodone
- propoxyphene

Ⓒ Narcotic agonist-antagonists

- [P] **pentazocine**
- buprenorphine
- butorphanol
- dezocine
- nalbuphine

The symbol Ⓒ indicates the **drug class.**
Drugs in **bold type** marked with the symbol [P] are prototypes.
Drugs in blue type are closely related to the prototype.
Drugs in red type are significantly different from the prototype.
Drugs in black type with no symbol are also used in drug therapy; no prototype

Pain is a multidimensional, subjective experience encompassing the physiologic, sensory, affective, cognitive, behavioral, and sociocultural dimensions of a patient's life. The International Association for the Study of Pain's definition of pain is the most widely used and emphasizes that pain is multidimensional; it defines pain as "an unpleasant sensory and emotional experience associated with actual or potential tissue damage, or described in terms of such damage." (National Pharmaceutical Council and Joint Commission on Accreditation of Healthcare Organizations, 2001; Merskey & Bugduk, 1994). Pain can truly be measured only by subjective data because no objective finding is present in all painful experiences. As early as 1968, the nurse-researcher Margo McCaffery defined pain as "whatever the experiencing person says it is, existing whenever s/he says it does" (McCaffery, 1968). Thus, the individual experiencing pain is the only person who can accurately state when pain is present and how it is being experienced. Pain may accompany disease or treatment and may change over time. Pain may result from multiple simultaneous causes. If unrelieved, pain can affect the patient's psychological, social, physiologic, and spiritual health and can prevent productive work and enjoyment of personal relationships. Despite the substantial effects that pain has on health status, multiple studies over the years have shown that health care providers undertreat pain, leading patients to suffer needlessly.

Pain may be a major indication for drug therapy, and you need knowledge of drug therapy based on core drug knowledge for prescribed drugs. Moreover, pain has an important bearing on multiple core patient variables, which you must consider during initial and ongoing assessments and evaluations of drug therapy.

PHYSIOLOGY

The peripheral nervous system and central nervous system (CNS) comprise an integrated system that provides a pathway for pain transmission. The physiologic mechanisms involved in the pain response are complex and are not yet completely understood. Transduction is the term used to describe the phenomena associated with the initiation of a pain signal. Pain receptors are found on the peripheral end plates of afferent neurons. Afferent neurons carry signals into the CNS, whereas efferent neurons carry signals from the CNS to the periphery. The sensation of peripheral pain begins in afferent neurons called nociceptors, which are found in the skin, muscle, connective tissue, circulatory system, and abdominal, pelvic, and thoracic viscera. Nociceptors may be stimulated by mechanical, thermal, hormonal (namely prostaglandins), or chemical (namely histamine, bradykinin, and serotonin, which are released during cellular destruction) stimuli. For example, when you stub your toe, pressure in the surrounding tissue causes direct mechanical activation of pain receptors. Potassium, which leaks from the damaged cells into the tissues, then activates the inflammatory response, sending chemical mediators to the site of injury. These mediators are chemically caustic to the nociceptors. Stimulation of the receptors at the end plates then promotes cellular depolarization and generates an action potential.

There are two types of nociceptors: delta fibers and C fibers. Delta fibers are fast traveling, myelinated, and responsive to mechanical stimuli. They sense sharp, stinging, cutting, or pinching pain. C fibers are slow traveling, unmyelinated, and responsive to mechanical, chemical, hormonal, or thermal stimuli. They sense dull, burning, or aching pain. During inflammation, nociceptors become sensitized, discharge spontaneously, and produce ongoing pain. Prolonged firing of the C-fiber nociceptors allows cells to release glutamate, which has a role in the conduction of nerve impulses. Glutamate acts on specialized receptors in the spinal cord, known as *N*-methyl-D-aspartate (NMDA) receptors. Stimulation of the NMDA receptors causes the spinal cord neurons to become more responsive to all incoming stimuli, leading to a central sensitization to pain impulses.

Once the nociceptor depolarizes, transmission of the pain signal has begun. Transmission is the process whereby the pain information is carried from the receptor end plate along the axon of the afferent neuron. Nociceptors enter the spinal cord and terminate in the dorsal horn, where they synapse in distinct regions. Substance P, a peptide in the unmyelinated fibers entering the dorsal horn, is released in response to painful stimuli. Substance P is a neurotransmitter and neuromodulator that activates special receptor sites. It appears to have a role in interpreting pain and regulating self-produced (endogenous) analgesic responses to nociceptor stimulation (Figure 23.1). The release of excitatory amino acids, such as glutamate and aspartate, also has an important role in carrying the painful stimulus to the brain.

From the dorsal horn, impulses are transferred, through the spinothalamic and spinoreticulothalamic tracts, to various higher brain areas for interpretation. Pain is mediated and modulated through forebrain mechanisms, which act at the spinal, brainstem, cerebral, and limbic levels. Stimulation of these various areas produces an affective response to the painful stimuli based on the individual's previous experience with pain as well as on social, environmental, and cultural influences. Thus, the response to any given painful stimulus will be different for different people. The forebrain has the greatest control over nociceptor functioning. Indeed, pathology of the forebrain can cause pain, even if the nociceptors have not been activated peripherally. Pain perception involves multiple cerebral structures. During clinical studies of pain, brain imaging with positron emission tomography (PET) has identified some of the principal structures of this central network activated by pain. PET imaging has shown synaptically induced increases in regional cerebral blood flow in several regions of the brain when a person is exposed to painful stimuli. The intensity of the blood flow response in the brain correlates parametrically with perceived pain intensity. The areas of the brain involved in interpreting pain include the contralateral insula and anterior cingulate cortex, frontal inferior cortex, posterior cingulate cortex, bilateral thalamus and premotor cortex, and cerebellar vermis. These brain regions are functionally diverse and are involved with sensation, motor control, affect, and attention.

Components That Influence Pain

Pain has sensory-discriminative (physical) components and affective-motivational (emotional) components. The sensory dimension of pain encompasses pain's location, intensity, and quality. The quality of pain is the way it feels to the patient, for example, burning or gnawing. Affective aspects

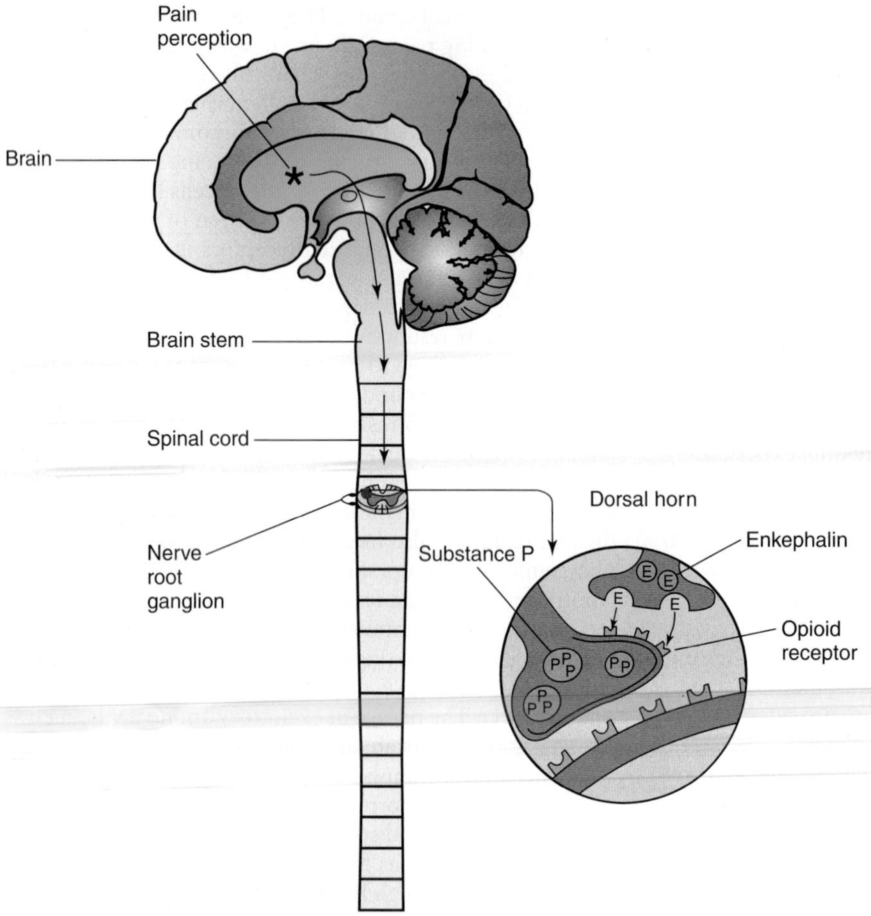

FIGURE 23.1 Inhibiting pain perceived over ascending pathways. Once the brain interprets a stimulus as pain, the nervous system responds along descending pathways. From the brain's perception of pain, an impulse is routed through the brain stem and into the spinal cord and travels through the dorsal horn to a dorsal root ganglion. Here, the impulses descending from the raphe nucleus system trigger the release of enkephalin (a peptide or endorphinlike substance). Enkephalin then stimulates the opioid receptors on the afferent neuron coming from the dorsal root ganglion. The release of enkephalin can excite or inhibit the release of the afferent neurotransmitters, which include substance P. If substance P is not released, the person will not sense pain. In some people, a sufficient release of endogenous enkephalin will change the membrane of the afferent neuron so that substance P cannot escape and cause pain. In others, exogenous opioids may be needed to achieve the same effect.

relate to the way that pain influences a patient's well-being, such as whether it is perceived as annoying, tortuous, or killing pain. Stimulation of the limbic system produces this emotional response to the physical stimulus of pain. Phenomena thought to influence the perception of pain are anxiety, fear, apprehension, attention, motivation, and other cognitive processes. For example, anxiety, fear, or apprehension appear to make the patient more sensitive to pain, allowing the patient to experience stimuli as painful when, under other circumstances, they might not be experienced this way. Conversely, the patient who is aware of his or her condition and wants to control pain may deliberately use techniques (e.g., distraction by talking to others) to cope and decrease the pain experienced. Inhibition of pain and the transmission of painful stimuli occur in various regions of the brain. Inhibitory substances such as endogenous opioids, serotonin, norepinephrine, and gamma-aminobutyric acid (GABA) are released into nerve synapses. These substances bind with receptors on primary afferent and dorsal horn neurons to prevent further transmission of painful stimuli. The ability to release these internal pain modulators varies from person to person; this variation partly explains why, when two people have a similar injury, one may feel a great deal of pain, whereas the other does not.

The peripheral and central nervous systems can become overly sensitized to nociceptive input. When the release of inflammatory mediators or the painful stimulus is intense, repeated, or prolonged, the nociceptors in the periphery generate more nerve impulses than usual and release the impulses more frequently. Central spinal neurons can become overexcited by substantial tissue or nerve injury and by recurrent input from the peripheral nervous system. When overexcitation occurs, the pain response may spread to additional areas in the brain. The patient can then experience an increased pain response to the same stimuli, a pain response to stimuli not previously experienced as painful, or pain from an uninjured area (referred pain). The overstimulation of the central spinal neurons may continue to produce a pain response long after the painful stimulus is gone.

Types of Pain

A number of different terms are used to describe and categorize pain. Pain can be categorized based on its presumed underlying pathophysiology as being either nociceptic or neuropathic. **Nociceptic pain** is caused by the activation of the delta and C nociceptors in response to painful stimuli, such as injury, disease, or inflammation. Pain perception and stimulus intensity are generally closely related to nociceptive pain. Nociceptic pain also indicates real or potential tissue damage. Nociceptic pain is further categorized as either somatic or visceral. Somatic pain results from ongoing activation of peripheral nociceptors found in structural tissues, such as bone, muscle, and soft tissue. It can be further divided as either deep or superficial. It is characterized as well-localized and intermittent, or as constant, aching, gnawing, throbbing, burning, or cramping. The bone and joint pain of arthritis is a common source of somatic pain. Muscle

strains after intense physical exertion also result in somatic pain. Both of these are examples of deep somatic pain. Sunburn is an example of superficial somatic pain.

Visceral pain results from stimulation within the deep tissues or organs and surrounding structural tissues. Common visceral pain syndromes include pain associated with cholecystitis, pancreatitis, uterine and ovarian disease, and liver disease. Patients often describe visceral pain as deep, boring, diffuse abdominal pain. Visceral pain is less circumscribed than somatic pain and often has a referred component (e.g., pain from the liver, which can be referred to the right shoulder) or neuropathic processes or causes. Additionally, pain can be described according to its duration (e.g., acute or chronic) or by its underlying pathophysiologic cause (e.g., cancer). Differentiation of pain serves a critical role in diagnostic and therapeutic planning. Adequate pain management is based on accurate pain assessments.

Neuropathic pain is the term used to represent pain in which the underlying pathology is abnormal processing of stimuli in the peripheral or central nervous systems. Thus, neuropathic pain is a result of some injury to the peripheral receptors, afferent fibers, or CNS, or an impairment of the nervous system. Neuropathic pain is unique in character and distribution. It can be described as shooting, burning, or stabbing and generally follows a radicular or radiating pattern. Neuropathic pain is often caused by trauma, inflammation, metabolic disease (e.g., diabetes), infections such as herpes zoster, toxins, and primary neurologic diseases. Several neuropathic pain syndromes may occur in patients with cancer. For example, direct tumor infiltration from adjacent soft tissues or lymph nodes or compression from metastases in the adjacent bony pelvis can damage the lumbosacral plexus. Postmastectomy syndrome is the result of nerve injury, with the development of a traumatic neuroma following surgery. It is characterized by a constricting, burning sensation in the posterior arm, axilla, and anterior chest and is aggravated by movement.

Acute pain, meaning the immediate phase of response to an insult or injury, results from tissue damage. It has cognitive, emotional, and sensory features. Acute pain resolves with the healing of the underlying injury. It is usually nociceptic but can be neuropathic. Acute pain may be related to the treatment of an underlying disease process or to an injury that is expected to resolve. Medical procedures, operations, and trauma are examples of types of treatments resulting in acute pain. Postsurgical pain is the most common treatment-related pain.

Chronic pain is no longer defined purely by how long it is present. In contrast to acute pain, chronic pain may persist well beyond actual tissue injury and healing. The level of identified pathology may be low or insufficient to account for the presence or extent of the pain experienced. Stress and other nonbiologic influences may exacerbate pain intensity, despite a reduction in the physiologic cause of the pain. Chronic pain will disrupt sleep and normal living; it does not have an adaptive or useful purpose, as acute pain does.

Cancer pain is one type of chronic pain. The pain may be related to the disease itself, or to diagnostic procedures or treatments for the cancer. The pain is usually progressive as the disease advances to end stage and can be severe and debilitating. Additionally, acute episodes may occur, either in response to movement or activity or secondary to therapy or treatment of cancer, such as surgical removal of the tumor or skin irritation from radiation. Cancer pain may also be intermittent. These acute and chronic components make it difficult to classify.

Chronic noncancer pain is another subtype of chronic pain. Chronic noncancer pain usually does not correspond well to identifiable levels of tissue pathology, and it frequently also does not respond well to standard treatments for pain. Chronic noncancer pain may arise from an acute injury that proceeds to chronic pain or from various chronic conditions such as osteoarthritis, migraine headaches, chronic abdominal pain from irritable bowel disease or other conditions, or from neuralgias. Chronic noncancer pain ranges from mild to excruciating.

Whatever the source or classification, pain may delay healing and rehabilitation, prolong other symptoms, and leave the patient immunocompromised. Every effort should be mobilized to manage pain effectively, including stepped pharmacologic intervention (i.e., predetermined, progressive levels of intervention).

DRUG THERAPY TO MANAGE PAIN

When drug therapy is prescribed to treat pain, the pharmacotherapeutics and pharmacokinetics of the drug and relevant core patient variables help to govern which drug will be selected. Drug therapy may be used to correct the underlying pathophysiologic cause of the pain (e.g., nitroglycerin, a vasodilator, will be selected to treat angina pectoris from narrowed coronary vessels), or it may be used to decrease the pain response itself (e.g., morphine for postsurgical pain). The degree of pain that the patient is experiencing affects the pharmacodynamics of **analgesics** (drugs used to treat pain). Nowadays, preventing pain is generally accepted to be easier than decreasing pain. It is also easier to treat pain at low levels than at severe levels. Pain that is allowed to escalate requires larger doses of drugs to obtain relief. These interrelationships between pain and core drug variables affect the therapeutic management of pain.

Drug classifications that are normally used for pain management are the **opioid** analgesics and the nonsteroidal anti-inflammatory drugs (NSAIDs). The opioids derive their name from opium because they are natural alkaloids, semisynthetic analogues, or synthetic compounds of opium. Opioids, or **narcotics,** as they are more commonly called, act on the CNS to interfere with the pain experience. Morphine is the standard drug of choice in this category, and all other opioids are compared with it when evaluating their efficacy. NSAIDs act in the peripheral nervous system, interfering with prostaglandin synthesis and preventing the transmission of pain impulses. Some drugs are combinations of these drug classes, and they act on both the CNS and peripheral nervous system simultaneously. NSAIDs and other nonopiate analgesics, such as acetaminophen (Tylenol), are used to treat mild to moderate pain. Opioids are used in the treatment of moderate to severe pain. For more information on NSAIDs and acetaminophen, see Chapter 24.

The dose and choice of analgesics must be individualized to meet the patient's need for pain relief. Adverse effects from any given drug may, however, place a ceiling on how large a daily dose can be.

Some other drug classes are used as secondary pain relievers, although their pharmacotherapeutics indicate that their primary uses are for other problems. When drugs are used secondarily for pain relief, they are known as **adjunct analgesics** or co-analgesics. Using multiple types of drugs to treat the exact symptoms of pain experienced is similar to using a combination of drugs (e.g., those that are cell cycle specific and those that are not cell cycle specific) to treat cancer. The outcome is more effective than that of any one drug alone. Adjuvant drugs can increase the efficacy of narcotics or provide independent analgesia for specific types of pain. Other CNS depressants that are primarily indicated for other diseases and disorders can be used as adjuncts. Included in this group are drugs that have antiemetic effects (effects against nausea) or mild tranquilizing effects. These CNS depressants are frequently used in acute pain (e.g., postsurgical pain). Classifications of other adjuvant drugs include antidepressants, corticosteroids, and anticonvulsants. Antidepressants are the treatment of choice for neuropathic pain described as burning or numbing. In clinical trials, tricyclic antidepressants are the only antidepressant drugs proved effective in managing neuropathic pain.

Steroids are useful for treating short-term, severe, episodic pain, such as that associated with nerve compression. They are also used in managing cancer pain to relieve chronic pressure-related pain states, such as progressive visceral distention, severe lymphedema, increased intracranial pressure, soft tissue infiltration unrelieved by NSAIDs and opioids, and continuing nerve compression.

Anticonvulsants are important adjuncts for neuropathic pain, particularly that described as stabbing or piercing. The anticonvulsants are used for conditions such as trigeminal neuralgia, sciatica, migraine headache, and various neuropathic pain states in patients with cancer. These agents directly affect the peripheral nerve conduction of pain impulses, which is completely separate from their central effect.

Finally, in addition to pharmacologic interventions to treat pain, nonpharmacologic methods may be used. These methods are not substitutes for analgesics, especially in moderate to severe pain, but they are valuable adjuncts to therapy. The effective use of nonpharmacologic measures may decrease the dose of narcotic that is required, thereby achieving pain control while minimizing adverse effects. Nonpharmacologic techniques include cognitive strategies for relaxation and physical strategies that interrupt pain transmission. Table 23.1 describes some of the nonpharmacologic techniques used in pain control.

The accepted standard plan for treating pain remains the World Health Organization's model of stepped progression from nonopioid to opioid use with increasing doses of the opioid until the pain is controlled. Nonopioids, including adjunct medications, may be added to an opioid regimen. Nonpharmacologic methods may also be added. Figure 23.2 illustrates the stepped-progression approach to pain control.

NARCOTIC ANALGESICS

Narcotic analgesics are required for conditions, disorders, or treatments that are accompanied by moderate to severe pain. The narcotic analgesics are the most effective drugs for pain management.

The degree of pain relief that is achieved may be expressed in analgesic equivalents, which is the dose of an analgesic required to produce the same analgesic effect as a 10-mg dose of morphine (the standard measure of pain relief). Some equianalgesic dosages are presented in Table 23.2.

The narcotic analgesics include opiate agonists, mixed agonist-antagonists, and antagonists based on their activity at opioid receptors. Although five types of opiate receptor sites (with the Greek names of mu, kappa, sigma, delta, and epsilon) are known to exist, activity occurs at only three sites (mu, kappa, and delta) with the narcotic analgesics available. From a nursing standpoint, comparing strong with mild to moderate analgesics within the opiate agonist classification may be helpful. This comparison will allow examination of two important opiate agonist prototypes: morphine (opiate agonist and strong analgesic) and codeine

TABLE 23.1 Nonpharmacologic Techniques Used in Pain Control

Technique	Summary Description
Relaxation therapy	Uses progressive muscle relaxation techniques, controlled breathing, and simple hypnosis strategies to help patient achieve physical and emotional relaxation
Guided imagery	Uses visual and auditory imagery selected by the patient and specific to pain-relieving or stress-reducing feelings
Biofeedback	Teaches control of stress through patient's ability to monitor and manipulate some aspects of the autonomic nervous system
Music distraction	Uses music that is selected by the patient for the purpose of distracting the patient from pain and focusing instead on rhythm, tone, harmony, and other aspects of the music
Exercise	Promotes blood flow and tissue oxygenation, prevents muscle atrophy and stiffness, assists in building muscle to stabilize painful joints. An exercise plan defined by a physiatrist is extremely helpful in very debilitated patients. Heat promotes increased blood flow to the affected part, whereas cold reduces swelling associated with the inflammatory response. Take care not to use excessive heat, which can cause burns. Try alternating heat with cold.
Transcutaneous electrical nerve stimulation	Attempts to "confuse" the pain signal by activating other sensory circuits
Massage (various types)	Alleviates muscle stiffness and pain by breaking up fibrous tissue in muscle, increasing circulation, and promoting normal elongation of muscle fibers

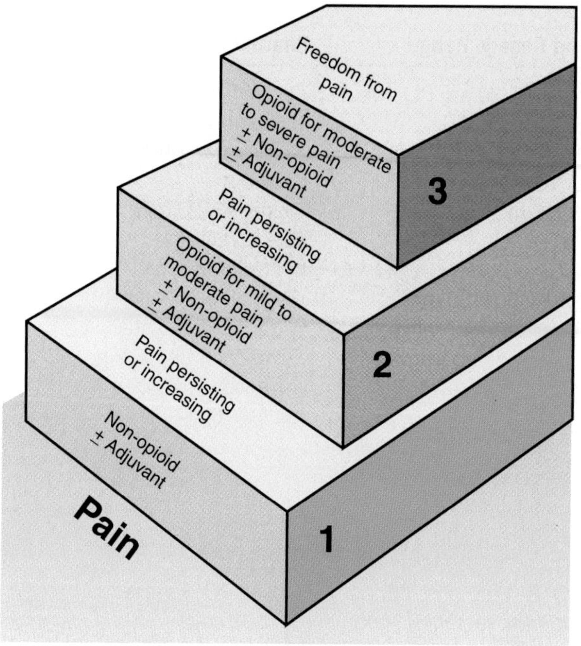

FIGURE 23.2 The World Health Organization's three-step analgesic ladder.

(opiate agonist and mild to moderate analgesic). Some narcotic analgesics have mixed opioid effects, being agonists at some receptors and antagonists at others. A mixed narcotic agonist-antagonist, pentazocine (Talwin), is the third prototype that is discussed in this chapter (Table 23.3).

Narcotics have an important role in pain management and control; however, they are typically underused. Research has repeatedly shown that major contributing factors to narcotic underuse are lack of knowledge on the part of health care professionals regarding pain and pain control and misinformation regarding the pharmacokinetics and pharmacodynamics of narcotics. Because patients' pain may be incorrectly assessed and improperly treated, you need to be aware of current advances in measuring, classifying, and managing pain.

TABLE 23.2 Equianalgesic Doses* (mg) of Selected Narcotic Analgesics

	Administration Route	
Drug	**Oral**	**Parenteral**
morphine	30	10
codeine	200	120–130
fentanyl	—	0.1–0.2
hydromorphone	7.5	1.3–1.5
meperidine	300**	75
methadone	20 (acute) 2–4 (chronic)	10 (acute) 2–4 (chronic)
oxycodone	30	—
pentazocine	180	60

*In measuring pain relief, the analgesic equivalent compares the degree of pain relief achieved with that obtained by a 10-mg dose of morphine (the standard dose), given parenterally.
** Not a recommended dose.

Ⓒ Strong Narcotic Agonists

Strong narcotic agonists include morphine, hydromorphone, levorphanol, oxycodone, oxymorphone, meperidine, fentanyl, alfentanil, sufentanil, methadone, and remifentanil. Table 23.3 presents a summary of selected narcotic analgesics and antagonists. The prototype strong narcotic agonist is morphine. The narcotic antagonist naloxone is significantly different from morphine.

NURSING MANAGEMENT OF THE PATIENT RECEIVING P MORPHINE

Core Drug Knowledge

Pharmacotherapeutics

The most important clinical indication for morphine is moderate to severe acute or chronic pain, including postoperative pain and pain that is nonresponsive to nonnarcotic analgesics. It can be used to treat chronic pain that is either cancer pain or noncancer chronic pain. Morphine is also used in dyspnea associated with acute left ventricular failure and pulmonary edema; it is the only narcotic agonist used to treat the pain of myocardial infarction (MI). Preoperatively, morphine can be used to sedate a patient, relieve anxiety, facilitate induction of anesthesia, or reduce the amount of anesthetic needed. Morphine can be administered by multiple routes: oral (PO), subcutaneous (SC), intramuscular (IM), intravenous (IV), epidural, rectal, and topical. Oral forms of morphine are preferred in treating cancer pain, unless the patient is unable to take medication by this route. The sustained-release form (MS Contin, Oramorph, or Kadian) is used only for patients who require an opioid analgesic for more than a few days and need around-the-clock pain control. Of the parenteral routes, the SC and IM routes should be limited to occasions when the drug is to be administered only one time. Repeated injections every 3 to 4 hours should be avoided because they cause additional discomfort, and repeated IM injections risk nerve and muscle injury. To provide continuous, 24-hour administration of morphine through a parenteral route, administer the drug by IV infusion regulated by an infusion-control pump. Topical forms of morphine have been found helpful in decreasing the pain associated with decubitus and other skin ulcers (Donnelly et al., 2002).

Pharmacokinetics

Onset of analgesic effect occurs within 15 to 30 minutes and lasts for about 3 to 7 hours. Morphine is metabolized in the liver and gut wall by conjugation to glucuronide, an active metabolite, which is excreted along with unchanged morphine in urine and breast milk. It is also excreted in the feces through biliary and enterohepatic recycling. It has a half-life of 1.5 to 2 hours.

Pharmacodynamics

Morphine is known to be an agonist at the mu, kappa, and possibly delta opiate receptors. Its actions are related to the distribution of opioid receptors; high densities of opioid receptors are found in the brainstem, medial thalamus, hypothalamus, limbic system, and spinal cord. Many other areas

TABLE 23.3 Summary of Selected Ⓒ Narcotic Analgesics and Antagonists in Adults

Drug (Trade) Name	Selected Indications	Route and Dosage Range	Pharmacokinetics
P morphine (Roxanol, RMS, *Canadian:* M-Eslon)	Moderate to severe acute and chronic pain, post-operative sedation, MI, pulmonary edema	*Adult:* q4h; 10–30 mg PO, IM, SC, 5–20 mg q4–6 h; IV, 2.5–15 mg diluted slow push; rectal, 10–20 mg q4h	*Onset:* PO, varies; IM, SC, rapid; IV, rapid *Duration:* 4–7 h $t_{1/2}$: 1.5 h
oxycodone (Roxicodone, Percodan, Percocet: *Canadian:* Supendol)	Moderate to moderately severe pain	*Adult:* PO, 5 mg q6h	*Onset:* 15–20 min *Duration:* 4–6 h $t_{1/2}$: Unknown
fentanyl (Sublimaze)	Analgesia during anesthesia, premedication, induction, maintenance and adjunct in anesthesia	*Adult:* IM/IV, 50–100 mg 30–60 min preoperative; adjunct or postoperative, 50–100 µg/kg; oral, 5–15 µg/kg as lollipop (oral transmucosal fentanyl citrate—OTFC)	*Onset:* IM/IV, 7–8 min; transdermal, gradual *Duration:* IM/IV, 1–2 h; transdermal, 72 h $t_{1/2}$: 1½–6 h
hydrocodone (Hycodan, Lortab)	Cough, analgesia	*Adult:* PO, 5–10 mg tid or qid for cough; 5–10 mg q4–6h for pain	*Onset:* 10–20 min *Duration:* Varies $t_{1/2}$: 3.8 h
hydromorphone (Dilaudid; *Canadian:* Hydromorph Contin)	Mild to moderate pain	*Adult:* PO, 2–4 mg q4h; IM, IV, 1–2 mg q6h; rectal, 3–6 mg q6–8h	*Onset:* PO, varies; IM, 15–30 min *Duration:* 4–5 h $t_{1/2}$: 2–3 h
levorphanol (Levo-Dromoran)	Anesthesia adjunct, moderate to severe pain	*Adult:* IM, slow IV, PO, 1–2 mg; may repeat in 3–8 h	*Onset:* 30–90 min *Duration:* 6–8 h $t_{1/2}$: 12–16 h
meperidine (Demerol)	Analgesia, PCA analgesia	*Adult:* PO, IM, SC, 50–150 mg q3–4h; PCA, 15–35 mg/h	*Onset:* PO, 15 min; IM, SC, 10–15 min *Duration:* 2–4 h $t_{1/2}$: 3–8 h
methadone (Dolophine; Canadian: Methadose)	Analgesia, narcotic detoxification and withdrawal	*Adult:* PO, IM, SC, 2.5–10 mg q3–4h for analgesia; PO, 40–120 mg/d as liquid for methadone maintenance	*Onset:* PO, 30–60 min; IM, SC, 10–20 min *Duration:* PO, 4–12 h; IM, SC, 4–6 h $t_{1/2}$: 25 h
Ⓒ Moderate Narcotic Analgesics			
P codeine	Cough, analgesia	*Adult:* PO, SC, IM, 15–60 mg q4h for pain, 10–20 mg q4h for cough	*Onset:* 15–20 min *Duration:* 4–6 h $t_{1/2}$: 3 h
Ⓒ Narcotic Agonist-Antagonist Analgesics			
P pentazocine (Talwin, Talacen)	Moderate to severe pain, anesthesia adjunct	*Adult:* PO, 50–100 mg q3–4h; IV, IM, or SC, 30 mg q3–4h	*Onset:* PO, 15–30 min; IM, SC, 10–20 min; IV, 2–3 min *Duration:* PO, 3–4 h; IM, SC, 1–3 h; IV, 60 min $t_{1/2}$: 2–3 h
buprenorphine (Buprenex)	Pain	*Adult:* IM, IV, 0.3 mg q6h	*Onset:* IM, 15 min; IV, 10 min *Duration:* 6 h $t_{1/2}$: 2–3h
butorphanol (Stadol)	Pain, anesthesia adjunct	*Adult:* IV, 0.5–2 mg q3–4h for pain; 0.5–4 mg for anesthesia; IM, 2 mg q3–4h for pain	*Onset:* Rapid *Duration:* 3–4 h $t_{1/2}$: 2.1–9.2 h
dezocine (Dalgan)	Pain	*Adult:* IM, 5–20 mg q3–6h, IV, 2.5–10 mg q2–4h	*Onset:* IM, 10–15 min; IV, 5 min *Duration:* Unknown $t_{1/2}$: 2.4 h
nalbuphine (Nubain)	Moderate to severe pain, anesthesia adjunct	*Adult:* IM, IV, SC 10 mg q3–6h for pain	*Onset:* IM, SC, <15 min; IV, 2–3 min *Duration:* 3–6 h $t_{1/2}$: 5 h

with opioid receptors are excitatory nociceptive pathways, which morphine inhibits. Morphine reduces the release of neurotransmitters in the presynaptic space and produces hyperpolarization of postsynaptic dorsal horn neurons; these actions prevent transmission of nociceptor pain. Morphine also decreases the release of substance P, which modulates pain perception. Some specific effects can be attributed to agonist action at specific opioid receptors. Generally, it is thought that mu receptors are responsible for supraspinal analgesia, respiratory and physical depression, euphoria, miosis, and reduced gastrointestinal (GI) motility. Kappa receptors are linked to spinal analgesia, miosis, and sedation. The delta receptors have been linked with dysphoria and psychotomimetic effects (effects, such as hallucinations, that mimic psychosis). The secondary pharmacologic effects of morphine, like those of other narcotic agonists, are related to various effects of receptor stimulation (Box 23.1).

Contraindications and Precautions

Morphine causes respiratory depression. The main contraindications to the use of morphine are hypersensitivity, preexisting respiratory depression, acute or severe bronchial asthma, and upper airway obstruction. Morphine should also be avoided in premature infants and during labor when delivery of a premature infant is anticipated.

Other contraindications for morphine given by injection or immediate-release oral solutions include heart failure secondary to chronic lung disease, cardiac arrhythmias, increased intracranial or cerebrospinal pressure, head injury, brain tumor, acute alcoholism, or delirium tremens. Because of its stimulating effects on the spinal cord, morphine should not be used during convulsions.

Caution must be used when administering morphine to patients receiving other CNS depressants because chances for respiratory depression increase. Morphine is generally considered contraindicated in cases of head injury and increased intracranial pressure; if it must be used in such cases, it must be given with extreme caution. Morphine, like all narcotics, may obscure clinical findings; the likelihood of respiratory depression and increased intracranial pressure is greater when morphine is given under these conditions. Caution should also be used when morphine is required for older or debilitated patients or those with renal or hepatic impairment. These patients may have altered pharmacokinetic processes and are more likely than other patients to exhibit adverse effects. Dose reduction may be necessary. Caution should also be used if morphine is given to patients who are sensitive to CNS effects because of concurrent alterations in their health status (e.g., respiratory compromise from chronic obstructive pulmonary disease).

Adverse Effects

The most hazardous adverse effects of morphine relate to excessive CNS depression; they include respiratory depression, hypoventilation, apnea, respiratory arrest, circulatory depression, cardiac arrest, shock, and coma. The most frequent adverse effects of morphine and other agonist narcotics are respiratory depression, apnea, bradycardia, lightheadedness, dizziness, sedation, nausea and vomiting, and sweating.

In addition, patients may experience cardiovascular adverse effects (e.g., hypotension, orthostatic hypotension, flushing, peripheral circulatory collapse); CNS effects (e.g., euphoria, dysphoria, delirium, agitation, anxiety, drowsiness, miosis, blurred vision, increased intracranial pressure); GI effects (e.g., abdominal pain, biliary tract spasm, anorexia, constipation); genitourinary (GU) effects (e.g., urinary retention or hesitancy, dysuria, decreased libido, impotence); and decreased cough reflex. Overdoses of morphine may be life threatening and should be treated with naloxone (Narcan), a narcotic antagonist.

Drug Interactions

Generally, providers can anticipate that concurrent therapy of morphine and any other CNS depressant may produce additive CNS adverse effects and substantial clinical effects. Increased respiratory and CNS depression effects are seen when morphine is given with barbiturate anesthetics, monoamine oxidase inhibitors (MAOIs), amitriptyline, cimetidine, clomipramine, and nortriptyline. Because morphine increases biliary tract pressure, levels of serum amylase or lipase may increase. One study showed that the bioavailability of oral morphine increased significantly following a high-fat meal. Parenteral mixtures of morphine with other drugs are often used when treating patients with a terminal

BOX 23.1 Secondary Pharmacologic Actions of Morphine and Other Narcotics

Provision of analgesia is the primary action of morphine and other narcotics. In addition, these drugs have a wide variety of other effects on the body.

- **Respiration:** Tidal volume is first decreased, then decreased because of reduced sensitivity of the respiratory center to carbon dioxide. Depression is dose related. Deaths from overdose usually result from respiratory arrest.
- **Cough reflex:** Cough reflex is reduced because of direct effects on the cough center in the medulla. This may be useful, or it may promote a buildup of secretions, atelectasis, and airway obstruction.
- **Hypotension and orthostatic hypotension:** These result from peripheral vasodilation, reduced peripheral resistance, and inhibition of baroreceptors. Effect is exaggerated in the presence of hypovolemia.
- **Euphoria, dysphoria, alterations in mood, feelings of relaxation, drowsiness, apathy, mental confusion:** These result from stimulation of opioid receptors.
- **Nausea and vomiting:** These develop from direct stimulation of emetic chemoreceptor trigger zone (CTZ) in the medulla.
- **Itching, flushing, red eyes:** These are produced by release of histamine.
- **Miosis (pinpoint pupils):** This results from stimulation of oculomotor nuclei, which increases parasympathetic stimulation of the eye. No tolerance develops to this effect.
- **Abdominal pain, cramps:** These occur from decreased gastric motility; prolonged gastric emptying time; decreased biliary, pancreatic, and intestinal secretions; and delays in food digestion in small intestine. Resting tone of small intestine increases.
- **Constipation:** This happens because of diminished peristalsis, increased tone of large intestine before spasms occur, and inattention to the normal stimuli for defecation reflex.
- **Biliary colic and epigastric distress:** These are due to the constriction of the sphincter of Oddi.
- **Urinary retention, urinary urgency, and difficulty urinating:** These develop from increased tone of smooth muscles in urinary tract and spasms.

disease who have severe pain. Studies of combinations of morphine with atropine, dexamethasone, scopolamine, metoclopramide, and ranitidine for physical and chemical compatibility showed that only morphine and ranitidine were incompatible, and that was only when the solution contained more than 40 mg/mL of morphine (Vermeire et al., 2002). Table 23.4 lists drugs that interact with morphine.

Assessment of Relevant Core Patient Variables

Health Status

Assess the patient for respiratory depression. Morphine should not be administered to any patient with respiratory depression because it may precipitate respiratory arrest. It should not be given to anyone with a previous hypersensitivity to morphine.

Assess for current alterations in health status that place the patient at risk for increased sensitivity to CNS depressant effects. These include cardiac, renal, hepatic, or pulmonary disease; hypothyroidism; Addison disease; prostatic hypertrophy; or urethral stricture.

Before therapy, perform a physical examination to establish a baseline in order to monitor the drug's effects. Evaluate orientation, affect, respiratory rate, adventitious sounds, and character of bowel sounds. If prolonged use is anticipated or the patient has a history of hepatic dysfunction, liver function tests should be done because morphine is metabolized in the liver.

Assess the patient for the presence and severity of pain. Pain is extremely subjective and unique for each person. The current health status can indicate whether pain might be expected. Physiologic changes that may bring on a pain response and indicate the need for drug therapy with morphine include decreased oxygenation of cardiac cells during an MI, inflamed or infected organs, or inappropriate cell growth from tumors pressing on nerves, vessels, or adjacent organs. Some health states are the source of pain for the patient, whereas others bring pain from their diagnosis or treatment. Postoperative pain is an example of pain caused by treatment.

Life Span and Gender

In using morphine or any other narcotic analgesic, assess for characteristics related to age, pregnancy, labor and delivery, and lactation.

For many years, experts believed that pain perception was absent or diminished in the very young and very old, but this belief isn't true. Pain is felt by all humans, regardless of age. Inability to express that pain is occurring, however, may impair assessment of pain in both very young and very old patients. The patient's age also influences the treatment of pain. Age-related factors are important when using morphine because it causes respiratory depression and hypotension.

The very young have impaired organ and system functioning because of immaturity. Dosages of pain-relieving drugs, therefore, need to be adjusted carefully to the child's body size and weight to prevent overdose and adverse effects.

Older adults are more likely to have age-related deterioration of organs, especially the liver and kidneys. Thus, they are more sensitive to adverse effects and can exhibit signs of overdosage unless dosage adjustments are made for them. Older adults should receive a reduced initial dose. Assess their response before additional doses are determined.

Morphine is assigned to pregnancy category C. Like other narcotics, morphine crosses the placenta rapidly. Pregnant women who abuse narcotics can cause fetal dependency; infant withdrawal will occur after delivery. If narcotics are given during labor, respiratory depression and psychophysiologic effects may appear in the neonate. Resuscitation equipment and the narcotic antidote, naloxone, should be available. The premature infant is at even greater risk for severe respiratory depression from exposure to morphine. For these reasons, morphine should not be given during labor if the delivery of a preterm infant is expected. Morphine has been shown to increase the length of labor. Morphine is secreted in breast milk. Although morphine in breast milk does not usually produce serious problems, withdrawal may be precipitated in breast-fed infants if maternal morphine is discontinued rapidly after prolonged exposure. Waiting 4 to 6 hours after dosing with morphine to breast-feed will decrease the amount transferred to the infant.

The sex of the patient may also have an effect on pain and the need for morphine. One study showed that women experienced more intense pain than men did after surgical procedures and required almost one third more morphine to achieve a similar degree of analgesia (Cepeda & Carr, 2003).

Lifestyle, Diet, and Habits

Morphine acts by depressing the CNS. Patients who use morphine to control chronic pain, such as that caused by cancer, or who receive morphine for an extended period will

TABLE 23.4 Agents That Interact With P Morphine

Interactants	Effect and Significance	Nursing Management
barbiturate anesthetics	Additive respiratory and CNS depression; apnea	Monitor respiratory function.
cimetidine	Additive CNS depression, respiratory depression	Monitor for excessive morphine response and toxicity.
esmolol	Esmolol toxicity—bradycardia, hypotension	Monitor cardiovascular function (may need to decrease esmolol dosage).
other CNS depressants (alcohol, other narcotic analgesics)	Additive CNC depression, respiratory depression	Avoid combinations if possible. Monitor respiratory function.

eventually need higher doses to control their pain as they become tolerant to the drug's therapeutic effects. **Tolerance** means that the body has become accustomed to the effects of a substance and that the patient must use more of it to achieve the desired effect. With morphine, chronic usage may result in a degree of tolerance up to 35-fold. Clearly, as patients develop tolerance to morphine, they will require larger doses to achieve adequate pain control. In addition to developing tolerance to therapeutic effects, patients also develop tolerance to adverse effects, including lethal effects, of morphine. Patients in whom drug tolerance develops can thus take dosages that would be potentially lethal in patients who are opioid naïve.

Patients who abuse alcohol, prescription drugs that suppress the CNS (e.g., opioid analgesics or benzodiazepines), or street or illicit drugs have special needs when they have pain. When a patient abuses such substances, he or she may develop a cross-tolerance to morphine's pain-relieving effects. Thus, these patients also require higher than normal doses to achieve the desired therapeutic effects of pain relief.

In morphine use that lasts longer than 3 months, physical **dependence** will also occur. Dependence is characterized by a withdrawal or abstinence syndrome when morphine is discontinued; it represents an exaggerated rebound from its acute effects. Dependence may occur during the treatment of cancer pain, and it is important in the clinical management of such pain to allow for proper agonist coverage during changes in drug dosages, schedules, or type of drug therapy. Otherwise, the patient may experience unnecessary pain and the discomfort of abstinence syndrome. Physical dependence is *not* the same as addiction. **Addiction** involves compulsive use of the drug for a secondary gain, not for pain control. The consensus document of the American Academy of Pain Medicine, American Pain Society, and the American Society of Addiction Medicine (2001) defines addiction as a neurobiologic disease characterized by one or more of these behaviors: impaired control over drug use, compulsive use, continued use despite harm, and craving. Patients who receive morphine for pain management, even over a long period, will not normally seek morphine once the pain stimulus is gone. They will, however, need their morphine doses to be decreased slowly before the drug is discontinued, to prevent withdrawal. Thus, they will develop dependence but not addiction. It is very rare for patients who are using morphine, or another narcotic, strictly for relief of pain to become addicted. Patients who currently abuse or have a history of abusing opioids do have a risk for addiction from drug therapy in pain management. This risk is not a reason to withhold morphine or any other opioid if the patient is experiencing pain. Instead, health care providers, in cooperation with the patient, can accomplish careful drug selection and dosage adjustment. If addiction does occur after therapy concludes, it must be addressed separately. Patients should be helped to wean themselves away from drug use before they are discharged from their providers' care.

Environment

Closely monitor patients receiving morphine as part of monitored anesthesia care (MAC) or postoperatively for signs of serious adverse effects, particularly respiratory depression. Health care providers or patients themselves may administer narcotic analgesics, as in patient-controlled analgesia (PCA). Morphine, like all narcotics, is a controlled substance, and by law every dose must be properly accounted for and documented, including partial doses that may be wasted. Although oral doses may be administered in any setting, doses given by IV infusion, injection, and epidural and intrathecal catheters are normally given only in the hospital where the patient can be closely monitored. The exception is IV infusions, which may be used in the home during hospice care.

Culture and Inherited Traits

The experience of pain is personal and subjective; however, how individuals respond to painful stimuli reflects what they have learned about pain from their families, society, and cultures of origin. Learned messages about pain are indirect, and people react to them subconsciously. These messages include reasons that people experience pain and what are considered appropriate responses to it. For example, some religions view pain as a punishment from God for sins. Others view pain as a test from God to develop inner strength and faith. Still others may believe that pain is merely an aspect of life like any other. Some stoic cultures believe that people should tolerate pain without verbal complaints. British, German, and Asian groups are thought of as stoic cultures. Other cultural groups are very expressive about pain, see such expressiveness as acceptable, and may encourage it. Spanish, Italian, and Latin groups are thought to be expressive cultures. Although not everyone who shares a cultural background reacts identically to pain, consider these generalizations when patients have pain. Validate the expressive patient's pain, or encourage stoic patients to take needed pain medication. For both types of patient, offer support as well as pain medication.

Nursing Diagnoses and Outcomes

- Ineffective Breathing Pattern, Hypoventilation, related to respiratory depression caused by the drug
  Desired outcome: *The patient maintains effective breathing despite respiratory depression.*
- Ineffective Airway Clearance secondary to cough suppression by the drug
  Desired outcome: *The patient's airway remains patent and clear.*

CRITICAL THINKING SCENARIO

Thinking critically about drug therapy in pain management

Mr. Schneider is 60 years old. He is a second-generation German American. He has worked for 35 years in a local steel mill. He had surgery for a bowel obstruction yesterday. When you assess him, he states he does not have pain, yet he is restless in the bed and moaning. He says he will take something for pain when the pain is very severe. He does not want to get out of bed to ambulate, and he will only cough superficially when asked to demonstrate coughing and deep breathing.

1. Discuss factors that may be contributing to the inconsistencies between the patient's verbal report and nonverbal behavior.
2. Why is appropriate pain management important for this patient?
3. Propose a teaching plan that you think would help this patient with effective pain management.

- Constipation secondary to activity of the drug
  Desired outcome: The patient remains free of constipation.
- Urinary Retention related to indirect anticholinergic effects of the drug on the urinary sphincters
  Desired outcome: The patient maintains normal urinary output.
- Risk for Injury related to orthostatic hypotension or sedation secondary to drug effects
  Desired outcome: The patient remains free of injury.
- Acute Pain related to trauma or disease process and insufficient analgesia
  Desired outcome: The patient remains free of pain.
- Deficient Knowledge related to morphine therapy
  Desired outcome: The patient has adequate knowledge of the drug and its adverse effects and their management.

Planning and Intervention

The key issue in morphine therapy is adequate control of pain balanced against the considerable adverse effects of respiratory depression and excessive sedation. Goals of treatment include adequate pulmonary ventilation, a respiratory rate within 12 to 20 breaths/minute, minimal effects of constipation and urinary retention, freedom from injury, and adequate family and patient education for managing drug therapy. It is also important to teach the patient possible adverse effects of morphine and how to manage them. Other goals relate to maintaining safety during potential episodes of orthostatic hypotension.

Maximizing Therapeutic Effects

Assessing Pain

The first step in maximizing the therapeutic effects of drug therapy with morphine or any other narcotic is to complete a full pain assessment. Pain has been greatly underassessed and undertreated. Many professional organizations, clinical guidelines, and accreditation bodies now recommend that pain be routinely assessed for all patients; this recommendation has been likened to making pain a fifth vital sign, which requires assessment whenever the other vital signs are assessed during patient care. Remember that pain is a subjective experience. It is whatever the patient says it is, occurring whenever the patient says it does. Objective data, such as elevated blood pressure or pulse rate, moaning, or grimacing, may accompany pain, but the absence of objective data does not indicate that pain does not exist. Many people actually cope with pain by using distraction techniques, such as smiling, talking, quiet rhythmic breathing, or watching television. Patients who experience chronic pain are especially likely to use distraction techniques. Every patient has a different level of tolerance for what he or she feels is an acceptable level of pain. Careful assessment enables you to assist the patient in identifying and achieving this level of control. Pain assessment tools allow the individual's pain to be tracked using the same scale or criteria. Although pain can be assessed by asking questions, this approach is not considered a true tool because a tool must be tangible. Verbal assessment may be necessary in a particular situation, but a true tool that has been shown to be valid and reliable is preferable.

To begin the pain assessment, first determine the location of the pain. Location gives possible clues to the source of the pain and can help identify whether the pain is acute or of a more chronic nature. Many pain assessment tools incorporate a representation of the human body from a frontal and posterior view. The tools ask patients to shade or circle on the diagram to show the location of the pain. Such identification helps the patient define what he or she is experiencing and provides a starting point for further assessment. Each pain location should be recorded in the patient's chart along with its associated intensity and quality.

The next step is to determine the pain intensity. Many assessment tools are available to rate pain intensity (Figure 23.3). Each tool provides a continuum in some form to represent a range from "no pain" to the "worst pain imaginable." Asking the patient to rate pain using an imaginary scale in his or her head is *not* considered a tool. One of the most widely recognized pain assessment tools for reliability and ease of use is the visual analogue scale, which is numeric. It may be a scale from 0 to 5 or 0 to 10, but both ranges allow patients to rate their pain by assigning a number that demonstrates greater pain as they move up the scale. The visual analogue scale may be printed, with the patient pointing to the appropriate number; or the scale may be on a hand-held device with a sliding pointer; with the patient sliding the pointer to the appropriate number to demonstrate his or her pain.

Because research findings indicate that approximately 7% to 11% of adults cannot conceptualize well enough to use the visual analogue pain scale, other pain assessment tools may be helpful. One alternative is a descriptive pain-intensity tool in which words replace the numbers 0 to 5, again with the two extremes being no pain or the worst imaginable pain. The FACES scale, used frequently with children, cognitively impaired adults, and those who do not speak English, shows a series of facial expressions ranging from very unhappy and crying to very happy and smiling (National Pharmaceutical Council and Joint Commission on Accreditation of Healthcare Organizations, 2001; Wong & Baker, 1988). The patient is then asked to pick the face that most resembles how he or she feels. In the poker chip tool, four poker chips are placed in front of the patient. Each one is a "piece of hurt," with one piece being "just a little hurt" and four pieces being "the most hurt." Patients are asked to show how many pieces of hurt they have. This tool is also frequently used with children.

Each patient may interpret the extremes of any of the scales differently based on his or her past experiences. With consistent use, however, the pain assessment tool gives the patient and the provider a common ground on which to plan treatment and understand the degree of relief from the treatments provided.

Intensity of pain is only one aspect of pain that should be assessed; pain quality and character (affective descriptions) should also be measured. Not all pain assessment tools currently available assess for all these parameters. Some of the well-tested tools include the Brief Pain Inventory, the McGill Pain Questionnaire, and the Memorial Pain Assessment Card (National Pharmaceutical Council and Joint Commission on Accreditation of Healthcare Organizations, 2001; Melzack, 1975; Daut et al., 1983; Cleeland & Ryan, 1994; Fishman et al., 1987).

Of these, the McGill Pain Questionnaire is the only one that is not a visual tool. Instead, it is a set series of questions

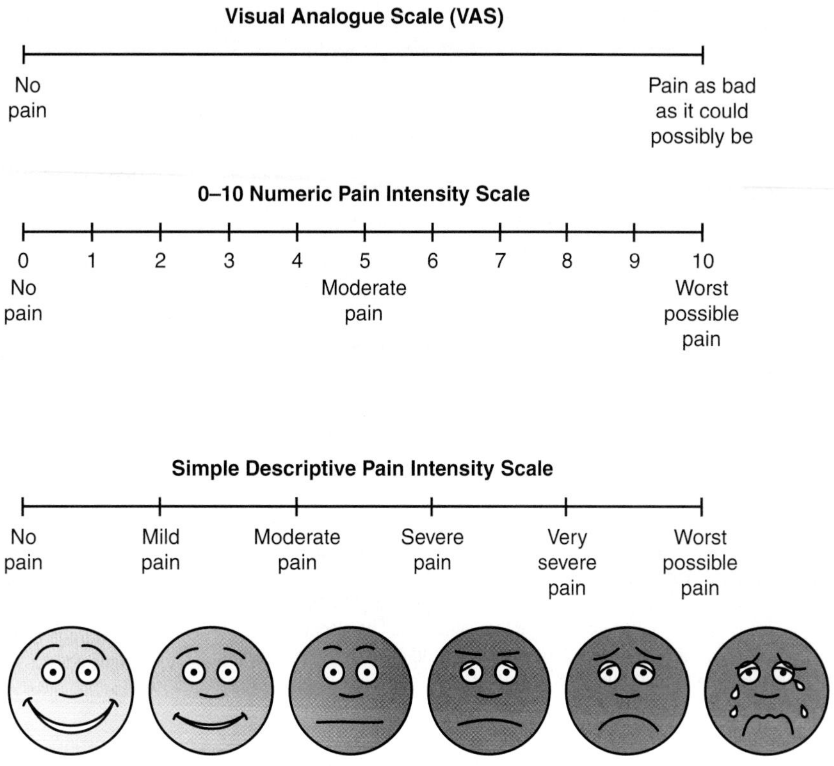

FIGURE 23.3 Pain assessment tools. Many pain intensity scales are available for ranking the pain of children and adults alike. Such scales as (**A**) the visual analogue, numeric pain intensity, and simple descriptive pain intensity rank pain from no pain to worst pain possible. Scales such as (**B**) the FACES pain rating scale are ideal for children and others who have difficulty with numeric concepts. To assist children with the FACES scale, the nurse explains that each face represents a person who feels happy because the person has no pain or a person who feels sad because the person has a lot of pain. Face 1 hurts a little bit, Face 2 hurts a little bit more, Face 3 hurts even more, Face 4 hurts a lot, and Face 5 has the biggest hurt you can have. Then, the nurse asks the child to choose the face that best describes his or her own pain and documents the selection. (From Wong, D. L., Hockenberry-Eaton, M., Wilson, D., et. al. [2001]. *Wong's Essentials of Pediatric Nursing.* [6th ed., p. 1301.]. St. Louis: Mosby. Copyrighted by Mosby, Inc. Reprinted by permission.)

to ask the patient, after which you record the patient's answers. This tool has long and short forms; the long form takes 5 to 15 minutes to complete, the short form can be completed in 2 to 3 minutes, making it preferable in an acute care setting. Assessment of pain intensity and all aspects of pain is an important part of treating pain effectively, especially for patients who are stoic, who use coping mechanisms to deal with pain, or whose pain may be undertreated if you offer drug therapy only to those who state that they are in pain.

Providing Analgesia

Morphine, like other drugs that relieve pain, is more effective when it is administered before the level of pain becomes severe. This is another reason why it is important to assess the patient's pain level frequently. When pain exists, analgesic dosages are best administered around the clock rather than as needed. Continual administration promotes a steady blood level of the drug, which prevents drug troughs that allow pain to escalate. In around-the-clock dosing, a baseline amount of the drug is administered over the 24-hour period when acute pain is expected or when severe, chronic pain occurs. Patients should be awakened for the analgesic if receiving it orally; however, they may refuse the drug at any time.

The appropriate dose of morphine must be given to control the patient's pain. No one dose will be appropriate for every patient. Titration of dosage is usually required when therapy begins and continues for as long as the patient receives care. To titrate the morphine dose means to increase it incrementally. Aggressiveness of titration depends on pain intensity and response. Remember that patients with a history of substance abuse or drug tolerance will need higher dosages of analgesics. Morphine is titrated until the desired therapeutic response, or efficacy, is achieved or until adverse effects occur. Efficacy is usually defined as a pain level below 4 out of 10 or a level determined by both the patient and health care provider. Nonopioids, such as NSAIDs, may be used in conjunction with morphine. Other adjunct drugs may be added to morphine if necessary for pain control. Finally, in addition to pharmacologic interventions, nonpharmacologic methods may be used in conjunction with morphine. These methods are not substitutes for morphine, but they are valuable adjuncts to therapy (see Table 23.1).

For patients with chronic pain, the use of a long-acting form of morphine may better manage the patient's pain. Recognizing the need for long-term control and facilitating the conversion from short-acting to long-acting morphine, or other opioid, is important. A thorough assessment is needed to best determine which particular drug and route would best meet the individual patient's needs. Make sure that a fast-acting rescue drug (see Minimizing Adverse Effects) is also prescribed to treat breakthrough pain (Vallerand, 2003).

Minimizing Adverse Effects

Minimizing the adverse effects of morphine requires frequent and astute assessment and implementation of basic nursing care (Box 23.2). Dosing the drug carefully to meet the needs posed by core patient variables can minimize adverse effects. In general, dosages will need to be lower for children, older adults, and patients with renal or hepatic impairment. Morphine should be administered before pain becomes severe. Because this dosing schedule is more effective, a smaller dose of the drug can be given, which helps to prevent or minimize adverse effects.

Breakthrough pain and incidental pain may occur during pain management with drug therapy. Clinicians use the term **breakthrough pain** to describe transitory flare-ups of pain

BOX 23.2 Minimizing Adverse Effects of Morphine

For All

- Consult with the physician and pharmacist to individualize dosage and dosing intervals based on the patient's weight, age, pain intensity, diagnosis, concurrent medical status, and use of other CNS depressants.
- Because ambulation may increase occurrence of the frequent adverse effects, have patient lie down after the dose has been taken.
- Because low pain levels may increase occurrence of the frequent adverse effects, consider a nonnarcotic analgesic for patients with mild to moderate pain.

Respiratory Depression

- Assess vital signs, especially respiratory function, on a regular, frequent basis.
- Measure the oxygen concentration of the blood with a pulse oximeter on a regular and as-needed basis.
- Have the patient perform turning, coughing, and deep breathing, and reposition the patient to remove secretions and maintain adequate pulmonary ventilation.
- Place the patient on the side, not flat on the back, to maintain an open airway until condition stabilizes. If the patient must be placed on the back, remove pillow, and tilt the patient's head back slightly to prevent the tongue from occluding the airway. Use an oral airway if necessary.
- Withhold the next dose and notify the physician if the patient is bradypneic.
- Administer oxygen as needed.
- Have emergency respiratory equipment available.
- Keep naloxone, the narcotic antidote, on hand. Administer as needed.

Hypotension

- Monitor blood pressure carefully in postoperative patients, patients who have low circulating blood volume, or patients who are simultaneously receiving a CNS depressant (e.g., phenothiazine) or general anesthetics. These conditions make such patients more prone to hypotension.
- Monitor for orthostatic hypotension, especially during transport, for patients with decreased circulating blood levels or impaired cardiac function and for those receiving sympatholytic (blocking the action of the sympathetic nervous system) drugs.
- Monitor intake and output and replace fluids for patients who are hypovolemic.
- Assess ambulatory patients carefully for orthostatic hypotension.

Constipation

- Encourage dietary fiber when taking morphine orally.
- Encourage oral fluids when tolerated; keep patient well hydrated with IV fluids if NPO.
- Promote ambulation (assisted as necessary) as much as possible.
- Administer stool softeners or laxatives PRN.

Urinary Retention and Decreased Urinary Output

- Monitor intake and output at least every work shift.
- Question to determine whether the patient self-reports difficulty voiding, lack of voiding, frequent voiding of very small amounts, or feelings of bladder fullness or tenderness.
- Palpate the bladder to differentiate urinary retention from oliguria.
- Encourage oral fluids if allowed; provide adequate hydration with IV fluids if NPO.
- Use noninvasive means to promote voiding (ensure female patient sits upright, ensure male patient stands, run water in sink, pour water over perineum, use sitz baths).
- Obtain order and perform urethral catheterization if needed.

Light-headedness, Dizziness, and Sedation

- Assist the patient who is ambulating and getting out of bed.
- Ensure the use of side rails when the patient is in bed.

Nausea and Vomiting

- Keep the patient NPO during acute episodes; maintain the patient on IV fluids for hydration.
- Offer ice chips and clear liquids as symptoms diminish.
- Obtain order and administer antiemetics if indicated.

over baseline in a patient receiving opioid therapy. Breakthrough pain is generally graded as moderate to severe in intensity. It may last from a few seconds to a few hours. It may or may not have a precipitating event. Spontaneous, or activity-related, pain is called incidental pain. An incident may be related to a specific movement or to all movements.

Factors to consider when assessing and treating breakthrough and incidental pain are those that relate to cause. When pain does occur, is it related to a specific time during the dosing schedule? If so, a change in the dosing interval or an increase in the drug dose may be beneficial. Does a certain movement cause pain, or is the pain unpredictable? Patients often have incidental or breakthrough pain associated with movement or activity. How long does the pain last? Although morphine has a fairly rapid onset, some severe pain may persist for less time than it takes for the analgesic to take effect.

All patients being treated for pain need access to **rescue doses** for breakthrough pain. The rescue dose should be equianalgesic to 10% to 30% of the dose the patient receives in 24 hours and is added to the established pain management. Patients who require more than three rescue doses in a day should have their analgesic dosage adjusted either by increasing the baseline dose or maximizing the co-analgesics. A thorough assessment will assist the health care provider to decide whether the best option is to increase the dosage or to incorporate other therapies. Rescue doses, sometimes referred to as "PRN" or bolus doses, may be administered by a PCA device if the patient is receiving IV or epidural analgesia. Program into the IV pump the dose that has been ordered for the rescue or bolus dose and the frequency that the patient may receive a dose. When patients experience pain, they press a button, similar to a call light, and the pump administers the correct dose if it is time. Some institutions, especially with older adults or others who are at risk for experiencing adverse effects from around-the-clock dosing, may use PCA without a basal rate. In other words, the pump administers medication only when patients request it. When the pump is used in this manner, patients need to request a dose as soon as they begin to experience pain.

Providing Patient and Family Education

- Patients being treated for pain need to know what the treatment plan will be for managing their pain and that

they are not expected to suffer. Ensure patients that health care providers will listen to them and act when they report that they have pain.
- Patients need to know that they have an important role to play in managing their pain. Review the following points with them:
  - Know how to use the pain assessment tools.
  - Report honestly how they feel during assessment.
  - Establish (with the health care team) what pain level will trigger automatic re-evaluation of the pain management plan. Ideally, re-evaluation should happen before pain develops or increases (e.g., in the preoperative period or early in the course of a disease).
- Teach the patient who is receiving PCA how to appropriately use this. Patients should be instructed to request a dose whenever they have pain; waiting for the pain to become severe before seeking a dose will make it more difficult for the drug to be effective and may require larger doses of the morphine. Emphasize to patients that they cannot overdose themselves because the computer in the pump will be programmed to administer only a prescribed dose at a prescribed interval (Box 23.3).
- Correct any fears or misconceptions, including the following:
  - Pain is inevitable.
  - Pain must be endured.
  - Patients will "lose control" of themselves if they take drugs for pain.
  - Patients will become addicted.
- Teach patients that drug therapy with morphine over a prolonged period (as in chronic or cancer pain) may produce physical dependence on the drug. Explain that physical dependence is not the same as addiction, nor is it a reason to withhold pain treatment. If the pain resolves, the patient can be weaned from the drug to prevent withdrawal. Weaning is not appropriate with cancer pain because the pain will not resolve on its own.
- If the patient is discharged home on morphine, teach the following:
  - Administration
  - Effects (adverse and otherwise)
  - Avoidance of driving and other hazardous activities during drug therapy
  - Avoidance of alcohol and concurrent CNS depressant therapy, unless a health care provider is managing the concurrent therapy
  - Placement of drug secure from children and anyone likely to abuse it

FOCUS ON RESEARCH

Box 23.3 Teaching to Meet Patients' Needs

Chumbley, G. M., Hall, G. M., & Salmon, P. (2002). Patient-controlled analgesia: What information does the patient want? *Journal of Advanced Nursing, 39*(5), 459–471.

The Study

In an effort to provide information on the use of patient-controlled analgesia that better met patients' needs, seven focus groups were created at a hospital in London, England. Patients told the researchers that they wanted to know a number of specific items. These included: what drug was being administered, what the adverse effects of the drug were, reassurance that the drug and delivery method were safe, reassurance that they could not overdose or become addicted, and specific detailed information (including pictures) of how to use the pump correctly to administer the drug. When this information was incorporated into the patient education materials, patients, who were part of a research study, reported that they felt more satisfaction with their patient education.

Nursing Implications

Patient-controlled analgesia is a common practice used in treating both acute and chronic pain. For all patient education to be effective, it needs to meet the learning needs of the individual patient. The findings from this small study are important to consider when teaching about this method of providing pain relief.

Ongoing Assessment and Evaluation

Documentation of pain management should include the following:

- The pain scale used by the patient
- The rating given by the patient
- The components, sensory and affective, of pain
- The amount of morphine, route, and the time each dose is administered
- The degree of pain relief obtained from morphine therapy
- The effectiveness of adjunct drug therapy and nonpharmacologic interventions used
- Any morphine-induced adverse effects

Increasing pain in a patient previously stabilized on a certain dose of morphine should not be automatically attributed to tolerance without investigating for evidence of disease progression or complications. Cancer pain, for example, changes constantly. It may increase or decrease secondary to anticancer treatment, infectious processes, spreading tumors, or natural degenerative body changes (arthritis). Postoperative pain that morphine does not relieve may indicate postoperative complications, such as compartment syndrome.

The patient should have adequate pain control with minimal adverse effects. Breakthrough pain should be minimal if the pain is adequately controlled. The patient should remain free from injury from orthostatic hypotension or sedation. The patient and family should show an understanding of adverse effects if discharged on morphine and should be able to describe how to manage those effects should they occur.

Drugs Closely Related to P Morphine

Hydromorphone

Hydromorphone (Dilaudid) is a semisynthetic analogue of opium. Its effects on the body are almost identical to those of morphine. As an analgesic, hydromorphone is equally effective as morphine, although more potent. Between 1 and 1.5 (1 to 1.50) mg of subcutaneous (SC) or intramuscular (IM) hydromorphone is equal to 10 mg of morphine given through the same routes. Hydromorphone is available in oral, parenteral, and rectal forms. Hydromorphone also has equal antitussive (cough suppression) effects; however, its ability to cause respiratory depression and physical dependency is less than that of morphine. Hydromorphone's ability to cause constipation, sedation, and emesis is unknown; thus,

MEMORY CHIP

P Morphine

- Narcotic analgesic used in moderate to severe pain
- Standard against which all other narcotic analgesics are measured for effectiveness
- Major contraindications: significant respiratory depression, increased intracranial pressure, and CNS depression
- Most common adverse effects: light-headedness, dizziness, sedation, nausea, and vomiting
- Most serious adverse effect: respiratory depression
- **Life span alert: Avoid use in premature infants or during labor when delivery of premature infant is expected.**
- Maximizing therapeutic effects: Assess pain thoroughly before and during therapy and titrate the dose until the desired pain-relieving effect is achieved.
- Minimizing adverse effects: Individualize dose based on patient-related variables; monitor vital signs, especially respiratory rate, frequently; and have the antidote, naloxone, on hand.
- Most important patient education: for long-term use in cancer pain, physical dependency will develop. This is not the same as addiction and not an appropriate reason to withhold the drug.

comparisons with morphine cannot be made. Unlike morphine, hydromorphone can cause transient hyperglycemia.

Levorphanol

Levorphanol (Levo-Dromoran), a synthetic compound, can be used to manage pain and as a preoperative agent. It has similar analgesic, constipating, respiratory-depressive, sedating, and physical dependency qualities to those of morphine. It has fewer antitussive and emetic effects. Like hydromorphone, levorphanol is more potent than morphine, with an SC dose of 2 mg equal to 10 mg of morphine.

Oxycodone

Oxycodone is a semisynthetic analogue of opium. Oxycodone is metabolized by the 2D6 isoenzyme. Unlike morphine, it is only available as an oral preparation. It is available in regular-release (Roxicodone), timed-release (OxyContin), and rapid-release formulas (OxyIR). Oxycodone has similar analgesic, antitussive, constipating, respiratory-depressive, sedating, emetic, and physical dependency effects to those of morphine.

The long-acting, timed-release forms are very helpful in managing severe chronic pain, either cancer pain or non-cancer chronic pain.

Although oxycodone has been a safe and effective therapy for patients with severe chronic pain, unfortunately, this drug has also been abused as a street drug. When abused, the drug is crushed before being taken, so that an extremely high dose of the narcotic is available all at once, instead of being released slowly over time. Severe adverse effects are possible when it is used in this manner. Those who abuse it are most probably addicted to the drug.

Oxycodone is often administered as a combination drug with either aspirin (Percodan, Roxiprin) or acetaminophen (Tylox, Percocet, Roxicet). One problem with using combination drugs is that the amount of these other drugs that can be administered daily is limited. When increasing the dosage to provide for adequate pain control, calculate the total daily intake of aspirin or acetaminophen because overdosage of either of these drugs can cause serious adverse effects (see Chapter 24 for more information).

Oxymorphone

Oxymorphone (Numorphan) is a semisynthetic analogue of opium. It is used in pain control, as a preoperative medication, to support anesthesia, as an obstetric analgesic, and for the relief of anxiety in patients with dyspnea associated with pulmonary edema secondary to acute left ventricular dysfunction. Oxymorphone is available in injection and rectal forms. It has analgesic and constipating effects similar to those of morphine; however, it causes more respiratory depression, emesis, and physical dependence. Oxymorphone has fewer antitussive effects than morphine; its sedating effects are unknown.

Meperidine

Meperidine (Demerol) is a synthetic compound used to treat pain as a preoperative medication, to support anesthesia, and during labor. Meperidine has similar analgesic and respiratory depressive effects and abilities to cause physical dependence as morphine. Meperidine has fewer sedative and constipating effects and substantially fewer antitussive effects than morphine. Meperidine has a longer half-life and is less potent than morphine, requiring 75 mg IM or SC to have an equianalgesic effect equal to that of 10 mg of morphine. A unique drug interaction occurs between meperidine and the hydantoins (anticonvulsants), which decreases the effectiveness of meperidine. This effect may result from an increased hepatic metabolism of meperidine.

The most important difference between morphine and meperidine is related to the pharmacokinetics of meperidine. Meperidine is metabolized to an active metabolite, normeperidine. Normeperidine has a long half-life (15 to 30 hours) and will accumulate in the body with chronic dosing. Half-life is further extended in patients with renal impairment, which slows excretion of normeperidine. Normeperidine is a CNS toxin. Accumulated doses in the body can cause tremors, seizures, and changes in level of consciousness. Older adults are especially sensitive to the adverse effects of normeperidine, which may be the result of impaired renal function. For these reasons, meperidine should normally be avoided in pain management when multiple doses will be given. The exception would be if the patient were allergic to morphine; however, the patient must have normal renal function.

Fentanyl

Fentanyl is a synthetic compound. Its major uses are as a preanesthetic, anesthetic, and analgesic. Fentanyl's analgesic properties are equal to those of morphine. It produces fewer respiratory and emetic effects. Its antitussive, constipating, sedating, and physical dependency effects are unknown in comparison with those of morphine. Fentanyl is much more potent than morphine, with 0.1 mg producing equianalgesia to that of 10 mg of morphine.

Fentanyl is available in various forms. Fentanyl as a liquid for injection (Sublimaze) is used as an anesthetic, an analgesic of short duration during anesthesia, and a supplement to general or regional anesthesia. An off-label use is pain control through epidural PCA, usually after surgery.

Fentanyl is also available in a transdermal system (Duragesic). It is used in chronic pain, usually related to cancer, when the patient requires continuous opioid analgesia for pain that other methods cannot control. When first used, it takes approximately 24 hours for the full pain-relieving effect to occur. The patient should be treated with short-acting opioids during this period. Short-acting opioids are not needed when changing the patch after 72 hours, except for rescue doses for breakthrough pain. The use of transdermal fentanyl in the treatment of noncancer chronic pain is continuing to gain acceptance. A recent study showed that, compared with oral sustained-release morphine, transdermal fentanyl was more effective in controlling pain and was cost effective (Frei et al., 2003). Other studies are supporting the use of transdermal fentanyl in treating chronic noncancer pain even in patients who have not previously received other opioids, such as morphine (Mystakidou et al., 2003). For more information, see Box 23.4.

There are two types of fentanyl transmucosal systems. Fentanyl Oralet is used only as a premedication to anesthesia or to induce conscious sedation before a procedure such as cardiac catheterization. Use of this form carries a risk for hypoventilation; thus, it is administered only in hospital settings where anesthesia care can be monitored (e.g., operating rooms [ORs], emergency departments [EDs], and intensive care units [ICUs]). Trained personnel must monitor the patient throughout therapy with Oralet; emergency equipment and a narcotic antagonist must be available. Oralet is frequently used in children, although it may be used in adults. The lozenge is manufactured with a handle, similar in appearance to a lollipop. Administration should begin 20 to 40 minutes before the need for the desired therapeutic effect. Instruct the patient to suck on the lozenge. Remove the handle from the patient's mouth when effectiveness is adequate or if the patient develops complications.

The other transmucosal form of fentanyl (Actiq) is used only for the management of breakthrough pain in patients with cancer who are already receiving and are already tolerant to opioid therapy. Only oncologists and pain specialists who are familiar with opioids should administer it to treat cancer pain. If used in the home, storage of the drug in a safe place is critical because the dose found in this form may be fatal to children. Neither transmucosal form of fentanyl is used for acute or chronic pain (other than cancer pain).

COMMUNITY-BASED CONCERNS

Box 23.4 Teaching About Transdermal Fentanyl

As more and more patients learn to manage their own health care and drug therapy at home, you will assume an even greater role in teaching patients and their caregivers about safe self-care and drug administration. For a patient who will be discharged while receiving transdermal fentanyl, some important drug administration teaching points for the patient or the caregiver follow.

1. Caregivers who administer a transdermal fentanyl patch should first put on gloves to avoid absorbing any of the drug themselves. They should also wear gloves when removing the patch.
2. Tear open a new patch packet carefully; never cut the patch with scissors.
3. Remove the liner on the sticky side of the patch.
4. Apply the fentanyl patch to nonirritated, smooth, hairless skin (clip hair; avoid shaving to avoid breaking the skin) on the chest, back, flank, or upper arm right after opening the patch package. If necessary, wash the skin with clear water and dry completely before applying the patch. Do not use soaps, creams, alcohol, oils, lotions, or anything else that might irritate the skin or alter its characteristics.
5. Hold the patch in place for 30 seconds to ensure firm adherence.
6. Wear the system continually for 72 hours and then replace with a new patch, placed in a different location.
7. To discard a used patch, fold it in half with the sticky sides together (to prevent any residual drug from touching the skin) and flush the patch down the toilet, because active drug remains in the patch. (Patches discarded in the trash may be attractive to and accidentally come in contact with children or pets.)
8. Use the short-acting drug prescribed as a rescue dose for any breakthrough pain. Keep a log of how often you need to use rescue doses and bring this information with you to your next appointment. This log provides valuable information about how the well the prescribed drug and dose are controlling your pain.

Alfentanil

Alfentanil (Alfenta) is used in the OR as an analgesic during anesthesia, to induce anesthesia when intubation and mechanical ventilation are required, and as the analgesic component of MAC. Its analgesic effects are similar to those of morphine. Its onset of action is immediate.

Sufentanil

Sufentanil (Sufenta) produces a greater analgesic effect than morphine. It is used as an anesthetic and analgesic adjunct to maintain balanced anesthesia when patients are intubated and on a ventilator. It is also used as an epidural analgesic during labor and vaginal delivery (when combined with low-dose bupivacaine).

Methadone

Methadone (Methadose, Dolophine) can be used for pain, to prevent withdrawal symptoms from heroin (detoxification), and as a maintenance treatment for narcotic abuse. Although its ability to produce analgesia and the duration of its analgesic effect (4–6 hours, compared with 3–7 hours) are similar to those of morphine, its half-life is much longer. The half-life of methadone is 15 to 30 hours, compared with 1.5 to 2 hours for morphine. Adverse effects and signs of overdose may occur when methadone is used as pain management because of these pharmacokinetic properties. Methadone may be initiated in a hospital setting only for prevention of withdrawal. Only approved treatment programs for narcotic abuse may initiate treatment with methadone for maintenance treatment of addiction. If a patient is already in a maintenance treatment program with methadone and requires hospitalization, the hospital may provide the methadone, after personnel confirm the dose with the treatment center that normally observes the patient.

Remifentanil

Remifentanil (Ultiva), although classified as a narcotic agonist-analgesic, is used as a general anesthetic and as part of monitored anesthesia care. Remifentanil has more anal-

gesic effects than morphine but similar respiratory depressive and emetic effects. Physical dependence and constipation occur less often than with morphine.

Drugs Significantly Different From P Morphine

Naloxone (Narcan) is a narcotic antagonist. It is believed to antagonize the effects of narcotics by competing for opioid receptor sites. It is used to reverse the effects of opiates (e.g., respiratory depression) and to treat opioid overdose. Naloxone is not effective for respiratory depression caused by anything other than narcotic agonist analgesics. Naloxone can be used in adults, children, and neonates.

Although it can be given by the IM, SC, or IV route, the most rapid onset is achieved with IV use, and this route is recommended in emergencies. IV onset is within 2 minutes; duration of action depends on the dose given and the route used, although it is quite short. Careful monitoring of the patient beyond initial response is warranted because the duration of action of the narcotic agonist may be longer than the duration of naloxone. Thus, the patient may relapse into respiratory arrest or depression. Repeated doses may be necessary to maintain reversal of the opiate's effects. Abrupt reversal of narcotic depression may result in the adverse effects of nausea, vomiting, sweating, tachycardia, increased blood pressure, and tremors. Administration of naloxone will precipitate withdrawal in persons physically dependent on narcotics. It will also reverse all the analgesic effects in those receiving morphine or other narcotic agonists for pain control if the dose is sufficient.

Naloxone's reversal of respiratory depression from buprenorphine (a mixed agonist and antagonist) may be incomplete, requiring mechanical assistance for respiration. Naloxone may be combined with subinguinal preparations of buprenorphine to treat drug addiction. (For further information on buprenorphine, see Drugs Closely Related to Pentazocine, below.)

C Mild Narcotic Agonists

The mild narcotic agonists include codeine, hydrocodone, and propoxyphene. Codeine is the prototype for the mild narcotic agonists.

NURSING MANAGEMENT OF THE PATIENT RECEIVING P CODEINE

• Core Drug Knowledge

Pharmacotherapeutics

Codeine is used to control mild to moderate pain in adults and children. For this purpose, it is available in oral tablets and an injectable form for parenteral use. Orally, it may be combined with acetaminophen. Codeine is also used for cough suppression. The dose needed to achieve an antitussive effect is less than the dose required for analgesia. Although codeine has fewer antitussive effects than morphine (when comparing similar weights of the drugs), it is more widely used to suppress coughs because it has low adverse effects at the antitussive doses. Codeine may be used alone, in the form of oral tablets, or in combination with other drugs that are expectorants (in a liquid or syrup form) to suppress coughs.

Pharmacokinetics

Codeine is well absorbed from the GI tract. Its peak effect occurs in 1 to 2 hours. (Other pharmacokinetic parameters are identified in Table 23.3). Codeine is metabolized in the liver by oxidative reactions through the P-450 isoenzyme system. Whether codeine is actually a prodrug, which requires changing by the P-450 system to be active, is the subject of some debate. Codeine is excreted in the urine. It crosses the placenta and is secreted in breast milk.

Pharmacodynamics

Codeine has pharmacologic effects similar to those of morphine, but its actions are milder. Codeine acts at specific opioid receptors in the CNS to produce analgesia, euphoria, and sedation. Codeine also acts directly on the medullary cough center to depress the cough reflex. It has a drying effect on mucous membranes and can increase the viscosity of respiratory tract secretions.

Contraindications and Precautions

Codeine should not be administered to patients receiving other narcotic analgesics for pain relief; such a combination can cause serious respiratory depression and sedation. Codeine should be used with caution in patients who need to cough to maintain the airways (postoperative patients and patients who have undergone major abdominal or thoracic surgery). Careful use is recommended for patients with asthma and emphysema because cough suppression in these patients can lead to accumulation of secretions and a loss of respiratory reserve. Codeine is used with caution in patients with pre-existing cardiac disease because of its potential to induce bradycardia and peripheral vasodilation.

Codeine is assigned to pregnancy category C. Like other opiate narcotics, it crosses the placenta, is secreted in breast milk, and can cause sedation and respiratory depression in the fetus or infant. Therefore, it should be used with caution during pregnancy and lactation. The closer it is given to delivery, the more likely it is for respiratory depression to occur in the newborn. Resuscitation equipment should be on hand if the mother has received codeine or other opiates during labor. Codeine should be avoided if the delivery of a premature infant is expected. Caution should also be used with patients who are hypersensitive to or have a history of addiction to narcotics; codeine is a narcotic and has a potential for addiction. Patients who need to drive or be alert should use codeine with extreme caution because it can cause sedation and drowsiness. Caution is important when codeine is used for patients who have experienced a head injury or undergone a craniotomy. Codeine can increase intracranial pressure, which can be detrimental to these patients.

Adverse Effects

As already stated, codeine has a low incidence of adverse effects when used at the appropriate dosage level as an antitussive. The most frequent adverse effects observed with the use of codeine as a cough suppressant include drowsiness, sedation, dry mouth, nausea and vomiting, and constipation. When dosed as an analgesic, the adverse effects are similar to those of morphine, although they are less severe. Allergic reactions, including rashes and urticaria, have been noted in highly sensitive people. Respiratory depression and cardiovascular effects have occurred with higher doses.

Drug Interactions

An increased likelihood of respiratory depression, hypotension, or profound sedation exists when codeine is given with any other drugs that cause CNS depression, such as antihistamines, phenothiazines, barbiturates, sedative-hypnotics, tricyclic antidepressants, and alcohol. Codeine may also interact with histamine-2 antagonists, such as cimetidine. Table 23.5 lists drugs that interact with codeine.

Assessment of Relevant Core Patient Variables

Health Status

Assess whether the patient needs to cough to maintain a patent airway. Such patients (e.g., postoperative patients) should not receive codeine. In this situation, the cough is a protective mechanism to rid the airways of potentially harmful substances that may lead to pneumonia. The same rationale is used when treating patients with asthma or emphysema. If they do not cough, they have the potential to retain secretions that may exacerbate their disease.

Before therapy, perform a physical examination to establish a baseline to monitor the effects of the drug. Parameters to evaluate include orientation, affect, respiratory rate, adventitious sounds, and character of bowel sounds. If prolonged use is anticipated or the patient has a history of hepatic dysfunction, ensure that liver function tests are done because codeine is metabolized in the liver.

Life Span and Gender

Consider the patient's age before administering codeine. Older adult patients are especially sensitive to respiratory depression with the use of narcotics. Therefore, a reduced dosage of codeine is advised. Codeine use is contraindicated in premature infants because of their sensitivity to respiratory depression. In addition, carefully assess whether a female patient is pregnant before administering codeine. The drug should not be given to women in labor unless absolutely necessary.

Lifestyle, Diet, and Habits

Codeine has less potential for causing physical dependence than morphine. Withdrawal symptoms from codeine dependency are similar to those seen in withdrawal from morphine, although the symptoms are less severe. Assess patients for a history of drug abuse and administer codeine cautiously in such patients.

Environment

If the patient will be taking codeine as an outpatient, assess his or her need to drive or operate potentially dangerous equipment. Patients must refrain from these activities until you have assessed the drug's sedative effects.

Nursing Diagnoses and Outcomes

- Disturbed Sensory Perception related to drowsiness and sedation
  Desired outcome: *The patient will be protected from injury related to sedation and drowsiness.*
- Risk for Ineffective Airway Clearance related to suppression of cough reflex
  Desired outcome: *The patient will maintain baseline respiratory function.*
- Constipation secondary to activity of the drug
  Desired outcome: *The patient remains free of constipation.*

Planning and Intervention

Maximizing Therapeutic Effects

Actions are similar to those for morphine.

Minimizing Adverse Effects

During therapy, ensure the use of safety precautions, such as raising side rails and assisting to walk if the patient is having CNS adverse effects. Monitor movement of air and respiratory status periodically during drug use. The use of codeine should be avoided in patients who need a strong cough reflex. Other actions are similar to those of morphine.

TABLE 23.5 Agents That Interact With P Codeine

Interactants	Effect and Significance	Nursing Management
antihistamines	Additive effects when given simultaneously, resulting in CNS depression	Monitor closely for CNS depression. Avoid coadministration if possible.
barbiturates	Additive effects when given simultaneously, resulting in CNS depression	Monitor closely for CNS depression. Avoid coadministration if possible.
histamine-2 receptor antagonists	Actions of narcotic analgesics enhanced, resulting in toxicity and increased risk for respiratory depression	Monitor for respiratory depression. Decrease dosage of narcotic analgesic as needed. Avoid coadministration if possible.
phenothiazines	Additive effects when given simultaneously, resulting in CNS depression	Monitor closely for CNS depression. Avoid coadministration if possible.

Providing Patient and Family Education

- Remind patients that drowsiness and impaired orientation can occur. Thus, patients should not drive or perform other tasks requiring alertness until the effects of the drug are known.
- Teach the patient to avoid combining use of codeine with alcohol or other CNS depressants.
- Instruct patients and their families to report respiratory difficulty at once to you or the prescriber.
- Provide general pain control information, similar to that given for morphine.

Ongoing Assessment and Evaluation

Monitor the drug's effect on motor control and sedation, and the patient's respiratory status. By the end of therapy, the patient should be free from injury related to sedation and have open and functioning airways manifested by breathing without difficulty. Assessment and evaluation of pain control are the same as for morphine.

Drugs Closely Related to P Codeine

Drugs similar to codeine include hydrocodone and propoxyphene.

Hydrocodone

Hydrocodone, although classified as a narcotic agonist and possessing the ability to produce some analgesia, is used only for its antitussive effects. It is available only in combination with an expectorant in a syrup or elixir formula for coughs. A recent phase II clinical trial examined the use of hydrocodone for treating cough in patients with advanced cancer. The study showed that 10 mg per day in divided doses was safe and effective for these patients. Dose escalation may be required for full effectiveness (Homsi et al., 2002). Like codeine, hydrocodone is metabolized through oxidative reactions by the P-450 isoenzyme system, and may possibly also be a prodrug, only active after metabolism through P-450.

MEMORY CHIP

P Codeine

- Used to treat mild to moderate pain and as a cough suppressant
- Major contraindications: same as for all narcotics (e.g., respiratory depression, use of other CNS depressants)
- Most common adverse effects: as a cough suppressant—drowsiness, sedation, dry mouth, nausea and vomiting, and constipation (all incidence is low at this dose); as an analgesic—similar to those of morphine, although less severe
- Most serious adverse effect: respiratory depression (in overdoses)
- **Life span alert: same as for morphine**
- Maximizing therapeutic effects: same as for morphine
- Minimizing adverse effects: Avoid use if patient's health status requires a strong cough; other considerations are the same as for morphine.
- Most important patient education: Provide general information on pain management as for all other narcotics.

Propoxyphene

Propoxyphene (Darvon) is used to treat mild to moderate pain. Compared with codeine, it has similar analgesic, respiratory-depressive, sedative, emetic, and physical dependency effects. Whether it shares codeine's antitussive and constipating effects remains unknown. Excessive doses of propoxyphene, either alone or in combination with other CNS depressants (including alcohol), are a major cause of drug-related death. For this reason, propoxyphene and products that include it should not be prescribed to suicidal patients or those with addictive tendencies. Warn patients strongly not to exceed the prescribed dosage.

C Narcotic Agonists-Antagonists

Some narcotic analgesics have mixed opioid effects, being an agonist at some receptors and an antagonist at others. Pentazocine (Talwin) is an example of a mixed narcotic agonist-antagonist and is also the prototype narcotic agonist-antagonist. Drugs similar to pentazocine include buprenorphine, butorphanol, dezocine, and nalbuphine.

NURSING MANAGEMENT OF THE PATIENT RECEIVING P PENTAZOCINE

Core Drug Knowledge

Pharmacotherapeutics

In patients not previously exposed to opioids, pentazocine can be used as an agonist to control pain. In normal doses, pentazocine is effective for moderate to severe pain, such as postoperative pain or pain during labor. It is also used as premedication for anesthesia and a supplement to surgical anesthetics.

Pharmacokinetics

Pentazocine is well absorbed orally and from SC and IM sites. When given orally, it undergoes a substantial first-pass effect of hepatic metabolism, and bioavailability is less than 20% of the dose given. The peak serum levels from oral doses occur within 1 to 3 hours, with a duration of action of 3 hours (see Table 23.3). Pentazocine's metabolites and the small proportion of drug not metabolized are excreted in urine. Pentazocine crosses the placenta.

Pharmacodynamics

Pentazocine is a mixed agonist-antagonist. It stimulates kappa receptors much as morphine does but also exhibits weak antagonist effects at the mu receptors, the primary morphine receptors. In patients who abuse opioids or are receiving narcotic agonists, such as morphine, for pain control, this drug may precipitate a withdrawal syndrome because of its antagonistic effects. Pentazocine may increase intracranial pressure. When pentazocine is given intravenously, it elevates systemic and pulmonary arterial pressure, systemic vascular resistance, and left ventricular end-diastolic pressure. These effects increase the workload of the heart.

Contraindications and Precautions

Pentazocine is contraindicated for patients with known hypersensitivity to it. Caution and low doses should be used if the drug is administered to patients with respiratory depression, severely limited respiratory reserves, severe bronchial asthma, obstructive respiratory conditions, and cyanosis. Pentazocine may cause allergic reactions in patients sensitive to sulfites. This event is uncommon in the general population but more likely in patients with asthma.

Adverse Effects

The most common adverse effects of pentazocine are nausea, vomiting, dizziness or lightheadedness, and euphoria. Pentazocine causes little respiratory depression because of its antagonist action at the mu receptors. Areas that may experience other possible adverse effects include cardiovascular (hypotension, hypertension, tachycardia, circulatory depression, and shock), CNS (sedation, headache, weakness, depression, disturbed dreams, insomnia, syncope, hallucinations, tremor, irritability, excitement, tinnitus, disorientation, and confusion), and dermatologic (soft tissue induration, nodules, cutaneous depression, ulceration with sloughing, sclerosis of the skin and subcutaneous tissues at site of injection, diaphoresis, stinging during injection, flushed skin, pruritus, and toxic epidermal necrolysis).

Drug Interactions

Pentazocine increases the action of alcohol and subsequently its accompanying CNS depressant effects. Barbiturate anesthetics increase the effect of respiratory and CNS depression from pentazocine because of additive pharmacologic activity. Table 23.6 lists drugs that interact with pentazocine.

Assessment of Relevant Core Patient Variables

Health Status

Assess the patient for conditions that are contraindications or precautions to drug therapy as well as for hepatic disease because decreased metabolism of the drug will occur, which predisposes the patient to greater adverse effects.

Because of the effect of increasing intracranial pressure, pentazocine may compound the clinical course of patients with head injuries. Its use in these patients should be avoided if at all possible; if pentazocine must be used, it should be done very cautiously and the patient carefully monitored. Because of the cardiac effects, IV pentazocine should not be given to patients with an MI. If oral forms are given, they must be administered cautiously, with the patient monitored carefully.

Life Span and Gender

Assess female patients for pregnancy before administration. Pentazocine is a pregnancy category C drug. Infants born to mothers who abuse pentazocine will exhibit neonatal withdrawal and have lower birth weights than normal. The safety and efficacy of pentazocine in children younger than 12 years have not been established; therefore, clarify that the pediatric patient is age 12 years or older before administration.

Lifestyle, Diet, and Habits

A common form of pentazocine abuse is called "T's and Blues." The "T's" refers to oral doses of pentazocine (under its trade name Talwin), and the "Blues" refers to tripelennamine (trade name, PBZ), a histamine-1 antihistamine. In this abused form, tablets are dissolved in tap water, filtered, and then injected intravenously as a substitute for heroin. The most frequent and serious complication of this form of addiction is pulmonary disease. Pulmonary disease results from blocking the pulmonary arteries and arterioles with unsterile particles of cellulose and talc from the tablets. Neurologic complications from "T's and Blues" may also occur, including seizures, strokes, and CNS infections. Pentazocine with naloxone (Talwin NX) has been produced in an effort to decrease the prevalence of this abuse. Giving pentazocine to patients who are dependent on opiates may induce withdrawal symptoms.

Environment

Pentazocine in parenteral form is administered in a hospital setting; oral forms may be administered in any setting by physicians, nurses, or patients themselves. Discuss any possible risks in the home or living environment with the patient.

TABLE 23.6 Agents That Interact With P Pentazocine

Interactants	Effect and Significance	Nursing Management
alcohol	Increased sedation	Avoid concurrent use. Caution against operating hazardous machinery or driving a motor vehicle.
thiopental	Increased CNS depression	Caution patient not to drive until effects subside completely. Avoid concurrent usage.
fluoxetine	Hypertension, diaphoresis, ataxia, flushing, nausea, dizziness, and anxiety	Monitor patient with caution if both drugs are used concurrently.
methohexital	Increased CNS depression	Consult prescriber about possible dosage adjustment.
zotepine	Increased risk of pentazocine-induced respiratory depression; enhanced sedation	Reduce dosage of pentazocine if necessary. Monitor for respiratory depression.
tobacco	Metabolism of pentazocine about 40% higher in smokers	Consult prescriber about increasing pentazocine dosage.

Nursing Diagnoses and Outcomes

- Disturbed Sensory Perception related to dizziness and lightheadedness
  Desired outcome: *The patient will not be injured from falls while taking pentazocine.*
- Imbalanced Nutrition secondary to nausea and vomiting
  Desired outcome: *The patient's nutrition will not be compromised while on pentazocine.*
- Ineffective Health Maintenance related to abuse of pentazocine
  Desired outcome: *The patient will use drug therapy appropriately.*
- Deficient Knowledge related to pentazocine therapy
  Desired outcome: *The patient has adequate knowledge of the drug and its adverse effects and their management.*

Planning and Intervention

Maximizing Therapeutic Effects

Be sure to provide environmental controls to reduce sensory stimuli and aid relaxation. For example, lights may be dimmed, noise reduced, and room temperature adjusted for greatest comfort. General actions for pain control are similar to those described for morphine.

Minimizing Adverse Effects

During therapy, ensure that safety precautions are used, such as raising side rails and assisting with ambulation. In cases of overdosage, naloxone is indicated. General principles for pain control are the same as those followed for morphine.

Providing Patient and Family Education

- Teach patients that pentazocine may cause drowsiness. They must use it with caution while driving or performing tasks that require mental alertness, physical dexterity, or coordination.
- Emphasize that patients must avoid concurrent use of pentazocine with alcohol and other CNS depressants.
- Instruct patients to notify their physician if skin rash, confusion, or disorientation develops.

Ongoing Assessment and Evaluation

Monitor the drug's effect on motor control, sedation, and pain. Adequate pain control should be achieved without adverse effects. Effectiveness of pain control is assessed similarly to morphine.

> **MEMORY CHIP**
>
> **P Pentazocine**
>
> - Used for moderate to severe pain
> - Is an agonist at some opioid receptors and a weak antagonist at others
> - May precipitate withdrawal in patients physically dependent on narcotics
> - Abused on the street (known as "T's and Blues")
> - Most common adverse effects: nausea, vomiting, dizziness, lightheadedness, and euphoria
> - Most serious adverse effects: respiratory depression and circulatory depression
> - Maximizing therapeutic effects: same as for all narcotics
> - Minimizing adverse effects: same as for all narcotics
> - Most important patient education: Avoid alcohol and CNS depressants while taking drug.

Drugs Closely Related to P Pentazocine

Buprenorphine

Buprenorphine (Buprenex), used in the treatment of moderate to severe pain, has a high affinity at the mu receptors and disassociates from these sites slowly. This characteristic may explain its long duration of action (6 hours versus 3 hours for pentazocine) and its low ability to cause physical dependence. When used as an analgesic, it is administered either by the IV or IM route. It also possesses very strong antagonist tendencies at opioid receptors, similar to the action of naloxone. Because of this, buprenorphine (either alone [Subutex] or combined with naloxone [Suboxone]) has been approved to use in the initial treatment of drug dependency. Naloxone is added to prevent against intravenous misuse of buprenorphine. This combination drug is used for maintenance treatment for drug abuse. Initiation of withdrawal symptoms, which could occur if administered parenterally, does not occur if the combination drug is used as intended. Buprenorphine and buprenorphine with naloxone are supplied in sublinguinal tablets prescribed only by physicians who have a special United States Drug Enforcement Agency (DEA) registration and have participated in the required education.

How buprenorphine, a narcotic analgesic with strong receptor antagonist action, produces pain relief is not specifically known.

Buprenorphine is metabolized by the hepatic enzyme CYP3A4. Drugs that inhibit this pathway, such as antifungals (e.g., ketoconazole), macrolide antibiotics (e.g., erythromycin), and human immunodeficiency virus (HIV) protease inhibitors (e.g., ritonavir, indinavir, and saquinavir), will increase the circulating volume of buprenorphine. Lower doses of Subutex or Suboxone will be required.

Sedation is the most frequently occurring adverse effect, affecting more than half of the patients receiving buprenorphine. The next most common adverse effects, although their prevalence is much lower than sedation, are dizziness and vertigo, hypotension, headache, sweating, nausea and vomiting, miosis, and hypoventilation. When given to treat substance abuse, the most common adverse effects from buprenorphine and buprenorphine with naloxone are cold or flu-like symptoms, headaches, sweating, sleeping difficulties, nausea, and mood swings. Adverse effects are most severe in the beginning of treatment and may last several weeks. Strong respiratory depression can occur with buprenorphine, especially if it is crushed and given intravenously. Several deaths have occurred with this type of drug abuse; these drugs are especially dangerous if taken concurrently with benzodiazepines because this combination increases CNS depression. Other CNS depressants, such as other narcotic analgesics, tranquilizers, or alcohol, will also potentiate the CNS depression that can occur, possibly with fatal results. Buprenor-

phine may also produce cytolytic hepatitis and hepatitis with jaundice. The amount of liver damage ranges from a transient asymptomatic elevation in liver enzymes to hepatic failure. It is unclear at this time whether the liver complications are related to the drug or to pre-existing liver problems secondary to IV drug abuse.

Because of these adverse effects, buprenorphine should be used cautiously in patients with compromised respiratory status and those receiving additional drugs that cause respiratory depression. Likewise, it should be used cautiously in those with hepatic disease. Like pentazocine, it is a pregnancy category C drug, and the safety of its use in children under the age of 16 years and during breast-feeding has not been established. Like pentazocine, if buprenorphine is given to a patient who is opioid dependent, withdrawal will occur. The likelihood of withdrawal is greater with buprenorphine than with pentazocine because buprenorphine has strong antagonist action, whereas pentazocine has only weak antagonist properties. Neonatal withdrawal will occur in those neonates whose mothers received buprenorphine during pregnancy.

When using buprenorphine to treat drug addiction, teach patients to place the tablet under their tongue and allow the tablet to dissolve, which will take 2 to 10 minutes. Tablets should not be swallowed because the medication is not effective this way, and opioid withdrawal may occur. If more than 2 tablets are prescribed and patients cannot get them all under the tongue at one time, they should place two under the tongue, and as soon as the tablets dissolve, place the additional tablets under the tongue. This medication must be taken regularly to be effective; it cannot be taken on an as-needed basis.

Patient education for those prescribed buprenorphine or buprenorphine with naloxone should include the warnings about the serious, and potentially fatal, adverse effects that can occur if the drug is intravenously abused. In addition, if buprenorphine with naloxone is used intravenously in the presence of other narcotics, it will induce severe withdrawal symptoms. Buprenorphine, both in Subutex and Suboxone, will cause dependency. The drug should not be stopped suddenly because withdrawal will occur.

Assess the patient for concurrent drug use of benzodiazepines, alcohol, and other CNS depressants that may increase the risk for serious CNS depression from buprenorphine. Patients should be instructed not to take any of these substances while on buprenorphine. Patients should not drive or operate heavy machinery or perform any other dangerous activity until they know whether they will have sedation from the buprenorphine. They should be cautioned about this possibility at the start of therapy and at each dose increase. Assess also for the use of drugs that are inhibitors of the CYP3A4 enzymatic pathway because these drugs will interact with buprenorphine.

Determine that liver function has been assessed before the beginning of therapy. Additionally, the patient needs to know that re-evaluation of liver function will be important throughout therapy.

Advise patients that they should keep the medication in a safe place and protect it from theft because it contains a narcotic painkiller, and that selling or giving this medication to another person is against the law. Finally, educate the patient's family that in case of an emergency, such as a drug overdose, the ER personnel need to be told that the patient is receiving buprenorphine.

Butorphanol

Butorphanol (Stadol) is used as an analgesic, preoperative medication, supplement to balanced anesthesia, and pain reliever during labor. An intranasal form was shown effective in clinical trials in treating the pain of migraine headaches. The analgesic potency of butorphanol, compared by weight, is 20 times that of pentazocine and 3.5 to 7 times that of morphine. Like pentazocine, butorphanol has both narcotic agonist and antagonist effects. Its antagonist activity is approximately 30 times that of pentazocine but only one fortieth that of naloxone. Its mechanism for pain relief is not completely understood. Like pentazocine, it produces the same cardiovascular effects when given intravenously, increases intracranial pressure, is metabolized in the liver (by the 3A4 isoenzyme), is a pregnancy category C drug, and has no known safety data relevant to its use in children. It may induce withdrawal in patients who abuse opiates, although whether it is an antagonist at the mu receptors is not definitely known. Unlike pentazocine, its most common adverse effect is somnolence. Common adverse effects similar to pentazocine include nausea and vomiting and dizziness. Other adverse effects that occur with regularity include confusion, sweating, dry mouth, headache, vasodilation, insomnia, constipation, and an unpleasant taste.

Dezocine

Dezocine (Dalgan), a strong, narcotic analgesic with agonist and antagonist effects, is used IM or IV in acute pain. Its analgesic potency, onset, and duration of action in the relief of postoperative pain are comparable with those of morphine. Its use and effectiveness in chronic pain have not been adequately studied. Its antagonist effects are greater than those of pentazocine. Dezocine depresses respiratory function in a way similar to that of morphine, which is much greater than that seen with pentazocine. In addition, unlike pentazocine, dezocine does not produce important cardiovascular effects. Dezocine has adverse effects similar to all strong analgesics. The most common are nausea and vomiting, sedation, dizziness, and reactions at the injection site. Dezocine is not recommended for patients who are physically dependent on narcotics because of its antagonist effects.

Nalbuphine

Nalbuphine (Nubain) is a potent analgesic with agonist and antagonist effects. Its analgesic potency is essentially the same as that of morphine and about three times greater than that of pentazocine. Its antagonist activity is approximately 10 times that of pentazocine. Nalbuphine is used for moderate to severe pain, as a preoperative analgesic, as a supplement to balanced anesthesia, and as an obstetric analgesic during labor and delivery. Unlike pentazocine, nalbuphine does not increase pulmonary artery pressure, systemic vascular resistance, or cardiac work. Nalbuphine produces respiratory depression similar to morphine. Unlike morphine, the depressive effects seem to have a ceiling effect, with increases beyond 30 mg of nalbuphine producing no further respiratory depression. Like pentazocine, nalbuphine can produce an allergic response in patients with sulfite sensitivity and also trigger withdrawal in patients dependent on narcotics. The most common adverse effect is sedation, which occurs in about one third of the patients who use the drug. Other fairly common adverse effects are sweating, nausea and vomiting, dizziness and vertigo, dry mouth, and headache.

CHAPTER SUMMARY

- Pain is a subjective experience. Objective signs may or may not accompany pain. Lack of objective data does not mean that the pain is not present.
- Pain, a complex physiologic phenomenon, is not clearly or completely understood at this time.
- Pain is mediated through the CNS by nociceptors and perceived by the opiate receptors. When the opiate receptors are stimulated, perception of pain decreases.
- Pain has many types or classifications, which are based on the pathophysiologic origin of the pain (nociceptive versus neuropathic), whether the pain reflects a current injury or period of healing or extends beyond this time (acute versus chronic), or a subgroup of one of these classifications (visceral, somatic, cancer, or noncancer chronic).
- Pain, to be treated appropriately, must be assessed with a pain assessment tool. Simply asking patients to rate their pain on a scale in their head is not the same as using an assessment tool.
- Pain is best controlled when patients take analgesics before pain becomes severe and doses are administered around the clock.
- Doses of analgesics should be titrated to obtain maximum efficacy with minimal adverse effects.
- Nonanalgesics and nonpharmacologic methods of pain management may be used to supplement drug therapy.
- Patients who have been receiving opioids for an extended period will develop tolerance to the pain relief from the analgesics and need increased doses. Patients who abuse substances will have cross-tolerance and need higher than expected doses to receive analgesia from drug therapy.
- Morphine is the standard narcotic analgesic. It is an agonist at the opioid receptors. All other narcotics are compared with morphine to measure their efficacy. Morphine is indicated in the treatment of moderate to severe pain.
- In addition to analgesia, morphine, like all narcotics, produces a wide variety of other effects on the body. The most serious of these is respiratory depression, which if severe, can be life threatening.
- The antidote to morphine overdosage and respiratory depression caused by any narcotic is naloxone, a narcotic antagonist.
- Morphine, like all narcotics, is a controlled substance. By law, every dose must be properly accounted for and documented. This rule includes partial doses that may be wasted.
- Relevant core patient variables are important to consider when providing morphine or other narcotics for pain control. The variables may alter the drug chosen, dose, frequency, route, patient's emotional response to pain, or frequency and depth of assessment made while the patient receives morphine or other narcotics.
- Codeine is another narcotic analgesic used for mild to moderate pain. It is also used to suppress coughs. Its effects are similar to those of morphine, but usually milder.
- Pentazocine, a different type of narcotic, is a combination of opioid agonists and opioid antagonists. Because of the antagonist effects at some receptors, it generally causes less respiratory depression than morphine and has less risk for inducing physical dependence. If given to a patient physically dependent on a narcotic, pentazocine may induce withdrawal.
- Patients and their families need education about the importance of pain control and what will be done when they report pain. Moreover, they need to know that they are not expected to suffer. Discuss with them any fears or misconceptions about analgesic use and dispel such mistakes with facts.
- Reassess patients for pain following changes in drug therapy, after every dose until a set dose controls pain, and periodically during the course of therapy.

QUESTIONS FOR STUDY AND REVIEW

1. Why should morphine not be administered to treat acute pain in a person with respiratory depression?
2. Can morphine be administered to treat chronic pain if the patient's respiratory rate is between 8 and 12 breaths/minute? Why?
3. Your patient has a history of opioid abuse, just came from surgery, and has a chest tube. Explain why he might need a larger dose of morphine to control his postoperative pain than other patients require.
4. What is a "rescue dose"?
5. Why might more than one dose of naloxone, a narcotic antagonist, be needed when a patient has severe respiratory depression from opiate overdose?
6. Why should codeine not be administered to anyone who needs to be able to cough to clear his or her airway?

Need More Help?

Chapter 23 of the study guide for *Drug Therapy in Nursing* 2e contains NCLEX-style questions and other learning activities to reinforce your understanding of the concepts presented in this chapter. For additional information or to purchase the study guide, visit *http://connection.lww.com/go/aschenbrenner.*

REFERENCES AND BIBLIOGRAPHY

American Academy of Pain Medicine, American Pain Society, and the American Society of Addiction Medicine. (2001). Consensus document. Definitions related to the use of opioids for the treatment of pain [Online]. Available: *http://www.asam.org/ppol/paindef.htm.*

Cepeda, M. S., & Carr, D. B. (2003). Women experience more pain and require more morphine than men to achieve a similar degree of analgesia. *Anesthesia and Analgesia, 97*(5), 1464–1468.

Chumbley, G. M., Hall, G. M., & Salmon, P. (2002). Patient-controlled analgesia: What information does the patient want? *Journal of Advanced Nursing, 39*(5), 459–471.

Cleeland, C. S., & Ryan K. M. (1994). Pain assessment: Global use of the Brief Pain Inventory. *Annals of Academic Medicine Singapore, 23*(2), 129–138.

Daut, R. L., Cleeland, C. S., & Flanery, R. C. (1983). Development of the Wisconsin Brief Pain Questionnaire to assess pain in cancer and other diseases. *Cancer, 17*(2), 197–210.

Donnelly, S., Davis, M. P., Walsh, D., et al., for the World Health Organization. (2002). Morphine in cancer pain management: A practical guide. *Supportive Care in Cancer: Official Journal of the Multinational Association of Supportive Care in Cancer, 10*(1), 13–35.

Fishman, B., Pasternak, S., Wallenstein, S. L., et al. (1987). The Memorial Pain Assessment Card: A valid instrument for the evaluation of cancer pain. *Cancer, 60*(5), 1151–1158.

Frei A., Andersen, S., Hole, P., et al. (2003). A one-year health economic model comparing transdermal fentanyl with sustained-release morphine in the treatment of chronic noncancer pain. *Journal of Pain and Palliative Care Pharmacotherapy, 17*(2), 5–26.

Homsi, J., Walsh, D., Nelson, K. A., et al. (2002). A phase II study of hydrocodone for cough in advanced cancer. *American Journal of Hospice and Palliative Care, 19*(1), 49–56.

McCaffery, M. (1968). *Nursing practice theories related to cognition, bodily pain and man-environmental interactions.* Los Angeles: UCLA Students Store.

Melzack, R. (1975). The McGill Pain Questionnaire: Major properties and scoring methods. *Pain, 1*(3), 277–299.

Merskey, H., & Bugduk, N. (1994). *Classification of chronic pain. Descriptions of chronic pain syndromes and definitions of pain terms* (2nd ed.). Seattle: IASP Press.

Mystakidou, K., Tsilika, E., Parpa, E., et al. (2003). Long-term cancer pain management in morphine pre-treated and opioid naïve patients with transdermal fentanyl. *International Journal of Cancer, 107*(3), 486–492.

National Pharmaceutical Council (NPC) and Joint Commission on Accreditation of Healthcare Organizations (JCAHO). Joint position paper. (2001). Pain: Current understanding of assessment, management, and treatments [Online]. Available: *http://www.jcaho.org/news+room/health+caare+issues/pain+mono_npc.pdf.*

Vallerand, A. H. (2003). The use of long-acting opioids in chronic pain management. *Nursing Clinics of North America, 38*(3), 435–445.

Vermeire, A., Remon, J. P., Schrijvers, D., et al. (2002). A new method to obtain and present complete information on the compatibility: Study of its validity for eight binary mixtures of morphine with drugs frequently used in palliative care. *Palliative Medicine, 16*(5), 417–424.

Wong, D., & Baker, C. (1998). Pain in children: Comparison of assessment scales. *Pediatric Nursing, 14*(1), 9–17.

Drugs Treating Mild to Moderate Pain, Fever, Inflammation, and Migraine Headache

chapter 24

Learning Objectives

At the completion of this chapter the student will:

1. Correlate the processes of inflammation, fever, and pain with the actions of salicylates, prostaglandin synthetase inhibitors, para-aminophenol derivative drugs, and antimigraine drugs.
2. Identify core drug knowledge pertaining to salicylates, prostaglandin synthetase inhibitors, para-aminophenol derivative drugs, and antimigraine drugs.
3. Identify the core patient variables pertaining to salicylates, prostaglandin synthetase inhibitors, para-aminophenol derivative drugs, and antimigraine drugs.
4. Relate the interaction of core drug knowledge to core patient variables for salicylates, prostaglandin synthetase inhibitors, para-aminophenol derivative drugs, and antimigraine drugs.
5. Generate a nursing plan of care from the interactions between core drug knowledge and core patient variables for salicylates, prostaglandin synthetase inhibitors, para-aminophenol derivative drugs, and antimigraine drugs.
6. Describe nursing interventions to maximize therapeutic and minimize adverse effects for salicylates, prostaglandin synthetase inhibitors, para-aminophenol derivative drugs, and antimigraine drugs.
7. Determine key points for patient and family education for salicylates, prostaglandin synthetase inhibitors, para-aminophenol derivative drugs, and antimigraine drugs.

KEY TERMS

cyclooxygenase

nonsteroidal anti-inflammatory drug (NSAID)

para-aminophenol derivative

prostaglandin synthetase inhibitors

Reye syndrome

salicylates

salicylate poisoning

salicylism

serotonin

triptans

FEATURED WEBLINK

http://www.ampainsoc.org
Need more information about the types of pain? Try the American Pain Society website for more information.

CONNECTION WEBLINK

Additional Weblinks are found on Connection:
http://www.connection.lww.com/go/aschenbrenner.

Drugs for Treating Mild to Moderate Pain, Fever, Inflammation, and Migraine Headache

Ⓒ Nonsteroidal Anti-inflammatory Drugs (NSAIDs)

Ⓒ Salicylates
- **[P] aspirin**
- diflunisal
- salsalate

Ⓒ Prostaglandin synthetase inhibitors
- **[P] ibuprofin**
- Proionic acids
  - fenoprofen
  - flurbiprofen
  - ketoprofen
  - naproxen
  - oxaprozin
- Acetic acids
  - diclofenac
  - etodolac
  - indomethacin
  - ketorolac
  - sulindac
  - tolmetin
- Fenamates
  - mefenamic acid
  - meclofenamate sodium
- Oxicams
  - meloxicam
  - piroxicam
- Alkanones
  - nabumetone
- COX-2 inhibitors
  - celecoxib
  - valdecoxib

Ⓒ Para-aminophenol derivatives
- **[P] acetaminophen**

Ⓒ Serotonin-selective agonists
- **[P] sumatriptan**
- almotriptan
- eletriptan
- frovatriptan
- naratriptan
- rizatriptan
- zolmitripan
- ergotamine
- dihydroergotamine

The symbol Ⓒ indicates the **drug class**.
Drugs in **bold type** marked with the symbol [P] are prototypes.
Drugs in blue type are closely related to the prototype.
Drugs in red type are significantly different from the prototype.
Drugs in black type with no symbol are also used in drug therapy; no prototype

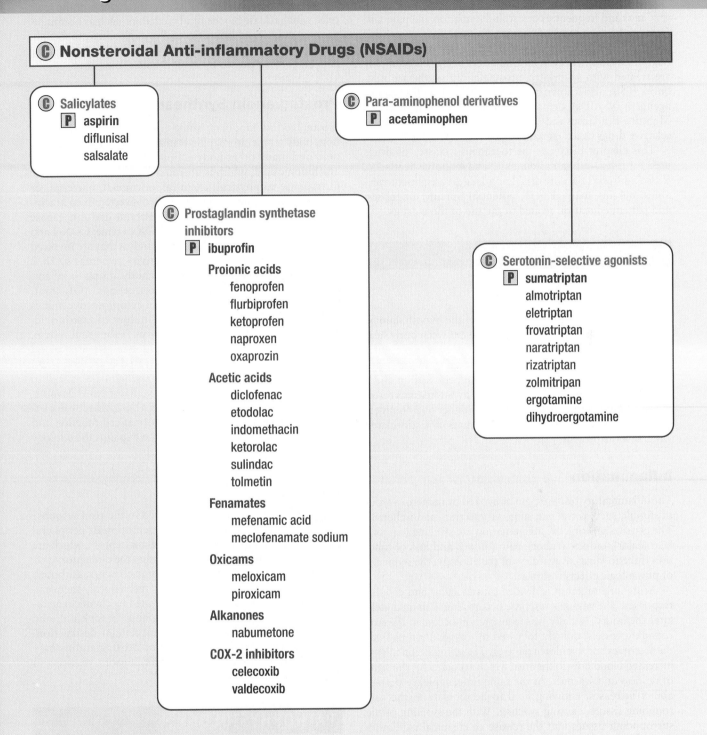

Fever, inflammation, and pain are symptoms of acute illness and frequently coexist. Inflammation and pain also can be symptoms of chronic diseases, such as arthritis and gout. Inflammation may also induce intense pain called migraine headache. Fever, inflammation, and pain commonly are treated with salicylates, prostaglandin synthetase inhibitors (PSIs; also known as nonsteroidal anti-inflammatory agents or NSAIDs), or para-aminophenol derivative drugs. Migraine headaches are commonly treated with serotonin-selective drugs called **triptans** or antimigraine agents.

This chapter discusses the therapeutic classes of drugs used for fever, inflammation, pain, and migraine headache. It also addresses the core drug knowledge, core patient variables, nursing management, potential nursing diagnoses, and patient education related to the use of these drugs.

PHYSIOLOGY

Fever

Temperature regulation is a function of the hypothalamus. Normally, a homeostatic balance exists between body heat generated and body heat lost. In excessive heat, the regulatory mechanism is activated, and the body responds with integumentary vasodilation, resulting in perspiration and a net heat loss. When fever is present, the hypothalamus resets the regulating mechanism to tolerate a higher body temperature. Additionally, prostaglandin formation is stimulated when fever is present.

Inflammation

The inflammatory response can be evoked by numerous types of stimuli, such as trauma, surgery, infection, and ischemia. The classic signs of local inflammation are swelling (tumor), heat (calor), redness (rubor), pain (dolor), and loss of function (functio laesa). Regardless of the etiology, the sequence of physiologic effects is similar.

Acute inflammation is divided into vascular and cellular responses. The vascular response occurs almost immediately after the injury. Initially, vasoconstriction occurs in the surrounding vessels, quickly followed by vasodilation of both the arterioles and venules in the area. The vasodilation allows increased blood flow to the area, which accounts for the signs of redness and warmth. At the same time, capillary permeability increases, allowing fluid to accumulate in the surrounding tissues, causing swelling. With the swelling of the surrounding tissues and the release of chemical mediators from the injured tissues, pain and impaired function occur.

The cellular response is divided into four phases:

1. Margination of white blood cells (WBCs)—WBCs move to the periphery of the blood vessels to prepare for emigration.
2. Emigration of WBCs—The WBCs pass through the capillary walls and migrate into the tissue spaces.
3. Chemotaxis—Cellular debris or bacteria become more "attractive" to the WBCs.
4. Phagocytosis—Neutrophils and monocytes engulf and degrade the cellular debris.

Inflammation also is enhanced by the rupture of the mast cells, which release biochemical mediators, such as histamine, prostaglandins, and leukotrienes. Prostaglandins are thought to be pivotal in the inflammatory response by potentiating pain and edema caused by other chemical mediators.

Prostaglandin Synthesis

Prostaglandins modulate some components of inflammation, body temperature, pain transmission, platelet aggregation, and many other body actions. They are derived from arachidonic acid, which is liberated from the cell membrane in response to physical, chemical, hormonal, bacterial, or other stimuli (Figure 24.1). They are converted from arachidonic acid to prostaglandins by the enzyme **cyclooxygenase** (COX). There are two forms of the COX enzyme: COX-1 and COX-2. COX-1 synthesizes prostaglandins that are involved in the regulation of normal cell activity, whereas COX-2 appears to produce prostaglandins mainly at sites of inflammation. For instance, in the gastrointestinal (GI) tract, COX-1 is responsible for secretion of cytoprotective mucus and bicarbonate, suppression of the output of gastric acid, and support for submucosal blood flow. In the renal system, COX-1 promotes vasodilation, resulting in increased blood flow to the kidneys. COX-2 is activated by arthritis and other stimuli and produces the prostaglandins that lead to inflammation, swelling, and joint pain. Most NSAIDs indiscriminately target both COX-1 and COX-2, thereby depleting the prostaglandins needed for normal cell function and protection. This lack of discrimination explains the etiology of many of these drugs' adverse effects.

Pain

The physiologic mechanisms involved in the pain response are complex (see Chapter 23). The sensation of peripheral pain begins in afferent neurons called nociceptors, which are found in skin, muscle, connective tissue, the circulatory system, and abdominal, pelvic, and thoracic viscera. Although these receptors may be activated by mechanical, chemical, or thermal stimuli, they also are activated by chemical mediators, such as prostaglandins, histamine, bradykinin, and serotonin, which are released during cellular destruction. It is theorized that the inhibition of prostaglandins may diminish activation of peripheral pain sensors, resulting in decreased pain.

PATHOPHYSIOLOGY

Migraine Headache

A migraine is a very bad headache that tends to recur. Although the cause of migraine may be a chemical or electrical stimulation, the key element of a migraine headache is blood flow changes in the brain. It is theorized that the nervous system responds to a trigger (Box 24.1) by inducing spasms in the arteries at the base of the brain. As these arteries constrict, the flow of blood to the brain is reduced. At the same time, platelets clump together and release serotonin. **Serotonin** is a powerful vasoconstrictor that further reduces

Physiology

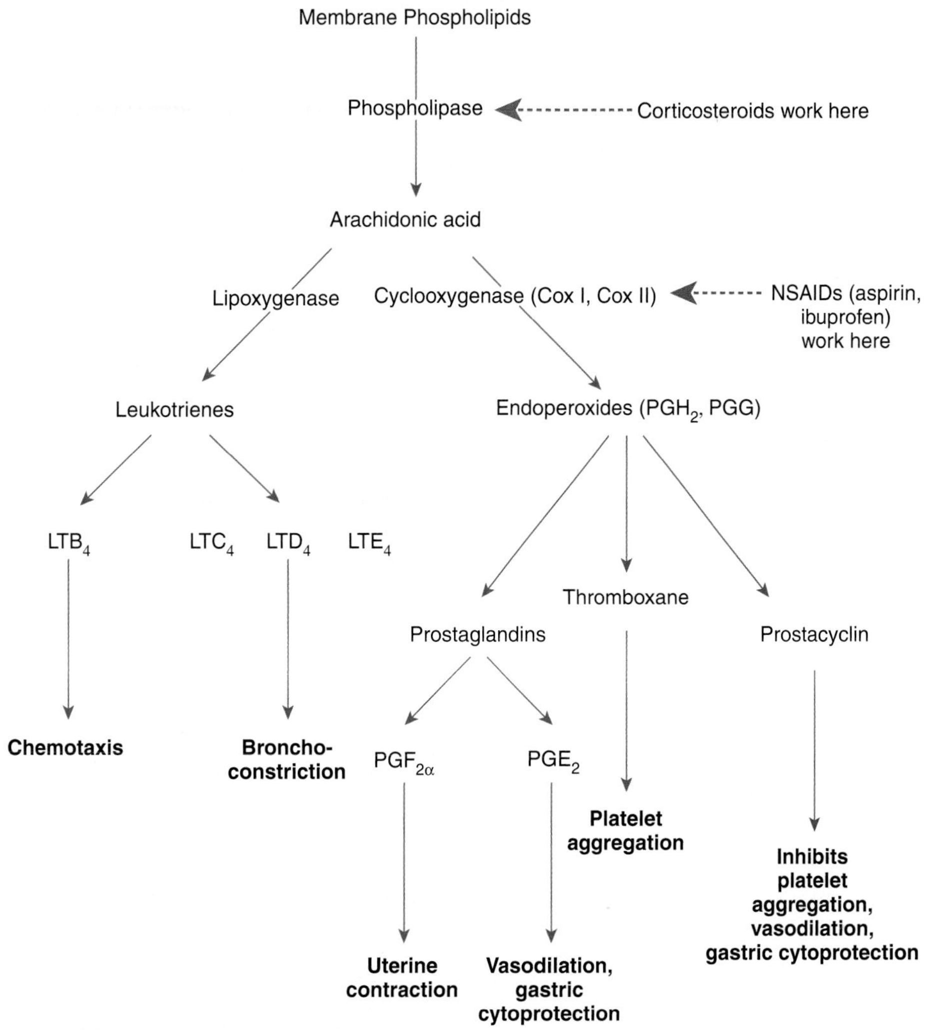

FIGURE 24.1 Synthesis of prostaglandins.

blood flow to the brain resulting in increased hypoxemia. In reaction to the hypoxemia, arteries within the brain dilate to meet the brain's oxygen needs. The pain associated with migraine is directly related to the spreading arterial dilation that allows blood to pump into the brain.

Although many types of migraine exist, the two major variations are classic and common migraine. The patient experiencing a classic migraine attack experiences an "aura." An aura is a group of neurologic symptoms that develop 10 to 30 minutes before the migraine headache occurs. These symptoms include temporary vision loss, wavy or zigzag lines, or flashing lights. Other symptoms of classic migraine include difficulty speaking, confusion, weakness in an arm or leg, and tingling face or hands. The pain associated with classic migraine is described as intense throbbing or pounding in the forehead or temple, ear or jaw, or around the eyes. It generally starts on one side of the head but can spread to the other side as well.

The common migraine is not preceded by an aura. During the headache phase of a common migraine, the patient may experience abdominal pain, diarrhea, increased urination, nausea, and vomiting. Both classic and common migraines can strike as often as several times a week or rarely as once every few years.

DRUGS TO TREAT INFLAMMATION AND FEVER

Salicylates, PSIs, and para-aminophenol derivative drugs are used to treat inflammation and fever in a variety of conditions. Salicylates are used in managing conditions ranging from a simple headache to acute myocardial infarction. PSIs are used primarily for their anti-inflammatory effects but are also used extensively as an analgesic. The newest PSIs have been approved for other conditions such as familial adenomatous polyposis (FAP) and are undergoing extensive research into their viability to affect disorders such as Alzheimer and kidney disease.

COMMUNITY-BASED CONCERNS

Box 24.1 Migraine Headache Triggers

Migraines sometimes can be prevented, which eliminates the need to treat them. Exactly what triggers a migraine differs from patient to patient, and many patients' migraines can be triggered by multiple factors. You can help patients to track and identify their personal triggers so that they can avoid them and, perhaps, forestall migraine headaches. Common migraine triggers include:

General Triggers

- Physical exertion
- Stress, worry, or anxiety
- Menstruation
- Pungent odors
- Sleep deprivation, fatigue, or excessive sleep
- Glare from the sun or fluorescent lights
- Weather or ambient changes
- High humidity
- High altitude
- Head trauma
- Drinking cold water

Physical Triggers

- Menstruation
- Ovulation
- Ovarian cycle disorders

Dietary Triggers

- Alcohol
- Tyramine (aged cheeses and fermented foods)
- Aspartame (artificial sweetener)
- Monosodium glutamate (MSG)
- Phenylethylamine (present in some OTC drugs and chocolate)
- Nitrates (preservatives used in sausage, bacon, and lunch meats)
- Citrus foods and products

Pharmacologic Triggers

- Oral contraceptives
- Glyceryl trinitrate
- Theophylline
- Reserpine
- Nifedipine
- Indomethacin
- Cimetidine

Ⓒ NONSTEROIDAL ANTI-INFLAMMATORY AGENTS

By definition, a **nonsteroidal anti-inflammatory drug** is any drug that decreases inflammation but is not a steroid. NSAIDs are conventionally categorized as **salicylates** and **prostaglandin synthetase inhibitors,** although some of the literature refers to PSIs as NSAIDs. This is a subdivision of convenience because both salicylates and PSIs work by inhibiting COX and decreasing prostaglandins and thromboxane. A major difference is that salicylates irreversibly inhibit COX, whereas the action of the PSIs is reversible. The irreversible effects of aspirin, a salicylate, for example, account for the longer duration of its antiplatelet action. Salicylates are discussed first, followed by PSIs.

Ⓒ Salicylates

Since salicylates were isolated from the bark of the willow tree in 1829, they have become one of the mainstays of drug therapy in a variety of diseases and disorders. The therapeutic uses of salicylates continue to be researched in all areas of medicine. The prototype salicylate is acetylsalicylic acid, commonly known as aspirin. Table 24.1 presents a summary of selected salicylates.

NURSING MANAGEMENT OF THE PATIENT RECEIVING [P] ASPIRIN

Core Drug Knowledge

Pharmacotherapeutics

Aspirin has a variety of therapeutic uses. It is indicated for mild to moderate pain, especially pain resulting from inflammation. It is used frequently to relieve headache, neuralgia, myalgia, arthralgia, postpartum pain, dental or oral surgery pain, and dysmenorrhea (painful menstruation).

Aspirin is the preferred agent for treating pain and inflammation associated with juvenile arthritis, rheumatoid arthritis, and osteoarthritis. It also is the preferred agent in treating fever, pleurisy, and arthritis. Other inflammatory conditions, such as tendonitis and bursitis, respond well to aspirin. In addition, it is used for treating pericarditis in patients with systemic lupus erythematosus (SLE).

Because of its antithrombotic and anti-inflammatory effects, aspirin is useful in preventing or reducing the risk for myocardial infarction (MI) and recurrent transient ischemic attacks (Box 24.2). It is considered the drug of choice for treating Kawasaki syndrome (mucocutaneous lymph node syndrome).

Pharmacokinetics

Aspirin absorption usually occurs within 30 minutes depending on the dosage form, GI pH, and the presence of food or antacids in the stomach. Although a portion of aspirin is absorbed in the stomach, most is absorbed in the small intestine. Aspirin suppositories are slowly and variably absorbed. Buffered aspirin does not delay absorption; however, enteric-coated and extended-acting preparations do delay absorption.

Aspirin is 99% metabolized into salicylate and other metabolites by the liver. Aspirin and its metabolites are widely distributed throughout the body and body fluids, including breast milk. Additionally, they cross the placental barrier. Peak plasma levels occur within 2 hours. The half-life of aspirin is 15 minutes, whereas the half-life of salicylate is 2 hours. Aspirin and its metabolites are excreted by the kidneys (see Table 24.1).

Pharmacodynamics

Aspirin is used for its analgesic, anti-inflammatory, antipyretic, and antithrombotic effects. It interferes with prostaglandin synthesis by irreversibly inhibiting COX. Antipyretic

TABLE 24.1 Summary of Selected (C) Salicylates

Drug (Trade) Name	Selected Indications	Route and Dosage Range	Pharmacokinetics
(C) Salicylates			
[P] acetylsalicylic acid (aspirin, Bayer Aspirin; *Canadian:* Apo-ASA)	Minor aches, pains, or temperature Anti-inflammatory Acute rheumatic fever Prevention of transient ischemic attacks Prevention of myocardial infarction	*Adult:* PO, dependent on indication, in order of indications listed to the left: 325–1,000 mg q4h; 2.6–5.2 g/d in divided doses; 7.8 g/d in divided doses; 325 mg–1.3 g/d in two to four divided doses; 325 mg/d *Child:* PO, <25 kg; 60–90 mg/kg/d; >25 kg, 2.4–3.6 g/d in divided doses	*Onset:* 15–30 min *Duration:* 3–6 h $t_{1/2}$: 2–3 h
diflunisal (Dolobid; *Canadian:* Apo-Diflunisal)	Arthritis Mild to moderate pain Headache	*Adult:* PO, 250–500 mg bid not to exceed 1.5 g/d *Adult:* PO, 1 g initially followed by 500 mg q12h (under 50 kg or elderly, 500 mg initially followed by 250 mg q12h) *Adult:* PO, 500 mg q12h *Child:* Safe dosage not established	*Onset:* 30–60 min *Duration:* 12 h $t_{1/2}$: 8–12 h
salsalate (Disalcid)	Arthritis Musculoskeletal inflammation	*Adult:* PO, initially 500 mg–1 g bid or tid; maintenance, 2–4 g in divided doses *Child:* Safe dosage not established	*Onset:* 10–30 min *Duration:* 3–6 h $t_{1/2}$: 2–3 h

FOCUS ON RESEARCH

Box 24.2 Is Aspirin the Answer?

Gum, P. A., Kottke-Marchant, K., Welsh, P. A., et al. (2003). A prospective, blinded determination of the natural history of aspirin resistance among stable patients with cardiovascular disease. *Journal of the American College of Cardiology, 41*(6), 961–965.

The Study

The researchers designed this study to determine whether aspirin resistance is a potential etiology for cardiovascular clinical events. The study involved 326 stable cardiovascular patients from 1997 to 1999 who were taking aspirin (325 mg/day for 7 days or longer) and no other antiplatelet agents. The researchers used optical platelet aggregation to test for aspirin sensitivity. Aspirin resistance was found in 5.2% of the study group. During follow-up, patients with aspirin resistance had a 24% risk for death, myocardial infarction (MI), or cerebrovascular accident (CVA), compared with a 10% risk among patients who were aspirin sensitive. The researchers concluded that aspirin resistance does occur in patients with stable cardiovascular disease and that patients in this population who are aspirin resistant have a threefold higher risk than others for major cardiovascular events.

Nursing Considerations

Aspirin is routinely given to patients as prophylaxis against new or recurring cardiovascular events. It is important to remember that despite the use of aspirin, patients are still at risk for these events. Instruct the patient to report chest pain or pressure, shortness of breath, headache, visual changes, decreased muscle movement, or changes in the ability to think or speak because these symptoms may indicate cardiovascular events such as angina, MI, or CVA.

effects of aspirin are a result of inhibited prostaglandin synthesis in the hypothalamus. Aspirin also may enhance peripheral vasodilation and sweating. Anti-inflammatory action is believed to be caused by peripheral inhibition of prostaglandin synthesis, but aspirin also may inhibit the action and synthesis of other mediators of inflammation. The antithrombotic effect of aspirin results from the inhibition of thromboxane A_2, a prostaglandin that induces platelet aggregation.

Contraindications and Precautions

Aspirin is contraindicated for patients with salicylate hypersensitivity. It also is contraindicated for patients with peptic ulcer disease, bleeding disorders, or patients on anticoagulation therapy because of its antiplatelet activity. Additionally, aspirin is contraindicated for patients with gout and for those with renal or liver impairment. Aspirin is contraindicated in children with varicella or flu-like illness because it is associated with the occurrence of **Reye syndrome,** a potentially fatal disease characterized by swelling in the brain, increased intracranial pressure, and seizures.

Aspirin is assigned to pregnancy category D and should be avoided by pregnant women because it can interfere with the prostaglandins that mediate uterine contraction, resulting in delayed or prolonged labor. In addition, aspirin's antiplatelet activity increases the risk for maternal or neonatal hemorrhage. Aspirin also should be avoided by lactating women because it is secreted in breast milk and may exert its antiplatelet action in the infant.

Aspirin should be avoided by patients who smoke cigarettes and by patients with a history of alcohol abuse; both

agents are known to be ulcerogenic. Aspirin should be given with caution to patients with asthma, nasal polyps, and hyperuricemia. Patients older than 60 years and those taking corticosteroids have a higher risk for aspirin's adverse effects.

Adverse Effects

Two adverse effects specific to aspirin therapy are salicylism and salicylate poisoning. **Salicylism** is mild aspirin toxicity, which may occur with long-term or high-dose aspirin therapy. Typical symptoms include headache, tinnitus, GI distress, paresthesias, and respiratory stimulation (i.e., increased respiratory rate secondary to stimulation in the central nervous system [CNS]). Patients may appear drowsy or confused. The only intervention needed for salicylism is to reduce the dose of aspirin or stop aspirin therapy.

Salicylate poisoning is a life-threatening event. The lethal dose of aspirin is 5 to 8 g for a child and 10 to 30 g for an adult. There is no antidote for salicylate poisoning. Treatment of salicylate poisoning includes gastric emptying, either with syrup of ipecac or gastric lavage; administration of activated charcoal; and life support, if indicated. Consequences of salicylate poisoning include respiratory alterations; fluid, electrolyte, and acid-base imbalances; seizures; high temperature; and shock leading to coma and death. Patients suspected of salicylate poisoning should be taken to an emergency department rather than a clinic or doctor's office for treatment. Children's aspirin has a pleasant flavor and may not be recognized as a drug by children. Therefore, it is important to keep aspirin in a safe place.

Common adverse effects related to aspirin are the result of prostaglandin inhibition. It is important to remember that prostaglandins are found in most body tissues and organs and frequently have opposing effects on the body. Adverse effects occur because of the inhibition of a particular prostaglandin necessary for normal cell function by inhibiting COX-1.

The most common adverse effects of aspirin are related to the GI system. Aspirin may irritate the gastric mucosa, resulting in nausea, vomiting, abdominal pain, ulcerations, perforation, and bleeding. These effects occur because of a direct irritating action to the mucosa of the GI tract and the inhibition of prostaglandin E_2 (PGE_2), which has a cytoprotective mechanism to the mucosa. Aspirin can be given with antacids to decrease its GI effects; however, antacids will also decrease the absorption of aspirin. Severe gastropathies occur most frequently in patients older than 60 years, those with a history of peptic ulcer disease, cigarette smokers, those who concomitantly use alcohol or corticosteroids, and those with dyspepsia during aspirin therapy.

Aspirin may cause hypersensitivity responses, such as rashes, hives, or bronchoconstriction, and possibly respiratory distress and anaphylaxis. Patients prone to these responses usually have severe corticosteroid-dependent asthma, nasal polyps, or chronic urticaria. High aspirin levels may induce ototoxicity manifested by tinnitus.

Another potentially serious adverse effect of aspirin is excessive or abnormal bleeding, especially in patients with hemophilia, anemias, or severe liver disease. Aspirin inhibits platelet aggregation by the inhibition of the prostaglandin thromboxane. Aspirin's antithrombotic action lasts for the life of the platelet (8–11 days). Other hematopoietic problems, such as agranulocytosis and aplastic anemia, have been reported infrequently.

Aspirin has been associated with hepatotoxicity in patients with juvenile arthritis, active SLE, rheumatic fever, or pre-existing hepatic impairment. The hepatotoxicity is thought to be a direct toxicity to the liver and is associated with high-dose therapy.

In the renal system, acute renal failure may occur in susceptible patients. Patients with conditions associated with diminished renal blood flow, such as congestive heart failure (CHF), cirrhosis, renal insufficiency, and advanced age are at the highest risk. Prostaglandins play a role in opposing potent renal vasoconstrictors. Therefore, when the action of these prostaglandins is inhibited, vasoconstriction occurs, and blood flow is diminished to the renal system, resulting in acute renal failure. Another problem inhibiting the renal prostaglandins is sodium and water retention. This inhibition is especially problematic for patients with conditions such as hypertension and CHF. Less common renal toxicities include interstitial nephritis and nephrotic syndrome. In addition to increased blood urea nitrogen (BUN) and creatinine levels, proteinuria occurs. Acute renal failure, water retention, interstitial nephritis, and nephrotic syndrome usually occur early in aspirin therapy and are reversible by stopping aspirin treatment.

Additionally, aspirin decreases uric acid excretion by the kidneys; therefore, aspirin may potentiate gout.

Drug Interactions

Aspirin is a highly protein-bound drug and may interact with other drugs that are also highly protein bound. Because aspirin displaces the other active drugs into the serum, the pharmacologic effects of the displaced drug are enhanced. Drugs such as anticoagulants, oral hypoglycemics, insulin, methotrexate, and alcohol may be enhanced enough to cause toxicity. Conversely, drugs such as antacids, urinary alkalizers, probenecid, and corticosteroids may decrease the effectiveness of salicylates.

In addition, aspirin can cause false-negative results on the glucose oxidase test (Tes-Tape) and a false-positive result on the copper reduction test (Clinitest). These false-positive results have become less important since use of home blood glucose monitoring systems has become widespread. A summary of drug–drug interactions for aspirin is provided in Table 24.2.

Assessment of Relevant Core Patient Variables

Health Status

Assess the patient for potential medical conditions or drugs that contradict the use of aspirin or require close patient monitoring. It is important to assess for potential hypersensitivities to salicylates or other NSAIDs and for a history of asthma or nasal polyps because patients with these conditions are prone to bronchospasm. Also, assess gross hearing as a baseline for possible ototoxicity.

For patients on long-term therapy, obtain a baseline complete blood count (CBC), platelet count, and test results for renal and hepatic function. It is important to assess the patient's knowledge concerning the potential adverse effects

TABLE 24.2 Agents That Interact With P Aspirin

Interactants	Effect and Significance	Nursing Management
antacids	Antacids increase urinary pH, thus reducing renal reabsorption of aspirin and increasing aspirin clearance. As more aspirin is cleared from the body, a potentially subtherapeutic aspirin level may result.	Monitor serum aspirin level when initiating or discontinuing antacid therapy.
anticoagulants	Aspirins inhibit platelet function, thus prolonging bleeding time. Aspirins displace anticoagulants from protein binding sites, thus increasing their effects. Both actions may result in hemorrhage.	Avoid administering aspirin or other salicylates if possible. If given, monitor prothrombin activity closely, and adjust the anticoagulant dose accordingly.
carbonic anhydrase inhibitors (CAI)	Aspirins displace CAI from protein binding sites and inhibit renal clearance. CAI accumulation and toxicity may result in central nervous system (CNS) depression and metabolic acidosis.	Coadministration should be avoided. When CAI is required, monitor plasma aspirin level and arterial blood gas (ABG) values. Monitor neurologic status.
corticosteroids	Corticosteroids stimulate metabolism of aspirins and increase renal elimination. Aspirin levels may become subtherapeutic.	Tailor aspirin dosage as needed. Monitor aspirin concentrations when adding or withdrawing corticosteroids.
ethanol (alcohol)	Both aspirin and alcohol damage the gastric mucosal barrier. The production of gastric acid stimulated by alcohol promotes the damage. Aspirin decreases the activity of gastric alcohol dehydrogenase, increasing bioavailability. Alcohol may potentiate aspirin-induced GI blood loss and prolong bleeding time.	Separate aspirin and alcohol intake by 12 h. Use buffered aqueous solutions or enteric-coated or extended-release aspirins.
insulin	Basal insulin concentrations are increased, and the acute insulin response to a glucose load is enhanced. This potentiates the serum glucose-lowering action of insulin and results in hypoglycemia.	Monitor blood glucose concentration, and tailor the insulin dosage regimen as needed.
methotrexate	Aspirins may decrease renal clearance and plasma protein binding of methotrexate, leading to methotrexate toxicity.	Decrease methotrexate dosage. Monitor methotrexate plasma level.
probenecid	Renal filtration of uric acid may be altered, leading to the inhibition of uricosuric action of either drug.	Avoid coadministration.
sulfonylureas	Hypoglycemic effect of sulfonylureas may be increased, but the mechanism of this action is not known.	Monitor blood glucose. If hypoglycemia occurs, consider decreasing the sulfonylurea dose.
urinary alkalizers	Aspirin excretion is enhanced in an increased pH environment, which results in decrease of therapeutic aspirin effect.	Anticipate need for possibly higher than expected aspirin doses.
valproic acid	Aspirin displaces valproic acid from protein binding sites. Coadministration may cause valproic acid toxicity.	Monitor serum valproic acid concentrations and liver enzyme levels.

and drug interactions associated with aspirin and to assess the patient for efficacy of the therapy.

Life Span and Gender

Determine whether the patient is pregnant. Aspirin should not be given to women in the last trimester of pregnancy because of an increased risk for maternal hemorrhage. In addition, taking aspirin during late pregnancy can result in adverse fetal effects, including low birth weight, increased intracranial hemorrhage, stillbirths, and neonatal death. Determine the patient's age before administering aspirin. Aspirin should never be given to children younger than 16 years with flu-like symptoms because of its association with Reye syndrome. Aspirin should be given with caution to patients older than 60 years because of an increased risk for adverse effects, especially gastropathies. Men may metabolize aspirin faster than women do, resulting in a decreased duration of action.

Lifestyle, Diet, and Habits

It is important to inquire about the patient's use of over-the-counter (OTC) drugs because many OTCs contain aspirin as an ingredient. Concomitant use will increase the risk for hepatic and renal toxicity. Assess for alcohol or drug abuse

because the patient may have undiagnosed pre-existing hepatic dysfunction. Assessing for cigarette smoking also is important because smoking increases gastric acid production. With the loss of the cytoprotective mechanisms in the stomach from aspirin therapy, the risk for GI bleeding is increased.

Environment

Assess the patient's understanding of aspirin therapy. Aspirin has become the cheapest and most common of all household remedies. Because of its OTC availability and low cost, many people do not understand the potentially life-threatening effects it may cause. Interestingly, because of these two facts (availability and low cost), many people also do not believe aspirin is an important therapeutic intervention and are offended by receiving instructions to take aspirin. For these reasons, patient education is vital.

Nursing Diagnoses and Outcomes

- Acute or Chronic Pain related to ineffectiveness of aspirin
  Desired outcome: *The patient will contact the prescriber if pain persists.*
- Risk for Injury: GI Bleeding, Hepatic or Renal Toxicity related to aspirin therapy
  Desired outcome: *The patient will avoid injury by contacting the prescriber if any signs of toxicity occur.*
- Ineffective Protection related to blood dyscrasias or rash
  Desired outcome: *The patient will contact the prescriber if any signs of blood dyscrasias or rash occur.*
- Deficient Fluid Volume related to nausea and vomiting
  Desired outcome: *The patient will avoid dehydration by contacting the prescriber if persistent nausea or vomiting occurs.*
- Disturbed Sensory Perception (visual and auditory) related to blurred vision or tinnitus
  Desired outcome: *The patient will contact the prescriber if blurred vision or tinnitus occurs.*
- Risk for Injury related to self-medication
  Desired outcome: *The patient will avoid injury by taking aspirin as prescribed.*

CRITICAL THINKING SCENARIO

Aspirin therapy for arthritis

Mrs. Tyler, age 55, has been a patient at your clinic for the past 5 years. She has severe persistent asthma and takes oral prednisone as well as beta-adrenergic agonists as needed. She intermittently has an elevated glucose and follows a 2,400-calorie diet. She was diagnosed with degenerative arthritis of her back today. The health care provider advised Mrs. Tyler to take 2 aspirin every 6 hours to relieve her discomfort and to increase the dose to 3 tablets every 6 hours if the pain continues. As Mrs. Tyler leaves, she turns to you and states, "Aspirin—what a joke—I could have gotten that advice from a website on my computer."

1. How would you respond to Mrs. Tyler?
2. What patient education would you do?
3. Does Mrs. Tyler's medical history predispose her to any problems with aspirin?

Planning and Intervention

Maximizing Therapeutic Effects

Give aspirin with milk or food to decrease gastric distress, as needed.

Minimizing Adverse Effects

Do not administer aspirin to a patient with a medical condition that contraindicates its use. It is important to monitor closely patients with pre-existing medical conditions or those on drug therapy that may interact with aspirin. Arrange for periodic laboratory testing, including a CBC, platelet count, and liver and renal function tests for patients on long-term therapy.

Providing Patient and Family Education

- Encourage the patient to take the drug exactly as prescribed by the health care provider to avoid adverse effects or overdose of aspirin.
- Caution patients not to take aspirin if they have problems with their kidney or liver, are asthmatic and have nasal polyps (aspirin can cause an asthma attack), or are in their last trimester of pregnancy (aspirin may cause hemorrhage during delivery and adverse fetal effects).
- It is important to teach the patient about the potential side effects and adverse effects of aspirin and the importance of contacting the prescriber if any occur. Advise the patient to contact the prescriber if any of the following serious adverse effects occur:
  - Confusion, dizziness, drowsiness
  - Seizures (convulsions)
  - Difficulty breathing, wheezing
  - Tinnitus (ringing in the ears)
  - Blurred vision
  - Black, tarry stools; unusual bleeding or bruising; red or purple spots on the skin; dark urine; prolonged bleeding from a cut; vomiting blood or what looks like coffee grounds
- Caution patients that if aspirin is taken for a long time or in high doses, it can cause problems with the blood, kidneys, or liver.
- Advise patients to avoid drinking alcohol and smoking when taking aspirin because these activities can increase the risk for gastric irritation and bleeding.
- Explain the importance of taking the drug exactly as prescribed to avoid potential GI distress or bleeding. For example, it is best to adhere to the following directions when taking different types of aspirin:
  - Chewable tablets can be chewed before swallowing, crushed and taken with food, or mixed in a drink.
  - Extended-release tablets should be swallowed whole, never crushed or chewed.
  - Tablets, caplets, or gel-caps should be swallowed with a full glass of water.
  - Suppositories should be removed from the foil, the tip moistened, and then placed in the rectum.
- It is important to caution the patient to contact the prescriber in the event of persistent nausea or vomiting to avoid fluid loss.
- Tell patients to take aspirin with food, milk, or antacid to prevent GI upset, and that if they miss a dose, the dose should be taken as soon as possible. If it is time for the

next dose, only that dose should be taken; double or extra doses should never be taken.

- It is important to encourage patients to read all OTC drug labels to avoid taking any drugs with aspirin or ibuprofen as an ingredient.
- Encourage patients with diabetes to use blood glucose monitoring rather than urine testing.
- Inform patients never to give aspirin to children younger than 16 years, unless directed to do so by the prescriber, and to keep aspirin out of the reach of children.
- Tell the patient to keep aspirin in a cool, dry place to maintain its potency and to discard any aspirin that smells like vinegar.
- Explain to patients that if the fever does not resolve in 3 days or pain does not go away in 10 days, they should see their health care provider.
- It is important to instruct patients on long-term aspirin therapy to see their health care provider every 6 months for blood work to avoid serious adverse effects.

Ongoing Assessment and Evaluation

Monitor for signs and symptoms of GI distress or bleeding, anemia, hepatotoxicity, and renal failure. It is important to discontinue aspirin if the patient develops a rash, unexplained fever, or angioedema. Monitor for tinnitus and contact the prescriber immediately if this symptom occurs. Also, monitor the patient for efficacy of aspirin therapy.

Therapy is considered effective if the patient is free of fever, pain, or inflammation and does not develop serious adverse effects. In addition, the patient realizes and can explain the importance of contacting the prescriber immediately if any adverse reactions occur.

Drugs Closely Related to P Aspirin

Diflunisal

Diflunisal (Dolobid) is similar to aspirin, but it does not metabolize into salicylic acid. It is used for acute or long-term relief of mild to moderate pain, acute and chronic rheumatoid arthritis, and osteoarthritis. It is not recommended for use as an antipyretic. Diflunisal has an onset of 1 hour, and peak action occurs in 2 to 3 hours. The half-life is 8 to 12 hours. Potential adverse effects are the same as for aspirin. The main advantage of diflunisal is its twice-a-day dosing schedule. The main disadvantage of diflunisal is its cost. Its efficacy for children has not been established.

Salsalate

Salsalate (Disalcid) is the ester of salicylic acid. Salsalate is absorbed completely from the GI tract. Absorption occurs in the small intestine because salsalate acid is practically insoluble in acidic gastric fluids. As an anti-inflammatory and analgesic drug, salsalate acid has the same efficacy as aspirin; however, it does not have antiplatelet or antipyretic effects. Salsalate is useful particularly for patients who cannot tolerate aspirin's GI effects or for patients at risk for anticoagulation. Peak action of salsalate occurs in 2 to 4 hours, and therapeutic levels may be maintained for up to 16 hours with twice-a-day dosing. Salsalate is not recommended for children.

MEMORY CHIP

P Aspirin

- Used for its analgesic, antipyretic, anti-inflammatory, and antiplatelet effects; irreversibly inhibits cyclooxygenase (COX)
- Major contraindications: peptic ulcer disease, gout, renal or hepatic impairment, bleeding disorders, and patients already on anticoagulation therapy
- Most common adverse effects: GI related
- Most serious adverse effects: hepatic and renal toxicity
- **Life span alerts: Aspirin should not be given to children with varicella- or flu-like illness; it should not be given during pregnancy, especially during the third trimester; *monitor patients over the age of 60 years carefully.***

C Prostaglandin Synthetase Inhibitors

The PSIs are a subgroup of NSAIDs, although some prescribers use the term NSAIDs instead of PSIs. PSIs are grouped by chemical classes—propionic acids, acetic acids, naphthylalkanones, fenamates, oxicams, and COX-2 inhibitors. Despite the chemical differences among PSIs, they all inhibit COX and prostaglandin synthesis. Different PSIs may inhibit specific isoenzymes of the COX group, which may explain the differences in efficacy and adverse effects among the PSIs when used in specific disease states. Therapeutic efficacy of a PSI in a particular patient is based on clinical response and usually cannot be predicted before use. As previously mentioned, there are two distinct forms of COX. It is proposed that PSIs should be classified as either COX-1 specific, COX nonspecific, COX-2 preferential, or COX-2 specific.

Ibuprofen, a COX-nonspecific agent, has had FDA approval since the mid-1970s and currently is available in prescription and nonprescription dosages. Ibuprofen is the prototype for PSIs. Table 24.3 presents a summary of selected prostaglandin synthetase inhibitors.

NURSING MANAGEMENT OF THE PATIENT RECEIVING P IBUPROFEN

Core Drug Knowledge

Pharmacotherapeutics

Labeled uses for ibuprofen include rheumatoid arthritis, osteoarthritis, mild to moderate pain, primary dysmenorrhea, and fever. Unlabeled uses for ibuprofen include ankylosing spondylitis, juvenile rheumatoid arthritis, acute gout, and sunburn. Table 24.4 presents labeled and unlabeled indications for selected PSIs.

Pharmacokinetics

Approximately 80% of ibuprofen is absorbed from the GI system after oral administration. Absorption is slower if the drug is taken with food; however, the extent of absorption

TABLE 24.3 Summary of Selected (C) Prostaglandin Synthetase Inhibitors

Drug (Trade) Name	Route and Dosage Range	Pharmacokinetics
(C) Prostaglandin Synthetase Inhibitors		
P ibuprofen (Motrin, Advil; *Canadian:* Actiprofen)	*Adult:* PO, 200–800 mg tid–qid not to exceed 3,200 mg/d *Child:* PO, 20–40 mg/kg/d in three to four divided doses	*Onset:* Rapid *Duration:* 24 h $t_{1/2}$: 2–4 h
diclofenac sodium (Voltaren; *Canadian:* Novo-Difenac)	*Adult:* PO, 100–200 mg/d in two to four divided doses *Child:* Safety and efficacy not established	*Onset:* 1 h *Duration:* 4–6 h $t_{1/2}$: 1.2–1.8 h
etodolac (Lodine; *Canadian:* Ultradol)	*Adult:* PO, 600–1,200 mg/d in two to four divided doses, not to exceed 1,200 mg/d *Child:* Safety and efficacy not established	*Onset:* 30 min *Duration:* 4–8 h $t_{1/2}$: 6–8 h
fenoprofen (Nalfon)	*Adult:* PO, 300–600 mg tid–qid not to exceed 3,200 mg/d *Child:* Safety and efficacy not established	*Onset:* 30 min *Duration:* 4–6 h $t_{1/2}$: 2–3 h
flurbiprofen (Ansaid)	*Adult:* PO, 50–100 mg bid–tid; maximum dose, 300 mg/d *Child:* Safety and efficacy not established	*Onset:* 1 h *Duration:* 4–8 h $t_{1/2}$: 2–4 h
indomethacin (Indocin; *Canadian:* Apo-Indomethacin)	*Adult:* PO, 25 mg bid or tid up to total 150–200 mg/d	*Onset:* 30 min *Duration:* 4–6 h $t_{1/2}$: 2.6–11 h
	Child: IV, 1.5–2.5 mg/kg/d in three to four divided doses	*Onset:* Immediate *Duration:* 15–30 min $t_{1/2}$: Same as above
ketoprofen (Orudis; *Canadian:* Apo-Keto)	*Adult:* PO, 150–300 mg/d single or divided doses; maximum 300 mg/d *Child:* Safety and efficacy not established	*Onset:* 30 min *Duration:* 4–8 h $t_{1/2}$: 2–4 h
ketorolac (Toradol; *Canadian:* Acular)	*Adult:* PO, 10 mg q4–6h for maximum of 2 wk; IM/IV, 30–60 mg, followed by 15–30 mg q6h for a maximum of 5 d	*Onset:* PO, varies; IM/IV; 30 min *Duration:* PO, IM/IV; 6 h $t_{1/2}$: 2.4–8.6 h
meclofenamate sodium (Meclomen)	*Adult:* PO, 50–400 mg tid–qid *Child:* Not indicated for children <14 y	*Onset:* 30 min–1 h *Duration:* 6 h $t_{1/2}$: 1–4 h
mefenamic acid (Ponstel; *Canadian:* Apo-Fenamic)	*Adult:* PO, initially 500 mg q6h, then decrease to 250 mg q6h; maximum dose, 1,000 mg/d, not to exceed 5–7 d *Child:* Not indicated for children <14 y	*Onset:* 1–2 h *Duration:* 6 h $t_{1/2}$: 2–4 h
meloxicam (Mobic)	*Adult:* 7.5 mg once daily	*Onset:* Rapid *Duration:* Unknown $t_{1/2}$: 15–20 h
nabumetone (Relafen; *Canadian:* Apo-Nabumetone)	*Adult:* PO, 1,000 mg/d, not to exceed 2,000 mg/d *Child:* Safety and efficacy not established	*Onset:* 1–2 h *Duration:* 24–48 h $t_{1/2}$: 24 h
naproxen (Naprosyn; *Canadian:* Naxen)	*Adult:* PO, 250–750 mg bid, not to exceed 1,500 mg/d; acute gout, 750–825 mg initially, followed by 250–275 mg qid; moderate pain or dysmenorrhea, 500–550 mg, followed by 250–275 mg *Child:* PO, 10 mg/kg in 2 doses	*Onset:* 1–2 h *Duration:* 7–12 h $t_{1/2}$: 12–15 h
oxaprozin (Daypro)	*Adult:* PO, 600–1,200 mg once daily *Child:* Safety and efficacy not established	*Onset:* 1 h *Duration:* 24–48 h $t_{1/2}$: 26–92 h
piroxicam (Feldene; *Canadian:* Fexicam)	*Adult:* PO, 10–20 mg/d or in divided dose *Child:* Safety and efficacy not established	*Onset:* 15–30 min *Duration:* 24–48 h $t_{1/2}$: 30–86 h
sulindac (Clinoril; *Canadian:* Apo-Sulindac)	*Adult:* PO, 150–200 mg bid, not to exceed 400 mg/d *Child:* Safety and efficacy not established	*Onset:* 1 h *Duration:* 7–16 h $t_{1/2}$: 7–8 h

(continued)

TABLE 24.3 Summary of Selected Ⓒ Prostaglandin Synthetase Inhibitors (continued)

Drug (Trade) Name	Route and Dosage Range	Pharmacokinetics
tolmetin (Tolectin; *Canadian:* Novo-Tolmetin)	*Adult:* PO, initial 200–400 mg tid–qid; maintenance, 600–1,800 mg in divided doses, not to exceed 1,800 mg *Child:* PO, initial 20 mg/kg/d in three to four divided doses; maintenance, 15–30 mg/kg/d in three to four divided doses	*Onset:* Rapid *Duration:* 6–8 h $t_{1/2}$: 1–1.5 h
COX-2 inhibitors		
celecoxib (Celebrex)	*Adult:* PO, 100–200 mg bid 200 mg qd 400 mg qd 400 mg bid	*Onset:* <1 h *Duration:* Unknown $t_{1/2}$: 11 h
valdecoxib (Bextra)	*Adult:* PO, 10–20 mg qd	*Onset:* Rapid *Duration:* Unknown $t_{1/2}$: 8–11h

TABLE 24.4 Indications for Prostaglandin Synthetase Inhibitors

	Celecoxib	Diclofenac	Etodolac	Fenoprofen	Flurbiprofen	Ibuprofen	Indomethacin	Ketoprofen	Ketorolac	Meclofenamate	Mefenamic acid	Meloxicam	Nabumetone	Naproxen	Oxaprozin	Piroxicam	Sulindac	Tolmetin	Valdecoxib
Rheumatoid arthritis	•		•	•	•	•	•	•		•	•	x	•	•	•	•	•	•	•
Osteoarthritis	•		•	•	•	•	•	•		•	•	•	•	•	•	•	•	•	•
Juvenile RA						•	x							•	•		x	•	
Ankylosing spondylitis	x	•		x	x	x	•	x					x	•			•		
Mild to moderate pain	•	•	•	•	•	•	•	•	•	•	•	x	x	•	x				x
Severe pain	•						•												x
Bone pain	•	x	•	x	x	x	x	x	x	x	x		x	x	x		x		x
Dental pain	•		•	x	x	•		•	x					•					x
Migraine		x		x	x	•			x					x			x		
Headache	•	x		x			x	•	x	x	x			•		x	x		
Dysmenorrhea	•	•			x	•		•		•	•			•					•
Gouty arthritis						x	•	x						•			•		
Tendonitis							•							•			•		
Bursitis							•							•			•		
Arthralgia		x	•	•	•	•	•	•	•	x	x			•	x		x		
Myalgia		x	•	•	•	•	•	•	•	x	x			•	x		x		
Ocular pain		•							•										
Patent ductus arteriosis						x	•												
Photophobia		•							•										
Postop ocular inflammation		•			x				•										
Actinic keratosis		•																	
Allergic conjunctivitis									•										
Cystic fibrosis						x													
Desmoid tumor																	x		
Miosis inhibition					•														
Pericarditis							x												
Familial adenomatous polyposis	•																x		

•, Labeled use; x, unlabeled use.

is not affected. Peak serum concentrations occur in 1 to 2 hours. Analgesic and antipyretic effects occur in 2 to 4 hours, whereas a therapeutic inflammatory response takes a few days to 2 weeks. Ibuprofen is highly protein bound and is metabolized in the liver. Plasma half-life is 2 to 4 hours with urinary excretion within 24 hours (see Table 24.4).

Pharmacodynamics

Ibuprofen's effects are believed to be secondary to inhibited synthesis or release of prostaglandins. Ibuprofen probably has a peripheral rather than a central action as an analgesic. Higher doses are required for an anti-inflammatory effect than for analgesia. Antipyretic activity may be the result of action on the hypothalamus, leading to increased peripheral blood flow, vasodilation, and subsequent heat dissipation.

Contraindications and Precautions

Because chronic use of ibuprofen can result in gastritis, ulceration with or without perforation, or GI bleeding, ibuprofen is contraindicated in patients with a history of or active GI disease, including peptic ulcer disease, ulcerative colitis, or GI bleeding. Other patients at high risk for GI adverse effects are those who routinely consume alcohol or smoke tobacco products because these behaviors are also conducive to ulcer development.

Ibuprofen should be used cautiously in patients with preexisting hepatic, renal, or hemopoietic dysfunction and in patients older than 60 years. Liver dysfunction can occur during therapy with PSIs, resulting in jaundice and fatal hepatitis. Ibuprofen is metabolized in the liver, and accumulation can occur with liver dysfunction, increasing the risk for toxicity. Ibuprofen and its metabolites are excreted renally. Again, accumulation may occur in patients with renal impairment, increasing the risk for toxicity. Additionally, reduced renal blood flow caused by inhibition of prostaglandin synthesis can result in overt renal decompensation. Patients with the highest risk for renal decompensation are those with renal disease, hepatic disease, CHF, diabetes mellitus, SLE, edema, or extracellular volume depletion; those taking diuretics or nephrotoxic drugs; and elderly patients.

Ibuprofen should be used cautiously in patients with preexisting coagulopathy or hemophilia, because of the effect of the drug on platelet function and vascular response to bleeding. Ibuprofen can prolong bleeding time. Anemia may be exacerbated with the use of ibuprofen.

Conditions associated with fluid retention, such as CHF, can be exacerbated with ibuprofen therapy. Hypertension may be exacerbated by ibuprofen-induced fluid retention.

Ibuprofen is classified as a pregnancy category B drug until the third trimester, when ibuprofen enters pregnancy category D because of the potential for PSIs to cause premature closure of the ductus arteriosus in utero. Additionally, persistent pulmonary hypertension arising from ductus arteriosus constriction is a potential complication. PSIs also have the potential to prolong pregnancy and inhibit labor if taken during the third trimester.

Adverse Effects

Ibuprofen, like salicylates, inhibits COX-1 and COX-2, resulting in adverse effects.

Gastropathies are commonly associated with ibuprofen. Nausea, vomiting, diarrhea, constipation, flatulence, and abdominal pain may be representative of minor adverse effects in some patients or serious GI toxicity in others. During long-term administration, the most serious effects are peptic ulcer disease or gastritis that leads to GI bleeding or even perforation. These events can occur at any time, with or without warning.

Ibuprofen also can induce blurred vision, decreased visual acuity, and corneal deposits. The mechanism for visual disturbances is unclear. Vision generally improves after the drug is discontinued. In addition, like aspirin, ibuprofen may induce tinnitus.

In the renal system, acute renal failure may occur in susceptible patients. Patients with conditions associated with diminished renal blood flow, such as CHF, cirrhosis, renal insufficiency, and advanced age, are at the highest risk. Vasodilatory renal prostaglandins and the potent vasoconstrictor angiotensin II work in concert to maintain renal blood flow. Inhibition of renal prostaglandins diminishes renal blood flow, leading to acute renal failure. Less common renal toxicities include interstitial nephritis and nephrotic syndrome. In addition to increased BUN and creatinine levels, proteinuria occurs. Another problem resulting from the inhibition of the renal prostaglandins is sodium and water retention. This effect is especially problematic for patients with conditions such as hypertension and CHF. Acute renal failure, water retention, interstitial nephritis, and nephrotic syndrome usually occur early in ibuprofen therapy and are reversible by stopping drug therapy.

Ibuprofen may cause excessive or abnormal bleeding, especially in patients with hemophilia, anemias, or severe liver disease. Ibuprofen diminishes platelet aggregation by inhibiting the prostaglandin thromboxane. This effect is transient and reversible. Other blood dyscrasias, such as agranulocytosis and aplastic anemia, have been infrequently reported.

Ibuprofen has been associated with hepatotoxicity, such as hepatitis or jaundice. Hepatotoxicity is uncommon, but patients should be monitored closely if on prolonged therapy.

Some patients taking ibuprofen may experience cross-sensitivity to aspirin or other PSIs, including those in a different chemical class. However, cross-sensitivities are not always complete, and patients may be able to take other PSIs, even those in the same chemical class.

Drug Interactions

Ibuprofen is highly protein bound and has many interactions similar to those produced by salicylates. In addition to the drugs listed in Table 24.5, ibuprofen should not be given along with salicylates. Giving these drugs together does not increase efficacy, but it does increase the risk for adverse effects. Ibuprofen should be discontinued 72 hours before adrenal function tests are performed. Ibuprofen also may elevate sodium and chloride levels. Table 24.5 lists drug interactions with ibuprofen.

Assessment of Relevant Core Patient Variables

Health Status

Assess the patient for potential contraindications to ibuprofen therapy. It is important to obtain a drug history to identify potential drug–drug interactions and to assess for potential

TABLE 24.5 Agents That Interact With P Ibuprofen

Interactants	Effect and Significance	Nursing Management
anticoagulants	Ibuprofen inhibits platelet function and possibly produces gastric erosion. Anticoagulation effect is increased; hemorrhage may develop.	Avoid coadministering salicylates if possible. Monitor prothrombin activity closely if appropriate. Adjust the anticoagulant dose accordingly.
beta blockers	Ibuprofen inhibits renal prostaglandin synthesis, allowing unopposed pressor systems to produce hypertension. It also impairs antihypertensive effect of beta blockers.	Avoid coadministering if possible. Monitor blood pressure. Adjust beta blocker dosage as needed.
diuretics	Ibuprofen reduces natriuresis and antihypertensive response, resulting in decreased diuretic effect.	May need to administer a salicylate instead of ibuprofen. Anticipate possible need for higher dose of diuretic.
lithium	Ibuprofen is suspected to reduce renal elimination of lithium. Interaction may cause lithium toxicity.	Monitor lithium levels every 4–5 d until they stabilize after ibuprofen is added or withdrawn from treatment. Adjust lithium dosage as needed.
methotrexate	Ibuprofen is suspected to reduce renal elimination of methotrexate and may cause methotrexate toxicity.	Monitor methotrexate levels. Consider longer duration leucovorin rescue therapy in patients receiving ibuprofen.
sulfonylureas	Hypoglycemic effect of sulfonylureas may be increased, although the mechanism is not understood.	Monitor blood glucose levels. Anticipate an order to decrease the sulfonylurea dose if hypoglycemia occurs.

hypersensitivities to salicylates or other PSIs. Assess for a history of asthma or nasal polyps because patients with these conditions are prone to bronchospasm.

In addition, it is important to assess a patient's baseline gross hearing because of the potential for ototoxicity from ibuprofen use. For patients on long-term therapy, obtain a baseline CBC, platelet count, and test results of renal and hepatic function. Assess the patient for efficacy of ibuprofen therapy; severe or visceral pain may not be affected by ibuprofen.

Life Span and Gender

Determine whether the patient is pregnant. Ibuprofen should not be given to women in the last trimester of pregnancy because it may cause premature closure of the ductus arteriosis. Determine the patient's age before administering ibuprofen. Although ibuprofen is considered safe for children, some of the other PSIs are contraindicated. Ibuprofen should be given with caution to patients older than 60 years because these patients have an increased risk for adverse effects, especially GI bleeding. Ibuprofen, like aspirin, is thought to be metabolized faster in men, which may result in a shorter duration of action than it has in women.

Lifestyle, Diet, and Habits

As with aspirin, it is important to inquire about the patient's use of OTC drugs because many OTCs contain ibuprofen or aspirin. Concomitant use of either or both will increase the risk for hepatic and renal toxicity.

Assess for alcohol or drug abuse because the patient may have undiagnosed pre-existing hepatic dysfunction. In addition, the patient should be assessed for a history of cigarette smoking because ibuprofen, like aspirin, decreases the cytoprotective mechanisms of the stomach.

Environment

Ascertain the setting in which ibuprofen will be administered. Ibuprofen may be self-administered at home or given in any health care setting. Because this drug first appeared on the market as a prescription drug, the lay public often believes that it is more effective than aspirin or acetaminophen. Because of ibuprofen's reasonable cost and high efficacy, some patients may take the drug at a higher dose than the labeling suggests or for a much longer duration without seeing a medical provider. This practice places the patient at a higher risk for adverse effects, or other problems, if the etiology of their symptoms is not addressed.

Nursing Diagnoses and Outcomes

- Acute or Chronic Pain related to ineffectiveness of ibuprofen
  Desired outcome: *The patient will contact the prescriber if pain persists.*
- Increased Risk for Injury related to incorrect self-administration or to drug-induced GI bleeding or hepatic and renal toxicity
  Desired outcome: *The patient will remain free of injury by taking the drug only as directed. In addition, the patient will be able to explain the importance of contacting the health care provider immediately if any adverse effects occur.*
- Increased Risk for Deficient Fluid Volume related to nausea and vomiting
  Desired outcome: *The patient will contact the prescriber immediately if intractable nausea or vomiting occurs.*
- Ineffective Protection related to blood dyscrasias
  Desired outcome: *The patient will contact the prescriber immediately if any signs and symptoms of blood dyscrasias occur.*

- Disturbed Sensory Perception (visual) related to blurred vision
  Desired outcome: *The patient will discontinue ibuprofen immediately and contact the health care provider if vision is affected.*

Planning and Intervention

Maximizing Therapeutic Effects

Give ibuprofen with milk or food to decrease gastric distress, if needed.

Minimizing Adverse Effects

Closely monitor patients with pre-existing medical conditions or drug therapy that may interact with ibuprofen. It is important to administer misoprostol to patients at high risk for developing gastropathies with ibuprofen (Box 24.3). Periodic CBC, platelet count, and liver and renal function tests should be obtained for patients on long-term therapy.

Providing Patient and Family Education

- Instruct patients to take the drug exactly as directed by the prescriber to avoid adverse effects or overdose with ibuprofen.
- Tell patients not to take ibuprofen if they have problems with their kidneys or livers, to use ibuprofen cautiously during the first two trimesters of pregnancy, and not to take it at all during the third trimester of pregnancy. In addition, patients should not take ibuprofen if they are asthmatic and have nasal polyps because ibuprofen could cause an asthma attack.
- Advise patients to take ibuprofen with food, milk, or possibly an antacid to prevent GI upset.
- Instruct patients that if a dose is missed, it should be taken as soon as possible. If it is almost time for the next dose, only that dose should be taken; double or extra doses should never be taken.
- Caution patients that the drug can cause problems with the blood, kidneys, or liver if taken for a long time or in high doses.
- Caution patients that drinking alcohol and smoking while taking ibuprofen can increase the risk for GI irritation and bleeding.
- Advise patients to contact their health care provider if minor adverse effects such as diarrhea, dizziness, drowsiness, heartburn, nausea, and vomiting do not subside or if they are bothersome.
- Warn patients about serious adverse effects of ibuprofen and to advise them to seek medical attention immediately if they occur. Adverse effects include the following:
  - Black, tarry stools; blood in urine; dark yellow or brown urine
  - Difficulty breathing, wheezing; skin rash, redness, blistering, peeling, or itching; swelling of eyelids, throat, lips, or feet
  - Rapid heartbeat
  - Blurred vision
  - Muscle aches and pains, fever, chills
  - Weight change
  - Unusual bleeding or bruising, unusual tiredness or weakness, prolonged bleeding from a cut, vomiting blood or what looks like coffee grounds
- Instruct patients to change position slowly to avoid dizziness. If dizziness occurs, the patient should refrain from driving a car or operating machinery.
- Tell patients to read the labels of all OTC drugs and to avoid any with aspirin or other NSAIDs as an ingredient.
- Warn patients to seek immediate medical assistance if they accidentally take too many tablets.
- Advise patients with diabetes to monitor their blood glucose levels rather than testing their urine.
- Instruct patients to keep ibuprofen in a cool, dry place to preserve its potency.
- Tell patients to see their health care provider if their fever does not resolve in 3 days or their pain does not go away in 10 days.
- Advise patients on long-term ibuprofen therapy to see their health care provider every 6 months for blood testing to make sure they are not having adverse effects from the drug.

Ongoing Assessment and Evaluation

The patient requires monitoring for signs and symptoms of GI distress or bleeding, anemia, tinnitus, hepatotoxicity, and renal failure. Monitor patients older than 60 years closely for these adverse effects. Arrange periodic laboratory tests for patients on long-term therapy or those at high risk for adverse effects. Monitor the patient for relief of pain and inflammation.

Therapy is considered effective if the patient is free of fever, pain, or inflammation and does not develop adverse effects.

BOX 24.3 Using Misoprostol to Reduce PSI Adverse Effects

Misoprostol (Cytotec) increases bicarbonate and mucus production in the gastrointestinal tract. It may also inhibit gastric acid secretion. To minimize possible gastropathies in patients on long-term prostaglandin synthetase inhibitor (PSI) therapy, consider prophylactic therapy with misoprostol for patients with any of the following:

- Age >60 years
- History of peptic ulcer disease
- Cigarette smoker
- Concomitant use of alcohol
- Concomitant use of corticosteroids
- Dyspepsia during salicylate or PSI use
- Poor surgical risk if ulcer complications occur

Drugs Closely Related to P Ibuprofen

Propionic Acids

In addition to ibuprofen, the following drugs are in the propionic class of PSIs: fenoprofen (Nalfon), flurbiprofen (Ansaid), ketoprofen (Orudis), naproxen (Naprosyn, Anaprox), and oxaprozin (Daypro). These drugs are similar to ibuprofen in action, indications, nursing management, and patient education. They differ only in their onset, peak, and duration of action. Although these drugs are chemically sim-

MEMORY CHIP

[P] Ibuprofen

- Used for its anti-inflammatory, analgesic, and antipyretic effects; reversibly inhibits cyclooxygenase (COX)
- Major contraindications: active GI diseases; used with caution in patients with renal or hepatic impairment, hemopoietic dysfunction, pre-existing coagulopathy, cardiac impairment, and age >60 years
- Most common adverse effects: GI related
- Most serious adverse effects: hepatic and renal toxicity
- **Life span alert: Ibuprofen is in pregnancy category D in the third trimester; *monitor patients over the age of 60 years carefully.***

ilar, patients may have relief of symptoms from one drug in this group but not another. Naproxen and ketoprofen, like ibuprofen, may be purchased OTC.

Acetic Acids

The acetic acids include diclofenac (Voltaren), etodolac (Lodine), indomethacin (Indocin), ketorolac (Toradol), sulindac (Clinoril), and tolmetin (Tolectin). They are potent PSIs, highly protein bound, and may displace other protein-bound drugs, which may cause toxicities. They are associated with a high incidence of GI distress and should be given with meals or milk. They also may increase blood pressure or cause sodium and water retention. This group of PSIs also has an increased risk for causing liver dysfunction. Patients should have periodic liver function tests evaluated.

Patients taking indomethacin have an increased risk for adverse effects. It may aggravate depression, other psychiatric disturbances, epilepsy, and parkinsonism. Indomethacin is also associated with a high incidence of severe frontal headaches.

Ketorolac is the only PSI administered both orally and intramuscularly. It is administered for its analgesic effect alone. The efficacy of its intramuscular administration is similar to that of morphine and opioid analgesics. Despite its intramuscular (IM) administration, ketorolac also may induce GI distress, including peptic ulcers and bleeding.

The advantage of acetic acids is their long half-life with resultant once-daily or twice-daily dosing. A major disadvantage is their high cost.

Fenamates

Mefenamic acid (Ponstel) and meclofenamate sodium (Meclomen) are the two fenamate drugs used in the United States. They have anti-inflammatory, analgesic, and antipyretic actions. They have no clear advantage over other PSIs and have an increased risk for adverse effects, especially diarrhea.

Oxicams

Meloxicam (Mobic) and piroxicam (Feldene) are the only oxicams currently available in the United States. They have anti-inflammatory, analgesic, and antipyretic effects. They are equivalent to aspirin, indomethacin, and naproxen in treating osteoarthritis and rheumatoid arthritis and are better tolerated. Meloxicam is as effective as piroxicam and has fewer GI adverse effects. The advantage of oxicams is their once-daily dosing. The high cost is a disadvantage.

Alkanones

Nabumetone (Relafen) is a new type of PSI indicated for osteoarthritis and rheumatoid arthritis. Despite its high efficacy, it has a relatively low incidence of side effects. It appears to cause less gastric damage than other PSIs. It is assumed that its decreased GI effects are related to its decreased inhibition of COX-1. Like other drugs with a long half-life, nabumetone is administered once a day. The disadvantage of this drug is its high cost.

Drugs Significantly Different From [P] Ibuprofen

COX-2 Inhibitors

The discovery of COX-2 has made possible the design of drugs that reduce inflammation without removing the protective prostaglandins in the stomach and kidney made by COX-1. Currently, two COX-2 inhibitors are available: celecoxib and valdecoxib. These drugs exhibit anti-inflammatory, analgesic, and antipyretic activities by selectively inhibiting COX-2 prostaglandin synthesis, but not platelet aggregation. These highly selective COX-2 inhibitors may not only be useful in conditions such as rheumatic and osteoarthritis but also in colon cancer, Alzheimer disease, and kidney disease.

In 2004, rofecoxib (Vioxx), a COX-2 inhibitor, was taken off the market due to an increased risk for cardiovascular and cerebral events. While it is unknown if other COX-2 inhibitors induce these adverse events, it is prudent to monitor patients on these drugs for signs and symptoms of cardiac or CNS adverse effects.

CELECOXIB

Celecoxib (Celebrex) was the first COX-2 inhibitor on the market. Its pharmacotherapeutics is similar to that of other PSIs. In addition, celecoxib also is approved to reduce the number of adenomatous colorectal polyps in patients with a rare genetic disease called familial adenomatous polyposis (FAP) (see Table 24.3). It is given as an oral tablet.

Celecoxib should not be given to patients who have experienced salicylate hypersensitivity evidenced by asthma, urticaria, or allergic-type reactions after taking aspirin or other PSIs. It is also contraindicated in patients with known sulfonamide hypersensitivity because it is structurally related to sulfonamides. Precautions are similar to those for ibuprofen, with the exception of hemophilia, because celecoxib does not inhibit platelet aggregation. Celecoxib is not approved for use in adolescents or children.

Potential adverse effects also are similar to ibuprofen. Theoretically, because of the specificity of celecoxib for the COX-2 pathway, it has the potential to cause less gastropathy and risk for GI bleeding. However, serious GI bleeding or obstruction has been reported in patients receiving celecoxib despite its cytoprotective properties.

Celecoxib may interact with multiple drugs. It can decrease the effectiveness of loop or thiazide diuretics and angiotensin-converting enzyme (ACE) inhibitors. Celecoxib decreases the excretion of methotrexate, vancomycin, and aminoglycosides, resulting in an increased risk for toxicity or adverse effects from these drugs. Celecoxib may increase the serum drug levels of warfarin and lithium, again placing the patient at risk for toxicity or adverse effects. When given with fluconazole, the serum concentration of celecoxib is increased. Celecoxib is a pregnancy category C drug. Like

other PSI drugs, it should not be given during the last trimester of pregnancy because it may cause premature closure of the ductus arteriosus.

VALDECOXIB

Valdecoxib (Bextra) is the latest COX-2 inhibitor approved by the FDA. Its FDA-approved pharmacotherapeutics are limited to rheumatoid arthritis, osteoarthritis, and dysmenorrhea. Like celecoxib, valdecoxib is structurally related to sulfonamides; thus it is contraindicated for use in patients allergic to sulfonamides. It is also used with extreme caution in patients who have recently undergone coronary bypass graft surgery, because of an increased risk for cardiovascular events. Also like celecoxib, valdecoxib is not approved for use in adolescents or children.

Adverse effects are also similar to those produced by celecoxib. Valdecoxib is associated with allergic reactions and, in rare circumstances, may induce severe skin reactions such as Stevens-Johnson syndrome and exfoliative dermatitis, which may be lethal. For that reason, valdecoxib should be discontinued at the first sign of rash. Drug-drug interactions are the same as those provoked by celecoxib. Valdecoxib is also a pregnancy category C drug and should be avoided in the last trimester of pregnancy.

(C) Para-aminophenol Derivatives

Acetaminophen (Tylenol), a widely used analgesic and antipyretic, is the only **para-aminophenol derivative** available in the United States. Although similar to an NSAID and often grouped as such, it does not have an anti-inflammatory effect. It was first used in clinical medicine in 1893, but widespread use began after it received FDA approval in 1950. It is available without a prescription as an individual agent and in combination with a variety of other drugs. Table 24.6 presents a summary of selected para-aminophenol derivatives.

NURSING MANAGEMENT OF THE PATIENT RECEIVING [P] ACETAMINOPHEN

Core Drug Knowledge

Pharmacotherapeutics

Acetaminophen is indicated for treating fever or mild pain. It is used for patients with a hypersensitivity to aspirin or PSIs or intolerance to their GI effects and for patients who are receiving anticoagulant therapy.

Pharmacokinetics

Acetaminophen is administered orally and absorbed rapidly and completely from the GI tract or rectal mucosa. Peak concentrations occur within 60 minutes. The half-life is 1 to 3.5 hours, and the duration is 3 to 5 hours. Acetaminophen is metabolized in the liver and eliminated by the kidneys. Acetaminophen crosses the placenta and is secreted in breast milk.

Pharmacodynamics

Acetaminophen possesses both antipyretic and analgesic effects, but it has no peripheral anti-inflammatory effects. Thus, it may be less effective than other drugs for pain related to peripheral inflammation.

Acetaminophen's exact mechanism of action is unknown. It is centrally acting primarily, has no effects on platelet aggregation, and is a reversible weak inhibitor of COX. The antipyretic activity is thought to be produced by blocking the effects of endogenous pyrogen on the hypothalamic heat-regulating center, possibly by inhibiting prostaglandin synthesis. Heat is lost by vasodilation, increased peripheral blood flow, and sweating. The analgesic effect is believed to result from inhibited prostaglandin synthesis or from inhibited synthesis or actions of chemical mediators that sensitize the pain receptors to mechanical or chemical stimulation.

Contraindications and Precautions

Acetaminophen is contraindicated in patients with hepatic disease, viral hepatitis, or alcoholism. In these diseases, metabolism of the drug may be decreased, resulting in a risk for hepatotoxicity. Because acetaminophen is excreted primarily by the kidneys, serum concentrations may increase in patients with renal impairment, again resulting in an increased risk for toxicity.

Acetaminophen is also used with caution in patients with pre-existing anemia because acetaminophen may exacerbate anemias. Patients who have phenylketonuria or who must restrict intake of phenylalanine should avoid acetaminophen products containing aspartame (Nutrasweet), such as Tempra chewable tablets, Alka-Seltzer Advanced Formula, Children's Anacin-3, Junior Strength Tylenol, Children's Tylenol, and Double-Strength Tempra.

Acetaminophen is assigned to pregnancy category B and therefore should be used cautiously in patients who are pregnant or lactating. However, it is the safest antipyretic analgesic drug to use, if necessary, during pregnancy or lactation.

Adverse Effects

Acetaminophen is generally well tolerated. Most adverse effects occur when the drug is taken in high doses or for prolonged periods. However, acetaminophen overdose is poten-

TABLE 24.6 Summary of Selected (C) Para-Aminophenol Derivatives

Drug (Trade) Name	Selected Indications	Route and Dosage Range	Pharmacokinetics
(C) Para-aminophenol Derivatives			
[P] acetaminophen (Tylenol; *Canadian:* Atasol)	Fever, analgesia	*Adult:* PO, 325–650 mg q3–4h, not to exceed 4g/d *Child:* PO, 10 mg/kg q4–6h	*Onset:* 10–30 min *Duration:* 3–5 h $t_{1/2}$: 1–3.5 h

tially fatal. Metabolites of acetaminophen can bind to tissue groups in either the kidney or liver, causing a loss of glutathione reserves and resulting in either nephrotoxicity or hepatotoxicity. Symptoms during the early stage of toxicity include anorexia, nausea, vomiting, pallor, and diaphoresis. During the intermediate stage (days 1–3), the patient may complain of right upper quadrant pain and experience decreased urine output. The late stage (days 3–5) is characterized by jaundice, elevated aspartate transaminase and alanine transaminase levels, and a dramatic rise in prothrombin time, indicating hepatic necrosis and symptoms of renal failure. During this stage, the patient also may experience CNS stimulation followed by CNS depression. Early administration of acetylcysteine, which replaces glutathione reserves, is the only antidote. Acetaminophen overdose is an emergency that must be treated in the hospital.

Acetaminophen may cause adverse effects in the hepatic, renal, hematologic, and GI systems. Hepatotoxicity and hepatic necrosis may occur in patients who are on high-dose or long-term therapy. Another potential adverse effect in patients with high-dose or long-term therapy is acute renal failure, renal papillary necrosis, or renal tubular necrosis. In the hematologic system, acetaminophen may cause anemia, leukopenia, thrombocytopenia, or pancytopenia. In the GI system, acetaminophen may cause GI bleeding. Bleeding occurs secondary to low prothrombin levels.

Drug Interactions

Acetaminophen may interact with activated charcoal, antacids, ethanol, hydantoins, and sulfinpyrazone. In rats, *S*-adenosyl-L-methionine (SAMe), an herbal product, decreases acetaminophen binding to hepatic microsomal proteins and has been shown to improve survival after acetaminophen overdose (Song et al., 2004). The utility of these findings in preventing acetaminophen hepatotoxicity is uncertain; more studies are needed to evaluate the role of SAMe in human acetaminophen toxicity. Table 24.7 presents additional information about drug interactions with acetaminophen.

Assessment of Relevant Core Patient Variables

Health Status

Assess the patient's pain level. Acetaminophen is effective for mild to moderate pain. Assess for pre-existing medical condition or drug therapy that contraindicates using acetaminophen or necessitates close monitoring of the patient. For patients expected to be on long-term therapy, obtain and document baseline CBC, platelet count, and renal and hepatic function values.

Life Span and Gender

Note the patient's age before administering acetaminophen. Acetaminophen is an excellent drug for treating children's fever and pain. Unlike aspirin, it is not associated with Reye syndrome. Elderly patients are more likely to develop hepatic and renal toxicity because of age-related decreases in hepatic and renal function. Also, note whether the patient is pregnant. Acetaminophen is the drug of choice for pregnant women because it does not have any antiplatelet activity.

TABLE 24.7 Agents That Interact With P Acetaminophen

Interactants	Effect and Significance	Nursing Management
activated charcoal	Charcoal reduces gastrointestinal (GI) absorption of ingested drugs and adsorbs enterohepatically circulated drugs. Charcoal may actually remove drugs from the systemic circulation. Depending on the clinical situation, this will reduce the effectiveness or toxicity of a given agent.	Administer activated charcoal as soon as possible, in a situation involving toxicity of acetaminophen. Do not administer activated charcoal within 2–3 h of acetaminophen administration, in any situation using acetaminophen therapeutically.
antacids	Antacids can delay and decrease the oral absorption of acetaminophen.	Administer antacids and acetaminophen at least 2 h apart.
ethanol (alcohol)	Induction of hepatic microsomal enzymes by chronic ethanol consumption may be associated with acetaminophen-induced hepatotoxicity. Chronic consumption of ethanol may increase the risk of acetaminophen-induced liver damage.	Caution patient who consumes ethanol chronically and in excess about the potential interaction. Advise patients to avoid ethanol ingestion while taking acetaminophen. Monitor suspected ethanol abusers closely for hepatotoxicity.
drugs that increase the risk of hepatotoxicity hydantoins sulfinpyrazone	Hydantoins and sulfinpyrazone may induce hepatic microsomal enzymes, which accelerate the metabolism of acetaminophen. An unusually high rate of acetaminophen metabolism could lead to abnormally high levels of hepatotoxic metabolites. The potential hepatotoxicity of acetaminophen may be increased and the therapeutic effects of acetaminophen may be decreased when administered with chronic doses of hydantoins or sulfinpyrazone.	At usual therapeutic doses of acetaminophen and hydantoins or sulfinpyrazone, no special dosage adjustment is required. Risk is greatest when acetaminophen overdose accompanies chronic use of hydantoins or sulfinpyrazone. Monitor patients closely.

Lifestyle, Diet, and Habits

It is important to inquire about the patient's use of OTC drugs because many of these products contain acetaminophen as an ingredient. Concomitant use will increase the risk for hepatotoxicity. Assess for alcohol or drug abuse because the patient may have undiagnosed pre-existing hepatic dysfunction.

Environment

Determine the patient's understanding of acetaminophen therapy. Acetaminophen is self-administered easily at home without medical supervision. Because of its low cost and availability, many people do not understand acetaminophen's potentially life-threatening adverse effects. Patient education is important to avoid unintentional overdose or long-term complications.

Nursing Diagnoses and Outcomes

- Acute or Chronic Pain related to ineffectiveness of acetaminophen
  Desired outcome: *The patient will contact the health care provider if pain persists.*
- Risk for Injury related to drug-induced hepatic and renal toxicity or to improper self-medication
  Desired outcome: *The patient will take drug as directed and contact the health care provider if any signs of toxicity occur.*
- Ineffective Protection related to potential blood dyscrasias
  Desired outcome: *The patient will contact the health care provider if any signs of blood dyscrasias occur.*

Planning and Intervention

Maximizing Therapeutic Effects

Acetaminophen can be administered without regard to meals. Monitor the patient for therapeutic effect of acetaminophen and relief of symptoms.

Minimizing Adverse Effects

It is important to assess patients for medical conditions that contradict the use of acetaminophen. Carefully monitor patients with pre-existing medical conditions or drug therapy that may interact with acetaminophen. Periodic CBC, platelet count, and liver and renal function tests should be performed for patients on long-term therapy.

Providing Patient and Family Education

- Tell patients to take the drug exactly as prescribed by the health care provider to avoid adverse effects or overdose.
- Warn patients not to take this drug if they have problems with their kidneys or livers.
- Teach patients exact directions for correct administration because acetaminophen is manufactured in a variety of formulations.
- Teach patients with diabetes to monitor their blood glucose level for signs of hypoglycemia.
- Instruct the patient to read all OTC drug labels and to avoid any with acetaminophen as an ingredient.
- Stress the potential for acetaminophen overdose and the importance of seeking medical attention should the patient accidentally take too many tablets.
- Advise patients to keep acetaminophen in a light-resistant container out of the reach of children.
- Encourage patients to contact the health care provider immediately if they have any adverse effects (e.g., signs of blood dyscrasias and signs of hepatic or renal toxicity), if fever does not subside within 3 days, or if pain is not relieved within 10 days.

Ongoing Assessment and Evaluation

Monitor the patient for sore throat, chills, easy bruising, and unusual bleeding because these signs may indicate blood dyscrasias. It also is important to monitor the patient for any signs and symptoms of hepatotoxicity and renal failure. Do not give acetaminophen if the patient develops a rash, unexplained fever, or angioedema. The patient needs to contact the health care provider immediately if any of these symptoms occur.

Therapy is considered effective if the patient is free of fever and pain. In addition, the patient should remain free of adverse effects and should be able to explain the importance of contacting the health care provider immediately if any adverse effects occur.

(C) Serotonin-Selective Drugs

Serotonin-selective drugs are used to relieve pain and inflammation related to migraine headache. They are not useful for other types of headache or inflammation that occur elsewhere in the body. These drugs are also known as "triptans" because the generic name of these drugs ends as such. Sumatriptan, the first 5-$HT_{1B/1D}$ agonist approved for use in the United States, is the prototype for this class of drugs. Table 24.8 presents a summary of selected serotonin receptor antagonists.

NURSING MANAGEMENT OF THE PATIENT RECEIVING [P] SUMATRIPTAN

Core Drug Knowledge

Pharmacotherapeutics

Sumatriptan is used to treat acute migraine headache with or without aura and to manage cluster headache. Because of its serotonin agonist properties, it is currently being studied for

MEMORY CHIP

[P] Acetaminophen

- Used for mild to moderate pain and fever; usually well tolerated; has no anti-inflammatory effect
- Major contraindications: hepatic disease, viral hepatitis, and alcoholism
- Most common adverse effects: rash, urticaria, and nausea
- Most serious adverse effects: Acetaminophen may cause hepatic or renal toxicity in susceptible patients.
- **Life span alert: Acetaminophen is the drug of choice for infants and children with flu or flu-like symptoms; analgesic of choice during pregnancy or lactation.**

TABLE 24.8 Summary of (C) Serotonin Receptor Agonists

Drug (Trade) Name	Selected Indications	Route and Dosage Range	Pharmacokinetics
P sumatriptan (Imitrex)	Migraine and cluster headache	*Adult:* PO, 50 mg; may be repeated every 2 h *Adult:* nasal spray, 5–20 mg; may be repeated in 2 h *Adult:* SC, 6 mg; may repeat in >1 h	*Onset:* PO, 30–60 min INH, 15–20 min SC: 10–15 min *Duration:* Short $t_{1/2}$: PO, 2.5 h Inh, 2 h SC, 115 min
almotriptan (Axert)	Migraine and cluster headache	*Adult:* PO, 6.25–12.5 mg	*Onset:* 30 min–2 h *Duration:* Short $t_{1/2}$: 3.1 h
eletriptan (Relpax)	Migraine and cluster headache	*Adult:* PO, 20–40 mg	*Onset:* 1 h *Duration:* Long $t_{1/2}$: 4 h
frovatriptan (Frova)	Migraine and cluster headache	*Adult:* PO, 2.5 mg; may repeat in 2 h	*Onset:* 2–3 h *Duration:* Long $t_{1/2}$: 26 h
naratriptan (Amerge)	Migraine and cluster headache	*Adult:* PO, 2.5 mg; may repeat once >4 h	*Onset:* 1–3 h *Duration:* Long $t_{1/2}$: 6 h
rizatriptan (Maxalt, Maxalt MLT)	Migraine and cluster headache	*Adult:* PO, 5 or 10 mg; may repeat in 2 h	*Onset:* 30 min–2 h *Duration:* Short $t_{1/2}$: 2–3 h
zolmitriptan (Zomig, Zomig ZMT)	Migraine and cluster headache	*Adult:* PO, 2.5 mg; may repeat in >2 h *Adult:* nasal spray, 5 mg; may repeat in 2 h	*Onset:* 15 min *Duration:* Short $t_{1/2}$: 3 h

the treatment of irritable bowel syndrome (IBS) when constipation is the primary symptom.

Pharmacokinetics

Sumatriptan may be administered orally, intranasally, or subcutaneously. When administered orally, pain relief begins within 1 hour and peak effects occur within 2 to 4 hours. Intranasal sumatriptan is rapidly absorbed, and peak concentration is achieved within 1 to 1.5 hours. The most effective route of administration is subcutaneous. With subcutaneous administration, onset of pain relief occurs within 10 minutes, and most patients have pain relief within 1 to 2 hours. Bioavailability of subcutaneous sumatriptan is 97%, whereas bioavailability of oral sumatriptan is approximately 15%. Sumatriptan is metabolized in the liver and excreted by the kidneys.

Pharmacodynamics

Sumatriptan is selective for 5-$HT_{1B/1D}$ receptors located on cranial blood vessels and sensory nerves of the trigeminal vascular system. Stimulation of these receptors results in vasoconstriction and inhibition of the release of proinflammatory neuropeptides. The end result is a decreased throbbing sensation in the head that often accompanies migraine and cluster headaches as well as decreasing vascular inflammation.

Contraindications and Precautions

Sumatriptan is contraindicated in patients with coronary artery disease (CAD), arteriosclerosis, and ischemic cardiac diseases such as uncontrolled hypertension, angina pectoris—especially vasospastic angina—and acute myocardial infarction (MI) or a history of myocardial infarction. In addition, it is contraindicated in patients with cerebrovascular diseases, such as stroke, intracranial bleeding, and transient ischemic attacks, and in peripheral vascular diseases, such as Raynaud disease.

It is strongly recommended that sumatriptan should not be given to patients with chronic diseases that increase the risk for CAD until those patients have had a cardiac workup. Those diseases include diabetes mellitus, hypertension, hypercholesterolemia, and obesity. Patients with a family history of CAD, those who smoke tobacco, postmenopausal women, and men older than 40 years should also have a cardiovascular workup before being prescribed sumatriptan.

Because sumatriptan is metabolized by the liver and excreted by the kidneys, use it cautiously in patients with hepatic or renal impairment, or in those patients at risk for hepatic or renal dysfunction, such as the elderly. Sumatriptan

should be used cautiously in patients with a history of seizures because it may induce them.

Adverse Effects

Adverse reactions are less likely to occur when sumatriptan is administered orally or intranasally. The most serious adverse effects of sumatriptan are cardiac events; however, they rarely occur. These events include coronary artery vasospasm, cardiac dysrhythmias such as ventricular tachycardia, or ventricular fibrillation, angina, myocardial ischemia including MI, and cardiac arrest. These events occur more frequently in patients with risk factors for CAD, especially if they had taken ergotamine within the previous 24 hours.

More frequently, cardiovascular adverse effects include hypotension or hypertension, palpitations, or syncope. Chest pressure syndrome also occurs frequently. This syndrome includes sensations of chest tightness or heaviness, jaw pain or tightness, and regional pain or pressure.

Sumatriptan can also induce cerebrovascular events such as cerebral vasospasm resulting in intracranial bleeding, subarachnoid hemorrhage, stroke, or seizures. Again, these events are rare and generally occur in patients with risk factors for, or a history of, cerebral vascular disorders.

More commonly, patients may feel weak, dizzy, or lightheaded. They may also experience myalgias, muscle cramps, and stiffness.

Patients receiving intranasal sumatriptan may experience atypical burning sensations in the ear, nose, throat, nasal cavity, or sinus. They may also experience throat discomfort or dysgeusia (a distortion of the sense of taste). Subcutaneous sumatriptan may induce flushing or a sensation of warmth, burning, or heat.

Drug Interactions

Sumatriptan interacts with drugs that contain ergotamine, other 5-HT_1 agonists, sibutramine, and antidepressants such as selective serotonin reuptake inhibitors (SSRIs) and monoamine oxidase inhibitors (MAOIs). Table 24.9 highlights these interactions.

Assessment of Relevant Core Patient Variables

Health Status

Assess the characteristics of the headache, including location, quality, intensity, and the presence or absence of an aura. Assess also for trigger factors that may have caused or may continue the headache.

Take a careful patient history, focusing on cardiovascular and cerebrovascular disorders or diseases. Question patients with diabetes mellitus, hypertension, hypercholesterolemia, or obesity for signs and symptoms that may suggest CAD. Evaluate available laboratory tests, especially liver and renal function tests, because dysfunction of the liver and kidneys may contribute to accumulation of sumatriptan, resulting in increased risk for adverse effects and toxicity. Communicate any positive findings to the health care provider before administering sumatriptan.

Life Span and Gender

Evaluate female patients for pregnancy, breast-feeding, or menopausal symptoms. Sumatriptan is a pregnancy category C drug and should not be given during pregnancy unless the benefits outweigh the risks. It is unclear whether sumatriptan is secreted in breast milk; therefore, it should not be taken by nursing mothers. Postmenopausal women and men older than 40 years should have a cardiovascular workup before receiving sumatriptan, to rule out the potential for CAD.

Lifestyle, Diet, and Habits

Identify trigger factors that may be part of the patient's lifestyle. Evaluate the patient for a history of smoking tobacco because smoking is a risk factor for the development of CAD.

Environment

Sumatriptan is routinely given in the outpatient area.

Nursing Diagnosis and Outcome

- Risk for Tissue Perfusion, Impaired, related to cardiovascular or cerebrovascular events

TABLE 24.9 Agents That Interact With P Sumatriptan

Interactants	Effect and Significance	Nursing Management
ergotamine-containing drugs ergotamine dihydroergotamine methysergide	Coadministration with ergotamine-containing drugs within 24 h may have additive vasospastic effects.	Do not administer sumatriptan within 24 h of ergotamine-containing drugs.
Monoamine oxidase inhibitors (MAOIs)	MAOIs inhibit the metabolism of oral sumatriptan.	Do not administer oral or intranasal sumatriptan within 14 d of MAOI use.
Serotonin receptor agonists	Coadministration with other serotonin receptor agonists increases the risk for vasospastic effects and serotonin syndrome.	Do not administer sumatriptan with other serotonin receptor agonists.
selective serotonin reuptake inhibitors (SSRIs)	Coadministering sumatriptan with SSRIs may cause rapid accumulation of serotonin in the CNS.	Avoid this combination Monitor for signs of serotonin syndrome.
sibutramine	Coadministering sumatriptan with sibutramine may have additive effects.	Avoid this combination Monitor for signs of serotonin syndrome.

Desired Outcome: The patient will recognize the signs and symptoms of cardiovascular or cerebrovascular events and seek medical assistance immediately.

- Risk for Injury related to weakness, dizziness or syncope, or lightheaded

  Desired Outcome: The patient will remain free of injury while taking sumatriptan.

Planning and Intervention

Maximizing Therapeutic Effects

Confirm that the patient has a diagnosis of migraine or cluster headache because sumatriptan is ineffective for other types of headache. Administer the medication at the first sign of pain, rather than waiting until the pain is intolerable. Decrease the environmental stimuli during the migraine attack.

Minimizing Adverse Effects

Assess the patient for a history of cardiovascular or cerebrovascular disorder that might induce adverse effects during sumatriptan therapy. After administering sumatriptan, monitor for signs and symptoms of vasospasm and allergy.

Administer sumatriptan as ordered—orally, intranasally, or subcutaneously. Use aseptic technique when administering subcutaneously.

Providing Patient and Family Education

- Teach the patient to take sumatriptan for migraine or cluster headache only. Emphasize that the patient should avoid the use of sumatriptan if the headache pain is not the same as his or her usual pain pattern.
- Explain the importance of avoiding sumatriptan if they have cardiovascular or cerebrovascular disorders or chronic medical condition that increases the risk for CAD.
- Teach the patient the signs and symptoms of vasospastic events and the importance of seeking medical care immediately if they occur.
- Instruct patients to take the sumatriptan exactly as directed by the health care provider to avoid adverse effects or toxicity. If the pain is not relieved with the first dose of sumatriptan, the patient should follow the instructions of the health care provider for subsequent dosing.
- Teach the patient that the headache may recur. It is important to take only the prescribed dose and not to exceed 200 mg of sumatriptan in a 24-hour period.
- Teach the patient the importance of avoiding smoking cigarettes.
- Teach the patient the correct way to administer sumatriptan. The oral medication should be taken with a full glass of water and not crushed or chewed. If using the intranasal inhaler, the head should be upright. Also, teach the patient aseptic technique to administer sumatriptan subcutaneously.
- Teach the patient to identify trigger factors that induce migraine. Once they are identified, help the patient develop a plan to avoid or eliminate the trigger factor from the patient's lifestyle.
- Teach the patient complementary interventions when taking sumatriptan. The patient should decrease environmental stimuli, rest in a darkened room, and place an ice bag at the back of the neck.

Ongoing Assessment and Evaluation

Evaluate the patient for the cessation of headache and for signs and symptoms of vasospastic events. Monitor the patient's blood pressure after administering sumatriptan. Evaluate the frequency of migraine attacks and refer the patient to the health care provider for prophylaxis as needed. The patient should be pain free after sumatriptan is administered. The patient should remain free of symptoms of vasospastic events and serotonin syndrome. Box 24.4 discusses serotonin syndrome.

Drugs Closely Related to P Sumatriptan

The other serotonin receptor agonists, also called triptans, which are used in managing migraine, are all very similar to sumatriptan. They have the same pharmacotherapeutics, pharmacodynamics, and adverse effects. They have very similar contraindications and precautions and drug–drug interactions (see Table 24.9). The major difference among the triptans is the pharmacokinetics. All of the triptans are pregnancy category C drugs and should be used only when the benefits outweigh the risks.

Almotriptan

Almotriptan (Axert) has a quick onset, short duration, and 70% to 80% bioavailability. It may be better tolerated than sumatriptan and may have a lower incidence of chest pain, tightness, or pressure. Almotriptan may be given with MAOIs.

Eletriptan

Eletriptan (Relpax) has a slower onset than almotriptan and longer duration, with a 50% bioavailability. Its bioavailability is increased when taken with a high-fat meal. Like almotriptan, it may be taken with MAOIs.

Frovatriptan

Frovatriptan (Frova) has a very slow onset and a very long duration of action, and it is only 20% to 30% bioavailable. It has the longest half-life of all the triptans; thus, rebound

MEMORY CHIP

P Sumatriptan

- Used for treatment of acute migraine or cluster headache
- Major contraindications: cardiovascular and cerebrovascular disorders
- Most common adverse effects: flushing, dizziness, weakness, nausea, drowsiness, stiffness, or feelings of tingling, heat, fatigue
- Most serious adverse effects: vasospasm resulting in ischemic events to the cardiovascular and cerebrovascular systems
- Maximizing therapeutic effects: Administer only to patients with documented migraine or cluster headaches.
- Minimizing adverse effects: Avoid administration to patients with cardiovascular or cerebrovascular disorders. Do not administer to patients with atypical headaches.
- Most important patient education: signs and symptoms of ischemic events and importance of seeking medical care should any occur

BOX 24.4 Serotonin Syndrome

Symptoms of serotonin syndrome include excitement, hypomania, restlessness, loss of consciousness, confusion, disorientation, anxiety, agitation, motor weakness, myoclonus, tremor, hemiballismus, hyperreflexia, ataxia, dysarthria, incoordination, hyperthermia, shivering, pupillary dilation, diaphoresis, emesis, and tachycardia.

headaches may occur less frequently. Like almotriptan and eletriptan, it may be given with MAOIs.

Naratriptan

Naratriptan (Amerge) has an onset similar to sumatriptan, but a longer duration and 70% bioavailability. It has a formulation that is dissolves in the mouth without the need for water. It has less headache recurrence than sumatriptan and may be given with MAOIs.

Rizatriptan

Rizatriptan (Maxalt) has a quick onset and duration, with a bioavailability of 45%. Like naratriptan, it has a formulation that dissolves in the mouth. Rizatriptan requires a dosage adjustment if taken with propranolol (Inderal).

Zolmitriptan

Zolmitriptan (Zomig) has the fastest onset of action, a short duration, and a bioavailability of 40%. It also has a dissolve-in-the-mouth formulation.

Drugs Significantly Different From P Sumatriptan

Ergotamine

Ergotamine (Ergomar) is another type of drug used to abort an acute migraine or cluster headache. It has a complex mechanism of action that is very different from sumatriptan. Like sumatriptan, ergotamine stimulates 5-$HT_{1B/1D}$ receptors. It also affects serotonergic, dopaminergic, and alpha-adrenergic receptors. In addition, it stimulates uterine contraction and has emetic properties.

Ergotamine has several routes of administration. It can be given orally, sublingually, rectally, or by inhalation. When given orally or rectally, it is often combined with caffeine, which increases its absorption. While pain relief occurs within 0.5 to 2 hours of administration, vasoconstriction may persist for up to 48 hours. Ergotamine is metabolized in the liver, and its major metabolites are excreted in bile.

Contraindications for the use of ergotamine include alkaloid hypersensitivity, history of cardiovascular or cerebrovascular disorders, and pre-existing hepatic dysfunction. Ergotamine is a pregnancy category X drug because it stimulates uterine contraction. It is also contraindicated for use when breast-feeding because it may cause ergotism (vomiting, diarrhea, weak pulse, and unstable blood pressure) in nursing infants. Ergotamine is used with caution in patients with chronic diseases that increase the risk for cardiovascular disorders.

The most serious adverse effect to ergotamine is overdose or ergotism. Overdose can cause ischemia to peripheral arteries and arterioles with resultant hypoxia to the extremities. As hypoxia continues, the extremities become cold, mottled, or numb. Untreated, the patient may develop gangrene and require amputation.

More common adverse effects include abdominal pain, nausea or vomiting, myalgias, leg weakness, and numbness or tingling in the extremities. Daily or frequent use of ergotamine may cause physical dependence.

Drug–drug interactions may occur with CYP3A4 inhibitors such as ritonavir, nelfinavir, indinavir, erythromycin, clarithromycin, ketoconazole, and itraconazole. Concurrent use of these drugs may cause vasospasm and cerebral or peripheral ischemia. Concurrent use of beta-blocking agents, hormonal contraceptives, vasoconstrictors, or nicotine increases the risk for peripheral vasoconstriction. The use of ergotamine and triptans should occur at least 24 hours apart.

Dihydroergotamine

Dihydroergotamine (DHE) is a semisynthetic ergot alkaloid administered parenterally or intranasally to treat migraine. Dihydroergotamine is generally reserved for treating severe migraine because less toxic agents are available for mild to moderate migraine and cluster headache relief. Its pharmacodynamics is similar to those of ergotamine; however, it causes less peripheral vasoconstriction, nausea, and vomiting.

Contraindications and drug–drug interactions are also similar to those with ergotamine. Dihydroergotamine is a pregnancy category X drug because it induces uterine contractions. Although it is not known whether dihydroergotamine is secreted in breast milk, it should not be used by nursing mothers because of its structural similarity to ergotamine.

DRUGS USED AS PROPHYLAXIS FOR MIGRAINE HEADACHE

Patients with severe debilitating or frequent migraine headaches are often prescribed medications to reduce the severity and frequency of attacks. It is important to remember that these drugs are ineffective for aborting an active migraine attack.

Beta-Adrenergic Blocking Agents

Beta blockers are used to prevent migraine headache because of their ability to relax blood vessels. The drug of choice is propranolol (Inderal), although nadolol (Corgard), atenolol (Tenormin), timolol (Blocadren), and metoprolol (Lopressor, Toprol) are also effective. Long-term therapy may induce sleep problems and vivid dreams, memory problems, fatigue, depression, and impotence. Beta blockers require close monitoring in patients with asthma, chronic obstructive pulmonary disease (COPD), diabetes, or high cholesterol because they may worsen symptoms of lung disease and asthma, may affect cholesterol levels, and may also affect how the body responds to low blood sugar. Beta-adrenergic blocking agents are discussed in Chapter 13.

Anticonvulsants

Anticonvulsants are increasingly recommended for migraine prevention. The exact mechanism of action is unclear; however, anticonvulsants are thought to prevent migraines by blocking sodium or calcium channels or by enhancing the

activity of gamma-aminobutyrate (GABA). Divalproex sodium (Depakote) and sodium valproate (Depakene) are the only anticonvulsants with FDA approval for migraine prophylaxis. Nausea, vomiting, and GI distress are the most common side effects and are generally self-limiting. Additional adverse effects include weight gain, hair loss, tremor or shakiness, and fetal neural tube defects during pregnancy. Rare but severe adverse effects include fatal pancreatitis and hepatitis.

Several studies have shown the efficacy of gabapentin (Neurontin) as well, although it is not FDA approved for this pharmacotherapy. The most common adverse events with gabapentin are dizziness or giddiness and drowsiness.

Two other anticonvulsants, tiagabine (Gabitril) and topiramate (Topamax) have been efficacious in small studies. However, the sample size in these studies was too small to generalize the conclusions of these studies. For a more thorough discussion of these anticonvulsants, see Chapter 19.

Antidepressants

Antidepressants are useful in treating many chronic pain states, including migraine headache. Although the actual mechanism of action is unknown, the pain response occurs sooner than the expected antidepressant effect. Amitriptyline (Elavil) is the most common antidepressant used for migraine prophylaxis. Although other antidepressants have been prescribed, only amitriptyline has been studied in clinical trials.

Common adverse effects to amitriptyline include dry mouth, constipation, blurred vision, urinary retention, weight gain, and orthostatic hypotension. Amitriptyline is discussed in Chapter 17.

Calcium Channel Blockers

Several calcium channel blockers are used as migraine prophylaxis. They include diltiazem (Cardizem), nifedipine (Procardia, Adalat), nimodipine (Nimotop), and verapamil (Calan). Calcium channel blockers are used to prevent migraine headache because of their ability to prevent vasoconstriction.

Constipation is the most frequent adverse effect of calcium channel blockers. Other adverse effects include dizziness, headache, facial flushing, and edema.

CHAPTER SUMMARY

- Prostaglandins are found in almost all body tissues and affect the body in a multitude of ways.
- Prostaglandins are subdivided into COX-1 and COX-2. COX-1 is involved in the maintenance of cells whereas COX-2 prostaglandins are generally found at the site of inflammation.
- Drugs for fever, inflammation, and pain include salicylates (aspirin), prostaglandin synthetase inhibitors (PSI) (ibuprofen), and para-aminophenol derivatives (acetaminophen). These drugs work by inhibiting the synthesis of prostaglandins.
- Aspirin and acetaminophen overdoses are common. Patients do not realize the potentially serious consequences of ingesting these drugs because they are easily obtained without a prescription.
- The most common adverse effects of aspirin and ibuprofen are GI in nature.
- The most serious adverse effects of aspirin and ibuprofen are hepatic dysfunction, renal dysfunction, and GI bleeding.
- COX-2 inhibitors decrease the potential for GI bleeding, although it may still occur in some patients.
- COX-2 inhibitors do not inhibit platelet aggregation.
- The most serious adverse effects of acetaminophen are hepatic and renal dysfunctions.
- Migraine headaches are caused by arterial dilation and the resultant blood flow to the brain.
- The drugs of choice for managing acute migraine headache are selective serotonin agonists, also known as "triptans" or antimigraine agents.
- Drugs used for prophylaxis of migraine headaches include beta-blocking agents, anticonvulsants, antidepressants, and calcium-channel blocking agents.

QUESTIONS FOR STUDY AND REVIEW

1. How do prostaglandins affect the processes of inflammation, pain, and fever?
2. How does prostaglandin inhibition induce adverse effects of salicylates, PSIs, and acetaminophen?
3. What are the most potentially serious adverse effects of salicylates, PSIs, and acetaminophen, and how might you decrease their occurrence?
4. Identify two major differences between nonselective PSIs and COX-2 inhibitors.
5. How do the triptans decrease migraine headache pain?
6. What is the key difference between serotonin receptor agonists and ergotamine-containing drugs in the management of migraine headache?

Need More Help?

Chapter 24 of the study guide for *Drug Therapy in Nursing* 2e contains NCLEX-style questions and other learning activities to reinforce your understanding of the concepts presented in this chapter. For additional information or to purchase the study guide, visit *http://connection.lww.com/go/aschenbrenner.*

REFERENCES AND BIBLIOGRAPHY

Clinical Pharmacology [Online]. Available: *http://cp.gsm.com.*

Facts and Comparisons. (2004). *Drug facts and comparisons.* Philadelphia: Lippincott Williams & Wilkins.

Hardman, J. G. (2001). *Goodman & Gilman's the pharmacological basis of therapeutics* (10th ed.). New York: McGraw-Hill Health Professions Division.

Katzung, B. (2004). *Basic and clinical pharmacology* (9th ed.). New York: McGraw-Hill/Appleton & Lange.

Silberstein, S. D., & McCrory, D. C. (2003). Ergotamine and dihydroergotamine: History, pharmacology, and efficacy. *Headache, 43*(2), 144–166.

Song, Z., McClain, C. J., & Chen, T. (2004). S-Adenosylmethionine protects against acetaminophen-induced hepatotoxicity in mice. *Pharmacology, 71*(4), 199–208.

Tatro, D. S. (2004). *Drug interaction facts.* Philadelphia: Lippincott Williams & Wilkins.

Tepper, S. J., Rapoport, A. M., & Sheftell, F. D. (2002). Mechanisms of action of the 5-HT1B/1D receptor agonists. *Archives of Neurology, 59*(7), 1084–1088.

Drugs Treating Arthritis and Gout

chapter 25

Learning Objectives

At the completion of this chapter the student will:

1. Correlate the processes of inflammation and pain with antirheumatic drugs, antigout drugs, and uricosuric drugs.
2. Identify core drug knowledge pertaining to antirheumatic drugs, antigout drugs, and uricosuric drugs.
3. Identify core patient variables pertaining to antirheumatic drugs, antigout drugs, and uricosuric drugs.
4. Relate the interaction of core drug knowledge to core patient variables for antirheumatic drugs, antigout drugs, and uricosuric drugs.
5. Generate a nursing plan of care from the interactions between core drug knowledge and core patient variables for antirheumatic drugs, antigout drugs, and uricosuric drugs.
6. Describe nursing interventions to maximize therapeutic and minimize adverse effects for antirheumatic drugs, antigout drugs, and uricosuric drugs.
7. Determine key points for patient and family education for antirheumatic drugs, antigout drugs, and uricosuric drugs.

KEY TERMS

ankylosis

antigout drugs

chrysotherapy

cytokine

disease-modifying antirheumatic drug (DMARD)

monoclonal antibody

nitritoid crisis

pannus

tophi

uricosuric drugs

FEATURED WEBLINK

http://www.medicinenet.com/Gout/article.htm
What are the differences between acute and chronic gout? Find out at this website.

CONNECTION WEBLINK

Additional Weblinks are found on Connection:
http://www.connection.lww.com/go/aschenbrenner.

Drugs Treating Arthritis and Gout

(C) Disease-Modifying Antirheumatic Drugs (DMARDs)

(C) **salicylates and prostaglandin synthetase inhibitors**
(see Chapter 24)

[P] **methotrexate**
anakinra
cyclophosphamide
cyclosporine
gold salts
- auranofin
- aurothioglucose
- gold sodium thiomalate

glucocorticoid steroids
hydroxychloroquine
leflunomide
penicillamine
sulfasalazine
TNF inhibitors
- etanercept
- infliximab
- adalimumab

(C) Antigout Drugs

Acute gout
[P] **colchicine**
(C) **salicylates and prostaglandin synthetase inhibitors**
(see Chapter 24)

Chronic gout
[P] **probenecid**
sulfinpyrazone
allopurinol

The symbol (C) indicates the **drug class.**
Drugs in **bold type** marked with the symbol [P] are prototypes.
Drugs in blue type are closely related to the prototype.
Drugs in red type are significantly different from the prototype.
Drugs in black type with no symbol are also used in drug therapy; no prototype

This chapter focuses on two inflammatory conditions, rheumatoid arthritis (RA) and gout. RA has been traditionally treated with a salicylate or prostaglandin synthetase inhibitors (PSIs), which are discussed in Chapter 24. Salicylates and PSIs are still used in managing RA, but they merely decrease the symptoms associated with RA and do not alter the progression of the disease. RA is not a wear-and-tear disease like osteoarthritis. Rheumatologists have discovered that joint damage begins very early in RA, even when symptoms are absent or minimal. Because of this new information, treatment protocols have changed to include disease-modifying antirheumatic drugs (DMARDs) within 3 months of a diagnosis of RA. Drugs within the DMARD class include the prototype methotrexate as well as anakinra, cyclophosphamide, cyclosporine, gold salts, hydroxychloroquine, leflunomide, penicillamine, sulfasalazine, and tumor necrosis factor (TNF) inhibitors.

For inflammation caused by acute gout, antigout drugs are used. The only drug in this class is colchicine. Salicylates and PSIs, which are discussed in Chapter 24, are also used. Chronic gout is treated with uricosuric drugs, which decrease the hyperuricemia associated with gout. Uricosuric drugs include probenecid, sulfinpyrazone (Anturane), and allopurinol (Zyloprim).

In addition to discussing the therapeutic classes of drugs used to treat RA and gout, this chapter also addresses the core drug knowledge, core patient variables, nursing management, potential nursing diagnoses, and patient education related to the use of DMARDs, antigout drugs, and uricosuric drugs.

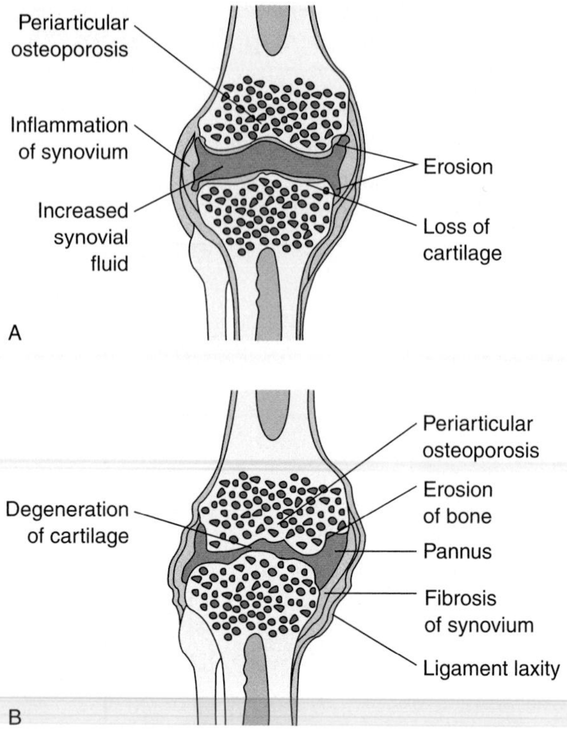

FIGURE 25.1 (**A**) Early rheumatoid arthritis with fluid accumulation and synovial swelling; (**B**) Late rheumatoid arthritis with pannus formation, eroded articular cartilage, and joint space narrowing.

PATHOPHYSIOLOGY

Rheumatoid Arthritis

RA is a systemic inflammatory disease that affects all age groups, although it is more prevalent in people in the age group between 40 and 60 years old. Women are three times more likely than men to have RA.

RA is thought to be an autoimmune disorder because 70% of patients have a substance in their blood, synovial fluid, and synovial tissue called rheumatoid factor (RF), which is an antibody to their own immunoglobulin G (IgG). RA interacts with IgG or other antibodies to form immune complexes. These immune complexes activate the complement system, resulting in an inflammatory response. Leukocytes, monocytes, and lymphocytes are attracted to the area and phagocytize the immune complexes. During that process, lysosomal enzymes are released. These enzymes are capable of destroying joint cartilage, resulting in an inflammatory process that starts the cycle again. As the disease progresses, a destructive granular tissue called **pannus** extends through the synovial space, damaging the articular cartilage. Continued progression destroys the entire joint space, resulting in reduced joint motion and possible **ankylosis** (extreme stiffness or joint fusion). See Figure 25.1.

The primary characteristic of RA is symmetric polyarticular inflammatory arthritis. The clinical course is highly variable. Symptoms include morning stiffness that lasts more than 1 hour, symmetric involvement of joints, and rheumatoid nodules over bony prominences or extensor surfaces. Joints commonly affected include the proximal interphalangeal (PIP), metacarpophalangeal (MCP), wrist, elbow, knee, ankle, and metatarsophalangeal (MTP) joints.

RA has a substantial effect on quality of life because of pain, fatigue, and depression. Because of these quality-of-life issues, RA can reduce the life span of people who have it.

Gout

Gout is a disease of purine metabolism. Uric acid is a metabolite of two purines, adenine and guanine. Hyperuricemia may result from overproduction or underexcretion of uric acid. However, hyperuricemia does not always result in gout. Gout occurs when the hyperuricemia forms monosodium urate crystals, which precipitate into the synovial fluid and initiate an inflammatory response. As in RA, the inflammatory response attracts leukocytes to phagocytize the crystals. When the leukocytes die, they release lysosomal nodules called **tophi.** These nodules can be found in bursae, synovium, tendons, and along the extensor surface of the forearm. Certain drugs, foods, or alcohol may precipitate an attack. Attacks are usually monoarticular and characterized by severe pain, erythema, and warmth in the affected joint (Figure 25.2). Recurrent attacks damage the joint space, resulting in gouty arthritis.

Ⓒ DISEASE-MODIFYING ANTIRHEUMATIC DRUGS

Disease-modifying antirheumatic drugs are used in conjunction with salicylates and PSIs, or as monotherapy when salicylates and PSIs are ineffective or not tolerated. They are

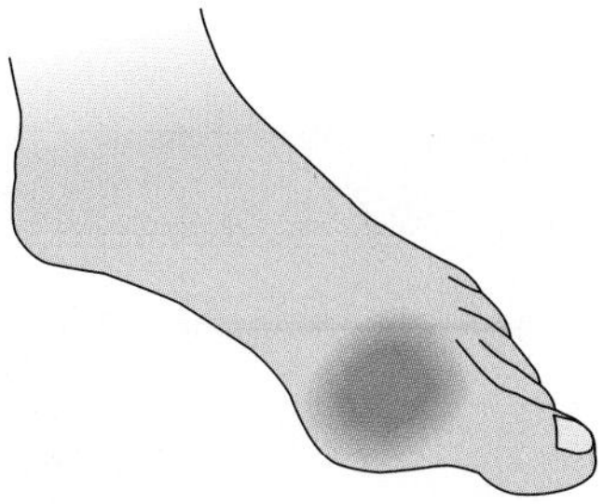

FIGURE 25.2 Gout in the first metatarsal phalangeal joint of the left foot.

so named because they are capable of arresting the progression of RA and can induce remission in some patients. The therapeutic class of DMARDs is a combination of several different pharmacologic classes of drugs, including alkylating agents, antimetabolites, antimalarials, gold salts, sulfonamide antibiotics, TNF inhibitors, monoclonal antibodies, interleukin antagonists, and immune response modifiers. Although the mechanism of action is different for each of these drugs, they are all similar in the fact that they slow the progression of RA. Table 25.1 provides a summary of selected antirheumatic drugs.

Methotrexate is often the first DMARD prescribed for RA. Rheumatologists often recommend that methotrexate be used with one or more other DMARD (combination therapy) because combination therapy enables lower doses of the individual drugs to be used, which may reduce the risk for adverse effects that can occur with higher doses. In addition, combination therapy has proved more effective than monotherapy with any DMARD.

People with RA are more likely to continue treatment with methotrexate than with other DMARDs because of favorable results and tolerable side effects. In fact, about half of people who take methotrexate for RA continue taking the medication for more than 5 years, which is longer than people with RA continue to take any other DMARD. Thus, methotrexate is the prototype for this therapeutic class.

NURSING MANAGEMENT OF THE PATIENT RECEIVING [P] METHOTREXATE

Core Drug Knowledge

Pharmacotherapeutics

Methotrexate (Rheumatrex) is a folate antimetabolite used in treating various malignancies, including osteosarcoma, non-Hodgkin lymphoma, Hodgkin disease, cutaneous T-cell lymphoma, head and neck cancer, lung cancer, and breast cancer. Because it also has immunosuppressive effects, it is used to treat adult and juvenile RA and psoriasis.

Pharmacokinetics

Methotrexate is given orally or parenterally to manage RA. Its absorption may be decreased in the presence of food. A small portion is metabolized in the liver; the drug is excreted in the urine mostly as unchanged drug (see Table 25.1).

Pharmacodynamics

Methotrexate induces folate depletion, which leads to inhibition of purine synthesis and results in the arrest of DNA, RNA, and protein synthesis. Because it targets rapidly proliferating cells, such as epithelial cells, it slows progression of psoriasis. It exerts immunosuppressive effects by inhibiting the replication and function of T lymphocytes that stimulate the production of cytokines, in particular interleukin-1 (IL-1), IL-6, and IL-8, as well as TNF-alpha.

Contraindications and Precautions

Methotrexate is contraindicated in patients with immunosuppression, pre-existing blood dyscrasia, or impaired bone marrow function, and during pregnancy and lactation. It is given cautiously to patients with pre-existing hepatic or renal dysfunction, malnutrition, or ulcerative colitis.

Adverse Effects

Common adverse effects include headache, nausea, stomatitis, gingivitis, and alopecia. Methotrexate can suppress bone marrow function and induce gastrointestinal (GI) ulceration, hepatitic fibrosis, or pneumonitis. Because relatively low doses are used to manage RA, the risk for severe adverse effects is decreased. However, this reduction does not change the need to monitor closely for potential adverse effects. Methotrexate can cause photosensitivity, and the patient should avoid direct sunlight.

Drug Interactions

Methotrexate may interact with many drugs. In general, methotrexate should not be given concurrently with other drugs associated with the development of nephrotoxicity, hepatotoxicity, or suppressed bone marrow function. Table 25.2 presents potential interactions with methotrexate.

Assessment of Relevant Core Patient Variables

Health Status

Assess the patient for comorbid states or drugs that contradict the use of methotrexate. Complete a thorough physical examination, carefully evaluating for signs of hepatic or renal insufficiency, suppressed bone marrow function, or adventitious lung sounds. Document the severity of joint inflammation and any restriction in range of motion as a baseline for later comparison to assess the efficacy of methotrexate therapy.

Before beginning therapy, evaluate the results of a complete blood count (CBC), renal and hepatic function tests, urinalysis, and a chest x-ray. Coordinate serial laboratory testing. The CBC, renal function, and liver-function tests should be repeated 2 weeks after therapy begins, again at 1 month, and then every 2 months thereafter throughout therapy. Assess the patient's willingness to adhere to this close monitoring. If the patient is female, evaluate for possible pregnancy and help the patient develop a plan for contraception during therapy.

Life Span and Gender

Methotrexate is given cautiously to very young and elderly patients because these patients' livers and kidneys may not

TABLE 25.1 Summary of Selected (C) Disease-Modifying Antirheumatic Drugs

Drug (Trade) Name	Selected Indications	Route and Dosage Range	Pharmacokinetics
P methotrexate (Rheumatrex)	RA	*Adult:* PO, 7.5–20 mg/wk in a single dose *Child:* PO/IM, 5–15 mg m^2/week	*Onset:* Varies *Duration:* Unknown $t_{1/2}$: 2–4 h
adalimumab (Humira)	RA	*Adult:* SC, 40 mg every other week. Patients not taking concomitant methotrexate, 40 mg SC every week	*Onset:* 1–7 d *Duration:* Unknown $t_{1/2}$: 14 d
anakinra (Kineret)	RA	*Adult:* SC, 100 mg daily	*Onset:* Slow *Duration:* Unknown $t_{1/2}$: 4–6 h
auranofin (Ridaura)	RA	*Adult:* PO, 5–9 mg/d in 1 or 2 doses *Child:* PO, 0.1 mg/kg/d initially, titrate up to 0.15 mg/kg/d; maximum dose, 0.2 mg/kg/d	*Onset:* Varies *Duration:* 6 mo $t_{1/2}$: 26 d
aurothioglucose (Solganal)	RA	*Adult:* IM, 10 mg initially, then 25 mg for the second and third doses, given at weekly intervals, followed by 50 mg weekly until a total dose of 0.8–1.0 g has been administered Maintenance dosage is 25–50 mg IM given at 3- to 4-wk intervals indefinitely *Child:* IM, 0.25 mg/kg the first week. Increase dosage by 0.25 mg/kg weekly up to a maintenance dosage of 0.75–1 mg/kg once per week. Doses are given once per week for a total of 20 doses, then continued every 2–4 wk	*Onset:* Slow *Duration:* 6 mo $t_{1/2}$: 26 d
cyclophosphamide (Cytoxan)	RA	*Adult and child:* PO, 1.5–2.5 mg/kg/d in combination with other agents	*Onset:* Rapid *Duration:* Unknown $t_{1/2}$: 4–6 h
cyclosporine (Neoral)	RA	*Adult:* PO, 100–200 mg/d in 2 doses	*Onset:* Varies *Duration:* 24–36 h $t_{1/2}$: 17.9 h
etanercept (Enbrel)	RA	*Adult:* SC, 25 mg 2× week or 50 mg given as two 25-mg injections on the same day administered in different sites *Child 4–17 y:* SC, 0.4 mg/kg 2× week	*Onset:* 2–4 wk *Duration:* Unknown $t_{1/2}$: 115 h
hydroxychloroquine (Plaquenil)	RA	*Adult:* PO, 200–600 mg/d in 1 or 2 doses *Child:* PO, 3–5 mg/kg/d PO divided in 1–2 doses. Maximum dose, 7 mg/kg/d or 400 mg/d PO	*Onset:* Rapid *Duration:* Unknown $t_{1/2}$: 3–5 d
infliximab (Remicade)	RA	*Adult:* IV, Dose is based on body weight and ranges from 200–400 mg per treatment. The initial dose is repeated at 2 and 6 weeks and once every 8 weeks thereafter	*Onset:* 3–7 d *Duration:* 6–12 wk $t_{1/2}$: 9.5 d
gold sodium thiomalate (Myochrysine)	RA	*Adult:* IM, 10 mg in a single injection the first week, 25 mg the following week, then 25–50 mg per week thereafter	*Onset:* Slow *Duration:* 6 mo $t_{1/2}$: 3–27 d
leflunomide (Arava)	RA	*Adult:* PO, 10–20 mg/d in a single dose	*Onset:* Varies *Duration:* Unknown $t_{1/2}$: 14 d
penicillamine (Cuprimine)	RA	*Adult:* PO, 125–250 mg/d in a single dose, increase q 2–3 months to a maximum of 1,500 mg/d *Child:* PO, Initially, 3 mg/kg × 3 mo, then 6 mg/kg in 2 divided doses for 3 mo. Continue to a maximum of 10 mg/kg/d in 3–4 divided doses.	*Onset:* Varies *Duration:* Unknown $t_{1/2}$: 1.7–3.2 h
sulfasalazine (Azulfidine EN-tabs)	RA	*Adult and elderly:* PO, 0.5–1 g PO per day for the first week. Increase the daily dose by 500 mg each week up to a maintenance dose of 3 g/d given in 2–3 divided doses. *Child >6 y:* PO, 30–50 mg/kg/day in 2 divided doses	*Onset:* 1 h *Duration:* 6–12 h $t_{1/2}$: 5–10 h

CRITICAL THINKING SCENARIO

DMARD therapy

Mrs. Spencer, a 68-year-old woman, has rheumatoid arthritis, which was diagnosed 8 years ago. Mrs. Spencer has been given four different types of prostaglandin synthetase inhibitors over the years, producing moderate pain relief in both her hands, knees, and elbows. She has been experiencing frequent flare-ups of her symptoms, so her primary doctor referred her to a rheumatologist, who prescribed DMARD therapy with methotrexate.

1. Why do you think Mrs. Spencer has had rheumatoid arthritis all these years without the benefit of DMARD therapy?
2. What assessments should you document before administering methotrexate?
3. Consider which laboratory tests you think should be done before administering methotrexate.
4. Prepare patient teaching about methotrexate for this patient.
5. What type of response to methotrexate therapy do you think Mrs. Spencer may achieve?
6. What would you anticipate if Mrs. Spencer does not respond to monotherapy with methotrexate?

be able to adequately clear the drug, and they therefore risk accumulation. It is a pregnancy category X drug because fetal abnormality has been documented. Planning pregnancy is essential: methotrexate treatment should be stopped 3 months before conception. This caution applies to males as well as females. Methotrexate is secreted in breast milk and may be toxic to the baby.

Lifestyle, Diet, and Habits

Evaluate for the use of alcohol or illicit drugs because these substances may predispose the patient to hepatic dysfunction. Also, evaluate the nutritional status of the patient; malnourished patients are more likely than others to be immunosuppressed or have blood dyscrasias. To minimize the potential for methotrexate photosensitivity, determine how frequently the patient must be in the sun.

Environment

Methotrexate as an oral medication for RA is routinely taken by the patient at home. In some circumstances, methotrexate may be given by the intramuscular route. In such cases, teach the patient the correct aseptic technique for self-administering an intramuscular injection. If you administer the intramuscular injection, you must handle methotrexate according to the facility's protocol because skin contact with methotrexate poses a risk for carcinogenicity, mutagenicity, or teratogenicity.

Nursing Diagnoses and Outcomes

- Comfort Impaired: Nausea related to drug therapy
  Desired outcome: The patient will eat small, frequent meals when nauseated to maintain nutritional balance.
- Risk for Infection related to potential depression of bone marrow function and blood dyscrasias
  Desired outcome: The patient will recognize signs of depressed bone marrow function and blood dyscrasias and contact the health care provider immediately for intervention if any appear.

TABLE 25.2 Agents That Interact With P Methotrexate

Interactants	Effect and Significance	Nursing Management
amiodarone	The mechanism of the interaction is unknown, but the risk for methotrexate toxicity may be increased.	Monitor for signs of methotrexate toxicity if amiodarone is initiated.
aspirin, prostaglandin synthetase inhibitors (PSIs), bismuth	Aspirin, PSIs, and bismuth decrease the renal clearance of methotrexate, resulting in an increased risk for methotrexate toxicity.	Less likely to occur in doses for RA. Monitor for signs of methotrexate toxicity.
digoxin	Methotrexate may reduce GI absorption of digoxin, resulting in decreased serum digoxin concentration.	Monitor for efficacy of digoxin therapy. Monitor serum digoxin levels frequently.
hydantoins	Methotrexate may decrease absorption or increase metabolism of hydantoins, resulting in subtherapeutic drug levels.	Monitor serum hydantoin levels. Monitor for seizure activity.
penicillins	Penicillins impair the renal excretion of methotrexate.	Obtain methotrexate serum concentration if penicillins are initiated. Monitor for signs of methotrexate toxicity.
probenecid	Probenecid impairs the renal excretion of methotrexate.	Obtain methotrexate serum concentration if probenecid is initiated. Monitor for signs of methotrexate toxicity.
proton-pump inhibitors (PPIs)	PPI drugs may decrease the renal clearance of methotrexate, resulting in increased serum methotrexate concentrations.	Monitor for methotrexate toxicity.
sulfonamides	Sulfonamides displace methotrexate from protein binding sites and decrease renal clearance of methotrexate.	Obtain methotrexate serum concentration if sulfonamides are initiated. Monitor for signs of methotrexate toxicity.

- Imbalanced Nutrition: Less than Body Requirements related to potential nausea, stomatitis, and gingivitis
  Desired outcome: *The patient will maintain nutritional balance throughout therapy.*
- Risk for Injury related to drug accumulation caused by hepatic or renal dysfunction
  Desired outcome: *The patient will remain injury free throughout therapy.*

Planning and Intervention

Maximizing Therapeutic Effects

Administer methotrexate weekly as ordered. Ensure that the patient drinks enough water to minimize the risk for nephrotoxicity. Encourage the patient to continue pharmacotherapy with methotrexate, even if the patient has not yet received any beneficial results.

Minimizing Adverse Effects

Vitamin B (folic acid), 5 mg every day, may decrease the potential for adverse effects of methotrexate. When the patient has mouth ulcers, consult with the prescriber to request an order for allopurinol, 300 mg. Dissolve the allopurinol in 50 mL of water. It is important to instruct the patient to use this solution to rinse the mouth, but not to swallow the solution. Remind the patient that methotrexate can cause photosensitivity. Patients should take care to remain out of the sun, wear protective clothing, and use a lotion with skin protection factor (SPF) 45 if they cannot avoid being in the sun.

Providing Patient and Family Education

- Assist patients in preparing a schedule for methotrexate because this drug is not taken daily.
- Instruct patients to administer intramuscular methotrexate as indicated.
- Teach patients to keep methotrexate in a safe place, out of the reach of children.
- Instruct patients to contact the prescriber immediately if they experience:
  - Symptoms of infection—fever or chills, cough, sore throat, pain, or difficulty passing urine
  - Symptoms of decreased platelets or bleeding—bruising, pinpoint red spots on the skin, black and tarry stools, blood in the urine
  - Symptoms of anemia—unusual weakness or tiredness, fainting spells, lightheadedness
  - Diarrhea
  - Difficulty breathing, a nonproductive cough
  - Mouth or throat ulcers
  - Redness, blistering, peeling or loosened skin, including inside the mouth
  - Skin rash, hives, or itching
  - Changes in vision
  - Vomiting
- Teach patients the importance of adequate nutrition and hydration to minimize the risk for adverse effects.
- Stress the effects of alcohol and drugs in precipitating adverse effects to the liver.
- Instruct patients to keep out of the sun or to wear protective clothing outdoors and use a sunscreen. Emphasize that they must not use sun lamps or sun tanning beds or booths.
- Instruct patients on the importance of serial laboratory testing and coordinate dates for testing to occur.
- Explain the importance of range-of-motion exercises in addition to pharmacotherapy.
- Advise patients that the beneficial effects from methotrexate do not occur immediately and that it is important to continue therapy to allow the benefits to begin.

Ongoing Assessment and Evaluation

Monitor patients for signs of blood dyscrasias, suppressed bone marrow function, pulmonary changes, and hepatic or renal dysfunction at each visit. Document the extent of joint inflammation and range of motion at each visit. Coordinate serial testing that includes CBC, urinalysis, and liver and renal function tests.

Effective treatment with methotrexate should decrease subjective symptoms such as perceived pain level, and objective symptoms, such as decreased joint inflammation and increased range of motion. The patient should be free of adverse effects or receiving appropriate interventions focused at ameliorating adverse effects.

Drugs Significantly Different From P Methotrexate

Anakinra

Anakinra (Kineret), a recombinant form of the human interleukin-1 receptor antagonist (IL-1Ra), is produced by recombinant DNA technology. It is approved for use in patients with moderate to severe active RA who have unsuccessfully tried therapy with one or more DMARDs.

Anakinra acts similarly to the native IL-1Ra. IL-1 and TNF are the primary proinflammatory cytokines associated with RA. IL-1 plays a dominant role in cartilage damage and bone resorption in rheumatoid arthritis, whereas TNF-alpha is more responsible for inflammation. By antagonizing IL-1, stimulation of osteoclasts is decreased, resulting in decreased bone resorption and joint destruction.

Anakinra is contraindicated in patients with hypersensitivity to *Escherichia coli* protein. It is also contraindicated

MEMORY CHIP

P Methotrexate

- Disease-modifying antirheumatic drug used as monotherapy or in combination with salicylates, prostaglandin synthetase inhibitors, or other DMARDS to decrease the progression of RA
- Major contraindications: immunosuppression, blood dyscrasias, pregnancy
- Most common adverse effect: nausea, headache, stomatitis, gingivitis, alopecia
- Most serious adverse effect: depressed bone marrow function
- Maximizing therapeutic effects: remain hydrated
- Minimizing adverse effects: take vitamin B, 5 mg every day
- Most important patient education: substantial adverse effects may occur. Be sure to contact the health care provider if they occur.

in immunocompromised patients because it further decreases the immune response. Anakinra is administered as a subcutaneous injection, and the needle cover contains latex, which may cause reactions in patients (and health care workers) with latex hypersensitivity. Anakinra should not be given to a patient with an active infection, because risk for infection is increased during therapy with anakinra. It should be given cautiously to patients with pre-existing renal dysfunction because it is renally excreted. Live-virus vaccines should not be administered during anakinra therapy because of anakinra's effects on the immune response.

Common adverse effects include headache, sinusitis, abdominal pain, diarrhea, upper respiratory infection, and injection site reactions. More serious adverse effects include neutropenia and severe infections.

Anakinra is administered as a subcutaneous injection. Teach the correct aseptic technique for subcutaneous injection and the importance of rotating the site of injection among the thigh, stomach, and upper arms and of making sure that each injection is a minimum of 1 inch away from the previous day's site. Also, teach the patient to avoid areas that are tender, hard, red, or bruised.

Anakinra is in pregnancy category B. It is unclear whether anakinra is secreted in breast milk. Safety and efficacy have not been established for children.

Cyclophosphamide

Cyclophosphamide (Cytoxan) is an alkylating agent used primarily for its antitumor activity. Because of the oncogenicity associated with alkylating agents, cyclophosphamide is used primarily in severe, refractory RA and RA vasculitis. Cyclophosphamide is presented as the prototype alkylating agent in Chapter 36.

Cyclosporine

Cyclosporine (Neoral, Sandimmune) is an oral and parenteral immunosuppressive agent used most frequently to prevent organ transplant rejection. It is also approved to treat severe RA in patients unresponsive to conventional therapy, alone or in combination with methotrexate when the disease has not adequately responded to methotrexate. Its immunosuppressive effects result from inhibiting proliferation of T lymphocytes, production and release of lymphokines, and release of IL-2. As the prototype immune modulator, cyclosporine is presented in depth in Chapter 34.

Gold Salts

AURANOFIN

The administration of gold salts is called **chrysotherapy.** Auranofin contains about 29% gold and is the only gold compound available for oral administration. It is used to treat early active cases of both adult and juvenile types of RA that have not responded to salicylates or PSIs. The drug is less effective against advanced, chronic cases of RA.

Auranofin exhibits antirheumatic, anti-inflammatory, and immunomodulating properties. The mechanism of action is unknown but may involve the inhibition of antigen processing by macrophages or the inhibition of lysosomal enzyme release, thus decreasing inflammation. Additionally, gold has a strong affinity for sulfur and may interfere with the cellular sulfhydryl system, which would inhibit the function of macrophages responsible for causing inflammation in rheumatic patients.

Auranofin is contraindicated for use in patients with Sjögren syndrome, severe debilitation, systemic lupus erythematosus (SLE), uncontrolled congestive heart failure (CHF), marked hypertension, urticaria, eczema, colitis, or a history of sensitivity to gold compounds. Auranofin is contraindicated in patients with a history of disorders induced by the use of gold-based drugs, such as exfoliative dermatitis, pulmonary fibrosis, necrotizing enterocolitis, and anaphylactic reactions. It also is contraindicated in patients who have experienced severe toxicity from previously administered gold compounds or other heavy-metal preparations.

Auranofin should be used with caution in patients with bone marrow aplasia, a history of blood dyscrasias, or depressed bone marrow function. Patients who have recently undergone radiation therapy are at high risk for blood dyscrasias because of radiation's depressant effect on the hematopoietic system. Patients receiving antimalarials, immunosuppressants, or phenylbutazone are at high risk for blood dyscrasias and should be monitored closely. Auranofin also should be used with caution in patients with pre-existing renal disease, inflammatory bowel disease, hepatic disease, or skin rash. These conditions indicate compromised organ systems, which could increase the risk for gold toxicity.

Chrysotherapy can produce severe toxic reactions. Therefore, patients receiving gold compounds must be monitored closely for early signs of adverse effects. The most serious adverse effect of auranofin is fatal suppression of bone marrow function. Other potential blood dyscrasias are leukopenia, thrombocytopenia, and anemia. The adverse effects of gold therapy may occur months after therapy discontinues.

The most common adverse effects of auranofin affect the GI tract. Diarrhea is an expected response to the initiation of auranofin treatment and, in some cases, may be severe. Other GI symptoms include nausea, vomiting, anorexia, abdominal cramps, and flatulence.

Chrysotherapy also can produce mucocutaneous reactions because of the deposits of gold in tissues. Pruritus, rash, skin pigment changes (to gray or blue), conjunctivitis, glossitis, stomatitis, and alopecia may occur.

Additional adverse effects from auranofin involve the renal system. Transient and mild proteinuria may occur in about 50% of patients at some time during therapy. Less common effects include nephrotic syndrome and glomerular nephritis. In rare instances, acute tubular necrosis and renal failure may occur. Gold therapy should be terminated if proteinuria does not resolve or hematuria occurs. Other rare but serious adverse effects include interstitial pneumonitis and fibrosis.

Auranofin should not be given to patients receiving penicillamine because of the possibility of causing potentially severe hematologic or renal effects. Although documentation of drug and auranofin interactions may not be available, drugs possessing toxic properties similar to those of auranofin should be avoided, if possible. Auranofin should be used cautiously in patients receiving drugs that can cause bone marrow toxicity or nephrotoxicity. Auranofin may enhance the response to a tuberculin skin test, resulting in a false-positive reaction.

Auranofin is a pregnancy category C drug. It crosses the placenta and is secreted in breast milk, and therefore should not be used by women who are pregnant or breast-feeding.

AUROTHIOGLUCOSE

Aurothioglucose (Solganal) is an intramuscular dosage form of gold therapy. Its pharmacodynamics and pharmacotherapy are the same as those of auranofin. It is in a sesame oil suspension, which causes erratic and slow absorption. Aurothioglucose is about 50% gold.

The onset and duration of action are difficult to quantify because the therapeutic effects may not begin for several weeks and may last long after the drug has been discontinued. Between 1 and 2 months of weekly injections are required to achieve a steady-state serum level. Like auranofin, aurothioglucose is distributed throughout the body; however, it is not associated with circulating cells in most patients. The metabolic fate of aurothioglucose is unknown. About 40% is excreted each week during a standard weekly dosing schedule, and the remainder is excreted more gradually. About 70% is excreted in urine and 30% in feces. The half-life can be as long as 160 days.

When administering aurothioglucose, be sure to have emergency life-support equipment available. Patients may experience anaphylactic shock, syncope, bradycardia, difficulty swallowing, and angioedema following an injection of aurothioglucose.

Another potential reaction of aurothioglucose is a **nitritoid crisis.** The symptoms of this reaction (e.g., flushing, feeling of warmth, lightheadedness, or hypotension) resemble the response to a large dose of nitroglycerin; hence, the term nitritoid. Patients are given a small test dose to assess for these responses. If they do not react to the test dose, a series of weekly or monthly injections may be given. Before each injection, a urinalysis and CBC are performed. Therapy must stop if the patient develops hematuria, proteinuria, or blood dyscrasias.

To administer the drug in uniform suspension, immerse the vial in warm water, remove the drug with a dry needle and syringe, and inject the drug in the gluteal muscle, taking care to avoid IV administration. The patient should then remain in a recumbent position and be monitored for an allergic or nitroid reaction for at least 15 minutes after administration.

Patients should be reevaluated after receiving a cumulative dose of 1 g of aurothioglucose. Contraindications, precautions, and adverse effects are the same as for auranofin.

GOLD SODIUM THIOMALATE

Gold sodium thiomalate (Myochrysine) is another aqueous solution of gold administered intramuscularly. Its pharmacodynamics and pharmacotherapeutics are similar to those of auranofin. Gold sodium thiomalate also may induce nitritoid or anaphylactic reactions. As with aurothioglucose, a urinalysis and CBC must be done before each injection. Contraindications, precautions, and adverse effects are similar to those of auranofin.

Glucocorticoid Steroids

Glucocorticoid steroids such as prednisone and prednisolone can be administered as oral or intravenous preparations for systemic effects and as an intra-articular injection for a local effect. They are generally given as "pulse therapy" for an acute exacerbation of RA. This approach allows a "resetting" of the inflammatory thermostat, improves the patient's symptoms, and allows other DMARDs to become active in suppressing joint destruction. Glucocorticoid steroids are discussed in depth in Chapter 51.

Hydroxychloroquine

Hydroxychloroquine (Plaquenil) is an antimalarial drug also used in managing RA and discoid LE. In treating malaria, the mechanism of action is the same as for chloroquine. In managing RA and discoid LE, the mechanism of action is unclear.

Hydroxychloroquine should be given with caution to infants or pregnant and lactating women because these patients are highly likely to develop toxicity. In children, the dose must be calculated properly, and pediatric patients must be monitored closely because toxicity has occurred with routine dosing. For patients on long-term therapy with hydroxychloroquine, the greatest concern is the development of irreversible retinal damage.

Drug–drug interactions, adverse effects, nursing management, and patient education are the same as for patients taking chloroquine (see Chapter 45).

Leflunomide

Leflunomide (Arava) is innovative DMARD that was designed specifically for RA. The pharmacologic activity of leflunomide is accomplished through its active primary metabolite A77 1725, also known as M1. M1 inhibits dihydro-orotate dehydrogenase (DHODH), an enzyme involved in the autoimmune process, which inhibits a key step in pyrimidine synthesis. Suppression of pyrimidine synthesis within T and B lymphocytes interferes with RNA and protein synthesis within the cells and prevents further cell cycle progression. Reduced lymphocyte activity leads to reduced cytokine and antibody-mediated destruction of the synovial joints and decreases the inflammatory process. Symptoms may abate in as little as 4 weeks. Additionally, because of its unique mechanism of action, leflunomide may be used in conjunction with other drugs such as PSIs and other DMARDs.

Leflunomide is contraindicated in patients with severe hepatic insufficiency and in patients with diagnosed hepatitis B or hepatitis C. Leflunomide may increase concentrations of liver enzymes such as aspartate aminotransferase (AST) and alanine aminotransferase (ALT) and has been associated with inducing hepatotoxicity. Leflunomide also is contraindicated for use during pregnancy or breast-feeding. Leflunomide is a category X drug because it has been shown to induce fetal deformity. Women who have received leflunomide and wish to become pregnant must undergo a drug elimination process before conception. Cholestyramine (8 g) is administered three times a day for 11 days. The days do not have to be consecutive, but they must total 11 days. Plasma leflunomide levels are then evaluated twice, at least 14 days apart. The plasma drug level should be less than 0.02 μg/mL before conception is attempted. Without this procedure, blood levels greater than 0.02 μg/mL may persist for up to 2 years, depending on individual variations in clearance.

Patients with bone marrow dysplasia, immunodeficiency, or severe uncontrolled infections are poor candidates for leflunomide therapy. Vaccinations with live vaccines are not recommended during therapy.

Common adverse effects include nausea, diarrhea, increased AST and ALT levels, alopecia, rash, headache, and increased risk for immunosuppression and infections.

Potential drug interactions include cholestyramine, charcoal, rifampin, and drugs that induce hepatotoxicity. Lefluno-

mide does not appear to interact with triphasic oral contraceptives. This fact is important because women of childbearing age must be taking a reliable contraceptive agent throughout leflunomide therapy.

Penicillamine

Penicillamine (Cuprimine) is used in treating patients with early, mild, and nonerosive RA. Its antirheumatic action may result from its ability to inhibit the formation of collagen. Penicillamine also appears to depress circulating levels of IgM rheumatoid factor and immune complexes in serum and synovial fluid. It also may decrease cell-mediated immune response by selectively inhibiting T-lymphocyte function.

In addition to its use as an antirheumatic drug, penicillamine is used as a chelating agent for removing excess copper from the blood of patients with Wilson disease and in reducing cystine excretion in patients with cystinuria.

Although penicillamine is a by-product of penicillin, it has no antibiotic activity. However, the possibility of cross-sensitization between penicillin and penicillamine exists; therefore, penicillamine should not be given to patients who are allergic to penicillin.

Penicillamine has potentially toxic adverse effects, including cutaneous lesions, blood dyscrasias, and a number of autoimmune disorders (Box 25.1). Penicillamine is associated with a high incidence of potentially life-threatening adverse hematologic reactions because it depresses bone marrow function. Patients with a history of hematologic disorders or previous penicillamine-induced dyscrasias could experience these adverse reactions, which include leukopenia, thrombocytopenia, aplastic anemia, pancytopenia, sideroblastic anemia, agranulocytosis, and leukopenia. Penicillamine should be discontinued when the platelet count decreases to less than 100,000/mm^3, the leukocyte count decreases to less than 3,000/mm^3, or neutropenia occurs.

Rare but serious adverse effects are myasthenia gravis (MG) syndrome and obliterative bronchiolitis. Penicillamine should be discontinued at the first sign of ptosis or diplopia (signifying MG syndrome) or exertional dyspnea, cough, or wheezing (signifying obliterative bronchiolitis). These symptoms should be reported immediately.

In the renal system, penicillamine can induce hematuria and proteinuria, which may indicate an impending immune complex membranous glomerulonephritis. This condition can degenerate into nephrotic syndrome. Penicillamine should be discontinued when proteinuria values exceed 1 g per 24 hours.

The most common adverse effects involve the integumentary system. Rash and pruritus occurring in the first few months (early rash) are generally typical of drug hypersensitivity. Early rash usually disappears when the drug is discontinued. Late rash during therapy may be accompanied by intense pruritus, fever, arthralgia, or lymphadenopathy. This rash may take weeks to disappear. Patients may also develop exfoliative dermatitis, increased skin friability, vesicular ecchymoses, and pemphigus.

Penicillamine also can cause GI upset such as nausea, vomiting, anorexia, abdominal pain, and diarrhea. Patients with a history of peptic ulcer, hepatic dysfunction, and pancreatitis may experience reactivation of the disorder.

Because of the potential for adverse effects from penicillamine, patients should be taught carefully about this drug, including the signs and symptoms of potentially serious consequences. Inform female patients that this drug should not be taken if they are pregnant or breast-feeding. It also should not be taken by patients who have severe renal dysfunction or severe anemia; have taken penicillamine before and developed a high fever; or are taking gold salts by mouth or injection. Moreover, patients allergic to penicillin should not take penicillamine.

Explain minor side effects, such as change in taste, diarrhea, loss of appetite, nausea, vomiting, and stomach pain, and advise patients to discuss these effects with the health care team if the effects do not subside or are particularly annoying. Patients should learn to take penicillamine at least 1 hour before or 2 hours after eating food. Patients taking penicillamine for Wilson disease must avoid foods that contain copper, such as chocolate, nuts, liver, and broccoli. In addition, patients should drink plenty of water to prevent kidney stones from forming. Patients should avoid taking antacids and iron preparations because they may prevent the drug from working properly.

A missed dose should be taken as soon as possible, but if it is almost time for the next dose, only that dose should be taken (double or extra doses should never be taken). Instruct patients to continue to take penicillamine even if it appears that it is not working. Penicillamine should be stored away from moisture (particularly away from a bathroom) and out of the reach of children. Urge patients to schedule monthly blood and urine tests to make sure they are not having any adverse reactions to penicillamine.

Sulfasalazine

Sulfasalazine (Azulfidine) is a sulfonamide antibiotic that is considered a first-line treatment for both adult and juvenile RA. Sulfasalazine is a prodrug of sulfapyridine and mesalamine. Mesalamine inhibits cyclooxygenase, resulting in decreased production of arachidonic acid metabolites and reducing inflammation.

COMMUNITY-BASED CONCERNS

Box 25.1 Danger Signs: Adverse Reactions to Penicillamine

When educating patients about the potential adverse effects of penicillamine, the nurse should alert them especially to signs and symptoms of a potentially life-threatening adverse reaction. Patients should contact their health care providers should any of the following occur:

- Bloody, black, or tarry stools
- Bloody or cloudy urine
- Cough or hoarseness
- Fever, chills, or sore throat
- Wheezing or difficulty breathing
- Eye pain or vision problems
- Joint pain
- Lower back or side pain
- Mouth ulcers, sores, or white spots on the lips or in the mouth
- Ringing in the ears (tinnitus)
- Swelling of face, feet, or lower legs
- Unusual bleeding, bruising, pinpoint red spots on skin
- Unusual tiredness or weakness
- Swollen or painful glands

Sulfasalazine is contraindicated in patients with salicylate hypersensitivity, sulfonamide hypersensitivity, furosemide hypersensitivity, thiazide diuretic hypersensitivity, sulfonylurea hypersensitivity, or carbonic anhydrase inhibitor hypersensitivity because it is broken down to a salicylate component and a sulfonamide component. It is also contraindicated for patients with intestinal or urinary obstruction and porphyria. It is given cautiously to patients with preexisting megaloblastic anemia or glucose-6-phosphate dehydrogenase (G6PD) insufficiency because, as a sulfonamide, it decreases folate absorption.

The most common adverse reactions associated with Azulfidine EN-tabs are rash, anorexia, headache, nausea, vomiting, gastric distress, and reversible low sperm count. Serious adverse effects include suppressed bone marrow function and hepatitis. These potentially serious adverse effects require that a baseline CBC, renal function, and liver function tests be completed before initiation of therapy and repeated periodically throughout therapy.

Sulfasalazine is a pregnancy category B drug. Although sulfasalazine is not secreted in breast milk, one of its metabolites, sulfapyridine, does enter the milk. Sulfapyridine is generally considered safe for a nursing baby except in stressed or ill infants, those with G6PD deficiency, and premature infants.

Tumor Necrosis Factor Inhibitors

ETANERCEPT

Etanercept (Enbrel) was the first TNF antagonist developed. It was produced by recombinant DNA technology. Etanercept is used in managing RA, to reduce signs and symptoms of the disease and delay structural damage in patients with moderately to severely active RA. It can be used in combination with methotrexate in patients who do not respond adequately to methotrexate alone. Etanercept also is indicated for reducing signs and symptoms of moderately to severely active polyarticular-course juvenile RA in patients who have had an inadequate response to one or more DMARDs.

In RA, activated T cells release inflammatory mediators called **cytokines**, including interleukins and tumor necrosis factor. TNF binds to TNF receptors on cellular membranes and triggers a cascade of inflammatory events that results in increased inflammation of the synovial membrane, the release of destructive lysosomal enzymes, and further joint destruction. Etanercept binds specifically to circulating TNF, prevents it from binding to TNF receptors on the cell membranes, and prevents the TNF-mediated cellular response.

The only absolute contraindication to etanercept is hypersensitivity. However, several cautions must be considered before using this drug. Etanercept has been associated with inducing sepsis and fatal infections in patients with predisposing diseases, such as advanced or poorly controlled diabetes. Therapy should be delayed until known infections have been resolved. In addition, etanercept may induce demyelinating disorders such as multiple sclerosis, myelitis, and optic neuritis and should be used cautiously in patients with these disorders.

Because etanercept blocks the biological activity of TNF, it could potentially affect host defenses against infections and neoplastic diseases. The safety and efficacy of etanercept in patients with suppressed bone marrow function or other types of immunosuppression are not known. Live vaccines should be avoided during etanercept therapy because definitive clinical data on potential effects are not yet available.

Common adverse reactions to etanercept include injection-site reactions, upper respiratory infections, headache, nausea, and rhinitis. Less common but very serious adverse effects include severe infections, induction of demyelinating diseases, and aplastic anemia.

Etanercept is a pregnancy category B drug. Whether it is secreted in breast milk is unknown. Etanercept is approved for use in children as young as 4 years old.

INFLIXIMAB

Infliximab (Remicade) is another TNF that is approved for managing RA and Crohn disease. In RA patients, it is given concurrently with methotrexate. Its off-label uses include psoriasis, psoriatic arthritis, and uveitis.

Infliximab differs from etanercept because it is a **monoclonal antibody** (a cell that is produced with the ability to recognize and bind to a specific antigen) that specifically inhibits the activity of TNF-alpha. TNF-alpha stimulates macrophages, which produce IL-1, IL-6, and IL-8. These interleukins then stimulate chondrocytes, osteoclasts, and fibroblasts that release the substances matrix metalloproteinase 1 (MMP1 or interstitial collagenase) and matrix metalloproteinase 3 (MMP3 or progelatinase), ultimately leading to erosion of bone and cartilage. Infliximab reduces inflammation in patients with RA by binding to and neutralizing TNF-alpha on the cell membrane and in the blood, thus stopping the cycle that damages bone and cartilage.

Infliximab should not be given to patients with known murine protein hypersensitivity. It is given cautiously to patients with CHF because it may exacerbate the symptoms. Other contraindications and precautions are similar to those for etanercept. The most common adverse effects associated with infliximab are abdominal pain, cough, dizziness, fainting, and headache. Infliximab increases the risk for developing tuberculosis or reactivating latent tuberculosis. It also increases the risk for serious or even fatal opportunistic infections, such as histoplasmosis, listeriosis, and pneumocystosis. Before therapy is initiated, the patient must be evaluated for the potential for tuberculosis (TB) and for immune status.

Infliximab is in pregnancy category B. As with etanercept, whether it is secreted in breast milk is unknown. Unlike etanercept, it is not approved for use in children.

ADALIMUMAB

Adalimumab (Humira) is the second TNF monoclonal antibody developed for managing RA. It is indicated for patients who have had an inadequate response to at least one DMARD; it can be given as monotherapy or in conjunction with other DMARDs. Its mechanism of action is the same as that of infliximab.

Patients with mannitol hypersensitivity should not receive adalimumab because the solution contains mannitol. The needle cover of the syringe contains latex; thus, patients (and health care workers with latex hypersensitivity) should not handle the needle cover without protective equipment. Other contraindications and precautions are similar to those for etanercept. Common adverse effects include injection-site reactions, infections, and neutropenia.

Adalimumab is a pregnancy category B drug. Whether it passes into breast milk is unclear. Safe and effective use in adolescents and children has not been established.

Ⓒ ANTIGOUT DRUGS

Antigout drugs are used to treat acute cases of gout and to prevent gout. As previously explained, gout is associated with hyperuricemia. Hyperuricemia occurs either because of increased uric acid production or by accumulation of uric acid related to decreased renal excretion. Antigout drug therapy focuses on either decreasing the inflammatory response caused by hyperuricemia or on reducing hyperuricemia itself. Table 25.3 summarizes drugs used to treat gout.

Drugs for Treating Acute Gout

The prototypical antigout drug is colchicine, which has been used since 1763. It is an alkaloid of a plant called *Colchicum autumnale*. It was originally found in several gout mixtures sold by charlatans; however, its use was popularized in the United States by Benjamin Franklin.

NURSING MANAGEMENT OF THE PATIENT RECEIVING [P] COLCHICINE

Core Drug Knowledge

Pharmacotherapeutics

The most common use of colchicine is for treating acute gouty arthritis. It is occasionally effective for other types of arthritis. Non–FDA-approved uses of colchicine include treating amyloidosis, Behçet syndrome, biliary cirrhosis,

TABLE 25.3 Summary of Selected Ⓒ Antigout and Ⓒ Uricosuric Drugs

Drug (Trade) Name	Selected Indications	Route and Dosage Range	Pharmacokinetics
Ⓒ Antigout Agent			
[P] colchicine	Acute gouty arthritis Non-FDA approved uses: amyloidosis, Behçet syndrome, biliary cirrhosis, hepatic cirrhosis, mediterranean fever, Paget disease, pericarditis, pseudogout	*Adult:* PO, 1–1.2 mg initially, followed by 0.5–0.6 mg/h, or 1–1.2 mg q2h until pain is relieved or adverse effects occur; maintenance, 0.5–0.6 mg/d; IV, 2 mg infused over 12 h, followed by 0.5 mg q6h with a total 24 h dose not to exceed 4 mg *Child:* Safety and efficacy not established	*Onset:* PO, 0.5–2 h; IV, 30–50 min *Duration:* PO, unknown; IV, unknown $t_{1/2}$: PO, 20 min; IV, 20 min
Ⓒ Uricosuric Agents			
[P] probenecid (Benemid; *Canadian:* Benuryl)	Chronic gout, serum urate levels above 9 mg/d, combination with antibiotic therapy	*Adult:* PO, 250 mg bid for 1 wk then 500 mg bid to a maximum dose of 2–3 g/d; combined w/antibiotic therapy, 1 g concurrent with oral antibiotics or 30 min before IM antibiotic *Child:* Not for child <2 y; other dosages based on weight	*Onset:* 30 min *Duration:* 4–6 h $t_{1/2}$: 4–7 h
sulfinpyrazone (Anturane; *Canadian:* Anturan)	Chronic gout Inhibition of platelet aggregation	*Adult:* PO (in order of indications listed to the left), 100–200 mg bid for 1 wk then increase to 200–400 mg bid, may reduce to 100 mg/d after serum urate levels are controlled; 200 mg bid–tid *Child:* Safety and efficacy not established	*Onset:* 30 min *Duration:* 4–6 h $t_{1/2}$: 3 h
allopurinol (Zyloprim; *Canadian:* Purinol)	Prevention of acute gouty attacks Uric acid nephropathy hyperuricemia Recurrent calcium oxalate renal calculus Prevention of acute gouty attacks during treatment of myeloproliferative neoplastic disease	*Adult:* PO (in order of indications listed at left), 100 mg qd increased by 100 mg weekly until serum urate concentration decreases below 6 mg/d or until maximum dose of 800 mg is achieved; same as above; 200–300 mg/d in divided doses; 600–800 mg/d in divided doses *Child:* PO (prevention of acute gouty attacks during treatment of myeloproliferative neoplastic disease), 6–10 y: 10 mg/kg in divided doses, <6 y: 150 mg/d in divided doses	*Onset:* 30 min–1 h *Duration:* 18–30 h $t_{1/2}$: 1–2 h metabolite, 18–30 h

hepatic cirrhosis, Mediterranean fever, Paget disease, pericarditis, and pseudogout.

Pharmacokinetics

Colchicine can be given either orally or intravenously. However, parenteral use is avoided because of potential toxicity. Colchicine should never be injected subcutaneously or intramuscularly because such injections cause severe local irritation. Oral colchicine is rapidly absorbed, metabolized in the liver, and excreted primarily in the feces, with 10% to 20% eliminated unchanged in the urine. Patients with hepatic disease may have increased renal elimination. Enterohepatic recirculation occurs to a large extent and can lead to adverse GI effects with larger dosages. Colchicine distributes to the kidney, liver, spleen, and intestinal tissues and concentrates primarily in the leukocytes. It can be found in leukocytes for 10 days after administration.

Pharmacodynamics

Colchicine possesses anti-inflammatory properties. Although it is highly effective in treating acute gouty arthritis, it is not an effective analgesic for other types of pain, nor does it affect uric acid clearance. Colchicine inhibits the activity of leukocytes by decreasing their migration into the affected area, resulting in an interruption of the cyclic inflammatory response. Another action of colchicine is to prevent the release of an inflammatory glycoprotein from phagocytes, although it does not inhibit phagocytosis of uric acid crystals. Additional pharmacologic actions of colchicine include lowering body temperature, suppressing the respiratory center, and vasomotor stimulation, leading to hypertension. These actions can be extremely serious in cases of overdose.

Contraindications and Precautions

Colchicine is contraindicated in patients with severe cardiac disease, hepatic disease, and renal disease because these patients are at risk for developing cumulative toxicity. Other patients at risk for cumulative toxicity are elderly or debilitated patients. These patients should be monitored closely.

Patients with renal impairment or elevated plasma levels of colchicine because of renal disease can develop a myoneuropathy characterized by proximal weakness and elevated serum creatine kinase levels. This reaction usually occurs in patients who have been taking colchicine for several years; however, it is prudent to monitor all patients with renal insufficiency for this reaction.

Colchicine is eliminated primarily through the biliary pathway. Patients with hepatic disease should be monitored closely during treatment with colchicine. Additionally, patients at risk for hepatic disease, such as those with alcoholism, should be monitored closely.

Colchicine should be used cautiously in patients with preexisting GI disease or depressed bone marrow function. These patients are at a higher risk for adverse effects of colchicine.

Patients with myelosuppression are at risk for infections or bleeding. Dental work should be performed before initiating colchicine therapy or deferred until blood counts return to normal.

Oral colchicine is classified as a pregnancy category C drug and therefore should be avoided by pregnant or lactating women. Parenteral colchicine is in pregnancy category D and should never be administered to pregnant or breast-feeding women.

Adverse Effects

The most common adverse effects of colchicine affect the GI tract. Up to 80% of patients taking colchicine may experience nausea, vomiting, diarrhea, abdominal pain, and paralytic ileus. These reactions can indicate toxicity, and the drug should be discontinued until the symptoms resolve.

Long-term therapy with colchicine may depress bone marrow function, inducing aplastic anemia, pancytopenia, thrombocytopenia, leukopenia, or agranulocytosis. Patients receiving parenteral colchicine experience depressed bone marrow function more frequently than do patients receiving the drug orally. Signs and symptoms of serious adverse reactions that must be reported to the prescriber include fever, chills, or sore throat; wheezing or difficulty breathing; muscle weakness; numbness or tingling in hands and feet; skin rash, itching; stomach pain; swelling of face or mouth; unusual bleeding, bruising, and pinpoint red spots on skin; and unusual tiredness or weakness.

Other adverse effects include renal, integumentary, hematologic, and endocrinologic effects. In the renal system, potential adverse effects are bladder spasms, nephrotoxicity, proteinuria, hematuria, anuria, and acute renal failure. Integumentary effects include angioedema, urticaria, injection-site reaction, skin necrosis, tissue necrosis, and median nerve neuritis. Effects on the endocrine system can include hypothyroidism.

Drug Interactions

Colchicine can enhance the effects of radiation therapy or drugs that depress bone marrow function. Colchicine also may interact with cyanocobalamin (vitamin B_{12}), cyclosporine, erythromycin, and nonsteroidal anti-inflammatory drugs (NSAIDs). Colchicine use may interfere with certain test results, yielding a false-positive finding when assessing for hemoglobin in urine. Table 25.4 presents potential drug interactions with colchicine.

Assessment of Relevant Core Patient Variables

Health Status

Assess the patient for potential medical conditions or drugs that contradict the use of colchicine or require close patient monitoring. Assess the joints for edema, erythema, or increased warmth. In addition, assess for signs of hypothyroidism. Obtain a baseline CBC, platelet count, and tests for renal and hepatic function.

Life Span and Gender

Determine whether the patient is pregnant or breast-feeding before administering colchicine. Pregnant or breast-feeding women should not receive parenteral colchicine. They may, however, receive oral colchicine if absolutely necessary.

Lifestyle, Diet, and Habits

Evaluate the patient's diet. Foods such as organ meats, oily fish, seafood, beans, peas, oatmeal, spinach, asparagus, cauliflower, and mushrooms should be avoided because these foods are high in purines. Also, evaluate the patient's intake of alcohol. Alcohol can cause both overproduction and underexcretion of uric acid. Because dehydration can trigger acute

TABLE 25.4 Agents That Interact With P Colchicine

Interactants	Effect and Significance	Nursing Management
agents that cause bone marrow suppression: amphotericin B, antineoplastic agents, carbamazepine, chloramphenicol, clozapine, flucytosine, phenothiazines, zidovudine	Drugs possessing hematoxic properties similar to those of gold salts may potentiate the action of both agents, resulting in bone marrow suppression.	Avoid coadministration if possible. Monitor complete blood count (CBC) and platelet count frequently. Monitor patient for sore throat, chills, easy bruising, or bleeding tendencies.
cyanocobalamin	Administration of colchicine can result in a reversible decrease in the absorption of cyanocobalamin, resulting in anemia.	Monitor for signs and symptoms of anemia. Monitor CBC.
cyclosporine	Cyclosporine may cause hyperuricemia. Concomitant use of cyclosporine and colchicine may also increase cyclosporine concentrations, resulting in a high risk for nephrotoxicity.	Avoid coadministration, if possible. Monitor blood urea nitrogen, creatinine, and cyclosporine levels.
erythromycin	The addition of erythromycin to colchicine therapy may lead to colchicine toxicity.	Monitor for fever, gastrointestinal (GI) symptoms, myalgia, and leukopenia.
ethanol (alcohol)	Ethanol ingestion increases the risk of adverse GI effects and can increase serum urate concentration, thus decreasing the antigout effects of colchicine.	Avoid alcohol ingestion during therapy. Monitor for effectiveness of colchicine.
nonsteroidal anti-inflammatory drugs (NSAIDs)	Concomitant use of NSAIDs and colchicine increases the likelihood of developing adverse GI effects, especially ulceration or hemorrhage.	Avoid coadministration. Monitor for adverse GI effects. Monitor for easy bruising or bleeding.

gout attacks, it is important to ensure that the patient consumes adequate amounts of fluids. Plasma uric acid levels rise during starvation. Therefore, ensure that the patient eats at regular intervals throughout the day.

Environment

Be aware of the setting in which colchicine may be administered. Colchicine is self-administered most frequently by patients in the home environment. Patients are advised to take the drug hourly until GI symptoms occur, then to reduce the dosage. For severe attacks, colchicine can be given intravenously to avoid GI symptoms.

Nursing Diagnoses and Outcomes

- Acute Pain related to drug-induced abdominal cramps or paralytic ileus
  Desired outcome: *The patient will contact the prescriber if abdominal pain occurs.*
- Risk for Injury related to drug-induced renal toxicity or possible extravasation of IV colchicine
  Desired outcome: *The patient administering colchicine at home will contact the prescriber if urinary changes occur. The hospitalized patient will remain free of extravasation of IV colchicine.*
- Risk for Deficient Fluid Volume related to drug-induced nausea, vomiting, and diarrhea
  Desired outcome: *The patient will contact the prescriber if GI symptoms occur.*
- Ineffective Protection related to possible blood dyscrasias
  Desired outcome: *The patient will contact the prescriber if sore throat, easy bruising, or lethargy occurs.*

Planning and Intervention

Maximizing Therapeutic Effects

In an acute care setting, administer colchicine with a full glass of water at evenly spaced intervals throughout the day. The patient who self-administers the drug should learn to follow this regimen as well. Adherence to diet and alcohol restrictions decreases hyperuricemia, thus allowing colchicine to achieve its maximum effect.

Minimizing Adverse Effects

Closely monitor patients with pre-existing medical conditions or those on drug therapy that may interact with colchicine. The patient needs to be advised to take colchicine at the first sign of an acute gout attack.

It is important to question the female patient about the possibility of pregnancy before administering IV colchicine. Administer IV colchicine cautiously and monitor frequently for signs of extravasation.

Providing Patient and Family Education

- Advise patients not to take colchicine if they have severe cardiac disease, hepatic disease, or renal disease.
- Make sure that pregnant or breast-feeding patients are not given IV colchicine.
- Advise patients to take colchicine at the first sign of a gout attack and to follow the directions on the drug container.
- Tell patients that if they miss a dose, they should take it as soon as they can. If it is almost time for the next dose, only that dose should be taken; patients should not take double or extra doses.

- Emphasize that colchicine can cause minor side effects, such as loss of appetite and hair loss, and that patients should tell their health care teams if the adverse effects do not go away or if they are particularly annoying.
- Caution the patient to report GI adverse effects (e.g., nausea, vomiting, diarrhea, and abdominal pain) because these symptoms could indicate drug toxicity or lead to fluid loss over time.
- Stress to patients that colchicine can cause serious adverse effects and that they should call their prescribers immediately if any signs and symptoms occur, including sore throat, easy bruising, lethargy, or signs of renal toxicity.
- Advise patients to avoid alcohol because it can cause stomach problems and increase uric acid concentrations in the blood, making a gouty attack more likely. Review foods that are high in purines to decrease dietary intake of uric acid.
- Inform patients that colchicine may produce severe adverse effects when coadministered with many prescription and over-the-counter (OTC) drugs and advise them never to take any other drugs without consulting their prescribers.
- Tell patients to keep colchicine away from light and out of the reach of children.
- Stress that patients must see their health care teams every month for blood and urine tests to make sure that they are not experiencing adverse effects from colchicine.

Ongoing Assessment and Evaluation

Monitor for hematopoietic and renal toxicity, joint involvement, deformity, and range of motion. The patient needs to be monitored for efficacy of colchicine therapy.

Therapy is considered effective if the patient reports decreased frequency of acute gout attacks and remains free of adverse effects. The patient should understand and be able to explain the importance of contacting the health care team immediately if any adverse effects occur, of scheduling periodic hematologic and renal testing, and of contacting the prescriber before taking any other prescription or OTC drugs.

Drugs for Treating Chronic Gout

Uricosuric drugs increase urate excretion. Having no anti-inflammatory or analgesic activity, they are not useful in treating acute gout attacks. In fact, when first initiated, they can exacerbate an acute attack of gout. Uricosuric drugs include probenecid, sulfinpyrazone, and allopurinol. Probenecid (Benemid) is the prototype uricosuric drug.

MEMORY CHIP

P Colchicine

- Decreases the inflammatory reaction of **acute** gout
- Major contraindications: severe cardiac, hepatic, or renal diseases
- Most common adverse effects: related to gastrointestinal system
- Most serious adverse effects: blood dyscrasias, including bone marrow suppression
- Maximizing therapeutic effects: adherence to diet and alcohol restrictions to reduce hyperuricemia
- Minimizing adverse effects: Take colchicine at the first sign of an attack, then only until the symptoms start to resolve.
- Most important patient education: related to diet and alcohol restrictions

NURSING MANAGEMENT OF THE PATIENT RECEIVING P PROBENECID

Core Drug Knowledge

Pharmacotherapeutics

Probenecid is used in treating chronic gout. It keeps the uric acid level below the saturation point, thereby preventing the formation and deposition of urate crystals. Probenecid should be discontinued at the time of an acute attack because its use can prolong the inflammatory response. Probenecid also is used in patients with visible tophi, those with serum urate levels above 9 mg/dL, and those with a family history of tophi or decreased uric acid excretion. It also is used in combination with antibiotic therapy to increase or prolong the serum concentration of antibiotics, such as penicillin, by delaying their renal clearance.

Pharmacokinetics

Probenecid is administered orally and absorbed completely. The drug is distributed throughout the body tissues and is 75% to 95% bound to plasma protein, predominantly to albumin. Probenecid undergoes hepatic metabolism, resulting in active metabolites. Both parent drug and active metabolites have renal elimination. Small amounts of probenecid are excreted in the feces (see Table 25.3).

Pharmacodynamics

Probenecid interferes with tubular handling of organic acids within the nephron. It inhibits the active resorption of uric acid at the proximal convoluted tubules, resulting in increased excretion of uric acid.

Contraindications and Precautions

Probenecid is contraindicated in patients with depressed bone marrow function or uric acid kidney stones because the drug can exacerbate these conditions. Probenecid should not be administered to patients with severe renal impairment (glomerular filtration rate <50 mL/min) or to patients with medical conditions in which uric acid production can increase acutely, such as those undergoing cancer chemotherapy or radiation therapy.

Probenecid should be administered cautiously to patients with peptic ulcer disease because it may increase GI adverse effects. Probenecid is assigned to pregnancy category C and therefore should be avoided, if possible, during pregnancy and while breast-feeding.

Adverse Effects

Therapeutic dosages of probenecid are generally well tolerated with few adverse effects. The most common adverse effects include headache, nausea, vomiting, and anorexia. Less common effects include dizziness, flushing, alopecia, polyuria, nephrotic syndrome, interstitial nephritis, leukope-

nia, and anemia. Adverse effects signaling danger include blood in urine; fever, chills, or sore throat; wheezing or difficulty breathing; lower back or side pain; mouth sores; difficulty passing urine; rash and itching; swelling of feet, ankles, face, or lips; unusual bleeding, bruising, pinpoint red spots on the skin; or unusual tiredness or weakness.

Some patients with gout can experience an increased incidence of uric acid stones or of acute gouty attacks during the first 6 to 12 months of therapy. These increases occur because of increased renal clearance of uric acid.

Drug Interactions

Uricosurics may interact with many drugs (Table 25.5). Probenecid reduces the renal tubular secretion of many drugs, which causes an increase in the serum concentration and increases the risk for adverse effects and toxicities. Conversely, the same action allows probenecid to be used as adjunct therapy with antibiotics. Because the antibiotics are not excreted, serum concentrations are elevated and prolonged.

Uricosuric actions of probenecid are inhibited by salicylates. When probenecid is used to treat hyperuricemia or gout, salicylates should not be administered. Anticoagulant effects of heparin can be increased by concomitant administration of probenecid. Probenecid also can interfere with hepatic conjugation. This effect may prolong the elimination half-life of lorazepam, thus risking toxicity. Probenecid interferes with laboratory tests for urinary 17-ketosteroids and may cause false-positive Clinitest results for patients with diabetes.

Assessment of Relevant Core Patient Variables

Health Status

Assess the patient for potential medical conditions or drug therapies that contraindicate the use of probenecid or require close patient monitoring. Obtain baseline CBC, platelet count, and renal function test values. Neurologic functioning must be evaluated and pregnancy status ascertained. It is important to assess the patient's knowledge concerning the potential adverse effects and drug interactions associated with probenecid. Finally, assess the efficacy of probenecid therapy.

Life Span and Gender

Determine whether the patient is pregnant or breast-feeding before administering probenecid. Probenecid should not be given to pregnant or breast-feeding women. Discover the age of the patient before administering probenecid. Probenecid is not indicated for children younger than 2 years. Elderly patients taking probenecid must be monitored closely because they are at increased risk for developing uric acid stones related to decreased renal function.

Lifestyle, Diet, and Habits

Assess the patient's usual dietary patterns. Patients should be advised to limit their intake of vitamin C or cranberry juice. These substances tend to acidify the urine, which decreases probenecid excretion. Risk for toxicity is increased when probenecid remains in the body.

Note whether the patient taking probenecid has diabetes and, if so, advise him to monitor the blood glucose levels with capillary blood monitoring systems instead of Clinitest strips. This approach will help to ensure an accurate glucose level determination.

Nursing Diagnoses and Outcomes

- Increased Risk for Injury related to probenecid-induced renal toxicity
  Desired outcome: *The patient will contact the prescriber if any urinary changes occur.*
- Deficient Fluid Volume related to nausea and vomiting
  Desired outcome: *The patient will contact the prescriber if nausea and vomiting persist.*
- Ineffective Protection related to drug-induced blood abnormalities
  Desired outcome: *The patient will contact the prescriber if sore throat, easy bruising, or lethargy occurs.*

Planning and Intervention

Maximizing Therapeutic Effects

Do not administer probenecid with vitamin C or cranberry juice. Probenecid is excreted more easily in alkaline urine.

Minimizing Adverse Effects

Advise the patient to take probenecid with milk or food to decrease the potential for GI effects. Fluid intake should range between 2 and 3 L/day (unless contraindicated) to minimize potential for uric acid stone formation.

Providing Patient and Family Education

- Advise patients not to take probenecid if they have depressed bone marrow function, severe renal dysfunction, or uric acid kidney stones, or if they are pregnant or breast-feeding.
- Emphasize to patients that if they miss a dose, they should take it as soon as they can. If it is almost time for the next dose, however, only that dose should be taken; they should never take double or extra doses.
- Tell patients that probenecid can cause minor side effects, such as dizziness, flushing, hair loss, headache, loss of appetite, nausea, vomiting, and painful or swollen joints, and that they should let their health care teams know about these side effects if they do not go away or if they are particularly annoying.
- Be sure patients understand that probenecid can cause serious adverse effects, and that they should call their health care teams immediately if they observe signs of renal toxicity (urinary changes) or signs of blood abnormalities (e.g., sore throat, easy bruising, or lethargy).
- Tell patients that several months may elapse before the full effect of probenecid is seen.
- Stress to patients that they should avoid alcohol because it can cause stomach problems and increase uric acid levels in the blood, which makes a gouty attack more likely.
- Tell patients to avoid aspirin and drugs such as ibuprofen because they can make probenecid less effective.

TABLE 25.5 Agents That Interact With P Probenecid

Interactants	Effect and Significance	Nursing Management
allopurinol	The antihyperuricemic effects of allopurinol and probenecid are additive when administered together.	Interaction may be therapeutic.
Antiviral Agents		
acyclovir famciclovir ganciclovir	Probenecid reduces the renal tubular secretion of antiviral agents, which increases the serum concentration and elimination regular half-life of antiviral agents. This results in an increased risk of adverse effects and toxicity.	Monitor serum concentration of antiviral agents. Assess patient for signs of antiviral toxicity.
Antibiotics		
penicillin cephalosporins aztreonam ciprofloxacin clofibrate imipenem cilastatin	Probenecid reduces the renal tubular secretion of antibiotic agents, which increases the serum concentration and elimination regular half-life of selected antibiotics. This results in an increased risk of adverse effects and toxicity.	Monitor serum concentration of antibiotic agents. Assess patient for signs of antibiotic toxicity.
Drugs That Cause Hyperuricemia		
ethacrynic acid diazoxide ethanol ethambutol thiazide diuretics triamterene pyrazinamide	Drugs that cause hyperuricemia decrease the effectiveness of probenecid.	Monitor for effectiveness of probenecid. Anticipate possible need for dosage adjustment.
Diuretics		
bumetanide furosemide indapamide	Probenecid can interfere with the natriuresis and plasma renin activity increases caused by certain diuretics. These diuretics can, in turn, increase the levels of serum uric acid, antagonizing the effects of probenecid.	Monitor for effectiveness of probenecid. Anticipate potential probenecid dosage adjustment.
dyphylline	Uricosurics directly affect the kidneys to decrease the active tubular secretion of dyphylline. May increase the half-life and decrease the total body clearance of dyphylline.	Consider use of theophylline in place of dyphylline. Monitor for signs of toxicity, such as nausea, tachycardia, and nervousness.
methotrexate	Probenecid is suspected to reduce renal elimination of methotrexate and may cause methotrexate toxicity.	Decrease methotrexate dosage. Monitor serum methotrexate concentration.
Prostaglandin Synthetase Inhibitors (PSIs)		
indomethacin ketoprofen ketorolac naproxen	Probenecid reduces the renal tubular secretion of selected nonsteroidal anti-inflammatory drugs (NSAIDs), which increases the serum concentration and elimination half-life of selected NSAIDs. This results in an increased risk of adverse effects and toxicity.	Do not coadminister ketoprofen and probenecid. Monitor for adverse reactions or toxicity to NSAIDs. Anticipate NSAID dose reduction.
salicylates	Salicylates inhibit actions of either drug alone.	Avoid coadministration. Advise patient to use acetaminophen for analgesic or antipyretic needs.
zidovudine	Probenecid may inhibit zidovudine glucuronidation. This may result in cutaneous eruption accompanied by systemic symptoms, including malaise, myalgia, or fever.	Coadminister with caution. Observe for possible rash and systemic symptoms.

- Tell patients to drink at least 10 glasses of water a day to prevent kidney stones.
- Patients with diabetes should be instructed to use blood glucose monitoring.
- Warn patients to keep this drug out of the reach of children.
- It is important to tell patients to see their health care team every month for blood and urine tests to make sure that they are not having any adverse reactions to probenecid.

Ongoing Assessment and Evaluation

It is important to obtain periodic CBC, platelet count, and renal function tests. Monitor for signs and symptoms of renal toxicity, headache, or dizziness and contact the prescriber immediately if any of these symptoms occur. Monitor the patient needs for efficacy of probenecid therapy.

Therapy is considered effective when the patient reports increased comfort or reduced pain and inflammation and remains free of adverse effects. In addition, the patient should express an understanding of the need to contact the health care team immediately if adverse effects occur, and of the advantages of increasing fluid intake and avoiding alcohol, aspirin, and PSIs.

Drug Closely Related to P Probenecid

Sulfinpyrazone is an active metabolite of the PSI phenylbutazone, so it has some anti-inflammatory effects. Its action is the same as that of probenecid; however, it is longer acting and more potent. In addition to increasing uric acid excretion, sulfinpyrazone inhibits platelet aggregation and thus can be used in MI prophylaxis. Because of its antiplatelet action, monitor the patient for signs of bleeding and do not administer sulfinpyrazone with other drugs, such as salicylates or anticoagulants (warfarin) that affect platelet aggregation. Sulfinpyrazone may induce GI distress; thus, administering the drug with meals or milk may be helpful.

Drug Significantly Different From P Probenecid

Allopurinol is a uricosuric agent and a xanthine oxidase inhibitor. It differs from probenecid and sulfinpyrazone by its mechanism of action. Allopurinol works by inhibiting uric acid formation, whereas probenecid and sulfinpyrazone work by increasing uric acid excretion. Like the other agents, allopurinol is not recommended for use during an acute gouty attack because the decrease in plasma uric acid levels mobilizes urate deposits in the body, resulting in exacerbation of the acute attack. Allopurinol works best for patients who overproduce uric acid and for those with excessive tophi. In some critical care units, cardiothoracic surgeons use allopurinol with antioxidants preoperatively to prevent reperfusion-induced injury when blood flow is re-established.

Potential adverse effects include skin rash, fever, GI distress, and liver toxicity. Drug interactions may occur with drugs that are metabolized by the hepatic microsomal enzymes, such as theophylline. Close monitoring is needed to avoid toxicity.

MEMORY CHIP

P Probenecid

- Used for the management of **chronic** gout
- Major contraindications: bone marrow depression or uric acid kidney stones
- Most common adverse effects: headache, nausea, vomiting, and anorexia
- Most serious adverse effects: blood dyscrasias
- Maximizing therapeutic effects: Do not administer with Vitamin C or cranberry juice.
- Minimizing adverse effects: Take with milk or food to decrease gastrointestinal distress.
- Most important patient education: Taking the drug during an acute attack may worsen the symptoms.

CHAPTER SUMMARY

- Arthritic inflammatory diseases are initially treated with salicylates and PSIs.
- DMARDs (disease-modifying antirheumatic drugs) delay joint destruction and should be initiated within 3 months of diagnosis of rheumatoid arthritis.
- DMARDs have a common goal of reducing the progression of rheumatoid arthritis, but have different mechanisms of action to achieve that goal.
- Pharmacologic classes of DMARDs include alkylating agents, antimetabolites, antimalarials, gold salts, sulfonamide antibiotics, tumor necrosis factor (TNF) inhibitors, monoclonal antibodies, interleukin antagonists, and immune response modifiers.
- Methotrexate is the DMARD of choice for most rheumatologists. Its efficacy is enhanced when given in combination with other DMARDs.
- Gout is a disease of altered purine metabolism resulting in hyperuricemia. However, hyperuricemia alone does not always result in gout.
- Antigout drugs resolve symptoms in two different ways: colchicine opposes leukocyte phagocytosis, which inhibits further urate deposits; whereas uricosuric agents reduce hyperuricemia.

QUESTIONS FOR STUDY AND REVIEW

1. What advantage do DMARDs have over salicylates, PSIs, and acetaminophen?
2. What is the major disadvantage of using DMARDs?
3. What is the advantage of using DMARDs within 3 months of diagnosis of RA?
4. Why are so many different classes of medications under the umbrella term DMARD?
5. What is TNF?
6. What contraindication and potential adverse effect is common to all TNF inhibitors? Why?
7. Compare colchicine and probenecid.

Need More Help?

Chapter 25 of the study guide for *Drug Therapy in Nursing* 2e contains NCLEX-style questions and other learning activities to reinforce your understanding of the concepts presented in this chapter. For additional information or to purchase the study guide, visit *http://connection.lww.com/go/aschenbrenner.*

REFERENCES AND BIBLIOGRAPHY

Clinical Pharmacology [Online]. Available: *http://cp.gsm.com.*

Facts and Comparisons. (2004). *Drug facts and comparisons.* Philadelphia: Lippincott Williams & Wilkins.

Genovese, M. C., Cohen, S., Moreland, L., et al. (2004). Combination therapy with etanercept and anakinra in the treatment of patients with rheumatoid arthritis who have been treated unsuccessfully with methotrexate. *Arthritis and Rheumatology, 50*(5), 1412–1419.

Hardman, J. G. (2001). *Goodman & Gilman's the pharmacological basis of therapeutics* (10th ed.). New York: McGraw-Hill Health Professions Division.

Katzung, B. (2004). *Basic and clinical pharmacology* (9th ed.). New York: McGraw-Hill/Appleton & Lange.

Keystone, E. C., Kavanaugh, A. F., Sharp, J. T., et al. (2004). Radiographic, clinical, and functional outcomes of treatment with adalimumab (a human anti-tumor necrosis factor monoclonal antibody) in patients with active rheumatoid arthritis receiving concomitant methotrexate therapy: A randomized, placebo-controlled, 52-week trial. *Arthritis and Rheumatology, 50*(5), 1400–1411.

Korpela, M., Laasonen, L., Hannonen, P., et al. (2004). Retardation of joint damage in patients with early rheumatoid arthritis by initial aggressive treatment with disease-modifying antirheumatic drugs: Five-year experience from the FIN-RACo study. *Arthritis and Rheumatology, 50*(7), 2072–2081.

Micromedex Healthcare Series [Online]. Available: *http://healthcare.micromedex.com.*

Tatro, D. S. (2004). *Drug interaction facts.* Philadelphia: Lippincott Williams & Wilkins.

Cardiovascular and Renal System Drugs

unit 7

Drugs Affecting Cardiac Rhythm

chapter 26

Learning Objectives

At the completion of this chapter the student will:

1. Identify core drug knowledge about drugs that affect cardiac rhythm.
2. Identify core patient variables relevant to drugs that affect cardiac rhythm.
3. Relate the interaction of core drug knowledge to core patient variables for drugs that affect cardiac rhythm.
4. Differentiate Class I, II, III, and IV antiarrhythmic drugs.
5. Describe the varied therapeutic effects of beta blockers and calcium channel blockers.
6. Generate a nursing plan of care from the interactions between core drug knowledge and core patient variables for drugs that affect cardiac function.
7. Describe nursing interventions to maximize therapeutic and minimize adverse effects for drugs that affect cardiac rhythm.
8. Determine key points for patient and family education for drugs that affect cardiac rhythm.

KEY TERMS

action potential
arrhythmia
atrial fibrillation
atrial flutter
automaticity
cardiac cycle
depolarization
dysrhythmia
ectopic foci
electrocardiogram
proarrhythmia
re-entry phenomenon
refractory period
repolarization
resting membrane potential
transmembrane potential
ventricular fibrillation
ventricular tachycardia

FEATURED WEBLINK

http://www.arcmesa.com/pdf/cardsys/cardsys_struc.htm
This web page, at the ArcMesa Educators website, shows the anatomy and physiology of the cardiovascular system.

CONNECTION WEBLINK

Additional Weblinks are found on Connection:
http://www.connection.lww.com/go/aschenbrenner.

Drugs Affecting Cardiac Rhythm

Ⓒ Class I Antiarrhythmics

Class 1-A
- [P] **quinidine**
- procainamide
- dysopyramide

Class 1-B
- lidocaine
- tocainide
- mexiletine
- moricizine
- phenytoin

Class 1-C
- flecainide
- propafenone

Ⓒ Class II Antiarrhythmics (Beta Blockers)

Beta blockers approved as antiarrhythmics
- [P] **propanolol** (see also Chapter 13)
- acebutolol
- esmolol

Beta blockers not approved as antiarrhythmics
- atenolol
- bisoprolol
- metoprolol
- nadolol
- prindolol
- timolol

Ⓒ Class III Antiarrhythmics

- [P] **amiodarone**
- sotalol
- bretylium
- ibutilide
- dofetilide

Ⓒ Class IV Antiarrhythmics (Calcium Channel Blockers)

Calcium channel blockers approved as antiarrhythmics
- [P] **verapamil**
- IV diltiazem

Non-calcium channel blockers
- adenosine

Calcium channel blockers approved as antiarrhythmics
- amlodipine
- bepridil
- felodipine
- isradipine
- nicardipine
- nifedipine
- nimodipine
- nisoldipine

Ⓒ Potassium Removing Resins

- [P] **sodium polystyrene sulfonate**

The symbol Ⓒ indicates the **drug class.**
Drugs in **bold type** marked with the symbol [P] are prototypes.
Drugs in blue type are closely related to the prototype.
Drugs in red type are significantly different from the prototype.
Drugs in black type with no symbol are also used in drug therapy; no prototype

The heart is the muscle responsible for pumping blood through the circulatory system. The contraction of the heart depends on changes in electrical stimulation in cardiac muscle cells. These changes in electrical activity occur at regular, set intervals. This pattern establishes a normal rhythm for the beating heart. When pathologic processes interfere with these normal changes in stimulation, the rhythm of the heart is altered. These alterations may be severe enough to stop the heart. Arrhythmia is the term used to describe these alterations. **Arrhythmia,** meaning "no rhythm," occurs any time the normal rate or rhythm of the heart is altered. The heart continues to beat, but not in the expected pattern or manner. The term **dysrhythmia,** meaning "abnormal rhythm," is used interchangeably with arrhythmia and is preferred by many clinicians. This chapter identifies drugs that are used to treat alterations in the rhythm of the heart.

Drugs to treat cardiac arrhythmias are grouped by class: I, II, III, and IV. There are three subclasses of Class I antiarrhythmic drugs. The prototype for Class IA antiarrhythmics is quinidine (Quinaglute Dura-Tabs). Other drugs in this class are procainamide (Procan SR) and disopyramide (Norpace). Drugs significantly different from the Class IA drugs are the Class IB antiarrhythmics, which include lidocaine (Xylocaine), tocainide (Tonocard), mexiletine (Mexitil), moricizine (Ethmozine), and phenytoin (Dilantin); and the Class IC antiarrhythmics, which include flecainide (Tambocor) and propafenone (Rythmol).

Class II antiarrhythmics are the beta blockers. The prototype beta blocker is propranolol (Inderal). Of the other numerous drugs in this class, only acebutolol (Monitan) and esmolol (Brevibloc) are approved as Class II antiarrhythmics. Any of the other beta blockers may be used based on the clinical judgment of the physician.

Class III antiarrhythmics include the prototype amiodarone (Cordarone). Drugs similar to amiodarone are sotalol (Betapace), bretylium, ibutilide, and dofetilide.

Class IV antiarrhythmics are the calcium channel blockers; the prototype is verapamil (Calan). The other calcium channel blocker approved for treating arrhythmias is intravenous diltiazem (Cardizem). A drug significantly different from verapamil is adenosine (Adenocard). Calcium channel blockers used to treat cardiac and circulatory pathologies other than arrhythmias are amlodipine (Norvasc), bepridil (Vascor), felodipine (Plendil), isradipine (DynaCirc), nicardipine (Cardene), nifedipine (Procardia), nimodipine (Nimotop), and nisoldipine (Sular).

Because hyperkalemia is an electrolyte imbalance that may cause potentially lethal arrhythmias, drugs to prevent arrhythmias are the potassium-removing resins. The prototype potassium-removing resin is sodium polystyrene sulfonate (Kayexalate).

PHYSIOLOGY

The heart is composed of four chambers: the left and right atria and the left and right ventricles. Blood is returned from the body to the right atrium of the heart. It progresses from the right atrium to the right ventricle to the lungs to be reoxygenated and have carbon dioxide removed. The reoxygenated blood returns to the left atrium, then to the left ventricle. The contraction of the left ventricle pushes the blood into the aorta, thus back into systemic circulation.

Blood is circulated throughout the body by a coordinated sequence of chamber contractions and valve openings and closings known as the **cardiac cycle.** The two phases of the cardiac cycle are systole and diastole. Together they describe the timeframe from the beginning of one heartbeat to the beginning of another. During systole, the ventricles contract, and the aortic and pulmonic valves open, allowing blood to be ejected into the aorta and pulmonary artery. During diastole, the ventricles relax, and the mitral and tricuspid valves open; at the same time, blood flows into the atria. This blood is propelled into the ventricles by atrial contraction, which occurs at the end of diastole. As systole begins again, the increased pressure from ventricular contraction causes the mitral and tricuspid valves to shut.

Contractions of the heart are dependent on the unique electrical conduction system of the cardiac muscle. The conduction system connects to highly specialized cardiac cells that allow the heart to beat predictably and rhythmically. The system is composed of the sinoatrial (SA) node, the atrioventricular (AV) node, the bundle of His, the bundle branches, and the Purkinje fibers. The SA node, influenced by both the sympathetic and the parasympathetic nervous systems, is known as the pacemaker of the heart. The progression of the electrical impulse that produces the heartbeat starts in the SA node. This electrical impulse, called the action potential, leaves the SA node, travels through the atria, and causes them to contract. The impulse then travels through the bundle of His to the bundle branches and then through the Purkinje fibers (Figure 26.1A). This electrical activity (depolarization and repolarization, explained in more detail later) is captured on an **electrocardiogram** (ECG or EKG) (see Figure 26.1B). During each phase of the cardiac cycle, a distinct wave pattern is produced on the ECG.

The first wave you see is the P wave, which represents atrial depolarization. After the impulse leaves the atria, it is slowed at the AV node so that the atria and the ventricles do not contract simultaneously. On the ECG, this slowing is translated into a period of inactivity called the PR segment: a straight line between the beginning of the P wave and the start of the first deflection of the next wave. All of the electrical activity in the heart that takes place before the impulse reaches the ventricles is seen in the PR interval, which includes the P wave and the PR segment. The ventricle depolarization is shown by a large complex of three waves: The Q, the R, and the S, called the QRS complex. After the ventricles depolarize, they begin the repolarization phase, which results in another wave on the ECG called the T wave. The atria also repolarize, but their repolarization usually occurs at the same time as ventricular depolarization; thus, the atrial repolarization wave is usually hidden in the QRS complex.

Figure 26.2A shows a normal-rate ECG. Compare this normal rate to the slow heart rate (bradycardia: a resting heart rate less than 60 beats per minute [bpm]) shown in Figure 26.2B and to the fast heart rate (tachycardia: a resting heart rate higher than 100 bpm) shown in Figure 26.2C. To best comprehend how this unique conduction system works, it is important to understand how potassium, sodium, and calcium ions bring about electrical changes in the cardiac cells that stimulate contraction of

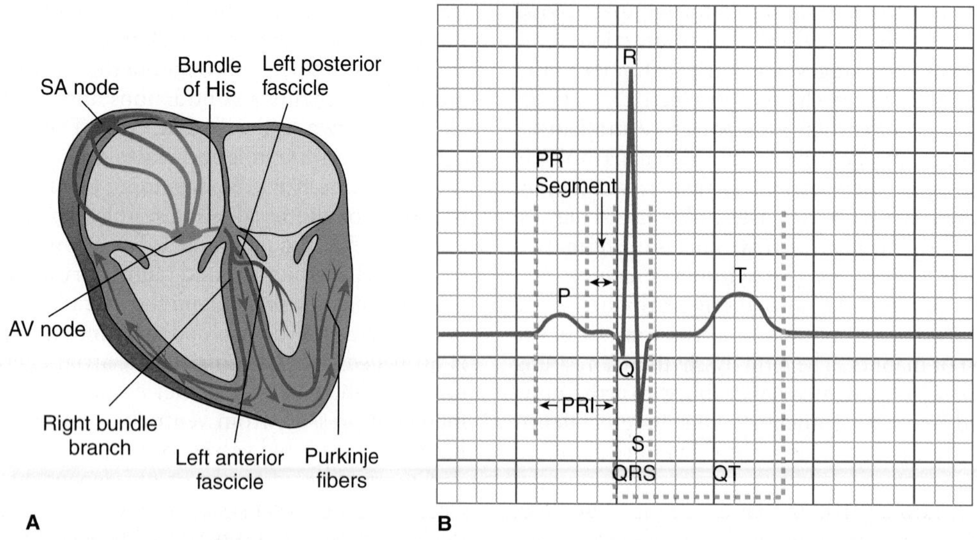

FIGURE 26.1 Cardiac conduction. The heart's electrical circuitry (**A**) has a profound effect on efficient blood flow to the tissues. An electrical impulse from the sinoatrial (SA) node travels over the atrial tracks to produce atrial contraction. The impulse slows slightly as it nears the ventricles at the atrioventricular (AV) node (the AV junction). After passing through the bundle of His, the impulse descends along the left and right bundle branches to the Purkinje fibers, stimulating ventricular contraction and proceeding on to the SA node to continue the cycle. The efficiency of the conduction system has a major influence on cardiac rhythm and output reflected by blood flow. (**B**) This is the pattern of one cardiac cycle on an EKG. Note the components of the complex, including the waves and intervals. PRI, PR interval; QRS, QRS complex; QT, QT interval.

the cardiac cells. The fibers of the heart muscle alternate between resting and contracting; this contraction is caused by electrical and chemical changes within the cell. Potassium is predominantly an intracellular (within the cell) ion, and sodium and calcium are predominantly extracellular (outside the cell) ions (Figure 26.3). Calcium is also stored in special places within the cell, but it is not active as long as it is stored.

These ions (potassium, sodium, and calcium) all flow following the normal concentration gradient (moving from areas of high concentration to areas of low concentration). Because of the different concentrations of intracellular and extracellular ions, an electrical gradient exists across the membrane of the cell. This electrical gradient is called the **transmembrane potential.** All changes that occur in the transmembrane potential during an entire cycle of contraction and relaxation are, as a unit, called the **action potential.** At rest, the electrical charge of the transmembrane potential,

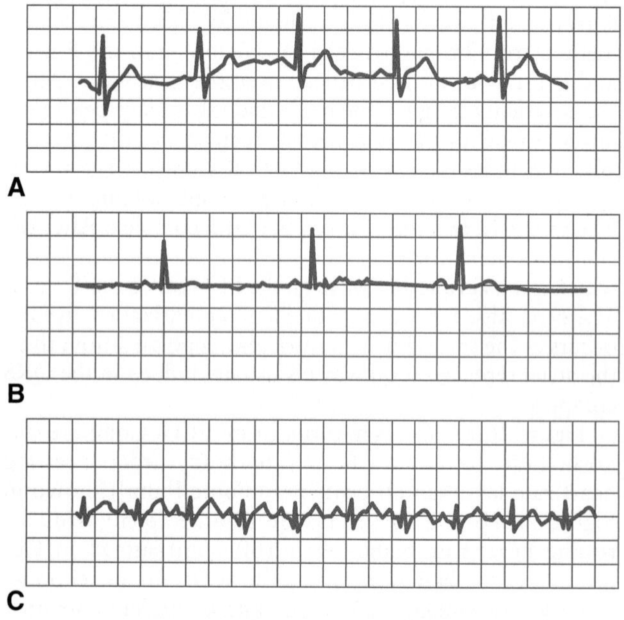

FIGURE 26.2 (**A**) Normal sinus rhythm, ECG. (**B**) Bradycardia, slow heart rate. (**C**) Tachycardia, fast heart rate.

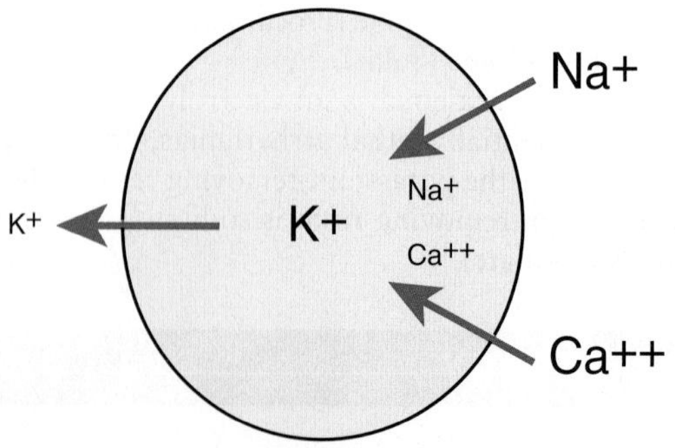

FIGURE 26.3 Intracellular and extracellular ions. Potassium is the predominant intracellular ion. It will move to the outside of the cell, following its concentration gradient. Sodium and calcium are predominantly extracellular ions; they will move into the cell.

also known as the **resting membrane potential,** is –90 millivolts (mV). This means that there is a 90-mV difference between the electrical charge inside and outside of the cell, and that the charge is negative inside the cell. As sodium moves into the cell, **depolarization** occurs. At this point, the transmembrane potential changes from negative to positive. Depolarization occurs rapidly and is called phase 0 of the action potential. During this rapid depolarization, the sodium channels open quickly for only a brief period. While these "fast channels" are open, sodium rushes into the cell. The influx of sodium ions into the cell increases the transmembrane potential to about +30 (meaning that the charge is now positive inside the cell relative to outside the cell). As soon as this positive charge is achieved, the voltage-regulated sodium channels close, and the cell begins to return to a negative state. This movement of the transmembrane potential away from a positive value and toward the negative resting potential is called **repolarization.** The initial downward movement toward zero is phase 1 of the action potential. As the charge reaches 0 mV, a plateau occurs. This plateau is what differentiates the action potential of cardiac muscle from the action potential of skeletal muscle. In this plateau phase, called phase 2, the calcium channels open slowly. These "slow channels" allow calcium ions to enter the cell. The positively charged calcium channels close, potassium channels open, and potassium again moves into the cell. The cell then begins a rapid acceleration of repolarization: phase 3 of the action potential. When full polarization is achieved once more, the cell is in phase 4 of the action potential and will remain there until stimulated again to depolarize. In other words, the cycle will start over (Figure 26.4).

After the cell depolarizes, and until it restores its normal electrical charge, it cannot be stimulated to fire again. This interval is termed the **refractory period.** Initially after depolarization, the cell cannot be stimulated to fire, no matter how great the stimulus. This state is the absolute refractory period. As repolarization continues, the cell eventually responds, even though it is not at the resting state. However, the intensity of the stimulus needed to depolarize the cell is greater than when the cell is in the resting state. This ability to respond, but only to a larger than normal stimulus, is termed the relative refractory period.

Calcium is required for contraction of the heart. In contracting cells of the heart, calcium links excitation (from polarization) to contraction. The contraction of cardiac and vascular smooth muscle tissues is dependent on the movement of extracellular calcium into these cells. The influx of calcium, however, is approximately 20% of the calcium needed to initiate a contraction. The calcium that enters the cell stimulates the release of calcium that is stored inside the sarcoplasmic reticulum. This process is called calcium induced calcium release. The process occurs during the plateau phase of the action potential. This additional release of calcium is what actually induces a contraction. Contraction will occur as long as calcium and energy are present.

The plateau phase is unique to the cardiac muscle. In contrast, repolarization of skeletal muscle occurs rapidly after depolarization, allowing the muscle to be stimulated to contract again almost immediately. Tetany, or constant contractions, may occur in skeletal muscles. This process would be life threatening if it occurred in the heart because no effective contractions would be present. Thus, this plateau phase can be considered a protective mechanism of the heart muscles to promote effective contractions (Figure 26.5).

Imbalances of the electrolytes involved in the action potential, either greater than or less than normal serum levels, may produce changes in the action potential and cause various cardiac arrhythmias. Contractility of the heart is also affected by the concentration of catecholamines in the heart muscle—the more catecholamines, the greater the rate of contraction and the greater the force of contraction will be.

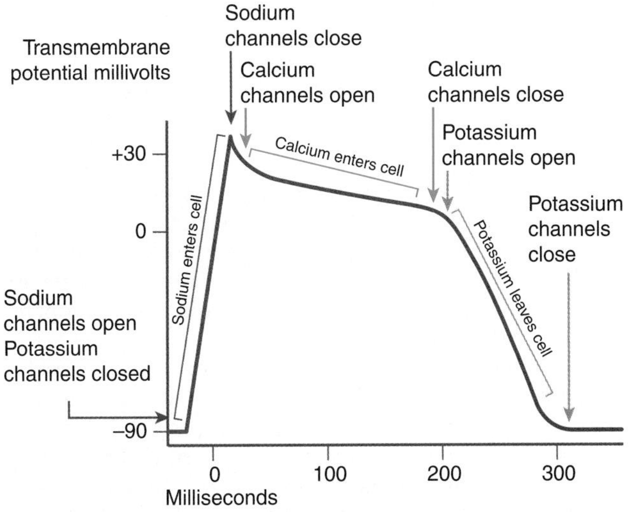

FIGURE 26.4 Movement of electrolytes during the action potential. As sodium enters the cell, rapid depolarization occurs. Once sodium channels close, the process of repolarization slowly begins. When calcium enters the cell, a plateau occurs. When the calcium channels close and potassium channels open, rapid repolarization occurs.

PATHOPHYSIOLOGY

Arrhythmias, also called dysrhythmias, are a disturbance in the electrical activity of the heart. Some arrhythmias are insignificant and do not create any problems for the patient. Others disrupt the function of the heart, increase the oxygen demand of the heart, and interfere with cardiac output. Some are considered life threatening or lethal.

Changes in the ionic currents through ion channels of the myocardial cell membrane are the main cause of cardiac arrhythmia. The ions are sodium, potassium, and calcium. These ionic changes allow arrhythmias to develop in one of three ways: through a disorder with impulse formation, through a disorder of the impulse conduction system, or through a combination of both. When a disorder of impulse formation is present, the rate of SA nodal discharges is altered, allowing changes in the **automaticity** (ability to generate an impulse spontaneously) of the heart. Decreased automaticity results in sinus bradycardia; increased automaticity results in sinus tachycardia. These changes may be the result of drug toxicity, such as from digoxin, or of excessive sympathetic activity. Eliminating the contributing factor controls the arrhythmia. A different problem with automaticity occurs when the SA nodal rate decreases excessively and other

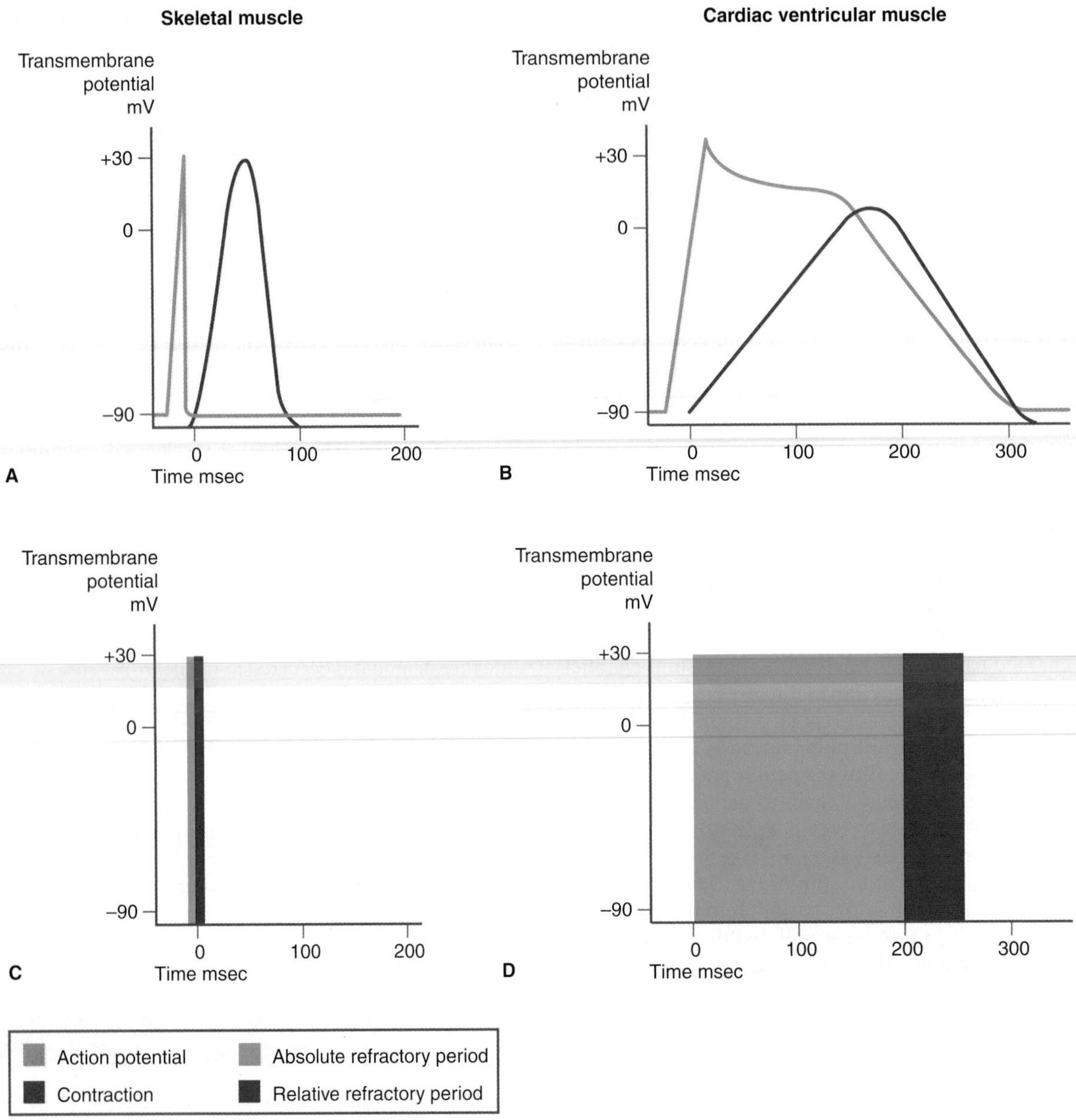

FIGURE 26.5 Comparisons of action potential, contraction, and refractory periods in skeletal and cardiac muscle.

excitable heart tissue reaches the threshold potential earlier than the SA node, thus generating an impulse. These abnormal sites of impulse formation are **ectopic foci.** These ectopic pacemakers may result from hypokalemia, myocardial ischemia, emotional stress, or hypoxia. Ectopic foci may arise in atrial, nodal, Purkinje, or ventricular muscle.

Disorders of impulse conduction may result from an alteration in either the rate or the pathway of impulse conduction. When conduction of the impulses through the AV node is delayed, heart block occurs.

Re-entry phenomenon is a more common source of alterations of impulse formation. Electrical impulses normally travel along a Purkinje fiber and divide at the small branch points in the fiber. When they meet each other in the connecting branch, they normally extinguish each other. However, where there is a temporary block in one of the branches because of an alteration in nerve impulse conduction, the impulse cannot continue to travel in its normal forward path, canceling itself out in the common branch. Instead, the impulse is carried through the unopposed side and re-enters the branch from the opposite direction. Re-entry or the **re-entry phenomenon** causes repetitive cardiac stimulation, firing, and arrhythmias (Figure 26.6).

Arrhythmias can occur in the atria or in the ventricles. **Atrial flutter** (Figure 26.7A) is an arrhythmia originating in the atria: rapid atrial beating (approximately 300 times per minute) but a slower, usually regular, ventricular beating. **Atrial fibrillation** (AF) (see Figure 26.7B) is the most commonly seen arrhythmia in clinical practice. This arrhythmia is caused by rapid, irregular discharges from multiple atrial ectopic foci. The result is quivering of the atria without any true diastole occurring. Impulses are transmitted irregularly through the AV node, producing an irregular ventricular response, which is often rapid. The incidence of atrial fibrilla-

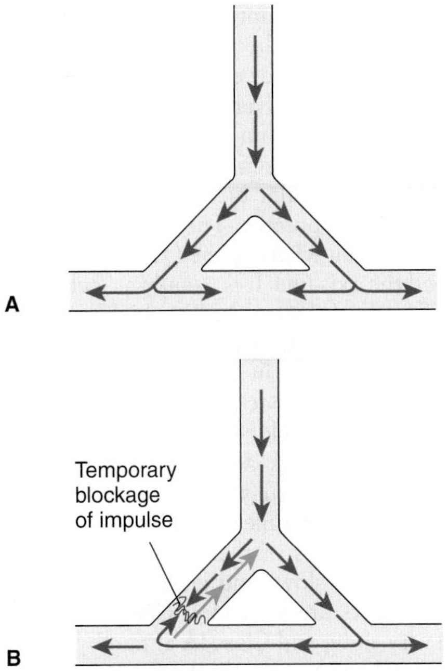

FIGURE 26.6 Reentry phenomenon. In normal cardiac conduction (**A**), electrical impulses cancel each other out. In reentry phenomenon, conduction is altered by a temporarily blocked impulse (**B**), allowing the impulse coming from the other direction to recycle and stimulate the Purkinje fibers to contract again. The result is a disturbance in cardiac rhythm. Antiarrhythmic drugs are used to treat these disturbances.

tion is increasing; it produces a great deal of morbidity and some mortality, although it is not directly life threatening. The American College of Cardiology (ACC), the American Heart Association (AHA), and the European Society of Cardiology (ESC) have defined four classifications of atrial fibrillation:

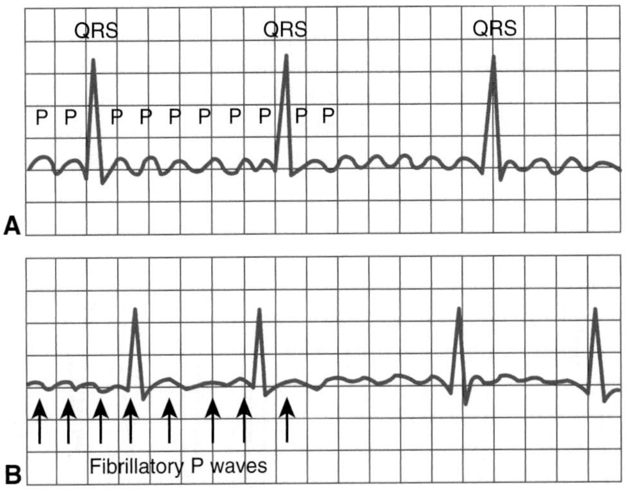

FIGURE 26.7 (**A**) Atrial flutter. Note rapid P waves with occasional QRS complexes. (**B**) Atrial fibrillation. Note small, irregular waves. QRS complexes can be an irregular rate but appear normal.

- *Acute causes of AF,* such as surgery, pulmonary diseases, and electrocution
- *AF without associated cardiovascular disease,* such as in younger patients
- *AF with associated cardiovascular disease,* such as coronary vascular disease
- *Neurogenic AF,* in which the autonomic nervous system can trigger fibrillation in susceptible patients through heightened vagal tone (Fuster et al., 2001)

The classification can make a difference in the drug regime a patient is given. In the past, the goal of atrial fibrillation treatment was to slow the rate but not correct the rhythm. However, in a recent study that compared rate control and rhythm control in 4,060 patients, rhythm-controlled strategy offered no survival advantage over the rate-controlled strategy. One advantage of using the rate-control strategy was that it produced fewer adverse drug effects than did the rhythm-controlled strategy (Wyse et al., 2002). The implication from the study is that rate control should be considered a primary approach to therapy and that rhythm control, if used, may be abandoned early if it is not fully satisfactory (see Box 26.1). A substudy of the AFFIRM group looked at maintenance of sinus rhythm in patients with atrial fibrillation using antiarrhythmic drugs. The results of this investigation showed that amiodarone was more effective at 1 year than either sotalol or class I agents for the strategy of maintaining sinus rhythm without cardioversions (AFFIRM First Antiarrhythmic Drug Substudy Investigators, 2003). Exactly which drug is best at

FOCUS ON RESEARCH

Box 26.1 Treatment Options With Atrial Fibrillation

Wyse, D. G., Waldo, A. L., DiMarco, J. P., et al., Atrial Fibrillation Follow-up Investigation of Rhythm Management (AFFIRM) Investigators. (2002). A comparison of rate control and rhythm control in patients with atrial fibrillation. *New England Journal of Medicine, 347*(23), 1825–1833.

The Study

In this randomized, multicenter trial, 4,060 patients were enrolled in a comparison of the two approaches to treating atrial fibrillation (AF): cardioversion and treatment with antiarrhythmic drugs, such as amiodarone and flecainide, to maintain sinus rhythm; or rate-controlling drugs, such as verapamil and diltiazem, without cardioversion (allowing atrial fibrillation to persist). The conclusions showed that managing atrial fibrillation with the rhythm-control strategy offers no survival advantage over management with the rate-control strategy, and that the rate-control strategy has potential advantages, such as lower risk for adverse drug effects.

Nursing Implications

You need to understand that the choice of medications prescribed to a patient with AF will be based on one of these two treatment approaches. The ventricular rate is controlled with beta blockers and calcium channel blockers. Because the use of anticoagulant drugs is recommended in both approaches, you can expect that these patients will also be taking anticoagulants. Studies concerning these drugs are ongoing, so you must be aware of new findings that can affect practice. Education for the patient is a must, including information about how to take medications, how to take an accurate pulse, how to recognize signs and symptoms of CHF, and when the patient should call the prescriber.

maintaining sinus rhythm while causing the fewest adverse effects is not known at this time. The AFFIRM study does provide direction. Treatment of atrial fibrillation patients should always include stroke risk assessment and close follow-up if anticoagulation is discontinued (Prasun & Kocheril, 2003).

Ventricular tachycardia is rapid ventricular beating (greater than 100 bpm; usually 150–200 bpm) arising from ventricular ectopic foci. **Ventricular fibrillation** is quivering of the ventricle without a systolic beat. If not terminated rapidly (2–3 minutes) with defibrillation, brain damage will occur because the brain is not receiving oxygen. Ventricular tachycardia and ventricular fibrillation are serious and potentially life-threatening arrhythmias. They may occur after an acute myocardial infarction. These arrhythmias must be corrected within a relatively short timeframe or the patient is likely to die because these contraction patterns do not allow the ventricle to fill appropriately; thus, when the ventricle contracts, not enough blood is pushed out into the general circulation. Cardiac output therefore drops dramatically, and blood pressure falls. Once the patient has been converted to normal rhythm, there may be a tendency to revert to ventricular tachycardia or ventricular fibrillation later. Patients who are deemed most at risk for reverting may be placed on long-term drug therapy, receive an implantable cardioverter defibrillator (ICD), or both.

DRUGS AND OTHER THERAPIES TO TREAT ARRHYTHMIAS

Drug therapy has been the mainstay for treating arrhythmias; however, the latest research studies show it has become possible to prevent the recurrence of some arrhythmias with the use of ICDs (Rao & Saksena, 2003). ICDs have an established and definitive role in preventing sudden cardiac death; technologic innovations and refinements in therapeutic capabilities of these devices have widened the spectrum of patients who can benefit from ICD. This therapy can improve myocardial function with physiologic atrioventricular sequential pacing, treat life-threatening ventricular tachyarrhythmias with electrical therapies, and prevent bradycardia with support pacing (Rao & Saksena, 2003). Drug therapy no longer remains the sole source of therapy for atrial fibrillation. Concomitant use of drug therapy with ICDs is often the rule for chronic atrial fibrillation. Antiarrhythmics are agents used to prevent, suppress, or treat a disturbance in cardiac rhythm. The primary outcomes are to decrease automaticity, decrease speed of conduction, and decrease reentry. Clinical trials are providing new information on the effectiveness of different drugs in treating various arrhythmias. Selection of an antiarrhythmic drug is based on outcomes from these clinical trials, not solely on the electrophysiologic changes related to the drug class, such as the AFFIRM study. Catheter ablation is being used to treat supraventricular arrhythmias with a highly successful and often curative intervention (Blomstrom-Lundqvist et al., 2003). The ablative procedure is done in an electrophysiology laboratory with electrode catheters positioned in the area of the AV node to apply radiofrequency energy to the slow conducting pathway. The slow pathway is ablated, and the patients' conduction then uses the fast pathway, as it should with normal rhythm (Gilbert, 2001).

One problem with all antiarrhythmics is that, because of their ability to modify the rhythm of the heart, they can cause a new arrhythmia or exacerbate the arrhythmia that they are treating. This adverse effect is termed **proarrhythmia.** Such effects range from an increase in frequency of premature ventricular contractions (PVCs) to the development of more severe ventricular tachycardia, ventricular fibrillation, or torsades de pointes. The latter is a rapid, unstable form of tachycardia whereby the QRS complexes appear to twist around the axis line. It is usually associated with a prolonged Q-T interval (Figure 26.8), which may lead to death.

When antiarrhythmic drugs were developed, a system of classification was sought in an attempt to organize the complex information into a conceptually meaningful fashion. The classification system developed was fairly comprehensive and was grouped by the drugs' actions (not by the drugs, per se). Class I antiarrhythmic drugs block sodium channels. Several subtypes of sodium channels have been discovered, which depend on the kinetics of their sodium-channel properties (i.e., very fast, very slow, and intermediate). Class IB antiarrhythmic agents are very fast; Class IC antiarrhythmic agents are very slow; and Class IA antiarrhythmic agents are intermediate. Class IA antiarrhythmic agents also are known to suppress sodium-channel activity in all cardiac tissues, whereas Class IB antiarrhythmic agents suppress sodium-channel action only in diseased or depolarized tissue.

Class II antiarrhythmic drugs block adrenergic receptors (beta blockers), producing antisympathetic effects that slow the heart rate, lengthen the time needed for conduction, and increase the force of contraction. The effect seen with Class II antiarrhythmic drugs is depression of phase 4 of depolarization. Class III antiarrhythmic drugs lengthen the duration of the action potential. This effect prolongs phase 3 of repolarization. Class IV antiarrhythmic drugs block calcium channels. This action depresses phase 4 of depolarization and lengthens phases 1 and 2 of repolarization (Figure 26.9).

Although this classification system is widely used, it has substantial limitations. Some drugs have characteristics of more than one class; other drugs (such as digoxin and adenosine) used in specific types of arrhythmias do not fit within any of the classes within the system. Despite these limitations, the antiarrhythmics discussed in this chapter are presented in the traditional groupings of Class I, II, III, and IV.

The major goals of antiarrhythmic therapy are to alleviate symptoms (e.g., palpitations, lightheadedness, shortness of breath), improve quality of life, and prolong survival in patients with cardiac arrhythmias. The relief of symptoms in most patients can be achieved either by slowing the rate

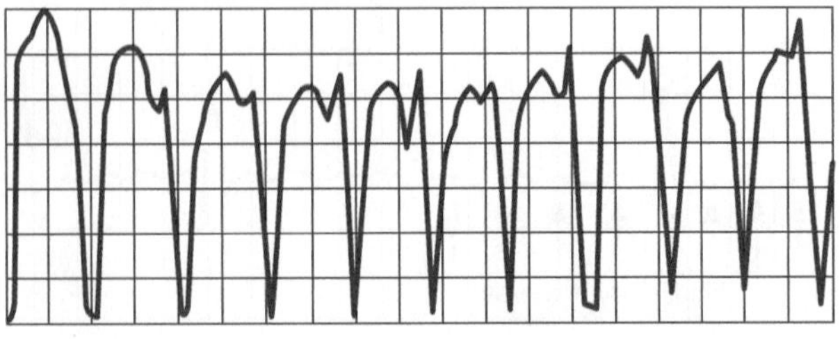

FIGURE 26.8 Torsade de pointes. A rapid, unstable form of tachycardia where the QRS complexes appear to twist around the axis line. It is usually associated with a prolonged Q-T interval.

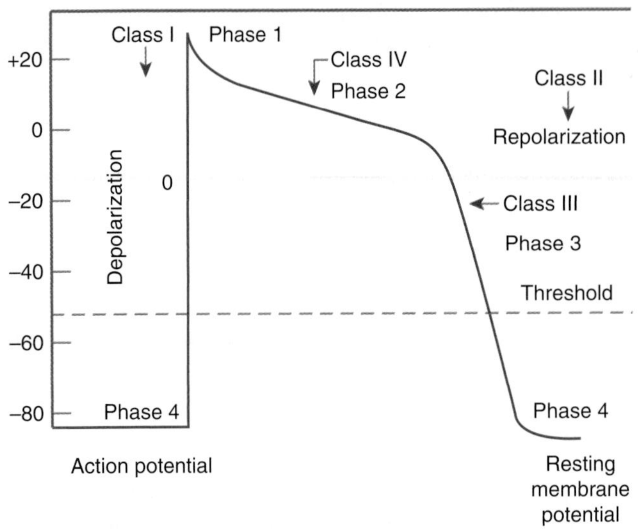

FIGURE 26.9 Action potential and antiarrhythmic drugs. The change in the charge of the myocardial cell that occurs when sodium (Na+) and calcium (Ca++) flow into the cell and potassium (K+) flows out is called the action potential. Different antiarrhythmic drugs act at different phases of polarization and repolarization. Class I drugs (quinidine) act during depolarization, class II drugs (propranolol) act during the resting period of repolarization, class III drugs (amiodarone) act during rapid repolarization, and class IV drugs (verapamil) act during early repolarization.

or by preventing recurrence. However, relief of the arrhythmia is not always associated with decreases in mortality.

C CLASS I ANTIARRHYTHMIC DRUGS

Class I antiarrhythmics are local anesthetics or membrane-stabilizing agents that depress phase 0 in depolarization. The drugs in subgroups of A, B, and C are not interchangeable because they have different pharmacotherapeutics. Class IA antiarrhythmics include quinidine (Quinora, Quinidex Extentabs, Quinaglute Dura Tabs, Quinalan, quinidine sulfate, quinidine gluconate, Cardioquin), procainamide (Procan SR), disopyramide (Norpace), and moricizine (Ethmozine). Drugs similar to quinidine are the Class IB drugs lidocaine (Xylocaine), tocainide (Tonocard), mexiletine (Mexitil), moricizine, and phenytoin (Dilantin) and the Class IC drugs flecainide (Tambocor) and propafenone (Rythmol). Table 26.1 presents a summary of selected Class IA antiarrhythmic drugs. The prototype Class IA antiarrhythmic is quinidine.

NURSING MANAGEMENT OF THE PATIENT RECEIVING P QUINIDINE

Core Drug Knowledge

Pharmacotherapeutics

Quinidine is used primarily to treat atrial arrhythmias, including premature atrial, AV junctional, paroxysmal atrial (supraventricular) tachycardia, paroxysmal AV junctional rhythm, atrial flutter, paroxysmal and chronic atrial fibrillation but has decreased in use during the past decade for maintaining sinus rhythm, being replaced by amiodarone (Fang et al., 2004). It can be used as maintenance therapy after electrical conversion of atrial fibrillation or flutter, but again is being replaced by amiodarone for this use. Other uses of quinidine include treating premature ventricular contractions and paroxysmal ventricular tachycardia not associated with complete heart block. A noncardiac use of quinidine (quinidine gluconate only) is in treating life-threatening *Plasmodium falciparum* malaria. Normally given orally, quinidine may be given parenterally when oral therapy is not possible or when more rapid therapeutic effects are required (see Table 26.1).

Pharmacokinetics

Quinidine is rapidly absorbed from the gastrointestinal (GI) tract. The concentration of quinidine varies among the different quinidine salts. Quinidine gluconate contains 62% active quinidine, whereas quinidine polygalacturonate contains 80% active quinidine, and quinidine sulfate contains 83% active quinidine. Quinidine distributes to all body tissues except the brain. It is fairly highly protein bound at 80% to 90% and is metabolized by the liver and excreted unchanged by the kidneys. The influence of renal dysfunction on the disposition of quinidine is controversial; volume of distribution and renal clearance may be reduced. Acid urine promotes elimination of quinidine. Patients with cirrhosis may have a prolonged half-life and an increased volume of distribution. In congestive heart failure (CHF), total clearance and volume of distribution are decreased. In elderly patients, elimination half-life may be increased.

Pharmacodynamics

Quinidine depresses myocardial excitability, conduction velocity, and contractility. The effective refractory period is prolonged, increasing conduction time. Re-entry phenomenon is therefore prevented. Quinidine also exerts an indirect anticholinergic effect; it decreases vagal tone and may promote conduction in the AV junction.

It is important to examine the relationship of Class I antiarrhythmics to mortality. In patients without structural heart disease, the use of Class I drugs rarely causes proarrhythmia serious enough to be life threatening. However, in studies of patients with ventricular tachycardia and ventricular fibrillation, no controlled study has produced decisive evidence demonstrating that Class I antiarrhythmics have the potential for prolonging survival of patients at high risk for dying suddenly. In fact, data from meta-analysis of several studies show that most, if not all, Class I antiarrhythmics are inclined to increase mortality (Singh, 1999). Thus, drugs that prolong the action potential only (Class I) are not the answer for decreasing mortality in patients with arrhythmias and structural heart disease. Class I agents are still widely used to decrease the number of shocks that patients with implantable cardioversion defibrillators receive. The efficacy for this use is unknown.

Contraindications and Precautions

Quinidine is contraindicated in the presence of hypersensitivity or a history of idiosyncratic reaction to quinidine or other cinchona derivatives. Hypersensitivity and idiosyncratic reac-

TABLE 26.1 Summary of Selected (C) Class I Antiarrhythmics

Drug (Trade) Name	Selected Indications	Route and Dosage Range	Pharmacokinetics
[P] quinidine (Quinaglute Dura-Tabs; *Canadian:* Quinate)	Premature atrial and ventricular contractions	*Adult:* PO, 200–300 mg three or four times daily *Child:* PO, 30 mg/kg/24 h or 900 mg/m^2/24 h in five divided doses	*Onset:* PO, 1–3 h; IM; 30–90 min; IV, rapid *Duration:* 6–8 h $t_{1/2}$: 6–7 h
	Paroxysmal supraventricular tachycardias	*Adult:* PO, 400–600 mg every 2 or 3 h until the paroxysm is terminated, administer after digitalization, dosage individualized *Child:* PO, 30 mg/kg/24 h or 900 mg/m^2/24 h in five divided doses	
	Atrial flutter	*Adult:* After digitalization dosage is individualized	
procainamide (Procan SR; *Canadian:* Apo-Procainamide)	Arrhythmia	*Adult:* PO, initially 50 mg/kg/d in divided doses every 3 h; PO maintenance 50 mg/kg/d in divided doses q6h; IV, loading (initial), 1 mL/min of 20 mg/mL solution or 100 mg every 5 min direct IV, up to 1 g total; maintenance 1–3 mL/min of 2 mg/mL solution *Child:* PO, 15–50 mg/kg/d divided every 3–6 h; max of 4 g/d; IV, initial 3–6 mg/kg/dose over 5 min; maintenance, 20–80 µg/kg/min continuous infusion; maximum, 100 mg/dose or 2 g/d	*Onset:* PO, 30 min; IM, 10–30 min; IV, immediate *Duration:* 3–4 h $t_{1/2}$: 2.5–4.7 h
lidocaine (Xylocaine HCl IV for cardiac arrhythmias)	Arrhythmia	*Adult:* Initial IV bolus 50–100 mg at rate of 25–50 mg/min; one-third to one-half the initial dose may be given after 5 min; do not exceed 200–300 mg in 1 h. Continuous infusion 20–50 mg/kg/min *Child:* AHA recommends bolus of 1 mg/kg IV, followed by 30 µg/kg per min w/caution	*Onset:* IM, 5–10 min; IV, immediate *Duration:* IM; 2 h; IV, 10–20 min $t_{1/2}$: 10 min, then 1.5–3 h
flecainide (Tambocor)	PSVT and PAF	*Adult:* Starting dose of 50 mg every 12 h; increase in 50-mg increments twice a day every fourth day until efficacy is achieved. Max dose is 300 mg per day. *Child:* Not recommended	*Onset:* 30–60 min *Duration:* 24 h $t_{1/2}$: 20 h
	Sustained ventricular tachycardia	*Adult:* 100 mg every 12 h; increase in 50-mg increments twice a day every fourth day until efficacy is achieved. Max dose is 400 mg per day. *Child:* Not recommended.	

PSVT, paroxysmal supraventricular tachycardia; PAF, paroxysmal atrial flutter.

tion are manifested by thrombocytopenia, skin eruption, or fever. Sparfloxacin, gatifloxacin, and moxifloxacin may result in additional prolongation of the QT interval; concurrent use is contraindicated. Quinidine also is contraindicated in patients with the following conditions or findings:

- Myasthenia gravis
- A history of thrombocytopenic purpura associated with quinidine administration
- Digitalis intoxication manifested by arrhythmias or AV conduction disorders
- Complete heart block
- Left bundle branch block or other severe intraventricular conduction defects exhibiting marked QRS widening or bizarre ECG complexes
- Complete AV block with an AV nodal or idioventricular pacemaker
- Aberrant ectopic impulses and abnormal rhythms due to escape mechanisms
- Drug-induced torsades de pointes (ventricular tachycardia associated with QT prolongation)
- Long QT syndrome

Quinidine should be used with extreme caution in patients with incomplete AV block because complete block may develop. Caution also must be used in digitalis toxicity because unpredictable arrhythmias may result. Quinidine is used cautiously in patients with partial bundle branch block, severe CHF, and hypotension because quinidine will further depress myocardial contractility and arterial pressure. Caution must also be used when giving quinidine to patients with renal, hepatic, or cardiac insufficiency because toxicity is more likely to occur.

Quinidine crosses the placenta and achieves fetal serum levels similar to maternal levels. It is in pregnancy category C, indicating that safety has not been established. Quinidine also is excreted in breast milk. Milk-to-serum ratios have been found to be 0.71. Although safe use during breast-feeding has

not been established clearly, the American Academy of Pediatrics considers the drug compatible with breast-feeding. Safety and efficacy in children have not been established.

Adverse Effects

The most common adverse effects involve the GI system and include nausea, vomiting, abdominal pain, diarrhea, and anorexia. These may occur after a fever. Arrhythmias also occur commonly, but most are not life threatening. Another common adverse effect is a syndrome of cinchonism, related to the tree bark source of quinidine, usually associated with chronic toxicity but also described after a brief exposure to a moderate dose in sensitive patients. The symptoms of cinchonism include tinnitus, high-frequency hearing loss, deafness, headache, nausea, dizziness, vertigo, lightheadedness, and disturbed vision.

The most serious adverse effect is cardiotoxicity, which is manifested by increased PR and QT intervals, 50% widening of the QRS complex, ventricular tachyarrhythmias (including ventricular tachycardia, fibrillation, and torsades de pointes), frequent ventricular ectopic beats, or tachycardia. If signs of cardiotoxicity are present, quinidine should be discontinued at once, and the ECG of the patient should be monitored closely.

Other cardiovascular (CV) adverse effects include cardiac asystole, arterial embolism, ventricular extrasystole occurring at the rate of one or more for every six normal beats, complete AV block, ventricular flutter, and hypotension. Although large oral doses cause peripheral vasodilation that decreases blood pressure, the most serious hypotension is more likely to occur when quinidine is given intravenously.

Hepatic toxicity can occur, including granulomatous hepatitis. This reaction is believed to be the result of quinidine hypersensitivity. Fever occurs, and liver enzymes are elevated. Other hypersensitivity reactions, which are rare but may occur, are angioedema, acute asthma, vascular collapse, respiratory arrest, and purpura vasculitis. Other adverse effects that may occur include:

- Hematologic: acute hemolytic anemia, hypoprothrombinemia, thrombocytopenia, thrombocytopenic purpura, agranulocytosis, leukocytosis, neutropenia, and shift to left in white blood cell differentials
- Central nervous system (CNS): headache, fever, vertigo, apprehension, excitement, confusion, delirium, syncope, dementia, ataxia, and depression
- Ophthalmic: mydriasis and blurred vision, disturbed color perception, reduced vision field, photophobia, diplopia, night blindness, and optic neuritis
- Dermatologic: rash, urticaria, cutaneous flushing with intense pruritus, photosensitivity, exfoliative eruptions, psoriasis, and abnormalities of pigmentation
- Development of lupus erythematosus, which resolves after drug therapy stops

Quinidine overdosage may be associated with depressed mental function even if the patient is hemodynamically stable. In addition, CNS symptoms (e.g., lethargy, confusion, coma, respiratory depression or arrest, seizures, headache, paresthesia, and vertigo) may occur after the onset of CV toxicity. GI effects include vomiting, abdominal pain, diarrhea, and nausea. The CV effects are tachyarrhythmias, depressed automaticity and conduction, hypotension, syncope, and heart failure.

Some of the adverse effects of quinidine may be similar to reasons the drug is prescribed. For this reason, it is important to monitor blood levels to determine whether the drug is in therapeutic range or is elevated excessively.

Drug Interactions

Quinidine interacts with many other antiarrhythmic and cardiac drugs. It also interacts with anticoagulants and several drugs that affect the CNS. Sparfloxacin, gatifloxacin, and moxifloxacin may result in additional prolongation of the QT interval; concurrent use is contraindicated. Table 26.2 lists drugs that interact with quinidine.

Assessment of Relevant Core Patient Variables

Health Status

The health care team must determine whether the patient has a type of atrial arrhythmia that is an indication for therapy. It also is important to determine whether the patient has any of the following contraindications to quinidine therapy:

- Hypersensitivity to quinidine
- Myasthenia gravis
- A history of thrombocytopenic purpura from quinidine use
- Arrhythmias or AV conduction disorders from digitalis toxicity
- Complete heart block
- Left bundle branch block or other severe intraventricular conduction defects that exhibit marked widening of QRS complex
- Complete AV block with an AV nodal or idioventricular pacemaker
- Aberrant ectopic impulses and arrhythmias due to escape mechanisms
- A history of drug-induced torsades de pointes
- A history of long QT syndrome

The patient with renal, hepatic, or cardiac insufficiency is at greater risk for toxicity. If the patient has cirrhosis, the elimination half-life may be prolonged and the volume of distribution increased. This effect increases the risk for adverse events. If the patient has CHF, total clearance and volume of distribution will be decreased. This decrease may result in greater risk for adverse effects or in less substantial therapeutic effects than expected.

Determine whether the patient is on or has orders for cholinergic drugs. When these drugs are administered with quinidine, paroxysmal supraventricular tachycardia (SVT) may not be stopped. Also, assess which other drugs the patient is receiving to determine whether a drug interaction is likely to occur.

Review the patient's potassium level because potassium enhances the effect of quinidine, and hypokalemia will reduce the effectiveness. The risk for quinidine-induced torsades de pointes is also increased with hypokalemia.

Life Span and Gender

The assessment should focus on whether the patient is pregnant or breast-feeding because safety and efficacy have not been established in these circumstances. Likewise, quinidine

TABLE 26.2 Agents That Interact With P Quinidine

Interactants	Effect and Significance	Nursing Management
antacids	Increases urinary pH affecting the rate of drug elimination	Stagger administration times of quinidine and antacids by at least 2 h.
barbiturates	May reduce serum level and half-life of quinidine	Monitor therapeutic effect of quinidine, and consult with prescriber about dosage adjustment.
cholinergic drugs	May result in failure to terminate paroxysmal supraventricular tachycardia (PSVT)	Use cautiously, if at all, in patients with myasthenia gravis.
cimetidine	Increased serum levels and risk of quinidine toxicity	Monitor serum levels of quinidine. Assess for signs of adverse effects.
hydantoins, nifedipine, rifampin, sucralfate, disopyramide	Decreased levels and effectiveness of quinidine	Monitor drug effectiveness.
sparfloxacin, gatifloxacin, and moxifloxacin	May result in additional prolongation of the QT interval	Concurrent use is contraindicated.
verapamil	May cause hypotension, bradycardia, atrioventricular block, pulmonary edema	Monitor electrocardiogram. Check quinidine serum levels.
anticholinergics	Concurrent use may cause additive vagolytic effect	Consistently monitor and check quinidine serum levels.
anticoagulants	Potentiation of anticoagulation; hemorrhage possible	Assess coagulation times and patient for signs of bleeding.
beta blockers (metoprolol, propranolol)	Effects of metoprolol or propranolol may be increased in extensive metabolizers	Assess for adverse effects.
procainamide	Increased pharmacologic effects of procainamide and elevated NAPA (a major metabolite of procainamide) plasma levels	Watch for signs of toxicity.
succinylcholine	Prolonged neuromuscular blockade	Monitor drug levels, and attempt to stagger doses.
tricyclic antidepressants (TCA)	TCA clearance possibly reduced, thereby increasing effects	Same as above.

has not been proved safe or effective for children. If the patient is elderly, elimination half-life may be increased for quinidine.

Lifestyle, Diet, and Habits

Assess the patient's normal dietary patterns for adequate potassium intake because hypokalemia decreases effectiveness and increases the risk for some adverse effects. Administer with food or milk to decrease GI irritation.

Environment

Know the setting in which quinidine may be administered. Oral quinidine may be taken at home, in an acute care setting, or in a long-term care facility. Parenteral quinidine is given in a hospital where the patient can be closely observed and ECG and blood pressure can be monitored.

Nursing Diagnoses and Outcomes

- Imbalanced Nutrition: Less than Body Requirements related to nausea, vomiting, abdominal pain, anorexia, and diarrhea secondary to adverse effects of drug therapy
  Desired outcome: *The patient will not develop adverse effects substantial enough to alter nutrition.*
- Decreased Cardiac Output related to cardiac changes secondary to adverse effects of drug therapy
  Desired outcome: *The patient will not develop deleterious cardiac changes that alter cardiac output.*
- Risk for Injury, such as hepatic toxicity, related to adverse effects of drug therapy
  Desired outcome: *The patient will not incur hepatic toxicity while on drug therapy.*

Planning and Intervention

Maximizing Therapeutic Effects

To maximize the therapeutic effects of quinidine, adjust the dose to achieve a serum plasma drug concentration of 2 to 6 mg/mL. Additionally, monitor the serum potassium level and maintain it in a normal range to promote action of quinidine. Give medication at the same time daily to maintain blood levels.

Minimizing Adverse Effects

Administer oral quinidine with food to prevent GI upset and thus avoid altered nutrition. Give a test dose of a single 200-mg tablet or 200 mg intramuscularly to determine whether the patient has an idiosyncratic reaction to quinidine. It is important to connect the patient to a cardiac monitor and monitor rhythm continuously (when given intravenously) or obtain frequent ECGs (when quinidine is given orally).

Stop the quinidine and notify the prescriber if any of the following events occurs:

- Increase exceeding 25% in duration of QRS complex
- Disappearance of P waves
- Restoration of sinus rhythm

When using an intravenous (IV) infusion pump, it is important to dilute 800 mg of quinidine with 50 mL of D_5W and infuse slowly at 1 mL/min. Monitor serum quinidine levels to detect excessively high values and frequently monitor arterial blood pressure (when given intravenously). If blood pressure falls substantially, therapy should be discontinued, and the prescriber should be notified.

Monitor blood counts and liver and kidney function tests. Discontinue if blood dyscrasias develop or if liver or renal function tests disclose elevated values.

Treatment of a drug overdose may include gastric lavage, emesis, or administration of activated charcoal. Other management includes symptomatic management of CNS and GI effects and checking ECG tracings, blood gases, serum electrolytes, and blood pressure. It also is important to institute measures to acidify the urine. Mechanical ventilation and other supportive measures may be needed. IV infusion of 1/6 molar sodium lactate may be used to reduce the cardiotoxic effects of quinidine.

Providing Patient and Family Education

- Explain the purpose of the drug and the potential adverse effects.
- Teach the patient to take the medication at the same time each day.
- Explain the rationale for ECG monitoring and frequent blood testing, which is that these are methods used to detect early onset of adverse effects.
- Emphasize the importance of returning for follow-up tests.
- Teach patients not to chew oral, sustained-release tablets.
- Instruct patients to take oral doses with food to prevent GI upset.
- Emphasize the importance of notifying the prescriber or the nurse in the hospital if tinnitus, visual disturbances, dizziness, headache, nausea, skin rash, or breathing difficulty is experienced.

Ongoing Assessment and Evaluation

The patient's ECG will be monitored throughout therapy. Quinidine blood levels are checked to ensure that they are therapeutic, not toxic. Periodically, liver enzymes, renal function, and complete blood counts also are monitored. Drug therapy is considered effective if the arrhythmia is converted and does not recur and if the patient does not develop serious adverse effects from the drug.

Drugs Significantly Different From P Quinidine

Class IB Antiarrhythmics

The Class IB drugs are similar to quinidine (Class IA) and Class IC drugs because they depress phase 0 (although not as much). Unlike quinidine, they also suppress automaticity. Like quinidine, these drugs also may cause arrhythmias in addition to treating them. Unlike quinidine, they are used primarily with ventricular arrhythmias, and they may shorten the action potential duration (see Table 26.1). Class IB drugs have little hemodynamic effect and do not suppress left ventricular function (Haugh, 2002). The most important of these drugs are discussed below.

MEMORY CHIP

P Quinidine

- Class I antiarrhythmic used in atrial arrhythmias, such as atrial flutter and fibrillation
- Decreases myocardial excitability, conduction velocity, and contractility
- Prevents re-entry phenomenon
- Exerts an indirect anticholinergic effect
- Major contraindications: cardiac arrhythmias related to conduction abnormalities (complete heart block, left bundle branch block, complete atrioventricular block, long QT syndrome, and drug-induced torsades de pointes)
- Most common adverse effects: GI related
- Most serious adverse effect: cardiotoxicity
- Maximizing therapeutic effects: Adjust dose until reaching therapeutic range and maintain potassium at normal levels.
- Minimizing adverse effects: Monitor electrocardiogram and use an IV infusion pump if given intravenously.
- Most important patient education: Take oral doses with food.

LIDOCAINE

Lidocaine (Xylocaine) may be used with all acute ventricular arrhythmias that are related to cardiac surgery or acute myocardial infarction because these may be life threatening. In other strengths and routes, lidocaine also is used as a local and topical anesthetic. Lidocaine used to treat arrhythmias will, in therapeutic levels, weaken phase 4 diastolic depolarization, decrease the automaticity, and decrease or cause no change in the excitability and membrane responsiveness. Additionally, it decreases the action potential duration and the effective refractory period of Purkinje fibers and ventricular muscle. However, the ratio of the effective refractory period to the action potential duration is increased. The effective refractory period of the AV node may increase, decrease, or remain unchanged; the atrial effective refractory period remains unchanged. Lidocaine raises the ventricular fibrillation threshold, which is why it is effective in treating ventricular fibrillation.

Clinical electrophysiologic studies have demonstrated no change in sinus node recovery time, sinoatrial conduction time, and His-Purkinje fibers conduction time. AV node conduction time is either unchanged, or it may be shortened. Lidocaine does increase the electrical stimulation threshold of the ventricle during diastole. This increase enables a longer diastole because the ventricle requires a longer time before it can be receptive to depolarization and contract again. This effect is helpful in treating ventricular arrhythmias. In therapeutic doses (serum levels of 1.5 to 6 μg/mL), lidocaine has no effect on the contractility of the heart, blood pressure, or the absolute refractory period.

Lidocaine is usually administered intravenously because it is ineffective orally. Under certain circumstances, it may be administered intramuscularly. Single IM doses are justified

in the following exceptional circumstances: ECG equipment not available to verify diagnosis (but the potential benefits must outweigh the possible risk) and when the facilities for IV administration are not readily available. When given intramuscularly, higher and more rapid serum levels are achieved by injection into the deltoid muscle over the gluteus or vastus lateralis. However, lidocaine given intramuscularly may increase creatine phosphokinase (CPK) levels. CPK is an enzyme used as a diagnostic test for acute myocardial infarction (MI). Lidocaine is about 50% protein bound. Lidocaine is metabolized extensively in the liver into at least two active metabolites. These metabolites have both antiarrhythmic and convulsant (inducing convulsions) effects. Metabolism of this drug is impaired substantially by any condition that impairs liver function. Although renal elimination only processes about 10% of the dose given, it is highly involved in the excretion of the metabolites. Accumulation of one of the metabolites (known as GX) because of renal disease or impaired renal function contributes to lidocaine toxicity.

Lidocaine has a biphasic half-life. The half-life involved with the distribution phase is less than 10 minutes. This brevity accounts for the short duration of action when an IV bolus is given. Because of the drug's very short half-life, repeated boluses may be required to quickly achieve therapeutic level when a continuous IV infusion is required to maintain the therapeutic effects (see Table 26.1 for dosing information). The elimination half-life is 1.5 to 2 hours. It may be 3 hours or more if the lidocaine infusion has lasted longer than 24 hours.

Lidocaine is a pregnancy category B drug. However, caution should be used because no adequate and well-controlled studies have been done in pregnant women. Although safety and efficacy have not been established with children from clinical studies, the American Heart Association's Standards and Guidelines recommend using lidocaine when needed in children (see Table 26.1). Caution should be used, and lower doses are recommended, for patients who have CHF, reduced cardiac output, digitalis toxicity accompanied by AV block, hypovolemia and shock, in all forms of heart block, and when used in older adults.

Adverse effects of lidocaine are seen particularly in the CV system and CNS. CV effects are related to serum levels, with the most severe cardiac depression coinciding with toxic levels of lidocaine. The most common CV effects are cardiac arrhythmias and hypotension. Other effects include bradycardia and CV collapse, which may lead to cardiac arrest. CNS adverse effects also are related to blood concentrations of lidocaine. The most common CNS effects are dizziness, lightheadedness, fatigue, and drowsiness. These common, mild effects are seen with low blood levels of lidocaine and resolve rapidly. As blood levels of lidocaine rise, nervousness, confusion, mood changes, hallucinations, euphoria, tinnitus, blurred or double vision, and a sensation of heat, cold, or numbness may occur. In common health care jargon, these CNS effects are referred to as the "lidocaine crazies." With excessively high serum levels of lidocaine (>6 µg/mL), toxicity is present, and the patient develops seizures and loses consciousness.

It is very important to continually monitor the ECG of the patient receiving IV lidocaine. Emergency resuscitative equipment and drug therapy should be on hand in case the patient develops serious adverse effects. As soon as the patient is clinically stable, she or he should be switched to another antiarrhythmic that can be given orally.

TOCAINIDE

Tocainide (Tonocard) is used to treat life-threatening ventricular arrhythmias. As a Class IB antiarrhythmic, it is similar to lidocaine, producing dose-dependent decreases in sodium and potassium conduction and thereby decreasing the excitability of the cardiac cells. Most patients who respond to lidocaine will respond to tocainide. Failure to respond to lidocaine usually indicates that the patient will not respond to tocainide either. The electrophysiologic effects of tocainide are similar to those seen with lidocaine. Tocainide does not prolong the QRS duration or QT intervals. Tocainide slightly depresses the left ventricular function and left ventricular end-diastolic pressure. Usually, this effect produces no changes in the cardiac output. It does slightly, but significantly, increase aortic and pulmonary arterial pressures. This effect is most likely related to increases in vascular resistance. Tocainide has been used safely in patients with acute MI, post-MI, and various degrees of CHF.

Tocainide is given orally because it does not have the high metabolism of lidocaine. Bioavailability of tocainide is nearly 100%; peak serum levels are reached in 0.5 to 2 hours after oral dosing. Protein binding is very low at 10% to 20%. It is inactivated by conjugation in the liver. About 40% of the drug is excreted in the urine unchanged. Half-life is increased in severe renal dysfunction.

It is important to use tocainide cautiously in patients with known heart failure or minimal cardiac reserve, or when beginning or continuing antiarrhythmic therapy in the presence of signs of increasing depression of cardiac conductivity. Like all antiarrhythmics, tocainide can be proarrhythmic. The most common adverse effects are dizziness, vertigo, nausea, paresthesia, and tremor. These reactions are generally mild, transient, and dose related; they are reversible by reducing the dose, by taking the drug with food, or by discontinuing the therapy. The most serious adverse effect, although not common (less than 1% of patients), is the occurrence of blood dyscrasias (e.g., agranulocytosis, depressed bone marrow function, leukopenia, neutropenia, aplastic or hypoplastic anemia, and thrombocytopenia). These effects, which usually occur during the first 12 weeks of therapy, can be fatal in about one fourth of patients who experience them. Monitor blood work weekly during this period for signs of any of these effects. If any of these disorders are diagnosed, discontinue the tocainide immediately. Blood work should return to normal within 1 month.

Fatalities also have occurred with patients who develop severe pulmonary disorders (such as pulmonary fibrosis, interstitial pneumonitis, fibrosing alveolitis, pulmonary edema, and pneumonia). Instruct patients to report immediately any pulmonary symptoms, such as shortness of breath on exertion, cough, or wheezing. Discontinue tocainide if any of these disorders develop.

Other potential adverse effects include:

- CV: ventricular fibrillation, extension of acute MI, cardiogenic shock, angina, AV block, hypertension, increased QRS duration, pericarditis, prolonged QT interval, right bundle branch block, syncope, vasovagal episodes, cardiomegaly, sinus arrest, vasculitis, and orthostatic hypotension

- CNS: coma, convulsions/seizures, depression, psychosis, agitation, decreased mental acuity, dysarthria, impaired memory, increased stuttering, slurred speech, insomnia, sleep disturbances, local anesthesia, dream abnormalities, myasthenia gravis, and malaise
- Dermatologic: Stevens-Johnson syndrome, exfoliative dermatitis, erythema multiforme, urticaria, alopecia, pruritus, and pallor or flushed face
- GI: abdominal pain, constipation, stomatitis, dysphagia, dyspepsia, thirst, and dry mouth
- Hepatic: hepatitis and jaundice
- Respiratory: respiratory arrest and pulmonary edema or embolism

MEXILETINE

Mexiletine (Mexitil) is another Class IB drug. It also is used in life-threatening ventricular arrhythmias and, like all antiarrhythmics, may produce arrhythmias. It only is administered orally. It has pharmacologic and electrophysiologic properties similar to those of lidocaine.

MORICIZINE

Moricizine (Ethmozine) is used in documented life-threatening arrhythmias. Compared with quinidine, it has a longer time until onset of action and a longer duration of action. It shares some of the characteristics of other drugs in Class 1A, 1B, and 1C. Because of its strong proarrhythmic effects, its use is limited.

PHENYTOIN

Although treatment of arrhythmias is not a labeled use of phenytoin (Dilantin), it is used commonly in treating digitalis-induced arrhythmias. It, like other Class IB drugs, depresses phase 0 slightly and may shorten the action potential. A full discussion of phenytoin and its use in treating seizures can be found in Chapter 19.

Class IC Antiarrhythmics

Class IC drugs are flecainide (Tambocor) and propafenone (Rythmol) (see Table 26.1). These drugs depress phase 0 considerably. In addition, they have a slight effect on repolarization and decrease conduction substantially. Flecainide can be in paroxysmal SVTs, including AV nodal re-entry tachycardia and AV re-entry tachycardia. The proarrhythmic effects of flecainide range from an increase in frequency of PVCs to the development of more severe ventricular tachycardias. Propafenone is used to treat life-threatening ventricular arrhythmias and has similar proarrhythmic actions to flecainide. Both of these Class IC drugs can be given orally. The use of Class IC drugs is limited to patients with life-threatening arrhythmias.

C CLASS II ANTIARRHYTHMIC DRUGS

Antiarrhythmic Class II drugs (beta blockers) depress phase 4 depolarization. They slow the heart rate and reduce contractility. The prototype class II drug is propranolol (Inderal). Other drugs in this class are acebutolol (Monitan) and esmolol (Brevibloc). It is important to keep in mind that only some of the beta blockers are approved for use as antiarrhythmics. What follows is a brief discussion of propranolol when it is used solely as an antiarrhythmic. Propranolol is discussed in more depth in Chapter 13. Other uses of beta blockers relevant to CV function are found in Chapters 27, 28, and 29.

NURSING MANAGEMENT OF THE PATIENT RECEIVING P PROPRANOLOL

Propranolol is used for treating cardiac arrhythmias, specifically supraventricular tachycardia, ventricular, and tachyarrhythmias secondary to digoxin toxicity. Propranolol also is used alone or in combination to treat hypertension. Other uses include treating angina, MI, and hypertrophic subaortic stenosis.

Propranolol blocks the beta-adrenergic receptor sites; thus, it is classified as a beta blocker. This blockage of the receptor sites occurs as the drug competes with beta-adrenergic agonists for available beta receptor sites. Propranolol blocks both the beta-1 sites, which are located chiefly in the cardiac muscle, and beta-2 receptors, which are located chiefly in the bronchial and vascular musculature.

Several mechanisms have been proposed by which propranolol achieves its effects on the CV system. One mechanism is that propranolol competitively blocks catecholamines at non-CNS adrenergic neuron sites, especially in the heart, thereby leading to decreased cardiac output. A second mechanism is a central effect that leads to reduced sympathetic outflow to the periphery. Third, because stimulation of beta receptors is responsible for the release of renin from the kidneys, beta blockade with propranolol prevents renin from being released. Total peripheral resistance initially increases slightly because of these mechanisms. However, it readjusts to the pretreatment level or lower with chronic use. Because the decrease in cardiac output is greater than the increase in peripheral resistance, blood pressure is lowered. Propranolol also has a membrane-stabilizing effect, like that of anesthetics, which depresses the cardiac action potential. This effect is what causes the antiarrhythmic response.

Propranolol is contraindicated in sinus bradycardia, greater than first-degree heart block, cardiogenic shock, CHF (unless secondary to a tachyarrhythmia treatable with beta blockers), overt cardiac failure, diabetes, bronchial asthma or bronchospasm, severe chronic obstructive pulmonary disease, and hypersensitivity to beta blockers. For a full discussion of propranolol, refer to Chapter 13.

C CLASS III ANTIARRHYTHMIC DRUGS

Class III antiarrhythmics produce a prolongation of phase 3 (repolarization). Action potential duration and refractory periods are prolonged, leading to reduction in membrane excitability of all myocardial tissue. The drugs in this class include amiodarone (Cordarone), sotalol, bretylium (bretylium tosylate, Bretylol), ibutilide (Corvert), and dofetilide (Tikosyn). Table 26.3 presents a summary of selected drugs

TABLE 26.3 Summary of Selected (C) Class III Antiarrhythmics

Drug (Trade) Name	Selected Indications	Route and Dosage Range	Pharmacokinetics
[P] amiodarone (Cordarone)	Ventricular fibrillation	*Adult:* PO, 800–1,600 mg/d in divided doses for 1–3 wk; reduce to 600–800 mg/d in divided doses for 1 mo *Child:* Not established	*Onset:* 2–3 q *Duration:* 6–8 h $t_{1/2}$: 2.5–10 d, then 40–55 d
sotalol (Betapace; *Canadian:* Sotacor)	Ventricular arrhythmias	*Adult:* PO, 80 mg bid; adjust gradually q2–3d; may require 240–320 mg/d	*Onset:* Varies *Duration* and $t_{1/2}$: 12 h
bretylium (Bretylol; *Canadian:* Bretylate)	Ventricular fibrillation	*Adult:* IV, 5 mg/kg by rapid bolus *Child:* IV, 5 mg/kg per dose followed by 10 mg/kg at 15–30 min intervals, maximum 30 mg/kg	*Onset:* IM, varies; IV, min *Duration:* IM, IV, 24 h $t_{1/2}$: 6.9–8.1 h
	Ventricular arrhythmias	*Adult:* IV, infuse diluted solution of 5–10 mg/kg >8 min, and repeat q1–2h; IM, 5–10 mg/kg undiluted, repeated at 1–2 h intervals if arrhythmias persist *Child:* IV, 5–10 mg/kg per dose q6h	
ibutilide (Covert)	Atrial fibrillation Atrial flutter	*Adult (≥60 kg):* IV, 1 mg infused over 10 min (<60 kg): 0.01 mg/kg infused over 10 min; may repeat 1 ×	*Onset:* Within 10 min *Duration:* Variable $t_{1/2}$: 2–12 h

in this class. The prototype Class III antiarrhythmic is amiodarone.

NURSING MANAGEMENT OF THE PATIENT RECEIVING [P] AMIODARONE

Core Drug Knowledge

Pharmacotherapeutics

Because of severe and potentially lethal adverse effects, amiodarone is only approved for use in life-threatening arrhythmias. Orally, amiodarone (Cordarone, Pacerone) is used in treating only the following documented life-threatening ventricular arrhythmias that do not respond to documented adequate doses of other antiarrhythmics or when alternative agents are not tolerated:

- Recurrent ventricular fibrillation
- Recurrent, hemodynamically unstable ventricular tachycardia

If the patient is nonresponsive to other therapy, intravenous amiodarone is used in the initiation of treatment and as prophylaxis for frequently recurring ventricular fibrillation and hemodynamically unstable ventricular tachycardia. Intravenous amiodarone also can be used in patients who meet the requirements for oral amiodarone but who cannot take oral medication.

Amiodarone is not specifically FDA approved for treating AF; it has been found to be effective in patients with paroxysmal or persistent AF (VerNooy & Mounsey, 2004). For chronic maintenance therapy of AF, Amiodarone has been established as the antiarrhythmic with the highest efficacy (VerNooy & Mounsey, 2004).

Pharmacokinetics

With oral administration, amiodarone is absorbed slowly, and the absorption is highly variable. The bioavailability of a single dose of the drug (oral or IV) is about 50% of the dose given, although it can range from 35% to 65%. Some researchers suggest that the incomplete bioavailability is caused by incomplete absorption related to amiodarone's high lipid solubility. Incomplete bioavailability has ramifications for dosing when the patient is being switched from oral to IV (or vice versa). The patient may require a smaller IV dose than the oral dose.

Amiodarone is widely distributed throughout the body, with much variability. It is extensively distributed in some sites, such as adipose tissue and highly perfused organs (e.g., liver, lung, and spleen). Variability in distribution contributes to variability in response to drug therapy, which is exhibited by the patient. The drug is highly protein bound (96%). This high protein binding also complicates the distribution of amiodarone. Individual variability in protein levels may cause some of the variability of drug action. Free drug levels are difficult to measure in extensive protein binding. Because of its high lipid solubility, amiodarone and its metabolite are thought to concentrate in cell membranes, especially of the liver, heart, and fat cells.

Research supports the idea that the slow distribution of amiodarone into tissue sites is an important component of the drug's unusual pharmacokinetic and pharmacodynamic activities.

Metabolism occurs in the liver, apparently by cytochrome P-450 3A4, forming an active metabolite, diethanolamine (DEA). DEA accumulates in most tissues to an even greater extent than the parent, amiodarone. DEA has pharmacologic properties similar to amiodarone. Like amiodarone, DEA is highly protein bound, although its distribution is concentrated in the heart.

The actual route of amiodarone elimination is not well understood. Amiodarone has a biphasic elimination with

an initial one-half reduction of plasma levels after 2.5 to 107 days. A much slower terminal plasma elimination has a mean half-life of 53 days for amiodarone and 61 days for DEA. Thus, it takes almost a year for the drug to reach steady state with chronic oral administration. Because of this, a loading regimen of the drug is needed to achieve an initial pharmacologic effect. With prolonged administration, serum concentrations of amiodarone and DEA are similar. The main route of excretion is hepatic into the bile. Some enterohepatic recirculation may occur (see Table 26.3).

Pharmacodynamics

Although amiodarone produces electrophysiologic changes characteristic of all four antiarrhythmic classes, it predominantly has Class III effects. Amiodarone has two major properties: prolongation of the refractory period, and noncompetitive alpha- and beta-adrenergic inhibition. It also modulates thyroid function (one molecule of amiodarone contains two iodine atoms, and amiodarone shares some structural similarities to thyroid hormones), phospholipid metabolism, and production of certain cytokine (extracellular factors that are important in controlling the inflammatory response).

Like Class I antiarrhythmic drugs, amiodarone blocks the fast sodium channel. It may do this when the channel is in the inactivated state. Unlike Class I antiarrhythmic drugs, amiodarone also blocks potassium channels. These activities contribute to the slowing of conduction and increased refractory period. Amiodarone blocks multiple potassium channels, including inward and outward currents. Like Class II antiarrhythmic drugs, amiodarone has a noncompetitive antisympathetic action. Like Class IV antiarrhythmic drugs, it has a negative chronotropic effect (slowing heart rate) from blocking the slow calcium channel. All these actions (blocking sodium, potassium, and calcium channels, and inhibition of sympathetic action) have an effect on slowing conduction (negative dromotropic effect) at the SA node and on slowing conduction and increasing the refractory period at the AV node. Amiodarone does have some vasodilating effects, which decrease the oxygen needs of the heart.

The effect on sodium channels appears to be limited to acute dosing (by IV) and is not present in chronic dosing. The effect on calcium and potassium channels may be both acute and chronic. However, unlike oral dosing, IV dosing has little or no effect on the length of the sinus cycle, the refractoriness of the right atrium or right ventricle, repolarization, intraventricular conduction, and infranodal (below or beneath the nodes) conduction. These differences suggest that the initial acute effects of amiodarone IV are focused predominantly on the AV node (because of sodium channel blockade).

Several electrophysiologic effects occur with the administration of amiodarone. An increased cardiac refractory period occurs, usually without influencing the resting membrane potential. Sinus rate decreases by 15% to 20%. The PR and QT intervals increase by about 10%. U waves appear, and T waves are altered. These changes do not usually require discontinuation of amiodarone, although marked sinus bradycardia or sinus arrest and heart block can occur. QT prolongation can be associated with worsening of the arrhythmia, but this event is rare.

After IV dosing, amiodarone relaxes the vascular smooth muscle, reduces peripheral vascular resistance (decreasing afterload), and slightly increases the cardiac index (ratio of cardiac output per minute to the body surface area). With oral dosing, amiodarone produces no appreciable change in left ventricular ejection fraction. After acute IV dosing, amiodarone may have a mild negative inotropic effect on left ventricular ejection fraction, decreasing the force of contractility. Oral dosing, however, produces no meaningful change in left ventricular ejection fraction.

Because of its ability to lengthen repolarization and refractoriness in atria and ventricles, while also blocking adrenergic stimulation, amiodarone is a potentially valuable drug in treating atrial fibrillation. One reason that amiodarone's use in atrial fibrillation is attractive to researchers is its ability to increase the action potential duration in atrial and ventricular tissues following chronic drug administration, while producing lesser effects in Purkinje fibers and M cells (special cardiac cells). Additionally, its effect on repolarization is not influenced by heart rate. Despite producing marked slowing of the heart rate and substantial increases in the QT interval, the drug only seldom produces torsades de pointes (see Adverse Effects). Amiodarone is known to be effective in maintaining normal sinus rhythm, which is now considered crucial in treating atrial fibrillation. Low doses of amiodarone have been found to maintain sinus rhythm in patients with paroxysmal or chronic atrial fibrillation who were previously nonresponsive to other drug therapies. Furthermore, amiodarone has been found to effectively treat and prevent atrial fibrillation in patients who have CHF. Few other drugs have this benefit, yet almost 40% of patients with CHF develop atrial fibrillation.

Contraindications and Precautions

Contraindications for giving the drug orally include severe sinus-node dysfunction producing marked sinus bradycardia, second- and third-degree AV block, and a history of episodes of bradycardia that have caused syncope (unless the drug is used with a pacemaker). Contraindications for giving the drug intravenously are similar and include marked sinus bradycardia, second- and third-degree AV block (unless the patient has a functioning pacemaker), and cardiogenic shock. Additionally, if patients have a known hypersensitivity response to the drug, it should be avoided.

Amiodarone inhibits peripheral conversion of thyroxine (T_4) to triiodothyronine (T_3), prompting increased T_4 levels, increased levels of inactive reverse T_3, and decreased levels of T_3. It also is a potential source of large amounts of inorganic iodine. Because it releases inorganic iodine, and perhaps for other unknown reasons, amiodarone can cause hypothyroidism or hyperthyroidism. Because of the slow elimination of amiodarone and its metabolite, high plasma iodide levels, altered thyroid function, and abnormal thyroid function tests may persist for several weeks or months after the drug is discontinued.

Amiodarone is in pregnancy category D. It can cause congenital goiter/hypothyroidism or hyperthyroidism. Amiodarone is excreted into breast milk. In animal studies, nursing offspring are less viable and have reduced body weight gains.

Adverse Effects

Amiodarone has several adverse effects that are potentially fatal. Pulmonary toxicity is the most important of these serious adverse effects. The frequency of pulmonary toxicity with

amiodarone is between 2% and 17%. About 10% of the patients who develop pulmonary toxicity will die. The syndrome, seen frequently with oral dosing, is cough, progressive dyspnea, and test findings (e.g., radiographic, gallium scan, or pulmonary function tests) consistent with pulmonary toxicity. Phospholipidosis (foamy cells, foamy macrophages) will be present in most cases of amiodarone-induced pulmonary toxicity. However, this finding is not a specific marker for amiodarone toxicity; these changes are also present in about 50% of patients taking the drug.

Any new changes in the respiratory system warrant the patient being re-examined to determine whether pulmonary toxicity is present. Amiodarone is prescribed to patients with life-threatening arrhythmias. Therefore, the drug must be discontinued cautiously if pulmonary toxicity is suspected because more patients die from sudden cardiac death (the most common cause of death for these patients) than from pulmonary toxicity. Before discontinuing amiodarone because of suspected pulmonary toxicity, other causes of respiratory impairment (e.g., infection) should be ruled out.

Another potentially fatal adverse effect of amiodarone is exacerbation of the arrhythmia it is treating. It also may make the arrhythmia more difficult to reverse. This event occurs in about 2% to 5% of patients treated. The risk for exacerbation is increased if more than one type of arrhythmia is present. Exacerbation can include new ventricular fibrillation, incessant ventricular tachycardia, increased resistance to cardioversion, and polymorphic (more than one form) ventricular tachycardia associated with QT prolongation (torsades de pointes). Amiodarone also has caused symptomatic bradycardia, heart block, and sinus arrest with suppression of escape foci (ectopic foci picking up as pacemaker when SA is not functioning to maintain a heartbeat) in 2% to 4% of patients. Drug-related bradycardia does not appear to be dose related.

A final potentially lethal adverse effect is liver disease. This effect is very rare, however. Some liver injury, evidenced only by elevated liver enzyme levels, is common with amiodarone, but such injury is normally mild and not serious.

Optic neuritis or optic neuropathy, although not a fatal adverse effect, can be a potentially serious adverse effect because visual impairment can occur and may result in permanent blindness. This adverse effect is rare, however.

Other adverse effects include common CNS effects (e.g., malaise, dizziness, paresthesia, tremor, headache, and insomnia). These can occur in 20% to 40% of patients. The effects are not serious, rarely require discontinuing the drug, and often are alleviated with dosage reduction or dividing the dose. GI complaints (e.g., nausea, vomiting, constipation, anorexia, and abdominal pain) also are common; about 25% of patients have these complaints. The drug rarely needs to be discontinued because of these effects. The GI effects are seen mostly with high doses and usually are alleviated with dose reduction or divided doses.

Photosensitivity is a problem for about 10% of patients taking amiodarone. With long-term treatment, a blue-gray discoloration of the exposed skin may be seen. The risk, which may be increased in patients with fair complexions or excessive sun exposure, may be related to cumulative dose and the duration of therapy. It will reverse slowly after the drug is discontinued, although sometimes it is irreversible. Hypothyroidism or hyperthyroidism may occur, as may edema, coagulation abnormalities, flushing, epididymitis, vasculitis, pseudotumor cerebri, thrombocytopenia, and angioedema.

When amiodarone is given intravenously, hypotension is its most frequent adverse effect, although it is not normally serious. Clinically significant hypotension occurs in the first few hours of drug administration and appears to be related to the rate of infusion, not the drug concentration. Blood pressure should return to normal if the rate is slowed down.

Drug Interactions

Amiodarone increases the plasma concentration of digoxin. This effect is believed to be caused by amiodarone's inhibition of P-glycoprotein. P-glycoprotein pumps drugs entering the enterocyte back into the intestinal lumen. It also is active on the tubular side of the renal epithelium and the biliary side of hepatocytes and serves to promote drug excretion at these sites. By inhibiting P-glycoprotein excretion, the elimination of digoxin is decreased, increasing blood levels of this drug.

Amiodarone also decreases the clearance of many other drugs, including flecainide and warfarin. Most likely, multiple mechanisms underlie these effects. Amiodarone's impairment of flecainide elimination appears to be mostly renal. Its impairment of warfarin clearance is most likely related to amiodarone being an inhibitor of CYP2C9 (another major isoenzyme of metabolism); warfarin relies solely on CYP2C9 for metabolism. Research on amiodarone's effects on metabolism and elimination of other drugs is continuing. Table 26.4 provides additional information on drug interactions. Amiodarone also interferes with laboratory tests. It alters thyroid function tests because of its effects on T_3 and T_4 and also may alter liver function tests (alanine aminotransferase [ALT], aspartate aminotransferase [AST]).

Assessment of Relevant Core Patient Variables

Health Status

Determine the patient's cardiac status using an ECG. This check will verify whether the patient has an arrhythmia that is responsive to amiodarone and ensure that none of the pathologic conditions that contraindicate amiodarone's use are present. Also, obtain baseline results of thyroid function tests and liver function tests. It is important to assess respiratory status through chest x-ray, pulmonary function studies (including diffusion capacity), and auscultation of breath sounds before treatment.

Life Span and Gender

Determine the patient's age because safety and efficacy have not been established in children. The benzyl alcohol that is contained in some of these products as a preservative has been associated with a fatal "gasping syndrome" in premature infants. In older adults, amiodarone has a lower clearance rate and an increased half-life. It also is important to determine whether the patient is pregnant because amiodarone is a pregnancy category D drug. The drug should only be used if the potential benefits outweigh

TABLE 26.4 Agents That Interact With P Amiodarone

Interactants	Effect and Significance	Nursing Management
anticoagulants	Potentiation of anticoagulant response; prothrombin may be increased	Dose decrease usually needed; monitor prothrombin
beta blockers	May increase risk of bradycardia and hypotension from additive effect	Monitor pulse and blood pressure
calcium channel blockers	Increased risk of atrioventricular block or hypotension	Monitor for electrocardiographic (ECG) changes; monitor blood pressure
cyclosporine	Increased plasma levels of cyclosporine resulting in elevated creatinine	Reduce dose; monitor creatinine levels
dextromethorphan	Impairs metabolism of dextromethorphan	Assess for adverse effects
digoxin	Increased digoxin serum levels	Monitor digoxin levels; decrease dose of digoxin; consider stopping digoxin
disopyramide	Increases QT prolongation; may cause arrhythmias	Monitor for ECG changes
fentanyl	Increases effect of fentanyl and may cause hypotension and bradycardia	Monitor blood pressure and pulse
flecainide	Increases the effect of flecainide	Decrease the dose of flecainide, therapeutic levels will be maintained
hydantoins	Impairs metabolism of hydantoins; elevated serum levels of hydantoins may occur; amiodarone level also may be decreased	Monitor blood levels; assess for adverse effects
lidocaine	Increased levels of lidocaine	Monitor blood pressure (rare complications)
methotrexate	Impairs metabolism of methotrexate	Assess for adverse effects
procainamide	Increased procainamide serum levels may occur	Monitor for adverse effects
quinidine	Increased quinidine levels; potential for fatal arrhythmias	Assess ECG for changes
theophylline	Increased theophylline levels with toxicity	Monitor levels; assess for adverse effects
cholestyramine	Increased enterohepatic elimination of amiodarone, reduced serum levels and half-life may occur	Monitor for therapeutic effects
cimetidine	Increased serum levels of amiodarone may occur	Assess for adverse effects
ritonavir	Large increases in amiodarone blood levels may occur, increasing the risk of adverse effects	Assess for adverse effects; monitor ECG

the substantial risks to the fetus. If the patient is breast-feeding, she should be advised to discontinue nursing while on amiodarone.

Environment

Be aware of the setting in which amiodarone is administered. IV amiodarone is given in an intensive care unit (ICU) where the patient can receive continuous cardiac monitoring. Oral doses can be given in any environment, except when giving a loading dose; during this time, the patient needs to be hospitalized. While the patient is taking oral doses, assess the patient's exposure to sunlight because photosensitivity can occur.

Culture and Inherited Traits

Variations in response to amiodarone may be genetically related. However, little is yet known about this genetic variation.

Nursing Diagnoses and Outcomes

- Decreased Cardiac Output related to cardiac arrhythmia.
  Desired outcome: *Cardiac rhythm will return to normal, allowing for normal cardiac output.*
- Risk for Injury related to adverse effects of drug therapy
  Desired outcome: *The patient will not suffer permanent injury or death as a result of drug therapy.*

Planning and Intervention

Maximizing Therapeutic Effects

To maximize the therapeutic effect of amiodarone, administer the prescribed loading doses. When giving amiodarone intravenously, mix the drug in glass bottles or polyolefin bags of 5% dextrose in water (D_5W). Although some of the amiodarone dose is lost during administration because it is absorbed by polyvinyl chloride tubing, this tubing should be used because the clinical trials that established dosage used this particular type of tubing, and recommended doses account for this loss. Surface properties of solutions of amiodarone are altered so that drop size may be reduced. This size reduction can account for an underdosage of up to 30%. Use a volumetric infusion pump to prevent underdosage.

Minimizing Adverse Effects

Oral and Intravenous Doses

It is important to correct electrolyte disturbances before beginning therapy. Hypokalemia and hypomagnesemia can exaggerate the degree of QT prolongation and increase the

potential for torsades de pointes. Assess for proarrhythmic changes. Use pulse oximetry or arterial blood gases to assess for changes in respiratory function, including breath sounds, dyspnea, and oxygen delivery to the tissues. If changes occur, it is important to repeat the chest x-ray, physical examination, gallium scan, and pulmonary function tests to rule out pulmonary toxicity.

Assess for symptoms of visual impairment. Regular eye examinations are recommended throughout therapy. Ophthalmic examination should be sought immediately if impairment occurs. It also is important to assess T_3 and T_4 levels to determine thyroid function. Assess for signs of hyperthyroidism or hypothyroidism. Liver function studies also should be monitored.

Oral Doses

Monitor the patient closely during the loading phase until the risk for recurrent ventricular tachycardia or fibrillation has abated. It is important to attempt to discontinue prior antiarrhythmic drugs gradually. Reduce the dose of these other drugs by 30% to 50% several days after initiating amiodarone, when arrhythmias should be suppressed.

In patients whose arrhythmias are not well controlled on amiodarone alone, introduce other agents, using half of the usual recommended dosage. It is a good idea to divide the dose or give amiodarone with food to minimize or prevent nausea, vomiting, and other GI effects.

Intravenous Doses

Adjust the starting dose to suppress life-threatening arrhythmias based on individual response to therapy. Monitor the patient continuously during therapy, using a cardiac monitor. It is important to monitor blood pressure carefully because hypotension is most likely to occur in the early period, and to reduce the infusion rate if hypotension occurs.

Avoid administering amiodarone with aminophylline, cefamandole, cefazolin, mezlocillin, heparin, and sodium bicarbonate because these agents are incompatible with amiodarone and will form a precipitate. If possible, administer amiodarone using a central venous catheter to prevent phlebitis.

Use an in-line filter. It is important to use IV therapy until the ventricular arrhythmia is stabilized. Transfer the patient to oral therapy either during or after IV treatment, and adjust the IV dose to a new lower, oral dose. If the patient is treated with IV infusion for less than 1 week, give an oral dose of 800 to 1,600 mg/day initially. If the patient is treated with IV for 1 to 3 weeks, give an oral dose of 600 to 800 mg per day initially. If the patient is treated with IV for longer than 3 weeks, give an oral dose of 400 mg/day initially. When adequate arrhythmia control is achieved, decrease to 600 to 800 mg/day (orally) in one to two doses for 1 month; the maintenance dose is 400 mg/day.

Providing Patient and Family Education

- Explain the purpose of the drug and possible adverse effects of the drug.
- Emphasizes the importance of returning for follow-up blood work and ECGs.
- Teach the patient to use appropriate protection when out in the sun and to limit sun exposure.
- Instruct the patient to notify the physician for new onset of cough, shortness of breath, and changes in visual acuity.

Ongoing Assessment and Evaluation

The patient's ECG should be monitored intermittently throughout therapy and after the initial stabilization and loading dose period for new arrhythmias or worsening of the current arrhythmia being treated. Make recurrent assessments of respiratory function, visual acuity, thyroid function, and liver function. Amiodarone therapy is considered effective if the arrhythmia is corrected and the patient does not develop serious adverse effects.

Drugs Closely Related to P Amiodarone

Sotalol

Sotalol also is categorized as a Class IC antiarrhythmic. Like amiodarone, it prolongs repolarization (phase 3). These Class III effects are seen in doses greater than 160 mg/day. Additionally, like amiodarone, sotalol decreases automaticity at the SA node and ectopic pacemakers. It also decreases conduction velocity at the AV node, although unlike amiodarone, it does not decrease it at the atrium, bundle of His, or Purkinje fibers. ECG changes are similar except that sotalol does not lengthen the QT interval. Although sotalol and amiodarone both have antiadrenergic effects, they work by different mechanisms. Sotalol is actually a beta blocker, blocking both beta-1 and beta-2 sites. It is used in treating life-threatening ventricular arrhythmias. Because of its multiple sites of

MEMORY CHIP

P Amiodarone

- Class III antiarrhythmic used to treat life-threatening ventricular arrhythmias and prevent their recurrence
- Produces prolonged phase of repolarization (phase 3)
- Has properties of Classes I, II, and IV
- Has extremely long half-life and great variability in pharmacodynamics and pharmacokinetics
- Major contraindications: severe sinus bradycardia and second- or third-degree atrioventricular heart block
- Most common adverse effects: central nervous system effects (e.g., malaise, dizziness, paresthesia, tremor, headache, and insomnia); GI effects (e.g., nausea and vomiting); photosensitivity; and hypotension (IV use)
- Most serious adverse effects: pulmonary toxicity and cardiac arrhythmias
- **Life span alert: Drug is in pregnancy category D; use only if benefit outweighs risk.**
- Maximizing therapeutic effects: Use a loading dose.
- Minimizing adverse effects: Correct pre-existing electrolyte imbalances before giving the drug; adjust IV dose to control ventricular arrhythmia; monitor blood pressure (IV dosing); monitor electrocardiogram for changes; and assess for respiratory changes.
- Most important patient education: Take with food to minimize GI distress and notify the physician if cough or shortness of breath develops.

CRITICAL THINKING SCENARIO

Amiodarone therapy

Mr. Bowen is 74 years old. He was brought to the hospital emergency department by ambulance. He was diagnosed with myocardial infarction and was in ventricular fibrillation arrhythmia. He is cardioverted to sinus rhythm and started on amiodarone by IV infusion. When he is transferred to the intensive care unit, his blood pressure drops to 88/50 mmHg. The intensive care unit nurse examines Mr. Bowen's laboratory results; the only unexpected finding is that he has a low serum albumin level.

1. What possible causes may account for the hypotension?
2. What action should you take to manage Mr. Bowen's hypotension?
3. If you are unable to correct the hypotension, what might you do next?

action, it, like amiodarone, is being studied and recommended for use in treating atrial fibrillation. Sotalol has been shown to maintain sinus rhythm in about half the patients with atrial fibrillation after cardioversion to their normal rhythm. Like all other antiarrhythmics, sotalol may induce arrhythmias as well as treat them. Torsades de pointes, although possible, is not likely to occur if the dose is controlled, if the patient has normal renal function, and if the patient does not have severe CHF. Sotalol is administered orally after the patient has been on IV antiarrhythmics for ventricular arrhythmias. It is considered safe to begin therapy in the outpatient setting if given for atrial fibrillation (see Table 26.3).

Bretylium

Bretylium also is used in treating life-threatening ventricular arrhythmias when the patient has failed to respond to first-line drugs, such as lidocaine. Like amiodarone, bretylium prolongs phase 3 (repolarization) and the refractory period. Unlike amiodarone, bretylium increases the automaticity of the SA node and ectopic pacemakers and has no effect on the conduction velocity in the atrium and the AV node. Bretylium also does not produce the ECG changes that amiodarone does. Bretylium has a much shorter duration of action (6–8 hours) and half-life (5–10 days) than amiodarone. It is has a very low protein binding compared with that of amiodarone, which is very high. Bretylium is given only by IV infusion.

Transient tachycardia and elevated blood pressure may occur after administration of bretylium as a result of the initial release of norepinephrine. Subsequently, the release of norepinephrine is blocked, and orthostatic hypotension may occur.

The most frequent adverse effect is postural hypotension, occurring in about half the patients receiving the drug while they are supine. Other adverse effects include bradycardia, increased premature ventricular contractions, transient hypertension, initial increase in arrhythmias, and angina. Nausea and vomiting can occur, usually after rapid IV administration (see Table 26.3).

Ibutilide and Dofetilide

Ibutilide and dofetilide are both new drugs in the category termed the "pure" Class III antiarrhythmics. They are not as multifaceted as amiodarone. The goal of developing these new Class III drugs was to find a drug as effective as amiodarone but without its adverse effects.

Ibutilide was the first of the pure Class III drugs approved for use in the United States. It is approved only for IV use to convert atrial flutter and atrial fibrillation to normal sinus rhythm. It is about twice as effective in converting atrial flutter as atrial fibrillation. Ibutilide increases the atrial effective refractory period and prolongs the QT interval. This effect on the QT interval is dose dependent. Ibutilide also causes some blockade of potassium channels. As a result, duration of the action potential in the ventricles is also prolonged somewhat. Ibutilide is metabolized extensively in the liver; its high first-pass effect is the reason it must be given intravenously. Unlike amiodarone, ibutilide has a short half-life of 4 to 8 hours; its metabolites have a similar half-life. Ibutilide distributes rapidly to a large volume, and its electrophysiologic effects decrease quickly after IV administration. Proarrhythmia effects are therefore greatest within the first hour of administration. Ibutilide use is associated with an estimated 8% risk for torsades de pointes. When it occurs, it often is transient. However, if ibutilide is given concurrently with beta blockers or calcium channel blockers, torsades de pointes is more likely to occur.

Dofetilide is used to convert patients in atrial fibrillation to normal sinus rhythm and maintain them in sinus rhythm. Dofetilide delays repolarization in the atria, ventricles, and Purkinje fibers by blocking some of the potassium channels. It has no effect on sodium or calcium channels and thus little effect on conduction velocity, force of contraction, and systemic hemodynamics. It is not approved for managing ventricular arrhythmias, and its efficacy for these arrhythmias is under investigation (Khan, 2004). It increases repolarization and refractoriness in both atrial and ventricular tissue, although the predominant effect is on the atrial tissue. It is well absorbed orally and has a bioavailability of more than 90%. Most of the drug is excreted unchanged in the urine, and the rest is metabolized in the liver. Dofetilide has a reverse use-dependent effect, and at slow rates has the tendency to increase the QT interval. Dofetilide is not likely to cause torsades de pointes.

C CLASS IV ANTIARRHYTHMIC DRUGS

Class IV antiarrhythmics depress phase 4 depolarization and lengthen phases 1 and 2 of repolarization (see Figure 26.6). This class is composed of several calcium channel blockers, but only two have been approved specifically as antiarrhythmics: verapamil (Calan) and diltiazem (Alti-diltiazem [Canada], Apo-Diltiaz [Canada], Cardizem, Dilacor). Table 26.5 presents a summary of selected Class IV antiarrhythmics and other calcium channel blockers. The prototype Class IV antiarrhythmic calcium channel blocker is verapamil.

Calcium channel blockers prescribed for other purposes include amlodipine (Norvasc), bepridil (Vascor), felodipine (Plendil), isradipine (Dyna Circ), nimodipine (Nimotop), nisoldipine (Sular), nicardipine (Cardene), and nifedipine (Procardia, Adalat). Other uses of calcium channel blockers are described in Chapters 27 and 29. Adenosine is a non–calcium channel blocker drug that is significantly different from verapamil.

TABLE 26.5 Summary of Selected (C) Class IV Antiarrhythmics and Selected Other Calcium Channel Blockers

Drug (Trade) Name	Selected Indications	Route and Dosage Range	Pharmacokinetics
[P] verapamil (Calan, Isoptin)	Angina pectoris	*Adult:* PO, 80–120 mg tid, increase q1–2d as needed	*Onset:* PO, 30 min; IV, rapid *Duration:* PO, 3–7 h; IV, 2 h $t_{1/2}$: 3–7 h
	Supraventricular tachyarrhythmias	*Adult:* IV, 5–10 mg over 2 min; may repeat dose of 10 mg 30 min after first dose. Give dose over 3 min for elderly. *Child:* IV, >1 y, 0.1–0.2 mg/kg over 2 min; 1–15 y, 0.1–0.3 mg/kg over 2 min; do not exceed 5 mg; repeat after 30 min, if necessary.	
	Hypertension	*Adult:* PO, 240 mg qd; sustained-release form in morning; 80 mg tid. May need to individualize dose by titration.	
diltiazem (Cardizem, Tiazac; *Canadian:* Apo-Diltiaz)	Angina pectoris Essential hypertension Atrial fibrillation or flutter (IV only)	*Adult:* PO, 30 mg qid before meals and hs, increase gradually at 1–2 d intervals to 180–360 mg in three to four divided doses; SR, cardizem CD, 180–240 mg/d PO for hypertension; 120–180 mg/d PO for angina IV, 0.25 mg/kg over 2 min; second bolus of 0.35 mg/kg given over 2 min IV infusion: 5–15 mg/h for up to 24 h *Child:* Safety and efficacy not established	*Onset:* PO and SR, 30–60 min; IV, immediate *Duration:* Unknown $t_{1/2}$: 3½–6 h; SR, 5–7 h
Non-antiarrhythmic Calcium Channel Blockers			
amlodipine (Norvasc)	Angina pectoris Essential hypertension	*Adult:* PO, 5 mg qd, may increase over 10–14 d to a max dose of 10 mg/d *Child:* Safety and efficacy not established	*Onset:* PO, unknown *Duration:* Unknown $t_{1/2}$: 30–50 h
nicardipine (Cardene)	Stable angina	*Adult:* PO, 20 mg tid; range, 20–40 mg tid; allow 3 d before increasing dosage *Child:* Safety and efficacy not established	*Onset:* 20 min *Duration:* Unknown $t_{1/2}$: 2–4 h
	Hypertension	*Adult:* PO, 20 mg tid; range 20–40 mg tid. Adjust dosage based on BP response; allow 3 d before increasing *Child:* Safety and efficacy not established	

NURSING MANAGEMENT OF THE PATIENT RECEIVING [P] VERAPAMIL

Core Drug Knowledge

Pharmacotherapeutics

Verapamil and diltiazem, calcium channel blockers, are used as antiarrhythmics. Verapamil used in conjunction with digoxin controls ventricular rate in chronic atrial flutter or fibrillation. It also can be used prophylactically for repetitive paroxysmal SVT. IV verapamil also is used to treat supraventricular tachyarrhythmias.

Verapamil also is used in treating angina (including Prinzmetal angina) and hypertension. Unlabeled uses include preventing migraine headache, cluster headache, and exercise-induced asthma. Other unlabeled uses include treating hypertrophic cardiomyopathy, bipolar disorder (alternative therapy), and recumbent nocturnal leg cramps (see Table 26.5).

Verapamil can be given sublingually for treating the severely hypertensive patient with tachycardia or tachyarrhythmia (Zhang et al., 2002). Recent large-scale clinical trials have found no association between long-acting calcium channel blockers and adverse cardiovascular outcomes (Eisenberg et al., 2004).

Pharmacokinetics

Well absorbed after oral administration, verapamil undergoes a substantial first-pass effect, resulting in considerably less bioavailability. Verapamil is excreted by the kidneys. It crosses the placenta and appears in breast milk. When sustained-release verapamil is administered with food, it takes longer to reach maximum plasma levels. However, bioavailability is not affected appreciably; hence, verapamil may be administered without regard to meals.

Pharmacodynamics

Verapamil acts by inhibiting the movement of calcium ions across the cardiac and arterial muscle cell membrane. This action results in slowing conduction through the AV node

(conduction velocity), prolonging the effective refractory phase (automaticity), depressing myocardial contractility, and producing dilation of both coronary arteries and peripheral arterioles. Verapamil interrupts re-entry at the AV node and thus can restore normal sinus rhythm in paroxysmal SVT. The other outcomes of verapamil therapy are decreased oxygen demand, decreased cardiac effort, and increased oxygen to the myocardium.

Contraindications and Precautions

The drug is contraindicated in sick sinus syndrome or second- or third-degree heart block (except with a functioning pacemaker), hypotension (systolic pressure < 90 mm Hg), severe left ventricular dysfunction, cardiogenic shock, and severe CHF. Verapamil is in pregnancy category C. Verapamil may cause a greater hypotensive effect in elderly patients than in younger ones; thus, it should be administered cautiously to older patients. Caution should also be used in patients with cirrhosis of the liver (the half-life is greatly increased) and with renal disease. Caution should be used if the patient has Duchenne muscular dystrophy because verapamil may decrease neuromuscular transmission. IV verapamil can induce respiratory muscle failure in these patients.

Adverse Effects

The most common adverse effect of verapamil is constipation. Other common adverse effects include dizziness, lightheadedness, headache, nausea, hypotension, peripheral edema, bradycardia, AV block, pulmonary edema, rash, shortness of breath, and asthenia. Verapamil may produce potentially lethal ventricular arrhythmias.

Drug Interactions

Several drugs interact with verapamil. Verapamil may elevate serum transaminases with and without concomitant elevations in alkaline phosphatase and bilirubin. Usually, the elevations are transient, although several cases of hepatocellular injury have occurred. Verapamil will form a crystalline precipitate if administered into an infusion line containing 0.45% sodium chloride solution with sodium bicarbonate. A milky white precipitate forms when given IV push into the same line being used for nafcillin infusion. Table 26.6 lists drugs that interact with verapamil.

Assessment of Relevant Core Patient Variables

Health Status

Determine whether the patient has chronic atrial flutter or fibrillation, which is causing elevated ventricular rate, or chronic repetitive paroxysmal SVTs, both of which pose a need for therapy. Also, determine whether the patient has any of the following conditions because they are contraindications to treatment with verapamil: sick sinus syndrome or second- or third-degree heart block (except with a functioning pacemaker), hypotension (with systolic pressure under 90 mmHg), severe left ventricular dysfunction, cardiogenic shock, or severe CHF. It also is important to determine whether the patient has renal or liver impairment or Duchenne muscular dystrophy because verapamil must be used with caution in these patients.

Life Span and Gender

Determine whether the patient is pregnant, because verapamil is in pregnancy category C and must be used cautiously during pregnancy. Also, note the patient's age before administering verapamil: the safety and efficacy of verapamil have not been established in children, but experience has shown that treatment results in children are similar to those for adults. Intravenous verapamil is contraindicated in neonates and infants, but only when given to treat supraventricular tachycardia, because of a high risk for electromechanical dissociation. In children older than 5 years and in adolescents, IV verapamil may be administered with the same restrictions as in adult patients (a wide QRS complex tachycardia or substantial hemodynamic compromise) (Paul et al., 2000).

TABLE 26.6 Agents That Interact With P Verapamil

Interactants	Effect and Significance	Nursing Management
barbiturates	Clearance of verapamil possibly increased and bioavailability decreased	Monitor pulse, blood pressure, and respiration carefully. Monitor patient responses and blood levels.
calcium salts	Antagonism of effects of verapamil with calcium	Administer 2 h apart.
hydantoins	Serum verapamil levels possibly decreased	Monitor for therapeutic effect.
quinidine	Hypotension bradycardia, ventricular tachycardia, atrioventricular (AV) block, and pulmonary edema possible	Use concomitantly only when no other alternatives exist.
rifampin	Possible loss of clinical effectiveness of oral verapamil	Use of IV verapamil may circumvent the interaction.
vitamin D	Therapeutic efficacy of verapamil possibly reduced	Stagger dosage and monitor vital signs.
beta blockers	Coadministration, potential increased adverse effects due to depressant effects on myocardial contractility of AV conduction	Concurrent use normally avoided.
cardiac glycosides (digoxin)	Possible increased digoxin levels	Monitor for adverse effects of cardiac glycoside.

Verapamil may have greater hypotensive effects on older adults.

Lifestyle, Diet, and Habits

Patients should not drink alcohol or use aspirin while using this medicine. They should also avoid grapefruit and grapefruit juice because these foods will affect the verapamil level.

Environment

Know the setting in which verapamil may be administered. IV verapamil is administered only in the hospital, where the patient is monitored constantly using ECG and blood pressure measurements. Oral verapamil can be administered in any setting.

Nursing Diagnoses and Outcomes

- Risk for Constipation related to adverse effects of the drug
  Desired outcome: The patient will prevent or minimize constipation by increasing fluid intake and adding fruit and fiber to the diet.
- Decreased Cardiac Output related to decreased rate and force of contraction and return to normal rhythm related to therapeutic effects of drug
  Desired outcome: The patient's decreased cardiac output will reduce symptoms of cardiac alterations without developing adverse cardiac effects from drug therapy.

Planning and Intervention

Maximizing Therapeutic Effects

To maximize the therapeutic effects of verapamil, first verify that the IV line is patent before IV administration. Digoxin may be given with verapamil to achieve the additive effect of slowing at the AV node.

Minimizing Adverse Effects

When administering verapamil in an IV route, do not dilute it with a sodium lactate injection in polyvinyl chloride (PVC) bags, which may not be stable. It is important to administer IV slowly (bolus 5–10 mg over 2 minutes, 5 mg/hour infusion) and to use an IV pump to regulate the drip rate.

Do not administer IV verapamil simultaneously with (or within a few hours of) IV beta blockers because both drugs suppress contractility and AV conduction. Monitor the patient's ECG and blood pressure constantly during IV therapy. Throughout oral therapy too, monitor for ECG changes and hypotension. Encourage patients on oral verapamil therapy to increase fluid intake and include fresh fruit and fiber in their diets to help prevent constipation.

Providing Patient and Family Education

- Explain the purpose of the drug and its adverse effects.
- Stress the importance of adequate fluid intake and dietary fruit and fiber to help prevent constipation.
- Teach the patient how to take the pulse daily while on oral verapamil, instructing the patient to notify the prescriber if irregular beating (arrhythmias) occurs.
- Teach the patient how to take his own blood pressure, urging him to monitor the blood pressure on a regular basis. If the blood pressure falls below 90/60 mm Hg or any other parameter set by the prescriber, instruct the patient to contact a member of the health care team.
- Emphasize the importance of scheduling follow-up visits and blood studies.

Ongoing Assessment and Evaluation

Monitor the patient's ECG and blood pressure throughout therapy. It is important to monitor liver function periodically to detect elevated serum drug levels. Therapy is effective when normal rhythm is re-established without onset of new arrhythmias, hypotension, or other clinically important adverse effects.

Drug Significantly Different From P Verapamil

Adenosine, unlike verapamil, is not a calcium channel blocker. Adenosine is not related chemically to verapamil or any other antiarrhythmic. It is an endogenous nucleoside occurring in all cells of the body. Adenosine, like verapamil, decreases automaticity, decreases conduction velocity at the AV node, and increases the refractory period at the AV node. It may produce first-, second-, or third-degree heart block of short duration. Unlike verapamil, it increases heart rate. It is used in the conversion of paroxysmal supraventricular tachycardia (PSVT) to normal sinus rhythm, and only is given as a rapid IV bolus (see Table 26.5). The IV boluses should be

MEMORY CHIP

P Verapamil

- Class IV antiarrhythmic and a calcium channel blocker; may be given intravenously, orally, or sublingually
- Inhibits movement of calcium ions across the cardiac and arterial muscle cell membrane
- Slows conduction, depresses automaticity, depresses myocardial contractility, and dilates coronary arteries and peripheral arterioles
- Antiarrhythmic uses: controls ventricular rate in chronic atrial flutter or fibrillation; prophylactically with digoxin for repetitive paroxysmal supraventricular tachycardia; treat supraventricular tachyarrhythmias (IV administration)
- Also used in angina and hypertension
- Major contraindications: significantly depressed cardiac function, including second- or third-degree heart block, severe hypotension, severe left ventricular dysfunction, severe congestive heart failure, or cardiogenic shock
- Most common adverse effect: constipation
- Most serious adverse effect: ventricular arrhythmias
- **Life span alerts: IV routes are contraindicated in neonates and infants; and older adults are more sensitive to hypotensive effects.**
- Maximizing therapeutic effects: Shield drug solution from light; give with digoxin for additive effect of slowing at the atrioventricular node.
- Minimizing adverse effects: Monitor electrocardiogram and blood pressure constantly while on IV; and monitor periodically throughout oral therapy.
- Most important patient education: techniques to prevent constipation

administered directly into the vein, or as proximally to the vein as possible, and followed by a rapid saline flush. The bolus may be repeated if necessary.

Adenosine is removed from the circulatory system very rapidly. It is taken up by erythrocytes and vascular endothelial cells. Its half-life is estimated to be less than 10 seconds. Adenosine is metabolized primarily to inosine and adenosine monophosphate (AMP). Conversion to normal sinus rhythm frequently occurs within 1 minute after dosing.

Adenosine is contraindicated in second- or third-degree AV block, sick sinus syndrome (unless a previously inserted pacemaker is functional), atrial flutter, atrial fibrillation, and ventricular tachycardia because the drug does not convert these arrhythmias.

The most common adverse effects of adenosine are facial flushing and shortness of breath and dyspnea. Other adverse effects that may occur include:

- CV: sweating, palpitations, chest pain, hypotension (rare), prolonged systole, ventricular fibrillation, ventricular tachycardia, and transient increase in blood pressure
- CNS: headache, lightheadedness, dizziness, tingling in arms, numbness, apprehension, blurred vision, burning sensation, heaviness in arms, and pain in neck or back
- GI: nausea, metallic taste, tightness in throat, pressure in groin (rare)
- Respiratory: chest pressure, hyperventilation, and head pressure (rare)

C POTASSIUM-REMOVING RESINS TO PREVENT ARRHYTHMIAS

Because hyperkalemia may lead to cardiac arrhythmias, potassium-removing resins are drugs used to prevent arrhythmias from occurring. These resins bind with potassium and allow it to be excreted. The prototype and sole drug in this class is sodium polystyrene sulfonate (Kayexalate).

NURSING MANAGEMENT OF THE PATIENT RECEIVING P SODIUM POLYSTYRENE SULFONATE

Core Drug Knowledge

Pharmacotherapeutics

Sodium polystyrene sulfonate is a potassium-removing resin used in treating hyperkalemia. It can be given orally or as an enema. Table 26.7 presents a summary of information about this drug.

Pharmacokinetics

The exchange of potassium ions after administration of sodium polystyrene sulfonate occurs in the large intestine. The drug is not absorbed systemically and is excreted through the GI tract. The onset of action after oral administration is 2 to 12 hours; after rectal administration, onset of action takes more time, although exact numbers are unknown (see Table 26.7).

Pharmacodynamics

As sodium polystyrene sulfonate moves through the intestine or is maintained in the intestine, it releases sodium ions that are replaced with potassium ions. The efficiency of this process is limited and unpredictable. The ion exchange capacity is approximately 1 mEq potassium per 1 g of drug. Small amounts of calcium and magnesium also can be lost during the exchange process. Effective lowering of serum potassium may take several hours or days.

Contraindications and Precautions

Caution must be used when giving this drug to anyone who cannot tolerate a small increase in sodium intake, such as patients with severe CHF, hypertension, or marked edema. Because therapeutic effects are slow, this drug generally should not be used in patients with severe hyperkalemia in whom the hyperkalemia poses a medical emergency.

Adverse Effects

Hypokalemia may result from therapy and is the most serious adverse effect. Other electrolyte imbalances that may result include hypocalcemia and hypernatremia. Common adverse GI-related effects include gastric irritation, anorexia, nausea, vomiting, and constipation. The constipation occasionally may be severe and cause fecal impaction. Diarrhea occurs occasionally.

Drug Interactions

When administered with nonabsorbable cation-donating antacids and laxatives, such as magnesium hydroxide and aluminum carbonate, systemic alkalosis can occur.

Assessment of Relevant Core Patient Variables

Health Status

Monitor the patient's serum potassium level, and if it is severely elevated, the patient's total physiologic condition and ECG should be reviewed. Also, determine whether the patient has been receiving potassium supplements or replacements in IV fluids.

TABLE 26.7 C Potassium-Removing Resin

Drug (Trade) Name	Selected Indications	Route and Dosage Range	Pharmacokinetics
P sodium polystyrene sulfonate (Kayexalate)	Treatment of hyperkalemia	*Adult:* PO, 15 g 1–4 × day *Child:* PO 1 g/kg q6h *Adult:* Enema, 30–50 g q6h	*Onset:* PO, 2–12 h Enema, >12 h *Duration:* Unknown $t_{1/2}$: Unknown

Life Span and Gender

Note the patient's age before administering sodium polystyrene sulfonate. Large doses of sodium polystyrene sulfonate can cause fecal impaction in elderly patients.

Lifestyle, Diet, and Habits

It is important to investigate the patient's dietary history and preferences, particularly if the patient normally consumes a potassium-rich diet.

Environment

Be aware that sodium polystyrene sulfonate is administered in the hospital.

Nursing Diagnoses and Outcomes

- Risk for Constipation related to adverse effects of drug therapy
  Desired outcome: *Constipation will be prevented by administering sorbitol, orally or rectally, if warranted.*
- Potential complication: hypokalemia.
  Desired outcome: *The patient's potassium level will be lowered only to the normal range.*

Planning and Intervention

Maximizing Therapeutic Effects

Clear the GI tract with a cleansing enema before administering the drug by enema. For adults, insert a soft, large (28 French) rubber tube about 20 cm into the rectum. Mix the resin in an aqueous vehicle, such as 100-mL sorbitol or 20% dextrose to make a suspension; infuse the drug by gravity. During infusion, it is important to stir the fluid to keep the particles in suspension.

After the fluid has run into the patient, flush the tube with 50- to 100-mL fluid to make a total of 150- to 200-mL fluid as infused. It is important to clamp the tube and leave it in place for at least 30 minutes, but preferably several hours (keeping the solution in the colon allows the resin to work).

If back-leakage develops, elevate the patient's hips on pillows or have the patient assume a knee-chest position temporarily. These positions will help keep the solution in the sigmoid colon.

Irrigate the colon using a Y-tube connection with approximately 2 L of a nonsodium flushing solution at body temperature to remove the resin. The Y-tube allows the returns to drain as the colon is being irrigated.

When the drug is administered orally, create a suspension of the powdered formula with water or syrup for greater palatability.

Minimizing Adverse Effects

If the potassium serum level is severely elevated, use other methods to reduce potassium (sodium polystyrene sulfonate alone may be insufficient to correct an imbalance before a medical emergency occurs). Other methods include the use of IV calcium to antagonize the effect of hyperkalemia on the heart; IV sodium bicarbonate, glucose, insulin to cause an intracellular shift of potassium; and dialysis.

Monitor serum electrolytes for changes in potassium and other electrolytes. It also is important to monitor the ECG for changes indicative of hypokalemia (lengthened QT interval; widening, flattening, or inversion of the T wave; prominent U waves; or arrhythmias).

Monitor the pulse rate for arrhythmias and irregularities. It is a good idea to administer sorbitol, orally or rectally, to prevent constipation if warranted.

Providing Patient and Family Education

- Explain the therapeutic and possible adverse effects of the drug.
- It is important to emphasize the importance of repeated blood work to monitor blood electrolyte concentrations.

Ongoing Assessment and Evaluation

Monitor serum electrolytes throughout therapy. Assess for signs of hypokalemia and monitor the patient's pulse and ECG periodically throughout therapy. Sodium polystyrene sulfonate therapy is considered effective in patients whose serum potassium levels return to normal and who do not develop cardiac arrhythmias from hyperkalemia, hypokalemia, or other electrolyte imbalances.

CHAPTER SUMMARY

- Antiarrhythmics restore normal rhythm and rate by varied mechanisms.
- All drugs given to treat an arrhythmia also may cause an arrhythmia.
- Class I drugs block the influx of sodium in the myocardial membrane. They are local anesthetics or membrane stabilizing agents that depress phase 0 of the action potential.
- Quinidine, a Class I antiarrhythmic, is used for treating atrial fibrillation and flutter. Quinidine depresses myocardial excitability, conduction velocity, and contractility. The effective refractory period is prolonged, increasing conduction time. Re-entry phenomenon is therefore prevented. Quinidine also exerts an indirect anticholinergic effect; it decreases vagal tone and may promote conduction in the AV junction.
- Potassium enhances the effect of quinidine, and hypokalemia will reduce the effectiveness.

MEMORY CHIP

P Sodium Polystyrene Sulfonate

- Used to lower serum potassium levels
- Given orally or as enema
- Major contraindication: extremely high potassium levels
- Most common adverse effects: related to GI system
- Most serious adverse effect: hypokalemia
- Maximizing therapeutic effects: Give a cleansing enema first (if drug is given as enema); and leave resin in place at least 30 minutes after administering as enema.
- Minimizing adverse effects: Monitor serum electrolytes and electrocardiogram.

- Class IB antiarrhythmics depress phase 0 of the action potential, but not as much as Class IA drugs do. They also suppress automaticity. Like quinidine, these drugs may also cause arrhythmias, in addition to treating them. Unlike quinidine, they are used primarily with ventricular arrhythmias, and they may shorten the action potential duration. Lidocaine is a Class IB drug; it may be used with all acute ventricular arrhythmias that occur related to cardiac surgery or acute myocardial infarction.
- Class IC antiarrhythmics also depress phase 0 but markedly so. In addition, they have a slight effect on repolarization and decrease conduction substantially. They have been found to increase mortality significantly when used in patients who have had a myocardial infarction.
- All Class I antiarrhythmics have the potential to increase mortality; none have been proved to decrease mortality.
- Class II antiarrhythmics block the beta-1 and beta-2 adrenergic receptors and stabilize the cardiac cell membranes. They depress phase 4 depolarization.
- Propranolol, a beta blocker and Class II antiarrhythmic, is used to treat supraventricular, ventricular, and tachyarrhythmias secondary to digoxin toxicity or arising from excessive catecholamine action during anesthesia.
- Propranolol slows the sinus heart rate, depresses AV conduction, decreases cardiac output, reduces systolic and diastolic blood pressure at rest and on exercise, and reduces supine and standing blood pressure.
- Class II antiarrhythmics are the only antiarrhythmics that have been shown to decrease mortality.
- Class III drugs slow heart action by prolonging the action potential or myocardial repolarization (prolonged phase 3).
- Amiodarone, a Class III antiarrhythmic, is used to treat life-threatening ventricular arrhythmias. It also has actions from other classifications. These diverse actions of amiodarone are why the drug is being considered as potentially appropriate for treating atrial fibrillation as well.
- Amiodarone has unusual pharmacokinetic and pharmacodynamic properties. These unique effects include incomplete bioavailability, distribution to multiple tissue sites, extreme lipid solubility, biotransformation to an active metabolite, and extremely slow elimination of amiodarone and its metabolite. These effects may be attributable to genetic variations, although this possibility is not yet confirmed. Because of these unique effects, the effect on patients is variable.
- Adverse effects of amiodarone can be serious and potentially fatal. The patient needs to be monitored closely while receiving it.
- Class IV drugs alter the action potential, decrease AV conduction, and prolong repolarization by inhibiting the influx of calcium in cardiac muscle cells. A few calcium channel blocker drugs are in this class.
- Verapamil, a calcium channel blocker and Class IV antiarrhythmic, controls ventricular rate in chronic atrial flutter or fibrillation (used in conjunction with digoxin). It is also used prophylactically for repetitive paroxysmal SVT. IV verapamil is used to treat SVT.
- Verapamil also is used in treating angina (including Prinzmetal angina) and hypertension.
- Sodium polystyrene sulfonate is a potassium-removing resin used in treating hyperkalemia. Because hyperkalemia may lead to cardiac arrhythmias, this drug prevents arrhythmias from occurring.
- Sodium polystyrene sulfonate is given orally or as an enema.
- Although sodium polystyrene sulfonate is in the GI tract, sodium ions are exchanged for potassium ions, which are then excreted in the stool. Onset is slow and unpredictable. Therefore, if the serum potassium level is quite elevated, other mechanisms of lowering the potassium level should be used.

▲ QUESTIONS FOR STUDY AND REVIEW

1. Why are ventricular arrhythmias considered potentially life threatening?
2. What is meant by proarrhythmia?
3. Why do all antiarrhythmics have proarrhythmic qualities?
4. Describe the phase of the action potential affected by Class I, Class II, Class III, and Class IV antiarrhythmics.
5. Amiodarone, a Class III drug, is used to treat which type of arrhythmias?
6. What changes in the ECG do you commonly see with amiodarone?
7. Why is a loading dose (or doses) necessary to administer when using the Class III drug amiodarone?
8. What suggestions can you give to a patient taking verapamil, a Class IV antiarrhythmic, to prevent constipation?

? Need More Help?

Chapter 26 of the study guide for *Drug Therapy in Nursing* 2e contains NCLEX-style questions and other learning activities to reinforce your understanding of the concepts presented in this chapter. For additional information or to purchase the study guide, visit *http://connection.lww.com/go/aschenbrenner.*

■ REFERENCES AND BIBLIOGRAPHY

The AFFIRM First Antiarrhythmic Drug Substudy Investigators. (2003). Maintenance of sinus rhythm in patients with atrial fibrillation: An AFFIRM substudy of the first antiarrhythmic drug. *Journal of the American College of Cardiology, 42*(1), 20–29.

Blomstrom-Lundqvist, C., Scheinman, M. M., Aliot, E. M., et al., for the European Society of Cardiology Committee, NASPE-Heart Rhythm Society. (2003). ACC/AHA/ESC guidelines for the management of patients with supraventricular arrhythmias—executive summary. A report of the American College of Cardiology/American Heart Association Task Force on Practice Guidelines and the European Society of Cardiology Committee for Practice Guidelines (writing committee to develop guidelines for the management of patients with supraventricular arrhythmias) developed in collaboration with NASPE-Heart Rhythm Society. *Journal of the American College of Cardiology, 42*(8), 1493–1531.

Borchard, U., & Hafner, D. (2000). Ion channels and arrhythmias [original in German]. *Zeitschrift für Kardiologie, 89*(Suppl. 3), 6–12.

Eisenberg, M. J., Brox, A., & Bestawros, A. N. (2004). Calcium channel blockers: An update. *American Journal of Medicine, 116*(1), 35–43.

Fang, M. C., Stafford, R. S., Ruskin, J. N., et al. (2004). National trends in antiarrhythmic and antithrombotic medication use in atrial fibrillation. *Archives of Internal Medicine, 164*(1), 55–60.

Fuster, V., Ryden, L. E., Asinger, R. W., et al. American College of Cardiology/American Heart Association/European Society of Cardiology Board. (2001). ACC/AHA/ESC guidelines for the management of patients with atrial fibrillation: Executive summary.

A report of the American College of Cardiology/American Heart Association Task Force on Practice Guidelines and the European Society of Cardiology Committee for Practice Guidelines and Policy Conferences (committee to develop guidelines for the management of patients with atrial fibrillation): Developed in collaboration with the North American Society of Pacing and Electrophysiology. *Journal of the American College of Cardiology, 38*(4), 1231–1266.

Gilbert, C. J. (2001). Common supraventricular tachycardias: Mechanisms and management. *American Association of Critical-Care Nurses Clinical Issues, 12*(1), 100–113.

Haugh, K. (2002). Antidysrhythmic agents at the turn of the twenty-first century. *Critical care Nursing Clinics of North America, 14* (1), 53–69.

Khan, M. H. (2004). Oral class III antiarrhythmics: What is new? *Current Opinion in Cardiology, 19*(1), 47–51.

Paul, T., Bertram, H., Bokenkamp, R., et al. (2000). Supraventricular tachycardia in infants, children, and adolescents [in German]. *Paediatric Drugs, 2*(3), 171–181.

Prasun, M. A., & Kocheril, A. G. (2003). Treating atrial fibrillation: Rhythm control or rate control. *Journal of Cardiovascular Nursing, 18*(5), 369–373.

Rao, B. H., & Saksena, S. (2003). Implantable cardioverter-defibrillators in cardiovascular care: Technologic advances and new indications. *Current Opinion Critical Care, 9*(5), 362–368.

Singh, B. N. (1999). Overview of trends in the control of cardiac arrhythmia: Past and future. *American Journal of Cardiology, 84*(9A), 3R–10R.

VerNooy, R. A., & Mounsey, J. P. (2004). Antiarrhythmic drug therapy of atrial fibrillation. *Cardiology Clinics, 22*(1), 21–34.

Wyse, D. G., Waldo, A. L., DiMarco, J. P., et al., Atrial Fibrillation Follow-up Investigation of Rhythm Management (AFFIRM) Investigators. (2002). A comparison of rate control and rhythm control in patients with atrial fibrillation. *New England Journal of Medicine, 347*(23), 1825–1833.

Zhang, H., Zhang, J., & Streisand, J. B. (2002). Oral mucosal drug delivery: Clinical pharmacokinetics and therapeutic applications. *Clinical Pharmacokinetics, 41*(9), 661–680.

Drugs Affecting Blood Pressure

chapter 27

Learning Objectives

At the completion of this chapter the student will:

1. Describe therapy appropriate for prehypertension, stage 1 hypertension, and stage 2 hypertension.
2. Identify the core drug knowledge for drugs that affect blood pressure.
3. Differentiate the antihypertensive drug classes.
4. Identify core patient variables relevant to drugs that affect blood pressure.
5. Relate the interaction of core drug knowledge to core patient variables for drugs that affect blood pressure.
6. Generate a nursing plan of care from the interaction between core drug knowledge and core patient variables for drugs that affect blood pressure.
7. Describe nursing interventions to maximize therapeutic effects and minimize adverse effects for drugs that affect blood pressure.
8. Determine key points for patient and family education for drugs that affect blood pressure.

KEY TERMS

diastolic blood pressure
essential hypertension
hypertension
hypertensive crisis
primary hypertension
renin-angiotensin-aldosterone system
secondary hypertension
shock
sympatholytic
sympathomimetic
systolic blood pressure

FEATURED WEBLINK

http://www.guideline.gov/summary/summary.aspx?doc_id=4771&nbr=3450&string=Joint+AND+National+AND+Committee+AND+Hypertension
This website provides the complete Seventh Report of the Joint National Committee on Detection, Evaluation, and Treatment of High Blood Pressure (JNC VII) and current guidelines on hypertension management.

CONNECTION WEBLINK

Additional Weblinks are found on Connection:
http://www.connection.lww.com/go/aschenbrenner.

Drugs Affecting Blood Pressure

(C) Antihypertensives

(C) Diuretics
(see Chapter 32)

(C) Beta blockers
(see Chapter 13)

(C) Calcium channel blockers
(see Chapter 26)

(C) Angiotensin II receptor blockers (ARBs)
- [P] **losartan**

(C) Selective aldosterone receptor blockers
- [P] **eplerenone**
- spironolactone

(C) Direct acting vasodilators
- [P] **hydralazine**
- epoprostenol
- minoxidil

Adjuncts to hypertensive treatment
- (C) **antihyperlipidemics** (see Chapter 30)
- (C) **nitrates** (see Chapter 29)

(C) Angiotensin-converting enzyme inhibitors (ACE inhibitors)
- [P] **captopril**
- benazepril
- enalapril
- enalaprilat
- fosinopril
- lisinopril
- moexipril
- quinapril
- ramipril
- trandolapril
- perinatopril

(C) Alpha-beta blockers
- [P] **labetalol**
- carvedilol

(C) Drugs used in hypertensive crisis
- [P] **nitroprusside**
- diazoxide
- fenoldopam mesylate
- trimethaphan
- phentolamine
- phenoxybenzamine
- metyrosine

(C) Centrally acting alpha-2 agonists
- [P] **clonidine**
- methyldopa

Peripherally acting alpha-1 blockers
- prazosin
- terazosin
- doxazosin

Peripherally acting antiadrenergics
- reserpine
- guanethidine
- guanadrel

(C) Vasopressors

Drugs used in shock
- [P] **dopamine**
- dobutamine
- epinephrine
- norepinephrine
- isoproterenol
- ephedrine
- mephentermine
- metaraminol
- methoxamine
- phenylephrine
- midodrine

The symbol (C) indicates the **drug class.**
Drugs in **bold type** marked with the symbol [P] are prototypes.
Drugs in blue type are closely related to the prototype.
Drugs in red type are significantly different from the prototype.
Drugs in black type with no symbol are also used in drug therapy; no prototype

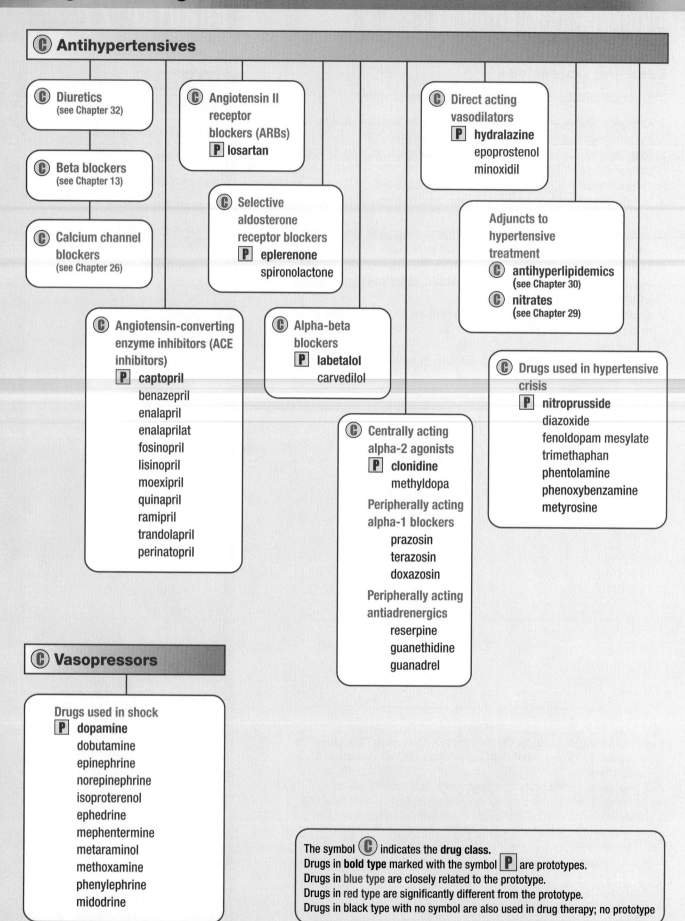

Hypertension occurs when systolic or diastolic blood pressure is elevated beyond normal ranges over time. Lifestyle changes and antihypertensive drugs may be used to restore blood pressure to normal levels and to prevent the adverse effects of hypertension. The main drug classes used to treat hypertension are diuretics, beta blockers, calcium channel blockers, angiotensin-converting enzyme (ACE) inhibitors, angiotensin II receptor blockers (ARB), selective aldosterone blockers, alpha-2 stimulators, alpha-beta blockers, and direct vasodilators. Although many of these drug classes have multiple therapeutic indications, this chapter focuses on their capacity as antihypertensives. Diuretics, beta blockers, and calcium channel blockers and their prototypes are discussed in greater depth elsewhere in the text. The prototype for ACE inhibitors is captopril (Capoten). The prototype angiotensin II receptor antagonist is losartan (Cozaar). The prototype selective aldosterone receptor blocker is eplerenone (Inspra). The prototype alpha-2 stimulator is clonidine. A drug in the same class as the prototype is methyldopa (Aldomet). Two groups of drugs are considered significantly different from the alpha-2 stimulator prototype, clonidine. These drugs are the peripherally acting alpha-1 blockers and the peripherally acting antiadrenergics. The category of peripherally acting alpha-1 blockers includes prazosin (Minipress), terazosin (Hytrin), and doxazosin (Cardura). The peripherally acting antiadrenergics are composed of reserpine (Serpalan), guanethidine (Ismelin), and guanadrel (Hylorel).

The prototype alpha-beta blocker is labetalol (Normodyne, Trandate). Another drug in the class, carvedilol (Coreg) is also used in the treatment of congestive heart failure (CHF) and is discussed further in Chapter 28. Hydralazine (Apresoline) is the prototypical direct-acting vasodilator. Drugs significantly different from the prototype are minoxidil (Loniten) and epoprostenol (Flolan).

This chapter also examines drugs used to treat hypertensive crises. The prototype drug used to treat hypertensive crises is nitroprusside. Drugs closely related to nitroprusside are diazoxide (Hyperstat), fenoldopam (Corlopam), and trimethaphan (Arfonad). Drugs significantly different are phentolamine, phenoxybenzamine, and metyrosine.

Finally, this chapter examines drugs used to raise blood pressure during shock, the vasopressors. The prototype vasopressor is dopamine (Intropin). Drugs similar to dopamine include dobutamine (Dobutrex), norepinephrine (Levophed), isoproterenol (Isuprel), epinephrine, ephedrine, mephentermine (Wyamine), and metaraminol (Aramine). Drugs significantly different from dopamine include phenylephrine (Neo-Synephrine) and midodrine (ProAmatine). Dopamine, isoproterenol, epinephrine, ephedrine, and phenylephrine all are discussed in more depth in Chapter 13.

PHYSIOLOGY

Contractions of the heart propel blood through the vascular system. Each contraction increases outflow from the heart and pushes along the volume of blood already in the systemic circulation. As the blood moves through the circulatory system, the tightness or constriction (tension) of the vessels provides resistance. Arterial pressure, which results from these forces, is measured as blood pressure. The highest pressure is achieved during systole (when the heart contracts and ejects blood into the circulation) and is known as **systolic blood pressure.** The lowest pressure that can be measured is achieved during diastole (when the heart relaxes and fills with blood and the vessels propel the blood already in circulation) and is known as **diastolic blood pressure.**

Blood pressure is measured in millimeters of mercury (mmHg) and is calculated by measuring the amount of blood leaving the heart multiplied by the amount of resistance in the peripheral vessels. The formula for measuring blood pressure is blood pressure = cardiac output × peripheral resistance, or BP = CO × PR. Figure 27.1 depicts the mechanisms involved in regulating blood pressure.

When cardiac output or peripheral resistance increases, blood pressure increases. When cardiac output or peripheral resistance decreases, blood pressure decreases. Several innate mechanisms regulate blood pressure by affecting either cardiac output or peripheral resistance.

Role of Adrenergic Receptors

Adrenergic receptors in the nervous system have a role in blood pressure management. Adrenergic receptors are grouped into receptor sites—alpha-1, alpha-2, beta-1, and beta-2. When alpha-1 receptors are stimulated, they cause peripheral constriction, and blood pressure increases as a result. This effect, which is similar to stimulation of the sympathetic nerves, is called a **sympathomimetic** effect (one that mimics the effect of the sympathetic system). Conversely, blockage of these receptor sites dilates resistance vessels (arterioles) and capacitance vessels (veins), thereby decreasing pressure.

Alpha-2 receptor sites are located within the brain. Stimulation of these receptors inhibits the sympathetic system, causing a **sympatholytic** effect (one that stops the effect of the sympathetic system). The resulting reduction in sympathetic outflow from the central nervous system (CNS) has two effects. It decreases the heart rate and, therefore, cardiac output. It also decreases vasoconstriction, which reduces peripheral resistance. The effect from both of these actions is a decrease in blood pressure.

Beta-1 receptor sites are located primarily in the heart. Stimulation of beta-1 receptor sites increases the heart rate, the speed of cardiac conduction, and the force of cardiac contraction. Cardiac output is increased, thereby increasing blood pressure.

Beta-2 receptor sites are located primarily in the bronchial and vascular musculature. Stimulation of these sites induces bronchial and peripheral dilation. The peripheral dilation contributes to decreased blood pressure by decreasing peripheral resistance. If both beta-1 and beta-2 receptor sites are stimulated equally and simultaneously, the effect on blood pressure is negligible. (See Chapter 13 for more information about adrenergic receptors.)

Role of Renin-Angiotensin-Aldosterone System

Another mechanism involved in blood pressure regulation is the **renin-angiotensin-aldosterone system.** Renin, which is synthesized by the kidneys, produces angiotensin I. Angiotensin I is a basically inactive substance until it is converted

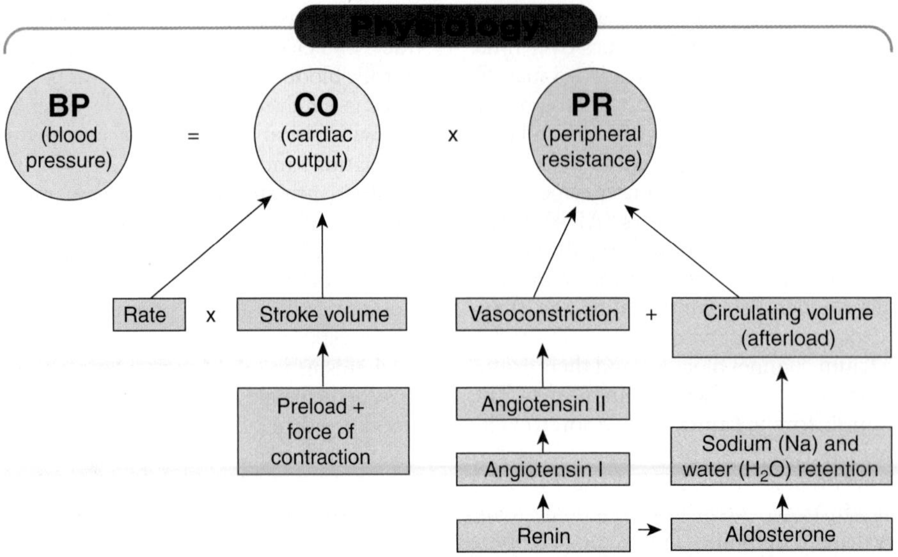

FIGURE 27.1 Mechanisms involved in regulating blood pressure. To alter blood pressure, either cardiac output or peripheral vascular resistance must change. The ideal is a balance between them. Some antihypertensive drugs alter cardiac output and some change vascular resistance.

to the active angiotensin II by a special enzyme, angiotensin-converting enzyme (ACE). Angiotensin II is formed from various alternative pathways and is also formed at the cellular level. Angiotensin II is a potent vasoconstrictor. It also stimulates secretion of aldosterone from the adrenal medulla. Aldosterone increases retention of sodium and water in the body, which, in turn, increases circulating volume. The resulting vasoconstriction and increased circulating volume raise blood pressure by increasing peripheral resistance and cardiac output. The effects on vasoconstriction and circulating volume have traditionally been viewed as the total effects of aldosterone and angiotensin II on hypertension. Recently, additional effects from angiotensin II and aldosterone have been recognized that also contribute to the pathologies seen with hypertension. These hormones also promote the growth of certain cells and stimulate increased mass in both the arterial wall and the left ventricle. Angiotensin II and aldosterone make the following more likely to occur: inflammation of the vessels, thrombosis, oxidative stress, congestive heart failure (CHF), cardiac arrhythmias, reduced fibrinolysis, and sudden cardiac death (O'Keefe et al., 2003; Stier et al., 2003). Aldosterone is also believed to play a role in structural renal injury, proteinuria, collagen synthesis, and myocardial fibrosis (Lakkis et al., 2003). Although the interruption of the renin-angiotensin-aldosterone system is target-organ protective, complete blockade is difficult to achieve because the body has some escape mechanisms. These escape mechanisms are not completely understood, but aldosterone has been identified as an important escape mediator (Lakkis et al., 2003).

PATHOPHYSIOLOGY

In the United States, hypertension is a chronic disorder that affects an estimated 50 million people aged 6 years and older, or 1 in 5 Americans (1 in 4 adults). Approximately one third of these people do not realize that they have high blood pressure. Hypertension killed 44,619 Americans in 2000 and contributed to the death of about 118,000 more. The death rate from hypertension increased more than 21% from 1990 to 2000 (American Heart Association, 2003). Hypertension is common to all racial groups, although some groups are more prone to hypertension than others. In the United States, American Indians have about the same, or a somewhat higher, incidence of hypertension than the general population. Hispanics have generally the same, or a lower, rate than non-Hispanic whites, but African Americans have the highest rate. Compared with white Americans, African Americans have an earlier onset, higher prevalence, and greater rate of stage 2 hypertension. This explains why African Americans also have a 1.3 times greater rate of nonfatal stroke, a 1.8 times greater rate of fatal stroke, a 1.5 times greater rate of dying from heart disease, and a 4.2 times greater rate of end-stage kidney disease. Rates of hypertension do vary within the African American population. Those African Americans with the highest rates are more likely to be middle aged or older, less educated, overweight or obese, physically inactive, and have diabetes. Death rates from hypertension are higher for African Americans than for whites and are higher for black males than black females (American Heart Association, 2003). Drug therapy that does not control hypertension may be especially problematic for African American males. One recent study showed that there was a higher prevalence of cardiac and renal abnormalities in young urban African American men (18–54 years of age) who received drug treatment for hypertension, but still had uncontrolled hypertension, than for those who were hypertensive but not on drug therapy (Post et al., 2003).

Women who take oral contraceptives have a small increase in both systolic and diastolic pressures, although the blood pressure usually continues to remain within the normal range. However, women who take oral contraceptives, smoke, are overweight, and are older than 35 years do experience

hypertension. It is three times more common in this group than in women without these risk factors. High blood pressure is extremely common in older adults. Depending on their race, between almost two thirds and nearly three fourths of older adult Americans have hypertension. Older adults often are responsive to lifestyle changes, which should be included as part of their treatment along with drug therapy. Hypertension is also now a problem in children and adolescents because of high rates of childhood obesity, with accompanying lack of exercise and the increasing prevalence of type I diabetes.

The American Heart Association defines hypertension as persistent elevation of systolic pressure equal to or greater than 140 mmHg or diastolic pressure equal to or greater than 90 mmHg. The diastolic pressure is based on the fifth Korotkov sound, which is the disappearance of sound. This criterion is now used for all age groups. Many factors, from exercise to stress to a variation in normal sodium intake, may increase blood pressure temporarily. Therefore, a definitive diagnosis of hypertension is not made until the average of two or more readings, each recorded at two or more visits, reveals persistent elevations (JNC VII, 2003). There are two main categories of hypertension: primary hypertension and secondary hypertension. **Primary hypertension,** also known as **essential hypertension,** is responsible for 90% to 95% of all hypertension; secondary hypertension accounts for the remaining percentage. Primary hypertension has no identified cause. However, it can be managed successfully with lifestyle changes and drug therapy to prevent the adverse effects of hypertension. Risk factors associated with the development of primary hypertension include elevated blood lipid levels, smoking, diabetes, age older than 60 years, gender (male and postmenopausal women), and family history of cardiovascular disease (women younger than 65 years or men younger than 55 years).

Secondary hypertension occurs secondary to another condition, such as renal stenosis or renal tumor. Therapy aims to correct or remove the underlying cause. If this therapy is successful, the secondary hypertension will be eliminated. However, when the cause cannot be treated successfully, antihypertensive agents are used to control the blood pressure.

Hypertension, if untreated, can lead to stroke, myocardial infarction (MI), kidney disease, CHF, and even death. These diseases and disorders result from several physiologic changes. Persistently elevated pressure constricts the arterioles, which increases peripheral vascular resistance. The increased peripheral vascular resistance in turn increases the workload of the left ventricle, which results in ventricular hypertrophy. The myocardium must work ever harder to overcome the increased resistance to outflow. Hence, the demand for oxygen increases. Eventually, the heart can compensate no longer, and CHF results. Hypertension is the most common risk factor for CHF in the population. At least 90% of the time hypertension will precede CHF. Yet, as stated before, many people do not realize they have high blood pressure and therefore do not seek any medical attention; thus, their hypertension remains uncontrolled.

Another change resulting from persistent hypertension is a sclerosing (thickening and hardening) of the blood vessel wall, which narrows the blood vessel's lumen. The narrowed lumen inhibits blood flow, leading to decreased organ perfusion and, possibly, arterial thrombosis and tissue ischemia. Tissues at the greatest risk for damage include the brain, heart, eyes, and kidneys. As mentioned earlier, angiotensin II and aldosterone are now believed to be associated with inflammation of the arteries and cell growth in the arteries and heart; these effects may contribute to narrowed arteries, increased ventricular size, and stiffening of the ventricle. Aldosterone's proposed effects on the kidney (structural renal injury, proteinuria) may account for the renal damage seen with hypertension.

Chronic hypertension produces changes, which may result in a stroke. However, hypertension can also develop after a stroke in patients who previously had normal blood pressure. Sudden and severe blood pressure increases after a stroke may indicate or cause intracerebral hemorrhage. This situation often warrants therapy to decrease blood pressure. To complicate matters somewhat, some degree of hypertension is physiologically necessary after a stroke to help maintain perfusion to the brain. Additionally, after a stroke, elevations in blood pressure may be related to other factors such as emotional stress, bladder distention, pain, or hypoxia (Harrington, 2003). For more information about hypertension and stroke, see Chapters 27 and 32.

Memory changes may be an outcome from narrowing of vessels that supply the brain. One study has shown recently that risk for late-age Alzheimer disease is increased if hypertension is present and untreated in mid-life. More than 3,700 Japanese American men were followed in the Honolulu Heart Program. Elevated, untreated blood pressure was found to be associated with dementia, although not if the blood pressure was treated with antihypertensives as a follow-up to the systolic hypertension (Launer et al., 2000). In Europe, trials also found that long-term hypertension therapy reduced the risk for dementia by 55% (Forette et al., 2002).

People with primary hypertension are relatively symptom free for a long time. Hypertension often is detected initially at an incidental blood pressure screening or during a routine physical examination. Because it is painless and symptom free, primary hypertension often remains undiagnosed until the symptoms of end-organ damage surface.

Hypertension is classified according to the degree of elevation. The risk for coronary vascular disease doubles with each increment of 20/10 above 115/75. The treatment guidelines for hypertension from the JNC VII, released in 2003, created a new category of hypertension, prehypertension. Individuals with a systolic reading of 120 to 139 mmHg or a diastolic blood pressure of 80 to 89 mmHg are considered prehypertensive, which means that they are at increased risk for becoming hypertensive later in life and should take steps to modify their lifestyles to minimize the risk for developing coronary vascular disease. Stage 1 hypertension occurs when the systolic pressure is 140 to 159 mmHg or the diastolic pressure is 90 to 99 mmHg. Stage 2 hypertension occurs when the systolic pressure is equal to or greater than 160 mmHg or the diastolic pressure is equal to or greater than 100 mmHg.

Table 27.1 shows the classifications of blood pressure for individuals 18 years and older. If the systolic and diastolic blood pressure readings are in different categories, then the classification is based on the higher values.

TABLE 27.1 Blood Pressure and Hypertension Categories*

Category	Systolic	Diastolic
Normal	<120 mm Hg	<80 mm Hg
Prehypertension	120–139 mm Hg	80–89 mm Hg
Stage 1 hypertension	140–159 mm Hg	90–99 mm Hg
Stage 2 hypertension	≥160 mm Hg	≥100 mm Hg
Hypertensive crisis	>210 mm Hg	>120 mm Hg

*In the categories of prehypertension, stage 1 hypertension, and stage 2 hypertension, diagnosis is made based on either the systolic or diastolic reading being at the specified level.

Hypertensive Crisis

When the patient's blood pressure is elevated acutely, the condition is termed a **hypertensive crisis.** This situation is defined as systolic blood pressure exceeding 210 mmHg and diastolic blood pressure exceeding 120 mmHg. When hypertensive crisis occurs, the patient is in danger of rapidly developing damage to one of the vital organs, such as the brain, heart, or kidneys, and it is considered an emergency. The situation requires immediate assessment and intervention. The priority is to reduce the blood pressure as quickly as can be managed safely to prevent injury. Blood pressure does not need to be reduced to a normal level immediately. Although the pressure must be reduced, it must stay high enough to maintain perfusion of vital organs. The initial goal of treatment in hypertensive emergencies is to reduce the blood pressure by no more than 25% within minutes and up to 2 hours. It should then be reduced toward 160/100 mmHg within 2 to 6 hours. The purpose of the gradual reduction is to avoid excessive falls in pressure that could induce renal, cerebral, or coronary ischemia. The exact level of pressure reduction depends on patient-related variables.

Hypertensive crisis may be caused by an ongoing condition, such as hypertensive encephalopathy, cerebral hemorrhage, eclampsia, pheochromocytoma (a tumor of the adrenal medulla), dissecting aortic aneurysm, unstable angina pectoris, acute MI, or acute left ventricular failure with pulmonary edema. It also could be induced from a drug–food interaction, for example, when monoamine oxidase inhibitors (MAOIs) are prescribed as drug therapy and tyramine-rich food is eaten. The symptoms manifested are acute and include decreased level of consciousness, neurologic deficits, decreased renal output, vomiting, and severe headache (cephalalgia). Emergencies initially are treated with intravenous (IV) administration of an appropriate agent for rapid onset.

A hypertensive crisis that is less serious occurs when it is desirable to reduce the blood pressure within a few hours, but risk for target organ damage is not imminent. This situation is called hypertensive urgency. Examples of hypertensive urgency are upper levels of stage 2 hypertension, hypertension with optic disc edema, and severe perioperative hypertension. Urgent situations may be treated with oral doses of drugs with relatively fast onset of action, including loop diuretics, beta blockers, ACE inhibitors, alpha-2 agonists, or calcium channel blockers.

LIFESTYLE MODIFICATION AND HYPERTENSION

In prehypertension, therapy usually consists of lifestyle changes, which include reducing weight and adopting the Dietary Approaches to Stop Hypertension (DASH). DASH recommends a diet rich in fruits, vegetables, and nonfat dairy, along with a reduced intake of saturated and total fat and sodium intake, but higher potassium and calcium intake. It also recommends moderate alcohol intake, regular exercise, and stopping smoking. Lifestyle changes also are believed to be essential in preventing hypertension, and patients should be encouraged to adopt them, especially if risk factors for cardiovascular disease are present.

Recent research from the American Heart Association indicates that the DASH diet promotes salt excretion and increases urine production, similar to the effects seen with diuretic drugs. These effects appear to be most prominent in those whose blood pressure is sensitive to the effects of sodium (e.g., African Americans or older adults). About half of the population with hypertension is salt sensitive. It is not known whether these effects are from specific foods in the diet or the combination of foods. Although potassium and calcium cause natural sodium loss and are found in high levels in this diet, the effects on salt excretion seem greater than either of these dietary sources of electrolytes can account for, thus suggesting a combination of factors is likely to be involved (American Heart Association, 2004).

Lifestyle modification remains an important aspect of therapy for patients in stage 1 or stage 2 hypertension. Lifestyle modifications may decrease the required drug therapy dosage.

DRUG THERAPY AND HYPERTENSION

Drug therapy is now recommended to be started with every patient who has been diagnosed as having hypertension, whether it is stage 1 or stage 2. Drug therapy is also recommended in prehypertension if the patient has compelling indications, such as type 1 diabetes with proteinuria, heart failure, isolated systolic hypertension (older adults), or myocardial infarction. Drug therapy for treating hypertension has proven efficacy in decreasing cardiovascular mor-

bidity and mortality. Additionally, the use of drug therapy has been found to be protective against stroke, coronary events, heart failure, progression of renal disease, progression to more severe hypertension, and deaths from all causes. Figure 27.2 provides an overview of how the various drug classes work to decrease blood pressure.

Drugs used to manage blood pressure primarily include those classified as diuretics, beta blockers, calcium channel blockers, ACE inhibitors, and angiotensin II receptor blockers. Additional therapy includes the alpha-2 stimulators, alpha-beta blockers, and direct vasodilators. Adjunct treatment includes the lipid lowering agents. Combination therapy is common.

A thiazide diuretic should be used in drug treatment for most patients with uncomplicated hypertension, either alone or with drugs from other classes. Thiazide diuretics have been shown to be as effective as, but less expensive than, other drug classes. Sometimes, hypertension occurs in conditions in which another complicating physiologic condition is present. These other conditions may respond best to other agents and are considered compelling reasons for starting single-agent drug therapy with a drug class other than a thiazide. Single-agent therapy is usually tried in stage 1 hypertension, although combination therapy (two or more drugs) may be used. Combination therapy is indicated for stage 2 hypertension. Most patients with hypertension will require two or more anti-hypertensive drugs to achieve a target blood pressure of more than 140/90 mmHg or a target of more than 130/80 mmHg if they have diabetes or chronic kidney disease. The exact combinations of drugs used to treat hypertension will vary, based on whether or not the hypertensive patient has comorbidities. As new information is acquired regarding pharmacodynamic effects of antihypertensives, the clinical guidelines concerning drug therapy choices are likely to change. Current recommendations are from the JNC VII. This information is found at the featured Weblink for this chapter.

The drug dosage should be started low and titrated up to what is considered the maximum dose for efficacy. Ideally, the drug should have a therapeutic effect for 24 hours, requiring a dose to be taken only once daily. Many antihypertensives are now available in combination with each other. Combination antihypertensives provide the patient with the benefits of both types of therapy and the added advantage of needing to take only one pill, thereby improving adherence. Table 27.2 lists health status considerations for selecting drugs as first-line therapy for hypertension.

Diuretics

Diuretics exert their effect in different areas of the renal tubules to promote excretion of sodium and water from the body. Because water is not reabsorbed to as great an extent as usual from the kidneys, the volume of circulating fluid decreases. Although the exact mechanism of how diuretics reduce blood pressure is not known, it is generally accepted that the resulting decrease in peripheral resistance, from decreased circulating volume, is what lowers blood pressure. Findings from the Antihypertensive and Lipid-Lowering Treatment to Prevent Heart Attack Trial (ALLHAT), a study of more than 33,000 North American hypertensive patients with at least one other coronary heart disease (CHD) risk factor, showed that thiazide-type diuretics are superior to ACE inhibitors or calcium channel blockers in preventing one or more major forms of CVD (ALLHAT Officers and Coordinators, 2002). Meta-analysis of 42 clinical trials (192,478 patients in all) also showed that low-dose diuretics were effective in reducing the incidence of CHD, CHF, cardiovascular disease events, cardiovascular disease mortality, and total mortality. Neither beta blockers, ACE inhibitors, calcium channel blockers, alpha blockers, or ARBs given as single drug therapy were significantly better than low-dose diuretics for any outcome (Psaty et al., 2003). When polypharmacy is indicated to achieve blood pressure control, thiazide diuretics can be combined with beta blockers, ACE inhibitors, angiotensin receptor blockers (ARBs), or calcium channel blockers. Diuretics are discussed in detail in Chapter 32.

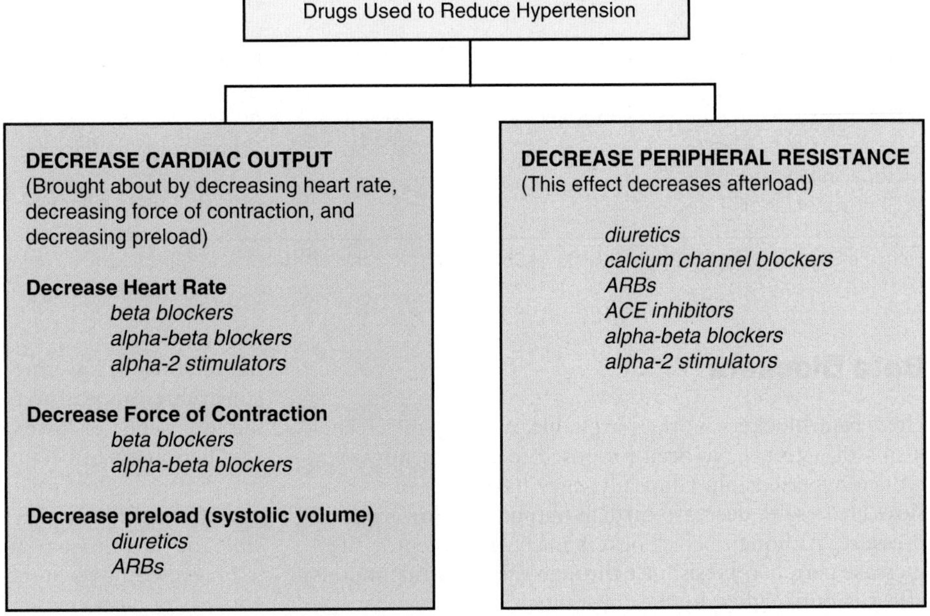

FIGURE 27.2 Focus of drug therapy in reducing hypertension.

TABLE 27.2 Health Status Considerations for Selecting Drugs as First-Line Therapy for Hypertension

Health Status	Drug Class
Compelling Indications (unless contraindicated by comorbidity)	
Diabetes mellitus (type 1)	ACE inhibitors, beta blockers, calcium channel blockers
Heart failure (asymptomatic)	ACE inhibitors, diuretics, beta blockers
Isolated systolic hypertension (older adults)	Diuretics (preferred), calcium channel blockers (long-acting dihydropyridine)
Myocardial infarction	Beta blockers (nonintrinsic sympathomimetic activity), ACE inhibitors (with systolic dysfunction)
Possible Indications	
Angina	Beta blockers, calcium channel blockers
Atrial tachycardia and fibrillation	Beta blockers, calcium channel blockers (nondihydropyridine)
Cyclosporine-induced hypertension (caution with the dose of cyclosporine)	Calcium channel blockers
Diabetes mellitus (types 1 and 2) with proteinuria	ACE inhibitors (preferred), angiotensin II receptor blockers
Diabetes mellitus (type 2)	Low-dose diuretics
Dyslipidemia	Alpha blockers
Essential tremor	Beta blockers (noncardioselective)
Heart failure (symptomatic)	Angiotensin II receptor blockers, aldosterone receptor blockers
Hyperthyroidism	Beta blockers
Migraine	Beta blockers (noncardioselective), calcium channel blockers (nondihydropyridine)
Myocardial infarction	Diltiazem, verapamil
Osteoporosis	Thiazides
Preoperative hypertension	Beta blockers
Benign prostatic hypertrophy (BPH)	Alpha blockers
Chronic kidney disease	ACE inhibitors, angiotensin II receptor blockers, loop diuretics
Possible Precautions (Needs Special Monitoring) and Contraindications	
Bronchospastic disease	Beta blockers (contraindicated)
Depression	Beta blockers, central alpha stimulants, reserpine (contraindicated)
Diabetes mellitus (types 1 and 2)	Beta blockers, high-dose diuretics (precaution)
Dyslipidemia	Beta blockers (nonintrinsic sympathomimetic activity), diuretics (high dose) (precaution)
Gout	Diuretics (precaution)
2nd- or 3rd-degree heart block	Beta blockers (contraindicated), calcium channel blockers (nondihydropyridine) (contraindicated)
Heart failure	Beta blockers (except carvedilol), calcium channel blockers (except amlodipine, felodipine) (precaution)
Liver disease	Labetalol, methyldopa (contraindicated)
Peripheral vascular disease	Beta blockers (precaution)
Pregnancy	ACE inhibitors (contraindicated), angiotensin II receptor blockers (contraindicated)
Renal insufficiency	Potassium-sparing diuretics (precaution)
Renovascular disease	ACE inhibitors, angiotensin II receptor blockers (precaution)

From the Seventh Report of the Joint National Committee on Prevention, Detection, Evaluation, and Treatment of High Blood Pressure. 2003. *JAMA, 289* (19), 2560–2571.

Beta Blockers

How beta blockers work is arguable, and several mechanisms of action have been proposed to explain how they reduce hypertension. Clinically, they have been proven to slow heart rate, decrease cardiac output, and lower blood pressure. Although beta blockers (at beta-2 receptor sites) increase peripheral resistance through vasoconstriction, this effect is outweighed by the substantial decrease in cardiac output, thereby lowering blood pressure. The peripheral vasoconstriction appears to be temporary, with resistance returning to baseline or lower levels with prolonged therapy. It is also believed that beta blockers have a central effect, which may decrease sympathetic outflow to the peripheral nervous system. Additionally, beta-adrenergic receptors are responsible for the release of renin from the kidneys. This release is prevented by using beta blockers. For more information about beta blockers, see Chapter 13.

Calcium Channel Blockers

Calcium channel blockers inhibit the movement of calcium ions across cell membranes, which decreases the mechanical contraction of the heart, reduces impulse formation (automaticity), and lessens conduction velocity. Calcium channel blockers also dilate coronary vessels and peripheral arteries, thereby decreasing peripheral resistance and blood pressure. Although decreased contractions of the heart usually result in decreased cardiac output, cardiac output is not decreased by calcium channel blocker therapy, most likely because of the reflex tachycardia that occurs secondary to vasodilation. Calcium channel blockers also are discussed in Chapter 26.

Angiotensin-Converting Enzyme Inhibitors

In the renin-angiotensin-aldosterone sequence, a special enzyme is needed to convert the inactive angiotensin I to the active angiotensin II. Angiotensin II is a potent vasoconstrictor. Its presence increases secretion of aldosterone. When aldosterone levels rise, sodium and water are retained, and other effects are exerted on the heart, vessels, and kidneys. The ACE inhibitors prevent the conversion of angiotensin I to angiotensin II, which in turn decreases peripheral arterial resistance and sodium and water retention. It is also likely to decrease the other negative effects from these hormones. The prototype ACE inhibitor is captopril.

Angiotensin II Receptor Blockers

Angiotensin II receptor blockers, or ARBs (sometimes referred to as angiotensin II receptor antagonists, or AIIRAs), are a fairly new class of drugs. They block the action of angiotensin II from all the different pathways where it is formed, not just the single substrate altered by ACE inhibitors. These drugs are effective in lowering blood pressure. In addition, they seem to block deleterious effects from angiotensin II at the end-organ stage, which is where serious complications of sustained hypertension occur. This effect seems to be independent of the antihypertensive effect produced by the drugs. For patients with diabetic renal disease, ARBs have been shown to reduce the rate of end-stage renal disease. Calcium channel blockers have not shown this benefit (Prisant, 2003). Another study showed that in patients with hypertension who did not currently have vascular disease, the ARB losartan was found more effective than the beta blocker atenolol in preventing cardiovascular morbidity and death (Devereux et al., 2003). The prototype for this class is losartan.

Selective Aldosterone Blockers

Selective aldosterone blockers are the newest class of drugs approved for use in treating hypertension. These drugs block the mineralocorticoid receptors while having little interaction with androgen and progesterone receptors (thus the term selective aldosterone blocker). Blockade of these selective aldosterone receptors lowers blood pressure and reduces the end-organ damage that occurs with hypertension. The use of ACE inhibitors and ARBs alone does not protect organs from damage completely because the body uses renin-angiotensin-aldosterone system escape mechanisms. Aldosterone blockers, when added to either ACE inhibitor therapy or ARB therapy, provide added benefit to the patient (O'Keefe et al., 2003); this benefit may be attributable to preventing the deleterious effects from renin-angiotensin-aldosterone system escape mechanisms (Lakkis et al., 2003). The prototype drug for this class is eplerenone.

Second-Line Antihypertensives

Centrally acting alpha-2 stimulators (also called agonists), peripherally acting alpha-1 blockers, peripherally acting alpha-beta blockers, peripherally acting antiadrenergics, and direct vasodilators are used in second-line treatment for hypertension in patients who have not responded sufficiently to the other drug classes. They are normally added to other drug therapy. These drug classes tend to cause substantial adverse effects in patients.

Clonidine (Catapres), the prototype alpha-2 stimulator, stimulates the alpha-2 receptors centrally in the medulla oblongata, thereby inhibiting the sympathetic nervous system. Reduced sympathetic outflow from the CNS occurs, resulting in decreased heart rate, decreased blood pressure, decreased vasoconstriction, and decreased renal vascular resistance. The other second-line agents are significantly different from the alpha-2 stimulator prototype, clonidine. These drugs are the peripherally acting alpha-1 blockers and the peripherally acting antiadrenergics. Peripherally acting alpha-1 blockers block postsynaptic alpha-1 adrenergic receptors, producing vasodilation of resistance vessels (arterioles) and capacitance vessels (veins), thereby decreasing blood pressure. Peripherally acting antiadrenergics either deplete the stores of norepinephrine or interfere with its release and distribution at the sympathetic neuroeffector junction. Therefore, less norepinephrine is available at the synaptic cleft, causing depression of sympathetic nerve function and decreasing the heart rate and blood pressure.

Drugs that are combinations of alpha-1 adrenergic blockers and nonselective competitive beta-adrenergic blockers are known as alpha-beta blockers. The alpha-1 and beta blocking properties decrease blood pressure.

The direct-acting vasodilators directly relax the arterioles, bringing about a decrease in peripheral resistance and lower blood pressure. These drugs are not suitable for monotherapy because of reflexive tachycardia and are used most frequently with two other drugs that each control blood pressure through different mechanisms.

Antihyperlipidemic Drugs

Antihyperlipidemic drugs reduce blood lipid levels. They are used as adjuncts to hypertensive drug therapy. Because hypertension can be caused or aggravated by the narrowed arterial passages when fat is deposited on the wall of the vessel, decreasing fat levels circulating in the blood is advantageous. Dietary modifications are a common first step for both hypertension and elevated cholesterol levels. Therefore, patient education should stress dietary modifications heavily for patients who are hypertensive and have elevated serum lipid levels. Antihyperlipidemic drugs are discussed in more detail in Chapter 30.

C ANGIOTENSIN-CONVERTING ENZYME (ACE) INHIBITORS

Captopril is the prototype ACE inhibitor.

NURSING MANAGEMENT OF THE PATIENT RECEIVING P CAPTOPRIL

Core Drug Knowledge

Pharmacotherapeutics

Captopril, like other ACE inhibitors, is used to lower blood pressure in hypertensive patients. Captopril is also used in treating CHF (usually in combination with diuretics and digitalis, although digitalis is not required for captopril to be effective). In addition, captopril is useful in treating diabetic nephropathy and left ventricular dysfunction after MI. Unlabeled uses include treating hypertensive crisis, neonatal and childhood hypertension, rheumatoid arthritis, hypertension related to scleroderma, renal crisis, idiopathic edema, Bartter syndrome (improves potassium metabolism and corrects hypokalemia), Raynaud syndrome (symptomatic relief), and hypertension of Takayasu disease. Captopril is also used to diagnose anatomic renal artery stenosis (captopril test) and primary aldosteronism. Table 27.3 provides a summary of selected antihypertensives.

Pharmacokinetics

Captopril is absorbed rapidly after oral ingestion. Food decreases absorption. Captopril has a rapid onset of action. The drug is metabolized (50%) by the liver. It crosses the placenta and also appears in breast milk. It is ranked in pregnancy risk category C in the first trimester and category D in the second and third trimesters. Captopril does not cross the blood–brain barrier. It is eliminated unchanged (50%) by the kidneys. Its half-life is less than 2 hours in normal renal function and 3.5 to 32 hours in renal impairment.

Pharmacodynamics

Captopril inhibits the ACE needed to change the inactive angiotensin I to the active form angiotensin II. This reduction of angiotensin II decreases the secretion of aldosterone, thus preventing sodium and water retention. Captopril, therefore, decreases peripheral vascular resistance and lowers blood pressure. Cardiac output increases, but the heart rate does not. However, peripheral vascular resistance is lowered more than cardiac output is increased, resulting in a substantial decrease in blood pressure. Captopril also increases renal blood flow but has no effect on the glomerular filtration rate. The serum potassium level may increase slightly as a result of decreased aldosterone levels.

ACE is similar to bradykinase (kinase II). Therefore, ACE inhibitors increase the levels of bradykinin, and bradykinin stimulates the synthesis of prostaglandins. It has been hypothesized that the prostaglandins contribute to the antihypertensive effect of the ACE inhibitors.

Contraindications and Precautions

Captopril and all other ACE inhibitors can cause injury and death to a developing fetus during the second and third trimesters. It is contraindicated in patients with hypersensitivity to the drug, and there may be a cross-sensitivity to other ACE inhibitors. Captopril should be administered cautiously to patients with hypovolemia (from aggressive diuretic use or dialysis), aortic stenosis (theoretically, patients treated with vasodilators are at risk for decreased coronary perfusion because they do not develop the afterload reduction as other patients do), children (safety and efficacy are not established), and breast-feeding women (concentrations of captopril in breast milk equal about 1% of maternal concentrations).

Adverse Effects

Chronic cough can occur with captopril and all ACE inhibitors, presumably because the drug inhibits the degradation of endogenous bradykinin. The cough is nonproductive and persistent. It resolves within 1 to 4 days after therapy stops but is a major reason for nonadherence to therapy. The next most common adverse effect is rash. Other adverse effects that may occur are first-dose hypotension (especially in severely salt- or volume-depleted patients, i.e., those treated aggressively with diuretics), and hypotension, although this effect usually is limited to patients with CHF and is transient. Although uncommon, captopril, like other ACE inhibitors, carries the risk for two serious life-threatening effects—angioedema and neutropenia. Angioedema can occur after the first dose of captopril, or at any other time during therapy. Angioedema confined to face and lips may resolve untreated. Angioedema associated with laryngoedema can be fatal and needs immediate emergency care. The risk for neutropenia depends on the patient's clinical status. Most at risk are patients with collagen vascular diseases, such as systemic lupus erythematosus (SLE), and impaired renal function. Also at risk are patients with heart failure. Neutropenia generally resolves quickly after captopril is discontinued. Fatalities have occurred, mostly in patients ill with the above-mentioned diseases.

Allergic reactions and anaphylaxis also are possible with captopril. Other adverse effects, which are not common, include:

- Proteinuria
- Cardiovascular (CV): chest pain, angina, MI, palpitations, orthostatic hypotension, tachycardia, and rhythm disturbances
- CNS: insomnia, paresthesia, dizziness, headache, fatigue, drowsiness, ataxia, confusion, depression, malaise, and nervousness
- Gastrointestinal (GI) and genitourinary (GU): abdominal pain, nausea and vomiting, diarrhea, constipation, anorexia, oliguria, dry mouth, dyspepsia, pancreatitis, and hepatitis
- Respiratory: asthma, bronchospasm, and dyspnea
- Dermatologic: alopecia, pruritus, flushing, photosensitivity, erythema multiforme, and exfoliative dermatitis
- Miscellaneous: impotence, syncope, asthenia, anemia, blurred vision, fever, myalgia, arthralgia, eosinophilia, and vasculitis

TABLE 27.3 Summary of Selected (C) Antihypertensives

Drug (Trade) Name	Selected Indications	Route and Dosage Range	Pharmacokinetics
(C) Angiotensin-Converting Enzyme (ACE) Inhibitors			
(P) captopril (Capoten; *Canadian:* Apo-Capto)	Hypertension Heart failure LVD after MI Diabetic neuropathy	*Adult:* PO, 25–150 mg bid or tid *Adult:* PO, 25–100 mg tid *Adult:* PO, 50 mg tid *Adult:* PO, 25 mg tid	*Onset:* 15 min *Duration:* Dose related $t_{1/2}$: <2 h
benazepril (Lotensin)	Hypertension	*Adult:* PO, 20–40 mg/d	*Onset:* 1 h *Duration:* 24 h $t_{1/2}$: 10–11 h
enalapril (Vasotec)	Hypertension	*Adult:* PO, 10–40 mg/d *Adult:* IV, 1.25 mg over 5 min every 6 h	*Onset:* 1 h *Duration:* 24 h $t_{1/2}$: 1.3 h *Onset:* 15 min *Duration:* 6 h $t_{1/2}$: 1.3 h
fosinopril (Monopril)	Hypertension CHF	*Adult:* PO, maintenance: 20–40 mg/d *Adult:* PO, 20–40 mg/d	*Onset:* 1 h *Duration:* 24 h $t_{1/2}$: 12 h
lisinopril (Prinivil, Zestril; *Canadian:* Apo-Lisinopril)	Hypertension CHF Acute MI	*Adult:* PO, maintenance: 20–40 mg/d *Adult:* PO, 5 mg/d with diuretics and digitalis *Adult:* PO, maintenance: 10 mg/d	*Onset:* 1 h *Duration:* 24 h $t_{1/2}$: 12 h
moexipril (Univasc)	Hypertension	*Adult:* PO, maintenance: 7.5–30 mg/d	*Onset:* 1 h *Duration:* 24 h $t_{1/2}$: 2–9 h
ramipril (Altace)	Hypertension	*Adult:* PO, 2.5–20 mg/d	*Onset:* 1–2 h *Duration:* 24 h $t_{1/2}$: 13–17 h
quinapril (Accupril)	Hypertension CHF	*Adult:* PO, 20–80 mg/d *Adult:* PO, 20–40 mg/d with diuretics and digitalis	*Onset:* 1 h *Duration:* 24 h $t_{1/2}$: 2 h
(C) Angiotensin II Receptor Antagonists			
(P) losartan (Cozaar)	Hypertension	*Adult:* PO, 25–100 mg/d	*Onset:* 1 wk (therapeutic effect) *Duration:* Unknown $t_{1/2}$: 2 h
(C) Selective Aldosterone Receptor Blockers			
(P) eplerenone (Inspra)	Hypertension	*Adult:* PO, 50–100 mg/d	*Onset:* 4 wk (full therapeutic) *Duration:* Unknown $t_{1/2}$: 4-6 h
(C) Alpha-Beta Adrenergic Blockers			
(P) labetalol (Normodyne, Trandate)	Hypertension	*Adult:* PO, maintenance: 200–400 mg bid *Adult:* IV, 20 mg over 2 min up to 300 mg/d	*Onset:* Unknown *Duration:* 8–12 h $t_{1/2}$: 6–8 h *Onset:* Rapid *Duration:* Unknown $t_{1/2}$: 5.5 h

(continued)

TABLE 27.3 Summary of Selected (C) Antihypertensives (continued)

Drug (Trade) Name	Selected Indications	Route and Dosage Range	Pharmacokinetics
(C) Centrally Acting Alpha-2 Stimulators and Others			
(P) clonidine (Catapres; *Canadian:* Apo-Clonidine)	Hypertension	*Adult:* PO, 0.2–0.6 mg/d in divided doses not to exceed 2.4 mg/d; transdermal, one, 0.1-mg–two 0.3-mg patches q7d	*Onset:* 30–60 min *Duration:* 12–24 h $t_{1/2}$: 12–16 h
		Child: PO, 0.05–0.4 mg bid	*Onset (transdermal):* Slow *Duration:* 7 d $t_{1/2}$: Unknown
prazosin (Minipress)	Hypertension	*Adult:* PO, maintenance, 6–15 mg/d in divided doses *Child:* PO, 0.5–7 mg tid	*Onset:* 2 h *Duration:* 6–12 h $t_{1/2}$: 2–3 h
terazosin (Hytrin)	Hypertension	*Adult:* PO, maintenance, 1–5 mg/d up to 20 mg/d	*Onset:* Up to 15 min *Duration:* 12–24 h
	Benign prostatic hypertrophy	*Adult:* PO, 10 mg/d	$t_{1/2}$: 9–12 h
doxazosin (Cardura)	Hypertension	*Adult:* PO, initially 1 mg/d, increasing to maximum of 16 mg/d, if needed	*Onset:* Unknown *Duration:* Unknown $t_{1/2}$: 22 h
	Benign prostatic hypertrophy	*Adult:* PO, 1–8 mg/d	
(C) Direct-Acting Vasodilators			
(P) hydralazine (Apresoline; *Canadian:* Apo-Hydralazine)	Hypertension	*Adult:* PO, 50 mg qid *Child:* PO, 7.5 mg/kg/d or 200 mg/d *Adult:* IV or IM, 20–40 mg, repeat as needed *Child:* IV or IM 0.1–0.2 mg/kg/dose every 4 to 6 h as needed	*Onset:* Unknown *Duration:* 6–8 h $t_{1/2}$: 3–7 h
	Hypertension in eclampsia	*Adult:* IV, 5–10 mg bolus every 20 min; after 20 mg, try another drug	*Onset:* 10–20 min *Duration:* 2–4 h

Overdosage of captopril most frequently results in hypotension. Vascular re-expansion with IV normal saline solution is the treatment of choice.

Drug Interactions

Captopril interacts with several other drugs, as presented in Table 27.4. Captopril may cause a false-positive test result with urine acetone. Food greatly decreases the bioavailability of captopril (by 30%–40%), but it remains unknown whether the therapeutic effects of captopril are affected to a similar degree.

Assessment of Relevant Core Patient Variables

Health Status

Blood pressure should be determined before captopril therapy begins. Patients receiving captopril to treat CHF are likely to be receiving concurrent diuretics. If the drug history reveals that the patient has received diuretics, especially high doses of diuretics, the patient should be assessed for signs of hypovolemia, which places the patient at increased risk for hypotension. Other factors that may cause hypovolemia include excessive perspiration, vomiting, and diarrhea. Watch for signs of dehydration and determine whether the patient has renal impairment because some patients have developed increases in blood urea nitrogen (BUN) and serum creatinine levels after blood pressure is reduced.

Patients with CHD may develop stable elevations of the BUN and serum creatinine with long-term captopril use, although discontinuation of treatment is not usually required. Electrolytes, especially potassium and sodium, should be in normal ranges to start therapy because hyperkalemia and hyponatremia may result from therapy.

A recent research study suggested a link between depression and poor adherence with hypertensive therapy in urban African American men (Box 27.1).

TABLE 27.4 Agents That Interact With P Captopril

Interactants	Effect and Significance	Nursing Management
antacids	Decreases bioavailability of captopril	Stagger drug administration by at least 2-h intervals.
capsaicin	Increases effect of captopril and may exacerbate coughing	Inform patient that coughing may attend coadministration, and suggest cough control measures. Assess for adherence to therapy.
indomethacin	Decreases effect of captopril, which may lead to an increase in blood pressure	Monitor blood pressure carefully to assess for therapeutic effect.
phenothiazines	Increases pharmacologic effects of captopril	Monitor blood pressure for hypotension.
probenecid	Increases effect of captopril, possibly raising serum levels and decreasing total clearance	Monitor blood pressure for hypotension.
allopurinol	Possibility for cross-sensitivity	Avoid concurrent administration. Monitor for signs of allergic reaction.
digoxin	Increases plasma digoxin levels	Monitor for possible bradycardia and other adverse effects.
lithium	Increases serum lithium levels	Monitor laboratory data for evidence of lithium level elevation and patient for symptoms of lithium toxicity.
potassium preparations or potassium-sparing diuretics	Increases serum potassium levels	Monitor electrolyte values. Observe patient for signs of hyperkalemia.

Life Span and Gender

The adverse effect of cough appears to affect women more than men. Determine whether the patient is pregnant. Patients who are pregnant should not receive captopril or other ACE inhibitors. If the patient becomes pregnant while taking captopril, therapy should be discontinued as soon as possible. Also, determine whether the patient is breast-feeding because captopril crosses into breast milk, and efficacy and safety have not been established in children.

Lifestyle, Diet, and Habits

Assess the patient's normal dietary habits before administering captopril. Poor oral intake and decreased sodium intake may predispose the patient to adverse effects of cap-

FOCUS ON RESEARCH

Box 27.1 Depression and Blood Pressure Control

Kim, M. T., Han, H. R., Hill, M. N., et al. (2003). Depression, substance use, adherence behaviors, and blood pressure in urban hypertensive black men. *Annals of Behavioral Medicine, 26*(1), 24–31.

The Study

The relationship between depression, alcohol and illicit drug use, adherence to recommended therapy, and blood pressure was studied in 190 urban hypertensive black men enrolled in an ongoing hypertension control clinical trial. More than one fourth of them were found to have a high risk for clinical depression, and depression was significantly associated with meeting criteria for alcohol abuse or dependence. The level of depression experienced by the men was found to be significantly correlated with poor adherence to medication and diet. Alcohol intake and illegal drug use were also found to be significantly correlated with poor dietary adherence and smoking. Descriptive analyses showed statistically significant associations among depression, substance use, poor adherence, and poor blood pressure outcomes.

Nursing Implications

Clinical depression may be a factor preventing urban black men from achieving successful outcomes from hypertensive treatment. The effectiveness of managing hypertension depends on the patient's willingness to make necessary lifestyle changes, including diet modifications, decreased alcohol intake, smoking cessation, and taking prescribed medication regularly. Patients who are depressed are not able to achieve these behavior changes easily. Although more study and research are indicated, and it is not known whether these findings can be generalized to nonurban black men, other races, or women, you should be attuned to the need to identify other conditions, like depression, that may be preventing patients from adhering to the lifestyle modifications recommended for hypertension management. Too often, nurses and other health care providers become discouraged and give up when their patients do not incorporate recommended behavior changes into their lives. When hypertension remains poorly controlled in these patients, the patient is faulted as being "noncompliant." If depression is the true source of the patient's inability to redirect his or her behavior, it can be treated. Screening and appropriate treatment for depression, as part of comprehensive high blood pressure care, may be the crucial nursing action to best help urban black hypertensive men control their hypertension.

topril. If the patient normally uses a salt substitute containing potassium or potassium supplements, these substances may need to be discontinued to avoid possible hyperkalemia. Also, explore with the patient lifestyle changes intended to decrease blood pressure, such as weight loss, smoking cessation, increased exercise, and limited salt intake.

Environment

Although captopril may be given in any environment, it is important to assess the safety of the patient's environment before taking the first dose because of the possibility of first-dose hypotension. One study found that patients living in the southeastern United States had significantly lower treatment success with captopril than patients living in other parts of the United States. Some unknown environmental factor has been hypothesized to cause this effect (Cushman et al., 2000).

Culture and Inherited Traits

Note the patient's ethnic and cultural background before administering captopril. Captopril is effective even in hypertensive patients with low renin levels. When captopril is used as monotherapy in African Americans who are "low-renin hypertensive," a smaller antihypertensive response occurs than that seen in the general population.

Nursing Diagnoses and Outcomes

- Risk for Injury from first-dose hypotension related to effect of drug therapy and from drug-induced neutropenia
  Desired outcome: *The patient will not sustain injury from hypotensive event or neutropenia.*
- Ineffective Therapeutic Regimen Management, Nonadherence, related to persistent dry cough secondary to drug therapy
  Desired outcome: *Adherence to drug therapy will be unaffected by chronic cough.*
- Disturbed Sensory Perception related to possible electrolyte imbalance, hyperkalemia, and hyponatremia, related to effects of captopril
  Desired outcome: *The patient's electrolyte levels will remain within normal ranges.*
- Risk for Impaired Skin Integrity related to drug-induced rash and pruritus
  Desired outcome: *Skin integrity will not be impaired.*

Planning and Intervention

Maximizing Therapeutic Effects

Administer captopril 1 hour before meals because food decreases absorption.

Minimizing Adverse Effects

First-Dose Hypotension

Monitor the patient for at least 2 hours after the initial dose and until blood pressure stabilizes. Transient hypotension does not indicate that captopril should be discontinued; the dose can be restarted after blood pressure stabilizes. It is important to assist the patient to a supine position and give normal saline solution IV if severe hypotension occurs. Assess patients receiving diuretic therapy, especially when the diuretic dose increases, because salt deficiency or volume depletion increases risk.

Hypotension

Assess patients with CHF very carefully. It is important to start therapy with low doses, to decrease the diuretic before starting captopril therapy, or to increase salt intake about 1 week before starting captopril therapy.

Altered Laboratory Results

Assess blood reports for hyperkalemia, hyponatremia, and neutropenia, and assess urine for proteinuria.

Allergic Reactions

If a polyacrylonitrile dialyzer is used, extreme care is needed during dialysis of a patient on captopril. Allergic reactions may occur suddenly with severe or fatal effects. Make sure that dialysis stops at the first sign of nausea, abdominal cramping, burning, angioedema, or shortness of breath leading to severe hypotension. Be prepared to intervene if the patient experiences anaphylactic reactions.

Providing Patient and Family Education

- Explain the purpose of the drug therapy and its possible adverse effects. If the patient is to start on captopril at home, advise the patient to take the first dose at bedtime to minimize the possibilities of injury from first-dose hypotension.
- Tell the patient to arise slowly from a lying or seated position in case of orthostatic hypotension and dizziness.
- Explain that the drug may produce a persistent dry cough, but that it is not serious. It is a good idea to encourage the patient to continue therapy and to provide ideas on minimizing the cough. However, tell the patient to consult the prescriber if the cough becomes intolerable.
- Advise the patient to notify the prescriber promptly about the following adverse effects: sore throat; fever; swollen hands or feet; irregular heartbeat; chest pain; swollen face, eyes, lips, and tongue; difficulty breathing; or hoarseness. A rash may also appear and should be reported, although this finding is not as urgent as the others are.
- Tell the patient not to use potassium supplements or salt substitutes containing potassium, because of the risk for hyperkalemia.
- Explain the importance of adhering to schedules for follow-up blood tests.
- Counsel the patient to make lifestyle changes (e.g., diet, weight loss, and exercise) to reduce blood pressure. Offer positive reinforcement for changes made, and encourage the patient to sustain these changes.
- Teach the patient how to self-monitor blood pressure to assess drug effectiveness.

Ongoing Assessment and Evaluation

Blood pressure should be monitored throughout captopril therapy. Blood pressure that decreases to a normal range is indicative of successful drug therapy. White blood cell counts, potassium and sodium levels, and urine protein values should be monitored throughout therapy as well. Levels that remain in the normal range demonstrate that adverse effects have not occurred. In patients with CHF, cardiac out-

put will increase because of decreased peripheral resistance, and the patient's exercise tolerance time will increase. These findings also indicate effective drug therapy. The decreased peripheral resistance (afterload) will improve ejection fraction in patients who have left ventricular dysfunction resulting from MI, reducing the incidence of overt heart failure that requires hospitalization.

Patients receiving captopril for diabetic nephropathy need to be monitored for renal insufficiency. Progressing renal insufficiency and serious clinical outcomes (need for dialysis, need for kidney transplantation, and death) should be slowed. Also, monitor these patients for proteinuria, even though captopril should decrease proteinuria.

C ANGIOTENSIN II RECEPTOR BLOCKERS

Losartan is the representative angiotensin II receptor blocker.

NURSING MANAGEMENT OF THE PATIENT RECEIVING P LOSARTAN

Core Drug Knowledge

Pharmacotherapeutics

Losartan, a monopotassium salt, is used to treat hypertension. Losartan is also used to treat kidney damage in people with type 2 diabetes. Losartan has been found to decrease the risk for fatal and nonfatal stroke in patients with hypertension and left ventricular hypertrophy, but there is evidence that this benefit does not apply to African American patients. Losartan is also indicated for treating diabetic nephropathy with an elevated serum creatinine and proteinuria in patients with type 2 diabetes and a history of hypertension. For these patients, losartan reduces the rate of progression of nephropathy, determined by the doubling of serum creatinine or end-stage renal disease requiring dialysis or renal transplantation. Valsartan can be used in treating heart failure, but this use is currently unlabeled. (See Chapter 28 for more about the use of ARBS in CHF.)

Pharmacokinetics

Losartan undergoes a substantial first-pass metabolism and is converted to an active metabolite, which performs most of the antagonism at the angiotensin II receptors. Cytochrome P-450 2C9 and 3A4 isoenzymes are involved in the metabolism of losartan. Both the drug and the active metabolite are highly protein bound. The peak concentration occurs in 1 hour for losartan and in 3 to 4 hours for its metabolite. The half-life is about 2 hours for the drug and 6 to 9 hours for the metabolite. Excretion occurs in the urine and stool (see Table 27.3).

Pharmacodynamics

Angiotensin II receptor blockers do not inhibit ACE. Instead, they block the vasoconstricting and aldosterone-secreting effects of angiotensin II by selectively blocking the binding of angiotensin II to the angiotensin I receptors in many tissues, especially in the vascular smooth muscle and adrenal gland tissues. Although an angiotensin II receptor exists, it does not seem to have an effect on the CV system. ARBs have a much greater affinity for angiotensin I than angiotensin II receptors. Losartan has about a 1,000-fold increase in affinity for angiotensin I. Losartan is a reversible, competitive inhibitor of the angiotensin I receptor. The active metabolite appears 10 to 40 times more potent by weight than losartan. It appears to be a reversible but not competitive inhibitor of the angiotensin I receptor.

Losartan, like other ARBs, inhibits the pressor effect of angiotensin II, removing the negative feedback that occurs normally. This effect causes a twofold to threefold increase in plasma renin activity and a rise in angiotensin II plasma levels. These increases are not enough to offset the positive effects that ARBs have on hypertension. Although aldosterone secretion decreases, potassium levels do not seem to be affected by losartan. There is a minimal decrease in serum uric acid when oral losartan is administered long-term.

Research indicates that losartan contributes to the regression of left ventricular hypertrophy that is associated with chronic hypertension. Additionally, losartan appears to increase exercise capacity in patients with either asymptomatic or symptomatic heart failure.

Contraindications and Precautions

The only contraindication to losartan is hypersensitivity to any component of the drug. Because of its anti–angiotensin II effect and risk for fetal and neonatal morbidity and death, losartan is in the same pregnancy category as captopril (cat-

MEMORY CHIP

P Captopril

- Inhibits the angiotensin-converting enzyme (ACE) needed to change angiotensin I (inactive) to angiotensin II (active). Angiotensin II is a potent vasoconstrictor, so that less angiotensin II means less vasoconstriction.
- Decreased angiotensin II also decreases secretion of aldosterone, which thus prevents retention of sodium and water
- Lowers blood pressure by decreasing peripheral vascular resistance; smaller antihypertensive response (monotherapy) in African Americans than whites
- Most common adverse effect: chronic cough
- Most serious adverse effects: angioedema and neutropenia
- **Life span alert: Captopril can cause injury and death to a developing fetus during the second and third trimesters.**
- Minimizing adverse effects: Monitor blood pressure for 2 hours after initial dose until stabilized; and monitor patient's blood pressure throughout therapy.
- Most important patient education: Urge continuation of lifestyle changes while on drug therapy; and teach the signs and symptoms of hypotension.

egory C for first trimester and category D for the second and third trimesters) and should not be used during pregnancy unless the benefit outweighs the risk.

Adverse Effects

A major advantage of losartan and other ARBs is that it does not cause the dry cough that occurs so frequently with ACE inhibitors.

Overall, ARBs are well tolerated, with only about 2% of patients receiving losartan experiencing adverse effects bothersome enough to warrant discontinuing the drug. Of the adverse effects that do occur, the most frequent is upper respiratory infection; dizziness and diarrhea are the next two most frequent adverse effects. Other effects that may occur, but are not common, include anxiety and nervousness; musculoskeletal pain, cramps, and myalgia; nasal congestion, sinus disorder, and sinusitis; rash; tachycardia; and urinary tract infection.

Overdosage of losartan may produce hypotension, dizziness, and tachycardia. Bradycardia may be produced from parasympathetic (vagal) stimulation. Hypotension should be treated with supportive therapy. Valsartan cannot be removed by dialysis.

Drug Interactions

Losartan is known to interact with two drugs; whether these interactions are clinically meaningful is not known. Administration with cimetidine appears to increase the availability of losartan somewhat, but the active metabolite is not affected. Administration with phenobarbital reduces by about 20% the activity of losartan and its active metabolite. Food will slow the absorption of losartan but has minimal effects on the activity of the drug. Losartan, when taken with either potassium supplements or drugs that spare potassium loss (e.g., triamterene), may lead to elevated serum potassium levels. Table 27.5 presents a summary of agents that interact with losartan.

Assessment of Relevant Core Patient Variables

Health Status

Patients who have pathologies that are dependent on the renin-angiotensin-aldosterone system (e.g., patients with severe CHF) should not use ARBs because oliguria, progressive azotemia, or (rarely) acute renal failure or death may result. Patients receiving ACE inhibitors who have renal artery stenosis have shown elevated serum creatinine or BUN, and it is hypothesized that ARBs would have the same effect. Assess patients for these conditions and monitor them for possible effects. Elevations in serum creatinine or BUN also may occur in other patients taking losartan. Of all patients who use losartan for hypertension, minor elevations in BUN and creatinine will occur in fewer than 1%. Although elevated serum levels of losartan have been found in patients with decreased creatinine clearance, the active metabolite is not affected. Therefore, no dose adjustment is required for these patients.

Determine whether the patient is taking a prescribed potassium supplement or a potassium-sparing diuretic, either of which can produce hyperkalemia when taken with losartan, because of the potassium in its chemical formulations.

TABLE 27.5 Agents That Interact With P Losartan

Interactants	Effect and Significance	Nursing Management
cimetidine	Increases area under the curve of losartan but does not affect the pharmacokinetics of the active metabolite; unlikely to be a significant reaction	Assess for increased hypertensive effect when first coadministered.
fluconazole	Metabolism of losartan via CYP2C9 may be inhibited; possibility of hypotension or adverse effects	Monitor blood pressure and assess for adverse effects if coadministered.
indomethacin	May decrease the effectiveness of losartan; blood pressure may not be as well controlled	Monitor blood pressure closely if coadministered; contact prescriber if loss of blood pressure control.
phenobarbital	Decreases available losartan and its active metabolite; blood pressure may not be as well controlled	Monitor blood pressure closely if coadministered; contact prescriber if loss of blood pressure control.
rifamycins	May increase the metabolism of losartan; blood pressure may not be as well controlled	Monitor blood pressure closely if coadministered; contact prescriber if loss of blood pressure control.
potassium-sparing diuretics; other potassium-sparing drugs; potassium supplements; salt substitutes containing potassium	Additive effects to increase potassium levels; serious elevations of serum potassium may occur	Avoid coadministration with losartan.

Patients who have impaired hepatic impairment do have increased bioavailability of losartan because metabolism is impaired. They should be given a lower starting dose of the drug and be monitored for therapeutic and adverse effects. Small decreases in hemoglobin and hematocrit will occur in patients taking losartan. Although the effect is normally not clinically important, monitor these patients.

Hypovolemia and salt depletion (usually from diuretic therapy) pose the same risk for hypotension to patients receiving losartan as to patients receiving captopril. It is important to correct these conditions before giving losartan.

Life Span and Gender

Determine whether the patient is pregnant or breast-feeding before administering losartan. Because of adverse effects on the fetus and neonate, losartan should not be used during pregnancy. Animal studies indicate that losartan passes into breast milk; it is not known whether losartan also passes into human milk. However, because of the serious effects that may occur, patients should not breast-feed while taking losartan. Additional concerns for women on losartan come from other animal studies showing that female rats receiving the drug have a slightly higher rate of pancreatic cancer and impaired fertility. Again, the effects in humans are not known. The safety and efficacy of losartan and other ARBs in children younger than 18 years is not known. No dosage adjustments seem to be necessary for older adults because losartan is equally safe and effective in this group compared with in younger adults. Older adults generally tolerate ARB therapy better than therapy with other antihypertensive drug classes. Because losartan has essentially no contraindications, older adults with hypertension and other comorbidities can still be prescribed losartan (McInnes, 2003).

Lifestyle, Diet, and Habits

Assess the patient's usual lifestyle. Lifestyle modifications that are general for all patients requiring hypertensive therapy should be followed for patients taking losartan. Assess whether the patient is taking an over-the-counter (OTC) potassium supplement or uses a salt substitute containing potassium because either one in combination with losartan may produce hyperkalemia.

Environment

Be aware of the setting in which losartan may be administered. Losartan may be administered in any setting.

Culture and Inherited Traits

It is a good idea to note the patient's racial background before administering losartan. Like captopril, losartan is less effective when used as monotherapy in hypertensive African Americans than in other racial groups. This effect may be because this racial group usually carries a low renin level.

Nursing Diagnoses and Outcomes

- Risk for Injury related to adverse effects on fetus and neonate.
  Desired outcome: *The patient receiving losartan will report pregnancy to prescriber as soon as possible.*
- Risk for Injury related to fall secondary to adverse effect of dizziness.
  Desired outcome: *The patient will not fall.*
- Risk for Infection (upper respiratory) related to adverse effects of drug therapy.
  Desired outcome: *The patient will not develop an upper respiratory infection, or if one develops, it will be managed appropriately to minimize complications.*

Planning and Intervention

Maximizing Therapeutic Effects

Like all drug therapy for hypertension, the use of losartan should be accompanied by the recommended lifestyle changes. Determine whether the patient has made these changes and provide encouragement to continue with them throughout drug therapy.

If losartan is ineffective alone, add a diuretic. Hydrochlorothiazide has been found to have an additive effect. A combination of losartan and hydrochlorothiazide is available. Consult with the physician or nurse practitioner for additional drug orders if indicated.

Minimizing Adverse Effects

Help the patient out of bed when he or she is first started on losartan therapy, in case dizziness occurs. It is important to treat the patient symptomatically for upper respiratory tract infections and diarrhea, if they are present. Monitor creatinine, BUN, hemoglobin, and hematocrit levels to verify that changes are not clinically meaningful. If the patient is currently prescribed a potassium supplement or a drug therapy that increases potassium levels indirectly, consult with the prescriber about changing this therapy before the start of losartan.

Providing Patient and Family Education

- If the female patient is of childbearing age, caution her about the adverse effects that losartan can have on the fetus and neonate. Urge the woman to notify the prescriber immediately if she becomes pregnant.
- Explain the importance of arising slowly until the effects of the drug are known or if dizziness is present.
- Teach the patient to avoid hazardous activities until effects of the drug are known.
- Teach the patient not to take OTC potassium supplements or use a salt substitute that has potassium in it.
- Tell the patient to notify the prescriber if upper respiratory infection occurs.
- Provide general teaching about hypertension, lifestyle changes, and losartan core drug knowledge.

Ongoing Assessment and Evaluation

Monitor blood pressure throughout therapy and determine whether the desired blood pressure goal has been achieved. Consider adding a diuretic if losartan is not effective in monotherapy. Verify that the patient continues with lifestyle changes. Treatment is effective if the desired reduction in blood pressure occurs in either monotherapy or multidrug therapy without the patient having serious adverse effects.

MEMORY CHIP

P Losartan

- Used to treat hypertension and kidney damage in people with type 2 diabetes
- Blocks vasoconstricting and aldosterone-secreting effects of angiotensin II by preventing angiotensin II from binding to receptor sites
- Does not produce ACE cough
- Most frequent adverse effects: upper respiratory infections, dizziness, and diarrhea
- No serious adverse effects in normal dosing
- **Life span alert: Do not give to women who are pregnant or breast-feeding.**
- Maximizing therapeutic effect: Continue with lifestyle changes.
- Minimizing adverse effects: Assist patient out of bed and with ambulation.
- Most important patient education: Use caution until it is known whether drug will cause dizziness; avoid OTC potassium supplements and salt substitutes containing potassium.

C SELECTIVE ALDOSTERONE BLOCKERS

Eplerenone is the prototype selective aldosterone blocker.

NURSING MANAGEMENT OF THE PATIENT RECEIVING P EPLERENONE

Core Drug Knowledge

Pharmacotherapeutics

Eplerenone is used to treat hypertension, either alone or with other antihypertensives. Eplerenone has been shown to lower blood pressure and reduce end-organ damage that can occur in hypertension. The full therapeutic effect of eplerenone takes 4 weeks to be evident. When given after myocardial infarction to patients with evidence of systolic left ventricular dysfunction and symptoms of heart failure, eplerenone reduced hospitalizations for cardiovascular problems and deaths from cardiovascular disease (Stier, 2003). Eplerenone has been approved for treatment of CHF after a myocardial infarction.

Pharmacokinetics

Eplerenone is well absorbed from the GI system and reaches mean peak plasma concentrations within 1.5 hours after administration. Absorption is not affected by food. Eplerenone is about 50% protein bound and is bound primarily to alpha1-acid glycoproteins. Metabolism of eplerenone is through the liver and CYP3A4 is the primary isoenzyme involved in its metabolism. Metabolism produces inactive metabolites. Elimination half-life is about 4 to 6 hours. Steady state is achieved within 2 days. Less than 5% of eplerenone is excreted unchanged. About two thirds of the drug is excreted by the kidneys through the urine, and about one third is excreted through the GI tract through stool.

Pharmacodynamics

Eplerenone binds selectively to the mineralocorticoid receptors, thereby blocking aldosterone from binding to these receptors. Eplerenone does not bind significantly to the glucocorticoid receptors, or to the progesterone or androgen receptors, which are also stimulated by aldosterone. By preventing aldosterone from binding to its receptors sites in the kidney, heart, blood vessels, and brain, eplerenone inhibits sodium and water retention as well as the other effects of aldosterone, which cause hypertension. By inhibiting aldosterone from attaching to its receptors, eplerenone also impairs the negative regulatory feedback mechanism of the renin-angiotensin-aldosterone system. Because the body does not receive the feedback message that aldosterone levels are sufficiently high, the body produces extra renin and aldosterone. Increasing renin activity and elevated plasma levels of aldosterone do not, however, offset the beneficial effects on blood pressure exerted by eplerenone.

Contraindications and Precautions

Eplerenone is contraindicated if the patient has a serum potassium level greater than 5.5 mEq/L; type 2 diabetes with microalbuminuria; serum creatinine greater than 2 mg/dL in men or greater than 1.8 mg/dL in women; or a creatinine clearance less than 50 mL/minute. Eplerenone is also contraindicated if the patient is currently taking any of the following medications: potassium supplements; potassium-sparing diuretics (amiloride, spironolactone, triamterene); or a strong inhibitor of CYP3A4 (e.g., ketoconazole or itraconazole). All of these conditions will increase the risk for developing hyperkalemia. No adequate and well-controlled studies have been conducted for eplerenone in pregnant women, although animal studies have not shown potential complications; it is considered a pregnancy category B drug.

Adverse Effects

Generally, the drug is well tolerated, and adverse effects are mild. Hyperkalemia is the primary adverse effect of eplerenone. The potassium levels may be high enough to cause serious or fatal arrhythmias. Another electrolyte imbalance that can occur, although not as frequently, is hyponatremia. Dizziness is another fairly common adverse effect, although its incidence is less than half that of hyperkalemia. Other adverse effects that can occur, but are rare or infrequent, include:

- GI: diarrhea, abdominal pain
- GU: albuminuria, painful breasts and gynecomastia (in men), abnormal vaginal bleeding
- Metabolic: hypercholesterolemia, hypertriglyceridemia, increased BUN, increased uric acid, increased serum creatinine, and increased ALT
- Miscellaneous: coughing, fatigue, flu-like symptoms

Drug Interactions

Eplerenone interacts with a few other drugs, mostly those that are ACE inhibitors, ARBs, or CYP3A4 potent inhibitors.

Administration with St. John's wort decreases the availability of eplerenone by about 30%. Grapefruit juice increases the availability of eplerenone by about 25%. Table 27.6 presents a summary of drugs that interact with eplerenone.

Assessment of Relevant Core Patient Variables

Health Status

Before administering eplerenone, verify that the patient has hypertension. Assess serum potassium, serum creatinine, and creatinine clearance for alterations that indicate a contraindication to the drug. Also, assess whether the patient is receiving any concurrent drug therapy that is considered a contraindication to eplerenone therapy. The safety and efficacy of eplerenone have not been established in severe liver disease.

Lifespan and Gender

Assess the lifespan status of the patient. Because the exact effect of eplerenone on pregnancy is not known, assess whether the patient is pregnant. The drug should be used only if potential benefits outweigh potential risks. Eplerenone passes into breast milk, but the exact concentration of the drug is unknown. The effects on the breast-fed infant are unknown at this time. Nursing mothers should most likely either discontinue the drug or discontinue nursing. The efficacy and safety of eplerenone are not known for children. Older adults may safely take eplerenone unless they have severe renal impairment.

Lifestyle, Diet, and Habits

Assess whether the patient uses an OTC potassium supplement or takes a salt substitute containing potassium; both are contraindications to drug therapy with eplerenone. Determine whether the patient uses St. John's wort or drinks grapefruit juice, both of which change the amount of drug available.

Environment

Eplerenone can be administered in any environmental setting and does not require special assessment of the environment.

Nursing Diagnoses and Outcomes

- Risk for Injury related to the adverse effect of dizziness
  Desired outcome: *The patient will not become injured from a fall caused by dizziness while on eplerenone therapy.*
- Potential Complication: Hyperkalemia related to eplerenone therapy
  Desired outcome: *The patient will maintain normal potassium levels while taking eplerenone therapy.*
- Deficient Knowledge related to avoiding potassium supplements and potassium-based salt substitutes

TABLE 27.6 Agents That Interact With P Eplerenone

Interactants	Effect and Significance	Nursing Management
ACE inhibitors, ARBs	Increased risk for hyperkalemia; may cause arrhythmias	Avoid coadministration if possible; monitor serum potassium levels closely if coadministered.
potent CYP3A4 inhibitors (eg., ketoconazole, itraconazole); weak CYP3A4 inhibitors (eg., erythromycin, saquinavir, verapamil, fluconazole)	Potent inhibitors increase circulating levels of eplerenone fivefold; weak inhibitors increase them twofold. This increases risk for adverse effects, especially hyperkalemia.	Avoid coadministration of potent CYP3A4 inhibitors. Give lower initial dose of eplerenone if weak inhibitors are coadministered; titrate slowly while monitoring serum potassium levels.
NSAIDs	Theoretical interaction; NSAIDs given with other potassium-sparing antihypertensives decrease antihypertensive effect and produce severe hyperkalemia in patients with impaired renal function. This interaction may possibly also occur with eplerenone.	Monitor blood pressure and potassium levels closely if these drugs are coadministered.
St. John's wort	Decreases available eplerenone by 30%	Avoid starting St. John's wort after dosage has been titrated to achieve therapeutic effect from eplerenone; alternately, monitor for therapeutic effect if herb is to be started. Increase dose of eplerenone if needed.
lithium	Theoretical interaction; coadministration of lithium and diuretics or ACE inhibitors has led to lithium toxicity	Monitor lithium levels if coadministered with eplerenone.

Desired outcome: *Patient will have adequate knowledge to make informed decisions when choosing OTC supplements and salt substitutes while taking eplerenone.*

Planning and Intervention

Maximizing Therapeutic Effects

Eplerenone is most effective if taken daily as directed. Encourage the patient to make lifestyle changes that are known to decrease hypertension, including following a DASH diet (although the recommendation for high potassium intake needs to be modified while taking eplerenone).

Minimizing Adverse Effects

Monitor the patient's serum potassium level periodically during eplerenone therapy. Monthly assessments throughout therapy are indicated for those at risk for hyperkalemia (including those on ACE inhibitors and ARBs); however, more frequent assessment (every other week) is warranted initially until the effects of the drug on the patient are known. Hyperkalemia occurs more frequently as renal function decreases, so that patients with deteriorating renal function need to be assessed carefully. If the patient is receiving drugs that are weak CYP3A4 inhibitors (e.g., erythromycin, saquinavir, verapamil, fluconazole), the initial dose should be half of what is normally given until the effect on the potassium level is known. Patients who are experiencing dizziness while on eplerenone therapy should be assisted in ambulation and protected from falls.

Providing Patient and Family Education

- Patients need to know to avoid salt substitutes that contain potassium. This advisory is especially important because many patients might use a salt substitute when they are limiting sodium intake as part of implementing the lifestyle changes recommended for hypertension. They should also avoid foods very high in potassium, such as bananas.
- Patients need to be taught to avoid potassium supplements and the contraindicated drugs while taking eplerenone.
- Teach the patient and the family the rationale for and importance of periodic blood tests to check potassium levels.
- Teach the patient that eplerenone may be taken either with or without food.
- Teach the patient and family to avoid using St. John's wort or drinking grapefruit juice without first contacting the patient's physician or nurse practitioner because these substances change the amount of eplerenone available in the bloodstream. For patients who use these substances, the dosage of eplerenone may need to be adjusted down with grapefruit juice consumption and upward with the start of St John's wort.
- Teach the patient who experiences dizziness to use handrails when going up and down stairs, to stand slowly from a sitting or a lying position, and to get assistance with walking to prevent falls.

Ongoing Assessment and Evaluation

Potassium levels and renal function should be assessed throughout therapy. Drug therapy with eplerenone is successful if the patient has a decrease in blood pressure and does not experience substantial adverse effects.

MEMORY CHIP

[P] Eplerenone

- Used in treating hypertension
- Works by selectively blocking aldosterone receptors
- Major contraindications: elevated potassium levels, severe renal failure, type 2 diabetes with microalbuminuria, concurrent administration of drugs that increase potassium levels either directly or indirectly
- Most common adverse effects: hyperkalemia, dizziness, hyponatremia
- Most serious adverse effect: hyperkalemia
- Maximizing therapeutic effect: Take regularly, implement or continue lifestyle changes along with drug therapy.
- Minimizing adverse effects: Monitor potassium levels and renal function.
- Most important patient education: Avoid potassium-based salt substitutes; avoid potassium supplements.

Drugs Significantly Different From [P] Eplerenone

Spironolactone

Spironolactone is a nonspecific aldosterone blocker. Like eplerenone, it can block the mineralocorticoid receptors for aldosterone, preventing sodium and fluid retention that contributes to hypertension. Unlike eplerenone, it also equally stimulates androgen and progesterone receptors, which is likely the cause of the frequent endocrine adverse effects, such as inability to achieve an erection, gynecomastia (in men), irregular bleeding or postmenopausal bleeding (in women), hirsutism, and deepening of the voice. The frequency of these adverse effects (compared with their rarity with eplerenone) makes spironolactone less desirable as an antihypertensive agent. More information about spironolactone is provided in Chapter 32.

[C] ALPHA-BETA BLOCKERS

Labetalol is the prototype alpha-beta blocker.

NURSING MANAGEMENT OF THE PATIENT RECEIVING [P] LABETALOL

Core Drug Knowledge

Pharmacotherapeutics

Labetalol is used for treating hypertension, usually with other agents, especially thiazide and loop diuretics, although it may be used alone. The parenteral form is used for managing severe hypertension and is given only in the hospital. Labetalol is often used to manage acute, severe hypertension that occurs after an acute ischemic stroke. Unlabeled uses include lowering hypertension associated with pheochromocytoma, although higher IV doses may be needed, and paradoxic hypertensive responses have been reported. Labetalol also has been used in clonidine-withdrawal hypertension (see Table 27.3).

Pharmacokinetics

Labetalol is completely absorbed orally, and the peak action occurs in 2 to 4 hours. Maximum steady-state blood pressure response occurs within 24 to 72 hours. The drug also can be administered parenterally, with the onset occurring rapidly and peaking in 5 minutes. After IV therapy is discontinued, blood pressure returns gradually to near-baseline levels in 16 to 18 hours. Labetalol has an extensive first-pass effect and is metabolized rapidly by the liver. It is excreted in the stool and urine. Labetalol penetrates the CNS, crosses the placenta, and appears in breast milk in minimal amounts (0.004% of maternal dose). It is a pregnancy category C drug.

Pharmacodynamics

Labetalol is an adrenergic blocking agent that has a nonspecific beta blocking action at both the beta-1 and beta-2 receptor sites, and a selective alpha-1 blocking action. The ratio of alpha-beta blocking action is 1:3 with oral use and 1:7 with IV use. The alpha blocking actions cause peripheral vasodilation. Because the alpha blocking action decreases standing blood pressure more than it decreases lying blood pressure, orthostatic hypotension may occur, although it is transient. The beta blocking action prevents reflex tachycardia. It also prevents exercise-induced tachycardia and elevations in blood pressure; however, it has no effect on respiratory rate. The beta blocking effect also results in a decrease in the plasma renin level. Labetalol reduces blood pressure while maintaining glomerular filtration rate and renal blood flow. Although labetalol can be parenterally administered as either repeated IV boluses or a continuous IV infusion, IV infusion has certain benefits, including greater control of antihypertensive action and a decrease in the severity and rate of adverse effects.

Contraindications and Precautions

Labetalol is contraindicated with severe bradycardia, second- or third-degree heart block, bronchial asthma, overt noncompensated heart failure, and cardiogenic shock from stimulation of beta-1 and beta-2 receptor sites. Caution should be used in patients with a history of heart failure (who are well compensated). Heart failure has been known to occur, even in patients with no history of it. Caution is used with patients with nonallergic emphysema, bronchitis, or diabetes mellitus, because of beta blockade. Labetalol must be used cautiously in pregnancy, because no adequate controlled studies have been conducted in pregnant women. Safety and efficacy in children have not been established. Labetalol should be administered with caution to patients with impaired hepatic function because drug metabolism may be diminished. When given to patients with hypertension after acute ischemic stroke, the drug must be titrated carefully to prevent too severe a drop in blood pressure, which can impair perfusion of the brain tissue (Harrington, 2003).

Adverse Effects

Labetalol usually is well tolerated, with the adverse effects being mild and transient. Orthostatic hypotension after oral dosage occurs in 2% of patients receiving labetalol. It is usually transient and unlikely to occur if the recommended starting dose and titration increments are followed closely. It is most likely to occur 2 to 4 hours after a dose, especially a large dose or dose change and if the patient is tilted or assumes an upright position within 3 hours of receiving the dose. The weakness, fatigue, and dizziness that can occur with administration are associated with postural hypotension. Other adverse effects include:

- GU: ejaculatory failure, impotence, priapism, difficulty in micturition, acute urinary bladder retention, and Peyronie disease
- GI: diarrhea, cholestasis with or without jaundice, and reversible increases in serum transaminase
- Respiratory: respiratory dyspnea and bronchospasm
- Miscellaneous: asthenia, muscle cramps, and toxic myopathy; rashes, reversible alopecia, bullous lichen planus, and facial reddening much like that of psoriasis; jaundice and hepatic dysfunction rarely are associated with labetalol, but if they occur, they are reversible when the drug is stopped.

Signs of overdosage include excessive hypotension that is posture sensitive and excessive bradycardia.

Drug Interactions

The major drug interactions involving labetalol are shown in Table 27.7. Labetalol interacts with beta-adrenergic agonists, cimetidine, glutethimide, halothane, and nitroglycerin. There are no drug–food interactions. The metabolite of labetalol in the urine may cause a false increase in urinary catecholamine levels. Reversible increases in serum transaminase have been noted in 4% of patients taking labetalol; more rarely, blood urea increases, which is also reversible.

Assessment of Relevant Core Patient Variables

Health Status

Assess whether pain, bladder distention, or hypoxia exists before initiating hypertension treatment with labetalol. These causes of hypertension should be treated with other drugs. Determine whether the patient has CHF, second- or third-degree heart block, cardiogenic shock, severe bradycardia, bronchospastic disease, or diabetes mellitus because the beta blocking action may be harmful to patients with these conditions. It is important to determine whether the patient has impaired hepatic function because metabolism may be decreased. Also, determine whether the patient is already receiving drug therapy with drugs that interact with labetalol.

Life Span and Gender

Determine the age of the patient because safety and efficacy have not been established in children. Because liver function may be deteriorated in the elderly, the first-pass effect may be diminished, increasing the absolute bioavailability of labetalol. Determine whether the patient is pregnant or breast-feeding because caution with administration is necessary.

Lifestyle, Diet, and Habits

Absolute bioavailability of labetalol increases when it is taken with food. Determine whether the patient has made lifestyle changes to decrease blood pressure, such as losing

TABLE 27.7 Agents That Interact With P Labetalol

Interactants	Effect and Significance	Nursing Management
beta-adrenergic agonists	Counteract the bronchodilatory effect of the agonists in patients with bronchospasm	Monitor therapeutic effects of the beta-adrenergic agonist and anticipate the need for increased dosage of beta adrenergic agonist to counteract interaction.
cimetidine	Increases bioavailability of oral labetolol, thereby increasing therapeutic or adverse effects of labetalol	Monitor for therapeutic and adverse effects, and anticipate dosage adjustment to offset adverse effect of interaction.
glutethimide	May decrease effects of labetolol (by microsomal enzyme induction); may continue for several days after glutethimide therapy stops	Monitor for therapeutic effect of labetalol.
halothane	Synergistic effects, leading to significant myocardial depression	Monitor for signs of myocardial depression throughout anesthesia. (Effects may be controlled by reducing halothane dosage.)
nitroglycerin	Blunts reflex tachycardia without preventing hypotensive effect	Monitor for hypotension.

weight, stopping smoking, increasing exercise, and limiting salt intake.

Environment

Be aware of the setting in which labetalol may be administered. Oral labetalol may be taken in any setting, but IV labetalol is administered only in the hospital. Withdrawal of beta blocking drug therapy before major surgery is controversial because hypersensitivity to catecholamines has been noted in patients after withdrawal. However, labetalol withdrawal has not been evaluated relevant to major surgery.

Nursing Diagnoses and Outcomes

- Decreased Cardiac Output related to effect of drug therapy
  Desired outcome: *The patient will not develop decreased cardiac output substantial enough to alter cardiac perfusion.*
- Risk for Injury related to orthostatic hypotension secondary to adverse effects of drug therapy
  Desired outcome: *The patient will not sustain injury if transient orthostatic hypotension develops.*

Planning and Intervention

Maximizing Therapeutic Effects

Administer oral labetalol with food to increase absolute bioavailability.

Minimizing Adverse Effects

Prepare IV infusions of labetalol carefully. Multiple concentrations may be ordered, and the required diluent varies depending on the desired concentration. Different manufacturers make different concentrations of labetalol, which also influences how much drug volume needs to be added to the diluent. Carefully read the labels and follow the manufacturer's instructions when preparing IV infusions of labetalol (Harrington, 2003).

Patients receiving IV infusions of labetalol need to have their blood pressure monitored closely throughout the infusion. Blood pressure should be monitored every 5 to 10 minutes during infusion. Orthostatic blood pressures should also be assessed. Verify that orthostatic blood pressure remains stable after an initial oral dose or after a dosage increase. Keep patients who receive IV labetalol flat during infusion to prevent orthostatic hypotension and assess the patient's tolerance to an upright position before allowing him or her to ambulate (Harrington, 2003).

When labetalol infusion is used to treat hypertension after acute ischemic stroke, it is imperative to reduce blood pressure gradually to reduce the risk for intracerebral hemorrhage while maintaining sufficient cerebral perfusion. IV infusions should always be regulated by an IV pump to maintain a steady infusion rate and prevent excessive rates of infusion. Once the targeted blood pressure has been achieved, labetalol may be discontinued, or it may be maintained for another 24 hours. Blood pressure should be carefully assessed after IV infusions have been stopped at a rate of every 5 minutes for 30 minutes, every 30 minutes for the next 2 hours, then hourly for at least 6 hours to confirm that the blood pressure remains stable. Orthostatic blood pressure should also be assessed after labetalol therapy is discontinued (Harrington, 2003).

Observe the patient closely for signs of heart failure. At any sign of cardiac failure, it is important to consult with the prescriber regarding administering a diuretic drug or fully digitalizing the patient, which are the recommended treatments for labetalol-induced CHF. If cardiac heart failure continues, labetalol may be withdrawn slowly, if possible. Exacerbation of angina and, in some cases, MI and ventricular arrhythmia, have occurred with abrupt discontinuation of beta blocking agents.

To discontinue labetalol that has been administered for a long time, reduce the dosage gradually over 1 week to 2 weeks and monitor the patient carefully. This practice applies to all patients receiving labetalol but especially to

those with ischemic heart disease. If angina markedly worsens or acute coronary insufficiency develops, the drug may need to be reinstituted temporarily.

It is important to consult with the surgeon and anesthetist before major surgery because labetalol may or may not be discontinued.

Monitor blood glucose levels in diabetic patients (hypoglycemia may be masked because of suppression of tachycardia; hyperglycemia is also possible because beta blockade reduces insulin release in response to elevated blood glucose). Dosage adjustments of insulin may be necessary.

It is important to stop labetalol therapy if the patient appears jaundiced or if laboratory tests indicate evidence of hepatic injury.

Providing Patient and Family Education

- Explain the purpose and adverse effects of labetalol.
- Caution the patient not to stop the drug suddenly.
- Teach the patient to take the drug with food.
- Explain the symptoms of heart failure and the importance of reporting symptoms to the prescriber immediately.
- Urge the patient to notify the prescriber if asthma or breathing problems occur.
- It is important that the diabetic patient does not exhibit tachycardia, which is a sign of hypoglycemia, while taking labetalol. Caution the patient to report any sign of tachycardia immediately to the prescriber.
- Teach the patient to lie down and remain flat if weakness, orthostatic hypotension, or syncope occurs. It also is important for the patient to change positions slowly after lying down by sitting on the edge of the bed for a few minutes before standing.
- Caution the patient to avoid standing in one position for any length of time (to prevent episodes of hypotension from venous pooling). If it is necessary to stand, the patient should contract the calf muscles while standing and wear support stockings.
- Caution the patient to avoid hot baths, showers, or becoming overheated, which may contribute to peripheral vasodilation and hypotensive episodes.
- Encourage continuing lifestyle changes.
- Teach the patient how to monitor blood pressure.
- Explain the importance of scheduling and keeping follow-up appointments to monitor drug effectiveness.

Ongoing Assessment and Evaluation

Monitor blood pressure throughout labetalol therapy. Measure orthostatic blood pressure after the initial dose or after large dosage increases. Blood pressure that returns to the normal range without continued hypotension is evidence of effective therapy. Also monitor the patient for symptoms of cardiac failure. In diabetic patients, it is important to regularly monitor liver function and blood glucose levels.

C CENTRALLY ACTING ALPHA-2 AGONISTS

The prototype centrally acting alpha-2 agonist is clonidine.

CRITICAL THINKING SCENARIO

Managing complications of labetalol therapy

Your patient, Mr. Parker, is receiving labetalol IV for hypertension. Today, for the first time, he has rales (crackles) in the mid and lower lobes of both lungs. He has gained 3 lb since he was last weighed 2 days ago. On checking, you note that his urinary output has decreased in the last 2 days also.

1. What do you conclude from these findings?
2. Based on your assessment, which type of orders might you seek from the physician or nurse practitioner?
3. Which nursing actions would you propose implementing independently?

NURSING MANAGEMENT OF THE PATIENT RECEIVING P CLONIDINE

Core Drug Knowledge

Pharmacotherapeutics

Clonidine is used to lower blood pressure. It is considered a secondary or supplemental antihypertensive because it usually is not appropriate for monotherapy. It is used in step 3 or 4 antihypertensive therapy. Unlabeled uses are varied but mostly relate to its sympathetic inhibition effects. Uses include preventing symptoms of alcohol, methadone, or opiate withdrawal during detoxification, constitutional growth delay in children, diabetic diarrhea, Gilles de la Tourette syndrome, menopausal flushing, diagnosis of pheochromocytoma (overnight clonidine suppression test), post-therapeutic neuralgia, reduction of allergen-induced inflammatory reactions in patients with extrinsic asthma, smoking cessation, and ulcerative colitis (see Table 27.3).

MEMORY CHIP

P Labetalol

- Used for hypertension most frequently with other agents, especially thiazide and loop diuretics
- An adrenergic-blocking agent that has a nonspecific beta-blocking action at beta-1 and beta-2 receptor sites and selective alpha-1 blocking action as well. Alpha-blocking actions cause peripheral vasodilation. Beta-blocking action prevents reflex tachycardia
- Parenteral form is for severe hypertension and is given only in the hospital
- Major contraindications: severe bradycardia; second- or third-degree heart block; bronchial asthma; overt, noncompensated heart failure; and cardiogenic shock due to stimulation of beta-1 and beta-2 receptor sites
- Adverse effects: uncommon and tend to be mild and transient. Orthostatic hypotension may occur
- Minimizing adverse effects: Discontinue long-term therapy gradually over 1 to 2 weeks with careful patient monitoring; and if given IV, keep the patient lying flat for 3 hours after administration.

Pharmacokinetics

Clonidine may be administered orally or transdermally and is well absorbed from the GI tract and skin. The onset of action is 30 to 60 minutes after an oral dose, with peak effect occurring within 3 to 5 hours. Clonidine is distributed widely, crosses the blood–brain barrier, and is secreted in breast milk in small amounts. Metabolism occurs in the liver, and 40% to 60% of clonidine is eliminated unchanged in urine.

When administered transdermally, the drug is released at a constant rate for 7 days. Therapeutic plasma levels are achieved 2 to 3 days after initial application, although these levels are lower than those achieved with oral dosing. Applying a new transdermal delivery system weekly maintains the plasma concentration. When the transdermal system is removed and not replaced, plasma levels will persist for about 8 hours and then decline slowly over several days. Elimination half-life is 19 hours (see Table 27.3).

Pharmacodynamics

Clonidine stimulates the alpha-2 receptors centrally in the medulla oblongata, thereby inhibiting the sympathetic nervous system. Reduced sympathetic outflow from the CNS occurs, resulting in decreased heart rate, decreased blood pressure, decreased vasoconstriction, and decreased renal vascular resistance. However, renal blood flow and glomerular filtration rate remain unchanged essentially. Initially, alpha receptors in the peripheries will be stimulated, producing vasoconstriction. However, the main effect is reduced sympathetic outflow (sympatholytic) and vasodilation. Clonidine also reduces renin activity and excretion of aldosterone and catecholamines. Because of these effects, blood pressure is reduced. Because standing and lying blood pressures are reduced almost equally, little orthostatic hypotension occurs. Coadministering a diuretic enhances the antihypertensive effect.

Clonidine also acutely stimulates growth hormone release in children and adults but does not produce a chronic elevation with long-term use.

Contraindications and Precautions

The drug is contraindicated in patients with a history of hypersensitivity to clonidine or to the base of the transdermal product. Clonidine is used cautiously in patients with severe coronary insufficiency, recent MI, cerebrovascular disease, and chronic renal failure. It also is used cautiously in pregnancy (it is a category C drug), breast-feeding patients, and children (for whom safety and efficacy have not been established).

Adverse Effects

Some adverse effects are fairly common. They are dry mouth, drowsiness, dizziness, sedation, and constipation. Dry mouth and drowsiness also occur frequently when clonidine is administered transdermally. Rebound hypertension can occur if the drug therapy is discontinued abruptly.

Other less common adverse effects include:

- GI: complaints of anorexia, malaise, nausea and vomiting, parotid pain and rarely parotitis, mild transient abnormalities in liver function tests, weight gain, rare transient elevation of blood glucose or serum creatine phosphokinase, and gynecomastia.
- CV: orthostatic hypotension, palpitations, tachycardia and bradycardia, Raynaud phenomenon, electrocardiogram (ECG) abnormalities, conduction disturbances, arrhythmias, sinus bradycardia, CHF, and rare atrioventricular block. Nightmares, insomnia, hallucinations, delirium, nervousness, agitation, restlessness, anxiety, depression, and headache have been reported, as have rash, angioneurotic edema, hives, urticaria, hair thinning and alopecia, and pruritus without rash.
- Other (rare): weakness, fatigue, muscle or joint pain, cramps of the lower limbs, increased sensitivity to alcohol, dryness, itching or burning eyes, dry nasal mucosa, pallor, fever, and weakly positive Coombs test. Transient localized skin reactions, allergic contact dermatitis, hyperpigmentation, localized vesiculations, and burning have occurred with the transdermal route as well.

Overdosage results in bradycardia, hypotension, CNS depression, respiratory depression, apnea, hypothermia, miosis, seizures, lethargy, agitation, irritability, vomiting, diarrhea, hypoventilation, reversible cardiac conduction defects, arrhythmias, and transient hypertension.

Drug Interactions

Clonidine can interact with two classes of drugs—beta-adrenergic blocking agents and tricyclic antidepressants. There are no major drug–food interactions. The drug–laboratory test interactions may result in temporary abnormalities in serum liver function tests. Table 27.8 lists common drug interactions with clonidine.

TABLE 27.8 Agents That Interact With P Clonidine

Interactants	Effect and Significance	Nursing Management
beta-adrenergic blocking agents	Severity of withdrawal hypertension from abrupt discontinuation of clonidine may be greater in patients taking beta-adrenergic blockers; may be due to unopposed alpha-adrenergic stimulation	Monitor blood pressure carefully.
tricyclic antidepressants	May block antihypertensive effect of clonidine	Monitor blood pressure carefully.

Assessment of Relevant Core Patient Variables

Health Status

You must determine whether the patient has severe coronary insufficiency, recent MI, or cerebrovascular disease, which may be affected adversely by decreased sympathetic outflow from the CNS. The patient also needs to be assessed for chronic renal failure because this condition increases the drug half-life, and a decreased dose may be needed.

Life Span and Gender

The patient's pregnancy status needs to be determined because clonidine is a pregnancy category C drug. It is also important to determine a patient's age before administering clonidine. Elderly patients may benefit from a decreased dose because they will have aging-related deterioration of their renal function. Safety and efficacy in children have not been established.

Lifestyle, Diet, and Habits

Explore the patient's lifestyle and suggest possible changes to decrease blood pressure, such as losing weight, stopping smoking, increasing exercise, and limiting salt intake. Owing to the decreased heart rate, vasodilation, and decreased blood pressure that result from clonidine, the drug effectively can control the symptoms of withdrawal from opiates and street drugs. Patients with hypertension who abuse opiates and are not seeking assistance to control their substance abuse should not be prescribed clonidine for their blood pressure. Box 27.2 presents clonidine use and abuse in the community.

COMMUNITY-BASED CONCERNS

Box 27.2 Clonidine Use and Abuse

Nurses need to be aware that clonidine is used not only as an antihypertensive agent, but also as an agent to alleviate severe discomforts associated with withdrawal from narcotic drug abuse. This has several implications for nursing management and the community.

- Nurses and other health care providers should always assess for possible substance abuse before a prescription for clonidine is given.
- Clonidine should not be prescribed routinely for hypertensive patients who also are substance abusers because the patient may not take the drug as prescribed for hypertension. Instead, the patient may reserve the clonidine to use for comfort in a time when a "fix" is not available.
- Because a black market exists for clonidine in some communities, the patient may be tempted to sell the prescription.
- Nurses and other health care providers should be alert to patients returning for a duplicate prescription of clonidine, claiming to have lost the original shortly after it was prescribed. This may indicate the patient has sold or stored the prescription. In such cases, the prescriber may be notified and consulted about a change in the prescription, particularly if it appears that the patient is not taking the clonidine.
- If regular monitoring suggests little or no therapeutic response and the patient claims to have used all of the prescribed drug and requests more, the prescriber should be notified and consulted about changing the drug.

Environment

Be aware of the setting in which clonidine may be administered. Clonidine can be administered in any environment. In the hospital before surgery, drug administration may continue for up to 4 hours before the procedure and be resumed as soon as possible thereafter to prevent hypertensive rebound from withdrawal. In the home, patients may self-administer clonidine with a transdermal patch. In such cases, patients should discard used patches with care so that children cannot find the patch, play with it, or suck on it and sustain severe hypotension. One study indicated that patients living in the southeastern United States had significantly lower treatment success with clonidine than did those who lived in other parts of the United States. An environmental cause for this statistic has been hypothesized (Cushman et al., 2000).

Nursing Diagnoses and Outcomes

- Acute Pain from dry mouth related to drug therapy
  Desired outcome: The patient's pain from dry mouth will be minimized or managed so that the patient continues to adhere to the therapeutic regimen.
- Risk for Injury related to drug-induced drowsiness, dizziness, and sedation
  Desired outcome: The patient will sustain no injury related to adverse effects of drug therapy.
- Constipation secondary to adverse effects of drug therapy
  Desired outcome: The patient will not become constipated while on drug therapy.

Planning and Intervention

Maximizing Therapeutic Effects

Oral Route

Give clonidine in combination with other antihypertensives; it is very occasionally used alone.

Transdermal

Apply the dosage patch to a hairless area of intact skin on the upper arm or torso every 7 days, and rotate application sites. If the patch loosens during the 7-day period, an adhesive overlay may be applied directly over the patch to ensure a good seal.

If used as monotherapy, additional antihypertensive agents, such as diuretics, may be indicated during the first 2 or 3 days after initial transdermal application.

Minimizing Adverse Effects

Reduce the dosage gradually to prevent rebound hypertension; do not stop clonidine abruptly. It is a good idea to offer ice chips or hard candy for dry mouth, if not contraindicated by physiologic status. Also, encourage oral fluids and moderate exercise to minimize constipation.

Caution patients not to drive, operate heavy machinery, or perform other actions requiring alertness until it is known whether drowsiness, dizziness, and sedation will occur. Sedation may be minimized by increasing the daily dosage slowly and by giving most of the dosage at bedtime.

Providing Patient and Family Education

- Explain the purpose of clonidine therapy and possible adverse effects.
- Caution the patient not to stop taking clonidine abruptly.
- Urge the patient to discard transdermal patches safely away from children and pets.
- Teach techniques that maximize therapeutic effects and minimize discomfort.
- Recommend lifestyle changes, reinforcing changes that are effective.
- Teach the patient how to monitor blood pressure and emphasize the importance of regular measurement.
- Schedule the patient for follow-up clinical care to assess drug effectiveness.

Ongoing Assessment and Evaluation

Monitor the patient's blood pressure regularly throughout therapy and assess the patient regularly for therapeutic and adverse effects.

Drugs Significantly Different From [P] Clonidine

Two groups of drugs, the alpha-1 blockers and the anti-adrenergic agents, are also secondary antihypertensives, like clonidine. Unlike clonidine, which acts centrally, these drugs act peripherally.

Peripherally Acting Alpha-1 Blockers

The alpha-1 blockers are composed of prazosin, terazosin, and doxazosin. These drugs block postsynaptic alpha-1 adrenergic receptors, producing vasodilation of resistance vessels (arterioles) and capacitance vessels (veins) and thereby decreasing blood pressure. Both standing and lying blood pressures are reduced, particularly the diastolic blood pressure. A substantial first-dose effect of hypotension, especially orthostatic hypotension, can occur with these drugs. Prazosin and doxazosin are both extensively metabolized in the liver, whereas terazosin circulates in the body mostly unchanged. Excretion of all three is mostly through the GI tract, with some excretion occurring through the renal system. Prazosin has the unique disadvantage of causing sodium and water retention and increasing plasma volume.

These drugs differ from clonidine in that they have unique therapeutic actions. Terazosin and doxazosin also are used in treating benign prostatic hypertrophy. The reduction of symptoms and increase in urine flow rate are attributed to relaxation of smooth muscle from the alpha-1 blockade in the bladder neck and prostate gland. Bladder contractility is not affected because there are few alpha receptors in the bladder body.

Unlabeled uses of these drugs include treating refractory CHF, managing Raynaud vasospasm, treating benign prostatic hyperplasia (prazosin), and treating CHF with concurrent digoxin and diuretics (doxazosin). Frequent adverse effects of these drugs are dizziness, asthenia, headache, palpitations, and nausea. Like clonidine, these drugs are in pregnancy category C.

MEMORY CHIP

[P] Clonidine

- Stimulates the alpha-2 receptors centrally, which reduces sympathetic outflow from the CNS and results in decreased heart rate, blood pressure, vasoconstriction, and renal vascular resistance
- Used as a second-line antihypertensive, also to relieve the discomfort of withdrawal symptoms from narcotics
- Most common adverse effects: dry mouth, drowsiness, dizziness, sedation, and constipation; dry mouth and drowsiness also occur with transdermal administration
- Most serious adverse effect: rebound hypertension (with abrupt stopping)
- Maximizing therapeutic effects: Give clonidine orally in combination with other antihypertensives; apply a new patch to a hairless area every 7 days (transdermal).
- Minimizing adverse effects: Do not stop therapy abruptly.
- Most important patient education: Teach the patient how to manage common adverse effects.

Peripherally Acting Antiadrenergics

Reserpine, guanethidine, and guanadrel are peripherally acting antiadrenergics. They have a different mechanism of action than clonidine.

RESERPINE

Like clonidine, reserpine (Serpalan) is used to treat hypertension as a secondary agent. Unlike clonidine, reserpine is also used to relieve symptoms in agitated psychotic states, such as schizophrenia, primarily if the patient cannot tolerate phenothiazides. Reserpine depletes the stores of norepinephrine. Therefore, less norepinephrine is available for release into the synaptic cleft, which causes depression of sympathetic nerve function and also decreasing heart rate and blood pressure. Reserpine also has sedative and tranquilizing effects believed to result from depletion of catecholamine and 5-hydroxytryptamine.

Reserpine has a slow onset of action and a prolonged duration of action after discontinuation. Plasma levels slowly decrease after IV administration with a mean half-life of 33 hours.

Contraindications and precautions for the use of this drug include active peptic ulcer disease, ulcerative colitis (reserpine increases GI motility and secretion), and renal impairment. Patients who are receiving electroconvulsive therapy, are pregnant (category C) or breast-feeding, or are children (safety and efficacy have not been established) should avoid reserpine.

Adverse effects associated with reserpine are serious. This drug can cause severe depression and therefore is contraindicated if the patient's emotional health record shows a history of depression. The drug should be discontinued at the first sign of depression. Depression may last for several months after discontinuing reserpine and may be severe enough to result in suicide. Besides depression, vomiting, diarrhea, arrhythmias, dyspnea, dizziness, headache, and rash may occur. These adverse effects are serious and clinically important enough to limit therapeutic usefulness of the drug. Therefore, this drug is used only if other drug therapies have been unsuccessful in controlling hypertension.

Major drug interactions are with MAOIs, tricyclic antidepressants, digitalis, quinidine, and sympathomimetics (direct and indirect acting).

GUANETHIDINE AND GUANADREL

Both guanethidine and guanadrel are used to treat hypertension. Guanethidine can also be used in treating renal hypertension. Guanethidine and guanadrel inhibit or interfere with the release and distribution of norepinephrine at the sympathetic neuroeffector junction, which leads to decreased sympathetic function and results in decreased heart rate and blood pressure.

Guanethidine has an extremely long half-life of 4 to 8 days, whereas guanadrel's half-life is similar to clonidine's at 10 hours.

Contraindications for both drugs are pheochromocytoma, frank CHF, use of MAOIs, and drug hypersensitivity. A major adverse effect is orthostatic hypotension, which can occur frequently with these drugs because they decrease the reflexive vasoconstriction that occurs when arising from a lying position.

C DIRECT-ACTING VASODILATORS

The representative direct-acting vasodilator is hydralazine.

NURSING MANAGEMENT OF THE PATIENT RECEIVING P HYDRALAZINE

Core Drug Knowledge

Pharmacotherapeutics

Hydralazine is normally used as an adjunct to other antihypertensives. Parenteral hydralazine is used for severe hypertension when the need to reduce the blood pressure is urgent or the patient cannot take oral drugs. It may also be given alone. In unlabeled use, hydralazine is used following valve replacement, for treating severe aortic insufficiency, and for reducing afterload to manage CHF.

Pharmacokinetics

Hydralazine is well absorbed orally, with the onset occurring soon after administration. The oral drug peaks in 1 to 2 hours; given parenterally, hydralazine peaks in 10 to 20 minutes (see Table 27.3). Hydralazine is metabolized by the liver and is excreted in urine. It crosses the placenta and may enter breast milk. It is compatible with breast-feeding according to the American Academy of Pediatrics. Hydralazine has increased bioavailability when the oral form is administered with food.

Pharmacodynamics

Hydralazine produces direct smooth muscle relaxation of the arterioles. Hydralazine alters cellular calcium metabolism, thereby interfering with calcium movement within the vascular smooth muscles responsible for venous contraction and dilation. Peripheral vasodilation results, promoting a decrease in arterial blood pressure and decreased peripheral resistance. As a reflexive action to the peripheral vasodilation, the body increases heart rate, stroke volume, and cardiac output. The reflex mechanism is caused by an increase in sympathetic stimulation. Because hydralazine preferentially dilates arterioles rather than veins, orthostatic hypotension does not occur as frequently as with other antihypertensives. However, this effect promotes an increase in cardiac output. Because of the reflexive increases in cardiac function, hydralazine is commonly given with drugs that decrease sympathetic activity, such as beta blockers or the alpha-2 stimulant, clonidine.

Hydralazine increases plasma renin activity, leading to production of angiotensin II. Angiotensin II increases aldosterone production, which increases sodium and water retention. Because of these changes, hydralazine is coadministered frequently with a diuretic.

Contraindications and Precautions

The drug is contraindicated with hypersensitivity to hydralazine, coronary artery disease, and mitral valvular rheumatic disease. It should be administered cautiously to patients with advanced renal damage, cerebral vascular accidents, suspected coronary artery disease, pulmonary hypertension, and sensitivity to tartrazine (FDC yellow dye #5) because some of the products contain this substance. Hydralazine is a pregnancy category C drug; safety and efficacy in children have not been established.

Adverse Effects

The adverse effects of hydralazine usually resolve when the dose is reduced. Occasionally, the drug will need to be discontinued because of adverse effects. Many of the adverse effects are related to increased cardiac output. The most common adverse effects include palpitations, tachycardia, angina, anorexia, nausea, and vomiting.

A serious adverse effect that may occur while taking hydralazine is the development of symptoms of SLE, such as arthralgia, dermatoses, fever, splenomegaly, and glomerular nephritis. The syndrome usually occurs after 6 months of drug therapy or more, and the likelihood of occurrence increases with larger doses and longer duration of therapy. Complete blood counts (CBCs) and antinuclear antibody titer will be affected. This simulation of SLE occurs more frequently in slow acetylators. It is more common in women and whites than in men and blacks. Symptoms usually resolve after the drug has been discontinued, but residual effects may last a long time. Some have been detected years later. Long-term treatment with steroids may be required.

Other adverse effects of hydralazine include peripheral neuritis with paresthesia, numbness, and tingling. This effect may result from an antipyridoxine effect. Reduction in hemoglobin and red cell count, leukopenia, agranulocytosis, and purpura have been reported with the use of hydralazine. In addition, serum sodium levels may rise.

Symptoms of drug overdose are hypotension, tachycardia, headache, and generalized skin flushing. If overdose occurs, cardiac function needs to be supported and volume expanders given. Gastric contents should be evacuated and a charcoal slurry administered, if possible, once cardiac function stabilizes.

Drug Interactions

Hydralazine interacts with the beta blockers metoprolol or propranolol and with indomethacin. Table 27.9 lists drugs that interact with hydralazine.

Assessment of Relevant Core Patient Variables

Health Status

Begin the assessment by measuring the patient's blood pressure and taking a drug history, particularly of other antihypertensives. Also, determine whether the patient has coronary artery disease or mitral valvular rheumatic heart disease because these conditions are contraindications to hydralazine therapy. Renal function must be assessed because dose adjustments may be necessary. Other assessments include determining whether the patient has pulmonary hypertension, a history of cerebral vascular accidents, or sensitivity to tartrazine (if the prescribed drug form contains this component). Administer this drug cautiously if any of these conditions are present. Baseline CBCs and antinuclear antibody tiers should be determined before starting therapy, and values should be within normal ranges.

Life Span and Gender

Determining the patient's pregnancy status is important because hydralazine is classified as pregnancy category C. The patient's age and gender are important as well. Safety and efficacy in children have not been established, and the incidence of hydralazine-induced SLE is higher in women.

Lifestyle, Diet, and Habits

Explore blood pressure–lowering lifestyle modifications with the patient, including losing weight, stopping smoking, increasing exercise, and limiting salt intake. Limiting salt intake especially is important with hydralazine because of the sodium reabsorption that occurs with the drug.

Environment

Be aware of the setting in which hydralazine may be administered. Parenteral hydralazine is administered in the hospital. Oral hydralazine may be given in any environment.

Culture and Inherited Traits

It is important to note the patient's genetic background before administering hydralazine. White people are more likely to develop hydralazine-induced SLE.

Nursing Diagnosis and Outcome

- Ineffective Therapeutic Regimen Management related to adverse effects of drugs
  Desired outcome: *The patient will not experience adverse effects severe enough to stop drug therapy.*

Planning and Intervention

Maximizing Therapeutic Effects

Administering hydralazine with food promotes bioavailability.

Minimizing Adverse Effects

Administer hydralazine with a beta blocker (preferably) or clonidine to decrease reflex tachycardia and with a diuretic to offset fluid retention. Consult with the physician or nurse practitioner if these drugs are not currently ordered.

Assess for signs of peripheral neuritis (numbness, tingling in hands and feet). If these signs are present, pyridoxine (a B vitamin) should be administered because the neuritis may be caused by the antipyridoxine effect of drug therapy. Inform the physician or nurse practitioner of signs of peripheral neuritis. Give a form of the drug that is not made with tartrazine if the patient is allergic to tartrazine (the incidence of sensitivity in the general population is low, but patients who are allergic are commonly allergic to aspirin as well).

Monitor the results of CBCs and the antinuclear antibody titer for indications of hydralazine-induced lupus. This monitoring is important especially if arthralgia, fever, chest pain, continued malaise, or other unexplained symptoms develop. Also, monitor blood pressure for hypotension.

Consult with the prescriber to individualize the drug dosage to achieve the desired goal of blood pressure. Typically, the patient begins with low divided doses, and the dosage is then increased gradually to minimize adverse effects. If hydralazine is given parenterally, administer it as soon as possible after drawing it into a syringe to promote stability of the drug. (Note: hydralazine changes color after contact with a metal filter.)

Providing Patient and Family Education

- Explain the purpose and adverse effects of hydralazine and the rationale for using multiple drugs to treat hypertension, if applicable.
- Teach the patient to recognize and report the following signs to the prescriber (especially if there is no apparent reason for these signs): prolonged generalized tiredness, fever, aching joints or muscles, or chest pain.

TABLE 27.9 Agents That Interact With P Hydralazine

Interactants	Effect and Significance	Nursing Management
beta blockers (metoprolol, propranolol)	Serum level of either the beta blockers or hydralazine may be increased by concurrent use	Monitor for therapeutic and adverse effects.
indomethacin	Pharmacologic effect of hydralazine may be decreased	Monitor blood pressure to ensure therapeutic response.

Ongoing Assessment and Evaluation

Monitor the patient's blood pressure throughout therapy. If hydralazine is given parenterally, blood pressure should be monitored closely because it will start to fall within a few minutes of administration, with an average maximal decrease occurring in 10 to 80 minutes. Use CBCs and the antinuclear antibody titers to monitor for signs of adverse effects.

Drugs Significantly Different From P Hydralazine

Minoxidil

Like hydralazine, minoxidil is a direct-acting vasodilator. It also does not create orthostatic hypotension because it does not affect vasomotor reflexes. It appears to block calcium uptake through the cell membrane. Like hydralazine, it is used with beta blockers to control reflex tachycardia and with a diuretic—preferably one acting in the ascending loop of Henle—to prevent substantial fluid accumulation.

Minoxidil differs in its serious adverse effects. It can cause pericardial effusion, occasionally progressing to cardiac tamponade, and it can worsen angina pectoris. Fluid retention and several hundred milliequivalents of salt accumulation can occur in a few days of use if the drug is not prescribed with a loop diuretic.

Hypertrichosis (excess hair growth) occurs in 3 to 6 weeks after starting therapy in 80% of patients receiving minoxidil. Elongation, thickening, and enhanced pigmentation of fine body hair develops. It is usually noticed first on the temples, between eyebrows, at the hairline, and in the eyebrows or sideburn area of the upper lateral cheek. It will progress down the back, arms, legs, and scalp. New hair growth stops when minoxidil use is discontinued, although it will take 1 to 6 months for appearance to return to normal. This adverse effect of hypertrichosis spawned a new therapeutic use for minoxidil—treating male pattern baldness and female hair loss or thinning of hair in the frontoparietal area. For growing hair, topical minoxidil (Rogaine) is the drug of choice. Oral usage to promote hair growth is not approved. At least 4 months of twice-daily treatments are necessary before evidence of hair regrowth is seen. Clinical trials showed 39% of the men achieved moderate to dense terminal hair regrowth by 12 months, although 48% of the men thought such growth had occurred. Clinical trials with women resulted in somewhat less improvement; between 12% and 13% achieved moderate growth, and between 32% and 50% showed minimal growth after 32 weeks of use. Additionally, more women thought they had minimal or moderate hair regrowth than the researchers' findings indicated. Accidental ingestion of topical minoxidil will produce severe systemic effects of hypotension because 5 mL of topical minoxidil contains as many milligrams of the drug as the maximum adult oral dose.

MEMORY CHIP

P Hydralazine

- Second-line antihypertensive drug
- Direct-acting vasodilator. Relaxes arterioles, which decreases peripheral resistance and lowers blood pressure
- Adverse effect of reflex tachycardia makes hydralazine unsuitable for monotherapy; usually given with two beta-blockers and diuretics, each of which controls blood pressure by different mechanisms
- Most common adverse effects: palpitations, tachycardia, angina, anorexia, nausea, and vomiting
- Most serious adverse effects: symptoms of systemic lupus erythematosus (SLE); the likelihood increases with larger doses and longer therapy; whites are more likely to develop hydralazine-induced SLE
- Minimizing adverse effects: Administer hydralazine with a beta blocker to decrease reflex tachycardia and a diuretic to prevent fluid retention.
- Most important patient education: Have patient learn to report signs of SLE (e.g., prolonged generalized tiredness, fever, and aching joints or muscles).

Epoprostenol

Like hydralazine, epoprostenol directly dilates peripheral vessels. Unlike hydralazine, epoprostenol also directly dilates pulmonary vascular beds and inhibits platelet aggravation. For these reasons, the sole clinical indication for epoprostenol is to treat primary pulmonary hypertension. IV infusions of 15 minutes' duration or less will produce dose-related increases in the cardiac index and stroke volume and dose-related decreases in pulmonary vascular resistance, total pulmonary resistance, and mean systemic arterial pressure. The effects on mean pulmonary artery pressure are variable and minor. Epoprostenol is hydrolyzed rapidly at neutral pH in blood and also is subject to enzymatic metabolism. The drug dose is titrated upward in small increments until adverse effects occur from the vasodilation effects of the drug. A chronic dose is then established. Abrupt withdrawal, including interruptions in the drug delivery (e.g., temporarily running out of drug), or sudden large dose reductions, may result in rebound pulmonary hypertension.

Adverse effects of epoprostenol are those seen during the acute phase of dosing, and during chronic administration. Those seen most commonly during the dosing phase of therapy are flushing, headache, nausea, and vomiting. The next most common are hypotension, anxiety, nervousness, restlessness, chest pain, bradycardia, and abdominal pain. Occasional adverse effects are musculoskeletal pain, dyspnea, back pain, sweating, dyspepsia, hyperesthesia and paresthesia, and tachycardia. Some patients have developed pulmonary edema during dose ranging; these patients should not receive long-term treatment with epoprostenol because this adverse effect is serious and potentially fatal.

Adverse effects during the chronic phase are often the same as clinical features of primary pulmonary hypertension. The following adverse effects are seen with epoprostenol therapy more frequently (more than 10%) than in pulmonary hypertension:

- CV: flushing and tachycardia
- GI: diarrhea, nausea, and vomiting
- Musculoskeletal: jaw pain, myalgia, and nonspecific musculoskeletal pain
- CNS: anxiety, nervousness, tremor, dizziness, headache, hyperesthesia, and paresthesia
- Miscellaneous: chills, fever, sepsis, and flu-like symptoms

Symptoms of overdosage are those that are seen in the acute phase of dosing (flushing, headache, nausea, and vomiting).

The drug is contraindicated in patients who have CHF with severe left ventricular systolic dysfunction and in those who are hypersensitive to the drug. The drug is in pregnancy category B; whether it is excreted in breast milk is unknown, and its effects on children are not known. Older adults should receive lower doses because they may not metabolize or excrete the drug optimally.

Epoprostenol is given intravenously by continuous infusion through a central line catheter, with the rate regulated by an infusion pump. It may be given through a peripheral line but only until central access is obtained. Treatment of primary pulmonary hypertension is chronic. Patients will be discharged with the drug and the infusion pump. The treatment may last up to several years. Patients should be aware of this fact before instituting therapy. Patients who will receive epoprostenol at home, and their families, need teaching regarding drug reconstitution, administration, and central catheter care in addition to information about the drug. A firm commitment to this treatment on the part of the patient and family is required for the drug therapy to be effective.

C DRUGS USED IN HYPERTENSIVE CRISIS

The prototype drug used in hypertensive crisis is nitroprusside. Table 27.10 presents a summary of selected drugs that are used to treat hypertensive crisis.

NURSING MANAGEMENT OF THE PATIENT RECEIVING P NITROPRUSSIDE

Core Drug Knowledge

Pharmacotherapeutics

Nitroprusside is the drug of choice when an immediate reduction of blood pressure is indicated in hypertensive crisis. It should be administered concurrently with longer-acting antihypertensives to minimize the duration of treatment. Other uses include reducing bleeding during surgery through the production of a controlled hypotensive state. It is also used for treating acute CHF. Unlabeled uses include treating MI

TABLE 27.10 Summary of Selected Drugs for C Hypertensive Crisis

Drug (Trade) Name	Selected Indications	Route and Dosage Range	Pharmacokinetics
P nitroprusside (Nitropress)	Hypertensive crisis	*Adult:* IV, 0.3 μg/kg/min with gradual upward titration until desired effect or maximum rate of 10 μg/kg/min occurs	*Onset:* 1–2 min *Duration:* 3–5 min $t_{1/2}$: 2 min
diazoxide (Hyperstat IV)	Hypertensive crisis	*Adult:* direct IV, 1–3 mg/kg to a maximum of 150 mg in a single injection; repeat every 5–15 min until blood pressure drops, then repeat at 4- to 24-h intervals to maintain blood pressure until oral drug can begin	*Onset:* 1–2 min *Duration:* <12 h $t_{1/2}$: 28 ± 8.3 h
phentolamine (Regitine; *Canadian:* Rogitine)	Preoperatively to prevent or control hypertension with pheochromocytoma	*Adult:* IV/IM, 5 mg 1 or 2 h before surgery, repeated if needed; 5 mg as needed during surgery *Child:* IV/IM, 1 mg	*Onset:* Immediate *Duration:* 3–10 min $t_{1/2}$: Unknown
	Prevent or treat dermal necrosis and sloughing resulting from administration or extravasation of IV norepinephrine	*Adult:* IV (prophylactic), 10 mg/L of norepinephrine solution; SC (treatment), 5–10 mg in 10 mL of saline solution into area of extravasation within 12 h *Child:* 0.1–0.2 mg/kg to maximum 10 mg	
	Diagnosis of pheochromocytoma	*Adult:* IV, 2.5 mg dissolved in 1 mL sterile water injected directly by syringe into vein *Child:* 1 mg as above	

(with coadministration of dopamine) and left ventricular failure (with coadministration of oxygen, morphine, and a loop diuretic).

Pharmacokinetics

Nitroprusside is administered parenterally (intravenously) for immediate onset. Maximum effects are observed in 1 to 2 minutes. Resting circulating half-life is about 2 minutes. When the drug is discontinued, the blood pressure may return to its previous level within minutes. The metabolism of nitroprusside is important to understand because it has bearing on dosing and adverse effects. Nitroprusside is metabolized rapidly to cyanide through a reaction with hemoglobin. Cyanide is poisonous. Thiosulfate, a sulfate derivative created through normal physiologic mechanisms, reacts with the cyanide to produce another element, thiocyanate. The thiocyanate thereby processed by the liver is then excreted in the urine. Cyanide that becomes thiocyanate and is excreted is prevented from producing poisonous effects in the patient. Cyanide that does not produce thiocyanate will bind with cytochromes. This binding prevents the cytochromes from participating in oxidative metabolism. Without oxidative metabolism, the cells cannot provide for their energy needs. Lactic acid is created, and eventually the cells die from hypoxia. Conversion of cyanide to thiocyanate occurs at a rate of 1 μg/kg per minute. This rate of cyanide clearance corresponds to steady-state processing when nitroprusside is infused at slightly more than 2 μg/kg per minute. If this rate is exceeded, cyanide will build up and poison the patient. The half-life of thiocyanate increases from about 3 days to double or triple this time in patients with renal failure.

Pharmacodynamics

Nitroprusside directly relaxes vascular smooth muscle, allowing dilation of peripheral arteries and veins. It is more active on veins than on arteries, thereby promoting peripheral pooling of blood. This effect decreases venous return to the heart, reducing left ventricular end-diastolic pressure and pulmonary capillary wedge pressure (preload). The arteriolar dilation that occurs reduces systemic resistance and decreases mean arterial pressure (afterload). Dilation of coronary vessels also occurs. These processes produce a marked reduction in blood pressure, a slight increase in pulse rate, a slight decrease in cardiac output, and an increased production of renin. The ability to decrease the blood pressure is seemingly unlimited.

Contraindications and Precautions

Nitroprusside is contraindicated for compensatory hypertension in which the primary hemodynamic lesion is aortic coarctation or arteriovenous shunting. Nitroprusside also is contraindicated for providing surgical hypotension in patients with known inadequate cerebral circulation or in moribund patients undergoing emergency surgery. Another contraindication is acute CHF associated with reduced peripheral vascular resistance, such as high output heart failure, which may be seen in endotoxic sepsis. Additionally, the drug is contraindicated in patients with the rare condition of congenital optic atrophy or tobacco amblyopia; these patients have unusually high cyanide-to-thiocyanate ratios.

Nitroprusside is used cautiously in older adults and in patients with renal and hepatic impairment, hypovolemia, and anemia. Nitroprusside given for its hypotensive effect during surgery may decrease the patient's ability to compensate for hypovolemia and anemia. Nitroprusside is a pregnancy category C drug.

Adverse Effects

Small, transient excesses in the infusion rate can result in excessive hypotension, sometimes compromising perfusion of vital organs. This hypotension is self-limiting after discontinuation of the drug. A too-rapid reduction of blood pressure can result in abdominal pain, apprehension, diaphoresis, dizziness, headache, muscle twitching, nausea, palpitations, restlessness, retching, and retrosternal discomfort. Symptoms quickly subside when the nitroprusside infusion slows or stops; they do not return when the infusion resumes at a slower rate. Cyanide toxicity can occur when the nitroprusside infusion rate exceeds the rate of cyanide excretion. Cyanide toxicity may manifest as venous hyperoxemia (in which bright-red venous blood appears as the cells become unable to extract the oxygen delivered to them), metabolic (lactic) acidosis, air hunger, confusion, and death.

Elimination of cyanide increases with the administration of thiosulfate. However, this effect also has risks. Thiosulfate increases the production of thiocyanate. Thiocyanate is mildly neurotoxic; neurotoxicity is signaled by tinnitus, miosis, and hyperreflexia at serum levels of 1 mmol/L (60 mg/L). Thiocyanate toxicity is life threatening when levels are three or four times higher (200 mg/L). Thiocyanate also interferes with iodine uptake by the thyroid.

Methemoglobin, derived from hemoglobin, can hide cyanide. After nitroprusside is administered, hemoglobin can convert to methemoglobin, leading to methemoglobinemia. This adverse effect is rare, occurring when a patient receives the maximum rate of nitroprusside infusion for a prolonged period (>16 hours). Methemoglobinemia is characterized by blood that appears chocolate brown and that does not change color after exposure to air.

Like other vasodilators, nitroprusside may increase intracranial pressure and cause adverse CV effects, such as bradycardia or tachycardia, and ECG changes. Platelet aggregation may be decreased, and flushing, venous streaking, irritation at the infusion site, rash, hypothyroidism, and ileus may be detected.

Drug Interactions

No drug interactions are associated with nitroprusside.

Assessment of Relevant Core Patient Variables

Health Status

The initial assessment includes determining the patient's blood pressure and physical states that are contraindications for nitroprusside use, such as compensatory hypertension, acute CHF associated with reduced peripheral vascular resistance, inadequate cerebral circulation before anesthesia, moribundity before emergency surgery, congenital optic atrophy, or tobacco amblyopia. You must also determine whether intracranial pressure is elevated.

Life Span and Gender

Determine the patient's age before administering nitroprusside. Nitroprusside is given with caution to children and the elderly who may be more sensitive to the hypotensive effects of the drug. Determine whether the patient is pregnant before administering nitroprusside. In patients who are pregnant, nitroprusside is given only if clearly indicated because it is a category C drug.

Environment

Be aware of the setting in which nitroprusside may be administered. Nitroprusside is administered in a hospital setting where blood pressure can be monitored continuously by a continually reinflated sphygmomanometer (automatic blood pressure cuff) or preferably by an intra-arterial pressure sensor. Once diluted, nitroprusside is sensitive to light. The solution should be protected from light by wrapping it in the supplied opaque sleeve, aluminum foil, or other opaque material. It is not necessary to cover the drip chamber or the IV tubing.

Culture and Inherited Traits

Nitroprusside has a prompt hypotensive effect on all populations.

Nursing Diagnoses and Outcomes

- Decreased Cardiac Output related to venous dilation, diminished preload, and severe hypotension secondary to therapeutic and adverse effects of drug therapy
  Desired outcome: *Hypotension will not occur to an extent that cardiac output cannot meet the perfusion needs of the vital organs.*
- Acute Pain related to decreased comfort from rapid blood pressure reduction secondary to too rapid drug infusion
  Desired outcome: *The patient's blood pressure will not drop so quickly that adverse effects result.*
- Risk for Injury related to increased intracranial pressure, cyanide poisoning, or thiocyanate toxicity secondary to adverse effects of drug therapy.
  Desired outcome: *The patient will not suffer injury while on drug therapy.*

Planning and Intervention

Maximizing Therapeutic Effects

The infusion rate must be titrated to reduce blood pressure without compromising organ perfusion. When it is given for CHF, titrate the nitroprusside infusion so that measured cardiac output does not increase and systemic blood pressure remains as low as possible without compromising organ perfusion or the maximum infusion rate has been reached—whichever comes first.

Nitroprusside can be inactivated by reactions with trace contaminants. If these reactions have occurred, the nitroprusside will appear blue, green, or red; it will be much brighter than its normal faint brownish color. If the solution appears discolored or if particulate appears, the solution should not be used.

After nitroprusside has been reconstituted in 2 to 3 mL of dextrose in water or sterile water, it must be further diluted in 250 mL to 1,000 mL of 5% dextrose in water (D_5W). Reconstituted nitroprusside should not be injected directly.

The nurse must protect the container of diluted solution (but not the tubing or drip chamber) from light by placing it in an opaque sleeve or wrapping it in aluminum foil for stability of the solution.

Minimizing Adverse Effects

To avoid extreme hypotensive effect, start nitroprusside at a low infusion rate (0.3 μg/kg per minute) and increase it gradually until the desired effect has been achieved or the maximum infusion rate (10 μg/kg per minute) is attained.

Do not adjust the infusion rate by gravity because slight variations in infusion rate can lead to substantial variations in blood pressure. An infusion pump, preferably a volumetric infusion pump, should always be used.

It is important to monitor the patient's blood pressure constantly during the infusion, either with a continually inflating sphygmomanometer or (preferably) with an intra-arterial pressure sensor.

The usual dosage rate is 0.5 to 10 μg/kg per minute. However, cyanide clearance occurs when the dosage rate is less than 2 μg/kg per minute. To prevent dangerous, possibly lethal, buildup of cyanide, the maximum infusion should never exceed 10 minutes.

If the blood pressure remains uncontrolled after 10 minutes at the maximum infusion rate, stop the infusion immediately. Cyanide level assay is technically difficult to perform, and cyanide levels in body fluids other than packed red blood cells are difficult to interpret. Therefore, it is difficult to determine cyanide toxicity directly from laboratory findings.

Monitoring the acid-base balance and venous oxygen concentrations may help indicate cyanide toxicity. However, these tests do not always accurately reflect cyanide levels. Clinical studies show that metabolic acidosis, although normally occurring with elevated cyanide levels, may lag behind peak cyanide levels by an hour or more. Therefore, monitor also for other signs of cyanide toxicity, such as red venous blood, air hunger, or confusion. It is also important to monitor for signs of thiocyanate toxicity (tinnitus, miosis, hyperreflexia) and methemoglobinemia (chocolate-brown blood).

Toxicity to nitroprusside can occur even if the dose is well within recommended limits. Toxicity may be evident by excessive hypotension, cyanide toxicity, or thiocyanate toxicity. Closely monitoring the patient throughout therapy is the key to safety.

Administer other longer-acting antihypertensives as needed during nitroprusside therapy to limit the dosage of nitroprusside as necessary. It is important to monitor for signs that blood pressure has been reduced too rapidly (e.g., abdominal pain, apprehension, diaphoresis, dizziness, headache, muscle twitching, nausea, palpitations, restlessness, retching, or retrosternal discomfort). Slow or discontinue the infusion until symptoms diminish. The infusion may then resume at a slower rate.

Also, assess for signs of increased intracranial pressure and other adverse effects; correct pre-existing anemia and hypovolemia before administration with anesthesia, if appropriate. Administer to a pregnant patient only if clearly indicated.

Providing Patient and Family Education

- Explain to the patient and family that the drug is being given to lower blood pressure quickly and that blood pressure will be monitored constantly to prevent it from dropping too low.
- Urge the patient to report adverse effects (such as abdominal pain, apprehension, diaphoresis, dizziness, headache, muscle twitching, nausea, palpitations, restlessness, retching, or retrosternal discomfort) immediately to the nurse.

Ongoing Assessment and Evaluation

Monitor blood pressure throughout therapy so that it is reduced without sacrifice to vital organs. Signs of increasing intracranial pressure and other adverse effects should be assessed as well. Drug therapy is effective when blood pressure falls to a safe level, organ damage is averted, and severe hypotension, cyanide toxicity, or thiocyanate toxicity does not develop.

Drugs Closely Related to P Nitroprusside

Diazoxide

Like nitroprusside, diazoxide reduces blood pressure by relaxing smooth muscle in the peripheral arterioles, although it does not affect the veins. It is used to treat hypertensive emergencies. The hypotensive effect of diazoxide also occurs quickly, beginning within 1 minute of IV administration. Maximum effect is in 2 to 5 minutes. Unlike nitroprusside, diazoxide is not a diuretic, but it is related structurally to the thiazides. The oral form of this drug is used to treat hyperinsulinism by increasing blood glucose levels. Consequently, transient elevations in blood glucose levels also occur with IV dosing in most patients receiving diazoxide.

The rapid reduction of severely elevated hypertension with 300 mg of IV diazoxide has been associated with angina and with myocardial and cerebral infarction. To avoid possible ischemia and optic nerve damage (rare adverse effects), the recommended dose is now 1 to 3 mg/kg IV up to 150 mg at one time. The dose may be repeated in 5 to 15 minutes until blood pressure stabilizes. IV diazoxide should be administered undiluted.

Diazoxide does not cause cyanide toxicity as nitroprusside does. The most common adverse effects are hypotension, nausea and vomiting, and dizziness.

Fenoldopam

Fenoldopam is a new drug for treating hypertensive emergencies. It also is a rapid vasodilator. It is a pregnancy category B drug. Fenoldopam is administered only as a continuous IV infusion, never as a bolus dose. The dose should be titrated up or down every 15 minutes until the desired blood pressure has been achieved. The most common adverse effects of fenoldopam are GI disturbances; dose-related tachycardia may also occur.

Trimethaphan

Trimethaphan differs from nitroprusside in its therapeutic action. Although it may be used short term to control hypertensive crisis, it is also used to induce a controlled hypotension during surgery and as emergency treatment for pulmonary edema in patients with pulmonary hypertension associated with systolic hypertension. Like nitroprusside, it is a direct vasodilator. Unlike nitroprusside, trimethaphan is also a short-acting ganglionic blocker. It blocks the transmission in autonomic ganglia (both sympathetic and parasympathetic) without producing a change in the membrane potential. It does not modify impulse conduction in the preganglionic or postganglionic neurons, or prevent acetylcholine release by preganglionic impulses. It occupies ganglionic receptors and stabilizes postsynaptic membranes from the action of acetylcholine, which is released by the presynaptic nerve endings (Facts and Comparisons, 2004).

Administered intravenously, trimethaphan has a quick onset and a short duration of action (no longer than 10–30 minutes). Tachyphylaxis may occur, requiring additional doses. The reverse Trendelenburg position (head up, feet down) enhances the action of the drug. Only physicians properly trained to use and monitor this drug therapy should attempt surgical hypotension with trimethaphan. The nurse assists in monitoring the patient closely during surgery for signs of complications. Severe hypotension, with its ramifications, may occur.

MEMORY CHIP

P Nitroprusside

- Drug of choice for hypertensive crisis when blood pressure must be reduced immediately
- Major contraindications: compensatory hypertension resulting from aortic coarctation or arteriovenous shunting, and surgical procedures on patients with inadequate cerebral circulation
- Most common adverse effect: hypotension from too rapid infusion
- Most serious adverse effects: severe hypotension and cyanide poisoning
- Maximizing therapeutic effects: Wrap diluted bag of drug in an opaque sleeve or aluminum foil to protect from light.
- Minimizing adverse effects: Always use an IV pump to regulate infusion; start the infusion at a low dose and slowly increase; once the maximum infusion rate has been achieved, do not continue for more than 10 minutes; and monitor blood pressure throughout therapy.

Drugs Significantly Different From P Nitroprusside

Phentolamine, phenoxybenzamine, and metyrosine are used only to treat the marked elevations in blood pressure associated with pheochromocytoma, a catecholamine-secreting tumor of the adrenal medulla. Phentolamine is also used in preventing and treating dermal necrosis and sloughing after IV extravasation of norepinephrine.

Phentolamine and phenoxybenzamine are both alpha-adrenergic blockers. They lower peripheral vascular resistance and therefore decrease blood pressure. Metyrosine inhibits tyrosine hydroxylase, which is the catalyst for the first transformation in catecholamine biosynthesis. Because of this blockade, endogenous levels of catecholamine decrease. Most patients receiving this drug experience decreased frequency and severity of hypertensive attacks. Patients who

respond to therapy normally experience a decrease in blood pressure within the first 2 days of therapy.

Cardiac stimulation occurs with phentolamine. The concomitant use of a beta blocker may be needed to control tachycardia. Tachycardia may occur with phenoxybenzamine but to a lesser extent. Cardiac responses do not occur with metyrosine. Orthostatic hypotension may occur with both phentolamine and phenoxybenzamine. Sedation, drooling, speech difficulty and tremor, and diarrhea are adverse effects unique to metyrosine.

PATHOPHYSIOLOGY OF SHOCK

Shock is the result of inadequate tissue perfusion, leaving the cells without the necessary oxygen and nutrients they need to have normal function and survive. When cell dysfunction is widespread, the result can be death for the patient. Shock has multiple causes. Hypovolemic shock results from a decrease in circulating blood volume from bleeding or hemorrhage. It occurs when intravascular volume decreases more than 15% to 25%. Cardiogenic shock is caused by the heart's inability to pump enough blood to adequately perfuse the vital organs, which may itself be caused by MI, ventricular arrhythmias, severe cardiomyopathy, or CHF. Septic shock occurs when a severe infection brings about circulatory insufficiency. Obstructive shock is caused by a massive blockage in blood flow and results in inadequate tissue perfusion. This event could be caused by a large pulmonary embolus, cardiac tamponade, restrictive pericarditis, or severe cardiac valve dysfunction. Neurogenic shock is uncommon. It occurs as a result of blockade of neurohormonal outflow. This event may be induced by drugs (e.g., spinal anesthesia) or trauma to the spinal cord.

Shock has two phases—early (or compensated) and late (or noncompensated). In early shock, the body tries to compensate for the decreased perfusion. The heart and respiratory rates increase, and blood pressure is generally maintained, or it may be low to normal. The body will begin to shunt some blood flow away from the skin, although the skin is still perfused. Urine output will decrease slightly as renal blood flow is reduced. Emotionally, the patient may be anxious or confused. When the body is no longer able to make up for changes brought on by shock, the patient develops late, or uncompensated, shock. Tachycardia persists, but the blood pressure falls dramatically, and respiration rates decrease. Venous constriction occurs; with the circulation shut off, the skin becomes cold and clammy. Urine output declines dramatically and may cease as the kidneys are no longer perfused. The patient becomes nonresponsive and unconscious.

DRUGS TO TREAT HYPOTENSION RESULTING FROM SHOCK

(C) Vasopressors

Drug therapy in shock is directed at increasing blood pressure to help support tissue perfusion. Drugs are given in addition to fluid volume. Vasopressors, drugs to increase the blood pressure, are sympathomimetic. They increase cardiac contractility and heart rate, constrict veins (vasoconstriction), and dilate arteries. The prototype vasopressor is dopamine.

NURSING MANAGEMENT OF THE PATIENT RECEIVING (P) DOPAMINE

Core Drug Knowledge

Pharmacotherapeutics

Dopamine (Intropin) is used to correct the hemodynamic imbalances present in shock caused by MI, trauma, endotoxic septicemia, open heart surgery, renal failure, and chronic cardiac decompensation (CHF). For the treatment to be most effective, the patient should not be experiencing severe disruptions in urine production, myocardial function, and blood pressure. In other words, the earlier the signs of shock are recognized and treatment is started with fluids and dopamine, the more successful the therapy will be. Table 27.11 gives a summary of selected vasopressors.

Pharmacokinetics

The onset of dopamine's action is within 5 minutes. Duration of action is less than 10 minutes. The drug is distributed widely in the body, but does not cross the blood–brain barrier. Dopamine is metabolized in the liver, kidneys, and plasma by monoamine oxidase (MAO) and catechol-*O*-methyltransferase to inactive compounds. About one fourth of it is taken up into adrenergic nerve terminals that are specialized neurosecretory vesicles. There, through hydroxylation, it becomes norepinephrine. Dopamine is excreted mainly by the kidneys.

Pharmacodynamics

Dopamine is a naturally occurring catecholamine and a precursor to norepinephrine. It stimulates alpha-1 and beta-1 receptors through direct and indirect (by releasing the stored epinephrine) methods. It also has dopaminergic effects. Beta-1 stimulation produces increased cardiac output by increasing the force of contraction and heart rate. Although there is an increase in the oxygen needs of the myocardium from dopamine, this effect is less pronounced than when isoproterenol is administered. Tachyarrhythmias usually do not occur. Systolic blood pressure increases, whereas diastolic pressure usually does not. Minimal increases in the diastolic pressure may occur. Total peripheral resistance (from alpha effects) are not changed substantially if dopamine is given at low or intermediate levels of dosing. Although blood flow to the peripheral beds may decrease, blood flow to the mesenteric beds increases. Dopamine dilates renal and mesenteric vasculature as well as cerebral and cardiac beds; this effect is believed to be caused by stimulation of dopaminergic receptors. An increase in renal blood flow, glomerular filtration rate, and urinary output is then seen. The dopaminergic effect of no change in the peripheral resistance is lost as the dose becomes high, with the alpha stimulation taking precedence. The alpha stimulation brings about increased peripheral resistance, raising blood pressure at higher doses of dopamine. The drug's dosage should be titrated upward until adequate perfusion of vital organs is achieved.

TABLE 27.11 Summary of Selected (C) Vasopressors

Drug (Trade) Name	Selected Indications	Route and Dosage Range	Pharmacokinetics
[P] dopamine (Intropin; *Canadian*: Revimine)	Hemodynamic imbalances	*Adult:* IV, 2–5 μg/kg/min *Seriously Ill Adult:* IV, 5 μg/kg/min; increase in increments of 5–10 μg/kg/min up to a rate of 20–50 μg/kg/min *Child:* Safety and efficacy not established	*Onset:* IV, 1–2 min *Duration:* IV, length of infusion $t_{1/2}$: 2 min
dobutamine (Dobutrex)	Cardiac decompensation due to decreased contractility	*Adult:* IV infusion, 2.5–10 μg/kg/min	*Onset:* 1–2 min *Duration:* Unknown $t_{1/2}$: 2 min
epinephrine (Adrenaline)	Cardiac arrest	*Adult:* IV, 0.5–1.0 mg *Child:* Injection, 1;1,000 solution, 0.01 mg/kg or 0.3 mg/m^2 SC q4 h	*Onset:* SC, IM, 5–10 min; IV, instant; inhalation, 3–5 min *Duration:* SC, IM, IV, short-acting inhalation, 1–3 h
	Respiratory distress	*Adult:* SC, 0.3–0.5 mg of 1;1,000 solution; inhalation, individualize dosage; wait 1–5 min between doses. *Child:* SC, 0.01 mg/kg; topical nasal solution, same as adult	
isoproterenol (Isuprel)	Bronchospasm (during anesthesia)	*Adult:* 0.01–0.02 mg of diluted solution IV	*Onset:* IV, immediate *Duration:* IV, 1–2 min $t_{1/2}$: Unknown
	Shock or cardiac standstill and arrhythmias	*Adult:* IV infusion, 5 μg/min of diluted solution; IV push, 0.02–0.10 mg of diluted solution; IM/SC, 0.2 mg of undiluted 1:5,000 solution	
mephentermine (Wyamine)	Hypotension attendant to spinal anesthesia	*Adult:* IM, 30–45 mg 10–20 min prior to procedure	*Onset:* IM, 10–15 min; IV, immediate *Duration:* IM, 1–2 h $t_{1/2}$: 15–20 min
	Hypotension following spinal anesthesia	*Adult:* IV, 30–45 mg as a single injection	
	Shock following hemorrhage	*Adult:* IV, 0.1% solution in 5% dextrose in water just until blood replacement achieved	
norepinephrine (levarterenol, Levophed)	Acute hypotension, shock	*Adult:* IV, 8–12 μg/min; maintenance rate, 2–4 μg/min	*Onset:* IV, rapid *Duration:* 1–2 min after discontinuation of infusion $t_{1/2}$: Unknown
	Cardiac arrest	*Adult:* IV, administer during cardiac resuscitation to restore and maintain BP after effective heart beat and ventilation established	
phenylephrine (Neo-Synephrine)	Mild/moderate hypotension	*Adult:* SC or IM, 2 to 5 mg; IV, 0.2 mg, do not repeat injections more often than every 10–15 min	*Onset:* IV, immediate; IM/SC, 10–15 min *Duration:* IV, 15–20 min; SC/IM, 1–2 h $t_{1/2}$: Unknown
	Severe hypotension/shock	*Adult:* IV, add 10 mg to 250 or 500 mL of dextrose injection; start at 100–180 μg/min; maintenance, 40–60 μg/min	
	Pediatric hypotension	*Child:* SC or IM, 0.5–1 mg/11.3 kg	

Contraindications and Precautions

Dopamine is contraindicated in pheochromocytoma, uncorrected tachyarrhythmias, and ventricular fibrillation. Any underlying hypovolemia should be corrected before the start of therapy. Acidosis decreases the effectiveness of dopamine and other vasopressors. It is important to correct acidosis before starting therapy or as soon as it occurs. Dopamine must be administered when blood pressure, cardiac output, urinary flow, and pulmonary wedge pressure can be monitored closely. Dopamine is a pregnancy category C drug.

Adverse Effects

The most frequent adverse effects from dopamine are ectopic beats, nausea and vomiting, tachycardia, angina, palpitation, dyspnea, headache, hypotension, and vasoconstriction. Infrequent effects are abnormal conduction, bradycardia, widened QRS complex, and piloerection. High doses may cause ventricular arrhythmias and dilated pupils. High doses given over a long time have caused gangrene. Gangrene has also occurred in patients receiving low doses who had occlusive vascular disease.

Overdosage is evidenced by excessive hypertension. If excessive hypertension occurs, reduce the rate or stop the infusion until the patient is stabilized.

Drug Interactions

A few drugs are known to interact with dopamine, as presented in Table 27.12.

Assessment of Relevant Core Patient Variables

Health Status

Determine that pheochromocytoma, uncorrected tachyarrhythmias, and ventricular fibrillation are not present because these conditions are contraindications to the use of dopamine. Verify that existing volume deficits have been corrected. Also, assess for drugs known to cause interaction, especially MAOIs. It is important to determine whether the patient has a history of occlusive vascular disease (e.g., arteriosclerosis, arterial embolism, Raynaud disease, or frostbite) because these patients may be more likely to have necrosis from vasoconstriction with dopamine. If possible, determine whether the patient has sulfite sensitivity because some of these products have sulfites in them. Patients with sulfite sensitivity (rare in the general population; most commonly seen in asthmatics and atopic nonasthmatics) may have allergic reactions, including anaphylactic symptoms and life-threatening or less severe asthmatic attacks.

Life Span and Gender

Assess for pregnancy because dopamine is a category C drug. Whether dopamine is excreted into breast milk is unknown. Note the patient's age before administering dopamine. Its effect and safety in children has not been established, although it has been used in a limited number of pediatric patients.

Environment

Be aware of the setting in which dopamine may be administered. Dopamine is administered intravenously only in acute care settings in which the patient's CV status can be continuously monitored.

Nursing Diagnoses and Outcomes

- Risk for Injury related to decreased perfusion of vital organs.
  Desired outcome: *Drug therapy will be titrated to provide sufficient perfusion of vital organs to prevent serious damage.*
- Risk for Injury related to adverse effects of drug therapy.
  Desired outcome: *Adverse effects of drug therapy will not occur or will be minimized to prevent injury.*

TABLE 27.12 Agents That Interact With P Dopamine

Interactants	Effect and Significance	Nursing Management
guanethidine	Partial or total reversal of the antihypertensive effects of guanethidine. This may be desirable if hypotension from shock is present.	Monitor blood pressure.
halogenated hydrocarbon anesthetics	May sensitize the myocardium to the effects from a catecholamine. This may cause a serious arrhythmia	Use a cardiac monitor and assess cardiac function carefully. Use extreme caution.
monoamine oxidase inhibitors; furazolidone (antimicrobial with MAOI action)	Increase the pressor effect of dopamine 6- to 20-fold as dopamine metabolism is inhibited	Avoid this combination. If given by mistake, administer phentolamine.
oxytocic drugs	Severe persistent hypertension	Avoid combination if possible. Monitor BP closely if must be given.
phenytoin	Simultaneous infusion has led to seizures, severe hypotension, and bradycardia	Discontinue phenytoin and provide supportive measures.
tricyclic antidepressants	The pressor response of dopamine may be decreased, causing it to be less effective	Increase dosage of dopamine if necessary

Planning and Intervention

Maximizing Therapeutic Effects

Administer IV dopamine using an IV pump to regulate flow. It is important to start at low doses and titrate up until the desired renal or hemodynamic response is attained. Do not add 5% sodium bicarbonate or other alkaline IV solution, oxidizing agents, or iron salts because these substances deactivate dopamine.

Minimizing Adverse Effects

Always dilute the drug (if not prediluted) because this is a potent drug; always use an IV administration pump. Before treatment, it is important to correct hypovolemia with whole blood or plasma as indicated. Monitor the blood pressure, urinary flow, cardiac output, and pulmonary wedge pressure closely throughout therapy.

Assess for a disproportionate rise in diastolic blood pressure (this event may be a sign of predominant vasoconstriction). It is important to monitor patients with a history of occlusive vascular disease closely for changes in temperature or color of skin or extremities. If you observe such changes, consult with the physician to determine whether the benefits of dopamine outweigh the risk for possible necrosis.

It is important to infuse into a large vein (antecubital fossa preferred to those in hands or feet) to prevent extravasation (which will cause necrosis and sloughing of tissue). Monitor the insertion site for patency and free flow. If extravasation does occur, it is important to treat immediately with phentolamine (causes sympathetic blockade), injecting into the subcutaneous (SC) space with a needle and syringe. Discontinue dopamine gradually to prevent hypotension.

Providing Patient and Family Education

- The administration of dopamine occurs during an acute medical crisis. Patient education is therefore limited at this time.
- If the patient is awake and alert, inform the patient that his or her blood pressure is low, and the medication will raise blood pressure to a normal level.
- Reassure the patient that he or she will be monitored closely during drug administration. This information would also be appropriate for family members.

Ongoing Assessment and Evaluation

Dopamine therapy is effective if blood pressure stabilizes, urinary output returns to normal, cardiac output returns to normal, and the patient does not have serious adverse effects from the drug.

MEMORY CHIP

P Dopamine

- Used to treat the hypotension resulting from shock as it stimulates alpha and beta receptors to increase cardiac output, blood pressure, and renal perfusion
- Correct hypovolemia prior to administering
- Major contraindications: pheochromocytoma, uncorrected tachyarrhythmias, and ventricular fibrillation
- Most common adverse effects: ectopic beats, nausea and vomiting, tachycardia, angina, palpitations, dyspnea, headache, hypotension, and vasoconstriction
- Most serious adverse effect: ventricular arrhythmias
- Maximizing therapeutic effects: Use an IV pump; titrate the dose upward until desired renal or hemodynamic response is achieved.
- Minimizing adverse effects: Monitor blood pressure, urinary output, cardiac output, and pulmonary wedge pressure throughout therapy.

Drugs Closely Related to P Dopamine

Dobutamine

Dobutamine is chemically similar to dopamine. Like dopamine, its primary influence is on beta-1 receptors with similar effects on the force of contraction. Dobutamine is somewhat less effective than dopamine at increasing the rate at the sinoatrial (SA) node. Also like dopamine, dobutamine's beta-2 effects on vasodilation are minimal. Unlike dopamine, dobutamine has almost no effect on alpha receptors to cause vasoconstriction. Although cardiac output and blood pressure are similarly increased with both drugs, dobutamine does not produce the increased renal output that dopamine does. Furthermore, its effect on peripheral resistance is always to decrease it, whereas dopamine may increase or decrease peripheral resistance. Dobutamine does not cause the release of endogenous norepinephrine that dopamine causes.

The pharmacotherapeutic uses of dobutamine differ from those of dopamine. Dobutamine is indicated in the short-term treatment and support of patients experiencing cardiac decompression caused by depressed contractility. The decreased contractility may be secondary to either organic heart disease or from cardiac surgery. Patients with atrial fibrillation and a rapid ventricular rate should be treated first with digoxin before dobutamine treatment to protect the ventricles.

Dobutamine is metabolized by two methods: methylation of the catechol and conjugation. By-products are excreted in the urine. Onset of action is 1 to 2 minutes but as long as 10 minutes may be needed to see the peak effect. A contraindication unique to dobutamine is the presence of idiopathic hypertrophic subaortic stenosis. Although elevated pulse usually does not occur when using dobutamine, tachycardia can occur with increases of 30 bpm or more. Accompanying the tachycardia is a rapid and substantial increase in blood pressure, with the systolic pressure rising 50% or greater. These adverse effects are usually dose related, and reducing the dose promptly corrects the problem. Interestingly, dobutamine also can cause substantial hypotension if given in excessive amounts; again, decreasing the dose usually corrects the problem. Dobutamine may cause or exacerbate ventricular ectopic beats, although ventricular tachycardia is rare. Other rare adverse effects include nausea, headache, anginal pain, nonspecific chest pain, palpitations, and shortness of breath. Phlebitis and local inflammation at the IV site may occur; a large vein should be chosen to administer the drug to minimize this possibility.

Patients receiving dobutamine, like dopamine, need to be monitored continuously on a cardiac monitor while receiving the drug. Blood pressures should be checked frequently.

Pulmonary wedge pressure and cardiac output should be checked whenever possible.

Isoproterenol

Like dopamine, isoproterenol has a strong effect on beta-1 receptors, producing similar increases in contractility. However, isoproterenol's effect on the heart rate and vasodilation is much greater than dopamine's. Isoproterenol does not stimulate the alpha receptors for vasoconstriction. Isoproterenol increases cardiac output like dopamine. Renal perfusion is also affected, although unlike dopamine, it can increase or decrease it. Peripheral resistance is always decreased, but blood pressure may be increased or decreased by isoproterenol. Although isoproterenol may be used to treat shock, this practice is not common because it can cause tachycardia. The other uses of isoproterenol and more complete information about it are found in Chapter 13.

Epinephrine

Epinephrine is also a vasopressor, as is dopamine. Epinephrine stimulates both alpha and beta receptors. Its effect on the contractility of the heart (beta-1) is similar to dopamine's effect, whereas its effects on SA node rate (beta-1), vasodilation (beta-2), and vasoconstriction (alpha-1) are stronger than dopamine's effects. Although epinephrine increases the cardiac output, its other pharmacodynamic effects differ from dopamine's. It decreases renal perfusion, decreases total peripheral resistance, and elevates systolic, while lowering diastolic blood pressures. Epinephrine is indicated in the treatment and prophylaxis of cardiac arrest and attacks of transitory atrioventricular (AV) heart block with syncopal seizures (Stokes-Adams syndrome). Epinephrine is discussed completely in Chapter 13.

Norepinephrine

Norepinephrine is another vasopressor that stimulates the adrenergic system. Its beta-1 effects on contractility are less than the effects of dopamine, whereas its effect on the SA node rate is similar. Similar to dopamine, norepinephrine has strong alpha receptor stimulation, producing vasoconstriction, but no effect on vasodilation from beta-2 receptors. Although peripheral resistance and blood pressure are raised, norepinephrine decreases renal perfusion and either has no effect on, or decreases, cardiac output. Norepinephrine is used to restore blood pressure when hypotension is caused by one of the following conditions: pheochromocytomectomy, sympathectomy, poliomyelitis, spinal anesthesia, MI, blood transfusion, and drug reactions. It also is used as an adjunct in treating cardiac arrest and severe hypotension. More information about norepinephrine is also found in Chapter 13.

Ephedrine

Ephedrine has less effect on contractility (beta-1 receptors) and less effect on vasoconstriction (alpha-1) than dopamine. Its effect on heart rate (beta-1) and vasodilation (beta-2) is similar to the effect of dopamine. Ephedrine's pharmacodynamic effects of increasing blood pressure, increasing cardiac output, and increasing or decreasing peripheral resistance are similar to those of dopamine. Unlike dopamine, ephedrine decreases renal perfusion. Ephedrine is used clinically in acute hypotension, especially that caused by spinal anesthesia, Stokes-Adams syndrome with complete heart block, use of a CNS stimulant in narcolepsy and depressive states, and acute bronchospasm (occasionally). It is also used as a vasopressor following sympathectomy or drug overdosage (from ganglionic blocking drugs, antiadrenergic drugs, *Veratrum* alkaloids, or other drugs used to lower blood pressure during treatment of hypertension). Ephedrine is also used in enuresis and myasthenia gravis.

Mephentermine

Mephentermine has a weaker effect on the beta-1 receptors, causing less increase in contractility and heart rate than does dopamine. However, it has a stronger effect on the beta-2 receptors, producing moderate vasodilation. It only has a weak effect on alpha-1 receptors, causing a small increase in vasoconstriction. Its pharmacodynamics, when compared with those of dopamine, are in some ways similar. It increases cardiac output and blood pressure. It may have no effect on peripheral resistance or it may increase it, and renal perfusion may increase or decrease. Mephentermine is used to treat hypotension from ganglionic blockade or spinal anesthesia. It can be used on an emergency basis to maintain blood pressure during hypovolemic shock, but only until blood or blood substitutes become available.

Metaraminol

Metaraminol is similar to mephentermine in that it has only minor effects on beta-1 receptors, creating mild increases in contractility and heart rate. It has more effect on vasoconstriction from alpha-1 stimulation than mephentermine, but less than dopamine. It has no effect on vasodilation from beta-2 stimulation. It primarily increases blood pressure by increasing peripheral resistance. Unlike dopamine, it lowers cardiac output and renal perfusion. Although the SA node is stimulated somewhat (which theoretically should increase the heart rate), the net effect on the heart is bradycardia, resulting from a strong reflexive response to the substantial vasoconstriction this drug achieves. Metaraminol is used to prevent and treat acute hypotensive states that occur with spinal anesthesia. It is an adjunct treatment for hypotension caused by hypovolemia, reactions to drug therapy, surgical complications, and shock associated with brain damage caused by trauma or tumor. Unlike dopamine, it can be given intramuscularly or subcutaneously as well as by IV infusion.

Drugs Significantly Different From [P] Dopamine

Phenylephrine

Unlike dopamine, the effects of phenylephrine are solely on alpha-1 receptors, producing strong vasoconstriction effects. Renal perfusion and cardiac output are decreased. Blood pressure is increased by the increase in peripheral resistance.

Phenylephrine is used to treat vascular failure in shock-like states, drug-induced hypotension, or hypersensitivity. It is also used to overcome paroxysmal supraventricular tachycardia, to prolong spinal anesthesia, as a vasoconstrictor in regional analgesia, and to maintain an adequate blood pressure during spinal and inhalation anesthesia. Phenylephrine is discussed completely in Chapter 13.

Midodrine

Midodrine raises blood pressure, but it is not used as a vasopressor in shock. Instead, it is used for symptomatic treat-

ment of orthostatic hypotension in those patients whose lives are impaired substantially by this condition, despite standard clinical treatment. An unlabeled use is treating urine incontinence. Midodrine is administered orally. It is a prodrug that becomes active when it changes into the metabolite desglymidodrine. The metabolite is an alpha-1 agonist that increases the tone of the arteriolar and venous vasculature, increasing peripheral resistance. It results in increased standing, sitting, and lying blood pressures in orthostatic hypotension. Because it increases supine blood pressure, it should not be given less than 4 hours before bedtime. Suggested dosing times are shortly before or just after arising in the morning, midday, and late afternoon. This dosing schedule should assist the patient to maintain his or her normal daytime activities and prevent supine hypertension during the night. If supine hypertension does occur, it may be controlled by preventing the patient from lying completely flat (e.g., lying with the head of the bed elevated).

CHAPTER SUMMARY

- Blood pressure is derived from the amount of blood leaving the heart times the resistance in the peripheries (blood pressure = cardiac output × peripheral resistance). When either cardiac output or peripheral resistance increases, the blood pressure will rise. Drug therapy to reduce hypertension is designed to decrease either cardiac output or peripheral resistance or both. Drug therapy to increase blood pressure increases cardiac output, peripheral resistance, or both.
- Hypertension is classified in 3 stages (from prehypertension to stage 2), according to the degree of blood pressure elevation.
- In prehypertension, blood pressure is usually managed by lifestyle changes alone. These changes include weight reduction, dietary restriction of saturated fat, moderation of alcohol intake, regular physical activity, reduction of sodium intake, increased intake of potassium and calcium rich foods, and smoking cessation. Lifestyle modifications continue even if the patient advances to stage 1 or 2 hypertension.
- Drug therapy may be initiated in prehypertension if the patient has certain other comorbidities. Drug therapy is always initiated in stage 1 or 2 hypertension. A thiazide diuretic is usually used as the drug of first choice. Other classes of drugs may be added if necessary. Most patients will require the use of at least two types of antihypertensives to achieve full therapeutic effect.
- Captopril, an ACE inhibitor, inhibits the angiotensin-converting enzyme needed to change the inactive angiotensin I to the active form angiotensin II, thereby preventing sodium and water retention, decreasing peripheral vascular resistance, and lowering blood pressure. A major adverse effect is a chronic cough, which may be so severe that the patient cannot tolerate or continue drug therapy. First-dose hypotension may occur.
- Losartan is an ARB (angiotensin receptor blocker); it does not inhibit ACE. Instead, it blocks the vasoconstricting and aldosterone-secreting effects of angiotensin II by selectively blocking the binding of angiotensin II to the angiotensin receptors in many tissues, especially in the vascular smooth muscle and adrenal gland tissues.
- Eplerenone is a selective aldosterone receptor blocker. It interferes with the renin-angiotensin-aldosterone system. By blocking the mineralocorticoid aldosterone receptors, it prevents sodium and fluid reabsorption that leads to hypertension.
- Labetalol is an adrenergic blocking agent that has a nonspecific beta blocking action at both the beta-1 and beta-2 receptor sites and a selective alpha-1 blocking action. The alpha blocking actions cause peripheral vasodilation. Because the alpha blocking action decreases standing blood pressure more than lying blood pressure, orthostatic hypotension may occur. The beta blocking action prevents reflex tachycardia.
- Clonidine, an alpha-2 stimulator, stimulates the alpha-2 receptors centrally. This stimulation inhibits sympathetic nervous system responses. Reduced sympathetic outflow from the CNS occurs, resulting in decreased heart rate, decreased blood pressure, decreased vasoconstriction, and decreased renal vascular resistance. Initially, alpha receptors in the peripheries will be stimulated, producing vasoconstriction. However, the main effects are sympatholytic (reduced sympathetic outflow and vasodilation). Because of the sympatholytic effects, the drug may be used to control withdrawal symptoms from substances of abuse. Therefore, clonidine generally is not prescribed for hypertensive patients who are known substance abusers unless they are in a drug treatment program.
- Hydralazine, a direct-acting vasodilator, acts directly on the smooth muscles of the arterioles to produce relaxation and, in turn, peripheral vasodilation. This effect promotes decreased arterial blood pressure and decreased peripheral resistance. As a reflex to peripheral vasodilation, the body increases heart rate, stroke volume, and cardiac output. The reflex mechanism is attributable to an increase in sympathetic stimulation.
- Nitroprusside, an agent used in hypertensive crisis, directly relaxes vascular smooth muscle. It is more active on veins than arteries, thereby promoting peripheral pooling of blood. This effect decreases venous return to the heart, reducing left ventricular end-diastolic pressure and pulmonary capillary wedge pressure (preload). The resultant arteriolar dilation reduces systemic resistance and decreases mean arterial pressure (afterload). The result is markedly reduced blood pressure. The ability to decrease the blood pressure is seemingly unlimited. Nitroprusside is rapidly metabolized to cyanide through a reaction with hemoglobin. Cyanide poisoning may occur during its use. If blood pressure remains uncontrolled after 10 minutes at the maximum infusion rate, stop the infusion immediately. The nitroprusside infusion should be controlled by an administration pump, and the blood pressure must be monitored constantly.
- Dopamine, a vasopressor, is used to correct the hemodynamic imbalances present in shock. Dopamine is a naturally occurring catecholamine and a precursor to norepinephrine. It stimulates alpha-1 and beta-1 receptors through direct and indirect (releasing the stored epinephrine) methods. It has either no or only a minimal effect on beta-2 receptors. It also has dopaminergic effects. The effects from dopamine are increased renal perfusion, increased cardiac output, increased or decreased peripheral resistance (depending on the dose), and increases in blood pressure. Dopamine is administered by IV continuous infusion. The patient must be monitored closely and continuously while on dopamine infusion.

QUESTIONS FOR STUDY AND REVIEW

1. What lifestyle changes constitute Step 1 in antihypertensive therapy?
2. Why are thiazide diuretics now the agent of first choice for most patients with hypertension?
3. How do ACE inhibitors like captopril lower the blood pressure?
4. Describe how an ARB works differently than an ACE inhibitor. What are the advantages of ARB therapy over ACE inhibitor therapy?
5. Why is clonidine *not* recommended for antihypertensive patients who currently abuse narcotics?

6. Which electrolyte imbalance is most likely to occur when the aldosterone receptor blocker eplerenone is administered?
7. Describe nursing actions that promote safety for the patient receiving nitroprusside.
8. Why is dopamine dosage determined by urinary output and CV response?

? Need More Help?

Chapter 27 of the study guide for *Drug Therapy in Nursing* 2e contains NCLEX-style questions and other learning activities to reinforce your understanding of the concepts presented in this chapter. For additional information or to purchase the study guide, visit *http://connection.lww.com/go/aschenbrenner.*

REFERENCES AND BIBLIOGRAPHY

American Heart Association. (2003). Journal Report 5/20/2003. DASH diet acts through diuretic effect to lower blood pressure [Online]. Available: *http://www.americanheart.org/presenter.jhtml?identifier=3011838.*

American Heart Association. (2004). High blood pressure statistics [Online]. Available: *http://www/americanheart.org/presenter.jhtml?identifier=2139.*

ALLHAT Officers and Coordinators for the ALLHAT Collaborative Research Group. Antihypertensive and Lipid-Lowering Treatment to Prevent Heart Attack Trial Collaborative Research Group. (2002). Major outcomes in high-risk hypertensive patients randomized to angiotensin-converting enzyme inhibitor or calcium channel blocker vs diuretic: The Antihypertensive and Lipid-Lowering Treatment to Prevent Heart Attack Trial (ALLHAT). *Journal of the American Medical Association, 288*(23), 2981–2997.

Antihypertensive and Lipid-Lowering Treatment to Prevent Heart Attack Trial Collaborative Research Group. (2003). Diuretic versus alpha-blocker as first-step antihypertensive therapy: Final results from the Antihypertensive and Lipid-Lowering Treatment to Prevent Heart Attack Trial (ALLHAT). *Hypertension, 42*(3), 239–246.

Cushman, W. C., Reda, D. J., Perry, H. M., et al. (2000). Regional and racial differences in response to antihypertensive medication use in a randomized controlled trial of men with hypertension in the United States. Department of Veterans Affairs Cooperative Study on Antihypertensive Agents. *Archives of Internal Medicine, 160*(6), 825–831.

Devereux, R. B., Dahlof, B., Kjeldsen, S. E., et al., Life Study Group. (2003). Effects of losartan or atenolol in hypertensive patients without clinically evident vascular disease: A substudy of the LIFE randomized trial. *Annals of Internal Medicine, 139*(3), 169–177.

Facts and Comparisons. (2004). *Drug facts and comparisons.* Philadelphia: Lippincott Williams & Wilkins.

Forette, F., Seux, M. L., Staessen, J. A., et al., Systolic Hypertension in Europe Investigators. (2002). The prevention of dementia with antihypertensive treatment: New evidence from the Systolic Hypertension in Europe (Syst-Eur) study. *Archives of Internal Medicine, 162*(18), 2046–2052.

Harrington, C. (2003). Managing hypertension in patients with stroke. Are you prepared for labetalol infusion? *Critical Care Nurse, 23*(3), 30–38.

Lakkis, J., Lu, W. X., & Weir, M. R. (2003). RAAS Escape: A real clinical entity that may be important in the progression of cardiovascular and renal disease. *Current Hypertension Report, 5*(5), 408–417.

Launer, L. J., Ross, G. W., Petrovistch, H., et al. (2000). Midlife blood pressure and dementia: The Honolulu-Asia aging study. *Neurobiological Aging, 21*(1), 49–55.

McInnes, G. T. (2003). The expanding role of angiotensin receptor blockers in the management of the elderly hypertensive. *Current Medical Research and Opinion, 19*(5), 452–455.

National Guideline Clearinghouse. (2003). The seventh report of the Joint National Committee on Detection, Evaluation and Treatment of High Blood Pressure (JNC VII) [Online]. Available: *http://www.guideline.gov/summary/summary.aspx?doc_id=4771&nbr=3450&string=Joint+AND+National+AND+Committee+AND+Hypertension.*

O'Keefe, J. H., Lurk, J. T., Kahatapitya, R. C., et al. (2003). The renin-angiotensin-aldosterone system as a target in coronary disease. *Current Atherosclerosis Reports, 5*(2), 124–130.

Post, W. S., Hill, M. N., Dennison, C. R., et al. (2003). High prevalence of target organ damage in young, African American inner-city men with hypertension. *Journal of Clinical Hypertension, 5*(1), 24–30.

Prisant, L. M. (2003). Diabetes mellitus and hypertension: A mandate for intense treatment according to new guidelines. *American Journal of Therapeutics, 10*(5), 363–369.

Psaty, B. M., Lumley, T., Furberg, C. D., et al. (2003). Health outcomes associated with various antihypertensive therapies used as first-line agents: A network meta-analysis. *Journal of the American Medical Association, 289*(19), 2534–2544.

Stier, C. T. Jr. (2003). Eplerenone: A selective aldosterone blocker. *Cardiovascular Drug Review, 21*(3), 169–184.

Stier, C. T. Jr., Koenig, S., Lee, D. Y., et al. (2003). Aldosterone and aldosterone antagonism in cardiovascular disease: Focus on eplerenone (Inspra). *Heart Disease, 5*(2), 102–118.

Drugs Treating Congestive Heart Failure

chapter 28

Learning Objectives

At the completion of this chapter the student will:

1. Understand the rationale for polypharmacy in treating congestive heart failure.
2. Identify core drug knowledge about cardiac glycosides.
3. Identify core patient variables relevant to cardiac glycosides.
4. Relate the interaction of core drug knowledge to core patient variables for drugs that are cardiac glycosides.
5. Generate a nursing plan of care from the interactions between core drug knowledge and core patient variables for drugs that are cardiac glycosides.
6. Describe nursing interventions to maximize therapeutic effects and minimize adverse effects for drugs that are cardiac glycosides.
7. Determine key points for patient and family education for drugs that are cardiac glycosides.

KEY TERMS

afterload

cardiac output

cardiomyopathy

chronotropic

contractility

digitalization

dromotropic

ejection fraction

heart rate

inotropic

loading dose

peripheral resistance

preload

stroke volume

FEATURED WEBLINK

http://www.ahcpr.gov/clinic/epcsums/hrtfailsum.htm
The website of the Agency for Healthcare Research and Quality provides the current American College of Cardiology and American Heart Association guidelines for treating heart failure.

CONNECTION WEBLINK

Additional Weblinks are found on Connection:
http://www.connection.lww.com/go/aschenbrenner.

Drugs Treating Congestive Heart Failure

(C) Angiotensin-Converting Enzyme Inhibitors (ACE Inhibitors)
(see Chapter 27)

(C) Diuretics
(see Chapter 32)

(C) Beta Blockers
(see Chapters 13 and 27)

(C) Cardiac Glycosides

- [P] **digoxin**
- inamrinone
- milrinone
- carvedilol

Other Drugs
(used selectively)

Angiotensin II receptor blockers (ARBs)

- valsartan
  (see Chapters 14 and 30)

hydralazine
(see Chapter 27)

spironolactone
(see Chapter 32)

nitroglycerin

The symbol (C) indicates the **drug class.**
Drugs in **bold type** marked with the symbol [P] are prototypes.
Drugs in blue type are closely related to the prototype.
Drugs in red type are significantly different from the prototype.
Drugs in black type with no symbol are also used in drug therapy; no prototype

The heart is the muscle responsible for pumping blood through the circulatory system. When disease processes interfere with the ability of the heart to pump blood effectively, the organs and tissues are affected and damage may occur. Congestive heart failure (CHF), sometimes referred to as heart failure, is one such disease process. In CHF, the heart does not pump effectively to meet the needs of the body.

The drug classes primarily used to treat CHF are angiotensin-converting enzyme (ACE) inhibitors, diuretics, beta blockers, and cardiac glycosides. This chapter briefly discusses the various drug classes used in treating CHF and presents a thorough discussion of the cardiac glycosides, drugs used to increase the force of contractility of the heart. The prototype cardiac glycoside is digoxin (Lanoxin). Drugs significantly different from digoxin are inamrinone (Inocor), milrinone (Primacor), and carvedilol (Coreg).

PHYSIOLOGY

As stated in Chapter 26, the heart is composed of four chambers—the left and right atria and the left and right ventricles. Blood is returned to the right atrium of the heart from the body. It progresses from the right atrium to the right ventricle to the lungs to be reoxygenated and to have carbon dioxide removed. The reoxygenated blood returns to the left atrium, then to the left ventricle. The contraction of the left ventricle moves the blood back into systemic circulation, as is seen in Figure 28.1.

Blood is circulated throughout the body by a coordinated sequence of chamber contractions and valve openings and closings known as the **cardiac cycle.** The two phases of the cardiac cycle are systole and diastole. Together, they describe the timeframe from the beginning of one heartbeat to the beginning of another. During **systole,** the ventricles contract and the aortic and pulmonic valves open, allowing ejection of blood into the aorta and pulmonary artery. During **diastole,** the ventricles relax, and the mitral and tricuspid valves open, allowing blood to flow into the atria. This blood is sent to the ventricles by passive flow; atrial contraction contributes to the volume sent to the ventricle. Atrial contraction occurs at the end of diastole. As systole begins again, the increased pressure from ventricular contraction causes the mitral and tricuspid valves to shut.

The volume of blood that leaves the left ventricle in 1 minute is the **cardiac output.** Cardiac output consists of two elements, stroke volume and heart rate, and is the product of these two elements (cardiac output = stroke volume × heart rate). **Stroke volume** is the amount of blood that leaves the left ventricle with each contraction. Stroke volume is normally about 75 mL. **Heart rate** is how fast the heart is beating, or the number of contractions per minute. The normal adult range is 70 to 80 bpm. Cardiac output is affected by factors that alter either stroke volume or heart rate.

Stroke volume is dependent on three factors: preload, contractility, and afterload. **Preload** is the passive stretching force exerted on the ventricular muscle created by the amount of blood that has filled the heart by the end of diastole. Preload will be affected by the amount of blood that has returned to the heart (venous return), the ability of the atria to contract forcefully enough to move blood into the ventricles, and how much blood was left in the ventricle during the last contraction. **Contractility** is the force of the squeezing that the ventricle is able to achieve to eject the blood into the systemic circulation. **Afterload** is the amount of pressure the ventricular muscles must overcome to eject the blood into the systemic circulation. Contractility also is affected by the concentration of catecholamines in the heart muscle; that is, the more catecholamines, the greater the contractility. Afterload is controlled by the diameter of the vessel and the pressure within the vessel, which is known as **peripheral resistance** (PR = pressure × diameter of vessel).

Contractions of the heart are dependent on the unique electrical conduction system of the cardiac muscle. The physiology of the conduction system of the heart is described within the physiology section of Chapter 26, Drugs Affecting Cardiac Rhythm.

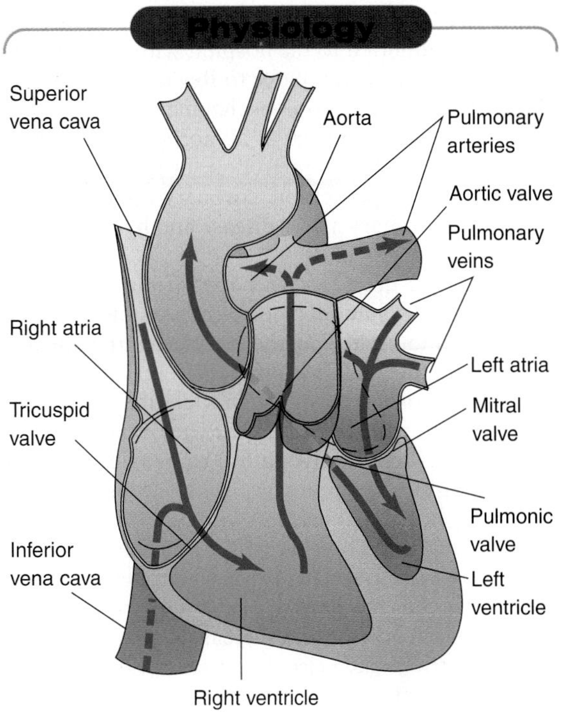

FIGURE 28.1 Cardiac circulation. The unoxygenated blood is returned through the superior and inferior vena cava to the right atrium, where it is removed to the right ventricle. Blood leaves the ventricle through the pulmonary artery to be reoxygenated in the lungs. The oxygenated blood returns to the left atrium via the pulmonary veins and then into the left ventricle. Blood is ejected from the ventricle to the body through the aorta.

PATHOPHYSIOLOGY

Congestive heart failure, a major pathologic problem in the United States, is associated with high morbidity and high mortality. Nearly 5 million people in the United States have CHF; 500,000 people are diagnosed with the condition

annually. CHF is primarily a disease of older adults; about 80% of those admitted to the hospital with CHF are older than 65 years of age (Committee to Revise the 1995 Guidelines, 2001). Pathologic processes that may cause CHF occur either in the heart itself, such as an aortic stenosis or myocardial deficiency after an infarction, or systemically, such as from systemic hypertension, coronary artery disease, or renal failure. Coronary artery disease and hypertension are the primary causes of CHF.

Cardiac output decreases when the left ventricle is unable to eject its normal volume of blood during systole; the **ejection fraction** (the amount leaving the ventricle with contraction compared with the total amount in the ventricle before contraction) is therefore decreased. For a while, the body attempts to compensate for the decreased cardiac output. The heart muscle enlarges (**cardiomyopathy**) to provide more contractile force to try to improve cardiac output. Eventually, however, the heart becomes less and less effective in contracting. As output becomes greatly diminished, the kidneys retain sodium and water to increase circulating volume. Unfortunately, this mechanism places more of a burden on the already overworked heart, increasing preload and afterload. The ventricles then eject less and less. As blood accumulates in the ventricles, the pressure in the vessels coming to the heart increases. Buildup of blood in the left ventricle causes pulmonary congestion or left-sided heart failure. Symptoms include rales, rhonchi, and shortness of breath. Buildup of fluid in the right ventricle causes systemic congestion or right-sided heart failure. Symptoms include peripheral edema, positive jugular vein distention, and a third heart sound (S_3).

In CHF, left-sided failure occurs first, then right-sided failure. This effect is sometimes called backward failure. In most patients, the compensatory hypertrophy of the heart muscle eventually leads to some degree of "stiffness," or loss of elasticity of the ventricle. This "stiffness" alters ventricular diastolic function and does not allow the ventricle to fill completely, further decreasing cardiac output. Although most patients develop systolic dysfunction first and then diastolic dysfunction, some patients do initially develop diastolic dysfunction. Diastolic dysfunction may also be caused by systemic hypertension and coronary artery disease. Additional causes of diastolic dysfunction are fibrosis from aging, infiltrative diseases (such as myocarditis), and constrictive pericarditis. Cardiac output is decreased with diastolic dysfunction, although the ejection fraction may be normal. The compensatory mechanisms of the body are identical in response to the diminished cardiac output. Initially with this type of failure, the body does not have a fluid overload; hence, the symptoms of fluid overload (e.g., S_3, jugular venous distention, and peripheral edema) are not present. For this reason, some practitioners believe the term heart failure is a more accurate description of the entire disease process than the term CHF, whereas other practitioners employ the term chronic heart disease. All of these terms may be used in practice.

Because patients with CHF vary in the severity of their symptoms with progression of the pathologies, a classification system is used to group patients by their functional abilities. Therapies are usually prescribed based on the classification. The most common classification used is the New York Heart Association (NYHA) groupings. Patients are placed into one of four classes depending on their functional abilities. Box 28.1 summarizes the NYHA classifications for CHF.

DRUGS TO TREAT CONGESTIVE HEART FAILURE

When the heart cannot achieve the normal cardiac output for various reasons, a backlog of blood, or congestion, occurs, and heart failure develops. Several drug classes are used to treat CHF, including ACE inhibitors, diuretics, beta blockers, and cardiac glycosides. These four drug groups form what is considered the standard basis of care for CHF (Committee to Revise the 1995 Guidelines, 2001). The use of ACE inhibitors combined with diuretics has been found to decrease the mortality associated with congestive heart disease. Beta blockers, such as carvedilol and metoprolol, have also been found to reduce mortality in patients with CHF who are already taking an ACE inhibitor and a diuretic (Poole-Wilson, 2003). Additionally, new research suggests that the clinical benefits of ACE inhibitors and beta blockers are related to modifying the changes that occur in the left ventricle with CHF. ACE inhibitors seem to prevent progression of left ventricular dilation, and beta blockers such as carvedilol may reverse hypertrophy and improve systolic function (Khattar, 2003). Cardiac glycosides, of which digoxin is the prototype, have been found useful in the symptom management of CHF. Although digoxin does not decrease mortality, it has been shown to decrease the need for hospitalization.

In some subsets of patients, other drugs may be added to the regimen. These drugs include hydralazine, a vasodilator and antihypertensive; spironolactone, a potassium-sparing diuretic; angiotensin II receptor antagonists (also known as angiotensin II blockers) such as valsartan; and nitrates, potent vasodilators such as isosorbide or nitroglycerin, which are used either alone or with hydralazine. Research into the effectiveness of these additional drug therapies is ongoing. Clinical studies with valsartan have shown a small reduction in morbidity and mortality overall when valsartan was added to other prescribed therapy for CHF. This effect was greater in those patients who did not also receive

BOX 28.1 New York Heart Association Classification for Congestive Heart Failure

- Class I: Patients are asymptomatic; patients have no limitation of their activities, they do not have symptoms from ordinary activities.
- Class II: Patients are short of breath or fatigued with moderate activity such as climbing two flights of stairs; they are comfortable at rest or with mild exertion, and have slight limitation of activity.
- Class III: Patients are short of breath or fatigued with very mild exertion activity, such as climbing one-half flight of stairs; are comfortable only with rest, and have marked limitation of their activity.
- Class IV: Patients are exhausted, short of breath, or fatigued at rest; any activity brings on discomfort and symptoms; they have severe limitations on their activity and are confined to bed or chair.

ACE inhibitors. There was no evidence that it provides added benefit when used with an adequate dose of an ACE inhibitor. For patients receiving both an ACE inhibitor and a beta blocker, there was an opposite finding: a statistically significant 42% increase in mortality when valsartan was added to these two drug therapies (Konstam, 2002; Cohn & Tognoni, 2001).

Currently, valsartan is the only angiotensin II receptor blocker that is approved for use in CHF. Its use is limited to those who cannot tolerate ACE inhibitors and possibly to those receiving an ACE inhibitor who cannot take beta blockers and need additional therapy (Shusterman, 2002; Poole-Wilson, 2003). More research is under way to determine whether angiotensin II receptor blockers might be either more effective or as effective but with fewer adverse effects than ACE inhibitors, when either agent is used alone to treat CHF.

Other research is being conducted to explore the role of aldosterone in CHF. Aldosterone receptors have now been identified in the brain, blood vessels, and heart, and aldosterone may be more important in cardiovascular disease than has been previously thought (Stier et al., 2003). Therefore, aldosterone antagonists (e.g., eplerenone, approved as an antihypertensive) are also being studied for possible effectiveness in treating CHF.

Drug therapy has been effective in increasing survival of those with CHF. Research has indicated that survival after 1 year of treatment had improved 10% for those admitted to a hospital for CHF treatment in the years 1999 to 2001, compared with those admitted from 1989 to 1991. Although the improvement is slight, it is statistically significant and is related to the effective use of polypharmacy, which became optimal after 1998 (Feinglass et al., 2003). Although the effective use of drug therapy with ACE inhibitors, diuretics, and beta blockers has been proved to decrease mortality from CHF, and clinical guidelines support their use, implementation of these therapies is still less than 100% in practice. One study of CHF patients in a managed care plan showed that almost half of the patients with CHF were not receiving ACE inhibitors, and three fourths of them were not receiving beta blockers (Schmedtje et al., 2003). One study that examined methods to increase beta blocker use in heart failure found that the use of a nurse facilitator, who used guidelines to initiate and titrate beta blockers, was more effective in initiating and maintaining patients on beta blockers than providing physician education or clinical reminders to physicians about beta blockers, or providing patient education about beta blockers (Ansari et al., 2003). Although drug therapy may be modified in the future, polypharmacy is, and will remain, the standard treatment of choice for CHF. Nurses have an important role in helping CHF patients receive drug therapy recommended by clinical practice guidelines.

Angiotensin-Converting Enzyme Inhibitors

As circulating volume to the kidneys decreases in CHF, the renin-angiotensin-aldosterone system is activated as the body attempts to "correct" for the low levels of circulating volume. Renin stimulates the production of angiotensin I. Angiotensin I is converted by a special enzyme into an extremely potent vasoconstrictor, angiotensin II. Angiotensin II also stimulates the production of aldosterone, which causes sodium and fluid retention, thereby increasing circulating blood volume. As a result, the already overworked heart must work harder. Vasoconstriction is designed to direct the diminished blood volume to vital organs. It also increases peripheral resistance, which decreases cardiac output and further increases the workload on the failing heart. ACE inhibitors prevent the conversion of angiotensin to the active vasoconstrictor form, thereby preventing the deleterious effects from the renin-angiotensin-aldosterone systems. There is growing evidence that ACE inhibitors prevent progressive left ventricular dilation (Khattar, 2003).

A meta-analysis of several studies examining the effect of ACE inhibitors on CHF (Agency for Healthcare Research and Quality, 2003) found that the drugs are effective in reducing mortality whether or not the patients have diabetes and are equally effective in black and white populations. Women who are symptomatic with CHF benefit from ACE inhibitor therapy, although the benefit may be somewhat less than that found in men. Women who are asymptomatic, however, do not appear to achieve a mortality benefit from ACE inhibitors.

Certain ACE inhibitors have been approved for use in CHF: captopril (Capoten), fosinopril (Monopril), lisinopril (Prinivil), enalapril (Vasotec), and quinapril (Accupril). A recent large clinical drug study of lisinopril (Assessment of Treatment with Lisinopril and Survival [ATLAS] study) found that the use of this drug with diuretics, digoxin, or both provided symptomatic relief of CHF. The study also showed that high doses of lisinopril reduced morbidity (fewer hospitalizations and hospital days) and mortality more than low doses of lisinopril (Simpson & Jarvis, 2000). Previously, low doses of ACE inhibitors have been used in CHF. Although the drug cost was higher in the high-dose group, the lower hospital costs for heart failure offset the drug costs. Therefore, improved clinical outcomes could be achieved without increased treatment costs (Schwartz et al., 2003). Adverse effects related to ACE inhibitors include hypotension, worsening renal function, potassium retention, cough, and angioedema. More information about ACE inhibitors is found in Chapter 27.

Diuretics

Diuretics act in the nephrons of the kidney to increase urinary output. This action decreases circulating volume and peripheral resistance, reducing the workload on the failing heart. Thiazide and loop diuretics are both frequently used to treat the edema that occurs in CHF. Occasionally, the potassium-sparing diuretic and aldosterone-blocking drug spironolactone is added to the drug regimen. As mentioned earlier, patients should receive diuretics until they have a normal fluid level before starting beta blockers. The potential adverse effects of diuretics include loss of electrolytes, especially potassium and magnesium, which can predispose a patient to serious cardiac arrhythmias, especially if the patient is also taking digoxin. Other adverse effects include hypotension and azotemia (increased urea in the blood). Diuretics are discussed fully in Chapter 32.

Beta Blockers

Beta blockers have been shown to be highly effective in the treatment of all grades of heart failure that are attributable to left ventricular systolic dysfunction (Cleland, 2003). Although beta blockers can decrease contractility of the heart, thereby decreasing cardiac output (which is detrimental initially in CHF), they also block the effect of the sympathetic nervous system and cause vasodilation and decreased peripheral vascular resistance (which is helpful to patients with CHF). Clinical studies now support the theory that beta blockers may actually reverse the remodeling process by reducing left ventricular volumes and improving systolic function (Khattar, 2003). These changes can produce long-term clinical benefits to patients with CHF, even if coronary artery disease is the cause of heart failure. Beta blockers are known to suppress renin release in patients taking ACE inhibitors. A small study suggests that the suppression of the plasma renin activity is only temporary (Fung et al., 2003).

Carvedilol (Coreg), which is a nonselective beta blocker that also has alpha blocking properties, was the first beta blocker approved for treating mild-to-moderate CHF. It was the first new drug approved for treating CHF in many years. Research has also examined the effectiveness of metoprolol (Lopressor), another beta blocker, in treating CHF, and its label has been modified to include CHF as an indicated use. Metoprolol and carvedilol have both been found to decrease the mortality associated with CHF, even for patients with more advanced CHF (Tangeman & Patterson, 2003; Hjalmarson et al., 2000; Eichhorn & Bristow, 2001; Goldstein et al., 2001). However, one study showed that carvedilol was more effective in decreasing mortality (Wikstrand et al., 2002). Metoprolol has the advantage of once-a-day dosing because it is available in a long-lasting form, whereas carvedilol is taken twice a day. Metoprolol has been found effective whether the dose is 100 mg/day or more or less than 100 mg/day (Wikstrand et al., 2002). One study has shown that carvedilol can reduce morbidity and mortality in dialysis patients with chronic heart failure (Cice et al., 2003). This finding is important because between one third and one half of patients with CHF have renal insufficiency, which is one of the strongest predictors of mortality for patients with CHF (Shlipak, 2003). More research is needed to determine the effectiveness of carvedilol compared with metoprolol, as well as the effect of ACE inhibitors in renal insufficiency that does not require dialysis. Meta-analysis of many research studies (Agency for Healthcare Research and Quality, 2003) shows that beta blockers reduce mortality for men and women with symptomatic heart failure as well as for diabetics and nondiabetics. Black and white patients have the same risk reduction whether they receive bisoprolol (Zebeta, another beta blocker), metoprolol, or carvedilol. Black people appear to have worse mortality outcomes if they receive bucindolol (a beta blocker not currently approved, but in phase 3 trials in the United States). These findings suggest that different beta blockers may produce different results when used to treat CHF and that prescription of beta blockers for this condition should be limited to those medications that have been used in clinical trials.

Beta blockers are not used during acute episodes of CHF but rather in chronic CHF. They are recommended to be started, along with an ACE inhibitor, in patients who are asymptomatic (NYHA class I). Patients who are symptomatic (NYHA classes II–IV) should have normal fluid volume, or only minimal evidence of fluid retention, when they begin beta blocker treatment. Pretreatment with diuretics is important for these patients to prevent an acute exacerbation of CHF caused by the slowing of the heart rate and decrease in contractile force that occurs with beta blockers. Diuretic therapy should continue once other therapy has begun. The patient should be started on a small dose and monitored carefully for signs of hypotension and worsening CHF. Dosage is increased gradually over several weeks until the therapeutic dosage range is reached. Full therapeutic effects may not occur for 1 to 3 months, although some immediate response can be seen with carvedilol. Treatment is most effective if begun in the early stages of the disease (Cleland, 2003). Potential adverse effects of beta blockers include fluid retention, worsening of heart failure, fatigue, bradycardia and heart block, and hypotension. With each new dose, the patient should be observed for dizziness or lightheadedness for 1 hour. Patients who have had initial difficulties with carvedilol are often successful on the drug when it is tried again.

For more information on beta blockers, see Chapters 13 and 27.

Cardiac Glycosides

The fourth drug that is included in CHF treatment is a cardiac glycoside. The cardiac glycosides also are known as digitalis preparations or digitalis glycosides. Currently, the only cardiac glycoside available in the United States is digoxin. Digoxin is used to maintain clinical stability and improve symptoms, quality of life, and exercise tolerance in patients with all phases of CHF; it does not decrease mortality from CHF. Digoxin is not used as the primary treatment for stabilizing patients with acute episodes of noncompensated heart failure; rather, it should be added after other drug therapy has stabilized the patient, as long as the patient is in normal sinus rhythm (Dee, 2003; Campbell & MacDonald, 2003).

Digoxin increases the force of cardiac contraction, increasing cardiac output, which in turn increases perfusion to the kidneys. Higher renal perfusion increases the production of urine. Thus, the drug reduces preload and afterload. Although this effect has been historically considered the main pharmacodynamic action of digoxin, there is evidence that its primary benefit actually occurs through neurohormonal modulation. Digoxin has been shown to enhance vagal tone, slowing ventricular rate and reducing sympathetic tone when abnormally high (as in CHF). It also slows heart rate (Campbell & MacDonald, 2003).

P CARDIAC GLYCOSIDES

The prototype cardiac glycoside drug is digoxin (Lanoxin). Inamrinone (Inocor) and milrinone (Primacor) are drugs significantly different from the cardiac glycosides.

NURSING MANAGEMENT OF THE PATIENT RECEIVING P DIGOXIN

Core Drug Knowledge

Pharmacotherapeutics

Digoxin (Lanoxin) is used in treating CHF. It is a second-line drug as long as the patient has normal sinus rhythm. If the patient with CHF has atrial fibrillation, it is used as a first-line drug. Digoxin appears to be most helpful in treating patients with severe heart failure, cardiomegaly, and a third heart sound (Campbell & MacDonald, 2003). Digoxin is also used in treating chronic atrial fibrillation to maintain a satisfactory resting ventricular rate. It is used either alone or with other agents such as beta blockers or the calcium channel blockers, diltiazem or verapamil (Campbell & MacDonald, 2003). It is no longer recommended to prevent paroxysmal (recurrent episodes) atrial fibrillation. Table 28.1 provides a summary of selected cardiac glycosides. (A complete discussion of drugs used to treat arrhythmias can be found in Chapter 26.)

The therapeutic range for digoxin is generally considered to be 0.5 to 2 ng/mL. Digoxin has been shown to improve symptoms, increase the quality of life, and increase the exercise tolerance of patients with CHF. These benefits occur regardless of the underlying heart rhythm (normal sinus or atrial fibrillation), the etiology of the heart failure, or other drugs used in therapy (e.g., ACE inhibitors, beta blockers) (Dee, 2003).

Pharmacokinetics

Absorption of digoxin varies with the type of preparation. Tablet absorption is about 60% to 80%; elixirs, 70% to 85%; and solution-filled capsules, 90% to 100%. Taking digoxin with food slows down absorption, but total absorption usually is unchanged. The exception is when digoxin is taken with a meal that is very high in bran fiber, which may reduce absorption. Digoxin also may be administered intravenously. Digoxin is distributed widely in the tissues. High concentrations are found in the myocardium, skeletal muscle, liver, brain, and kidneys. Digoxin crosses the blood–brain barrier and the placenta. Serum drug levels are not affected significantly by changes in fat tissue weight; thus, dosing is best calculated on lean (ideal) body weight rather than actual weight if the patient is obese. Metabolism takes place in the liver. However, much of the drug, 50% to 75%, is excreted unchanged by the kidneys. Digoxin is not removed by dialysis. Because of digoxin's long half-life, several days are required for a steady state to be achieved and for optimal clinical effects to be seen.

To speed the onset of therapeutic effects, a dose higher than normal, a **loading dose,** may be given to raise the blood level quickly to the desired range. This practice is known as **digitalization.** The total dose needed for digitalization is divided into several doses, with roughly half the loading dose given as the first dose. The remainder is divided and given at 6-hour to 8-hour intervals for oral dosage and 4-hour to 8-hour intervals for parenteral dosage. The dose is lower if the loading dose is given intravenously instead of orally. To avoid cumulative and toxic effects, dosage adjustments must be made when there is renal failure or suspected age-related deterioration of renal function.

Pharmacodynamics

The effect of digoxin on the heart is dose related. It exerts an indirect effect on the heart from stimulation of the autonomic nervous system and a direct action on both the cardiac muscle and the specialized electrical conduction system of the heart. The indirect effect of digoxin is to create a vagomimetic effect, one that mimics the action of stimulating the vagus nerve. The increase in the vagal tone is now believed to be the central effect of digoxin, which is primarily responsible for the therapeutic effects of the drug. Stimulating the vagus nerve depresses the sinoatrial (SA) node and

TABLE 28.1 Summary of Selected C Cardiac Glycosides

Drug (Trade) Name	Selected Indications	Route and Dosage Range	Pharmacokinetics
P digoxin (Lanoxin; *Canadian:* Novo-Digoxin)	Congestive heart failure (CHF), atrial fibrillation, atrial flutter	*Adult:* PO, loading dose, 0.75–1.25 mg in divided doses; maintenance of 0.125–0.25 mg/d; IV, loading, 0.4–1.0 mg in divided doses; maintenance, 0.063–0.25 mg *Child:* Dosage individualized	*Onset:* PO, 30–120 min; IV, 5–30 min *Duration:* PO, 6–8d; IV, 4–5 d $t_{1/2}$: 30–40 h
inamrinone (Inocor)	CHF	*Adult:* IV, initially 0.75 mg/kg bolus slowly over 2–3 min with dose repeated in 30 min, if needed; maintenance infusion, 5–10 mg/kg/min; not to exceed 10 mg/kg daily *Child:* Safety and efficacy not established	*Onset:* Immediate *Duration:* 2h $t_{1/2}$: 3–6 h
milrinone (Primacor)	CHF	*Adult:* IV, loading dose, 50 mg/kg bolus over 10 min; maintenance, 0.375–0.75 mg/kg/min, not to exceed 1.13 mg/kg daily *Child:* Safety and efficacy not established	*Onset:* Immediate *Duration:* 8 h $t_{1/2}$: 2–3 h

prolongs conduction to the atrioventricular (AV) node. This decrease in conduction is known as a negative **dromotropic** effect. Because of the prolonged conduction time, heart rate slows. This effect is termed a negative **chronotropic** effect. Cardiac output is increased as a result of these factors. The improved cardiac output results in an increase in renal perfusion, causing mild diuresis. Digoxin also inhibits sympathetic tone, especially when it is abnormally high, as it is in CHF. Inhibiting sympathetic tone decreases sympathetic stimulation of the heart rate and thereby slows the heart rate. This effect on sympathetic tone is partly from vagotonic action and is partly a direct effect.

The direct effect of digoxin is to strengthen the contractile force of the heart, which is called a positive **inotropic** effect. This effect is believed to be caused by digoxin increasing the movement of calcium ions across the myocardial cell membrane during depolarization discharge. Because calcium is needed for contraction, a stronger contraction can occur with more calcium. The way digoxin increases calcium in the cell is by directly blocking a special enzyme, Na^+-K^+-ATPase, on cell membranes. Because of the blockade, Na^+ concentration increases in the cell. The increased Na^+ concentration causes increases in intracellular Ca^{2+} levels because of the Na^+-Ca^{2+} exchanger. Digoxin competes with potassium to attach to Na^+-K^+-ATPase. When digoxin is attached, potassium cannot be attached at the same site. Digoxin also directly increases the refractory period at the AV node. During this time, the heart muscles cannot be stimulated into contracting again. Digoxin also is known to increase total peripheral resistance.

Contraindications and Precautions

Digoxin is contraindicated in heart block, ventricular fibrillation, certain cases of ventricular tachycardia, some cases of sick sinus syndrome, beriberi-related heart disease, hypersensitivity to digoxin, and allergies (although allergies are rare), and in the presence of digitalis toxicity. Caution must be used when administering digoxin over the long term to patients with CHF who are difficult to regulate or who have a greater than normal risk for developing toxicity (e.g., those with unstable renal function or a tendency toward hypokalemia). For these patients, the physician may consider a cautious withdrawal of digoxin. Monitor these patients very carefully for signs of returning or recurrent heart failure.

Also use caution when giving digoxin to patients with severe carditis, acute myocardial infarction (MI), severe pulmonary disease, and severe heart failure because these patients may be more sensitive to digoxin-induced arrhythmias. Patients with renal insufficiency are more likely to have adverse effects and develop digoxin toxicity. Use caution in patients who have thyroid disorders because plasma levels of digoxin are inversely proportional to thyroid status. In untreated hypothyroidism, digoxin requirements are reduced; in thyrotoxic patients, larger doses of digoxin may be necessary. Patient response to digoxin is unchanged in compensated thyroid disease. The electrolyte imbalances of hypokalemia, hypomagnesemia, and hypercalcemia potentiate the effect of digoxin, and the patient may develop signs of toxicity even with normal drug serum levels. Remember that digoxin competes with potassium for Na^+-K+-ATPase receptor sites on cell membranes. Therefore, low potassium levels allow digoxin to occupy more receptors, increasing the risk for adverse effects. Hypocalcemia may nullify the effects of digoxin because digoxin creates its effect by increasing intracellular calcium to increase contraction. Serum calcium levels will need to be rectified to achieve therapeutic effects of digoxin.

Digoxin is a pregnancy category C drug, and its safety for use in breast-feeding women has not been established. Children may receive digoxin; however, premature and immature infants are very sensitive to its effects. Dosage must be titrated carefully in children, and they should be monitored closely for signs of toxicity.

Adverse Effects

Adverse effects are dose related and are signs of digoxin toxicity. Adverse effects occur in 5% to 20% of patients receiving digoxin, with between 1% and 4% experiencing serious reactions. The most common adverse effects are cardiac toxicity, followed by gastrointestinal (GI) disturbances and CNS toxicity. The cardiac toxicities include bradycardia, AV block, complete heart block, ventricular tachycardia, premature ventricular contractions, ventricular fibrillation, paroxysmal and nonparoxysmal nodal rhythms, AV dissociation, accelerated junctional nodal rhythm, paroxysmal atrial tachycardia, and atrial fibrillation. Almost any type of arrhythmia can be stimulated by digoxin toxicity. It may seem paradoxical that digoxin slows the rate of the ventricles but can allow ventricular arrhythmias to occur. When digoxin slows down the normal pacemaker of the heart, ectopic pacemakers in the ventricle can take over, producing serious arrhythmias.

GI effects are anorexia, nausea, vomiting, diarrhea, and abdominal pain. CNS effects are headache, weakness, apathy, drowsiness, visual disturbances (e.g., blurred, yellow vision; halo effect in vision), confusion, restlessness, disorientation, seizures, electroencephalogram abnormalities, delirium, hallucinations, neuralgia, and psychosis.

When toxicity is suspected, an electrocardiogram (ECG) may help identify whether digoxin toxicity has occurred. Digoxin causes a normal slowing of heart rate, a narrower QRS complex, and a depressed T wave. However, toxicity results in a prolonged P-R interval and a shortened Q-T interval. In the event of toxicity, the drug must be discontinued until all signs of toxicity are gone. Occasionally, if severe arrhythmias have occurred, additional treatment may be necessary. Potassium chloride may be given to help correct the arrhythmia, especially if hypokalemia is present. It may be given orally or intravenously if the need is urgent. Women appear to achieve higher serum levels on the same dose compared with men, which may increase their risk for developing toxicity (Campbell & Macdonald, 2003). Digoxin toxicity is usually associated with serum levels greater than 2 ng/mL; however, it can occur with lower serum levels if hypokalemia, hypomagnesemia, or hypothyroidism is also present. Evidence exists that higher doses of daily digoxin (>0.25 mg/day) or trough (the low point) serum levels greater than 1 ng/mL increase the risks for digoxin toxicity, including death (Campbell & MacDonald, 2003). Digibind (digoxin immune Fab) is used as the antidote to digoxin toxicity.

Some concern exists that the long-term effects of digoxin, even with serum levels within the accepted therapeutic range, may include an increased frequency of hospitalization for

cardiovascular events other than heart failure and an increased risk for death from arrhythmias or myocardial infarction (Committee to Revise the 1995 Guidelines, 2001). Still, at this time, digoxin is considered an important drug in the treatment of CHF.

Drug Interactions

Digoxin interacts with many drugs. The interactions usually relate to decreased or increased serum levels of digoxin or increased incidence of adverse effects as can be seen in Table 28.2.

Assessment of Relevant Core Patient Variables

Health Status

Determine whether the patient has ventricular fibrillation, ventricular tachycardia, heart block, sick sinus syndrome,

TABLE 28.2 Agents That Interact With P Digoxin

Interactants	Effect and Significance	Nursing Management
alprazolam, aminoglycosides (oral), amiodarone, anticholinergics, benzodiazepines, bepridil, captopril, cyclosporine, diltiazem, erythromycin, esmolol, felodipine, flecainide, hydroxychloroquine, ibuprofen, indomethacin, itraconazole, nifedipine, omeprazole, propafenone, propantheline, quinidine, quinine, tetracycline, tolbutamide, verapamil	Increased serum digoxin levels resulting from various mechanisms, such as altered GI flora, increased absorption, decreased clearance; may increase patient's risk for excessive levels and effects of digoxin	Monitor patient and blood tests for signs of digitalis toxicity.
aminoglutethimide, aminoglycosides (oral), aminosalicylic acid, antacids, antihistamines, antineoplastics, barbiturates, cholestyramine, colestipol, hydantoins, hypoglycemics (oral), kaolin/pectin, metoclopramide, neomycin, penicillamine, rifampin, sucralfate, sulfasalazine	Decreased serum digitalis level	Monitor patient to assess effects of drug therapy. Effect of digoxin may be reduced.
albuterol	Possibly enhanced skeletal muscle binding of digoxin	Monitor for therapeutic effect of digoxin.
beta blockers	Possibly complete heart block resulting from atrioventricular nodal conduction	Monitor ECG regularly.
disopyramide	Altered pharmacologic effect of digoxin	Monitor for therapeutic effect of digoxin.
nondepolarizing muscle relaxants and succinylcholine	Increased potential for toxic levels of either digoxin or interactant	Monitor patient and laboratory test values for signs of toxicities.
potassium-sparing diuretics	Unpredictable	Monitor patient, electrolyte levels, and laboratory values to detect signs of toxicities and decreasing therapeutic drug effects.
spironolactone	Increased or decreased serum digoxin level	Monitor patient, electrolyte levels, and laboratory values to detect signs of toxicities and decreasing therapeutic drug effects.
amiloride	Decreased inotropic effects of digoxin	Monitor for therapeutic effects of digoxin.
triamterene	Increased pharmacologic effects of digoxin	Monitor for adverse effects of digoxin.
sympathomimetics	Enhanced pacemaker activity, leading to increased risk for cardiac arrhythmias	Monitor pulse for arrhythmias, and evaluate ECG as indicated.
thiazide and loop diuretics and amphotericin B	Increased urinary potassium and magnesium loss, leading to increased effect and toxic levels of digoxin	Assess patient's electrolyte values. Replace electrolytes as needed.
thyroid hormones and thioamines	Decreased effect of digoxin with thyroid hormones; increased effect with thioamines	Report changes in laboratory and diagnostic test values to the prescriber in anticipation of need for dosage adjustment.

beriberi-associated heart disease, or hypersensitivity to digoxin because these conditions are contraindications to its use. Obtain a baseline ECG for comparison in case digoxin toxicity is later suspected. Also determine whether the patient is on drug therapy that promotes the loss of potassium, such as thiazide or loop diuretics, because hypokalemia increases the net effect of digoxin, placing the patient at increased risk for digoxin toxicity. Examine laboratory findings for indications of hypokalemia, hypomagnesemia, or hypercalcemia, all of which predispose the patient to digoxin toxicity. Determine thyroid function, which can alter the dosage requirement of digoxin. Also determine whether the patient has renal impairment because poor renal excretion may allow digoxin levels to build up to toxic levels. Patients with renal impairment may require a lower dose of digoxin. Assess the patient's weight before beginning digoxin therapy because along with renal function, weight is considered in determining dosage. Serum concentrations are not affected by large changes in fat tissue weight; therefore, to prevent potential overdose, calculate and use the obese patient's ideal body weight, instead of true weight, to determine proper dosage.

Life Span and Gender

Determine whether the patient is pregnant. Digoxin is administered with caution during pregnancy because 50% to 83% of the maternal serum concentration of digoxin affects the fetus. Also determine whether the patient is breast-feeding because safety in infants has not been established. Carefully monitor women receiving digoxin because they may be at increased risk for toxicity (Rathore et al., 2002).

It is a good idea to note the patient's age before administering digoxin. A small study (Ratnapalan et al., 2003) showed that digoxin can interact with the beta blocker carvedilol, which is coadministered frequently in children with severe ventricular failure. In the study, the combined effect of the two drugs was a 50% decrease in the clearance of digoxin and increased serum concentrations of digoxin. These factors increased the risk for adverse effects and digoxin toxicity in the children. Accidental poisoning of children in the home is common with digoxin. In these cases, digoxin usually had been prescribed for a parent or grandparent, not for a child. Elderly patients must be given digoxin carefully because they tend to have low body mass and decreased renal functioning, making them more prone to adverse effects of the drug. A lower maintenance dosage (0.125–0.25 mg per day) should be used. Noncardiac signs of digoxin toxicity may be difficult to identify in older adults because the signs are often vague. Also, the older adult may be confused because of adverse effects from other drug therapies or the confusion may be mistakenly believed to be caused by changes from aging. Additionally, some of the signs, such as nausea and weakness, can also occur with uncontrolled CHF.

Lifestyle, Diet, and Habits

Determine the patient's normal dietary intake of potassium, calcium, and magnesium because intake may have a bearing on the serum levels of these electrolytes. Low serum levels of potassium or magnesium increase the risk for toxicity, whereas low calcium decreases the effectiveness of digoxin. St. John's wort, an herbal preparation, should not be started after digoxin therapy is begun because it has been known to reduce the serum level of digoxin by about 25% and to decrease therapeutic activity. Patients already using St. John's wort who stop using it after digoxin therapy has been regulated are at risk for having adverse effects from the higher serum levels of digoxin (Baede-van Dijk, et al., 2000). A recent study showed that hawthorn extract may provide significant benefit to patients with CHF when used as an adjunct to standard drug therapy (Box 28.2). Other complementary medicines can trigger digoxin toxicity. These substances include squill, strophanthus, and oleander, which contain cardiac glycosides. Senna and cascara may increase potassium loss, leading to digoxin toxicity (Campbell & MacDonald, 2003).

FOCUS ON RESEARCH

Box 28.2 Complementary Therapies in Congestive Heart Failure

Pittler, M. H., Schmidt, K., & Ernst, E. (2003). Hawthorn extract for treating chronic heart failure: Meta-analysis of randomized trials. *American Journal of Medicine; 114*(8), 665–674.

The Study

Crataegus monogyna Jacq (Lindm), *C. laevigata* (Poir) DC, or related *Crataegus* species, collectively known as hawthorn, have been investigated as an adjunct treatment for CHF. This study was a meta-analysis of eight clinical trials that were all randomized, double-blinded, and placebo-controlled studies of the use of single preparations of hawthorn extract as adjunct treatment for 632 patients with CHF. Patients received hawthorn in addition to standardized CHF drug therapy. Symptoms such as dyspnea and fatigue were significantly improved with the use of hawthorn treatment compared to the use of placebo. Exercise tolerance was also increased for patients taking hawthorn. Adverse effects of hawthorn in the studies were infrequent and mild, and usually transient. Most frequent adverse effects were nausea, dizziness, and cardiac and gastrointestinal complaints. The authors concluded that hawthorn extract appears to provide a significant benefit when used in addition to standardized drug therapy.

Nursing Implications

With the use of complementary medication growing among American adults, reliable scientific clinical trials are needed to test whether a true benefit can be obtained from these preparations. This meta-analysis of several studies shows that hawthorn is effective as an adjunct therapy. You can use this information to provide better patient education when patients ask about the effectiveness of hawthorn extract. You might also ask patients if they are interested in adding complementary therapies to their prescribed drug treatment. Although it is not clearly stated by the study, it can be inferred that a therapy that increases the effectiveness of other therapies, without having significant adverse effects, may be appealing for several reasons. First, the patient's quality of life would improve. Second, achieving more therapeutic effect without having to increase the dosage of the prescription drugs helps to minimize the risk for adverse effects from those therapies. Third, the cost of the over-the-counter hawthorn may be less than the cost of increasing the prescription drug dosage. When nurses teach interested patients about the potential addition of hawthorn, they must be careful to strongly emphasize that hawthorn cannot replace the prescription therapy, only supplement it. Lack of symptom control and worsening of CHF is likely to occur if prescribed drug therapy is stopped.

Environment

Be aware of the environment in which digoxin will be administered. Digitalization of a patient most often occurs in the hospital where the patient can be monitored closely for adverse effects. In addition, IV doses of digoxin are administered in the hospital. Once the patient is stabilized and on an oral maintenance dose, administration of digoxin may be performed in any setting, including self-administration at home.

Nursing Diagnoses and Outcomes

- Decreased Cardiac Output related to altered cardiac function
  Desired outcome: *The patient's CHF will be well controlled.*
- Risk for Injury related to drowsiness, confusion, disorientation, seizures, delirium, hallucinations, and psychosis secondary to adverse effects of drug therapy
  Desired outcome: *The patient will not sustain an injury related to adverse drug events while on drug therapy.*

Planning and Intervention

Maximizing Therapeutic Effects

To achieve rapid onset of therapeutic effects, the patient is digitalized with an IV or PO loading dose. Roughly half the loading dose is given in the first increment, and the remainder is given in divided doses at appropriate intervals. Assess for therapeutic and adverse effects before each dose.

Minimizing Adverse Effects

Digoxin has a narrow therapeutic index, which means that there is not much difference between the dosage needed to produce therapeutic effects and the dosage that will produce toxic effects. It is important to monitor the serum levels of digoxin to help prevent serious drug toxicity. The safe therapeutic serum level is 0.5 to 2.0 ng/mL. Unfortunately, some patients exhibit signs of digoxin toxicity even when their serum levels are within a "normal" range. Therefore, it is important to monitor for signs of digoxin toxicity. Box 28.3 provides guidelines for minimizing adverse effects from digoxin toxicity.

Providing Patient and Family Education

- Explain the reason for taking digoxin and the adverse effects of digoxin.
- Teach the patient how to check his or her own radial or carotid pulse. Instruct the patient to take the pulse for a full minute before taking digoxin. If the pulse is below 60 bpm (or another parameter set by the prescriber for the patient), the patient should not take the drug without consulting with the prescriber.
- Caution the patient not to discontinue digoxin without approval from the prescriber.
- Tell the patient to avoid over-the-counter antacids and cough, cold, allergy, and diet drugs, except on the advice of the prescriber, because these drugs frequently contain antihistamines that may interact with digoxin.
- Explain the importance of notifying the prescriber if any of the following occur while taking digoxin: loss of appetite, nausea, vomiting, diarrhea, stomach pain, unusual tiredness or weakness, drowsiness, headache, blurred or yellow vision, skin rash or hives, or mental depression.
- It is important to instruct the patient to return for requested laboratory work to check the serum digoxin level and electrolyte levels.
- Caution the patient to keep digoxin out of the reach of children (Box 28.4).

Ongoing Assessment and Evaluation

Monitor the patient's pulse rate throughout therapy. Assess serum digoxin levels after the drug is first started and has reached a steady state, at each dosage change, and whenever signs of digoxin toxicity are present. Renal function is monitored periodically throughout therapy by measuring blood urea nitrogen, creatinine, and electrolyte levels (potassium, calcium, and magnesium). Again, blood work will need to be monitored when digoxin is first started; recurrent blood work will be done based on the individual's response to therapy.

Symptoms of CHF should improve, and the patient should have increased urinary output, less edema, less shortness of breath, and fewer rales. When digoxin is given for atrial fibrillation, the arrhythmia should be corrected. The nurse will assess for development of arrhythmias. Development of arrhythmias may be a sign of digoxin toxicity. When the patient's CHF or arrhythmia is controlled without injury to the patient from adverse effects or toxicity, the drug therapy is considered effective.

CRITICAL THINKING SCENARIO

Multiple drug therapy for congestive heart failure

Ms. Mahoney, a 65-year-old woman who lives alone in a two-story home, comes to the emergency department complaining of difficulty breathing. She reports increased shortness of breath, especially when climbing the stairs and walking; weakness; and ankle swelling. A diagnosis of congestive heart failure is made. She is hospitalized and stabilized. Her discharge medications include the ACE inhibitor lisinopril, the loop diuretic furosemide (Lasix), the beta blocker carvedilol, digoxin, and an oral potassium supplement.

1. What is the desired therapeutic effect of this combination drug therapy?
2. Why should hypokalemia be prevented in Ms. Mahoney?
3. What blood work needs to be carefully monitored in Ms. Mahoney?

Drugs Significantly Different From [P] Digoxin

Inamrinone

Inamrinone (Inocor) was previously known as amrinone. The name was officially changed in the United States by the U.S. Pharmacopeia (USP) and the United States Adopted Names Council in July 2000 because of several drug errors that occurred when the drug was confused with a similar sounding drug, amiodarone, which is an antiarrhythmic.

BOX 28.3 Minimizing Adverse Effects From Digoxin Toxicity

Monitor serum digoxin levels

- Measure levels at least 8 hours following the last oral dose and preferably 24 hours after the last dose if the patient is receiving maintenance therapy. Following this procedure will prevent reading falsely elevated digoxin blood levels.
- Monitor most closely when digoxin is first started, when the dose is changed, or when the patient has signs of toxicity.
- Periodic monitoring is needed when digoxin is used in long-term maintenance. The frequency of monitoring is based on patient response to drug therapy.

Assess for bradycardia

- Take the patient's apical pulse for 1 full minute to determine heart rate accurately before administering each dose of digoxin. If the pulse is below 60 beats/min, do not administer the dose without approval from the health care provider.

Correct electrolyte imbalances

- Monitor for low levels of potassium and magnesium and high levels of calcium because these altered levels place the patient at risk of developing digoxin toxicity.
- If potassium and magnesium levels are low, seek an order for replacement of the electrolyte.
- Electrolytes should not be administered rapidly. Calcium and potassium, especially, may bring on serious arrhythmias when administered by IV.
- Encourage the patient to follow a diet of potassium-rich foods while taking digoxin to prevent hypokalemia and digoxin toxicity. However, potassium intake should just be normal if the patient is on a potassium-sparing diuretic, ACE inhibitor, or a potassium chloride supplement.

Assess for other symptoms of digoxin toxicity

- Monitor for anorexia, nausea, vomiting, diarrhea, headache, blurred vision, confusion, and drowsiness
- Anorexia, nausea, vomiting, and diarrhea may also be evident when CHF is uncontrolled. This makes the assessment for digoxin toxicity more difficult.

Treatment of digoxin-induced arrhythmias

- Oral or slow IV potassium often is used as a treatment. IV doses are for more urgent problems.
  - Divided oral doses for adults should total 3 to 6 g (40 to 80 mEq), as long as normal renal function exists.
  - When given to adults by IV, 40 to 80 mEq are diluted in 5% dextrose and water (D_5W) to a concentration not greater than 40 mEq/100 mL. The drug should be administered at a rate not exceeding 20 mEq/h and more slowly if the patient reports pain at the catheter insertion site.
  - For children, oral doses totaling 1 to 1.5 mEq/kg or about 0.5 mEq/kg/h IV are given with careful ECG monitoring.
  - The ECG should be monitored for potassium toxicity (peaking of T waves). If the arrhythmia is corrected, the infusion should be stopped.
  - Potassium should not be used when renal failure exists or when complete heart block is secondary to digoxin toxicity and not related to tachycardia.
- Phenytoin, an anticonvulsant, may be used to treat atrial and ventricular arrhythmias.
  - Give 50 to 100 mg of phenytoin every 5 minutes. Total dose should not exceed 600 mg.
  - Phenytoin is used when potassium is *not* effective
- Lidocaine, an antiarrhythmic, is used to treat ventricular arrhythmias
  - Give IV for a dose of 1 mg/kg over 5 minutes, then 15 to 50 µg/kg per minute to maintain rhythm.
  - Lidocaine is used when potassium is not effective
- Atropine, an anticholinergic, may be used symptomatically to treat severe sinus bradycardia or slow ventricular rate due to secondary AV block.
  - Give 0.01 mg/kg IV
- Cholestyramine, colestipol (both are antilipids), or activated charcoal may be used to bind with digoxin in the intestine and prevent enterohepatic recirculation.

Use of the digoxin antidote

- The drug digoxin immune fab (Digibind) is considered the antidote to digoxin. This drug, used to treat potentially life-threatening toxicity, is given in approximately the same dosage as the digoxin in the patient's body. It combines with digoxin to make it unable to bind at its receptor site, therefore inactivating it.
- Improvement generally begins within 30 minutes of IV administration.
- Give digoxin immune fab over 15 to 30 minutes through a 0.22-mm filter, although it may be given as a bolus when cardiac arrest is imminent. This may be given to children or adults.
- Serum digoxin levels will remain high after administration of digoxin immune fab. Therefore, serum digoxin levels should not be used as a guideline of the antidote's effectiveness. Instead, the nurse should evaluate the patient's response to determine the antidote's effectiveness.

Miscellaneous

- Avoid administration of IM digoxin because it causes site pain.

COMMUNITY-BASED CONCERNS

Box 28.4 Digoxin

Digoxin can cause fatal effects if taken accidentally by children. Adults prescribed digoxin should be aware of these risks and take the following precautions in their homes:

- Store digoxin out of the reach of children.
- Have a child-safety cap placed on the medication container.
- Do not leave loose pills out where children can see them.
- Do not tell children that digoxin is "candy."

This name change has not yet been adopted internationally. The International Nonproprietary Name (INN) is still amrinone. If this drug is purchased from a source outside of the United States the label will list the ingredient as amrinone, not inamrinone. United States health care workers need to be very careful if faced with this situation to prevent making a drug error.

Like digoxin, inamrinone is used in treating CHF. However, it is used only for short-term management of those patients who have not responded positively to treatment with digoxin, diuretics, and vasodilators. Unlike digoxin, inamrinone is *not* a cardiac glycoside. Inamrinone has a

MEMORY CHIP

[P] Digoxin

- Used in treating CHF, atrial fibrillation, and atrial flutter
- Direct effect is to strengthen force of cardiac contraction (positive inotropic effect)
- Indirect effect is to depress the SA node and slow conduction to the AV node (negative dromotropic effect), thus slowing heart rate (negative chronotropic effect)
- Can cause the same arrhythmias it is used to treat
- Antidote for digoxin overdose is digoxin immune fab
- Major contraindications: heart block, ventricular fibrillation, certain cases of ventricular tachycardia, some cases of sick sinus syndrome, and presence of digitalis toxicity
- Most common adverse effects: cardiac toxicity; hypokalemia, hypomagnesemia, and hypercalcemia increase the risk of toxicity
- Most serious adverse effect: ventricular fibrillation
- **Life span alert: Older adults tend to have increased risk for adverse effects due to decreased renal function. Children are often poisoned accidentally by digoxin.**
- Maximizing therapeutic effects: achieve rapid onset of therapeutic effects with a loading dose ("digitalization")
- Minimizing adverse effects: Monitor serum digoxin levels, assess for bradycardia (take apical pulse minute before giving drug), monitor and correct electrolyte imbalances, and assess for noncardiac signs of digoxin toxicity.
- Most important patient education: Teach how to take pulse and to avoid taking the dose if pulse is below 60; keep digoxin out of the reach of children.

positive inotropic effect and a vasodilatory effect similar to digoxin. However, inamrinone has a different structure and mode of action from digoxin. It is also different from catecholamines. Its mechanism of action is believed to be related to its ability to inhibit phosphodiesterase, which inactivates cyclic adenosine monophosphate (cyclic AMP) and alters calcium, resulting in the contraction of myocardial muscle cells. Afterload and preload are reduced by the direct relaxant effect of inamrinone on the vascular smooth muscle, creating vasodilation. These effects produce a prompt increase in cardiac output from the failing heart. Inamrinone is administered by IV infusion. The peak of action of inamrinone is within 10 minutes; duration of action varies with the size of the dose. Duration of action is about 2 hours when larger doses are given. The main route of elimination is in urine.

Many of the adverse effects of inamrinone are common to those seen with digoxin. Inamrinone may cause supraventricular and ventricular arrhythmias, nausea, and, less frequently, vomiting, abdominal pain, and anorexia. Unlike digoxin, inamrinone may cause two serious adverse effects—thrombocytopenia and hepatoxicity. Thrombocytopenia occurs in about 2.5% of patients receiving the drug, although it is more common in patients receiving prolonged therapy. Thrombocytopenia and hepatoxicity may be fatal, which is why the drug is not considered first-line therapy and is limited to short-term use.

Milrinone

Milrinone (Primacor) is also used to treat CHF. It is used for short-term IV use in patients already receiving digoxin and diuretics. Unlike digoxin, it is not a cardiac glycoside, but it increases the force of contraction similarly to digoxin. Like inamrinone, milrinone increases the force of contraction, is a vasodilator, and is different in structure and mode of action from digoxin and catecholamines. Milrinone works in the same way as inamrinone; it inhibits phosphodiesterase, which inactivates cyclic AMP and alters calcium, resulting in the contraction of myocardial muscle cells. Like milrinone, it also has vasodilating effects. In addition to improving cardiac contractility, milrinone improves left ventricular diastolic relaxation. Milrinone produces a prompt increase in cardiac output and decreases pulmonary capillary wedge pressure and vascular resistance. Milrinone is excreted primarily in the urine.

Adverse effects of milrinone are ventricular arrhythmias (the most common adverse effect, occurring in about 12% of patients), hypotension, angina, and ventricular tachycardia, which all occur in a small percentage of patients. Life-threatening arrhythmias are infrequent. Milrinone can cause headache. It also can cause thrombocytopenia, but much less frequently than inamrinone does.

CHAPTER SUMMARY

- CHF occurs when the heart is unable to effectively contract and pump out the volume of blood in the left ventricle.
- CHF is treated with combinations of drug therapy. Primary drug therapy includes the use of an ACE inhibitor, a beta blocker, and a diuretic. Digoxin is added after the patient's CHF is stable.
- The combination of an ACE inhibitor and a diuretic has been shown to decrease mortality from CHF. The addition of a beta blocker also has been shown to decrease mortality. Digoxin does not decrease mortality from CHF, but it decreases symptoms and improves exercise tolerance, thereby improving the quality of life.
- Digoxin strengthens the force of contraction of the heart (positive inotropic effect), prolongs conduction to the AV node (negative dromotropic effect), and slows the heart rate (negative chronotropic effect).
- Adverse effects of digoxin are dose related and are signs of digoxin toxicity. The most common adverse effects are cardiac toxicity, GI disturbances, and CNS toxicity.
- A low potassium level, low magnesium level, or a high calcium level potentiates the effect of digoxin, and digoxin toxicity may occur. This effect can occur even if the serum level of digoxin is in "normal" range.
- Bradycardia is a clinical sign of excessive digoxin. Always check an apical pulse for 1 full minute to detect for bradycardia before administering digoxin. Notify the physician and do not give the drug if the pulse is less than 60 bpm unless approved by the physician.
- Digoxin can be used to treat an arrhythmia, but it also may cause an arrhythmia.
- Inamrinone and milrinone also strengthen the force of contraction of the heart and are used in treating CHF. These drugs are only given intravenously and for short periods, never for chronic maintenance.

QUESTIONS FOR STUDY AND REVIEW

1. What are digoxin's primary effects on the heart?
2. What is the rationale for initially giving a larger than therapeutic dose (digitalization) for the first few doses of digoxin therapy?

Drugs Treating Angina

chapter 29

Learning Objectives

At the completion of this chapter the student will:

1. Differentiate drug therapy for chronic stable angina from unstable angina.
2. Identify core drug knowledge about drugs used to treat angina.
3. Identify core patient variables relevant to drugs used to treat angina.
4. Relate the interaction of core drug knowledge to core patient variables for drugs used to treat angina.
5. Generate a nursing plan of care based on interactions between core drug knowledge and core patient variables for drugs used to treat angina.
6. Describe nursing interventions to maximize therapeutic and minimize adverse effects for drugs used to treat angina.
7. Determine key points for patient and family education for drugs used to treat angina.

KEY TERMS

angina

microvascular angina

myocardial infarction

Prinzmetal angina

stable angina

unstable angina

variant angina

FEATURED WEBLINK

http://www.guideline.gov/summary/summary.aspx?doc_id=3588&nbr=2814&string=angina

The American College of Cardiology and American Heart Association provide this guideline update for the management of patients with chronic stable angina.

CONNECTION WEBLINK

Additional Weblinks are found on Connection: **http://www.connection.lww.com/go/aschenbrenner.**

Drugs Treating Angina

Ⓒ Nitrates

- Ⓟ **nitroglycerin**
- isosorbide

Ⓒ Beta Blockers
(see Chapter 13)

- Ⓟ **propranolol**
- atenolol
- metoprolol
- nadolol

Ⓒ Calcium Channel Blockers
(see Chapter 26)

- Ⓟ **verapamil**
- amlodipine
- bepridil
- diltiazem
- nicardipine
- nifedipine

Adjunct Treatment for Angina

Ⓒ Anticoagulants/antiplatelets

- Ⓟ **aspirin** (see Chapters 24 and 31)
- Ⓟ **clopidogrel** (see Chapter 31)
- Ⓟ **heparin** (see Chapter 31)
- glycoprotein IIb-IIIa inhibitors (see Chapter 31)

Other

- antihyperlipidemics (see Chapter 30)
- ACE inhibitors (see Chapter 27)

The symbol Ⓒ indicates the **drug class.**
Drugs in **bold type** marked with the symbol Ⓟ are prototypes.
Drugs in blue type are closely related to the prototype.
Drugs in red type are significantly different from the prototype.
Drugs in black type with no symbol are also used in drug therapy; no prototype

Angina is pain in the chest that occurs because the heart muscle is not receiving enough oxygen. Drug therapy to treat angina allows more oxygen to be delivered to the heart or decreases the oxygen needs of the heart, or both, which stops the pain. This chapter discusses the three main drug therapies used in angina—beta blockers, calcium channel blockers, and nitrates. Because the prototypes for beta blockers and calcium channel blockers are presented in Chapters 13 and 26, respectively; only the nitrates are presented in this chapter.

PHYSIOLOGY

The heart is a muscle in the chest that pumps oxygenated blood to the organs, muscles, tissues, and cells of the body. The heart itself requires oxygen delivered to its cells. The coronary arteries deliver oxygenated blood to the heart. Oxygen requirements of the heart increase as the heart pumps faster and works harder. Oxygen demands of the heart also increase if the heart has to overcome a greater peripheral resistance in the vessels to eject blood from the left ventricle.

PATHOPHYSIOLOGY

When the oxygen requirements of the heart are greater than the supply of oxygen it is getting, the heart muscle becomes ischemic. The oxygen imbalance may be from a reduced coronary blood flow or from a need for increased oxygen. Ischemia of the heart muscle will produce symptoms of chest pain in the patient. Chest pain that results from ischemia is termed **angina.** Angina is usually intermittent and substernal, although the pain may radiate elsewhere, often to the left arm or left shoulder. The pain is usually described as pressure on the chest. Additionally, the following symptoms may be present: nausea, sweating, weakness, loss of appetite, shortness of breath or difficulty breathing, upper back pain, and pain that feels knife-like.

The four major risk factors associated with coronary heart disease and angina are cigarette smoking, diabetes, elevated blood lipid levels, and hypertension. A recent large study re-evaluated the presence of these risk factors in 122,458 people enrolled in 14 international randomized clinical trials of coronary heart disease. Their findings confirm that each of those patients had at least one of the four main risk factors. (Khot et al., 2003)

There are four types of angina:

- Stable angina
- Unstable angina
- Prinzmetal or variant angina
- Microvascular angina

In **stable angina,** oxygen need exceeds the ability of the body to supply oxygen. This disparity may be caused by a narrowing of the coronary arteries from atherosclerosis (deposits of fat in the vessel) or from an activity that increases the oxygen needs of the heart temporarily. Stable angina occurs during exercise, stress, or periods of increased physical exertion and is normally reversed with rest. No permanent damage to the heart usually occurs after an episode of stable angina. An episode of stable angina does not indicate that the patient is about to have a **myocardial infarction** (MI), a complete blockage of one of the vessels supplying blood and nutrients to the muscle of the heart. An episode of stable angina does not place the person at a greater risk for having an MI later.

Unstable angina is caused by severely decreased coronary blood flow. Pain in unstable angina occurs when the patient is resting; it can even occur during sleep and awaken the patient. Unstable angina may develop suddenly on exertion, which may be the first time the patient has had anginal pain. It also can occur in patients who have previously had stable angina. For these patients, unstable angina is a marked increase in the frequency or the severity of their pain. Other presentations of unstable angina include non–Q-wave MI, or post-MI onset of angina (more than 24 hours after the MI). Unstable angina results most frequently from plaque rupture in the vessel, followed by a local thrombus formation. Plaque rupture is caused by a complex sequence of events, including local inflammatory activity. Because of this etiology, unstable angina is considered a critical phase of coronary heart disease and places the patient at high risk for having an MI. For this reason anticoagulants, antiplatelets, and antilipids are used in treatment. Special cardiac markers, not normally found in the blood, have been found in those with unstable angina. These regulatory contractile proteins are called cardiac troponin T and cardiac troponin I. Their presence has been shown to be a sensitive and specific marker for myocardial cell damage. Troponins T and I, which can be measured by a special blood test, appear to be better indicators of damage and early risk from unstable angina than the traditionally used creatine kinase myocardial band (isoenzyme M). Both fatal and nonfatal MIs were more frequent in patients with unstable angina who had elevations of one or both of these markers. Patients who have had angina at rest within the last 48 hours and are troponin positive are considered to have a 20% risk for MI, death, or both within the next 30 days. Patients who have had angina at rest within the last 48 hours but who are troponin negative are believed to have only a less than 2% chance for MI, death, or both (Hamm, 2000). There appears to be a direct relationship between the extent that the troponin level is elevated and mortality (Cannon & Turpie, 2003; Antman et al., 1996) The updated guidelines for management of patients with unstable angina and non–ST-segment elevation MI (ACC/AHA, 2002) states that testing for biomarkers of cardiac injury should be done in all patients who present with chest discomfort that is consistent with acute coronary syndrome; cardiac troponins T and I are the preferred marker, although creatine kinase–cardiac muscle isoenzyme by mass assay is acceptable.

Other cardiac markers currently being studied are the C-reactive protein (a systemic sign of inflammation, associated with atherosclerosis) and B-type natriuretic peptide, a neurohormone produced mostly in the ventricular myocardium. These have both been associated with increased mortality and recurrent cardiac problems in patients with acute coronary syndromes. (Cannon & Turpie, 2003; Rosenson & Koenig, 2003; deLemos et al., 2001).

Prinzmetal angina, also called **variant angina,** is caused by sudden coronary artery spasms that induce ischemia in the

heart muscle. These spasms, if lengthy, can lead to sudden death. However, this type of angina is rare. Prinzmetal angina may be precipitated by emotional stress, medications, street drugs (e.g., cocaine), or exposure to cold temperatures.

Microvascular angina is a newly discovered form of angina. Patients with this type of angina experience chest pain but have no apparent coronary blockages. The pain results from impaired function of the tiny blood vessels that perfuse the heart, arms, and legs. Microvascular angina can be treated with some of the same drugs used to treat stable angina (Box 29.1).

DRUGS TO TREAT ANGINA

Three main drug groups are used to treat angina—beta blockers, calcium channel blockers, and nitrates. Beta blockers prevent the beta-adrenergic receptors from being stimulated. These drugs have multiple effects on the heart and cardiovascular system, including slowing the heart rate, depressing atrioventricular (AV) conduction, decreasing cardiac output, and reducing systolic and diastolic blood pressure at rest and during exercise. These effects decrease the oxygen demands of the heart and thereby decrease angina. Beta blockers used commonly for treating angina are propranolol, atenolol, metoprolol, and nadolol. Other beta blockers that may be used in treating angina are bisoprolol (Zebeta), carteolol (Cartrol), and esmolol (Brevibloc), although this is an off-label use of these drugs. The beta blockers are discussed fully in Chapter 13.

Calcium is needed in the automatic and conducting cells of the heart to help create an action potential. In the cells of the heart that contract, calcium links excitation with contraction and controls energy storage and use. Calcium travels to these cells through special channels. Calcium-channel blockers inhibit calcium from moving across cell membranes. The effects of this inhibition on the cardiovascular system are decreased contraction, depression of impulse formation (automaticity), and slowing of conduction velocity. These have the effect of decreasing the oxygen needs of the heart. Calcium channel blockers also cause arteriolar dilation, decreasing afterload. Calcium-channel blockers are used in chronic stable angina when the patient cannot tolerate beta blockers, or if the symptoms are not adequately controlled while on this therapy (ACC/AHA, 2002). The calcium channel blockers used for chronic stable angina are verapamil (Calan), amlodipine (Norvasc), bepridil (Vascor), diltiazem (Cardizem), nicardipine (Cardene), and nifedipine (Procardia). The calcium channel blocker used in unstable angina is verapamil. Amlodipine, nifedipine, verapamil, and diltiazem are used in treating Prinzmetal angina. The calcium channel blockers are discussed more fully in Chapter 26.

Nitrates dilate vascular smooth muscle and both venous and arterial vessels (although more relaxation occurs on the venous side). Venous dilation decreases the returning flow of blood to the heart (preload). Arterial dilation reduces systemic vascular resistance and arterial pressure (afterload). These effects decrease the workload on the heart and its oxygen needs. Nitrates also improve the circulation to the heart itself by redistributing blood flow to the collateral vessels.

Some other drug therapies are used as adjuncts to the main drug therapies for treating angina. These therapies are not designed to decrease oxygen demands on the heart. Rather, these therapies are used to slow down the progression of coronary artery disease or prevent complications that may arise with angina. As mentioned earlier, thrombus formation is an important concern with unstable angina and some of these therapies specifically target this problem. Aspirin is one drug that is used in chronic stable angina and unstable angina. Aspirin has anticoagulant properties, which are helpful in preventing thrombus formation and a potentially resulting MI. Aspirin's use as an antiplatelet agent is further discussed in Chapter 31, and the description of aspirin as a prototype drug for pain is in Chapter 24. Clopidogrel, an antiplatelet drug, can be used in place of or in addition to aspirin in some patients with unstable angina. Glycoprotein IIb/IIIa receptor antagonists are a new class of platelet inhibitors that are more potent than aspirin because they target the final common pathway of platelet aggregation (Weitz & Bates, 2000). One of these drugs should be added to acetylsalicylic acid (ASA) and heparin therapies if the patient with unstable angina is to have percutaneous coronary intervention and cardiac catheterization (ACC/AHA, 2002). One small study showed that one of these drugs, tirofiban, when given in addition to heparin, provided earlier clinical stability and prevented major in hospital cardiac events in patients with unstable angina and non–Q-wave MI as compared with those on heparin therapy alone (Okmen et al., 2003).

Heparin, an anticoagulant given by the intravenous (IV) or subcutaneous (SC) route, is used in conjuncture with antiplatelets (aspirin, clopidogrel, or both) in unstable angina to prevent thrombus formation. The use of low-molecular-weight heparin is being proposed instead of unfractionated heparin because it provides a more stable pharmacodynamic response and is easier to use. Low-molecular-weight heparin has been shown to be as effective as traditional, unfractionated heparin and appears to be most beneficial to

COMMUNITY-BASED CONCERNS

Box 29.1 Chest Pain

Many community groups request health education topics for their members. Nurses are often the health care professionals who respond to these requests. If called on to discuss consumer response to chest pain be sure to include the following points when teaching families and the public how to respond appropriately when someone is experiencing an angina attack:

- Instruct them to have the person rest (sit or lie down).
- If the person is known to take nitroglycerin tablets, give one and have the person place it under the tongue.
- Repeat in 5 minutes and again in another 5 minutes if chest pain does not go away.

If after three tablets of nitroglycerin the pain does not go away, the person should be considered to be having a heart attack. Call the emergency medical number, and get the person to the nearest hospital.
OR
If the person with chest pain does not take nitroglycerin, have him or her sit or lie down If the pain does not go away within 5 minutes, assume that the person is having a heart attack. Call the medical emergency number and get the person to the nearest hospital.

patients who are at the highest risk for complications from unstable angina (Kaul & Shah, 2000). Heparin is discussed in Chapter 31. Lipid-lowering agents often are used in conjuncture with drugs to treat angina to slow the progression of coronary heart disease. Decreasing circulating fats in the blood will decrease the rate at which fatty deposits are deposited on the walls of the vessels. These fatty deposits narrow the vessel and block the blood flow, causing angina. Such blockages are especially problematic in the coronary arteries. In one recent study, the antilipid drug atorvastatin was given to patients in the first 5 days of an acute coronary syndrome; C-reactive protein was found to decrease in this group but not for those on a placebo (Correia et al., 2003) Lipid-lowering agents are discussed in Chapter 30. An ACE inhibitor is used in patients with coronary artery disease if they also have diabetes, systolic dysfunction, or both (ACC/AHA, 2002). ACE inhibitors are discussed in detail in Chapter 27. If the pain of unstable acute angina is not controlled by nitrates or anti-ischemic therapy, morphine, a narcotic, may be used. Morphine is discussed in Chapter 23.

New drug classes being examined in Europe for potential use in treating angina include potassium-channel openers and blockers and direct thrombin inhibitors. No clinical trials of these drugs are currently underway in the United States, although some other research is being done. Potassium-channel openers are a novel class of vasodilators. By opening the potassium channel, the conductivity of potassium ions into the cells is increased, which results in hyperpolarization of smooth muscle membranes and produces vasodilation (Lawson, 2000). Potassium blockers inhibit the cellular cardiac repolarization of potassium currents and multiple neuronal and vascular currents. This effect exerts an anti-ischemic and an antiarrhythmic effect on the body (Mitrovic et al., 2000). Finally, direct thrombin inhibitors are being studied because they appear to inhibit thrombin-mediated platelet aggregation and fibrin deposits (Weitz & Bates, 2000). Table 29.1 presents a summary of selected antianginal drugs.

C NITRATES

Nitrates include nitroglycerin (Nitrostat), which is the prototype, and isosorbide (Sorbitrate).

NURSING MANAGEMENT OF THE PATIENT RECEIVING P NITROGLYCERIN

Core Drug Knowledge

Pharmacotherapeutics

Therapeutic uses of nitroglycerin vary by the route of administration. Given sublingually or by transmucosal or translingual spray, nitroglycerin is used to treat acute angina. It also is used through topical, transdermal, translingual spray, and transmucosal or oral sustained-release methods to prevent chronic recurrent angina. When given intravenously, nitroglycerin is used to treat hypertension secondary to surgical procedures; to create controlled hypotension during anesthesia; to treat congestive heart failure (CHF) associated with acute MI; and to treat angina unresponsive to organic nitrates or beta blockers. Unlabeled uses for nitroglycerin include reducing cardiac workload in patients with acute MI and CHF (sublingual and topical), providing adjunctive treatment of Raynaud disease and other peripheral vascular diseases (topical), and managing hypertensive crisis (IV).

Pharmacokinetics

Nitroglycerin is absorbed rapidly sublingually; it also is absorbed through the skin. Metabolism occurs in the liver, and the drug has an extensive first-pass effect when given orally. It is excreted in the urine. Absorption of sublingual products depends on salivary secretion; dry mouth will decrease absorption. The drug is absorbed directly into the vascular system through this route; it is not swallowed and absorbed through the gastrointestinal (GI) tract. Thus, it bypasses the first-pass effect. Absorption of transdermal products is through the skin and into the vascular system. Ointments and transdermal systems provide a gradual release of drug into the circulatory system. The drug reaches its target organs before it is inactivated by the liver. Transdermal absorption will be increased with physical exercise, elevated external temperatures (e.g., saunas), and if the drug is applied to broken skin (see Table 29.1).

Pharmacodynamics

Nitroglycerin relaxes vascular smooth muscle and dilates both arterial and venous vessels. Dilation of veins is more predominant than dilation of arteries, resulting in peripheral pooling of blood and decreased preload. Blood pressure will decrease as a result of venous dilation. Reflex tachycardia may follow the drop in blood pressure. Arteriolar dilation reduces systemic vascular resistance and arterial pressure, thus reducing afterload. Myocardial oxygen consumption is decreased. Nitroglycerin redistributes blood flow in the heart, improving circulation to ischemic areas.

Tolerance to the vascular and antianginal effects may develop. Tolerance is minimized by starting with as small a dose as possible and removing the nitroglycerin (paste or transdermal patches) from the patient for 10 to 12 hours a day. The sublingual and translingual spray forms of the drug are the least likely to produce tolerance. The transmucosal form also appears to produce minimal tolerance.

One recent small study of the effects of transdermal nitroglycerin on ventricular function after myocardial infarction showed that, during the 6-month study period, patients on transdermal nitroglycerin had a significantly larger increase in systolic pulmonary venous flow velocity, and an improved ejection fraction, when compared with those not receiving nitroglycerin. The authors concluded that long term use of nitrates after an MI may help preserve diastolic left ventricular function (Kiraly et al., 2003)

Contraindications and Precautions

Nitroglycerin is contraindicated in hypersensitivity or idiosyncratic reactions to nitrates, severe anemia, closed-angle glaucoma (intraocular pressure may increase), orthostatic

TABLE 29.1 Summary of Selected ○C Antianginal Drugs

Drug (Trade) Name	Selected Indications	Route and Dosage Range	Pharmacokinetics
○C Nitrates			
P nitroglycerin (Nitrostat, Nitrobid IV, Nitrol, Nitro-Dur, Nitrolingual)	Acute angina	*Adult:* SL, 1 tablet under tongue, every 5 min; total of 3 tablets	*Onset:* IV: 1–2 min; sublingual, 1–3 min; TL spray, 2 min; topical and transdermal, 30–60 min
	Prophylaxis	*Adult:* Topical (transdermal paste or patch), apply ½ inch q8h; increase by ½ inch to achieve desired results; translingual spray, 0.4 mg/metered dose into oral mucosa, not to exceed 3 doses/15 min	*Duration:* IV, 3–5 min; SL, 30–60 min; topical/transdermal, up to 24 h
	Hypertension	*Adult:* IV, 5 mg/min by infusion pump; increase by 5-mg increments every 3–5 min as needed	$t_{1/2}$: 1–4 min (IV)
		Child: Safety and efficacy not established	
isosorbide dinitrate (Sorbitrate, Isordil; *Canadian:* Apo-ISDN)	Treatment and prevention of angina pectoris	*Adult:* SL, 2.5–5 mg; PO, 5–40 mg tablets or capsules	*Onset:* PO, 20–40 min; SL, 2–5 min
		Child: Safety and efficacy not established	*Duration:* PO, 4–6 h; SL, 1–2 h
			$t_{1/2}$: Unknown
○C Beta Blocker			
atenolol (Tenormin; *Canadian:* Apo-Atenol)	Hypertension	*Adult:* PO, 50 mg/d; after 1–2 wk, dose may be increased to 100 mg	*Onset:* PO, varies; IV, immediate
		Child: Dose has not been established	*Duration:* PO and IV, 24 h
	Angina pectoris	*Adult:* PO, 50 mg qd. If optimal response not achieved in 1 wk, increase to 100 mg/d, up to 200 mg/d	$t_{1/2}$: 6–9 h
	Acute myocardial infarction	*Adult:* IV, 5 mg over 5 min; follow with 5 mg, 10 min later; switch to 50 mg PO 10 min after last IV dose; follow with 50 mg PO 12 h later; administer 100 mg PO qd or 50 mg PO bid for 6–9 d	
		Child: Safety and efficacy not established	
○C Calcium Channel Blocker			
nifedipine (Adalat, Procardia; *Canadian:* Apo-Nifed)	Angina pectoris Stable angina Hypertension	*Adult:* PO, 10 mg tid, titrate over 7–14 d; SR: PO, 30–60 mg/qd; titrate over 7–14 d	Onset: PO and SR, 20 min
		Child: Safety and efficacy not established	Duration: 8–24 h
			$t_{1/2}$: 2–5 h

hypotension, first hours to days of acute diagnosed MI (sublingual forms), head trauma or cerebral hemorrhage (may increase intracranial pressure), and allergy to adhesives (transdermal). Caution also is advised when using nitroglycerin to treat patients with open-angle glaucoma. The IV route is contraindicated in hypotension, uncorrected hypovolemia, inadequate cerebral circulation, increased intracranial pressure, constrictive pericarditis, and pericardial tamponade. Caution also is advised when administering IV nitroglycerin to patients with hepatic disease and severe renal disease. Nitroglycerin is in pregnancy category C, and it is not known whether nitrates are excreted in breast milk; therefore, cautious use is advised.

Adverse Effects

The most common adverse effect of nitroglycerin is headache, which may be persistent and severe. Cardiovascular effects may include hypotension, postural hypotension, tachycardia, palpitations, and syncope. Other effects on the central nervous system (CNS) include dizziness, vertigo, anxiety, and weakness. These adverse effects are related to the vasodilation and cardiovascular effects that occur with nitroglycerin use. Dermatitis can occur from topical application. Local burning under the tongue can occur with sublingual administration. Alcohol intoxication can develop in patients receiving high doses of IV nitroglycerin because many of the IV products contain alcohol as a diluent.

Overdosage will result in hypotension, tachycardia, flushing, perspiring skin turning cold and cyanotic, headache, vertigo, palpitations, visual disturbances, diaphoresis, dizziness, syncope, nausea, vomiting, and anorexia. Other signs and symptoms of overdose include initial hyperpnea, dyspnea and slow breathing, heart block, and increased intracranial pressure exhibited by cerebral symptoms of confusion, moderate fever, and paralysis. These signs and symptoms are related to excessive cardiovascular action.

Drug Interactions

A few drugs interact with nitroglycerin (Table 29.2). Nitroglycerin may interfere with the Zlatkis-Zak color reaction, causing a false report of decreased serum cholesterol levels.

Assessment of Relevant Core Patient Variables

Health Status

Ascertain whether the patient has acute angina or chronic recurrent angina. Assess the patient's pulse rate and blood pressure. Determine whether the patient has any of the following conditions, which are contraindications to nitroglycerin use: closed-angle glaucoma, orthostatic hypotension, severe anemia, head trauma or cerebral hemorrhage, first hours to days of acute confirmed MI, hypersensitivity to nitrates, or allergy to adhesives (if the patient is receiving a transdermal dosage form). If the patient is to receive IV nitroglycerin, first be sure that the patient does not have hypotension or uncorrected hypovolemia, inadequate cerebral circulation, increased intracranial pressure, constrictive pericarditis, or pericardial tamponade because these are contraindications for this route. If hepatic or severe renal disease exists, caution must be used with IV administration.

Life Span and Gender

Nitroglycerin is in pregnancy category C, so determine whether the patient is pregnant. Assess whether the patient is breast-feeding because cautious use is advised in that case. Safety and efficacy in children have not been established; note the age of the patient (Box 29.2).

Lifestyle, Diet, and Habits

If the patient has chronic stable angina, it is important to determine how much or what type of activity precipitates an anginal attack, or if angina occurs at rest, which may indicate unstable angina. In patients who smoke cigarettes, smoking constricts the blood vessels and may cause angina. Patients whose diet is high in cholesterol or saturated fats risk developing fatty deposits within the vessels, which contribute to narrowing the vessels.

Environment

Be aware of the environment in which the drug will be administered. Nitroglycerin can be administered in any environment, with the exception of IV nitroglycerin, which is administered in the hospital while on continuous monitoring for blood pressure and heart rate. Sublingual tablets are likely to lose effectiveness if exposed to light, excessive heat, or moisture. Between 40% and 80% of the IV nitroglycerin dose will migrate into many plastics. Therefore, the drug is diluted only into glass parenteral solution bottles and administered with IV tubing not made from polyvinyl chloride (PVC) that is provided by the manufacturer.

Nursing Diagnoses and Outcomes

- Acute Pain, Chest, related to cardiac disease
  Desired outcome: *Acute chest pain will be resolved with the use of drug therapy without injury to the heart occurring.*
- Decreased Cardiac Output related to therapeutic effects of drug
  Desired outcome: *Patient's blood pressure will decrease to therapeutic levels but will not decrease to the level of hypotension.*
- Risk for Injury related to orthostatic hypotension and dizziness secondary to adverse effects of drug therapy
  Desired outcome: *Patient will not sustain injury because of orthostatic hypotension and dizziness.*
- Acute Pain, Headache, related to adverse effects of drug therapy
  Desired outcome: *Patient's headache, if it occurs, will be managed successfully by analgesics so that patient will adhere to drug therapy.*

Planning and Intervention

Maximizing Therapeutic Effects

Sublingual Tablets

Place one tablet under the patient's tongue, where it should be allowed to dissolve. It is important to administer a tablet every 5 minutes, up to three in 15 minutes if necessary, to achieve full therapeutic effect. Have the patient sit or lie down to allow for rest and decrease the oxygen needs of the heart.

It is a good idea to keep tablets in the original dark bottle and keep the lid on when not in use to prevent deterioration and loss of efficacy. Avoid exposure of tablets to high temperatures.

Topical Ointment and Transdermal Patches

Apply to areas that do not have excessive hair, to promote absorption. Apply to the chest, upper arm, or upper thigh to promote absorption and increase onset of systemic action. Do not apply to distal parts of extremities (i.e., near the hands or feet).

CRITICAL THINKING SCENARIO

Nitroglycerin

Peter Riley, 4 years old, is staying at his grandparents' house for the weekend. He finds his grandfather's nitroglycerin ointment in the bathroom. He squeezes some out and spreads it over his entire left arm. When his grandparents realize what he has done, they call the Advice Nurse hotline for their HMO.

1. If you were the Advice Nurse, what would you tell the grandparents to do?
2. What is the major risk to Peter?

TABLE 29.2 Agents That Interact With P Nitroglycerin

Interactants	Effect and Significance	Nursing Management
alcohol	Severe hypotension and cardiovascular collapse	Ensure patient does not consume alcohol. Educate patient about risks of interaction.
heparin	Decreased pharmacologic effects of heparin	Monitor for therapeutic effect of heparin.
fentanyl	Severe hypotension or increased fluid volume requirements that may cause decreased antimanic controls	Monitor hypotension and fluid levels.
lithium	Possible lithium toxicity and neurotoxic and psychotic symptoms	Give with caution and daily monitor serum lithium levels. Give drug with food or milk or after meals.
theophylline	Pharmacologic actions of theophylline potentially enhanced, particularly drug interactions	Have frequent blood tests to monitor drug effects, and ensure safe and effective dosage.
sildenafil tadalafil vardenafil	Potentiation of vasodilation from nitrates resulting in significant hypotension	Educate patients not to use these drugs for erectile dysfunction.

Translingual Spray

Spray nitroglycerin onto or under the tongue to promote absorption. Do not allow the patient to inhale the drug. If used to treat acute angina, spray one or two metered doses. The dose may be repeated but not more than three times in 15 minutes. If used prophylactically, administer one metered dose 5 to 10 minutes before onset of activity that may precipitate angina.

FOCUS ON RESEARCH

Box 29.2 FRT Sexual Variations in Angina

DeVon, H. A., & Zerwic, J. J. (2003). The symptoms of unstable angina: Do women and men differ? *Nursing Research, 52*(2), 108–118.

The Study

Based on the knowledge that the epidemiology, presentation, and outcomes of coronary heart disease differ between men and women, this study's purpose was to determine whether the symptoms of unstable angina also differ between men and women. A convenience sample of 50 men and 50 women with unstable angina were asked to complete three instruments to assess their symptoms of angina: the Unstable Angina Symptoms questionnaire, the Hospital Anxiety and Depression Scale, and the Canadian Cardiovascular Society classification of angina. Analysis of the data, after controlling for age, diabetes, anxiety, depression, and functional status, showed that women were more likely to experience weakness, difficulty breathing, nausea, loss of appetite, upper back pain, stabbing pain, and knifelike pain than men with unstable angina; although a higher percentage of the women experienced these symptoms, the differences were not statistically significant. Women did have a significantly higher incidence of depression than men.

Nursing Implications

Although this study did not show any differences among men and women, it does show that patients may present with other symptoms than substernal chest pain when they are experiencing unstable angina. Many of these symptoms are somewhat vague and nonspecific. It is important to assess for these other symptoms and to recognize that taken together they may help confirm the diagnosis of unstable angina as opposed to representing other disease entities or pathological problems.

Transmucosal Tablets

Place one tablet between lip and gum above incisors or between cheek and gum to promote slow dissolving and extended absorption.

Intravenous

Use only the non-PVC IV administration tubing supplied by the manufacturer and glass IV bottles for the diluted drug solution to prevent loss of active drug into the tubing or bag.

Minimizing Adverse Effects

All Routes

Assess the patient's pulse and blood pressure before administering drug therapy. It also is important to monitor for orthostatic hypotension and to assist the patient to a standing position gradually when arising. Treat any headache that develops with aspirin or acetaminophen until tolerance to this adverse effect occurs. When withdrawing nitroglycerin as a treatment for angina, it is important to reduce the dosage gradually to prevent withdrawal reactions.

Sublingual

Do not give more than three tablets—one every 5 minutes—to relieve acute angina. If three tablets do not alleviate angina, the patient is considered to be having an acute MI, and it is urgent to obtain emergency help immediately.

Transdermal

This route is not appropriate for acute angina. Do not apply the drug to broken or irritated skin. It is important to remove the patch for 10 to 12 hours every 24 hours to prevent nitrate tolerance from developing. If anginal symptoms develop at night, the use of a beta blocker or calcium channel blocker should be considered. Patients who normally have angina only during daytime hours are not at substantial risk for developing nighttime angina with a nightly nitrate-free period.

Do discharge a cardioversion or defibrillation paddle through a transdermal system. Arcing may develop, which may concentrate local current, damaging the paddles and burning the patient.

Intravenous

Monitor the patient's blood pressure and heart rate while IV therapy continues. It is important to assess for alcohol intoxication if giving high doses for a prolonged period. Use an IV pump to regulate the infusion rate.

Providing Patient and Family Education

All Routes

- Explain the purpose and adverse effects of nitroglycerin.
- Instruct the patient to sit or lie down when experiencing angina.
- Explain that postural hypotension may occur (especially if standing still after a dose). If feelings of dizziness, weakness, or fainting occur, the patient should lie down or place the head in a low position (if sitting), and take deep breaths.

Sublingual Tablets

- Teach the patient to place a sublingual tablet under the tongue at the first sign of an anginal attack, and not to wait for the pain to become severe.
- Explain that if angina is not relieved, up to two more tablets may be taken; one 5 minutes after the first tablet and the other 5 minutes after the second tablet. Instruct the patient to go the nearest emergency department if angina is not relieved after the above measures are taken.
- Teach the patient to keep the sublingual tablets in their original bottle and to keep the cap on the bottle. It also is important to explain the importance of not storing the bottle in the sun.

Translingual Spray

- Instruct the patient on proper administration—spraying it onto or under the tongue, not inhaling it.
- Explain that the drug may be used prophylactically or to treat the onset of angina.

Transmucosal Tablets

- Instruct the patient on the proper placement of the tablet—under the upper lip between the lip and gum above the incisor, or in the pouch between the cheek and gum. It is important to explain that it will dissolve slowly over a 3- to 5-hour period.
- Emphasize the importance of not chewing or swallowing the tablet.
- Explain that the rate of dissolution may be increased by touching the tablet with the tongue or by drinking hot fluids.

Sustained-Release Tablets

- Instruct the patient to swallow these tablets, not to chew them or place them sublingually because doing so alters onset of the drug effects.

Ointment

- Explain that ointments do not provide immediate relief of acute angina pain and should only be used prophylactically.
- Instruct the patient to use an applicator or dose-measuring papers, not the hands, to measure and apply the prescribed amount of nitroglycerin ointment.
- Instruct the patient not to rub the drug into the skin.
- Teach the patient to choose a different area on the skin when applying a new dose. Tell the patient to use a tissue to remove any old ointment left on the skin before applying a new dose.
- Instruct the patient to wipe off any ointment that gets on the outside of the tube to prevent it from getting on the hands, and to recap the tube securely.

Transdermal

- Teach the patient to apply the patch to as hairless a skin area as possible. The chest or upper arm are used typically; avoid placing the patch in the distal portion of the extremities.
- Instruct the patient to remove the patch for 10 to 12 hours as prescribed.
- Explain the importance of avoiding saunas and other environments that increase the external temperature.
- If the adhesive becomes loose during the "on" period, instruct the patient to place additional tape over the patch to guarantee contact with the skin.
- A discarded patch still contains active nitroglycerin, which can be a hazard for children and pets. Therefore, it is important to advise the patient to flush used patches down the toilet.

Ongoing Assessment and Evaluation

The patient's blood pressure and heart rate will be monitored throughout therapy. If given intravenously, this monitoring should be continuous. Assess for relief of angina or control of chronic angina. Therapy is effective when angina is controlled or prevented without the development of hypotension or damage to the heart.

MEMORY CHIP

P Nitroglycerin

- Used in treating angina; IV route is used to decrease blood pressure (BP)
- Usually given sublingually topically, sometimes IV in acute care setting
- Relaxes smooth muscles and dilates vascular beds
- Most common adverse effect: headache followed by hypotension
- Most serious adverse effect: can be hypotension
- Maximizing therapeutic effects: Keep tablets out of sunlight (keep in original dark bottle), moisture (keep cap sealed tightly when drug not in use), and excessive heat; give one tablet every 5 minutes, up to 3 in 15 minutes; and have patient rest or lie down during anginal attacks.
- Minimizing adverse effects: Take BP before and during therapy; to prevent orthostatic hypotension, keep the patient lying down during therapy.
- Most important patient education: If three sublingual tablets do not alleviate pain, seek immediate emergency medical treatment; utilize prophylactic doses prior to activities that may precipitate angina; and remove patches or ointment for 10 or 12 hours out of every 24 to prevent tolerance.

Drug Closely Related to P Nitroglycerin

Isosorbide (Isordil) is a nitrate, like nitroglycerin, and is used for treating and preventing angina. It is not used to treat hypertension. Isosorbide is given sublingually or orally. Sublingual isosorbide has a slower onset and a longer duration of action compared with sublingual nitroglycerin. Because sublingual isosorbide does not relieve chest pain as rapidly as nitroglycerin, isosorbide is limited to treating acute angina in patients intolerant of or unresponsive to sublingual nitroglycerin. Oral preparations include tablets, sustained-release tablets, and chewable tablets. Oral sustained-relief routes of isosorbide also have a slower onset and longer duration than comparable forms of nitroglycerin. Although nitroglycerin may be used occasionally with adequate monitoring during the early phases of an acute MI, isosorbide should never be used, because of its greater sustained effects.

● CHAPTER SUMMARY

- Nitroglycerin is used to treat angina and to prevent angina. When given intravenously, it also is used to reduce hypertension.
- Nitroglycerin relaxes vascular smooth muscle and dilates both arterial and venous beds. Dilation of veins is more predominant than dilation of arteries, resulting in peripheral pooling of blood and decreased preload.
- Blood pressure will decrease as a result of venous dilation. Reflex tachycardia may follow the drop in blood pressure. Thus, the patient's blood pressure is assessed before each dose and during drug therapy with nitroglycerin, and the pulse should be assessed during therapy.
- Arteriolar dilation reduces systemic vascular resistance and arterial pressure, thus reducing afterload. Reduced afterload decreases the work the heart must perform to eject blood from the left ventricle and thereby decreases the oxygen needs of the heart.
- The most common adverse effect of nitroglycerin is headache.
- When nitroglycerin is given intravenously because of elevated blood pressure, the patient must be continually monitored in an intensive care setting. For safety, the drug should be administered by pump.

▲ QUESTIONS FOR STUDY AND REVIEW

1. If the patient is taking nitroglycerin through a transdermal patch to prevent recurrent angina, why should he or she wear the patch only 12 to 14 hours a day?
2. How often should a tablet of sublingual nitroglycerin be administered to treat an episode of angina? How many tablets can be administered?
3. Why should you take the patient's blood pressure before administering a dose of nitroglycerin ointment topically?
4. When measuring the dose of nitroglycerin ointment, you get some on your hands. Later, you experience a throbbing headache. What is the explanation for this headache?
5. How does nitroglycerin decrease anginal pain?

? Need More Help?

Chapter 29 of the study guide for *Drug Therapy in Nursing* 2e contains NCLEX-style questions and other learning activities to reinforce your understanding of the concepts presented in this chapter. For additional information or to purchase the study guide, visit *http://connection.lww.com/go/aschenbrenner.*

■ REFERENCES AND BIBLIOGRAPHY

ACC/AHA. (2002). Guideline update for the management of patients with chronic stable angina: A report of the American College of Cardiology/American Heart Association Task Force on Practice Guidelines [Online]. Available: *http://www.guideline.gov/summary/summary.aspx?doc_id=3588&nbr=2814&string=angina.*

ACC/AHA. (2002). Guideline update for the management of patients with unstable angina and non-ST-segment elevation myocardial infarction: A report of the American College of Cardiology/American Heart Association Task Force on Practice Guidelines [Online]. Available: *http://www.guideline.gov/summary/summary.aspx?doc_id=3190&nbr=2416&string=angina.*

Antman, E. N., Tanasijevic, M. J., Thompson, B., et al. (1996). Cardiac-specific troponin I levels to predict the risk of mortality in patients with acute coronary syndromes. *New England Journal of Medicine, 335*(18), 1342–1349.

Cannon, C. P., & Turpie, A. G. G. (2003). Unstable angina and non-ST-elevation myocardial infarction: Initial antithrombotic therapy and early invasive strategy. *Circulation, 107*(21), 2640–2645. Available: *http://circ.ahajournals,org/cgi/content/full/107/21/2640.*

Correia, L. C., Sposito, A. C., Lima, J. C., et al. (2003). Anti-inflammatory effect of atorvastatin (80 mg) in unstable angina pectoris and non-Q-wave acute myocardial infarction. *American Journal of Cardiology, 92*(3), 298–301.

deLemos, J. A., Morrow, D. A., Bentley, J. H., et al. (2001). The prognostic value of B-type natriuretic peptide in patients with acute coronary syndromes. *New England Journal of Medicine, 345*(14), 1014–1021.

Hamm, C. W., & Braunwald, E. (2000). A classification of unstable angina revisited. *Circulation, 102*(1), 118–122.

Kaul, S., & Shah, P. K. (2000). Low molecular weight heparin in acute coronary syndrome: Evidence for superior or equivalent efficacy compared with unfractionated heparin? *Journal of the American College of Cardiology, 35*(7), 1699–1712.

Khot, U. N., Khot, M. B., Bajzer C. T., et al. (2003). Prevalence of conventional risk factors in patients with coronary heart disease. *Journal of the American Medical Association, 290*(7), 898–904.

Kiraly, C., Kiss, A., Timar, S., et al. (2003). Effects of long-term transdermal nitrate treatment on left ventricular function in patients following myocardial infarction. *Clinical Cardiology, 26*(3), 120–126.

Lawson, K. (2000). Potassium channel openers as potential therapeutic weapons in ion channel disease. *Kidney International, 57*(3), 838–845.

Mitrovic, V., Oehm, E., Thormann, J., et al. (2000). Potassium channel openers and blockers in coronary artery disease. Comparison to beta blockers and calcium antagonists. *Herz, 25*(2), 130–142.

Okmen, E., Cakmak, M., Tartan, Z., et al. (2003). Effects of glycoprotein IIb/IIIa inhibition on clinical stabilization parameters in patients with unstable angina and non-Q-wave myocardial infarction. *Heart Vessels, 18*(3), 117–122.

Richards, S. B., Funck, M., & Milner, K. A. (2000). Differences between black and whites with coronary heart disease in initial symptoms and delay in seeking care. *American Journal of Critical Care, 9*(4), 237–244.

Rosenson, R. S., & Koenig, W. (2003). Utility of inflammatory markers in the management of coronary artery disease. *American Journal of Cardiology, 92*(1A), 10i–18i.

Weitz, J. I., & Bates, S. M. (2000). Beyond heparin and aspirin: New treatments for unstable angina and non-Q-wave myocardial infarction. *Archives of Internal Medicine, 160*(6), 749–758.

Drugs Affecting Lipid Levels

chapter 30

Learning Objectives

At the completion of this chapter the student will:

1. Identify the core drug knowledge for drugs that affect lipid levels.
2. Differentiate the drug classes that affect lipid levels.
3. Identify core patient variables relevant to drugs that affect lipid levels.
4. Relate the interaction of core drug knowledge to core patient variables for drugs that affect lipid levels.
5. Generate a nursing plan of care from the interaction between core drug knowledge and core patient variables for drugs that affect lipid levels.
6. Describe nursing interventions to maximize therapeutic effects and minimize adverse effects for drugs that affect lipid levels.
7. Determine key points for patient and family education for drugs that affect lipid levels.

KEY TERMS

arteriosclerosis

atherosclerosis

hyperlipidemia

lipids

FEATURED WEBLINK

http://circ.ahajournals.org/cgi/content/full/110/2/227

This site features the issue of the journal *Circulation* that has the complete 2004 updates to the National Cholesterol Education Program Treatment Panel III Guidelines.

CONNECTION WEBLINK

Additional Weblinks are found on Connection: **http://www.connection.lww.com/go/aschenbrenner.**

Drugs Affecting Lipid Levels

Ⓒ Antihyperlipidemics

- Ⓒ Statins
  - [P] **lovastatin**
  - atorvastatin
  - fluvastatin
  - pravastatin
  - rosivastatin
  - simvastatin
- Ⓒ Fibric acid derivatives
  - fenofibrate
  - gemfibrozil
  - clofibrate
- Ⓒ Nicotinic acid
  - niacin
- Ⓒ Bile acid sequestrants
  - cholestyramine
  - colestipol
- Ⓒ Thyroid hormone
  - dextrothyroxine sodium

The symbol Ⓒ indicates the **drug class.**
Drugs in **bold type** marked with the symbol [P] are prototypes.
Drugs in blue type are closely related to the prototype.
Drugs in red type are significantly different from the prototype.
Drugs in black type with no symbol are also used in drug therapy; no prototype

This chapter discusses drugs used to lower serum lipid levels. The prototype drug is lovastatin (Mevacor). Other drugs in this class, known as statins, include atorvastatin (Lipitor), fluvastatin (Lescol), pravastatin (Pravachol), simvastatin (Zocor), and rosuvastatin (Crestor). Drugs similar to lovastatin include the fibric acid derivatives (gemfibrozil [Lopid], clofibrate [Atromid-S]), (fenofibrate [Tricor]), nicotinic acid (niacin), the bile acid sequestrants (cholestyramine [LoCholest, Questran, Prevalite] and colestipol [Colestid]), and dextrothyroxine sodium (Choloxin).

PHYSIOLOGY

Serum **lipids** are fats found in the bloodstream. These lipids include cholesterol, cholesterol esters (compounds), phospholipids, and triglycerides. They are transported in the blood as part of large molecules called lipoproteins. The five major families of blood (plasma) lipoproteins are:

- Chylomicrons
- Very-low-density lipoproteins (VLDLs)
- Intermediate-density lipoproteins (IDLs)
- Low-density lipoproteins (LDLs)
- High-density lipoproteins (HDLs)

Cholesterol is a soft, waxy substance found among the lipids in the bloodstream and in all of the body's cells. The body, mostly in the liver, produces essentially all of the cholesterol needed for normal functioning—about 1,000 mg a day. Cholesterol plays a role in forming cell membranes, some hormones, and other needed tissues. LDL is the major cholesterol carrier in the blood; about two thirds to three quarters of blood cholesterol is carried by LDL. LDL has a structure that can vary, based on its size and density. LDL includes VLDL and IDL. (IDL is considered an abnormal lipoprotein.) Lipoprotein a (Lp[a]) is a type of LDL and is considered a genetic variation. About one third to one fourth of blood cholesterol is carried by HDL. Chylomicrons are the largest and least dense of the lipoproteins. Triglycerides are transported primarily by the chylomicrons and VLDL, a subgroup of LDL.

PATHOPHYSIOLOGY

Hyperlipidemia is an elevation of blood lipid levels. Hyperlipidemia is considered a risk factor for the following disorders: **atherosclerosis** (also called **arteriosclerosis**), a narrowing of the arterial interior caused by buildup of hard, thick deposits, and a hardening and loss of elasticity of the arterial wall; coronary artery disease (CAD); and production of thromboses. Patients with narrowed arteries from atherosclerotic cardiovascular disease are more likely to have hypertension because the blood must be pushed harder to get through the narrowed lumen. The narrowness of the vessels increases peripheral resistance. Myocardial infarction and stroke are likely sequelae from hypertension and atherosclerosis, which contribute to morbidity and mortality. (See Chapter 27 for a complete discussion of hypertension and its treatments.)

Blood work to evaluate lipid levels should include a total cholesterol level, an LDL level, and an HDL level. Sometimes, the ratio of HDL to LDL is also given (Box 30.1). A high level of LDL cholesterol (more than 130 mg/dL) reflects an increased risk for heart disease, which is why LDL cholesterol is often called "bad" cholesterol. Lower levels of LDL cholesterol reflect a lower risk for heart disease. A high level of Lp(a) is an important risk factor for developing atherosclerosis prematurely. The way an increased Lp(a) level contributes to disease is not understood. The lesions in artery walls contain substances that may interact with Lp(a), leading to the buildup of lipids in atherosclerotic plaques. Medical experts think HDL tends to carry cholesterol away from the arteries and back to the liver, where it is passed from the body. Some experts believe HDL removes excess cholesterol from atherosclerotic plaques and thus slows their growth. HDL cholesterol is known as "good" cholesterol because a high level of HDL seems to protect against heart attack. The opposite is also true: a low HDL level (less than 35 mg/dL) indicates a greater risk for heart disease.

In most patients with cardiovascular disease, the underlying disorder is atherosclerosis, for which LDL is known to be a major risk factor. Elevated lipid levels are also a risk factor for CAD included in a group of atherosclerotic risk factors, known collectively as metabolic syndrome. The other risk factors include insulin resistance, obesity, and hypertension. Forty-seven million people in the Untied States are estimated to have metabolic syndrome (Scott, 2003). Data from epidemiologic studies and from clinical trials have shown that lowering cholesterol levels is associated with a lower overall risk for morbidity and mortality because of coronary heart disease. Additionally, aggressive reduction of cholesterol can yield more clinical benefits than can be achieved with less aggressive therapy (Third Report of the NCEP, 2004). Left ventricular mass is also a powerful predictor for future cardiovascular events; hyperlipidemia is associated with higher left ventricular mass. The healthy endothelium usually provides an anticoagulant, vasodilatory, and antiinflammatory array of functions, which are basic to vascular homeostasis. Dysfunction of the endothelium is a common pathologic feature evident in all phases of atherosclerosis. Hypercholesterolemia (elevated LDL levels) provokes many aspects of endothelial dysfunction, both

BOX 30.1 Interpreting Blood Lipid Levels

Total cholesterol

- Less than 200 mg/dL: desirable blood cholesterol level
- 200 to 239 mg/dL: borderline-high blood cholesterol level
- 240 mg/dL and over: high blood cholesterol level

High-density lipoprotein (HDL) cholesterol

- 40–59 mg/dL: desired HDL level
- Less than 35 mg/dL: low HDL level

Low-density lipoprotein (LDL) cholesterol

- Less than 100 mg/dL optimum: desired LDL level
- More than 130 mg/dL: elevated LDL level

before and during the thickening of the walls of the larger arteries in atherosclerosis. Guidelines from the Third Report of the National Cholesterol Education Program (NCEP), Adult Treatment Panel (ATP III) (2004) recommend that total cholesterol levels be less than 200 mg/dL; LDL cholesterol levels optimally should be less than 100 mg/dL, and HDL levels should be between 40 and 59 mg/dL. The recommended LDL levels have been shifted downward considerably from previous recommendations as studies continue to show that lower LDL levels decrease risk for CHD. Many Americans have cholesterol levels that greatly exceed these recommendations. Estimates are that 102.3 million American adults have total blood cholesterol values of 200 mg/dL and higher, and that about 41.3 million American adults have levels of 240 or higher (see American Heart Association website given under Featured Weblink). Unfortunately, several studies and literature analyses have shown that practitioners undertreat elevated cholesterol levels, either by not prescribing drug therapy or by not prescribing a dose high enough to aggressively and effectively bring the total cholesterol and LDL levels down to recommended levels. In these studies, only between 6% and 38% of patients had their lipid levels lowered to the level recommended in current clinical guidelines (Pearson, 2000; Kristianson et al., 2003; Ballantyne, 2003; Fonarow & Watson, 2003).

Triglyceride levels have also been shown to be an independent risk factor for coronary heart disease. It has been hypothesized that triglyceride-rich lipoproteins move into macrophages in the bloodstream and then interact with small, dense LDL and HDL particles to form arterial thromboses. So far, however, clinical studies have not been able to demonstrate that lowering triglycerides alone will decrease the rate of myocardial infarctions (MIs). The effect of lowering triglyceride levels may therefore be linked to lowering cholesterol, or to some other, unknown, process.

Patients who have combined hyperlipidemia (elevation of more than one lipid) exhibit a set lipid profile; it is hypothesized that such patients have an atherogenic lipoprotein phenotype. This phenotype is associated with elevated triglyceride levels, low levels of HDL, and a preponderance of small, dense, atherogenic LDL particles. These patients are at an increased risk for coronary heart disease, regardless of their total LDL. Research suggests that when plasma triglycerides exceed a critical level, approximately 133 mg/dL, the formation of small, dense LDL from larger, less dense LDL particles is more likely to occur. Lipid-lowering drugs that are also capable of lowering triglyceride levels below this critical level will thus cause a shift to a less dense, and therefore less atherogenic, LDL profile.

Patients with diabetes are considered to be at high risk from elevated lipid levels because a link has been established between elevated cholesterol levels and diabetic nephropathy. High serum cholesterol levels seem to have the same effect on glomerular mesangial cells as on the endothelial cells in the vasculature. Thus, an atherosclerotic-like process appears to occur in the cells of the kidneys because the mesangial cells possess binding sites for LDL and oxidized LDL. Cholesterol lowering has been shown to have a beneficial effect on renal function in patients with diabetes.

Lifestyle and Reduction of Low-Density Lipoprotein Levels

The NCEP ATP III recommends a multipronged approach in reducing LDL levels. They title this approach *therapeutic lifestyle changes* (TLC). These lifestyle changes include reduced intake of saturated fats, trans fats, and cholesterol; minimum intake of fatty acids; weight reduction; increased physical activity; increased intake of soluble fiber; and possibly increased intake of plant stanols and sterols (Table 30.1). Drug therapy is added if lipid levels are substantially elevated, if the patient has major risk factors for coronary heart disease even if lipid levels are not elevated, or if the patient has been diagnosed with coronary heart disease.

C ANTIHYPERLIPIDEMICS

Lowering serum lipid levels decreases the risk for atherosclerosis, hypertension, and coronary heart disease. Lowering cholesterol levels can stop or reverse atherosclerosis in

TABLE 30.1 Daily Recommendations in Therapeutic Lifestyle Changes Diet

Food Element	Recommended Daily Intake
Saturated fat	Less than 7% of total calories
Trans fatty acids	No percentage established, should be kept low
Polyunsaturated fat	Up to 10% of total calories
Monounsaturated fat	Up to 20% of total calories
Cholesterol	Less than 200 mg
Carbohydrate (predominantly complex sources including whole grains, fruit, and vegetables)	50% to 60% of total calories
Fiber	20–39 g
Protein	Approximately 15% of total calories
Total calories	Balance intake with expenditure to maintain desirable body weight and prevent weight gain

From: Third Report of the National Cholesterol Education Program (NCEP) Expert Panel on Detection, Evaluation, and Treatment of High Blood Cholesterol in Adults (Adult Treatment Panel III). (2004). Executive Summary [Online]. Available: *http://www.nhlbi.nih.gov/guidelines/cholesterol/atp3xsum.pdf.*

all vascular beds. Each 10% reduction in cholesterol levels is associated with a reduction of approximately 20% to 30% in the incidence of coronary heart disease. Because most cholesterol is carried by the LDL and VLDL, it is important to target these lipoproteins, especially in drug therapy. The antihyperlipidemics are composed of the statins (also referred to as 3-hydroxy-3-methyl-glutaryl coenzyme A [HMG CoA] reductase inhibitors), the fibric acid derivatives, nicotinic acid, the bile acid sequestrants, and dextrothyroxine sodium. Although these types of antihyperlipidemics work in slightly different ways, they all decrease cholesterol levels; most decrease triglyceride levels, most decrease LDL and VLDL levels, and most also increase HDL levels.

(C) Statins

Statins lower blood cholesterol levels and thus decrease the uptake of modified lipoproteins by vascular cells. Evidence exists that statins work in other ways besides lowering cholesterol levels to decrease the occurrence of cardiovascular events. Statins appear to have a positive effect on the vascular endothelium, by restoring it or improving its function. Statins seem to exert this effect by increasing the bioavailability of nitric oxide, promoting re-endothelialization, reducing oxidative stress (antioxidant effect), and inhibiting the inflammatory response (Wolfrum et al., 2003; Shishehbor et al., 2003).

Long-term statin use has been found to decrease mortality by 24% to 42% in patients with CAD. Statins are as effective or more effective than other secondary prevention medications used in CAD (aspirin, beta blockers, and angiotensin-converting enzyme [ACE] inhibitors; in patients with diabetes, they are better than any treatment for diabetes or tight glycemic control) (Fonarow & Watson, 2003). They provide additional effectiveness when used jointly with these therapies (Heart Protection Study Group, 2002). In addition to treatment for those known to have CAD, statin therapy was found in the Heart Protection Study to be effective in preventing CAD in those at high risk (those with cerebrovascular disease, peripheral arterial disease, or diabetes), even if their blood lipid levels were not elevated when therapy was started. In fact, this study suggests that the target level of less than 100 mg/dL, recommended by the Third Report of the National Cholesterol Education Program Expert Panel, should be even lower, such as below 77 mg/dL. The Heart Protection Study also showed that statins prevented not only coronary events but also ischemic strokes. Older adults, as well as middle-aged adults, benefit from aggressive statin use in hypercholesteremia (Heart Protection Study Group, 2002; Law et al., 2003; Aronow, 2003). Thus, aggressive use of statin therapy has been found to be effective in primary and secondary prevention of a variety of cardiac complications. Unfortunately, research shows that statins are underutilized (Box 30.2).

Further research is indicating that statins may have a role in preventing Alzheimer's disease, treating multiple sclerosis and other neuroinflammatory disorders, reducing morbidity and mortality associated with peripheral arterial disease and end-stage renal disease, and improving or moderating diabetes (Crisby et al., 2002; Stuve et al., 2003; McKenney, 2003; Rockwood et al., 2002). More research is needed on these potential future uses of statins.

FOCUS ON RESEARCH

Box 30.2 Statins Are Underprescribed

Kristianson, K., Fyhrquist, F., Devereux, R. B., et al. (2003). An analysis of cholesterol control and statin use in the Losartan Intervention for Endpoint Reduction in Hypertension Study. *Clinical Therapeutics, 25*(4), 1186–1199.

The Study

A large multicenter research study, the Losartan Intervention for Endpoint Reduction in Hypertension Study, was conducted with 9,193 patients aged 55 to 80 years with hypertension and left ventricular hypertrophy. The goal of the study was to compare the effectiveness of two types of drug therapy, losartan and atenolol, in reducing the incidence of morbidity and mortality in this population. Although statin therapy is known to lower the risk for cardiovascular complications, it was not the primary goal of this study, and the use of statin therapy was left to the discretion of the cardiologist who was the investigator at each trial center location. After the primary study was completed, a secondary study examined the baseline and the end-of-study mean total cholesterol and high-density lipoprotein cholesterol levels and the use of statins. At baseline, only 6.1% of the patients were receiving statins; total cholesterol levels were above levels recommended by clinical guidelines for more than 72% of those who were receiving statin therapy. More than 84% of patients who were not receiving statin therapy at baseline had cholesterol levels above that recommended by the clinical guidelines. At the end of the study, only approximately 22% of the patients had been started on statin therapy, and almost 60% of these patients still had cholesterol levels above guideline recommendations. Of those not receiving statins by the end of the study, nearly 79% had cholesterol levels in excess of those recommended. In this large study, statins were not optimally administered, and cholesterol levels were poorly controlled.

Nursing Implications

Elevated cholesterol levels have been known for some time to be a risk factor for cardiovascular events in patients with severe hypertension and left ventricular hypertrophy. It has also been known for some time that lipid levels are undertreated, even with effective drug therapy available. The results of this study confirm that even cardiologists, who work with patients known to have high cholesterol and high-risk factors for cardiovascular events, tend to undertreat patients. Clearly more aggressive therapy is warranted to help reduce morbidity and mortality from elevated lipid levels. The most recent research also indicates that lowering lipid levels, even when the baseline reading is not elevated, continues to decrease mortality from cardiovascular events.

What can nurses do to help patients with elevated cholesterol levels? First, nurses need to be knowledgeable about current guidelines for lipid management. Nurse practitioners should aggressively treat lipid levels in their patients with elevated lipid profiles by prescribing statin therapy and making sure that the prescribed drug and dose effectively lowers lipid levels. Nurses who do not prescribe drug therapy should monitor patients' lipid levels carefully and consult with either the physician or nurse practitioner when the levels are above guideline recommendations and indicate that drug therapy is warranted. Nurses in a hospital setting may also participate in hospital-wide, multidisciplinary committees or quality-improvement projects that are charged with setting drug protocols and standards to ensure that the institution is following the current clinical guidelines. Nurses in all practice settings need to be active in patient education to help patients and their families understand the importance of reducing blood cholesterol and lipid levels and the role that drug therapy can play in achieving this goal. Additionally, nurses should include diet modification information and stress the importance of exercise in their patient teaching about reducing blood lipid levels.

Although all the statins are considered to act similarly, some pharmacologic differences exist among them. The most notable difference is metabolism by the P-450 3A4 isoenzyme. All of the statins, with the exception of pravastatin, are primarily metabolized by this pathway. Coadministration of drugs that inhibit this pathway will therefore decrease the metabolism of these statins and increase their circulating blood levels. This increase may contribute to adverse effects, especially myalgia (muscle aches or weakness without creatine kinase [CK] elevations), myositis (muscle symptoms with elevated CK levels), and rhabdomyolysis (a potentially lethal event with muscle symptoms with high CK levels and creatinine elevations). Individual, innate differences in the amount of P-450 3A4 isoenzyme available are also a factor in the metabolism of these statins. These differences can account for why some patients can tolerate a particular dose of a statin, or tolerate a statin in combination with an inhibitor of P-450 3A4 without complications, whereas others cannot. There is no way to predict inherited variability to increases in drug concentration from drug–drug interactions. Thus, patients need to be assessed for individual response to therapy. Certain fibric acid derivatives, another drug class used to alter lipid levels, which may be combined with statins, have been found to have their own independent adverse effect of myopathy. When combined with some statins, but again not with pravastatin, elevations of statin levels may occur in some individuals, increasing the risk for myopathies (Pasternak et al., 2002; Bottorff, 2002).

Because so much research has shown the superior effectiveness of the statins, they are the most used antihyperlipidemic agents. Lovastatin is the prototype. The other classes of antihyperlipidemic drugs will be discussed as drugs similar to lovastatin. Table 30.2 displays a summary of selected antihyperlipidemics.

TABLE 30.2 Summary of Selected (C) Antihyperlipidemics

Drug (Trade) Name	Selected Indications	Route and Dosage Range	Pharmacokinetics
(C) Statins			
[P] lovastatin (Mevacor; *Canadian:* Apo-Lovastatin)	Reduce serum cholesterol levels	*Adult:* PO, 20–80 mg/d in single or divided dose	*Onset:* 1–2 wk *Duration:* Length of therapy $t_{1/2}$: 3–4 h
simvastatin (Zocor)	Reduce serum cholesterol and triglyceride levels	*Adult:* PO, 5–40 mg/d as single dose in the evening	*Onset:* 1–2 wk *Duration:* Length of therapy $t_{1/2}$: 3 h
pravastatin (Pravachol)	Reduce serum cholesterol and triglyceride levels	*Adult:* PO, 10–40 mg/d at bedtime	*Onset:* 1–2 wk *Duration:* Length of therapy $t_{1/2}$: 1.8 h
fluvastatin (Lescol)	Reduce serum cholesterol and triglyceride levels	*Adult:* PO, 20–80 mg/d single dose in the evening	*Onset:* 1–2 wk *Duration:* Length of therapy $t_{1/2}$: 1.2 h
Other Antihyperlipidemics			
cholestyramine (Questran; *Canadian:* Novo-Cholamine)	Lower serum cholesterol levels	*Adult:* PO, powder, 4 g, one to two times daily mixed in 60–180 mL of water or noncarbonated drink	*Onset:* Unabsorbed *Duration:* 1 mo after therapy concludes $t_{1/2}$: Unknown
colestipol (Colestid)	Lower serum cholesterol levels	*Adult:* PO, granules, 5–30 g/d mixed in about 90 mL of liquid; tablets, 2–16 g/d; may be divided	*Onset:* Unabsorbed *Duration:* Same as above $t_{1/2}$: Unknown
dextrothyroxine (Choloxin)	Lower serum cholesterol levels	*Adult:* PO, 1–2 mg/d to 4–8 mg/d *Child:* PO, 0.05 mg/kg/d up to 0.4 mg/kg/d or 4 mg/d	*Onset:* Unknown *Duration:* Length of therapy $t_{1/2}$: Unknown
clofibrate (Atromid-S; *Canadian:* Claripex)	Reduce serum cholesterol and triglyceride levels	*Adult:* PO, 2 g/d in divided doses	*Onset:* Unknown *Duration:* Length of therapy $t_{1/2}$: 15 h (up to 110 h in renal impaired)
nicotinic acid (niacin, vitamin B_3)	Reduce serum cholesterol and triglyceride levels	*Adult:* PO, 1–2 g tid with meals; maximum 8 g/d; dietary supplement, 100–500 mg/d	*Onset:* Up to several days *Duration:* Length of therapy $t_{1/2}$: Unknown
gemfibrozil (Lopid; *Canadian:* Apo-Gemfibrozil)	Reduce serum cholesterol and triglyceride levels	*Adult:* PO, 1,200 mg/d in two divided doses, 30 min before meals	*Onset:* Unknown *Duration:* Length of therapy $t_{1/2}$: 1.5 h (plasma)

NURSING MANAGEMENT OF THE PATIENT RECEIVING P LOVASTATIN

Core Drug Knowledge

Pharmacotherapeutics

Lovastatin (Mevacor) is used in the treatment of primary hypercholesterolemia and combined hyperlipidemia (also referred to as mixed dyslipidemia). It is also used in the secondary prevention of coronary events (e.g., MI). Unlabeled uses of lovastatin include the treatment of diabetic dyslipidemia, nephrotic hyperlipidemia, neck artery disease, familial dysbetalipoproteinemia (alterations of the beta or LDL lipoproteins in the blood), and familial combined hyperlipidemia. Lovastatin is available in both rapid-release and extended-release forms.

Pharmacokinetics

Although about 35% of the drug is absorbed, lovastatin has a high first-pass effect because metabolism by the isoenzyme CYP3A4 (an important subset of the CYP450 family) allows less than 5% of the oral dose to reach the general circulation. An active metabolite, lovastatin acid, is formed from metabolism. The drug is highly protein bound (more than 95%). It is excreted primarily through the gastrointestinal (GI) tract in the feces, but about 10% is eliminated in the urine. Severe renal disease will increase plasma concentration of lovastatin (see Table 30.2). Immediate-release forms are best absorbed after a meal. In contrast, extended-release forms have their absorption impaired by food.

Pharmacodynamics

Lovastatin, as well as the other statins, competitively inhibits HMG-CoA reductase, which is the enzyme that catalyzes the early rate-limiting step in cholesterol biosynthesis. The effect is to increase HDL and to decrease LDL, total cholesterol, VLDL, and plasma triglycerides. The mechanism that lowers LDL may involve both reduction of VLDL concentrations and increased catabolism of LDL. In clinical trials, lovastatin reduced total cholesterol between 16% and 29%, decreased LDL levels between 21% and 40%, decreased triglyceride levels between 6% to 30%, and increased levels of HDL between 2% and 9.5%.

This drug, as well as the others in the class, is highly effective in reducing total cholesterol and the LDL level in heterozygous familial and nonfamilial forms of hypercholesterolemia.

The lipid lowering that occurs with the statins, such as lovastatin, is known to reduce the progression of atherosclerosis, reduce blood thrombogenicity, prevent myocardial infarction and stroke, and prolong survival in patients with atherosclerosis.

Contraindications and Precautions

Contraindications include active liver disease, unexplained persistently elevated results of liver function tests, pregnancy (lovastatin is in pregnancy category X), and breast-feeding. Precaution should be used if lovastatin is coadministered with drugs that inhibit the CYP3A4 hepatic pathway or with drugs that also can produce myopathy, such as fibric acid derivatives.

Adverse Effects

Adverse effects of lovastatin are usually mild and transient; the drug is generally well tolerated. Two adverse effects that have potentially serious consequences are myopathies (diseases of the muscles) and elevated liver enzymes. A fairly common complaint is nonspecific muscle aches or joint aches, which are not associated with any signs of muscle damage. Serious skeletal muscle effects may result from lovastatin. Although rare, rhabdomyolysis (occurring in 0.1% of patients on statins as monotherapy) is the most serious. Rhabdomyolysis is an acute, sometimes fatal disease, in which direct injury to the plasma membrane of the skeletal muscle occurs (manifested by CK, also known as creatine phosphokinase [CPK], levels, which are elevated beyond 10 times the upper normal limit). The damage to the muscle causes leakage of the skeletal muscle components (myoglobin) into the blood or the urine. Brown urine usually occurs. Rhabdomyolysis can lead to acute renal failure and death. The risk is increased if the patient is also taking drugs that share the same common metabolic path, such as cyclosporine or nicotinic acid. Transient, mildly elevated CK levels are common, especially in the first 3 months of therapy. These levels do not indicate a serious problem. Myopathy should be considered in any patient who receives this drug and who shows diffuse myalgia, muscle tenderness or weakness, and substantial elevation of CPK levels. The rate of serious myopathy appears to be equivalent among all the statins (Pasternak et al., 2002).

The elevation in hepatic enzyme levels is another adverse effect that may occur fairly frequently and is usually dose related. Although some sources question whether the elevation of hepatic enzymes (transaminase) from statin use is truly hepatic toxicity, progression to liver failure is possible, although only rarely reported. A reversal of hepatic enzyme elevations is frequently noted with a decreased dose or temporary discontinuation of the statin; elevations do not commonly reoccur with either reintroducing the drug to the patient or switching to another statin (Pasternak et al., 2002). Marked persistent elevations of liver enzymes occur in about 2% of patients taking lovastatin. Although these elevations are not normally accompanied by other signs of liver damage, such as jaundice, elevations more than three times the normal limit may occur within 3 to 12 months of starting lovastatin. If this elevation persists, the dose should be reduced or the drug discontinued.

Adverse effects that can occur but are not considered serious include effects in the central nervous system (CNS), such as headache, dizziness, insomnia, and paresthesia. GI complaints include nausea and vomiting, diarrhea, abdominal pain and cramps, constipation, flatulence, heartburn, dyspepsia, and altered taste. Other adverse effects are chest pain, rash, blurred vision, and alopecia. Photosensitivity may occur.

Drug Interactions

Because lovastatin is metabolized through the hepatic enzyme CYP3A4, all inhibitors of this pathway have the potential to interact with the drug, decreasing its metabolism and elevating, sometimes dramatically, its level in the blood

(Bottorff, 2002; Pasternak et al., 2002). Examples of CYP3A4 inhibitors are itraconazole (an antifungal), erythromycin (an antimicrobial), and grapefruit juice, which has been shown to substantially increase the serum levels of lovastatin and lovastatin acid (the active metabolite). Drugs that compete with lovastatin for metabolism by CYP3A4 also have the potential to interact with lovastatin. Rhabdomyolysis has been reported in heart transplant recipients who were treated with both lovastatin and cyclosporine (an antirejection drug used in the process of organ transplantation that is also metabolized by CYP3A4). Table 30.3 lists drugs that interact with lovastatin.

Food appears to increase drug absorption and elevate blood levels of lovastatin.

Laboratory tests that are altered by lovastatin use include increased serum transaminases aspartate transaminase (AST), alanine aminotransferase (ALT), CPK, alkaline phosphatase, bilirubin, γ-glutamyl transpeptidase, and thyroid function test abnormalities.

Assessment of Relevant Core Patient Variables

Health Status

Before lovastatin therapy begins, the patient's serum cholesterol and lipid levels should be determined and a health history of diseases that contribute to increased blood cholesterol and LDL levels taken. These conditions include hypothyroidism, poorly controlled diabetes mellitus, nephrotic syndrome, dysproteinemia, obstructive liver disease, and alcoholism. These conditions should be investigated and treated before starting lovastatin. Assess for active liver disease because it is a contraindication for taking lovastatin. Also, determine liver function through liver enzyme measurements for baseline knowledge. Lovastatin, as well as other statins, should not be given if the patient has active liver disease or unexplained persistently elevated liver function test results (e.g., liver enzymes greater than three times the upper normal limit) because additional elevation of liver enzyme levels occurs during therapy with lovastatin and all statins. A baseline CK level should be drawn; many patients routinely have asymptomatic CK elevations, and knowing of such elevations at baseline assists in clinical decision making later in therapy.

Be aware that patients who have undergone organ transplantation and who require lifelong multidrug therapy are at increased risk for experiencing drug–drug interactions when also receiving lovastatin. Patients with chronic disease states such as diabetes and hypothyroidism are also at risk.

Determine whether the patient is receiving other drugs that are metabolized by (i.e., are substrates of) CYP3A4 or that inhibit metabolism by CYP3A4 because there may be potential drug interactions when starting lovastatin.

Assess the patient's body frame because a small body frame and frailty pose an increased risk for drug-related myopathy.

TABLE 30.3 Agents That Interact With P Lovastatin

Interactants	Effect and Significance	Nursing Management
azole antifungals itraconazole ketoconazole	Increases lovastatin levels about 20-fold. May increase risk of adverse effects, including myopathy.	Consult with provider regarding temporarily stopping or reducing the dose of lovastatin while on the antifungal.
bile acid sequestrants	Decreases the bioavailability and effect of lovastatin and other statins.	Give the bile acid sequestrant 4 hours after lovastatin.
cyclosporine	Increases circulating levels of lovastatin and increases risk of severe myopathy or rhabdomyolysis.	Consult with provider about stopping lovastatin or decreasing the dose. Monitor closely for adverse effects.
erythromycin	Increases circulating levels of lovastatin and increases risk of severe myopathy or rhabdomyolysis.	Consult with provider about stopping lovastatin or decreasing the dose. Monitor closely for adverse effects.
gemfibrozil	Increases circulating levels of lovastatin; severe myopathy or rhabdomyolysis reported.	Avoid this combination if at all possible.
isradipine	May increase clearance of lovastatin and its metabolites by increasing hepatic blood flow. This decreases the effect of lovastatin.	Increased dose for lovastatin may be needed, consult with provider if patient is not achieving desired cholesterol goals.
nicotinic acid	Increases circulating levels of lovastatin and increases risk of severe myopathy or rhabdomyolysis.	Consult with provider about stopping lovastatin or decreasing the dose. Monitor closely for adverse effects.
digoxin	Elevates digoxin levels slightly.	Monitor digoxin levels. Assess for signs of digoxin toxicity.
warfarin	Increases prothrombin time. Bleeding has occurred in some patients receiving both drugs.	Monitor for bleeding. Consult with provider regarding adjusting dose of warfarin downward as needed to keep prothrombin time in therapeutic range.

Life Span and Gender

Determine whether the patient is pregnant or considering becoming pregnant because lovastatin is a pregnancy category X drug. Animal studies have shown skeletal malformations, but no such data exist for humans. However, fetal harm is likely because of the decrease in cholesterol synthesis and possibly other products in the cholesterol biosynthesis pathway. Lovastatin is excreted in the breast milk; thus, breast-feeding should be avoided while taking this drug.

Older adults, because they are likely to have more drugs prescribed to them than younger people, are more at risk for drug interactions when receiving lovastatin. Adults older than 80 years, especially women, seem most at risk for statin-associated myopathy. However, information gleaned from clinical trials indicates that older adults benefit from lipid-lowering therapy as much as younger adults; therefore, treatment with lipid-lowering drugs is worthwhile in older adults and is recommended.

Safety and efficacy in patients younger than 18 years have not been determined. Treatment in this age group is not recommended at this time.

Lifestyle, Diet, and Habits

Before starting drug therapy, patients should be treated with nonpharmacologic methods of controlling cholesterol and lipids, including dieting to reduce cholesterol levels and LDL levels, exercising, and normalizing weight if needed. Diet therapy usually continues for 12 weeks before drug therapy starts and should be continued even after drug therapy is started.

Determine whether the patient has alcoholism, which may be a secondary cause of hyperlipidemia. Determine whether the patient regularly drinks grapefruit juice and how much is usually consumed because grapefruit juice is a major inhibitor of the CYP3A4 isoenzyme necessary for lovastatin metabolism.

Environment

Lovastatin may be started in any environment. Because therapy extends over a prolonged period, the drug is usually taken by the patient at home or in a long-term care facility. Assess the patient's exposure to sunlight because photosensitivity may occur.

Culture and Inherited Traits

Explore whether the patient observes cultural or religious dietary practices that promote high intake of fats and cholesterol.

Nursing Diagnoses and Outcomes

- Risk for Injury related to elevated blood lipid levels
  Desired outcome: *The patient's blood lipid levels will be controlled without the patient's sustaining an injury.*
- Risk for Injury to skeletal muscles related to adverse effects of drug therapy
  Desired outcome: *The patient will not incur serious skeletal muscle injury while on drug therapy.*
- Risk for Altered Nutrition: Less than Body Requirements related to adverse effects of drug therapy
  Desired outcome: *The patient will not have GI adverse effects serious enough to alter meeting the body's nutritional needs.*

Planning and Intervention

Maximizing Therapeutic Effects

Lovastatin is most effective when administered in the evening, possibly because evening is also when most cholesterol synthesis occurs. Immediate-release lovastatin should be administered after the evening meal; extended-release lovastatin is administered at bedtime without food to be most effective. The patient should be advised to continue a cholesterol-reducing diet.

Minimizing Adverse Effects

Liver function test (AST and ALT) results should be monitored before starting therapy, at 12 weeks after starting therapy or after each dose adjustment, and then yearly or as indicated. Consult with the prescriber about reducing the dose or stopping the drug if the increased (more than three times the upper limits of normal) liver enzyme levels persist.

Evaluate the patient carefully for muscle soreness, tenderness, or pain and CK levels before starting therapy. Reassess for muscle symptoms after 6 to 12 weeks of therapy and at each follow-up visit. CK levels may be monitored more frequently and on a regular basis depending on the patient's risk factors for myopathy and physician preference.

Rule out common causes of muscle aches, such as exercise or strenuous work, if the patient is experiencing muscle symptoms. Encourage the patient to avoid strenuous physical activity. Obtain a CK measurement when the patient has unexplained muscle symptoms and compare to baseline levels. If the CK levels are moderately elevated (3 to 10 times the upper limit of normal), continue with drug therapy but follow the patient's symptoms and CK levels weekly until either symptoms disappear or the CK levels return within normal range. If CK levels reach above 10 times the upper limit of normal and the patient has symptoms, therapy should be stopped.

Monitor the older adult who receives polypharmacy carefully for drug interactions with lovastatin (see the Critical Thinking Scenario: Managing Adverse Effects of Lovastatin Therapy). Also, carefully monitor adults older than 80 years, especially women, who have small body frames and are frail because they are more at risk for myopathies.

Providing Patient and Family Education

- Stress the importance of following a low-cholesterol and low-saturated-fat diet while on drug therapy (Box 30.3).
- Instruct patients to report any unexplained muscle pain, tenderness, or weakness at once.
- Because of the risks for fetal harm, advise female patients to avoid taking this drug if they become pregnant.
- In some patients taking lovastatin, photosensitivity may occur. Urge all patients to avoid prolonged exposure to sunlight and other ultraviolet light until their response to therapy is known.

Ongoing Assessment and Evaluation

The patient should have liver function tests and CK measurement performed periodically throughout drug therapy with lovastatin. Monitor the results of these tests for elevations. Assess the patient for muscle pain throughout ther-

CRITICAL THINKING SCENARIO

Managing adverse effects of lovastatin therapy

Janice Klinefelter, age 64 years, has been taking the statin lipid-lowering drug lovastatin for 9 months. She has tolerated the drug therapy well and up to this point has had no major adverse effects. Her cholesterol and LDL levels are close to reaching the desired goal. During an office follow-up visit, she complains that she must be getting old because she feels stiff and her leg muscles are cramping and painful, problems she has never complained of before. Her blood work, drawn the day before the office visit, shows that her liver function enzyme levels (AST and ALT) are mildly elevated, and her creatine kinase levels are four times upper normal levels. At baseline, both blood tests were within the normal range. She denies having started any new medication.

1. What questions would you ask Ms. Klinefelter as part of your assessment?
2. What course of action would you choose now?
3. What teaching would you provide to Ms. Klinefelter?

COMMUNITY-BASED CONCERNS

Box 30.3 Diet Teaching to Lower Cholesterol Levels

An important role of the nurse is to provide health education. Because heart disease is a leading cause of death in the United States, teaching the benefits of a low-cholesterol diet is an important nursing action—not just for patients with elevated cholesterol levels and their families, but also for the population at large.

Encourage a diet that is low in saturated fats, which would include the following foods:

- Fruits and vegetables
- Whole grains, such as cereal, rice, and pasta
- Lean red meats and poultry (no skin)
- Low-fat or skim milk dairy products
- Lean fish and shellfish
- Beans and peas
- Unsaturated oils such as olive oil, corn oil, and safflower oil

Encourage a diet that limits foods that are high in saturated fat and cholesterol. This means avoiding or limiting the following foods:

- High-fat dairy products, such as whole milk, cream, ice cream, butter, and cheese
- Egg yolks
- Saturated oils such as coconut oil, palm oil and palm kernel oil
- Solid fats such as shortening, soft margarine, and lard
- Organ meats such as liver, sweetbreads, kidneys, and brain
- High-fat processed meats such as hot dogs, sausage, bologna, and salami
- Fatty red meats that have not been trimmed
- Duck and goose meat
- Fried foods

Emphasize that patients should avoid not only highly saturated foods, but also foods that are made with them.

apy. Blood work that monitors the complete lipid profile should be obtained periodically throughout therapy. Therapy is considered effective when the total cholesterol level is below 200 mg/dL, LDL is lower than 100 mg/dL, and HDL is above 40 mg/dL and the patient has not incurred any serious adverse effects.

Drugs Closely Related to P Lovastatin

C Fibric Acid Derivatives

Like lovastatin and the other statins, the fibric acid derivatives gemfibrozil (Gemcor, Lopid), clofibrate (Atromid-S), and fenofibrate (Tricor) work to lower triglyceride levels and increase HDL cholesterol. These drugs can reduce triglyceride levels between 20% and 55%. However, unlike lovastatin and other statins, their effect on LDL cholesterol may be either to lower or raise it slightly. These fibric acid derivatives are available as oral tablets or capsules. Although in certain patients these drugs might be used alone, most frequently they are used in combination with statins. Some patients, such as those with diabetes or metabolic syndrome, need to lower triglycerides and increase HDL, and a combination of a fibric acid derivative (also known as a fibrate) and a statin such as lovastatin may be the drug therapy of choice. Although the combined used of a fibrate and a moderate-dose statin carries a somewhat increased risk for myopathy, the incidence continues to be low, especially if used in populations without multisystem diseases or currently taking multiple medications. Gemfibrozil may substantially increase the circulating blood levels of some statins, like lovastatin. Fenofibrate has not been linked as strongly, but the potential exists for a drug interaction with lovastatin or other statins. Because of its adverse effects, clofibrate is the least seldom used.

FENOFIBRATE

Fenofibrate (Tricor) is used to treat hypertriglyceridemia. It is chemically similar to clofibrate and gemfibrozil. Exactly how fenofibrate works has not been clearly established. The metabolite of fenofibrate, fenofibric acid, lowers plasma triglycerides apparently by inhibiting the synthesis of

MEMORY CHIP

P Lovastatin

- Used to treat hyperlipidemia. It lowers LDL, triglycerides, and total cholesterol, and raises HDL.
- Major contraindications: active liver disease, unexplained persistent elevated liver function tests results, and pregnancy
- Most common adverse effect: elevated liver enzyme levels
- Most serious adverse effects: rhabdomyolysis and myopathy
- **Life span alert: pregnancy category X; avoid lovastatin if the patient is breast feeding. Older adults are more likely to have drug interactions.**
- Minimizing adverse effects: Monitor liver enzymes levels for at least first year of therapy.
- Most important patient education: Teach patients to continue on a low-fat diet and to report any unexplained muscle pain, tenderness, or weakness at once.

triglycerides, which reduces the amount of VLDL that is released into the circulation. It also stimulates the catabolism of triglyceride-rich VLDL. Additionally, fenofibrate reduces the serum uric acid levels in patients with normal and elevated uric acid levels by increasing the urinary excretion of uric acid. Treatment of some patients with hyperlipoproteinemia may result in an increase of LDL cholesterol.

Fenofibrate is well absorbed from the GI tract; food increases absorption. Peak levels occur within 6 to 8 hours. Fenofibrate is highly protein bound (99%). It is rapidly hydrolyzed by esterases to the active metabolite, fenofibric acid. Fenofibric acid is primarily conjugated with glucuronic acid and then excreted in the urine. Fenofibrate has a half-life of 20 hours. It is excreted, in the form of its metabolites, in the urine.

Fenofibrate is contraindicated in hepatic or severe renal dysfunction (including primary biliary cirrhosis and patients with unexplained persistent liver function abnormality), pre-existing gallbladder disease, and hypersensitivity.

Serious adverse effects of fenofibrate include pancreatitis, cholelithiasis, myopathy, myositis, and hepatic impairment. These adverse effects are similar to those for gemfibrozil and clofibrate, the fibric acid derivatives. Rash, the most common adverse effect, requires discontinuation of the drug. Other possibly adverse effects on the CNS vary. Effects include dizziness, increased appetite, insomnia, and paresthesia. Dermatologic reactions include pruritus. GI complaints such as dyspepsia, nausea and vomiting, diarrhea, abdominal pain, constipation, flatulence, and excessive burping may occur. Genitourinary effects include polyuria and vaginitis. Common respiratory symptoms include rhinitis, cough, and sinusitis. Eye irritation, blurred vision, conjunctivitis, earache, and eye floaters may be present. Miscellaneous effects include flu-like symptoms, pain, headache, asthenia and fatigue, arthralgia, and arrhythmia. Increases in blood urea and creatinine and decreases in hemoglobin and uric acid have occurred.

GEMFIBROZIL

Gemfibrozil (Gemcor, Lopid) is used to treat hypertriglyceridemia and to reduce coronary heart disease risk in some patients who have not responded to other forms of treatment. It inhibits peripheral lipolysis and decreases the hepatic extraction of free fatty acids, thus reducing hepatic triglyceride production. It also leads to a decrease in VLDL production and an increase in HDL concentration for most patients. The exact mechanism of action for raising HDL levels is unknown. In addition, the drug may reduce the incorporation of long-chain fatty acids into new triglycerides. It may also increase the turnover and removal of cholesterol from the liver and increase excretion of cholesterol in the feces.

Gemfibrozil is well absorbed from the GI tract. Peak levels occur 1 to 2 hours after administration of the dose. Gemfibrozil is primarily oxidized to hydroxymethyl and a carboxyl metabolite. Excretion is mostly renal.

Contraindications include hepatic or severe renal dysfunction, including primary biliary cirrhosis, pre-existing gallbladder disease, or hypersensitivity. This drug is in pregnancy category C and is not recommended for use in pregnant or breast-feeding women.

Gemfibrozil may increase the risk for hepatic malignancy and cholelithiasis. It also may occasionally be associated with muscle inflammation, which may be severe.

GI problems are the most common adverse effects of both gemfibrozil and clofibrate, with nausea and diarrhea most common with clofibrate, and dyspepsia very common with gemfibrozil. Abdominal pain and diarrhea are also fairly common with gemfibrozil, whereas nausea, vomiting, and constipation are possible. Like lovastatin, this drug may produce abnormal elevations of liver function enzyme levels. The effects are usually reversible when the drug is discontinued. A large variety of miscellaneous adverse effects is also possible with the fibric acid derivatives. Gemfibrozil produces a moderate hyperglycemic effect; special monitoring will be necessary for patients with diabetes who are receiving gemfibrozil.

CLOFIBRATE

Clofibrate (Atromid-S) is used to treat hyperlipidemia with high triglyceride levels. Clofibrate primarily lowers serum triglyceride and VLDL levels. The exact mechanism of action is unknown, but it may increase the catabolism of VLDL to LDL and decrease hepatic synthesis of VLDL. Most of the effectiveness is seen in type III hyperlipidemia.

Clofibrate is hydrolyzed to chlorophenoxy isobutyric acid (CPIB), which is the active form of the drug. Peak action is seen within 3 to 6 hours after administration. Excretion occurs primarily through the kidneys.

Like gemfibrozil, contraindications for clofibrate include hepatic or severe renal dysfunction, including primary biliary cirrhosis, pre-existing gallbladder disease, or hypersensitivity. This drug is also in pregnancy category C, and its use should be avoided by patients who are pregnant or breast-feeding.

Clofibrate has caused hepatic tumors (benign and malignant) in test animals and is associated with increased risk for cancer in humans. It has also been shown to substantially increase the risk for cholelithiasis and to increase the mortality from cholecystectomy surgery (while on clofibrate therapy). Other serious adverse effects of clofibrate include cardiac arrhythmias and reactivation of peptic ulcers. Like gemfibrozil, this drug may occasionally be associated with severe muscle inflammation.

As already noted, adverse effects for clofibrate are similar to those for gemfibrozil. Clofibrate may also cause flu-like symptoms.

(C) Nicotinic Acid

Nicotinic acid (niacin or vitamin B_3) is used to treat hyperlipidemia. Like lovastatin, nicotinic acid reduces levels of triglycerides and LDL cholesterol levels and raises levels of HDL cholesterol. Triglycerides and VLDL levels are reduced by 20% to 40% in 1 to 4 days. LDL level reductions may be seen in 5 to 7 days, with the maximal effect seen in 3 to 5 weeks. The effect on LDL is dose dependent. The decrease will be greater if the patient is also receiving bile acid sequestrants (40%–60% decrease). HDLs are increased by 20%. Niacin is the most effective drug for increasing HDL levels while lowering levels of LDL and triglycerides, and improving other lipid risk factors, such as Lp(a) (Miller, 2003). Although the exact mode of action is unknown, nicotinic acid is known to inhibit lipolysis in adipose tissue, to decrease esterification of triglyceride in the liver, and to increase lipoprotein lipase activity.

Nicotinic acid is rapidly absorbed from the intestine, with peak effects achieved 45 minutes after administration. It is excreted, mostly unchanged, in the urine. The newer sustained-release forms have fewer adverse effects, making them more tolerable for patients and, therefore, excellent choices to elevate HDL levels.

Contraindications for this drug are hepatic dysfunction, active peptic ulcer, severe hypotension, and hemorrhaging.

Doses that are larger than those used to treat niacin deficiency (pellagra) are needed to achieve the lipid-lowering effects of nicotinic acid. These larger doses produce peripheral vasodilation, mostly in the cutaneous vessels of the face, neck, and chest. Vasodilation results in flushing of the skin, which is usually transient. Vasodilation and increased blood flow from niacin administration are attributable to histamine release. Myalgias are possible when nicotinic acid is combined with statins, although they are uncommon. Other adverse effects of nicotinic acid include GI effects such as activation of peptic ulcer, nausea, vomiting, abdominal pain, diarrhea, and dyspepsia. An increase in uric acid levels can also occur. The most serious adverse effect is hepatotoxicity, although it is uncommon. Liver enzyme levels should be closely monitored in patients who are receiving niacin.

C Bile Acid Sequestrants

The bile acid sequestrants cholestyramine (LoCholest, Questran, Prevalite) and colestipol (Colestid) are now used occasionally for reducing elevated serum cholesterol levels in patients who have primary hypercholesterolemia and have not responded to other drug therapy. Cholestyramine and colestipol are also used to relieve pruritus associated with partial biliary obstruction.

Bile acid sequestrants are not absorbed orally but work in the GI tract. The reduction in LDLs is apparent in 4 to 7 days and may total 20%. A decline in serum cholesterol levels is usually apparent after 1 month of treatment. Once drug therapy is discontinued, cholesterol levels will return to baseline within 1 month.

A major difference between the bile acid sequestrants and lovastatin is how they achieve a decrease in the cholesterol levels. Unlike lovastatin, which works by decreasing the synthesis of cholesterol, the bile acid sequestrants promote the oxidation of cholesterol to bile acids. Cholesterol is the major, and perhaps the only, precursor to bile acids. Bile acids are secreted from the gallbladder and liver into the intestine during digestion. In the intestine, bile acids emulsify the fat and lipid particles from food, promoting absorption. Much of the bile acid that is secreted is reabsorbed and returned to the liver by hepatic circulation.

The bile acid sequestrants cholestyramine and colestipol bind with the bile acids in the intestine to make them nonresorbable. The bile acids are then eliminated in the stool. The decrease in available bile acid causes the body to increase the oxidation of cholesterol to bile acids, which in turn decreases the LDL and serum cholesterol levels. Although hepatic synthesis of cholesterol rises, serum cholesterol levels fall because of an increased clearance of cholesterol-rich lipoproteins from the plasma. Serum triglyceride levels may increase somewhat initially but will then gradually fall below pretreatment levels within 4 weeks.

Patients with partial biliary obstruction have an increased bile acid concentration. Cholestyramine and colestipol, by decreasing circulating bile acid, reduce bile acid deposits in the skin tissues with a resultant decrease in pruritus.

The most common adverse effect of cholestyramine and colestipol is constipation, which can be severe and may lead to fecal impaction. Less frequently experienced are abdominal pain, distention, and cramping; GI bleeding; belching; bloating; flatulence; nausea and vomiting; diarrhea and loose stools; indigestion and heartburn; anorexia; and steatorrhea. Chronic use of cholestyramine can result in prolonged bleeding resulting from vitamin K deficiency. Headache can also occur with both cholestyramine and colestipol. In addition, dizziness, anxiety, vertigo, drowsiness, and fatigue have been noted with colestipol.

Absorption of fat-soluble vitamins such as A, D, E, and K may be impaired because cholestyramine interferes with the normal fat absorption and digestion. Because cholestyramine is a chloride anion exchange resin, prolonged use may cause hyperchloremic acidosis.

Because of their effect in the GI tract, the bile acid sequestrants interact with many different drugs and may impair the absorption of those drugs. Consult a drug guide to determine whether a drug interaction is likely before giving the bile acid sequestrants with any other drug therapy.

Before starting therapy with cholestyramine or colestipol, determine whether both the patient's serum cholesterol and triglyceride levels are elevated. If so, elevated triglyceride levels should be treated first with other drug therapy because triglycerides may rise initially from the treatment with cholestyramine.

Consideration should be given to the patient's life span before treatment with either of the bile acid sequestrants. Younger and smaller patients are more at risk for developing hyperchloremic acidosis. In adults older than 60 years, constipation is more likely to develop with ongoing cholestyramine therapy. Cholestyramine and colestipol come in a powdered form, which needs to be diluted with fluid. These preparations are considered unpalatable by some patients, and therefore adherence with therapy may be limited. Colestipol also comes in tablet form. Cholestyramine and colestipol should be administered before meals.

The bile acid sequestrants are no longer frequently used because of their GI adverse effects, cumbersome administration, and poor palatability.

C Thyroid Hormone

DEXTROTHYROXINE SODIUM

A thyroid hormone, dextrothyroxine sodium (Choloxin) is also used to decrease serum cholesterol levels. It stimulates the liver to increase catabolism and excretion of cholesterol by way of the biliary route into the GI tract. Synthesis of cholesterol is unaffected. The predominant effect is the reduction of serum LDL cholesterol levels. Elevated beta lipoprotein levels and triglyceride fractions may also be reduced.

Dextrothyroxine sodium is contraindicated in patients who have abnormal thyroid function and any of the following conditions: organic heart disease, angina pectoris, history of MI, history of cardiac arrhythmia (including tachycardia), rheumatic heart disease, history of congestive heart failure, decompensated or borderline compensated cardiac status, hypertension (other than mild, labile systolic hypertension), advanced liver or kidney disease, and history of iodism (a condition induced by prolonged and excessive use of iodine or its compounds; iodine poisoning).

Increased serum thyroxine levels indicate absorption and distribution of the drug throughout the body and should not be interpreted as drug toxicity. If signs or symptoms of iodism develop, the drug should be discontinued. Some forms of this drug are prepared with tartrazine and should not be given to patients who are sensitive to this dye. This sensitivity is more frequently seen in patients who also have aspirin hypersensitivity.

Adverse effects of dextrothyroxine sodium are mainly attributable to the increase in body metabolism from elevated thyroid levels. Patients who are least affected by adverse effects are those who have normal thyroid function and who also have no signs or symptoms of organic heart disease. Adverse effects are varied. Cardiovascular effects include angina, arrhythmias, electrocardiographic evidence of ischemic myocardial changes, increase in heart size, and both fatal and nonfatal MI. CNS effects are insomnia, nervousness, tremors, headache, tinnitus, dizziness, psychic changes, and altered sensorium paresthesia. Dermatologic problems include hair loss, skin rash, and itching. GI effects such as dyspepsia, nausea, vomiting, constipation, diarrhea, decreased appetite, weight loss, gallstones, and cholestatic jaundice may occur. Ophthalmic problems include visual disturbances, exophthalmos, retinopathy, and lid lag. Other reported effects are sweating, flushing, hyperthermia, diuresis, menstrual irregularities, changes in libido, hoarseness, peripheral edema, malaise, tiredness, muscle pain, and worsening of peripheral vascular disease.

CHAPTER SUMMARY

- Hyperlipidemia is a known risk factor for atherosclerosis and the problems and complications associated with atherosclerosis. The blood lipids include the total cholesterol, HDL cholesterol, the LDL cholesterol, VLDL cholesterol, and triglycerides.
- Use of statins decreases primary and secondary risk for cardiac disease and stroke. In addition to lowering lipid levels, statins appear to have protective and healing effects on the endothelium. Cardiovascular disease risk is cut with statin use even if the LDL baseline is not considered elevated when therapy is started.
- Many patients being treated for elevated cholesterol levels do not achieve the recommended treatment goals of total cholesterol under 200 mg/dL, LDL under 100 mg/dL, and HDL above 40 mg/dL.
- Lovastatin, the prototype statin, lowers LDL, VLDL, triglyceride levels, and total cholesterol levels, and raises HDL levels. It has been shown to decrease mortality from cardiovascular complications associated with elevated cholesterol levels and LDL levels.
- Lovastatin is metabolized through the hepatic enzyme CYP3A4. All other drugs or agents that are inhibitors of this pathway may have a drug interaction with lovastatin, decreasing lovastatin metabolism and sometimes dramatically raising blood levels of lovastatin.
- All lipid-lowering drugs can elevate liver enzyme levels. This elevation is not normally serious, although the patient's liver enzyme levels should be monitored closely for up to the first year of therapy. Liver enzyme levels usually return to normal with either a dose reduction or discontinuation of the drug.
- Dietary modifications to limit fat and cholesterol intake should be implemented before starting any drug to lower lipid levels. These modifications need to be continued once drug therapy has begun.
- The fibric acid derivatives, gemfibrozil, clofibrate, and fenofibrate, lower triglyceride levels and increase HDL cholesterol. Their effect on LDL cholesterol can be either to lower it slightly or to increase it slightly. They are usually co-prescribed with a statin. Gemfibrozil reduces hepatic triglyceride production. The mechanisms of clofibrate and fenofibrate are not clear.
- Nicotinic acid (niacin or vitamin B_3) reduces triglycerides, reduces LDL cholesterol, and increases HDL. Although the exact mode of action is unknown, nicotinic acid is known to inhibit lipolysis in adipose tissue, decrease esterification of triglyceride in the liver, and increase lipoprotein lipase activity.
- The bile acid sequestrants, cholestyramine and colestipol, decrease LDL. They work differently than other lipid-lowering drugs by binding with the bile acids in the intestine so that the bile acids are nonresorbable and are eliminated in the stool. The decrease in available bile acid causes the body to convert cholesterol to bile acids.
- Dextrothyroxine, a thyroid hormone, reduces LDL. It stimulates the liver to increase catabolism and excretion of cholesterol by way of the biliary route into the GI tract. Synthesis of cholesterol is unaffected.

QUESTIONS FOR STUDY AND REVIEW

1. Which of the forms of cholesterol is believed to provide some protective mechanism for the body and is termed "good" cholesterol?
2. How do elevated cholesterol levels contribute to hypertension?
3. Why is it important to determine whether other drugs received by a patient taking lovastatin are metabolized by CYP3A4 or are inhibitors of CYP3A4?
4. Why is it important to monitor liver enzymes while a patient is receiving lovastatin or other lipid-lowering drugs?
5. Why do CK levels greater than 10 times the upper limit of normal require that lovastatin therapy be discontinued?

Need More Help?

Chapter 30 of the study guide for *Drug Therapy in Nursing* 2e contains NCLEX-style questions and other learning activities to reinforce your understanding of the concepts presented in this chapter. For additional information or to purchase the study guide, visit *http://connection.lww.com/go/aschenbrenner.*

REFERENCES AND BIBLIOGRAPHY

ALLHAT Officers and Coordinators for the ALLHAT Collaborative Research Group. The Antihypertensive and Lipid-Lowering Treatment to Prevent Heart Attack Trial. (2002). Major outcomes in moderately hypercholesterolemic hypertensive patients randomized to pravastatin vs usual care: The Antihypertensive and Lipid Lowering Treatment to Prevent Heart Attack Trial (ALLHAT-LLT). *Journal of the American Medical Association, 288*(23), 2998–3007.

American Heart Association [Online]. Available at: *http://www.americanheart.org/presenter.jhtml?identifier=1516.*

Aronow, W. S. (2003). Hypercholesterolemia. The evidence supports use of statins. *Geriatrics, 8*(8), 18–20, 26–28, 31–32.

Ballantyne, C. M. (2003). Current and future aims of lipid-lowering therapy: Changing paradigms and lessons from the Heart Protection Study on standards of efficacy and safety. *American Journal of Cardiology, 92*(4B), 3K–9K.

Bottorff, M. B. (2002). Statin safety: New insights into myopathy and rhabdomyolysis. Cardiology Review. *Preventive Cardiology Clinic Newsletter,* August.

Braun, L. T., & Davidson, M. H. (2003). Cholesterol-lowering drugs bring benefits to high-risk populations even when LDL is normal. *Journal of Cardiovascular Nursing, 18*(1), 44–49; quiz, 75–76.

Crisby, M. (2003). Modulation of the inflammatory process by statins. *Drugs Today (Barc), 39*(2), 137–143.

Crisby, M., Carlson, L. A., & Winblad, B. (2002). Statins in the prevention and treatment of Alzheimer disease. *Alzheimer Disease and Associated Disorders, 16*(3), 131–136.

Fonarow, G. C., & Watson, K. E. (2003). Effective strategies for long-term statin use. *American Journal of Cardiology, 92*(1A), 27i–34i.

Grundy, S. M., Cleeman, J. I., Merz, C. N., et al. (2004). NCEP Report. Implications of recent clinical trials for National Cholesterol Education Program Adult Treatment Panel III guidelines. *Circulation, 110*(2), 227–239.

Heart Protection Study Group. (2002). MRC/BHF Heart Protection Study of cholesterol lowering with simvastatin in 20,536 high-risk individuals: A randomized placebo-controlled trial. *Lancet, 360*(9326), 7–22.

Kristianson, K., Fyhrquist, F., Devereux, R. B., et al. (2003). An analysis of cholesterol control and statin use in the Losartan Intervention for Endpoint Reduction in Hypertension Study. *Clinical Therapeutics, 25*(4), 1186–1199.

Law, M. R., Wald, N. J., & Rudnicka, A. R. (2003). Quantifying effect of statins on low density lipoprotein cholesterol, ischaemic heart disease, and stroke: Systematic review and meta-analysis. *British Medical Journal, 326*(7404), 1423.

McKenney, J. M. (2003). Potential nontraditional applications of statins. *Annals of Pharmacotherapy, 37*(7–8), 1063–1071.

Miller, M. (2003). Niacin as a component of combination therapy for dyslipidemia. *Mayo Clinic Proceedings, 78*(6), 735–742.

Pasternak, R. C., Smith, S. C., Bairey-Merz, C. N., et al. (2002). ACC/AHA/NLBI Clinical Advisory on the Use and Safety of Statins. *Journal of the American College of Cardiology, 40*(3), 567–572.

Pearson, T. A. (2000). The undertreatment of LDL-cholesterol: Addressing the challenge. *International Journal of Cardiology, 74*(Suppl. 1), S23–S28.

Rockwood, K., Kirkland, S., & Hogan, D. B. (2002). Use of lipid lowering agents, indication bias, and the risk of dementia in community-dwelling elderly people. *Archives of Neurology, 59*(2), 223–227.

Scott, C. L. (2003). Diagnosis, prevention, and intervention for the metabolic syndrome. *American Journal of Cardiology, 92*(1A), 35i–42i.

Shishehbor, M. H., Brennan, M. L., Aviles, R. J., et al. (2003). Statins promote potent systemic antioxidant effects through specific inflammatory pathways. *Circulation, 108*(4), 426–431.

Stuve, O., Youssef, S., Steinman, L., et al. (2003). Statins as potential therapeutic agents in neuroinflammatory disorders. *Current Opinion in Neurology, 16*(3), 393–401.

Third Report of the National Cholesterol Education Program (NCEP) Expert Panel on Detection, Evaluation, and Treatment of High Blood Cholesterol in Adults (Adult Treatment Panel III). (2004). Executive Summary [Online]. Available: *http://www.nhlbi.nih.gov/guidelines/cholesterol/atp3xsum.pdf.*

Wolfrum, S., Jensen, K. S., & Liao, J. K. (2003). Endothelium-dependent effects of statins. *Arteriosclerosis, Thrombosis, and Vascular Biology, 23*(5), 729–736.

Drugs Affecting Coagulation

chapter 31

Learning Objectives

At the completion of this chapter the student will:

1. Identify core drug knowledge about drugs affecting coagulation.
2. Differentiate between the anticoagulants heparin and warfarin.
3. Understand the differences between anticoagulants and thrombolytics.
4. Differentiate antiplatelet drugs from hemorheologic drugs.
5. Differentiate clotting factors from hemostatic agents.
6. Identify core patient variables relevant to drugs affecting coagulation.
7. Relate the interaction of core drug knowledge to core patient variables for drugs affecting coagulation.
8. Generate a nursing plan of care from the interactions between core drug knowledge and core patient variables for drugs affecting coagulation.
9. Describe nursing interventions to maximize therapeutic and minimize adverse effects for drugs affecting coagulation.
10. Determine key points for patient and family education for drugs affecting coagulation.

KEY TERMS

anticoagulants

clotting cascade

clotting factors

coagulation

embolus

fibrin

fibrinolysis

hemophilia

hemostasis

International Normalized Ratio (INR)

plasmin

platelets

thrombin

thromboembolus

thrombus

FEATURED WEBLINK

http://www.stroke.ahajournals.org/cgi/reprint/34/4/1056
Visit this American Heart Association site for the complete Guidelines for the Early Management of Patients With Ischemic Stroke, a scientific statement from the stroke council of the American Stroke Association.

CONNECTION WEBLINK

Additional Weblinks are found on Connection:
http://www.connection.lww.com/go/aschenbrenner.

Drugs Affecting Coagulation

Hypercoagulation

C Anticoagulants

Parenteral

- **P** **heparin**
  - enoxaparin
  - ardeparin
  - dalteparin

Oral

- **P** **warfarin**

C Antiplatelets

- **P** **clopidogrel**
  - aspirin
  - cilostazol
  - ticlopidine
  - abciximab
  - anagrelide
  - dipyridamole
  - eptifibatide
  - tirofiban

C Hemorheologics

- **pentoxifylline**

C Thrombolytics

- **P** **alteplase, recombinant**
  - reteplase, recombinant
  - tenectaplase
  - streptokinase
  - anistreplase
  - urokinase
  - drotrecogin alfa

Hypocoagulation

C Clotting factors

- **P** **antihemophilic factor**
  - human factor IX complex
  - coagulation factor VIIa, recombinant
  - anti-inhibitor coagulant factor

C Hemostatics

- **P** **aminocaproic acid**
  - aprotinin
  - tranexamic acid

The symbol **C** indicates the **drug class.**
Drugs in **bold type** marked with the symbol **P** are prototypes.
Drugs in blue type are closely related to the prototype.
Drugs in red type are significantly different from the prototype.
Drugs in black type with no symbol are also used in drug therapy; no prototype

This chapter examines drugs used to treat **coagulation** (blood aggregation, or clotting) disorders. Disturbances in the coagulation balance cause abnormalities in the body's ability to transport blood through the vessels to the cells or to form blood clots. Pathophysiologic effects may result from an excess of or a deficit in coagulation factors. When the body begins bleeding, a series of events occurs to slow blood flow, stop blood loss at the injury site, and prevent extensive blood loss. This process is known as **hemostasis.** Excessive coagulation, or hypercoagulation, will result in a **thrombus** (blood clot).

Several drug classes that are used to treat hypercoagulation disorders are discussed in this chapter. The first class is **anticoagulants** (substances that keep blood from clotting). Existing naturally and in drug form, anticoagulants prevent thrombus formation and the extension of existing thrombi. There are two types of anticoagulants—those that are given parenterally and those that are given orally. The prototype parenteral anticoagulant is heparin (Lipo-Hepin, Hep-Lock). Drugs similar to heparin are the low-molecular-weight heparins (enoxaparin [Lovenox], ardeparin [Normiflo], and dalteparin [Fragmin]). The prototype oral anticoagulant is warfarin (Coumadin).

Other drug classes used to treat hypercoagulability include the antiplatelet agents, the hemorheologics, and the thrombolytics. Antiplatelet agents interfere with platelet membrane function and platelet aggregation. The prototype for the antiplatelets is clopidogrel (Plavix). Drugs in the same class are cilostazol (Pletal) and ticlopidine (Ticlid). A drug closely related to clopidogrel is aspirin. Drugs that are significantly different from clopidogrel are dipyridamole (Persantine), the glycoprotein IIb/IIIa inhibitors (tirofiban [Aggrastat], eptifibatide [Integrilin], abciximab [Reo Pro]), and anagrelide (Agrylin).

Hemorheologics reduce blood viscosity, increase the flexibility of red blood cells (RBCs), and decrease platelet aggregation. Pentoxifylline (Trental) is the prototype for the hemorheologics.

Thrombolytics, unlike anticoagulants and other drugs that are used to treat hypercoagulation, actually dissolve existing clots. They are used to treat medical emergencies resulting from thrombus formations' blocking blood flow to the heart, lung, or deep veins of the legs. The prototype thrombolytic is alteplase, recombinant (Activase).

Other drugs in this class are reteplase, recombinant (Retavase). Drugs closely related to alteplase recombinant are the thrombolytic enzymes: streptokinase (Streptase, Kabikinase), anistreplase (Eminase), and urokinase (Abbokinase, Abbokinase Open-Cath). A drug that is significantly different from alteplase is drotrecogin alfa (activated) (Xigris).

This chapter also describes drug classes used when hypocoagulation, or subnormal coagulation, is a problem. These drug classes include clotting factors and hemostatic agents. Clotting factors are replacements for genetic deficiencies of normal clotting factors, which lead to **hemophilia** (uncontrollable bleeding). The prototype drug is antihemophilic factor (AHF, factor VIII). Other drugs in this class include coagulation factor VIIa (recombinant), anti-inhibitor coagulant complex, and human factor IX complex.

Hemostatics inhibit **fibrinolysis,** the process of breaking down a formed clot. They are either systemic or topical. The prototype systemic hemostatic drug is aminocaproic acid (Amicar). Other drugs in this class include tranexamic acid (Cyklokapron) and aprotinin (Trasylol). Topical hemostatics are used to control minor bleeding, usually after surgery. The various agents work differently. No prototype is identifiable for topical hemostatics.

This chapter also discusses drugs used to treat overactive bladder and decrease frequency of urination. These drugs are antimuscarinics. The prototype is tolterodine (Detrol).

PHYSIOLOGY OF COAGULATION

Normal circulation requires blood to circulate freely through large and small blood vessels. However, blood must also be able to form clots to prevent excessive blood loss from injuries. To perform both of these functions requires the body's ability to balance coagulation and anticoagulation.

Blood Components and Balanced Blood Flow

Blood is composed of various cells and substances, each with a specific purpose that assists in maintaining a balance of coagulation and anticoagulation. Present in blood are **platelets** (also called thrombocytes), which are fragmented cells that assist in blood clotting and clot formation. In addition, the blood contains a number of other substances that promote coagulation but are inactive. These substances are the procoagulants (precursors to clotting factors) and **clotting factors,** which are plasma proteins that cause blood clotting. The clotting factors are inactive in the blood until an injury mobilizes them.

Circulating in an active form are the anticoagulants, which dominate the procoagulants, unless an injury to a blood vessel occurs that disrupts the dominance of the anticoagulants.

When a blood vessel is injured initially, the vessel goes into spasm (vasoconstriction), which decreases blood flow and limits blood loss. Because platelets have a surface composed of glycoprotein, they adhere to the endothelial surface of the damaged blood vessel. Next, with the help of enzymatic action, the platelets release a substance called adenosine diphosphate, which in turn is converted to thromboxane A_2. This activity attracts other platelets to the damage site. Together, the platelets form a temporary plug that seals the injured vessel. Normally, this plug is effective because it is stabilized with **fibrin,** an insoluble protein.

Clotting Cascade

Fibrin is a product of the **clotting cascade.** The cascade is initiated by the tissue damage and platelet activation, which mobilize the clotting factors circulating in the blood. Once active, these clotting factors work with calcium to form fibrin. At this point, blood coagulation is completed and blood loss stops.

The clotting cascade occurs over two pathways, intrinsic and extrinsic, to achieve hemostasis. The intrinsic pathway—so named because all of the clotting factors are present in the blood—is activated by damage to the blood vessel. In the extrinsic pathway, the clotting factors are activated by the damaged tissue. One or both pathways may be activated in response to injury. Figure 31.1 depicts the intrinsic and extrinsic pathways in the clotting cascade.

Physiology

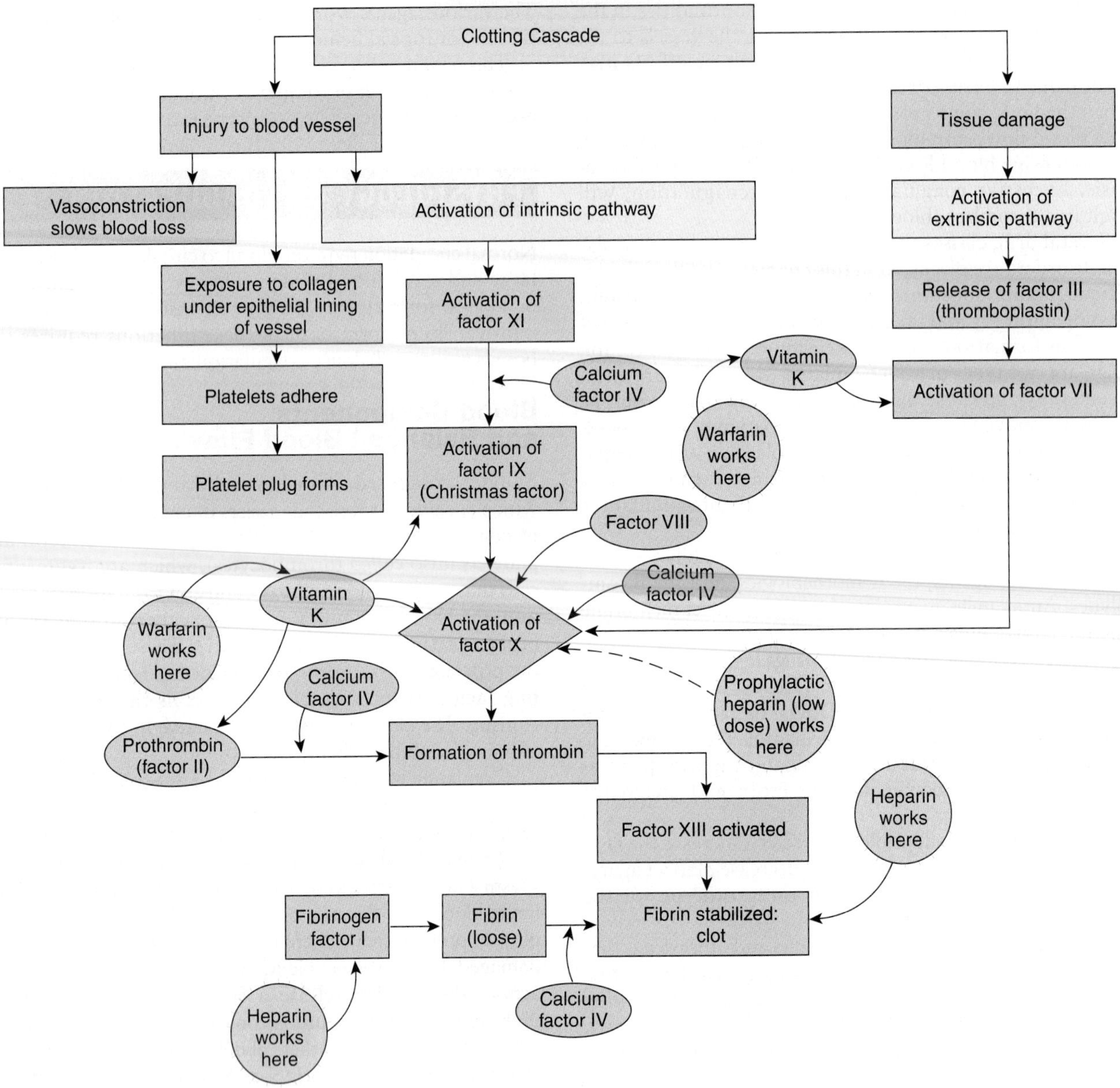

FIGURE 31.1 Events in the clotting cascade.

Intrinsic Pathway

Activity in the intrinsic pathway begins with an enzyme reaction that modifies factor XII from its inactive to active form. In turn, factor XII helps modify factor XI so that it can activate factor IX. Factor IX acts on factor VIII, and factor VIII activates factor X. Activated factor X affects factor V and promotes the conversion of prothrombin (factor II) to **thrombin.** Thrombin in turn converts factor I (fibrinogen) to fibrin. Thrombin also activates factor XIII, a fibrin-stabilizing factor. The fibrin threads that are produced trap the clotting factors that remain in the injured area, preventing the extension of the blood clot beyond the injury. The cascade thus ends in the formation of a stable blood clot.

Extrinsic Pathway

Activity in the extrinsic pathway begins with the activation of factor III followed by the activation of factor VII, then factor X. The remaining steps in this process follow those of the intrinsic pathway and are referred to as the final common pathway. The prevention of clot extension, which occurs at the end of the clotting cascade, is assisted by the release of heparin. Heparin, a naturally occurring anticoagulant normally found in small amounts in the blood, is released from mast cells at the time of the initial injury.

Hemolysis

After a blood clot forms, the blood has a removal system that begins to lyse (decompose or break down) the clot

about 1 to 2 days after bleeding stops. Plasma protein contains a substance known as plasminogen, which, along with other plasma proteins, is trapped in the blood clot. The damaged tissue releases tissue plasminogen activators, which change plasminogen to its active form, **plasmin.** Activated plasmin is the substance that lyses the blood clot.

PATHOPHYSIOLOGY

When blood flow is impeded and slowed in an area, coagulation occurs, leading to formation of a thrombus. Any excessive action from the coagulating factors may also produce a thrombus that obstructs blood flow. A thrombus can form anywhere in the cardiovascular system. The components of a thrombus vary, depending on whether the thrombus is arterial (formed under high flow conditions) or venous (formed from stasis). Arterial thrombi consist mostly of platelet aggregates held together with thin fibrin strands, whereas venous thrombi are mostly red cells, a large amount of fibrin, and only a few platelets. An **embolism (embolus)** is any undissolved matter carried in a blood or lymph vessel to another location where it lodges and occludes the vessel. When a portion of a thrombus breaks off, the fragment may travel through the bloodstream and lodge in a vessel (**thromboembolus**), again occluding blood flow. When the thromboembolus is lodged in a coronary vessel, a myocardial infarction (MI) occurs. When it is lodged in the brain, a stroke, or cerebrovascular accident (CVA), occurs. When the thromboembolus is lodged in the pulmonary vessels it is called a pulmonary **embolus.** When a thromboembolus lodges in a blood vessel, blood flow through the vessel decreases or stops, depending on the size and position of the thrombo-embolus and the degree of obstruction. With decreased blood flow, tissues and cells do not receive necessary oxygen and nutrients, and necrosis (cell death) occurs.

Arterial thrombi produce negative effects on blood flow either from directly obstructing blood flow or by producing embolisms that lodge in the microcirculation. Venous thrombi most often occur in the deep vessels of the lower limbs (referred to as deep vein thrombosis [DVT]) and produce their serious effects from inflaming the vessel wall, direct obstruction of blood flow, or through pulmonary embolism (Hirsch et al., 2001). DVT may be secondary to surgery, trauma, malignancy, hereditary thrombotic disorders, stroke, spinal cord injury, or unexplained causes. The exact mechanism of the relationship between cancer and thrombosis is not known; however, it is known that cancer patients have an increased risk for developing thrombosis. Patients who present with thromboembolism of unknown causes are believed to have a higher risk for developing cancer, although no data support thorough cancer screening with these patients (Valente & Ponte, 2000).

Acute coronary syndromes are also related to thrombus. Acute coronary syndromes include unstable angina, non–ST-elevation MI, and ST-elevation MI. All of these conditions have an underlying pathology of unstable coronary plaque on a coronary vessel, with an overlying intracoronary thrombus. Thrombus formation can also be a problem in atrial fibrillation. In this condition, the blood is not moving, which may lead to coagulation of the blood into clots.

Some conditions of hypercoagulability result from increased platelet activity. Constriction of, or fatty deposits in, a blood vessel narrows its lumen, leading to decreased or slowed blood flow through the vessel. The decreased flow causes stasis, which results in blood coagulation. Platelet activity is responsible for the formation of the blood clot. This is a particular problem for patients with chronic, obstructive vascular disease because blood clots further impair or entirely block an already diminished blood flow, thereby posing a risk for tissue death from lack of oxygen and nutrients.

In peripheral vascular disease, the blood vessels in the extremities, particularly the legs, are narrowed. This narrowing prevents the flow of oxygenated blood to the tissues. Lack of oxygenation causes pain, especially with use of the extremity. This condition is known as intermittent claudication. Rest relieves the pain because it decreases the oxygen needed by the tissue. With the impaired circulation, venous stasis occurs, which in turn leads to platelet aggregation and thrombus formation. This thrombus further impairs circulation through the vessel to the tissue.

DRUG THERAPY FOR HYPERCOAGULATION

In general, disorders of hypercoagulability result from either an increase in platelets or an increase in the activity of the clotting system, or combinations of both. Treatment is aimed at interfering with the clotting cascade. The desired effect is to lengthen the time necessary for blood to clot, to alter platelet aggregation preventing clotting, or to do both. Anticoagulant drug therapy is used to prevent new clots from forming, to avoid extension of the thrombus, or to deter a thromboembolus. Antiplatelet therapy decreases the ability of platelets to stick together.

When an existing clot may be fatal to the patient because of blocked blood flow to vital organs, thrombolytic agents are used to break it up. When the clot or obstruction blocks a coronary artery, the heart is affected; damage to the heart from an MI can be permanent or fatal. When the clot blocks the pulmonary artery, the blood supply to the lungs is altered; this alteration in turn decreases the oxygenation of blood to be circulated. This is a life-threatening condition. If the clot is in the brain, ischemia of the tissue will result in brain cell death with loss of brain function and permanent neurologic deficits or disabilities in the patient. If the injury is severe or an extensive portion of the brain is affected, death can result. Because brain cells are highly dependent on sufficient oxygen for survival, rapid treatment to break apart a thrombus and relieve hypoxia is crucial. When the thrombus is large and blocks the great veins in the legs, circulation is impaired in the limb. If the circulatory impairment is severe enough, the patient may risk losing the limb as a result of tissue death. This event also is considered a medical emergency. Thrombolytic agents are indicated in these emergency situations to prevent severe damage to the body or death.

When the patient has a less urgent need for therapy, has a high risk for developing arterial thrombi, or requires additional treatment after the use of thrombolytic drugs, antiplatelet drugs are used. Antiplatelets decrease clumping or aggregating of platelets. Platelet aggregation is also affected by hemorheologic drugs. In addition, the hemorheologics increase the flexibility of RBCs and decrease the blood viscosity.

C ANTICOAGULANT DRUGS

Heparin, a naturally occurring anticoagulant, is produced by mast cells located in connective tissue throughout the body. The blood cells known as basophils produce a small amount as well. The areas that produce the largest amount of heparin are the lungs and, to a lesser degree, the liver. This fact reflects a natural protective mechanism of the body because these two areas receive the smallest emboli.

All anticoagulants interfere with the clotting cascade and prolong blood clotting time. They vary by their route and their method of action. There are two types of anticoagulants, those that can only be administered parenterally and those that can only be administered orally. The parenteral anticoagulants work by preventing the conversion of fibrinogen to fibrin. The oral anticoagulants work by preventing the synthesis of factors dependent on vitamin K for synthesis, factors II (prothrombin), VII, VIII, IX, and X. Two different laboratory tests, one for drugs administered orally and one for those administered parenterally, are therefore used to measure the therapeutic effects of these anticoagulants.

The prototype parenteral anticoagulant is heparin, which is unfractionated (containing both low-molecular and high-molecular weights) and stabilized with either sulfate (Lipo-Hepin, Liquaemin Sodium) or calcium (Calciparine). Table 31.1 presents a summary of selected drugs used to treat hypercoagulability.

NURSING MANAGEMENT OF THE PATIENT RECEIVING P HEPARIN

Core Drug Knowledge

Pharmacotherapeutics

Heparin is the prototype parenteral anticoagulant. It interferes with the final steps of the clotting cascade. It is used to prevent the extension of a blood clot, particularly in patients with deep vein thrombosis (DVT) or pulmonary embolism. It is also used prophylactically in patients with short-term increased risk for thrombus formation, such as in the post-

TABLE 31.1 Summary of Selected Drugs for Hypercoagulability

Drug (Trade) Name	Selected Indications	Route and Dosage Range	Pharmacokinetics
P heparin (*Canadian:* Hepalean)	Anticoagulation	*Adult:* IV, 5,000 U bolus (or 35–70 U/kg) followed by 20,000–40,000 U/24 h or 15–25 U/kg/h *Child:* IV, 50 U/kg bolus, followed by 100 U/kg/4 h or 20,000 U/m2/24 h	*Onset:* Immediate *Duration:* 2–6 h $t_{1/2}$: 30–180 min
	Prophylaxis	*Adult:* SC, 5,000 U q8–12h	*Onset:* 20–60 min *Duration:* 8–12 h
enoxaparin (Lovenox)	Prophylaxis	*Adult:* SC, 30 mg, bid or 40 mg/d	*Onset:* 20–60 min *Duration:* 12 h $t_{1/2}$: 4.5 h
P warfarin (Coumadin; *Canadian:* Warfilone)	Prophylaxis and treatment	*Adult:* PO, 5–10 mg/day for 2–4 d, then adjust according to results of PT or INR values	*Onset:* 24 h *Duration:* 2–5 d $t_{1/2}$: 1–2.5 d
P clopidogrel (Plavix)	Reduction of atherosclerotic events	*Adult:* PO, 75 mg/d	*Onset:* Rapid *Duration:* Unknown $t_{1/2}$: 8 h
aspirin (Bayer; *Canadian:* APO-ASA)	Prophylaxis for MI Decrease risk of TIA in men	*Adult:* PO, 300–325 mg/d *Adult:* PO, 1,300 mg/d divided into two to four doses	*Onset:* 5–30 min *Duration:* Varies $t_{1/2}$: 15–20 min
P pentoxifylline (Trental)	Intermittent claudication	*Adult:* PO, 400 mg tid†	*Onset:* Rapid *Duration:* Unknown $t_{1/2}$: 0.4–0.8 h
P alteplase, recombinant (Activase)	Acute MI	*Adult (>67 kg)*: 100 mg total: 15 mg bolus, 50 mg infusion over 30 minutes, then 35 mg infusion over 60 min	*Onset:* Rapid *Duration:* Unknown $t_{1/2}$: Unknown
	Acute ischemic stroke	*Adult:* IV, 0.9 mg/kg (max 90 mg) 10% given as bolus over 1 min, 90% infused over 60 min	
	Pulmonary embolism (PE)	*Adult:* IV, 100 mg infusion over 2 h	

operative period after a total hip replacement. When treating disseminated intravascular coagulation (DIC), heparin prevents further clotting in the microcirculation, leaving the procoagulants available to work at other sites in the body. Heparin is not recommended as adjunct therapy for patients who have received thrombolytic therapy for an ischemic stroke. Neither has it been found to be particularly helpful in preventing a second stroke or in preventing further neurologic impairment after a stroke (Adams et al., 2003).

The heparin dosage is tailored to the patient and the severity of the condition. Continuous intravenous (IV) infusion of heparin is used to achieve full anticoagulation. In adults, a heparin IV drip is usually started by giving an IV bolus of the drug followed by continuous infusion. Selecting heparin dosage from a weight-based nomogram was found to achieve a therapeutic range more rapidly than methods of estimating the appropriate dose based on clinical experience alone or combined with general guidelines (Balcezak et al., 2000). Other ways to achieve full anticoagulating effects from heparin include using intermittent IV boluses or subcutaneous injections of heparin. In adults, subcutaneous administration of heparin may also prevent thromboembolic events (see Table 31.1).

The duration of anticoagulation therapy for venous thromboembolism is based on the patient's level of risk for thrombosis if anticoagulation is stopped, as well as the patient's risk for bleeding if drug therapy is continued. Risk for recurrent thrombosis is considered low if it was precipitated by a reversible risk factor, such as surgery (because the surgery and the postoperative period are past, so that risk is no longer present). Risk for recurrence is high if the thromboembolism occurred with no apparent risk factors, or if the patient has persistent risk factors (e.g., cancer). Patients at low risk for recurrence should receive anticoagulation therapy for 3 months. Those at higher risk should receive anticoagulation therapy for 6 months to indefinitely, depending on the patient's variables.

Pharmacokinetics

Heparin is not absorbed from the gastrointestinal (GI) tract because it is destroyed by gastric acid; hence, it must be administered parenterally. When administered IV, heparin has an immediate onset of action. When administered subcutaneously, heparin's onset of action is 20 to 60 minutes. After administration, the drug is widely distributed in the body, although it does not cross the placenta, nor is it found in breast milk. Metabolism occurs in the liver, where it is inactivated. It is eliminated from the body in the urine.

Pharmacodynamics

Heparin, along with antithrombin III, rapidly promotes the inactivation of factor X, which, in turn, prevents the conversion of prothrombin to thrombin. Heparin also has an effect on fibrin, limiting the formation of a stable clot. In blood tests measuring activated partial thromboplastin time (aPTT), heparin prolongs the clotting time without affecting the bleeding time. Low-dose heparin therapy, which is prophylactic dosing, deactivates factor X but has minimal effect on already produced thrombin; thus, it does not normally alter aPTT levels. However, full anticoagulation effects can occur in some individuals. Heparin has no effect on blood clots that have already formed.

Contraindications and Precautions

Heparin is contraindicated in patients who are hypersensitive to beef or pork because some heparin products are derived from the intestinal mucosa of pigs and others from beef lung. Heparin is also contraindicated in patients with thrombocytopenia, bleeding disorders, and active bleeding other than DIC.

This drug should be used with caution in patients with the potential for hemorrhage, for example, immediately after surgery and in those with peptic ulcer disease and liver disease.

Adverse Effects

The most common adverse effect of heparin is bleeding. Although heparin-induced thrombocytopenia (HIT) occurs rarely, it is potentially life threatening. Treatment for HIT includes discontinuing heparin, allowing the platelet count to return to normal, and treating any thrombosis. Two agents are currently approved to treat HIT-related thrombosis: lepirudin (Refludan) and argatroban (Argatroban). Other adverse effects of heparin, although uncommon, include hepatitis, rashes, urticaria, hypersensitivity, and fever.

If a patient receives an overdose of heparin or shows signs of bleeding, protamine sulfate, the antagonist for heparin, may be administered. Protamine sulfate, a strong base, reacts with heparin, a strong acid, to form a stable salt, thereby neutralizing the anticoagulant effects of heparin. The protamine sulfate dose is based on the heparin dose: 1 mg of protamine sulfate per 100 U of heparin, or 0.5 mg of protamine sulfate per 100 U of heparin if the heparin was administered more than 30 minutes before the protamine sulfate. No more than 100 mg of protamine sulfate should be given within a 2-hour period because this drug can cause anticoagulation in its own right. Administering protamine sulfate too rapidly may result in hypotension, bradycardia, dyspnea, and anaphylaxis. Hypersensitivity reactions may occur in some patients because of the fish base of protamine sulfate. Symptoms include flushing and feelings of warmth.

If the patient is not actively bleeding after heparin overdosage, the patient is usually monitored closely, and the protamine sulfate is not administered because heparin has a short half-life. The patient will recover from the overdosage without the added risk for complications from the protamine sulfate.

Drug Interactions

Several different drugs affect the action of heparin. Table 31.2 identifies these drugs and the significance of the reaction.

Assessment of Relevant Core Patient Variables

Health Status

Before administering the first dose of heparin, review the patient's record for evidence of allergy or a pre-existing prolonged bleeding time that would contraindicate administering heparin.

Life Span and Gender

Be aware that heparin is safe for pregnant women, although it places other patients at risk for injury, particularly those

TABLE 31.2 Agents That Interact With P Heparin

Interactants	Effect and Significance	Nursing Management
cephalosporins	Additive effect with heparin is possible, which increases risk of bleeding.	Monitor for signs of bleeding. Monitor activated partial thromboplastin time carefully. Use drug cautiously when it is required.
nitroglycerin	Information is conflicting, but effect of heparin may be increased, increasing risk of bleeding.	Same as above.
penicillins	Parenteral administration can alter platelet aggregation and coagulation test findings. They may have additive effect with heparin to increase the risk of bleeding.	Same as above.
salicylate	Antiplatelet effect increases risk of bleeding.	Concurrent use is normally avoided.

who are confused, cognitively impaired, unable to modify behavior to prevent injuries, or incapable of complying with requests to modify behavior.

Lifestyle, Diet, and Habits

Because heparin prolongs both internal and external bleeding, slight injuries may potentially cause serious adverse effects. Ask patients about their activity level. Patients who normally engage in active behaviors in which bumping or body injuries frequently occur are more at risk for injury when receiving subcutaneous heparin therapy at home.

Environment

Be aware of the environment in which the drug will be administered. Heparin is normally administered in an acute care setting.

Nursing Diagnosis and Outcome

- Risk for Injury, Hemorrhage, related to heparin therapy
  Desired outcome: Hemorrhage will not occur.

Planning and Intervention

Maximizing Therapeutic Effects

Monitor laboratory values (e.g., the aPTT) to confirm that a therapeutic lengthening of the clotting time has been achieved. The therapeutic lengthening of the clotting time is generally measured as one and one half to two times the control aPTT. Because control times vary from laboratory to laboratory depending on the test equipment used, the difference between the two times is used to measure effectiveness. For example, if the aPTT control time is 30 seconds, a therapeutic level for the patient would be 45 to 60 seconds. Guidelines vary according to individual patients, who may require aPTT values of less than one and one half times the control or more than two times the control to be therapeutic.

Heparin levels should be allowed to reach steady state before measuring aPTT, usually 6 to 8 hours after the infusion starts. If the aPTT is less than one and one half to two times the control, contact the prescriber to seek new drug therapy orders. If the aPTT is below the desired therapeutic range, the dosage needs to be increased. Repeated testing is needed after each dosage change has reached steady state (6–8 hours after the dosage change). In institutions with established protocols for adjusting heparin infusion rates to meet therapeutic levels, the rate may be changed by a registered nurse. If aPTT values deviate from the protocol limits, the prescriber must be notified.

IV heparin therapy should not be interrupted because interruption lowers the blood levels of heparin and affect the therapeutic response. If occlusion or infiltration necessitates changing the IV site, the new IV line should be inserted as soon as possible to minimize the disruption of the infusion.

Doses of subcutaneous (SC) heparin should not be missed; they should be administered at the regularly prescribed times to maintain blood levels.

Minimizing Adverse Effects

Before initiating therapy, review such laboratory values as aPTT, hematocrit, and platelet count. These tests provide baseline information regarding clotting abilities and identify patients with conditions that contraindicate heparin therapy. However, these tests are not usually performed for prophylactic heparin use.

If the aPTT during treatment exceeds the desired range, the dosage should be decreased. Contact the prescriber to seek new drug therapy orders, or act on the standard protocol (if one is used).

An IV controller or pump should be used for continuous IV drip heparin to promote a steady rate of delivery and prevent rapid overdosage, which may occur when IV flow rates are regulated by gravity. Use of a pump is a standard safety precaution.

Administration of IV heparin should not be interrupted to give another drug. Doing so increases the risk for thrombus formation because therapeutic levels may not be maintained.

Other drugs should not be administered through the same tubing as heparin because heparin is incompatible with many other drugs and fluids. An additional peripheral IV line or a multilumen central venous catheter should be used instead.

The patient should be monitored for bleeding from the gums, nose, vagina, or wounds. Urine and stools should be examined to detect blood as well. The skin should be inspected for ecchymoses or hematomas that indicate bleeding into the tissues. If the patient develops active bleeding from an orifice or a wound, the prescriber needs to be notified immediately. Protamine sulfate is administered if active bleeding occurs.

IM injections should be avoided to prevent bleeding into the muscle. Pressure should be placed on IV sites when removing the line until bleeding stops. For SC administration of heparin, a 25-gauge or finer needle should be used (Box 31.1). Do not aspirate or massage the area after administration.

To protect the patient from injury or falls, side rails should be raised or padded, particularly if the patient is confused, disoriented, restless, or unable to comprehend or follow activity restrictions during therapy.

Providing Patient and Family Education

- Before heparin therapy begins, inform the patient why the drug is needed and what it is expected to accomplish. Heparin should be described as an anticoagulant, not a blood thinner. Although this is a common description, it is not correct.
- Explain that frequent blood samples will need to be analyzed to measure the patient's clotting time and determine whether the patient is receiving a safe amount of heparin.
- Instruct the patient to report any blood in urine or stools and any bleeding from the gums, nose, vagina, or wounds.
- Educate the patient to use a soft toothbrush and an electric razor during therapy to prevent bleeding and to follow activity restrictions to prevent bruising and internal bleeding from injuries.

If the patient will be receiving heparin at home, some additional instructions apply, as outlined in Box 31.2.

Ongoing Assessment and Evaluation

Throughout therapy, monitor for signs of bleeding and review aPTT values to maintain drug levels in the therapeutic range. Drug therapy is considered effective when a thrombus or extension of an existing thrombus is avoided.

Drugs Closely Related to P Heparin

Low-molecular-weight heparin is derived from standard heparin through either chemical or enzymatic depolymerization (breakdown of polymers into monomers, their basic building block). Whereas standard heparin has a molecular weight of 5,000 to 30,000 daltons, low-molecular-weight heparin ranges from 1,000 to 10,000 daltons, resulting in properties that are distinct from those of traditional heparin. Low-molecular-weight heparin binds to protein (although less strongly than traditional heparin), has enhanced bioavailability, interacts less with platelets, and yields a very predictable dose response, eliminating the need to monitor the aPTT. Low-molecular-weight heparin, like standard heparin, binds to antithrombin III; however, low-molecular-weight heparin also inhibits thrombin to a lesser degree (and actual factor X to a greater degree) than standard heparin.

Low-molecular-weight heparins also have prolonged half lives compared with unfractionated heparin (standard heparin that has not been depolymerized). This characteristic, in combination with the increased bioavailability, allows the drug to be dosed once daily SC. Such dosing enables treatment for stabilized patients in their own homes, while they are followed as outpatients.

Low-molecular-weight heparins cause less bleeding when given in therapeutic doses, compared with unfractionated

BOX 31.1 Research-Based Subcutaneous Administration Techniques for Heparin

Traditionally, the abdomen, 2 inches from the umbilicus, was the preferred site for injection because it was believed that this site carried less risk for developing hematoma. Research has shown, however, that site selection of the arm or thigh, as opposed to the abdomen, does not increase bruising or alter APTT (Fahs & Kinney, 1991). Research further indicates that technique affects hematoma formation. As early as 1988, Wooldridge found that changing the needle after drawing the drug into the syringe, having an air bubble in the syringe to follow the dose and lock the drug into the subcutaneous space, injecting at a 90-degree angle, and avoiding aspiration and massage after injection helped to prevent hematoma formation. The use of a 3-cc syringe rather than a 1-mL syringe has been found to cause smaller bruises when administering heparin (Hadley, Chang, & Rogers, 1996).

COMMUNITY-BASED CONCERNS

Box 31.2 Enoxaparin at Home

Patients receiving subcutaneous injections of enoxaparin at home are typically responsible for self-administering the medication. These patients need information on the following topics:

- Locating appropriate injection sites and rotating injection sites
- Performing subcutaneous injections using appropriate technique
- Disposing of used syringes and needles in an impervious container, such as a plastic milk jug or a coffee can. The lid should be taped shut before placing the container in the regular home trash.
- Recapping needles: Patients may recap their own used needle. If a family member is administering the medication, the needle and syringe should be placed in the container uncapped.

MEMORY CHIP

P Heparin

- Anticoagulant that prevents formation or extensions of blood clots
- Has no effect on existing blood clots
- Parenteral administration (IV or SC)
- Major contraindications: thrombocytopenia, bleeding disorders, and active bleeding other than DIC
- Most common adverse effect: bleeding (antidote for heparin overdose is protamine sulfate)
- Most serious adverse effect: thrombocytopenia
- **Life span alert: heparin is the anticoagulant that can be used during pregnancy**
- Maximizing therapeutic effects: Monitor APTT for therapeutic range; adjust dose till therapeutic range achieved.
- Minimizing adverse effects: Use IV pump; assess for signs of bleeding.
- Most important patient education: Instruct patients to report any blood in urine or stools or bleeding from gums, nose, vagina, or wounds.

heparin, as well as less heparin induced thrombocytopenia and osteoporosis.

In multiple clinical trials and in meta-analyses of trials, low-molecular-weight heparin treatment for DVT and pulmonary embolism resulted in decreased recurrent thromboembolism, major bleeding, and death when compared with standard, unfractionated heparin (Mukherjee et al., 2002). Other studies indicate that low-molecular-weight heparins are as safe and effective as unfractionated heparin in treating pulmonary embolism, as prophylaxis of venous thromboembolism, and in treatment for DVT.

Enoxaparin

Enoxaparin (Lovenox), which is considered safer and equally effective as heparin, has an effect on activated factor X and has limited effect on thrombin. Thus, its effect on aPTT is decreased. Enoxaparin also affects clotting factor C and antithrombin. Most enoxaparin is absorbed after SC administration and is widely distributed. Enoxaparin has been found to be superior to unfractionated heparin in reducing death, MI, and emergency revascularization in patients with Q-wave MI. Enoxaparin appears to have similar efficacy and safety compared with unfractionated heparin when used to treat ST-segment elevation myocardial infarction (Cohen et al., 2003). Low-molecular-weight heparins, like enoxaparin, appear to be safe and effective for treating acute coronary syndrome when combined with platelet glycoprotein IIB/IIIa inhibitors (Mukherjee et al., 2002; Ferguson et al., 2003).

Patients who are to receive enoxaparin by SC injection after discharge should be taught how to administer the drug to themselves. It is important that they understand the reason for therapy, the necessity of taking the drug on time, and the importance of following a regular dosage schedule and having follow-up blood analyses done as recommended. They should also be advised about scheduling and keeping appointments with the prescriber.

Other important teaching points focus on safety, for example, clearing pathways, removing loose scatter rugs, wearing nonskid footwear, obtaining adequate lighting, and using handrails on stairways in bathtubs. Additional teaching and management concerns are similar to those for heparin therapy.

Ardeparin

Ardeparin (Normiflo) is a low-molecular-weight heparin like enoxaparin. It is used to prevent DVT after knee replacement surgery. An unlabeled use is for secondary prophylaxis for recurrent thromboembolic events. Like enoxaparin, it should be administered only by deep SC injection. In contrast to enoxaparin, which is a pregnancy category B drug, ardeparin is a category C agent. One unique characteristic of ardeparin is its ability to increase lipoprotein lipase activity. However, it has been found to cause a paradoxic elevation of serum triglyceride levels in clinical trials. Another unique feature of ardeparin is that it contains metabisulfite, a sulfite that may cause allergic reactions, including anaphylaxis, in susceptible people. Adverse effects of ardeparin are similar to those of enoxaparin.

Dalteparin

Dalteparin (Fragmin), another low-molecular-weight heparin, is used to prevent DVT. It is also used in treating unstable angina and non–Q-wave MI for preventing ischemic complication in patients on concurrent aspirin therapy. A unique feature of dalteparin is that the multiple-dose vial contains benzyl alcohol as a preservative; benzyl alcohol has been associated with "fatal gasping" syndrome in premature infants. Because of this possibility, dalteparin should not be used in infants or in pregnant women (because it crosses the placenta). Other characteristics of dalteparin are similar to those of enoxaparin.

NURSING MANAGEMENT OF THE PATIENT RECEIVING [P] WARFARIN

Core Drug Knowledge

Pharmacotherapeutics

Warfarin is an oral anticoagulant. It is administered after heparin therapy to complete treating a thrombus or embolism. Warfarin is also used prophylactically for patients with a long-term risk for thrombus formation, for example, when the mitral valve has been replaced or when hypercoagulability is a chronic concern related to venous stasis. It is also used prophylactically in patients with atrial fibrillation who are at high risk for a cardioembolic stroke; about one third of patients with atrial fibrillation are at such risk. Women with atrial fibrillation especially seem to benefit from preventative treatment (Hart et al., 2003).

Dosage is based on achieving a therapeutic level as measured by changes in the prothrombin time (PT). The patient's PT is measured against a control PT. PT control times vary with laboratory test methods and equipment, so that a standardized unit, known as the **International Normalized Ratio (INR)**, has been developed to measure therapeutic levels of warfarin. The INR is determined by a mathematical equation and reflects the patient's PT compared with the standardized PT value. Some institutions use one or the other laboratory test to measure warfarin effect. Others use both. For treatment or prophylaxis of a thrombus or embolus, the patient's PT should be 1.4 to 1.6 times the control time; the INR should be equal to 2 to 3. For prophylaxis in patients with mechanical heart valves, the PT should be 1.5 to 1.7 times the control or the INR should be 2.5 to 3.5.

Pharmacokinetics

After absorption, warfarin is bound to albumin in the plasma. The drug action peaks in 1 to 9 hours; however, the anticoagulant effects do not begin for 24 hours. Maximum effect occurs 3 to 4 days after dosing starts, which is the time required for the drug to reach a steady state in the blood. The time factor is related to previously activated factors that are still circulating in the blood. Each time the dose changes, another 3 to 4 days are needed for the drug to reach its full effect. The effects of warfarin persist for 4 to 5 days after discontinuation. The drug crosses the placenta but is not present in breast milk. It is metabolized in the liver and excreted in the bile.

Patients receiving heparin therapy will begin taking warfarin before they discontinue heparin. This overlap allows the warfarin to reach a therapeutic level before heparin is discontinued. The practice is safe because the two drugs affect different clotting factors (see Table 31.1).

Pharmacodynamics

Warfarin works by competitively blocking vitamin K at its sites of action. Thus, it prevents the activation of factors II (prothrombin), VII, IX, and X. It has no effect on factors that have already been activated. When warfarin is given immediately, the pharmacodynamic response to the drug is affected by the preoperative hemoglobin level. Lower preoperative hemoglobin has been associated with an increased response to warfarin therapy (Messieh, 2000).

Contraindications and Precautions

Warfarin is contraindicated for patients with active bleeding, open wounds or ulcerations of the GI tract, or bleeding disorders, such as hemophilia or thrombocytopenia. It is not recommended for use in patients with subacute endocarditis, pericarditis, or pericardial effusions. Warfarin is also contraindicated for patients who are undergoing surgery in which hemorrhage is possible (spinal, eye, GI, cranial, and arterial bypass grafting). Usually, the drug is discontinued 7 days before elective surgery.

Cautious use is recommended in patients with renal and hepatic impairment. Warfarin use is primarily determined by comparing the risks of the drug with the benefits to the patient.

Adverse Effects

The most frequent adverse effects of warfarin are bleeding and hemorrhage. Nausea, vomiting, diarrhea, and abdominal cramps can occur as well. Tissue necrosis is a rare adverse effect. A fetal warfarin syndrome has been identified when warfarin is given to pregnant women. (See discussion under Life Span and Gender.)

Drug Interactions

Several drug–drug and drug–food interactions must be considered when a patient begins warfarin therapy (Table 31.3). Many of these drug interactions may be related to effects on the P-450 system. Many herbal preparations also interact with warfarin (Table 31.4). Because drug and herbal interactions are numerous, a complete assessment of all other drug therapies should be conducted when starting a patient on warfarin.

Assessment of Relevant Core Patient Variables

Health Status

Because deficiencies of vitamin K increase the bleeding risk in patients receiving warfarin, the availability of vitamin K should be assessed. Besides the body's production of vitamin K in the GI tract, one source of vitamin K is food. Vitamin K is a fat-soluble vitamin and depends on the absorption of fat for its own absorption. Bile is necessary for fats to be digested and absorbed. A patient with decreased available bile, from obstructed bile ducts for example, absorbs less vitamin K. Patients with poor dietary intake of vitamin K will also be deficient in the vitamin.

Vitamin K deficiency may occur in adults whose normal GI flora has been affected by long-term antibiotic therapy or whose dietary intake consists of parenteral nutrition without vitamin K supplements.

Life Span and Gender

Patients with vitamin K deficiency experience decreased synthesis of normal clotting factors and are at greater risk for hemorrhage if they receive warfarin. Because vitamin K is continually produced in the GI tract, deficiencies are rare in healthy adults. Newborns, however, may have a vitamin K deficiency because intestinal flora is not active at birth. Warfarin should not be used during pregnancy and is in FDA pregnancy category X because it is associated with a described syndrome of fetal defects; therefore, it is important to determine the stage of the reproductive cycle for women.

Consider the patient's age before therapy begins. Bleeding complications with anticoagulant drugs appear to occur more frequently in older adults (those older than 75 years) than in younger adults. Older adults also have an increased sensitivity to the effects of warfarin, in both the early induction phase and the maintenance phase of drug therapy.

Lifestyle, Diet, and Habits

Obtain information about the patient's dietary habits. Because vitamin K competes with warfarin, high vitamin K levels decrease the effectiveness of warfarin. Diets rich in vitamin K, therefore, should be avoided. If the diet was normally rich in vitamin K when the warfarin dosage was adjusted, restricting these foods is not as important. However, if the patient's diet does not normally include vitamin K–rich foods, these foods should be avoided. Consider lifestyle behaviors that place the patient taking heparin at increased risk for falls and injuries for the patient taking warfarin, as well. Many herbal medications interact with warfarin: assess for their use.

Environment

Be aware that warfarin therapy may be started in the hospital, but most treatment is self-administered by the patient at home. Explore with the patient potential risks in the home environment.

Nursing Diagnosis and Outcome

- Risk for Injury, Bleeding, related to adverse effects of warfarin
  Desired outcome: *The patient will not experience bleeding.*

Planning and Intervention

Maximizing Therapeutic Effects

Warfarin dosage should be individualized until PT or the INR is in therapeutic range. An initial loading dose is given to attain a rapid therapeutic level. This dose is then followed by a maintenance dose. Doses are usually given in the evening at 6:00 PM. This timing allows for early morning blood draws for PT or INR by hospital laboratory personnel.

Minimizing Adverse Effects

The patient's response to warfarin therapy is measured by using either the ratio of the patient's PT compared with the control PT, or the INR. The prescriber needs to be notified if the patient's clotting time is greater than the therapeutic level. Usually, drug dosage will be decreased if clotting time exceeds this level. Skipping one dose may be all that is required to lower the PT to the therapeutic level. In case of

TABLE 31.3 Agents That Interact With P Warfarin

Interactants	Effect and Significance	Nursing Management
acetaminophen, androgens, beta blockers, clofibrate, corticosteroids, cyclophosphamide, dextrothyroxine, disulfiram, erythromycin, fluconazole, gemfibrozil, glucagon, hydantoins, influenza virus vaccine, isoniazid, ketoconazole, miconazole, moricizine, propoxyphene, quinolones, sulfonamides, tamoxifen, thioamines, thyroid hormones, urokinase	They may increase the effect of warfarin by unknown or complicated mechanism, increasing risk of bleeding.	Monitor for bleeding carefully. Monitor PT or INR carefully. Anticipate dose adjustments of warfarin if these drugs are started after titrating the dose of warfarin.
amiodarone, chloramphenicol, cimetidine, ifosfamide, lovastatin, metronidazole, omeprazole, phenylbutazones, propafenone, quinidine, quinine, sulfamethoxazole-trimethoprim (SMZ-TMP), sulfinpyrazone	The effect of warfarin may be increased by inhibiting its metabolism, increasing the risk of bleeding.	Same as above.
chloral hydrate, loop diuretics, nalidixic acid	The effect of warfarin may be increased because of displacement from binding sites, increasing the risk of bleeding.	Same as above.
aminoglycosides, mineral oil, tetracyclines, vitamin E	The effect of warfarin may be increased because of interference with vitamin K, increasing the risk of bleeding.	Same as above.
cephalosporins, diflunisal, NSAIDs, penicillins, salicylate	The effect of warfarin may be increased because of effects on platelets and GI irritation (from NSAIDs), increasing the risk of bleeding.	Avoid administering NSAIDs and salicylates if possible. Other considerations are the same as above.
ascorbic acid, dicloxacillin, ethanol, ethchlorvynol, griseofulvin, nafcillin, sucralfate, trazodone	The effect of warfarin may be decreased by an unknown action.	Be aware that dose of warfarin may need to be adjusted to be in therapeutic range. Monitor PT or INR to assess drug effectiveness.
aminoglutethimide, barbiturates, etretinate, carbamazepine, glutethimide, rifampin	The effect of warfarin may be decreased by induction of the anticoagulant's hepatic microsomal enzymes.	Avoid variation in vitamin K–rich food after titrating warfarin dose. Vitamin K is considered antidote to warfarin. Otherwise nursing considerations are the same as above.
cholestyramine, contraceptives, oral estrogens, thiazide diuretics, thiopurines, spironolactone, vitamin K	The effect of warfarin may be decreased by various mechanisms.	Same as above.

warfarin overdose, the antidote, vitamin K (phytonadione), is administered.

Falls may cause internal bleeding. The patient's home should be assessed for factors that may lead to falls. Encourage the use of proper lighting and handrails on stairways, which may help prevent falls.

Providing Patient and Family Education

- Teach the patient signs of bleeding and methods to prevent bleeding (which are the same as for heparin).
- Instruct the patient to take the drug at the same time each day because this dosing schedule helps prevent a drop in warfarin blood levels. After the drug level is stabilized and daily PT is not needed, the patient may switch to morning dosing. Doing so may increase absorption and improve adherence to drug therapy. The patient should be advised to return for follow-up blood work.
- Teach the patient that skipping a dose of warfarin could alter therapeutic levels. If patients forget a dose, they should take it as soon as they remember. However, they should not double up on the next dose to prevent bleeding.
- Instruct the patient that taking aspirin, large doses of acetaminophen, or other over-the-counter drugs with these ingredients can affect warfarin's action.
- Warn women to avoid becoming pregnant while on this drug.

TABLE 31.4 Interactions of Herbs and Warfarin*

Effect	Herbs
Increase the effects of warfarin	Boldo, bromelains, dan shen, dong quai (*Angelica sinensis*), garlic, ginkgo (*Ginkgo biloba*), *Lycium barbarum* L
Decrease the effects of warfarin	Coenzyme Q_{10}, green tea, ginseng (*Panax*), St. John's wort
Additive bleeding effects with warfarin	Herbs with potential anticoagulant effects:
	Alfalfa, dong quai (*Angelica sinensis*), aniseed, arnica, asafoetida, bladder wrack (*Fucus*), bogbean, boldo, buchu, capsicum, cassia, celery, chamomile (German and Roman), dandelion, fenugreek, horse chestnut, horseradish, licorice, meadowsweet, nettle, parsley, passion flower, pau d'arco, prickly ash (Northern), quassia, red clover, sweet clover, sweet woodruff, tonka beans, wild carrot, wild lettuce
	Herbs that contain salicylate or have antiplatelet properties:
	Agrimony, aloe gel, aspen, black cohosh, black haw, bogbean, cassia, clove, dandelion, feverfew, garlic, German sarsaparilla, ginger, ginkgo (*Ginkgo biloba*), ginseng (*Panax*), licorice, meadowsweet, onion, policosanol, poplar, senega, tamarind, willow, wintergreen
	Herbs with fibrinolytic properties:
	Bromelains, capsicum, garlic, ginseng (*Panax*), inositol nicotinate, onion
May decrease the effectiveness of warfarin	Herbs with coagulant properties:
	Agrimony, goldenseal, mistletoe, yarrow

*Other herbal interactions are possible.

- Dietary teaching should focus on the need to avoid increased intake of foods rich in vitamin K, primarily green vegetables.
- Emphasize the importance of informing other health care providers (e.g., dentist, podiatrist) that they are taking warfarin. Patients should also be instructed to wear or carry medical identification stating that they are receiving warfarin.

Ongoing Assessment and Evaluation

To determine the therapeutic effects of warfarin, the patient's PT or INR is monitored. Therapy is effective when a thrombus is prevented and bleeding does not occur (Box 31.3).

CRITICAL THINKING SCENARIO

Solving problems related to anticoagulant therapy

Melanie Graves is diagnosed with a left leg deep vein thrombosis (DVT). She is started on heparin 1,000 U/h by intravenous infusion. After 3 days, she will start taking warfarin in addition to the heparin.

1. Explain the rationale for starting warfarin while the patient is receiving heparin. Three days have passed. The first dose of warfarin (5 mg) is given at 6 pm. The following morning, blood is drawn to evaluate the PT. The control is 30 seconds, Ms. Graves' PT is 30 seconds, and the INR is 1.
2. Discuss the information about the dosage of the warfarin that can be obtained from this initial blood work. Explain how you arrived at this conclusion.

Ms. Graves complains that she doesn't like having her blood drawn so frequently. She says she cannot wait to go home so that she does not have to have any more blood work.

3. What elements will you develop in the initial teaching plan for her?

C ANTIPLATELET DRUGS

Drugs that prevent platelet aggregation are called antiplatelet drugs. They are used when overactive platelets pose long-term risks for hypercoagulability. The drugs differ in their modes of action and adverse effects. Although aspirin may be the most frequently prescribed antiplatelet drug, it is also used frequently for other clinical reasons. It is a prototype nonsteroidal anti-inflammatory drug (NSAID) and is discussed in Chapter 24. Ticlopidine was previously identified as the prototype antiplatelet, but clopidogrel has replaced it because it has fewer adverse effects and is now more widely used.

NURSING MANAGEMENT OF THE PATIENT RECEIVING P CLOPIDOGREL

Core Drug Knowledge

Pharmacotherapeutics

Clopidogrel is used to reduce the occurrence of atherosclerotic events (MI, stroke, and vascular death) in patients who have atherosclerosis and have had a recent MI or stroke, or who risk having one of these events because they have peripheral arterial disease. It is also used for medical management of patients with acute coronary syndrome and for those undergoing percutaneous coronary intervention (PCI) or coronary artery bypass graft (CABG).

Pharmacokinetics

Clopidogrel is rapidly absorbed by the GI tract. At least 50% is absorbed. The bioavailability is not changed from food. The drug is metabolized in the liver to an active form and then eliminated by the kidneys and GI tract. The drug

FOCUS ON RESEARCH

Box 31.3 How Chronic Conditions and Drug Therapies Affect Older Adults' Risk for Car Accidents

McGwin, G. Jr., Sims, R. V., Pulley, L., et al. (2000). Relations among chronic medical conditions, medications, and automobile crashes in the elderly: A population-based case-control study. *American Journal of Epidemiology, 152*(5), 424–431.

The Study

Older drivers are known to have elevated crash rates and are more likely to be injured or die if they are involved in a crash. This study sought to identify medications and chronic conditions that are associated with a risk for at-fault crashes in older drivers. One study examined 901 drivers 65 years or older who were selected in a population-based case-controlled study in 1996 from Alabama Department of Public Safety driving records. More than half (497) had not been in car accidents. The rest had been involved in crashes; 244 were found at fault in the accident. Older drivers with heart disease or a history of stroke were more likely to be in car crashes and be the at-fault driver than older drivers without heart disease or stroke history. Women with arthritis were also more likely to be found at fault in car crashes. Drug therapies in older adults associated with an increased risk for being at fault in a car crash included nonsteroidal anti-inflammatory drugs, angiotensin-converting enzyme inhibitors, benzodiazepines, and anticoagulants. Calcium channel blockers and vasodilators were associated with a reduced risk for crash involvement.

Nursing Implications

Patient education about factors that increase the risk for car crashes has relevance for improving the health and safety of older adults. Caution older patients that certain chronic conditions or drug therapies may increase their risk for having a car crash. It is not clear yet exactly how these factors are related to increasing the risk for car crashes. More research is needed in this area.

MEMORY CHIP

P Warfarin

- Anticoagulant used to complete treatment with heparin after clot formation; is used prophylactically in patients at high risk of thrombus formation
- Administered orally
- May be given with heparin until therapeutic level of warfarin is obtained
- Major contraindications: active bleeding, ulcerations of the GI tract, or bleeding disorders
- Most common adverse effect: bleeding (vitamin K is the antidote for warfarin toxicity)
- Most serious adverse effect: fetal warfarin syndrome
- **Life span alert: Warfarin is not for use in pregnancy because it causes fetal defects.**
- Maximizing therapeutic effects: Monitor PT for therapeutic range; adjust dosage until therapeutic range is attained.
- Minimizing adverse effects: Monitor for signs of bleeding.
- Most important patient education: Teach patients to monitor for bleeding, modify behavior to avoid injuries, and to avoid greatly increased vitamin K intake.

and metabolite are both highly protein bound. Steady state occurs between 3 and 7 days with daily dosing. Platelet aggregation and bleeding time gradually return to baseline levels generally within 5 days after drug therapy is stopped. For more information, see Table 31.1.

Pharmacodynamics

Clopidogrel inhibits the binding of adenosine diphosphate (ADP) to its platelet receptor and the subsequent ADP-mediated activation of the glycoprotein IIb/IIIa complex and thus inhibits platelet aggregation. It thus prolongs the bleeding time. Clopidogrel must be metabolized to an active metabolite to produce this effect, although the active metabolite has not been isolated. This effect is thought to be mediated by the CYP3A4 isoenzyme. Clopidogrel irreversibly modifies the platelet ADP receptor so that platelets exposed to the drug are affected for the remainder of their life span. The inhibition of platelet aggregation is dose dependent, and effects can be seen within 2 hours after a single oral dose of clopidogrel. By the time the drug is at steady state, the average inhibition of platelet aggregation is between 40% and 60% of normal.

Contraindications and Precautions

Clopidogrel is contraindicated in patients with hypersensitivity and in those with active bleeding disorders such as peptic ulcers or intracranial hemorrhage. Caution should be used when administering clopidogrel to patients with severe hepatic dysfunction because knowledge regarding the effects on such patients is limited. Caution should be used if the patient is at risk for increased bleeding from trauma, surgery, or other pathologic conditions. Assigned to pregnancy risk category B, clopidogrel should be used only if absolutely necessary during pregnancy. The drug is not recommended for use in breast-feeding mothers; it is not known whether the drug is excreted in breast milk.

Adverse Effects

Adverse reactions to clopidogrel are similar to aspirin. The most common adverse effect is GI distress, which can include abdominal pain, indigestion, diarrhea, nausea, GI bleeding, and ulcers. Clopidogrel is similar in chemical structure to ticlopidine, which is associated with a small (0.8%) risk for severe neutropenia. Clopidogrel appears to have a much smaller risk than ticlopidine for producing severe neutropenia. The possibility of neutropenia should be considered if the patient develops a fever or other sign of infection while taking clopidogrel.

Drug Interactions

At high concentrations in laboratory studies, clopidogrel inhibits the hepatic isoenzyme P-450 2C9. A drug interaction is possible whereby clopidogrel interferes with the metabolism of drugs metabolized through this pathway, such as phenytoin, tamoxifen, tolbutamide, warfarin, torsemide, fluvastatin, and many NSAIDs. Because the exact reaction cannot be predicted, the patient should be observed for potential changes in drug efficacy if any of these drugs are coadministered with clopidogrel. Because clopidogrel increases bleeding risk, especially from GI ulcers, caution should be used if clopidogrel is coadministered with other drugs that can cause GI ulcers and bleeding, such as aspirin or NSAIDs, because additive effects are likely.

Because the active metabolite of clopidogrel is mediated by the CYP3A4 isoenzyme system, drug–drug interactions could theoretically occur with drugs that inhibit or induce CYP3A4. Additionally, clopidogrel may interact with numerous herbs. Patients taking herbal remedies or multiple prescription drugs should be monitored closely for either toxic or subtherapeutic effects of clopidogrel.

Assessment of Relevant Core Patient Variables

Health Status

Review the patient's history and physical examination for any contraindications to the use of this drug. The patient should have a baseline complete blood count (CBC) with differential to determine platelet functioning. Liver function studies should also be done. A baseline cardiovascular assessment is indicated when starting therapy. Neurologic status should also be assessed when clopidogrel is given to prevent stroke.

Life Span and Gender

Determine the patient's age before therapy begins. Caution must be used in children younger than 18 years because safety has not been established. The exact effects of clopidogrel on pregnancy and lactation are not known, and caution must be used. In older adults, no differences in platelet aggregation and bleeding time have been noted; thus, no dosage adjustment is needed.

Lifestyle, Diet, and Habits

Lifestyle behaviors that would place the patient at increased risk for bleeding while taking this drug should be discussed with the patient. Because patients take clopidogrel to decrease the risk for atherosclerotic events (such as MI and stroke), assess whether the patient is following a heart-healthy diet that is low in fat and cholesterol.

Environment

Be aware of the environment in which the drug will be administered. Clopidogrel may be administered in the hospital. However, most of the time, it is self-administered by the patient at home. Discuss with the patient potential risks in the home environment. Falls and activities that are likely to produce internal or external bleeding should be avoided while taking clopidogrel.

Nursing Diagnoses and Outcomes

- Risk for Injury: Increased Risk for Bleeding related to decreased platelet aggregation from drug therapy
  Desired outcome: *The patient will suffer no injury related to bleeding while on clopidogrel.*
- Risk for Nausea related to adverse effects of clopidogrel.
  Desired outcome: *Nausea and GI distress will not be extreme enough to warrant stopping clopidogrel therapy.*

Planning and Intervention

Maximizing Therapeutic Effects

Clopidogrel should be administered routinely to achieve its maximum therapeutic effects.

Minimizing Adverse Effects

Clopidogrel can be taken with food to decrease GI problems if they occur. The home environment should be assessed for safety hazards that may contribute to falls or other accidents. Remember that severe neutropenia is a potential risk, and evaluate patient's white blood cell count if the patient develops signs of infection.

Providing Patient and Family Education

- Inform patients and families about laboratory tests that are needed on a regular basis and the reasons for their frequency.
- Emphasize to patients and families the importance of informing all health care providers (e.g., dentists and other physicians) of the drug regimen. If surgery is needed, and the antiplatelet effect is not desired, drug therapy should be discontinued 7 days before the procedure to prevent excessive bleeding.
- Instruct patients and families to apply pressure on wounds until bleeding stops.
- Emphasize to the patient that behaviors that may lead to injury should be avoided (e.g., roller-blading, ice skating, motorcycle riding, use of nonmotorized scooters, walking on icy patches).
- Instruct patients and families to make the home environment more "fall proof" by removing scatter rugs, placing handrails on stairs, and fastening any loose carpet edges.

Ongoing Assessment and Evaluation

Periodic measurement of bleeding time and platelet function is needed throughout therapy. Neutrophil counts should be assessed if the patient develops signs of infection to rule out severe neutropenia. Therapy is evaluated as effective when the outcomes are achieved and atherosclerotic events have been prevented.

MEMORY CHIP

P Clopidogrel

- Used to prevent atherosclerotic events in patients who have had myocardial infarction or stroke, or who are at risk for having these events
- Prevents platelet aggregation and prolongs bleeding time
- Major contraindication: active bleeding disorders
- Most common adverse effects: GI distress
- Most serious adverse effect: neutropenia
- Maximizing therapeutic effects: Administer regularly.
- Minimizing adverse effects: Take with food to decrease GI distress; assess for risk for falls and injuries.
- Most important patient education: Avoid activities that increase risk for falls or injury, remove scatter rugs or other hazards that may contribute to falls in the home; apply pressure to any bleeding cut.

Drug Closely Related to P Clopidogrel

Aspirin

Aspirin, a drug used for its antiplatelet properties, has a mechanism of action that differs from that of clopidogrel in that it irreversibly inhibits platelet cyclo-oxygenase and the subsequent synthesis of thromboxane A_2 for the life of the platelet. Thromboxane A_2 is a vasoconstrictor that facilitates platelet aggregation. Inhibiting its synthesis, therefore, inhibits platelet aggregation. Aspirin is recommended to be given within 24 to 48 hours of the onset of a stroke. It is not recommended to use aspirin concurrently or within 24 hours of the use of thrombolytic agents, such as alteplase (Adams et al., 2003). Aspirin is also used to decrease the incidence of coronary heart disease in adults who are at increased risk for heart disease. Men older than 40 years, postmenopausal women, and younger adults with risk factors for coronary heart disease (hypertension, diabetes, smoking, elevated lipid levels, obesity, family history) are examples of patients who should be considered for cardiac preventive therapy with aspirin (Berg et al., 2002). Aspirin is used in prophylaxis against thromboembolic complications in cardiovascular disease, including MI and transient ischemic attack (TIA). Aspirin in low doses is recommended after MI to prevent future infarcts, and in patients with atrial fibrillation to prevent stroke. Aspirin has been found to be an effective prophylactic treatment against stroke in patients with atrial fibrillation, unless strong risk factors are present, in which case warfarin would be used instead. Aspirin prevents noncardioembolic strokes primarily. One third of patients with atrial fibrillation are at low risk for stroke and should be treated with aspirin (Hart et al., 2003). In diabetic patients, low-dose aspirin is a primary prevention therapy if the patient has cardiovascular risk factors (family history of coronary heart disease, cigarette smoking, hypertension, obesity, albuminuria, elevated lipid levels, and age older than 30 years). Aspirin is a secondary prevention strategy in patients with diabetes with large vessel disease; indications would include history of MI, vascular bypass surgery, stroke or TIAs, peripheral vascular disease, claudication, angina, or any combination of these factors (American Diabetic Association, 2003). A major adverse effect of aspirin is its ability to cause GI bleeding, and it may increase the risk for hemorrhagic stroke. These adverse effects may limit the use of aspirin in some patients. Aspirin may pose a risk for neutropenia, but compared with clopidogrel, aspirin poses a much smaller risk for this complication. For more information on aspirin, see Chapter 24.

Cilostazol

Cilostazol (Pletal) is a platelet aggregation inhibitor with vasodilating activity. It is used to treat the symptoms of intermittent claudication. Intermittent claudication occurs in about one third of patients who have peripheral arterial disease. Cilostazol improves pain-free walking distance. In addition to its antiplatelet activity, cilostazol also decreases triglycerides and increases high-density lipoprotein cholesterol. Cilostazol is contraindicated for use in patients with congestive heart failure (CHF), acute MI, or severe renal impairment. Cilostazol is extensively metabolized in the liver by the CYP3A4 and, to a lesser extent, CYP2C19 isoenzymes; thus, potential drug–drug interactions are similar to those of clopidogrel. Cilostazol is a pregnancy category C drug. Breast-feeding should be ceased during cilostazol therapy, to avoid potential harm to the infant.

Drugs Significantly Different From P Clopidogrel

Dipyridamole

Unlike clopidogrel, dipyridamole is primarily a coronary vasodilator that increases functional levels of adenosine, which produces vasodilation. It also inhibits the enzyme phosphodiesterase, which increases cyclic adenosine monophosphate (cAMP). Although the substance cAMP is another coronary vasodilator, it also has an antiplatelet effect. Dipyridamole dilates coronary arteries, increasing flow in narrowed vessels. It does not usually produce much systemic vasodilation. A mild positive inotropic effect has also been documented.

Dipyridamole is used with anticoagulants and other antiplatelets in patients after surgery, such as prosthetic heart valve placement and vascular grafting procedures, to prevent thrombus formation. Investigational uses include post-MI treatment and prevention of TIAs. It is used diagnostically during thallium myocardial perfusion imaging. Dipyridamole has not been found to reduce the risk for vascular death in patients with arterial vascular disease, although it may reduce the risk for further vascular events (De Schryver et al., 2003).

Dipyridamole is moderately absorbed after oral administration. Its distribution is widespread, crossing the placenta and entering breast milk. It is metabolized in the liver and excreted by the GI tract. It should be used cautiously in patients with hypotension because some vasodilation occurs.

The most frequent adverse effects are headache, dizziness, and nausea. After IV administration, MI, arrhythmias, and bronchospasm may occur, although they are uncommon.

Dipyridamole has additive effects on platelet aggregation when given with aspirin. Bleeding risk is increased when dipyridamole is used concurrently with anticoagulants, thrombolytics, NSAIDs, or sulfinpyrazone. Ingesting alcohol increases the risk for hypotension. Theophylline may negate the effects of dipyridamole during diagnostic thallium imaging.

Glycoprotein IIb/IIIa Inhibitors

Tirofiban (Aggrastat), eptifibatide (Integrilin), and abciximab (ReoPro) are all antagonists of the platelet glycoprotein IIb/IIIa receptor, the major platelet surface receptor involved in platelet aggregation. This receptor is found only on platelets and their progenitors. Activation of the glycoprotein IIb/IIIa receptors leads to the binding of fibrinogen and von Willebrand factor to platelets and thus to platelet aggregation. Tirofiban and eptifibatide reversibly prevent fibrinogen and von Willebrand factor from binding to the glycoprotein IIb/IIIa receptor, thereby inhibiting platelet aggregation. Both tirofiban and eptifibatide are used in treating acute coronary syndrome (unstable angina or non–Q-wave MI), and they have been found to be safe and effective when combined with the low-molecular-weight heparin, enoxaparin, for this purpose (Ferguson et al., 2003; Mukherjee et al., 2002). Tirofiban may also be used in patients undergoing percutaneous transluminal coronary angioplasty; eptifibatide may also be used in treating patients undergoing

percutaneous coronary intervention. Both of these drugs are administered by IV infusion.

One difference between these two drugs is their rate of ability to bind with protein in the blood. Tirofiban is moderately protein bound (65%), whereas eptifibatide has low protein binding (25%).

Contraindications for the two drugs are the same and include active internal bleeding or a history of bleeding within the last 30 days; a history of thrombocytopenia following a prior exposure to tirofiban; history of stroke within 30 days or any history of hemorrhagic stroke; a major surgical procedure or severe physical trauma within the last 30 days; severe hypertension; concomitant use of another parenteral glycoprotein IIb/IIIa inhibitor; any history of intracranial hemorrhage, intracranial neoplasm, arteriovenous malformation, or aneurysm; history, symptoms or findings suggestive of aortic dissection, acute pericarditis; platelet counts less than 1,000,000/mm^3; a serum creatinine level of 2 mg/dL or higher; or dependency on renal dialysis.

The most frequent adverse effect for both tirofiban and eptifibatide is bleeding, which can be a minor or major event. Nonbleeding adverse effects for tirofiban (when coadministered with heparin) include nausea, fever, and headache. The only nonbleeding adverse effect of eptifibatide is hypotension, which may be serious.

Abciximab is used as adjunct to percutaneous transluminal coronary angioplasty or atherectomy, to prevent acute cardiac ischemic complications in patients at high risk for abrupt closure of the treated coronary vessel. It is used with aspirin and heparin. Like tirofiban and eptifibatide, bleeding is the major adverse effect of abciximab.

Anagrelide

Anagrelide (Agrylin) is another antiplatelet agent that is significantly different from clopidogrel. It is used in treating essential thrombocythemia (ET) to reduce the elevated platelet count and the risk for thrombosis and to reduce the associated symptoms of the disorder. Exactly how anagrelide reduces platelet counts is unknown at this time. It is hypothesized that dose-related reduction in platelet production results from a decrease in megakaryocyte hypermaturation. White blood cell counts and other coagulation factors are not affected. RBC counts may be altered, but these alterations are not clinically important. The most common adverse effects of anagrelide are headache, diarrhea, edema, palpitations, and abdominal pain. Serious potential adverse effects include CHF, MI, cardiomyopathy, cardiomegaly, complete heart block, atrial fibrillation, CVA, pericarditis, pulmonary infiltrates, pulmonary fibrosis, pulmonary hypertension, pancreatitis, gastric or duodenal ulcers, and seizures. None of these serious adverse effects is common.

G HEMORHEOLOGIC DRUGS

The hemorheologic drugs differ from the antiplatelet drugs in that they act on RBCs to reduce blood viscosity and increase the flexibility of RBCs. This effect helps to prevent thrombus formation and allows the RBCs to enter the microcirculation, thereby increasing oxygenation at the cellular level. These effects are helpful in treating peripheral vascular disease. The prototype hemorheologic drug is pentoxifylline.

NURSING MANAGEMENT OF THE PATIENT RECEIVING P PENTOXIFYLLINE

Core Drug Knowledge

Pharmacotherapeutics

Pentoxifylline is used to manage the symptoms of intermittent claudication from peripheral vascular disease. Using this drug improves the patient's ability to walk for longer distances without pain. It has also been used to treat acute and chronic cerebral vascular disease because it improves the psychopathologic symptoms. Unlabeled uses include treating diabetic angiopathies, neuropathies, TIAs, chronic leg ulcers, Raynaud disease, and disorders of the circulation of the eye (see Table 31.1).

Pharmacokinetics

Pentoxifylline is absorbed readily from the GI tract. It undergoes first-pass effect in the liver with about 50% of the drug remaining. It is widely distributed. Onset of therapeutic effects takes 2 to 4 weeks. Full therapeutic effects are not evident, however, until 4 to 8 weeks after therapy starts. The drug is metabolized by RBCs and the liver and is excreted in urine.

Pharmacodynamics

Pentoxifylline increases the flexibility of RBCs by increasing cAMP levels. In turn, this effect decreases platelet aggregation and promotes vasodilation. Blood fibrinogen concentration is lowered. In addition, the drug increases cellular adenosine triphosphate levels, which stabilizes the cell membrane and reduces the RBC aggregation, thus lowering blood viscosity (see Table 31.1).

Contraindications and Precautions

Because pentoxifylline is derived from the methylxanthines (caffeine and theophylline), it is contraindicated in patients who have an intolerance to it or to the methylxanthines. Patients with impaired renal function may require a reduced dose to prevent toxicity. Pentoxifylline should be used cautiously in pregnant or nursing women. The drug is in pregnancy risk category C and is excreted in breast milk. Caution should also be used in children younger than 18 years because safety has not been established. Pentoxifylline should also be used with caution in patients with coronary artery or cardiovascular disease, such as angina, arrhythmias, or severe hypotension.

Adverse Effects

Pentoxifylline's adverse effects occur primarily in the central nervous, cardiovascular, and GI systems. The effects on these systems may result from this drug's similarity to caffeine and theophylline.

Headache, dizziness, tremor, dyspepsia, nausea, and vomiting are all common adverse effects. Other adverse effects can occur occasionally. These effects include agitation, nervousness, insomnia, angina, chest pain, arrhythmia, tachycardia, edema, hypotension, abdominal discomfort, bloating, belching, flatus, diarrhea, blurred vision, epistaxis, bad taste, rash, urticaria, pruritus, and brittle fingernails.

Drug Interactions

There may be an increased risk for bleeding when pentoxifylline is given with warfarin. Risk for theophylline toxicity may increase as well because pentoxifylline is a methylxanthine like theophylline. Smoking may decrease the effect of pentoxifylline. When caring for patients receiving pentoxifylline and warfarin, monitor PT and INR values carefully.

Assessment of Relevant Core Patient Variables

Health Status

Determine whether the patient is hypersensitive to the drug or to methylxanthines before beginning therapy. Assess the patient's baseline walking tolerance, circulation, and pulses in the affected extremities. Ask the patient to describe any pain experienced with activity and the effect of rest on the pain.

Life Span and Gender

Determine whether the patient is pregnant or breast-feeding.

Lifestyle, Diet, and Habits

Find out whether the patient smokes tobacco. Usual patterns of exercise and activity should be compared with desired level of exercise and activity.

Environment

Be aware that pentoxifylline is generally self-administered in the home, although it may also be administered in the hospital. Discuss potential risks in the home environment with the patient.

Nursing Diagnosis and Outcome

- Risk for Injury related to adverse pentoxifylline effects (dizziness, drowsiness, blurred vision)
  Desired outcome: The patient will remain injury free while on pentoxifylline.

Planning and Intervention

Maximizing Therapeutic Effects

Pentoxifylline must be taken for several weeks before the full therapeutic effects are evident.

Minimizing Adverse Effects

Pentoxifylline may be given with food to minimize GI upset.

Providing Patient and Family Education

- Inform patients that pentoxifylline does not have an immediate effect and that they should not stop taking the drug before the therapeutic effects are achieved.
- Instruct patients to avoid driving or operating machinery until it is known whether dizziness or blurred vision will occur from the drug. If these problems continue after the initial phase of drug therapy, the prescriber should be contacted in case the dosage needs to be decreased.
- Advise patients not to smoke because smoking constricts the blood vessels.
- Instruct patients to keep all follow-up visits with the prescriber.

Ongoing Assessment and Evaluation

Peripheral circulation should be reassessed periodically to measure improvement. Throughout pentoxifylline therapy, the patient's exercise tolerance should be assessed, with improvement being noted over time if therapy is effective. For patients also taking antihypertensive drugs, blood pressure should be monitored throughout therapy.

C THROMBOLYTIC DRUGS

Thrombolytic drugs assist in breaking down formed blood clots. These drugs are used for patients who are diagnosed with an evolving, acute MI; a pulmonary embolism; or acute ischemic stroke. They may also be given to unclog central venous catheters. These drugs may be given systemically or directly at the site of the blood clot. Although these drugs are given during emergency situations and can save lives, their adverse effects can be life threatening. Therefore, these drugs should be administered by clinicians who are familiar with them and skilled in using them. Patients receiving these drugs need to be monitored carefully for adverse effects. The prototype of the thrombolytic drugs is alteplase, recombinant (Activase). A review of the research indicates that alteplase, recombinant is associated with more benefit and less risk for adverse effects than other thrombolytic therapies (Wardlaw et al., 2003). Other drugs in this class, the tissue plasminogen activators, are reteplase, recombinant (Retavase) and tenecteplase (TNKase). Drugs closely related to alteplase, recombinant, are drotrecogin alfa (activated) (Xigris), streptokinase (Streptase), urokinase (Abbokinase), and anistreplase (Eminase).

NURSING MANAGEMENT OF THE PATIENT RECEIVING [P] ALTEPLASE, RECOMBINANT

Core Drug Knowledge

Pharmacotherapeutics

Alteplase, recombinant is indicated in a number of thromboembolic conditions considered medical emergencies, for example, acute evolving MI from an acute coronary artery

MEMORY CHIP

[P] Pentoxifylline

- Hemorheologic agent that reduces blood viscosity and increases flexibility of red blood cells
- Used to manage symptoms of intermittent claudication
- Needs to be taken for several weeks before full therapeutic effect is seen
- Major contraindication: sensitivity to methylxanthines
- Most common adverse effects: headache, dizziness, tremor, dyspepsia, nausea, and vomiting
- Most serious adverse effect: tachycardia

thrombus. Therapy for this condition is most effective when it is initiated as soon as possible after the onset of symptoms. Alteplase, recombinant is also indicated to treat acute ischemic stroke. It is the only drug therapy approved for treating ischemic stroke. Treatment must be initiated within 3 hours after the onset of stroke and after intracranial bleeding (hemorrhagic stroke) has been ruled out by a computed tomography (CT) scan. Box 31.4 describes management of patients who are receiving alteplase, recombinant, for ischemic stroke. Patients should be at least 18 years old and have a clinical diagnosis of stroke with clinically meaningful neurologic deficit to receive this drug after ischemic stroke. Alteplase, recombinant is also indicated to treat massive pulmonary embolism (PE). For these uses, alteplase, recombinant is administered by IV infusion. Unlabeled uses for alteplase, recombinant are treating unstable angina to provide coronary thrombolysis and reduce ischemic events; clearing clots that have formed in central venous catheters; treating small vessels occluded by microthrombi; managing peripheral arterial thromboemboli; and restoring blood flow to frostbitten limbs. Low doses are used for all of these indications (see Table 31.1).

Pharmacokinetics

Alteplase is infused intravenously so that distribution begins immediately. Steady state is higher if accelerated infusion of alteplase is used. Alteplase is rapidly cleared from the plasma, primarily by the liver. About 80% of the drug is cleared within 10 minutes after the infusion has completed (see Table 31.1).

Pharmacodynamics

Alteplase, recombinant is a tissue plasminogen activator (tPA) synthesized by recombinant DNA technology. It acts in the same way as endogenous tPA. Alteplase, recombinant is actually an enzyme that, when fibrin is present, converts plasminogen to plasmin. It has limited effect if fibrin is not present. When administered, alteplase, recombinant binds to the fibrin in a clot and converts the trapped plasminogen to plasmin. Fibrinolysis, or break down of the clot, then occurs.

Contraindications and Precautions

Alteplase, recombinant should be used only in clinical settings where hematologic function and clinical response can be adequately monitored. It should be administered by a clinician with experience and knowledge in treating the thromboembolic disorders.

Contraindications to the use of alteplase include active internal bleeding, evidence of intracranial bleeding on pretreatment evaluation; suspicion of subarachnoid hemorrhage; recent (within the last 2 months) stroke; intracranial surgery or severe head trauma; intraspinal surgery or trauma; intracranial neoplasm; seizure at onset of stroke; arteriovenous malformation or aneurysm; conditions (including other prescribed drug therapy) that makes the patient likely to bleed; and severe uncontrolled hypertension (systolic blood pressure, ≥180 mmHg; or diastolic blood pressure ≥110 mmHg).

Risks of alteplase, recombinant therapy, when used to treat acute ischemic stroke, may be increased if the patient has severe neurologic deficits or major early infarct signs visible in the CT scan (e.g., substantial edema, mass effect of midline shift).

Certain conditions may increase the risk for bleeding from alteplase, recombinant therapy. If any of the following are present, the benefits to the patient must be weighed against this increased risk:

- Recent (≤10 days) major surgery (e.g., CABG, obstetrical delivery, organ biopsy, previous puncture of noncompressible vessels such as internal jugular)
- Cerebrovascular disease
- Recent (≤10 days) GI or genitourinary (GU) bleeding
- Recent (≤10 days) trauma
- Hypertension (systolic blood pressure ≥180 mmHg; diastolic blood pressure ≥110 mmHg)
- Likelihood of left heart thrombus (e.g., mitral stenosis with atrial fibrillation)
- Acute pericarditis
- Subacute bacterial endocarditis
- Hemostatic defects including secondary to severe hepatic or renal disease
- Serious liver dysfunction
- Pregnancy
- Diabetic hemorrhagic retinopathy or other ophthalmic hemorrhaging
- Septic thrombophlebitis or occluded arteriovenous cannula at seriously infected site

BOX 31.4 Management of Patients Receiving Alteplase, Recombinant, for Treatment of Ischemic Stroke

- Infuse 0.9 mg/kg (maximum, 90 mg) over 60 minutes with 10% of the dose given as a bolus over 1 minute.
- Admit the patient to an intensive care unit or stroke unit for monitoring.
- Perform neurologic assessment every 15 minutes during infusion, and every 30 minutes for the next 6 hours, and then every hour until 24 hours from treatment.
- Delay placing nasogastric tubes, indwelling bladder catheters, or intra-arterial pressure catheters.
- If the patient develops severe headache, acute hypertension, nausea, or vomiting, discontinue infusion (if still being administered), and obtain computed tomography scan of brain immediately.
- Monitor blood pressure every 15 minutes for the first 2 hours, every 30 minutes for the next 6 hours, and then every hour until 24 hours after treatment.
- Increase frequency of blood pressure monitoring if systolic is equal to or greater than 180 mm Hg or diastolic is equal to or greater than 105 mm Hg. Administer antihypertensive drug therapy to maintain blood pressure below these levels.
- If diastolic is 105–140 mm Hg or systolic is 180 mm Hg or greater, give IV labetalol, 10 mg over 1 to 2 minutes. Repeat or double the dose every 10 to 20 minutes to a maximum dose of 300 mg. Or, give initial bolus of labetalol followed by continuous IV infusion of 2–8 mg/minute. If this approach does not control blood pressure and diastolic is 121–140 mm Hg or systolic is greater than 230 mm Hg, consider starting nitroprusside infusion.
- If diastolic is greater than 140 mm Hg, start nitroprusside infusion at 0.5 mg/kg/minute.

From Adams, H. P., Adams, R. J., Brott, T., et al. (2003). Guidelines for the early management of patients with ischemic stroke: A scientific statement from the Stroke Council of the American Stroke Association. *Stroke, 34*(4), 1056–1083. Available: *http://www.stroke.ahajournals.org/cgi/reprint/34/4/1056.*

- Older adult (>75 years)
- Currently receiving oral anticoagulants
- Any other condition in which bleeding would pose a major hazard or would be very difficult to manage because of its location

Adverse Effects

Bleeding is the most frequently occurring adverse effect. It can be internal, involving GI, GU, or respiratory tracts or the retroperitoneal or intracranial areas. On the other hand, it can be surface or superficial bleeding at puncture sites (e.g., IV sites or arterial punctures) or surgical incisions. Nausea, vomiting, hypotension, and fever can occur with alteplase use; however, these are common sequela after an MI and therefore may or may not be related to drug therapy. Other adverse effects that are possible with alteplase, although not common, include occasional, mild hypersensitivity reactions; urticaria; fat embolism (which can occur with any thrombolytic); cerebral edema with fatal brain herniation (if administered when ≥3 hours have elapsed since onset of ischemic stroke); and cardiovascular complications (bradycardia, cardiogenic shock, arrhythmias, pulmonary edema, heart failure, cardiac arrest, recurrent ischemic reinfarction, myocardial rupture, mitral regurgitation, pericardial effusion, pericarditis, cardiac tamponade, venous thrombosis and embolism, and electromechanical dissociation).

Drug Interactions

Anticoagulant therapy, such as with heparin or antiplatelet therapy, such as aspirin, increases the risk for bleeding. Aminocaproic acid, an antifibrinolytic agent, decreases the effects of alteplase. Heparin is sometimes used after treatment with alteplase, although this use is not recommended in current guidelines because it increases the risk for bleeding from a drug interaction. Most of the research studies of the coadministration of these therapies have not found significant benefit to outweigh the increased incidence of bleeding. Aspirin therapy may also follow alteplase therapy. The use of heparin or aspirin within 24 hours of alteplase use is not recommended (Adams et al., 2003; Hirsh et al., 2001). The use of nitroglycerin should be avoided during alteplase therapy because it may decrease antithrombotic effects.

Assessment of Relevant Core Patient Variables

Health Status

Assess the patient for conditions that contraindicate administering, or are precautions for administering, alteplase. If the patient has an acute ischemic stroke, confirm that the onset was less than 3 hours ago because this is the recommended time frame for starting alteplase therapy. Laboratory values, such as hematocrit, hemoglobin level, platelet count, PT, and aPTT, can provide baseline clotting information. Assess the patient's skin for old puncture sites or incisions from which bleeding may likely occur during alteplase therapy. Determine whether the patient is receiving or will be receiving other drug therapy that increases the risk for bleeding from alteplase treatment.

Life Span and Gender

When considering life span and gender variables, determine the patient's age and whether pregnancy is an issue. If the patient is currently pregnant or has delivered a child within 10 days, the risk for bleeding with alteplase is increased. Alteplase is a pregnancy category C drug. Assess whether the woman is breast-feeding because it is not known whether alteplase is secreted in breast milk. Safety and efficacy in children have not been established. Although increasing age (>76 years) decreases the benefits received from alteplase therapy, treatment is still effective in reducing death rates from these cardiovascular events. Older adults have an increased risk for intracranial bleeding when they are treated for acute ischemic stroke, but treatment is still beneficial and should be provided. Accelerated infusion of alteplase (within 90 minutes) slightly increases the risk for stroke for older adults.

Environment

Alteplase must be administered in an acute care setting because the patient needs close monitoring.

Nursing Diagnosis and Outcome

- Risk for Injury related to drug-induced bleeding from alteplase
  Desired outcome: *The patient will not suffer injury from alteplase.*

Planning and Intervention

Maximizing Therapeutic Effects

The drug should be reconstituted in sterile water for injection without preservatives. Do not use bacteriostatic water for injection. The reconstituted solution is colorless to pale yellow and transparent. The 50-mg vial is diluted using a large-bore (e.g., 18-gauge) needle. Direct the sterile water without preservatives at the dry drug. The 100-mg vial does not have a vacuum, unlike the 50-mg vial. Use the transfer device provided to reconstitute the alteplase. Mix the drug and diluent by gentle swirling; avoid shaking or excessive agitation. Once reconstituted, it may be administered intravenously, or it may be further diluted in either 0.9% normal saline or 5% dextrose for IV infusion. The drug may be infused by either accelerated infusion, over 90 minutes (current recommended method), or by a 3-hour infusion. Make yourself familiar with the protocol of the institution as to which method is to be used or ensure that the order specifies the preferred administration technique. With both methods, more of the dose is administered in the first part of the infusion. Check the manufacturer's instructions for exact information about drug administration.

Minimizing Adverse Effects

Throughout the time the drug is administered, closely and continually monitor vital signs and observe for signs of active bleeding. Frank bleeding may occur at access sites, such as old intramuscular (IM) injection or arterial puncture sites; or from orifices such as the vagina or rectum. Internal bleeding may be signaled by abdominal pain with coffee grounds–like emesis; black, tarry stools; joint pain; and changes in level of consciousness.

Closely assess for possible bleeding throughout therapy. If it is necessary to perform an arterial puncture during therapy, the site chosen should be one in which external pressure can be applied, such as the femoral artery. A pressure

dressing should be applied to the site and checked carefully for evidence of bleeding. Venipuncture, if it must be done, should be done carefully to prevent bleeding. IM injections and unnecessary handling of patients should be avoided to prevent internal injury while they are receiving alteplase. If bleeding occurs and is not controllable with pressure, the infusion should be stopped and the prescriber notified.

Multiple IV lines are usually indicated to enable administration of the alteplase and other drugs and to provide a route for obtaining blood samples during therapy. These lines should be started before initiating alteplase therapy.

The patient should be connected to a cardiac monitor, both during the treatment and afterward, if alteplase is given as treatment for an MI. Arrhythmias may occur, especially after the clot has dissolved and the heart has been reperfused. Antiarrhythmic therapy should be on hand when starting alteplase therapy. Notify the prescriber if substantial arrhythmias occur.

When therapy is given to treat a pulmonary embolism, monitor respiratory status carefully. Note respiratory rate, dyspnea, pulse oximetry, and arterial blood gas findings in addition to all the assessments described previously.

When alteplase is given to treat acute ischemic stroke, the blood pressure should be monitored closely during therapy. Avoid starting alteplase if 3 hours or more have elapsed from the onset of the stroke because the benefits of treatment during this time frame are not known, and this timing increases the risk for cerebral edema with fatal brain herniation and may increase the risk for cerebral hemorrhage.

Providing Patient and Family Education

- Emphasize to patients and families the need for frequent assessment, pressure dressings, and activity limitations.
- Instruct patients to notify you if they experience signs of adverse reactions.

Ongoing Assessment and Evaluation

Vital signs, evidence of bleeding, and laboratory test results should be assessed throughout therapy as described previously. Therapy is judged effective if the patient sustains no injury or adverse effects of alteplase, the clot dissolves, and circulation is restored.

MEMORY CHIP

P Alteplase, Recombinant

- Used to break up blood clots posing acute medical emergencies such as acute myocardial infarctions, acute ischemic strokes, and pulmonary embolus
- Works by binding to the fibrin in a clot and converting the trapped plasminogen to plasmin. Fibrinolysis then occurs.
- Major contraindications: current internal bleeding, especially intracranial; recent surgeries or medical events in which patient bled or which put patient at increased risk for bleeding now; seizure at onset of stroke; or severe uncontrolled hypertension
- Most common adverse effect: bleeding
- Most serious adverse effect: bleeding
- **Life span alert: Current pregnancy or delivery of a child within the last 10 days increases risk for bleeding; older adults are more likely to have intracranial bleeding.**
- Maximizing therapeutic effects: Avoid vigorous shaking or agitation when reconstituting; administer IV over 90 minutes to 3 hours.
- Minimizing adverse effects: Monitor for bleeding; avoid venipuncture and arterial puncture if possible, use pressure dressings when needed; handle patient gently; when treating ischemic stroke, give within 3 hours of onset of symptoms.
- Most important patient education: need for frequent assessment and limitations on activity

Drugs Closely Related to P Alteplase, Recombinant

Thrombolytic Enzymes: Streptokinase, Urokinase, and Anistreplase

Streptokinase is used in treating acute evolving MI, pulmonary embolism DVT, arterial thrombosis, or embolism, and to open occluded arteriovenous cannulas. Unlike alteplase, which works by attaching to the fibrin in a thrombus and converting the trapped plasminogen to plasmin, streptokinase works indirectly to activate plasminogen. Streptokinase acts with plasminogen to produce an "activator complex" that converts plasminogen to plasmin. Because fibrin is not necessary for streptokinase to activate plasminogen, streptokinase can produce more systemic bleeding than alteplase, recombinant. Allergic reactions are more common in streptokinase than with alteplase because it is not produced from DNA recombinant technology. Fever and chills are the common allergic reactions. Hypotension is also more common in streptokinase and may be severe. Because adverse effects are more common with streptokinase, its use has become more limited, and alteplase, recombinant is the drug most frequently used.

Urokinase is used in treating pulmonary embolism, lysis of coronary artery thrombi, and re-establishing patency of occluded IV catheters. Anistreplase is used in treating acute MI. It has a longer half-life than streptokinase or urokinase, but otherwise possesses similar characteristics.

Drugs Significantly Different From P Alteplase, Recombinant

Drotrecogin Alfa (Activated)

Drotrecogin alfa, activated (Xigris) is an activated protein C used to reduce mortality in adults with severe sepsis who are at high risk for death. It has an antithrombotic effects and works by inhibiting factors Va and VIIIa. It breaks down clots by an indirect method; it inhibits plasminogen activator inhibitor and limits the creation of activated thrombin-fibrinolysis inhibitor. In other words, it prevents processes that are involved in creating stable clots. As an activated protein C, it also has anti-inflammatory effects. As with alteplase, recombinant, bleeding is the most common adverse effect.

C CLOTTING FACTORS

In addition to preventing blood coagulation, drug therapy may also be used to promote coagulation when the patient has a deficiency of normal blood clotting factors. These defi-

ciencies, which are associated with prolonged bleeding and clot formation times, result from an inherited absence of the factor (hemophilia) or from a decreased synthesis of the factor or factors.

Replacement of these factors is the treatment of choice. The prototype drug for this class is antihemophilic factor (AHF). Other drugs in the class include anti-inhibitor coagulant complex and factor IX complex. AHF is from pooled human blood sources. It is screened for hepatitis antibodies and heated to prevent the transmission of hepatitis. Blood donors are screened for human immunodeficiency virus (HIV) as well, and positive sources are screened again. The chance of disease transmission, therefore, still exists but is quite small.

Table 31.5 presents a summary of information about drugs used to treat hypocoagulation.

PATHOPHYSIOLOGY OF HEMOPHILIA

When clotting factors are deficient, blood clotting does not occur in a timely manner. A minor injury or trauma can cause prolonged bleeding, or hemorrhage, either internally or externally. Bleeding may occur into a joint, such as the elbow or knee, and cause serious damage.

Inherited deficiencies of specific clotting factors produce three major hemophilic conditions: hemophilia A (classic hemophilia), hemophilia B (Christmas disease), and von Willebrand disease. Hemophilia A results from lack of factor VIII. Hemophilia B results from lack of factor IX. Hemophilias A and B are transmitted on recessive, sex-linked genes. The genes are carried by women and transmitted to male children. Von Willebrand disease results from deficiency of factor VIII, factor VIII antigen, and von Willebrand factor. It is transmitted by an autosomal dominant gene and inherited by both sexes.

Decreased synthesis of clotting factors is characteristic of diseases that affect the liver, such as cirrhosis and hepatitis, because most clotting factors are produced in the liver. A second cause of decreased synthesis is an absence of vitamin K, which is necessary for the formation of four of the clotting factors: II (prothrombin), VII, IX, and X.

NURSING MANAGEMENT OF THE PATIENT RECEIVING P ANTIHEMOPHILIC FACTOR

Core Drug Knowledge

Pharmacotherapeutics

In patients with a demonstrated deficiency of clotting factor VIII, hemophilia A, AHF is used to prevent and control excessive bleeding. The drug effect is short term because the factor is used up in the clotting process (see Table 31.5).

Pharmacokinetics

Administered intravenously, AHF is totally absorbed. It is rapidly removed from the plasma because it is used in the clotting process. Its half-life is from 4 to 24 hours, with a 12-hour average half-life (see Table 31.5).

Pharmacodynamics

Factor VIII is an essential component of blood clotting. It is required for the conversion of prothrombin to thrombin.

TABLE 31.5 Summary of Selected Drugs for Hypocoagulation

Drug (Trade) Name	Selected Indications	Route and Dosage Range	Pharmacokinetics
P antihemophilic factor (Alphanate, Bioclate, Helixate, Hemofil M, Humate-P, Koate-HP, Kogenate, Monoclate-P, Profilate HP, Recombinate)	Temporarily replaces clotting factors missing because of hemophilia Prevents or corrects bleeding episodes Prophylaxis Mild to severe hemorrhage	*Adult:* administered so that factor VIII level assay is 20–40% of normal or up to 80–100% of normal after trauma or major surgery*	*Onset:* Immediate *Duration:* Unknown $t_{1/2}$: 12 h
anti-inhibitor coagulant complex (Autoplex T, Feiba VH)	Controls bleeding in patients with factor VIII inhibitors Joint hemorrhage	*Adult:* IV, 50–100 U/kg at 12-h intervals (Feiba VH) 25–100 U/kg, may repeat in 6 h (Autoplex I)	*Onset:* Immediate *Duration:* Unknown $t_{1/2}$: Unknown
P aminocaproic acid (Amicar)	Controls fibrinolysis and stops bleeding	*Adult:* PO or IV, 4–5 g over the first hour followed by 1–1.25 g/h for 8 h	*Onset:* PO, rapid; IV immediate *Duration:* IV, 2–3 h $t_{1/2}$: IV, 3 h

*Dosing is highly individualized to achieve desired results. See manufacturer's instructions.

Patients with factor VIII deficiencies have markedly prolonged bleeding and clotting times.

Contraindications and Precautions

A contraindication to AHF is a hypersensitivity to mouse protein (limited to products that contain monoclonal antibodies). Considered a pregnancy risk category C drug, AHF should be used only if necessary. The pooled blood product may contain minute amounts of blood types A or B. If the patient receives a large quantity of the preparation, the risk for hemolysis from blood type incompatibility exists. In patients who have not previously received multiple infusions of blood or plasma products, signs or symptoms of some viral infections, especially hepatitis C, are likely to develop. These patients, particularly those with mild hemophilia, should receive single-donor products. AHF also carries risk for HIV transmission, although current viral-depleting processes and donor-screening practices have reduced the potential for transmission considerably.

Adverse Effects

Several adverse effects may result from AHF, although none is common. Allergic reactions include anaphylaxis, urticaria, nausea, and chills. Other adverse effects include tachycardia, hypotension, headache, drowsiness, lethargy, vision disturbances, loss of consciousness, vomiting, hepatitis, intravascular hemolysis, back pain, chest constriction, and wheezing.

Drug Interactions

No important interactions are associated with AHF.

Assessment of Relevant Core Patient Variables

Health Status

Important assessments for patients with hypocoagulation problems include determining factor VIII level assays and reviewing test results, such as CBC, direct Coombs test, urinalysis, PTT, thromboplastin generation test, and prothrombin generation test. These test results provide data regarding current clotting times and serve as baseline information to determine whether reactions are occurring during therapy. In the physical examination, be alert for signs of active bleeding and extent of the bleeding.

Life Span and Gender

Because the safety of AHF during pregnancy has not been established, determine whether the patient is pregnant.

Lifestyle, Diet, and Habits

During assessment, any patient behaviors likely to result in injury, such as participation in contact sports, should be investigated.

Environment

AHF is generally self-administered at home by the patient or family.

Culture and Inherited Traits

Patients with religious views that forbid receiving blood products may be opposed to receiving AHF. Discuss with the patient beliefs that may have an impact on drug therapy.

Nursing Diagnosis and Outcome

- Risk for Injury, Hemorrhage, related to deficiency of clotting factor VIII
  Desired outcome: *The patient will receive enough factor VIII to prevent injury.*

Planning and Intervention

Maximizing Therapeutic Effects

Refrigeration is required for AHF until it is used. Before reconstitution, warm the concentrate and the diluent provided by the manufacturer to room temperature. Only plastic syringes are used for the infusion because the AHF solution can stick to glass surfaces.

The diluent is added to the concentrate in the vial, and the vial is rotated carefully until the contents dissolve. To help prevent gel formation, the vial should not be shaken. If a gel forms during reconstitution of AHF, the pharmacy or blood bank is notified, and the AHF is withheld.

Monitor coagulation studies during therapy to assess the effectiveness of AHF.

Minimizing Adverse Effects

After dilution, AHF must be administered within 3 hours to prevent bacterial growth. Only the IV route can be used. Apply pressure to all venipuncture sites for at least 5 minutes. IM injections are avoided to prevent bleeding into the muscle. Other measures include monitoring intake and output ratios and inspecting urine for color. If you note discrepancy in ratios or if urine becomes red or orange, a sign of hemolytic reaction, notify the prescriber.

Monitor for decreased hematocrit and increased Coombs test, both of which are indications of hemolytic anemia, and assess for allergic reaction. If present, the infusion should be stopped and the prescriber notified.

Providing Patient and Family Education

- Instruct patients and families to observe for bleeding from gums, skin, urine, stools, or emesis.
- Caution patients to avoid products containing aspirin or ibuprofen because they may further impair clotting.
- Discuss strategies to prevent bleeding, such as using a soft toothbrush, avoiding IM and subcutaneous injections, and avoiding behaviors and activities that are likely to cause injury.
- Advise patients to wear medical identification that identifies their disease.
- Emphasize that improved screening factors have decreased the risk for transmission of hepatitis or HIV substantially, although a slight risk for disease transmission remains.

Ongoing Assessment and Evaluation

Blood studies are monitored as previously described. Therapy is effective when prolonged bleeding is prevented or stopped.

MEMORY CHIP

P Antihemophilic Factor

- Provides factor VIII for those with hemophilia; made from pooled human sources
- Temporarily meets needs for clotting factor to prevent or stop bleeding
- Dosage is individualized to needs of patient
- No common adverse effects
- Most serious adverse effects: slight risk of hemolytic anemia and transmission of hepatitis or HIV
- Minimizing adverse effects: monitor hematocrit and Coombs test result (hemolytic anemia)
- Most important patient education: Teach patients to avoid injury to prevent bleeding, and to carry or wear identification of the disease.

Drugs Closely Related to P Antihemophilic Factor

Human factor IX complex is used to treat hemophilia B (Christmas disease), although it is not a substitute for fresh-frozen plasma used in mild factor IX deficiency. The complex contains factors II (prothrombin), VII, IX, and X. Factors II (prothrombin), VII, and X are required for converting prothrombin to thrombin, and factor IX is necessary for prothrombin production. The complex prevents or controls bleeding in hemophilia B, controls bleeding episodes in patients with factor VIII inhibitors, and reverses oral anticoagulant-induced hemorrhage. Human factor IX complex (Konyne 80, Profilnine SD, Proplex T, and AlphaNine SD) has one variant, mononine. Mononine contains factor IX, but after reconstitution, it has undetectable levels of factors II (prothrombin), VII, and X. It also contains histidine, mannitol, and mouse protein.

Factor IX, human contains only factor IX. Human factor IX complex and factor IX are administered intravenously. Dosage depends on the condition of the patient and the manufacturer's instructions, which vary according to the manufacturer. For additional information, refer to Table 31.6.

Anti-Inhibitor Coagulant Factor

Made from pooled human plasma, anti-inhibitor coagulant factor is a concentrate of activated and precursor clotting factors. It differs from AHF in that it is useful in treating patients with hemophilia who have significant levels of factor VIII inhibitors. It therefore allows clotting to occur in patients with hemophilia who are not responsive to AHF (see Table 31.6).

C HEMOSTATIC DRUGS

Hemostatics stop blood loss by enhancing blood coagulation. There are two types of hemostatic agents: systemic and topical. Systemic agents interfere with the breakdown of clots. Topical agents are used to control small amounts of bleeding or oozing, usually following surgery. The prototype systemic hemostatic drug is aminocaproic acid (Amicar). Tranexamic acid is also a hemostatic drug. Additional topical hemostatic drugs are presented in Table 31.6.

PATHOPHYSIOLOGY

Fibrinolysis normally occurs in balance with blood coagulation. A clot forms to prevent extensive blood loss. When the vessel heals, the clot is broken down (fibrinolysis) by activating plasminogen so that it becomes plasmin. Plasmin breaks down fibrin, fibrinogen, and other plasma proteins. When fibrinolysis is not in balance with the other phases of coagulation (i.e., an excess of plasmin exists), excessive bleeding occurs because the body cannot form a stable clot in response to injury.

NURSING MANAGEMENT OF THE PATIENT RECEIVING P AMINOCAPROIC ACID

Aminocaproic acid is the prototype systemic hemostatic drug.

Core Drug Knowledge

Pharmacotherapeutics

Aminocaproic acid treats severe, life-threatening hemorrhage from systemic hyperfibrinolysis or urinary fibrinolysis. Systemic hyperfibrinolysis has occurred with heart surgery, abruptio placentae, cirrhosis of the liver, and neoplastic disorders. Urinary hyperfibrinolysis is associated with severe trauma, shock, prostatectomy, nephrectomy, and renal cancers.

An unapproved use of aminocaproic acid is in preventing recurrent subarachnoid hemorrhage. Aminocaproic acid is also used to treat overdoses of fibrinolytic drugs, such as streptokinase.

Pharmacokinetics

Aminocaproic acid is administered orally or by IV infusion. After oral administration, the drug is quickly absorbed; through both routes, it is widely distributed. Most of the drug is excreted unchanged in the urine.

Pharmacodynamics

Aminocaproic acid prevents fibrinolysis in two ways. First, it blocks the action of plasminogen activators, thus interfering with the formation of active plasmin. Second, it interferes with the binding of active plasmin to fibrin, thus preventing breakdown of fibrin. The result is stabilization of the blood clot and control of bleeding.

Contraindications and Precautions

Aminocaproic acid should be used only in life-threatening situations and then only when overactivity of the fibrinolytic system is verified by laboratory testing. The drug is not to be used in patients with active intravascular clotting, such as DIC.

This drug is used with caution in patients with uremia or hepatic disease. Cautious use is recommended in patients with upper renal tract bleeding and in those with cardiac, liver, or renal disease. Cautious use is also recommended in pregnancy or lactation because safety has not been established.

TABLE 31.6 Topical Hemostatic Agents

Hemostatic Agent and Action	Indication	Dosage	Contraindications and Adverse Effects	Nursing Management
Topical thrombin (Thrombinar, Thrombogen, Thrombostat) When applied directly on the wound, thrombin converts fibrinogen to fibrin.	Used in oozing wounds after dental surgery, plastic surgery, neurosurgery, epistaxis, and graft procedures Also used with absorbable gelatin sponges for hemostasis during surgery	The amount of bleeding determines the strength of solution, 100 to 2,000 U/mL.	This is included in pregnancy risk category C. The drug may cause a hypersensitivity reaction. If the drug enters the bloodstream, intravascular coagulation occurs and may result in death. Reported adverse effects include febrile episodes and allergic reaction when used to treat epistaxis.	Clean blood from affected area with gauze pads. Apply solution soon after it is reconstituted (within 3 h of reconstitution if it has to be refrigerated). Monitor the application site frequently to detect any recurrence of blood loss.
Microfibrillar collagen hemostat (Avitene Hemostat, Hemotene, Hemoped) Attracts platelets when applied to a bleeding area. Platelet aggregation fills the space with a fibrin clot.	Adjunct in controlling bleeding when traditional methods are not effective or useful	The dose is impregnated into a web or sponge form. The amount used depends on the amount of bleeding.	The drug should not be resterilized after use; its use in infected wounds is not recommended. Its effect during pregnancy is not known. Excess drug should be removed after use to prevent complications. Adverse effects include increase in infection, formation of adhesions, and hypersensitivity.	Avoid handling the substance with wet gloves or instruments, because it will adhere to a wet surface. After application to the wound, apply pressure using a dry gauze sponge. Discard any unused material; this agent may not be resterilized.
Absorbable gelatin sponge (Gelfoam). Product absorbs and holds many times its weight in whole blood. Wound may be closed over sponge, which will dissolve slowly.	Used in dental and oral surgery, neurosurgery, and prostatectomy to control bleeding	It is supplied in several different sizes to match size of the wound and the amount of bleeding.	The preparation should not be resterilized using heat, because heat may alter the product's effectiveness. The sponge should not be used on incisions. It has no indication for use in postpartum bleeding. It should be used sparingly in areas where expansion may be detrimental to surrounding structures. Adverse effects include potential for infection or abscess formation.	Assess wound frequently for bleeding. Apply during surgery as recommended by the surgeon—either dry or saturated in saline solution. Squeeze sponge to remove any air bubbles when the sponge is to be moistened on application. After application, apply pressure with a gauze pad for 10 to 15 s.

(continued)

TABLE 31.6 Topical Hemostatic Agents (continued)

Hemostatic Agent and Action	Indication	Dosage	Contraindications and Adverse Effects	Nursing Management
Absorbable gelatin film (Gelfilm, Gelfilm Ophthalmic) Cellophane-like material that becomes rubbery when wet and may be implanted into body tissue will be slowly absorbed.	Used in neurosurgery, thoracic surgery, and ocular surgery	This is supplied in a standard size and cut to fit the area	Using this film in contaminated wounds is contraindicated.	Soak the film in a sterile saline solution until pliable. The surgeon will cut the film to the desired size.
Oxidized cellulose (Oxycel, Surgicel) Exact mechanism of action is unknown but provides hemostasis when applied directly on bleeding area. It does not affect normal blood clotting, but in contact with blood, this product forms an artificial clot.	Used to control bleeding when sutures or clipping are not possible Primarily for bleeding from capillaries, venioles, or arterioles Used for oral and dental surgery	This is supplied impregnated into pads, pledgets, and strips. Number used depends on amount of bleeding and size of wound.	This product is contraindicated for use as wound packing. Product should not be used in fractures or spinal surgery because it may interfere with bone regrowth or cause cyst formation. It is not recommended for use in bleeding from large arteries or with serous oozing. This drug product should not be used if it has been autoclaved because this method of sterilization causes it to break down. The product may be left in the wound, but its removal once hemostasis is achieved is recommended. If used during a laminectomy, it must be removed. Adverse effects include nasal burning, encapsulation of fluid, antibody reactions.	Use a surgical clamp to remove substance from its container. Do not wet the product; instead, apply it dry. Monitor wounds of patients using oxidized cellulose for signs of bleeding.

Adverse Effects

The most common adverse effect of aminocaproic acid is GI distress (anorexia, nausea). Life-threatening or serious adverse effects are rare; these include convulsions, rhabdomyolysis (acute, sometimes fatal disease with destruction of the skeletal muscle), and renal failure. Other adverse effects that may occur include headache, dizziness, seizures, malaise, thrombophlebitis, hypotension (after IV administration), arrhythmias, tinnitus, nasal congestion, vomiting, abdominal cramps, diarrhea, and diuresis. Symptoms of overdosage include nausea, diarrhea, delirium, hepatic necrosis, and thromboembolism.

Drug Interactions

An increase in clotting factors leading to hypercoagulation may occur if aminocaproic acid is administered concurrently with oral contraceptives or estrogen (Table 31.7).

Assessment of Relevant Core Patient Variables

Health Status

Initial assessments include identifying contraindications to the drug by determining clotting factor levels and platelet counts to assess the severity of the patient's condition.

Life Span and Gender

During assessment, the patient's possible pregnancy or breast-feeding status should be evaluated. If the patient is a child, his or her weight should be measured so that a correct dosage can be calculated.

Environment

Be aware of the environment in which the drug will be administered. Aminocaproic acid is administered in an acute care setting, such as a hospital.

Nursing Diagnosis and Outcome

- Risk for Altered Cardiovascular Perfusion related to volume loss secondary to uncontrolled bleeding or thrombophlebitis secondary to adverse effects of aminocaproic acid
  Desired outcome: Adequate perfusion will be maintained as evidenced by presence of pulses, normal skin color and warmth, and capillary refill.

Planning and Intervention

Minimizing Adverse Effects

Monitor vital signs at start of therapy and throughout therapy at intervals appropriate to the patient's condition. Every 15 to 30 minutes, the patient should be assessed for bleeding, particularly at incision and old injection sites.

To administer aminocaproic acid, an IV infusion pump is used to regulate the flow rate. The IV site and line are assessed for patency. Verify that the line is secured to prevent thrombophlebitis. Do not mix aminocaproic acid with other drugs.

The patient is connected to a cardiac monitor to detect arrhythmias and is observed for signs of thromboembolic complications, such as chest pain, dyspnea, changes in skin color and temperature, pain in an extremity, or changes in peripheral pulses. The prescriber is notified if these changes occur.

Additional ways to guard against adverse drug effects include monitoring intake and output and monitoring neurologic status in patients with subarachnoid hemorrhage. The prescriber should be notified of major discrepancies or changes.

To combat nausea, patients should be encouraged to eat small, frequent meals.

Providing Patient and Family Education

- Teach patients and families about the role of aminocaproic acid in controlling bleeding. They also must understand the importance of reporting any bleeding or symptoms of thromboembolism immediately.
- Instruct patients to change positions slowly to prevent orthostatic hypotension.

Ongoing Assessment and Evaluation

The patient should be monitored throughout treatment and recovery for signs and symptoms of bleeding or embolism or any other untoward event.

Drugs Closely Related to P Aminocaproic Acid

Tranexamic acid (Cyklokapron) is another systemic hemostatic agent. It competitively inhibits activation of plasminogen. It is used to reduce or prevent hemorrhage during and after tooth extraction in patients with hemophilia.

After oral administration, between 30% and 50% of the drug is absorbed. The drug remains in serum for 7 to 8 hours and is excreted from the body in the urine.

The drug is contraindicated for patients with subarachnoid hemorrhage. It should be used cautiously in patients with acquired defective color vision because altered color vision is an early sign of visual toxicity. Caution should be

TABLE 31.7 Agents That Interact With P Aminocaproic Acid

Interactants	Effect and Significance	Nursing Management
oral contraceptives	Increase in clotting factors may lead to hypercoagulant state and may possibly increase risk of thrombus formation.	Monitor for signs of thrombus.
estrogens	Same as above.	Same as above.

MEMORY CHIP

P Aminocaproic Acid

- Used to treat life-threatening bleeding from systemic hyperfibrinolysis or urinary fibrinolysis
- Prevents breakdown of the stable clot and controls bleeding
- Major contraindications: Use only in life-threatening situations and only when the overactivity of the fibrinolytic system is verified by laboratory testing; DIC.
- Most common adverse effect: GI distress
- Most serious adverse effects: renal failure (rare), rhabdomyolysis (rare), thromboembolism, and arrhythmias
- Minimizing adverse effects: Use IV pump, assess for bleeding or signs of thromboembolism, and place patient on cardiac monitor to detect arrhythmias.
- Most important patient education: Teach patients to report symptoms of thromboembolism.

used in pregnant or lactating women and in patients with renal insufficiency.

Aprotinin, also a systemic hemostatic agent, is indicated to reduce perioperative blood loss and the need for blood transfusion in patients undergoing cardiopulmonary bypass in the course of CABG surgery. It has also been studied for use in other types of surgery. The exact mechanism by which it reduces bleeding is unclear.

CHAPTER SUMMARY

- Anticoagulants do not break down existing clots; they prevent clots from forming.
- The parenteral anticoagulant heparin and the oral anticoagulant warfarin are used in treating thrombus or thromboembolic disorders to prevent extension of the clot or formation of an embolism. They are also used in high-risk patients to prevent formation of an initial clot. Patients may be taking both drugs at the same time during dose regulation of warfarin.
- Education for patients on anticoagulant therapy should include safety measures to prevent bleeding, instructions to be alert for signs of bleeding, and directions for what to do if bleeding occurs.
- Antiplatelet drugs prevent platelet aggregation and thereby prevent thrombus formation. They are used prophylactically to prevent CVAs (also called strokes) and MIs (also called heart attacks). They are used as part of treatment for ischemic strokes, after thrombolytic therapy.
- Hemorheologic agents promote the flexibility of the RBCs and decrease blood viscosity to prevent thrombus formation.
- Thrombolytic drugs break down existing clots. They are used in acute medical emergencies, such as evolving MI, pulmonary embolism, and acute ischemic stroke. Although they can save lives, these drugs carry a risk for inducing hemorrhage. The patient must be closely monitored during this drug therapy.
- Clotting factors are administered when the patient has a deficiency of clotting factors resulting from heredity or disease. These drugs allow natural clotting to occur and prevent massive blood loss.
- Hemostatics are drugs used to promote blood coagulation. Hemostatics come in systemic and topical forms. Systemic hemostatics also interfere with the breaking down of clots.

QUESTIONS FOR STUDY AND REVIEW

1. Describe how heparin and warfarin differ in their effects on the clotting cycle.
2. What interventions would promote safety while the patient is receiving heparin by continuous IV infusion?
3. Describe which laboratory values need to be monitored if the patient is receiving heparin and warfarin. What criteria will you use to determine whether these drugs are in a therapeutic range?
4. Why is it important to assess the usual vitamin K intake for a patient who will be receiving warfarin, but not for the patient who will be receiving heparin?
5. What assessment should be performed if the patient is receiving the antiplatelet drug clopidogrel and the antilipid drug fluvastatin?
6. What is the difference between an anticoagulant and a thrombolytic drug?
7. What drug therapy would be used for a patient who has hemophilia and who requires an inguinal hernia repair?

? Need More Help?

Chapter 31 of the study guide for *Drug Therapy in Nursing* 2e contains NCLEX-style questions and other learning activities to reinforce your understanding of the concepts presented in this chapter. For additional information or to purchase the study guide, visit *http://connection.lww.com/go/aschenbrenner.*

REFERENCES AND BIBLIOGRAPHY

Adams, H. P., Adams, R. J., Brott, T., et al. (2003). Guidelines for the early management of patients with ischemic stroke: A scientific statement from the Stroke Council of the American Stroke Association. *Stroke, 34*(4), 1056–1083. Available: *http://www.stroke.ahajournals.org/cgi/reprint/34/4/1056.*

Albers, G. W., Amarenco, P., Easton, J. D., et al. (2001). Guideline for antithrombotic and thrombolytic therapy for ischemic stroke. Sixth ACCP Consensus Conference on Antithrombotic Therapy. *Chest, 119*(1 Suppl.), 300S–320S.

American Diabetes Association. (2003). Clinical Practice Guidelines: Aspirin therapy in diabetes. [Online.] Available: *http://diabetes.org/professional/CPR_home.jsp.*

Balcezak, T. J., Krumholz, H. M., Getnick, G. S., et al. (2000). Utilization and effectiveness of a weight-based heparin nomogram at a large academic medical center. *American Journal of Managed Care, 6*(3), 329–338.

Berg, A. O., Allan, J. D., Frame, P. S., et al.; United States Preventive Services Task Force-Independent Expert Panel. (2002). Aspirin for the primary prevention of cardiovascular events: Recommendation and rationale. *Annals of Internal Medicine, 136*(2), 157–160.

Cohen, M., Gensini, G. F., Maritz, F., et al.; TETAMI Investigators. (2003). The safety and efficacy of subcutaneous enoxaparin versus intravenous unfractionated heparin and tirofiban versus placebo in the treatment of acute ST-segment elevation myocardial infarction patients ineligible for reperfusion (TETAMI): A randomized trial. *Journal American College of Cardiology, 42*(8), 1348–1356.

Colwell, J. A. (2003). Aspirin therapy in diabetes. *Diabetes Care, 26*(Suppl. 1), S87–S88.

De Schryver, E. L., Algra, A., & van Gijn, J. (2003). Dipyridamole for preventing stroke and other vascular events in patients with vascular disease. *Cochrane Database System Review,* (1):CD001820.

Ferguson, J. J., Antman, E. M., Bates, E. R., et al.; NICE-3 Investigators. (2003). Combining enoxaparin and glycoprotein IIb/IIIa antagonists for the treatment of acute coronary syndromes: Final results of the national investigators collaborating on enoxaparin-3 (NICE-3) study. *American Heart Journal, 146*(4), 628–634.

Hart, R. G., Halperin, J. L., Pearce, L. A., et al.; Stroke Prevention in Atrial Fibrillation Investigators. (2003). Lessons from the stroke prevention in atrial fibrillation trials. *Annals of Internal Medicine, 138*(10), 831–838.

Hirsh, J., Anand, S. S., Halperin, J. L., et al. (2001). Guide to anticoagulant therapy: Heparin. A statement for healthcare professionals from the American Heart Association. *Circulation, 103*(24), 2994–3018.

Messieh, M. (2000). Preoperative haemoglobin and warfarin response. *Journal of Bone and Joint Surgery, British, 82*(5), 728–730.

Mukherjee, D., Mahaffey, K. W., Moliterno, D. J., et al. (2002). Promise of combined low-molecular-weight heparin and platelet glycoprotein IIb/IIIa inhibition: Results from platelet IIb/IIIa antagonist for the reduction of acute coronary syndrome events in a global organization network B (PARAGON B). *American Heart Journal, 144*(6), 995–1002.

Valente, M., & Ponte, E. (2000). Thrombosis and cancer. *Minerva Cardioangiologica, 48*(4–5), 117–127.

Wardlaw, J. M., Zoppo, G., Yamaguchi, T., et al. (2003). Thrombolysis for acute ischemic stroke. *Cochrane Database System Review,* (3):CD000213.

Drugs Affecting Urinary Output

chapter 32

Learning Objectives

At the completion of this chapter the student will:

1. Describe normal kidney function and explain how diuretics work in the kidney.
2. Identify core drug knowledge about drugs that affect diuresis.
3. Identify core patient variables related to drugs that affect diuresis.
4. Relate the interaction of core drug knowledge to core patient variables for drugs that affect diuresis.
5. Generate a nursing plan of care from the interactions between core drug knowledge and core patient variables for drugs that affect diuresis.
6. Describe nursing interventions to maximize therapeutic and minimize adverse effects for drugs that affect diuresis.
7. Determine key points for patient and family education for drugs that affect diuresis.

KEY TERMS

- diuresis
- diuretic
- edema
- glomerular filtration
- hyperkalemia
- hypertension
- hypervolemia
- hypokalemia
- oliguria
- osmolality
- renal tubular reabsorption
- renal tubular secretion

FEATURED WEBLINK

http://circ.ahajournals.org/cgi/content/full/104/24/2996
The website of the American Heart Association Journals has the complete ACC/AHA guidelines for the evaluation and management of chronic heart failure in adults, including the use of diuretics.

CONNECTION WEBLINK

Additional Weblinks are found on Connection:
http://www.connection.lww.com/go/aschenbrenner.

DRUGS PRODUCING DIURESIS

(C) Diuretics

(C) Thiazide diuretics
- [P] **hydrochlorothiazide**
- bendroflumethiazide
- benzthiazide
- chlorothiazide
- chlorthalidone
- hydroflumethiazide
- indapamide
- methyclothiazide
- metolazone
- polythiazide
- quinethazone
- trichlormethiazide

(C) Loop diuretics
- [P] **furosemide**
- bumetanide
- torsemide
- ethacrynic acid

(C) Osmotic diuretics
- [P] **mannitol**
- glycerin
- urea
- isosorbide

(C) Potassium-sparing diuretics
- [P] **triamterine**
- amiloride
- spironolactone

(C) Carbonic anhydrase inhibitors
- [P] **acetazolamide**
- dichlorphenamide
- methazolamide

DRUGS THAT AFFECT BLADDER CONTRACTION

(C) Muscarinic stimulants

- [P] **bethanocol** (see Chapter 14)

(C) Muscarinic antagonists

- [P] **tolterodine**

The symbol (C) indicates the **drug class**.
Drugs in **bold type** marked with the symbol [P] are prototypes.
Drugs in blue type are closely related to the prototype.
Drugs in red type are significantly different from the prototype.
Drugs in black type with no symbol are also used in drug therapy; no prototype

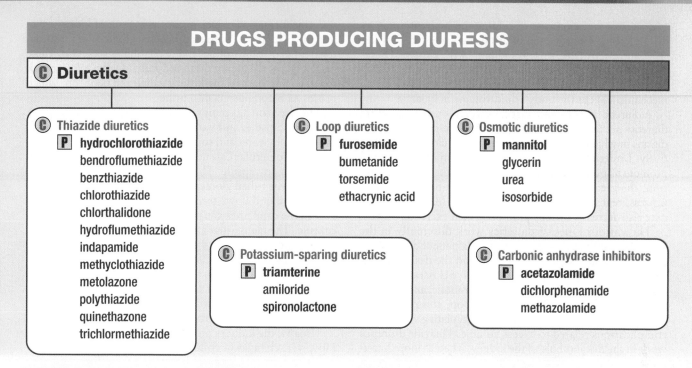

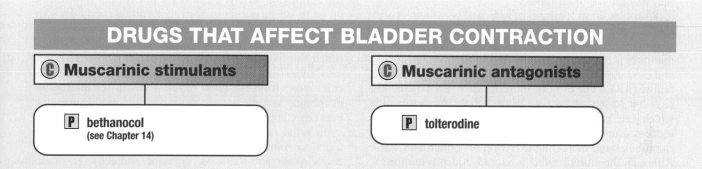

Diuresis is the process of ridding the body of fluids by increasing production of urine and excretion of water and electrolytes, such as sodium, by the kidneys. Diuresis occurs naturally if fluid intake has exceeded the body's normal requirements. This self-regulating or homeostatic mechanism keeps the body's fluid volume in balance.

A **diuretic** is a substance that causes diuresis. Drugs that are diuretics are used to decrease fluid volume in pathologic conditions in which the body cannot regulate fluid volume effectively. Diuretics decrease renal reabsorption of sodium and promote its excretion in water. The greater the sodium excretion, the greater the water excretion will be. During this process, reabsorption of other electrolytes (e.g., potassium) may also decrease, thereby promoting their excretion as well.

The various types of diuretics work differently in the body. Which diuretic is prescribed for a patient depends on the patient's underlying pathologies and the desired therapeutic effects. This chapter discusses five classes of diuretics: thiazide, loop, potassium-sparing, osmotic, and carbonic anhydrase inhibitors. The thiazide, loop, and potassium-sparing classes all are used to decrease circulating volume and complications related to excess volume. Thiazide diuretics work in the distal tubule of the kidney, whereas loop diuretics work in the loop of Henle. Potassium-sparing diuretics are used commonly in combination with other diuretics, and they work in the distal tubule.

Prototype drugs for thiazide, loop, and potassium-sparing classes are hydrochlorothiazide (HCTZ), furosemide, and triamterene, respectively. The osmotic diuretics, for which mannitol is the prototype, are used to decrease intraocular and intracranial pressure and to treat or prevent acute renal failure (ARF). The osmotic diuretics are filtered by the kidneys but poorly reabsorbed in the tubule. Acetazolamide, which is the prototype for the carbonic anhydrase inhibitors, induces diuresis by decreasing hydrogen ion secretion by the tubules and increasing excretion of sodium and water. Although the diuretic effect is limited, aqueous humor formation is reduced, thereby making these drugs useful for reducing intraocular pressure in glaucoma. This chapter also discusses nursing management strategies for patients on diuretic therapy.

PHYSIOLOGY

The renal system is a complex mechanism that has several important functions in maintaining health. It is the body's filtering and purifying center, ridding the body of impurities and waste by producing urine and excreting water, electrolytes, and other substances. Other functions of the renal system include regulating the body's acid-base balance, maintaining blood pressure, influencing circulating fluid volume, assisting in the production of red blood cells, and contributing to calcium metabolism (Figure 32.1).

The renal system consists of the kidneys, ureters, and bladder. The kidneys are a pair of intricate, bean-shaped organs located behind the upper abdomen outside the peritoneal cavity. They are active in filtering, reabsorbing, and excreting fluid, electrolytes, and waste products. The ureters are tubes that transport waste products and excess fluid from the kidneys to the bladder, a balloon-like receptacle, for later excretion.

Urine formation, which occurs as a result of kidney function, involves three complex processes: glomerular filtration, renal tubular reabsorption, and renal tubular secretion. These mechanisms, which are discussed individually below, work together in a part of the kidney called the nephron, which processes blood plasma into urine.

The nephron has many parts, including the glomerulus, Bowman capsule, and various tubules and membranes. In the nephron, water and solutes move from the blood plasma across a glomerular capsular membrane into an area known as a Bowman capsule. This movement across the capsular membrane is called **glomerular filtration.**

As the blood flows through the kidney capillaries, pressure in the capillaries causes fluid to filter into the Bowman capsule. The glomerular capsular membrane (the basement membrane), which lies between the glomerulus and the Bowman capsule, allows fluid and electrolytes but not blood cells and plasma proteins to pass into the Bowman capsule. The average glomerular filtration rate is 125 mL/min (or about 180 L of plasma in 24 hours). More than 99% of the plasma filtered is reabsorbed in the tubules.

Usually, the kidneys produce less than 2 L of urine daily. However, changes in colloid osmotic pressure or capsular hydrostatic pressure can alter glomerular filtration. For example, a decrease in colloid osmotic pressure may increase filtration. Conversely, an increase in capsular hydrostatic pressure, which occurs in obstructive disease, may decrease filtration.

The conversion of the filtrate into urine occurs in the renal tubule by processes known as renal tubular reabsorption and renal tubular secretion. In **renal tubular reabsorption,** molecules move from the renal tubule across a semipermeable membrane into the peritubular blood (the blood surrounding the renal tubule).

In **renal tubular secretion,** molecules move from the blood surrounding the renal tubule into the tubule. In both reabsorption and secretion, diffusion and active transport are key mechanisms.

The strength, or concentration, of the urine produced is known as **osmolality,** which is the density of active particles in solution or the osmotic concentration determined by the ionic concentration of dissolved substances per unit of solution. Urine osmolality depends on the volume and composition of extracellular fluids. It also depends on a countercurrent mechanism in the renal medulla (a part of the kidney), which controls the flow of water and solute so that water is kept out of the area around the tubule and so that sodium and urea are retained. An important contributor to this process is antidiuretic hormone (ADH), which is released when the osmolality of the extracellular fluid increases.

To enable water to move out of the tubule and into the surrounding capillaries, ADH increases the permeability of the collecting tubule to water; from the capillaries, it returns to the vascular system for circulation. As a result of increased water reabsorption, urine osmolality (concentration) increases. Without ADH, the renal tubules are impermeable to water, water is not reabsorbed, and dilute urine is produced.

The kidneys play a major role in regulating acid-base balance and maintaining a normal blood pH (7.35–7.45) by excreting hydrogen ions or reabsorbing bicarbonate. The kidneys regulate hydrogen ion secretion so that bicarbonate

Physiology

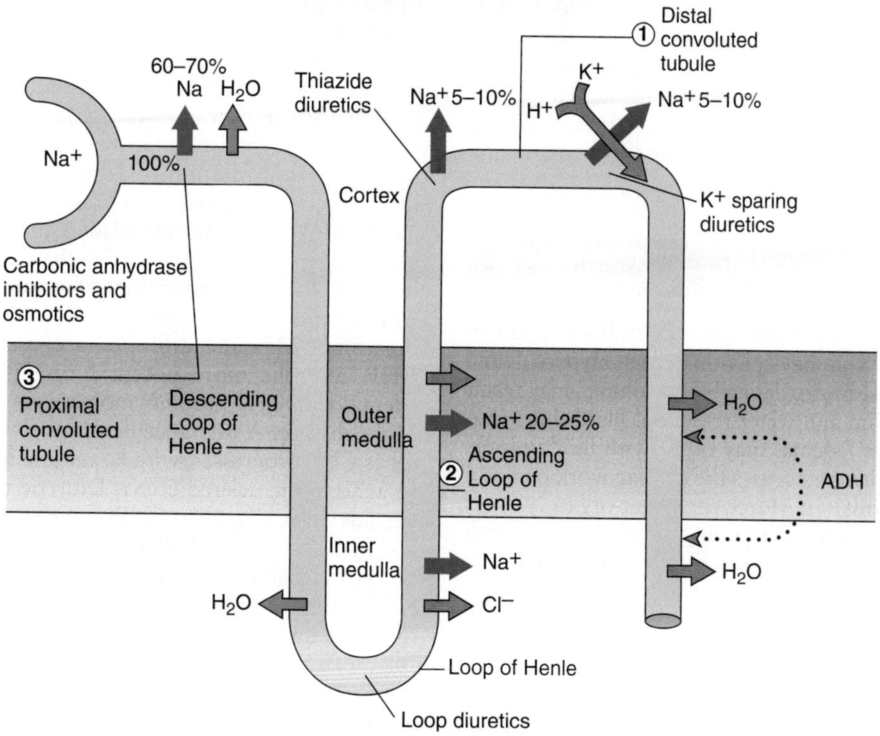

FIGURE 32.1 Diuretics work in the nephron. The main organ of the renal system is the kidney, which houses a tangled mass of nearly 1 million nephrons. The nephron is the structure known for its role in urine production. Different diuretic drugs work in different parts of the nephron: thiazide, thiazide-like, and potassium-sparing diuretics work in the distal convoluted tubule (**1**), loop diuretics in the ascending loop of Henle (**2**), and carbonic anhydrase inhibitors and osmotic diuretics in the proximal convoluted tubule (**3**). Fluid and electrolyte alterations depend on where the specific diuretic works in the kidney.

levels remain within normal limits. Most of the hydrogen ions excreted in the urine are secreted into the tubular fluid. Tubular fluid pH is acidic, and the kidney depends on buffers in the urine to combine with the hydrogen ion for excretion. The three buffers are bicarbonate (HCO_3), phosphate (HPO_4), and ammonia (NH_3).

The first step in bicarbonate reabsorption is the movement of carbon dioxide (CO_2) into a tubular cell where the CO_2 combines with water to form a hydrogen ion and a bicarbonate ion. The hydrogen ion is then secreted into the tubular fluid, and a sodium ion is reabsorbed. The sodium ion and bicarbonate ion pass into the extracellular fluid. The free hydrogen ion then combines with a filtered bicarbonate ion to form carbon dioxide and water. The water is eliminated in the urine, and the CO_2 diffuses into the tubular cell to combine with water, thereby forming a hydrogen ion and a bicarbonate ion to begin the process again.

Additional hydrogen ions are excreted in the urine in combination with a phosphate or ammonium buffer. The phosphate ion is filtered into the tubular fluid, where it combines with a free hydrogen ion and is excreted. Ammonia is synthesized in the tubular cells and diffuses into the tubular fluid, where it combines with a hydrogen ion to form an ammonium ion (NH_4), which is excreted.

Normally, the number of hydrogen ions secreted by the tubules is about equal to the number of bicarbonate ions filtered in the glomerulus. In metabolic acidosis, however, the number of hydrogen ions secreted exceeds bicarbonate filtration, and the urine becomes acidic. In metabolic alkalosis, bicarbonate filtration exceeds hydrogen ion secretion, and the urine becomes alkaline.

Additional work of the kidneys includes endocrine functions, whereby chemicals are produced to exert action elsewhere in the body. In this regard, the kidneys help maintain and regulate blood pressure and vascular resistance, red blood cell production, and calcium metabolism.

Blood pressure is affected by the kidneys' role in the renin-angiotensin-aldosterone mechanism. Renin, an enzyme, is synthesized and stored in the kidney and released in response to decreased blood flow or a change in the composition of fluid in the distal tubule. The release of renin plays a role in converting angiotensin I, a substance in the blood, into the powerful vasopressor angiotensin II. In response, the kidney decreases sodium and water excretion, causing blood pressure to increase. Angiotensin II also stimulates the adrenal cortex to secrete the hormone aldosterone, which promotes sodium and water reabsorption and increases blood pressure.

The kidney produces erythropoietin, which stimulates the bone marrow to produce and release red blood cells, particularly in response to hypoxia (oxygen deprivation). In kidney failure, loss of this ability contributes to anemia.

The kidneys play a vital role in the chemical transformation of compounds that are precursors to the active form of vitamin D, which is needed to absorb calcium from the gastrointestinal (GI) tract. Vitamin D also helps to regulate calcium deposition in the bones.

PATHOPHYSIOLOGY

When the body cannot maintain a balance of body fluid levels, fluid overload or volume depletion occurs. **Hypervolemia** (an abnormal increase in circulating blood volume) may result from excessive sodium and water retention. Fluid shifts into the interstitial spaces (**edema**) may occur with fluid volume excess. Peripheral edema increases the cardiac workload and decreases tissue perfusion. Moreover, other organ systems may be affected adversely by the congestion associated with edema. When systemic edema is severe, the congestion backs up into the lungs, affecting breathing and gas exchange.

Diuretic drugs are used in treating pathologic conditions in which fluid overload, and frequently edema, has occurred. These conditions include congestive heart failure (CHF), pulmonary edema, hypertension, and kidney disorders. Additionally, diuretics are used for treating adverse effects from long-term steroid or antiepileptic drug therapy, and such symptoms of fluid overload as increased intracranial and intraocular pressure and premenstrual syndrome.

Ineffective pumping of the heart can result in CHF because the heart does not empty well, and cardiac output is diminished. Increased demands placed on the heart by other systemic problems can also cause the heart to fail. When the heart chambers do not empty well with each contraction, blood backs up into the body, and congestion occurs in the body tissues. Edema in CHF usually results from increased sodium and water retention and venous congestion, which increases capillary pressure in the peripheral and pulmonary circulation. As a result of the ineffective pumping ability of the heart, the kidneys receive a diminished blood supply. Impaired glomerular filtration and reduced blood flow to the renal tubules then occur. The kidney interprets these findings as signs of hypovolemia (insufficient circulating fluid or volume depletion) and activates mechanisms to retain sodium and water and increase circulating volume. Thus, volume is increased in an already congested system, and CHF actually worsens.

Drug therapy for CHF is now focused on improving survival. Drugs proven to reduce morbidity and mortality in CHF are angiotensin-converting enzyme inhibitors (ACE inhibitors), diuretics, and beta blockers. In fact, a meta-analysis of 18 randomized clinical trials indicated that diuretics may be even more effective than other active drug therapy in reducing the risk for worsening disease and improving exercise capacity (Faris et al., 2002). For a complete discussion of CHF and its treatment, see Chapter 28.

The increased urinary output resulting from diuretic therapy is useful in CHF because it reduces edema and circulating volume and prevents further fluid retention by the kidneys. These actions have a net effect of decreasing preload (volume returned to the heart) and afterload (resistance exerted by the vessels to blood pumped by the heart) and easing the heart's workload. Pulmonary edema, characterized by fluid-filled lungs, is a life-threatening condition. It commonly results from CHF, but it also can result from infections, exposure to toxic gases, and reactions to drugs. However, the pulmonary edema associated with CHF occurs because pulmonary capillary pressure is greater than capillary osmotic pressure (because of increased left ventricular end-diastolic pressure). In addition, the capillary permeability of the pulmonary capillary membrane increases, thereby allowing fluid to leak into the lungs' interstitial spaces and the alveoli. This leakage impairs gas exchange, which stiffens the lungs and impairs expansion. Diuretics return fluid to the vascular space and increase fluid excretion, which eases breathing. Thiazide diuretics are used initially to treat CHF, and the more potent loop diuretics are used as edema from CHF becomes more severe with the progression of the disease. A tolerance develops to the effects of diuretics as CHF progresses, with larger and larger doses required to achieve the desired effect. Diuretic resistance should be considered a sign that CHF is worsening to the point at which the patient is likely to die (Neuberg et al., 2002).

Hypertension (blood pressure that is chronically elevated above normal), one of the most common cardiovascular disorders in the United States, is closely associated with kidney function. Renin is released by the kidneys. The outflow of renin activates several mechanisms that lead to activation of angiotensin II, a potent vasoconstrictor. Angiotensin II stimulates secretion of aldosterone, which promotes sodium retention. Sodium retention promotes water retention. The resulting increased vascular resistance and the increased fluid volume elevate blood pressure.

Although hypervolemia is not necessarily present in the hypertensive patient, the action of diuretics effectively lowers the blood pressure. Blood pressure (BP) is cardiac output (CO) multiplied by peripheral resistance (PR) ($BP = CO \times PR$). By reducing circulating volume, diuretics decrease cardiac output and reduce blood pressure. In reducing circulating volume, fluid is pulled back into the vascular space, reducing edema and the symptoms associated with it. Peripheral vascular resistance is thus decreased, further promoting reduction in blood pressure and decreasing the workload on the heart. Diuretics have been found to be at least as effective as other antihypertensives, and findings from the Antihypertensive and Lipid-Lowering Treatment to Prevent Heart Attack Trial (ALLHAT) indicate that they, and specifically the thiazides, should be used as first-line therapy in hypertension. In fact, findings from ALLHAT, in a study of more than 33,000 North American hypertensive patients with at least one other CHF risk factor, showed that thiazide-type diuretics are superior to ACE inhibitors or calcium channel blockers in preventing one or more major forms of cardiovascular disease (CVD) (ALLHAT Officers and Coordinators, 2002).

The kind of diuretic drug prescribed depends on the patient's condition and the severity of the hypertension. Diuretics may be used alone or with antihypertensive drugs to lower blood pressure. For more information on hypertension and its treatment, refer to Chapter 27.

A kidney disorder characterized by generalized edema is nephrotic syndrome. This condition alters glomerular permeability to protein, allowing massive proteinuria as plasma proteins are lost by way of the kidney. This loss causes hypoalbuminemia (a lower-than-normal blood level of the pro-

tein albumin). Low albumin levels decrease colloid osmotic pressure, which allows fluid to move out of the vascular system. This movement results in edema and decreased circulating volume. The kidneys attempt to compensate for the decreased blood volume by retaining sodium and water, which contributes to additional edema. Diuretics promote excretion of sodium and water, and therefore decrease the circulating blood volume.

A potentially reversible condition, ARF results from acutely reduced kidney function. Chronic renal failure, an irreversible and progressive reduction of kidney function, results from various conditions, including hypertension, diabetes mellitus, systemic lupus erythematosus, recurrent urinary tract infections, and obstruction. Renal failure is characterized by **oliguria** (abnormally reduced urine output, less than 400 mL/d); azotemia; sodium and water retention, leading to hypertension, CHF, and edema; metabolic acidosis; electrolyte imbalances; abnormalities of calcium, phosphorus, and vitamin D metabolism; and uremia in end-stage renal disease.

The effectiveness and safety of diuretics in treating ARF and chronic renal failure depend on kidney functioning. Osmotic diuretics are helpful in the early phases of ARF. Loop diuretics may be used in the early stages of chronic renal failure; thiazides are normally avoided in patients with decreased renal function because they decrease the glomerular filtration rate (GFR). Once end-stage renal failure sets in, however, diuretics are of little value and may be harmful. Diuretics should be used cautiously in patients with renal impairment.

C THIAZIDE DIURETICS

The thiazides comprise the largest group of diuretics. They are related structurally to the antibacterial sulfonamides, although a few drugs in the class differ slightly in chemical structure. These drugs are called thiazide-like diuretics and include indapamide (Lozol) and quinethazone (Aquamox). They exhibit the same diuretic mechanism of action, efficacy, and adverse reactions as the thiazides. Thiazide diuretics include hydrochlorothiazide (HydroDIURIL), benzthiazide (Exna), chlorothiazide (Diuril), chlorthalidone (Hygroton), and metolazone (Zaroxolyn). Additional thiazide diuretics include bendroflumethiazide (Naturetin), hydroflumethiazide (Diucardin), trichlormethiazide (Diurese), polythiazide (Renese), and methyclothiazide (Aquatensen, Enduron). The prototype thiazide diuretic is hydrochlorothiazide. Table 32.1 presents a summary of selected diuretic drugs.

NURSING MANAGEMENT OF THE PATIENT RECEIVING P HYDROCHLOROTHIAZIDE

Core Drug Knowledge

Pharmacotherapeutics

Hydrochlorothiazide (HCTZ) is used widely in managing hypertension, either alone or with other drugs. Several days are required to see the antihypertensive effects, and full therapeutic effects may not occur for 2 to 4 weeks. Hydrochlorothiazide also is used in treating edema resulting from CHF, hepatic cirrhosis, renal disease, and long-term steroid or estrogen therapy. Paradoxically, hydrochlorothiazide is used in diabetes insipidus as an antidiuretic, possibly because it enhances the action of ADH as a consequence of sodium depletion.

In investigational use, hydrochlorothiazide may be used alone or with amiloride or allopurinol to prevent formation and recurrence of calcium stones in hypercalciuria by promoting reabsorption of calcium. In addition, these drugs have been used to prevent osteoporosis in postmenopausal women. One study showed that thiazide diuretics help protect against hip fracture in adults older than 55 years of age because they decrease the age-related bone loss by decreasing urinary calcium wasting (Schoofs et al., 2003).

Pharmacokinetics

Administered orally, hydrochlorothiazide is absorbed rapidly from the GI tract, and more than 50% of the circulating drug is bound to plasma proteins. Action begins within a few hours. The drug crosses the placental barrier and is secreted in breast milk. Hydrochlorothiazide is metabolized by the liver and excreted in the urine.

Pharmacodynamics

Hydrochlorothiazide acts in the distal tubule and possibly in the diluting segment of the ascending loop of Henle. It increases excretion of sodium and chloride in the distal convoluted tubule by slightly inhibiting the ion pumps that work in sodium and chloride reabsorption. This action also inhibits water reabsorption. Because most of the sodium is reabsorbed before the distal tubule, hydrochlorothiazide has a weak diuretic effect. It also increases the excretion of potassium, bicarbonate, and magnesium and decreases the excretion of calcium. Water-soluble vitamins also are lost with the increased urine elimination from hydrochlorothiazide, as well as other diuretics (Suter et al., 2000). Hydrochlorothiazide decreases GFR and increases blood urea nitrogen (BUN).

Contraindications and Precautions

Important contraindications to hydrochlorothiazide therapy include severe renal impairment or anuria (urine output >250 mL daily), hepatic coma, and hypersensitivity to the drug or to sulfonamide antibiotics, which are similar chemically to hydrochlorothiazide and therefore increase the risk for cross-sensitivity. Thiazides should be used with caution in patients with renal disease, lupus erythematosus, liver disease, fluid and electrolyte imbalances, diabetes, gout, elevated cholesterol levels, elevated triglycerides, bronchial asthma, advanced arteriosclerosis, and heart disease. Hydrochlorothiazide is an FDA pregnancy category B drug.

Adverse Effects

Adverse effects are due mostly to the effects of fluid loss or imbalance or from the effects of electrolyte imbalances, which may include hypokalemia, hyponatremia, hypochloremia, and hypercalcemia. The most common adverse effects occur in various systems as follows: cardiovascular (hypotension), central nervous system (CNS; dizziness, lightheadedness, and vertigo), GI (anorexia, nausea, and vomiting), and genitourinary (GU; polyuria and nocturia).

TABLE 32.1 Summary of Selected Diuretic Drugs

Drug (Trade) Name	Selected Indications	Route and Dosage Range	Pharmacokinetics
C Thiazide Diuretics			
P hydrochlorothiazide (Esidrix, HydroDIURIL, Oretic; *Canadian:* Apo-Hydro)	Hypertension	*Adult:* PO, 12.5–50 mg/d; increase to 25–100 mg/d as a single or two divided doses *Child:* PO, infants up to 6 mo, 3.3 mg/kg/d in two doses; 6 mo–2 y, 12.5–37.5 mg/d in two doses, depending on body weight; 2–12 y, 37.5–100 mg/d in two doses depending on body weight	*Onset:* 2 h *Duration:* 6–12 h $t_{1/2}$: 5.6–14.8 h
	Edema	*Adult:* PO, 25–200 mg/d initially, then 25–100 mg/d *Child:* PO, 2.2 mg/kg/d in two doses	
C Loop Diuretics			
P furosemide (Lasix; *Canadian:* Apo-Furosemide)	Edema	*Adult:* PO, 20–80 mg/d in a single dose, may repeat 6 to 8 h later, titrate up to 600 mg/d in severe edema *Adult:* IM, IV, 20–40 mg, may repeat 2 h later	*Onset:* PO, within 1 h; IV, within 5 min *Duration:* PO, 6–8 h; IV, 2 h $t_{1/2}$: 2 h
	Hypertension	*Adult:* PO, 40 mg bid *Child:* PO, 2 mg/kg, may increase by 1–2 mg/kg, not to exceed 6 mg/kg	
	CHF, CRF	*Adult:* PO, IV, 2–2.5 g/d	
	Pulmonary edema	*Adult:* IV, 40 mg over 1–2 min, may increase to 80 mg *Child:* IV, 1 mg/kg, may increase by 1 mg/kg but not more than 6 mg/kg	
C Potassium-Sparing Diuretics			
P triamterine (Dyrenium)	Hypertension	*Adult:* PO, 100 mg bid when used alone; decrease starting dose when given with other diuretics; decrease dose of each, adjust to need; not to exceed 300 mg/d	*Onset:* PO, 2–4 h *Duration:* 12–16 h $t_{1/2}$: 3 h
amiloride (Midamor)	Hypertension	*Adult:* PO, add 5 mg/d to usual anti-hypertensive or other diuretic therapy; increase up to 10 mg/d	*Onset:* 2 h *Duration:* 24 h $t_{1/2}$: 6–9 h
spironolactone (Aldactone; *Canadian:* Novo-Spiroton)	Hyperaldosteronism	*Adult:* PO, 100–400 mg/d	*Onset:* 24–48 h *Duration:* 48–72 h $t_{1/2}$: 20 h
	Edema	*Adult:* PO, 100 mg/d (range: 25–200 mg/d) *Child:* PO, 3.3 mg/kg/d in single or divided doses	
	Hypertension	*Adult:* PO, 50–100 mg/d, single or divided doses *Child:* PO, 1–2 mg/kg bid	
	Diuretic-induced hypokalemia	*Adult:* PO, 25–100 mg/d	
C Osmotic Diuretics			
P mannitol (Osmitrol)	Acute renal failure	*Adult:* IV, 50–100 g of 5%–25% solution (preventative) or 50–100 g of 15%–25% solution (treatment)	*Onset:* 0.5–1 h *Duration:* 6–8 h $t_{1/2}$: 15–100 min

(continued)

TABLE 32.1 Summary of Selected Diuretic Drugs (continued)

Drug (Trade) Name	Selected Indications	Route and Dosage Range	Pharmacokinetics
	Intracranial pressure	*Adult:* IV, 1.5–2 g/kg as 15%–25% solution infused over 30–60 min	
	Intraocular pressure	*Adult:* IV, 1.5–2 g/kg as 15%–20% solution infused over 30 min	
	Diuresis in intoxications	*Adult:* IV, Up to 200 g	
	Urologic irrigation	*Adult:* Bladder catheter, 2.5% solution; add two 50-mL vials (25% mannitol) to 900-mL sterile water	
(C) Carbonic Anhydrase Inhibitors			
(P) acetazolamide (Diamox; *Canadian:* Apo-Acetazolamide)	Chronic open-angle glaucoma	*Adult:* PO, 250 mg–1 g daily in divided doses	*Onset:* PO, 1–1.5 h; IV, 2 min *Duration:* PO, 8–12 h; IV, 4–5 h $t_{1/2}$: Unknown
	Secondary glaucoma/preoperative acute congestive closed-angle glaucoma	*Adult:* PO, IV, 250 mg q4h or 250 mg bid or 500 mg followed by 125 or 250 mg q4h *Child:* IM, IV 5–10 mg/kg/dose q6h; PO, 10–15 mg/kg/d in divided doses	
	CHF	*Adult:* PO, 250–375 mg (5 mg/kg)/d	
	Drug-induced edema	*Adult:* PO, 250–375 mg qd, give every other day or 2 d on then 1 d off *Child:* PO, IV 5 mg/kg/dose	
	Epilepsy	*Adult and child:* PO, IV, 8–30 mg/kg/d in divided doses	
	Mountain sickness	*Adult:* PO, 500–1,000 mg/d in divided doses; may use sustained-release preparation	
(C) Antimuscarinic Agents			
(P) tolterodine (Detrol)	Overactive bladder	*Adult:* IR, 2 mg 2 x day ER, 4 mg 2 x day	*Onset:* Unknown *Duration:* Unknown

Other adverse effects related to fluid and electrolyte imbalances include CNS effects, such as paresthesia (numbness and tingling), headache, and drowsiness. Cardiovascular effects include orthostatic hypotension, volume depletion, cardiac arrhythmias, and chest pain. GI disturbances include diarrhea, constipation, jaundice, and pancreatitis. Dermatologic effects include poor skin turgor and dry mucous membranes. Finally, the musculoskeletal system may be prone to weakness and muscle cramps or spasms resulting from potassium loss, and possibly gout resulting from increased uric acid levels.

Drug Interactions

Hydrochlorothiazide and other thiazide diuretics increase the effect of many drugs or drug classes, including allopurinol, anesthetics, antineoplastics, calcium salts, diazoxide, digitalis, lithium, loop diuretics, methyldopa, nondepolarizing muscle relaxants, and vitamin D. Thiazide diuretics decrease the effectiveness of anticoagulants and antigout agents. The effect of thiazides is increased by amphotericin B, corticosteroids, and anticholinergics. The effect of thiazides is decreased by cholestyramine, colestipol, methenamines, and nonsteroidal anti-inflammatory drugs (NSAIDs). Although no major drug–food interactions are associated with hydrochlorothiazide, some blood test findings may be altered. For example, decreased protein-bound iodine levels may occur without the patient showing signs of thyroid disturbance. Table 32.2 lists agents that interact with hydrochlorothiazide.

Assessment of Relevant Core Patient Variables

Health Status

Determine whether the patient is allergic to sulfa or to other thiazides because these allergies are contraindications for use. Renal status must be assessed because severe renal impairment is a contraindication for hydrochlorothiazide use. Patients who have pre-existing renal disease, a creatinine clearance rate of 40 to 50 mL/min, a GFR of 25 mL/min, or a history of nonresponsiveness to thiazides most likely should be treated with loop diuretics instead of hydrochlorothiazide. If used, hydrochlorothiazide therapy in these patients must be monitored carefully.

Assess hepatic status because hepatic coma is a contraindication, and hepatic disease warrants cautious use. Other

TABLE 32.2 Agents That Interact With P Hydrochlorothiazide

Interactants	Effect and Significance	Nursing Management
allopurinol	May increase the incidence of hypersensitivity reactions to allopurinol	Monitor for allergic effects.
anesthetics	More anesthetic effect	Dosage may need to be decreased. Monitor/correct fluid imbalance prior to surgery if possible.
anticoagulants	Decreased anticoagulant effect	Monitor prothrombin time, partial thromboplastin time; dose may need adjustment.
antigout agents	Decreased effect with thiazides; increased uric acid levels	Monitor uric acid levels; dose may need to be adjusted.
antineoplastics	Induces leukopenia with prolonged use	Monitor white blood cell count.
calcium salts	Increased effect because thiazides promote calcium retention	Monitor calcium levels.
diazoxide	Hyperglycemia possible	Monitor blood glucose level.
digitalis glycosides	Hypokalemia from thiazides, which may induce digitalis toxicity	Monitor potassium level. Monitor for digitalis toxicity. Provide potassium in diet or supplements.
lithium	Sodium possibly lost instead of lithium ions, inducing lithium toxicity	Monitor blood lithium levels.
loop diuretics	Profound diuresis and serious electrolyte imbalance	Monitor electrolyte levels.
methyldopa	Rare occurrences of hemolytic anemia with concurrent use	Monitor complete blood chemistry.
nondepolarizing muscle relaxants	Possible prolonged neuromuscular blocking effects and respiratory depression	Assess respiratory status.
sulfonylureas, insulin	Increased blood glucose	Dose may need adjusting.
vitamin D	Biologic actions of vitamin D enhanced; hypercalcemia may have role	Monitor calcium levels.
amphotericin B, corticosteroids	Electrolyte depletion intensified	Monitor electrolyte levels, particularly potassium.
anticholinergics	Increased absorption of thiazides	Monitor blood pressure, electrolyte levels.
bile acid sequestrants (cholestyramine, colestipol)	Bind thiazides, reduce absorption	Give thiazides at least 2 h before resin.
methenamines	Possible decreased effect of thiazides due to alkalinization of urine	Monitor blood pressure, electrolyte levels; may need to adjust dosage.
nonsteroidal anti-inflammatory drugs	Reduced diuretic, natriuretic, and antihypertensive effect	Observe for therapeutic effect.

problems include a history of systemic lupus erythematosus, diabetes, gout, bronchial asthma, arteriosclerosis, heart disease, or elevated triglyceride or cholesterol levels. In diabetic patients, blood glucose levels must be assessed; in patients with gout, uric acid levels must be assessed; and in patients with kidney disease or kidney failure, creatinine levels must be assessed because hydrochlorothiazide elevates blood glucose, lipid, and uric acid levels.

Before therapy begins, it is important to assess fluid and electrolyte status because hydrochlorothiazide causes fluid and electrolyte losses. If the patient has fluid and electrolyte deficiencies before therapy, additional losses will increase the risk for serious adverse effects. Additional baseline measurements should include blood pressure and other vital signs; body weight; edema in the ankles, sacrum, and abdomen; and urinary elimination patterns and output volume.

Because many drugs interact with hydrochlorothiazide, assess the patient's drug history, particularly the current drug regimen. Drug therapy that also causes electrolyte loss or that may be affected adversely by the electrolyte loss induced from hydrochlorothiazide therapy should be most closely assessed. For example, hydrochlorothiazide causes potassium loss (**hypokalemia**). Hypokalemia increases the effect of the drug digoxin. Therefore, patients receiving digoxin for CHF have an increased risk for digoxin toxicity if they become hypokalemic during hydrochlorothiazide therapy.

Life Span and Gender

It is important to determine whether the patient is pregnant or breast-feeding. Hydrochlorothiazide must be used with caution by pregnant or breast-feeding women. Determine the patient's age before administering hydrochlorothiazide therapy. Efficacy and safety of hydrochlorothiazide have not been established in children. Hyponatremia is more likely to occur in older adults (>65 years) who receive thiazide diuret-

ics. The use of thiazide diuretics greatly increases the older adult's risk for becoming hyponatremic. Sodium deficiency may develop slowly, and the patient may have been on the drug for a year or more before hyponatremia is clearly present. Older women seem to be more at risk than older men for hyponatremia (Rosholm et al., 2002; Sharabi et al., 2002). Older adults also appear to be at increased risk for vitamin B_1 deficiency while taking hydrochlorothiazide or other diuretics. This deficiency is caused by vitamin loss with increased urination (Suter et al., 2000).

Lifestyle, Diet, and Habits

Assess the patient's normal fluid intake and dietary sources of electrolytes, particularly potassium, to evaluate whether the patient's nutritional intake can compensate adequately for electrolytes lost during drug therapy.

Environment

Some assessment factors related to hydrochlorothiazide therapy include whether the patient can get easily to a toilet, especially in the beginning of therapy when urine output increases. The patient's home must be set up for safety because falls may occur as a result of adverse effects of therapy. Hydrochlorothiazide can be self-administered at home or administered in acute care, long-term care, or subacute care settings.

Culture and Inherited Traits

Note the patient's ethnic background. In black American patients, hydrochlorothiazide therapy is somewhat more effective than in patients who are of European descent. It is believed that hypertensive black Americans have features that are consistent with a theory of corrected volume status where the sodium and potassium pump is inhibited. Because hydrochlorothiazide stimulates excretion of sodium and potassium, it exerts an additional effect in hypertensive black Americans.

Nursing Diagnoses and Outcomes

- Risk for Deficient Fluid Volume related to action and adverse effects of hydrochlorothiazide
  Desired outcome: *The patient will not experience fluid imbalance while on hydrochlorothiazide therapy.*
- Risk for Injury, Falls, related to adverse effects of hydrochlorothiazide
  Desired outcome: *The patient will not suffer injury from falls while taking hydrochlorothiazide.*
- Risk for Injury, Drug Interactions, related to multiple drug therapies
  Desired outcome: *The patient will not have adverse effects from drug interactions while taking hydrochlorothiazide.*

Planning and Intervention

Maximizing Therapeutic Effects

Administer hydrochlorothiazide in the morning so that the maximum diuretic effect will not disturb sleep (assuming the patient is awake days and sleeps nights). It is important to provide ready access to a bathroom (or bedside urinal, bedpan, or commode) to ensure comfort during peak drug action.

Monitor fluid intake, urine output, and body weight for changes. It is important to encourage the patient to avoid foods high in sodium content and not to increase sodium intake greatly after hydrochlorothiazide dosage has been regulated because that increase could counteract the effect of drug therapy. Encourage continued efforts at lifestyle changes that lower blood pressure (when used to treat hypertension). Work with the patient to identify and correct lifestyle factors that can affect adherence, as described in Box 32.1.

Minimizing Adverse Effects

Monitor serum electrolyte levels for hypokalemia, hyponatremia, hypomagnesemia, hypercalcemia, hyperglycemia, and hyperuricemia. Also, monitor serum triglyceride, cholesterol, and creatinine levels. Administer potassium supplements as indicated to maintain normal potassium levels. Older adults should be monitored closely throughout therapy for hyponatremia. Assess the older adult for signs of water-soluble vitamin deficiencies; a multivitamin may be

COMMUNITY-BASED CONCERNS

Box 32.1 Factors That Can Decrease Adherence to Diuretic Therapy

Older adults are often prescribed diuretic therapy as part of their drug regimen to treat hypertension or congestive heart failure. Sometimes, therapeutic or adverse effects from the drug therapy cause older adults to choose not to take their prescribed diuretic regularly. Here are some common reasons patients give for not wanting to take a diuretic, and some suggestions for how you can help the patient minimize these problems.

- *I have to get up and go to the bathroom several times during the night.* Encourage the patient to take the drug early in the morning. If he is to take it twice a day, have him take the second dose before 6 PM. If timing the dose this way still does not minimize the problem, consult with the prescriber to see if the dose can be given as one daily dose instead of two daily doses.
- *I can't get to the bathroom quick enough, and I wet myself.* The problem may not be the diuretic itself, but impaired mobility or fine motor skills required to unzip a pants zipper or manipulate clothing. If the patient has difficulty moving quickly, suggest that he empty his bladder routinely throughout the day so that he doesn't ever get an extremely full bladder, which may contribute to feelings of urgency. A bedside commode might be helpful if the patient is having trouble getting to the bathroom in the middle of the night. Clothing modifications, such as Velcro closures, might make manipulating clothing easier. A consultation with an occupational therapist may be helpful.
- *I can't go anywhere, because if I can't find a bathroom right away, I might have an accident.* Time the dosing of the diuretic so that it will have had a chance to reach full effect before the patient wants to go out. For example, if the patient wishes to go out at 10 AM, he might want to vary the time he takes his medication, taking it earlier in the morning that day. If he takes the drug at 6 AM and the drug's peak effect occurs in 2 hours, by 10 AM, the effect on urinary output would be less. He might also prefer to wear an absorbent pad or briefs when he goes out to give him a feeling of security that he won't accidentally wet his clothing.

indicated, especially if the patient does not eat a nutrient-rich diet.

It is important to assess the complete blood count (CBC) to detect blood abnormalities, and to inspect the skin for rashes or hives to detect sensitivity responses. Observe the patient for related signs and symptoms of fluid and electrolyte abnormalities. It also is important to weigh the patient regularly to determine extraordinary fluid loss (reflected in weight loss) and complications (reflected in weight gain). The patient might be weighed daily during the initial period of therapy and then weekly or biweekly once therapy is stabilized. A weight gain exceeding 3 pounds in 1 day—a sign of fluid retention and complications—should be reported to the prescriber.

Caution the patient to avoid rapid position changes that may intensify orthostatic hypotension and precipitate falls. As needed, elderly or debilitated patients should be assisted with walking to the bathroom to prevent injury. Hydrochlorothiazide can be administered with meals or milk to prevent or minimize GI upset. It is important to assess for signs of drug interactions if the patient is currently receiving other drug therapies known to interact with hydrochlorothiazide.

Providing Patient and Family Education

- Explain the importance of follow-up blood work to monitor electrolyte levels.
- Urge patients to report signs and symptoms of hypokalemia (irregular pulse rate, muscle weakness or cramps, constipation, or abdominal pain).
- Tell the patient to take his or her pulse and compare the rate with former or normal rates. (You may need to teach the patient how to take a pulse.)
- Encourage the patient to consume potassium-rich foods, such as bananas, apricots, and orange juice, and other electrolyte-rich beverages and food to counter electrolyte losses, especially potassium.
- Teach older adults and their family members to report signs and symptoms of hyponatremia (weakness, nerve disorders, loss of weight, "salt hunger," cramps, problems with digestion).
- Teach the patient to avoid injury from falls by rising slowly and balancing carefully to counter orthostatic hypotension.
- Instruct the patient to take hydrochlorothiazide with food if he or she has problems with GI discomfort.
- Explain the importance of wearing sunglasses, sunscreen, wide-brimmed hats, and cover-up clothing to avoid a possible photosensitivity reaction.
- Store hydrochlorothiazide safely to prevent accidentally poisoning children, elderly or forgetful adults, or others.

Ongoing Assessment and Evaluation

The effects of therapy and the degree to which expected outcomes have been achieved should be evaluated. Most patients receiving hydrochlorothiazide can expect to have a reduction in fluid retention, edema, and blood pressure. To that end, edema and blood pressure may be compared with baseline values. Fluid balance may be evaluated by weighing the patient at the same time of day on the same scale, ideally with the patient wearing the same weight of clothing. Laboratory tests may be reviewed regularly to detect electrolyte imbalances and blood abnormalities.

MEMORY CHIP

P Hydrochlorothiazide

- Widely used alone or with other agents to reduce blood pressure; also used to treat edema from CHF, hepatic or renal disease, or secondary to drug use
- Works in the distal tubule to promote excretion of sodium, chloride, potassium, and water
- Major contraindication: severe renal disease
- Most common adverse effects: from fluid and electrolyte loss (dizziness, light-headedness, vertigo, nausea, and vomiting)
- Most serious adverse effects: aplastic anemia and thrombocytopenia (although not normally life-threatening)
- Minimizing adverse effects: Monitor blood pressure, weight, intake and output, and serum electrolyte levels while on this drug.
- Most important patient education: Explain the importance of periodic blood work to monitor electrolytes.

C LOOP DIURETICS

The loop diuretics work in the loop of Henle to inhibit reabsorption of sodium and chloride. They exert a powerful effect on fluid and electrolyte balance. Loop diuretics are sometimes referred to as high-ceiling diuretics because the maximum diuretic effect that can be achieved is higher than with other diuretics. Loop diuretics include furosemide (Lasix), bumetanide (Bumex), ethacrynic acid (Edecrin), and torsemide (Demadex) (see Table 32.1.) The prototype drug in this class is furosemide.

NURSING MANAGEMENT OF THE PATIENT RECEIVING P FUROSEMIDE

Core Drug Knowledge

Pharmacotherapeutics

Furosemide is a potent diuretic that is effective in reducing peripheral edema from CHF and hepatic and renal diseases, including nephrotic disease (Box 32.2). It is highly effective in treating pulmonary edema. It also is effective in treating hypertension and is the first choice over thiazides in patients with pre-existing renal disease because, unlike thiazides, it does not decrease GFR. Some research indicates that inhaled furosemide reduces dyspnea. Further research is needed in this area, however, before inhaling furosemide to reduce dyspnea becomes a common, accepted therapeutic use (Nishino et al., 2000).

Pharmacokinetics

After oral administration, furosemide is absorbed rapidly and well from the GI tract. However, after intravenous (IV) administration, furosemide acts even more rapidly—within 10 minutes. Duration of action is 2 hours. The drug is about 95% bound to plasma proteins. Furosemide is metabolized in the liver and excreted by the kidneys. It crosses the placenta and may be excreted in breast milk.

FOCUS ON RESEARCH

Box 32.2 Furosemide Infusion in Refractory Congestive Heart Failure (CHF)

Paterna, S., Di Pasquale, P., Parrinello, G., Amato, P., Cardinale, A., Follone, G., Giubilato, A., & Licata, G. (2000). Effects of high-dose furosemide and small-volume hypertonic saline solution infusion in comparison with a high dose of furosemide as a bolus in refractory congestive heart failure. *European Journal of Heart Failure, 2*(3), 305–313.

The Study

A study of hospitalized patients with CHF who were unresponsive to high oral doses of furosemide, ACE inhibitors, digitalis, and nitrates was performed. The patients also all had an ejection fraction <35%, serum creatinine <2 mg/dL, BUN <60 mg/dL, a reduced urinary volume, and a low natriuresis. The patients either received an IV push bolus of furosemide (500 to 1,000 mg) bid or an IV infusion of furosemide (500 to 1,000 mg) in 150 mL of NaCl, bid over 30 minutes, over 6 to 12 days. Both groups also received KCL (20 to 40 mEq) IV to prevent hypokalemia. The group that received an IV push furosemide was hospitalized longer than the group that received an IV infusion of furosemide (11.67 ≤1.8 days versus 8.57 ± 2.3 days; p <.001). Both groups achieved a lower class rating of CHF (based on New York Heart Association [NYHA] classification) at discharge (this is an improvement). In a follow-up visit at 6 to 12 months, none of the patients who received the IV infusion of furosemide required readmission to the hospital and their NYHA classification remained as it was at discharge. This is contrasted with 40% of the patients who received IV push furosemide. These patients also reverted to a higher NYHA classification than they had achieved prior to discharge.

Nursing Implications

Patients with CHF who have been unresponsive to high doses of oral furosemide and other drugs may benefit from administration of furosemide as an IV infusion rather than an IV push, which is not diluted, when they are hospitalized for recurrent exacerbations of CHF. Nurses should consult with the other health care team members (nurse practitioners, physicians, and pharmacists) about this possibility of drug therapy for appropriate patients.

Pharmacodynamics

Furosemide inhibits the reabsorption of sodium, chloride, and water in the ascending loop of Henle. It also has some effect in the proximal and distal tubules. As a result, excretion of sodium, chloride, potassium, and water increases. Magnesium and calcium are excreted as well. Furosemide can increase blood glucose, low-density lipoprotein, total cholesterol, and triglyceride levels. In addition, furosemide decreases excretion of uric acid, which may raise uric acid levels.

Furosemide influences the activity of vagally mediated mechanoreceptors in the airways. It is hypothesized that the vagal afferent fibers may play an important role in modulating the feeling of dyspnea, which would be the mechanism for inhaled furosemide alleviating dyspnea. One small study was able to alleviate the sensation of dyspnea that was induced experimentally by breath-holding and by a combination of inspiratory resistive loading and hypercapnia (Nishino et al., 2000).

Contraindications and Precautions

Furosemide should not be used in anuria or if hypersensitivity to the compounds or to sulfonylureas exists. Cautious use must be exercised in patients with poor renal function and lupus erythematosus. Furosemide is a pregnancy category C drug.

Adverse Effects

Most of furosemide's adverse effects relate to fluid or electrolyte imbalance. The most common adverse effects are CNS (dizziness, vertigo, paresthesias, xanthopsia, and weakness); GI (nausea, anorexia, vomiting, oral and gastric irritation, and constipation); cardiovascular (orthostatic hypotension); hematologic (leukopenia, anemia, and thrombocytopenia); GU (glycosuria and urinary bladder spasm); dermatologic (photosensitivity, rash, pruritus, and urticaria); and musculoskeletal (muscle cramps and muscle spasms).

Other adverse effects are CNS (headache, blurred vision, hearing loss [may be permanent], restlessness, and fever); GI (diarrhea, cramping, pancreatitis, jaundice, and ischemic hepatitis); cardiovascular (chronic aortitis); hematologic (purpura and aplastic anemia); dermatologic (necrotizing angiitis, interstitial nephritis, exfoliative dermatitis, erythema multiforme, rash, local irritation, and pain with parenteral use); and miscellaneous (hyperuricemia, hyperglycemia, and activation or exacerbation of systemic lupus erythematosus [SLE]).

Excessive diuresis from furosemide can result in dehydration, reduction in blood volume with circulatory collapse, and the possibility of vascular thrombosis and embolism, particularly in the elderly. Patients with hepatic cirrhosis and ascites must be monitored carefully because rapid electrolyte shifts resulting from furosemide therapy may induce hepatic encephalopathy and coma.

Ototoxicity can occur with rapid IV therapy, especially in patients with poor renal function and in those patients receiving high doses of furosemide. Although usually transient, ototoxicity may result in permanent damage. The Na-K-Cl cotransport system exists, not only in the kidney, but also in the marginal and dark cells of the stria vascularis, which are responsible for endolymph secretion. Ototoxicity has been hypothesized to be an indirect effect on the body, related to changes in ionic composition and fluid volume within the endolymph (Humes, 1999).

Patients with SLE may have exacerbations of the illness when receiving furosemide. If increasing azotemia, oliguria, or BUN or creatinine levels occur in patients with renal impairment, furosemide therapy should be discontinued.

Drug Interactions

Furosemide increases the effect of aminoglycosides, anticoagulants, beta blockers, chloral hydrate, digitalis, and lithium. Furosemide decreases the effect of sulfonylureas and has an undetermined effect on nondepolarizing muscle relaxants and theophyllines. Thiazide diuretics, cisplatin, and clofibrate increase the effect of furosemide. Phenytoin, NSAIDs, probenecid, and salicylates all decrease the effect of furosemide. Bioavailability and degree of diuresis are reduced when furosemide is administered with food. Table 32.3 lists agents that interact with furosemide.

Assessment of Relevant Core Patient Variables

Health Status

Initially, assess for allergies to furosemide or other contraindications. A baseline assessment is then performed. This

TABLE 32.3 Agents That Interact With P Furosemide

Interactants	Effect and Significance	Nursing Management
aminoglycosides	Increased auditory toxicity; possible hearing loss	Monitor BUN and creatinine; adverse effects will increase if drugs are not excreted well. Assess for hearing problems. When giving furosemide IV, give very slowly.
anticoagulants	Enhanced anticoagulant action possible	Monitor PT, PTT.
beta blocker (propranolol)	Increased plasma levels of propranolol	Monitor therapeutic effect of propranolol.
chloral hydrate	Rare transient diaphoresis, hot flashes, hypertension, tachycardia, weakness, and nausea	Consider drug interaction if these effects occur.
digitalis glycosides	Furosemide-induced hypokalemia, possibly increasing digitalis toxicity	Monitor serum potassium level. Supply potassium in diet or as supplement. Monitor for signs of digitalis toxicity.
lithium	Possible increased plasma lithium levels and toxicity	Monitor lithium levels.
nondepolarizing muscle relaxants	Antagonized or potentiated action of muscle relaxants, perhaps depending on furosemide dose	Monitor for therapeutic effect.
sulfonylureas	Hyperglycemia	Sulfonylurea dosage may need adjustment.
theophylline	Theophylline effect enhanced or inhibited	Monitor for therapeutic effect of theophylline.
charcoal	Decreased absorption of furosemide	Monitor for therapeutic effect. May be antidote in case of furosemide overdose.
cisplatin	Additive ototoxicity	Monitor for hearing loss, tinnitus. Administer IV furosemide slowly.
clofibrate	Exaggerated diuretic response	Monitor intake and output, BP, edema, and fluid and electrolyte levels.
phenytoin	Decreased diuretic response	Monitor for therapeutic response.
NSAID	Decreased diuretic response	Monitor for therapeutic response.
probenecid	Decreased diuretic response	Monitor for therapeutic response.
salicylates	Diuretic response impaired in patients with cirrhosis and ascites	Monitor for therapeutic response.
thiazides	Profound diuresis and serious electrolyte levels	Monitor BP, edema, and fluid and electrolyte levels.

assessment is much like the one for a patient receiving HCTZ. It begins with taking blood pressure and vital signs and reviewing relevant blood test results and electrolyte levels. To assess fluid status and obtain baseline data for therapy, weigh the patient. Apparent edema is inspected and palpated. It is important to auscultate breath sounds, particularly in patients with CHF or pulmonary edema. Assess skin turgor and mucous membranes and measure fluid intake and urinary output.

During assessment, keep the proposed route of administration in mind because IV furosemide may have a substantially more potent effect on blood pressure and vital signs (cardiac arrest has been reported) than oral furosemide. As with HCTZ, also assess for gout, diabetes, and high serum cholesterol and triglyceride levels.

Life Span and Gender

Determine whether the female patient is pregnant. Furosemide is classified as a pregnancy category C drug and should not be used during pregnancy. It also is important to determine the patient's age before administering furosemide. Furosemide may increase the risk for developing patent ductus arteriosus when given during the first few weeks of life to premature infants with respiratory distress syndrome. Development of renal calcifications (kidney stones) also has been reported when furosemide is used in severely premature infants. Furosemide can be used safely in children, but doses should not exceed 6 mg/kg of body weight.

If severe diuresis occurs from use of the drug, acute hypotensive episodes may occur, especially in elderly people. Elderly patients are at increased risk for rapid changes in fluid volume, which can lead to circulatory collapse. Moreover, elderly adults also are less tolerant of the rapid changes in blood pressure, which may occur with furosemide therapy. In older adults, the rapid loss of plasma volume and the resulting hemoconcentration are likely to cause thromboembolic episodes, such as cerebral vascular thromboses and pulmonary embolism.

Lifestyle, Diet, and Habits

Furosemide may promote severe electrolyte imbalances, especially in patients who have high dosages and who are on sodium-restricted diets. Therefore, normal fluid intake and dietary preferences should be determined and evaluated for the adequacy of electrolyte content, especially potassium.

Environment

Assess whether the patient can get to a toilet easily when needed, especially in the beginning of therapy when urine output increases. The patient's home should be assessed for risk factors that may contribute to injuries (falls) resulting from adverse effects of drug therapy. Furosemide can be self-administered at home or administered by others in acute care, long-term care, or subacute care environments. Parenteral dosing is more common in an acute care environment.

Nursing Diagnoses and Outcomes

- Risk for Deficient Fluid Volume related to action and adverse effects of furosemide
  Desired outcome: *The patient will not experience fluid and electrolyte imbalance while taking furosemide.*
- Risk for Injury, Falls, related to adverse effects of furosemide
  Desired outcome: *The patient will not suffer injury while taking furosemide.*
- Risk for Injury, Drug Interactions, related to multiple drug therapies
  Desired outcome: *The patient will not have adverse effects from drug interactions while taking furosemide.*

Planning and Intervention

Maximizing Therapeutic Effects

If therapy begins in the hospital, the patient will receive small doses that may increase gradually and incrementally. Otherwise, interventions are the same as for HCTZ.

Minimizing Adverse Effects

When giving furosemide, follow the same procedures used for minimizing adverse effects of HCTZ therapy. The drug administration route must be considered carefully because furosemide may be given intravenously or orally. Administer 20 to 40 mg of IV furosemide over at least 1 to 2 minutes to decrease the risk for ototoxicity. It is a good idea to give oral furosemide with food or milk to minimize possible GI upset. Report the adverse effects of rapid onset or worsening of edema and deterioration in breath sounds to the prescriber. These signs indicate that dosage may need to be adjusted or that a complication is developing.

Providing Patient and Family Education

The patient's and family's educational needs are similar to the needs of patients taking HCTZ.

Ongoing Assessment and Evaluation

To judge an identified therapeutic outcome, such as a reduction in edema and blood pressure, ongoing assessments of the following parameters are performed: CBC, serum electrolyte and uric acid levels, and other test values are compared with baseline values to measure progress or complications. For example, in a patient with diabetes mellitus, it is important to monitor regularly serum glucose levels because furosemide therapy may alter the amount of insulin or oral antidiabetic needed.

MEMORY CHIP

[P] Furosemide

- A potent diuretic used to treat edema from CHF, pulmonary edema, and in hepatic and renal disease; may be used as an antihypertensive
- First choice diuretic for treating hypertension with preexisting renal disease
- Works in the loop of Henle to promote excretion of large amounts of sodium, chloride, potassium, and water
- Most important contraindication: anuria in CRF
- Most common adverse effects: related to fluid and electrolyte loss, especially potassium loss
- Most serious adverse effects: permanent deafness and activation or exacerbation of SLE
- **Life span alert: Teach that older adults are more sensitive to effects of rapid fluid loss.**
- Minimizing adverse effects: Administer IV push slowly; and monitor blood pressure, edema, breath sounds, weight, intake and output, and serum electrolyte levels while therapy continues.

POTASSIUM-SPARING DIURETICS

The potassium-sparing diuretics promote sodium and water excretion in the distal tubule. At the same time, potassium is not excreted; rather, it is reabsorbed. This group of drugs produces weak diuresis and antihypertensive effects when used alone. However, the drugs are used more frequently in combination with loop and thiazide diuretics to minimize potassium loss because they work synergistically with other diuretics. Patients taking potassium-sparing diuretics are at risk for developing hyperkalemia. Potassium-sparing diuretics include triamterene (Dyrenium), amiloride (Midamor), and spironolactone (Aldactone) (see Table 32.1.) The prototype of the potassium-sparing diuretics is triamterene.

NURSING MANAGEMENT OF THE PATIENT RECEIVING [P] TRIAMTERENE

Core Drug Knowledge

Pharmacotherapeutics

Like furosemide, triamterene is used to manage edema and hypertension. The edema may be associated with CHF, cirrhosis, nephrotic syndrome, steroid use, or secondary hypoaldosteronism. It typically is used with other diuretics because it allows potassium to be reabsorbed and sodium to be excreted.

Pharmacokinetics

Triamterene is absorbed incompletely after oral administration. The drug is metabolized in the liver and excreted by the kidneys. Triamterene crosses the placenta and is excreted in small amounts in breast milk.

Pharmacodynamics

Triamterene achieves its diuretic effect by inhibiting transport of sodium in the distal tubules independent of aldosterone. This mechanism causes increased loss of sodium, chloride, water, bicarbonate, and calcium. The drug promotes retention of potassium and magnesium. Triamterene does not inhibit uric acid excretion and thereby elevates serum uric acid levels, as do the loop diuretics.

Contraindications and Precautions

Contraindications to triamterene include known hypersensitivity, use of other potassium-sparing diuretics, pre-existing **hyperkalemia** (serum potassium level >5.5 mEq/L), anuria, severe or progressive renal disease (except nephrosis), severe liver disease, and hepatic coma.

Precautions to its use include electrolyte imbalance, history of renal stone formation (it has been found in some renal calculi), diabetes (it can raise blood glucose), and when folic acid stores have been depleted (it is a weak folic acid antagonist). It is in pregnancy category B, and safety and efficacy have not been established in children.

Adverse Effects

Serious adverse effects include hyperkalemia (potentially fatal), electrolyte imbalance, and signs of fluid and electrolyte loss. Most common adverse effects are weakness, nausea, anorexia, vomiting, and dry mouth.

Other adverse effects include GI (diarrhea, jaundice, and liver enzyme abnormalities); renal (azotemia, elevated BUN and creatinine levels); hematologic (thrombocytopenia and megaloblastic anemia); CNS (fatigue, dizziness, and headache); and miscellaneous (anaphylaxis, photosensitivity, and rash).

Drug Interactions

Triamterene increases the effect of amantadine and potassium preparations. ACE inhibitors, cimetidine, and indomethacin all increase the effect of triamterene. Triamterene interferes with the fluorescent measurement of serum quinidine levels. Table 32.4 lists agents that interact with triamterene.

CRITICAL THINKING SCENARIO

Adding triamterene to hypertension therapy

Mr. Nixon is a 53-year-old white man being treated for hypertension with hydrochlorothiazide (Dyrenium). He also receives 20 mEq of potassium as a supplement daily. Mr. Nixon continues to have blood pressure readings slightly above the desired treatment goal, and his potassium levels remain low. Mr. Nixon's prescriber writes an order to add triamterene to his drug regimen.

1. Identify the major electrolyte imbalance that Mr. Nixon may now experience.
2. Suggest actions that you can take to prevent this electrolyte imbalance.

Assessment of Relevant Core Patient Variables

Health Status

Assessment activities include determining whether the patient has any known hypersensitivity to triamterene and carefully examining electrolyte values, especially potassium levels. As for other diuretic drugs, additional assessments include measuring blood pressure, edema, weight, and urine output; examining serum glucose and creatinine levels; and identifying pre-existing conditions, such as diabetes mellitus, that may affect triamterene therapy.

Life Span and Gender

Triamterene must be used cautiously in pregnancy (risk category B). Triamterene crosses into breast milk, and because safety has not been established for children, the drug should not be used in breast-feeding women.

Glomerular filtration decreases with age; consequently, elderly patients do not excrete as much potassium as younger adults. Therefore, triamterene should be given cautiously to older adults because of the increased risk for hyperkalemia.

Lifestyle, Diet, and Habits

Determine whether the patient normally eats a diet high in potassium, takes a potassium supplement, or uses a potassium chloride salt substitute.

TABLE 32.4 Agents That Interact With P Triamterene

Interactants	Effect and Significance	Nursing Management
amantadine	Increased amantadine plasma levels and decreased urinary excretion; more risk for adverse effects	Monitor for adverse effects.
potassium preparations	Severe hyperkalemia; possible cardiac arrhythmias or cardiac arrest	Avoid concurrent use.
ACE inhibitors	Elevated serum potassium from ACE inhibitors; hyperkalemia	Monitor serum potassium level.
cimetidine	Increased bioavailability and decreased renal clearance of triamterene	Monitor for increased therapeutic effect.
indomethacin	Rapid progress into acute renal failure with concurrent use	Use together only if truly necessary.

Environment

Assess whether the patient can get to a toilet easily when needed, especially in the beginning of therapy when urine output increases. The patient's home should be assessed for risk factors that may contribute to injuries (falls) resulting from adverse effects of drug therapy. Triamterene can be self-administered at home or administered by others in acute care, long-term care, or subacute care environments. Parenteral dosing is more common in an acute care environment.

Nursing Diagnoses and Outcomes

- Risk for Deficient Fluid Volume related to action and adverse effects of triamterene
  Desired outcome: *The patient will not experience fluid and electrolyte imbalance while taking triamterene.*
- Risk for Injury related to adverse effects of triamterene, including risk for hyperkalemia
  Desired outcome: *The patient will not suffer injury, and potassium levels will remain within normal limits while patient is on triamterene therapy.*
- Risk for Injury, Drug Interactions, related to multiple drug therapies
  Desired outcome: *The patient will not have adverse effects from drug interactions while taking triamterene.*

Planning and Intervention

Maximizing Therapeutic Effects

As with other diuretics, the drug dose should be administered in the morning so that increased diuretic effect occurs during waking hours.

Minimizing Adverse Effects

Monitor blood potassium levels and assess for signs of hyperkalemia (nausea, diarrhea, muscle weakness or cramping, oliguria, weak pulse, and cardiac arrhythmias). It is important to limit the patient's intake of potassium-rich foods and avoid potassium supplements. Monitor for signs of fluid and electrolyte imbalance. Oral triamterene should be given with food or milk to prevent GI upset. It is a good idea to have the patient get out of bed slowly; assist with ambulation to prevent falls from dizziness.

Providing Patient and Family Education

The main distinction between triamterene and other diuretics is the hyperkalemia that may develop with drug use. Because triamterene is usually added to therapy with other types of diuretics, patients may become accustomed to being at risk for hypokalemia. The patient needs to learn to cope with the different risks associated with triamterene (see the Critical Thinking Scenario: Adding Triamterene to Hypertension Therapy). Other patient and family education points are similar to those points provided for the other diuretics.

- Teach the patient to avoid potassium-rich foods, supplements, and potassium chloride–salt substitutes
- Teach the patient the signs and symptoms of hyperkalemia.

Ongoing Assessment and Evaluation

Monitor the patient's potassium and other electrolyte levels, blood pressure, edema, weight, and urine output. Drug therapy with triamterene is effective when blood pressure is reduced to therapeutic levels or edema is reduced without the patient developing hyperkalemia.

Drug Closely Related to P Triamterene

Amiloride, which has the same mechanism of action, efficacy, and adverse reactions as triamterene, has two additional uses. In inhalable form, amiloride may be used to treat cystic fibrosis. In patients taking lithium, amiloride can reduce lithium-induced polyuria without increasing lithium levels.

Drug Significantly Different From P Triamterene

Like triamterene, spironolactone works in the distal tubule to increase sodium and water loss and to retain potassium. Unlike triamterene, spironolactone is an aldosterone antagonist. It interferes with testosterone synthesis, which leads to altered estrogenic and androgenic activity. Like other potassium-sparing diuretics, spironolactone can be used as an adjunct therapy to treat hypertension and edema associated with CHF, nephrosis, and cirrhosis. In addition, it is used in preventing or treating hypokalemia in high-risk patients, particularly those patients also taking digitoxin for cardiac disease or those patients with cardiac arrhythmias. Because of its antialdosterone effects, a major use is in diagnosing and treating primary hyperaldosteronism. Spironolactone also has been used to treat hirsutism, familial male precocious puberty, symptoms of premenstrual syndrome, and acne vulgaris (short-term use).

The effect of spironolactone is delayed. Onset of action may not occur for 24 to 48 hours. This delayed onset occurs because the drug blocks the effect of aldosterone, which then blocks the synthesis of the proteins required for sodium and potassium transport. The existing proteins continue to

MEMORY CHIP

P Triamterene

- Potassium-sparing diuretic used to manage edema and hypertension
- Major contraindication: the patient already receiving a potassium-sparing diuretic
- Most common adverse effects: nausea, vomiting, anorexia, dry mouth, and headache
- Most serious adverse effect: hyperkalemia (electrolyte imbalance)
- **Life span alert: Older adults are especially at risk for hyperkalemia.**
- Most important patient education: Tell the patient to avoid eating potassium-rich food, taking potassium supplements, or using a salt substitute containing potassium chloride.

do their job, and diuretic effect does not occur until the existing proteins are inactive.

Nursing management unique to spironolactone therapy involves helping the patient understand and cope with such adverse effects as impotence, menstrual irregularities, and gynecomastia. Additionally, teach the patient about the drug interaction between spironolactone and salicylates, such as aspirin, which decreases the diuretic effect of therapy.

C OSMOTIC DIURETICS

Osmotic diuretics are filterable freely in the glomerulus and not reabsorbed by the tubules. They increase osmotic pressure and pull fluid into the vascular space. Because they are not reabsorbed by the tubules, they prevent water reabsorption as well. They also prevent reabsorption of sodium and chloride. Osmotic diuretics include mannitol (Osmitrol), glycerin, isosorbide, and urea (see Table 32.1).

The prototype osmotic diuretic is mannitol. Structurally, it is a sugar. Mannitol is not used to treat hypertension or peripheral edema. Instead, it is used in more acute situations.

NURSING MANAGEMENT OF THE PATIENT RECEIVING P MANNITOL

Core Drug Knowledge

Pharmacotherapeutics

Major uses of mannitol include preventing and treating ARF, reducing intracranial pressure in cerebral edema, reducing intraocular pressure when other drugs have not worked, and promoting excretion of toxic substances in urine.

In addition, mannitol is used diagnostically to measure GFR and postoperatively as an irrigant after transurethral procedures.

Pharmacokinetics

Mannitol usually is administered as an IV solution because it does not diffuse across the GI epithelium, nor is it distributed like other sugars. It can be administered as a urinary irrigant but only in transurethral prostatic resections or other transurethral surgical procedures. It is metabolized poorly, and most of it is excreted in the urine. When used as an irrigant, mannitol has a rapid onset and a short duration of action. Mannitol crosses the placenta and may enter breast milk.

Pharmacodynamics

Mannitol increases the concentration of molecules in the glomerular filtrate. This increased osmolality causes the osmotic pressure to rise. The increased pressure inhibits water reabsorption, which leads to an increased and faster flow of water in the tubules and therefore water loss. Mannitol also decreases reabsorption of sodium and chloride.

Contraindications and Precautions

Mannitol is contraindicated in severe renal disease, severe pulmonary congestion or frank pulmonary edema, active intracranial bleeding (except during craniotomy), severe dehydration, progressive renal damage or dysfunction after mannitol therapy, and progressive heart failure or pulmonary congestion after mannitol therapy.

Mannitol must be used very cautiously in CHF, hypovolemia, pseudoagglutination, and hemoconcentration. Mannitol is a pregnancy category C drug. Safety and efficacy for children 12 years and younger have not been established.

Adverse Effects

Several adverse effects result from mannitol use. They are related mostly to the fluid changes induced by its use. The most common adverse effects are CNS (dizziness) and GI (nausea, anorexia, dry mouth, and thirst). The most serious adverse effect is onset of acute CHF in susceptible patients resulting from the sudden expansion of the extracellular fluid.

Other adverse effects related to fluid changes include cardiovascular (edema, thrombophlebitis, hypotension, hypertension, tachycardia, and angina-like chest pains); CNS (headache, blurred vision, and convulsions); GI (urinary retention and osmotic nephrosis); metabolic (fluid and electrolyte imbalance, acidosis, and dehydration); and miscellaneous (pulmonary congestion, rhinitis, local pain, skin necrosis, chills, urticaria, and fever).

Fluid and electrolyte alterations may occur suddenly with the rapid expansion of extracellular fluid. Therefore, monitor for possible water intoxication and advise the patient to report chest pain or shortness of breath. These symptoms may occur when fluid or electrolyte losses induce hypotension or tachycardia.

Overdosage from larger than recommended doses may result in increased electrolyte loss, particularly sodium, chloride, and potassium. Electrolyte depletions may be severe enough to bring on hypotension and cardiac irregularities.

Drug Interactions

Mannitol does not interact with any foods, interfere with any laboratory test results, or create any major drug–drug interactions.

Assessment of Relevant Core Patient Variables

Health Status

Initially determine any contraindications to mannitol therapy, including anuria resulting from severe renal disease, pulmonary congestion, impaired cardiac function or CHF, active intracranial bleeding, or severe dehydration. These conditions contraindicate therapy because they may worsen with mannitol, which increases extracellular fluid volume. If urine output does not range between 30 and 50 mL/hour after two test doses of mannitol, the drug should not be used.

Assess blood pressure, pulse rate and character, respiratory rate and character, and breath sounds. Other general assessments include checking skin color and edema, hydration status, level of consciousness, reflexes, and muscle strength before and during the mannitol infusion to detect adverse effects.

Life Span and Gender

Assess the patient for pregnancy and breast-feeding. Pregnant patients should only receive mannitol (pregnancy category C)

if therapy is clearly warranted and the benefits outweigh potential fetal harm. Explain to breast-feeding patients that mannitol may or may not be secreted in breast milk. It also is important to note the patient's age before administering mannitol. Mannitol's effect on children younger than 12 years remains unknown. Elderly patients are at increased risk for developing dizziness, disorientation, and confusion caused by rapid fluid loss when receiving mannitol.

Environment

Note that mannitol is administered only in an acute-care setting.

Nursing Diagnosis and Outcome

- Risk for Deficient Fluid Volume related to the action of mannitol
  Desired outcome: The patient's fluid and electrolyte levels will remain in normal limits.

Planning and Intervention

Maximizing Therapeutic Effects

Concentrations of mannitol that exceed 15% have a tendency to crystallize. This crystallizing is a characteristic of the drug because it is a sugar; it is not a sign that the drug is old and should be discarded. Therefore, the drug vial should be warmed to no more than body temperature before administration to eliminate crystals. An in-line filter should be used for the infusion.

Minimizing Adverse Effects

Monitor the patient's hourly urine output. Accuracy is essential; therefore, an indwelling catheter normally is required. It is important to adjust the drug infusion rate to maintain the patient's urine output between 30 and 50 mL/hour.

Adequacy of renal function is determined in patients with renal impairment by administering one or two test doses of 0.2 g/kg over 3 to 5 minutes before beginning an infusion. If urine output is less than 30 mL/hour after the test doses, mannitol is usually withheld.

Monitor blood pressure, pulse rate, electrocardiographic (ECG) tracings, intake-to-output ratios, renal function test results, and serum electrolyte levels to monitor for rapid fluid and electrolyte alterations. It is important to assess for water intoxication as evidenced by nausea, chest pain, and shortness of breath. Breath sounds and respiratory rate and character should be assessed regularly to detect complications, such as pulmonary congestion.

Provide mouth care and ice chips for dry mouth or thirst. It also is important to assess for hives, itching, or pain at the IV site, and to provide comfort and corrective measures as needed. It is a good idea to assist patients in rising slowly from bed and provide assistance when the patient walks, if the patient must get out of bed. Treatment of overdosage includes discontinuing infusion therapy at once and institution of measures to normalize electrolyte levels. Hemodialysis may be needed to eliminate mannitol and reduce serum osmolarity.

Providing Patient and Family Education

- Explain the purpose of mannitol therapy.
- Urge the patient to report any difficulty breathing, chest pain, or peripheral swelling (edema).
- Tell the patient that blurred vision or a runny nose (if these findings occur) should subside when therapy is discontinued.

Ongoing Assessment and Evaluation

Monitoring is ongoing throughout therapy and includes measuring urine output and checking for signs of fluid or electrolyte imbalance. Therapy is effective when urine output increases and intracranial or intraocular pressure is decreased without complications to the patient.

Drugs Closely Related to [P] Mannitol

Glycerin (Glycerol)

Glycerin is an osmotic agent given orally to reduce intraocular pressure before ophthalmic surgery and during acute glaucoma attacks. It is metabolized and eliminated by the kidneys. Peak reduction of intraocular pressure occurs 1 hour after administration. Duration of action is about 5 hours. Contraindications are similar to those for mannitol and include well-established anuria, severe dehydration, frank or impending acute pulmonary edema, severe cardiac decompensation, and hypersensitivity to any ingredient. Caution should be used if the patient has acute urinary retention, hypervolemia, congestive heart disease, diabetes, or cardiac, renal, or hepatic disease. It can cause adverse reactions similar to those reactions caused by mannitol (e.g., nausea, vomiting, headache, confusion, and disorientation). Serious complications of severe dehydration, cardiac arrhythmias, and hyperosmolar nonketotic coma are possible and may be fatal. Glycerin is a pregnancy category C drug.

A suppository form (glycerin suppositories, Fleet Babylax, Sani-Sipp) also is available and is used as a hyperosmolar laxative for temporary relief of constipation.

Isosorbide

Isosorbide (Ismotic) also is used to provide short-term reduction of intraocular pressure before and after intraocular

MEMORY CHIP

[P] Mannitol

- Treats acute renal failure, increased intracranial pressure, and increased intraocular pressure
- A sugar that draws water into the vascular space through osmosis. Freely filtered but not reabsorbed; thereby causes diuresis
- Major contraindications: anuria due to severe renal disease, pulmonary edema, and intracranial bleeding
- Most common adverse effects: dizziness and GI problems
- Most serious adverse effects: worsening of CHF; serious imbalances of fluid and electrolytes; and obscure or worsened hypovolemia
- Maximizing therapeutic effects: Warm the drug vial in water before using if crystals are seen; and administer no warmer than body temperature using an in-line filter.
- Minimizing adverse effects: Give a test dose for patients with marked oliguria or inadequate renal function. If urine output does not increase after two test doses, discontinue use.

surgery and to interrupt acute attacks of glaucoma. Isosorbide causes less risk for nausea and vomiting, and it should be used in place of other osmotics when these adverse effects are undesirable for the patient. Like glycerin, it is only given orally. It is a good idea to pour the drug over cracked iced and have the patient sip the drug to improve its taste and acceptance. Contraindications and adverse effects are similar to those of mannitol. Isosorbide is a pregnancy category B drug.

Urea

Urea (Ureaphil), like mannitol, is administered by IV infusion and is used to decrease intracranial pressure (in the control of cerebral edema) and intraocular pressure. An unlabeled use has been to induce abortion. Contraindications are severely impaired renal function, active intracranial bleeding, marked dehydration, and frank liver failure. Urea is a pregnancy category C drug.

No serious adverse effects occur if urea is infused slowly, if renal function is adequate, and if intracranial bleeding is not present. Adverse effects that occur are similar to those effects seen with mannitol and include headache, nausea, vomiting, syncope, and disorientation.

Urea should be mixed with 5% or 10% dextrose solution to prevent the hemolysis produced by pure solutions of urea. Infusions should be slow because rapid infusion may be associated with hemolysis and a direct effect on the cerebral vasomotor centers, causing increased capillary bleeding. It is important to avoid using veins in lower extremities of older adults because phlebitis and thrombosis of superficial and deep veins may occur. Monitor the infusion site carefully because extravasation may cause mild irritation to tissue necrosis.

C CARBONIC ANHYDRASE INHIBITORS

Carbonic anhydrase is an enzyme that plays a role in renal excretion of acid urine and reabsorption of sodium and potassium in the proximal tubule. However, an agent that inhibits carbonic anhydrase promotes the excretion of sodium, potassium, bicarbonate, and water, resulting in an alkaline diuresis. Inhibition of carbonic anhydrase decreases aqueous humor formation and consequently decreases intraocular pressure. Carbonic anhydrase inhibitors include acetazolamide (Diamox), methazolamide (Neptazane), and dichlorphenamide (Daranide) (see Table 32.1). The prototype carbonic anhydrase inhibitor is acetazolamide.

NURSING MANAGEMENT OF THE PATIENT RECEIVING P ACETAZOLAMIDE

Core Drug Knowledge

Pharmacotherapeutics

Acetazolamide is used to treat chronic open-angle glaucoma. It also can be used in acute closed-angle glaucoma when delay of surgery is desired to reduce intraocular pressure; as an adjunct in treating edema resulting from CHF or use of drugs; as an adjunct in treating epilepsy; and in preventing and treating acute mountain sickness.

Pharmacokinetics

Acetazolamide is well absorbed from the GI tract and excreted unchanged by the kidneys.

Pharmacodynamics

Acetazolamide is a nonbacteriostatic sulfonamide that blocks the action of carbonic anhydrase, which is needed for active transport of ions across the proximal tubule. Inhibition of carbonic anhydrase results in decreased hydrogen ion secretion by the tubules and increased sodium, potassium, bicarbonate, and water excretion. Increased excretion of these electrolytes reduces the pH of body fluids. Another effect of carbonic anhydrase inhibition is decreased formation of aqueous humor, which thereby lowers intraocular pressure.

Contraindications and Precautions

Contraindications to acetazolamide therapy are hypersensitivity, depressed sodium or potassium serum levels, marked kidney and liver disease or dysfunction, suprarenal gland failure, hyperchloremic acidosis, adrenocortical insufficiency, severe pulmonary obstruction, cirrhosis, and long-term use in chronic noncongestive closed-angle glaucoma.

Acetazolamide should be administered cautiously to patients with adrenocortical insufficiency because patients with this disorder are susceptible to electrolyte imbalances. Acetazolamide is a pregnancy category C drug. It is secreted in breast milk, although dosage received by the infant is minute. Safety and efficacy in children, however, have not been established.

Adverse Effects

Sulfonamide-type adverse reactions may occur because of cross sensitivity. Adverse effects are varied. The most common are GI related and include anorexia, nausea, vomiting, and constipation. Other adverse effects include:

- GI: melena, taste alteration, and diarrhea
- Renal: hematuria, glycosuria, urinary frequency, renal colic, renal calculi, crystalluria, polyuria, and phosphaturia
- CNS: convulsion, weakness, malaise, fatigue, nervousness, drowsiness, depression, dizziness, disorientation, confusion, ataxia, tremor, tinnitus, headache, lassitude, and flaccid paralysis
- Hematologic: bone marrow depression, thrombocytopenia, thrombocytopenic purpura, hemolytic anemia, leukopenia, pancytopenia, and agranulocytosis
- Dermatologic: urticaria, pruritus, skin eruptions, rash, and photosensitivity
- Other: weight loss, fever, acidosis, absent libido, impotence, electrolyte imbalance, hepatic insufficiency, and transient myopia

Symptoms of overdose include drowsiness, anorexia, nausea, vomiting, dizziness, paresthesia, ataxia, tremor, and tinnitus. The electrolyte disturbance most likely to occur from overdosage is hyperchloremic acidosis. Treatment involves inducing vomiting or performing gastric lavage. Hyperchloremic acidosis may respond to bicarbonate administration. Potassium supplements may be required.

Drug Interactions

Acetazolamide increases the effect of cyclosporine but decreases the effect of primidone. Concurrent use of acetazolamide (or other carbonic anhydrase inhibitors) and salicylates increases the effect of both drugs. Diflunisal (Dolobid) increases the effect of acetazolamide (or other carbonic anhydrase inhibitors). Because acetazolamide promotes excretion of bicarbonate ions, the patient's urine will be alkaline, which may cause some laboratory test results to be false positive for urinary protein. Table 32.5 lists agents that interact with acetazolamide.

Assessment of Relevant Core Patient Variables

Health Status

Assessment should focus on whether the patient is allergic to acetazolamide or to the chemically similar sulfonamide anti-biotics and thiazide diuretics. Investigate any history of chronic closed-angle glaucoma, renal or hepatic diseases, respiratory acidosis, and chronic obstructive pulmonary disease.

Review blood tests for electrolyte and fluid disturbances because the drug should be used cautiously in patients with fluid and electrolyte imbalances, especially hyponatremia, hypokalemia, and hyperchloremic acidosis; hepatic disease; adrenocortical insufficiency; respiratory acidosis; or chronic obstructive pulmonary disease.

Life Span and Gender

Determine the patient's breast-feeding status and age before administering acetazolamide. Safety has not been established for breast-feeding women because safety and efficacy have not been established in children. Elderly patients do not tolerate excessive diuresis and may experience hypotension and orthostatic changes. In these patients, dosage may need to be reduced.

Environment

Note the setting in which acetazolamide may be administered. Acetazolamide may be administered in any environmental setting. However, IV administration is performed only in the hospital.

Nursing Diagnoses and Outcomes

- Risk for Deficient Fluid Volume related to therapeutic action of acetazolamide
  Desired outcome: *The patient will have desired fluid volume changes without experiencing complications from these changes.*
- Risk for Injury related to adverse effects of acetazolamide (blood dyscrasias, metabolic acidosis, paresthesia)
  Desired outcome: *The patient will not suffer injury while taking acetazolamide.*

Planning and Intervention

Maximizing Therapeutic Effects

Use acetazolamide with miotics or mydriatics for complementary effect when treating open-angle glaucoma. Best diuretic effects in CHF and drug-induced edema occur when the drug is given every other day or daily for 2 days, with the third day off. Palatability may be enhanced with honey or other sweet syrup for crushed oral tablets.

Minimizing Adverse Effects

It is important to allow the kidneys to recover and prevent overdosage when acetazolamide is used as diuretic to reduce edema. If reduction in edema ceases after first dose, do not increase the dose; instead, a day of medication should be skipped. Overdosage can be treated by gastric lavage or by inducing vomiting.

Monitor CBC and platelet counts during therapy; bone marrow suppression is rare but may occur. It also is important to monitor serum potassium levels (especially if severe cirrhosis is present or there is concurrent use of steroids or adrenocorticotropic hormones).

Administer orally or by IV injection; intramuscular (IM) administration is painful. Do not add to syrups containing glycerin or alcohol if the drug must be crushed.

Providing Patient and Family Education

- Explain the importance of returning for follow-up blood work to check CBC and electrolyte levels.
- Urge the patient to notify the prescriber if sore throat, easy bruising, petechiae, and mucosal ulcerations develop (signs of blood abnormalities).
- Tell the patient to notify the prescriber if nausea, fatigue, abdominal pain, tinnitus, hyperpnea, and numbness in extremities occur (signs of metabolic acidosis).

TABLE 32.5 Agents That Interact With [P] Acetazolamide

Interactants	Effect and Significance	Nursing Management
cyclosporine	Increased trough levels of cyclosporine; possible nephrotoxicity and neurotoxicity	Monitor for signs of nephrotoxicity and neurotoxicity.
primidone	Decreased concentrations of primidone in blood and urine	Monitor for therapeutic effect.
salicylates	Accumulation and toxicity of acetazolamide, including CNS depression and metabolic acidosis; CAI-induced acidosis may allow increased CNS penetration by salicylates	Monitor for therapeutic effects.
diflunisal	Significant decrease in intraocular pressure; increased adverse effects possible	Monitor for therapeutic response. Monitor for adverse effects.

- Encourage the patient to take acetazolamide with food if GI upset occurs.
- Caution the patient to avoid prolonged sunlight exposure.
- Tell the patient to use caution when performing activities requiring alertness until effects of the drug are known.

Ongoing Assessment and Evaluation

Throughout acetazolamide therapy, the patient should be alert for unusual vision problems and should maintain the follow-up schedule previously established. Drug therapy and nursing care are considered successful if ocular pressure remains controlled and the patient's fluid and electrolyte values stay within normal ranges.

C ANTIMUSCARINIC AGENTS

Antimuscarinic agents affect bladder contraction. Muscarinic receptors in the bladder produce bladder contractions when stimulated. A muscarinic agent that stimulates bladder function, bethanechol, is discussed in Chapter 14. When the receptors are blocked, bladder contraction cannot occur, and urinary output decreases. Antimuscarinics are used to treat overactive bladder. The prototype is tolterodine (Detrol). See Table 32.1.

NURSING MANAGEMENT OF THE PATIENT RECEIVING P TOLTERODINE

Core Drug Knowledge

Pharmacotherapeutics

Tolterodine is used in treating overactive bladder, to help manage the symptoms of urinary frequency, urgency, and urge incontinence. It is administered orally twice a day.

MEMORY CHIP

P Acetazolamide

- Used primarily in treating chronic, open-angle glaucoma because it prevents formation of aqueous humor and decreases intraocular pressure
- Inhibits hydrogen ion secretion in renal tubule, and therefore increases loss of sodium, potassium, bicarbonate, and water
- Major contraindications: severe renal or hepatic disease
- Most common adverse effects: related to gastrointestinal system
- Most serious (although rare) adverse effect: bone marrow suppression
- **Life span alert: Older adults may have hypotension and orthostatic changes; dosage may need to be reduced.**
- Maximizing therapeutic effects (of CHF diuresis): Give every other day or every 2 days, with the next day off.
- Minimizing adverse effects: Allow kidney to recover; and prevent overdosage when used to reduce edema.
- Most important patient education: Explain the importance of follow-up blood work.

Pharmacokinetics

Oral absorption of tolterodine is rapid, although the absolute bioavailability can vary a great deal. Maximum steady-state serum levels usually occur within 1 to 2 hours. Tolterodine is a highly protein-bound drug, although its active metabolite is not. Extensive, although variable, first-pass metabolism occurs after an oral dose. Several metabolites are formed, including an active one. This metabolite is formed from oxidation through the P-450 2D6 isoenzyme. Most hepatic metabolism is through P-450 3A4. Excretion of drug and metabolites are in the urine, primarily, and in the stool.

Pharmacodynamics

Tolterodine is a competitive cholinergic muscarinic antagonist. Although cholinergic muscarinic receptors exist in both the bladder and the salivary glands, tolterodine has relative selective preference for the muscarinic receptors in the bladder. Blockade of these muscarinic receptors decreases the ability of the bladder to contract. Tolterodine and its active metabolite do not have affinity for other neurotransmitter receptors or other potential cellular targets, such as the special channels for calcium ions. Tolterodine produces a pronounced effect on the bladder function. It can cause an increase in residual urine and a decrease in detrusor pressure.

Contraindications and Precautions

Tolterodine is contraindicated if the patient has urinary retention, gastric retention, uncontrolled narrow-angle glaucoma, or hypersensitivity to the drug. Patients with renal or hepatic impairment should receive doses that are half of what is normally prescribed. Use cautiously if the patient has bladder outflow obstruction or GI obstructive disorders (e.g., pyloric stenosis) as urinary retention or gastric retention may occur. Tolterodine is a pregnancy category class C drug.

Adverse Effects

The most frequent adverse effect of tolterodine is dry mouth, which is related to the anticholinergic effects from the drug. Headache is another fairly common adverse effect. Other adverse effects that are related to the antimuscarinic (anticholinergic) effects of the drug are constipation, abnormal vision (accommodation abnormalities), urinary retention, and xerophthalmia (conjunctival dryness).

Drug Interactions

A few drug interactions are known to occur with tolterodine; most are not clinically important. Fluoxetine, a potent inhibitor of P-450 2D6 interacts with tolterodine and increases unbound tolterodine drug concentrations, but no dosage changes are needed. Drugs that inhibit P-450 3A4 (e.g., macrolide antibiotics such as erythromycin and clarithromycin, and antifungal agents such as ketoconazole, itraconazole, and miconazole) increase levels of tolterodine and require smaller doses. Food increases the bioavailability of tolterodine, although not the levels of active metabolite. Dosage changes are not needed. Interactions that require nursing management are listed in Table 32.6.

TABLE 32.6 Agents That Interact With P Tolterodine

Interactant	Effect and Significance	Nursing Management
Cytochrome 3A4 inhibitors (erythromycin, clarithromycin, ketoconazole, itraconazole, miconazole)	Inhibition of this metabolic pathway may make hepatic function suboptimal and place the patient at increased risk for adverse effects.	Dosage should be limited to 1 mg/day (half usually prescribed).

Assessment of Relevant Core Patient Variables

Health Status

Assess for urinary retention, bladder outlet obstruction, gastric retention, GI obstructive disorders, renal impairment, hepatic impairment, and uncontrolled narrow-angle glaucoma, which are contraindications or precautions to using the drug.

Lifespan and Gender

The safety and efficacy of tolterodine has not been established in children. The drug is in pregnancy category C, meaning that animal studies produced teratogenetic effects. If the woman is pregnant or might become pregnant, the drug should only be used if the benefit to the mother is believed to outweigh the potential risk to the infant. It is not known whether tolterodine is excreted in human breast milk; hence, breast-feeding should be avoided.

Although older adults will have higher serum levels of tolterodine dosage, adjustments are not needed. Older adults may have decreased renal function or hepatic impairment, however, and should be checked for these problems. Men and women can achieve equal therapeutic effects from drug therapy.

Environment

Tolterodine is usually administered in the home environment.

Nursing Diagnosis and Outcomes

- Altered Urinary Elimination related to overactive bladder
  Desired outcome: *Urinary elimination will be normal with tolterodine drug therapy.*
- Risk for Urinary Retention related to adverse effects of tolterodine
  Desired outcome: *Urinary retention will not occur while taking tolterodine.*

Planning and Intervention

Maximizing Therapeutic Effect

Administer the drug on a regular prescribed basis.

Minimizing Adverse Effects

If the patient has renal or hepatic dysfunction, or is receiving drugs that are P-450 3A4 inhibitors, administer a dose of tolterodine that is no more than half of what is commonly administered daily.

Patient and Family Education

Teach the patient or family to be alert for problems with urinary retention, GI retention, or visual changes such as blurred vision. These adverse effects need to be reported to the prescriber. Maintenance of a diary that records the episodes of incontinence and frequency of urination may be helpful in determining whether drug therapy is effective. If dry mouth is a problem, tell the patient to suck on hard candies or ice chips to relieve the dryness.

Ongoing Assessment and Evaluation

Treatment with tolterodine is effective if urinary incontinence and frequency are decreased and the patient does not develop serious adverse effects.

CHAPTER SUMMARY

- Diuretics are used widely to treat conditions in which increased extracellular fluid and edema are problems. Examples include hypertension, CHF, cirrhosis, renal disorders, intracranial pressure, and intraocular pressure.
- Diuretics work along the renal tubule and inhibit sodium and water reabsorption to increase water loss. The degree of diuretic effect depends on the section of the tubule in which the drug works.

MEMORY CHIP

P Tolterodine

- Blocks cholinergic muscarinic receptors in the bladder, decreasing bladder function
- Used to treat overactive bladder, controlling symptoms of urinary frequency, urgency, or urge incontinence
- Major contraindications: urinary retention, gastric retention, and uncontrolled narrow-angle glaucoma
- Most common adverse effects: dry mouth and headache
- Minimizing adverse effects: Decrease the dose if patient has renal or liver disease.
- Most important patient education: Urinary retention, GI retention, or visual changes such as blurred vision may occur and need to be reported.

- Diuretic drugs affect the excretion and reabsorption of other electrolytes, especially potassium, leading to one of the major adverse effects of diuretic therapy, an electrolyte imbalance.
- Thiazide and loop diuretics are the two classes of diuretics most frequently used.
- To prevent hypokalemia, patients taking non–potassium-sparing diuretics may need to increase their dietary intake of potassium or take supplements. Conversely, patients taking potassium-sparing diuretics are at risk for hyperkalemia and need to avoid excess potassium intake.
- Osmotic diuretics work by increasing the osmotic pressure within the vascular space. They are used primarily in ARF, in increased intracranial pressure, in increased intraocular pressure, and to promote excretion in the urine of toxic substances.
- Carbonic anhydrase inhibitors work by a different mechanism to cause diuresis. They are used primarily in treating open-angle glaucoma.
- Tolterodine is an antimuscarinic used to treat overactive bladder disease. Tolterodine selectively blocks muscarinic receptors in the bladder to produce its effects.

QUESTIONS FOR STUDY AND REVIEW

1. Identify the physical assessments for health status that should be completed before a patient starts thiazide therapy for hypertension.
2. Identify at least three conditions treated by diuretic therapy.
3. Discuss at least three fluid and electrolyte problems likely to occur in patients receiving thiazide or loop diuretics.
4. Why is a patient more likely to develop hypokalemia when on loop diuretics than on thiazide diuretics?
5. How are osmotic diuretics different from thiazide or loop diuretics?
6. What is the primary therapeutic use of carbonic anhydrase inhibitors?
7. What is the effect on the bladder from excessive blockade of muscarinic receptors?

Need More Help?

Chapter 32 of the study guide for *Drug Therapy in Nursing* 2e contains NCLEX-style questions and other learning activities to reinforce your understanding of the concepts presented in this chapter. For additional information or to purchase the study guide, visit *http://connection.lww.com/go/aschenbrenner.*

REFERENCES AND BIBLIOGRAPHY

ALLHAT Officers and Coordinators for the ALLHAT Collaborative Research Group. Antihypertensive and Lipid-Lowering Treatment to Prevent Heart Attack Trial Collaborative Research Group. (2002). Major outcomes in high-risk hypertensive patients randomized to angiotensin-converting enzyme inhibitor or calcium channel blocker vs diuretic: The Antihypertensive and Lipid-Lowering Treatment to Prevent Heart Attack Trial (ALLHAT). *Journal of the American Medical Association, 288*(23), 2981–2997.

Faris, R., Flather, M., Purcell, H., et al. (2002). Current evidence supporting the role of diuretics in heart failure: A meta-analysis of randomized controlled trials. *International Journal of Cardiology, 82*(2), 149–158.

Humes, H. D. (1999). Insights into ototoxicity. Analogies to nephrotoxicity. *Annals of New York Academy of Science, 884,* 15–18.

Neuberg, G. W., Miller, A. B., O'Connor, C. M., et al.; Prospective Randomized Amlodipine Survival Evaluation (PRAISE) Investigators. (2002). Diuretic resistance predicts mortality in patients with advanced heart failure. *American Heart Journal, 144*(1), 31–38.

Nishino, T., Ide, T., Sudo, T., et al. (2000). Inhaled furosemide greatly alleviates the sensation of experimentally induced dyspnea. *American Journal of Respiratory and Critical Care Medicine, 161*(6), 1963–1967.

Rosholm, J. U., Nybo, H., Andersen Ranberg, K., et al. (2002). Hyponatremia in very old nonhospitalized people: Association with drug use. *Drugs and Aging, 19*(9), 685–693.

Schoofs, M. W., van der Klift, M., Hofman, A., et al. (2003). Thiazide diuretics and the risk of hip fracture. *Annals of Internal Medicine, 139*(6), 476–482.

Sharabi, Y., Illan, R., Kamari, Y., et al. (2002). Diuretic induced hyponatraemia in elderly hypertensive women. *Journal of Human Hypertension, 16*(9), 631–635.

Suter, P. M., Haller, J. & Hany, A. (2000). Diuretic use: A risk of subclinical thiamine deficiency in elderly patients. *Journal of Nutrition, Health, and Aging, 4*(2), 69–71.

Hematopoietic and Immune System Drugs

unit 8

Drugs Affecting Hematopoiesis

chapter 33

Learning Objectives

At the completion of this chapter the student will:

1. Identify core drug knowledge about drugs that affect hematopoiesis.
2. Identify core patient variables relevant to drugs that affect hematopoiesis.
3. Relate the interaction of core drug knowledge to core patient variables for drugs that affect hematopoiesis.
4. Generate a nursing plan of care from the interactions between core drug knowledge and core patient variables for drugs that affect hematopoiesis.
5. Describe nursing interventions to maximize therapeutic and minimize adverse effects for drugs that affect hematopoiesis.
6. Determine key points for patient and family education for drugs that affect hematopoiesis.

KEY TERMS

anemia
aplastic
biologic modifier
biologic modulator
erythrocytes
erythropoiesis
erythropoietin
granulocytes
hematopoiesis
leukocytes
lymphocytes
macrophages
monocytes
neutropenia
neutrophils
phagocytosis
platelets
thrombocytopenia
thrombopoietin

FEATURED WEBLINK

http://www.kidney.org/professionals/kdoqi/guidelines_updates/doqi_uptoc.html#an
The National Kidney Foundation provides complete guidelines for caring for patients with chronic kidney disease and anemia at this site.

CONNECTION WEBLINK

Additional Weblinks are found on Connection:
http://www.connection.lww.com/go/aschenbrenner.

Drugs Affecting Hematopoiesis

Ⓒ Erythropoiesis Stimulants

- P **epoetin alfa**
- darbepoetin alfa

Ⓒ Colony-Stimulating Factors

- P **filgrastim**
- pegfilgrastim
- sargramostim

Ⓒ Interleukins

- P **oprelvekin (interleukin-11)**

The symbol Ⓒ indicates the **drug class.**
Drugs in **bold type** marked with the symbol P are prototypes.
Drugs in blue type are closely related to the prototype.
Drugs in red type are significantly different from the prototype.
Drugs in black type with no symbol are also used in drug therapy; no prototype

Biologic modulators, or **biologic modifiers,** are a group of biopharmaceuticals that are naturally occurring proteins used to alter the body's hematologic or immunologic responses. These substances are sometimes called biologic therapies. The rapid growth of these therapies over the past decade is attributable to the refinement of recombinant DNA technology, which has enabled researchers to produce large quantities of these substances outside the body. Many agents enhance the body's ability to create new cells. Other agents stimulate immunologic activity to combat specific antigens (substances that induce the formation of antibodies). Similar drugs from this class may also be used to suppress the immune system to prevent rejection of foreign transplanted tissue or to prevent rejection of the body's own tissue, as in autoimmune disease. This chapter deals with drugs that stimulate cell growth. Drugs that stimulate or suppress the immune system are discussed in Chapter 34.

Hematopoiesis, the production and differentiation of blood cells, normally occurs within bone marrow. Hematopoietic growth factors are substances generated by the body to enhance production of blood cells. Some of these agents are actually classified as hormone substances (e.g., epoetin), whereas others are cytokine growth factors. For this text, epoetin alfa (Epogen, Procrit), a hematopoietic hormone, is the prototype drug for stimulating red blood cell production. A drug in the same class and represented by the prototype is darbepoetin alfa (Aranesp). The prototype drug for white blood cell production is the colony-stimulating factor filgrastim (Neupogen); drugs similar to the prototype are pegfilgrastim (Neulasta) and sargramostim (Leukine). The prototype drug for creating platelets is oprelvekin (also known as interleukin-1; brand name, Neumega).

PHYSIOLOGY

The immune system is composed of hematopoietic cells and multiple hematologic-immunologic production and storage sites. Hematopoietic tissue is found in the bone marrow, lymph nodes, and lymphatic channels of the body. Stem cells located in the red bone marrow, found in the long bones and vertebral skeleton, produce the three types of functional hematopoietic cells: **erythrocytes** (also called red blood cells [RBCs]), **leukocytes** (also called white blood cells [WBCs]), and **platelets,** which are small cells necessary for blood coagulation. The reticuloendothelial system includes immunologically active tissue and cells found in the lymph system, spleen, liver, lungs, gastrointestinal tract, and brain. An integrated immune response involving hematopoietic cells and immune tissues provides the body's nonspecific and specific response to invasion by antigens identified as nonself. The essential components of the immune system are hematopoietic cells, barrier defenses, the nonspecific immune response, the specific immune response, and immunity. Hematopoietic cells are discussed in this chapter; the other components of the immune system are further discussed in Chapter 34.

Hematopoietic Cells

Red blood cells (RBCs) are mainly composed of hemoglobin, which enables the cells to carry oxygen to the cells in the body. The biconcave disc shape of the RBCs makes them flexible enough to maneuver through the small capillaries to deliver oxygen to the tissues.

The major peptide hormone, or glycoprotein, that stimulates the production of RBCs (called **erythropoiesis**) is **erythropoietin.** Erythropoietin is produced by the kidneys in response to tissue hypoxia and reduced oxygen carrying capacity of the red blood cells. Chronic obstructive pulmonary disease (COPD) and anemia, which produce chronic hypoxic states, are examples of disorders that stimulate production of erythropoietin and, consequently, production of RBCs. When hemoglobin levels fall (as in anemia), erythropoietin production is stimulated. Erythropoietin in turn stimulates the progenitor stem cells to make RBCs, which live about 120 days. Plasma erythropoietin levels vary from 0.01 U/mL to 0.03 U/mL and increase from 100- to 1,000-fold during hypoxia or anemia. When hemoglobin levels are elevated, erythropoietin production is halted, ending the stimulation to produce new RBCs.

Iron, the primary ion reversibly bound to oxygen in the heme molecule, is necessary to support erythropoiesis. It is held stable in the ferrous form by the other atoms that are in heme. When iron deficiency exists, the final step in heme synthesis is interrupted.

Platelets are the formed element involved in blood coagulation. Platelets are small cells that arise from the bone marrow precursor cells called megakaryocytes. Platelet production, although stimulated by many cytokines, is mostly dependent on the action of interleukin-6 and a peptide called **thrombopoietin.** Thrombopoietin is produced in the liver. A low platelet count stimulates the production of thrombopoietin. Platelets are important in normal blood clotting. (For more information on blood clotting, see Chapter 31.)

Leukocytes (white blood cells or WBCs) are key components of all immune system responses. During maturation in the bone marrow, WBCs differentiate into three main cell types—**granulocytes, monocytes,** and **lymphocytes**—that respond to cell injury or foreign invaders (Figure 33.1). Granulocytes are the most common type of WBC. Production of granulocytes is regulated by colony-stimulating factors (CSFs), also known as growth factors. Granulocytes are further divided into neutrophils, eosinophils, and basophils. The formation of granulocytes (myelopoiesis) is stimulated by many cytokines. These cells are produced in response to infection, inflammation, and tissue necrosis.

Barrier Defenses

The human body has many physical barrier defense mechanisms to protect it from the outside environment. The skin is the first line of defense. Mucus is another barrier defense, providing protection for the respiratory and genitourinary tracts. A third barrier defense, the gastrointestinal (GI) tract, provides an acid protector that destroys many microorganisms.

Nonspecific Immune Responses

If a pathogen gets past one of the barrier defense mechanisms and injures a cell, the body activates the nonspecific inflammatory reaction, initiating granulocyte, monocyte, and macrophage activities to destroy the invader and repair the damage. **Neutrophils** are the most common granulocyte and are considered the first line of defense against pathogens

Physiology

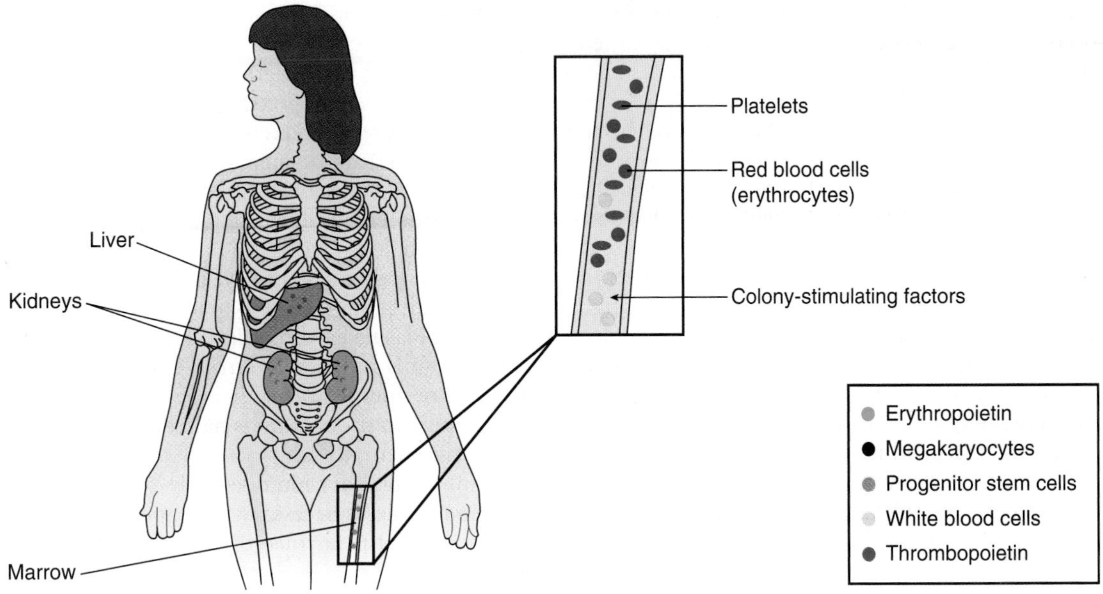

FIGURE 33.1 The kidney releases erythropoietin, which stimulates the progenitor cells in the bone marrow to produce red blood cells (erythrocytes). The liver produces thrombopoietin, which, along with interleukin-6, stimulates the production of platelets in the bone marrow. Colony-stimulating factors work on the developing white blood cells (leukocytes), allowing them to differentiate into granulocytes, monocytes, and lymphocytes. Granulocytes are further specialized as either neutrophils, eosinophils, or basophils.

that gain entry into the body. Neutrophils contain enzymes that kill bacteria in the bloodstream when the bacteria are ingested by the neutrophil. This process of engulfing and destroying bacteria is called endocytosis or **phagocytosis.** The life of the neutrophil is extremely short—only 6 to 8 hours. Normally, when an acute infection is present in the body, the numbers of both mature and immature neutrophils rise, producing neutrophilia. The immature neutrophils are called bands. When large numbers of bands are present in the blood count, it is termed a "shift to the left," and this event usually signals a bacterial infection. When the neutrophil level or count is low (**neutropenia**), infection is likely to occur. Basophils are granulocytes that are not capable of phagocytosis but contain chemical substances important for initiating and maintaining an immune response. These substances include histamine, heparin, and chemicals used in the inflammatory response. Monocytes differentiate into immunologically active cells called **macrophages.** Macrophages can be circulating phagocytes or can be fixed in specific tissues.

Specific Immune Responses

If an invader gets past the barrier and nonspecific immune systems and enters the tissues or bloodstream, a specific immune response involving lymphocytes is initiated.

Bone marrow stem cells develop into two types of lymphocytes: T lymphocytes, or T cells, and B lymphocytes, or B cells. These T and B lymphocytes may also differentiate into specialized cells such as natural killer cells and lymphokine-activated killer (LAK) cells, which have been identified as the cells that aggressively attack and destroy neoplastic cells. Because research in the area of lymphocyte identification is relatively new and ongoing, there may be other not-yet-identified lymphocytes taking part in the immune response. The specific immune response is discussed in detail in Chapter 34.

PATHOPHYSIOLOGY

The pathophysiologic consequence of hematologic failure is inadequate cell production to meet the body's demands for oxygen transportation, blood coagulation, or prevention of infection. Deficient cell production is named by the cell involved; when production of all cells is deficient, it is termed **aplastic.**

Anemia, a condition of reduced circulating RBCs, can be caused by deficient cell production (arising from folic acid deficiency, iron deficiency, or bone marrow failure), or abnormal hemolysis (as featured in sickle cell anemia and hemolytic anemia), or through loss of blood volume or cells, such as with overt bleeding. Anemia may also result from inadequate levels of the stimulating hormone erythropoietin. This effect most often occurs with chronic renal failure or bone marrow failure, conditions that cause insufficient production of erythropoietin. Anemias related to deficiency of erythropoietin have RBCs that are normal in size and color. Anemias related to iron deficiency or aluminum overload have smaller RBCs than normal, whereas anemias related to vitamin B_{12} or folate deficiency have RBCs that are larger than normal.

Anemias related to decreased erythropoietin levels can be treated with exogenous erythropoietin (epoetin alfa).

In chronic renal failure, hemoglobin levels that are below 10 g/dL induce the heart to work harder to meet the tissue's needs for oxygen. This phenomenon eventually leads to left ventricular hypertrophy and left ventricular dilation, creating greater morbidity with severely altered quality of life, as well as greater cardiac mortality. Early normalization of the hemoglobin level can prevent development of left ventricular dilation and improve quality of life. Additional physiologic abnormalities from the anemia of chronic kidney disease include impaired cognitive function, impaired immune response, growth retardation in pediatric patients, reduced quality of life, and decreased patient survival (Szromba et al., 2002; National Kidney Foundation, 2001).

To effectively manage early anemia in chronic renal failure, assume that an erythropoietin deficiency exists and rule out any iron deficiency that may be contributing to the problem. Assessment and evaluation of the anemia in a patient with chronic renal disease should occur when the hemoglobin (Hb) is less than 12 g/dL (hematocrit [Hct] < 37%) in men and postmenopausal women, or when it is less than 11 g/dL (Hct <33%) in premenopausal women and prepubertal patients. Therapy with replacement erythropoietin should begin if the evaluation determines that the patient has normal serum iron levels (National Kidney Foundation, 2001). Functional iron deficiency (normal ferritin levels but low transferrin saturation) is a common occurrence in patients who have started epoetin alfa therapy, even if they originally had normal iron levels. This deficiency occurs because stimulation of erythropoiesis increases the demand for iron, and eventually not enough iron is available (Szromba et al., 2002; National Kidney Foundation, 2000).

Abnormalities in WBC counts are fairly common, although abnormalities of WBC function are rare. Decreased numbers of neutrophils, called neutropenia, are related to two basic causes: decreased marrow activity and decreased neutrophil survival. When neutropenia is related to decreased marrow activity, it may be related to drug therapy (e.g., with antineoplastics, some antibiotics, gold, certain diuretics, antithyroid agents, antihistamines, and antipsychotics). Other causes include radiation exposure, megaloblastic anemia (anemia in which large nucleated abnormal RBCs are present in the blood), cyclic neutropenia (a benign disease), Kostmann (infantile) neutropenia, aplastic anemia (anemia from complete suppression, or loss of function, of the bone marrow), myelodysplastic syndrome, and marrow replacement by tumor.

A low platelet count is termed **thrombocytopenia.** Thrombocytopenia can result from decreased production, shortened survival, or loss of platelets. Decreased production is caused by aplastic anemia, marrow infiltration, deficiencies of vitamin B_{12} and folate, radiation, and hereditary factors. Decreased survival of platelets is related to immune-mediated factors (idiopathic, systemic lupus erythematosus, drug induced, neonatal from maternal immunoglobulin G [IgG]); hypersplenism, disseminated intravascular coagulation, thrombotic thrombocytopenic purpura, hemolytic uremic syndrome; and prosthetic valves.

Drugs that affect hematopoiesis include erythropoiesis stimulants, colony-stimulating factors, and interleukins. Table 33.1 provides a summary of selected hematopoietic agents.

C ERYTHROPOIESIS STIMULANTS

Hematopoietic growth factors are exogenous replacements of endogenous growth factors. They are used when the internal mechanism for producing sufficient blood cells does not meet the body's needs. The prototype drug used to create RBCs is epoetin alfa.

Epoetin alfa is a 165–amino acid glycoprotein manufactured by recombinant DNA technology. It is recombinant human erythropoietin. The product contains the same amino acid sequence as natural erythropoietin. The human erythropoietin gene is introduced into mammalian cells, which then produce erythropoietin that has the same biologic effects as endogenous erythropoietin.

NURSING MANAGEMENT OF THE PATIENT RECEIVING P EPOETIN ALFA

Core Drug Knowledge

Pharmacotherapeutics

Epoetin alfa (Epogen, Procrit), also referred to as erythropoietin or EPO, is used to treat anemia associated with chronic renal failure, to elevate or maintain the RBC level (assessed through the hematocrit or hemoglobin determinations) and to decrease the need for transfusion (see Table 33.1). Epoetin alfa is also used to treat anemia related to zidovudine therapy in human immunodeficiency virus (HIV)-positive patients (Box 33.1). It is used when the endogenous erythropoietin levels are 500 mU/mL or less and the dose of zidovudine is 4,200 mg/week or less. It is also used to treat chemotherapy-induced anemia in cancer patients. It is intended to decrease the need for transfusions in patients who will receive chemotherapy for at least 2 months. Improving hemoglobin levels in patients with cancers appears to also decrease the fatigue that often accompanies cancer (Nail, 2002). Finally, epoetin alfa is used in anemic patients who will be undergoing elective, noncardiac, or nonvascular surgery, and in patients who are at high risk for substantial blood loss during surgery, to reduce their need for postoperative blood transfusions. Two common but unlabeled uses for epoetin alfa are treating pruritus associated with renal failure and preventing the need for transfusions in premature infants.

Pharmacokinetics

Epoetin alfa can be administered either intravenously or subcutaneously. When epoetin alfa is given intravenously, its circulating half-life is 4 to 13 hours. Therapeutic levels are maintained for 24 hours or longer. After subcutaneous (SC) administration, peak levels are achieved within 5 to 24 hours and decline slowly afterward. Elimination is through the kidneys. Half-life is not affected by dialysis (see Table 33.1).

Pharmacodynamics

Epoetin alfa has the same effects on the body as endogenous erythropoietin. It stimulates production of RBCs. In patients with chronic renal failure, the first evidence that epoetin alfa

TABLE 33.1 Summary of Selected Hematopoietic Agents

Drug (Trade) Name	Selected Indications	Route and Dosage Range	Pharmacokinetics
(C) Erythropoiesis Stimulants			
(P) epoetin alfa or erythropoietin or EPO (Epogen, Procrit)	Anemia from chronic renal failure (CRF) Anemia related to ZDV therapy in HIV-associated illness Anemia related to chemotherapy in cancer patients	CRF: 50–100 U/kg 3 times/wk IV or SC injection to maintain Hct of 30%–36% HIV: 100 U/kg 3 times/wk for 8 wks IV or SC injection Cancer: 150 U/kg 3 times/wk SC injection (weekly injections under investigation)	*Onset:* IV, immediate SC within 5 to 24 h *Duration:* IV, ≥ 24 h SC levels fall slowly after 24 h $t_{1/2}$: 4–13 h
(C) Colony-Stimulating Factors			
(P) filgrastim, or granulocyte-colony stimulating factor (G-CSF) (Neupogen)	Neutropenia due to chemotherapy, after bone-marrow transplantation (BMT), or severe chronic neutropenia Prior to peripheral blood progenitor cell (PBPC) collection	Chemotherapy: 5 µg/kg/d SC injection, or infusion, or IV BMT: 10 µg/kg/d IV or SC infusion Chronic: congenital 6 µg/kg bid SC injection Idiopathic or cyclic: 5 µg/kg once/d SC injection PBPC collection: 10 µg/kg/d SC (injection or infusion) starting at least 4 d prior to procedure	*Onset:* IV, immediate *Duration:* Unknown $t_{1/2}$: 3.5 h
(C) Interleukins			
(P) oprelvekin or interleukin 11 (IL-11) (Neumega)	Thrombocytopenia from chemotherapy	*Adult:* 50 µg/kg/d SC injection *Child:* Safety and efficacy not established	*Onset:* Unknown *Duration:* Unknown $t_{1/2}$: 6.9 h

is producing a positive response is an increase in the reticulocyte (immature RBC) count within 10 days. Next seen, within 2 to 6 weeks, is an increase in the counts of RBCs, hemoglobin, and hematocrit. Once the target hematocrit (30%–36%) has been reached, it can be maintained by using epoetin alfa. The rate of hematocrit increase varies among patients and is dose dependent; however, doses over 300 U/kg three times weekly produce no additional biologic response. Other factors affecting rate and extent of response include the availability of iron stores, baseline hematocrit, and concurrent illnesses.

Responsiveness of HIV-positive patients to epoetin alfa therapy is based on their endogenous erythropoietin levels. Those with levels above 500 mU/mL do not appear to respond to therapy. An increased hematocrit and a decreased need for transfusion are evidence of a response. Cancer patients who receive epoetin alfa are most likely to respond to therapy if they have lymphoid and solid cancers that have not infiltrated the bone marrow.

Contraindications and Precautions

Avoid using epoetin alfa in uncontrolled hypertension and in cases of hypersensitivity to mammalian cell–derived products or human albumin. Although epoetin alfa therapy does not appear to have direct vasopressor effects, blood pressure may rise during therapy, especially during the early phase of treatment, when the hematocrit is rising. An elevation in blood pressure is especially problematic for patients with chronic renal failure, who are typically hypertensive already.

Increase the hematocrit level slowly, not more than four points in any 2-week period, because an excessive rate of increase may possibly exacerbate hypertension. Hypertension from increases in hematocrit has rarely been noted in patients with cancer receiving epoetin alfa. Hypertensive encephalopathy and seizures have occurred in patients with chronic renal failure who are treated with epoetin alfa.

Thrombotic events, such as myocardial infarction, transient ischemic attacks, cerebral vascular accident, or clotting of the artificial kidney during dialysis, can occur in patients with chronic renal failure who are receiving epoetin alfa. Patients receiving dialysis may need increased anticoagulation with heparin to prevent their artificial kidneys from clotting. The risk for thrombotic events is greatly increased in patients with ischemic heart disease or congestive heart failure when the prescriber is trying to increase the hematocrit to normal levels (42%) with epoetin alfa therapy.

In contrast, there does not seem to be any association between epoetin alfa therapy in HIV-positive patients and

FOCUS ON RESEARCH

Box 33.1 Epoetin Alfa Dosing in HIV-Positive Patients

Grossman, H. H., Goon, B., Bowers, P., et al.; 010 Study Group. (2003). Once-weekly epoetin alfa dosing is as effective as three-times-weekly dosing in increasing hemoglobin levels and is associated with improved quality of life in anemic HIV-infected patients. *Journal of Acquired Immune Deficiency Syndromes, 34*(4), 368–378.

The Study

A randomized, multicenter clinical trial of 272 HIV-positive adult patients receiving stable antiretroviral therapy compared the effectiveness of once-weekly epoetin alfa with traditional three-times-a-week dosing of epoetin alfa in treating drug-induced anemia. Both of the dosing schedules were effective in significantly increasing the hemoglobin levels. No difference existed in the final hemoglobin levels between the two groups. Quality of life also improved significantly in both groups, with no significant differences between the groups.

Nursing Implications

This study showed that once-weekly dosing of epoetin alfa was as effective in HIV-positive patients as thrice-weekly dosing. This study did not examine the use of weekly epoetin alfa for other population groups, such as those with chronic kidney disease. However, for patients with HIV infection or AIDS, this dosing option may be important. Once-weekly dosing will likely be perceived by patients and their families as more convenient than thrice-weekly dosing and may therefore promote adherence.

exacerbation of hypertension, seizures, or thrombotic events. Therapy should not be started, however, until blood pressure is controlled.

Do not use epoetin alfa therapy as a replacement for transfusion in patients with chronic renal failure who require correction for severe anemia. In HIV-positive patients with cancer, do not use epoetin alfa to treat anemia caused by iron or folate deficiencies, hemolysis, or GI bleeding.

Adverse Effects

Adverse effects occurring during epoetin alfa therapy appear to reflect the patients' underlying disease process or their postoperative state. It is difficult to determine, then, exactly what the adverse effects of epoetin alfa are. Hypertension may occur in patients with chronic renal failure who are on dialysis (see Contraindications and Precautions). Headache, nausea and vomiting, and tachycardia are all frequently reported. Seizures have been reported less often; they occur most commonly in patients with renal disease. Porphyria (excretion of nitrogen-containing compounds in the urine) may be exacerbated in patients with chronic renal failure, although this effect is rare.

Fever, headache, cough, rash, and nausea have been reported fairly frequently in HIV-positive patients. Patients with cancer often report fever, diarrhea, vomiting, and edema while on epoetin alfa therapy. Patients who receive epoetin alfa before surgery report fever, diarrhea, and vomiting. In clinical trials, all of these adverse effects were also reported by patients who received placebo instead of epoetin alfa.

Drug Interactions

No drug interactions are known to occur with epoetin alfa.

Assessment of Relevant Core Patient Variables

Health Status

Determine whether the patient has pre-existing uncontrolled hypertension, which is a contraindication for the use of epoetin alfa. If the patient does not have chronic renal failure, verify that the anemia is not caused by iron or folate deficiency, hemolysis, or GI bleeding, because these anemias should be treated differently. Determine whether the patient has pre-existing vascular disease because it may increase the patient's risk for developing thrombotic adverse effects. Before and during therapy, assess the patient's iron status, including transferrin saturation (serum iron divided by iron binding capacity) and serum ferritin (the iron-phosphorous-protein complex that is the form in which iron is stored in the tissues). Transferrin saturation should be at least 20%, and ferritin should be at least 100 ng/mL. Iron is needed to support erythropoiesis. Absolute or functional iron deficiency may develop during therapy. Functional iron deficiency, in which the ferritin level is normal but the transferrin saturation is low, is believed to be caused by the body's inability to mobilize iron stores rapidly enough to support increased erythropoiesis.

Life Span and Gender

Determine whether the patient is pregnant because epoetin alfa is a pregnancy category C drug. Adverse effects have occurred in rats given epoetin alfa in doses five times the comparable human dose; however, no adequate studies have been performed in humans. Use caution if administering epoetin alfa to a woman who is breast-feeding because it is not known whether the drug is excreted in breast milk. Ask the patient's age, which may affect the adverse effects from the drug. Safety and efficacy in children is not established. If giving epoetin alfa to premature infants, use the form without the benzyl alcohol (the preservative) because benzyl alcohol has been associated with a fatal "gasping syndrome" in premature infants. Carefully assess the older adult with cancer who is receiving epoetin alfa for adverse effects related to anemia because these patients are more sensitive to the anemia that results from chemotherapy. Older adults are also likely to experience

CRITICAL THINKING SCENARIO

Epoetin alfa and iron deficiency

Ada Greene, 65 years of age, has chronic kidney disease. Her blood work shows that her hemoglobin is 9 g/dL. An anemia evaluation shows that her serum iron levels are normal, and she is started on epoetin alfa. After 3 weeks of epoetin alfa therapy, her hemoglobin count is 10.5 g/dL, and her serum iron levels show normal ferritin levels but low transferrin saturation. She is diagnosed as having functional iron deficiency.

1. What would account for these changes in her iron levels?
2. What treatment would you expect to be ordered for Ms. Greene?

adverse effects from other, concurrent drug therapy. Some drugs bind to RBCs, and without adequate RBCs, epoetin alfa has no binding sites. In this case, levels of the drug will rise, increasing the incidence of adverse effects (Hood, 2003).

Lifestyle, Diet, and Habits

Verify that patients with chronic renal failure are continuing the dietary restrictions necessary in chronic renal failure. As the hematocrit rises and patients begin to feel better, they may feel that they no longer need a restrictive diet. Determine whether patients are at risk for iron deficiency; if so, encourage them to consume foods high in iron.

Environment

Epoetin alfa is administered in many ambulatory settings as well as in the hospital or dialysis center. For patients who receive home dialysis or intermittent ambulatory treatment (antiretroviral therapy, chemotherapy, or radiation therapy), therapy can be self-administered at home. Assess the patient factors in the home environment that may affect adherence to drug therapy. Be careful to review the re-imbursement policies of the patient's health care insurance because injectable medications are often not reimbursed as a home therapy.

Culture and Inherited Traits

No cultural barriers exist to the use of epoetin alfa. If your assessment reveals that the patient has a religious affiliation (such as the Jehovah's Witnesses) in which blood transfusions are forbidden, epoetin alfa may still be administered. Epoetin alfa is not considered a blood component by religious affiliations that object to transfusions and hence offers an excellent alternative to RBC transfusion for those individuals.

Nursing Diagnoses and Outcomes

- Impaired Tissue Oxygenation related to anemia
  Desired outcome: *Tissues will be oxygenated satisfactorily, and hematocrit will reach desired level with epoetin alfa therapy.*
- Risk for Injury related to adverse effects of epoetin alfa
  Desired outcome: *Adverse effects will be prevented or minimized to prevent injury.*

Planning and Intervention

Maximizing Therapeutic Effects

To maintain the biologic activity of epoetin alfa, do not shake the drug after reconstituting it. Vigorous shaking may denature the glycoprotein, making it biologically inactive. Allow time for the hematocrit to rise before seeking an order to adjust the dose. When epoetin alfa is given in chronic renal failure, the time required to elicit a clinically meaningful change in hematocrit is 2 to 6 weeks. The dose should not be adjusted more than once a month. After each dose adjustment, ensure that the patient has an appointment to have his or her hematocrit measured twice a week for at least 2 to 6 weeks to verify that the hematocrit is in the correct range, which will show that the drug is effective. If the hematocrit has not risen by 5 to 6 points in an 8-week period (and iron stores are adequate), the patient will require an increase in the dose. Seek orders and administer iron supplements intravenously, as needed, to help increase the effectiveness of the epoetin alfa.

When epoetin alfa is given to HIV-positive patients who are treated with zidovudine, give the initial dosage for 8 weeks. If the dosage does not produce the desired response, seek an order to increase it. Evaluate the patient's response every 4 to 8 weeks thereafter and seek new orders to adjust the dosage as needed. Monitor the hematocrit weekly during dosage adjustment (see Box 33.1).

When giving epoetin alfa to cancer patients on chemotherapy, give the initial dosage for 8 weeks. After that period, seek orders to adjust the dosage if needed. If patients still do not respond to therapy, they are unlikely to respond to higher doses.

When epoetin alfa is given to presurgical patients with anemia, it should be given subcutaneously for 10 days before surgery, on the day of surgery, and for 4 days postoperatively. Alternatively, epoetin alfa can be given in once-weekly doses at 21 days, 14 days, and 7 days before surgery, with a fourth dose on the day of surgery.

If response to epoetin alfa is delayed or diminished, assess for other reasons that may cause a low hematocrit (e.g., functional iron deficiency; underlying infectious, inflammatory, or malignant processes; occult blood loss; underlying hematologic diseases; folic acid or vitamin B_{12} deficiencies; hemolysis; aluminum intoxication; or osteitis fibrosa cystica [overactivity of the parathyroid gland that results in disturbances of calcium and phosphorus metabolism]).

Minimizing Adverse Effects

Remember that the single-dose 1-mL vials have no preservative. To prevent contamination, use only one dose per vial, do not re-enter the vial, and discard any unused portion. In contrast, the multidose 2-mL vial has preservative in it. Store it at 2° to 8°C after initial entry and between doses. Discard the vial 21 days after initial entry to prevent use of a possibly contaminated product.

Monitor the blood pressure of all patients receiving epoetin alfa throughout therapy to assess for hypertension.

In patients who have chronic renal failure and are receiving epoetin alfa, monitor the hematocrit to prevent adverse effects. Dosage adjustments to achieve the desired hematocrit are not uncommon. These adjustments, or titrations, may be stated in the original drug order or in a unit or hospital protocol. If neither guideline exists, contact the prescriber for further orders. You are responsible for verifying that the dose being administered is safe, based on the patient's current physiologic status, and will not promote serious adverse effects. If the hematocrit is approaching 36%, reduce the dose to maintain the suggested target hematocrit range. If the hematocrit rises above 36%, notify the prescriber and withhold administering doses until the hematocrit begins to decrease. Epoetin alfa should then be restarted with a lower dose. If the hematocrit increases by more than 4 points in a 2-week period, immediately seek orders to decrease the dose. After adjusting the dose, monitor hematocrit twice a week for 2 to 6 weeks.

In HIV-positive patients who are taking zidovudine while receiving epoetin alfa, monitor the hematocrit closely. If the hematocrit exceeds 40%, notify the prescriber and stop the dose until the hematocrit drops to 36%. When the prescriber orders epoetin alfa treatment resumed, the dose ordered should be decreased by 25%; titrate the drug based on orders or protocol until the desired hematocrit is obtained.

Finally, when giving epoetin alfa to patients with cancer who are receiving chemotherapy, the hematocrit also needs

to be monitored carefully. If the initial dose produces a rapid rise in hematocrit of more than 4% in 2 weeks, seek an order to reduce the dose. If the hematocrit exceeds 40%, notify the prescriber and stop administering the dose until the hematocrit drops to 36%. When resuming epoetin alfa therapy, the dose ordered should be 25% less than before. You may titrate the dose, based on orders or protocols, until the desired hematocrit is obtained.

Providing Patient and Family Education

- Teach the patient and family the purpose of the drug and the need for follow-up blood work to check the hematocrit.
- Instruct patients to maintain adequate iron intake, which may aid in the effectiveness of epoetin alfa. Foods high in iron include green leafy vegetables, beans, and organ meats. High-iron-content foods or supplements are best absorbed if taken with ascorbic acid, such as that found in citrus drinks.
- If the patient is to take an iron supplement, teach him or her that it is best taken without food or phosphate binders, and that the best time to take it is at bedtime.
- Explain to patients with chronic renal failure the importance of continuing with diet restrictions and dialysis (if used) while receiving epoetin alfa.
- For patients who will be self-administering epoetin alfa at home, teach proper SC injection technique and safe disposal of used needles and syringes.

Ongoing Assessment and Evaluation

Monitor patients' blood pressure and hematocrit throughout therapy. Check the hematocrit twice weekly until the target hematocrit has been achieved and the dose has been established. Monitor iron levels throughout therapy to verify that enough iron is available to support erythropoiesis. Therapy is effective when the hematocrit rises to a desired treatment level, the need for transfusions is reduced, and the patient does not have major adverse effects.

MEMORY CHIP

P Epoetin Alfa

- Recombinant human erythropoietin works exactly as endogenous erythropoietin; it stimulates the production of RBCs (erythropoiesis)
- Used to treat anemia in chronic renal failure, HIV infection (when zidovudine is used), and cancer (when chemotherapy is used), and in preoperative anemic patients (when high blood loss and transfusion are anticipated)
- Major contraindication: uncontrolled hypertension
- Difficult to determine true adverse effects because those reported are also present in disease process or post procedure
- Most common adverse effects: hypertension (in chronic renal failure [CRF]); fever (all other uses)
- Most serious adverse effects: thrombotic effects (in CRF)
- Maximizing therapeutic effects: Consult with prescriber about dose adjustment and verify iron availability.
- Minimizing adverse effects: monitor hematocrit
- Most important patient education: Advise patients of the need for follow-up blood work and the importance of dietary iron.

C COLONY-STIMULATING FACTORS

Colony-stimulating factors are glycoproteins that assist in the production of blood cells by binding to specific cell surface receptors and stimulating proliferation, differentiation commitment, and some end-cell functional activation. Filgrastim, a granulocyte colony-stimulating factor (G-CSF), is the prototype drug for stimulating white blood cell production. Drugs that are closely related are pegfilgrastim and sargramostim. Sargramostim is a granulocyte-macrophage colony-stimulating factor (GM-CSF). All are produced by recombinant DNA technology.

NURSING MANAGEMENT OF THE PATIENT RECEIVING P FILGRASTIM

Core Drug Knowledge

Pharmacotherapeutics

Filgrastim is licensed for use in patients with cancer, to increase their neutrophil count. For cancer patients with nonmyeloid malignancies (cancers that are not related to blood cell components) who are receiving myelosuppressive chemotherapy (which suppresses the production of blood cells in the bone marrow), it is used to decrease the incidence of infection, as manifested by febrile neutropenia. Primary administration of CSF as prophylaxis should be reserved for patients expected to experience febrile neutropenia at an incidence equal to or greater than 40%. It is also used for those patients with cancer who receive chemotherapy following bone marrow transplantation to reduce the duration of neutropenia and neutropenia-related clinical sequelae (e.g., febrile neutropenia). Filgrastim is also used in cancer patients before leukapheresis (removal of WBCs from blood, which are saved and then later transfused back into the patient). Filgrastim is also used in patients with severe, chronic neutropenia that is congenital, cyclic, or idiopathic in origin. For these patients, the goal is to reduce the incidence and duration of sequelae of neutropenia (e.g., fever, infections, and oropharyngeal ulcers).

Unlabeled uses of filgrastim include treating suppressed bone marrow function in patients with acquired immunodeficiency syndrome (AIDS), aplastic anemia, hairy cell leukemia, myelodysplasia, drug-induced and congenital agranulocytosis, and alloimmune neonatal neutropenia.

Filgrastim is administered as a single daily SC injection bolus, by short intravenous (IV) infusion (15–30 minutes), or by continuous SC or IV infusion.

Pharmacokinetics

Filgrastim begins to work as soon as it can bind with its receptor sites. Metabolism is not understood, but the elimination half-life is about 3.5 hours.

Pharmacodynamics

Filgrastim (Neupogen) is produced by *Escherichia coli* bacteria that have had the human G-CSF gene inserted. G-CSF

regulates the production of neutrophils within the bone marrow. Recombinant DNA G-CSF (filgrastim) acts the way that endogenous G-CSF does.

Filgrastim stimulates and mobilizes the cells that are the progenitor cells for neutrophils into the peripheral circulation. When this additional volume of progenitor cells is infused back into the patient by leukophoresis, the neutrophil count rises more rapidly.

Contraindications and Precautions

The only contraindication to administration of this agent is hypersensitivity to *E. coli*–derived proteins, filgrastim, or any of the product components. Caution should be used when a patient has a myeloid malignancy or requires concomitant cytotoxic (destructive to cells) chemotherapy or radiotherapy because the rapidly dividing myeloid cells may be sensitive to these substances.

Do not use filgrastim from 24 hours before to 24 hours after chemotherapy with cytotoxic substances because extremely elevated WBC counts have occurred as a result. Although no specific adverse effects have been noted with this use, monitor the WBC count closely during therapy. Be careful not to discontinue treatment with filgrastim prematurely. Although a transient increase in neutrophil count occurs 1 to 2 days after starting therapy, don't mistake this increase for the full therapeutic effect of drug therapy. Administer this agent throughout the time when the marrow-suppressing therapy's full nadir (lowest level) of neutrophils should have occurred before discontinuing therapy. Filgrastim is an FDA pregnancy category C drug and should be used with caution.

Adverse Effects

Determining the adverse effects of filgrastim in patients receiving chemotherapy is difficult because all of the effects recorded during clinical trials with the drug can also be consequences of the malignancy or the cytotoxic chemotherapy. In other words, adverse effects may mimic the disease being treated or other treatments for the disease. Medullary bone pain (pain within the marrow) is the only consistently observed adverse effect that can be attributed to drug therapy; it is mild to moderate in severity and is reported in 24% of patients taking filgrastim.

In patients receiving intensive chemotherapy or total body irradiation followed by bone marrow transplantation, few unique adverse effects have been attributable to the G-CSF therapy.

In patients in whom filgrastim is used during collection of peripheral blood progenitor cells, adverse effects have included decreased platelet count (although it usually remains in the normal range), anemia, mild to moderate musculoskeletal symptoms, medullary bone pain, headache, and increases in alkaline phosphatase levels. Patients with severe chronic neutropenia have also experienced mild to moderate bone pain.

Drug Interactions

Drug interactions with filgrastim have not yet been fully evaluated. Use drugs (e.g., lithium carbonate) that can potentiate the release of neutrophils with caution because a synergistic effect may result.

Assessment of Relevant Core Patient Variables

Health Status

Determine that the patient has nonmyeloid cancer, has neutropenic fevers or severe chronic neutropenia, has had a bone marrow transplantation, or is a candidate for peripheral blood progenitor cell collection because these states are indications for the use of filgrastim.

Life Span and Gender

Determine whether the patient is pregnant or breast-feeding; caution is warranted in these patients because filgrastim is a pregnancy category C drug. Whether the drug is excreted in breast milk is unknown. Ask the patient's age. Filgrastim has been used in pediatric patients aged 4 months to 17 years, and no long-term risks have been identified. Safety and efficacy in neonatal autoimmune neutropenia have not been established, however, and long-term effects of this agent have not been evaluated in neonates. Older adults with cancer are especially sensitive to adverse effects from neutropenia; the more severe and the longer the duration of the neutropenia, the more likely the older adult will develop a fatal infection. Neutropenia can also require that a lower dose of chemotherapy be given to older adults, thus making them less likely to receive the full therapeutic effect from chemotherapy. Prophylactic administration of filgrastim or pegfilgrastim (see below) to prevent febrile neutropenia is as effective for older adults as for younger adults in reducing the severity and duration of neutropenia. Administering filgrastim during the first cycle of chemotherapy may be especially valuable for older adults (Hood, 2003).

Environment

Determine the environment in which filgrastim is to be administered. IV infusions of filgrastim are administered in either a hospital or outpatient setting. SC injections may be administered in the hospital, outpatient center, or by the patient at home. Assess whether the patient will be able to return for daily injections or whether they have the ability to self-administer the drug. The drug should be kept refrigerated but not allowed to freeze. Determine that there is a refrigerator at home if the patient is to self-administer the drug.

Nursing Diagnoses and Outcomes

- Risk for Altered Body Temperature related to neutropenia
  Desired outcome: *Febrile neutropenia will be avoided while receiving filgrastim.*
- Risk for Caregiver Role Strain related to need to bring patient daily to clinic for treatment with filgrastim
  Desired outcome: *Caregiver role strain will not develop.*
- Risk for Infection related to neutropenia
  Desired outcome: *The patient will not develop an infection while receiving filgrastim.*
- Risk for Pain, Medullary Bone, related to adverse effect of filgrastim
  Desired outcome: *Bone pain will not develop or will not be unmanageable if it develops while the patient is taking filgrastim.*

- Management of Individual, Effective Therapeutic Regimen as evidenced by using correct technique daily to administer filgrastim subcutaneously and returning for all follow-up appointments
  Desired outcome: *Patient will be adept at self-administering filgrastim before discharge home and will be able to demonstrate technique when he or she returns for first follow-up appointment.*

Planning and Intervention

Maximizing Therapeutic Effects

To achieve the maximum therapeutic effect from the filgrastim, take the following actions:

- Keep it refrigerated. Allow the drug to reach room temperature before administering it.
- If giving the drug intravenously, dilute it in 5% dextrose solution with albumin added, to prevent absorption by plastic materials.
- Do not dilute the drug in saline because it may precipitate.
- Avoid shaking the drug, which can damage the protein.
- Administer filgrastim with the first cycle of chemotherapy for those at high risk for febrile neutropenia, including older adults.

Minimizing Adverse Effects

To prevent adverse effects, be careful not to decrease the dose prematurely (before the expected neutrophil nadir, or lowest point, is expected). Additionally, discard any vial that has been at room temperature for more than 24 hours, use only one dose per vial, and never re-enter a used vial. Because filgrastim is preservative free, these actions will guard against bacterial growth. If the absolute neutrophil count remains above 1,000/mm^3 for three consecutive days, discontinue filgrastim to prevent excessively high neutrophil counts.

Providing Patient and Family Education

Patients with neutropenia are at increased risk for contracting an infection. When providing patient education, instruct the patient and those in contact with the patient to wash their hands frequently, avoid crowds, and avoid people with illnesses (Box 33.2).

Ongoing Assessment and Evaluation

Monitor the patient's temperature closely throughout therapy for fever indicating infection. Monitor the WBC count throughout therapy. The WBC count should rise and return to a normal level but should not become unduly elevated. If patients must use drugs that potentiate neutrophil release, monitoring the WBC is especially important, because a synergistic effect may occur. Once the absolute neutrophil count remains above 1,000/mm^3 for 3 consecutive days, discontinue filgrastim. The other components of a complete blood count should also be monitored to detect any adverse effects from filgrastim. Filgrastim therapy is effective when infection is avoided (or is minimal if it occurs) and the WBC count rises to a normal level.

COMMUNITY-BASED CONCERNS

Box 33.2 Neutropenia and Infection

Patients who are neutropenic are at increased risk if they contract an infection, because they cannot defend themselves against the infecting organism. The infection may become severe or even life threatening. This is true for even "common" infections, which most people can overcome fairly easily on their own. Patients who are immunocompromised by either disease or drug therapy should be taught how to minimize their risk of becoming sick with an infection, as follows:

- Wash hands frequently. Family members and others in the household should also wash their hands frequently.
- Avoid people with acute illnesses.
- Avoid going out in crowds, especially during cold and flu season. This precaution would include such places as malls, movie theaters, and worship services.
- Handle food safely. Cook meats to an appropriately high temperature to kill bacteria. Clean thoroughly all surfaces that have come into contact with raw food products. Refrigerate leftover food as soon as possible.

Drugs Closely Related to P Filgrastim

Pegfilgrastim

Like filgrastim, pegfilgrastim is used in myelosuppressive chemotherapy to decrease the incidence of infection manifested as febrile neutropenia in patients who have nonmyeloid cancer and are receiving chemotherapy that suppresses the WBC count. Pegfilgrastim is filgrastim that has been chemically altered by attaching a polyethylene glycol (PEG) molecule to the filgrastim molecule. Although this change in molecular size does not alter the way the drug acts to increase the WBC count, it does have substantial effects on the pharmacokinetics and thus on the dosing of the drug. Pegfilgrastim, unlike filgrastim, has poor renal excretion. Its sole

MEMORY CHIP

P Filgrastim

- Used in patients with cancer to increase their neutrophil counts
- A DNA recombinant granulocyte colony-stimulating factor (G-CSF) that stimulates white blood cell development just as endogenous G-CSF does
- Administered by IV infusion or daily SC injections
- Most common adverse effects: medullary bone pain
- Most serious adverse effects: none
- **Life span alert: Older adults are more at risk from complications with neutropenia; prophylactic use of G-CSF is usually appropriate.**
- Maximizing therapeutic effects: Do not dilute in saline; avoid shaking; administer with the first cycle of chemotherapy in those at high risk for febrile neutropenia, including older adults.
- Minimizing adverse effects: Do not decrease the dose before the expected neutrophil nadir; keep refrigerated and use aseptic technique to minimize risk for bacterial growth.
- Most important patient education: how to decrease risk for infection

mechanism of elimination is related to binding on receptors of neutrophils. When mature neutrophil counts remain low (as a result of myelosuppression from chemotherapy), unbound, circulating levels of pegfilgrastim remain high, stimulating more neutrophil development. Once the mature neutrophil cell count has increased sufficiently, receptors are present to enable binding and elimination of the pegfilgrastim (Bedell, 2003). The advantage of this pharmacokinetic change is that pegfilgrastim has to be given only once per chemotherapy cycle, instead of daily like filgrastim. This difference may increase patients' adherence to therapy because they do not need to return daily for injections. Patients may also prefer this therapy because they receive fewer injections.

Effectiveness, contraindications, precautions, drug interactions, and adverse effects of pegfilgrastim are similar to those of filgrastim. One study that compared pegfilgrastim and filgrastim in treating patients with stage II to IV breast cancer showed that patients receiving pegfilgrastim had a significantly lower risk for febrile neutropenia (Siena et al., 2003). Pegfilgrastim comes in prefilled syringes and should be protected from light. Although it is kept refrigerated, it should be allowed to come to room temperature before administration. Like filgrastim, it should not be shaken. Because the solution is preservative free, only one injection should be administered per syringe; any remaining medication should be discarded.

As with filgrastim, the patient's complete blood cell count must be monitored after pegfilgrastim therapy. However, because patients are not seen as frequently when they receive pegfilgrastim as when they receive filgrastim, it is especially important that they are taught the signs of infection and know when to contact the clinic or the prescriber (Bedell, 2003).

Sargramostim

Sargramostim (Leukine) is produced by recombinant DNA technology in a yeast expression system. Sargramostim is a glycoprotein of 127 amino acids. The amino acid sequence differs from the natural human GM-CSF by substituting leucine at position 23; the carbohydrate portion may also be different than in the native protein. Unlike G-CSF (filgrastim), which induces production only of granulocytes, specifically neutrophils, GM-CSF induces partially committed progenitor cells to divide and differentiate into the granulocyte and the macrophage pathways. Sargramostim increases the cytotoxicity of monocytes toward certain neoplastic cell lines and activates neutrophils to inhibit the growth of pathogens or tumor cells.

Sargramostim is used to treat patients with non-Hodgkin lymphoma, acute lymphoblastic leukemia, and Hodgkin disease who are undergoing autologous bone marrow transplantation (transplantation of their own bone marrow that was previously collected). It accelerates myeloid recovery in these patients. Sargramostim is also used in bone marrow transplant failure or when engraftment delays occur. It can be used after the induction of chemotherapy in older adults with acute myelogenous leukemia to shorten their neutrophil recovery time and reduce severe, life-threatening infections. Sargramostim can also be used to mobilize the hematopoietic progenitor cells into the peripheral circulation, where they can be collected by leukapheresis. The additional progenitor cells are later returned after chemotherapy, enabling more rapid engraftment and decreasing the need for supportive care. The drug is administered after collection and transplantation of peripheral blood progenitors, to rapidly increase monocyte production. Sargramostim is also used after allogenic (from a matched donor) bone marrow transplantation to accelerate the myeloid recovery.

Unlabeled uses of sargramostim include increasing WBC counts in patients with myelodysplastic syndromes and in patients with AIDS who are receiving zidovudine; limiting the duration of leukopenia secondary to myelosuppressive chemotherapy and decreasing myelosuppression in preleukemic patients; correcting neutropenia in aplastic anemia; and decreasing transplantation-associated organ system damage, particularly liver and kidney disease (neutropenia correlates with organ system injury). Other potential uses for sargramostim that are being investigated are decreasing the course of mucositis, stimulating dendritic cells, preventing infection, acting as a vaccine adjuvant, promoting wound healing, and facilitating immunologic tumor control (Buchsel et al., 2002).

Sargramostim is administered by IV infusion for most applications. It may be given subcutaneously when used after peripheral blood progenitor cell transplantation.

Contraindications to sargramostim use include presence of excess leukemic myeloid blasts in the bone marrow or peripheral blood, known hypersensitivity to the drug, simultaneous administration of chemotherapy or radiotherapy, or administration of sargramostim 24 hours preceding or following chemotherapy or radiotherapy. Like filgrastim, sargramostim is a pregnancy category C drug. Whether it is excreted into breast milk is unknown. It does not appear to produce any greater toxicity in children than in adults.

Although most of the adverse effects that occur with sargramostim can also be attributed to the disease process or the chemotherapy used to treat it, be alert for unique events that may occur with sargramostim. Bone pain can occur, as with filgrastim. Administer sargramostim in the evening to minimize this problem; administration of acetaminophen 20 to 30 minutes before injection is also helpful. Site reactions are possible. Special attention to injection technique, as recommended by Buchsel and colleagues (2002), will minimize site pain. These steps include:

- Allowing enough time for the drug to come to room temperature before administration
- Choosing a short length (5/8-inch) and fine gauge (25–27) needle
- Icing the injection site before and after injection
- Avoiding pinching the skin if possible
- Injecting no more than 2 mL into any injection site
- Injecting the medication slowly into the subcutaneous space, avoiding IM injections
- Not rubbing after injection
- Rotating injection sites among the upper arms, abdomen, and thighs

Occasional transient supraventricular arrhythmias may occur during administration of sargramostim, especially if the patient has a history of cardiac arrhythmias. These arrhythmias are reversible when the drug is discontinued. Trapping of granulocytes in the pulmonary circulation has occurred following sargramostim infusion, sometimes producing dyspnea. The recommended treatment for patients who become dyspneic is to reduce the rate of infusion by half.

In patients with pre-existing pleural and pericardial effusions, sargramostim may aggravate fluid retention. This condition is usually reversible with dose interruption or reduction, although occasionally a diuretic is needed.

A first-dose effect has occurred rarely following the first dose of sargramostim. In this syndrome, respiratory distress, hypoxia, flushing, hypotension, syncope, or tachycardia occurs. The patient should be monitored for these problems for the first 20 minutes after the first injection, and the first dose should be administered in a clinical setting where the patient can be observed. The syndrome should be treated by stopping the infusion and treating the patient according to symptoms. Oxygen, methylprednisone, and diphenhydramine may be indicated. When symptoms have resolved, the infusion is resumed at half the rate. These effects do not usually happen again with future doses.

Excessively high WBC counts have sometimes rapidly occurred with sargramostim therapy (absolute neutrophil count [ANC] above 20,000 cell/mm^3 or platelets above 500,000/mm^3). If this effect occurs, the dose should be reduced or temporarily stopped.

In some patients with pre-existing renal or hepatic dysfunction, sargramostim has induced elevation of serum creatinine or bilirubin and hepatic enzymes.

Ⓒ INTERLEUKINS

Unlike other interleukins, oprelvekin (also known as interleukin-11) primarily alters hematopoietic activity and stimulates the production of platelets. Other interleukins are presented in Chapter 34. Interleukin-11, the sole drug in this class, is by necessity also the prototype for the class.

NURSING MANAGEMENT OF THE PATIENT RECEIVING [P] OPRELVEKIN

Core Drug Knowledge

Pharmacotherapeutics

Oprelvekin (Neumega) is used to prevent severe thrombocytopenia and to reduce the need for platelet transfusions following myelosuppressive chemotherapy in patients with nonmyeloid malignancies who are at high risk for severe thrombocytopenia. An unlabeled use is in the treatment of Crohn disease. It is administered as an SC dose once daily.

Pharmacokinetics

The peak serum level of oprelvekin is reached 3.2 hours after it is given subcutaneously. Although the drug is thought to be metabolized, the exact mechanism is not known. It is eliminated by the kidney.

Pharmacodynamics

Oprelvekin is produced in *E. coli* by recombinant DNA technology. The resultant polypeptide is 177 amino acids long and differs from the 178 amino acid length of endogenous interleukin-11 by a missing amino-terminal proline residue. Bone-forming and bone-resorbing cells are potential targets of interleukin-11. Its primary hematopoietic activity is to directly stimulate the production of megakaryocyte progenitor cells and thrombopoietin. This action stimulates production of platelets that are structurally and functionally the same as those platelets produced by endogenous interleukin-11. Platelet counts begin to rise 5 to 9 days after starting drug therapy with oprelvekin. When treatment with oprelvekin is stopped, platelet levels continue to rise for about 7 days; they fall toward baseline in about 14 days.

Contraindications and Precautions

Oprelvekin is contraindicated only if the patient has hypersensitivity to the drug or any of its components. Caution should be used if oprelvekin is used in patients with pre-existing cardiomyopathy or congestive heart failure because fluid retention is a common effect of therapy. Use caution if the patient has a history of atrial arrhythmia, which may increase the risk for developing an atrial arrhythmia from oprelvekin use. Do not use this drug with or immediately following cytotoxic chemotherapy. Oprelvekin is a pregnancy category C drug and has caused increased rates of fetal death in animal studies.

Adverse Effects

Fluid retention with weight gain is the most common adverse effect of oprelvekin. This condition may be evidenced by peripheral edema, dyspnea on exertion, an increase in pleural effusion (if effusion was present before therapy), and decreases of about 10% to 15% in hemoglobin concentration, hematocrit, and RBCs (dilutional anemia caused by increase in plasma volume). The cardiovascular adverse effects of oprelvekin may also be related to fluid retention (tachycardia, vasodilation, palpitations, syncope, and atrial fibrillation and flutter). Transient, mild blurred vision and papilledema have occasionally been reported. Antibody production and transient rashes have occasionally been observed at the injection site after administration but have not been associated with anaphylactic reactions or loss of clinical responsiveness to oprelvekin therapy.

The following adverse effects that are unique to oprelvekin (those that are not likely to be associated with the cancer or its therapy) have been noted occasionally: dimmed vision, paresthesia, dehydration, skin discoloration, exfoliative dermatitis, and eye hemorrhage.

Drug Interactions

There are no known drug interactions with oprelvekin.

Assessment of Relevant Core Patient Variables

Health Status

Assess for congestive heart failure, pleural or pericardial effusion, or susceptibility to developing congestive heart failure (CHF) because fluid retention is possible from oprelvekin. Assess also for a history of atrial fibrillation or flutter, other cardiac disorders, or cardiac medications because these factors may increase the risk for atrial arrhythmia during drug therapy. Determine that at least 6 hours has elapsed after the completion of chemotherapy before starting oprelvekin. The patient should not have received myeloablative therapy

(therapy in which myelocytes are destroyed) because this therapy is not an indication for oprelvekin use.

Life Span and Gender

Determine whether the patient is pregnant because oprelvekin is a pregnancy category C drug. Ask the patient's age and whether she is breast-feeding. Whether oprelvekin crosses into breast milk is unknown, and the safety and dosage for children under 12 years of age is also not known. Older adults may be more likely to develop atrial arrhythmias while taking oprelvekin.

Lifestyle, Diet, and Habits

Assess for moderate to heavy habitual alcohol intake, which may increase the risk for atrial arrhythmias.

Environment

Determine that refrigeration is available for storing oprelvekin. Oprelvekin must be kept refrigerated because neither it nor its diluent contains preservatives. The drug is also sensitive to light and must be stored accordingly.

Nursing Diagnoses and Outcomes

- Risk for Injury related to bleeding secondary to low platelet counts
  Desired outcome: *Injury will not occur while treating low platelet counts with oprelvekin.*
- Risk for Fluid Volume Excess related to adverse effects of oprelvekin
  Desired outcome: *Retention of fluid will not occur or will be controllable while on oprelvekin therapy.*
- Risk for Infection related to lack of medical asepsis in storage, preparation, and administration of subcutaneous oprelvekin
  Desired outcome: *The patient will remain free of infection.*
- Risk for Caregiver Role Strain related to the need to bring patient daily to clinic for treatment with oprelvekin
  Desired outcome: *Caregiver role strain will not occur.*

Planning and Intervention

Maximizing Therapeutic Effects

Store the powdered drug and the diluent in the refrigerator but do not freeze it. Keep the drug out of direct light. Reconstitute oprelvekin with the sterile water for injection (without preservative) that is provided with the medication. When injecting the sterile water into the vial, direct the spray of fluid toward the glass wall. To prevent excessive agitation, do not aim it directly into the powdered drug. Do not shake or excessively agitate the vial, which can denature the protein. To fully reconstitute the powder, gently swirl the vial.

Administration of oprelvekin should begin 6 to 24 hours after chemotherapy is completed. Continue until the postnadir platelet count is greater than or equal to 50,000 cells/mm^3. Clinical trials showed the need to dose for 10 to 21 days; the effect of giving oprelvekin for more than 21 days is not known. Discontinue oprelvekin treatment at least 2 days before starting the next round of chemotherapy.

Minimizing Adverse Effects

Because neither oprelvekin nor the sterile water used to dilute it contains preservatives, care should be taken to maintain aseptic technique when reconstituting and drawing up the medication. Do not re-enter or reuse the single-dose vial. Be certain to use the reconstituted drug within 3 hours of reconstitution.

Monitor fluid intake and output carefully. Diuretics may be indicated if the patient is experiencing fluid retention from oprelvekin therapy.

Providing Patient and Family Education

If the patient will self-administer at home, teach the patient how to administer the drug safely and correctly into the subcutaneous tissue. Patient education should emphasize the importance of telling the physician or nurse when fluid retention occurs and should also emphasize the need to avoid activities that may cause bleeding until platelet counts are in the normal range.

Ongoing Assessment and Evaluation

Monitor the patient's platelet count throughout therapy. Continue with oprelvekin therapy until the post-nadir platelet count is greater than or equal to 50,000 cells/mm^3. Also monitor the other components of the CBC to detect any adverse effects. Until the platelet count is adequate, monitor the patient for bleeding. Therapy with oprelvekin is effective if the platelet count rises to normal and severe bleeding is prevented.

MEMORY CHIP

P Oprelvekin (Interleukin-11)

- Used to prevent severe thrombocytopenia in cancer patients
- A recombinant DNA polypeptide that stimulates production of platelets in the same way that endogenous interleukin-11 does
- Administered daily by SC injection
- Major contraindication: Do not use with or immediately following cytotoxic chemotherapy.
- Most common adverse effects: fluid retention
- Most serious adverse effects: CHF or pulmonary edema from fluid retention; atrial arrhythmias
- **Life span alert: Older adults may be more likely to develop atrial arrhythmias.**
- Maximizing therapeutic effects: Do not shake or excessively agitate the vial; begin administration 6 h to 24 hours after the completion of chemotherapy; continue until the postnadir platelet count is greater than or equal to 50,000 cells/mm^3.
- Minimizing adverse effects: Monitor fluid intake and output; maintain aseptic technique.
- Most important patient education: Contact prescriber if fluid retention occurs; avoid activities that increase risk for bleeding.

CHAPTER SUMMARY

- The immune system is a complex system of cells and chemical mediators that prevents foreign pathogens or cells from invading the body.
- The mature blood cells differ in structure and function, but all develop from a common progenitor cell, or stem cell, from within the bone marrow.
- WBCs are active in the surveillance and initiation of inflammatory reactions to specific stimuli. WBCs include neutrophils, which digest foreign material; basophils, which release chemicals to initiate the immune response; mast cells, located in the skin and the respiratory and GI tracts; macrophages, which release chemicals to initiate the immune response; and eosinophils, which seem to be active in allergic reactions.
- Lymphocytes include T cells, which are important in modifying the immune response and in protecting the body from nonself cells, and B cells, which produce antibodies to specific antigens. The antibodies stimulate an immune and inflammatory reaction to the antigen and cause its destruction.
- Blood cell components may be altered because of pathophysiology or drug therapy to treat a disease process.
- Drugs that stimulate the immune system are hematopoietic growth factors, cytokines, and immune modulators. They are used to keep viral particles from replicating and to inhibit tumor growth.
- Recombinant human erythropoietin, also known as epoetin alfa, is used to treat anemias that result from decreased production of RBCs (erythropoiesis). Tissue oxygenation cannot occur optimally with anemia.
- Iron is also needed to form RBCs. Epoetin alfa therapy that is not effective or has a diminished effect is likely attributable to iron deficiency, which may be absolute or functional. Most patients with chronic renal failure will need iron transfusions at some time for RBCs to be produced following epoetin alfa administration.
- The colony-stimulating factors are the granulocyte (G-CSF) and the granulocyte-macrophage (GM-CSF). They stimulate WBC production. Low WBC counts, especially low neutrophil counts, place the patient at increased risk for contracting an infection.
- Unlike other interleukins, interleukin-11 (oprelvekin) has hematopoietic properties and stimulates the production of platelets. Without an adequate number of platelets, proper blood clotting cannot take place.
- Drugs that promote production of blood cells should not be given at the same time as chemotherapy because the rapidly producing cells are likely to be killed by the drug therapy.

QUESTIONS FOR STUDY AND REVIEW

1. What are the principal polypeptides and glycoproteins involved in hematopoiesis?
2. Why are people with chronic renal failure anemic?
3. What is the major risk to people who are neutropenic after chemotherapy?
4. How are platelets produced?
5. Why does the patient with CHF require close monitoring of their intake and output of fluids when they are started on oprelvekin?
6. Your patient has CHF and chronic renal failure and is receiving epoetin alfa. Why should the target range for hemoglobin and hematocrit be set lower than what is usually considered "normal"?

? Need More Help?

Chapter 33 of the study guide for *Drug Therapy in Nursing* 2e contains NCLEX-style questions and other learning activities to reinforce your understanding of the concepts presented in this chapter. For additional information or to purchase the study guide, visit *http://connection.lww.com/go/aschenbrenner.*

REFERENCES AND BIBLIOGRAPHY

Bedell, C. (2003). Pegfilgrastim for chemotherapy-induced neutropenia. *Clinical Journal of Oncology Nursing, 7*(1), 55–58.

Buchsel, P. C., Gorgey, A., Grape, F. B., et al. (2002). Granulocyte macrophage colony-stimulating factor: Current practice and novel approaches. *Clinical Journal of Oncology Nursing, 6*(4); 1–8.

Hood, L. E. (2003). Chemotherapy in the elderly: Supportive measures for chemotherapy-induced myelotoxicity. *Clinical Journal of Oncology Nursing, 7*(2), 185–190.

Nail, L. M. (2002). Fatigue in patients with cancer. *Oncology Nursing Forum, 29*(3), 537–544.

National Kidney Foundation. (2000). Guidelines for anemia of chronic kidney disease [Online.] Available: *http://www.kidney.org/professionals/kdoqi/guidelines_updates/doqi_uptoc.html#an.*

Siena, P., Piccart, M. J., Holmes, F. A., et al. (2003). A combined analysis of two pivotal randomized trials of a single dose of pegfilgrastim per chemotherapy cycle and daily filgrastim in patients with stage II-IV breast cancer. *Oncology Reports, 10*(3), 715–724.

Szromba, C., Thies, M. A., & Ossman, S. S. (2002). Advancing chronic kidney disease care: New imperatives for recognition and intervention. *Nephrology Nursing Journal, 29*(6), 547–559.

Drugs Affecting the Immune Response

chapter 34

Learning Objectives

At the completion of this chapter the student will:

1. Identify core drug knowledge about drugs that affect the biologic responses.
2. Relate the interaction of core drug knowledge to core patient variables for drugs that affect biologic responses.
3. Generate a nursing plan of care from the interactions between core drug knowledge and core patient variables for drugs that affect biologic responses.
4. Describe nursing interventions to maximize therapeutic effects and minimize adverse effects for drugs that affect the immunologic system.
5. Determine key points for patient and family education for drugs that affect the immune system.

KEY TERMS

active immunity
antibodies
antigens
autoimmune disease
B lymphocytes
biologic modulator
cellular immune response
chemotaxis
complement
cytokines
immunoglobulins
interferon
interleukins
immune modulators
immunotoxins
leukocytes
lymphokines
T lymphocytes

FEATURED WEBLINK

http://theoncologist.alphamedpress.org/cgi/content/full/6/4/374
The Oncologist CME Online Journal site contains an article on the fundamentals of cancer medicine, titled "The Molecular Perspective: Interferons," by Dr. David S. Goodsell.

CONNECTION WEBLINK

Additional Weblinks are found on Connection:
http://www.connection.lww.com/go/aschenbrenner.

Drugs Affecting the Biologic Response

Ⓒ Cytokines

- **P** **interferon alfa-2a**
- interferon alfa-2b
- interferon alfa-n3
- interferon-n1
- interferon alfacon-1
- interferon beta-1a
- interferon beta-1b
- interferon gamma-1b
- aldesleukin (interleukin-2)

Ⓒ Antibodies

- **P** **rituximab**
- abciximab
- alemtuzumab
- palivizumab
- trastuzumab
- basiliximab
- daclizumab
- gemtuzumab
- infliximab
- Iodine^{131}
- muromonab-CD3
- satumomab pendetide
- tositumomab + ^{90}Y ibritumomab tiuxetan

Ⓒ Immume Modulators

- **P** **cyclosporine**
- mycophenolate mofetil
- sirolimus
- tacrolimus
- azathioprine
- bacillus of Calmette and Guerin (BCG)
- bexarotene
- 9-cis transretinoic acid
- denileukin diftitox
- glatiramer
- levamisole
- thalidomide
- transretinoic acid (ATRA)

The symbol Ⓒ indicates the **drug class**.
Drugs in **bold type** marked with the symbol **P** are prototypes.
Drugs in blue type are closely related to the prototype.
Drugs in red type are significantly different from the prototype.
Drugs in black type with no symbol are also used in drug therapy; no prototype

Biologic modulators, or biologic modifiers, are a group of biopharmaceuticals that are naturally occurring proteins used to alter the body's immunologic responses. The use of biologic modulators is also called biologic therapy. The rapid growth of these therapies is attributable to the refinement of recombinant DNA technology, which has enabled researchers to produce large quantities of these substances outside the body. Agents are classified by their specific biologic mechanism of activity and by whether they stimulate or suppress immune processes. Some stimulate specific immunologic activity to combat unique **antigens** (substances that induce formation of antibodies). Similar drugs from this class may also be used to suppress the immune system to prevent rejection of foreign transplanted tissue, or when the body is inappropriately rejecting self, as in **autoimmune disease.** Moreover, some agents may at once stimulate some parts of the immune system and depress other parts of the immune system.

This chapter discusses three classifications of agents used to alter biologic responses: cytokines, antibodies, and immune modulators. Active and passive antibody-conferred vaccinations are addressed in Appendix G rather than in this chapter. **Cytokines** are immunologic toxins produced by white blood cells (WBCs, also called leukocytes) in response to foreign antigens such as microorganisms, transplanted tissue, or malignant cells. The prototype cytokine is interferon alfa-2a (Roferon-A). Drugs in the same class represented by the prototype are interferon alfa-2b (Intron-A), interferon alfa-n3 (Alferon N), interferon-n1 (Wellferon), interferon alfacon-1 (Infergen), interferon beta-1a (Avonex), interferon beta-1b (Betaseron), and interferon gamma-1b (Actimmune). A drug significantly different from the prototype interferon alfa-2a is aldesleukin (also known as interleukin-2 [IL-2]; brand name, Proleukin).

Antibodies (complex proteins produced in response to the presence of antigens) are a heterogeneous class of agents that can contain multiple genetic clones (polyclonal) or a single genetic design (monoclonal). Polyclonal antibodies are nonspecific in their action and are now used less frequently because technology has permitted specific targeting of cells using the monoclonal agents. Using hybridoma technology, monoclonal antibodies (MoAbs) can be engineered to attach to tumor cells for diagnosis or treatment of malignancies or target T lymphocytes, also called T cells, to prevent or suppress T-cell recognition of tissue from outside the body. You will find more information about T cells later in this chapter under the heading, Specific Immune Responses. The prototype antibody is rituximab (Rituxan). Drugs in the same class and represented by the prototype are trastuzumab (Herceptin) and alemtuzumab (Campath). Monoclonal antibodies closely related to the prototype rituximab include abciximab (ReoPro) and palivizumab (Synagis). Monoclonal antibodies significantly different from rituximab include muromonab CD3 (Orthoclone), daclizumab (Zenapax), infliximab (Remicade), and basiliximab (Simulect). Gemtuzumab (Mylotarg) is also a significantly different monoclonal antibody because it is a monoclonal antibody fused with an antineoplastic agent. Three radiolabeled monoclonal antibodies exist and are considered very different from the prototype. Satumomab pendetide (OncoScint CR/OV) is a radiolabeled monoclonal antibody that targets ovarian or colorectal cancer cells but does not have properties to initiate cell lysis. Tositumomab plus iodine-131 (^{131}I) (Bexxar) and yttrium-90 (^{90}Y) ibritumomab tiuxetan (Zevalin) are also significantly different antibodies because they are composed of both a monoclonal antibody and radioactive substances that have antineoplastic properties. The only available polyclonal antibodies are antilymphocyte globulin (lymphocyte immune globulin, Atgam) and rabbit antithymocyte globulin (RATG). Because of these agents' multiple clonal features, they are pharmacokinetically very different from other antibodies and are classed as significantly different antibodies.

The **immune modulators** are a group of several agents with distinctly different structures that alter T-cell or B-cell activity. The prototype is cyclosporine (Sandimmune, Neoral, SangCya). Drugs in the same class and represented by the prototype are tacrolimus (Prograf), sirolimus (Rapamune), and mycophenolate mofetil (CellCept). Drugs significantly different from cyclosporine are the retinoids (e.g., all-transretinoic acid [ATRA], tretinoin [Vesanoid]), 9-cis-transretinoic acid (Panretinide, isomer ATRA), and bexarotene (Targretin gel), levamisole (Ergamisol), azathioprine (Imuran), thalidomide (Thalomid), glatiramer (Copaxone). Bacille Calmette-Guérin (BCG) (ImmuCyst/TheraCys) is an inactivated microbial toxin that is classified as a biologic agent as well. Clinical investigators have also combined cytokines, enzymes, or microbes with antibodies to create a group of agents called fusion proteins, of which only denileukin diftitox (Ontak [diphtheria toxin and IL-2]) is currently a licensed agent (Kinzler & Brown, 2001; Pennell & Erickson, 2002). Research is now being conducted to determine whether other essential cell proteins, nutrients, and growth factors (e.g., dendritic cells, epidermal growth factor inhibitors) can be manipulated to provide a clinical benefit (Lotze et al., 1999; Wu & Lanier, 2003; Cho & Bhardwaj, 2003; Luo & Prestwich, 2002). Agents targeted against cellular enzymes that are essential for tumor replication include tyrosine kinase inhibitors (e.g., imatinib mesylate [Gleevec], gefitimib [Iressa]), and proteosome inhibitors (e.g., bortezamib [Velcade]). These agents are included in the chapter on cell cycle–nonspecific antineoplastics (see Chapter 36).

The body of knowledge about the components and actions of the immune system is developing daily. As researchers make new discoveries and better understand biologic interactions, they will find more ways to modify immune systems and treat a variety of viral, autoimmune, hematologic, and neoplastic disorders.

PHYSIOLOGY

The immune system is composed of hematopoietic cells and multiple hematologic-immunologic production and storage sites. Hematopoietic physiology and pharmacologic agents are described in greater detail in Chapter 33. The reticuloendothelial system includes immunologically active tissue and cells found in the lymph system, spleen, liver, lungs, gastrointestinal (GI) tract, and brain. An integrated immune response involving hematopoietic cells and immune tissues provides the body's nonspecific and specific response to invasion by antigens identified as nonself. The essential components of the immune system are hematopoietic cells, barrier defenses, the nonspecific immune response, the specific

immune response, and immunity. **Leukocytes** (or WBCs) are key components of all immune system responses. (See Chapter 33 for an overview of hematopoiesis and a discussion of leukocytes' primary actions relating to combating invasion by microbes, and establishing an initial barrier and inflammatory response.) This chapter will focus on pharmacologic agents that affect other aspects of the immune response.

Specific Immune Responses

If an invader gets past the barrier and nonspecific immune systems and enters the tissues or bloodstream, a specific immune response involving lymphocytes is initiated (Figure 34.1).

Bone marrow stem cells develop into two types of lymphocytes: **T lymphocytes,** or T cells, and **B lymphocytes,** or B cells. These T and B lymphocytes may also differentiate into specialized cells, such as natural killer cells and lymphokine-activated killer (LAK) cells, which have been identified as the cells that aggressively attack and destroy neoplastic cells. Because research in the area of lymphocyte identification is relatively new, other lymphocytes not yet identified may also take part in the immune response.

T cells are "programmed" in the thymus gland to develop into at least three different cell types. Effector or cytotoxic T cells are found in various areas of the body and aggressively attack nonself cells by releasing chemicals called **lymphokines.**

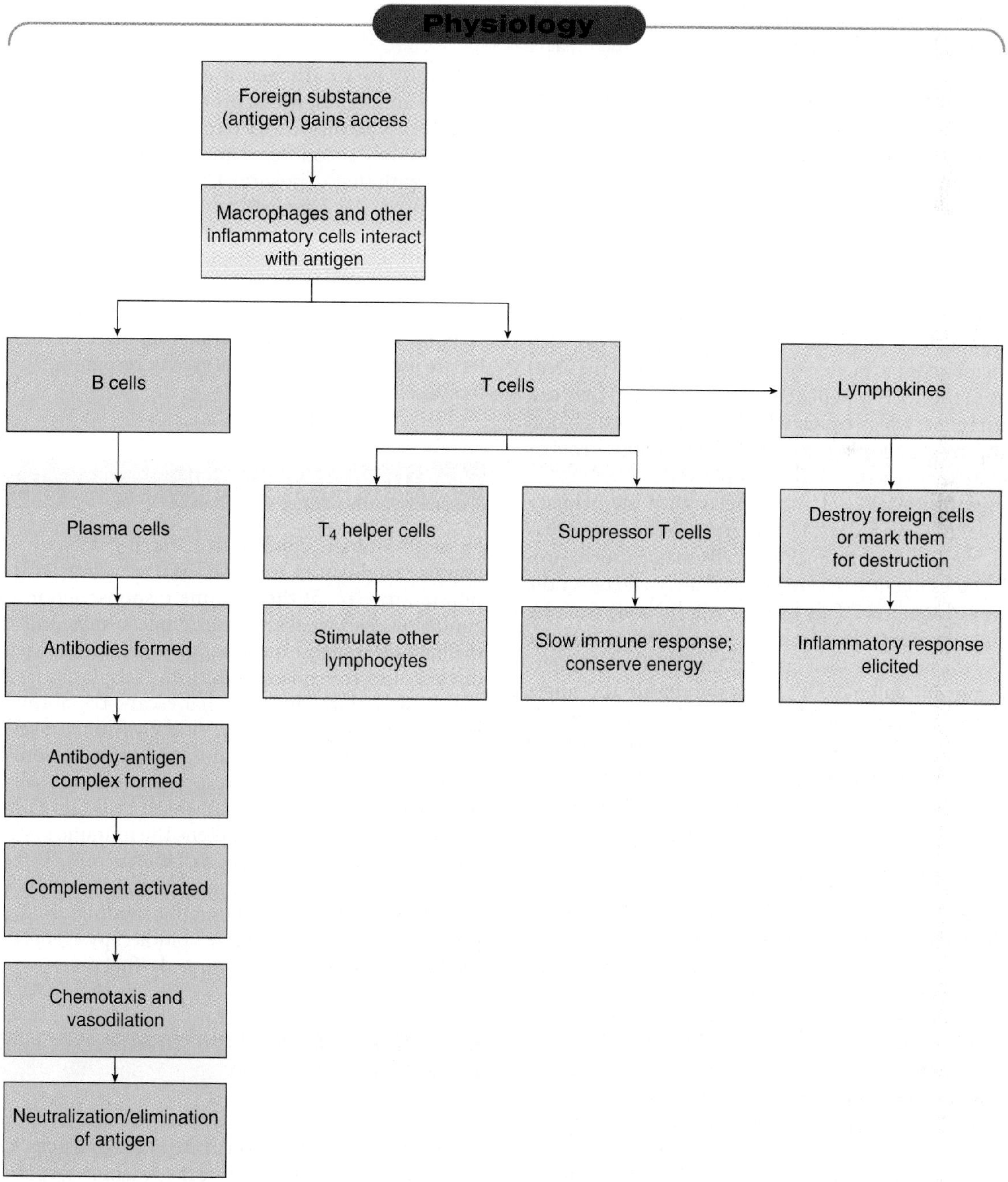

FIGURE 34.1 Response of T and B cells to invasion by foreign cells.

These chemicals either directly destroy a foreign cell or mark it for destruction by phagocytes and elicit an inflammatory response. This effect is termed the **cellular immune response.** Foreign or nonself cells have different membrane-identifying antigens called histocompatibility leukocyte antigens (HLAs). Helper T cells respond to the chemical indicators of immune activity and stimulate other lymphocytes to be more aggressive and responsive. Suppressor T cells respond to rising levels of chemicals associated with an immune response and suppress or slow the reaction. The balance between these two systems permits a rapid response that destroys invaders immediately, followed by a slowing reaction if the invasion continues. This slowing conserves energy and the components of the immune and inflammatory reaction.

B cells are found throughout the reticuloendothelial system in like groups called clones. These cells are "programmed" to identify specific antigens. When a B cell reacts with its specific antigen, it changes into a plasma cell. Plasma cells produce antibodies, or **immunoglobulins,** that circulate in the body and react with their specific "destiny" antigen when encountered. This effect is called a receptor–receptor site reaction and constitutes the humoral immune response. When the antigen and antibody react, they form an antigen–antibody complex, which reveals a new receptor site on the antibody that activates a series of plasma proteins in the body called **complement.** Complement proteins can destroy the antigen by altering the membrane and allowing osmotic inflow of fluid that bursts the cell. These proteins can also induce **chemotaxis** (attraction of phagocytic cells to the area) and increase the activity of phagocytes. In addition, they can release histamine, which causes vasodilation, increases blood flow to the area, and brings together all the components of the inflammatory reaction to destroy the antigen.

The initial formation of antibodies, called the primary response, takes several days. However, once the response is activated, the B cells form memory cells that, in turn, produce antibodies that are released immediately whenever the antigen is encountered. This process is a lifelong reaction called **active immunity.** B cells cluster in areas where they are most likely to encounter their specific antigen. For example, airborne antigens will meet B cells in the tonsils and upper respiratory tract. Experts believe that B cells are programmed genetically and are formed before birth. The introduction of a new and unusual antigen can result in widespread disease because the body is unable to recognize the foreign protein and mount an immune response.

Chemical factors also play an important role in the specific immune reaction, acting as communicators within the immune system to coordinate the immune response. For example, **interferons** are chemicals secreted by cells that have been invaded by viruses and possibly other stimuli. They prevent viral replication and suppress malignant cell replication and tumor growth. **Interleukins** are chemicals secreted by active WBCs to influence other WBCs. Interleukin-1 (lymphocyte-activating factor) stimulates T cells to initiate an immune response. Interleukin-2 (T-cell growth factor) is released from active T cells to stimulate the production of more T cells and to increase the activity of B cells, cytotoxic cells, and natural killer cells. Interleukin-2 also causes fever, arthralgia, myalgia, and slow-wave sleep-energy-conserving measures that help the body fight off invaders.

Several other factors released by lymphocytes and basophils have been identified. These include B-cell growth factor, macrophage-activating factor, macrophage-inhibiting factor, platelet-activating factor, eosinophil-chemotactic factor, and neutrophil-chemotactic factor. The presence or absence of these factors can influence the immune response.

The thymus gland, located in the mediastinal cavity, also releases a number of types of hormones that circulate in the body to stimulate and communicate with T cells. Thymosin, a thymus hormone, is important in the maturation of T cells and cell-mediated immunity. Research is currently under way to evaluate the use of exogenous thymosin in treating certain leukemias and melanomas (Goldstein, 2003; Wilkes et al., 1999).

Immunity

Immunity to a pathogen is achieved when the body has formed antibodies, which protect the body from developing an illness. Vaccines are used to stimulate an active immunity to commonly encountered antigens that could cause serious illness with first exposure. These vaccines are discussed in Appendix G. Sera are used to provide preformed antibodies, or passive immunity, in situations of acute exposure that could prove serious. In other words, giving an antibody permits an immediate immune response, whereas giving an antigen would require time to produce antibodies and a later response against illness. Several drugs discussed in this chapter are used to affect immune system recognition or reaction to nonself proteins.

PATHOPHYSIOLOGY

Pathophysiologic conditions requiring drug therapy with immune modulators are varied and are related to a dysfunction in any part of the immune response. Four abnormal conditions can weaken the immune system and stimulate the immune response: neoplasms, viral invasion, autoimmune disease, and transplant rejection. Neoplasms result from the growth of mutant cells that escape the normal surveillance of the immune system. Viral invasion of a cell changes the cell's membrane and antigenic presentation. In autoimmune disease, the body responds to specific self-antigens by producing antibodies against self-cells (autoantibodies). Organ transplantation weakens the immune system as the body reacts to the introduction of foreign cells. Three types of biotherapy agents are used to combat immune dysfunction: cytokines, antibodies, and immune modulators. Table 34.1 provides a summary of selected biotherapy agents that affect the biologic response to immune dysfunction.

C CYTOKINES

Cytokines are chemical mediators released by WBCs in response to antigenic invasion of the blood or tissues. Cytokines serve to enhance and accelerate the inflammatory and specific responses that will destroy the invading antigen. Cytokines are generally proinflammatory, but many also have antiviral,

TABLE 34.1 Summary of Selected Biotherapy Agents

Drug (Trade) Name	Selected Indications	Route and Dosage Range	Pharmacokinetics
(C) Cytokines			
[P] interferon alfa-2a (Roferon-A)	Hairy cell leukemia in patients >18 years, AIDS-related Kaposi sarcoma (KS), chronic myelogenous leukemia (CML)	Hairy cell leukemia: *Adult:* IM/SC, 3 million IU/d for 16–24 wk, then 3 million IU three times/wk AIDS-related KS: IM/SC, 36 million IU/d for 10–12 wk, then 36 million IU 3 times/wk CML: IM/SC, 1 million IU/d *Child for any disorder:* safety and efficacy not established	*Onset:* IM, rapid; PO, slow *Duration:* Unknown $t_{1/2}$: 3.7–8.5 h
interferon alfa-2b (Intron A)	Hairy cell leukemia, intralesional treatment of Condylomata acuminata, AIDS-related KS, malignant melanoma (adjuvant therapy with interleukin-2, or alone for localized disease), chronic hepatitis (non A/ non-B/C)	Hairy cell leukemia: IM/SC, 2 million units/m^2 3 times/wk Condylomata acuminata: intralesionally 1 million IU/lesion 3 times/wk AIDS-related KS: IM/SC, 30 million IU/m^2 3 times/wk Malignant melanoma: IV, 20 million IU/m^2 for 4 wk, maintenance 10 million IU/m^2 3 times/wk for 48 wk Chronic hepatitis: IM/SC, 3 million IU/m^2 3 times/wk *Child for any disorder:* Safety and efficacy not established	*Onset:* IM/SC/IV rapid *Duration:* IM/SC 3–12 hr, IV end of infusion $t_{1/2}$: 2–3 h
interferon beta-1b (Betaseron)	Decrease exacerbations in relapsing or remitting multiple sclerosis (MS)	*Adult:* SC, 0.25 mg qod, discontinue if disease is unremitting longer than 6 mo *Child for any disorder:* Safety and efficacy not established	*Onset:* Slow *Duration:* Hours $t_{1/2}$: 8 min–4.3 h
IL-2	Metastatic renal cell carcinoma or malignant melanoma; adjuvant therapy with IFN alfa-2a for high risk of recurrence malignant melanoma	Metastatic renal cell and malignant melanoma: *Adult:* IV, short infusion 600,000 IU/kg every 8 h for a total of 14 doses, separated into two 5-d cycles with 9-d rest between *Child:* Safety and efficacy not established	*Onset:* 5 minutes *Duration:* 180–240 min $t_{1/2}$: 85 min
(C) Monoclonal Antibodies			
[P] rituximab (Rituxan)	Relapsed or refractory low grade or follicular CD20-positive B-cell non-Hodgkin lymphoma	*Adult:* IV, 375 mg/m^2 once weekly for four doses *Child:* Safety and efficacy not established	*Onset:* Unknown *Duration:* 3–6 mo after completion of treatment $t_{1/2}$: 59.8 h after first dose, and 174 h after fourth dose
muromonab cd3 (Orthoclone OKT3)	Acute allograft rejection in renal transplantation, steroid-resistant acute allograft rejection in liver lung, cardiac, and bone marrow transplantation	*Adult:* IV (bolus only; <1 minute), 5 mg/d with diagnosed rejection *Child:* Safety and efficacy not established	*Onset:* Minutes *Duration:* 7 d $t_{1/2}$: 47–100 h

(continued)

TABLE 34.1 Summary of Selected Biotherapy Agents (continued)

Drug (Trade) Name	Selected Indications	Route and Dosage Range	Pharmacokinetics
C Immune Modulators			
P cyclosporine (Sandimmune IV and oral Neoral oral)	Prophylaxis of organ rejection in kidney, liver, heart, and bone marrow transplantation; solid organ transplantation regimen is concomitant with that of corticosteroids	*Adult and child:* PO, 15 mg/kg/d initially within 4–12 wk of transplantation, continued for 1–2 wk then tapered by 5% wk to maintenance level of 5–10 mg/kg/d; IV ⅓ of PO dose given 4–12 h before transplantation and infused over 2–6 hr; switch to PO form as soon as possible	*Onset:* PO, varies; IV, rapid *Duration:* 24–36 h $t_{1/2}$: 17.9 h
all-transretinoic acid (ATRA, Tretinoin, Vestanoid)	Induction therapy for acute promyelocytic leukemia; topical therapy for acne vulgaris, used investigationally for other skin disorders	Promyelocytic leukemia: *Adult:* PO, 45–60 mg/m² d in evenly divided doses bid to be continued for 30–90 d until complete remission is achieved Acne vulgaris: Topical cream (0.1%, 0.05%, 0.025%), gel (0.025%, 0.01%) or liquid (0.05%) applied once daily at bedtime to areas of skin where acne 1 form lesions appear	*Onset:* 1–2 h *Duration:* Approximately 2–3 wk $t_{1/2}$: 0.5–2 h
levamisole (Ergamisol)	Adjunct to fluorouracil for adjuvant postoperative treatment in surgically resected colorectal carcinoma, or with metastatic disease	*Adult:* PO, 50 mg 98 h for 3 d in conjunction with fluorouracil 450 mg/m²/d for 5 d starting 7–30 d after surgery, or when presenting for treatment, maintenance dose is the same, but given every 2 wk during 1x/wk FU therapy	*Onset:* Varies *Duration:* Unknown $t_{1/2}$: 3–4 h
azathioprine (Imuran)	Adjunct therapy with corticosteroids or cyclosporine for prevention of allograft rejection in renal, heart, and lung transplantation	Transplantation: *Adult and child:* PO/IV, 3–5 mg/kg as a single dose on the day of organ transplantation; PO maintenance, 1–2 mg/kg/d Rheumatoid arthritis: *Adult:* PO, 1 mg/kg/d as a single or double dose; may be increased to 2.5 mg/kg/d	*Onset:* PO, varies; IV, immediate *Duration:* 6–8 h $t_{1/2}$: 5 h

antiproliferative, and antineoplastic properties. Interferons and interleukins are cytokines produced by activated lymphocytes. The prototype is interferon alfa-2a (Roferon-A). Drugs in the same class as interferon alfa-2a include interferon alfa-2b, interferon alfa-n3, interferon-n1, interferon alfacon-1, interferon beta-1a, and interferon beta-1b. A drug that is significantly different from interferon alfa-2a is aldesleukin (also known as IL-2). One must recognize that these cytokines have considerable differences from the prototype in both actions and adverse effects.

The interferons available for pharmacologic use are produced by recombinant DNA technology from harvested human or animal WBCs. As stated, the prototype is interferon alfa-2a, produced by recombinant DNA technology using *Escherichia coli* bacteria.

NURSING MANAGEMENT OF THE PATIENT RECEIVING P INTERFERON ALFA-2A

Core Drug Knowledge

Pharmacotherapeutics

Interferon alfa-2a is licensed to treat hairy cell leukemia in selected patients 18 years and older, acquired immunodeficiency syndrome (AIDS)-related Kaposi sarcoma in selected patients 18 years and older, chronic myelogenous leukemia in chronic-phase Philadelphia chromosome–positive patients, and metastatic renal cell carcinoma, and it is used as adjuvant therapy after resection of high-risk malignant melanoma or

in patients with metastatic malignant melanoma. Substantial antineoplastic activity has been noted when this agent has been used to treat superficial bladder cancer, carcinoid tumors, cutaneous T-cell lymphoma, and low-grade non-Hodgkin lymphoma (see Table 34.1). It has also been widely used to treat select viral diseases such as hepatitis C, condylomata acuminata, cutaneous warts, and cytomegalovirus. It is normally administered subcutaneously or intramuscularly, although intravenous administration is preferred in some regimens.

Pharmacokinetics

Interferon alfa-2a must be given by injection. If given intramuscularly, it is absorbed rapidly with peak effects in 3.8 hours; if given subcutaneously, absorption is slower, with peak effects in 7.3 hours. Intravenous infusion may be intermittent or continuous. The drug is metabolized in the liver and kidneys with a half-life of 3.7 hours to 8.5 hours. Direct lesional injection or instillation (as in the bladder) is indicated for some disorders. Interferon alfa-2a crosses the placenta and may be secreted in breast milk. It is excreted in the urine.

Pharmacodynamics

Interferon alfa-2a inhibits the growth of tumor cells, prevents these cells from multiplying, and modulates the host immune response to help protect the body from tumor cells. It blocks specific viral infection by preventing viral replication in the body.

Contraindications and Precautions

Interferon alfa-2a is an FDA pregnancy category C drug, so its use during pregnancy may be risky to the fetus. It should also be avoided during lactation and in patients with known allergies to interferon or its components. Caution should be used when administering the drug to patients with pancreatitis, hepatic or renal disease, depressed bone marrow function, cardiac disease or a history of cardiac disease, or compromised central nervous system (CNS) function.

Adverse Effects

The most common adverse effects of interferon alfa-2a are dizziness, confusion, lethargy, flu-like symptoms, anorexia, nausea, and changes in taste. Depression, anxiety, and suicidal ideation have been reported in a substantial number of cases. Disease processes that exacerbate these symptoms warrant careful monitoring. Hypothyroidism may occur in up to 10% of the patients treated with interferon alfa-2a. Long-term therapy increases the risk for this complication. Other adverse effects include hypotension or hypertension, edema, arrhythmias, depression of bone marrow function, increased liver enzymes, rash, dry skin, and partial alopecia.

Drug Interactions

An increased risk for theophylline toxicity occurs when theophylline is administered concomitantly with interferon alfa-2a. This effect is caused by a decrease in theophylline clearance through the liver. Monitor patients to evaluate theophylline levels and adjust their theophylline dosages appropriately. Interferon alfa-2a can also cause increased effects and toxicity when combined with other neurotoxic, hematotoxic, and cardiotoxic drugs. Neurologic and hematologic toxicity has been particularly problematic for patients with human immunodeficiency virus (HIV) receiving concomitant antiretroviral therapy. Renal toxicity is more likely if interferon alfa-2a is given with IL-2 than if either is given alone. Anyone receiving drugs with overlapping toxicities must be carefully monitored. Table 34.2 lists drugs that interact with interferon alfa-2a.

Assessment of Relevant Core Patient Variables

Health Status

Before administering interferon alfa-2a, review the patient's record to see whether the drug is contraindicated. Cardiovascular, pulmonary, and neurologic disorders may escalate the adverse effects of this agent. Glucose intolerance is a common effect of interferon alfa therapies, and patients with diabetes mellitus are at particular risk for hyperglycemic crises. Assess and monitor patients with borderline thyroid function carefully for potential hypothyroidism. Perform a complete physical examination to establish a baseline for monitoring therapy. Next, record the patient's weight, temperature, skin condition, orientation, reflexes, pulse, and blood pressure. Because bone marrow depression and liver damage can be very serious, obtain a complete blood count (CBC) and hepatic profile at least monthly during therapy.

Life Span and Gender

Determine whether the patient is pregnant or lactating because interferon alfa-2a is a pregnancy category C drug and the drug enters breast milk. Assess the age of the patient because the drug is not approved for patients who are younger than 18 years.

TABLE 34.2 Agents That Interact With P Interferon Alfa-2a

Interactants	Effect and Significance	Nursing Management
theophylline/ aminophylline	Decreased theophylline clearance in patients with hepatitis. This may raise theophylline levels	Monitor theophylline levels. If they increase significantly, dosage adjustments may be required.
cimetidine	May amplify the effects of interferon when used in treating melanoma; significance unknown	Monitor effects of interferon.
vinblastine	Enhances interferon toxicity in some patients	Monitor for adverse effects of interferon.

Lifestyle, Diet, and Habits

Assess whether the patient consumes alcohol or other unprescribed mood-altering drugs that might increase the neurotoxicities of this agent.

Environment

Be aware of the environment in which the drug will be administered. Interferon alfa-2a may be given at home or in a clinic. If it is given at home, the patient needs a refrigerator so that the reconstituted drug can be stored. Explore with the patient any factors in the home setting that may affect adherence to drug therapy.

Nursing Diagnoses and Outcomes

- Risk for Infection related to possible suppression of bone marrow function, injections
  Desired outcome: *The patient will be protected from exposure to infection and will remain infection free.*
- Altered Nutrition: Less than Body Requirements related to GI effects and flu-like symptoms
  Desired outcome: *The patient will maintain nutritional status.*
- Risk for Injury related to CNS changes from drug therapy
  Desired outcome: *The patient will not sustain injury while on drug therapy.*
- Potential for Maladaptive Coping related to fatigue, mental status changes from medication
  Desired outcome: *Patient shows effective coping strategies and acceptance of therapy independently or with the assistance of mental health professionals.*
- Activity Intolerance attributed to treatment-related fatigue, flu-like syndrome
  Desired outcome: *Activity intolerance is mediated, and no therapy break is required.*

FOCUS ON RESEARCH

Box 34.1 Fatigue and Biologic Modifying Therapy

Fu, M. R., Anderson, C. M., McDaniel R., et al. (2002). Patients' perceptions of fatigue in response to biochemotherapy for metastatic melanoma: A preliminary study. *Oncology Nursing Forum, 29*(6), 961–966.

The Study

Few recent nursing research articles have focused on the management of patients receiving biologic therapy. Fu and colleagues (2002) published a preliminary study addressing patients' perceptions of fatigue during biochemotherapy treatment for metastatic malignant melanoma. Fatigue is the most commonly reported adverse effect of biotherapy and is of great concern because it can be so intense as to constitute a dose-limiting toxicity in some patients. In therapy in which dose intensity is essential for administrating optimal biologic doses, fatigue is an important nursing concern. In this pilot study, 12 patients in a Midwestern cancer center, aged 28 to 70 years, were asked to complete a demographic form and the Revised Piper Fatigue Scale at a single time after at least 1 cycle of biochemotherapy. All patients experienced moderate to severe fatigue, some reporting that it lasted up to 12 months after treatment. Female patients reported more intense fatigue than male patients.

Nursing Implications

Although the small sample size and collection of data at a single point make this a less-than-optimal study, it clearly demonstrated that fatigue is a common and important adverse effect of biochemotherapy. Patients should be taught to anticipate this effect and plan proactive measures to minimize fatigue or the ways in which it affects their quality of life. Many previous nursing studies have demonstrated that patients who are given information about expected effects find them easier to cope with when they occur. Such knowledge could lead you to believe it is possible to abate some of the negative clinical effects of fatigue by providing targeted education.

Planning and Intervention

Maximizing Therapeutic Effects

Following the manufacturer's guidelines for reconstitution and storage increases the therapeutic effectiveness of the drug. Obtaining baseline blood counts and chemistries before therapy and at least monthly during therapy helps direct therapy and ensures accurate dosage and treatment guidelines. Other nonpharmacologic strategies, such as adequate sleep and proper nutrition, may assist patients in coping with therapy and enhance their immunologic function.

Minimizing Adverse Effects

Most clinical experts recommend premedicating patients with drugs such as acetaminophen or diphenhydramine to reduce the flu-like adverse effects and administering interferon injections in the late evening to allow patients to sleep through most of the adverse effects. Encourage the patient to rest if he or she is experiencing fatigue with drug therapy (Box 34.1). Observe how the patient and family members use sterile technique, perform the injection, and rotate injection sites. Advise the patient to avoid crowds and people with known infections and to wash and treat injuries immediately to prevent infection. Warn the patient that interferon alfa-2a can cause confusion and dizziness, making falls and injury a risk. Consequently, stress the need for adequate lighting, bedside rails, assistance with walking, and avoidance of dangerous activities and driving. Severe GI effects may warrant a nutritional consultation, and small, frequent meals or nutritional supplements may be prescribed.

Providing Patient and Family Education

- Explain that interferon alfa-2a inhibits the growth of tumor cells.
- Teach the patient or a family member how to reconstitute the powder into a solution and to date and refrigerate the reconstituted solution.
- For maximum therapeutic effects, advise the patient to use reconstituted solution within 30 days and to mark drug days on the calendar so that the drug is taken when prescribed.
- Teach the patient and family how to administer the drug, use sterile technique, and rotate injection sites. Review injection technique periodically to ensure effectiveness and decrease adverse effects.
- Advise any women of childbearing age to whom this drug is prescribed to use barrier contraception to avoid pregnancy.
- Because hypotension can occur for several days after drug administration, advise patients to slowly move from a sit-

ting to standing position and to avoid operating machinery or driving while adjusting to the therapy's adverse effects.
- Teach patients to avoid infection and injury, maintain good nutrition, get regular blood tests and medical follow-up care, and watch for adverse effects.
- Emphasize the importance of calling the prescriber if fever, chills, sore throat, unusual bleeding or bruising, chest pain, palpitations, or changes in mental status occur.

Ongoing Assessment and Evaluation

Monitor the patient's CBC and white cell differential and liver and renal function before therapy and at least monthly during therapy to gauge the drug's effectiveness and to check for adverse effects.

Drug Significantly Different From [P] Interferon Alfa-2a

Interleukins are cytokines produced by T cells to communicate between WBCs. Aldesleukin (Proleukin) is approved for treating metastatic renal cell carcinoma and metastatic malignant melanoma, although many additional indications are emerging. The agent's immunostimulatory effects have been useful to stabilize helper T-cell counts in HIV disease and for bone marrow engraftment protection after bone marrow transplantation, and its antiviral effects have been promising in treating hepatitis.

This agent has been administered subcutaneously, intravenously, and intralesionally. It is paradoxically more potent when given by continuous infusion than by bolus injections, and the adverse effect profile is widely variable because of dose ranges from 20,000 IU daily after bone marrow transplantation to 72,000,000 IU daily for treating metastatic renal cell carcinoma. The drug may be contraindicated in lactating patients, those with known allergies to aldesleukin, those with an abnormal thallium stress test or abnormal pulmonary function tests, and those with organ homografts. Aldesleukin should be used cautiously in patients with renal, liver, or CNS impairment. Its adverse effect profile is very similar to that of high-dose interferon, but effects are potentially more acute in onset and severe in intensity. Even severe adverse effects resolve when the agent is discontinued, although hepatic, endocrine, and neurologic effects can persist for months after the conclusion of therapy. Concomitant administration of corticosteroids is not recommended based on preclinical data suggesting that steroids may abrogate the immunostimulatory effects of this agent (Cuaron & Thompson, 2001).

CRITICAL THINKING SCENARIO

Interferon Alfa-2a in hairy cell leukemia

Marla Barker, age 68, planned to spend her retirement years traveling, visiting her children and grandchildren, and playing golf. But 4 months ago, she was diagnosed with hairy cell leukemia. She was immediately started on interferon alfa-2a therapy. According to blood tests, the therapy is effective and her CBC is acceptable. When Mrs. Barker talks with you about treatment options, she reports that she feels depressed about her illness and fearful that she will never be able to travel or see her daughter get married next month. She also complains of stomatitis, exhaustion, anorexia, and continuing weight loss.

1. Consider the emotional and medical issues involved with this patient. Can she achieve emotional balance and a satisfactory quality of life within the limits set by her disease and drug therapy?
2. What restrictions on activity are imposed by interferon alfa-2a therapy? What special environmental needs will Mrs. Barker have when traveling?

MEMORY CHIP

[P] Interferon Alfa-2a

- Inhibits growth of tumor cells, prevents their multiplication, and heightens the host immune response to help protect the body from tumor cells. Blocks specifically viral infection by preventing viral replication
- Used to treat some types of leukemia, AIDS-related Kaposi sarcoma, and various cancers
- Most common adverse effects: dizziness, confusion, lethargy, flu-like symptoms, anorexia, nausea, and altered taste
- Most serious adverse effects: depression and suicidal ideation
- **Life span alert: Usually avoided during pregnancy and breast feeding**
- Maximizing therapeutic effects: Reconstitute and store following manufacturers' instructions.
- Minimizing adverse effects: Premedicate patient with other drugs to reduce the flu-like adverse effects.
- Most important patient education: Teach patients about the importance of avoiding infection.

C ANTIBODIES

The earliest antibody preparations were general agents directed toward destruction of lymphoid cells (antilymphocyte globulins). They were derived from animals (horses and rabbits) that were injected with human thymocytes (the thymus gland is the source of T cells in humans) and RBCs; the injections stimulated the animal to produce nonspecific immunoglobulin G (IgG) antibodies. The most common preparations were equine antithymocyte globulin (ATG, Atgam), antilymphocyte globulin (ALG), and antilymphocyte serum (ALS). These polyclonal antibodies are so named because they react to more than one antigen. The term antilymphocyte immunoglobulin (ALG; lymphocyte immune globulin) implies a product raised against all lymphocytes, and antithymocyte immunoglobulin (antithymocyte gammaglobulin; antithymocyte globulin; ATG) implies specificity for T cells. Despite what appear to be substantial differences in levels of immune suppression, in clinical practice, these agents show few differences in action. These agents have historically been administered to graft recipients, so that the foreign antibodies directly attack the host's T cells and reduce their circulating number.

Because these agents are derived from nonhuman sources, they have caused the production of atypical antibodies, and

individuals easily become resistant to their beneficial effects. Because of production shortages, difficulties in purification, and scientific advances in specific antibody development, these agents are now rarely used. Instead, targeted antibodies called monoclonal antibodies are used, which suppress one cell subtype or receptor site. Monoclonal antibodies can react with specific tumor receptor sites for diagnosis or treatment of malignancy. As the body of knowledge regarding specific cellular defects with particular diseases grows, so does our ability to develop cell-targeted antibody therapy for abnormal cells, genes, or receptor sites. Several agents are in human clinical trials at the time of this publication.

Antibody therapy has rapidly progressed in recent years, with increasingly greater specificity of the newly developed agents. Monoclonal antibodies target specific receptor sites of cells, causing varied immunologic effects depending on the cell to which they attach themselves. Monoclonal antibodies may be created from animal antibodies (almost always murine fused), animal-human antibodies (chimeric), or totally humanized antibodies. The nonhumanized antibodies produce more allergic and rejection reactions, caused by human antimurine antibodies (HAMA), which can contraindicate future therapy with a specific monoclonal antibody or any other with a murine component. These antibody responses manifest as allergic or anaphylactic reactions in patients receiving the antibody product. Polyclonal antibodies have a more global action that primarily affects T-lymphocyte recognition of foreign proteins. Because of the rapidly developing practice of using antibodies to target tumor cell receptor sites, the antibody prototype is a monoclonal antitumor antibody called rituximab (Rituxan). Monoclonal antibodies available for use as immunosuppressants are considered significantly different from the prototype, as are the monoclonal antibodies fused to radioactive substances or antineoplastic medications. All antibodies can produce allergic reactions, and most administration guidelines suggest premedicating the patient with acetaminophen and diphenhydramine and having emergency equipment, corticosteroids, and adrenaline readily available. All antibody products also carry the risk for cross-reactivity with other vaccine products, necessitating careful consideration before administering any other antibody or vaccine to these patients after monoclonal antibody therapy.

NURSING MANAGEMENT OF THE PATIENT RECEIVING P RITUXIMAB

Core Drug Knowledge

Pharmacotherapeutics

This agent is used to treat relapsed or refractory low-grade or follicular CD20-positive B-cell non-Hodgkin lymphoma. New applications for other tumors expressing the CD20-positive receptor have led to studies using rituximab to treat chronic leukemia, multiple myeloma, post-transplantation lymphoproliferative disorder, solid organ transplantation, and a variety of autoimmune diseases (Grillo-Lopez, 2003).

Pharmacokinetics

Rituximab is given as a slow IV infusion at 375 mg/m^2 weekly for 4 to 8 weeks, with a possible additional 4 weeks for responsive patients. The serum half-life is 59.8 hours after the first infusion (375 mg/m^2) and 174 hours after the fourth infusion, although the drug is detectable for 3 to 6 months after treatment is completed. The actual drug infusion is calculated based on the total dose the patient is to receive, not exceeding 50 mg/hour for the first half-hour of the initial infusion. If no reactions are apparent after 30 minutes, the dose may be escalated every 30 minutes by 50 mg/hour until a maximum infusion rate of 400 mg/hour is reached. All subsequent infusions begin at 100 mg/hour and can be escalated by 100-mg/hour increments every 30 minutes until the maximum infusion rate of 400 mg/hour is reached.

Pharmacodynamics

Rituximab is a type of monoclonal antibody that binds specifically to the CD20 antigen found on the surface of normal and malignant B lymphocytes and causes cell lysis. The CD20 antigen is expressed in more than 90% of B-cell non-Hodgkin lymphoma cells but not on normal bone marrow cells, pre-B cells, or other normal tissues. One section of the drug binds to CD20 antigen and another section of the drug calls other immune activators to assist in cell lysis. Cell lysis is possibly caused by complement-dependent cytotoxicity or antibody-dependent cytotoxicity. Decreased IgG and IgM serum levels are evident for 5 to 11 months after the last infusion.

Contraindications and Precautions

The only contraindication to rituximab therapy is type 1 hypersensitivity or anaphylaxis to murine proteins or any components of the product. Safety in children or in pregnant or lactating women has not been tested. Experience with older adults is limited; rituximab use must be carefully monitored in those patients.

Adverse Effects

Infusion-related effects occur in 80% of patients within 30 minutes to 2 hours after beginning the first rituximab infusion, although only 7% have severe reactions. Although response is less common with subsequent infusions (40%), its severity is unchanged. Reactions may be related to dose because most of the reaction dissipates when the infusion rate is slowed or interrupted. The most common infusion-related reactions include fever, flushing, chills, and rigors. Other reported symptoms include nausea, urticaria, fatigue, headache, pruritus, bronchospasm, dyspnea, hypotension, angioedema, dyspnea, rhinitis, vomiting, flushing, pain at disease sites, and throat swelling. Respiratory distress and hypotension are reportedly more common when tumors are larger than 10 cm (Wilkes et al., 1999). As much as 16% of patients experience asthenia on retreatment. Other possible effects include tachycardia, arrhythmias, anorexia, peripheral edema, dizziness, and depression. Bone marrow effects such as leukopenia, thrombocytopenia, and anemia can be present for up to 30 days after the last dose.

About 1% of patients will develop antibodies to human antimurine or chimeric antibodies, producing severe aller-

gic reactions and limiting their future treatment with any antibody.

Drug Interactions

Concomitant vaccines of any type are not recommended because of theorized potential interactions; no research has been done on these potential interactions.

Assessment of Relevant Core Patient Variables

Health Status

Assess for pre-existing cardiac and respiratory problems. Rituximab should be used cautiously in patients with pre-existing cardiac conditions such as arrhythmias or coronary artery disease because ventricular tachycardia, supraventricular tachycardia, angina, hypotension, and hypertension are common adverse effects. Patients with pre-existing pulmonary conditions may also experience exacerbated symptoms, particularly if the patient's tumor burden is larger than 10 cm.

Assess for other concurrent drug therapy use before giving rituximab. Rituximab has such potential for infusion reactions that concomitantly administering other agents that may cause severe allergic or anaphylactic reactions should be avoided during infusion and within 2 hours before or after infusion. Agents to avoid include amphotericin, blood products, or first doses of antibiotics.

Life Span and Gender

Consider the patient's age. This agent is not recommended for use in children or in pregnant or lactating women. Experience with elderly patients is limited; thus, careful evaluation for contraindications is strongly recommended before starting therapy with this agent.

Environment

Be aware of the environment in which rituximab will be administered. Rituximab is usually given in the ambulatory care oncology clinic, although patients with specific risk factors for cardiac or pulmonary adverse effects may be admitted to the hospital for the first dose.

Nursing Diagnoses and Outcomes

- Altered Comfort related to fever, chills, or headache
  Desired outcome: *Symptoms will be abrogated with premedications or relieved with mild analgesics or antipyretics.*
- Potential Altered Cardiac Output related to drug infusion
  Desired outcome: *Cardiac symptoms will not occur.*
- Potential Alteration in Nutrition (fluids and electrolytes) because of cytotoxicity and tumor lysis syndrome
  Desired outcome: *Normal fluid and electrolyte balance will be maintained throughout the treatment period.*
- Potential Impaired Oxygenation caused by infusion-related adverse effects
  Desired outcome: *The patient will maintain normal a breathing pattern, oxygen saturation will be adequate, and adventitious breath sounds will be absent.*

Planning and Intervention

Maximizing Therapeutic Effects

Mix rituximab in normal saline or dextrose solutions within a plastic bag, not in glass. The antibody sticks to glass, diminishing the amount of drug administered.

Minimizing Adverse Effects

Because infusion-related adverse effects are common, many clinicians administer premedications to reduce their severity. Premedications often include antipyretics (e.g., acetaminophen) and antihistamines (e.g., diphenhydramine and ranitidine). If patients experience infusion-related adverse effects, stop rituximab until symptoms resolve, then restart it at half the dose that produced adverse effects. Subsequent infusions should begin slowly and can be escalated in the same manner, with temporary discontinuation if infusion effects reoccur. Patients are usually observed in the ambulatory area for several hours after the initial dose.

For patients with hypertension, all antihypertensive agents are usually held for 12 hours before rituximab administration and for 12 to 24 hours afterward. Patients with cardiac or pulmonary risk factors should have continuous cardiac monitoring and frequent vital sign assessment. Stop the infusion at the first sign of adverse effects, which may worsen before resolving. To reduce the risk for recurrence, medications such as nitrates or magnesium can be administered. After symptoms have resolved, resume the infusion at a slower infusion rate, with continuous monitoring.

Providing Patient and Family Education

- Teach the patient and family about the purpose of the drug and common adverse effects. Instruct patients to notify the prescriber if they begin to experience adverse effects.
- Assure patients that they will be closely monitored while receiving rituximab. Doing so may require prolonged visits in the clinic, even after the infusion is complete, or frequent follow-up visits after initial therapy to permit monitoring clinical and laboratory parameters for tumor lysis syndrome.
- Because immunologic effects persist for many weeks or months, instruct patients to use birth control for 12 months after completing treatment and to avoid breast-feeding for the same amount of time.

Ongoing Assessment and Evaluation

Given the high rate of infusion reactions after the first dose, patients require premedication and close monitoring of vital signs for all rituximab infusions, unless no reactions have occurred.

Drugs Closely Related to P Rituximab

Trastuzumab (Herceptin)

Trastuzumab is a humanized monoclonal antibody that targets cells overexpressing the HER2 protein. This protein is overexpressed in as many as 25% to 30% of breast cancers (Slamon et al., 2001). Patients are tested at the time of diagnosis or disease recurrence for amplification of HER2/neu

MEMORY CHIP

P Rituximab

- Binds specifically to CD20 antigen on the surface of malignant B lymphocytes and causes cell lysis.
- Used in non-Hodgkin lymphoma
- Most common adverse effects: infusion-related effects (fever, flushing, chills, and rigors)
- Most serious adverse effects: respiratory distress and hypotension (more common when tumors are larger than 10 cm)
- **Life span alert: Use birth control during therapy and for 1 year afterward and avoid breast-feeding during this time; use with caution in older adults.**
- Maximizing therapeutic effects: Administer in saline or dextrose stored in plastic bags, not glass.
- Minimizing adverse effects: Premedicate patient with other drug therapies.
- Most important patient education: Instruct patient to notify nurse of adverse effects.

or p185-HER2 protein. Patients whose breast cancer cells overexpress either protein then are clinically evaluated for eligibility based on their ability to tolerate the expected adverse effects. A focused cardiopulmonary physical examination in addition to a test of cardiac function (echocardiogram [ECG] or MUGA scan) screens patients for adequate cardiovascular reserve or for lung diseases that predispose the patient to adverse effects. Patients treated previously or concurrently with anthracyclines (e.g., doxorubicin, epirubicin), cyclophosphamide, or radiation to the chest have enhanced risk for the most common cardiac toxicity—congestive heart failure. Congestive heart failure with or without persistent cardiomyopathy occurs most commonly as reversible congestive heart failure that occurs hours to days after a dose of trastuzumab. Although usually self-limiting, it is a relative indication for discontinuing trastuzumab therapy, especially if independent risk factors such as older age, heavy pretreatment anthracyclines, or chest irradiation are present. Pulmonary toxicity may overlap with cardiac symptoms, making it difficult to tell which is which. Infusion-related allergic reactions and cases of acute lung injury have been known to occur. Taxanes have also been reported to increase serum blood levels of trastuzumab that may enhance toxicities. Other clinical effects include suppression of bone marrow function (especially anemia and leukopenia), diarrhea, and rare nephrotic syndrome or acute pneumonitis/respiratory distress syndrome. Trastuzumab is administered as an initial loading dose of 4 mg/kg over 90 minutes, with subsequent weekly doses of 2 mg/kg over 30 minutes. The clinical benefit of prolonged therapy (beyond planned chemotherapy dosing) is currently being studied to ascertain whether disease-free survival can be extended because patients who overexpress the her2 protein have a high risk for relapse (Horton, 2002).

Cetuximab

Cetuximab (Erbitux) is a chimeric monoclonal antibody, licensed early in 2004, that targets the epidermal growth factor receptor (EGRF) site of both malignant and normal tissues. Competitive binding of this site with this MoAb can deprive cells of cytokines and ligands that are necessary for cellular growth and metabolism. Certain tumor cells overexpress this receptor, often connoting a poorer prognosis, and are more reliant on activation of this receptor, thus making them prone to apoptosis when the receptor is blocked. The FDA has approved this agent to treat colorectal cancer refractory to irinotecan for antitumor response rates of about 10%, although EGRF is also overexpressed in gastric, head and neck, lung, and pancreatic malignancies. Patients must overexpress the EGRF receptor and have immunohistochemistry testing in order to be eligible to receive this agent. It is administered as a 2-hour loading dose of 400 mg/m^2, followed by a 1-hour weekly infusion of 250 mg/m^2, and is well tolerated by most recipients. The most common adverse effect is an acne-like rash with dry or cracking skin, and potential skin infections. A severe infusion-related reaction with bronchospasm, stridor, urticaria, and hypotension has been reported in 3% of patients. Although test dosing was reported in clinical trials, it is not part of the licensed administration procedures. Potentially fatal interstitial lung disease has been reported, but extremely infrequently. Safety of this agent in children, pregnant or lactating women, and the elderly has not been established. An in-line filter is used for administration.

Alemtuzumab (Campath 1-H)

This humanized monoclonal antibody is directed against the CD52 cell surface antigen of the lymphocytic cells of patients with B- and T-cell chronic lymphocytic leukemia. This medication is indicated in alkylating-agent or fludarabine-refractory chronic leukemias or low-grade lymphoma because many of these diseases are histopathologically difficult to differentiate from one another. It is administered as a daily 2-hour infusion with dose escalation until toxicity is reached, then therapy is begun 3 times weekly on alternate days. The first dose is 3 mg, and when this dose is tolerated with minimal toxicity, the dose is increased to 10 mg daily, until tolerated. Once 10 mg per day is tolerable, the patient is given the planned maintenance dose of 30 mg 3 times a week for a 12-week course. The most common adverse effects are related to lymphopenia and infections associated with suppressed lymphocytes (e.g., *Pneumocystis carinii* or cytomegalovirus). Other bone marrow components may also be suppressed, and infusion-related allergic reactions may also occur. Lymphocyte counts can be monitored weekly to determine the need to discontinue therapy early, and many patients receive antimicrobial prophylaxis against viruses (acyclovir) or *Pneumocystis* species (e.g., sulfamethoxazole-trimethoprim).

Abciximab

Abciximab (ReoPro) is a monoclonal antibody and is actually a fragment called the Fab fragment. Unlike the prototype, rituximab, it does not have an antitumor function. It binds to a glycoprotein receptor on human platelets and inhibits their aggregation, leading to reduced hemostasis. The circulating half-life after IV bolus injection is 30 minutes, although clinical effects are evident for about 48 hours. In some patients, antiplatelet activity persists for up to 10 days. Many patients receive a 6- to 12-hour continuous IV infusion after the initial bolus to maintain optimal antiplatelet activity. This agent is used with a number of cardiovascular conditions, such as

ischemic heart disease, or after percutaneous coronary interventions in which antiplatelet activity is desired. It is administered as an IV infusion before planned procedures or at the onset of unstable angina. It may be contraindicated in patients with a recent history of stroke, major surgery or trauma, GI or genitourinary bleeding, vascular deformities, or uncontrolled hypertension. The primary adverse effect associated with abciximab is increased risk for bleeding.

Palivizumab

Palivizumab (Synagis) is a monoclonal antibody like rituximab; unlike rituximab, it has a unique function. This monoclonal antibody has been developed by recombinant DNA technology to be directly cytotoxic to the respiratory syncytial virus (RSV), reducing the number of viral organisms in the lower respiratory tract. It is administered as prophylaxis in neonates at high risk for developing life-threatening pulmonary disease if infected with RSV (e.g., premature infants, children with cystic fibrosis). Its use in treating confirmed RSV infection has not been established. It is contraindicated in adults in whom serious illness with RSV infection has not been documented. It is administered as a monthly IM injection given fall through spring and has a half-life of 18 to 20 days. The reconstituted drug does not contain a preservative and should be administered within 6 hours of reconstitution. Common adverse effects include infection with other organisms, worsening respiratory symptoms, GI upset, hepatic dysfunction, injection site erythema, and flu-like syndrome. The serum blood levels of alanine aminotransferase and aspartate transaminase may be elevated as a consequence of treatment with this agent.

Drugs Significantly Different From P Rituximab

Monoclonal antibodies significantly different from rituximab include muromonab-CD3, infliximab, basiliximab, and daclizumab. These drugs are significantly different because unlike the prototype rituximab, which targets the B lymphocytes, they target T lymphocytes to produce therapeutic immune suppression.

Muromonab-CD3

Muromonab-CD3 (Orthoclone OKT3) is used to prevent allograft rejection in patients who have undergone renal transplantation and to treat steroid-resistant acute allograft rejection in heart and liver transplants. Muromonab-CD3 is a murine monoclonal antibody to the T3 complex of T cells. It acts on the T cell as an antigen and disables it. Muromonab-CD3 is available only for IV use.

Muromonab-CD3 is assigned to pregnancy category C. It is contraindicated in patients with known allergies to the drug or any murine product and in cases of fluid overload. It should be used cautiously in patients with fever (give antipyretics before drug administration) and in those previously on muromonab-CD3 because serious reactions can occur.

The most common adverse effects of muromonab-CD3 are nausea, vomiting, diarrhea, tremor, fever, chills, dyspnea, and chest pain. Potentially serious adverse effects include acute pulmonary edema and cytokine-release syndrome (flu-like symptoms progressing to shock).

Muromonab-CD3 combined with other immunosuppressants poses a serious risk for infection and lymphoma. To decrease this risk, the dosage of other immune suppressants should be reduced and then returned to previous levels 3 days before muromonab-CD3 treatment is finished. Encephalopathy and CNS effects are risks when muromonab-CD3 is combined with indomethacin (Indometh); therefore, this combination should be avoided.

Daclizumab

Daclizumab (Zenapax) saturates a subunit of the IL-2 receptor (Tac subunit), thus inhibiting IL-2–mediated cellular responses known to be important in allograft rejection. It is indicated as part of a three- or four-drug regimen for prophylaxis of acute organ rejection in adults receiving their first cadaveric kidney transplant. It is currently undergoing human trials for prevention and treatment of allograft rejection with other solid-organ and bone marrow transplants. It is dosed at 1 mg/kg and administered within 24 hours before transplantation, then every 14 days for a total of 5 doses. It effectively binds at the Tac subunit for as much as 120 days when the serum levels are 5 to 10 μg/mL. It has the same precautions and gender and age recommendations as basiliximab. Immunosuppression is the most important adverse effect; however, as with other immunosuppressive monoclonal antibodies, GI distress is common. Hypertension is agent specific and reported in both children and adults.

Infliximab

Infliximab (Remicade) is a monoclonal antibody, a chimeric human-murine IgG antibody that acts by blocking tumor necrosis factor (TNF). It is licensed for treating moderate to severe Crohn disease. Its safety and efficacy have not been established in children or in pregnant or lactating women, or beyond three doses. It is also licensed for use with methotrexate to treat rheumatoid arthritis in patients who do not respond to methotrexate alone. In studies with RA, more than 50% of patients achieved clinical remission, with a tolerable toxicity profile. Infliximab is administered once as a short IV infusion; in severe Crohn disease, it is readministered on a monthly basis for a total of three doses. Because of its low toxicity profile, many allogeneic bone marrow transplantation protocols have been established to evaluate the efficacy of this agent in this population. The most common adverse effect is an infusion-related allergic-type reaction that includes fever, chills, pruritus, dyspnea, chest pain, and hypotension. Skin reactions such as rash, eczema, dry skin, acne, sweating, and flushing are also common. Autoimmune antibodies that produce a lupus-like syndrome have been reported and warrant discontinuing the drug. Infliximab is incompatible with polyvinyl chloride tubing and should be mixed in glass bottles and administered through polyethylene line infusion sets.

Basiliximab

Basiliximab (Simulect) is a monoclonal antibody that is an IL-2 receptor antagonist. It acts by binding to and blocking the CD25 antigen receptor site; this site is active in the cellular immune response involved in allograft rejection. Basiliximab is licensed as part of an immunosuppressive regimen that includes cyclosporine and corticosteroids for preventing organ transplantation rejection in patients receiving renal transplantation. It is administered as an IV infusion over 20 to 30 minutes, 2 hours before transplantation surgery

and 4 days after surgery. The average duration of immunosuppressive IL-2 receptor blockade activity is 36 days. Readministration after initial therapy with basiliximab has not been studied, but excess immunosuppression or hypersensitivity reactions are projected. Pediatric patients in whom it has been used have demonstrated slower renal clearance, although no appreciable differences have been noted between adults and the elderly. This agent has not been tested with pregnant or lactating women because IL-2 is known to cross the placenta, and great risk to the fetus has been suspected. The most common adverse effects relate to the infection risk associated with the immunosuppressive regimen; however, GI symptoms such as nausea, vomiting, and diarrhea have also been common. Occasional reports of headache, tremors, insomnia, and electrolyte disorders warrant careful assessment within 48 hours of therapy.

Gemtuzumab

Gemtuzumab (Mylotarg) is also a significantly different monoclonal antibody because it is a monoclonal antibody fused with the antineoplastic agent calicheamicin targeted against CD33-positive cells commonly found in acute leukemia. It is indicated for treating CD33-positive acute myeloid leukemia in first relapse, for which no other appropriate therapies exist. Gemtuzumab is administered as a 2-hour infusion of 9 mg/m^2 that is repeated once, 14 days after the initial dose. The second dose is held if bone marrow recovery and normal hepatic function tests are not evident. The agent is light sensitive and must be given in an ultraviolet (UV)-protected bag. Premedication with acetaminophen and diphenhydramine reduces the incidence of infusion-related hypersensitivity reactions. Patients with high white blood cell counts are at greater risk for acute hypersensitivity reactions, including respiratory compromise. The postulated mechanism for this reaction is tumor-specific cytotoxicity. Nausea and vomiting within hours of the infusion are also common complaints, and most patients are given at least one loading dose of antiemetic, with a prescription for several additional doses as needed in the first 48 hours after therapy. Patients experience a rapid drop in their blood counts as early as 2 days after administration, requiring supportive care such as antimicrobial or blood component therapy. Patients may receive therapy as outpatients but need to return for frequent laboratory assessment of hematology profiles and hepatic function tests. Transient increases in bilirubin and transaminases often occur, but severe hepatotoxicity, including hepatic veno-occlusive disease, has been reported in a small number of cases. Hepatotoxicity may be detected as asymptomatic abnormalities in laboratory studies or may present with more dramatic symptoms of weight gain, right upper quadrant pain, ascites, and hepatomegaly.

The following three agents are monoclonal antibodies attached to radioactive substances that attach to tumor cells and either target them for recognition on scan or enhance tumor-specific cell lysis. All agents require special handling procedures appropriate to radiopharmaceutical use by professionals. Reasonable limitations on exposure of bodily fluids with others are advised, although all radiolabeled monoclonal antibodies emit beta rather than gamma emissions; hence, fewer precautions are necessary. Patients may be advised to wash their dishes or clothes separately, or to flush the toilet two times after use, or to use condoms for sexual relations (Hendrix, 2003). These measures are suggested to avoid exposing family members to the small amount of radioactive substance that may be emitted.

Satumomab Pendetide

Indium-111 (^{111}In) satumomab pendetide (OncoScint CR/OV) is a murine monoclonal antibody that is unlike the prototype because it is bound to indium and targets tumor-associated glycoprotein but does not have properties that initiate cell lysis. This agent is used during lymphoscintigraphy to detect microscopic extrahepatic colorectal or ovarian cancer, although tumor types (e.g., breast, non–small cell lung, esophageal, gastric, pancreatic cancers) have also shown some sensitivity to its actions. It is not indicated as a screening tool for any of these diseases. After intravenous injection, serial nuclear scans detect the distribution of this radiolabeled monoclonal antibody. It is eliminated by natural metabolic pathways, with about 10% cleared through the kidneys over approximately 56 hours, but in some cases, it can be detectable for up to 120 hours. This agent has not been studied in children or in pregnant or lactating women, and it is therefore not recommended for use in these groups. Data are limited, but no clear contraindication exists for using this agent in the elderly. Common adverse effects are similar to those for other monoclonal antibodies, but because satumomab pendetide is a murine-based product, allergic and late antibody reactions may also occur. Preparation to administer this agent includes a laxative or enema to prevent nuclear localization in stool within the colon that could interfere with interpretation of the scans performed after injection of the antibody.

Tositumomab Plus Iodine-131

Tositumomab plus ^{131}I (Bexxar) is a murine antibody directed against the CD20 antigen found on the surface of normal and malignant B lymphocytes. It is indicated to treat CD20-positive follicular non-Hodgkin lymphoma that has relapsed after chemotherapy and has been refractory to rituximab. Treatment with this radiolabeled monoclonal antibody involves a two-step plan involving a dosimetric step, in which a priming dose of 450 mg tositumomab is administered intravenously over 1 hour, followed by administration of ^{131}I tositumomab (5 millicurie [mCi] ^{131}I combined with 35 mg tositumomab) intravenously over 20 minutes. Whole body scans for biodistribution must be obtained within 1 hour of the end of infusion of ^{131}I tositumomab and before the patient voids. This process is repeated once between days 2 and 4, with scans after the patient voids, and again on day 6 to 7. These serial scans verify biodistribution of the monoclonal antibody carrier before a therapeutic dose of radiation is administered. At about the seventh day, tositumomab is again administered as a 450-mg dose, followed this time by ^{131}I and tositumomab 35 mg, designed to deliver 75 cGy of whole body radiation. Because hypothyroidism is a common clinical effect with this agent, all eligible patients must receive thyroid-blocking agents from 24 hours before the dosimetric dose until 14 days after the therapeutic dose, to protect against permanent thyroid destruction. Prolonged myelosuppression has been reported, particularly if the patient's disease involves the bone marrow. Consequently, baseline and weekly complete blood counts are monitored for bone marrow tolerance. Because most of the tositumomab plus ^{131}I is

renally cleared, serum blood urea nitrogen (BUN) and creatinine levels are checked before administration, and creatinine clearance is calculated if renal function is potentially impaired. As with other murine proteins, severe or persistent hypersensitivity reactions may occur. The safety of future vaccines and antibody therapy may be compromised in the patient who receives this drug, because of the creation of antimurine antibodies. This therapy is not recommended for children and pregnant or lactating women.

Yttrium-90 Ibritumomab Tiuxetan

^{90}Y ibritumomab tiuxetan (Zevalin) is licensed as a two-step therapy similar to tositumomab, but rituximab is used as the monoclonal antibody carrier. In the dosimetric phase, rituximab is administered as a 250 mg/m^2 dose by intravenous infusion with a graduated infusion rate, as is done routinely with this agent. Four hours after the administration of rituximab, ^{111}In ibritumomab tiuxetan is administered intravenously over 10 minutes (dose of 5 mCi [1.6 mg total antibody dose]). Imaging for biodistribution is performed within the first 2 to 24 hours, between 48 and 72 hours, and optionally between 90 and 120 hours after the infusion. Initially, it was recommended that if biodistribution is acceptable, a therapeutic infusion should be administered between days 7 and 9, with the rituximab dose unchanged, but the ^{111}In ibritumomab tiuxetan administered as 0.4 mCi/kg (14.8 megabecquerels/kg [actual body weight of ^{90}Y ibritumomab tiuxetan; maximum dose is 32 mCi, or 1184 MBq]). More recent studies have shown that the dosimetry step is unnecessary in heavily pretreated patients, and patients may safely move straight to therapeutic doses. Infusion-related reactions are prevented by administering premedications. The most common adverse reactions involve suppression of bone marrow function and its clinical effects. Infection and bleeding caused by leukopenia or thrombocytopenia are more common when the patient's disease involves the bone marrow. Patients are cautioned to implement radiation precautions for 3 days after tositumomab is administered.

C IMMUNE MODULATORS

Immune modulators appear to act directly on the function of T cells and B cells, stimulating or suppressing the immune response. Lymphocytic modulators are divided into subcategories according to their primary chemical structure and pharmacologic properties. Immune modulators may suppress or stimulate immune function. Some of these agents stimulate certain functions of the cell response and suppress others.

For this text, the immune suppressant cyclosporine (Sandimmune, Neoral) is used as the prototype. Cyclosporine is in the subclass of polypeptide antibiotics. Drugs that are also immune modulators and polypeptide antibiotics and are represented by the prototype include tacrolimus (Prograf), sirolimus (Rapamune), and mycophenolate mofetil (CellCept). Drugs that are also immune modulators but are significantly different from cyclosporine are the retinoids (all-transretinoic acid [ATRA], 9-cis-transretinoic acid, and bexarotene); levamisole; azathioprine; thalidomide; glatiramer; BCG, and denileukin diftitox (Ontak) [diphtheria toxin and IL-2]. These drugs have a variety of immunologic actions and targets, making many of them more a group of miscellaneous agents rather than members of the same category.

The polypeptide antibiotics are a group of agents that were developed as antibiotics but were determined to be too toxic to hematopoietic cells for that use. What has evolved is a group of agents that destroys cells in the G_0 or G_1 phase of cell cycling, a long phase that is common for all lymphocytes. The first drug of this class to be licensed for use was cyclosporine. Immune modulators that act as immune suppressants block the normal effects of the immune system in the body. This action is beneficial in organ transplantation, in which the body destroys foreign tissue, and in autoimmune diseases, in which the body destroys its own cells.

NURSING MANAGEMENT OF THE PATIENT RECEIVING P CYCLOSPORINE

Core Drug Knowledge

Pharmacotherapeutics

Cyclosporine (Sandimmune, Neoral) is used as an adjunct treatment to prevent rejection in solid organ transplantation and to prevent graft-versus-host disease in allogeneic bone marrow or stem cell transplants. Adjunct therapy with corticosteroids is recommended. The two brands of the drug are different, and dosage adjustment may be required for patients who switch. Other labeled uses (for the Neoral form only) include severe rheumatoid arthritis and extensive, refractory psoriasis. Unlabeled uses include treating alopecia areata, atopic dermatitis, biliary cirrhosis, Crohn disease, ulcerative colitis, dermatomyositis, Graves ophthalmopathy, lupus nephritis, multiple sclerosis, myasthenia gravis, nephrotic syndrome, pemphigus, polymyositis, and pulmonary sarcoidosis. It is used with corticosteroids to prevent rejection in kidney, liver, and heart transplantation and to treat chronic rejection in patients previously taking other immunosuppressants. The drug is being studied for use in pancreas, bone marrow, and heart and lung transplantation. Sandimmune formulations are available as soft gelatin capsules, an oral solution, and as an IV solution. The IV form should be administered at one third of the oral dose. Neoral formulations are available as soft gelatin capsules and an oral solution.

Pharmacokinetics

The absorption of cyclosporine from the GI tract is incomplete and variable; the lipid formulation has improved absorption characteristics. The absolute bioavailability of oral cyclosporine varies widely among patients. Factors that affect bioavailability include food, enterohepatic recirculation, and the type of assay used to measure levels. Ingesting conventional cyclosporine with food high in fat may increase bioavailability. Sandimmune and Neoral are not bioequivalent and cannot be exchanged one for another without dose adjustments. Sandimmune capsules and oral solution have decreased bioavailability compared with Neoral. Cyclosporine is extensively metabolized by the cytochrome P-450 enzyme system in the liver, and to a lesser degree in the GI tract and the kidneys. Many metabolites have been identified

in the bile, feces, blood, and urine. Fortunately, these metabolites contribute little to drug toxicity. Excretion is primarily biliary, with less than 6% excreted in the urine. Neither dialysis nor renal failure substantially alters cyclosporine clearance. Children often need a larger oral dose, probably because of the limited absorptive area of their intestines. Patients with malabsorption may have difficulty achieving therapeutic levels with oral use. The IV dose is not significantly related to age, body surface area, or bowel length.

Pharmacodynamics

Cyclosporine is a potent immunosuppressant that is produced as a metabolite by the fungus *Beauvaria nivea.* It suppresses some humoral immunity, but to a greater extent, it suppresses cell-mediated immune reactions. The exact mechanism of action is not known, but experimental evidence suggests that cyclosporine acts by specific, reversible inhibition of immunocompetent T lymphocytes that target their cytotoxic effects to lymphocytes in the G_0 and G_1 phases of the cell cycle. The helper T cell is the main target, but the suppressor T cell may also be suppressed. It also inhibits lymphokine production and release, including IL-2 or T-cell growth factor. Cyclosporine does not suppress bone marrow function.

Contraindications and Precautions

Cyclosporine that is injected (Sandimmune) is contraindicated in patients with hypersensitivity to polyoxyethylated castor oil. Oral cyclosporine (Neoral) should not be used concomitantly with psoralen UV A range or UV B light therapy in patients with psoriasis. It is assigned to pregnancy category C and is used during pregnancy only if the potential benefit justifies the possible risk to the fetus. It readily crosses the placenta and is secreted in breast milk.

A substantial risk for nephrotoxicity exists with this drug. A form of chronic, progressive cyclosporine-associated nephrotoxicity is characterized by deterioration in renal function and morphologic changes in the kidney, which may persist even if the drug is discontinued. Oversuppression of the immune system can increase susceptibility to infection. Hepatotoxicity is also possible. Liver and renal function tests should be monitored closely. If a severe reaction occurs, dosage should be decreased, or the drug should be discontinued.

Adverse Effects

The most common adverse effects of cyclosporine are renal dysfunction, tremor, hirsutism, hypertension, and gum hyperplasia. As mentioned previously, the dose may have to be decreased if nephrotoxicity occurs. Hepatotoxicity is also possible. The risk for malignancies in cyclosporine recipients is higher than in the healthy population but similar to that of patients receiving immunosuppressive therapies. Lymphoproliferative and skin malignancies are most commonly reported. Other, less common adverse effects primarily involve the CNS and include confusion, lethargy, headache, ataxia, blurred vision, depression, encephalopathy, and convulsions. Studies have associated these symptoms with low cholesterol, low magnesium, aluminum overload, high-dose methylprednisolone, nephrotoxicity, and hypertension. Miscellaneous adverse effects include brittle nails, pruritus, anorexia, gastritis, hiccups, mouth sores, swallowing difficulty, pancreatitis, constipation, hypomagnesemia, anemia, conjunctivitis, hearing loss, edema, tinnitus, thrombocytopenia, joint pain, night sweats, hyperkalemia, and hyperuricemia.

Drug Interactions

Concomitant use of medications that affect the hepatic microsomal enzymes (P-450 system) requires monitoring and dose adjustment of cyclosporine. Drugs that can produce nephrotoxicity have an increased risk for producing renal dysfunction when used concomitantly with cyclosporine. Administering oral cyclosporine (Neoral) within 30 minutes of consuming food, particularly a high-fat meal, may decrease levels. Patients should not take cyclosporine with grapefruit juice unless instructed to do so; trough concentrations may be increased. Table 34.3 lists drugs that interact with cyclosporine.

Assessment of Relevant Core Patient Variables

Health Status

Before administering cyclosporine, review the patient's record to see whether the drug is contraindicated. If it can be administered safely, a physical examination should be performed to establish a baseline for monitoring therapy. Assess the patient's skin color, temperature, and texture, and note the appearance of any lesions to monitor for allergic reactions and signs of rejection. Hepatic function should be reviewed because the drug is metabolized primarily by the liver. Renal function should be evaluated because nephrotoxicity is a fairly common and irreversible adverse effect of the drug. A CBC and differential should be done as a baseline for potential hematologic changes that might occur during therapy. Vital signs should be assessed because hypertension is the most common adverse effect associated with cyclosporine administration. Because the associated hypertension is believed to be vasospastic in nature, calcium channel blockers are the antihypertensive treatment of choice. Acute tremors, seizures, mental status changes, or visual disturbances are indicative of neurologic toxicities. These toxicities usually are related to high serum blood cyclosporine levels and are an indication to discontinue the medication.

Life Span and Gender

Assess whether female patients are of childbearing age because the drug is in pregnancy category C. Children may require higher doses of medications because of decreased drug absorption.

Lifestyle, Diet, and Habits

Determine whether the patient is frequently in crowds, where he or she could be exposed to infection. Assess whether the patient has a lifestyle that involves frequent sun exposure. Determine whether the patient eats a high-fat diet because doing so increases the bioavailability of one form of the drug (Sandimmune) but decreases the bioavailability of another form (Neoral).

Environment

Be aware of the environment in which cyclosporine will be given. Cyclosporine is usually started in the hospital after

TABLE 34.3 Agents That Interact With P Cyclosporine

Interactants	Effect and Significance	Nursing Management
rifampin, phenytoin, phenobarbital	Decrease plasma concentrations of cyclosporine. May decrease therapeutic effectiveness of cyclosporine	Monitor for effectiveness of cyclosporine.
azithromycin, clarithromycin, diltiazem, erythromycin, fluconazole, itraconazole, ketoconazole, nicardipine, verapamil, and grapefruit juice	Increases the concentrations of cyclosporine through altering metabolism. May increase risk of adverse effects	Monitor for adverse effects of cyclosporine.
aminoglycosides, amphotericin B acyclovir, SMZ-TMP, melphalan, ketoconazole, diclofenac, naproxen, sulindac, cimetidine, ranitidine, tacrolimus	These nephrotoxic drugs may increase cyclosporine nephrotoxicity.	Monitor for signs of nephrotoxicity; dosage adjustment may be required.
HMG-Co A reductase inhibitors (atorvastatin, cerivastatin, fluvastatin, lovastatin, simvastatin)	Increased risk of myositis, rhabdomyolysis, and acute renal failure from cyclosporine	Monitor for adverse effects carefully. The HMG-Co A reductase inhibitor may need to be stopped if serious adverse effects occur.
nifedipine	Increased risk of gingival hyperplasia.	Provide good oral hygiene to minimize risk of gingival hyperplasia.

solid organ or bone marrow transplantation and then continued at home. Explore with the patient any factors in the home setting that might affect adherence to drug therapy. For special teaching when the drug is used at home, see Box 34.2.

Nursing Diagnoses and Outcomes

- Risk for Infection related to suppression of the immune system
  Desired outcome: *The patient will be protected from exposure to infection, and infections will be prevented or decreased.*
- Altered Perfusion related to hypertension caused by the medication
  Desired outcome: *Blood pressure will remain within normal limits or be controlled to normal limits with antihypertensive medications.*
- Altered Renal Function related to nephrotoxic and hypertensive effects of the medication
  Desired outcome: *The patient will be monitored closely for deterioration in renal function, and permanent renal damage will be prevented.*
- Altered Mental Status related to neurotoxic effects of cyclosporine (tremors, seizures, mental status changes, visual defects)
  Desired outcome: *The patient will maintain normal orientation, reasoning ability, and motor activity.*
- Deficient Knowledge related to multiple drug interactions and adverse effects
  Desired outcome: *The patient will be instructed in potential drug interactions, including both prescription and over-the-counter medications. The patient will be instructed in potential adverse effects of medications and the need for close monitoring after discharge.*

COMMUNITY-BASED CONCERNS

Box 34.2 Cyclosporine at Home

Patients who receive cyclosporine at home need to have the following points emphasized in their teaching:

- This drug must be taken at the same time every day and consistently in relation to meals to maximize the immunosuppressive activity of the drug.
- Oral preparations of the two forms of cyclosporine cannot be substituted for each other without dosage adjustments. Be familiar with the form you take and check each prescription refill to make sure you have the same product.
- Oral solutions should be measured using the dosing syringe provided with the medication, not a household teaspoon or tablespoon. Do not rinse the syringe with water either before or after measuring a dose because any water that is accidentally mixed into the drug will cause a variation in the dose provided.
- To improve the flavor, the cyclosporine can be mixed with orange or apple juice (preferably at room temperature). Avoid using grapefruit juice because it interacts with the P-450 system and changes drug metabolism. Sandimmune can be mixed with milk or chocolate milk, but the combination of Neoral and milk is unpalatable.
- Use a glass container, not plastic, to prevent possible chemical interactions.
- Stir the oral solution into the diluent and drink immediately, all at once. Do not allow the drug to sit in the diluent.
- After drinking the medication and diluent, pour more of the same type of diluent into the glass to rinse it. Drink this glass also to ensure that you have received the entire dose.

Planning and Intervention

Maximizing Therapeutic Effects

Ensure that cyclosporine therapy is started soon after transplantation. Medication should be administered as prescribed and according to recommendations to ensure therapeutic drug levels. Drug levels should be appropriately monitored to ensure adequate dosing. Although cyclosporine can be given intravenously, the oral form should be used as soon as possible. It can be mixed with juice (other than grapefruit juice) to increase palatability but should not be refrigerated. Cyclosporine should not be taken with foods, particularly those that are high in fat.

Minimizing Adverse Effects

Arrange for periodic blood tests to monitor for renal, hepatic, and hematologic effects of the medication. The drug should be held, and the physician should be notified, if signs of toxicity occur. Avoid mixing the drug with grapefruit juice. The patient should be protected from exposure to infection; immediate action must be taken at the first sign of infection. Patients should be assessed for adverse effects to the CNS, and vital signs should be monitored for hypertension.

Providing Patient and Family Education

- Teach patients how to take the oral form of this agent to maximize absorption.
- Caution patients not to discontinue taking this drug without consulting with their prescribers.
- Discuss with women of childbearing age the potential adverse effects on the fetus (most commonly, premature birth).
- Teach patients receiving cyclosporine to avoid exposure to infection by avoiding crowds and to promptly report injuries or signs of infection.
- Advise patients to avoid sun exposure to decrease the risk for skin malignancies.

Ongoing Assessment and Evaluation

Cyclosporine is an agent with many drug interactions, issues of bioavailability, and considerable adverse effects. It is important to follow cyclosporine serum drug levels and have the dose adjusted appropriately to achieve maximal immune suppression without excess adverse effects.

> **MEMORY CHIP**
>
> **[P] Cyclosporine**
>
> - Immunosuppressant that inhibits T-lymphocytes by causing cytotoxicity during the G_0 and G_1 phase.
> - Used as an adjunct treatment to prevent rejection in solid organ transplantation and to prevent graft versus host disease in allogeneic bone marrow or stem cell transplants.
> - Major contraindication: hypersensitivity to polyoxyethylated castor oil
> - Most common adverse effects: renal dysfunction, tremor, hirsutism, hypertension, and gum hyperplasia.
> - Most serious adverse effects: renal toxicity and hepatic toxicity
> - **Life span alert: Children may need higher doses; therapy usually avoided during pregnancy.**
> - Maximizing therapeutic effects: Start as soon after transplantation as possible.
> - Minimizing adverse effects: Monitor blood work.
> - Most important patient education: Teach patients about the importance of preventing infection.

Drugs Significantly Different From [P] Cyclosporine

Retinoids

The retinoids are a group of naturally occurring compounds that are derivatives of preformed (dietary) vitamin A or provitamin A carotenoid. Preformed vitamin A is primarily found in food substances, and the provitamin A group involves precursors of retinol. Retinol has long been recognized for its importance in vision, growth, reproduction, and epithelial cell differentiation. We now know that retinoids exert most of their effects through their influence on gene expression. They are essential for controlling growth and differentiation of normal cells during embryonic development. Because of their ability to influence differentiation of some cells while arresting development of others, they have become an important part of chemoprevention protocols aimed at preventing cancer in high-risk individuals. Retinoids are known to enhance humoral and cell-mediated immune responses as well. The agent that has been used the longest and most extensively is all-transretinoic acid (ATRA). Other similar retinoids include 9-cis-transretinoic acid (panretinide) and bexarotene.

All-Transretinoic Acid

This natural retinol metabolite is licensed for treating acute progranulocytic leukemia refractory to or relapsed from anthracycline chemotherapy; some unlabeled uses include treating myelodysplasia and providing chemoprevention against cervical dysplasia and precancerous skin lesions. The pharmacokinetics of ATRA (Tretinoin, Vesanoid) are poorly defined. For its licensed use, ATRA is given intravenously as an infusion. Chemoprevention protocols use oral formulations, and some research protocols use a topical formulation.

Like all retinoids, ATRA is teratogenic and in pregnancy category D; this classification precludes pregnancy during therapy and for an undefined period afterward. Egg or sperm donation before therapy is recommended for patients of childbearing age.

Acute hypervitaminosis A toxicity is a commonly described phenomenon with treatment doses of this agent. CNS symptoms prevail and include drowsiness, irritability, headache, and vomiting. More commonly are the dermatologic symptoms that include alopecia, dry desquamation, pruritus, and increased pigmentation. Constitutional symptoms are arthralgia, hepatosplenomegaly, and eye irritation. Symptoms are not usually life threatening and resolve 1 to 4 weeks after the conclusion of therapy. Other major toxicities of retinoids are hypercholesterolemia, teratogenesis, visual disturbances, and hyperleukocytosis.

Hyperleukocytosis with fever, respiratory distress, pulmonary infiltrates, and fluid retention are the characteristics of a syndrome called retinoic acid syndrome, which occurs in 20% to 30% of patients receiving therapy for progranulo-

cytic leukemia. It so closely mimics infection and sepsis that it may be difficult to differentiate from them. High-dose steroids and leukapheresis have been used to supplement supportive care, to help resolve the symptoms without discontinuing therapy. ATRA has no known drug interactions.

9-Cis-Transretinoic Acid (Panretinide, Isomer ATRA)

Like ATRA, this agent is a naturally occurring retinol derivative that acts on several sites. It is licensed for topical treatment of Kaposi sarcoma lesions. Administration guidelines and adverse effects are similar to those of ATRA except for the absence of retinoic acid syndrome, which is unique to ATRA.

Bexarotene (Targretin Gel)

This naturally occurring retinol derivative is available in both a systemic and topical form to treat cutaneous T-cell lymphoma (mycosis fungoides). This agent is also used to treat acne (Accutane).

Levamisole

Levamisole (Ergamisol) is used as an adjunctive therapy in patients being treated with fluorouracil (Adrucil) after surgical resection of Duke stage C colon cancer. The exact mechanism of synergy is unclear, but therapy responses are nearly doubled when the two agents are administered concomitantly. Levamisole restores depressed immune function, stimulating antibody formation, enhancing T-cell response, and potentiating monocyte and macrophage activity. Levamisole is readily absorbed when given orally.

Levamisole is assigned to pregnancy category C and should also be avoided with lactation. Common adverse effects include dizziness, headache, depression, paresthesias, changes in taste, nausea, stomatitis, diarrhea, dermatitis, alopecia, fatigue, fever, arthralgia, myalgia, and infection. Depression of bone marrow function is a potentially serious but infrequent complication.

Increased phenytoin (Dilantin) levels and phenytoin toxicity can occur if this drug is combined with levamisole. Patients on this combination should be monitored closely and have their phenytoin levels checked regularly, with changes in dosage made as appropriate. Because disulfiram (Antabuse)-like reactions can occur if levamisole is combined with alcohol, patients should be warned not to drink alcohol.

Azathioprine

Azathioprine (Imuran) is an intravenously infused antimetabolite that splits into a precursor, mercaptopurine. It is a unique antimetabolite agent because it is exclusively an immunosuppressant and not an antineoplastic. Because of its action, it is highly mutagenic and has been associated with the development of secondary malignancies. It is indicated as part of a multidrug regimen to prevent rejection in renal transplantation and to treat rheumatoid arthritis not responsive to conventional management. Unlabeled uses include treating Crohn disease and myasthenia gravis and preventing rejection after cardiac transplantation. Notable drug interactions occur with allopurinol, angiotensin-converting enzyme (ACE) inhibitors, and anticoagulants. The most common and severe adverse event is infection, although GI distress may be great enough to warrant limiting the dose. Azathioprine is given cautiously with other immunosuppressants because of increased risk for infection, and dose reduction is necessary in hepatic dysfunction.

Thalidomide

Thalidomide (Thalomid) has been used for many years for various purposes. As a result of its early use in pregnant women and the resulting severe birth defects, it is classified as a pregnancy category X drug. It is possible that severe birth defects can occur with only one dose. In the United States, it is marketed under a special distribution program called "System for Thalidomide Education and Prescribing Safety," which means that it is a restricted drug that may only be prescribed by registered individuals. Male and female patients who are prescribed thalidomide must receive oral and written instruction about the need to use two methods of contraception; they must use the contraception for 1 month before starting thalidomide, during treatment, and for 1 month after stopping thalidomide. Periodic pregnancy testing is required while receiving thalidomide. Breast-feeding must also be avoided. It is believed that thalidomide's most promising features for treating malignancy lie in its "antiangiogenesis" properties, yet its actions on autoantibodies have also made it a useful agent for treating autoimmune diseases.

Licensed uses for thalidomide include treating cutaneous manifestations of erythema nodosum leprosum (a complication of the treatment for leprosy), rheumatoid arthritis, multiple myeloma, bone marrow transplantation, and graft-versus-host disease refractory to standard therapy. It is an oral or intramuscular (IM) injected agent given once daily.

Common adverse effects include thrombotic problems, drowsiness, photosensitivity, and peripheral neuropathies. Skin disorders, GI distress, secretory disorders (e.g., decreased lacrimation, dry mouth), and fluid retention have also been reported with some frequency. Patients taking thalidomide are advised to immediately report neurologic symptoms because toxicity may not be reversible if the agent is not promptly stopped.

Glatiramer

Glatiramer acetate (Copaxone) is a synthetic copolymer of essential amino acids. It suppresses the specific immune processes involved in the pathogenesis of multiple sclerosis and reduces the frequency of relapses. Although the exact mechanism of action is unknown, it is thought to act by modulating T-cell autoimmune responses to myelin. The drug is given by daily SC injections and must be reconstituted and used immediately. A set of postinjection reactions—including chest pain, palpitations, anxiety, dyspnea, and urticaria—occurs in about 10% of patients with injection and is usually transient. Transient chest pain separate from the postinjection reaction has also been reported by about 20% of patients, but the symptom is self-limiting and not associated with other life-threatening symptoms. This drug may interfere with normal immune function while blocking the mechanism that causes multiple sclerosis; therefore, the patient should be protected from infection and injury. Photosensitivity is also common, necessitating use of sunscreen and protective clothing when outdoors.

Bacille Calmette-Guérin

BCG in the form of ImmuCyst is a suspension of an attenuated strain of *Mycobacterium bovis* that has been used as immunoadjuvant since the 1960s. TheraCys is live BCG. This agent in either of its forms is currently licensed to treat carcinoma in situ of the urinary bladder with or without papillary

tumors, although its unlabeled uses also include hematologic malignancies. It has been given intradermally, although it is more frequently administered intravenously or instilled into the bladder. Acting as a nonspecific immunomodulatory agent, it stimulates both nonspecific and specific immune responses, although the precise mechanism of action is not known.

Denileukin Diftitox

Denileukin diftitox (Ontak) [diphtheria toxin and IL-2] is an **immunotoxin** that combines an inactivated microbe (diphtheria toxin) and a cytokine (IL-2); it is licensed for treating persistent or relapsed cutaneous T-cell lymphoma whose malignant cells express the CD25 component of the IL-2 receptor. It is administered at either 9 mg/kg/day or 18 mg/kg/day for a 5-day course every 21 days. Denileukin diftitox is administered over at least 15 minutes while observing the patient for infusion-related reactions such as fever, chills, urticaria, or respiratory distress. Although no clear guidelines exist regarding the length of treatment, most individuals receive approximately 4 cycles of therapy. Two acute reactions have been reported with this agent: acute hypersensitivity and a flu-like syndrome complex. Acute hypersensitivity reactions within hours of infusion are common (67%). These reactions may be prevented by administering acetaminophen or diphenhydramine, although many clinicians also administer nonsteroidal anti-inflammatory agents or corticosteroids to these patients. A more delayed flu-like syndrome often has the typical fever and chills, but also GI distress, myalgias, and asthenia. In addition to these hypersensitivity toxicities, vascular leak syndrome with weight gain, edema, hypoalbuminemia, and hypotension occurs in up to 27% of patients. This agent has not been studied and established safe for administration to children or to women who are lactating or pregnant.

CHAPTER SUMMARY

- The immune system is a complex system of cells and chemical mediators that prevents foreign pathogens or cells from invading the body.
- WBCs are active in the surveillance and initiation of inflammatory reactions to specific stimuli. WBCs include neutrophils, which digest foreign material; basophils, which release chemicals to initiate the immune response; mast cells, which are located in the skin and the respiratory and GI tracts; macrophages, which release chemicals to initiate the immune response; and eosinophils, which seem to be active in allergic reactions.
- Lymphocytes include T cells, which are important in modifying the immune response and in protecting the body from nonself cells, and B cells, which produce antibodies to specific antigens. The antibodies stimulate an immune and inflammatory reaction to the antigen and cause its destruction.
- Interferons are produced by WBCs in response to viral invasion and other stimuli. They block viral replication and inhibit tumor cell growth. Interferons are used to treat various malignant and viral diseases.
- Interleukins are chemicals secreted by active WBCs to influence other WBCs.
- Antibodies can be used to target malignant cell clones or to modify T or B lymphocytes. Antibodies may be polyclonal or monoclonal.
- Current licensed monoclonal antibodies originate from murine antibodies, modified part-murine (chimeric) antibodies, or humanized antibodies. Antibodies without murine proteins produce fewer adverse effects and less risk for eliciting human antimurine antibodies (HAMAs) that preclude future therapy with other antibodies.
- Monoclonal antibodies can also be fused to antineoplastic medications, radioactive agents, or cytokines.
- Immune modulators may restore depressed immune function, stimulate immune function, stimulate antibody formation, or enhance T-cell response.
- Drugs that suppress the immune system are used to block T-cell activity in organ transplant patients when the immune system tries to destroy the foreign cells, and to treat autoimmune diseases when the immune system is mistakenly trying to destroy self cells.
- Patients taking drugs that modify the immune system need protection against infection, injury, and neoplasms because their susceptibility is increased.
- These drugs often cause adverse GI effects; therefore, efforts must be made to maintain nutritional status. A nutritional consultation, supplemental feedings, and small, frequent meals are often necessary.

QUESTIONS FOR STUDY AND REVIEW

1. What effects do cytokines have on the immune response?
2. What are interferons and interleukins?
3. Why are interferons used against malignant cells?
4. How do the adverse effects of IL-2 differ from those of interferons?
5. How does rituximab produce its therapeutic effect?
6. What is the most common adverse effect of rituximab?
7. What are the labeled indications for cyclosporine?
8. What are the dose-limiting toxicities of cyclosporine?

? **Need More Help?**

Chapter 34 of the study guide for *Drug Therapy in Nursing* 2e contains NCLEX-style questions and other learning activities to reinforce your understanding of the concepts presented in this chapter. For additional information or to purchase the study guide, visit *http://connection.lww.com/go/aschenbrenner.*

REFERENCES AND BIBLIOGRAPHY

Armstrong, A. C., Eaton, D., & Ewing, J. C. (2002). Cellular vaccine therapy for cancer. *Expert Review of Vaccines, 1*(3), 303–316.

Baselga, J., O'Dwyer, P. J., Thor, A. D., et al. (2000). *Epidermal growth factor receptor: Potential target for antitumor agents.* Dallas, TX: Center for Biomedical Continuing Education.

Brown, K. A., Esper, P., Kelleher, L. O., et al. (Eds). (2001). *Chemotherapy and biotherapy guidelines and recommendations for practice.* Pittsburgh, PA: Oncology Nursing Society.

Bruner, R. J., & Farag, S. S. (2003). Monoclonal antibodies for the prevention and treatment of graft-versus-host disease. *Seminars in Oncology, 30*(4), 509–519.

Bush, S. (2002). Monoclonal antibodies conjugated with radioisotopes for the treatment of non-Hodgkin's lymphoma. *Seminars in Oncology Nursing, 18*(1 Suppl. 1), 16–21.

Buzaid, A. C., & Atkins, M. (2001). Practical guidelines for the management of biochemotherapy-related toxicity in melanoma. *Clinical Cancer Research, 7*(9), 2611–2619.

Camacho, L. H. (2003). Clinical applications of retinoids in cancer medicine. *Journal of Biological Regulators and Homeostatic Agents, 17*(1), 98–114.

Cersosimo, R. J. (2003a). Monoclonal antibodies in the treatment of cancer, Part 1. *American Journal of Health-System Pharmacy, 60*(15), 1531–1548.

Cersosimo, R. J. (2003b). Monoclonal antibodies in the treatment of cancer, Part 2. *American Journal of Health-System Pharmacy, 60*(16), 1631–1641.

Cheng, J. D., Rieger, P. T., von Mehren, M., et al. (2000). Recent advances in immunotherapy and monoclonal antibody treatment of cancer. *Seminars in Oncology Nursing, 16*(4 Suppl. 1), 2–12.

Cheson, B. D. (2003). *Ibritumomab tiuxetan (Zevalin) in non-Hodgkin's lymphoma: Clinical background, practical considerations, and case studies*. New York: The Oncology Group, Division of SCP Communications, Inc.

Cho, H. J., & Bhardwaj, N. (2003). Against the self: Dendritic cells versus cancer, *APMIS: Acta pathologica, microbiologica, et immunologica Scandinavica, 111*(7–8), 805–817.

Coleman, C. (1998). Overview of biotherapy and nursing considerations. *Journal of Intravenous Nursing, 21*(6), 367–373.

Cuaron, L., & Thompson, J. (2001). The interferons. In P. T. Rieger (Ed.), *Biotherapy: A comprehensive overview* (2nd ed., pp. 125–194). Boston: Jones and Bartlett.

Cumisky, S. (2000). BCG immunotherapy for carcinoma of the urinary bladder. *Nursing Standard, 14*(37), 45–47.

Dereure, O. (2003). Skin reactions related to treatment with anticytokines, membrane receptor inhibitors and monoclonal antibodies. *Expert Opinion on Drug Safety, 2*(5), 467–473.

DiJulio, J. E. (2001). Monoclonal antibodies: Overview and use in hematologic malignancies. In P. T. Rieger (Ed.), *Biotherapy: A comprehensive overview* (2nd ed., pp. 283–316). Boston: Jones and Bartlett.

Food and Drug Administration. (2004). Cetuximab- Erbitux™ FDA labeling. [Online.] Available: *http://www.fda.gov/foi/label/2004/125084lbl.pdf*.

Frankel, C. (2000). Nursing management considerations with trastuzumab (Herceptin). *Seminars in Oncology Nursing, 16*(4 Suppl. 1), 23–28.

Fu, M. R., Anderson, C. M., McDaniel, R., et al. (2002). Patients' perceptions of fatigue in response to biochemotherapy for metastatic melanoma: A preliminary study, *Oncology Nursing Forum, 29*(6), 961–966.

Gale, D. M., & Sorokin, P. (2001). The interleukins. In P. T. Rieger (Ed.), *Biotherapy: A comprehensive overview* (2nd ed., pp. 195–244). Boston: Jones and Bartlett.

Gemmill, R., & Idell, C. S. (2003). Biological advances for new treatment approaches. *Seminars in Oncology Nursing, 19*(3), 162–168.

Goldstein, A. L. (2003). Thymosin beta4: A new molecular target for anti-tumor strategies. *Journal National Cancer Institute, 95*(22), 1646–1647.

Gong, J., Avigan, D., & Kufe, D. (1999). Dendritic-tumor cell fusions. In M. T. Lotze, & A. W. Thomson (Eds.), *Dendritic cells: Biology and clinical applications* (pp. 617–630). San Diego: Academic Press.

Grillo-Lopez, A. J. (2003). Rituximab (Rituxan/MabThera): The first decade (1993–2003). *Expert Reviews in Anticancer Therapeutics, 3*(6), 767–779.

Hendrix, C. (2003). Radiation safety guidelines for radioimmunotherapy with yttrium 90 ibritumomab tiuexetan. *Clinical Journal of Oncology, 8*(1), 31–34.

Hendrix, C. S., de Leon, C., & Dillman, R. O. (2002). Radioimmunotherapy for non-Hodgkin's lymphoma with yttrium 90 ibritumomab tiuxetan. *Clinical Journal of Oncology Nursing, 6*(3), 144–148.

Hoffman, R. L., & Reeder, S. J. (1998). Mycophenolate mofetil (CellCept): The newest immunosuppressant. *Critical Care Nurse, 18*(3), 50–57.

Horton, J. (2002). Trastuzumab use in breast cancer: clinical issues, *Cancer Control, 9*(6), 499–507.

Janmaat, M. L., & Giaccone, G. (2003). The epidermal growth factor receptor pathway and its inhibition as an anticancer therapy. *Drugs Today, 39*(Suppl C), 61–80.

Kahan, B. D., Kirken, R. A., & Stepkowski, S. M. (2003). New approaches to transplant immunosuppression. *Transplantation Proceedings, 35*(5), 1621–1623.

Kennedy, R. C., & Shearer, M. H. (2003). A role for antibodies in tumor immunity. *International Review of Immunology, 22*(2), 141–172.

Kinzler, D. M., & Brown, C. K. (2001). Cancer vaccines. In P. T. Rieger (Ed.), *Biotherapy: A comprehensive overview* (2nd ed., pp. 357–382). Boston: Jones and Bartlett.

Lazar, G. A., Marshall, S. A., Plecs, J. J., et al. (2003). Designing proteins for therapeutic applications. *Current Opinion in Structural Biology, 13*(4), 513–518.

Lotze, M. T., Farhood, H., Cara, C. W., et al. (1999). Dendritic cell therapy of cancer and HIV infection. In M. T. Lotze, & A. W. Thomson (Eds.), *Dendritic cells: Biology and clinical applications* (pp. 459–486). San Diego: Academic Press.

Luo, Y., & Prestwich, G. D. (2002). Cancer-targeted polymeric drugs. *Current Cancer Drug Targets, 2*(3), 209–226.

Malaguarnera M., Ferlito L., Gulizia G., et al. (2001). Use of interleukin-2 in advanced renal carcinoma: Meta-analysis and review of the literature. *European Journal of Clinical Pharmacology, 57*(4), 267–273.

Mavroukakis, S. A., & Muehlbauer, P. M. (2001). Clinical pathways for managing patients receiving interleukin-2. *Oncology Nursing Forum, 5*(5), 207–216.

Mitchell, M. S. & Kast, W. M. (2003). Combinations of anticancer drugs and immunotherapy. *Cancer Immunology and Immunotherapy, 52*(10), 655–660.

Pennel, C. A., & Erickson, H. A. (2002). Designing immunotoxins for cancer therapy. *Immunology Research, 25*(2), 177–191.

Pillon, L. R. (1991). Cyclosporine: A nursing focus on immunosuppressive therapy. *Dimensions of Critical Care Nursing, 10*(2), 68–73.

Poole, P., & Greer, E. (2000). Immunosuppression in transplantation: A new millennium in care. *Critical Care Nursing Clinics of North America, 12*(3), 315–321.

Rieger, P. T. (2001). Patient management. In P. T. Rieger (Ed.), *Biotherapy: A comprehensive overview* (2nd ed., pp. 461–506). Boston: Jones and Bartlett.

Reiger, P. T., Green, M., & Murray, J. L. (2001). Monoclonal antibodies: Applications in solid tumors and other diseases. In P. T. Rieger (Ed.), *Biotherapy: A comprehensive overview* (2nd ed., pp. 317–356). Boston: Jones and Bartlett.

Rieger, P. T., & Khuri, F. R. (2001). The retinoids. In P. T. Rieger (Ed.), *Biotherapy: A comprehensive overview* (2nd ed., pp. 407–430). Boston: Jones and Bartlett.

Riley, M. B. (2003). Ibritumomab tiuxetan. *Clinical Journal of Oncology Nursing, 7*(1), 110–112.

Schmidt, K. V., & Wood, B. A. (2003). Trends in cancer therapy: Role of monoclonal antibodies. *Seminars in Oncology Nursing, 19*(3), 169–179.

Schwartz, R. N., Stover L., & Dutcher J. (2002). Managing toxicities of high-dose interleukin-2. *Oncology, 16*(11 Suppl. 13), 11–20.

Seeley, K., & DeMeyer, E. (2002). Nursing care of patients receiving Campath™. *Clinical Journal of Oncology Nursing, 6*(3), 138–143.

Slamon, D. J., Leyland-Jones, B., Shak, S., et al. (2001). Use of chemotherapy plus a monoclonal antibody against HER2 for metastatic breast cancer that overexpresses HER2. *New England Journal of Medicine, 344*(11), 783–792.

Solomon, S., & Komanduri, K. (2001). The immune system. In P. T. Rieger (Ed.), *Biotherapy: A comprehensive overview* (2nd ed., pp. 39–64). Boston: Jones and Bartlett.

Sorokin, P. (2001). Campath-1H. *Clinical Journal of Oncology Nursing, 5*(2), 65–66.

Vieweg, J., & Dannull, J. (2003). Tumor vaccines: From gene therapy to dendritic cells—the emerging frontier. *Urology Clinics of North America, 30*(3), 633–643, x.

Waldmann, H. (2003). The new immunosuppression. *Current Opinion in Chemical Biology, 7*(4), 476–480.

White, C. A., Weaver, R. L., & Grillo-Lopez, A. J. (2001). Antibody-targeted immunotherapy for treatment of malignancy. *Annual Reviews in Medicine, 52,* 125–145.

Wilkes, G. M., Ingwersen, K., & Burke, M. B. (1999). *1999 Oncology nursing drug handbook*. Boston: Jones and Bartlett.

Wu, J., & Lanier, L. L. (2003). Natural killer cells and cancer. *Advances in Cancer Research, 90,* 127–156.

Antineoplastic Drugs

unit 9

Drugs That Are Cell Cycle–Specific

chapter 35

Learning Objectives

At the completion of this chapter the student will:

1. Identify core drug knowledge about cell cycle–specific drugs.
2. Understand the goals of treatment and the strategies used in chemotherapy.
3. Identify the phases of the cell life cycle and describe what happens at each phase.
4. Differentiate a normal from a malignant cell.
5. Explain the difference between a cell cycle–specific and a cell cycle–nonspecific chemotherapeutic agent.
6. Identify the different routes of administration for the various chemotherapeutic agents.
7. Describe precautions and practices to ensure safety, minimize exposure, and deal with untoward effects of chemotherapy to the patient, health care provider, and the environment.
8. Identify core drug knowledge about cell cycle–specific drugs.
9. Identify core patient variables relevant to cell cycle–specific drugs.
10. Relate the interaction of core drug knowledge to core patient variables for cell cycle–specific drugs.
11. Generate a nursing plan of care from the interactions between the core drug knowledge and core patient variables for cell cycle–specific drugs.
12. Describe nursing interventions to maximize therapeutic effects and minimize adverse effects for cell cycle–specific drugs.
13. Identify the potential effects of herbal medicine on chemotherapy.
14. Determine key points for patient and family education for cell cycle–specific drugs.

FEATURED WEBLINK

http://www.ons.org
The Oncology Nursing Society website provides links to online courses and tutorials about cancer and chemotherapy, information on conferences and seminars, and resources on cancer prevention, detection, treatment, symptom management, survivorship, and palliative care.

CONNECTION WEBLINK

Additional Weblinks are found on Connection:
http://www.connection.lww.com/go/aschenbrenner.

KEY TERMS

adjuvant therapy
cell cycle
cell cycle–specific
cell cycle–nonspecific
chemotherapy
consolidation therapy
cytokinesis
first-order kinetics
G_0 phase
G_1 phase
G_2 phase
generation time
growth fraction
induction therapy
intensification
irritant
maintenance
mitosis
M phase
nadir
neoadjuvant therapy
palliative therapy
radiation recall
salvage therapy
S phase
vesicant

Drugs That Are Cell Cycle–Specific

Ⓒ Antimetabolites

- **P 5-fluorouracil (5-FU)**
- methotrexate

Ⓒ Mitotic Inhibitors

Ⓒ Vinca alkaloids
- **P vincristine**
- vinblastine

Ⓒ Podophyllotoxins
- **P etoposide**
- teniposide

Ⓒ Taxanes
- **P paclitaxel**
- docetaxel

Ⓒ Camptothecines

- **P topotecan**
- irinotecan

Miscellaneous Cell Cycle-Specific Drugs

- **P hydroxyurea**
- L-asparaginase

The symbol Ⓒ indicates the **drug class.**
Drugs in **bold type** marked with the symbol P are prototypes.
Drugs in blue type are closely related to the prototype.
Drugs in red type are significantly different from the prototype.
Drugs in black type with no symbol are also used in drug therapy; no prototype

Today, the treatment options for cancer include more choices than ever before. Novel agents that function differently from the familiar cancer regimens of radiation, chemotherapy, surgery, and biotherapy have generated a lot of research initiatives and hopes for cure. Chemotherapy remains a vital part of the cancer armamentarium, however. **Chemotherapy** is the term that describes the use of cytotoxic agents that inhibit the growth, development, and proliferation of malignant cells. Sometimes the term antineoplastics is used instead of the term chemotherapy. Chemotherapy dates back to the 1500s, when heavy metals were used to treat cancers. Severe toxicities and few cures were reported. Since then, a vast spectrum of chemotherapeutic drugs has been discovered to achieve the goals of chemotherapy: cure, control, and palliation.

Unlike two other methods of treating cancer, surgery and radiation, chemotherapy produces a systemic effect. The chemotherapeutic drugs are transported by the bloodstream to different parts of the body, although most of these drugs do not cross the blood–brain barrier and therefore cannot reach the central nervous system (CNS).

Chemotherapy plays an important role in cancer therapy. It is the primary treatment for some cancers (Box 35.1) and serves as an adjunct to the other treatment methods. Chemotherapeutic agents may be administered as single agents or in combination regimens. They are used in the following treatment strategies:

- **Adjuvant therapy:** This therapy involves a short course of high-dose drug therapy (usually with a combination of drugs) administered after radiation or surgery to destroy residual tumor cells or prevent recurrence.
- **Induction therapy:** This term refers to the start of chemotherapy. As commonly used in treating hematologic cancers, induction consists of high-dose drug therapy (usually with a combination of drugs) given to induce a complete response when initiating a curative regimen.
- **Consolidation therapy:** This strategy consists of chemotherapy given after induction therapy has achieved a complete remission; the regimen is repeated to increase the probability of cure or to prolong patient survival.
- **Intensification:** After complete remission is achieved, the same agents used for induction therapy are given at higher (intensified) doses, or different drugs are given (also at high doses) to improve the chances of cure or longer remission.
- **Maintenance:** This therapy involves using low-dose cytotoxic drugs, singly or in combination, on a long-term basis in patients who are in complete remission, to delay regrowth of residual cancer cells.
- **Neoadjuvant therapy:** Chemotherapy is administered to reduce the tumor burden before surgery or radiation, to improve the outcomes of these methods.
- **Palliative therapy:** This therapy involves the use of chemotherapeutic drugs to control symptoms, provide comfort, and improve the patient's quality of life if cure is not achievable.
- **Salvage therapy:** This strategy involves the use of a potentially curative high-dose drug regimen given to a patient whose symptoms have recurred or whose treatment by another regimen has failed.

You need to be equipped with a clear knowledge of cell physiology, cancer pathophysiology, routes of administration for chemotherapeutic drugs, safety guidelines for handling chemotherapeutic drugs, classifications of antineoplastic drugs, and the therapeutic and adverse effects (toxicities) of antineoplastic drugs so that patient's needs can be anticipated early. Armed with this knowledge and set of skills, you will be able to assist the patient in navigating the often overwhelming challenges that the various treatment options offer. You can then offer the best education for the patient so that the patient can be managed well within any clinical setting and be able to participate in his or her care and adhere to a treatment regimen with a clear understanding of the goals and expectations of treatment.

BOX 35.1 Role of Chemotherapy in Various Cancers

Primary Treatment

Chemotherapy is the primary treatment for the following localized cancerous neoplasms:

Burkitt's lymphoma
CNS lymphomas
Hodgkin disease (of childhood and some adult stages)
Embryonal rhabdomyosarcoma
Wilms tumor
Small-cell lung cancer
Large-cell lymphomas

Future as a Primary Treatment

Chemotherapy holds promise as a future primary treatment for the following cancers:

Breast cancer
Esophageal cancer
Non–small-cell lung cancer
Nasopharyngeal cancer and other cancers of the head and neck
Pancreatic cancer
Prostate cancer
Cervical carcinoma
Gastric carcinoma

Treatment Before Surgery

Sometimes chemotherapy is the treatment used to shrink a tumor so that surgery can be less extensive and therefore less mutilating. Some cancers for which chemotherapy is used as a pretreatment include the following:

Soft-tissue sarcomas
Laryngeal cancer
Anal carcinoma
Bladder cancer
Breast cancer
Osteogenic sarcoma

PHYSIOLOGY

A knowledge of cellular kinetics and the life span of the **cell cycle** is needed to understand how chemotherapy works. The cell is the basic structure of the human organism. Normally, cell growth is strictly regulated. The process by which a cell replicates itself, forming two identical daughter cells,

is called cell division. Cell division, which is rare, occurs only to replace worn-out or dying cells and as part of the process of wound healing. Cell death is controlled, and when cells die, they are replaced in an orderly fashion. In cancer, however, the mechanisms for cell growth are disrupted, resulting in uncontrolled proliferation of cells. The time span over which a cell reproduces is called the cell cycle. The cell cycle has five phases: G_0, G_1, S, G_2, and M. All cells, whether normal or abnormal, progress through these different phases of the cell cycle. The complete cycle is illustrated in Figure 35.1.

The cell cycle is the cornerstone of cell cycle division and proliferation. Both normal and malignant cells undergo this process, which can last for approximately 25 to 30 hours. In the first phase, **Gap 0 (G_0) phase,** a cell can stay in a dormant or latent state for months or even years until stimulated to move forward in the cycle. Because certain cells divide more rapidly than others, some rest in the G_0 phase for a brief period, whereas others bypass the G_0 phase and directly enter the second phase, **Gap 1 (G_1) phase,** if the body needs a certain cell immediately. During the G_1 phase, the cell increases in size and synthesizes ribonucleic acid (RNA) and the proteins needed for deoxyribonucleic acid (DNA) synthesis. The time a cell spends in this phase varies and can last from hours to days, depending on the cell type.

After RNA and protein synthesis occur, the cell enters the third phase, **synthesis (S) phase.** During the S phase, RNA, proteins, and enzymes necessary for deoxyribonucleic acid (DNA) synthesis are formed. DNA contains the genetic code necessary for the growth and replication of the cell. DNA is an essential nucleic acid composed of deoxyribose, a phosphate, and four nitrogenous bases: adenine, guanine, cytosine, and thymine. Adenine and guanine are purines, and cytosine and thymine are pyrimidines. Chemical reactions occur between the two purines and between the two pyrimidines, leading to the formation of the double-stranded DNA helix, which serves as the genetic template of the cell. Generally, the synthesis phase lasts 8 to 12 hours.

The cell then enters the fourth phase, **Gap 2 (G_2) phase,** during which more RNA and protein synthesis takes place in preparation for mitosis (cell division). In this phase, the cellular apparatus called the mitotic spindle is constructed. The G_2 phase lasts for approximately 2 hours. After the G_2 phase, the cell is ready to undergo cell division.

The fifth phase of the cell cycle is **mitosis (M) phase,** which consists of the following orchestrated subphases: prophase, metaphase, anaphase, and telophase (see Figure 35.1). As the cell progresses through these subphases, the cytoplasm and nucleus divide, so that replication of the cell results in the birth of two daughter cells. When the nucleus divides, the cell's genetic material (chromosomes) is duplicated and distributed into the two daughter cells. The remainder of the

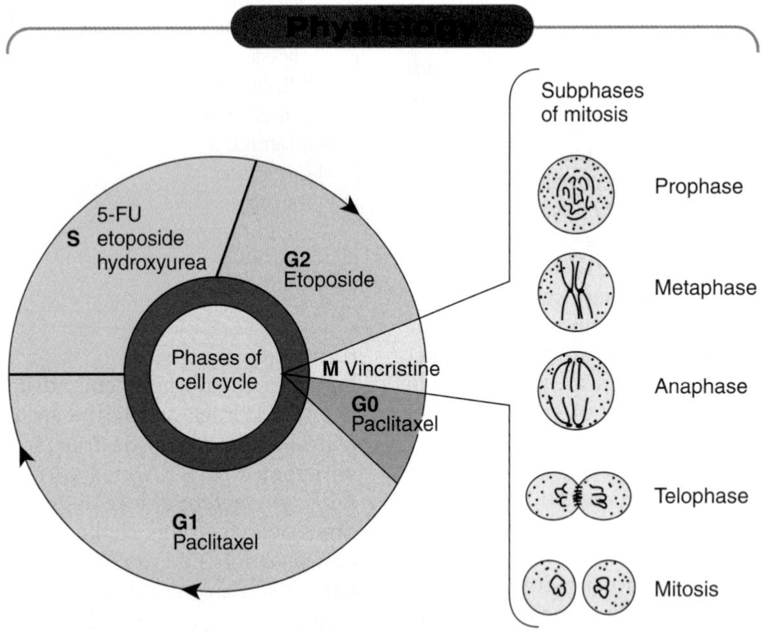

FIGURE 35.1 Cell cycle. The cell cycle has five phases through which it passes in reproducing itself. The phases represented include G_0 (resting, nonreproductive phase), G_1 (waiting for reproductive stimulus), S (stimulus received; DNA and RNA assembled), G_2 (mitotic spindles constructed and RNA synthesized), and M (mitosis; cell division). Antineoplastic drugs with actions that occur in a particular phase of the cycle are known as cell cycle-specific drugs. Among these drugs are 5-fluorouracil, which affects the S phase of the cell cycle; vincristine, which affects the M phase (mitosis); etoposide, which affects the S and G_2 phases; paclitaxel, which affects the G_0 and possibly the G_1 phases; and hydroxyurea, which affects the S phase.

cell (its cytoplasm) is also divided into the new daughter cells; this process is called **cytokinesis.** Each of these two new daughter cells will either pass through a new reproductive cycle or become arrested in G_0 and perform other cellular activities.

The time needed to complete the cell cycle, which varies with each type of cell, is called **generation time.** Tumors consisting of cells that have a short generation time or rapid mitotic rate are most sensitive to antineoplastic agents. Tumors that have cancer cells with a long generation time or slow mitotic rate are often resistant to chemotherapy.

Exactly how the body maintains normal cellular homeostasis is not clearly understood. The body is thought to possess a feedback system that signals a cell to enter the G_1 phase of the cell cycle in response to a neighboring cell's death. In individuals with cancer, this feedback system is dysfunctional, and the cancer cell enters the G_1 phase without prompting from the body's feedback system.

PATHOPHYSIOLOGY

Every cell in the body has a genetically programmed clock that directs the timing of its reproductive activity. Cancer is a disease in which the cells fail to respond to this clock, the homeostatic mechanism that controls the normal cellular birth and death processes.

Four basic features differentiate the cancer cell from the normal cell:

- Uncontrolled cell proliferation
- Decreased cellular differentiation
- Inappropriate ability to invade surrounding tissue
- Ability to establish new growth at ectopic sites

Although cancer cells have the same chemical structures as normal cells and undergo the same phases of the cell life cycle, the critical difference appears to be in their altered response to mechanisms that control growth and differentiation. Cell production in a cancer is not proportional to cell loss; production of new cells occurs at a faster rate than is needed to compensate for the loss of cells.

CELLULAR KINETICS OF CHEMOTHERAPY DRUGS

Most chemotherapy drugs exert cytotoxic activity primarily on macromolecular synthesis or function. In other words, they interfere with the synthesis of DNA, RNA, or proteins or with the appropriate functioning of the preformed molecule. When this interference happens, a proportion of the cells die. Chemotherapy works on the principle of **first-order kinetics:** the number of tumor cells killed by an antineoplastic drug is proportional to the dose used. The proportion of cells killed after chemotherapy administration is a constant percentage of the total number of malignant cells present. For example, if a tumor containing 1 million (1,000,000) cells is exposed to a chemotherapeutic drug that has a 90% cell kill rate, the first dose of chemotherapy will destroy 90% (900,000) of the cancer cells, and 100,000 cells will survive. The second dose will kill another 90% of the remaining cells (90,000 cells), and 10,000 cells will survive. Because only a portion of the cells die, doses of chemotherapy must be repeated to reduce the population of cancer cells until just one cell remains. The hope is that the body's immune response will kill the final cell. Figure 35.2 gives a visual explanation of the cell-kill theory.

ROUTES OF CHEMOTHERAPY ADMINISTRATION

As advances in chemotherapy occur, variations in the routes of administration continue to evolve. The choice of drug route depends on the therapeutic intent. Drug administration intravenously through peripheral or central lines (or both) is the method most commonly used for chemotherapy. Alternate routes of drug delivery to specific sites within the body, using devices or catheters, are becoming more popular in clinical practice. More oral formulations of cytotoxic agents are now available, making it very convenient for patients to receive treatment at home less expensively, because less cost is incurred for health care personnel. This route presents different challenges for the clinician

Physiology

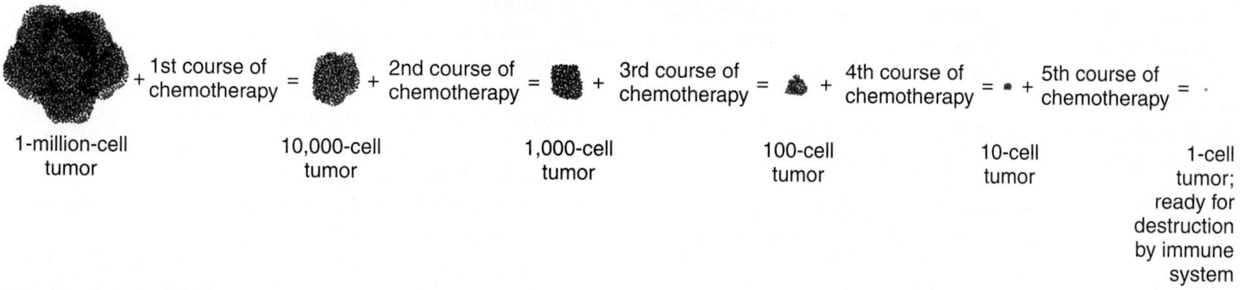

FIGURE 35.2 Cell kill theory. A set percentage of cells is killed after each dose of chemotherapy. The percentage killed is dependent upon the drug therapy. In the above example, each course of chemotherapy kills 90% of cells in a cancerous tumor.

because adverse effects may be different or the ability of the patient to tolerate the therapy may vary. Table 35.1 lists the different methods of drug delivery, including traditional and alternate routes, and outlines the practice implications for nurses who participate in the care of patients using these various routes and treatment methods in cancer therapy.

HANDLING AND PROPER DISPOSAL OF CHEMOTHERAPY AGENTS

Over the past decade, more health care professionals than ever before have handled chemotherapy agents. The mutagenic and carcinogenic effects known to occur from repeated exposure have raised great concern regarding the potential long-term risks to health care professionals who are exposed to antineoplastic drugs. For health care professionals of childbearing age, potential teratogenic risks and fertility impairment are another concern. Genotoxicity involving chromosomal changes has been documented following exposure to chemotherapy agents. Some drugs are also known to cause organ damage to the skin, mucous membranes, and corneas. Accidental exposure in poorly ventilated areas has resulted in acute symptoms, including headache, nausea, dizziness, and skin, throat, or eye irritation.

Conflicting research findings regarding the suspected and unknown potential long-term effects on individuals exposed to chemotherapeutic agents led to the establishment of advisory bodies that address exposure issues and recommend safe practice techniques for handling and disposing of these drugs. These advisory bodies are as follows:

- Occupational Safety and Health Administration (OSHA)
- American Society of Hospital Pharmacy (ASHP)
- Oncology Nursing Society (ONS)
- National Study Commission on Cytotoxic Exposure

These advisory bodies maintain that if professionals follow their recommendations while handling and disposing of these drugs, teratogenic risk is unlikely. The potential risk to health care professionals who handle chemotherapy agents and the body excreta of patients who have received these agents is unknown. Therefore, health care professionals must know the recommended precautions and implement them to minimize their potential exposure. According to the ONS guidelines, cancer chemotherapy should be administered by registered nurses who have successfully completed a course in chemotherapy administration. Exposure to chemotherapy can occur through the following routes: skin and mucous membrane absorption, inhalation, injection by needlestick, and ingestion.

Skin and mucous membrane absorption and inhalation can occur during the following activities:

1. Opening a chemotherapy vial or ampule
2. Eliminating air from a syringe filled with a chemotherapy agent
3. Disposing of intravenous (IV) bags, bottles, syringes, and tubing used in administering these agents
4. Disposing of the body excreta of patients who have received these drugs

Ingestion can occur through hand-to-mouth contact with the following items:

1. Food
2. Cosmetics
3. Cigarettes
4. Equipment contaminated with chemotherapy agents

The recommendations made by these advisory bodies serve as guidelines, and therefore institutional policies for handling, administering, and disposing of chemotherapeutic agents may vary. Employees must be familiar with their own institution's policies and procedures and use them as precautionary measures to minimize their potential exposure.

Recommendations to Minimize Exposure During Preparation, Transport, Disposal, and Storage of Chemotherapeutic Agents

To minimize exposure during preparation, transport, disposal, and storage of chemotherapeutic agents, adhere to the following recommendations:

1. Prepare these agents using a Class II or Class III Biological Safety Cabinet (also referred to as a vertical laminar airflow hood). These cabinets contain high-efficiency particulate air filters that pull and filter air away from the face of the person preparing the drug. It is recommended that these cabinets remain functioning 24 hours a day, 7 days a week, that they be vented to the outside, that they be cleaned daily with a 70% alcohol solution, and that they be serviced every 6 months to ensure adequate performance.
2. During drug preparation, wear disposable, lint-free, long-sleeved, nonabsorbent gowns made with a low-permeability fabric. The gowns should have a solid front with tight-fitting elastic at the wrists and back closure.
3. Wear a plastic mask and goggles in settings without biologic safety cabinets, such as a physician's office or whenever there is a possibility of splashing.
4. Use a plastic absorbent pad to cover the work surface preparation area so that any droplet contamination is absorbed.
5. Prime IV lines for chemotherapy administration with 5% dextrose in water (D_5W) or normal saline before the actual drug administration. Do not prime with the chemotherapy drug.
6. Use hydrophobic filter needles to draw antineoplastic drugs from vials and ampules.
7. Use a sterile gauze pad to purge air from a chemotherapy-filled syringe, connect and disconnect IV tubing containing antineoplastic drugs, and open chemotherapy vials and ampules; remove syringes from IV lines used for IV push administration; and remove empty chemotherapy bags or bottles from IV spikes.
8. Use a needleless delivery system or Luer-Lok connection to prevent accidental disconnection.
9. Use powder-free latex gloves at least 0.007 inch thick when handling chemotherapy agents and the body excreta of patients who have received these drugs within a 48-hour period. Personnel who have latex allergy should use alternative products made with nitrile.

TABLE 35.1 Administration Routes for Antineoplastic Drugs

Route	Advantages	Disadvantages	Potential Complications	Nursing Implications
Oral	Ease of administration	Inconsistency of absorption	Drug-specific complications	Evaluate compliance with medication schedule. Teach patient handling techniques.
Subcutaneous, Intramuscular	Ease of administration Decreased side effects	Requires adequate muscle mass and tissue for absorption Pain	Infection, bleeding	Evaluate platelet count (>50,000). Use smallest needle gauge possible. Prepare injection site with an antiseptic solution. Assess injection site for signs and symptoms of infection.
IV	Consistent absorption Required for vesicants	Sclerosing of veins over time	Infection, phlebitis	Check for blood return before and after administration of drugs
Intra-arterial*	Increased doses to tumor with decreased systemic toxic effects	Requires surgical procedure or special radiography for device placement	Bleeding, embolism	Monitor for signs and symptoms of bleeding. Monitor partial thromboplastin time, prothrombin time.
External pump	With intra-arterial port, patient freedom increased	Patient lies flat for 3–7 d during drug infusion	Pump occlusion, malfunction	Extensive patient education is needed.
Internal (implanted) pump	Greater mobility	Cost-effective only with long-term therapy (i.e., 3–6 mo)	Pump occlusion malfunction	Specialized nursing skills is needed.
Intrathecal,* intraventricular	More consistent drug levels in cerebrospinal fluid	Requires lumbar puncture or surgical placement of reservoir or implanted pump for drug delivery	Headaches, confusion, lethargy, nausea and vomiting, seizures	Observe site for signs of infection. Monitor functioning of reservoir or pump. Assess patient for headache or signs of increased intracranial pressure.
Intraperitoneal*	Direct exposure of intra-abdominal metastases to drug	Requires placement of Tenckhoff catheter or intraperitoneal port	Abdominal pain, abdominal distention, bleeding, ileus, intestinal perforation, infection	Warm chemotherapy solution to body temperature. Check patency of catheter or port. Instill solution according to protocol—infuse, dwell, and drain or continuous infusion.
Intrapleural	Sclerosing of pleural lining to prevent recurrence of effusions	Requires insertion of a thoracotomy tube	Pain, infection	Monitor for complete drainage from pleural cavity before instillation of drug. Following instillation, clamp tubing and reposition patient every 10–15 min for 2 h. Attach tubing to suction for 18 h. Assess patient for pain or anxiety. Provide analgesia and emotional support.

(continued)

TABLE 35.1 Administration Routes for Antineoplastic Drugs (continued)

Route	Advantages	Disadvantages	Potential Complications	Nursing Implications
Intravesicular	Direct exposure of bladder surfaces to drug	Requires insertion of Foley catheter	Urinary tract infections, cystitis, bladder contracture, urinary urgency, allergic drug reactions	Maintain sterile technique when inserting Foley catheter. Instill solution, clamp catheter for 1 h, and unclamp to drain.

* Note: Specialized nursing education may be required for certain administration methods. Refer to individual state nurse practice acts and agency policies and procedures.

Data from: Oncology Nursing Society. (1998). *Cancer chemotherapy guidelines and recommendation for practice.* Pittsburgh, PA: Oncology Nursing Press, Inc.

10. Wash hands before and after handling antineoplastic agents.
11. Never store food or beverages in a refrigerator used for chemotherapy storage.
12. Avoid eating, drinking, applying cosmetics, or chewing gum in the vicinity of drug preparation.
13. Transport chemotherapeutic drugs in sealed bags to prevent spilling. Spill kits should be readily available to personnel who have been properly instructed in chemotherapy handling and exposure procedures.
14. Institute universal (standard) precautions when handling the blood, vomitus, stool, or bed linens of a patient who has received chemotherapy within the past 48 hours. Wear protective equipment when necessary.
15. Flush the toilet twice after disposing of body fluids from patients who have received cytotoxic agents within the past 48 hours.
16. Dispose of all chemotherapy waste in impervious, leakproof containers dedicated for chemotherapy waste and not used for other hospital waste.
17. Instruct patients who receive chemotherapy at home to label drugs to indicate hazardous content and to store the drugs in areas where proper temperature will be maintained and where children cannot reach them.
18. Cover the toilet with a waterproof shield or pad before flushing.
19. All equipment contaminated with antineoplastic drugs must be disposed of in distinctly labeled hazardous waste receptacles. These chemotherapy wastes should be disposed of in Environmental Protection Agency permitted landfill waste sites or incinerators.

Management of Chemotherapy Spills

To manage spills of chemotherapeutic agents, adhere to the following recommended sequence:

1. Post a sign immediately to warn people away from the exposed area.
2. Don two pairs of powder-free latex gloves, a disposable gown, and a face shield.
3. Wear a NIOSH-approved respirator.
4. Place an absorbent pad over the spill to contain it.
5. Pick up glass fragments with a scoop and dispose of in a puncture-proof container.
6. Clean the area with a detergent three times from the least contaminated to the most contaminated areas.
7. Rinse the absorbed spill area with clean water. Repeat the washing and rinsing.
8. Dispose of all cleanup equipment according to institutional policy for chemotherapy waste.
9. Document the spill according to institutional policy; usually, spills of 5 mL or more are reportable. The following data should be included in the documentation: name of chemotherapy agent and approximate volume spilled, how spill occurred, procedures followed to contain and clean up spill, names of people who were exposed and of those who were notified of spill.

To expedite the handling of a spill and to minimize undue patient and employee exposure, well-equipped chemotherapy spill kits should be readily available (Box 35.2).

BOX 35.2 Contents of a Chemotherapy Spill Kit

1	Gown with cuffs and back closure*
1 pair	Shoe covers
2 pairs	Gloves
1 pair	Utility gloves
1 pair	Chemical splash goggles
1	Rebreather mask†
1	Disposable dust pan (to collect broken glass)
1	Plastic scraper (to scoop materials into dust pan)
2	Plastic-backed absorbable towels
1 each	250-mL and 1-L spill control pillows
2	Disposable sponges (to clean up spill, to clean up floor after spill removal)
1	Container for sharps
2	Large, heavy duty waste disposal bags for cleaning soiled area

*Made of water nonpermeable fabric.

†To meet National Institute of Occupational Safety and Health standards.

From Controlling occupational exposure to hazardous drugs. (1995). OSHA Instruction CPL2-2.20B. Washington, DC: Author. (© 1995), 21-1–21-34.

Measures for Accidental Exposure to Chemotherapy

To manage accidental exposure to chemotherapy, implement the following measures:

1. Eye contact: Immediately rinse the affected eye or eyes with copious amounts of water for no less than 15 minutes.
2. Skin contact: Immediately wash the area with soap and water.
3. Clothing contact: Immediately remove the contaminated clothing; if skin contact occurred, wash all such areas with soap and water. Place soiled clothing in a plastic bag until it is laundered, and then wash it twice, separately from all other clothing. After laundering the clothing twice, put the machine through a separate wash-rinse cycle.
4. Bed linen contact: Immediately remove the linens and place them in a contaminated linen receptacle; then clean the mattress using a 70% alcohol solution. Once the alcohol dries, the bed may be remade with clean linens.

CLASSIFICATION OF ANTINEOPLASTIC DRUGS

Antineoplastic drugs are classified according to their mode of action and the phase of the cell cycle in which the drug is active. However, rapidly dividing cells are the most sensitive to these drugs. Chemotherapeutic drugs that are most effective during a particular phase of the cycle are known as **cell cycle** (or cell phase) **specific,** whereas drugs that act independently of a specific cell cycle (or cell phase) are **cell cycle nonspecific.** This classification is not absolute; the cytotoxic mechanisms of the drugs likely involve more than one mechanism. Multiple intracellular sites might be affected, and the drugs' effects might not be confined to specific cycle events.

This chapter discusses the cell cycle–specific group of drugs (Table 35.2), the prototype or a representative drug from each classification, and the nursing management for each drug. Chapter 36 discusses the cell cycle–nonspecific group of drugs. The cell cycle–specific drugs consist of the antimetabolites (prototype, 5-fluorouracil) and mitotic inhibitors. These drugs exert the greatest killing effect on tumors when given as a continuous infusion or in divided doses with a short cycle. The mitotic inhibitors are subdivided into the vinca alkaloids (prototype, vincristine), the podophyllotoxins (prototype, etoposide), and the taxanes (prototype, paclitaxel). A new category of cell cycle–specific drugs called camptothecines (prototype, topotecan) and a miscellaneous group of antineoplastic drugs, such as the prototype drug hydroxyurea and L-asparaginase, are also included in this chapter.

C ANTIMETABOLITES

Antimetabolites are synthetic products that mimic the naturally produced metabolites, purines, pyrimidines, and folates that are essential for DNA and RNA synthesis. When the cell uses antimetabolites instead of the naturally occurring metabolites for these processes, cell death results. Because antimetabolites exert their cytotoxic activity during the S phase of the cell's life cycle, they are most effective against tumors that have a high **growth fraction.** The growth fraction of a tumor is the fraction of its cell population that is in any active phase of the cell cycle. Relatively quiescent tumors found in organs such as the pancreas and the uterus have low growth fractions, whereas rapidly proliferating tumors, such as those of the gastrointestinal (GI) mucosal epithelium and the hair follicles, have high growth fractions. The drugs in the antimetabolite category include 5-fluorouracil (5-FU), cytarabine (ARA-C), floxuridine (FUDR), fludarabine (Fludara), 6-mercaptopurine (Purinethol), methotrexate (MTX), thioguanine (6-thioguanine), gemcitabine (Gemzar), and capecitabine (Xeloda). The drug 5-FU, a pyrimidine antagonist that is a mainstay in chemotherapy, is discussed as the representative antimetabolite drug.

NURSING MANAGEMENT OF THE PATIENT RECEIVING P 5-FLUOROURACIL

Core Drug Knowledge

Pharmacotherapeutics

The drug 5-FU interferes with DNA synthesis and, to a lesser extent, inhibits the formation of RNA. It has proved to be clinically effective against a wide spectrum of solid tumors, particularly malignant GI tumors. It is indicated for the palliative management of carcinoma of the colon, breast, liver, ovary, pancreas, rectum, head and neck, and stomach. It has been used in combination with cisplatin and most often with levamisole or leucovorin.

Preclinical studies show that its cytotoxic activity can be potentiated by concomitantly administering reduced folates, such as leucovorin calcium. However, be vigilant in monitoring for severe adverse effects resulting from this combination. Dosage adjustments (see Table 35.2) are imperative for patients who are poorly nourished or are otherwise poor risks for tolerating treatment and having a successful outcome from therapy.

In addition to being administered intravenously (the most common route), 5-FU is also given by intra-arterial infusion into the hepatic artery through a surgically implanted pump. The goal of this type of delivery is to supply a high concentration of the antineoplastic drug directly to the tumor and surrounding area while sparing the normal tissues from toxic effects. A topical form of 5-FU is also available and has been curative for basal cell carcinomas and other malignant skin cancers.

Pharmacokinetics

After infusion, 5-FU distributes into tumors, intestinal mucosa, bone marrow, liver, and tissues throughout the body. It diffuses readily across the blood–brain barrier and distributes into cerebrospinal fluid (CSF) and brain tissue. The drug is extensively metabolized in the liver and excreted by the kidneys and lungs. The mean half-life of elimination from plasma is about 16 minutes, with a range of 8 to 20 minutes. The clearance of 5-FU is substantially lower in women than in men, whereas age has no appreciable effect on clearance in either gender.

TABLE 35.2 Summary of Selected (C) Cell Cycle–Specific Antineoplastic Drugs

Drug (Trade) Name	Selected Indications	Route and Dosage Range	Pharmacokinetics
(C) Antimetabolites			
[P] 5-fluorouracil (5-FU, Adrucil)	Carcinoma of colon, rectum, stomach, pancreas, breast, and ovary; hepatocellular carcinoma	*Adult:* IV, 12–15 mg/kg daily for 4 d/wk (maximum daily dose: 800 mg), then 6 mg/kg on days 6, 8, 10, and 12; maintenance, repeat first course every 30 d	*Onset:* IV, immediate *Duration:* IV, 6 h $t_{1/2}$: IV, 18–20 min
	Skin cancer, superficial basal cell cancer	*Adult:* Topical, apply sufficient drug to cover affected area bid	*Onset:* Minimal absorption in topical use *Duration:* Unknown $t_{1/2}$: Unknown
cytarabine (Ara-C)	Acute myelocytic leukemia, acute lymphocytic leukemia (ALL), Hodgkin disease, non-Hodgkin lymphoma	*Adult:* IV, 100 mg/m^2 d by continuous infusion for 7 d; then 100 mg/m^{2}q 12h for 1–3 wk; intrathecal, 20–30 mg/m^2	*Onset:* Rapid *Duration:* 12–18 h $t_{1/2}$: 1–3 h
floxuridine (FUDR)	Gastrointestinal (GI) adenocarcinoma with metastasis to liver, gallbladder, or bile ducts	*Adult:* Intra-arterial only, 0.1–0.6 mg/kg/d	*Onset:* Immediate *Duration:* 3 h $t_{1/2}$: 20 h
fludarabine (Fludara)	Chronic lymphocytic leukemia, non-Hodgkin lymphoma (investigational)	*Adult:* IV, 25 mg/m^2 d for 5 d, every 28 d	*Onset:* Rapid *Duration:* Unknown $t_{1/2}$: 10 h
6-mercaptopurine (Purinethol)	Acute leukemia, chronic myelogenous leukemia (CML)	*Adult and child:* PO (induction and consolidation), 2.5 mg/kg/d; maintenance, 1.5–2.5 mg/kg/d	*Onset:* Varies *Duration:* Unknown $t_{1/2}$: 20–50 min
methotrexate (Mexate, Folex)	Hodgkin disease; lymphomas; acute lymphoblastic and myelocytic leukemia; CNS metastasis; carcinoma of ovary, lung, cervix, testicle, breast; sarcomas; epidermoid carcinoma of head and neck	*Adult:* Trophoblastic neoplasms, PO/IM, three to five cycles of 15–30 mg/d for 5 d; leukemia maintenance, IV, 2.5 mg/kg every 14 d or 15 mg/m^2 PO/IM two times a wk; lymphoma, PO, 10–25 mg/d	Onset: PO, varies; IV rapid *Duration:* Unknown $t_{1/2}$: 2–4 h
6-thioguanine (Tabloid)	Acute myelocytic leukemia, chronic granulocytic leukemia	*Adult:* PO, 1–3 mg/kg/d	*Onset:* Slow *Duration:* 8 h $t_{1/2}$: 11 h
(C) Vinca Alkaloids			
[P] vincristine (Oncovin)	Acute lymphocytic leukemia (ALL), Hodgkin and non-Hodgkin lymphoma, CML, sarcomas, breast and small-cell lung cancers	*Adult:* IV, 1.4 mg/m^2/wk *Child:* 2.0 mg/m^2/wk; total single dose of 2 mg is seldom exceeded	*Onset:* Varies *Duration:* Not available $t_{1/2}$: 5 min, then 2–3 h, then 85 h
vinblastine (Velban)	Hodgkin disease, lymphocytic and histiocytic lymphomas, mycosis fungoides, advanced testicular cancer, breast cancer, squamous cell carcinoma of head and neck, Kaposi sarcoma	*Adult:* IV, 0.1 mg/kg–6 mg/m^2 weekly; continuous infusion, 1.4–1.8 mg/d for 5 d	*Onset:* Slow *Duration:* Unknown $t_{1/2}$: 3.7 min, then 16 h, then 24.8 h
vinorelbine (Navelbine)	Non–small-cell lung cancer, breast cancer combination with cisplatin	*Adult:* IV, 30 mg/m^2 weekly	*Onset:* Slow *Duration:* Unknown $t_{1/2}$: 22–66 h

(continued)

TABLE 35.2 Summary of Selected (C) Cell Cycle–Specific Antineoplastic Drugs (continued)

Drug (Trade) Name	Selected Indications	Route and Dosage Range	Pharmacokinetics
(C) Podophyllotoxins			
[P] etoposide (VePesid)	Refractory testicular tumors	*Adult:* IV, testicular cancer, 50–100 mg/m² d for 5 d every 3–4 wk or 100 mg/m² on days 1, 3, and 5	*Onset:* IV, 30 min; PO 30–60 min *Duration:* IV/PO, 20–30 h $t_{1/2}$: 4–11 h
	Small-cell lung cancer	*Adult:* IV, 35 or 50 mg/m² d for 5 d every 3–4 wk	
	Other cancers	*Adult:* PO, twice the IV dose	
teniposide (VM-26, Vumon)	Childhood acute lymphoblastic leukemia	*Adult:* IV, 165 mg/m² with cytarabine 300 mg/m² two times a wk for eight to nine doses	*Onset:* 30 min *Duration:* Unknown $t_{1/2}$: 5 h
(C) Taxanes			
[P] paclitaxel (Taxol)	Metastatic carcinoma of the breast, ovary, small-cell lung cancer	*Adult:* IV, 135–175 mg/m² over 24 h every 3 wk	*Onset:* Rapid *Duration:* 6–12 h $t_{1/2}$: 5.3–17.4 h
docetaxel (Taxotere)	Same as paclitaxel	*Adult:* IV, 60–100 mg/m² every 3 wk	*Onset:* Unknown *Duration:* Unknown $t_{1/2}$: 11 h
(C) Camptothecines			
[P] topotecan (Hycamtin)	Metastatic carcinoma of the ovary	*Adult:* IV, 1.5 mg/m² for 5 days every 3 wk	*Onset:* Unknown *Duration:* Unknown $t_{1/2}$: 3 h
irinotecan (Camptosar, CPT-11)	Metastatic carcinoma of the colon or rectum in patients whose disease has progressed or recurred after 5-FU therapy	*Adult:* IV, 125 mg/m²/wk × 4wk fld. By 2wk rest	*Onset:* Unknown *Duration:* Unknown $t_{1/2}$: 6 h
(C) Miscellaneous			
[P] hydroxyurea (Hydrea)	CML, malignant melanoma, inoperable carcinoma of ovary, squamous-cell carcinoma of head and neck (excluding lip)	*Adult:* PO, for CML, 20–30 mg/kg as continuous therapy; for solid tumors, 80 mg/kg every 3 d or 20–30 mg/kg/d	*Onset:* Varies *Duration:* 18–20 h $t_{1/2}$: 2–3 h
l-asparaginase (Elspar)	ALL, CLL, Hodgkin disease, lymphosarcoma	*Adult:* IV/IM, 200 IU/kg for 28 d; dosage varies with protocol	*Onset:* IM, varies; IV 30–40 min *Duration:* Unknown $t_{1/2}$: 8–30 h

* Note: Antineoplastic drug dosages are calculated specifically for each patient based on his/her body surface area (BSA). The BSA is calculated from height and weight measurements and determined by using a nomogram as illustrated in Chapter 6 or by using an electronic conversion calculator. There is a separate nomogram for the adult and pediatric populations.

Pharmacodynamics

During the S phase, 5-FU exerts its maximum cytotoxic effects. It acts as a "false" antimetabolite, causing a thymine deficiency. This deficiency deprives the cell of DNA and RNA, which are essential for cell division and growth. The result is unbalanced growth and death of the cell. The deprivation of DNA and RNA is most marked in rapidly growing cells because these cells take up 5-FU at a faster rate.

Contraindications and Precautions

5-FU is a pregnancy category D drug. Whether it is excreted in human milk is not known, so caution should be exercised by women who are breast-feeding. The drug has demonstrated mutagenic and teratogenic properties. The use of 5-FU is contraindicated in patients with poor nutritional status, depressed bone marrow function, and any known serious infection. This drug should not be administered to patients

who have a known sensitivity to the drug. Because 5-FU is known for its toxicity, patients who are poor risks should be monitored vigilantly. Death from toxicity can result even in patients who are in relatively good condition. Patients with familial pyrimidinemia should not receive 5-FU because of the potential for severe neurotoxicity.

Adverse Effects

Myelosuppression, evidenced by anemia, leukopenia, and thrombocytopenia, is the dose-limiting side effect of 5-FU. The **nadir** is the period during which the maximum cytotoxic effect of the drug is exerted on the bone marrow, causing the lowest blood cell count. The white blood cell (WBC) nadir occurs within 10 to 14 days after the drug is given; recovery is within 21 days.

Other dose-dependent toxicities are nausea, vomiting, anorexia, diarrhea, and stomatitis. GI ulceration and hemorrhage can lead to death. Cutaneous changes can also occur: alopecia (hair loss; thinning of the hair); hyperpigmentation of the skin, hands, and vein along the site of infusion; brittle and cracking nails; maculopapular rash; and painful, erythematous desquamation and fissures of the palms and soles. Cardiotoxicity is also an important toxicity of 5-FU. Cardiac events occur during the first 72 hours of the initial treatment cycle, manifested by chest pain, electrocardiogram (ECG) changes, arrhythmias, pulmonary edema, myocardial infarction, and (rarely) cardiac arrest.

Patients may also develop an acute cerebellar syndrome (which may persist after the drug is stopped) characterized by headache, disorientation, and nystagmus. Photophobia and ocular changes, such as increased lacrimation and blurred vision, may occur as well.

Drug Interactions

5-FU is incompatible with diazepam, droperidol, metoclopramide, ondansetron, and other chemotherapeutic drugs such as cytarabine, gallium nitrate, methotrexate, and vinorelbine. Leucovorin calcium may enhance the toxicity of 5-FU. Some drug–laboratory test interferences can occur with 5-FU administration, such as increased excretion of 5-hydroxyindoleacetic acid (5-HIAA); plasma albumin levels may decrease as a result of protein malabsorption. Table 35.3 lists drugs that interact with 5-FU.

Assessment of Relevant Core Patient Variables

Health Status

Before treatment begins, assess the patient's hematologic profile and document baseline neurologic status. Because GI alterations may occur with 5-FU dosing, check the patient's oral mucosa, bowel elimination patterns, and dietary habits. Review the patient's drug and hypersensitivity history, especially to 5-FU. Because of potential cutaneous changes, assess the condition of the patient's skin, nails, and hair. Monitor patients with a pre-existing cardiac disease closely.

Life Span and Gender

Explore the reproductive goals of the patient and assess women of childbearing age for pregnancy and lactation. Chemotherapy with 5-FU may cause fetal harm when administered to pregnant women. The drug has been found to be mutagenic and teratogenic in laboratory animals. It is not known whether 5-FU is excreted in the breast milk; therefore, breast-feeding may be hazardous. Compare the benefits and risks to children. The safety and efficacy of 5-FU in children are not established.

Lifestyle, Diet, and Habits

One adverse effect of 5-FU is skin sensitivity to the sun. Ask the patient whether he or she engages in activities that cause undue exposure to the sun and what methods of sun protection are used. Assess the patient's feelings regarding hair loss—the major visible reminder that the patient is undergoing chemotherapy—and consider its effect on the patient's sexuality and body image. The possibility and actuality of hair loss can be very distressing to the patient, particularly if he or she has an active social and work life. Because of 5-FU's deleterious effects on the GI mucosa, obtain information on normal dietary intake and eating patterns, which might necessitate dietary modifications.

Environment

5-FU is given in both inpatient and ambulatory care settings. In some situations, 5-FU may be given as a continuous infusion through an ambulatory pump in the home setting. In these instances, explore whether the patient or significant other is ready to take on this responsibility and knows how to troubleshoot problems with the pump, should they arise.

Nursing Diagnoses and Outcomes

- Risk for Infection related to drug-induced suppression of bone marrow function
  Desired outcome: The patient will be free from infection and exercise caution to avoid exposure to sources of infection.
- Risk for Injury: Bleeding related to drug-induced suppression of bone marrow function

TABLE 35.3 Agents That Interact With P 5-Fluorouracil

Interactants	Effect and Significance	Nursing Management
thiazide diuretics: hydrochlorothiazide, chlorothiazide, chlorthalidone, benzthiazide, metolazone	Possible blood abnormalities	Notify physician for possible dose modification. Monitor hematopoietic status of the patient.
cimetidine	Increased pharmacologic effect of 5-fluorouracil (5-FU)	Same as above.
leucovorin	Potentiates toxicity of 5-FU	Same as above.

Desired outcome: The patient will attain pretreatment hematologic status and learn to recognize, monitor, and manage situations that might induce bleeding.
- Imbalanced Nutrition: Less than Body Requirements related to drug-induced nausea, vomiting, stomatitis, and diarrhea
  Desired outcome: *The patient will maintain adequate nutrition with good emetic control and less frequent passage of stools. Oral mucosa will remain intact, and the patient will not experience pain or discomfort in the GI mucosa.*
- Disturbed Body Image related to loss of cutaneous integrity, as evidenced by alopecia and changes in skin and nails
  Desired outcome: *The patient will develop coping strategies (use of wigs, hair covering) to enhance appearance that may be distorted because of hair loss. In addition, cutaneous integrity will be sustained.*
- Disturbed Sensory Perception related to ocular changes, photophobia, and cerebellar ataxia
  Desired outcome: *The patient will be free from adverse effects resulting from oculomotor dysfunction.*

Planning and Intervention

Maximizing Therapeutic Effects

The daily dose of 5-FU should not exceed 800 mg. The dosage should be reduced if the patient has impaired liver function or poor nutritional status. The drug should be protected from light and should be inspected for precipitates before infusion. The solution should be stored at controlled temperature. If a precipitate caused by low-temperature storage is noted, the solution can be restabilized by heating it to 140°F, shaking it vigorously, and allowing it to cool down to body temperature before administration. A slight discoloration may happen during storage, which does not affect the drug's potency and safety.

Minimizing Adverse Effects

Monitor the patient closely because hematologic and GI toxicities can be fatal despite dosage reductions. A WBC differential count should be obtained before each drug course. Treatment should be withheld if laboratory test values are below safe levels. The drug should not be administered to patients with familial pyrimidinemia because of the risk for severe neurotoxicity.

If any of the following conditions occur, the drug should be discontinued:

- Stomatitis and esophagopharyngitis (first visible sign)
- Leukopenia (WBC <3,500 cells/mm^3) or a rapidly dropping WBC
- Thrombocytopenia (platelet count <100,000 cells/mm^3)
- Intractable vomiting
- Diarrhea
- GI ulceration and bleeding
- Bleeding from any site

Providing Patient and Family Education

- Follow the guidelines described in Box 35.3.
- Explain that 5-FU, like most chemotherapeutic drugs with a narrow margin of safety, is highly toxic.
- Give troubleshooting instructions if an alternative access device or an ambulatory infusion device is used at home.

COMMUNITY-BASED CONCERNS

Box 35.3 General Patient and Family Education for Chemotherapy

The nurse plays a pivotal role in providing adequate information to assist the patient/family with the new roles so that treatment outcomes will be achieved. After diagnosis, the treatment modality is discussed and chosen. For most cancers, chemotherapy plays a significant benefit. The talking points for the nurse when called on to educate patients, irrespective of the type of chemotherapeutic agent used, include:

- Instruct patient about the significant side effects and reportable signs and symptoms of the chemotherapeutic agent(s).
- Emphasize self-management measures to be undertaken to prevent or decrease the side effects:
  Practice good personal hygiene, wash hands frequently, and avoid sources of infection
  Maintain dietary intake of food and fluids. Refer to dietician for consultation.
  Avoid trauma or injury and potential sources of bleeding by shaving with an electric razor, avoiding aspirin and other nonsteroidal anti-inflammatory drugs, and avoiding unnecessary injections, use of rectal thermometers, and venipunctures.
  Check urine, stool, skin for signs of bleeding.
  Practice good oral hygiene, use of soft toothbrush, noncommercial (i.e., alcohol-based) mouthwashes, use of lubricants.
  Schedule appointments for blood tests and follow-up visits for chemotherapy and related medications.
- If the patient goes to other physicians, dentists, or another health care provider, patient should inform them of chemotherapy treatment.
- Teach patients the importance of relaxation techniques and other forms of complementary medicine from which they might benefit.
- Referrals to other agencies and support groups might be helpful. Provide patient with a list of these resources.
- Instruct patients in the importance of maintaining a balance between rest and exercise to avoid fatigue.
- Explain to patient that some of side effects of treatment are reversible and are thus not a sign of disease progression.
- If patients are using chemotherapy drugs at home, teach the patient how to properly handle, store, and dispose of the agents and related materials.
- Teach patient to accept a "new" baseline especially in activities and responsibilities imposed by demands of disease and treatment. Teach patients to learn how to delegate and ask for assistance with activities of daily living.

The patient should also know whom to call in case of problems.
- Explain that nausea and vomiting may occur 3 to 6 hours after drug therapy is administered; provide an appropriate antiemetic regimen. The metallic taste of the drug may be minimized by sucking on hard candy.
- If loose stools exceed normal bowel patterns by more than three movements daily, instruct the patient to observe the stools and notify the prescriber if stools are black or if blood is visible.
- Mouth sores may develop 5 to 8 days after drug administration. Offer helpful strategies such as practicing daily oral hygiene after meals and at bedtime, using $NaHCO_3$ rinses (1½ teaspoon of sodium bicarbonate to 1 quart of

water), brushing with a soft toothbrush, avoiding commercial mouthwashes, and gently flossing with unwaxed dental floss. If bleeding occurs, flossing should be stopped until bleeding subsides.
- Caution the patient not to use aspirin or any pain-relieving drugs containing aspirin without consulting the prescriber.
- Carefully monitor patients with pre-existing cardiac conditions.
- Teach the patient to self-assess for signs and symptoms of potential infection, check temperature, and report temperature spikes higher than 101°F.
- Suggest that the patient apply moisturizer to the lips and to avoid irritating, very hot, cold, or spicy foods and beverages. Bland, cool, soft foods, such as yogurt, custards, gelatins, and puddings, may be less irritating choices.
- Help the patient to understand that drug therapy produces photosensitivity. Instruct the patient to avoid the sun or protect the skin by applying a sunscreen (skin protection factor [SPF] ≥15) and wearing protective clothing year round.
- Encourage the patient to express his or her concerns about the effects of cutaneous changes on body image and assist in developing strategies to minimize the emotional impact. You might offer cosmetic strategies, such as wearing nail polish to cover darkened, dry, brittle nails and using wigs, hats, and scarves to hide hair loss.
- Instruct the patient to notify the physician if confusion or any visual disturbances occur.
- Advise women of childbearing potential about the possibility of harm to the fetus and about methods of contraception.

Ongoing Assessment and Evaluation

The main adverse effects of 5-FU therapy are alterations in the patient's hematopoietic system and GI functions. Therefore, monitor the patient's complete blood counts (CBCs) closely during each drug administration cycle to make sure that bone marrow recovery has occurred before another dose of the drug is given. Likewise, assess the patient's nutritional status. Stomatitis or other problems related to the gastric mucosa should be kept under control to avoid putting the patient at risk for poor nutrition.

MEMORY CHIP

P 5-Fluorouracil

- Indicated for treating carcinoma of the colon, rectum, breast, stomach, and pancreas
- Major contraindications: poor nutritional status, decreased bone marrow reserve or a potentially serious infection
- Most common adverse effects: alopecia and other cutaneous changes, such as photosensitivity, and increased pigmentation of the skin
- Dose-limiting effects: mainly on the bone marrow manifested by myelosuppression and the gastrointestinal mucosa, causing nausea, vomiting, diarrhea, and stomatitis
- **Life span alert: Advise women of child-bearing age of the potential for harm to the fetus and so that they practice contraception. It is not known whether the drug is excreted in breast milk; therefore, explain that breast-feeding is not advised.**
- Maximizing therapeutic effects: Potentiate antineoplastic activity of 5-FU by reduced folates such as the addition of leucovorin calcium.
- Minimizing adverse effects: Monitor CBC and assess for signs and symptoms of myelosuppression, which include infection and bleeding.
- Most important patient education: Teach patient good oral care and to monitor for signs and symptoms of stomatitis and infection. Advise patient of the possibility of transient alopecia reversed after chemotherapy is finished.

Drug Significantly Different From P 5-Fluorouracil

Methotrexate (MTX) is a folate antimetabolite that induces folate depletion, leading to the inhibition of purine synthesis and resulting in arrested DNA, RNA, and protein synthesis. MTX is indicated in managing Hodgkin disease; trophoblastic neoplasm; acute leukemia; meningeal leukemia; breast carcinoma; head, neck, and lung neoplasms; Burkitt lymphoma; osteosarcoma; lymphosarcoma; and mycosis fungoides. It may be given in a variety of doses and schedules through various routes of administration, such as oral, intramuscular, intravenous, intrathecal (in preservative-free solution) and intra-arterial. A small portion is metabolized in the liver; the drug is excreted in the urine mostly as unchanged drug. Because the drug is secreted by the renal tubules, certain drugs that follow the same pathway, such as salicylates, sulfonamides, phenytoin, and penicillin, may compete with MTX excretion, resulting in accumulation and increased toxicity. Therefore, these drugs should be discontinued 2 days before and restarted 2 days after MTX therapy. MTX toxicity includes nausea and vomiting, diarrhea, cumulative myelosuppression, neurotoxicity (at high doses), photosensitivity, rashes, and acute hepatotoxicity manifested by elevated liver enzyme levels. With high-dose regimens, the following important considerations should be undertaken:

- Emetogenic potential is high; initiate an appropriate antiemetic regimen.
- Monitor urine specific gravity, urine output, and urinary pH. Administer sodium bicarbonate and hydrate the patient to maintain urinary alkalinization (pH >7) and urinary output of more than 100 mL/hour.
- Obtain orders for leucovorin rescue. Leucovorin is given to bypass the inhibitor action of MTX and supplies the form of folic acid needed by the normal cells for DNA synthesis. Leucovorin is usually initiated 24 to 36 hours after MTX, according to a prescribed schedule based on serum MTX and creatinine levels. No doses of leucovorin should be missed because missed doses may increase toxicity.
- Monitor MTX blood levels for 72 hours until the nontoxic level of less than 0.1 micromolar is reached.

C MITOTIC INHIBITORS

The mitotic inhibitors interfere with the formation of the mitotic spindle, causing metaphase arrest. They are primarily known as M-phase active drugs, but they may also have

some activity in the G_2 and S phases. These drugs are the vinca alkaloids, the podophyllotoxins, and the taxanes.

Ⓒ Vinca Alkaloids

Vinca alkaloids are extracts of the periwinkle plant *Vinca rosea*. They bind to microtubular proteins, which are key to forming the mitotic spindle of the dividing cells. This binding arrests mitosis and eventually causes cell death. The vinca alkaloids act mainly in the M phase. However, high doses of the vinca alkaloids vincristine (Oncovorin, Oncovin, Vincasar PFS) and vinblastine (Velban, VLB) can also disrupt RNA and protein synthesis. Drugs in this category include vincristine, vinblastine, and vinorelbine (Navelbine). The drug vincristine is discussed as the representative vinca alkaloid drug.

NURSING MANAGEMENT OF THE PATIENT RECEIVING P VINCRISTINE

Core Drug Knowledge

Pharmacotherapeutics

The major clinical use of vincristine is in treating acute lymphoblastic leukemia. It is used in combination therapy for Hodgkin disease, non-Hodgkin malignant lymphomas, sarcoma, breast cancer, small cell lung cancer, rhabdomyosarcoma, neuroblastoma, and Wilms tumor. The recommended dosage of vincristine for an adult is discussed in Table 35.2. For children weighing less than 10 kg, or with body surface areas (BSAs) of less than 1 square meter, the dose is 0.05 mg/kg per week.

Pharmacokinetics

Following IV administration, vincristine binds extensively to both the plasma proteins and the blood elements, particularly the platelets. Its penetration across the blood–brain barrier is poor. Vincristine is metabolized by the hepatic system, and 70% of the drug is excreted in the bile or feces. A small fraction is excreted in the urine.

Pharmacodynamics

The mechanism of action of vincristine is attributed to mitotic inhibition, which arrests cell division in the metaphase stage of mitosis. The drug interferes with a protein called tubulin, which is required for formation of microtubules and the mitotic spindle. The depolymerized tubulin proteins do not allow the spindle proteins to assemble, and cell division is halted in the metaphase.

Contraindications and Precautions

Vincristine is a pregnancy category D drug. Neurotoxicity from vincristine may be more pronounced in patients with underlying neurologic problems. Vincristine is contraindicated in patients with the demyelinating form of Charcot-Marie-Tooth syndrome, a neurologic disease characterized by absence of deep tendon reflexes. Because liver disease may alter the elimination of vincristine, dosage modifications may be needed in patients with elevated bilirubin levels. Care must be taken to prevent accidental contamination of the eyes, especially when the drug is administered intravenously under severe pressure, because the drug can cause severe eye irritation, including corneal ulceration if it splashes into the eye. If eye contamination happens, the eyes must be washed immediately and thoroughly.

Vincristine is administered by IV routes only. Given intrathecally, vincristine may be fatal. Drug delivery may be by IV push directly over 1 minute or given by IV sidearm through a running IV line. It can also be given by continuous infusion, but only through a central line. Vincristine is a **vesicant.** Vesicants are extremely acidic drugs that may cause substantial tissue damage when accidental infiltration occurs. Therefore, extravasation precautions should be exercised during their infusion (Box 35.4).

Adverse Effects

The most common dose-limiting adverse effects with vincristine are neurologic, including motor, sensory, and autonomic neuropathies. Signs and symptoms of these neurologic deficits include loss of deep tendon reflexes, numbness and tingling of the hands and feet, foot drop, myalgias, weakness, and jaw pain. Constipation, which is a forerunner of paralytic ileus, can be serious and bothersome to the patient. The neurotoxic signs and symptoms appear weeks or months after drug administration and are long lasting and slow to resolve. The severity of the neurotoxicity is related to the cumulative dose of the drug.

Drug Interactions

The toxicity of vincristine may be potentiated by drugs that act on the peripheral nervous system. Vincristine has been reported to increase the uptake of high-dose MTX by cancer cells. When given concomitantly with digoxin, vincristine may decrease serum digoxin levels and, consequently, the effects of digoxin. Mitomycin used together with vincristine may cause acute pulmonary reactions. Table 35.4 summarizes interactions with vincristine.

Assessment of Relevant Core Patient Variables

Health Status

Careful consideration should be given to administering vincristine to patients with pre-existing neuromuscular disease or when other neurotoxic drugs are given. Clinical evaluation, including a thorough history and physical examination, may be needed for dose adjustments. Monitor the patient's hematologic profile. Concurrent use of drugs that cause constipation, such as narcotic analgesics and cholinergic drugs, should also be taken into account.

Life Span and Gender

Vincristine may affect sexual function. Explore the patient's sexual patterns. Assess women of childbearing age for pregnancy and lactation. Vincristine may cause fetal harm; therefore, pregnant patients should be apprised of this possibility if the drug is used in pregnancy. Whether vincristine is excreted in breast milk is unknown. Because of the potential for adverse effects in breast-feeding infants, the patient

BOX 35.4 Managing Peripheral Extravasation

Extravasation is the inadvertent infiltration of the chemotherapeutic drug into the subcutaneous tissues surrounding the site of infusion. Because a vesicant drug is very acidic, it can cause severe damage depending on the tissue it infiltrates, the amount of drug the tissue absorbs, and the length of the tissue's exposure to the infiltrated drug.

Extravasation over joint spaces, tendons, or neuromuscular bundles increases the risk of tissue damage. When a drug extravasates, the patient typically complains of pain, burning, or discomfort at the injection site. Sometimes pain might be a delayed reaction with other signs, such as reddening of the skin and blistering, which may progress to severe tissue involvement. The best cure for extravasation is prevention.

The nurse should be familiar with the institutional policies for managing extravasation. Although specific protocols for managing extravasation may vary among health care settings, general guidelines for managing extravasation include the following:

- Stop the infusion immediately and restart the infusion at a new site.
- Apply warm or cold compresses as indicated to the extravasation site, and if prescribed, administer a local antidote, such as hyalurodinase, to minimize any tissue damage.
- Notify the health care provider.
- Rest and elevate the affected extremity for 48 hours.
- Apply a sterile dressing that allows the extravasation area to remain visible. Avoid any pressure to the site.
- Obtain a photograph of the site for baseline comparisons
- Document the following: patient's name, date and time of extravasation, name of drug, approximate volume of infiltrate, needle gauge, site of extravasation, symptoms reported by the patient and assessed by the nurse, nursing measures implemented, name of health care provider notified, patient education provided, and nurse's signature.
- Consult physician regarding need for referral to plastic surgeon, if appropriate.

FLOWSHEET FOR SUSPECTED/ACTUAL CHEMOTHERAPY EXTRAVASATION

addressograph stamp

Date:__________ Date extravasation occurred:__________

INITIAL EVALUATION (Day 0)

DESCRIPTION OF EXTRAVASATION
Name and Volume of drug given:__________
IV site location: (indicate on diagram and describe):
____
Needle type and gauge:__________
Patient complaints:__________
Physician notified (name):__________
R.N. (name):__________

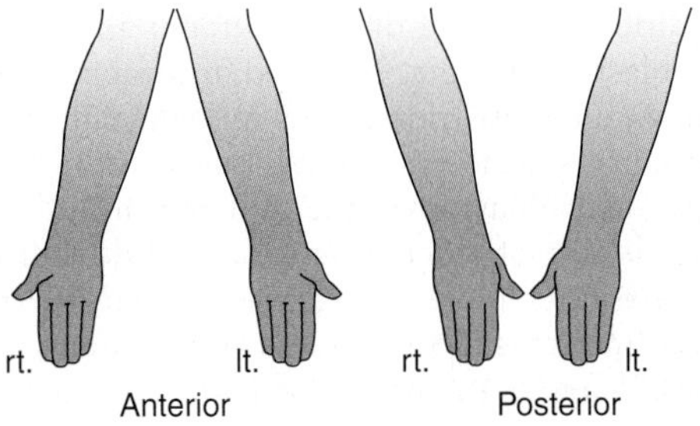

INITIAL INTERVENTIONS
Date
______ Antidote admin. (specify)______
______ Cold compresses
______ Warm compresses
______ 1% Hydrocortisone cream applied
______ Baseline photo

ADDITIONAL INTERVENTIONS
Date
______ Dermatology Consult
______ Plastic Surg. Consult
______ Wound care (described)
______
______
______ Follow-up photo

PATIENT TEACHING
Date
______ Extravasation fact card given and reviewed
______ Follow-up schedule reviewed

TABLE 35.4 Agents That Interact With P Vincristine

Interactants	Effect and Significance	Nursing Management
digoxin	Decreased serum level and therapeutic effect	Monitor digoxin level.
methotrexate (MTX)	Increased cellular uptake of MTX when given sequentially	Notify physician for dosage modification. Monitor for signs and symptoms of neurotoxicity.

should decide either to stop breast-feeding or to stop drug therapy. Note the patient's age and developmental status. Vincristine therapy may cause azoospermia and amenorrhea in postpubertal patients, although recovery occurs after therapy is completed. Risk for potential motor and sensory dysfunction associated with vincristine is greater in elderly patients than among younger ones.

Lifestyle, Diet, and Habits

Before drug administration, determine the patient's sensory, motor, and perceptual functions, because of the potential dysfunctions associated with vincristine. Consider bowel elimination patterns and food and fluid intake.

Environment

Be aware of the environment in which the drug will be administered. Vincristine may be given in an inpatient or ambulatory care setting.

Nursing Diagnoses and Outcomes

- Disturbed Sensory Perception related to perceptual neuropathies, as evidenced by absent deep tendon reflexes, numbness, weakness, and myalgias
  Desired outcome: *The patient will be able to function safely without injury. Optimal sensory and perceptual function will be maintained.*
- Risk for Constipation related to adverse effects of vincristine
  Desired outcome: *The patient will have a regular bowel elimination pattern and will pass soft stools.*
- Risk for Infection and Bleeding related to depression of bone marrow function
  Desired outcome: *Bone marrow recovery will be attained; rare and mild myelosuppression might occur. The patient will verbalize and also implement self-care measures to prevent infection.*
- Impaired Skin Integrity related to potential for vesicant extravasation
  Desired outcome: *The skin will remain intact, without cutaneous breakdown. The patient and health care provider will be able to recognize signs and symptoms of suspected extravasation and initiate prompt measures that will prevent further tissue damage.*
- Disturbed Body Image related to drug-induced hair loss
  Desired outcome: *The patient will be accepting of changes in physical appearance and will develop strategies to cope with hair loss.*
- Ineffective Sexuality Patterns: Impotence related to adverse effects of vincristine
  Desired outcome: *The patient will understand that this effect of the drug is reversible and will exhibit behavior changes that will result in more satisfying sexual functioning.*

Planning and Intervention

Maximizing Therapeutic Effects

Before each drug administration, monitor the patient's complete blood count (CBC) to ensure that it is within safe limits. The drug is light sensitive and should be protected from light. It should also be refrigerated. An initial bolus should be given through a new and patent free-flowing IV access, noting patient's response during and after drug instillation. If the drug is given as a continuous infusion, a central line should always be used. Vincristine (Oncovin) is only given intravenously. Intrathecal administration can result in death.

Minimizing Adverse Effects

The occurrence of peripheral neuropathies is a major concern with vincristine therapy. Its toxicity to the nerve fibers can induce severe motor, sensory, and autonomic deficits. Conduct a neurologic evaluation of the patient before each cycle to assess for major changes. Report any changes in perceptual or sensory functioning and consult the oncologist immediately regarding dosage modifications or discontinuation of the drug.

Because vincristine has vesicant properties, careful attention should be given to prevent extravasation (see Box 35.4). You should be thoroughly familiar with appropriate antidotes and protocols for the use of vesicants (Table 35.5).

Providing Patient and Family Education

- Follow the guidelines described in Box 35.3.
- Discuss and explain precautionary measures to the patient to lessen further insult to the hematologic and cutaneous systems.
- Advise the patient to promptly report problems resulting from the IV infusion—for example, pain, redness, swelling, or blistering at the infusion site.
- Instruct the patient and caregiver to observe and monitor the infusion site for early extravasation and cutaneous reactions.
- Teach the patient and caregiver how to care for suspected extravasation at home until medical attention can be obtained, if needed.
- Discuss methods for coping with adverse effects, such as a metallic taste sensation during drug administration, nausea or appetite loss, or constipation accompanied by cramping.
- Encourage the patient to maintain adequate nutrition. A high-fiber diet and plenty of fluids should be consumed to help relieve constipation. Stool softeners, laxatives, or both may be given for severe constipation. The usual constipation regimen consists of Colace, 100 mg once a day; and Senokot, two tablets at bedtime.
- Instruct the patient to avoid injury related to drug-related altered sensory and perceptual changes manifested by muscle weakness and neuropathy, numbness of the fingers and toes, tingling sensation, or absence of deep tendon reflexes. These changes may be temporary or permanent.
- Review with the patient strategies for taking care of hair and skin because thinning or loss of hair may occur 2 or 3 weeks after treatment. Teach the patient techniques to provide gentle care by avoiding heat or chemical irritants, and wearing wigs or hair coverings. You can help the patient recognize that hair will regrow within a few months after therapy stops.
- Emphasize to the patient and caregiver the importance of scheduling and keeping appointments for laboratory tests and medical checkups.
- Explore with the patient and significant other sexuality issues and discuss strategies for maintaining sexual health. Reassure the patient that impotence, should it occur, is usually reversible after drug is discontinued.

TABLE 35.5 Common Vesicants and Known Antidotes

Vesicant	Antidote	Nursing Management
vincristine (Oncovin, Vincasar PFS) vinblastine (Velban) vindesine (Eldisine)	Hyaloronidase	Stop infusion of drug. Inject antidote locally to extravasation site. Apply warm compress to extravasation site for 15–20 min at least qid for the first 2 days.
vinorelbine (Navelbine)	No known antidote	Stop infusion of drug. Use institutional or ONS guidelines.
mechlorethamine hydrochloride (nitrogen mustard)	Thiosulfate	Stop infusion of drug. Rapid administration of antidote is crucial. Prepare antidote as prescribed. The solution should be ⅙ molar. Inject solution through IV cannula–2-mL solution for each mL of vesicant extravasated.
Others:	No known antidotes	Stop infusion of drug. Use institutional or ONS guidelines. Institute comfort measures.
cisplatin (Platinol) dactinomycin (Actinomycin) daunorubicin (Cerubidine) doxorubicin (Adriamycin) epirubicin (Ellence) idarubicin (Idamycin) fluorouracil (5-FU, rare vesicant potential), mitomycin (Mitomycin-C) mitoxantrone (Novantrone)	Isotonic sodium	Rapid administration of antidote is crucial. Apply cold compresses as indicated. Teach patient how to prevent infection.

Ongoing Assessment and Evaluation

Acute elevation of uric acid may occur during induction of remission for leukemic patients. Measure uric acid levels during the first 3 to 4 weeks of treatment and undertake measures to prevent the occurrence of uric acid nephropathy. Assess the patient's bowel function and motor and sensory functions daily.

Drug Closely Related to P Vincristine

Vinblastine (Velban) is another vinca alkaloid derived from the periwinkle plant. Although its chemical structure, pharmacokinetics, and mechanism of action are similar to those of vincristine, this drug has markedly more clinical indications than vincristine does. Like vincristine in its efficacy in treating malignant lymphomas and Hodgkin disease, vinblastine is also used for chemotherapy in mycosis fungoides, testicular carcinoma, Kaposi sarcoma, choriocarcinoma, squamous cell cancer of the head and neck, and breast cancer.

The toxicity profile of vinblastine differs from that of vincristine. The dose-limiting toxicity of vinblastine is myelosuppression, whereas that of vincristine is neurotoxicity. Neurotoxicity occurs less frequently; although with high doses, this side effect can occur. Vincristine is considered more potent than vinblastine because it rarely affects the bone marrow. The mildly myelosuppressive action of vincristine makes it more attractive than vinblastine for combination chemotherapy.

C Podophyllotoxins

The podophyllotoxins were isolated from the mandrake plant (May crab apple). Examples of drugs in this group are etoposide (VP-16) and teniposide (VM-26), both of which

MEMORY CHIP

P Vincristine

- Primarily indicated for acute leukemia and for other cancers such as Hodgkin disease, breast cancer, neuroblastoma, and multiple myeloma
- Major contraindications: demyelating form of CharcotMarie syndrome
- Most common adverse effect: tissue necrosis if the drug, which is a vesicant, accidentally extravasates
- Most serious adverse effects: neurotoxic deficits manifested by paresthesias, myalgias, loss of deep tendon reflexes, and jaw pain. Paralytic ileus as evidenced by constipation may also occur.
- **Life span alert: Caution elderly patients regarding the potential for motor and sensory deficits that may compromise their safety and sensory acuity. Vincristine may cause fetal harm or risk to mothers who are breast-feeding. Apprise patients of these side effects.**
- Maximizing therapeutic effects: the drug is light sensitive; protect it from light. Infuse it slowly over approximately 1 minute.
- Minimizing adverse effects: Always assess bowel elimination pattern because of the danger of paralytic ileus.
- Ensure good vascular access and monitor for signs and symptoms of extravasation.
- Most important patient education: Instruct the patient to obtain a prescription for a prophylactic stool regimen.

are semisynthetic derivatives extracted from the American mandrake, *Podophyllum peltatum.* They act in the premitotic, G_2, and S phases and interfere with the topoisomerase II enzyme reaction. The drug etoposide is discussed as the representative podophyllotoxin drug.

NURSING MANAGEMENT OF THE PATIENT RECEIVING P ETOPOSIDE

Core Drug Knowledge

Pharmacotherapeutics

Etoposide is the prototype drug of the subgroup of alkaloids called podophyllotoxins. This drug is used in combination therapy for refractory testicular tumors and small cell lung cancer. It is also effective in treating Hodgkin and non-Hodgkin lymphoma, acute lymphocytic leukemia (ALL), breast cancer, and multiple myeloma. Etoposide is usually administered intravenously but is also available in an oral formulation (see Table 35.2). The recommended dose for oral use is twice the IV dose rounded to the nearest 50 mg.

Pharmacokinetics

Etoposide binds to serum albumin and becomes extensively bound to tissues (see Table 35.2).

It is predominantly excreted in the urine and to a lesser extent in the bile. About 30% of the drug is excreted unchanged. The drug's half-life is 4 to 11 hours.

Pharmacodynamics

Etoposide acts by inhibiting a DNA enzyme called topoisomerase II, causing breaks in the double strands of protein-linked DNA. This action inhibits DNA synthesis in the S and G_2 phases so that cells do not enter mitosis and prophase.

Contraindications and Precautions

Etoposide should not be given to patients with a known hypersensitivity to this drug or teniposide, the other podophyllotoxin derivative. The drug should never be administered by IV push or rapid IV infusion because doing so can cause hypotension. It should be infused over 30 to 60 minutes or longer, depending on the volume of the infusion. If the patient is taking warfarin concomitantly with etoposide, the patient's prothrombin time should be monitored closely. Etoposide is a pregnancy category D drug and should not be used in pregnant women.

Adverse Effects

Hypersensitivity or anaphylaxis-like reactions manifested by hypotension, chills, fever, facial flushing, bronchospasm, dyspnea, and tachycardia can occur during an etoposide infusion. However, these signs are not related to any cardiorespiratory pathology but rather to the rapid infusion of the drug itself. They can be ameliorated by stopping the infusion and giving the patient IV fluids, corticosteroids, antihistamines, and volume expanders as ordered.

The major dose-limiting effect of etoposide is myelosuppression, manifested primarily by granulocytopenia, which reaches nadir in 7 to 14 days; the platelet nadir is 9 to 16 days after parenteral administration. Recovery is noted in 20 days. When etoposide is given orally, the nadir granulocyte counts occur between 21 and 28 days, with recovery in 35 days. The other adverse effects of note are mild to moderate nausea and vomiting, which can be controlled by antiemetics. GI toxicities are more pronounced with the oral form of the drug. Hepatic toxicity, shown by elevated liver enzyme levels, results from administering higher than recommended doses.

Drug-induced alopecia is reversible when the drug is discontinued. Patients who have had radiation therapy might get **radiation recall,** which is characterized by erythematous rash in the irradiated area. This condition may progress to desquamation, vesicle formation, and permanent hyperpigmentation of the affected area.

Etoposide is classified as an **irritant.** As such, it may produce pain, urticaria, redness, and inflammation along the path of the vein into which the drug is infusing. Unlike vesicants, irritants do not generally cause tissue damage. Etoposide is also associated with the development of secondary malignancies.

Drug Interactions

Etoposide has a synergistic effect with cisplatin. It is incompatible with gallium nitrate and MTX. Table 35.6 presents more information about these interactions.

Assessment of Relevant Core Patient Variables

Health Status

Assess the patient for prior extensive myelosuppressive chemotherapy or irradiation to marrow-bearing areas of the skeleton. Knowing such a history is important so that dose reduction can be considered, if indicated, to avoid the potential for more severe myelosuppression. The patient's CBC should be determined before and during etoposide therapy. The patient's renal and hepatic functions should also

TABLE 35.6 Agents That Interact With P Etoposide

Interactants	Effect and Significance	Nursing Management
warfarin	Increases prothrombin time (PT)	Monitor PT closely. Monitor for signs of increased bleeding.
gallium-nitrate and methotrexate	Incompatible combinations	Avoid combined therapy.

be monitored, so that dose adjustments may be made in case these systems malfunction.

Life Span and Gender

Document the age and gender of the patient. The safety and efficacy of etoposide have not been established in children. Explore the patient's sexual patterns and reproductive goals. Assess women of childbearing age for pregnancy. This drug has mutagenic, carcinogenic, and teratogenic properties. Secondary malignancies have been reported with the use of this drug.

Lifestyle, Diet, and Habits

Alopecia affects 20% to 90% of patients who receive etoposide. Explore with the patient the likely effect of therapy on sexuality and body image. Hair loss could be complete and may be more distressing for socially active, working, or female patients.

Environment

Be aware of the environment in which the drug will be administered. Etoposide can be given in an acute care or ambulatory setting where the necessary clinical support is available in case hypotension or an anaphylactic reaction develops.

Nursing Diagnoses and Outcomes

- Risk for Injury related to etoposide-induced hypotension or anaphylactic reaction
  Desired outcome: *The patient will not experience hypotension or anaphylactic reaction.*
- Risk for Infection related to bleeding resulting from suppression of bone marrow function
  Desired outcome: *The patient will recover adequate hematologic function. The patient will undertake self-care measures to prevent infection and bleeding.*
- Imbalanced Nutrition: Less than Body Requirements related to nausea, vomiting, and anorexia from drug therapy
  Desired outcome: *The patient will maintain proper nutritional status and good emetic control.*
- Disturbed Body Image related to drug-induced alopecia
  Desired outcome: *The patient will implement coping strategies to alleviate feelings associated with loss of hair.*
- Sexual Dysfunction related to disease process and drug therapy
  Desired outcome: *The patient will increase knowledge about the effects of chemotherapy on sexual function and will continue functioning without interfering with sexual patterns and reproductive goals.*
- Impaired Skin Integrity resulting from irritation to infusion site and possible radiation recall
  Desired outcome: *The patient's skin will remain intact without breakdown from irritant chemotherapy. Patient will demonstrate competence in wound management if radiation recall occurs.*

Planning and Intervention

Maximizing Therapeutic Effects

The stability of etoposide depends on the concentration. To prevent crystallization, it should be diluted in 5% dextrose for injection or in 0.9% sodium chloride solution to reach a final concentration of 0.2 to 0.4 mg/mL. At a concentration of 0.2 mg/mL, etoposide is stable in a glass container for 96 hours and in plastic for 48 hours.

Minimizing Adverse Effects

Because of dose-limiting myelosuppression, WBC counts should be monitored before chemotherapy and at the expected WBC nadir. The patient receiving etoposide therapy should be observed closely for hypotension or anaphylactic reactions. The drug should be given by slow infusion, never by rapid infusion, over 30 to 60 minutes and possibly longer, depending on the volume of the infusion. Cardiopulmonary resuscitation equipment should be present at the patient's bedside. During drug administration, help allay the patient's fears about possible anaphylactic reactions by staying with the patient and infusing the solution slowly through a patent IV line to prevent hypotension and chemical phlebitis. Warm compresses should be applied to the affected site. Monitor the patient's hepatic and renal function before and during therapy. Assess for signs and symptoms of infection and teach the patient to monitor and self-report the same. If the oral formulation of etoposide is given, also give the patient adequate antiemetics.

Providing Patient and Family Education

- Follow the guidelines described in Box 35.3.
- Focus education for patients receiving etoposide on the importance of minimizing risks related to infection and injury, which are major concerns of patients with cancer.
- Discuss what to expect during the infusion (e.g., metallic taste, which may last a while but can be relieved by sucking on hard candy). If the oral formulation is used, the drug should be taken on a full stomach.
- Explain to the patient that an allergic reaction may occur during infusion or after it and that this reaction is signaled by facial flushing, shortness of breath, or feeling faint.
- Help the patient explore ways to manage adverse effects of mild nausea, loss of appetite, and mouth sores, which may develop in 4 to 7 days.
- Offer helpful oral hygiene practices, such as brushing the teeth at least four times daily with a soft brush and avoiding commercial mouthwashes containing alcohol, which can be irritating to the mucous lining.
- Provide nutritional guidelines, such as taking antiemetics as prescribed, eating many small meals rather than a few full meals, and avoiding highly seasoned food.
- Explain the importance of regular laboratory examinations, such as blood tests at certain intervals, to detect any decreases in blood counts (usually within 1 to 2 weeks after treatment).
- Stress guidelines for avoiding infection resulting from suppressed bone marrow function.
- Demonstrate methods to cope with hair loss and tingling in the hands and feet.
- Teach the patient how to avoid injury resulting from drug-related neuropathy.
- Instruct the patient to contact the prescriber about serious adverse effects, such as a temperature higher than 100.5°F, excessive vomiting, painful mouth sores with inability to eat or drink for 24 hours, black stools, or uncontrolled bleeding.

- Discuss with the patient and the patient's significant other both reproductive goals and birth control, because of the possible mutagenic and teratogenic properties of the drug.

Ongoing Assessment and Evaluation

Before each dose of drug therapy, check the WBC and platelet counts; platelet levels less than 50,000 cells/mm^3 or an absolute neutrophil count less than 500 cells/mm^3 are indications for withholding the drug until the bone marrow recovers sufficiently.

Drug Closely Related to P Etoposide

Teniposide (VM-26, Vumon) and etoposide possess basic similarities in their pharmacologic makeup, toxicities, and clinical applications. The chemical structures of etoposide and teniposide differ only by the substitution of a methyl group (etoposide) for the thenylidene (teniposide) on the glucopyranoside sugar.

For teniposide administration, only nondiethylhexylphthalate (non-DEHP) containers, such as glass or polyolefin plastic containers, can be used. This precaution prevents DEHP from leaching out of polyvinyl containers and into the solution. Administration with heparin is contraindicated because heparin causes a precipitate to form.

C Taxanes

The taxanes arrest mitosis by promoting the formation of abnormal spindle fibers and mitotic asters. Paclitaxel (Taxol), the first drug in this category, was isolated from the bark of the Pacific yew, *Taxus brevifolia.* Because the demand for this drug exceeded the supply of bark available, a semisynthetic form was developed. Docetaxel (Taxotere) is the other taxane, a semisynthetic derivative of the European yew, *Taxus baccata.* Both taxanes have similar structures and pharmacologic properties: long half-lives, substantial hepatic metabolism, biliary excretion, and large volumes of distribution. These drugs are given intravenously. They differ somewhat in their toxicity profile, particularly in the nonhematologic adverse effects. Paclitaxel is discussed as the representative taxane drug.

MEMORY CHIP

P Etoposide

- Indicated for the treatment of testicular carcinoma, small-cell and non–small-cell lung cancer, lymphoma, Hodgkin disease, and multiple myeloma
- Major contraindications: known hypersensitivity to etoposide or to any podophyllotoxin derivative
- Most common adverse effect: hypersensitivity or anaphylaxis evidenced by orthostatic hypotension, chills, dyspnea, or bronchospasm (wheezing) when given rapidly
- Dose-limiting effect: myelosuppression
- **Life span alert: Radiation recall may happen. The safety and efficacy of VP-16 have not been established in children.**
- Maximizing therapeutic effects: Always infuse slowly over 30–60 minutes; never by IV push.
- Minimizing adverse effects: Monitor results of complete blood count before chemotherapy and at expected nadir, approximately 10–14 days after the drug dose. Monitor for signs and symptoms of myelosuppression, which include infection and bleeding.
- Most important patient education: Forewarn the patient that the infusion causes a metallic taste. Advise the patient that sucking on hard candy may alleviate the metallic taste.

NURSING MANAGEMENT OF THE PATIENT RECEIVING P PACLITAXEL

Core Drug Knowledge

Pharmacotherapeutics

The most important cytotoxic activity of paclitaxel has been in treating ovarian and breast cancers. It is approved for use after failure of first-line or subsequent therapy in metastatic ovarian cancer. In breast cancer, it is given to patients who have metastatic breast cancer that has progressed or relapsed during anthracycline-based therapy. It is also used for adjuvant treatment of node-positive breast cancer, administered sequentially to standard doxorubicin-containing combination chemotherapy. Clinical studies have shown that it is effective against a diverse range of solid tumors that are refractory to conventional chemotherapy. It has recently been approved for second-line treatment of acquired immunodeficiency syndrome (AIDS)-related Kaposi sarcoma. Several administration regimens are used, such as 1-, 3-, 6-, and 24-hour infusions with varying doses (see Table 35.2).

Pharmacokinetics

Paclitaxel crosses the placenta and enters breast milk. The liver is the principal organ responsible for paclitaxel metabolism. The drug is excreted into the bile; less than 10% of the intact drug is excreted in the urine.

Pharmacodynamics

Paclitaxel inhibits the normal dynamic reorganization of the microtubular network during interphase and mitosis. Microtubules are cellular elements that appear to play an important role in the initiation of DNA synthesis, mitosis, and other cellular functions. The interference with the microtubules prevents depolymerization, which triggers apoptosis, or cell death, in rapidly dividing cells. It also prevents transition from the G_0 phase to the S phase by blocking cellular response to protein growth factors.

Contraindications and Precautions

Paclitaxel is a pregnancy category D drug. Patients who have a history of hypersensitivity to drugs formulated in Cremophor EL—an excipient used as a vehicle for paclitaxel because the drug is not water soluble—should not be challenged with paclitaxel because of the possibility of hypersensitivity reaction. Taxanes are not used in children.

Adverse Effects

About 10% of patients experience a hypersensitivity reaction. In nearly 80% of patients, this reaction occurs during the first

10 minutes of the infusion and happens on the first or second exposure to the drug. Whether the hypersensitivity reaction is caused by the drug itself or by Cremophor EL is debated. The manifestations of this anaphylactoid reaction are dyspnea, hypotension, tachycardia, wheezing, and chest pain.

Myelosuppression is dose limiting; neutrophils reach nadir at day 11, and platelets reach nadir by day 8. Fever is associated with low WBC counts. Neurotoxicity is another important problem, which generally begins 2 or 3 days after infusion. Patients complain of numbness, tingling, and pain in the hands and feet, which may progress to painful paresthesias, loss of deep tendon reflexes, arthralgia, and diffuse myalgia. The GI manifestations are mucositis, diarrhea, mild nausea and vomiting, and elevated liver enzyme levels. The cutaneous reactions are alopecia, facial flushing, and chemical phlebitis.

Paclitaxel has irritant properties. It also appears to be cardiotoxic: bradyarrhythmias, including heart block, have been reported. Severe conduction abnormalities have been observed in less than 1% of patients receiving paclitaxel, in some cases necessitating pacemaker insertion.

Drug Interactions

The most substantial drug interaction is between paclitaxel and cisplatin. When given in combination, they can cause synergistic myelosuppression and neurotoxicity. Table 35.7 presents other drugs that might have substantial interactions with paclitaxel. Additionally, paclitaxel infusion must be administered in glass, or in polyolefin or polypropylene containers with polyethylene-lined administration sets. Polyvinyl chloride containers and tubing cause the plasticizer DEHP to leach into the fluid and should not be used. An inline filter of less than 0.22 microns should also be used because particulates can form.

Assessment of Relevant Core Patient Variables

Health Status

Before administering the first dose of paclitaxel, ensure that baseline CBC, electrocardiogram, and vital signs are recorded. Assess the patient's hepatobiliary function, particularly serum bilirubin levels. Patients with existing neuropathies resulting from diabetes mellitus or alcohol ingestion could experience potentiated neurotoxicity resulting from paclitaxel administration. Investigate hypersensitivity to other drugs with a Cremophor EL base.

Life Span and Gender

Assess women of childbearing age for pregnancy and lactation. This drug is believed to be embryotoxic; therefore, its use should be avoided in pregnancy. It may be excreted in milk; breast-feeding should be stopped while on paclitaxel therapy. The clinical efficacy of the taxanes in children has not been evaluated.

Lifestyle, Diet, and Habits

Discuss the impact of alopecia and other adverse effects on the patient's sexuality, body image, and activities of daily living. Alopecia, which may include loss of eyebrow, eyelash, pubic, and axillary hair, may be devastating to a patient who leads an active social life. Similarly limiting are the neurotoxic effects of pain, burning, sensory loss, paresthesia, and loss of deep tendon reflexes. These symptoms might be more pronounced in patients with a history of alcohol abuse.

Environment

Be aware of the environment in which paclitaxel will be administered. It may be administered on either an inpatient or outpatient basis. However, for precautionary measures, the first paclitaxel dose is often administered in an inpatient setting because severe reactions—manifested by hypotension, bronchospasm, tachycardia, and chest pain—can occur. In any setting where the drug is given, resuscitation equipment and adequate supportive drugs should always be present, so that prompt intervention can be implemented if necessary.

Nursing Diagnoses and Outcomes

- Risk for Injury related to hypersensitivity or anaphylactic reactions from paclitaxel
  Desired outcome: *The patient will not suffer any injury resulting from hypersensitivity reaction to paclitaxel.*
- Risk for Infection and bleeding related to depressed bone marrow function
  Desired outcome: *The patient will be free from infection and bleeding, evidenced by normal vital signs and recovery from neutropenia and anemia, demonstrated by blood counts.*
- Disturbed Sensory Perception related to neuropathy
  Desired outcome: *The patient will be able to function safely within limitations of lessened perceptual and sensory acuity caused by paclitaxel.*
- Imbalanced Nutrition: Less than Body Requirements related to drug-induced nausea, vomiting, and diarrhea

TABLE 35.7 Agents That Interact With P Paclitaxel

Interactants	Effect and Significance	Nursing Management
quinidine, cyclosporine, quinine, verapamil	Reversal of multidrug resistance	Administer medications as ordered.
cisplatin (CDDP)	Myelosuppression more severe when CDDP is given before paclitaxel	Give paclitaxel first when these two drugs are ordered sequentially.
ketoconazole	Inhibits metabolism of paclitaxel	Monitor for paclitaxel toxicity.

Desired outcome: The patient will maintain adequate nutritional intake and be able to gain adequate control over emesis and diarrhea.

- Impaired Skin Integrity and Disturbed Body Image related to drug-induced alopecia
  Desired outcome: The patient will understand that the loss of hair is reversible and will initiate strategies to minimize body image distortion stemming from alopecia.

Planning and Intervention

Maximizing Therapeutic Effects

Store diluted paclitaxel in glass bottles or plastic bags and administer polyethylene-lined administration sets using an inline 0.22 micron filter. Do not allow the undiluted concentrate to come in contact with polyvinyl chloride equipment or devices. When used to treat breast cancer, paclitaxel should be part of a multidrug regimen that includes doxorubicin. Paclitaxel may be used as part of combination therapy with cisplatin to treat certain types of cancer, such as non–small cell lung cancer. The cytotoxicity from these two drugs is sequence dependent; for optimal results, paclitaxel should be given first.

Minimizing Adverse Effects

Measure and closely monitor the patient's baseline vital signs during the first 15 minutes of the paclitaxel infusion, and continue monitoring the patient for the first hour. Stay with the patient because most hypersensitivity reactions occur within the first 10 minutes of the first infusion. These reactions may also happen during a later cycle, even after an uneventful first infusion. If the reaction is severe, the infusion should be discontinued immediately; patients who develop a mild reaction can be rechallenged after the clinical manifestations have subsided. To prevent severe reactions, premedication is necessary. Premedication usually consists of corticosteroids (dexamethasone) taken 11 hours and 7 hours before treatment. Diphenhydramine 50 mg and an H_2-antagonist (cimetidine, 300 mg, or ranitidine, 150 mg) are given intravenously half an hour before the paclitaxel infusion. Current experience indicates that longer infusions and an adequate premedication regimen, such as the one mentioned previously, minimize this adverse effect. If a severe hypersensitivity reaction or anaphylaxis occurs, the drug should be discontinued immediately and supportive measures instituted (Box 35.5). Under these circumstances, the patient must not be rechallenged.

Patients with baseline neutrophil counts of less than 1,500 cells/mm^3 should not be treated. High-dose regimens of 250 mg/m^2 of paclitaxel have been combined with colony-stimulating factors, such as filgrastim. The use of growth factors is critical because they accelerate bone marrow recovery and prevent severe WBC nadir from occurring. Filgrastim is given subcutaneously at a dose of 5 µg/kg every day for 10 days, starting 1 day after the chemotherapy is given.

Providing Patient and Family Education

- Follow the guidelines described in Box 35.3.
- The first treatment is usually stressful for the patient and family because of the fear of the possible anaphylactic reaction. Reassure the patient that the health care team will be present during the first 20 minutes of the infusion when most of these reactions occur. Teach the patient to report the first symptoms of anaphylaxis, so that supportive measures can be undertaken.
- Explain drug delivery methods; for example, say that an IV drug can be given as a continuous infusion or intra-abdominally by a catheter placed in the abdomen.
- Review premedication regimens for preventing allergic reactions, including regimens for dexamethasone (Decadron), diphenhydramine (Benadryl), and cimetidine or ranitidine.
- Discuss medications to relieve adverse effects (nausea, joint pain, body aches), such as acetaminophen (Tylenol) or ibuprofen (Motrin, Advil) for pain.
- Offer methods to enhance appearance when alopecia sets in, such as wearing wigs and hats.
- Explain signs and symptoms of peripheral neuropathy, such as numbness, tingling in the hands and feet, impairment of fine motor skills, and difficulty in ambulating, and explore their potential effects on the patient's activities of daily living; for example, suggest moving carefully to avoid injury.
- Discuss measures to alleviate fatigue by getting rest, sleep, and exercise; pacing activities; and obtaining help with activities and chores of daily living.

BOX 35.5 Managing a Generalized Hypersensitivity Reaction and Anaphylaxis

Hypersensitivity or anaphylactic-like reactions manifested by hypotension, chills, fever, facial flushing, bronchospasm, dyspnea, and tachycardia can occur during a chemotherapeutic infusion. Hypersensitivity reactions usually occur within the first 10 minutes of the first infusion, but they may also happen during a later cycle, even after an uneventful first infusion. Because hypersensitivity reactions can be life threatening, the nurse needs to know what to do should one occur:

1. Stop the infusion immediately.
2. Stay with the patient.
3. Ask for medical support.
4. Maintain a good IV line with normal saline solution.
5. Administer emergency drugs as prescribed: epinephrine 1:10,000 IV or 1:1,000 SC given as 0.1 mg IV push every 10 minutes as needed for adults, and for children, 0.01 mg/kg SC or 0.2 mg–0.5 mg every 10–15 minutes; diphenhydramine 25–50 mg IV; methylprednisolone 30–60 mg or dexamethasone 10–20 mg IV; aminophylline 5 mg/kg IV over 30 minutes; and dopamine 2–20 mg/kg/min for hypotension.
6. Place the patient in a supine position.
7. Measure vital signs every 2–5 minutes until they stabilize.
8. Maintain a patent airway, and administer oxygen as needed.
9. Provide emotional support to the patient and family.
10. Document all nursing measures and patient responses.
11. Consult with the health care provider about a change in treatment plans or the need to rechallenge the patient. If the drug needs to be given, the following measures should be implemented: desensitization with the health care provider's support, a premedication regimen, prolongation of infusion time or an increase in the volume of diluent and, if appropriate, substitution of a similar drug.

- Explain how to self-administer a prescribed drug (e.g., granulocyte colony-stimulating factor [G-CSF]) by subcutaneous injection to minimize a severe drop in WBC count.
- Review the danger signs of infection and blood abnormalities that should be reported, such as a temperature higher than 100.5°F.
- Explain the importance of oral hygiene and careful nutrition to relieve the discomfort of mouth sores.

Ongoing Assessment and Evaluation

Depression of bone marrow function, primarily neutropenia, is a dose-limiting toxicity of paclitaxel. Monitor the patient's CBCs frequently. Patients should not be given subsequent courses until the neutrophils reach a level exceeding 1,500 cells/mm^3 and platelets recover to above 100,000 cells/mm^3. Perform cardiac monitoring during subsequent drug administration to ensure that patients do not develop severe cardiac abnormalities.

Drug Closely Related to P Paclitaxel

Docetaxel (Taxotere) is the only other drug in the taxane family. It is used in patients with locally advanced or metastatic breast carcinoma after disease progression with an anthracycline-based therapy or relapse during anthracycline-based adjuvant treatment. It is approved for the treatment of patients with head and neck malignancies, ovarian cancer, and non–small cell lung cancer that is locally advanced or has metastasized and has not responded to cisplatin. The FDA has just approved docetaxel in combination with prednisone for patients with hormone-refractory prostate cancer. An adverse effect unique to docetaxel administration is fluid retention syndrome. This syndrome is manifested by edema, weight gain, and third-space fluid retention. The fluid retention is cumulative and is believed to be caused by increased capillary permeability and by the vehicle used to increase docetaxel's solubility, *Tween 80*. Prophylactic measures include the use of corticosteroids, such as dexamethasone, 8 mg orally twice daily for 5 days, before docetaxel, with or without H_1- and H_2-receptor antagonists given intravenously 30 minutes before the drug; these measures appear to be effective in reducing the fluid retention. Other measures include the use of diuretics, such as spironolactone or furosemide, if ordered by the prescriber.

CRITICAL THINKING SCENARIO

Implementing paclitaxel therapy

Mrs. A. S., a 55-year-old woman with diagnosed breast cancer, is going to receive paclitaxel for the first time. The dose that is prescribed is 175 mg/m^2 to be given as a 3-hour infusion every 3 weeks for four cycles.

Describe the nursing responsibilities before the start of the infusion.

MEMORY CHIP

P Paclitaxel

- Indicated for patients who have metastatic carcinoma of the ovary after failure of first-line or subsequent chemotherapy; breast carcinoma after failure of combination chemotherapy for metastatic disease or relapse within 6 months of adjuvant treatment
- Major contraindications: hypersensitivity to Cremophor El, baseline neutropenia of <1,500/mm^3, pregnancy and lactation
- Most common adverse effects: nausea, vomiting, alopecia, and joint pains
- Dose-limiting effect: depression of bone marrow function, particularly neutropenia
- Most serious adverse effects: Severe hypersensitivity reactions occur during the first 10–15 minutes of drug infusion.
- Maximizing therapeutic effects: Use glass or polyolefin containers, non-DEHP administration sets, and in-line filtration for drug administration.
- Minimizing adverse effects: Administer paclitaxel first when given in combination with cisplatin or carboplatin to prevent profound myelosuppression. Premedicate patients with corticosteroids at 11 and 7 hours before drug administration; administer diphenhydramine 50 mg and an H_2-antagonist IV 30 minutes before paclitaxel to avoid anaphylactic reactions.
- Most important patient education: Because the premedication regimen is started at home, ensure that patient will understand the importance of complying with the dosing schedule and will have enough medications (dexamethasone) at home.

C CAMPTOTHECINES (TOPOISOMERASE-I INHIBITORS)

Topoisomerase-I is a nuclear enzyme needed for maintaining DNA structure during replication, transcription, and translation of genetic materials. Inhibition of this enzyme causes single-stranded DNA breaks and, subsequently, cell death. Topoisomerase-I inhibitors are a new category of cell cycle–specific agents, semisynthetic agents derived from the Chinese tree *Camptotheca acuminata*. The parent compound, camptothecin, was isolated in 1966 and was found to have antitumor activity in animal models. However, further testing was not pursued because of unpredictable toxicities, such as hemorrhagic cystitis and myelosuppression. In the early 1980s, inhibition of topoisomerase-I activity was found to be an important anticancer strategy. The two drugs in this category are topotecan hydrochloride (Hycamtin) and irinotecan (CPT-11).

NURSING MANAGEMENT OF THE PATIENT RECEIVING P TOPOTECAN

Core Drug Knowledge

Pharmacotherapeutics

Topotecan HCl (Hycamtin), a semisynthetic derivative of camptothecin, was approved in 1996 to treat patients with metastatic ovarian cancer after failure of initial or subsequent

chemotherapy. It has also demonstrated clinical efficacy in treating small cell lung cancer and ALL. It is administered intravenously.

Pharmacokinetics

The half-life of topotecan is about 3 hours. The drug has minimal protein binding, which may contribute to its ability to cross the blood–brain barrier. Topotecan is metabolized in the liver. The drug is primarily excreted by the kidneys, with approximately 30% to 40% excreted unchanged. Renal clearance is an important determinant of topotecan elimination.

Pharmacodynamics

Topotecan inhibits the activity of topoisomerase-I, an enzyme involved in gene transcription and DNA replication. This enzyme causes nicks and breaks along DNA strands, relieving stresses that build up as the DNA molecule unwinds in preparation for cell division and protein synthesis. Normally, the nicks would then be repaired by topoisomerase-I. Topotecan, by attaching to the enzyme, prevents it from repairing the nicks in the DNA, and the cell is unable to repair them efficiently.

Contraindications and Precautions

This drug is myelosuppressive and is contraindicated in patients who have poor bone marrow reserves. It should only be administered when the baseline neutrophil count is at least 1,500 cells/mm^3 and the platelet count is at least 100,000 cells/mm^3. Whether the drug is excreted in human milk is unknown. It should not be administered to patients who are pregnant or breast-feeding.

Adverse Effects

The dose-limiting toxicity of topotecan is myelosuppression, especially neutropenia, with a median time to nadir of 11 days. Thrombocytopenia is also dose-limiting in some regimens; median time to nadir is 15 days, with resolution after 5 days. Growth factor support has not been necessary for most patients. The nonhematologic adverse effects are nausea and vomiting, which are usually relieved with the appropriate antiemetic regimen. Other GI side effects are diarrhea and abdominal pain, which are managed symptomatically. Headache is a common neurologic complaint. Alopecia, fever, and flu-like symptoms have also been reported.

Drug Interactions

No known interactions with other drugs occur that might affect the potency of topotecan. Concomitant use of topotecan and cisplatin or other cytotoxic drugs worsens myelosuppression; concomitant use of G-CSF can prolong neutropenia.

Assessment of Relevant Core Patient Variables

Health Status

Assess the adequacy of the patient's bone marrow reserve. Because severe neutropenia is most common with the first course of treatment, topotecan should only be given to patients who have a baseline neutrophil count of at least 1,500 cells/mm^3 and a platelet count of at least 100,000 cells/mm^3.

Life Span and Gender

This drug falls into pregnancy category D. Explore the patient's reproductive goals. Assess women of childbearing age for pregnancy and lactation. Because it is not known whether the drug is excreted in human milk, this drug should not be administered to patients who are pregnant or breast-feeding. The safety and efficacy of topotecan have not been established in children.

Lifestyle, Diet, and Habits

Assess the patient's activities of daily living, including rest and exercise patterns. Fatigue is frequently reported. Obtain information on the patient's normal dietary intake to plan necessary antiemetic measures.

Environment

Be aware of the environment in which topotecan will be administered. It is usually given in an ambulatory setting. There are no acute risks that necessitate inpatient hospitalization. Clinical trials are currently in progress with an oral form of the drug. Home therapy, an attractive alternative, will make drug administration convenient and cost effective for the patient.

Nursing Diagnoses and Outcomes

- Risk for Infection and Bleeding related to depression of bone marrow function
  Desired outcome: *The patient will be free from infection and bleeding evidenced by normal vital signs and recovery from neutropenia and anemia as shown in the blood counts.*
- Imbalanced Nutrition: Less than Body Requirements related to drug-induced nausea, vomiting, and stomatitis
  Desired outcome: *The patient will maintain adequate nutritional intake and be able to gain adequate control of emesis and diarrhea.*
- Disturbed Body Image related to alopecia
  Desired outcome: *The patient will develop strategies to minimize body image distortion from loss of hair.*
- Altered Self-Image related to fatigue
  Desired outcome: *The patient will understand the etiology of fatigue and will implement fatigue management strategies that will minimize level of fatigue.*

Planning and Intervention

Maximizing Therapeutic Effects

A minimum of 4 courses (topotecan, 1.5 mg/m^2 intravenously for 5 days, given every 21 days) is recommended because the median time to response as shown in three ovarian clinical trials was 9 to 12 weeks and median time to response in four small cell lung cancer trials was 5 to 7 weeks. Unopened vials of the drug should be protected from light and kept at a controlled temperature of 68°F to 79°F. Reconstituted solutions should be used immediately.

Minimizing Adverse Effects

Because of dose-limiting myelosuppression, monitor WBC counts before chemotherapy and at the expected nadir. If the nadir is especially low, hematopoietic growth factors

such as G-CSF may be given to decrease the depth and duration of the nadir. These substances should not be given concomitantly with topotecan, however, because doing so will prolong the duration of the neutropenia. Growth factors should be administered 24 hours after the fifth dose of topotecan or on day 6 of the cycle.

Providing Patient and Family Education

- Follow the guidelines described in Box 35.3.
- Advise the patient of ways to lessen the fatigue level by conserving energy; engaging in moderate exercise and activity; observing good sleep hygiene; and talking to the physician about other possible underlying causes. Emphasize to the patient that fatigue is a side effect rather than a sign of disease progression or treatment failure.
- Teach the patient to eat small and frequent meals and take antiemetics if needed. Emphasize good oral hygiene.
- Review the signs and symptoms of infection and bleeding and instruct the patient about which ones should be reported to a prescriber.
- If G-CSF injections are necessary, ensure that the patient or patient's significant caregiver knows how to administer the drug.
- Reassure the patient that alopecia is a reversible process and teach the patient techniques for enhancing his or her appearance.

Ongoing Assessment and Evaluation

Undertake frequent monitoring of the patient's blood counts when subsequent therapy is planned. Neutrophil recovery to more than 1,000 cells/mm^3, platelet count to more than 100,000 cells/mm^3, and hemoglobin levels of 9.0 mg/dL are safe parameters to maintain for follow-up cycles.

MEMORY CHIP

P Topotecan

- Approved for use in patients with advanced or metastatic ovarian cancer after failure of initial or subsequent chemotherapy, small cell lung cancer, neuroblastoma, and sarcoma
- Major contraindications: severe depression of bone marrow function particularly when the neutrophil count is <1,500 cells/mm^3; known hypersensitivity to the drug or its components
- Most common adverse effects: nonhematologic adverse events including nausea and vomiting, diarrhea or constipation, alopecia, and fatigue
- Most serious adverse effect: depression of bone marrow function, particularly neutropenia
- Maximizing therapeutic effects: A minimum of four courses (topotecan 1.5 mg/m^2 intravenously for 5 days given every 21 days) is recommended, because the median time to response as shown in three ovarian clinical trials was 9 to 12 weeks and median time to response in four small-cell lung cancer trials was 5 to 7 weeks.
- Minimizing adverse effects: To minimize severe neutropenia, reduce subsequent doses by 0.25 mg/m^2. Growth factor support may be necessary for neutrophil recovery.
- Most important patient education: Teach the patient the importance of careful monitoring of blood counts and the avoidance of risk factors that might expose patient to sources of bleeding and infection.

CRITICAL THINKING SCENARIO

Implementing irinotecan therapy

Mr. J is a 65-year-old patient with colon cancer whose disease has progressed after 5-FU therapy. He was started on irinotecan monotherapy using a starting dose of 125 mg/m^2 administered by IV. The patient will return each week for 4 consecutive weeks. He will have a 2-week rest period between cycles. Diarrhea is a principal adverse effect. What are the important nursing considerations to review regarding this problem?

Drug Closely Related to P Topotecan

Irinotecan (CPT-11) is the second topoisomerase-I inhibitor. First synthesized in Japan in 1984, it was found to have activity against many tumor models, both in vitro and in animals. This drug is effective in treating metastatic carcinoma of the colon or rectum that has recurred or progressed following therapy with 5-FU; more recently, it has been useful as first-line therapy in combination with 5-FU and leucovorin in metastatic colon or rectal cancer (Box 35.6). The principal adverse effects associated with irinotecan are GI and hematologic. Diarrhea occurs early and late in treatment

FOCUS ON RESEARCH

Box 35.6 Improved Response Rates in Metastatic Colorectal Cancer with the Addition of Irinotecan to 5-FU/Leucovorin

Bankhead, C. (2000). "Metastatic colorectal cancer: Big survival gain adding irinotecan to 5-FU/leucovorin." *Oncology Times, 12* (12).

The Study

The three-drug regimen mentioned in this study showed significant increase in overall and progression-free survival and response among patients with metastatic colorectal cancer when compared with the standard 5-FU and leucovorin. The findings of this multicenter trial (2000) were reported in the *New England Journal of Medicine 343,* 905–914. The trial involved 683 patients randomized to one of three treatment arms:

1. irinotecan (125 mg/m^2), 5-FU (500 mg/m^2), and leucovorin (20 mg/m^2) administered daily for 4 weeks every 6 weeks.
2. 5-FU (425 mg/m^2) and leucovorin (20 mg/m^2) daily for 5 consecutive days every 4 weeks.
3. Irinotecan alone at 125 mg/m^2 weekly for 4 weeks every 6 weeks. Analysis showed a longer progression-free survival with the first regimen—7.0 versus 4.3 months with the second regimen. Tumor response rates were 39% with the three-drug regimen and 21% with the two-drug combination. The median overall survival was 14.8 months with the irinotecan, 5-FU/leucovorin and 12.6 months with the two-drug therapy. Results with irinotecan alone regimen were similar to those in the two-drug regimen. The modest improvement from this important study shows promise as the "new" standard of care for the metastatic colon cancer population. Multicenter trials are underway to explore its clinical utility in patients who have less advanced disease.

and can be dose limiting, depending on the time of onset. Early-onset diarrhea, which happens within 24 hours of drug administration, is thought to be caused by inhibition of anticholinesterase by irinotecan. It is characterized by sweating, flushing, abdominal cramping, hyperlacrimation, and sudden diarrhea. It responds to intravenous or subcutaneous injection of atropine, 0.25 to 1.0 mg. Late-onset diarrhea, which can be dose limiting, usually occurs between days 5 and 12 of the treatment cycle but can happen as early as day 2. Management of this type of diarrhea consists of giving loperamide, 4 mg every 2 hours, until the patient has not experienced diarrhea for 12 hours. Most patients also experience nausea and vomiting, which can be ameliorated with suitable antiemetic therapy. Other toxicities include leukopenia, anemia, and neutropenia, alopecia, and fatigue. Irinotecan is usually given in an ambulatory setting, with follow-up telephone calls to patients to ensure proper control of side effects, particularly diarrhea, which can cause nutritional deficits. For colon cancer, the initial dose of irinotecan is 125 mg/m^2 given intravenously over 90 minutes every week for 4 consecutive weeks, followed by a 2-week rest period. The optimal dosage for ovarian cancer has not been established.

MISCELLANEOUS CELL CYCLE-SPECIFIC DRUGS

Several antineoplastic drugs, which are believed to be cell cycle–specific but have unclear modes of action, are classified in the miscellaneous group. Hydroxyurea (Hydrea) and L-asparaginase (Elspar) are in this category. Hydroxyurea is the representative miscellaneous cell cycle–specific drug discussed in this chapter.

NURSING MANAGEMENT OF THE PATIENT RECEIVING P HYDROXYUREA

Core Drug Knowledge

Pharmacotherapeutics

Hydroxyurea is used in managing hematologic cancers, such as acute lymphoblastic or chronic myelogenous leukemia. It is also used in other hematologic conditions, such as essential thrombocytopenia, polycythemia vera, and hyperleukocytosis caused by acute leukemia. It is used in combination chemotherapy or with radiation and has shown some clinical efficacy against renal cancer, malignant melanoma, ovarian cancer, head and neck tumors, and prostate cancer. It is given orally (see Table 35.2) until the WBC count falls to 50,000 cells/mm^3, after which dosage is reduced gradually or discontinued.

Pharmacokinetics

Hydroxyurea is well absorbed from the GI tract. It penetrates the blood–brain barrier, achieving peak levels in the CSF within 3 hours. About 50% of the drug is metabolized in the liver, excreted in the urine as urea, and eliminated in the respiratory tract as carbon dioxide. The remainder is excreted intact in the urine.

Pharmacodynamics

The exact mechanism of action of hydroxyurea remains unestablished. It is a potent inhibitor of the enzyme ribonucleotide reductase, and it causes inhibition of DNA without inhibiting RNA or protein synthesis. It is S-phase specific and may hold other cells in the G_1 phase of the cell cycle.

Contraindications and Precautions

This drug is contraindicated in patients with severe anemia, severely depressed bone marrow function with WBC count of less than 2,500 cells/mm^3, or platelet count less than 100,000 cells/mm^3. Megaloblastosis unrelated to vitamin B_{12} or folic acid deficiency is often seen during chronic hydroxyurea therapy. Because the drug is excreted in the urine, it should be used with caution in patients with marked renal problems.

Adverse Effects

Hydroxyurea is a pregnancy category D drug. The major toxicity of hydroxyurea is dose-related myelosuppression. Leukopenia is common, with an onset of 10 days. Thrombocytopenia and anemia are less common and have a later onset. CNS effects, such as drowsiness, headache, dizziness, hallucinations, and disorientation, have been reported with high-dose therapy. GI problems, such as nausea, vomiting, diarrhea, and stomatitis, are less common. Combined therapy with radiation can increase the severity and incidence of side effects. If the reactions are severe, interruption of treatment might be indicated; this action is rarely necessary. Increases in serum uric acid, blood urea nitrogen (BUN), and creatinine levels have been noted.

Drug Interactions

No important drug interactions with hydroxyurea are known to exist.

Assessment of Relevant Core Patient Variables

Health Status

Before treatment, assess the patient's hematologic profile, including a CBC and, if indicated, a bone marrow biopsy, especially if the patient has previously received antineoplastic or radiation therapy. Ask the patient about adverse effects from these treatments. Order tests to determine adequate renal and hepatic function.

Life Span and Gender

Document the age of the patient. Because elderly patients may be more sensitive than young patients to the drug, dose reductions may be indicated. The dosage regimens for children have not been established. Assess women of childbearing age for pregnancy and lactation. Hydroxyurea has shown teratogenic effects in animals and may be mutagenic. Therefore, women should be cautioned about possible fetal harm if they are or may become pregnant.

Lifestyle, Diet, and Habits

Because hydroxyurea is an oral formulation, ensure that the patient will adhere to the dosing schedule at home and will incorporate this schedule into his or her daily activities. No dietary restrictions apply to the ingestion of hydroxyurea.

Environment

Hydroxyurea is self-administered at home. No emergency adverse effects of the drug are known that might require hospitalization. Patients taking long-term hydroxyurea therapy should be monitored closely because of the possibility of severe depression of bone marrow function. If appropriate, assess the home for potential sources of infection and bleeding risk (Box 35.7).

Nursing Diagnoses and Outcomes

- Risk for Infection and Bleeding related to suppressed bone marrow function
  Desired outcome: *The patient will recover adequate hematologic function. Patient will undertake self-care measures to prevent infection and bleeding.*
- Imbalanced Nutrition: Less than Body Requirements related to nausea and vomiting, anorexia, stomatitis, and hepatic dysfunction
  Desired outcome: *The patient will maintain a proper nutritional state and good emetic control. The patient will maintain intact oral mucosa and practice a good oral hygiene regimen. The patient will have normal hepatic function.*
- Disturbed Sensory Perception: Drowsiness, disorientation, confusion, or headache related to adverse effects of drug therapy
  Desired outcome: *The patient will be free from injury. The patient will maintain sensory acuity and orientation to time and environment.*
- Ineffective Sexuality Patterns related to effects of hydroxyurea
  Desired outcome: *The patient will increase knowledge about the effects of chemotherapy on sexual function and will initiate behaviors that will not interfere with sexual patterns and reproductive goals.*

COMMUNITY-BASED CONCERNS

Box 35.7 Home Therapy With Hydroxyurea

Some patients receive hydroxyurea (Hydrea) at home. They need to learn about safe, effective self-care. Some considerations to cover in patient education include the following:

- Because hydroxyurea is taken PO, problems with swallowing capsules can present difficulties. To counteract swallowing problems, hydroxyurea capsules can be mixed with applesauce, water, or juice and swallowed in liquid form.
- Taken in large doses, hydroxyurea may cause moderate drowsiness; patients should be cautioned to prevent risk of injury.
- Early side effects of nausea, vomiting, diarrhea, and loss of appetite may interfere with drug effectiveness. Antiemetic medications should be taken as prescribed. In some cases, taking hydroxyurea before bedtime helps to decrease nausea.
- The health care provider should be notified if foods or liquids cannot be retained for more than 24 hours after taking hydroxyurea.
- If the physician recommends blood testing, appointments should be scheduled so that the blood count can be monitored closely. A temporary decrease may occur within 7 to 14 days after treatment, but the blood counts will recover.
- Ways to prevent infection include avoiding people who have colds or any infection during the drug therapy period and avoiding injury, such as cuts from razor blades or kitchen knives.
- The health care provider should be notified if a severe skin rash or facial redness develops, although a less severe rash may occur in 1 to 2 weeks after treatment.
- Because hydration is important for therapeutic effect, the patient should drink plenty of fluids to prevent any problems with kidney function.
- Proper handling of cytotoxic agents particularly avoidance of contact with skin should be observed.

Planning and Intervention

Maximizing Therapeutic Effects

When hydroxyurea is given concomitantly with irradiation, hydroxyurea should be given 1 week before initiating radiation therapy. It can then be continued during radiotherapy and given indefinitely. The maximum therapeutic radiation dosage indicated for the clinical condition should be given. Modifying the radiation dosage is not usually necessary with concurrent hydroxyurea administration, as long as the patient is closely monitored and does not experience severe adverse effects.

Minimizing Adverse Effects

The dosage of hydroxyurea should be based on the patient's actual or ideal weight, whichever is less. Hydroxyurea therapy should be interrupted if the WBC falls below 2,500 cells/mm^3 or the platelets fall below 100,000 cells/mm^3. Hematopoietic count rebounds promptly; only a few doses might be missed. Anemia does not necessitate interrupting hydroxyurea therapy because whole blood replacement can be given. Dose modifications may be indicated in patients who have received prior radiation therapy or other cytotoxic drugs. Assess the patient's renal function because hydroxyurea can impair renal tubular function, an event manifested by elevated uric acid, BUN, and creatinine levels. Because tumor lysis can occur, the patient may need to be pretreated with allopurinol.

Providing Patient and Family Education

- Follow the guidelines described in Box 35.3.
- Before initiating drug therapy, review the common side effects of hydroxyurea with the patient and caregiver.
- Emphasize the importance of monitoring blood counts, particularly the WBC and platelets, at the prescribed intervals.
- If the patient will be managed from home, teach self-care measures to prevent risks for infection and bleeding. Also, instruct the patient on which signs and symptoms to report when they become pronounced. For more information, see Box 35.7.

Ongoing Assessment and Evaluation

Throughout therapy with hydroxyurea, assess the patient for signs of bleeding disorders and infection. Closely monitor CBCs to make sure that they are within safe treatment parameters. If the patient is receiving concomitant radiation therapy, check the oral mucosa to ensure that severe reactions, which can cause pain and difficulty with food intake, do not compromise the patient. Because radiation recall may occur with concomitant treatment, dermatologic changes should be reported to the prescriber and managed appropriately.

MEMORY CHIP

P Hydroxyurea

- Indicated for managing hematologic cancers, such as acute blastic or chronic myelogenous leukemia. It is used in combination chemotherapy or with radiation and has shown some clinical efficacy against malignant melanoma, ovarian cancer, and head and neck tumors.
- Major contraindication: depressed bone marrow reserve
- Most common adverse effects: gastrointestinal effects manifested by anorexia, nausea and vomiting, stomatitis, and diarrhea or constipation
- Most serious adverse effects: depression of bone marrow function including leukopenia, anemia, and thrombocytopenia. Rapid decrease in white blood cell counts may occur within a short period, which is the desired effect for leukemia patients.
- Minimizing adverse effects: Monitor the patient's blood count before, during, and after treatment. If anemia occurs, the patient may receive blood transfusion without interrupting treatment cycles. Premedicate the patient with the appropriate antiemetic regimen.
- Most important patient education: Hydroxyurea is administered orally. If the patient has difficulty swallowing, instruct the patient to empty the contents of the capsule into a glass of water, mix, and drink immediately. The contents may not be dissolved completely because of the drug formulation. Advise the patient on careful handling of a cytotoxic agent, particularly to avoid contact with the skin or mucous membrane.

Drug Significantly Different From P Hydroxyurea

L-Asparaginase (Elspar) belongs to the group of miscellaneous drugs that are cell cycle-specific. The inhibitory action of this drug occurs in the postmitotic (G_1) phase of the cell cycle. L-asparaginase is indicated in patients with acute lymphocytic leukemia (ALL). In this condition, the tumor cells depend on exogenous asparagine for survival. When L-asparaginase is administered to the leukemic patient, the serum asparagine is hydrolyzed to nonfunctional aspartic acid and ammonia, depriving malignant cells of the required amino acid. Absence of asparagine causes rapid inhibition of DNA and RNA synthesis. Normal cells are able to synthesize asparagines and therefore are less affected than tumor cells by depletion of this enzyme.

L-Asparaginase does not appear to cross the blood–brain barrier and is not excreted in the urine. It is administered by the intramuscular or IV routes. Patients receiving this drug should be treated in the hospital because anaphylactic reactions can occur. Toxicity is more common in adults than in children. A modified version of L-asparaginase, pegaspargase, is given to patients who are hypersensitive to the native form. In addition to anaphylaxis, other common side effects are hepatotoxicity, which occurs in most patients, and decreased clotting factors, which may lead to bleeding problems such as intracranial hemorrhage and fatal bleeding associated with low fibrinogen. Depression of bone marrow function is rare and transient. Mild to severe CNS effects, manifested by somnolence, lethargy, drowsiness, and malaise, have been noted. These effects are usually reversible with discontinuation of L-asparaginase.

HERBAL MEDICINE AND CHEMOTHERAPY

Plants and herbs have been used for medicinal purposes in both Eastern and Western cultures for thousands of years. In the United States, the use of herbal medicine is increasingly popular. Six herbs received FDA approval before the Dietary Supplement and Health Education Act (DSHEA) was passed in 1994. These herbs are *aloe* (a laxative); *capsicum* (a topical analgesic); *cascara, psyllium,* and *senna* (all laxatives); and *witch hazel* (an astringent). The DSHEA allows herbal medicines and dietary supplements to be marketed without testing for efficacy, safety, or quality control standards for production and without claims for how they affect the body. Herbs do not have to pass through standard rigorous FDA requirements. Because of the lack of quality control, the purity of these products is of concern. Studies have shown that some herbs are contaminated with heavy metals, nondeclared ingredients, poisonous substances, and pesticide residue. For these reasons, ask patients about the use of herbs, document their use, and tell patients that they may have to discontinue herbal medicines when they initiate therapy with antineoplastic agents. Provide accurate, objective information, so that the patient can make informed choices about herbal use. *St. John's wort,* commonly known as "nature's Prozac," has been studied, and potential interactions with certain chemotherapy agents (Table 35.8) have been found.

CHAPTER SUMMARY

- All cells, normal and malignant, progress through the different phases of the cell life cycle.
- In general, antineoplastic drugs are most effective on cells in the proliferative phases.
- Cell cycle–specific drugs exert their cytotoxicity at a particular phase or phases of the cell cycle and cause no substantial harm during the remaining phases.
- The major toxicities of antineoplastic drugs act on rapidly dividing cells, such as the bone marrow, GI mucosa, hair follicles, and gonadal cells.

TABLE 35.8 Agents With Potential Interactions With St. John's Wort

Chemotherapeutic agents	
anastrozole (Arimidex)	paclitaxel (Taxol)
cyclophosphamide (Cytoxan)	teniposide (VM-26)
docetaxel (Taxotere)	tretinoin (retinoic acid)
etoposide (VP-16)	vinblastine (Velban)
ifosfamide (Ifex)	vincristine (Oncovin)
Antiemetic agents	
dolasetron (Anzemet)	
granisetron (Kytril)	
ondansetron (Zofran)	

- Hypersensitivity, anaphylactic reactions, and extravasations are the most common immediate reactions associated with chemotherapy administration.
- Health care workers can be exposed to chemotherapy through the following routes: skin and mucus membrane absorption, inhalation, and ingestion.
- The major teaching points to emphasize with a patient receiving chemotherapy are to (1) practice good body and oral hygiene; (2) eat a nutritious diet and drink plenty of fluids; (3) avoid injury, especially cuts to the skin; (4) avoid possible sources of infection, such as animal excrement or people with colds, chickenpox, and herpes; and (5) pace activities of daily living to provide adequate rest and exercise.
- Medicinal herbs have the potential to interact with chemotherapeutic drugs, and their consumption should be discussed with the prescriber before initiating treatment.

▲ QUESTIONS FOR STUDY AND REVIEW

1. What are the goals of chemotherapy?
2. What are the different strategies undertaken in the use of chemotherapeutic agents?
3. What are the basic features of a malignant cell?
4. How do you clean up a chemotherapy spill?
5. How are health care workers exposed to chemotherapy?
6. Why is vincristine preferred over vinblastine for combination chemotherapy?
7. What are the nursing measures to take when an extravasation occurs?
8. What causes hypotension during an etoposide infusion?
9. What are the signs and symptoms of a hypersensitivity reaction?
10. Before starting a paclitaxel infusion, what should you check for?
11. What are examples of neoplastic agents that may potentially interact with St. John's wort?

? Need More Help?

Chapter 35 of the study guide for *Drug Therapy in Nursing* 2e contains NCLEX-style questions and other learning activities to reinforce your understanding of the concepts presented in this chapter. For additional information or to purchase the study guide, visit *http://connection.lww.com/go/aschenbrenner.*

REFERENCES AND BIBLIOGRAPHY

American Society of Hospital Pharmacists. (1990). *ASHP technical assistance bulletin on handling of cytotoxic and hazardous drugs.* Bethesda, MD: Author.

Aventis Pharmaceuticals. (1997). *Taxotere (docetaxel)* [Prescribing information insert]. Collegeville, PA: Author.

Baquiran, D. C. (2001). *Lippincott's cancer chemotherapy handbook* (2nd ed.). Philadelphia: Lippincott Williams & Wilkins.

Berg, D. (1998a). Irinotecan hydrochloride: Drug profile and nursing implications of a topoisomerase-I inhibitor in patients with advanced colorectal cancer. *Oncology Nursing Forum, 25,* 535–543.

Berg, D. (1998b). Managing the side effects of chemotherapy for colorectal cancer. *Seminars in Oncology, 25*(Suppl. 11), 53–59

Camp-Sorrell, D. (2000). Chemotherapy: Toxicity management. In C. H. Yarbro, M. H. Frogge, M. Goodman, et al. (Eds.), *Cancer nursing: Principles and practice* (5th ed., pp. 444–486). Boston: Jones and Bartlett.

Camptosar (irinotecan HCI) prescribing information. (2000). Kalamazoo, MI: Upjohn Pharmaceuticals.

Cassileth, B. (1999). Evaluating complementary and alternative therapies for cancer patients. *CA: A Cancer Journal for Clinicians, 49,* 362–375.

DeVita, V. T., Hellman, S., & Rosenberg, S. A. (2005). *Cancer: Principles and practice of oncology* (7th ed.). Philadelphia: Lippincott Williams & Wilkins.

Dorr, R. T., & Von Hoff, D. D. (1994). *Cancer chemotherapy handbook* (2nd ed.). Norwalk, CT: Appleton and Lange.

Eisenberg, D. M., Kessler, R. C., Foster, C., et al. (1993). Unconventional medicine in the United States, prevalence, costs and patterns of use. *New England Journal of Medicine, 328,* 246–252.

Eisenberg, D. M., Davis, R. B., Ettner, S. L., et al. (1998). Trends in alternative medicine use in the United States 1990–1997. *Journal of the American Medical Association, 280*(18), 1569–1575.

Groenwald, S., Frogge, M., Goodman, M., et al. (1995). *Comprehensive cancer nursing review* (2nd ed.). Boston: Jones and Bartlett.

Guy, J. L., & Ingram, B. A. (1996). Medical oncology: The agents. In R. McCorkle, M. Grant, M. Frank-Stromborg, et al. (Eds.), *Cancer nursing: A comprehensive textbook* (2nd ed., pp. 359–394). Philadelphia: W. B. Saunders.

Kummar, S., Noronha, V., & Chu, E. (2005). Antimetabolites. In V. T. De Vita, S. Hellman, & S. A. Rosenberg (Eds.), *Cancer: Principles and practice of oncology* (7th ed., pp 358–374). Philadelphia: Lippincott Williams & Wilkins.

Lederle Laboratories. (1997). *Methotrexate* [Package insert]. Pearl River, NY: Author.

Mead Johnson Oncology Products. (2000). *Taxol (paclitaxel)* [Package insert]. Princeton, NJ: Author.

Oncology Nursing Society. (2001). *Chemotherapy and biotherapy: Guidelines and recommendations for practice.* Pittsburgh, PA: Oncology Nursing Press.

Sasson, Z., Morgan, C., Wang, B., et al. (1994). 5-Fluorouracil related toxic myocarditis: Case reports and pathologic confirmation. *Canadian Journal of Cardiology, 10*(8), 861–864.

Tatro, D. S. (1999). Drug interactions with herbal products. In R. M. Short & T. H. Burnham (Eds.), *Facts and comparisons: The review of natural products.* St. Louis: Facts and Comparisons.

SmithKline Beecham Oncology. (2000). *Hycamtin* [Package insert]. Philadelphia: Author.

chapter 36

Drugs That Are Cell Cycle–Nonspecific

Learning Objectives

At the completion of this chapter the student will:

1 Differentiate a cell cycle–specific from a cell cycle–nonspecific agent.
2 Identify core drug knowledge about cell cycle–nonspecific drugs.
3 Identify core patient variables relevant to cell cycle–nonspecific drugs.
4 Relate the interaction of core drug knowledge to core patient variables for cell cycle–nonspecific drugs.
5 Generate a nursing plan of care based on the above interactions between core drug knowledge and core patient variables for cell cycle–nonspecific drugs.
6 Describe the nursing interventions to maximize therapeutic and minimize adverse effects of cell cycle–nonspecific drugs.
7 Determine key points for patient and family education for cell cycle–nonspecific drugs.
8 Discuss the treatment options for chemotherapy-induced nausea and vomiting.
9 State the rationale for using a combination of drugs in chemotherapy.
10 Identify the characteristics of drugs that are useful for combination chemotherapy.

KEY TERMS

acute emesis
alkylating agent
antitumor antibiotics
cell cycle–nonspecific
combination chemotherapy
delayed emesis
disease flare
emetogenics
hormones
hormone antagonists
liposomes
nitrosoureas
radiomimetic
tumor burden

FEATURED WEBLINK

http://breast-cancer-research.com/home
This Breast Cancer Research site has up-to-date research on breast cancer. The articles are free, free with registration, or available with a subscription.

CONNECTION WEBLINK657

Additional Weblinks are found on Connection:
http://www.connection.lww.com/go/aschenbrenner.

Drugs That Are Cell Cycle–Nonspecific

Ⓒ Alkylating Agents

- **P cyclophosphamide**
- cisplatin

Ⓒ Nitrosureas

- **P carmustine**
- streptozocin

Ⓒ Antitumor Antibiotics

- **P doxorubicin**
- bleomycin

Ⓒ Hormones and Hormone Antagonists

Ⓒ Adrenal corticosteroids

- betamethasone
- dexamethasone
- prednisone (see also Chapter 51)

Ⓒ Estrogens (see also Chapter 54)

- diethylstilbestrol
- estradiol

Ⓒ Antiandrogens

- bicalutamide
- flutamide
- nilutamide

Ⓒ Aromatase inhibitor

- anastrozole

Ⓒ Androgens (see also Chapter 53)

- testolactone
- fluoxymesterone

Ⓒ Gonadotropin-releasing hormone analogues

- goserelin acetate
- leuprolide

Ⓒ Progestins (see also Chapter 54)

- megestrol acetate
- medroxyprogesterone

Ⓒ Antiestrogens

- **P tamoxifen**

The symbol Ⓒ indicates the **drug class.**
Drugs in **bold type** marked with the symbol P are prototypes.
Drugs in blue type are closely related to the prototype.
Drugs in red type are significantly different from the prototype.
Drugs in black type with no symbol are also used in drug therapy; no prototype

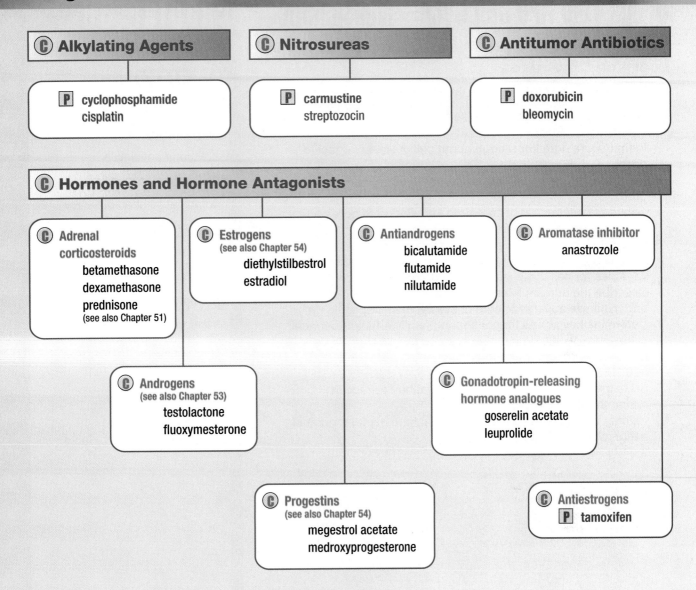

Cancer chemotherapy agents that are effective at specific phases in the cell's life cycle are classified as cell cycle specific. Drugs that are effective through all phases of the cell cycle and are not limited to a specific phase are classified as **cell cycle nonspecific.** This chapter focuses on the cell cycle–nonspecific antineoplastic drugs and the various management strategies used to ameliorate toxicities and maximize optimal therapeutic efficacy. Cell cycle–nonspecific drugs act on cells both in the proliferative and nonproliferative phases of the cell cycle. They directly affect the deoxyribonucleic acid (DNA) molecule and do not display any specificity for cells that are dividing. They are considered more toxic than the cell cycle–specific drugs because their destructive action does not differentiate between normal and malignant cycling cells. Additionally, their toxicities are felt throughout the cell cycle. This chapter also discusses the role of cytoprotectants and antiemetic agents, which have advanced the use of this group of chemotherapeutic agents. Included in the cell cycle–nonspecific class of drugs are the alkylating agents, antitumor antibiotics, and hormonal drugs (hormones and hormone antagonists). Nonspecific agents are given in bolus doses because they cause cell death independently of the proliferative state of the cell. These agents also reduce the number of cells that make up a patient's tumor or tumors, which is known as the **tumor burden.**

This chapter also focuses on the important role of combination therapy: cell cycle–specific or cell cycle–nonspecific drugs, or both, used together to combat malignant neoplasms. The combination of a cell cycle–nonspecific and a cell cycle–specific drug can kill cells that are slowly dividing and those that are actively dividing. Cell cycle–nonspecific drugs can also help recruit cells into a more actively dividing state, which then makes them more sensitive to cell cycle–specific drugs. This chapter also discusses the rationale for implementing single drug therapy and for designing effective combinations. Finally, it includes some of the most common drug combinations in clinical use today.

C ALKYLATING AGENTS

The **alkylating agents** attack cells in any phase of the cell cycle, including (for some agents) the resting phase. They exert their toxic effects by transferring their alkyl groups to various intracellular components, including nuclear DNA. Once the nucleotides have been alkylated, abnormal base pairing may occur, leading to DNA breakage (scission) and cross-linking. The damaged DNA molecule cannot replicate itself, and cell death results. The alkylating drugs are described as **radiomimetic,** so named because they mimic the actions of radiation therapy on the cells.

The alkylating drugs, the first modern chemotherapeutic agents, are a product of the secret wartime gas programs in the first and second World Wars. The exposure of seamen to mustard gas in World War II led to the discovery that alkylating drugs cause marrow and lymphoid hypoplasia, which led to their use in treating hematopoietic neoplasms such as Hodgkin disease and lymphocytic lymphoma.

Alkylating agents include nitrogen mustard and its derivatives (busulfan, chlorambucil, cyclophosphamide, and melphalan); the nitrosoureas (carmustine, lomustine, and streptozocin); and the platinum compounds (carboplatin, cisplatin, and oxaliplatin). Table 36.1 summarizes these drugs. The prototypical alkylating agent is cyclophosphamide (Cytoxan).

NURSING MANAGEMENT OF THE PATIENT RECEIVING P CYCLOPHOSPHAMIDE

Core Drug Knowledge

Pharmacotherapeutics

Cyclophosphamide (Cytoxan), a nitrogen mustard derivative, is the most widely used alkylating agent. It has a broad spectrum of antitumor activity and plays a major role in the treatment of hematologic malignancies such as Hodgkin disease, non-Hodgkin lymphoma, and multiple myeloma. It is the only alkylating agent that is effective against acute as well as chronic leukemias. Cyclophosphamide is an important component of regimens used in stem cell transplantation. It is also effective against solid tumors, such as those associated with breast cancer, small-cell lung cancer, and endometrial cancer, and with ovarian tumors. Cyclophosphamide is given intravenously or orally.

Pharmacokinetics

Cyclophosphamide and its active and inactive metabolites are well distributed throughout the body, including the brain and cerebrospinal fluid. The drug also distributes into breast milk and saliva. Most of the drug is metabolized in the liver, and about 60% of some metabolites bind extensively to plasma protein. It is exclusively excreted by the kidneys primarily as metabolites; however, because of avid tubular reabsorption, only about 5% to 25% of the drug is excreted unchanged in the urine.

Pharmacodynamics

Cyclophosphamide exerts its toxic effects by transferring alkyl groups to nuclear DNA, leading to abnormal base pairing, DNA breakage and cross-linking, and cell death. During extensive first-pass hepatic metabolism, cyclophosphamide undergoes hydroxylation and is converted into a cytotoxic agent with wide clinical utility in the treatment of various tumors. It is particularly effective with leukemias because the lymphocytes are very sensitive to this drug's effects.

Contraindications and Precautions

Patients with severely compromised bone marrow function and with known hypersensitivity to the drug should not be treated with cyclophosphamide. If the patient has poor renal or hepatic function, dose modification should be considered.

Adverse Effects

The dose-limiting toxicity associated with this drug (at high dosage) is leukopenia. Leukocytes reach nadir within 2 weeks, with recovery after 3 to 4 weeks. At standard doses, the drug is more platelet sparing. At very high doses, cyclophosphamide has a propensity for inducing sterile hemorrhagic cystitis. This problem is manifested by hematuria, pain, and burning on urination caused by the irritation of the bladder wall by acrolein, a metabolic by-product

TABLE 36.1 Summary of Selected (C) Cell Cycle–Nonspecific Antineoplastic Drugs

Drug (Trade) Name	Selected Indications	Route and Dosage Range	Pharmacokinetics
(C) Alkylating Agents			
(P) cyclophosphamide (Cytoxan; *Canadian:* Procytox)	Neck, genitourinary, advanced ovarian, and cervical cancers; also recurrent brain tumors in children	*Adult:* IV, single agent 360 mg/m² on d 1 every 4 wk, depending on platelet count; in combination with cyclophosphamide, 300 mg/m² on d 1 every 4 wk	*Onset:* Rapid *Peak:* 1 h *Duration:* Unknown $t_{1/2}$: 4–6 h
cisplatin (Platinol, CDDP)	Testicular cancer and other genitourinary tumors (bladder, prostate, metastatic ovarian, cervical, and endometrial)	*Adult:* IV, low level, 20–49 mg/mg²; moderate level, 50–75 mg/m²; and high level, 75–120 mg/m² or 3 mg/kg over 20–30 min or continuous 24-h infusion	*Onset:* 8–10 h *Peak:* 18–23 d *Duration:* 20–35 d $t_{1/2}$: 25–49 min; then 58–73 h
carboplatin (Paraplatin)	Ovarian cancer	*Adult:* IV, 360 mg/m² on d 1 given q 4 wk	*Onset:* Rapid *Peak:* Unknown *Duration:* 48–96 h $t_{1/2}$: 1.1–2h, then 2.6–5.9 h
ifosfamide (Ifex)	Testicular cancer	*Adult:* 1–2 g/d × 5 d	*Onset:* Rapid *Peak:* Unknown *Duration:* Unknown $t_{1/2}$: 3–10 h for low dose; 13.8 h for high dose
busulfan (Myleran)	Chronic granulocytic leukemia	*Adult:* PO, 4–8 mg/d until WBC decreases by half, then maintenance doses up to 4 mg/d	*Onset:* 0.5–2 h *Peak:* 2–3 h *Duration:* 4 h $t_{1/2}$: Unknown
chlorambucil (Leukeran)	Hodgkin disease, chronic lymphocytic leukemia, non-Hodgkin lymphoma, breast and ovarian cancer	*Adult:* 0.1–0.2 mg/kg for 3–6 wk then a maintenance dose not to exceed 0.1 mg/kg/d	*Onset:* Varies *Peak:* 1 h *Duration:* 15–20 h $t_{1/2}$:1 h
mechlorethamine (nitrogen mustard, Mustargen)	Lung cancer, chronic lymphocytic leukemia, chronic myelocytic leukemia, Hodgkin disease, lymphosarcoma, malignant effusions	*Adult:* IV, 0.4 mg/kg; intracavitary, 0.2–0.4 mg/kg	*Onset:* Immediate *Peak:* Seconds *Duration:* Minutes $t_{1/2}$: Minutes
melphalan (Alkeran)	Multiple myeloma	*Adult:* PO, 0.25 mg/kg/d × 7 d, followed by 3 wk drug free, then maintenance dose of 2 mg/d; IV, 16 mg/m² q 3 wk × 4 doses then q 4 wk	*Onset:* Varies (PO), Rapid (IV) *Peak:* 2 h (PO), 1 h (IV)
(C) Nitrosureas			
(P) carmustine (BCNU)	Palliative therapy of brain tumors, multiple myeloma, Hodgkin disease, and non-Hodgkin lymphoma as single-drug or combination therapy	*Adult:* IV, 150–200 mg/m² q 6 wk as a single dose or given in 2 d in divided doses as a slow infusion over 1–2 h	*Onset:* Immediate *Peak:* 15 min *Duration:* Unknown $t_{1/2}$: 15–30 min
streptozocin (Zanosar)	Pancreatic cancer, colon cancer, carcinoid tumors	*Adult:* IV, 500 mg/m² d for 5 d every 6 wk or 1 g/m² wk for 2 wk; dosages not to exceed 1.5 g/m² wk	*Onset:* Varies *Peak:* Unknown *Duration:* 24 h $t_{1/2}$: 35 min
lomustine (CCNU)	Hodgkin disease, brain tumors	*Adult:* 130 mg/m² q 6 wk	*Onset:* 10 min *Peak:* 5 h *Duration:* 48 h $t_{1/2}$: 16–72 h

(continued)

TABLE 36.1 Summary of Selected (C) Cell Cycle–Nonspecific Antineoplastic Drugs (continued)

Drug (Trade) Name	Selected Indications	Route and Dosage Range	Pharmacokinetics
(C) Antitumor Antibiotics			
[P] doxorubicin (Adriamycin)	Hematologic cancers (leukemias, Hodgkin disease, lymphomas, multiple myeloma); solid tumors (breast, ovarian, prostate, stomach, thyroid, liver, small-cell lung, and head and neck cancers)	*Adult:* IV, 60–75 mg/m^2 as single injection every 21 d; alternate schedule, 30 mg/m^2 on each of 3 successive d 4 wk; administered by slow IV push through a free-flowing IV line over 3–5 min or as a continuous 24-h infusion through a central venous access device	*Onset:* Rapid *Peak:* 2 h *Duration:* 24–36 h $t_{1/2}$: 12 min; then 3.3 h
doxorubicin HCl liposome (Doxil)	AIDS-related Kaposi sarcoma	*Adult:* IV, 20 mg/m^2 q 3 wk	*Onset:* Unknown *Peak:* Unknown *Duration:* Unknown $t_{1/2}$: 55 h
bleomycin (Blenoxane)	Lymphomas, squamous cell carcinoma, and testicular cancers	*Adult:* IV/IM/SC, 10–20 U/m^2 weekly or twice weekly	*Onset:* Immediate *Peak:* IV, 10–20 min; IM/SC, 30–60 min *Duration:* Unknown $t_{1/2}$: 2 h
daunorubicin hydrochloride (Cerubidine, DNR,)	Acute myelogenous leukemia, acute lymphocytic leukemia	*Adult:* 30–60 mg/m^2/d for 3 d IV *Child:* 25–45 mg/m^2 IV	*Onset:* Slow *Peak:* Unknown *Duration:* 8 d $t_{1/2}$: 20 h
daunorubicin citrate liposome (Daunoxome)	Advanced AIDS related Kaposi sarcoma	*Adult:* IV 40 mg/m^2 q 2 wk	*Onset:* Unknown *Peak:* Unknown *Duration:* Unknown $t_{1/2}$: 5.9–43.6 h
dactinomycin (Actinomycin, Cosmegen)	Testicular cancer, Ewing sarcoma trophoblastic tumor, rhabdomyosarcoma, trophoblastic neoplasms	*Adult:* 500 μg/d for a maximum 5 d *Child:* 15 μg/d to a max of 500 μg/d for 5 d	*Onset:* Rapid *Peak:* Unknown *Duration:* 9 d $t_{1/2}$: 36 h
idarubicin (Idamycin)	Acute myeloid leukemia	*Adult:* 12 μg/m^2 d × 3 d in combination with cytarabine	*Onset:* Rapid *Peak:* Minutes *Duration*: Unknown $t_{1/2}$: 6–9.4 h
mitoxantrone (Novantrone)	Acute monocytic leukemia, acute myelocytic leukemia, acute promyelocytic leukemia, breast cancer	*Adult:* 12 mg/m^2 d × 2–3 d in combination with cytosine arabinoside	*Onset:* Varies *Peak*: 10–14 d *Duration:* 28 d $t_{1/2}$: 5.8 d (median)
pentostatin (Nipent)	Alfa-interferon refractory hairy cell leukemia	*Adult:* IV, 4 mg/m^2 q other week	*Onset:* Rapid *Peak:* 11 min *Duration:* Unknown $t_{1/2}$: 5.7 h
plicamycin (Mithramycin)	Testicular tumors, severe hypercalcemia	*Adult:* IV, 25–30 μg/kg/d for 8–10 doses; severe hypercalcemia: 25 μg/kg/d × 3–4 d	*Onset:* Rapid *Peak:* 4 h *Duration:* Unknown $t_{1/2}$: Unknown

(continued)

TABLE 36.1 Summary of Selected (C) Cell Cycle–Nonspecific Antineoplastic Drugs (continued)

Drug (Trade) Name	Selected Indications	Route and Dosage Range	Pharmacokinetics
(C) Hormones and Hormone Antagonists			
(C) Adrenocorticosteroids			
prednisone (Meticorten; *Canadian:* Apo-Prednisone)	Adjunct for palliation of symptoms in acute leukemia, Hodgkin disease, lymphoma, complications of cancer such as thrombocytopenia, hypercalcemia	Individualize dosage depending on severity of condition and patient's response	*Onset:* Varies *Peak:* 1–2 h *Duration:* 1–1.5 d $t_{1/2}$: 3.5 h
(C) Androgens			
fluoxymesterone (Halotestin)	Advanced breast cancer in premenopausal women	*Adult:* 10–40 mg/d PO in divided doses	*Onset:* Rapid *Peak:* 2 h *Duration:* Unknown $t_{1/2}$: 9.5 h
testolactone (Teslac)	Advanced breast cancer	*Adult:* PO, 250 mg qid	*Onset:* Rapid *Peak:* Unknown *Duration:* Unknown $t_{1/2}$: Unknown
(C) Estrogens			
diethylstilbestrol diphosphate (Stilphostrol; *Canadian:* Hanvol)	Inoperable prostate cancer, postmenopausal metastatic breast cancer	*Adult:* PO, 50 mg tid increasing to 200 mg with maximum daily dose no greater than 1 g; IV, 0.5 g for 5 d, then 0.25–0.50 g once or twice wk	*Onset:* Rapid *Peak:* Unknown *Duration:* Unknown $t_{1/2}$: Not available
estradiol (Estinyl)	Advanced breast cancer in postmenopausal women, prostate cancer	*Adult:* Breast cancer: PO, 0.5 mg/d initially, gradually increased to 3 mg/d in three divided doses; prostate cancer: PO, 0.15–2 mg/d	*Onset:* Slow *Peak:* Days *Duration:* Unknown $t_{1/2}$: Unknown
(C) Progestins			
medroxyprogesterone (Provera, Depo-Provera)	Advanced endometrial carcinoma	*Adult:* IM, 400–800 mg twice/wk; PO, 200–300 mg/d	*Onset:* Slow, weeks *Peak:* Unknown *Duration:* Unknown $t_{1/2}$: Unknown
megestrol acetate (Megace)	Advanced endometrial carcinoma, breast cancer	*Adult:* PO, 40–320 mg/d	*Onset:* Slow *Peak:* Weeks *Duration:* Unknown $t_{1/2}$: Unknown
(C) Antiandrogens			
bicalutamide (Casodex)	Advanced prostate cancer	*Adult:* PO, 500 mg once daily	*Onset:* Slow *Peak:* 31.3 h *Duration:* Days $t_{1/2}$: 5.8 d
flutamide (Eulexin)	Advanced prostate cancer	*Adult:* PO, 250 mg q8h	*Onset:* Varies *Peak:* 2 h *Duration:* 72 h $t_{1/2}$: 6 h
nilutamide (Nilandron)	Advanced breast cancer in postmenopausal women with disease progression after tamoxifen	*Adult:* PO, 300 mg/d × 30 d, then 150 mg/d	*Onset:* Varies *Peak:* Unknown *Duration:* Unknown $t_{1/2}$: Unknown

(continued)

TABLE 36.1 Summary of Selected (C) Cell Cycle–Nonspecific Antineoplastic Drugs (continued)

Drug (Trade) Name	Selected Indications	Route and Dosage Range	Pharmacokinetics
(C) Gonadotropin-Releasing Hormone (GnRH) Analogues			
goserelin (Zoladex)	Advanced prostatic cancer, advanced breast cancer, endometriosis	*Adult:* SC 3.6 mg q 28 d	*Onset:* Slow *Peak:* 12–15 d *Duration:* Unknown $t_{1/2}$: 4.2 h
leuprolide (Lupron), Lupron Depot	Advanced prostatic cancer	*Adult:* SC, 1 mg/d *Depot:* 7.5 mg IM monthly q28–33d	*Onset:* Slow *Peak:* Unknown *Duration:* Unknown $t_{1/2}$: Unknown
(C) Aromatase Inhibitors			
anastrozole (Arimidex)	Advanced breast cancer in postmenopausal women whose disease progressed after tamoxifen therapy	*Adult:* PO, 1 mg daily	*Onset:* Rapid *Peak:* Unknown *Duration:* Unknown $t_{1/2}$: 7 d
(C) Antiestrogens			
(P) tamoxifen (Nolvadex; *Canadian:* Apo-Tamoxifen)	Breast cancers	*Adult:* PO, 20–40 mg/d	*Onset:* Varies *Peak:* 4–7 h *Duration:* Unknown $t_{1/2}$: 7–14 h

of cyclophosphamide. Other adverse effects of high-dose therapy (120 to 270 mg/kg) include syndrome of inappropriate antidiuretic hormone (SIADH). High doses can also cause cardiomyopathy in the form of congestive heart failure (CHF) and hemopericardium secondary to hemorrhagic myocarditis and myocardial necrosis. Hypersensitivity has been observed in both untreated and pretreated patients. Cyclophosphamide is an FDA pregnancy category D drug. Reproductive effects such as amenorrhea, gonadal suppression, sterility, and ovarian fibrosis can occur. Secondary malignancies have been reported with drug use. Other adverse effects include cutaneous problems manifested as alopecia and as transverse ridging and hyperpigmentation of the nails. Nausea, vomiting, and anorexia may also occur. On rapid infusion of the drug, patients may complain of dizziness, nasal stuffiness, and rhinorrhea.

Drug Interactions

Table 36.2 notes the effects of cyclophosphamide on other drugs. It is compatible with other common antineoplastic agents such as melphalan, paclitaxel, vinorelbine, idarubicin, cisplatin, and bleomycin. It can interact with some herbal medicines (see Chapter 35).

Assessment of Relevant Core Patient Variables

Health Status

Assess any organ system that could be potentially compromised by cyclophosphamide therapy. Before initiating treatment, baseline tests to determine sufficient hematopoietic and renal function should be performed. Cyclophosphamide

TABLE 36.2 Agents That Interact With (P) Cyclophosphamide

Interactants	Effect and Significance	Nursing Management
doxorubicin	Potentiates doxorubicin-induced cardiotoxicity	Dose modification is advised. Monitor cardiac function.
succinylcholine	Prolongs neuromuscular blocking activity	Administer with caution.
digoxin	Decreases pharmacologic effect	Digoxin dosage may need to be increased.
halothane and nitrous oxide	When used in conjunction, has produced mortality	Notify anesthesia department.
corticosteroids	Decreases conversion of cyclophosphamide to its active metabolites, decreasing activity	Notify health care provider for dose adjustment.

should not be given to patients who have impaired renal function, myelosuppression, or a known hypersensitivity to the drug. Patients who have had prior radiation to the pelvis or bladder are at increased risk for hemorrhagic cystitis.

Life Span and Gender

Document the age and developmental status of the patient. Cyclophosphamide can cause secondary malignancies such as bladder cancer, nonlymphocytic leukemia, and non-Hodgkin lymphoma, which generally occur later in the patient's life. Long-term therapy increases the risk for a secondary malignancy, although secondary malignancies have been known to occur several years after treatment with cyclophosphamide has been stopped. Patients should be counseled about this long-term risk. Patients who develop bladder cancer usually have a history of hemorrhagic cystitis. Adolescent patients who received cyclophosphamide for cancer treatment as children seem to be at higher risk than other populations for secondary cancers. This increased risk may be because these patients are more likely to experience hemorrhagic cystitis, but the exact etiology of these cancers is unclear (Cancer Care, 2004). Because of possible reproductive side effects, discuss reproductive goals with patients of childbearing potential who are considering high-dose therapy. Also, assess the woman of childbearing age for pregnancy and explore contraceptive methods because cyclophosphamide is a pregnancy category D drug.

Lifestyle, Diet, and Habits

Assess the daily dietary habits and elimination patterns of patients taking the oral formulation of the drug. The metabolites of the drug should be excreted during the day. If metabolite-rich urine stagnates, it can erode the bladder wall. To promote diuresis and ameliorate this potential adverse effect of drug administration, the patient must drink as much as 2 L of liquid a day. Activities of daily living should also be assessed because the patient may have difficulty getting to the bathroom if he or she has impaired mobility.

Environment

Be aware of the environment in which the drug will be administered. High-dose intravenous cyclophosphamide therapy is usually given in an acute care facility where patients can be adequately managed for potential major and acute toxicities, such as severe nausea and vomiting or hemorrhagic cystitis. However, pretreatment hydration with vigorous oral intake can be accomplished in the home setting if the patient and caregiver are well instructed and adhere to the hydration regimen.

Nursing Diagnoses and Outcomes

- Risk for Infection related to suppression of bone marrow function
  Desired outcome: *The patient will be free from infection and exercise caution to avoid exposure to infection.*
- Risk for Injury associated with depression of bone marrow function and related bleeding and hypersensitivity reaction (anaphylaxis)
  Desired outcome: *The patient will attain pretreatment hematologic status, learn to monitor and manage situations that may induce bleeding, and recognize and immediately report signs and symptoms associated with a hypersensitivity reaction.*
- Imbalanced Nutrition: Less than Body Requirements related to nausea, vomiting, and taste alterations
  Desired outcome: *The patient will experience adequate emetic control using pharmacologic and nonpharmacologic measures.*
- Impaired Urinary Elimination related to cyclophosphamide-induced nephrotoxicity
  Desired outcome: *The patient will maintain fluid balance and be free from signs and symptoms of hemorrhagic cystitis as evidenced by adequate fluid intake and output. In addition, renal function will not be compromised as shown by normal renal and blood count values and absence of hematuria, pain, and dysuria.*
- Impaired Skin Integrity and Disturbed Body Image related to alopecia and changes in skin pigmentation and nail condition.
  Desired outcome: *The patient will be able to recognize and report any changes in the skin and integuments and will undertake measures to enhance appearance and body image.*

Planning and Intervention

Maximizing Therapeutic Effects

Before administering cyclophosphamide, ensure that the test results disclose good renal function and adequate hematopoietic reserves to achieve the intended therapeutic effects.

Minimizing Adverse Effects

The incidence of hemorrhagic cystitis can be reduced by a vigorous hydration regimen of at least 2 to 3 L of fluid a day and, in high-dose therapy, administering the uroprotectant agent mesna. This drug is not routinely given to children. Prehydrate the patient orally and intravenously with at least 1 to 2 L of normal saline solution with potassium and magnesium additives several hours before and after infusing mesna. Monitor urine output vigilantly to ensure an output of at least half of the intake. Mannitol can be used to increase urine output. Aminoglycoside antibiotics, which carry a high risk for renal toxicity, should be avoided to prevent compromising renal function.

Providing Patient and Family Education

- Emphasize methods of preventing the major toxicities of cyclophosphamide therapy.
- Encourage the patient to drink large amounts of fluid, at least 2 to 3 L daily, to induce diuresis. Some of the pretreatment hydration can be accomplished at home; thus, if the patient understands the reason for it, his or her adherence to the regimen the night before drug administration will be improved. Additional hydration will be given in the hospital to augment previous oral intake.
- Advise the patient that temporary and reversible hair loss will occur. Refer the patient to a wig specialist before treatment is initiated, and educate the patient to refrain from using chemical treatments on the hair and from vigorous brushing. Teach the patient to use mild shampoos and, if the patient has long hair, suggest that it be cut before chemotherapy starts to avoid the trauma of seeing the gradual loss of hair.

- Review signs and symptoms of a hypersensitivity reaction with the patient to alleviate the patient's anxiety. Ask the patient for other known sensitivity to drugs and determine whether the patient is asthmatic.
- Instruct the patient to notify the prescriber about other serious adverse effects. Signs and symptoms to report include lower volume of urine or less frequent urination than usual; a temperature of 100.5°F or higher; excessive vomiting, diarrhea, or inability to keep food and fluids down that persists for more than 24 hours; and the presence of black stools, red rash, or unusual bruising, which are signs of bleeding.
- Reassure the patient that nausea and vomiting can be relieved with antiemetic drug therapy and emphasize that the patient should request these agents when needed. Teach nonpharmacologic measures such as relaxation and always ask the patient to initiate practices that have helped alleviate these symptoms in the past. Good emesis management is important because either acute or delayed emesis has distressing effects on physical and psychological functioning (see discussion below on the types of chemotherapy-induced emesis).
- Counsel the patient about the long-term risks of secondary malignancies (e.g., bladder and skin cancers) associated with prolonged low-dose cyclophosphamide therapy.
- If taking an oral formulation of the drug, instruct the patient to ingest the drug early in the morning on an empty stomach, to drink at least 10 to 12 glasses of water daily, and to empty the bladder frequently. These practices will ensure that the metabolites of the drug are excreted during the day and do not stagnate to erode the bladder wall.
- Discuss the need for sperm and egg banking with patients who are on high-dose therapy and are considering having children in the future.

Ongoing Assessment and Evaluation

When patients undergo subsequent courses of chemotherapy, assess renal function and hematopoietic reserve. Assess the patient's hematologic status every week during the first months of therapy and until maintenance therapy is set, and then at intervals of 2 to 3 weeks. For high-dose regimens, also monitor cardiac function. Dose modification should be considered in patients with impaired renal, hematologic, or hepatic function.

Drug Significantly Different From P Cyclophosphamide

Cisplatin (Cisplatinum, CDDP) is a widely used heavy metal that acts as a bifunctional alkylating agent. It produces intrastrand and interstrand linking in DNA through covalent bonds with the platinum molecule, leading to breaking of DNA strands during cell replication. It is clinically used to treat almost every solid tumor and lymphoma. The pharmacokinetics show rapid distribution of the drug to the tissues after intravenous (IV) infusion. Most of it bonds to protein. The drug is believed to be metabolized in the liver and excreted in the urine.

Cisplatin belongs to a group of antineoplastic drugs called **emetogenics**, which have high potential for causing severe nausea and vomiting (Box 36.1). Approximately 75% of chemotherapy patients experience this distressing adverse effect, which can drastically affect their physical functioning and quality of life. The risk factors that predispose the patient to this problem are illustrated in Box 36.2.

MEMORY CHIP

P Cyclophosphamide

- Indicated for testicular, ovarian, and bladder cancers
- Major contraindications: severe depression of bone marrow function, serious infections, nursing mothers, and women and men with child-bearing potential
- Most common adverse effect: hemorrhagic or nonhemorrhagic cystitis
- Dose-limiting effect: leukopenia
- **Life span alert: Patients on long-term therapy should be counseled about risks of secondary malignancy.**
- Maximizing therapeutic effects: Ensure that patient has adequate bone marrow reserve and good renal function
- Minimizing adverse effects: Promote vigorous hydration and diuresis to prevent cystitis.
- Most important patient education: Instruct the patient to drink plenty of fluids and empty the bladder every 2 hours.

BOX 36.1 Ranking Chemotherapeutic Drugs According to Emetogenic Potential

The following antineoplastic drugs are listed according to their emetogenic potential. Highly emetogenic drugs begin the list; mildly emetogenic drugs complete it.

Cisplatin
Dacarbazine
Streptozocin
Nitrogen mustard
Hexamethylmelamine
Actinomycin D
Cyclophosphamide*
Carboplatin*
Lomustine
Carmustine
Anthracyclines
Ifosfamide
Cytosine arabinoside
Procarbazine
Taxanes
Mitomycin-C
Etoposide
Methotrexate
Irinotecan
Topotecan
Gemcitabine
Bleomycin
Vinca alkaloids
5-Fluorouracil
Hormones
Chlorambucil

*Late onset of nausea and vomiting.

BOX 36.2 Risk Factors for Nausea and Vomiting

Anxiety, expectations of severe side effects, and previous chemotherapy experience are predisposing factors to the adverse effects of nausea and vomiting. Certain patient characteristics and prognostic factors also affect the incidence of nausea and vomiting:

- Age: younger patients experience nausea and vomiting more than older patients.
- Gender: a higher incidence of nausea and vomiting in women is thought to result from administration of more highly emetogenic drugs to women than to men and lower alcohol consumption among women.
- Alcohol intake: high alcohol consumption has a positive effect on emetic control.
- Performance status and motivation: patients who have a better physical, emotional, and functional status have a better tolerance of emesis.
- History of motion sickness or severe emesis during pregnancy: these patients are more susceptible to chemotherapy-induced episodes of nausea and vomiting.

The pathophysiology of chemotherapy-induced nausea and vomiting is well characterized. The emetic center contains the chemoreceptor trigger zone and is stimulated through peripheral and central pathways. Peripheral stimulation happens when chemotherapy causes damage to the gastrointestinal mucosa, activating afferent input through the vagus nerve. Serotonin is the neurotransmitter for peripheral stimulation. Emesis associated with cytotoxic agents occurs in different patterns: acute, delayed, anticipatory, breakthrough, and refractory (Box 36.3). Cisplatin therapy can be associated with any of these patterns of nausea and vomiting, but it is primarily associated with **acute emesis** (vomiting within 24 hours after chemotherapy) and **delayed emesis** (nausea and vomiting 24 hours after chemotherapy). In cisplatin therapy, severe nausea and vomiting occur within 1 to 4 hours after treatment and usually last for 24 hours. The drugs that are most effective in treating acute emesis from cisplatin therapy are the serotonin receptor antagonists. These first-line agents act by blocking serotonin from binding to receptors in the gastrointestinal (GI) tract. Delayed emesis from cisplatin therapy may persist for up to 5 days after treatment. The mechanism for delayed emesis is unclear. This type of emesis is usually treated with corticosteroids in combination with metoclopramide. Guidelines for treating various emetic patterns and adjunct nonpharmacologic treatments are found in Box 36.4 and Box 36.5. Antiemetics are discussed fully in Chapter 48; ondansetron is the prototype serotonin receptor antagonist drug presented. Appendix H: Antiemetic Drugs also provides more information on various drug therapies to treat nausea.

The major dose-limiting adverse effect of cisplatin is nephrotoxicity, which is dose related and cumulative. Pretreatment hydration and forced diuresis are required to prevent nephrotoxicity. Amifostine, the most recently approved cytoprotectant, is indicated for minimizing the nephrotoxic effects of cisplatin in advanced ovarian cancer or non–small-cell lung cancer as well as the peripheral toxicities. Neurotoxicity and ototoxicity may also limit the dose or the length of therapy of cisplatin because these adverse effects more commonly occur with larger doses or after repeated use. Peripheral neuropathy is common and painful. Neurotoxicity may also occur or worsen after cisplatin therapy has been discontinued, and some forms are irreversible. Ototoxicity, which may be bilateral or unilateral and possibly permanent, is more severe in children treated with cisplatin. Cumulative ototoxicity is common, although deafness has occurred

BOX 36.3 Types of Emesis and Their Treatments

Acute: Occurs within 24 hours after chemotherapy

Delayed: Occurs more than 24 hours after chemotherapy. Delayed emesis is not as distressing as acute emesis, but it may severely affect a patient's food intake and prolong hospitalization.

Anticipatory emesis: Learned response; happens after poorly controlled first experience with acute emesis. Usually unresponsive to antiemetic agents, although corticosteroids may be helpful. Can be prevented by effectively managing first chemotherapy cycle and educating patients about adverse effects.

Breakthrough emesis: Occurs during a treatment cycle despite prophylaxis

Refractory emesis: Occurs after at least 1 cycle of chemotherapy; can persist despite attempts to prevent it

BOX 36.4 Guidelines for Managing Chemotherapy-Induced Emesis

1. Determine the emetogenic potential of the drug: high, intermediate, or low.
2. When combination agents are given, give the antiemetic appropriate for the chemotherapeutic agent with the highest risk.
3. For acute emesis, the agents with the highest therapeutic index are the serotonin antagonists. At equivalent doses, they have the same safety and efficacy profiles and can be used interchangeably.
4. The oral route is as effective and safe as the intravenous route.
5. For acute emesis with high-risk agents, the combination of a serotonin antagonist with a corticosteroid is recommended. A corticosteroid is suggested for patients treated with intermediate emetic risk agents, whereas for low-risk agents, no antiemetic is needed. Antiemetics should be given for each day of the chemotherapy.
6. For delayed emesis, in patients receiving high-risk cisplatin, a corticosteroid plus metoclopramide or plus a serotonin antagonist is recommended. For high-risk agents without cisplatin, a corticosteroid as a single agent, a corticosteroid plus metoclopramide, or plus a serotonin antagonist are suggested regimens.
7. For intermediate and low-risk agents, no preventive agent for delayed emesis is recommended.
8. Prevention of chemotherapy-induced emesis by using the most active antiemetic agents appropriate for the drug to prevent acute or delayed emesis is suggested. Such regimens should be used with the **first** chemotherapy treatment to avoid the patient's "anticipating" poor emetic response on subsequent cycles. If anticipatory emesis occurs, behavioral therapy with systematic desensitization is effective and suggested.

Adapted from Gralla, R. J., Osoba, D., Kris, M. G., et al. (1999). American Society of Clinical Oncologists Recommendations for the Use of Antiemetics: Evidence-Based, Clinical Practice Guidelines. *Journal of Clinical Oncology, 17*(9), 2971.

BOX 36.5 Nonpharmacologic Treatments for Chemotherapy-Induced Emesis

Nonpharmacologic methods for managing nausea and vomiting are adjuncts to antiemetic therapy, not substitutes for it. These include:

1. Music therapy
2. Moderate aerobic exercise
3. Acupressure wristbands
4. Behavioral interventions such as hypnosis, biofeedback, guided imagery, and cognitive distraction*

*Effectiveness believed to be from producing relaxation, giving the patient a sense of control, reducing feelings of helplessness, and diverting the patient's attention away from the acute situation to more neutral and relaxing images.

rarely after an initial dose. Audiometry should be performed before the initial dose of cisplatin therapy and then before each subsequent dose to assess for ototoxicity. Coadministration of cisplatin with other drugs that produce ototoxicity, such as loop diuretics, may produce additive ototoxicity and should be avoided. Another serious adverse effect that can occur with cisplatin is an anaphylaxis-like reaction.

Other potential adverse effects of cisplatin are electrolyte imbalances. Cisplatin therapy can cause hypomagnesemia, hypocalcemia, hyponatremia, hypokalemia, and hypophosphatemia; these electrolyte imbalances are believed to be related to renal tubular damage that occurs with cisplatin therapy. Hypomagnesemia may be severe in high-dose cisplatin therapy, and this effect appears to contribute to some of the vascular toxicities caused by cisplatin, such as Raynaud phenomenon. Patients with low magnesium levels may need a diet high in magnesium to help offset losses from cisplatin therapy. Examples of these foods are nuts, chocolate, whole-wheat breads and cereals, instant coffee and tea, oatmeal, beans, and peas. Calcium and magnesium compete to gain entrance into the intestines, so calcium-rich foods increase the body's requirements for magnesium. Calcium-rich foods, such as dairy products, should be limited when eating foods high in magnesium during cisplatin therapy.

When administering cisplatin, be careful not to use needles or administration sets containing aluminum because these devices will result in precipitate formation or loss of drug potency because the drug reacts with aluminum.

C NITROSOUREAS

The **nitrosoureas** are alkylating drugs that are frequently classified separately from the others because they also have additional mechanisms of cytotoxicity. Like the alkylating agents, they cause breaks and cross-linking in DNA strands. They also inhibit DNA repair. Nitrosoureas are highly lipid-soluble drugs. As such, they cross the blood–brain barrier. They have broad clinical activity in treating lymphomas and certain solid tumors. Examples of frequently used nitrosoureas are carmustine and streptozocin, which are discussed in this chapter. Carmustine is the prototype of the nitrosoureas.

NURSING MANAGEMENT OF THE PATIENT RECEIVING P CARMUSTINE

Core Drug Knowledge

Pharmacotherapeutics

Carmustine (BCNU) is a nitrosourea used in the palliative therapy of brain tumors, multiple myeloma, Hodgkin disease, and non-Hodgkin lymphoma. It may be administered as a single drug or in combination with other antineoplastic agents. It is given as a slow infusion to prevent severe pain and burning at the IV site.

Pharmacokinetics

After IV administration, carmustine is rapidly degraded. Most of the drug is excreted by the renal system in 96 hours, and about 10% is excreted by the respiratory system as carbon dioxide. This drug crosses the blood–brain barrier because of its high lipid solubility.

Pharmacodynamics

The mechanism of action of carmustine is similar to that of an alkylating drug. It alkylates DNA and ribonucleic acid (RNA), thereby blocking synthesis and repair. It also inhibits essential enzymes by carbamylation of the amino acids.

Contraindications and Precautions

This drug is contraindicated in patients who are hypersensitive to it. It should be used cautiously in those with impaired respiratory or bone marrow function. Accidental skin contamination can cause hyperpigmentation and brown discoloration of the affected area. The drug should be dispensed in glass; plastic containers should be avoided. Carmustine is a pregnancy category D drug.

Adverse Effects

The major toxic effect of carmustine is suppression of bone marrow function, which generally occurs 6 weeks after drug administration. This delayed suppression is cumulative and is manifested as thrombocytopenia and leukopenia. Nausea and vomiting occur frequently. Pulmonary toxicity in the form of irreversible pulmonary fibrosis is associated with prolonged therapy and cumulative doses of more than 1,400 mg/m^2. The patient may complain of local reactions, such as intense pain and discomfort in the vein used for drug administration, flushing of the skin, and suffusion of the conjunctiva within 2 hours that can last for 4 hours after administration of the drug.

Drug Interactions

When given concomitantly with other drugs, carmustine exhibits certain effects, as shown in Table 36.3.

Assessment of Relevant Core Patient Variables

Health Status

Because the major carmustine-induced toxicities are related to bone marrow and pulmonary functions, assess patients for adequate bone marrow reserve and pulmonary function.

TABLE 36.3 Agents That Interact With P Carmustine

Interactants	Effect and Significance	Nursing Management
cimetidine	Increased toxicity and myelosuppression	Monitor blood counts.
digoxin, phenytoin	Decreased serum level	Measure serum level. Consult health care provider about dose modification if needed.

Patients at risk are those with a history of lung disease, patients receiving a greater cumulative dose than 1,400 mg/m^2 of carmustine, and children treated with cumulative doses of 770 mg/m^2 to 1,800 mg/m^2 and cranial irradiation.

Life Span and Gender

If the patient is on prolonged therapy, regularly perform pulmonary assessments to monitor for pulmonary dysfunction and disease. The onset of pulmonary problems is usually delayed, and disease is chronic. Pulmonary fibrosis has been reported to occur up to 15 years later in patients who received cumulative doses of as much as 1,800 mg/m^2, concomitantly with irradiation, as adolescents. Among adults, the same outcome has been noted with prolonged therapy and large cumulative doses. Assess women of childbearing age for pregnancy and lactation because carmustine is a pregnancy category D drug. It is not known whether carmustine is excreted in breast milk; hence, breast-feeding women should be cautioned.

Lifestyle, Diet, and Habits

Forewarn patients about the acute onset of nausea and vomiting associated with carmustine therapy. Assess the effect that nausea and vomiting will have on the patient's diet and activities of daily living. Nausea and vomiting usually occur 2 to 4 hours after drug administration. Because the signs and symptoms of myelosuppression are delayed, explore whether the patient's activities of daily living might expose him or her to risks for infection and bleeding.

Environment

Be aware of the environment in which carmustine will be administered. It is usually given in an acute care setting so that medical and nursing support are easily available should a hypersensitivity reaction or anaphylaxis occur.

Nursing Diagnoses and Outcomes

- Pain related to discomfort of drug administration
  Desired outcome: *The patient will be free from discomfort along the infusion route.*
- Risk for Infection and Injury, especially bleeding related to suppression of bone marrow function
  Desired outcome: *The patient will take steps to prevent exposure to potential sources of infection and bleeding, minimize risks for infection and bleeding, and comply with requirements for periodic blood counts.*
- Impaired Gas Exchange related to drug-related pulmonary fibrosis
  Desired outcome: *The patient will learn to recognize and report signs and symptoms of respiratory dysfunction. The patient will comply with the need to have pulmonary function tests during the course of treatment.*
- Imbalanced Nutrition: Less than Body Requirements because of drug-induced nausea and vomiting
  Desired outcome: *The patient will expect emetic episodes and ask for antiemetics as needed. The patient will learn how to manage dietary intake and patterns to ensure adequate nutritional intake.*
- Sexual Dysfunction related to mutagenic and teratogenic properties of the drug
  Desired outcome: *The patient will accept the impact of carmustine on reproductive and sexual functions. The patient will take steps to participate in counseling and accept emotional support to cope with these effects and achieve a satisfying sexual experience.*

Planning and Intervention

Maximizing Therapeutic Effects

After reconstitution, the solution is stable in a glass container for 24 hours at 4°C or for 8 hours at 25°C when protected from light.

Minimizing Adverse Effects

Monitor hematologic indices regularly, especially because myelotoxicity is delayed. Also monitor renal, hepatic, and pulmonary function tests to forestall any impending problems that might compromise the patient. If long-term therapy is planned, the prescriber should discuss the possible use of a venous access device (e.g., an implanted port through which to deliver the drug). During drug administration, the patient may experience intense discomfort. Exercise care to use a large vein for infusion if a port is not used. To minimize the pain, slow the infusion, and prolong the duration of administration. An ice compress can also help relieve the pain. You can control nausea and vomiting, which may occur within 2 hours of the treatment, with an adequate antiemetic regimen. Assess the patient for concurrent medication use because drug interactions can occur with phenytoin (Dilantin) or cimetidine. If the patient cannot be switched from these drug therapies, additional monitoring may be warranted.

Providing Patient and Family Education

Once the patient can be treated safely in an outpatient setting, develop an education plan that includes both the patient and significant caregivers.

- Teach the patient about general adverse effects and adverse signs and symptoms specific to carmustine therapy, including infection and bleeding (which might have delayed

onset) and pulmonary fibrosis if the patient will receive long-term therapy.

- Inform patients about IV drug delivery and describe reportable signs and symptoms that might signal possible extravasation.
- Discuss the potential for nausea and vomiting and provide the appropriate antiemetic regimen.
- Identify reportable problems, such as inability to eat or drink for more than 24 hours or respiratory problems.
- Explain the need for regular blood counts and pulmonary testing.
- Advise the patient to avoid taking aspirin or drugs that contain aspirin unless ordered by the prescriber and to report signs of bleeding, such as black stools, bloody gums, bruises, and red rash.
- Discuss the patient's concerns and the impact of the adverse effects on her reproductive and sexual functions and her quality of life.
- Teach patients which problems are most important to report to the health care team. Make sure the patient has phone numbers or beeper numbers to use when appropriate.

Ongoing Assessment and Evaluation

Closely monitor complete blood counts every week for 6 weeks to ensure that they are adequate before retreatment. You may need to monitor pulmonary function tests during the course of therapy so that patients at risk for pulmonary toxicity can be managed appropriately.

Drug Closely Related to P Carmustine

Streptozocin (Zanosar) is another drug that belongs to the nitrosourea group. It is the product of the organism *Streptomyces achromogenes*. It is well known for its efficacy in treating malignant islet cell tumors of the pancreas. Streptozocin is given intravenously. Patients may complain of pain and burning during the infusion. You can relieve this discomfort by slowing the infusion, increasing the volume used for dilution, and increasing the total volume of the primary IV infusion.

The most frequently reported adverse effect is severe nausea and vomiting. Another GI reaction is hepatotoxicity, manifested by an increase in liver enzyme and bilirubin levels, hypoalbuminemia, and jaundice. The development of renal toxicity is dose limiting and may be fatal. The mechanism of nephrotoxicity is unclear. Early manifestations include hypophosphatemia, glycosuria, proteinuria, azotemia, and renal tubular acidosis. Patients with pre-existing renal disease are at risk. Closely monitor renal, hematopoietic, and hepatic functions at baseline and periodically during therapy so that the patient's organ systems are not severely compromised. Additionally, streptozocin has shown diabetogenic activity evidenced by altered glucose metabolism, decrease in insulin levels, and elevated fasting blood glucose levels. This activity is thought to result from an increased uptake of the drug into the islets, which may occur in some patients. Clinical trials suggest that this activity can be reduced by pharmacologic intervention with nicotinamide.

MEMORY CHIP

P Carmustine

- Indicated for treating brain tumors, multiple myelomas, Hodgkin and non-Hodgkin lymphomas, and malignant melanoma
- Major contraindications: poor pulmonary function, which places the patient at risk of developing pulmonary toxicity, and known hypersensitivity to the drug
- Most common adverse effects: acute nausea and emesis
- Dose-limiting effect: delayed myelosuppression
- Most serious adverse effect: pain and burning at the site during drug infusion
- Maximizing therapeutic effects: after reconstitution, solution is stable in a glass container for 24 hours at 4°C or for 8 hours at 25°C when protected from light.
- Minimizing adverse effects: To decrease pain and burning during drug administration, infuse the IV slowly over 1 to 2 hours, increase the primary IV volume, and apply an ice pack over the site.
- Most important patient education: Instruct patient to comply with the prescribed hematologic monitoring.

C ANTITUMOR ANTIBIOTICS

Most **antitumor antibiotics** are isolated from fermented broths of various *Streptomyces* bacteria. Antitumor antibiotics interfere with DNA-directed RNA synthesis by inserting between the base pairs of DNA, binding to DNA, and changing the normal structure of the DNA and RNA chains. This action prevents the normal duplication and separation of these chains and inhibits further synthesis. The antitumor antibiotics are dactinomycin, bleomycin, doxorubicin, daunorubicin, mitomycin, idarubicin, pentostatin, epirubicin, plicamycin, and mitoxantrone. Liposomal versions of doxorubicin and daunorubicin are available (see Table 36.1). Several of these antibiotics, because they also induce double-stranded DNA breaks, are considered topoisomerase II inhibitors. These drugs include doxorubicin, daunorubicin, and idarubicin, which are anthracycline based (i.e., red pigmented), as well as mitoxantrone, a synthetic anthracenedione that is structurally similar to the anthracyclines. Their major dose-limiting toxicity is cardiotoxicity. Daunorubicin was the original prototype for the antitumor antibiotic class; however, doxorubicin (Adriamycin) is currently the most useful and popular antitumor antibiotic. Therefore, doxorubicin is described here as the prototype drug for this class.

NURSING MANAGEMENT OF THE PATIENT RECEIVING P DOXORUBICIN HCL

Core Drug Knowledge

Pharmacotherapeutics

Doxorubicin was isolated from the soil fungus *Streptomyces peucetius var caesius*. Although doxorubicin is the most recently discovered anthracycline, it has gained the distinction

of being the most commonly prescribed. It has wide clinical activity, particularly against hematologic cancers, such as the leukemias, Hodgkin disease, various lymphomas, and multiple myeloma, and solid tumors, such as carcinoma of the breast, ovary, prostate, stomach, thyroid, liver, and small-cell lung and head and neck cancers.

Doxorubicin may be used as a single drug or in combination with other drugs, such as vinblastine, cyclophosphamide, and paclitaxel. It is administered intravenously. Dose adjustments are necessary for patients who have poor bone marrow reserve because of age, prior therapy, or neoplastic marrow infiltration. Dose reductions are also recommended for patients with impaired liver function, as evidenced by elevated serum bilirubin levels and transaminases.

Pharmacokinetics

Doxorubicin is rapidly distributed in body tissues. It is metabolized in the liver and is primarily excreted in the bile. A small percentage is excreted in the renal system and may produce reddish discoloration of the urine. The pharmacokinetic profile of doxorubicin appears in Table 36.1. Recent advances in pharmaceutical technology led to the approval by the FDA of two anthracycline antibiotics, daunorubicin and doxorubicin, in **liposomes.** Liposomes are microscopic spherical vesicles that encapsulate the drug molecules. This novel drug formulation enhances the therapeutic efficacy of the drug by increasing the concentration, delaying clearance, retarding metabolism, decreasing the volume of distribution of the drug, and shifting its distribution to the diseased tissues with increased capillary permeability.

Pharmacodynamics

Doxorubicin acts mainly by intercalation between specific base pairs within the cancer cell's DNA. This action results in blocking the synthesis of new RNA or DNA or preventing DNA strand scission. Normal proliferating cells are also affected by doxorubicin, which accounts for such adverse effects as myelosuppression, alopecia, and stomatitis.

Contraindications and Precautions

Doxorubicin is contraindicated in severe CHF or any existing cardiomyopathy or marked myelosuppression from irradiation or chemotherapy. Precautions should be observed in patients with hepatic insufficiency because concentrations of active metabolites may be increased. Doxorubicin is a pregnancy category D drug.

Adverse Effects

The adverse effects of doxorubicin may be grouped into acute, chronic, and local reactions. Acute toxicities include nausea, vomiting, suppression of bone marrow function, and mucositis. Alopecia is reversible; other cutaneous reactions are hyperpigmentation of the nailbeds and dermal creases.

Cardiotoxicity is chronic and is the major toxicity that limits the use of doxorubicin. This toxicity is cumulative and may manifest weeks or months after the initial treatment. Doxorubicin shows an affinity for myocytes, which are the cells of the heart muscle. The damaged myocytes are not easily replaced because they have a slow mitotic rate. The decreased number of myocytes and the ensuing interstitial edema weaken the pumping capacity of the heart muscle. Cardiac damage may range from insignificant electrocardiographic changes to more serious and potentially fatal complications, such as CHF.

Local adverse effects include cutaneous effects, which can have devastating consequences to the patient. These include extravasation injury and radiation recall reaction. Anthracyclines such as doxorubicin are the most dreaded vesicants. Extravasation is especially problematic with these drugs because anthracyclines bind to nucleic acids, causing destructive and prolonged tissue injuries. They form free radicals that are toxic to the tissues and especially impede wound healing. The DNA–doxorubicin complex is retained and recirculates in the tissues, setting up a pattern for continuous tissue damage (refer to Chapter 35 for extravasation management).

Radiation recall is exhibited as erythematous changes that appear at a previously irradiated site. The phenomenon can occur weeks or months—even years—after radiation but appears more frequently with short intervals between sessions and high-dose chemotherapy. These reactions are manifested by erythema (redness), blisters, hyperpigmentation, edema (swelling), vesicle formation, exfoliation (skin loss), and sometimes ulcer formation. They can occur in the skin, lung, heart, and GI tract.

Drug Interactions

Drug interactions with doxorubicin are summarized in Table 36.4. Doxorubicin should not be mixed with the following drugs in solution because of incompatibility: aminophylline, cephalothin sodium, dexamethasone sodium phosphate, diazepam, hydrocortisone, furosemide, heparin, and fluorouracil.

Assessment of Relevant Core Patient Variables

Health Status

The risk for cardiotoxicity in patients receiving doxorubicin can be potentiated by concurrent therapy with cyclophosphamide and mediastinal irradiation. Ensure that initial car-

TABLE 36.4 Agents That Interact With P Doxorubicin

Interactants	Effect and Significance	Nursing Management
digoxin	Decreased serum levels and therapeutic effect of digoxin.	Monitor serum digoxin levels.
heparin	Precipitate formation if mixed together.	Administer doxorubicin and heparin separately.
barbiturates	Increased plasma clearance of doxorubicin.	Notify health care provider for dosage considerations.

diac evaluations, which might include an electrocardiogram (ECG) and a multigated radionuclide angiogram (MUGA), are made to establish a safe baseline for treatment. Before initiating treatment, obtain a careful history to ascertain that the patient does not have existing cardiomyopathy or hepatic insufficiency that might put him or her at risk during treatment.

Life Span and Gender

Document the age and gender of the patient. The risk for cardiac damage increases with age. Age influences cardiac tolerance to anthracycline therapy. Children and the elderly are more susceptible than young adults to adverse cardiac effects at low cumulative doses. Children especially suffer more from the synergistic cardiotoxicities of mediastinal irradiation and doxorubicin. However, they have a better chance of recovering from CHF-related problems than adults do. Women, especially those younger than 50 years, are more likely to experience nausea and vomiting. Assess the woman of childbearing age for pregnancy and explore her reproductive goals. Doxorubicin is a pregnancy category D drug and its potential effect on fertility is not known.

Lifestyle, Diet, and Habits

Assess the client for adequate nutritional intake. Malnutrition, particularly in children, potentiates cardiotoxicity. Also, assess the patient's anxiety about chemotherapy-related nausea and vomiting, which can substantially impair quality of life.

Environment

Be aware of the environment in which the drug will be administered. Doxorubicin is given either in an inpatient or outpatient setting because of the need to monitor adverse effects, especially the potential for extravasation, which requires prompt medical attention and necessitates patient education.

Nursing Diagnoses and Outcomes

- Risk for Infection related to suppressed bone marrow function
  Desired outcome: *The patient will be free from infection and will exercise caution to avoid exposure to sources of infection.*
- Risk for Injury related to cardiotoxicity, depressed bone marrow function, and associated bleeding
  Desired outcome: *The patient will not suffer from any acute or chronic cardiotoxicity and will be able to recognize and promptly report any of its clinical manifestations. In addition, the patient will attain pretreatment hematologic status. The patient will learn to monitor and manage situations that may induce bleeding.*
- Imbalanced Nutrition: Less than Body Requirements related to nausea, vomiting, and taste alterations
  Desired outcome: *The patient will remain adequately nourished because emesis control will be achieved by pharmacologic and nonpharmacologic means.*
- Impaired Skin Integrity related to possible extravasation and radiation recall
  Desired outcome: *The patient will recognize and report signs and symptoms that suggest an extravasation or recall reaction. Ideally, the patient will receive the doxorubicin dose without vascular or tissue damage.*

Planning and Intervention

Maximizing Therapeutic Effects

Recent advances in drug development have made possible the use of cardioprotectants in conjunction with anthracycline therapy. One such drug is dexrazoxane (Zinecard). Dexrazoxane is a potent intracellular chelating drug that interferes with iron-mediated free radical generation thought to be responsible for anthracycline-induced cardiotoxicity. It is indicated to reduce the severity and incidence of cardiomyopathy associated with doxorubicin in women with metastatic breast cancer who have received a cumulative dose of 300 mg/m^2 and who, in their prescriber's opinion, would benefit from continuing treatment with doxorubicin. Dexrazoxane and doxorubicin may be used concurrently in children. The recommended dose of dexrazoxane to doxorubicin is at a ratio of 10:1 (e.g., dexrazoxane, 500 mg, to doxorubicin, 50 mg). It should be given by slow IV push or rapid IV infusion before administering doxorubicin. The total elapsed time from the beginning of the dexrazoxane infusion to the initiation of doxorubicin should not be more than 30 minutes. The side effects of dexrazoxane using the recommended dose are mild; however, dexrazoxane could add to the myelotoxic effects of doxorubicin.

Minimizing Adverse Effects

Before initiating therapy, carefully assess the patient's cardiac and hematopoietic functions, because of the extensive effect of doxorubicin on the systems involved. Implement strategies using dose administration and scheduling to modify the risk for cardiotoxicity. The recommended maximum cumulative lifetime dose of doxorubicin is 550 mg/m^2. However, if the patient has previously had myocardial irradiation or cytotoxic drug therapy, the cumulative lifetime dose should be lowered to 400 mg/m^2. Modifying the dose and dosing schedule of the patient can ameliorate the cardiotoxic adverse effects. Multiple daily doses rather than large single boluses of the drug can also minimize cardiac damage.

Dose reduction to a cumulative dose of 400 mg/m^2 is advocated for patients who have had or who are receiving concurrent radiation therapy or cyclophosphamide (Cytoxan). With regard to extravasation, prevention is the key. Prevention requires that medical and nursing personnel be skilled in venous access techniques, perform meticulous monitoring during drug administration, and know actions to undertake promptly in case extravasation occurs. Large veins should be used, with a new peripheral line for vesicant administration. Extravasation can occur even with a good venous return and without the usual initial complaint of stinging at the injection site (see Chapter 35).

Providing Patient and Family Education

- Reassure the patient that reddish urine after doxorubicin injection is a harmless and expected response to the drug. This reaction may happen within 1 to 2 days postinfusion.
- Explain that a substantial fraction of patients who receive this drug complain of acute nausea and vomiting. Reassure the patient that proper antiemetics will be available and the patient should ask for them if needed. Carefully review nonpharmacologic interventions, such as relaxation techniques, with the patient and caregiver.

- Review signs and symptoms of extravasation. If a suspected extravasation occurs, provide and review a teaching card with directions for caring for an extravasation site, so that the patient can best participate in care. Reassure the patient that adequate monitoring and follow-up, through telephone triage by the health care team, will be undertaken even in the home setting.
- Discuss with the patient the signs and symptoms of other adverse effects, particularly cardiotoxicity and depressed bone marrow function, and encourage appropriate precautions. For example, encourage the patient to keep appointments for cardiac function tests and caution against taking aspirin or drugs that contain aspirin, which may promote bleeding during suppression of bone marrow function.
- Remind the patient who has had irradiation that recall reactions, manifested by redness, blistering, and hyperpigmentation, can have a delayed onset.

Ongoing Assessment and Evaluation

Advise the patient who continues on doxorubicin to have periodic examinations of cardiac functions as ordered. Radionuclide ventriculography and echocardiography are useful methods to detect impending myocardial damage. Look for any significant changes in the ECG readings that might indicate potential problems, such as irreversible cardiac damage. Also assess the patient frequently for weight gain, presence of ankle edema, dyspnea, elevated blood pressure, and nonproductive cough, which are typical clinical signs of CHF.

Drug Significantly Different From P Doxorubicin

Bleomycin (Blenoxane) is an antitumor antibiotic. Unlike doxorubicin, it is not an anthracycline, nor is it a cell cycle–nonspecific drug. It is used in treating lymphomas, squamous cell carcinoma, and testicular cancers. It is given by IV, subcutaneous, or intramuscular routes. The recommended dosage is expressed in either units or milligrams (1 U = 1 mg). Bleomycin is known for its pulmonary toxicity. For this reason, use of this drug has become limited. The early clinical features of bleomycin toxicity are dyspnea and rales, which can progress to pneumonitis and pulmonary fibrosis and might be fatal.

The treatment of bleomycin-induced toxicity consists of discontinuing the drug and administering corticosteroids. The practitioner should review pulmonary function tests and chest radiographs at baseline and periodically thereafter to monitor for adequate pulmonary reserve. Advise the patient to notify health care providers—especially the anesthesiologist—that he or she has received bleomycin therapy because pulmonary toxicity is enhanced by a high intraoperative fraction of inspired oxygen.

Other adverse effects are cutaneous toxicity, which is often seen as urticaria or erythematous swelling and phlebitis at the injection site caused by the irritant properties of bleomycin. Following drug administration, patients may complain of fever and chills. Patients may also have nausea and vomiting, general weakness, and rare instances of hypotension. These symptoms are considered to be an idiosyncratic reaction, similar to anaphylaxis, and are noted rarely and mostly in lymphoma patients. This problem could be prevented by administering a test dose of 2 U of bleomycin before the first two treatments. Premedication with acetaminophen and diphenhydramine is also helpful.

MEMORY CHIP

P Doxorubicin HCl

- Indicated for treating acute leukemias, soft tissue and bone sarcoma, Hodgkin and non-Hodgkin lymphoma, breast and ovarian cancers, bronchogenic carcinoma
- Major contraindication: severe depression of bone marrow function
- Most common adverse effects: alopecia and nausea with vomiting
- Most serious adverse effects: cardiac damage, bone marrow depression, and extravasation
- Maximizing therapeutic effects: Administer dexrazoxane cardioprotectant therapy, if indicated.
- Minimizing adverse effects: Maintain maximum lifetime dose of 550 mg/m^2; if patient is receiving radiation or concurrent myelotoxic therapy, dose is 400 mg/m^2.
- Most important patient education: Warn patient of the appearance of red urine discoloration after administration (harmless) and of the reality of alopecia, which is reversible.

C HORMONES AND HORMONE ANTAGONISTS

The **hormones** and **hormone antagonists** (antihormones) are a diverse group of drugs that are beneficial in treating neoplasms. Their use predates the first chemotherapeutic agent (nitrogen mustard) as the oldest form of cancer treatment. Hormones are hormonal or hormone-like drugs that inhibit tumor proliferation by blocking or antagonizing the naturally occurring substances that stimulate tumor growth.

Some hormones alter the cellular environment and affect the permeability of the cell membrane in ways that affect cell growth. This group (see Table 36.1) consists of adrenocorticosteroids, androgens, estrogens, progestins, antiestrogens, antiandrogens, gonadotropin inhibitors, and aromatase inhibitors. Hormonal therapy is recognized mostly for its efficacy in treating neoplasms that originate from tissues in which growth is hormonally mediated, notably prostate and breast cancers. The clinical responsiveness of breast tumors to hormonal manipulations was demonstrated more than 100 years ago. Over time, hormonal treatment of breast cancer has been accomplished by ablative surgery (oophorectomy, adrenalectomy, and hypophysectomy) or pharmacologically by using hormonal and antihormonal therapy.

C Adrenocorticosteroids

In addition to their cytotoxic effects, adrenocorticosteroids are used for their palliative benefits. For example, adrenocorticosteroids such as betamethasone, dexamethasone, and prednisone have anti-inflammatory properties and are use-

ful in reducing the edema and associated symptoms in brain tumors. Adrenocortical steroids are effective in leukemias and lymphomas because of their suppressant effect on lymphocytes. Many of their side effects, such as increased appetite and a feeling of well-being, are an extension of their normal physiologic activity and are considered beneficial and palliative. Some of their adverse effects are glucose intolerance, peptic ulceration, manic psychosis, and suppression of cellular immunity, which predisposes patients to infection.

(C) Androgens, Estrogens, and Progestins

Androgens, estrogens, and progestins are used to treat cancers of tissues that have specific hormone receptors—for example, mammary tissue and the prostate gland. Because these drugs have a greater degree of specificity for these tissues, their effects will inhibit proliferation of the tumor.

Androgens

Androgens control the growth and development of the male sex organs and maintain secondary sex characteristics. This group affects the release of various endogenous hormones, namely testosterone, follicle-stimulating hormone (FSH), and luteinizing hormone (LH). The two androgenic agents fluoxymestrone and testolactone are used palliatively for androgen-responsive recurrent breast cancer in postmenopausal women. These drugs are well tolerated, although they may exhibit adverse effects similar to those produced by the estrogens, including fluid retention, hypercalcemia, and liver impairment. Their most profound side effect is virilization in women, manifested by hirsutism, alopecia, acne, clitoral hypertrophy, and increased libido.

Estrogens

Estrogens are necessary to develop and maintain secondary sexual characteristics, control the female menstrual cycle, and affect the maturation of long bones. They diffuse through the membrane of estrogen-responsive cells and bind to and activate receptors in the cell nucleus. They are believed to change the hormonal milieu of the cells, making them less conducive to growth. Estrogen responsive cells (those that are sensitive to estrogen) are located in the reproductive system, breast, pituitary, hypothalamus, liver, and bone. However, not all of the tumors that arise in these organs are estrogen sensitive. In many patients, after the initial hormonal manipulation, even as the estrogen responsive cells are being destroyed, the cells that are not responsive to estrogen will continue to proliferate. Therefore, the response is neither complete nor permanent. Diethylstilbestrol (DES) and estradiol are estrogens. Both are given orally to treat advanced prostate cancer, adenocarcinoma, and metastatic breast cancer. Estradiol is also available as a vaginal cream that is well absorbed through the skin and mucous membranes. The adverse effects of these agents include gynecomastia, voice changes, hirsutism, change in libido, fluid retention, nausea, vomiting, and thrombophlebitis. During the first 2 weeks of DES therapy, hypercalcemia has been reported in women with breast cancer and bone metastases. Deaths from cardiovascular events or thromboembolic adverse effects have also been reported with long-term use of DES and high doses.

Progestins

Progestins are natural or synthetic substances that affect the actions of progesterone, a steroid that counteracts the actions of estrogens. Megestrol acetate (Megace) is a progestin indicated for treating carcinoma of the breast, endometrium, and kidney. It is also used for the treatment of anorexia and cachexia associated with cancer. Medroxyprogesterone is the other agent used in patients with advanced endometrial cancer. These agents are contraindicated during pregnancy because they have been found to cause fetal genital abnormalities.

(C) Antiandrogens

Antiandrogens compete with testosterone for androgen receptor binding sites on target cells. The most frequently used antiandrogenic agents are bicalutamide (Casodex), flutamide (Eulexin), and nilutamide (Nilandron). These agents are used for advanced stages of prostate cancer. Side effects are gynecomastia, diarrhea, hot flashes, breast pain, impotence, loss of libido, and abnormal liver function test results. Monitor the patient's liver function if the patient is on prolonged therapy.

(C) Gonadotropin-Releasing Hormone Analogues

The gonadotropin-releasing hormone (GnRH) analogues are goserelin acetate (Zoladex) and leuprolide (Lupron). LH and FSH are gonadotropins that stimulate hormone secretion by the gonads. They play an important role in the maturation of the germ cell. GnRH regulates the release of these hormones from the pituitary gland. Goserelin inhibits the secretion of gonadotropin. When patients are on prolonged therapy with this drug, their serum testosterone level is decreased to a level equivalent to that associated with surgical castration. This drug is an alternative treatment for males with advanced prostatic cancer who do not wish to undergo orchiectomy or estrogen therapy. It is also used in advanced breast cancer. Goserelin is well tolerated. In men, the adverse effects are hot flashes, sexual dysfunction, and fewer erections. Women suffer from decreased bone mineral density, vaginal bleeding, and breast tenderness. Goserelin is available as a preloaded, disposable syringe with a 14-gauge needle that is injected subcutaneously into the upper abdominal wall. The other drug, leuprolide, has similar indications and also causes chemical orchiectomy in men who have metastatic prostate cancer. Leuprolide has fewer side effects than goserelin does. It is available in three formulations: a subcutaneous injection, a depot suspension, and a suspension given intramuscularly. With both these medications, it is important to teach the patient the correct administration technique appropriate to the drug formulation and emphasize to the patient the importance of adhering to the dosage schedule.

(C) Aromatase Inhibitor

As tamoxifen became the mainstay for antiestrogen therapy in breast cancer, the role of aromatase was increasingly explored. Many breast cancers have estrogen receptors; the growth of these tumors is stimulated by estrogen. In postmenopausal women, the main source of estrogen is the conversion of precursors to estrogen (primarily estradiol) to estrogen; this conversion occurs through an enzyme called aromatase. Anastrozole (Arimidex) inhibits aromatase, thus decreasing the eventual levels of available estrogen. Anastrozole is a nonsteroidal aromatase inhibitor that is also considered an antiestrogen, similar to tamoxifen. It is indicated for the treatment of postmenopausal women who have advanced breast cancer that has progressed after tamoxifen therapy. It is given orally and is well tolerated. Discuss the patient's reproductive goals and warn patients that this drug can cause fetal harm. Anastrozole can interact with some herbal preparations; see Chapter 35.

(C) Antiestrogens

Antiestrogens are first-line therapy for treating breast cancer in postmenopausal women. They act as agonists by binding to the estrogen receptors in the target cells, making the estrogen unavailable to the tumor. Tamoxifen is the most widely recognized antiestrogen. However, tamoxifen is not a pure antiestrogen. Tamoxifen is a selective estrogen receptor modulator (SERM), one of a group of pharmacologic agents, often called "designer drugs," that produce estrogenic effects, alone or combined with antiestrogenic agents, at various sites in a woman's body. These sites include the breast, endometrium, cardiovascular, brain, and bone.

Tamoxifen possesses agonistic properties that stimulate endometrial proliferation, and it is known to induce estrogenic effects that are linked with thromboembolic events. These adverse effects have led to the search for pure antiestrogens, called selective estrogen receptor downregulators (SERDs). Fulvestrant (Faslodex), an SERD, is indicated as second-line therapy in postmenopausal women with metastatic breast disease. Because of its effectiveness and first-line use in treating advanced breast cancer, tamoxifen is the prototype antiestrogen drug.

NURSING MANAGEMENT OF THE PATIENT RECEIVING [P] TAMOXIFEN

Core Drug Knowledge

Pharmacotherapeutics

Tamoxifen (Nolvadex) is indicated as a first-line drug for treating advanced breast cancer in premenopausal and postmenopausal women. It is used in adjuvant therapy for the treatment of axillary node-negative breast cancer in women after mastectomy or segmental mastectomy, axillary dissection, and breast irradiation. In premenopausal women with metastatic breast cancer, tamoxifen is an alternative to oophorectomy and irradiation. It is the only drug approved to prevent breast cancer in high-risk women and to reduce the risk for contralateral breast cancer.

Pharmacokinetics

Tamoxifen is well absorbed, highly protein bound, and extensively metabolized in the liver after oral administration. It undergoes enterohepatic circulation, prolonging blood levels. It is taken up by tissues such as the lung, uterus, breast, brain, pancreas, and liver. It has a half-life of 7 to 14 days. Most tamoxifen is excreted in the bile and feces.

Pharmacodynamics

Tamoxifen, a potent nonsteroidal antiestrogenic drug, competes with estrogen for binding sites in tissues high in estrogen receptors, such as breast tissue. This mechanism deprives estrogen-sensitive tumors of estrogen. It may also stimulate the production of transforming growth factor-beta, which inhibits the growth of most breast cancer and other epithelioid cells.

Other favorable consequences of tamoxifen treatment have been reported; namely, increased bone mineral density in postmenopausal women and reduced cholesterol levels, which may account for a lower incidence of fatal myocardial infarction in women receiving adjuvant tamoxifen.

Contraindications and Precautions

Tamoxifen is contraindicated in patients with known hypersensitivity. Precautions should be observed when administering the drug to patients with myelosuppression and during pregnancy and lactation. Tamoxifen is a pregnancy category D drug. An increased incidence of endometrial changes, including hyperplasia, polyps, and endometrial cancer, has been reported with long-term tamoxifen therapy.

Adverse Effects

Short-term tamoxifen therapy is rarely associated with toxicity. Most patients taking this drug experience no toxicity whatsoever. These adverse effects, although they occur infrequently, are most common: hot flashes, particularly in premenopausal women, and mild nausea, which is transient and unaccompanied by vomiting. The severity of hot flashes diminishes with continued use of the drug. Other, less common adverse effects are headache, lightheadedness, weight gain, vaginal bleeding and discharge, menstrual irregularities, fluid retention, visual side effects, and skin rash, all of which are reported in fewer than 1% to 2% of patients. Increased bone and tumor pain and a local **disease flare** (worsening of the disease) have been observed; they indicate that the tumor is responding to treatment. Hypercalcemia may occur but is infrequent. Data from long-term studies have clearly established the serious long-term effects of tamoxifen use, which include endometrial cancer, thromboembolic events, and cataract formation requiring cataract surgery. Patients receiving long-term therapy should be monitored regularly. Adverse hematopoietic reactions are transient and uncommon, usually exhibited by thrombocytopenia.

Drug Interactions

Drug–laboratory test interactions have been reported with tamoxifen therapy, including elevated serum calcium and thyroxin levels. Other interactions are discussed in Table 36.5.

TABLE 36.5 Agents That Interact With P Tamoxifen

Interactants	Effect and Significance	Nursing Management
oral anticoagulants	Increased risk of bleeding	Monitor prothrombin time. Notify health care provider for dose modifications. Monitor for signs of bleeding.
bromocriptine	Increased serum levels	Monitor tamoxifen serum levels.

Assessment of Relevant Core Patient Variables

Health Status

Even though the adverse effects of tamoxifen are fairly mild, evaluate baseline hematopoietic test results, particularly platelet counts, to make sure that bone marrow function is adequate. Assess the tumor receptor status of the patient because the measurement of estrogen receptors provides important information for planning treatment. Also, screen the patient for a history of thrombophlebitis or endometrial cancer, which may modify the treatment plan. A baseline vision test may also be necessary.

Life Span and Gender

One of the most important issues confronting women receiving hormonal therapy is its effect on their sexual and reproductive health. Explore these concerns and discuss the various changes associated with tamoxifen therapy. You can explain that tamoxifen is a promising therapy for breast cancer and is the preferred adjuvant treatment for postmenopausal women with nodal involvement and estrogen receptor–positive tumors. Assess the patient for pregnancy and explore the contraceptive practices of the patient because the drug can cause fetal harm.

Lifestyle, Diet, and Habits

Women taking tamoxifen experience no limitations in their functional capacities. Lifestyle is not normally affected, except possibly by physical changes, such as hot flashes, menstrual irregularities, weight gain, and vaginal bleeding. You might explore how these changes could affect the woman's lifestyle. Although visual side effects are rare, caution patients about driving and performing tasks requiring visual acuity.

Environment

Be aware of the environment in which the drug will be administered. Tamoxifen is a fairly mild oral drug that does not usually require close monitoring. Patients take this drug at home and are instructed to have periodic checkups with their health care provider. Hematologic screenings can be done at an accredited laboratory that will send the findings to the prescriber for comparison with baseline values.

Nursing Diagnoses and Outcomes

- Pain related to discomfort produced by a flare reaction to drug therapy
  Desired outcome: *The patient will learn to recognize the signs and symptoms of a flare reaction and appreciate it as a positive response to tamoxifen therapy.*
- Sexual Dysfunction resulting from drug therapy
  Desired outcome: *The patient will be aware of the physical changes to reproductive and sexual functions. The patient will be accepting of these changes and will explore ways to enhance sexual and reproductive health.*
- Risk for Infection and Bleeding related to suppression of bone marrow function
  Desired outcome: *The patient will learn to recognize and report symptoms related to infection and bleeding and will implement measures to prevent unnecessary risks or injury that will compromise the hematopoietic and immune systems.*
- Risk for Impaired Skin Integrity related to skin rash and pedal edema
  Desired outcome: *The patient will report the appearance of skin rash and monitor peripheral edema from fluid retention. The patient will take steps to reduce edema from fluid retention, such as eating a low-salt diet.*
- Disturbed Sensory Perception (Vision and Balance) related to adverse effects of drug therapy
  Desired outcome: *The patient will recognize and report changes in visual acuity and other related symptoms, such as headache, dizziness, and lightheadedness, to the caregiver. The patient will take the necessary precautions to avoid injury resulting from altered visual acuity.*
- Risk for Injury related to drug-induced hypercalcemia
  Desired outcome: *The patient will be knowledgeable about clinical manifestations of hypercalcemia, such as nausea, vomiting, constipation, decreased urine volume, malaise, and loss of muscle tone. The patient will also know to report these signs and symptoms immediately to the prescriber, who might consider the need for hospitalization. The patient's calcium level will normalize.*

Planning and Intervention

Maximizing Therapeutic Effects

Tamoxifen is very effective in treating metastatic breast tumors identified as estrogen receptor positive. This criterion is an important determinant in the patient's response to tamoxifen therapy. Ensure that the necessary testing is done to determine patient's estrogen receptor status.

Minimizing Adverse Effects

Tamoxifen's adverse effects are generally mild and rare. Ensure monthly monitoring of blood counts, annual Papanicolaou smears, and regular visual function tests, to determine whether adverse effects occur. The changes noted most often are those related to the menopausal symptoms and can be very bothersome, especially to premenopausal women. Teach these patients to implement comfort measures such as wearing absorbent cotton clothing, lowering the thermostat

CRITICAL THINKING SCENARIO

Making decisions related to combination chemotherapy

Ms. J. M. is a 30-year-old patient with recurrent cancer of the tongue. The patient is being admitted to the hospital to start a combination treatment with cisplatin and paclitaxel. The prescribed dosage is paclitaxel 135 mg/m² by IV continuous infusion over 24 hours and cisplatin 75 mg/m² by IV piggyback one time.

1. Explain how you would sequence the delivery of these two drugs, and propose the rationale for this sequence.
2. Identify and prioritize the important nursing considerations to keep in mind when faced with this drug combination.

at home, avoiding caffeine and spicy foods, and exercising regularly. You may need to discuss the patient's concerns and the effect of the adverse events on her reproductive and sexual functions and her quality of life. The occurrence of a disease flare is actually a positive sign of tumor response to the therapy. Advise the patient that she might experience initial bone and tumor pain and an increase in tumor size. If these symptoms are bothersome, you can obtain a prescription for pain medication.

Providing Patient and Family Education

- Instruct the patient to report signs and symptoms of a disease flare to the prescriber. If signs and symptoms distress the patient, obtain the necessary supportive medications for her.
- Teach the patient to recognize and report changes in visual acuity and other related symptoms, such as headache, dizziness, and lightheadedness. If periodic vision checkups are ordered, emphasize their importance.
- Remind the patient to report immediately any clinical manifestations of hypercalcemia, such as nausea, vomiting, constipation, decreased urine output, malaise, and loss of muscle tone. Hypercalcemia may require hospitalization.
- Teach the patient to recognize and report the appearance of skin rash and peripheral edema.
- Educate the patient regarding likely changes in reproductive or sexual function, such as irregular or missed menstrual periods or unscheduled vaginal bleeding.
- Reassure the patient that all of the above symptoms are mild and rarely occurring adverse effects of tamoxifen therapy. These symptoms do not usually require discontinuing the drug.
- Counsel the patient about contraception and warn her that the drug can cause fetal harm.
- Advise the patient taking long-term tamoxifen therapy to have annual pelvic examinations and Papanicolaou screening and to note and report any unusual vaginal bleeding.

Ongoing Assessment and Evaluation

Throughout treatment, monitor the patient's blood count regularly. Although hypercalcemia is uncommon, evaluate serum calcium levels during therapy to make sure that appropriate measures are initiated to correct this condition should it occur. Also assess the patient's vision, because of the possibility for corneal changes and decreased visual acuity.

MEMORY CHIP

P Tamoxifen

- Indicated for advanced breast cancer in postmenopausal women and cancers of tissues having specific hormone receptors, such as the prostate gland
- Major contraindications: allergy to the drug, pregnancy, and lactation
- Most common adverse effect: occurrence of hot flashes, especially among premenopausal women
- Most serious adverse effects: risk of endometrial cancer and thromboembolic events associated with long-term therapy
- Maximizing therapeutic effects: Instruct the patient to take his/her pills bid, in the morning and evening. Drug should not be discontinued without consulting the physician or nurse
- Minimizing adverse effects: Teach the patient to regulate the home environment to a cooler temperature, wearing loose, cotton, layered clothing (for hot flashes); to eat small, frequent meals and to stay away from spicy foods (for nausea and vomiting); to notify the physician immediately if symptoms of muscle weakness, pain and swelling of legs and ankles, mental confusion, and constipation are noted.
- Most important patient education: Counsel women about the possible risks of endometrial cancer and to have regular gynecologic check-ups.

MAXIMIZING CELL KILL: COMBINATION THERAPY

With rare exceptions, monotherapy in cancer is not curative because of drug resistance. Most cancers contain cells that are resistant to any single agent. In tumors that initially respond to an agent, further drug resistance may develop during treatment as a result of proliferation of pre-existing drug-resistant cells or because of increased mutations that lead to drug resistance. If a combination of drugs is used, cells that are resistant to one chemotherapy agent may be killed by another agent in the combination. Furthermore, many antineoplastic drugs are dose limited because of their cytotoxicity. The limits imposed by toxicities to the different organ systems is another rationale for using combination drugs to achieve better therapeutic outcomes. **Combination chemotherapy,** first developed in the 1960s and 1970s, is one of the major advances in cancer therapy. It continues to guide the development of new treatment protocols for various malignancies. Combination therapy involves using two or more drugs proven effective against a tumor type (Box 36.6). It is considered superior to single-drug therapy because of higher tumor response rates and increased duration of remissions. The effectiveness of a particular antineoplastic drug is measured by objective criteria and tumor response (Box 36.7).

Many regimens in current use have proved to increase the response rate two to four times (Table 36.6). Two or more drugs can be administered simultaneously or in a preplanned sequence. In combination therapy, the response rates and survival are more dramatic because they accomplish the following objectives:

- Maximum cell kill within the range of toxicity tolerated by the patient
- A broader range of coverage against resistant cell lines in the heterogenous tumor population
- Minimal or slow development of new resistant cell groups

FOCUS ON RESEARCH

Box 36.6 Combination Therapy for Patients with Breast Cancer

Sledge, G. (2000). Update of the National Surgical Adjuvant Breast and Bowel Project (NSABP-28). Highlights of the 2000 NIH Consensus Conference on Adjuvant therapy for breast cancer. pp. 4–5

The Study

Results were presented of the third interim analysis of a phase III trial, NSABP B-28 using adriamycin and cyclophosphamide (AC) with or without sequential paclitaxel in 3,060 patients with node-positive breast cancer. Patients were randomized into two treatment arms that consisted of the following regimens: adriamycin 60 mg and AC 600 mg given every 21 days for four cycles or AC with paclitaxel 225 mg/m^2 over 3 hours every 21 days × four cycles. Tamoxifen 20 mg daily for 5 years was given concurrently with chemotherapy in patients > 50 years old and in patients < 50 years old with estrogen receptor or progesterone receptor–positive tumors in both arms. Toxicities reported among the first treatment group consisted of granulocytopenia (8%), febrile neutropenia (7%), nausea (6%), and infection (3%). Patients receiving paclitaxel with AC manifested neurosensory problems (15%), arthralgias/myalgias (12%), neuromotor disorders (7%), and granulocytopenia on day 1 (5%). The study concluded that patients receiving paclitaxel following the AC regimen did not benefit in terms of disease-free and overall survival rates compared with those receiving AC alone. Although there appeared to be a trend that patients who did not receive tamoxifen benefited from the addition of paclitaxel, the difference for either disease-free or overall survival was not statistically significant.

Nursing Implications

Nurses play a pivotal role in teaching patients and helping them understand risks and benefits of treatment. To do this, the nurse should have a thorough knowledge of the drugs involved, including their side effects and appropriate symptom management. The nurse should also be versed in the design and goals of the treatment plan, to clarify issues and respond to patients learning needs, thus helping the patient make an informed decision.

In designing successful drug combinations, the choice of drugs follows these principles:

- Selected drugs should be proven partially effective against the tumor when used alone.
- Ideally, the drugs used in combination are best if they do not have overlapping toxicities.
- The dosages and schedules for the various drugs should be maximized.
- Drugs should be administered at consistent intervals.
- Drugs should be selected to produce synergy.

TARGETED CANCER THERAPIES

Targeted cancer therapies are new types of drug therapy to treat cancer. Targeted cancer therapies use drugs that block the growth and spread of cancer. They interfere with specific molecules involved in carcinogenesis (the process by which normal cells become cancer cells) and tumor growth. These molecules are sometimes referred to as molecular targets; therefore, targeted therapies are sometimes called "molecular-targeted drugs," "molecularly targeted therapies," or other similar names. Targeted cancer therapies interfere with cancer cell growth and division in different ways and at various points during the development, growth, and spread of cancer. Many of these therapies focus on proteins that are involved in the signaling process. By blocking the signals that tell cancer cells to grow and divide uncontrollably, targeted cancer therapies can help stop the growth and division of cancer cells. By focusing on molecular and cellular changes that are specific to cancer, targeted cancer therapies may be more effective than current treatments and less harmful to normal cells so that they may produce fewer adverse effects.

Most targeted cancer therapies are still being studied in animals and are not ready yet for human use, but some are in clinical trials. Whether these drug therapies are best if used alone, in combination with each other, or in combination with other chemotherapy drugs is still to be determined.

A few targeted therapies have been approved by the FDA for specific cancer uses. These therapies include:

- "Small-molecule" drugs that block specific enzymes and growth factor receptors (GFRs) involved in cancer cell growth. These drugs are also called signal-transduction inhibitors. Two small-molecule drugs that have been approved are imatinib mesylate (Gleevec) and gefitinib (Iressa). Imatinib mesylate is approved by the FDA to treat GI stromal tumor (a rare cancer of the GI tract) and certain kinds of chronic myeloid leukemia. Imatinib mesylate targets abnormal proteins, or enzymes, that form

BOX 36.7 Rating Tumor Response

How well a tumor responds to chemotherapy can be rated by the categories below.

Complete Response

All evidence of tumor (physical examination and radiologic studies) has disappeared and no new lesions have developed. Response must last for at least 4 weeks. The patient must have no cancer-related symptoms and all abnormal biochemical parameters must have returned to normal.

Partial Response

The sum of the product of the diameters of measured lesions decreases 50% or more for at least 4 weeks without cancer-related symptoms or weight or performance deteriorations. If there is no change in tumor size but the biochemical parameters decline by 80% or more, the patient is considered stable.

Stable Disease

Patients who do not meet the criteria for partial response but who are without signs and symptoms of progressive disease for at least 3 months comprise this category.

Progressive Disease

An increase exceeding 25% in the total area of the bidimensionally measured lesions, the appearance of new lesions, or greater or significant deterioration that cannot be attributed to treatment or medical conditions is considered disease progression.

TABLE 36.6 Common Combination Regimens

Acronym	Regimen	Indications
ABVD	Doxorubicin, bleomycin, vinblastine with dacarbazine	Hodgkin lymphoma
AC	Doxorubicin, cyclophosphamide	Breast cancer
BEP	Bleomycin, etoposide, cisplatin	Testicular cancer
BIP	Bleomycin, ifosfamide, cisplatin, mesna	Cervical cancer
CAF	Cyclophosphamide, doxorubicin, fluorouracil	Breast cancer
CAP	Cyclophosphamide, doxorubicin, cisplatin	Non–small-cell lung cancer
CHOP	Cyclophosphamide, doxorubicin, vincristine	Non-Hodgkin lymphoma
CHOP-BLEO	Add bleomycin to CHOP	Non-Hodgkin lymphoma
CMF	Cyclophosphamide, methotrexate, fluorouracil	Breast cancer
CP	Cyclophosphamide, cisplatin	Ovarian cancer
DHAP	Cisplatin, cytarabine, dexamethasone	Hodgkin lymphoma
EAP	Etoposide, doxorubicin, cisplatin	Gastric cancer
EC	Etoposide, carboplatin	Small-cell lung cancer
FAC	Fluorouracil, doxorubicin, cyclophosphamide	Breast cancer
FAM	Fluorouracil, doxorubicin, mitomycin	Gastric cancer
FAMTX	Fluorouracil, doxorubicin, methotrexate, leucovorin	Gastric cancer
ITP	Ifosfamide, taxol, cisplatin	Genitourinary cancer
IVAC	Ifosfamide, vincristine, doxorubicin, cyclophosphamide	Multiple myeloma
ICE	Ifosfamide, carboplatin, etoposide	Lung cancer
MAID	Mesna, adriamycin (doxorubicin), ifosfamide, dacarbazine	Sarcoma
MOPP	Mechlorethamine, vincristine, procarbazine	Hodgkin lymphoma
MVAC	Vincristine, doxorubicin, cyclophosphamide	Lung cancer
MVP	Mitomycin, vinblastine, cisplatin	Lung cancer

inside cancer cells and stimulate uncontrolled growth. Gefitinib is approved by the FDA to treat advanced non–small-cell lung cancer. This drug targets the epidermal growth factor receptor (EGFR), which is overproduced by many types of cancer cells.

- The first approved apoptosis-inducing drug is bortezomib (Velcade). Bortezomib is approved by the FDA to treat multiple myeloma that has not responded to other treatments. Apoptosis-inducing drugs cause cancer cells to undergo apoptosis (cell death) by interfering with proteins involved in the process. Bortezomib causes cancer cells to die by blocking enzymes called proteasomes, which help to regulate cell function and growth. Another apoptosis-inducing drug called oblimersen (Genasense), which is only available in clinical trials, is being studied to treat leukemia, non-Hodgkin lymphoma, and solid tumors. Oblimersen blocks the production of a protein known as BCL-2, which promotes the survival of tumor cells. By blocking BCL-2, oblimersen leaves the cancer cells more vulnerable to anticancer drugs.
- Monoclonal antibodies, cancer vaccines, and angiogenesis inhibitors can be considered targeted therapies because they interfere with the growth of cancer cells. Monoclonal antibodies and other biologic response modifiers are discussed fully in Chapter 34. Angiogenesis, the formation of new blood vessels, is a process controlled by chemicals produced in the body that stimulate cells to repair damaged blood vessels or form new ones. Other chemicals, called angiogenesis inhibitors, signal the process to stop. Angiogenesis plays an important role in the growth and spread of cancer. New blood vessels "feed" the cancer cells with oxygen and nutrients, allowing these cells to grow, invade nearby tissue, spread to other parts of the body, and form new colonies of cancer cells. Because cancer cannot grow or spread without the formation of new blood vessels, angiogenesis inhibitors can be valuable tools in treating cancer. These drugs are currently being researched.

As research provides more information on targeted therapies, more drugs will be approved for use in treating cancers. These therapies are likely to drastically alter the future of cancer treatment.

CRITICAL THINKING SCENARIO

Implementing MAID Therapy

T. M. is a 53-year-old woman who was admitted for chemotherapy for a sarcoma on her right leg. The oncologist has just ordered for the patient to receive the MAID regimen. Because this is the patient's first treatment, she has a lot of questions to ask. Some of the questions are:

1. Which drugs are included in MAID?
2. Name three important clinical considerations for this treatment.

CHAPTER SUMMARY

- Cell cycle–nonspecific drugs exert their cytotoxic activity irrespective of the phase of the cell life cycle.
- Cell cycle–nonspecific drugs are considered more toxic than cell cycle–specific drugs.

- Alkylating drugs are radiomimetic.
- The nitrosoureas are alkylating agents that are highly lipid soluble.
- The antitumor antibiotics that are considered both anthracyclines and topoisomerase II inhibitors are daunorubicin, doxorubicin, and idarubicin. Mitoxantrone is a synthetic anthracenedione.
- The most feared adverse effect of anthracycline therapy is cardiotoxicity.
- Some prognostic factors relating to a patient's tolerance to acute emesis are age, gender, and method of drug administration.
- The different groups of hormones used in cancer therapy are the adrenal corticosteroids, androgens, antiandrogens, estrogens, antiestrogens, gonadotropin-releasing hormone analogues, progestins, and aromatase inhibitors.
- Combination chemotherapy is superior to single-drug therapy because it kills a maximum number of cancer cells within a toxicity range tolerated by the patient, it provides a broader range of coverage against resistant cells in the heterogenous tumor population, and it is characterized by minimal or slow development of new resistant cancer cells.
- Targeted therapies are being developed that will work directly to prevent cancer cell development and growth. Because they have an effect on only cancer cells, these therapies should have fewer adverse effects than other chemotherapies.

QUESTIONS FOR STUDY AND REVIEW

1. What are anthracyclines, and which of the antitumor antibiotics are they?
2. Which cell cycle–nonspecific drugs are highly lipid soluble? What can they do?
3. What are the different groups of drugs used to control acute emesis?
4. What is the role of dexrazoxane in anthracycline therapy? How is it administered?
5. What are the characteristics of drugs that are useful for combination therapy?
6. Why is combination chemotherapy superior to single-drug therapy?

Need More Help?

Chapter 36 of the study guide for *Drug Therapy in Nursing* 2e contains NCLEX-style questions and other learning activities to reinforce your understanding of the concepts presented in this chapter. For additional information or to purchase the study guide, visit *http://connection.lww.com/go/aschenbrenner.*

REFERENCES AND BIBLIOGRAPHY

Allen, T. M. (1997). Liposomes: Opportunities in drug delivery. *Drugs, 54* (Suppl. 4), 8–14.

American Society of Clinical Oncology (1999). Clinical Practice guidelines for the use of chemotherapy and radiotherapy protectants. *Journal of Clinical Oncology, 17,* 3333–3335.

American Society of Hospital Pharmacists. (1990). Technical assistance bulletin on handling cytotoxic and hazardous drugs. *American Journal of Hospital Pharmacy, 47,* 1033–1049.

American Society of Health-System Pharmacists (ASHP). (1999). ASHP therapeutic guidelines on the pharmacologic management of nausea and vomiting in adult and pediatric patients receiving chemotherapy or radiation therapy or undergoing surgery. *American Journal of Health-System Pharmacists, 56,* 729–764.

Armstrong, T., Rust, D., & Kohts, J. (1997). Neurologic, pulmonary, and cutaneous toxicities of high-dose chemotherapy. *Oncology Nursing Forum, 24* (Suppl. 1), 23–39.

Baquiran, D. C. (2001). *Lippincott's cancer chemotherapy handbook* (2nd ed.). Philadelphia: Lippincott Williams & Wilkins.

Cancer Care. (2004). Drug information: cyclophosphamide [Online]. Available: *http://www.cancercare.on.ca/pdfdrugs/CYCLOPHO.pdf.*

DeForni, M., & Armand, J. (1994). Cardiotoxicity of chemotherapy. *Current Opinions in Oncology, 6,* 340–344.

DeVita, V. T., Hellman, S., & Rosenberg, S. A. (2005). *Cancer: Principles and practice of oncology* (7th ed.). Philadelphia: Lippincott Williams & Wilkins.

Gralla, R. J., Osoba, D., Kris, M. G., et al. (1999). Recommendations for the use of antiemetics: Evidence-based, clinical practice guidelines. *Journal of Clinical Oncology, 17*(9), 2971.

Fisher, B., Constantino, J. P., Redmond, C., et al. (1994). Endometrial cancer in tamoxifen-treated breast cancer patients: Findings from the National Surgical Adjuvant Breast and Bowel Project (NSABP) B-14. *Journal of the National Cancer Institute, 86,* 527–537.

Joint Commission on Accreditation of Healthcare Organizations. (2000). *Patient and family education, accreditation manual for hospitals* (Vol. 1). Oak Brook, IL: Author.

Lamb, M. (1995). Effects of cancer on the sexuality and fertility of women. *Seminars in Oncology Nursing, 11*(2), 120–127.

Lipshultz, S., Sanders, S., Gorin, A., et al. (1994). Monitoring for anthracycline cytotoxicity. *Pediatrics, 93*(3), 433–437.

National Library of Medicine. (2004). MedlinePlus drug information: Cyclophosphamide (Systemic) [Online]. Available: *www.nlm.nih.gov/medlineplus/druginfo/uspdi/202174.html.*

National Cancer Institute. (2004). Targeted cancer therapies: Questions and answers [Online]. Available: *http://cis.nci.nih.gov/fact/7_49.htm.*

National Comprehensive Cancer Network. (2001). *Nausea and vomiting: Treatment guidelines for patients with cancer, version I.* Washington, DC: American Cancer Society and Author.

National Study Commission on Cytotoxic Exposure. (1987). *Recommendations for handling cytotoxic agents.* Providence, RI: Author.

Occupational Safety and Health Administration. (1986). *Work practice guidelines for personnel dealing with cytotoxic (antineoplastic) drugs.* (OSHA Instruction Publication #8-1.1). Washington DC: Department of Labor.

Oncology Nursing Society. (2001). *Chemotherapy and biotherapy: Guidelines and recommendations for practice.* Pittsburgh, PA: Oncology Nursing Press.

Pharmacia & Upjohn (2000). *Zinecard (dexrazoxane)* [Package insert]. Kalamazoo, MI: Author.

Pritchard, K. I. (2001). Selective estrogen receptor modulators in the prevention and treatment of breast cancer. *Clinical Oncology Updates, 3*(4), 1–15.

Wilkes, G. M., Ingwersen, K., & Burke, M. B. (2000). *Oncology nursing drug handbook.* Boston: Jones and Bartlett.

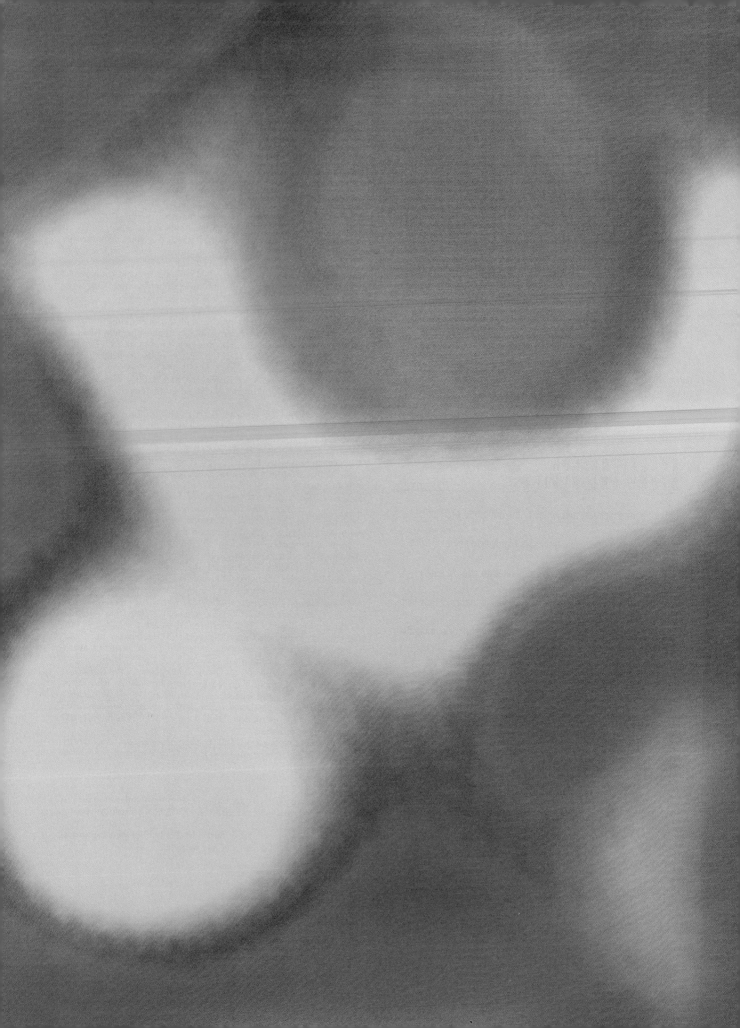

Antimicrobial Drugs

unit 10

Principles of Antibiotic Therapy

chapter 37

Learning Objectives

At the completion of this chapter the student will:

1 Describe the way that antimicrobial drugs are classified.
2 Explain how the principle of selective toxicity applies to antimicrobial therapy.
3 Explain the emergence of drug-resistant microbes.
4 Identify and discuss the four most common drug-resistant pathogens.
5 Distinguish between drug of choice and alternative drugs used to manage infections.
6 Discuss the procedures used to identify pathogens.
7 Relate the principle of drug susceptibility to antimicrobial therapy.
8 Identify patient care variables that influence the choice of antimicrobial agents.
9 Describe appropriate laboratory tests to monitor antimicrobial therapy.

KEY TERMS

anthelminthic
antibacterial
antifungal
anti-infectives
antimicrobials
antiprotozoal
antiviral
bacteriocidal
bacteriostatic
conjugation
culture
empiric therapy
F factor
Gram stain
microbe
pathogen
postantibiotic effect
R factor
selective toxicity
sensitivity
spectrum
spontaneous mutation
superinfection

FEATURED WEBLINK

http://members.tripod.com/MED_MOE/Antimicrobial.htm
This site provides an overview of antimicrobial therapy.

CONNECTION WEBLINK

Additional Weblinks are found on Connection:
http://www.connection.lww.com/go/aschenbrenner.

Drugs used to manage infections are called **antimicrobials** or **anti-infectives.** The first effective antimicrobial drug was penicillin. Since its introduction, morbidity and mortality from infections have steadily declined. However, as we grow in our knowledge of how specific types of microbes work and how to eradicate them, microbes also continue to develop ways to mutate or to secrete enzymes that make current antimicrobials ineffective.

This chapter focuses on the basics of antimicrobial therapy, including classification of antimicrobial drugs, selective toxicity, antimicrobial resistance, general considerations of antimicrobial therapy, and monitoring of antimicrobial therapy. Although this chapter discusses all antimicrobial drugs, antibiotics are emphasized because these drugs have multiple mechanisms of action, require more specificity to the microbe than other drugs do, and are associated with a higher incidence of resistance. Additional information on specific antimicrobial agents is provided in the individual chapters in this unit.

CLASSIFICATION OF ANTIMICROBIAL DRUGS

Two popular ways to classify antimicrobial drugs are by susceptible organism and by mechanism of action.

Classification by Susceptible Organism

A **microbe** is a unicellular or small multicellular organism. Microbes that are capable of producing disease are called **pathogens.** Types of microbes include bacteria, viruses, protozoa, some algae and fungi, and some worms (helminths). Drugs used to treat infection can be classified according to the type of microbe they affect. The major classifications include **antibacterial** drugs, **antiviral** drugs, **antifungal** drugs, **antiprotozoal** drugs, and **anthelminthic** drugs. Antibacterial drugs are subdivided into narrow-spectrum, broad-spectrum, or antimycobacterial drugs. As the name implies, a narrow-spectrum drug is effective against a few types of bacteria, whereas a broad-spectrum drug is effective against many types of bacteria. The antiviral classification also has a subdivision: antiretroviral agents. Box 37.1 outlines these classifications.

BOX 37.1 Classifications of Antimicrobial Drugs by Susceptible Organism

Antibacterial drugs

Narrow-spectrum
Broad-spectrum
Mycobacterium

Antiviral drugs

Antiretroviral

Antifungal drugs

Antiparasitic drugs

Anthelmintic drugs

Classification by Mechanism of Action

Antimicrobial drugs work in a variety of ways:

- Inhibition of bacterial cell wall synthesis
- Inhibition of protein synthesis
- Inhibition of nucleic acid synthesis
- Inhibition of metabolic pathways (antimetabolites)
- Disruption of cell wall permeability
- Inhibition of viral enzymes

These classifications, with examples of antibiotics for each group, are outlined in Table 37.1. In addition to being classified by their mechanisms of action as already listed, antibiotic drugs are further classified as bacteriostatic or bacteriocidal. **Bacteriostatic** drugs inhibit bacteria, but their effect is reversible if the drug is removed, unless the host defense mechanisms have eradicated the organism. Sulfonamides, erythromycin, and tetracyclines are examples of bacteriostatic drugs. Antibiotics that actually kill bacteria are **bacteriocidal.** They depend less on the body's defense mechanisms than bacteriostatic drug do. Examples include beta-lactam antibiotics such as the penicillins and cephalosporins or aminoglycosides. Additionally, some antibiotics exhibit a **postantibiotic effect:** organisms may not resume growing for several hours after exposure to the drug, despite undetectable drug levels.

Inhibition of Bacterial Cell Wall Synthesis

Unlike human cells, bacteria have rigid cell walls containing complex macromolecules, which are formed through biosynthetic pathways. The osmotic pressure within the cell is

TABLE 37.1 Classification of Antimicrobial Drugs by Mechanism of Action

Antibiotics	Mechanism of Action
Cephalosporins Daptomycin Penicillins Vancomycin	Inhibit cell wall synthesis
Aminoglycosides Chloramphenicol Clindamycin Erythromycin Tetracyclines	Inhibit protein synthesis
Fluoroquinolones Rifampin	Inhibit nucleic acid synthesis
Polymyxins Polyene antimicrobials Imidazole antifungal agents	Disrupt cell membrane permeability
Sulfonamides Trimethoprim	Work as an antimetabolite
Acyclovir Saquinavir	Inhibit viral enzymes

very high and relies on the integrity of the cell wall to resist the absorption of water. Without the rigid cell wall, the bacteria would absorb water, swell, and then lyse. Several antimicrobial drugs weaken the cell wall, allowing the cell to absorb water, a process that causes bacterial death. Penicillins and cephalosporins bind to specific proteins located within the bacterial cytoplasmic membrane, the portion of the cell wall that borders the cytoplasm. Binding to these proteins causes inhibition of transpeptidase, an enzyme needed for the final step of cell wall synthesis. The result is decreased cell wall synthesis. These antibiotics also activate autolytic enzymes that are destructive to the cell wall. Another antibiotic, vancomycin, interferes with bacterial cell wall synthesis by inhibiting the synthesis of precursors of murein or by preventing the formation of linear peptidoglycan chains. These chains are polysaccharides and polypeptides that are cross-linked to form the bacterial cell wall.

Inhibition of Protein Synthesis

Both human and bacterial cells require ribosomes to synthesize protein for use by the cell (see Chapter 39). However, ribosomes from human cells and those from bacterial cells are structurally different. Because of this difference, many of the commonly used antimicrobial drugs are able to disrupt bacterial protein synthesis without affecting protein synthesis in human cells.

Tetracyclines bind to the 30S subunit of the bacterial ribosome and block the attachment of aminoacyl-tRNA. Aminoglycoside antibiotics also interact with the 30S ribosomal subunit but bind to different receptors, blocking formation of the 70S initiation complex.

Erythromycin and clindamycin inhibit the formation of the complex and interfere with translocation reactions by binding to the 50S subunit of bacterial ribosomes. Chloramphenicol also binds to the 50S ribosomal subunit and inhibits peptidyl transferase activity.

Inhibition of Nucleic Acid Synthesis

Many bacteria use enzymes for replication that do not exist in human cells. For instance, fluoroquinolones inhibit deoxyribonucleic acid (DNA) gyrase, an enzyme needed for bacterial DNA replication. Although human cells contain an enzyme that functions in the same manner, the human enzyme is not affected by fluoroquinolones.

Inhibition of Metabolic Pathways (Antimetabolites)

Nucleic acid synthesis is dependent on folic acid (folate), which acts as a coenzyme in many biosynthetic reactions. Humans obtain folate in the diet, but many microorganisms must synthesize folate. Sulfonamides inhibit bacterial folate synthesis by acting as an antimetabolite of the precursor to folate, para-aminobenzoic acid (PABA). Similarly, trimethoprim is an antimetabolite of folic acid that selectively inhibits dihydrofolate reductases of bacteria and protozoa.

Disruption of Cell Wall Permeability

Drugs that disrupt the integrity of the bacterial cell wall cause the cell to leak components that are vital to its survival. The polymyxins disrupt the membranes of the bacterial cell wall by inserting themselves into the lipid bilayer and forming artificial pores. The polyene antimicrobials bind to membrane components that are present only in microbial cells. The imidazole antifungal agents act as selective inhibitors of enzymes involved in the synthesis of sterols that are essential components of fungal membranes.

Inhibition of Viral Enzymes

The replication of viruses requires multiple enzymatic activities. Nucleoside analogues, such as acyclovir, and protease inhibitors, such as saquinavir, interrupt important enzymes required for viral replication.

SELECTIVE TOXICITY

An important principle of antimicrobial therapy is **selective toxicity,** which is the ability to suppress or kill an infecting microbe without injury to the host. Selective toxicity is achievable because the drug accumulates in a microbe at a higher level than in human cells; the drug has a specific action on cellular structures or biochemical processes that are unique to the microbe; or an action of a drug on biochemical processes is more harmful to the microbe than to host cells. For example, differences in the chemical compositions of the cell walls of microbes and human cells permit the selective toxicity of polymyxins, polyene antimicrobials, and imidazole antifungal agents. Tetracycline and chloramphenicol do not have absolute selective toxicity: they are able to inhibit protein synthesis in some human cells as well. Understanding selective toxicity has made antimicrobial drugs safe and effective for managing infection in humans.

ANTIMICROBIAL RESISTANCE

Despite the large number of antimicrobial agents available, pharmaceutical companies are constantly looking for new ways to eradicate old microbes. This endless search is necessary because of antimicrobial resistance. This resistance is derived from the microbe—not from the patient.

Contributing Factors

Antimicrobial resistance may occur for several reasons: production of drug-inactivating enzymes, changes in receptor structure, changes in drug permeation and transport, development of alternative metabolic pathways, emergence of drug-resistant microbes, or factors that facilitate the development of resistance.

Production of Drug-Inactivating Enzymes

This common mechanism causes resistance to many beta-lactam antibiotics. The microbe synthesizes hydrolytic beta-lactamases, enzymes that are specific for certain penicillin and cephalosporin structures called beta-lactams. The beta-lactam structure must remain intact for the antibiotic to be effective; thus, when these enzymes affect the beta-lactam structure, the antibiotic becomes ineffective. To date, more than 100 beta-lactamases have been identified. Pathogens such as *Staphylococcus aureus,* *Haemophilus* species, and *Escherichia coli* have specificity to affect penicillins but not cephalosporins. *Pseudomonas aeruginosa* and *Enterobacter* species have a broader spectrum and may affect cephalosporins as well as penicillins.

Changes in Receptor Structure

Bacteria contain molecules that act as targets, or receptors, for antimicrobial drugs. These molecules may undergo changes in their structures. These structural changes make the microbe less susceptible to the toxic action of antibiotics. For example, alteration in penicillin-binding proteins (PCBs) decreases the affinity for binding beta-lactam antibiotics.

Changes in Drug Permeation and Transport

The antimicrobial action of many drugs depends on their ability to penetrate the cell membranes of an organism and reach effective intracellular concentrations. The organism's defense starts in the efficiency of its cell wall. If an antibiotic reaches the interior structures of the cell rapidly, the cell is unable to overcome the activity of the drug. If the antibiotic has difficulty passing through the cell wall, however, the bacteria are able to hydrolyze the antibiotic as it slowly enters the cell. Another bacterial defense mechanism is the production of an efflux pump, which effectively extrudes certain drugs, such as tetracycline, from the cell.

Development of Alternative Metabolic Pathways

Some bacteria are affected by antibiotics, such as sulfonamides, that act as antimetabolites by interrupting their metabolic pathway for replication. In the case of sulfonamides, the antibiotic inhibits dihydropteroate synthase, the enzyme necessary to metabolize folic acid. Resistant bacteria may produce levels of PABA, the precursor to folic acid, high enough to overcome the inhibition of dihydropteroate synthase. Additionally, certain bacteria are able to use preformed folic acid from their environment, thus bypassing the inhibitory actions of the sulfonamides.

Emergence of Drug-Resistant Microbes

All antimicrobials have the ability to promote the emergence of drug-resistant microbes. However, resistance is more likely to occur in organisms exposed to broad-spectrum drugs. Although the use of antimicrobials promotes the potential for drug resistance to occur, they do not directly cause the resistance. Drug-resistant microbes develop in two ways: by spontaneous mutation and by conjugation.

SPONTANEOUS MUTATION

Spontaneous mutation is exactly what the name infers: a change in the genetic composition of the microbe that may just be a random occurrence, or the microbe may have mutated by acquiring DNA from an external source. The resistance developed is drug specific.

CONJUGATION

Conjugation is a form of sexual reproduction in which two individual microbes join in temporary union to transfer genetic material. An important element of conjugation is a microbial structure composed of DNA, called a plasmid. Essentially, the plasmid can hold additional information, more than is in the usual genome for the organism, which codes for proteins that can sometimes be used by the host. Because polymerases work nonspecifically, information can be transcribed from them and used by any host, including bacteria. DNA on plasmids can code for any protein. Among the many things plasmids can code for is for the ability to conjugate. Most plasmids that have this ability are considered F positive (F+) and are said to have the **F factor** (F = fertility). For the plasmid to propagate, it must come in contact with another plasmid with the F factor.

Conjugation may occur between two microbes of the same species or between different species. For drug resistance to occur, the plasmid must come in contact with another plasmid that not only has the F factor but also possesses information necessary to deactivate an antibiotic. These two DNA segments together are known as **R factor** (R = resistance). More and more of our body's natural flora contain R factor. Thus, acquired bacteria with F factor may combine with natural flora that contains R factor and transfer antibiotic resistance to the invading pathogen. Conjugation frequently results in multiple drug resistance.

Factors That Facilitate the Development of Resistance

Several factors facilitate the development of resistance. Drug concentrations in tissues that are too low to kill resistant organisms contribute to the development of resistance. The minimum inhibitory concentration (MIC) of a drug must be present to stop or slow the replication of the microbe. When a tissue does not reach MIC, the microbe can become resistant to the antimicrobial. Inadequate tissue concentrations may occur because of an improper dose of drug or improper length of time between doses. Insufficient duration of therapy may allow resistant organisms to repopulate and re-establish an infection. Patients frequently stop taking antibiotics when they feel better "to save some in case the infection comes again." Treatment must be continued beyond clinical improvement, especially if there is any problem with host defenses.

Prophylactic use of antibiotics may also contribute to the development of resistant organisms. Prophylactic use of antimicrobial drugs means that the drug is given to prevent an infection rather than to treat an infection. This practice increases the risk for the development of resistant microbes; therefore, antimicrobial prophylaxis should be reserved for appropriate indications. Such indications include:

- Exposure to sexually transmitted diseases
- Recurrent urinary tract infections
- Neutropenia
- Surgery
- Bacterial endocarditis

COMMON ANTIBIOTIC-RESISTANT MICROBES

Although any microbe may become drug resistant, four important microbes are likely to: methicillin-resistant *Staphylococcus aureus* (MRSA), penicillin-resistant *Streptococcus pneumoniae,* vancomycin-resistant *Enterococci,* and multiple drug–resistant *Mycobacterium tuberculosis* (MDR-TB).

Methicillin-Resistant *Staphylococcus Aureus* (MRSA)

The abbreviation MRSA is commonly used for this infection; however, the abbreviation is somewhat misleading. In actuality, the pathogen is widely resistant to all of the antistaphylococcic penicillins, not just methicillin. In MRSA,

penicillin-binding proteins are altered, reducing the ability of penicillins to inhibit cell wall synthesis, except at very high drug concentrations that may not be achievable because of poor tissue penetration and toxicity concerns. Many strains of MRSA are also resistant to aminoglycosides, tetracyclines, erythromycin, and clindamycin.

Closely related to MRSA is methicillin-resistant *Staphylococcus epidermidis* (MRSE). MRSE frequently colonizes the nasal passages of health care workers, resulting in the spread of nosocomial infections, especially in critical care units.

Vancomycin is the drug of choice to manage infections caused by MRSA and MRSE. Because vancomycin is also used for many other drug-resistant microbes, vancomycin resistance is emerging. New drugs with different mechanisms of action, such as linezolid (Zyvox), dalfopristin-quinupristin (Synercid), and daptomycin (Cubicin), have been developed to treat vancomycin-resistant microbes.

Penicillin-Resistant *Streptococcus Pneumoniae*

In the past, penicillins have successfully treated pneumococcal infections such as otitis media in children, community-acquired pneumonia, and meningitis. Because they are used so frequently, particularly in children and the elderly, strains of penicillin-resistant *Streptococci* are emerging. To decrease penicillin resistance among *Streptococcus pneumoniae,* the Centers for Disease Control and Prevention (CDC) suggested that clinicians stop using penicillins and cephalosporins as prophylaxis for otitis media and that patients over the age of 65 years or those under the age of 2 years, who have an increased risk for pneumococcal infections, be immunized.

Vancomycin-Resistant *Enterococci* (VRE)

Enterococci are generally treated with a combination of antibiotics: an aminoglycoside with a penicillin or an aminoglycoside with a cephalosporin. The penicillin or cephalosporin damages the bacterial cell wall and allows the aminoglycoside to penetrate the cell. Strains of *Enterococci* have developed resistance to penicillin, gentamicin, and vancomycin, however. Potential alternative drugs for VRE include teicoplanin (Targocid), minocycline (Minocin), ciprofloxacin (Cipro), quinupristin-dalfopristin (Synercid), and daptomycin (Cubicin).

Multiple Drug–Resistant Tuberculosis (MDR-TB)

Multiple drug–resistant TB is increasingly common. Although some of the bacilli are inherently resistant, others develop resistance over the long course of TB treatment, which can last as long as 2 years. The cause of MDR-TB is inadequate drug therapy, a category that includes a duration of therapy that is too short; a dose that is too low; or, more commonly, patient adherence that is only intermittent. To decrease the incidence of MDR-TB, multiple drug therapy is implemented at the onset of treatment, followed by a decrease in the number of drugs, but no less than four drugs are given at any time.

GENERAL CONSIDERATIONS FOR SELECTING ANTIMICROBIAL THERAPY

The most important factor in managing infections is to "match the drug with the bug." Each pathogen has a "drug of choice" and "alternative drugs." Several factors must be considered when choosing the drug of choice or an alternative:

1. Identification of the pathogen
2. Drug susceptibility
3. Drug spectrum
4. Drug dose
5. Time to affect the pathogen
6. Site of infection
7. Patient assessment

Identification of the Pathogen

To eradicate an infection, drugs must be specific to the type of pathogen involved. An antiviral agent will not eradicate bacteria, nor will an antibacterial agent eradicate fungi. Thus, effective treatment requires identification of the pathogen.

The first step in the identification of the pathogen is viewing a Gram-stained preparation under a microscope. A **Gram stain** is a simple test done with a dye and a glass slide. A sample of the pathogen is obtained from body fluids, sputum, blood, or exudates. Visualization under the microscope shows the shape of the pathogen, which aids in identifying it (Figure 37.1). The Gram stain indicates whether the pathogen is gram-positive or gram-negative type. Gram-positive bacteria absorb Gram stain and are often aerobic. Aerobic bacteria need a fresh and continuous supply of oxygen to reproduce. Gram-negative bacteria do not absorb Gram stain and tend to be anaerobic. Anaerobic bacteria are much more difficult to eradicate than aerobic bacteria because anaerobes can reproduce in an environment that is oxygen free. Some drugs affect only gram-positive microbes; some affect only gram-negative microbes; and some affect both, but not to the same extent. In some cases, the pathogen must be grown in a culture medium for identification.

Drug Susceptibility

To choose the right drug for the infection, a drug susceptibility test is optimal. However, it is not always required. The site of infection is frequently a clue to the causative

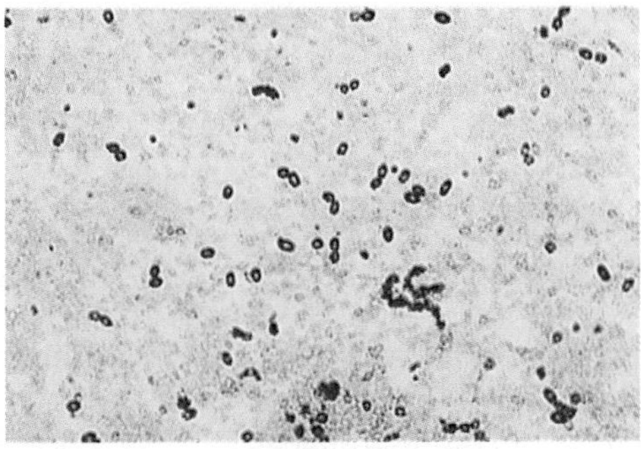

FIGURE 37.1 Gram-stained slide. This slide contains a type of gram-positive bacilli.

agent. For instance, *E. coli* causes most urinary tract infections. The health care practitioner therefore initially chooses a drug that can eradicate *E. coli.* Prescribing antibiotic treatment before the pathogen has been definitively identified is called **empiric therapy.** When multiple microbes may be the causative agent, empiric therapy may be started, but a culture of the infected area should be taken before treatment with antimicrobial agents is started because antimicrobial use may make identification of the microbe difficult. The culture is then used to determine drug susceptibility.

The most common test to identify drug susceptibility is called a culture and sensitivity. A sample of the exudate, body fluids, or serum is sent to the laboratory. The **culture** determines the identity of the microbe, and the **sensitivity** determines which antimicrobial agent will be therapeutic. Check the sensitivity test result of a patient receiving empiric therapy and notify the prescriber immediately if the current antibiotic is rated as "resistant." Sensitivity testing can be done by a disk diffusion test or broth dilution procedure.

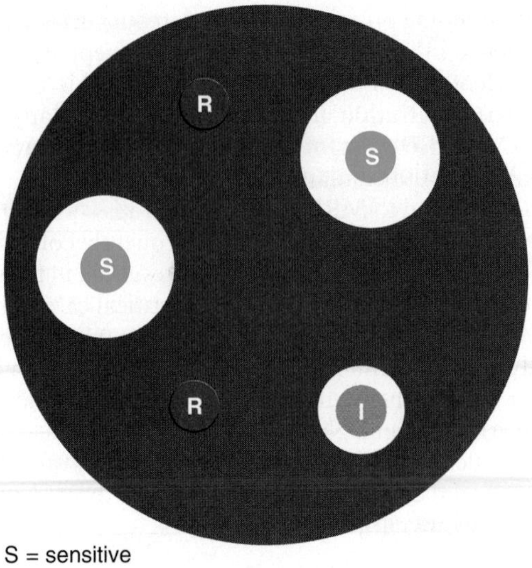

FIGURE 37.2 Disk diffusion test. In the disk diffusion test, samples of antibiotics are placed on a plate of the infecting organism. The organism is "sensitive" to the antibiotic if there is a bacteria-free zone around the antibiotic and "resistant" if the bacteria remain around the antibiotic.

Disk Diffusion Test

This is the most commonly performed test to determine drug susceptibility. In the disk diffusion method, disks containing a standardized amount of an antimicrobial agent are placed on an agar plate inoculated with the infecting organism. The plate is placed in an incubator, and the bacterial lawn is allowed to grow. A growth inhibition zone will appear around each antibiotic that affects the microbe (Figure 37.2). The diameter of the visible growth inhibition zone correlates with the minimum inhibitory concentration (MIC), which is the lowest concentration of an antibiotic that prevents visible growth of a microbe. Organisms are rated as sensitive (S) to a particular antibiotic if they are affected by it and resistant (R) if they are not.

Broth Dilution Procedure

In the broth dilution procedure, the bacteria are inoculated into a liquid medium containing graduated concentrations of the test antimicrobial. This method directly determines the MIC (Figure 37.3). The broth dilution procedure also determines the minimum bactericidal concentration (MBC), that is, the lowest concentration that will kill more than 99.9% of the original inoculum of the microbe. The broth dilution procedure is particularly helpful in managing difficult infections because it demonstrates both MIC and MBC.

Drug Spectrum

Choosing a drug with the narrowest possible **spectrum** is important. The range of microbes against which a drug is active is its spectrum. Narrow-spectrum drugs affect only a few microorganisms, whereas broad-spectrum drugs affect many microorganisms. The benefit of a narrow-spectrum antimicrobial agent is that it limits the potential for adverse effects, such as superinfection. A **superinfection** is one that occurs during the course of treatment for a primary infection. For example, an antibiotic suppresses all susceptible microbes, including the body's natural flora, which may keep other microbes in check. In the absence of these bacteria, nonsusceptible microbes can proliferate because they no longer have other microbes secreting toxins in their proximity and because they no longer need to compete for available nutrients. Two consequences may occur: secondary infections and the development of drug-resistant microbes.

An alternative to the use of broad-spectrum antimicrobials is combination therapy. Combination therapy is used fre-

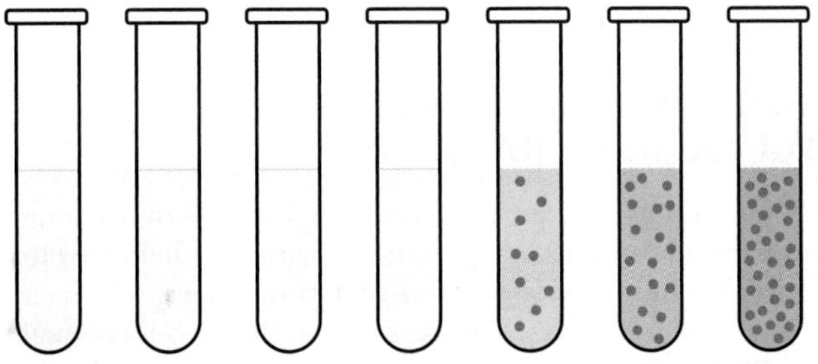

FIGURE 37.3 Broth dilution procedure. Bacteria are inoculated into a liquid medium containing graduated concentrations of the test antimicrobial. A clear test tube indicates that the concentration of the antimicrobial is sufficient to eradicate the microbe.

CRITICAL THINKING SCENARIO

Working with culture and sensitivity reports

Your patient has been receiving IV ciprofloxacin (Cipro) for a pulmonary infection, and you are about to hang a new infusion. The culture and sensitivity report has just arrived and shows an "R" next to ciprofloxacin. What should you do?

quently for an initial severe infection in which the pathogen is unknown. Once the pathogen is known, the appropriate drug can be administered. Another use for combination therapy is to treat an infection that is caused by more than one pathogen. This kind of infection is known as a mixed infection. Combination therapy is also used to prevent resistant microbes from developing. For instance, drug resistance occurs frequently during TB treatment as a result of its duration. When multiple drugs are given at the same time, the pathogen is less likely to be able to become resistant to all of the drugs employed. Another benefit of combination therapy is enhanced antibacterial action. For instance, some bacteria are capable of secreting enzymes that inhibit the action of the antibacterial agent. Combining beta-lactam inhibitors such as tazobactam with a penicillin allows the destruction of the enzyme by tazobactam, thus allowing penicillin to penetrate the cell wall and destroy the microbe.

Although combination therapy has many benefits, it also has many disadvantages compared with monotherapy. These disadvantages include an increased risk for toxic or allergic reactions, an increased risk for the development of resistant bacteria, and an increased risk for superinfection.

Drug Dose

Choosing the antimicrobial agent with the lowest effective dose is important. The dose of the antimicrobial agent is adjusted to affect the MIC at the site of infection. Pediatric doses are calculated as mg/kg per day.

Duration

Choosing the antimicrobial agent that takes the shortest time to affect the pathogen is equally important. The drug must remain at the site of infection at drug concentrations equal to or greater than MIC. The duration of treatment depends on the type of pathogen, the site of infection, and the presence or absence of host defenses. The duration of antimicrobial treatment is generally 7 to 10 days, but it may be extended to 30 days or more for infections such as prostatitis.

It is important to instruct the patient to take antimicrobial medication until all the medication is gone. Stopping therapy early may result in reinfection with the same pathogen, which will have become more drug resistant as a result of inadequate treatment.

Site of Infection

To be effective, a drug must be able to reach the site of infection at a concentration equal to or greater than the MIC. Achieving this concentration is a particular problem when the infection is in the meninges because many drugs do not cross the blood–brain barrier. Another difficult site is within an abscess because abscesses are poorly vascularized, and the presence of pus impedes drug concentrations. Specific types of infections, such as endocarditis, are difficult to treat because the vegetative growths are hard to penetrate.

Infections that occur in foreign objects such as pacemakers or prosthetic joints are also difficult to treat. When a foreign object enters the body, the immune system attempts to destroy the object by phagocytosis. While the phagocytes are busy attacking the foreign object, they are less able to attack bacteria that are multiplying at the site. Frequently, the infected foreign object must be removed to eradicate the bacterial infection.

Patient Assessment

Prescribers need to evaluate the individual patient before starting antimicrobial drugs. Important core patient variables include health status, life span, gender, environment, and culture.

Health Status

The type of antimicrobial agent chosen must reflect the immune status of the patient. Remember that most antimicrobial agents cannot eradicate infection without the assistance of the immune response. Immunocompetent patients may receive either bacteriocidal or bacteriostatic drugs because their immune systems can function with adequate response from phagocytic cells such as macrophages and neutrophils. Immunocompromised patients should receive drugs that are quickly bacteriocidal because such patients' immune responses are limited.

The patient must also be assessed for previous allergic responses to a particular drug class. When the patient states she or he has an allergy to a certain drug, find out what symptoms occurred when they took the drug. Many patients think that nausea, diarrhea, or headaches reflect an "allergy" to a certain drug. True allergic symptoms reflect an antigen–antibody reaction and are characterized by symptoms such as rash, itching, hives, periorbital swelling, and shortness of breath.

Life Span and Gender

Infants and the elderly are the populations most vulnerable to drug toxicity. In the infant, the liver and kidneys are still immature and may have difficulty metabolizing or excreting the drug, which results in accumulation. The same process in the elderly is related to the age of their liver and kidneys, which may no longer be functioning at an optimal level.

Prescribers may request lower doses of antimicrobial agents for these two populations to minimize the risk for toxicity.

During pregnancy, antimicrobial drugs may cross the placenta and cause damage to the developing fetus. For instance, tetracycline binds to developing teeth, producing a gray mottled discoloration.

Most antimicrobial agents enter breast milk, resulting in injury to the nursing child. For example, sulfonamide drugs may cause kernicterus, a type of brain damage caused by hyperbilirubinemia in the neonate.

Environment

The severity of the infection may influence the environment in which the antimicrobial is administered. The highest serum drug concentration is achieved when the antimicrobial is administered intravenously.

Another aspect to consider for intravenous (IV) therapy is the potential for severe adverse effects. For instance, amphotericin B, a powerful antifungal agent, causes an infusion reaction when administered. For that reason, most patients receiving amphotericin B are admitted to a facility that employs licensed nurses to administer the drug.

Culture and Inherited Traits

Certain cultures have genetic factors that are influenced by antimicrobial therapy. For example, some cultures have a predisposition to glucose-6-phosphate deficiency (G6PD). This deficiency tends to lyse red blood cells. Patients with this deficiency should not receive antimicrobials such as sulfonamides, which may induce red blood cell lysis.

MONITORING ANTIMICROBIAL THERAPY

Successful antimicrobial therapy eradicates the infection. Some antimicrobial agents have the ability to induce toxic adverse effects. Serum drug levels should be monitored for drugs that have a high potential for severe adverse effects. In addition, serum peak and trough levels may be measured. Blood for a peak level is drawn 30 to 45 minutes after IV administration or 1 hour after IM administration. The goal is to keep the serum drug level within the therapeutic margin.

For patients receiving long-term or high-dose antimicrobial therapy, other laboratory testing may be indicated. For instance, if an antimicrobial is known to cause anemia, the patient should be monitored using serial complete blood counts (CBCs).

The very young and the very old should also be monitored closely. Immaturity or advanced maturity may affect liver and kidney functioning. Appropriate testing would include hepatic and renal function tests.

The bottom line for patient monitoring is that it must be individualized according to the type of pathogen, site of infection, potential for adverse effects during therapy, and the patient care variables associated with each patient.

CHAPTER SUMMARY

- Bacteriocidal drugs kill bacteria, whereas bacteriostatic drugs inhibit bacterial growth but rely on the immune system to eradicate the pathogen.
- Antimicrobial therapy is effective because of the principle of selective toxicity: the ability of the drug to harm the pathogen without injuring the host.
- Drug resistance is an ever-present danger to effectively managing infection.
- Prophylactic use of antimicrobial drugs must be limited to appropriate indications to decrease the potential development of drug-resistant microbes.
- There are four major drug-resistant pathogens in the United States: methicillin-resistant *Staphylococcus aureus* (MRSA), penicillin-resistant *Streptococcus pneumoniae,* vancomycin-resistant *Enterococci* (VRE), and multiple drug–resistant *Mycobacterium tuberculosis* (MDR-TB).
- The most important principle in managing infection is to use the right drug for the right bug.
- A culture determines which pathogen is present, whereas a sensitivity test determines the susceptibility of the pathogen to a particular antibiotic.
- The antimicrobial agent used should be the one with the narrowest spectrum, at the lowest dose, that needs to be taken for the shortest time to affect the pathogen.
- Narrow-spectrum drugs affect only a few microorganisms, whereas broad-spectrum drugs affect many microorganisms.
- The minimum inhibitory concentration (MIC) is the minimum concentration of an antibiotic that completely suppresses bacterial growth.
- The minimum bactericidal concentration (MBC) is the concentration of an antibiotic that kills 99.9% of the initial inoculum in a broth dilution.
- Treatment with the drug of choice to eradicate a particular pathogen may have to be changed to an alternate drug because of specific core patient variables such as health status, life span, gender, environment, and culture and inherited traits.
- The most important element of patient education is to advise the patient to complete the entire course of therapy, taking the prescribed dose at the prescribed intervals.

QUESTIONS FOR STUDY AND REVIEW

1. What is the most important principle of antimicrobial therapy?
2. How are antimicrobials classified?
3. How do most antimicrobials work?
4. What is the principle of selective toxicity?
5. How does a superinfection occur?
6. In the United States, what microbes have developed substantial resistance to antimicrobials?

Need More Help?

Chapter 37 of the study guide for *Drug Therapy in Nursing* 2e contains NCLEX-style questions and other learning activities to reinforce your understanding of the concepts presented in this chapter. For additional information or to purchase the study guide, visit *http://connection.lww.com/go/aschenbrenner.*

REFERENCES AND BIBLIOGRAPHY

Facts and Comparisons. (2004). *Drug facts and comparisons.* Philadelphia: Lippincott Williams & Wilkins.

Hardman, J. G. (2001). *Goodman & Gilman's the pharmacological basis of therapeutics* (10th ed.). New York: McGraw-Hill Health Professions Division.

Loeffler, J., & Stevens, D. A. (2003). Antifungal drug resistance. *Clinical Infectious Diseases, 36*(Suppl. 1), S31–41.

Katzung, B. (2004). *Basic and clinical pharmacology* (9th ed.). New York: McGraw-Hill/Appleton & Lange.

McKeegan, K. S., Borges-Walmsley, M. I., & Walmsley, A. R. (2002). Microbial and viral drug resistance mechanism. *Trends in Microbiology, 10*(10 Suppl.), S8–14.

Rice, L. B. (2003). Do we really need new anti-infective drugs? *Current Opinions in Pharmacology, 3*(5), 459–463.

Tatro, D. S. (2004). *Drug interaction facts.* Philadelphia: Lippincott Williams & Wilkins.

Antibiotics Affecting the Bacterial Cell Wall

chapter 38

Learning Objectives

At the completion of this chapter the student will:

1. Identify the antibiotic drug classes that affect the bacterial cell wall and name at least one drug in each class.
2. Describe the primary therapeutic uses for each antibiotic drug class that affects the bacterial cell wall.
3. Identify core drug knowledge pertaining to antibiotics that affect the bacterial cell wall.
4. Identify core patient variables pertaining to antibiotics that affect the bacterial cell wall.
5. Relate the interaction of core drug knowledge to core patient variables for antibiotics that affect the bacterial cell wall.
6. Generate a nursing plan of care from the interactions between core drug knowledge and core patient variables for antibiotics that affect the bacterial cell wall.
7. Describe nursing interventions to maximize therapeutic and minimize adverse effects for antibiotics that affect the bacterial cell wall.
8. Determine key points for patient and family education for antibiotics that affect the bacterial cell wall.

KEY TERMS

bacterial cell envelope

beta-lactam

beta-lactamases

cephalosporinases

cyclic lipopeptide

penicillinases

penicillin-binding proteins (PBPs)

FEATURED WEBLINK

http://www.nlm.nih.gov/medlineplus/druginfo
New drugs enter the market every month. For up-to-date information that you can trust, log on to this drug information website.

CONNECTION WEBLINK

Additional Weblinks are found on Connection:
http://www.connection.lww.com/go/aschenbrenner.

Antibiotics Affecting the Bacterial Cell Wall

Ⓒ Penicillins

Narrow spectrum penicillins
- **P** **penicillin G**
- penicillin V
- procaine penicillin
- benzathine penicillin

Broad spectrum penicillins (aminopenicillins)
- ampicillin
- amoxicillin
- bacampicillin

Extended spectrum penicillins (antipseudomonal penicillins)
- carbenicillin indanyl
- mezlocillin
- piperacillin
- ticarcillin

Penicillinase-resistant penicillins (antistaphylococcal penicillins)
- cloxacillin
- dicloxacillin
- methicillin
- nafcillin
- oxacillin

Beta-lactamase inhibitors
- bacitracin
- clavulanic acid
- sulbactam
- tazobactam

Ⓒ Monobactam Antibiotics

- aztreonam

Ⓒ Carbapenems

- ertapenem
- imipenem
- meropenem

Ⓒ Cephalosporins

P **cefazolin**

First generation
(cefadroxil, cephalexin, cephradine, cephalothin, cephapirin)

Second generation
(cefaclor, cefprozil, loracarbef, cefuroxime, cefoxitin, cefonicid, cefotetan)

Third generation
(cefdinir, cefixime, cefpodoxime, ceftibuten, cefoperazone, cefotaxime, ceftizoxime, ceftriaxone, ceftazidime)

Fourth generation
(cefepime)

Ⓒ Vancomycins

- **P** vancomycin

Ⓒ Cyclic Lipopeptides

- **P** daptomycin

The symbol Ⓒ indicates the **drug class.**
Drugs in **bold type** marked with the symbol **P** are prototypes.
Drugs in blue type are closely related to the prototype.
Drugs in red type are significantly different from the prototype.
Drugs in black type with no symbol are also used in drug therapy; no prototype

Drugs affecting the bacterial cell wall include penicillins, monobactams, carbapenems, cephalosporins, vancomycin, and cyclic lipopeptide antibiotics. Penicillin G is the prototype drug for the penicillin drug class; drugs significantly different from penicillin are the beta-lactamase inhibitors and bacitracin. Other prototype drugs discussed in this chapter include aztreonam for the monobactam drug class; imipenem for the carbapenem drug class; cefazolin for the cephalosporin drug class; and vancomycin and daptomycin, which are the only drugs in their respective classes.

In addition to explaining how these drugs work, this chapter discusses nursing management related to evaluating the patient's condition, monitoring the patient's response, and teaching the patient and family about antibiotic therapy.

PHYSIOLOGY

Bacteria are surrounded by a rigid cell wall that is responsible for maintaining the integrity of the internal cellular environment. The interior of the cell has a high osmotic pressure. If the bacterial cell wall is not intact, the internal osmotic pressure will draw fluid into the cell until it bursts.

Even when the cell wall is breached by an antibiotic, bacterial death may not occur because of bacterial resistance. Bacterial resistance occurs for one of two reasons: the drug is unable to reach binding sites within the cell, or the bacteria produced an enzyme that inactivated the drug.

Bacterial Cell Envelope

Drugs that affect the bacterial cell wall must be able to penetrate the cell wall to bind to molecular targets on the cytoplasmic membrane within the cell. Gram-positive bacteria have only two layers to their **cell envelope:** a thick cell wall and cytoplasmic membrane. Despite the thickness of the cell wall, many drugs are capable of penetrating this wall and attaching to the targets on the cytoplasmic membrane. Gram-negative bacteria have an additional outer membrane to their cell envelope, and the cell wall is much thinner. Although the cell wall can be penetrated easily, the outer membrane cannot. Only drugs that can pass through the very small pores of the outer membrane can reach the target sites on the cytoplasmic membrane (Figure 38.1).

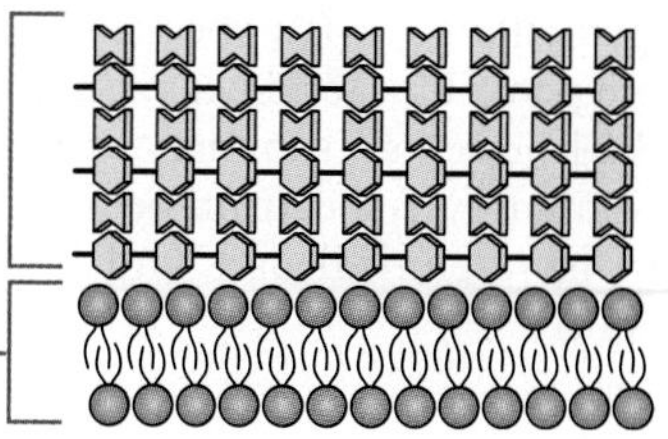

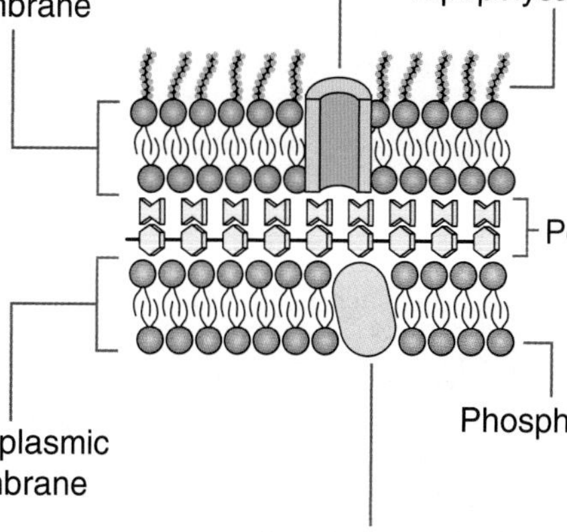

FIGURE 38.1 Although the gram-positive cell wall is much thicker than the gram-negative cell wall, antibiotics can attach to targets on the cytoplasmic membrane. In the gram-negative cell, the wall is thinner, but the cell also contains an outer membrane that makes it difficult for antibiotics to permeate the cell.

Bacterial Enzymes

Beta-lactamases are enzymes that disrupt the beta-lactam ring. This mechanism inactivates **beta-lactam** drugs, such as penicillins and cephalosporins, because their antibiotic activity is derived from characteristics of the beta-lactam ring. Enzymes that affect penicillins are called **penicillinases,** whereas enzymes that affect cephalosporins are called **cephalosporinases.**

PATHOPHYSIOLOGY

Bacteria may cause infections in any body organ, structure, or fluid. In addition to the original bacterial infection, the loss of certain "good" bacteria may result in a superinfection, such as that caused by *Candida* species.

C PENICILLINS

Penicillins were the first antibiotics introduced for clinical use. Alexander Fleming derived them from *Penicillium* molds in 1929. Developing penicillin was so important that its inventors won the Nobel Prize. Subsequent versions of penicillin have been developed to decrease the adverse effects of the drug and to modify its ability to act on resistant bacteria. Penicillins are also called beta-lactam antibiotics because their chemical structure contains a beta-lactam ring that is essential for antibacterial activity. All penicillins contain this essential beta-lactam ring; however, adding a side chain to specific types of penicillins influences their pharmacokinetic properties, binding capabilities, penicillinase resistance, and resistance to stomach acids. Penicillins are most effective against cells undergoing active growth and division. Penicillins are classified as narrow-spectrum penicillins,

aminopenicillins (broad-spectrum penicillins), extended-spectrum penicillins, and penicillinase-resistant penicillins. Table 38.1 presents a summary of selected penicillins. Penicillin G, a narrow-spectrum penicillin, was the first penicillin to have clinical uses and is the prototype for the penicillin class.

NURSING MANAGEMENT OF THE PATIENT RECEIVING [P] PENICILLIN G

Core Drug Knowledge

Pharmacotherapeutics

Penicillin G is indicated for use in infections caused by susceptible gram-positive bacteria, anaerobes, and spirochetes, including streptococci, non–penicillinase-producing staphylococci, and *Treponema pallidum.* Although penicillin G is generally ineffective for gram-negative bacteria, it is indicated for use in a few gram-negative infections, such as those caused by *Neisseria meningitidis* and non–penicillinase-producing strains of *Neisseria gonorrhoeae.* Clinically, these bacteria cause infections such as pneumonia, pharyngitis, tonsillitis, endocarditis, and scarlet fever. Other clinical uses include therapy for tetanus, anthrax, meningitis, syphilis, diphtheria, rat-bite fever, and fusospirochetal infections.

Penicillin G may also be used as prophylaxis in special patient populations to prevent bacterial endocarditis prior to procedures likely to produce temporary bacteremia, such as dental procedures. These patients include those with prosthetic heart valves, mitral valve prolapse, most congenital heart diseases, and acquired valvular heart disease. It may also be used as prophylaxis in patients with recurrent rheumatic fever or rheumatic heart disease.

Penicillin G may sometimes be used for gram-negative infections.

Pharmacokinetics

Penicillin G is absorbed rapidly from the gastrointestinal (GI) tract but is unstable in gastric acid. This instability means that the amount of penicillin G that is actually absorbed with any given dose varies with the acidity of stomach contents. The development of more stable penicillins, such as penicillin V, has led prescribers to discontinue using oral penicillin G.

Four forms of parenteral penicillin G are commercially available: salts of potassium, sodium, benzathine, and procaine. The potassium and sodium salts are referred to as the aqueous and crystalline forms of the drug and may be administered intravenously or intramuscularly. Benzathine and procaine penicillin are referred to as repository forms of penicillin because they provide tissue depots from which the drug is absorbed over several hours (procaine penicillin) or days (benzathine penicillin). As such, benzathine and procaine penicillins are administered only intramuscularly.

Penicillin G binds to plasma proteins and circulates in the blood to be released at various tissue sites. The average peak drug effect is 4 hours after administration. Penicillin G crosses the placenta and is secreted in breast milk. It does not penetrate the blood–brain barrier very well except in the presence of meningeal inflammation, a fact that makes it somewhat useful in treating meningitis.

Penicillin G is rapidly cleared unchanged from the plasma by the kidneys (by glomerular filtration and renal tubular secretion). Because this rapid clearance of the drug makes it somewhat difficult to maintain therapeutic levels, around-the-clock administration is needed for therapy to be truly effective.

Pharmacodynamics

Penicillin G inhibits the third and final stage of bacterial cell wall synthesis by binding to specific **penicillin-binding proteins** (PBPs) located inside the bacterial cell wall. After binding with specific PBPs, penicillin inhibits transpeptidase, an enzyme that is responsible for developing cross-bridges within the cell wall. These cross-bridges give the cell wall its strength. Additionally, penicillin affects autolytic enzymes (autolysins) that promote active cell wall destruction. The relationship between PBPs and autolysins is unclear; possibly, penicillin interferes with an autolysin inhibitor. As the cell wall weakens, the internal osmotic pressure of the bacteria changes, allowing the cell to swell, then burst. The body's immune system completes the process of fighting the infection and cleans up debris from ruptured bacteria.

Penicillin has selective toxicity to bacteria because human cells do not use the biochemical process that the bacteria use to form a cell wall and are thus protected from destruction.

Contraindications and Precautions

Penicillin G is contraindicated in the presence of known allergies to penicillin, cephalosporins, or imipenem. Penicillin sensitivity tests are available if the patient's history of allergy is unclear and penicillin is the drug of choice. Caution should be exercised in the presence of renal disease, pregnancy, and lactation.

Adverse Effects

The most serious adverse effect of penicillin G is allergic reaction: rash, fever, and wheezing, and possibly anaphylaxis and death. More common adverse effects of penicillin therapy involve the GI tract: nausea, vomiting, diarrhea, abdominal pain, glossitis, stomatitis, gastritis, sore mouth, and furry tongue. These effects are primarily related to the loss of normal flora (naturally occurring bacteria in the body) and subsequent opportunistic infections. Other adverse effects include superinfections (e.g., yeast infections) and local pain or inflammation at the injection site. Other, less common effects include lethargy, hallucinations, anemia, thrombocytopenia, nephritis, and sodium overload (especially with the sodium salt of penicillin G).

Drug Interactions

The effectiveness of penicillin G is decreased when taken concurrently with tetracyclines. Parenteral aminoglycosides (amikacin, gentamicin, kanamycin, neomycin, netilmicin, streptomycin, tobramycin) are inactivated when these drugs are administered with penicillin G. Table 38.2 lists agents that interact with penicillin G.

Oral probenecid is sometimes given with intravenous (IV) penicillin G because it slows the excretion of the drug by competing with the penicillin molecule for excretion sites

(text continues on page 675)

TABLE 38.1 Summary of Selected Ⓒ Penicillins and Other Beta-Lactam Antibiotics

Drug (Trade) Name	Selected Indications	Route and Dosage Range	Pharmacokinetics
Ⓒ Penicillins			
P penicillin G (Pfizerpen, *Canadian:* Falapen)	Pneumococcal infections Streptococcal infections (Group A) Bacterial endocarditis Diphtheria Neurosyphilis Congenital syphilis	Penicillin G is administered IV as penicillin G potassium or sodium and IM as penicillin G potassium, sodium, procaine, or benzathine. Dosages highly individualized by disorder. *Adult:* IM, 300,000–8 million units qd in divided doses; IV, 6–20 million units qd by continuous or intermittent infusion (q2–4 hours) *Child:* IM/IV, 25,000–250,000 units/kg/d in divided doses	*Onset:* IM, rapid; IV, rapid *Duration:* Varies $t_{1/2}$: 30–60 min
penicillin G benzathine (Bicillin, Bicillin Long-Acting, Permapen)	Streptococcal Early syphilis Syphilis of > 1 y duration	*Adult:* IM, 1.2 million U q4wk *Adult:* IV, 2.4 million U in one single dose *Adult:* Parenteral, 2.4 million U once weekly for 3 wk *Child:* >27 kg, parenteral, 900,000–1.2 million U in one dose; >27 kg, 300–600,000 U in one dose	*Onset:* IM, slow *Duration:* 1–4 wk $t_{1/2}$: 30–60 min
penicillin G procaine (Wycillin)	Pneumococcal infections Staphylococcal infections	*Adult and child:* IM, 600,000–1.2 million U/d in one or two doses for 10 d–2 wk	*Onset:* IM, slow *Duration:* 15–20 h $t_{1/2}$: 30–60 min
penicillin V (Pen V-K Veetids; *Canadian:* Apo Pen V-K, Nadopen-V, Novopen-VK, Nu-Pen-VK)	Fusospirochetal infections Streptococcal infections	*Adult:* PO, 250–500 mg q6–8 h *Adult:* PO, 125–250 mg q6–8 h for 10 d *Child:* PO, 25–50 mg/kg/d q6–8h	*Onset:* Rapid *Duration:* Varies $t_{1/2}$: 30–60 min
Ⓒ Aminopenicillins			
ampicillin (Omnipen; Prinupen, *Canadian:* Apo-Ampi, Novo-Ampicillin, Nu-Ampi)	Septicemia	*Adult:* IV, 150–200 mg/kg/d for 3 d, then IM q3–4h *Child:* Same as adult	*Onset:* PO, 30 min; IM, 15 min; IV, immediate *Duration:* 6–8 h $t_{1/2}$: 1–2 h
	Bacterial meningitis	*Adult:* IV, 150–200 mg/kg/d by continuous infusion and then IM injections q3–4h *Child:* Same as adult	
	Respiratory/soft-tissue infections	*Adult:* PO, 40 kg or more; IV or IM, 250–500 mg q6h; <40 kg, IV or IM, 25–50 mg/kg at 6–8 h intervals; <20 kg, PO, 50 mg/kg/d in equal doses q6–8h	
amoxicillin (Amoxil; Moxilan; *Canadian:* Apo-Amoxi, Gen-Amoxicillin, Lin-Amnox, Novamoxin)	URI, GU infections	*Adult:* PO, 250–500 mg q8h *Child:* Same as adult	*Onset:* Varies *Duration:* 6–8 h $t_{1/2}$: 1–1.4 h
	Lower respiratory tract infections	*Adult:* PO, 500 mg q8h *Child:* Same as adult	

(continued)

TABLE 38.1 Summary of Selected (C) Penicillins and Other Beta-Lactam Antibiotics (continued)

Drug (Trade) Name	Selected Indications	Route and Dosage Range	Pharmacokinetics
bacampicillin (Spectrobid; *Canadian:* Penglobe)	URI, UTI	*Adult:* PO, 400 mg q12h *Child:* PO, 25 mg/kg/d in two doses q12h	*Onset:* Varies *Duration:* 8–10 h $t_{1/2}$: 1.5 h
	Lower respiratory tract infections	*Adult:* PO, 800 mg q12h *Child:* 50 mg/kg/d in two doses q12h	
(C) Extended-Spectrum Penicillins			
carbenicillin (Geopen, Geocillin; *Canadian:* Carbapen, Gripenin)	UTI	*Adult:* PO, 382–764 mg PO qid *Child:* PO, 30–50 mg/kg/d in divided doses q6h	*Onset:* Varies *Duration:* 6–8 h $t_{1/2}$: 60–70 min
	UTI due to *Pseudomonas, Enterococcus,* or prostatitis	PO, 764 mg qid	
ticarcillin (Ticar)	Bacteremia, septicemia Intraabdominal infections Intraabdominal abscess Bone and joint infections Gynecologic infections Lower respiratory tract meningitis Skin and skin structure infections Pulmonary infection secondary to complications of cystic fibrosis	*Adult and child ≥40 kg:* IV/IM, 200–300 mg/kg/d in divided doses q4–6h *Child <40 kg:* (serious infection): IM/IV, 200–300 mg/kg/d in divided doses q4–6h *Child <40 kg:* (uncomplicated infection): IM/IV, 50–100 mg/kg/d in divided doses q6–8h	*Onset:* IM/IV, rapid *Duration:* 4–6 h $t_{1/2}$: 0.8–1.4 h
	Uncomplicated UTI	*Adult and child:* ≥ 40 kg: IM/IV, 1 g q6h *Child ≥1 mo and <40 kg:* IM/IV, 50–100 mg/kg in divided doses q6–8h	
	Complicated UTI	*Adult and child:* IV, 150–200 mg/kg in equally divided doses q4–6 h	
piperacillin (Pipracil)	Lower respiratory tract infections Skin and skin structure infections Bone and joint infections Intraabdominal infections Gynecologic infections Bacteremia Septicemia	*Adult:* IV, 3–4 g infusion over 20–30 min q4h *Child:* Although safety and efficacy in children have not been fully established, pediatric patients have received 76–100 mg/kg/day IV or IM in divided doses q4h	*Onset:* IV, rapid *Duration:* 4–6 h $t_{1/2}$: 0.7–1.3 h
mezlocillin (Mezlin)	Same as piperacillin	*Adult:* IM/IV, 3g q4h or 4 g q6h *Child:* IV, 50 mg/kg over 30 min q4h or IM q4h	*Onset:* IM, rapid; IV, immediate *Duration:* 8–10 h $t_{1/2}$: 50–55 min
	Endocarditis due to *Pseudomonas aeruginosa* or *Serratia sp.*	*Adult:* IV, 5 g IV q8h in combination with an aminoglycoside	
	Uncomplicated UTI	*Adult:* IM/IV, 1.5–2g q6h	
	Complicated UTI	*Adult:* 3 g IV q6h	
	Uncomplicated gonorrhea	*Adult:* IM/IV, 1–2 g as a single dose with probenecid	
(C) Penicillinase-Resistant Penicillins			
dicloxacillin (Dynapen; *Canadian:* Dycill, Pathocil)	Infections due to penicillinase-producing staphylococci	*Adult and child >40 kg:* PO, 125 mg q6h; up to 250 mg q6h in severe infections *Child <40 kg:* PO, 12.5–25 mg/kg/d in equally divided doses q6h; up to 25 mg/kg/d in equally divided doses q6h in severe infections	*Onset:* Varies *Duration:* 6–8 h $t_{1/2}$: 30–90 min

(continued)

TABLE 38.1 Summary of Selected Ⓒ Penicillins and Other Beta-Lactam Antibiotics (continued)

Drug (Trade) Name	Selected Indications	Route and Dosage Range	Pharmacokinetics
nafcillin (Unipen; *Canadian:* Nallpen)	Infections due to penicillanase-producing staphylococci Infections caused by group A beta-hemolytic streptococci, *Streptococcus viridans*	*Adult:* IV, 0.5–2 g q4h *Child:* IV, 50–100 mg/kg/d in equally divided doses q6h; for severe infections 100–200 mg/kg/d *Adult:* IM, 500 mg q4–6h *Child:* IM, 50–100 mg/kg/d in equally divided doses q6h; for severe infections 100–200 mg/kg/d *Adult:* PO, 0.25–1 g q4–6h *Child:* PO, 50–100 mg/kg/d in divided doses q6h	*Onset:* PO, varies; IM, rapid; IV, immediate *Duration:* PO and IV, 4 h; IM, 4–6 h $t_{1/2}$: 1 h
oxacillin (Prostaphlin)	Infections due to penicillinase-producing staphylococci Infections caused by streptococci	*Adult and child >40 kg:* IM/IV, 0.25–2 g, q4–6h; maximum daily doses is 23 g *Child <40 kg:* IM/IV, 50–100 mg/kg/d in equally divided doses q4–6h *Adult and child >40 kg:* PO, 0.5–1 g q4–6h *Child <40 kg:* PO, 50–100 mg/kg/d in equally divided doses q4–6h	*Onset:* PO, varies; IM/IV, rapid *Duration:* PO/IM, 4–6 h; IV length of infusion $t_{1/2}$: 0.5–1 h
Ⓒ Monobactams			
aztreonam (Azactam)	Moderately severe systemic infection *Pseudomonas aeruginosa* Urethritis Endocervicitis Proctitis Gonorrhea	*Adult:* IV, 0.5–2 g IV q6–12h *Infant and child ≥1 mo of age:* IV, 30 mg/kg q6–8h; for patients with cystic fibrosis, 50 mg/kg q6–8 h *Infant and child ≥1 mo of age:* IV, 50 mg/kg q4–6h *Adult:* IM, 1 g as a single dose	*Onset:* IM, varies; IV, rapid *Duration:* 6–8 h $t_{1/2}$: 1.5–2 h
Ⓒ Carbapenems			
imipenem/cilastatin (Primaxin)	Intra-abdominal infections gynecologic infections Gynecologic infections Lower respiratory tract infections Skin and skin structure infections Bone and joint infections Bacteremia or septicemia Endocarditis Febrile neutropenia	*Adult:* IV, 250–500 mg q 6h to a maximum of 4 g/d *Adult:* IM, 500–750 mg q 12h depending on severity of infection *Child >3 mo:* 15–25 mg/kg IV q6h to a maximum dose of 2 g/day	*Onset:* IM rapid IV immediate *Duration:* 6–12 h $t_{1/2}$: 90–120 min
meropenem (Merrem)	Intra-abdominal infections Bacterial meningitis	*Adult and child >50 kg:* IV, 1–2 grams q8h *Child <50 kg:* IV, 20–40 mg/kg q8h	*Onset:* immediate *Duration:* 10–12 h $t_{1/2}$: 1 h
ertapenem (Invanz)	Community-acquired pneumonia Skin and skin structure infections Complicated GI infections Complicated intra-abdominal infections Acute pelvic infections	*Adult:* IM/IV, 1 gram per day *Child:* Safety in children not established	*Onset:* IM, 10 min IV, rapid *Duration:* unknown $t_{1/2}$: 4 h

(continued)

TABLE 38.1 Summary of Selected C Penicillins and Other Beta-Lactam Antibiotics (continued)

Drug (Trade) Name	Selected Indications	Route and Dosage Range	Pharmacokinetics
C Combination Drugs			
ampicillin/sulbactam (Unasyn)	Skin and skin structure infections Soft tissue infections Otitis media Sinusitis Respiratory tract infections GU infections Septicemia	*Adult and child >40 kg:* IV/IM, 1.5–3 grams q6–8h *Child >1 year:* IV, 75 mg/kg q6h	*Onset:* IM, rapid IV, immediate *Duration:* 6–8 h $t_{1/2}$: 1–1.5 h
amoxicillin/clavulanic acid (Augmentin)	Otitis media Respiratory tract infections Skin and skin structure infections Urinary tract infections Community acquired pneumonia SARS	*Adult:* PO, 250–500 q8h *Child <40 kg:* PO, 20–40 mg/kg in divided doses q8h	*Onset:* 30 min *Duration:* 8 h $t_{1/2}$: 1–1.5 h
ticarcillin/clavulanic acid (Timentin)	Skin and skin structure infections Bone and joint infections Septicemia Respiratory tract infections Intra-abdominal infections Gynecologic infections Urinary tract infections	*Adult and child >40 kg:* IV, 3 g q4h or 4 g q6h *Child <40 kg:* IV, 33.3–50 mg/kg q4h or 50–75 mg/kg q6h *Neonate >2 kg:* IV, 75 mg/kg q8h *Neonate <2 kg:* IV, 75 mg/kg q12h	*Onset:* IM/IV, rapid *Duration:* 4–6 h $t_{1/2}$: 1 h
piperacillin/tazobactam (Zosyn)	Intra-abdominal infections Skin and skin structure infections Gynecologic infections Respiratory tract infections	*Adult:* IV, 3–4 g q6–8h	*Onset:* IM/IV, rapid *Duration:* 4–6 h $t_{1/2}$: 0.7–1.5 h

TABLE 38.2 Agents That Interact With P Penicillin G

Interactants	Effect and Significance	Nursing Management
aminoglycosides	GI absorption of penicillins may be impaired by aminoglycosides.	Avoid combination therapy if possible. Administer at least 2 h apart. Tailor dose of penicillin as needed.
anticoagulants	Large IV doses of penicillin may prolong bleeding time.	Monitor for signs of bleeding.
food	GI absorption of penicillins are impaired by the presence of food.	Administer at least 1 h before or 2 h after meals.
oral contraceptives	Penicillins may suppress intestinal flora, which provide an enzyme essential for enterohepatic recirculation for certain oral contraceptives. This may result in a decreased contraceptive plasma level.	Advise patients taking oral contraceptives to use an additional method of birth control while taking penicillins.
methotrexate	Coadministration may increase serum methotrexate levels resulting in toxicity.	Avoid if possible. Monitor signs and symptoms of methotrexate toxicity.
tetracyclines	The bacteriostatic action of tetracyclines may impair the bactericidal activity of penicillins.	Avoid combination therapy.

in the renal tubule. The result is that penicillin levels stay high for a longer time, achieving a greater effect. When the supply of penicillin G is adequate, probenecid is not required. However, when supplies of penicillin G are low, probenecid can be used to prolong the action of IV penicillin.

Assessment of Relevant Core Patient Variables

Health Status

Take a careful health history to assess for any known reactions to antibiotics. Examine the skin for any rash or lesions to provide a baseline to avoid misdiagnosis of an allergic reaction. Assess the respiratory status of the patient as a baseline for possible wheezing associated with an allergic reaction.

For patients with a questionable history of allergic reaction to penicillin, a skin test may be performed to determine current allergic status. Because the skin test itself may cause an anaphylactic response in susceptible patients, it should be done only in a setting that can respond to the potential emergency. In rare situations, a penicillin-allergic patient may need to be given penicillin. In these rare cases, penicillin is administered according to a desensitization schedule. Desensitization does not always stop an allergic response; therefore, it must be done in an acute care setting. Epinephrine and respiratory support must be immediately available for either skin testing or desensitization.

For elderly patients or patients with kidney disease, evaluate kidney function (including blood urea nitrogen [BUN] and creatinine clearance) to determine baseline functioning. Patients with decreased kidney functioning may need a reduced dose of penicillin G. For long-term therapy, baseline liver function tests should also be performed. In addition, assess for previously prescribed drugs that may interact with penicillin to cause undesired effects.

When penicillin G is used for gram-negative infections, culture and sensitivity tests should always be performed to be sure that the causative bacteria are sensitive to penicillin G.

Life Span and Gender

Document the method of birth control used by a woman of childbearing age because antibiotics, such as penicillin G, can counteract the effects of an oral contraceptive. Assess women of childbearing age for pregnancy and lactation. Pregnant and lactating women should be given penicillin G with caution because superinfections may occur in the fetus or infant, or the infant may develop diarrhea. If the patient is elderly, he or she may need a reduced dose because of decreased kidney function.

Lifestyle, Diet, and Habits

Instruct patients self-administering penicillin G to administer the drug around the clock, to ensure that drugs levels stay within a therapeutic range. Assess the patient's daily schedule to ensure that the patient who is self-administering penicillin G can complete the therapy as prescribed.

Environment

Be aware of the environment in which the drug will be administered. Whether administered at home or in an acute care setting, penicillin G solution should be mixed and stored in a refrigerator between 2° and 8°C (36° and 46°F) for up to 7 days. It should never be frozen. Commercially prepared infusion solutions may be kept at room temperature for 24 hours. Oral penicillin does not require specific environmental requirements.

Nursing Diagnoses and Outcomes

- Risk for Injury related to drug-related allergic reactions
  Desired outcome: *The patient will recognize symptoms of allergy and contact the prescriber immediately to minimize ill effects.*
- Imbalanced Nutrition: Less than Body Requirements related to drug-induced GI effects, such as diarrhea, GI upset, altered taste sensation, or superinfection
  Desired outcome: *The patient will maintain consistent body weight and consult prescriber about persistent adverse effects that affect nutritional status.*
- Diarrhea related to drug therapy
  Desired outcome: *The patient will avoid dehydration, maintain fluid intake, and contact prescriber about persistent diarrhea.*
- Risk for Infection related to overgrowth of nonsusceptible organisms.
  Desired outcome: *The patient will report signs of superinfection to the prescriber.*

Planning and Intervention

Maximizing Therapeutic Effects

Review culture and sensitivity reports to make sure that penicillin G is appropriate for the patient, especially for gram-negative infections. Administer penicillin G as prescribed, spaced evenly around the clock to increase effectiveness. For oral preparations, administer the dose on an empty stomach. Optimally, drug therapy should continue for at least 7 to 10 days, but it may continue for 2 weeks.

In acute care settings, retrieve the antibiotic from the refrigerator approximately 15 minutes before administration, and evaluate the IV site for signs of phlebitis before and after administration.

Intramuscular (IM) penicillin should be administered deep into the muscle mass. Aspirate the syringe to avoid accidental injection into the vasculature. Assess landmarks for IM administration to avoid injection into a nerve.

Minimizing Adverse Effects

Provide small, frequent meals; mouth care; and ice chips for the patient to suck if stomatitis and sore mouth are problems. Monitor the patient to ensure that adequate fluids are given to replace fluid lost with an adverse effect such as diarrhea. Monitoring fluid intake and output is especially important. Notify the prescriber if a substantial change develops in the intake-to-output ratio because such a change may be the first indication of kidney dysfunction.

When penicillin is administered parenterally (IM or IV), the patient should be monitored for a minimum of 30 minutes. Epinephrine and respiratory support should be immediately available whenever parenteral penicillin is administered.

COMMUNITY-BASED CONCERNS

Box 38.1 Taking Antibiotics Safely

Every year, families in the community face colds, sore throats, flu, and other types of infections. Should all of these conditions be treated with antibiotics? Even as a new member of the health care team, you can answer questions concerning antibiotic safety with ease. Be sure to emphasize these key points:

- Illnesses with very similar symptoms may be caused by entirely different types of microbes.
- Illnesses caused by microbes other than bacteria are generally not affected by antibiotics.
- Overuse, including inappropriate use of antibiotics, leads to bacterial resistance (super-strains of microbes that are very difficult to kill).
- Antibiotics take time to work, so it will take a couple of days to feel better.
- Take the medication exactly as prescribed—don't take fewer pills per day to make the prescription last longer.
- Never take medication from a previous illness—if its expiration date has passed, it might not work.
- Never take medication prescribed for another person, even if your symptoms are similar to theirs.
- All medications can cause adverse effects, especially nausea or diarrhea, but these effects are not signs of allergy.
- Signs of allergy include reddened skin, rash, itching, hives, swelling of one or more body parts, shortness of breath, wheezing, or chest palpitations. If you have these symptoms, do not take any more of the drug! Call the person who prescribed the medication immediately.

Providing Patient and Family Education

- Explain to patients with penicillin allergy the importance of wearing some form of identification (e.g., Medic Alert necklace or bracelet) to alert health care personnel of the allergy in an emergency.
- Stress the importance of completing the full course of antibiotics, explaining the purpose of the drug and stating that it may not work for other types of infection.
- Emphasize the need to take penicillin G exactly as prescribed at evenly spaced intervals around the clock. Instruct the patient that oral drugs should be taken on an empty stomach 1 hour before or 2 hours after a meal.
- Instruct the patient to take missed doses as soon as remembered but not at the time that the next dose is scheduled.
- If the patient must mix the solution, instruct the patient to do so just before administration. When premixed solutions are used, they should be kept in the refrigerator and retrieved approximately 15 minutes before administration.
- Advise the patient to contact the prescriber if no improvement occurs within 3 days.
- Because any patient may develop sensitivity to penicillin G at any time, discuss the signs and symptoms of allergic reaction and instruct the patient to stop the drug and call the prescriber if a rash, welts, itching, or shortness of breath develops.
- One of the most important features of patient and family education is to teach the patient that penicillin is one drug within a class of drugs. Advise the patient who has ever had any type of allergic reaction to penicillin never to take any other drug with a name that ends with "cillin."
- Review common adverse effects and home interventions that may relieve discomfort. Patients who experience abdominal cramps or GI distress may try eating small, frequent meals. To relieve a sore mouth or throat, sucking on ice chips may help. If diarrhea occurs, teach the patient to increase fluid intake and to contact the prescriber if symptoms do not resolve in 24 hours.
- Teach the patient about other adverse effects, such as a change in tongue color, fatigue, easy bruising, and vaginal discharge. Instruct the patient to report these signs and symptoms of superinfection to the prescriber immediately.
- Advise women of childbearing age to use a backup method of birth control for the duration of therapy.
- Explain the importance of sterile technique if family members administer IV therapy at home.

Ongoing Assessment and Evaluation

Monitor for signs of allergic reaction and for resolution of the presenting symptoms of infection (e.g., fever, lethargy, or hot and reddened or inflamed skin). Failure of these symptoms to resolve may indicate a treatment failure. Monitor for signs of superinfection and notify the prescriber immediately to arrange for treatment. For patient comfort, provide warm compresses and gentle massage to painful or swollen injection sites and observe for signs of phlebitis or abscess formation.

Monitor patients receiving parenteral sodium penicillin G for potential fluid overload. Monitoring is especially important in patients with cardiac disease or hypertension. Monitor patients receiving potassium penicillin G for signs of hyperkalemia that may result in cardiac arrhythmias. Arrange for periodic electrolyte studies for patient receiving either preparation.

When treatment ends, the initial infection should be resolved. The patient should be adequately nourished and hydrated, and any adverse drug effects should be resolved.

MEMORY CHIP

P Penicillin G

- Used for infections caused by gram-positive bacteria, anaerobes, and spirochetes. Also used as prophylaxis to prevent bacterial endocarditis.
- Major contraindications: hypersensitivity to penicillin, cephalosporins, or imipenem
- Most common adverse effects: nausea, vomiting, diarrhea
- Most serious adverse effect: hypersensitivity
- **Life span alert: Elderly patients may need reduced dosage because of decreased kidney function.**
- Maximizing therapeutic effects: Oral preparations should be given on an empty stomach. When using for gram-negative infections, be sure culture and sensitivity tests are done before administration.
- Minimizing adverse effects: Monitor intake and output because it may be the first sign of kidney dysfunction. Blood levels may become toxic if the kidneys cannot excrete penicillin.
- Most important patient education: Take the medication exactly as prescribed until the entire prescription is completed, despite the absence of symptoms. Monitor for signs and symptoms of allergic response and stop the medication if any occur.

Drugs Closely Related to P Penicillin G

Other Narrow-Spectrum Penicillins

In addition to penicillin G, other narrow-spectrum penicillins include penicillin V, procaine penicillin, and benzathine penicillin.

PENICILLIN V

Penicillin V (Pen-Vee-K, V-cillin-K) is the acid-stable oral form of penicillin G. It has replaced the need for oral penicillin G. It is indicated for the same infections as penicillin G and for prophylaxis during dental and upper respiratory procedures for patients who are immunocompromised or who are prone to bacterial endocarditis.

Contraindications, precautions, drug interactions, and adverse effects are the same as those associated with penicillin G.

Penicillin V should be given only on an empty stomach, 1 hour before or 2 to 3 hours after meals, with a full glass of water. Advise the patient to continue the drug for the full course of the drug therapy, usually 7 to 10 days. Advise the patient neither to save the drug for self-medication at a later date nor to share the drug with any other person.

PROCAINE PENICILLIN

Procaine penicillin is the procaine salt of penicillin G. Because it is given by IM injection only, its use has been limited by the advent of IV antibiotics and newer broad-spectrum IM antibiotics. This drug must be stored in the refrigerator. Because it is viscous, it must warm at room temperature for approximately 15 minutes before being injected. Patients may react to procaine with confusion or agitation. This response is sometimes mistaken for a penicillin allergy.

BENZATHINE PENICILLIN

Benzathine penicillin is the benzathine salt of penicillin G. It has low solubility and provides an IM reservoir for low levels of penicillin over a long time. It can be detected in serum for up to 12 weeks after injection. It is used primarily for treating syphilis and preventing rheumatic fever.

Broad-Spectrum Penicillins (Aminopenicillins)

Aminopenicillins include ampicillin, amoxicillin, and bacampicillin. The aminopenicillins have a slightly altered side chain that makes them effective against many gram-negative microorganisms, including *Haemophilus influenzae, Escherichia coli, Salmonella* and *Shigella* species, and indole-positive *Proteus mirabilis.* Aminopenicillins are ineffective against most infections caused by *Staphylococcus aureus* because they are easily inactivated by penicillinase produced by this species.

The benefits of these drugs include their higher oral absorption, higher serum levels, and longer half-lives (amoxicillin and bacampicillin). Within this group, ampicillin is the only drug that may be administered both orally and intravenously.

Because these drugs are available for oral use and are effective against some of the most serious pediatric infections, they are frequently used to treat otitis media, upper respiratory infections, tonsillitis, skin infections, and pneumonia in children. Aminopenicillins should be used only for infections that are not sensitive to penicillin G or penicillin V because they have a broader spectrum of activity and therefore pose a greater opportunity for resistant strains to develop and adverse effects to occur.

Teach parents or other caregivers to follow storage and administration instructions exactly, to discard leftover drug and not save it for later use, to report frequently occurring rash or diarrhea, and to watch for superinfections.

Extended-Spectrum Penicillins (Antipseudomonal Penicillins)

This group of penicillins, including carbenicillin indanyl, mezlocillin, piperacillin, and ticarcillin, have an even broader spectrum than the aminopenicillins. They are effective against all of the organisms susceptible to the aminopenicillins, plus *Pseudomonas aeruginosa, Enterobacter* species, *Bacteroides fragilis,* many *Klebsiella* species, *Proteus vulgaris, Proteus morganii,* and *Proteus rettgeri.* Like the aminopenicillins, extended-spectrum penicillins are easily inactivated by penicillinase produced by *S. aureus.* They are available for oral or parenteral administration.

When given to combat *Pseudomonas,* extended-spectrum penicillins are frequently given concurrently with aminoglycoside antibiotics. Although this combination is highly effective, remember to administer these two antibiotics at least 2 hours apart to avoid an antagonist drug–drug interaction.

The extended-spectrum penicillins should be reserved for use in serious infections by susceptible organisms. Again, caution patients to take oral preparations on an empty stomach, to complete the full course, and to monitor for side effects.

Penicillinase-Resistant Penicillins (Antistaphylococcal Penicillins)

With the use of penicillins over the years, increasing numbers of bacterial species are developing the enzyme penicillinase to counteract the effects of penicillin. The penicillinase-resistant drugs were developed to remain effective against bacteria that produce penicillinase and thus are resistant to penicillin. Although the penicillinase-resistant antibiotics are highly effective against strains of staphylococci, they are inactive against many other bacteria that secrete penicillinase, especially gram-negative bacteria. Culture and sensitivity tests are mandatory when using a penicillinase-resistant drug. The drugs in this group include cloxacillin and dicloxacillin, which are oral preparations, and nafcillin and oxacillin, which are IV preparations. Methicillin is no longer available in the United States.

Certain strains of staphylococci are resistant to the drugs in this class. A patient infected with these strains of staphylococci may have an infection known as methicillin-resistant *Staphylococcus aureus* (MRSA). Resistance to methicillin

---

CRITICAL THINKING SCENARIO

Implementing penicillin V therapy

You have a patient who has been taking penicillin V for 2 days to "cure" an infection. You find out that this antibiotic was left over from an upper respiratory infection for which it had been prescribed 2 years earlier. The patient states that he stopped the drug when he felt better and kept it around just in case he got sick again. Describe how you would explain the dangers of taking antibiotics in this manner in a way that will make sense to the patient and lead to his adherence to antibiotic therapy in the future.

implies resistance to any drug in this class. Methicillin is used infrequently because it can cause interstitial nephritis, whereas nafcillin and oxacillin are equally effective and do not have this adverse effect. The oral use of these drugs is now recommended for treating all gram-positive infections because staphylococci are almost entirely penicillin resistant. Again, urge the patient to complete the full course of drug therapy, to take oral drugs on an empty stomach, and not to self-medicate with this drug at another time.

Drugs Significantly Different From P Penicillin G

Beta-Lactamase Inhibitors

Resistance to beta-lactams may occur because of the bacteria's ability to produce beta-lactamase. Clavulanic acid, tazobactam, and sulbactam are combined with other beta-lactam antibiotics to act as competitive "suicide" inhibitors of bacterial beta-lactamases. They accomplish this feat by binding to the enzyme's active site, thus allowing the penicillin to reach its target site. Clavulanic acid, tazobactam, and sulbactam do not alter the actions of the beta-lactam antibiotics. They simply prevent penicillins from being destroyed. On their own, they exhibit only weak antibacterial effects.

Bacitracin

Bacitracin is an oral, parenteral, and topical polypeptide antibiotic. It acts principally against gram-positive bacteria. Thus, it is combined frequently with drugs such as neomycin and polymyxins, which are active against gram-negative bacteria. The most common use of bacitracin is as a topical agent to prevent superficial skin and eye infections following minor injuries. It is available as a cream or ointment as well as ophthalmic drops or ointment.

Oral bacitracin is designated as an orphan drug to treat pseudomembranous colitis caused by *Clostridium difficile.* IM bacitracin is used rarely because of the risk for serious nephrotoxicity. However, IM bacitracin may be used to treat infants with pneumonia or empyema. Oral or parenteral bacitracin is used only in clinical situations in which less toxic drugs have not been effective.

Bacitracin is bacteriostatic, but it may also be bacteriocidal. Whether it is bacteriostatic or bacteriocidal depends on the antibiotic concentration and the specific susceptibility of the organism. It inhibits bacterial cell wall synthesis by preventing transfer of mucopeptides into the growing cell wall.

To avoid systemic absorption of bacitracin, it should not be applied to serious burns, deep wounds, animal bites, over large areas of the body, or into a perforated tympanic membrane. Although topical bacitracin has few adverse effects, ophthalmic bacitracin may cause blurred vision that resolves spontaneously.

C MONOBACTAM ANTIBIOTICS

Aztreonam is a monobactam with a mechanism of activity similar to that of penicillin: it inhibits bacterial cell wall synthesis. It is used to manage infections caused by gram-negative aerobic bacteria. These organisms include *Klebsiella, Pseudomonas, Proteus, Serratia, Shigella, Salmonella,* and *Neisseria* species. It has no activity against gram-positive bacteria or anaerobes. The structure of aztreonam differs substantially from the structures of other beta-lactam antibiotics; this drug may be given safely to penicillin-allergic patients because there is little cross-sensitivity.

Aztreonam is administered IV or IM and is eliminated by renal tubular secretion. Half-life is prolonged in patients with renal failure. It is widely distributed throughout the body, including the central nervous system (CNS).

Hypersensitivity is the only contraindication to aztreonam therapy. Common adverse effects include vertigo and headache. Serious, but rare, adverse effects include GI distress with possible superinfection, hepatotoxicity, seizures, and blood dyscrasias, including neutropenia.

Important drug–drug interactions include synergistic effects when aztreonam is given with aminoglycosides and other beta-lactam antibiotics. Antagonistic effects may occur when it is given with cefoxitin or imipenem. Toxic aztreonam levels may occur when probenecid is given at the same time.

When aztreonam is given intravenously, check frequently for signs of thrombophlebitis at the IV insertion site. For long-term therapy, monitor laboratory studies, such as complete blood count (CBC), liver function test (LFT), prothrombin time (PT), partial thromboplastin time (PTT), and platelet count.

C CARBAPENEMS

Like monobactams, carbapenems are chemically different from penicillins but retain the beta-lactam ring structure. They are very broad-spectrum antibiotics with activity against gram-positive cocci, gram-negative cocci, and bacilli, and they are the most effective beta-lactam antibiotics for use against anaerobes. Imipenem (Primaxin), meropenem (Merrem), and ertapenem (Invanz) are the carbapenems approved for use in the United States.

Imipenem

Imipenem is rapidly inactivated by renal dehydropeptidase 1. Therefore, imipenem is always administered with cilastatin, a drug that inhibits this enzyme. Cilastatin-imipenem given IV or IM has a high affinity for bacterial PBPs and thus penetrates the cell wall efficiently. It also has a high resistance to bacterial enzymes, making it a very effective antibiotic. Imipenem is used to treat severe resistant infections, especially nosocomial infections.

Cilastatin-imipenem is structurally similar to penicillin and cephalosporins. For that reason, patients with a severe hypersensitivity to either of these agents should not be given cilastatin-imipenem. Cilastatin-imipenem is given cautiously to patients with head trauma, brain lesions, and pre-existing seizure disorders because these patients have a high risk for cilastatin-imipenem–induced seizures. Because cilastatin-imipenem is substantially excreted by the kidneys, patients with renal insufficiency, including the elderly, need a reduced dose. Cilastatin-imipenem is an FDA pregnancy category C drug; however, whether it is excreted in human milk is unknown.

Drug–drug interactions include cyclosporine, ganciclovir, or theophylline: the CNS effects of these drugs may be additive. Serious adverse effects include seizures, pseudomembranous colitis, and blood dyscrasias. More common adverse effects include GI distress, superinfections such as candidiasis, injection-site reactions, phlebitis, and elevations of LFT, BUN, and creatinine.

Meropenem

Meropenem is an IV antibiotic that is similar to cilastatin-imipenem. It is used to manage abdominal infections, such as appendicitis and peritonitis, and bacterial meningitis. It is also useful in managing nosocomial infections that are resistant to other antibiotics.

Meropenem is not degraded by renal dipeptidases and can therefore be given as a single agent. It is excreted substantially unchanged; thus, a reduced dose is necessary for patients with renal insufficiency. It belongs to FDA pregnancy category B; whether it is excreted into breast milk is unknown.

As with cilastatin-imipenem, hypersensitivity is the only contraindication. Precautions to meropenem use are the same as for cilastatin-imipenem.

Meropenem may interact with valproic acid; thus, patients receiving valproic acid should be monitored to ensure that their treatment is effective. Adverse effects are similar to those of cilastatin-imipenem; however, seizures are less likely to occur.

Ertapenem

Ertapenem is the newest carbapenem approved for use in the United States. It is administered either intramuscularly or intravenously. Its spectrum of activity is less than that of cilastatin-imipenem or meropenem. Most importantly, ertapenem has little or no activity against *P. aeruginosa* or *Acinetobacter* species. Ertapenem is indicated to manage moderate to severe complicated intra-abdominal infections, skin and skin structure infections, pyelonephritis, acute pelvic infections, and community-acquired pneumonia.

Like meropenem, ertapenem is administered as a single agent. It is also excreted primarily by the kidneys, and reduced doses are required for patients with renal compromise. It belongs to FDA pregnancy category B and is secreted in breast milk. Ertapenem is the only carbapenem not indicated for use in children.

Contraindications and precautions are similar to those for cilastatin-imipenem and meropenem. Probenecid decreases the renal clearance of ertapenem. Adverse effects are similar to those of other carbapenems, and although seizures may occur, they are less likely to occur with ertapenem.

C CEPHALOSPORINS

The cephalosporins were first introduced in the 1960s. They are similar to the penicillins in structure and in activity and are also considered beta-lactam antibiotics. Four generations of cephalosporins have been introduced, each group with its own spectrum of activity. Selecting an antibiotic from this class depends on the sensitivity of the involved organism, the preferred route of administration, and sometimes the cost of therapy. The major differences between the generations include their activity against gram-negative bacteria, their resistance to beta-lactamases, and their ability to distribute into cerebrospinal fluid. The first-generation cephalosporins have the least activity against gram-negative bacteria, and the fourth-generation cephalosporins have the most. The first-generation cephalosporins have little resistance to beta-lactamases; resistance increases in second and third generations, with the fourth generation having the most resistance. First- and second-generation cephalosporins have poor distribution into cerebrospinal fluid, and third- and fourth-generation cephalosporins have good distribution. Cefazolin (Ancef, Kefzol), a first-generation agent, is the prototypical cephalosporin. See Table 38.3 for a summary of selected cephalosporins.

NURSING MANAGEMENT OF THE PATIENT RECEIVING P CEFAZOLIN

Core Drug Knowledge

Pharmacotherapeutics

Cefazolin can be used to treat many kinds of infections: skin, bone, heart, blood, respiratory tract, GI tract, sinus, ear, and urinary tract. It is used to treat respiratory infections caused by *Streptococcus pneumoniae, S. aureus, Klebsiella* species, *H. influenzae,* and group A beta-hemolytic streptococci; skin infections caused by *S. aureus* and strains of streptococci; GI infections caused by *E. coli, P. mirabilis, Klebsiella* species, sensitive strains of *Enterobacter,* and *Enterococci;* biliary tract infections caused by *E. coli, P. mirabilis, S. aureus,* and streptococci; septicemia caused by *S. pneumoniae, S. aureus, E. coli, P. mirabilis,* and *Klebsiella* species; bone and joint infections caused by *S. aureus;* and endocarditis caused by *S. aureus* and beta-hemolytic streptococci. Cefazolin is also used for perioperative prophylaxis in surgeries involving the GI or genitourinary tracts, bone, and skin.

Pharmacokinetics

Cefazolin is rapidly absorbed after IM injection. Peak effect occurs within 1.5 to 2 hours. It is also administered IV, with immediate onset and peak effect in 5 minutes. Only two of the first-generation cephalosporins are available exclusively for oral use: cephalexin and cefadroxil.

Cefazolin is widely distributed to body fluids and tissues, including bone. It does not cross the blood–brain barrier, but it does cross the placenta and enters breast milk. It is excreted unchanged in the urine.

Pharmacodynamics

Cefazolin, like penicillin G, has no direct effect on the body. Cefazolin produces its bactericidal effects by binding with PBPs, which disrupts bacterial cell wall synthesis. Like penicillin, it also activates autolysins, which results in additional damage to the cell wall, allowing the cell to swell and then burst from the osmotic pressure within the cell. Like penicillins, it is most effective against cells undergoing active growth and division.

(*text continues on page 683*)

TABLE 38.3 Summary of Selected (C) Cephalosporins

Drug (Trade) Name	Selected Indications	Route and Dosage Range	Pharmacokinetics
First-Generation Cephalosporins			
(P) cefazolin (Kefzol, Ancef)	Respiratory tract infections Skin, joint, biliary, genital infections Endocarditis Surgical prophylaxis Septicemia	*Adult:* IM/IV Life-threatening infections 1–2 g every 6 h Moderate infections 250 mg–1 g every 8 h *Child:* IM/IV Life-threatening infections 100 mg/kg in 3–4 divided doses Moderate infections 25–50 mg/kg in 3–4 equal doses	*Onset:* IM, 30 min; IV, 10 min *Duration:* 6–12 h $t_{1/2}$: 90–120 min
cefadroxil (Duricef; *Canadian:* Apo-Cefadroxil, Novo-Cefadroxil)	Respiratory tract infections Skin infections Otitis media Tonsillitis/pharyngitis UTI Endocarditis prophylaxis	*Adult:* PO, 1–2 g qd or q12h in divided doses Loading dose of 1 g initially Endocarditis prophylaxis: *Adult:* 2 g 1 h before procedure *Child:* PO, 30 mg/d divided twice daily up to a maximum of 2 g/d Endocarditis prophylaxis: *Child:* 50 mg/kg 1 h before procedure	*Onset:* rapid *Duration:* 12–24 h $t_{1/2}$: 1½–2 h
cephalexin (Keflex, Biocef; *Canadian:* Apo-Cephalex, Keftab, Novo-Lexin, Nu-Cephalex)	Respiratory tract infections Skin, bone infections Otitis media UTI	*Adult:* PO Severe infections 500 mg–1 g every 6 h Moderate infections 250–500 mg every 6 h *Child:* PO Severe infections 50–100 mg/kg in 4 equal doses Moderate infections 25–50 mg/kg day in 4 equal doses	*Onset:* 15–30 min *Duration:* 6–12 h $t_{1/2}$: 50–80 min
cephalothin (Keflin)	Lower respiratory tract infections Skin and bone infections Septicemia Endocarditis Bacterial peritonitis	*Adult:* IM/IV Severe infections 1–2 g every 4 h Moderate infections 500–1 g every 4–6 h *Child:* Severe infections 80–160 mg/kg/d in divided doses every 4 h Moderate infections 14–27 mg/kg every 4 h	*Onset:* IM, rapid; IV, immediate *Duration:* unknown $t_{1/2}$: ½–1 h
cephradine (Velosef)	Serious respiratory tract infections UTI Skin infections Otitis media	*Adult:* PO, 250 mg–500 mg every 6–12 h *Child >1y:* PO, 25–50 mg/kg every 6 h	*Onset:* PO/IM, rapid; IV, immediate *Duration:* 6–12 h $t_{1/2}$: 1–2 h
cephapirin (Cefadyl)	Lower respiratory tract infections UTI Skin infections Septicemia Endocarditis Bacterial peritonitis	*Adult:* IM/IV, 500 mg–1 g every 4–6 h *Child:* IM/IV, 40–80 mg/kg/d in divided doses every 6 h	*Onset:* IM, rapid; IV, immediate *Duration:* 4–6 h $t_{1/2}$: ½–1 h

(continued)

TABLE 38.3 Summary of Selected Ⓒ Cephalosporins (continued)

Drug (Trade) Name	Selected Indications	Route and Dosage Range	Pharmacokinetics
Second-Generation Cephalosporins			
cefaclor (Ceclor; *Canadian:* Apo-Cefaclor, Novo-Cefaclor, Nu-Cefaclor, PMS-Cefaclor)	Respiratory tract infections UTI Skin, bone, joint infections Gynecologic infections Septicemia Otitis media	*Adult:* PO, 250–500 mg every 8 h *Child:* PO, 20–40 mg/kg/d in divided doses every 8 h	*Onset:* 15 min *Duration:* 6–12 h $t_{1/2}$: 30–60 min
cefprozil (Cefzil)	Respiratory tract infections UTI Skin infections Otitis media	*Adult:* PO, 250–500 mg 1–2 times per day *Child:* PO, 7.5–15 mg/kg every 12 h	*Onset:* Varies *Duration:* 12–24 h $t_{1/2}$: 1–1½ h
cefuroxime (Ceftin, Zinacef; *Canadian:* Apo-Cefuroxime, Kefurox)	Severe respiratory tract infections Skin infections Otitis media Surgical prophylaxis	*Adult:* PO, 250–500 mg PO every 12 h *Adult:* IM/IV, 750 mg IV or IM every 8 h *Child:* PO, 125 mg PO every 12 h *Child and infant ≥ 3 mo:* IM/IV, 50–100 mg/kg/d in equally divided doses every 6–8 h *Neonate:* IM/IV, 20–100 mg/kg/d in equally divided doses every 12 h	*Onset:* PO: varies; IM: 20 min; IV: rapid *Duration:* 18–24 h $t_{1/2}$: 1–2 h
cefoxitin (Mefoxin)	Lower respiratory tract infections Skin and bone infections Gynecologic infections Gonococcal infections Septicemia Peritonitis	*Adult:* IM/IV, 1–2 g every 6–8 h *Child >3 mo:* IM/IV, 80–160 mg/kg/d in divided doses every 4–6 h	*Onset:* IM: 5–10 min; IV: immediate *Duration:* 6–8 h $t_{1/2}$: 40–60 min
cefonicid (Monocid)	Lower respiratory tract infections UTI Septicemia Skin infections Surgical prophylaxis	*Adult:* IM/IV, 0.5–2 g/d Surgical prophylaxis: 1 g 1 h prior to procedure *Child:* safety not established	*Onset:* IM, 5–10 min; IV, immediate *Duration:* 6–8 h $t_{1/2}$: 4½ h
cefotetan (Cefotan)	Respiratory tract infections UTI Gynecologic infections Skin, bone, joint infections Gonococcal infections Intra-abdominal infections	*Adult:* IM/IV, 1–2 g every 4–6 h *Child >3 mo:* IM/IV, 20–40 mg/kg/d in divided doses every 4–6 h	*Onset:* IM: 30–60 min; IV: 15–20 min *Duration:* 18–24 h $t_{1/2}$: 3–4½ h
loracarbef (Lorabid)	Respiratory tract infections UTI Skin infections Otitis media Pharyngitis/tonsillitis	*Adult:* PO, 200–400 mg every 12 h *Child:* PO, 15–30 mg/kg/d in divided doses every 12 h	*Onset:* IV, rapid *Duration:* 6–12 h $t_{1/2}$: 1.2 h
Third-Generation Cephalosporins			
Cefdinir (Omnicef)	Pneumonia CAL exacerbations Otitis media Maxillary sinusitis Pharyngitis/tonsillitis Skin infections	*Adult:* PO, 600 mg/d *Child:* PO, 14 mg/kg/d *Infants ≥ 6 mo:* PO, 14 mg/kg/d Note: All may be divided into 2 doses given every 12 h	*Onset:* 2 h *Duration:* 8–10 h $t_{1/2}$: 1.7 h

(continued)

TABLE 38.3 Summary of Selected Ⓒ Cephalosporins (continued)

Drug (Trade) Name	Selected Indications	Route and Dosage Range	Pharmacokinetics
cefpodoxime (Vantin)	Respiratory tract infections UTI Skin infections Otitis media STDs	*Adult:* PO, 200–400 mg every 12 h *Child:* PO, 5 mg/kg every 12 h	*Onset:* Varies *Duration:* 12 h $t_{1/2}$: 2–3 h
ceftibuten (Cedax)	Respiratory tract infections Otitis media	*Adult:* PO, 400 mg every day *Child >6 mo:* 9 mg/kg to a max of 400 mg/d	*Onset:* Rapid *Duration:* 24 h $t_{1/2}$: 1–1½ h
cefoperazone (Cefobid)	Lower respiratory tract infections UTI Skin and bone infections Bacterial septicemia Peritonitis PID Endometritis	*Adult:* IM/IV, 1–2 g IV/IM every 12 h Maximum dose is 12 g/d *Child:* IM/IV, 100–150 mg/kg/d IV/IM, in divided doses every 8–12 h Maximum dose is 12 g/d *Neonate:* IM/IV, 50 mg/kg/dose IV given every 12 h	*Onset:* IM, 1 h; IV, 5–10 min *Duration:* 6–12 h $t_{1/2}$: 2 h
cefotaxime (Claforan)	Serious lower respiratory tract infections UTI Skin and bone infections Gonococcal infections Bacteremia Septicemia Meningitis	*Patient ≥50 kg:* IM/IV, 1 g IV or IM every 12 h Moderate to severe infections: 1–2 g every 8 h Severe infections: 2 g every 6–8 h Life-threatening infections: 2 g every 4 h Maximum dosage is 12 g/d *Child and infant 1 mo–12 y, <50 kg:* 75–100 mg/kg/d given in 3–4 divided doses Severe infections: 150–225 mg/kg/d given in 3–4 equally divided doses *Neonate 1–4 wk:* IM/IV, 50 mg/kg every 6 or 8 h *Neonate <7 d, ≤2 kg:* 50 mg/kg IV or IM every 8 or 12 h in neonates weighing >2 kg	*Onset:* IM, 30 min; IV, 5–10 min *Duration:* 4–12 h $t_{1/2}$: 1 h
ceftizoxime (Cefizox)	Serious lower respiratory tract infections UTI Skin, bone, joint infections Intra-abdominal infections Septicemia Meningitis PID caused by GC	*Adult:* IM, 1–2 g every 8–12 h *Adult:* IV, 500 mg every 12 h *Child >6 mo:* IM/IV, 50 mg/kg every 6–8 h	*Onset:* IM, 30 min; IV, immediate *Duration:* 6–12 h $t_{1/2}$: 1½–2 h
ceftriaxone (Rocephin)	Serious lower respiratory tract infections UTI Skin, bone, joint infections Gonococcal infections Intra-abdominal infections	*Adult:* IM/IV, 1–2 g IV or IM every 12–24 h Maximum dosage is 4 g/d *Child and infant ≥1 mo:* IM/IV, 50–75 mg/kg/d divided every 12—24 h Maximum dose is 2 g/d *Neonate >7 d, >2000 g:* IM/IV, 50–75 mg/kg/d every 24 h	*Onset:* IM, 30 min; IV, immediate *Duration:* 12–24 h $t_{1/2}$: 5–8 h

(continued)

TABLE 38.3 Summary of Selected Ⓒ Cephalosporins (continued)

Drug (Trade) Name	Selected Indications	Route and Dosage Range	Pharmacokinetics
		Neonate ≤7 d, <2000 g: IM/IV, 50 mg/kg/d every 24 h *Neonate ≤7 d:* IM/IV, 50 mg/kg/d given every 24 h	
ceftazidime (Fortaz, Ceptaz, Tazidime, Tazicef, Tazidime)	Serious respiratory tract infections UTI Skin, bone, joint infections Gynecologic infections Intra-abdominal infections Septicemia Meningitis	*Adult:* IM/IV, 1–2 g every 8 h Maximum 6 g/d *Child and infant ≥1 mo:* IV, 30–50 mg/kg every 8 h Maximum dose is 6 g/d *Neonate 0–4 wk:* IV, 30 mg/kg every 12 h	*Onset:* IM, 30 min; IV, immediate *Duration:* 6–12 h $t_{1/2}$: ½–1 h
Fourth-Generation Cephalosporins			
cefepime (Maxipime)	Lower respiratory tract infections UTI Skin and bone infections Gonococcal infections Septicemia Peritonitis	*Adult and adolescent >16 y:* IV, 2 g IV every 8 h *Infant and child ≤40 kg:* IV, 50 mg/kg/dose every 8 h	*Onset:* IM, 30 min; IV, immediate *Duration:* 10–12 h $t_{1/2}$: 2–2.3 h

Contraindications and Precautions

Cefazolin is contraindicated in anyone with a known allergy to cephalosporins. Caution must be used in patients with renal failure and in pregnant or lactating patients. Because of the structural similarities between cephalosporins and penicillins, patients who are allergic to one type of drug may experience cross-sensitivity to the other. Cephalosporin hypersensitivity occurs in 5% to 10% of patients with penicillin allergy. Patients with a history of severe allergic reactions to penicillins should not receive cephalosporins because of the increased risk for cross-sensitivity reactions in these patients.

Adverse Effects

Hypersensitivity reactions occur frequently with cephalosporin drugs. Severe immediate reactions are rare. Hypersensitivity presents most frequently as a maculopapular rash that develops several days after the onset of therapy.

Other common adverse effects of cefazolin involve the GI tract. Nausea, vomiting, diarrhea, anorexia, abdominal pain, and flatulence are common side effects. Pseudomembranous colitis, a potentially dangerous disorder, has also been reported with cefazolin. The drug should be discontinued immediately at any sign of violent, bloody diarrhea and abdominal pain.

CNS symptoms include headache, dizziness, lethargy, and paresthesias. Nephrotoxicity is also associated with the use of cefazolin, most particularly with patients who have predisposing renal insufficiency. Superinfections are also common with cephalosporin use. As with the penicillins, this adverse effect is related to the normal flora having been destroyed. Thrombophlebitis and an abscess at the injection site are potential adverse effects of administering cephalosporins intravenously.

Serum sickness–like reactions, such as erythema multiforme or skin rashes accompanied by polyarthritis, arthralgia, and fever, may occur following a second course of therapy. Symptoms resolve after the patient stops taking the drug.

Drug Interactions

Risk for nephrotoxicity is greater when cefazolin is given concurrently with aminoglycoside antibiotics. Patients receiving oral anticoagulants may experience increased bleeding when also given cefazolin. Like penicillin, cefazolin may have prolonged effects when given concurrently with probenecid. Table 38.4 presents agents that interact with cefazolin. A disulfiram-like reaction may occur in patients taking cephalosporins with a chemical structure similar to that of disulfiram (see Chapter 9). These drugs include cefamandole (Mandol), cefonicid (Monocid), cefoperazone (Cefobid), and cefotetan (Cefotan). Symptoms of a disulfiram-like reaction include flushing, shortness of breath, nausea and vomiting, chest pains, palpitations, dizziness and faintness, confusion, sweating, blurred vision, and possibly respiratory depression, seizures, and unconsciousness.

Effects on Test Results

False-positive results may occur in tests of urine glucose using Benedict solution, Fehling solution, and Clinitest tablets. Blood glucose monitoring is therefore recommended in patients with diabetes who are receiving cefazolin. False-positive results have also been noted in direct Coombs tests and measurements of urinary 17-ketosteroids. These tests should be avoided in patients receiving any cephalosporins.

TABLE 38.4 Agents That Interact With P Cefazolin

Interactants	Effect and Significance	Nursing Management
aminoglycosides	Increased risk of nephrotoxicity, although the mechanism of action is unknown.	Monitor aminoglycoside levels frequently. Monitor kidney function closely. Reduce dosage or discontinue one or both drugs if signs of kidney dysfunction occur.
oral anticoagulants	Some cephalosporins may have a warfarin-like activity and antiplatelet effects. This results in an augmentation of the action of oral anti-coagulants and an increased risk of bleeding.	Advise patients of the signs and symptoms of overanticoagulation. Monitor oral anticoagulant levels. Reduce oral anticoagulant dosage accordingly.

Assessment of Relevant Core Patient Variables

Health Status

Follow the same guidelines used for evaluating the health status of a patient receiving penicillin.

Life Span and Gender

Document the age of the patient and, if appropriate, assess for pregnancy and lactation. In elderly patients who have any degree of renal insufficiency, cefazolin should be used cautiously, and the dosage should be adjusted. Adjusted dosage recommendations are based on creatinine clearance levels. Cefazolin is not recommended for infants younger than 1 month because of their immature renal and hepatic functioning.

Lifestyle, Diet, and Habits

Assess the patient's lifestyle and dietary practices to ensure that the drug can be taken consistently, completely, and on an empty stomach, if possible. Assess for the patient's use of alcoholic beverages. Although all cephalosporins do not cause a disulfiram-like reaction, it is preferable to refrain from drinking alcohol while on cephalosporin therapy.

Environment

Be aware of the environment in which the drug will be administered. After dilution, cefazolin can be kept at room temperature for 24 hours or in a refrigerator between 2° and 8°C (36° and 46°F) for 96 hours (4 days). In acute care settings, retrieve the antibiotic from the refrigerator and let it warm at room temperature for about 15 minutes before administering it. The IV site should be evaluated for signs of phlebitis before and after drug administration. Premixed solutions should be kept in the refrigerator and retrieved approximately 15 minutes before administration as well.

Nursing Diagnoses and Outcomes

- Diarrhea related to drug effects
  Desired outcome: *The patient will avoid dehydration, maintain fluid intake, and contact the prescriber if diarrhea persists.*
- Imbalanced Nutrition: More or Less than Body Requirements related to GI effects, alteration in taste, superinfections
  Desired outcome: *The patient will maintain body weight and contact the prescriber if persistent adverse effects alter nutritional status.*
- Risk for Infection related to overgrowth of nonsusceptible organisms
  Desired outcome: *The patient will report signs of superinfection to the prescriber.*

Planning and Intervention

Maximizing Therapeutic Effects

Review culture and sensitivity tests to evaluate the efficacy of treatment. Oral suspensions of cephalosporins should be kept in the refrigerator. Be sure that the patient receives injections of cefazolin as prescribed around the clock for increased effectiveness. Monitor the site of infection and presenting signs and symptoms throughout the course of drug therapy. Failure of the signs and symptoms of infection to resolve may indicate the need to repeat culture and sensitivity testing. For optimal effect, drug therapy should continue for at least 2 days after all signs and symptoms resolve.

Minimizing Adverse Effects

Cefazolin may be taken with food or fluids to decrease GI distress. Provide small, frequent meals; mouth care; and ice chips to suck on if stomatitis and sore mouth are problems. Monitor the patient's hydration status and ensure that adequate fluids are given to replace fluid lost with diarrhea. Evaluate the patient for CNS effects and use safety precautions, such as elevating side rails.

Administer IM cefazolin deep into a large muscle. Forewarn the patient that the injection may be uncomfortable. The patient receiving IM cefazolin should be monitored for an abscess at the injection site. IV administration may be as an IV push or IV piggyback. Administer IV cefazolin exactly as prescribed by the prescriber. The patient receiving IV cefazolin should also be monitored for the possibility of thrombophlebitis.

The patient receiving combination therapy with aminoglycoside antibiotics should be monitored (serum blood urea nitrogen and creatinine levels) frequently for nephrotoxicity. The patient receiving oral anticoagulants in addition to cefazolin should receive instructions to monitor for signs of blood loss, for example, bleeding gums and easily bruised skin. Dosage of the oral anticoagulant may have to be reduced.

Providing Patient and Family Education

- Because cefazolin and the other cephalosporins are similar to penicillins, follow the same guidelines for providing patient and family education to a patient receiving penicillin.
- In addition, inform patients about possible interactions between cephalosporins and alcohol, urging the patient to refrain from drinking alcohol for 72 hours after drug therapy stops.
- Educate patients on hidden sources of alcohol, such as over-the-counter cough and cold preparations.

Ongoing Assessment and Evaluation

Monitor the patient for any signs of superinfection and notify the prescriber immediately to arrange for treatment if superinfection does occur. Monitor also for signs of allergic or serum sickness-like reactions (fever, hives, swollen glands, neutropenia, arthralgia, and edema). Implement comfort measures as needed and monitor for signs of phlebitis, abscess formation, and other complications. When treatment ends, the initial infection should be resolved. The patient should be adequately nourished and hydrated, and any adverse drug effects should be resolved.

Drugs Closely Related to P Cefazolin

First-Generation Cephalosporins

Similar to cefazolin are these other first-generation cephalosporins: oral cefadroxil and cephalexin; cephradine, which is available in oral, IV, and IM preparations; and cephalothin and cephapirin, which are available for IM and IV administration only. All of these drugs cover basically the same spectrum of pathogens. They are most active against gram-positive bacteria, especially staphylococci and nonenterococcal streptococci. They have minor activity against gram-negative bacteria. Most first-generation cephalosporins are destroyed by beta-lactamases and have minimal ability to concentrate in the cerebrospinal fluid (CSF). Oral forms are not affected by food and are best taken with food to decrease the GI upset that accompanies their use.

MEMORY CHIP

P Cefazolin

- Used for infections caused by gram-positive bacteria, anaerobes, and spirochetes. Also used as prophylaxis in patients having GI or GU surgery.
- Major contraindication: hypersensitivity to cephalosporins or penicillin
- Most common adverse effects: nausea, vomiting, diarrhea
- Most serious adverse effect: hypersensitivity
- **Life span alert: Cefazolin should be used cautiously and the dosage adjusted in elderly patients who have any degree of renal insufficiency.**
- Maximizing therapeutic effects: When using for gram-negative infections, be sure culture and sensitivity tests are done before administration.
- Minimizing adverse effects: Inject IM preparations into a large muscle mass. Be sure IV preparations are administered according to the health-care prescriber's orders, either IV push or IV piggyback.
- Most important patient education: Take the medication exactly as prescribed until the entire prescription is completed, despite the absence of symptoms. Monitor for signs and symptoms of allergic response and stop the medication if any occur.

Second-Generation Cephalosporins

Second-generation cephalosporins include cefaclor, cefprozil, and loracarbef, which are available for oral administration; cefuroxime, which is available in oral, IM, or IV preparations; and cefoxitin, cefonicid, and cefotetan, which are available for IM or IV administration. These drugs are less sensitive to destruction by beta-lactamases than first-generation drugs but still cannot achieve effective concentrations in the CSF.

The second-generation cephalosporins have broader coverage against gram-negative bacteria than first-generation cephalosporins because they are better able to penetrate the gram-negative cell envelope and have an increased affinity for the PBPs of gram-negative bacteria.

In addition to the same uses as first-generation cephalosporins, second-generation cephalosporins are used to treat lower respiratory tract infections caused by *Bacteroides* species; dermatologic infections caused by *Staphylococcus epidermidis* and *Bacteroides, Clostridium, Peptococcus,* and *Peptostreptococcus* species; urinary tract infections (UTIs) caused by *Morganella morganii, Proteus vulgaris;* uncomplicated gonorrhea caused by *N. gonorrhoeae;* intra-abdominal infections caused by *E. coli* and *Klebsiella, Bacteroides,* and *Clostridium* species; gynecologic infections caused by *E. coli, N. gonorrhoeae,* and *Bacteroides, Clostridium, Peptococcus,* and *Peptostreptococcus* species; and septicemia caused by *Bacteroides* species.

Cefotetan may induce two additional adverse effects: bleeding or disulfiram-like reactions. Cefotetan has been associated with reduced prothrombin levels because it interferes with vitamin K metabolism, an effect that may induce bleeding. Patients receiving cefotetan should be monitored for signs and symptoms of bleeding. Advise the patient to stop the drug immediately if any signs of bleeding occur and notify the prescriber. Advise the patient to avoid aspirin, other nonsteroidal anti-inflammatory drugs, or other anticoagulants throughout therapy.

Patients who consume alcohol during therapy with cefotetan may experience a disulfiram-like reaction (see Chapter 9). Symptoms include flushing, shortness of breath, nausea and vomiting, chest pains, palpitations, dizziness and faintness, confusion, sweating, blurred vision, and possibly respiratory depression, seizures, and unconsciousness. Advise patients who take cefotetan to avoid alcohol for 72 hours after completing therapy.

Third-Generation Cephalosporins

Third-generation cephalosporins include the oral drugs cefdinir, cefixime, cefpodoxime, and ceftibuten and the IM and IV drugs cefoperazone, cefotaxime, ceftizoxime, ceftriaxone, and ceftazidime. These drugs are highly resistant to destruction by beta-lactamases and are highly effective against gram-negative aerobes. Ceftazidime is especially effective for bacterial strains resistant to aminoglycosides and is also

effective against *P. aeruginosa.* This generation of cephalosporins is used for severe infections or in immunocompromised patients. The exception is ceftriaxone, which is the drug of choice for gonorrhea. With the exception of cefoperazone and cefixime, third-generation cephalosporins can penetrate the blood–brain barrier to treat CNS infections caused by *E. coli, H. influenzae, N. meningitidis, S. pneumoniae,* and *Klebsiella pneumoniae.* They are also effective against *Serratia marcescens* and *Citrobacter* species.

Cefoperazone, a third-generation cephalosporin, is similar to the second-generation cephalosporins cefotetan and cefmetazole. Like them, it may induce bleeding tendencies. Educate the patient as described in the section on second-generation cephalosporins.

Fourth-Generation Cephalosporins

Cefepime is the first fourth-generation cephalosporin. It is active against both gram-positive and gram-negative organisms. It has a greater spectrum than third-generation drugs, is more active against organisms such as *P. aeruginosa* or Enterobacteriaceae that have developed resistance to third-generation drugs, and has good penetration into the CSF. Like third-generation cephalosporins, cefepime is highly resistant to destruction by beta-lactamases.

C VANCOMYCIN

Vancomycin (Vancocin) is a complex and unusual tricyclic glycopeptide antibiotic. It is the only drug in its class. The use of vancomycin is limited by its ability to produce toxic effects. Because of its toxicity, vancomycin is used only when other antibiotics fail to resolve an infection. It has been touted as able to eradicate most gram-positive pathogens; however, the emergence of vancomycin-resistant enterococci (VRE) has become problematic.

NURSING MANAGEMENT OF THE PATIENT RECEIVING P VANCOMYCIN

Core Drug Knowledge

Pharmacotherapeutics

Vancomycin is used in treating bacterial septicemia, endocarditis, bone and joint infections, and pseudomembranous colitis caused by *C. difficile.* It is effective for most strains of *S. aureus* and *S. epidermidis;* streptococci, including enterococci, *Corynebacterium* species, and *Clostridium* species. Vancomycin is exceptionally effective for treating gram-positive infections in penicillin-allergic patients. It is also used for penicillin- and methicillin-resistant staphylococcal infections.

Vancomycin is used with aminoglycosides to combat *Streptococcus faecalis* and methicillin-resistant organisms. However, this synergism also increases possible toxicity.

Gram-negative bacteria and mycobacteria are resistant to vancomycin. Vancomycin is not used in treating meningitis because of poor penetration into CSF.

Pharmacokinetics

Oral bioavailability of vancomycin is extremely low; therefore, it is generally administered intravenously. Oral administration is used in treating some GI infections, such as pseudomembranous colitis. Some patients, especially those with renal impairment, have developed detectable vancomycin serum levels following oral administration.

After intravenous administration, plasma concentrations reach a peak approximately 1 hour after infusion. In patients with normal renal function, vancomycin has a serum half-life of 4 to 6 hours, but in elderly patients or those with renal impairment, half-life can be as long as 146 hours.

Vancomycin is distributed widely into most body tissues and fluids, including pericardial, pleural, ascitic, and synovial fluids, and the meninges if they are inflamed. It is not known whether any metabolism takes place. Excretion is mainly by glomerular filtration; only small amounts are excreted in the feces. With oral administration, excretion is mainly fecal.

Pharmacodynamics

Vancomycin is bactericidal because it inhibits cell wall synthesis by altering the cell's permeability. Vancomycin also inhibits the synthesis of ribonucleic acid (RNA). Because of this dual mechanism of action, resistance to vancomycin has been limited to strains of group D streptococci. The body is not directly affected.

Contraindications and Precautions

Vancomycin is contraindicated for patients with hypersensitivity to it and for pregnant patients. Although it is excreted into breast milk, vancomycin is not contraindicated for breast-feeding women. Breast-feeding neonates and infants, however, should be monitored for vancomycin serum concentration to avoid potential toxicities. Use it with caution in patients with renal disease, such as renal failure or renal impairment, and in patients receiving other drugs with the potential for nephrotoxicity, such as aminoglycosides.

Oral vancomycin should be used with caution in patients with inflammatory bowel disease because this disorder increases absorption of oral vancomycin, thereby increasing the risk for toxicity.

Adverse Effects

The most serious toxicities caused by vancomycin are ototoxicity and nephrotoxicity. Ototoxicity can take the form of cochlear toxicity (tinnitus, hearing loss) or vestibular toxicity (ataxia, vertigo, nausea and vomiting, nystagmus).

Nephrotoxicity can also occur with vancomycin, although its incidence has decreased. Nephrotoxicity and elevated serum concentrations are more likely to occur in patients receiving other nephrotoxic drugs, such as aminoglycosides. Cases of interstitial nephritis, a hypersensitivity reaction, have been reported.

Vancomycin can cause histamine release, resulting in anaphylactoid reactions. Symptoms include fever, chills, sinus tachycardia, and pruritus. Paresthesias, flushing, rash, or redness in the face, neck, upper body, arms, or back are also symptoms of histamine release. In some cases, hypotension occurs. Because of the presenting symptoms, this

histamine-release reaction is often called the "red man" or "red neck" syndrome. Other adverse reactions include phlebitis or other injection-site reactions, leukopenia, and thrombocytopenia.

Drug Interactions

Orally administered vancomycin should be avoided in patients receiving antihyperlipidemic drugs (HMG-CoA reductase inhibitors, statins). Vancomycin should be used with caution in combination with other drugs that have potential nephrotoxic or ototoxic effects and in patients receiving nondepolarizing muscle relaxants. Table 38.5 presents drugs that interact with vancomycin.

Assessment of Relevant Core Patient Variables

Health Status

Assess the patient for contraindications or precautions to the use of vancomycin, including other drugs with potential nephrotoxicity and ototoxicity. Lower doses of vancomycin are recommended for patients with renal dysfunction or for patients receiving other ototoxic or nephrotoxic drugs. Assess gross hearing in patients with preexisting hearing impairment. Periodic audiograms may be necessary during therapy. For patients with expected long-term therapy, a baseline CBC and hepatic and renal function tests should be performed. Consult with the prescriber about any laboratory abnormalities before vancomycin therapy begins.

Life Span and Gender

Ask women of childbearing age about their contraceptive methods and assess for pregnancy and lactation. Vancomycin should not be given to pregnant women and should be given cautiously to breast-feeding women. Note whether patient is elderly because such patients are at higher risk for toxicity and drug accumulation because of their age-related decreases in renal function.

Environment

Be aware of the environment in which the drug will be administered. Vancomycin is generally administered in an inpatient setting because of its potentially serious toxicities and the need to closely monitor vancomycin serum concentrations.

Nursing Diagnoses and Outcomes

- Risk for Injury related to drug-induced histamine-release reactions
  Desired outcome: *The patient will experience no preventable reaction related to vancomycin.*
- Disturbed Sensory Perception (auditory) related to drug-induced ototoxicity
  Desired outcome: *The patient will report any unusual auditory sensations and have periodic audiograms to detect early ototoxicity.*
- Excess Fluid Volume related to nephrotoxicity from drug therapy
  Desired outcome: *The patient will remain normovolemic throughout therapy.*

TABLE 38.5 Agents That Interact With P Vancomycin

Interactants	Effect and Significance	Nursing Management
antihyperlipidemic drugs cholestyramine colestipol	These antihyperlipidemic agents are anion-exchange resins and can bind with vancomycin, resulting in a decreased effectiveness.	Separate administration of these drugs by 3–4 h. Monitor efficacy of vancomycin therapy.
nephrotoxic drugs aminoglycosides amphotericin B bacitracin cisplatin cyclosporine polymyxin B	Parenteral vancomycin with other nephrotoxic drugs can lead to additive risks for nephrotoxicity.	Monitor renal function closely. Consider lower doses of vancomycin.
nondepolarizing muscle relaxants atracurium gallamine metocurine pancuronium pipecuronium tubocurarine vecuronium	Vancomycin may affect presynaptic and postsynaptic myoneural function and act synergistically with nondepolarizing muscle relaxants. This may result in additive neuromuscular blockade.	Avoid this combination when possible. When given, monitor neuromuscular function closely, and be prepared to initiate mechanical ventilation.
ototoxic drugs aminoglycosides salicylates ethacrynic acid furosemide paromomycin	Parenteral vancomycin with other ototoxic drugs can lead to additive risks for ototoxicity.	Monitor sensory/hearing functions closely. Consider lower doses of vancomycin.

- Risk for Infection related to overgrowth of nonsusceptible organisms.
  Desired outcome: The patient will report signs of superinfection to the prescriber.

Planning and Intervention

Maximizing Therapeutic Effects

Ensure that the patient receives the full course of vancomycin as prescribed, divided around the clock to increase effectiveness. Coordinate administering drugs to decrease potential drug–drug interactions. In addition, culture and sensitivity results should be monitored to be sure that vancomycin is the drug of choice for this patient.

Minimizing Adverse Effects

Administer vancomycin over at least 60 minutes. This rate will diminish effects such as flushing, tachycardia, hypotension, or rashes that occur when administration is too fast.

Ototoxicity after IV administration is believed to be associated with serum concentration ranges above 60 to 80 μg/mL, which may occur when doses are too large or infused too rapidly. Administering IV vancomycin too rapidly may also lead to red man syndrome. In addition, take care to avoid extravasation because vancomycin is extremely irritating to tissues.

Peak and trough levels are terms associated with serum concentration measurements. Obtain the peak serum level 1 hour after initiating the infusion and the trough serum level 30 minutes before beginning the next infusion. The risk for nephrotoxicity is minimized if trough serum concentrations are kept below 10 μg/mL, although nephrotoxicity can still occur in patients with therapeutic concentrations.

Providing Patient and Family Education

- Advise the patient of the importance of completing therapy.
- Explain the potential adverse effects and need for periodic blood monitoring.
- Advise the patient to report symptoms such as tinnitus, hearing loss, vertigo, or nausea and vomiting.
- Teach the patient the importance of accurate fluid intake and output measurements.

Ongoing Assessment and Evaluation

Elderly patients may need vancomycin concentration monitoring because age-related decreases in renal function put them at risk for toxicity and drug accumulation.

Monitor for signs of ototoxicity. Factors that may increase the risk for developing ototoxicity include excessive dose, serum concentrations above 60 μg/mL, prolonged exposure to the drug, multiple ototoxic drugs, dehydration, excessive noise, and bacteremia. Assess for symptoms, such as ataxia and nystagmus, that may indicate ototoxicity. Monitor fluid intake and output to assess for potential nephrotoxicity.

For patients receiving long-term or high-dose therapy, coordinate periodic audiometric testing and serial CBCs, LFTs, and kidney function tests. As with other potent antibiotics, monitor for signs of superinfection. When treatment ends, the initial infection should be resolved. The patient should be adequately nourished and hydrated, and any adverse drug effects should be resolved.

MEMORY CHIP

P Vancomycin

- Used for serious gram-positive infections, especially *Clostridium difficile* and methicillin-resistant *Staphylococcus aureus.*
- Major contraindications: hypersensitivity and pregnancy
- Most common adverse effects: histamine release resulting in "red-man" syndrome
- Most serious adverse effects: ototoxicity and nephrotoxicity
- **Life span alert: Elderly patients may need vancomycin concentration monitoring because of a higher risk of toxicity and drug accumulation secondary to age-related decreases in renal function.**
- Maximizing therapeutic effects: Obtain culture and sensitivity report before administration.
- Minimizing adverse effects: Administer over 60 minutes.
- Most important patient education: Need for periodic CBC when taking for prolonged period or high doses. Need to advise the health care team for changes in hearing.

C CYCLIC LIPOPEPTIDES

Daptomycin (Cubicin) is the only drug in a new class of antibiotics called **cyclic lipopeptides.** This class of antibiotics has a substantially different mechanism of action than other antibiotic drugs. Another benefit of daptomycin is its ability to retain potency against antibiotic-resistant gram-positive bacteria.

NURSING MANAGEMENT OF THE PATIENT RECEIVING P DAPTOMYCIN

Core Drug Knowledge

Pharmacotherapeutics

Daptomycin is used to manage complicated skin and skin structure infections caused by aerobic gram-positive *Enterococcus faecalis, S. aureus* (including MRSA), *Streptococcus agalactiae, Streptococcus dysgalactiae,* and *Streptococcus pyogenes.* Daptomycin is also effective against gram-positive bacteria that are resistant to vancomycin and linezolid (see Chapter 39). Additionally, studies have shown that daptomycin is effective against bacterial endocarditis.

Pharmacokinetics

Daptomycin is a once-daily IV medication. It reaches maximum serum concentration within 1 hour and has a half-life of 9.4 hours. The usual dosing range is 4 to 8 mg/kg per day. Although the exact method of metabolism is unclear, 78% of daptomycin is excreted as unchanged drug by the kidneys. For that reason, a patient with severe renal impairment should receive a lower dose of medication.

Pharmacodynamics

Daptomycin is a bacteriocidal antibiotic that has a unique mechanism of action. It works by binding to the bacterial

membrane and interfering with the integrity of the cell wall. This disruption causes a rapid depolarization of the membrane potential that leads to inhibition of protein, DNA, and RNA synthesis and, eventually, bacterial cell death. Daptomycin also has a postantibiotic effect that lasts approximately 6 hours.

At this time, no mechanism of resistance to daptomycin has been identified, there are no known transferable elements (plasmids) that confer resistance, and cross-resistance has not been reported.

Contraindications and Precautions

The only contraindication to the use of daptomycin is hypersensitivity. Precautions to its use include pre-existing GI disorders, myopathy, and peripheral neuropathy. It should be used cautiously in elderly people, in women who are breast-feeding and in patients with pre-existing renal dysfunction.

Like other antibiotics, daptomycin may alter the normal flora of the GI tract. Patients with pre-existing GI disorders have a higher risk for developing pseudomembranous colitis. Daptomycin has been associated with inducing muscle weakness and pain. For that reason, patients with pre-existing myopathy and peripheral neuropathy should be monitored closely during daptomycin therapy. Whether daptomycin enters breast milk is unclear; therefore, it should be given cautiously to women who breast-feed.

Adverse Effects

Daptomycin is generally well tolerated. The most common adverse effects are constipation, diarrhea, nausea and vomiting, and dyspepsia. In the CNS, daptomycin may induce headache, insomnia, or dizziness. Cardiovascular adverse effects include hypotension or hypertension and unspecified chest pain. Metabolic and nutritional adverse reactions such as electrolyte disturbance, hyperglycemia, hypoglycemia, hypokalemia, hypomagnesemia, and increased serum bicarbonate have been reported. Additionally, hematopoietic effects such as anemia, eosinophilia, leukocytosis, and thrombocytopenia may occur.

Daptomycin may induce problems with the musculoskeletal system, including arthralgia, back pain, limb pain, muscle cramps, muscle weakness, myalgia, and osteomyelitis.

Elevations of creatine kinase (CK), hepatic enzymes, alkaline phosphatase, and international normalized ratio (INR) may also occur.

Drug Interactions

No clinically important drug–drug interactions have been identified. Theoretically, daptomycin may interact with other drugs that have the ability to cause myopathy, such as HMG-CoA reductase inhibitors. Another theoretical drug–drug interaction is warfarin because daptomycin may elevate INR.

Assessment of Relevant Core Patient Variables

Health Status

Assess the patient for contraindications or precautions to the use of daptomycin. Be especially vigilant for a history of renal insufficiency or current medications that may induce myopathy, such as HMG-CoA reductase inhibitors. Review the culture and sensitivity report to ensure that daptomycin is recommended for the invading organism. Review the CBC, renal function tests, liver function tests, comprehensive metabolic panel, and a baseline CK. Alterations in these laboratory values should be discussed with the prescriber before starting therapy.

Life Span and Gender

Daptomycin is in FDA pregnancy category B. The patient should be cautioned to avoid breast-feeding while taking daptomycin as it is unclear if it enters breast milk. Dosing for the elderly should be adjusted if the patient has renal insufficiency. Daptomycin is not approved for use in children.

Environment

Daptomycin is used for serious infections that have not responded to other types of medications; thus, the patient will most likely be admitted to an acute care hospital. In rare circumstances, daptomycin may be administered in the home environment by a home health nurse.

Nursing Diagnoses and Outcomes

- Acute Pain related to myopathy
  Desired outcome: *The patient will contact the health care provider should pain or tingling in the extremities occur.*
- Imbalanced Nutrition: Less than Body Requirements related to drug-induced GI effects, such as nausea, vomiting, diarrhea, or dyspepsia
  Desired outcome: *The patient will maintain consistent body weight and consult prescriber about persistent adverse effects that affect nutritional status.*
- Diarrhea related to drug therapy
  Desired outcome: *The patient will avoid dehydration, maintain fluid intake, and contact prescriber about persistent diarrhea.*
- Risk for Infection related to overgrowth of nonsusceptible organisms
  Desired outcome: *The patient will report signs of superinfection to the prescriber.*
- Fatigue related to metabolic and hematopoietic alterations
  Desired outcome: *The patient will immediately report signs of fatigue to the health care provider.*

Planning and Intervention

Maximizing Therapeutic Effects

Review the culture and sensitivity report to ensure that daptomycin is an appropriate drug. Before administration, visually inspect daptomycin for particulate matter and discoloration. Administer daptomycin with 0.9% sodium chloride injection or lactated Ringer's solution because daptomycin is not compatible with dextrose-containing solutions. It should be administered over 30 minutes without any other intravenous substances, additives, or other medications. The primary line should be flushed with a compatible solution before and after daptomycin infusion.

Minimizing Adverse Effects

Evaluate the IV site before administering daptomycin. Teach the patient the importance of reporting diarrhea, muscle pain or tingling, and fatigue immediately because these signs and symptoms signal potentially severe adverse effects.

Providing Patient and Family Education

- Advise the patient of the importance of completing therapy.
- Explain the potential adverse effects and need for periodic blood monitoring.
- Teach the patient the importance of reporting diarrhea, muscle pain or tingling, and fatigue to the prescriber immediately.
- Advise the patient to stop taking HMG-CoA reductase inhibitors until advised to resume the medication by the prescriber.

Ongoing Assessment and Evaluation

Evaluate for resolution of the presenting infection. Question the patient frequently concerning the onset of musculoskeletal pain or tingling. Arrange for a weekly CK to be drawn. Should the patient have symptoms of myopathy, the drug should be discontinued if the CK is 5 times the upper limit of normal. The drug should be discontinued, even if the patient is asymptomatic, if the CK elevates to 10 times the normal limit.

By the end of daptomycin therapy, the initial infection should be resolved. Any adverse effects should be resolved or at least should be addressed. The patient should have normal laboratory values or be receiving appropriate electrolyte or hematopoietic replacement.

MEMORY CHIP

P Daptomycin

- Used for serious aerobic gram-positive complicated skin and skin structure infections caused by *enterococcus faecalis, Staphylococcus aureus*, methicillin-resistant *S. aureus, Streptococcus agalactiae, Streptococcus dysgalactiae,* and *Streptococcus pyogenes.*
- Major contraindications: hypersensitivity
- Most common adverse effects: nausea, vomiting, diarrhea, dyspepsia
- Most serious adverse effects: myopathy
- **Life span alert: Elderly patients may need a reduced dose of daptomycin because of renal insufficiency.**
- Maximizing therapeutic effects: Obtain culture and sensitivity report before administration
- Minimizing adverse effects: Administer over 30 minutes. Monitor weekly CK.
- Most important patient education: Notify prescriber if diarrhea, muscle pain, or tingling occurs.

CHAPTER SUMMARY

- Penicillins are classified as narrow-spectrum, penicillinase-resistant, aminopenicillins (broad-spectrum) and extended-spectrum (antipseudomonal) penicillins. They are also known as beta-lactam antibiotics.
- Penicillins may be inactivated by beta-lactamase, an enzyme produced by the bacteria. Penicillinase-resistant penicillins or penicillin–beta-lactamase combination drugs decrease the effects of penicillinase.
- Penicillins are most effective against gram-positive bacteria because they have difficulty penetrating the gram-negative cell envelope.
- Penicillins are the safest antibiotics available, except in patients with a hypersensitivity to penicillin.
- Penicillins can be administered orally, intramuscularly, or intravenously.
- Patients with a possible history of penicillin allergy should receive skin testing before administration.
- Patients with hypersensitivity to any penicillin should be considered allergic to all penicillins.
- Monobactam and carbapenem antibiotics are also beta-lactam antibiotics. Imipenem has the broadest spectrum of activity of all antibiotics.
- Cephalosporins are the antibiotics most widely used today.
- Cephalosporin antibiotics are structurally similar to penicillins. Between 5% and 10% of patients with hypersensitivity to penicillin will also react to cephalosporins.
- Cephalosporin antibiotics are grouped according to "generations."
- As cephalosporin generations progress, the drugs have increased activity against gram-negative bacteria and anaerobes, increased resistance to destruction by beta-lactamases, and increased ability to reach the CSF.
- Most of the cephalosporins are administered parenterally. Only 11 of 23 cephalosporins currently on the market may be given orally.
- Cefotetan (a second-generation cephalosporin) and cefoperazone (a third-generation cephalosporin) may induce bleeding.
- Cefotetan (a second-generation cephalosporin) and cefoperazone (a third-generation cephalosporin) may induce a disulfiram-like reaction if combined with alcohol.
- Vancomycin is very effective against most gram-positive infections; however, its use is limited by its potential to cause severe adverse effects.
- Vancomycin is the drug of choice for pseudomembranous colitis caused by *Clostridium difficile,* infections caused by methicillin-resistant *Staphylococcus aureus,* and serious infections in patients who are allergic to penicillin.
- Daptomycin, a cyclic lipopeptide, is the only member of this new class of antibiotics.
- To decrease the possibility that antibiotic resistance will develop, daptomycin should be reserved for infections that do not respond to other antibiotics.
- Patients with an antibiotic allergy should wear a Medic Alert necklace or bracelet.

QUESTIONS FOR STUDY AND REVIEW

1. How do penicillins work?
2. Why are most penicillins ineffective against gram-negative bacteria?

3. Why are there four classifications of penicillins?
4. Why are clavulanic acid, tazobactam, and sulbactam added to some penicillin preparations?
5. Compare and contrast the carbapenem antibiotics.
6. What is the difference between the generations of cephalosporins?
7. What classes of antibiotics are called beta-lactam antibiotics? Why?
8. Why is vancomycin reserved for serious infections?
9. What are the characteristics of daptomycin that are different from other antibiotics? Why is one of its characteristics so important?

? **Need More Help?**

Chapter 38 of the study guide for *Drug Therapy in Nursing* 2e contains NCLEX-style questions and other learning activities to reinforce your understanding of the concepts presented in this chapter. For additional information or to purchase the study guide, visit *http://connection.lww.com/go/aschenbrenner.*

REFERENCES AND BIBLIOGRAPHY

Carpenter, C. F., & Chambers, H. F. (2004). Daptomycin: Another novel agent for treating infections due to drug-resistant gram-positive pathogens. *Clinical Infectious Diseases, 38*(7), 994–1000.

Cottagnoud, P. H., & Tauber, M. G. (2004). New therapies for pneumococcal meningitis. *Expert Opinion on Investigational Drugs, 13*(4), 393–401.

Clinical Pharmacology [Online]. Available: *http://cp.gsm.com.*

Eliopoulos, G. M. (2004). Current and new antimicrobial agents. *American Heart Journal, 147*(4), 587–592.

Facts and Comparisons. (2004). *Drug facts and comparisons.* Philadelphia: Lippincott Williams & Wilkins.

Fenton, C., Keating, G. M., Curran, M. P., et al. (2004). Daptomycin. *Drugs, 64*(4), 445–455.

Hardman, J. G. (2001). *Goodman & Gilman's the pharmacological basis of therapeutics* (10th ed.). New York: McGraw-Hill Health Professions Division.

Katzung, B. (2004). *Basic and clinical pharmacology* (9th ed.). New York: McGraw-Hill/Appleton & Lange.

Micromedex Healthcare Series [Online]. Available: *http://healthcare.micromedex.com.*

Romano, A., Gueant-Rodriguez, R. M., Viola, M., et al. (2004). Cross-reactivity and tolerability of cephalosporins in patients with immediate hypersensitivity to penicillins. *Annals of Internal Medicine, 141*(1), 16–22.

Tatro, D. S. (2004). *Drug interaction facts.* Philadelphia: Lippincott Williams & Wilkins.

Antibiotics Affecting Protein Synthesis

chapter 39

Learning Objectives

At the completion of this chapter the student will:

1. Identify core drug knowledge pertaining to drugs affecting protein synthesis.
2. Identify core patient variables pertaining to drugs affecting protein synthesis.
3. Relate the interaction of core drug knowledge to core patient variables for drugs affecting protein synthesis.
4. Generate a nursing plan of care from the interactions between core drug knowledge and core patient variables for drugs affecting protein synthesis.
5. Describe nursing interventions to maximize therapeutic and minimize adverse effects for drugs affecting protein synthesis.
6. Determine key points for patient and family education for drugs affecting protein synthesis.

KEY TERMS

azotemia

cylindruria

hyposthenuria

nephrotoxicity

ototoxicity

peak and trough

proteinuria

pyuria

xeroderma

xerophthalmia

FEATURED WEBLINK

http://www.cfsan.fda.gov/~mow/intro.html

Most of the drugs in this chapter treat infections caused by *Staphylococcus* and *Streptococcus* species. Not familiar with these microbes? Log on to this website for more information.

CONNECTION WEBLINK

Additional Weblinks are found on Connection: **http://www.connection.lww.com/go/aschenbrenner.**

Antibiotics Affecting Protein Synthesis

(C) Aminoglycosides

- [P] **gentamicin**
- amikacin
- kanamycin
- neomycin
- netilmicin
- tobramycin
- paromomycin
- streptomycin

(C) Licosamides

- [P] **clindamycin**
- lincomycin

(C) Macrolide Antibiotics

- [P] **erythromycin**
- azithromycin
- clarithromycin
- dirithromycin
- troleandomycin
- telithromycin

(C) Oxazolidinones

- [P] **linezolid**

(C) Streptogramins

- [P] **quinupristin/dalfopristin**

(C) Tetracyclines

- [P] **tetracycline**
- demeclocycline
- doxycycline
- minocycline

Miscellaneous Antibiotics That Affect Protein Synthesis

- [P] **chloramphenicol**
- spectinomycin

The symbol (C) indicates the **drug class.**
Drugs in **bold type** marked with the symbol [P] are prototypes.
Drugs in blue type are closely related to the prototype.
Drugs in red type are significantly different from the prototype.
Drugs in black type with no symbol are also used in drug therapy; no prototype

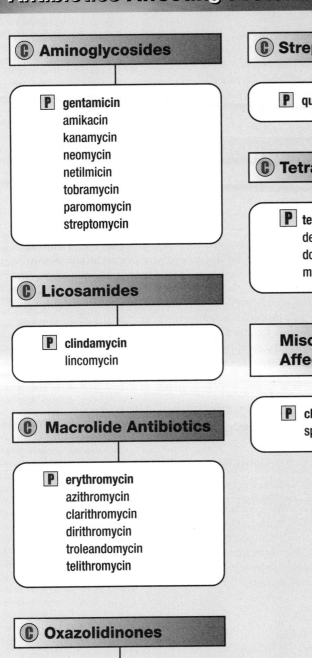

Drugs affecting protein synthesis include aminoglycoside agents, lincosamide agents, macrolide agents, oxazolidinones, streptogramins, tetracyclines, and miscellaneous antibiotics. The prototype drug for the aminoglycosides is gentamicin; drugs significantly different from gentamicin are paromomycin and streptomycin. The prototype lincosamide is clindamycin. Erythromycin is the prototype macrolide antibiotic; a drug significantly different from erythromycin is telithromycin. The oxazolidinone prototype is linezolid, the streptogramin prototype is quinupristin/dalfopristin, and the tetracycline prototype is tetracycline. The miscellaneous antibiotics are represented by the prototype chloramphenicol; a drug significantly different from chloramphenicol is spectinomycin.

In addition to explaining how these drugs work, this chapter discusses nursing management related to evaluating the patient's condition, monitoring the patient's response, and teaching the patient and family about antibiotic therapy.

PHYSIOLOGY

In all cells, the process of protein synthesis is divided into two sections: transcription and translation. Initially, transcription occurs within the nucleus, producing messenger ribonucleic acid (mRNA). This mRNA migrates from the nucleus to the cytoplasm. During this step, mRNA goes through different types of maturation, including one called splicing, during which the noncoding sequences are eliminated. The coding mRNA sequence is a unit of three nucleotides, called a codon.

Translation occurs in the cytoplasm. The ribosome binds to the mRNA at the start codon (AUG) that is recognized only by initiator tRNA (transfer ribonucleic acid). The ribosome proceeds to the elongation phase of protein synthesis. During this stage, complexes composed of an amino acid linked to tRNA bind sequentially to the appropriate codon in mRNA by forming complementary base pairs with the tRNA anticodon. The ribosome moves from codon to codon along the mRNA. Amino acids are added one by one, translated into polypeptide sequences dictated by DNA and represented by mRNA. At the end, a release factor binds to the stop codon, terminating translation and releasing the completed polypeptide from the ribosome. Figure 39.1 illustrates the process of protein synthesis.

C AMINOGLYCOSIDES

The aminoglycosides have been in use since 1944. They are extremely effective antibiotics for treating severe infections. Their general use, however, is limited because of the potential for serious adverse effects, especially ototoxicity and nephrotoxicity. Aminoglycosides include gentamicin, amikacin, kanamycin, netilmicin, neomycin, tobramycin, paromomycin, and streptomycin. The most frequently used aminoglycosides are gentamicin, tobramycin, and amikacin. Gentamicin is the most widely used, possibly because of its availability as a generic formulation, and is the prototype drug for the aminoglycoside family. Table 39.1 presents a summary of selected aminoglycoside agents.

NURSING MANAGEMENT OF THE PATIENT RECEIVING P GENTAMICIN

Core Drug Knowledge

Pharmacotherapeutics

Clinically, gentamicin is useful for urinary tract infections (UTIs), such as pyelonephritis; gynecologic infections; peritonitis; endocarditis; pneumonia; bacteremia and sepsis; respiratory infections, including those associated with cystic fibrosis; osteomyelitis; and foot and other soft tissue infections associated with diabetes.

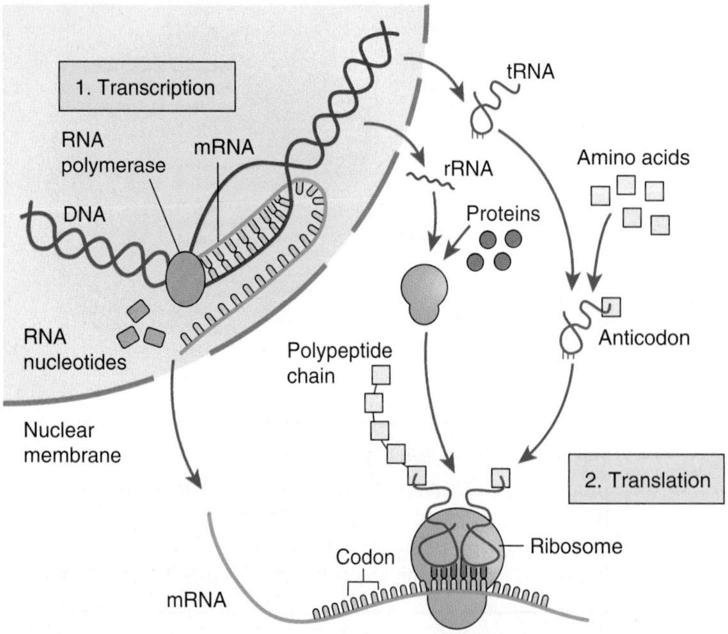

FIGURE 39.1 Protein synthesis.

TABLE 39.1 Summary of Selected (C) Aminoglycoside Antibiotics

Drug (Trade) Name	Selected Indications	Route and Dosage Range	Pharmacokinetics
[P] gentamicin (Garamycin; *Canadian:* Alcomicin)	Gram-negative infections Staphylococcal infections	*Adult:* IM/IV, 3–5 mg/kg/d in divided doses *Child:* 6–7.5 mg/kg in divided doses *Infants and neonates:* 7.5 mg/kg in divided doses q8h	*Onset:* Rapid *Duration:* 6–8 h $t_{1/2}$: 2–3 h
amikacin (Amikin)	Gram-negative infections Staphylococcal infections	*Adult:* IM/IV, 15 mg/kg/d *Child:* Same as adults *Neonate:* IM/IV, 10 mg/kg initially then 7.5 mg/kg q12h	*Onset:* IM, varies; IV, immediate *Duration:* 6–8 h $t_{1/2}$: 2–3 h
kanamycin (kantrex)	*Escherichia coli* and other infectious agents Suppression of intestinal flora	*Adult:* IM, 15 mg/kg/d; IV, dilute 500-mg vial with 100–200 mL sterile diluent per day PO, 1 g every hour for 4 h then 1 g q6h for 36–72 h	*Onset:* IM/IV, rapid *Duration:* 8–12 h $t_{1/2}$: 2–3 h
netilmicin (Netromycin)	Complicated urinary tract infections Septicemia Intra-abdominal infections	*Adult:* IM/IV, 4–6.5 mg/kg q8–12h *Child 6 wk–12 y:* IM/IV, 5.5–8 mg/kg q8–12h *Neonate < 6 wk:* 4–6.5 mg/kg q12h	*Onset:* IM, rapid; IV, immediate *Duration:* 12–16 h $t_{1/2}$: 2.0–2.5 h
neomycin (Mycifradin Sulfate)	Preoperative suppression of intestinal bacteria Hepatic coma	*Adult:* 1 g at 19, 18 and 9 h before surgery *Adult:* 4–12 g/d	*Onset:* PO, varies *Duration:* 6–8 h $t_{1/2}$: 3 h
tobramycin (Nebcin; *Canadian:* Tomycine)	Gram-negative infections especially *Pseudomonas* staphylococcal infections, burns Soft tissue wounds	*Adult and child:* 3–5 mg/kg every 12 h *Neonate < 1 w:* IM/IV: up to 4 mg/kg every 12 h	*Onset:* Rapid *Duration:* 8–12 h $t_{1/2}$: 2–3 h
streptomycin	Nontuberculosis infections Tuberculosis	*Adult:* IM, 1–2 g/d in divided doses *Child:* IM, 20–40 mg/kg/d q12h *Adult:* IM, 15 mg/kg 2–3 times a week (max 1.5 g per dose)	*Onset:* Rapid *Duration:* 8–12 h $t_{1/2}$: 2.5 h
paromomycin (Humatin)	Intestinal amebiasis Hepatic coma	*Adult and child:* 25–35 mg/kg/d in three divided doses *Adult:* 4 g/d in divided doses	*Onset:* Poorly absorbed *Duration:* Excreted $t_{1/2}$: Unchanged in feces
telithromycin (Ketek)	Acute exacerbation of chronic bronchitis Acute bacterial sinusitis Community-acquired pneumonia Not approved for children	*Adult:* 800 mg PO × 5 d 800 mg qd 7–10 d	*Onset:* 1 h *Duration:* unknown $t_{1/2}$: 10 h

Gentamicin is effective in managing infections caused by gram-negative bacilli. Susceptible organisms include *Pseudomonas aeruginosa, Proteus mirabilis, Escherichia coli; Klebsiella, Enterobacter, Serratia,* and *Citrobacter* species; and staphylococci. Gentamicin must be transported across the cell membrane in order to enter the cell and disrupt protein synthesis. This process requires oxygen; therefore, gentamicin and other aminoglycosides are ineffective against anaerobes. Gentamicin is not considered useful in treating meningitis unless it is administered intrathecally.

Gentamicin is also indicated for topical treatment of eye or skin infections caused by susceptible organisms. It is used as a liposome injection for treating disseminated *Mycobacterium avium-intracellulare* infection, and it has an orphan drug indication as drug-impregnated polymethylmethacrylate (PMAA) beads on surgical wire for treating chronic osteomyelitis.

Pharmacokinetics

Parenteral gentamicin is widely distributed through the body in extracellular fluids; however, it does not penetrate appreciably into the central nervous system (CNS). It crosses the placenta and is secreted in breast milk. Gentamicin concentrates in the kidney, reaching levels 50 times higher than those in serum. It also concentrates in the endolymph and perilymph of the inner ear. High concentrations of gentamicin in these fluids are associated with its major adverse effects—**nephrotoxicity** and **ototoxicity.** Parenteral gentamicin is excreted unchanged in urine, whereas oral gentamicin is excreted unchanged in feces.

Because it is poorly absorbed when taken orally, gentamicin is usually reserved for parenteral or topical use. It may, however, be given orally to exert a local decrease in gastrointestinal (GI) tract bacteria before surgical or other invasive procedures.

Pharmacodynamics

Gentamicin, like all antibiotics, has no direct effect on the cells of the body. It exerts its effect by entering the bacterial cell and binding to the 30S ribosomal subunit (see Chapter 37). This event leads to a misreading of the information used within the cell to form proteins. The cell then produces amino acids that do not link correctly. The result is a change in metabolic function that in turn prevents bacterial reproduction and weakens the cell wall, leading to cell wall rupture and death. Many strains of bacteria are resistant to the aminoglycosides and do not allow them to enter the cell. Because of this, aminoglycosides are often given with synergistic antibiotics to increase their effectiveness or to alter the cell wall so that the aminoglycoside can enter.

Contraindications and Precautions

Gentamicin is contraindicated during pregnancy and lactation. It is also contraindicated in patients with known allergy to any aminoglycoside. It is used cautiously in patients with renal or hepatic disease, dehydration, pre-existing hearing loss, myasthenia gravis, parkinsonism, and infant botulism.

Adverse Effects

Many serious side effects are associated with gentamicin, limiting its usefulness. The most well-known adverse effects are nephrotoxicity, ototoxicity, and neuromuscular blockade. Ototoxicity occurs most frequently when serum trough levels are elevated, in infants or elderly patients, or with prolonged or high-dose therapy. Nephrotoxicity occurs most frequently in infants or the elderly or with prolonged or high-dose therapy. Neuromuscular blockade may result in profound respiratory depression. It occurs most frequently in patients with myasthenia gravis and in patients receiving general anesthetics or nondepolarizing skeletal muscle relaxants.

In the CNS, gentamicin therapy may induce confusion, depression, disorientation, numbness, tingling, and weakness. Leukemoid reactions and depressed bone marrow function are potential adverse effects in the hematologic system. GI symptoms include nausea, vomiting, diarrhea, weight loss, stomatitis, and hepatic toxicity. Gentamicin may induce palpitations, hypotension, and hypertension in the cardiovascular system. Hypersensitivity reactions include purpura, rash, urticaria, and exfoliative dermatitis. Other adverse effects such as superinfections, fever, apnea, and joint pain may also occur.

Drug Interactions

Gentamicin may interact with other drugs that are known to be ototoxic, nephrotoxic, or neurotoxic such as acyclovir, amphotericin B, cephalothin, cisplatin, cyclosporine, loop diuretics (especially ethacrynic acid), prostaglandin synthetase inhibitors, and vancomycin. Additionally, gentamicin may interact with biophosphate derivatives, indomethacin, nondepolarizing skeletal muscle relaxants, extended penicillins, and cephalosporins. Table 39.2 lists drugs that interact with gentamicin.

Assessment of Relevant Core Patient Variables

Health Status

In assessing the health status of the patient taking gentamicin, elicit a thorough health history, particularly the renal history. Because gentamicin is excreted unchanged by glomerular filtration, patients with renal dysfunction or dehydration are at risk for nephrotoxicity. Evaluate patients for a history of hearing impairment and eighth cranial nerve impairment because these patients have an elevated risk for ototoxicity.

Investigate any history of myasthenia gravis or parkinsonism. Gentamicin may cause severe neuromuscular weakness, lasting hours to days, because of its potential curare-like effect, and it may aggravate muscle weakness in patients with these disorders.

Perform a baseline gross hearing test before administering gentamicin. Evaluate laboratory test results that indicate the renal and hepatic function of the patient.

Life Span and Gender

Evaluate women for potential pregnancy. Although gentamicin is not absolutely contraindicated during pregnancy, it has been found to be ototoxic to the fetus. Evaluate neonates (younger than 1 month) and patients older than 65 years frequently because these patients have immature or decreased renal function, which increases their risk for ototoxicity and nephrotoxicity.

Lifestyle, Diet, and Habits

Assess the nutritional status of the patient. Patients whose oral intake is restricted and patients who eat poorly are at increased risk for hypomagnesemia during gentamicin therapy. Dehydrated patients have an increased risk for nephrotoxicity.

Environment

Be aware of the environment in which gentamicin will be administered and, if appropriate, assess the home or living environment for potential risk factors. Parenteral gentamicin is usually administered in the acute hospital setting; however, it may also be given in the home environment by a home health care nurse. Oral or topical gentamicin may be given in any environment.

In the hospital setting, store gentamicin in the refrigerator and be sure that it does not freeze. Before administration, gentamicin solution should be inspected for discoloration or particulates. After administration, any unused solution should be discarded.

TABLE 39.2 Agents That Interact With P Gentamicin

Interactants	Effect and Significance	Nursing Management
Ototoxic, nephrotoxic, and neurotoxic drugs • acyclovir • amphotericin B • cephalothin • cisplatin • cyclosporine • loop diuretics, especially ethacrynic acid • prostaglandin synthetase inhibitors • vancomycin	Risk for ototoxicity, nephrotoxicity, or neurotoxic effects is increased when these drugs are coadministered with gentamicin.	Avoid these combinations if possible. Monitor serum gentamicin levels. Monitor for hearing change daily. Monitor fluid intake and output. Monitor kidney function tests. Reduce dose of one or both drugs as needed.
Bisphosphonate derivatives • alendronate • etidronate • pamidronate • risedronate • tiludronate • zoledronic acid	Gentamicin may enhance the hypocalcemic effect of bisphosphonate derivatives.	Monitor calcium and magnesium levels.
indomethacin	Indomethacin may increase serum gentamicin concentration in premature infants receiving indomethacin for patent ductus arteriosus.	Monitor serum gentamicin levels. Monitor for adverse effects or signs of toxicity.
"Azole" antifungal agents	Coadministration may decrease serum concentration of gentamicin.	Monitor serum gentamicin levels. Monitor therapeutic effects of gentamicin.
Nondepolarizing muscle relaxants	The actions of nondepolarizing muscle relaxants may be enhanced.	Mark patient's chart and arrange for extended monitoring and support following anesthesia. Monitor respirations and other vital signs following anesthesia.
Extended penicillins • carbenicillin • ticarcillin	Extended penicillins may inactivate gentamicin.	Avoid combination when possible. Administer these drugs at least 2 h apart.
Penicillin and cephalosporins	Synergic bacterial activity.	This is a beneficial interaction.

Nursing Diagnoses and Outcomes

- Risk for Injury related to potential drug-related allergic reactions or neuromuscular blockade or suppression of bone marrow function
  Desired outcome: *The patient will remain free of injury and will contact the prescriber if unusual adverse effects occur.*
- Diarrhea related to drug effects
  Desired outcome: *The patient will avoid dehydration, maintain fluid intake, and contact the prescriber if diarrhea persists.*
- Imbalanced Nutrition: Less than Body Requirements related to drug-induced GI effects or superinfection
  Desired outcome: *The patient will maintain body weight and report to the health care provider any persistent adverse effects that affect nutritional status.*
- Risk for Injury related to CNS effects
  Desired outcome: *The patient will remain free of injury and contact the provider if confusion, disorientation, or depression occurs.*
- Disturbed Sensory Perception related to potential ototoxicity
  Desired outcome: *The patient will report sensory or perceptual changes to the prescriber.*
- Excess Fluid Volume related to potential nephrotoxicity
  Desired outcome: *The patient will report any weight gain exceeding 3 lb to the health care prescriber.*

Planning and Intervention

Maximizing Therapeutic Effects

Make sure that patients receive the full course of gentamicin as prescribed at around-the-clock intervals; coordinate the administration of drugs to decrease potential drug interactions; and evaluate culture and sensitivity reports to make sure that gentamicin is the appropriate drug.

Because gentamicin may be inactivated by extended penicillins, such as carbenicillin or ticarcillin, administer these drugs at least 2 hours apart to ensure the efficacy of gentamicin.

Minimizing Adverse Effects

To reduce the occurrence of adverse effects, it is imperative to maintain blood levels of gentamicin within a therapeutic margin that is very narrow. To do this, **peak and trough** drug levels are monitored throughout therapy. Blood for peak levels is drawn 30 minutes after the completion of intravenous (IV) administration and 1 hour after intramuscular (IM) administration. Blood for trough levels is drawn just before the next dose.

Monitor for signs of ototoxicity. Before administering each dose, assess the patient's balance and gross hearing.

Monitor for signs of nephrotoxicity. Assess the hydration status of the patient and be alert for dilute urine or proteinuria. Monitor the patient for gentamicin-induced diarrhea because diarrhea may also cause dehydration.

If CNS effects occur, safety measures should be instituted to protect the patient. Small, frequent meals can be arranged for patients with GI effects, and frequent mouth care and ice chips can be offered to relieve stomatitis and sore mouth.

If a patient receiving gentamicin requires surgery, the chart should indicate prominently that gentamicin has been given. Remember that gentamicin may interact with neuromuscular blocking agents commonly used during surgery, resulting in prolonged neuromuscular blockade. The patient will require extended monitoring and support after surgery to detect problems and intervene if they occur.

Monitor laboratory tests such as renal and hepatic function tests, peak and trough levels of gentamicin, and the fluid intake and output status of the patient.

Providing Patient and Family Education

- One of the most important features of patient and family education is to teach the patient that gentamicin is one drug within a class of drugs.
- Advise patients that they should not take this drug if they are pregnant or breast-feeding.
- Advise the patient to take oral gentamicin on an empty stomach, 1 hour before or 2 hours after any meal or other drugs. Patients should also be instructed to take forgotten doses as soon as they remember, not to double the dose, and to contact the prescriber if symptoms do not improve in 3 days.
- Teach the patient how to identify, report, and manage signs and symptoms of allergic reaction and adverse effects.
- Teach the patient signs of ototoxicity such as persistent headache, nausea, balance difficulties, dizziness, vertigo, tinnitus, or high-frequency hearing loss. The patient should be instructed to contact the prescriber immediately if any of these symptoms occur.
- Teach the patient signs of nephrotoxicity, such as frequent or diminished urinary excretion. The patient should be instructed to contact the prescriber immediately if such signs occur.
- Teach the patient how to recognize superinfection and to watch for CNS effects such as confusion, depression, numbness, tingling, or weakness. Explain the importance of contacting the prescriber if any of these symptoms occur.
- Help the patient develop strategies for minimizing GI upset and oral soreness.
- Show patients how to use gentamicin eye drops correctly, making sure to stress the importance of keeping the dropper portion of the bottle from touching the eye to avoid contamination.

Ongoing Assessment and Evaluation

Coordinate the care of the patient to ensure that other potentially nephrotoxic or ototoxic drugs are not added to the treatment plan. The primary prescriber should be notified if any such drugs are added. Monitor peak and trough levels of gentamicin. Although maintaining gentamicin serum concentrations within traditional ranges is believed to minimize the risk for nephrotoxicity, some patients may still develop ototoxicity or nephrotoxicity. Acute tubular necrosis is the most common gentamicin-induced nephrotoxicity. Monitor for **azotemia** (excessive urea levels in the blood), decreased creatinine clearance, **hyposthenuria** (loss of the ability to concentrate urine), **pyuria** (increased white blood cell count), **proteinuria,** and **cylindruria** (cells or casts in the urine).

Evaluate for signs of ototoxicity. Gentamicin may induce both cochlear and vestibular damage to the inner ear. Cochlear damage, a high-frequency hearing loss, may be preceded by high-pitched tinnitus. Cochlear damage may be subtle; therefore, coordinate referrals for audiologic testing for patients who receive repeated or prolonged courses of gentamicin therapy. Vestibular damage is characterized by a headache followed by vertigo, dizziness, or nausea. To avoid permanent ototoxic damage, the drug should be withdrawn at the first sign of tinnitus or persistent headache.

Evaluate patients for signs of neuromuscular blockade, such as muscle weakness, especially of the respiratory muscles.

Observe the injection site regularly because IM injection of gentamicin can cause irritation.

When therapy ends, the presenting infection should be resolved. The patient should be adequately nourished and hydrated and free from adverse drug effects.

MEMORY CHIP

P Gentamicin

- Used for serious gram-negative infections
- Major contraindications: hypersensitivity, pregnancy, and breast-feeding
- Most common adverse effects: nausea, vomiting, diarrhea, and weight loss
- Most serious adverse effects: nephrotoxicity, ototoxicity, and neuromuscular blockade
- Maximizing therapeutic effects: Administer at least 2 hours before or after extended infusions of penicillins.
- Minimizing adverse effects: Monitor peak and trough levels throughout therapy.
- Most important patient education: Teach the patient the signs and symptoms of both nephrotoxicity and ototoxicity and also the importance of contacting the health care provider immediately if any symptoms should occur.

Drugs Closely Related to [P] Gentamicin

Amikacin

Amikacin (Amikin) is a parenteral aminoglycoside with a broader spectrum of activity than gentamicin for gram-negative bacilli. Amikacin is also less likely to induce bacterial resistance. Although some hospitals use amikacin as the first-line treatment for systemic infection because of an increased resistance to gentamicin, many others reserve its use for infections that do not respond to other aminoglycoside antibiotics. Its contraindications, adverse effects, drug interactions, and patient management are similar to those of gentamicin.

Kanamycin

Kanamycin (Kantrex) is used orally to reduce ammonia-forming bacteria in hepatic coma and as an adjunctive therapy to decrease GI flora. Its use for systemic infections is limited by the number of bacteria that are resistant to it and the availability of gentamicin in its less expensive generic formulation. Its contraindications, adverse effects, drug interactions, and patient management are similar to those of gentamicin.

Neomycin

Neomycin (Mycifradin Sulfate) has the highest risk for toxicity of all the aminoglycosides. Because it is so toxic, it is not administered parenterally. It is available orally to decrease GI flora as a preparation for bowel surgery and to treat hepatic encephalopathy. Because it is not absorbed from the GI tract, it frequently causes superinfection within the bowel. Neomycin is also available in over-the-counter (OTC) drugs as a topical antibiotic. Contraindications, adverse effects, drug interactions, and patient management are the same as those for gentamicin.

Netilmicin

Netilmicin (Netromycin) is another parenteral aminoglycoside, used to manage both gram-negative and gram-positive infections. It is inactive against most streptococci and some aerobic and most anaerobic bacteria. Netilmicin induces less resistance than gentamicin does and is less likely to produce ototoxicity in patients with normal renal function. However, in patients with compromised renal function, netilmicin increases the risk for both ototoxicity and nephrotoxicity. Contraindications, adverse effects, drug interactions, and patient management are the same as those for gentamicin.

Tobramycin

Tobramycin (Nebcin) is similar to gentamicin in its antibacterial spectrum; however, it is more active than gentamicin against *Pseudomonas* species. It is given parenterally, topically to treat superficial ophthalmic infections, or by nebulization to treat respiratory infections. Tobramycin has a low therapeutic index. Using ideal body weight to determine the mg/kg per dose appears to be more accurate than dosing on the basis of total body weight. Peak and trough levels should be closely monitored in patients with serious infections or in disease states known to substantially alter aminoglycoside pharmacokinetics, such as cystic fibrosis, burns, or major surgery. Contraindications, adverse effects, drug interactions, and patient management are the same as those of gentamicin.

Drugs Significantly Different From [P] Gentamicin

Paromomycin

Paromomycin (Humatin) is an aminoglycoside antibiotic that differs from gentamicin because of its amebicidal and anthelminthic activity. Paromomycin has poor oral bioavailability; thus, it is used to treat intestinal amebiasis and various intestinal parasites by its local activity. It is also useful in managing hepatic encephalopathy or coma because it inhibits bacteria in the gut that produce urease, an enzyme that breaks down urea into carbon dioxide and ammonia.

Paromomycin is contraindicated in patients with renal failure or intestinal obstruction. Adverse GI effects of paromomycin include anorexia, nausea, vomiting, gastric burning and pain, abdominal cramps, and diarrhea.

The only important drug–drug interaction with paromomycin occurs with succinylcholine. When they are given in combination, paromomycin may potentiate the neuromuscular effects of succinylcholine.

Coordinate follow-up appointments for the patient. Stool cultures should be done weekly for 6 weeks after therapy, then monthly for 2 years.

Streptomycin

Streptomycin is a parenteral aminoglycoside. It is used as part of combination therapy for both active tuberculosis and for treating streptococcal or enterococcal endocarditis. As a single agent, it is used for mycobacterial infections, plague, tularemia, and brucellosis. In addition to ototoxicity and nephrotoxicity, streptomycin may induce neurotoxicity.

(C) LINCOSAMIDES

The lincosamides include clindamycin (Cleocin, Cleocin Pediatric) and lincomycin (Lincocin). They are very toxic drugs, so their use must be monitored and limited to situations with infections by bacteria with known sensitivity. Although lincomycin was the first drug developed in this class, it is rarely used. Clindamycin is discussed as the prototype lincosamide. Table 39.3 presents a summary of lincosamide antibiotics.

NURSING MANAGEMENT OF THE PATIENT RECEIVING [P] CLINDAMYCIN

Core Drug Knowledge

Pharmacotherapeutics

Clindamycin is active against a wide range of aerobic gram-positive cocci and several anaerobic gram-negative and gram-positive organisms. Many species of streptococci (except enterococci) and staphylococci are extremely susceptible. Most anaerobes, both gram positive and gram negative, are also susceptible. Clindamycin is indicated for treating serious to life-threatening infections caused by susceptible strains of anaerobes; streptococci; staphylococci; pneumococci, including septicemia; and acute hematogenous osteomyelitis. Topical forms are used to treat acne vulgaris. A vaginal preparation is available for treating bacterial vaginosis.

TABLE 39.3 Summary of Selected (C) Lincosamide Antibiotics

Drug (Trade) Name	Selected Indications	Route and Dosage Range	Pharmacokinetics
[P] clindamycin (Cleocin; *Canadian:* Dalacin-c)	Serious infections from streptococci, pneumococci, and staphylococci	*Adult:* PO, 150–450 mg q6h; IM/IV, 600 mg–2.7 g q6–12h up to 4.8 g/d for life-threatening infections *Child:* PO, 8–12 mg/kg/d in three divided doses; 10 kg, maximum of 37.5 mg tid; IM/IV, 15–40 mg/kg q6–12h up to 40 mg/kg/d for severe infection	*Onset:* PO, varies; IM, 20–30 min; IV, immediate *Duration:* 8–12 h $t_{1/2}$: 2–3 h
lincomycin (Lincocin)	Serious infections from streptococci, pneumococci, and staphylococci	*Adult:* PO, 500 mg q8h; IM, 600–1,200 mg/d; IV, 600–1,000 mg q8–12 h	*Onset:* PO, varies; IM, 20–30 min; IV, immediate *Duration:* PO, 6–8 h; IM, 0.5 h; IV, 14 h $t_{1/2}$: 5 h

Pharmacokinetics

The oral absorption of clindamycin varies greatly, depending on the presence of food in the stomach. Peak levels are achieved in about 1 to 2 hours. Given intramuscularly, clindamycin is rapidly absorbed within 20 to 30 minutes, with peak levels occurring at 1 to 3 hours. IV administration produces a peak effect within minutes. Topical clindamycin is only minimally absorbed.

Clindamycin crosses the placenta and enters breast milk and cerebrospinal fluid (CSF). It is readily carried to most body tissues. Metabolized in the liver, it is excreted through the bile and urine.

Pharmacodynamics

Clindamycin is either bacteriostatic or bactericidal, depending on its concentration at the site of action and on the specific susceptibility of the organism being treated. It enters the bacterial cell and binds to bacterial ribosomes, suppressing protein synthesis and leading to cell death in susceptible bacteria. It has no direct effect on the body.

Contraindications and Precautions

Clindamycin is contraindicated in pregnancy and lactation and in patients with a known allergy to lincosamides, history of asthma or other allergies, allergy to tartrazine (a component of several oral preparations of clindamycin), or hepatic or renal dysfunction. Caution should be exercised in patients with a history of antibiotic-associated colitis, regional enteritis, or ulcerative colitis.

Adverse Effects

The most common adverse effects of clindamycin are nausea and vomiting and abdominal pain following oral delivery. Diarrhea, abdominal cramps, and abdominal tenderness may suggest antibiotic-associated colitis, also known as pseudomembranous colitis or *Clostridium difficile* colitis.

Thrombocytopenia, neutropenia, and eosinophilia have been reported during clindamycin therapy. Sore throat or fever may indicate neutropenia.

Maculopapular rash, erythema, and pruritus can develop from systemic or topical use of clindamycin. Pathologic dryness of the skin (**xeroderma**), conjunctiva (**xerophthalmia**), or mucous membranes is the most common effect of topical application. Alcohol in some topical formulations may irritate the eyes, mucous membranes, or abraded skin if allowed to come into contact with them.

Hypersensitivity reactions range from skin rashes and urticaria to anaphylactoid reactions. After injection, pain, abscess, and phlebitis are relatively common.

Drug Interactions

Neuromuscular blockers, aluminum salts, erythromycin, and pyrimethamine interact with clindamycin. Topical preparations containing benzoyl peroxide, tretinoin, salicylic acid, or other topical preparations for acne, when used with clindamycin preparations, can cause a cumulative irritant effect, leading to excessive drying and peeling of the skin. Table 39.4 lists agents that interact with clindamycin.

Assessment of Relevant Core Patient Variables

Health Status

Assess patients for allergy to lincosamides or predisposition to such allergy as shown by a previous reaction to tartrazine. Some clindamycin preparations contain tartrazine dye, which can precipitate bronchial asthma or other allergic reactions in sensitive patients. Patients sensitive to clindamycin may also be sensitive to doxorubicin.

Next, investigate any history of GI disease because clindamycin predisposes patients to the overgrowth of nonsusceptible organisms and hence may induce pseudomembranous colitis.

TABLE 39.4 Agents That Interact With P Clindamycin

Interactants	Effect and Significance	Nursing Management
antibiotics erythromycin chloramphenicol	Coadministration antagonizes the effects of clindamycin.	Avoid coadministration.
aluminum salts or kaolin	Marked decreased GI absorption of lincosamides if taken with these.	Administer absorbent antidiarrheal product 2 h before or 3–4 h after administering oral clindamycin.
neuromuscular blockers	Lincosamides potentiate the action of neuromuscular blockers, resulting in increased neuromuscular blockade, respiratory depression, and extended paralysis.	Mark patient's chart with warning of the drug combination. Arrange for extended monitoring and support of patient after surgery or procedure. Monitor respiration and other vital signs.
opiate agonists	Coadministration enhances the effect of opiates, resulting in increased respiratory depression.	Monitor respiration and other vital signs.
pyrimethamine	Synergistic effects in treating toxoplasmic encephalitis in patients with AIDS.	This is a beneficial interaction.

Any previous renal or hepatic disease must be explored because the half-life of clindamycin is prolonged in patients with hepatic dysfunction, and toxicity can occur. Hepatic and renal function should be tested at baseline, and the results should be evaluated before beginning therapy. For patients with severe renal impairment, dose reduction should be considered.

Patients on long-term therapy should have a baseline complete blood count (CBC) because of clindamycin's potential to induce blood dyscrasias.

Life Span and Gender

Explore the benefits of treatment versus potential risks with the pregnant or lactating woman. In general, clindamycin is prescribed for pregnant or lactating women only if the benefits outweigh the potential risks.

Assess the growth and developmental level of the child or infant. Clindamycin should be used cautiously in children. Neonates younger than 1 month (and premature infants) have a prolonged plasma half-life for clindamycin, probably because of an immature hepatic system.

Lifestyle, Diet, and Habits

Assess the patient's lifestyle to determine the likelihood that the patient will take the drug around the clock.

Environment

Be aware of the environment in which gentamicin will be administered and, if appropriate, assess the home or living environment for potential risk factors. Parenteral solutions of clindamycin must be used within 24 hours of reconstitution. Oral or topical clindamycin may be administered in any environment.

Nursing Diagnoses and Outcomes

- Risk for Injury related to allergic reactions
  Desired outcome: *The patient will stop drug therapy and immediately report symptoms of allergic reaction to the prescriber.*
- Diarrhea related to drug effects
  Desired outcome: *The patient will avoid dehydration and report persistent diarrhea to the provider.*
- Imbalanced Nutrition: Less than Body Requirements related to drug-related GI effects, alteration in taste, superinfections
  Desired outcome: *The patient will maintain body weight and report persistent symptoms affecting nutritional status.*
- Risk for Injury related to possible blood dyscrasias
  Desired outcome: *The patient will remain injury free throughout drug therapy.*

Planning and Intervention

Maximizing Therapeutic Effects

Make sure that the patient receives the full course of clindamycin as prescribed, at around-the-clock intervals for maximal effectiveness. Coordinate the administration of drugs to decrease potential undesired interactions. Culture and sensitivity reports may be reviewed periodically to confirm that clindamycin is the appropriate drug for the patient.

Minimizing Adverse Effects

Clindamycin should be administered on an empty stomach with a full glass of water. For patients with GI effects, provide a small meal with administration. Provide frequent mouth care and ice chips to suck if stomatitis and sore mouth are problems. It is also important to keep this drug out of the reach of children to avoid accidental overdose.

Providing Patient and Family Education

- Patients should understand that they should not take clindamycin or any other lincosamide antibiotic if they have ever had a reaction to a drug with a generic name that ends with "mycin" or "micin."
- Advise patients to contact the prescriber immediately if they experience substantial diarrhea.
- Advise pregnant or breast-feeding patients to avoid clindamycin.

- Discuss general dosage and safe storage recommendations.
- Advise the patient to take clindamycin on an empty stomach with a full glass of water. If GI distress occurs, take with food.
- The patient should be urged to contact the prescriber if clindamycin therapy does not improve symptoms in 3 days.
- Teach the patient to recognize and report symptoms of allergic reaction and superinfection (sore throat, easy bruising or bleeding, and fatigue) or allergic reaction.
- Advise women of childbearing age who are taking birth control pills to use a backup method of contraception while taking clindamycin.
- Advise patients using clindamycin lotion that dry skin may occur. Instruct the patient to drink plenty of fluids and keep the skin moisturized.

Ongoing Assessment and Evaluation

Monitor the patient for the onset of diarrhea. If it occurs, the prescriber should be notified immediately because diarrhea may be the presenting sign of pseudomembranous colitis. Obtain an order for the stool to be evaluated for white blood cells (WBCs), blood, and mucus. Arrange for a proctoscopy to be performed.

During therapy, monitor for potential procedures that would require the use of neuromuscular blocking agents. If a procedure is scheduled, note prominently on the patient's chart the current use of clindamycin. After the procedure, the patient should be monitored and supported for an extended period once the neuromuscular blocker is discontinued.

Monitor for sore throat and fever, which may be signs of thrombocytopenia, neutropenia, or eosinophilia.

When treatment ends, the initial infection should be resolved. The patient should be adequately nourished and hydrated, and any adverse drug effects should be resolved.

Drug Closely Related to P Clindamycin

Lincomycin is an oral and parenteral lincosamide antibiotic. It is used for serious staphylococcal and streptococcal infections. Lincomycin is usually reserved for patients who cannot take penicillins or clindamycin. It is not a drug of choice because it has been associated with severe or fatal colitis. Like clindamycin, lincomycin is used with caution in patients with asthma, liver disease, GI disease, colitis, and tartrazine sensitivity. Adverse effects, drug interactions, and patient management are similar to those of clindamycin.

MEMORY CHIP

P Clindamycin

- Used for serious infections caused by gram-positive cocci and both gram-positive and gram-negative anaerobes.
- Major contraindications: hypersensitivity, pregnancy, breast-feeding, and renal or hepatic dysfunction
- Most common adverse effects: nausea, vomiting, abdominal pain, rash, and pruritus
- Most serious adverse effect: pseudomembranous colitis
- Maximizing therapeutic effects: Administer at evenly spaced intervals.
- Minimizing adverse effects: Give with food to minimize GI distress.
- Most important patient education: Teach the patient the signs and symptoms of superinfection, especially pseudomembranous colitis, and explain the importance of contacting the health care provider immediately if any symptoms occur.

C MACROLIDE ANTIBIOTICS

The macrolide antibiotics have been in use since 1952. They are characterized by molecules made up of large-ring lactones. Macrolides are bacteriostatic or bactericidal in susceptible bacteria. They include erythromycin and troleandomycin. Synthetic derivatives of erythromycin, also classified as macrolide antibiotics, include azithromycin, clarithromycin, and dirithromycin. Erythromycin was the first macrolide discovered and is the prototype for this class. Table 39.5 presents a summary of macrolide antibiotics.

NURSING MANAGEMENT OF THE PATIENT RECEIVING P ERYTHROMYCIN

Core Drug Knowledge

Pharmacotherapeutics

Erythromycin is commonly used in treating Legionnaire disease, *Mycoplasma pneumoniae* pneumonia, diphtheria, chlamydial infections, and chancroid, and as an alternative to beta-lactam antibiotics in patients who are allergic to penicillin. Erythromycin may have benefits in hypomotility conditions, such as diabetic gastroparesis, because it increases gastric motility and emptying.

Erythromycin is generally more effective against gram-positive organisms than against gram-negative organisms because of its ability to penetrate into gram-positive organisms. Gram-positive organisms susceptible to erythromycin include *Staphylococcus aureus, Streptococcus agalactiae, Streptococcus pyogenes, Streptococcus pneumoniae, Streptococcus viridans* species, and *Corynebacterium diphtheriae.*

Other susceptible organisms include *Chlamydia trachomatis, Entamoeba histolytica, Listeria monocytogenes, Borrelia burgdorferi* (the causative agent in Lyme disease), *Mycoplasma pneumoniae, Treponema pallidum,* and *Ureaplasma urealyticum.*

Pharmacokinetics

Erythromycin base (E-Mycin, Ery-Tab) is easily inactivated by gastric acid; therefore, several formulations have been developed to overcome this problem. Erythromycin stearate (Erythrocin) is the most likely to yield to gastric acid destruction. Erythromycin estolate (Ilosone) is more acid stable, dissociates in the upper intestine, and releases an inactive ester that is absorbed and hydrolyzed in the blood to produce free erythromycin. Erythromycin ethylsuccinate (EES, EryPed) is first absorbed and then hydrolyzed in the blood to free erythromycin. The newest formulation of oral erythromycin is encapsulated pellets that are small enough to pass through the pyloric sphincter independent of gastric emptying and are absorbed as the base. None of the oral forms, however, allows complete absorption. The drug reaches peak levels

TABLE 39.5 Summary of Selected (C) Macrolide Antibiotics

Drug (Trade) Name	Selected Indications	Route and Dosage Range	Pharmacokinetics
[P] erythromycin (E-Mycin, Ilosone, EES, Erythrocin stearate; *Canadian:* Apo-Erythro)	Urethral, endocervical, or rectal infections Syphilis Legionnaire disease Rheumatic fever Bacterial endocarditis *Mycoplasma* infections Bronchitis Pharyngitis Skin infections	*Adult:* PO, 250–500 mg q6h (maximum 4g) *Child:* PO, 30–50 mg q6–12h (maximum 100 mg/kg in divided doses) *(Note:* EES dosage is slightly higher)	*Onset:* 1–2 h *Duration:* 6–8 h $t_{1/2}$: 3–5 h
azithromycin (Zithromax)	Lower respiratory tract infection Nongonococcal urethritis and cervicitis Skin infections Acute otitis media Pharyngitis/tonsillitis *Helicobacter pylori* infection	*Adult:* PO, 500 mg/d on first day, then 250 mg for days 2 through 5 *Child 6 mo–2 y:* PO, 10 mg/kg on day 1, then 5 mg/kg on days 2–5; *> 2 y,* PO, 10 mg/kg as single dose (not to exceed 500 mg) first day; then 5 mg/kg (not to exceed 250 mg) once daily for 4 d	*Onset:* Rapid *Duration:* 24 h $t_{1/2}$: 11–48 h
	Mycobacterium avium (prevention or treatment)	*Adult:* PO, 500 mg q12h	
clarithromycin (Biaxin)	Respiratory infections Skin infections	*Adult:* PO, 250–500 mg q12h for 7–14 d *Child:* PO, 7.5 mg/kg bid to maximum of 500 mg bid	*Onset:* Rapid *Duration:* 8–12 h $t_{1/2}$: 3–7 h
troleandomycin (Tao)	Respiratory tract infections	*Adult:* PO, 250–500 mg q6h *Child:* PO, 125–250 mg q6h	*Onset:* Rapid *Duration:* 8–12 h $t_{1/2}$: 8–10 h
dirithromycin (Dynabac)	Bronchitis Skin infections Pharyngitis/tonsillitis Community-acquired pneumonia	*Adult:* 500 mg qd; duration depends on disorder *Child:* Not recommended	*Onset:* Rapid *Duration:* 24 h $t_{1/2}$: 2–36 h

1 to 4 hours after administration. Erythromycin is also available for IV use as erythromycin lactobionate or erythromycin gluceptate. Administration of IV erythromycin is painful and is used only when high serum levels of erythromycin are required. When given intravenously, erythromycin peak effect occurs within 1 hour. Erythromycin is also available in an ophthalmic preparation.

Erythromycin crosses the placenta and is secreted in breast milk. It does not cross the blood–brain barrier. It is metabolized in the liver and excreted in the bile and urine. Table 39.5 has additional information.

Pharmacodynamics

Erythromycin has no direct effect on the body. The macrolides are bactericidal or bacteriostatic. They exert their effect by inhibiting RNA-dependent protein synthesis at the chain elongation step. This action can prevent the cell from dividing, or it can cause cell death, depending on the sensitivity of the bacteria and the concentration of the drug.

Contraindications and Precautions

Erythromycin is contraindicated in patients who are allergic to it. Caution should be used in any patient with hepatic insufficiency because the ability to break down erythromycin for excretion may be compromised. Caution should be exercised during pregnancy or lactation and in patients with impaired hearing, biliary function, GI disease, and cardiac arrhythmias. Ocular preparations are contraindicated in patients with viral, fungal, or mycobacterial infections of the eye.

Adverse Effects

Adverse effects suggesting allergic reaction to erythromycin include urticaria, maculopapular rash, erythema, and interstitial nephritis. Pruritus is a possible reaction to topical application of erythromycin.

The most common adverse effects related to erythromycin occur in the GI tract. They include nausea or vomiting, abdominal pain, and diarrhea. These effects are often dose related and may occur regardless of the route of administration.

Rare potential adverse effects include hepatotoxicity, pseudomembranous colitis, QT interval prolongation and ventricular tachycardia of the torsades de pointes type, tinnitus, and reversible hearing loss.

Drug Interactions

Erythromycin interacts with many agents. Table 39.6 presents the most important potential drug interactions.

TABLE 39.6 Agents That Interact With P Erythromycin

Interactants	Effect and Significance	Nursing Management
Azole antifungal agents	Decreases the metabolism of antifungal agents	Monitor for toxic effect of antifungal agents.
Benzodiazepines	Decreases the metabolism of certain benzodiazepines, resulting in an increased CNS depression and prolonged effect	Monitor for sedation. Ensure safety precautions for patients. Reduce dosage of benzodiazepine as necessary.
Calcium channel blockers (CCBs)	Decrease the metabolism of certain CCBs, resulting in hypotension	Monitor vital signs. Ensure safety precautions for patients. Discuss changing to azithromycin or dirithromycin with the prescriber.
carbamazepine	Decreases the metabolism of carbamazepine, resulting in an increased risk for carbamazepine toxicity	Monitor carbamazepine levels closely. Reduce carbamazepine dose if necessary.
digoxin	Increases the serum concentration of digoxin, resulting in toxicity	Monitor digoxin levels carefully. Monitor for signs of toxicity. Adjust digoxin dose as necessary during erythromycin therapy.
clozapine	Decreases the metabolism of clozapine, resulting in an increased risk for clozapine toxicity	Avoid coadministration if possible. Monitor clozapine levels carefully. Monitor CBC. Discuss changing to azithromycin or dirithromycin with the prescriber.
Corticosteroids	Decreases the metabolism of systemic corticosteroids, resulting in an increased risk for adverse effects and toxicity	Monitor therapeutic effects of systemic corticosteroids. Monitor for adverse effects and toxicity. May be beneficial effect for patients with asthma.
cyclosporine	Decreases the metabolism of cyclosporine, resulting in an increased risk for adverse effects and toxicity	Avoid combination if possible. Monitor cyclosporine levels carefully. Monitor for cyclosporine toxicity. Adjust cyclosporine as needed.
Lincosamide antibiotics	Lincosamide antibiotics may decrease the therapeutic effect of erythromycin.	Avoid combination.
pimozide	Decreases the metabolism of pimozide, resulting in QT interval prolongation	Avoid combination.
repaglinide	Decreases the metabolism of repaglinide, resulting in hypoglycemia	Monitor serum glucose frequently. Monitor for signs and symptoms of hypoglycemia.
Selective serotonin reuptake inhibitor (SSRI) agents	Decreases the metabolism of SSRI drugs, resulting in an increased risk for adverse effects and toxicity	Monitor for toxic effects of SSRI drugs.
theophylline	Macrolides inhibit the metabolism of theophylline. Theophylline reduces the bioavailability and increases the renal clearance of erythromycin. These actions result in increased efficacy of theophylline and decreased efficacy of erythromycin.	Monitor theophylline levels closely. Monitor for theophylline toxic effects. Monitor for treatment failure of erythromycin.
warfarin	Decreases the metabolism of warfarin, resulting in an increased risk for warfarin toxicity	Monitor warfarin levels carefully. Monitor INR or PT frequently. Adjust warfarin dose as needed.

Assessment of Relevant Core Patient Variables

Health Status

In assessing a patient's health status before administering erythromycin, explore any history of hypersensitivity to erythromycin or other macrolide antibiotics because of the risk for cross-sensitivity.

Assess for hepatic or biliary dysfunction. Moreover, monitor hepatic function patients receiving prolonged treatment. Ilosone, the estolate salt of erythromycin, should not be used in patients with hepatic disease because of the potential for hepatotoxicity.

Review the patients' GI history, particularly because the normal flora of the colon may allow an overgrowth of *Clostridium* organisms. A toxin produced by *C. difficile* is a primary cause of antibiotic-associated colitis. Patients who develop diarrhea while taking or soon after taking erythromycin should be evaluated for potential antibiotic-associated pseudomembranous colitis.

Monitor the patient's hearing because high-dose therapy with erythromycin may cause a reversible loss of hearing, and patients with preexisting hearing impairment may be at especially great risk.

In addition, explore any possibility of cardiovascular disorder, specifically a history of torsades de pointes, because IV administration of erythromycin at a rate above 15 mg/min may place patients with such a history at risk for this arrhythmia.

Life Span and Gender

Evaluate the woman for pregnancy and lactation. Erythromycin should be used with caution in breast-feeding women because it is excreted in breast milk at about 50% of maternal plasma concentrations, which may induce diarrhea and superinfection in the infant. Consider the developmental level of the patient. Erythromycin lactobionate injection may contain benzyl alcohol as a preservative, which can cause toxicity in neonates. Infants less than 2 weeks of age are at risk for developing hypertrophic pyloric stenosis with erythromycin therapy.

Lifestyle, Diet, and Habits

Assess the patient's dietary habits to determine the likelihood that the patient will take erythromycin stearate at least 1 hour before or 2 hours after meals.

Environment

Be aware of the environment in which the drug will be administered. Oral or ophthalmic erythromycin may be given in any environment, whereas IV infusion should be given in a monitored setting.

Nursing Diagnoses and Outcomes

- Risk for Injury related to possible allergic reactions
  Desired outcome: *The patient will stop drug therapy and report any signs of allergic reaction immediately to the prescriber.*
- Diarrhea related to drug-induced GI upset
  Desired outcome: *The patient will avoid dehydration, maintain fluid intake, and contact the prescriber if diarrhea persists.*
- Risk for Infection related to potential for superinfection following drug therapy
  Desired outcome: *The patient will contact the provider if any signs of superinfection occur, for example, sore throat or fever.*

Planning and Intervention

Maximizing Therapeutic Effects

Reconstitute erythromycin with sterile water only. Diluents containing preservatives or organic salts should not be used. Prepared infusion solutions that are stored at room temperature must be used within 8 hours. Prepared solutions that are refrigerated must be used within 24 hours.

Evaluate culture and sensitivity reports to verify that erythromycin is the drug of choice. Moreover, administer erythromycin as prescribed, at around-the-clock intervals to increase effectiveness. Because food interferes with drug absorption, administer erythromycin stearate at least 1 hour before or 2 hours after meals. Other formulations of erythromycin may be given without regard to meals. If GI irritation occurs, however, erythromycin stearate may be administered with food. Each dose should be administered with a full glass of water, not with fruit juice.

Minimizing Adverse Effects

Provide small, frequent meals; mouth care; and ice chips to suck if stomatitis and sore mouth are problems. Additionally, regular monitoring is needed to ensure adequate hydration, with fluids provided to replace fluid lost with diarrhea. Because erythromycin can be very irritating to veins, it is important to administer IV infusions over 30 to 60 minutes. If pain persists, reduce the rate of infusion. If pain persists, ice may be applied and the prescriber notified.

Providing Patient and Family Education

- Encourage the patient to take the complete course of antibiotics.
- Explain safe drug handling and storage.
- Explain the importance of taking erythromycin around the clock to maintain a therapeutic drug level.
- Teach the patient the potential adverse effects and the measures to alleviate discomfort if such events occur.
- Advise the patient to take erythromycin on an empty stomach, unless GI distress is unbearable.
- Advise the patient to contact the prescriber if there is no improvement in 3 days.

Ongoing Assessment and Evaluation

Monitor for signs of allergic reactions, resolution of presenting signs and symptoms of infection, signs of superinfection, and for patients receiving IV erythromycin, signs of phlebitis or abscess formation. When therapy ends, the patient should be free of the initial infection. The patient will be adequately nourished and hydrated, and adverse effects will be resolved.

MEMORY CHIP

[P] Erythromycin

- Used for infections caused by gram-positive organisms. Less effective for gram-negative organisms.
- Major contraindication: hypersensitivity
- Most common adverse effect: GI distress
- Most serious adverse effects: Hepatotoxicity, QT prolongation, pseudomembranous colitis, and ventricular tachycardia
- Maximizing therapeutic effects: Administer on an empty stomach, unless GI distress is pronounced.
- Minimizing adverse effects: Provide small, frequent meals.
- Most important patient education: Complete the entire course of medication, even when feeling better.

Drugs Closely Related to [P] Erythromycin

Azithromycin

Azithromycin (Zithromax) is a semisynthetic macrolide antibiotic that is similar in structure to erythromycin. It is available in oral and IV formulations. Azithromycin is generally active against organisms that are also usually susceptible to erythromycin. It is not clear whether azithromycin, like erythromycin, is effective in treating diabetic gastroparesis. Azithromycin produces less GI intolerance than erythromycin does. It is unique in that it can reach exceptionally high levels in tissues, thus increasing its efficacy and duration of action. For this reason, it is administered only once a day.

Absorption of azithromycin *capsules* is decreased in the presence of food, and capsules should be given on an empty stomach. The absorption of azithromycin *suspension* is increased in the presence of foods, so much so that the serum concentration may be too high. For that reason, the suspension should be taken on an empty stomach. Conversely, azithromycin *tablets* have an increased absorption when given with a meal with high-fat content and may be given with or without food.

Because azithromycin is not metabolized, it should be used cautiously in patients with hepatic disease. Adverse effects, drug interactions, and patient management are similar to those for erythromycin.

Clarithromycin

Clarithromycin (Biaxin) is an oral macrolide antibiotic similar to erythromycin and azithromycin. Like azithromycin, clarithromycin penetrates tissues to a greater degree than erythromycin. Clarithromycin is generally active against organisms that are usually susceptible to erythromycin. These include most staphylococcal and streptococcal strains. In addition, clarithromycin is active against *Moraxella catarrhalis, Mycoplasma pneumoniae, Legionella* species, and *Chlamydia pneumoniae.* Clarithromycin inhibits *Mycobacterium avium* at concentrations achievable in lung tissue and is active against *Borrelia burgdorferi,* the cause of Lyme disease. Combined with omeprazole, clarithromycin is useful for *Helicobacter pylori*–associated peptic ulcer disease.

Clarithromycin is administered orally as a tablet or suspension. It is administered without regard to meals. To prepare the oral suspension, tap the bottle several times to loosen the powder, then add 5 mL distilled or purified water to bottles labeled as containing 125 mg/5 mL or 250 mg/5 mL, respectively, of clarithromycin. The preparation should be shaken vigorously before each administration. This drug is stable at room temperature for up to 14 days.

Clarithromycin is contraindicated during pregnancy. It is unknown whether clarithromycin is excreted in breast milk. It is used cautiously in patients with either hepatic or renal insufficiency because it is partially renally excreted.

Adverse effects, drug interactions, and patient management are similar to those associated with erythromycin.

Troleandomycin

Troleandomycin (Tao), a synthetic macrolide, is available only in oral form. It should not be used in any patient with hepatic impairment because it may cause hepatic injury. Troleandomycin inhibits cytochrome P-450 and thus can inhibit the metabolism of many drugs and increase their serum concentrations, resulting in increased risk for adverse or toxic effects. Adverse effects, drug interactions, and patient management are similar to those for erythromycin.

Dirithromycin

Dirithromycin (Dynabac), a newer oral macrolide, is also similar to erythromycin but is pharmacokinetically more effective. Dirithromycin's spectrum of activity is similar to that of erythromycin, and once-daily dosing is possible because of the extensive tissue distribution of the active dirithromycin metabolite, erythromycylamine. Adverse effects, drug interactions, and patient management are similar to those of erythromycin.

Drug Significantly Different From [P] Erythromycin

Telithromycin (Ketek) is the first drug in a new class of antibiotics called ketolides. A semisynthetic drug structurally similar to macrolides, telithromycin is approved to treat acute bacterial exacerbation of chronic bronchitis or acute bacterial sinusitis caused by *Streptococcus pneumoniae, Haemophilus influenzae,* or *Moraxella catarrhalis;* acute bacterial sinusitis caused by *Staphylococcus aureus;* and community-acquired pneumonia caused by *S. pneumoniae* (including multidrug-resistant isolates [MDRSP]), *H. influenzae, M. catarrhalis, Chlamydophila pneumoniae,* and *Mycoplasma pneumoniae.* Its advantages include once-daily dosing, short duration of administration (5 to 10 days), and its ability to accumulate rapidly in white blood cells, inflammatory fluid, and cells and tissues of the upper and lower respiratory tract at concentrations above the minimum inhibitory concentration (MIC) of these major respiratory pathogens.

Telithromycin is metabolized primarily by the liver. It is excreted by several pathways: 37% is metabolized by the liver, whereas 7% is excreted unchanged in feces, and 13% is excreted unchanged by the kidneys.

Contraindications to telithromycin use include a history of hypersensitivity to macrolide antibiotics. Telithromycin is also contraindicated for patients taking cisapride or pimozide, because coadministration may increase peak plasma concentrations of these drugs, resulting in clinically important increases in the QT interval. Telithromycin is also contra-

indicated for patients receiving certain antiarrhythmic agents. Telithromycin is contraindicated in cases of congenital prolongation of the QT interval, uncorrected hypokalemia and hypomagnesia, and clinically important bradycardia because these are considered prodysrhythmic conditions. Finally, telithromycin is contraindicated for patients with myasthenia gravis because the drug may induce a severe exacerbation, including life-threatening acute respiratory failure.

The adverse effect profile for telithromycin is similar to that for erythromycin, mainly nausea, diarrhea, headache, and dizziness. A potent CYP3A4 inhibitor, telithromycin has a long list of potential drug–drug interactions. Telithromycin is a pregnancy category C drug and is not recommended for patients under the age of 18 years.

C OXAZOLIDINONES

Oxazolidinones are the first new class of antibiotics developed specifically for treating methicillin-resistant *Staphylococcus aureus* (MRSA) infections. Linezolid (Zyvox) is the prototype for this new class of drugs.

NURSING MANAGEMENT OF THE PATIENT RECEIVING P LINEZOLID

Core Drug Knowledge

Pharmacotherapeutics

Linezolid is approved for use in treating bacteremia associated with vancomycin-resistant *Enterococcus faecium* or *E. faecalis* (VRE); complicated skin infections and nosocomial or community-acquired pneumonia caused by MRSA; and bacteremia associated with nosocomial or community-acquired pneumonia caused by penicillin-susceptible *Streptococcus pneumoniae.* Many hospitals require approval by the Infectious Diseases Committee before linezolid can be administered.

Pharmacokinetics

Linezolid is available in both oral and parenteral formulations. Oral linezolid is 100% bioavailable. This means that the IV and oral forms are interchangeable without making dosage adjustments. Oral linezolid is rapidly absorbed from the GI tract and is widely distributed. Food delays absorption but does not decrease peak plasma concentrations. Linezolid is partly metabolized in the liver and is excreted in urine. The half-life is approximately 5 hours.

Pharmacodynamics

Linezolid attacks bacteria by blocking the early stages of the process bacteria use to make proteins, whereas other antibiotics act at later stages of protein synthesis. This unique mechanism of action suggests that bacteria may not be able to develop resistance as quickly and that cross-resistance between linezolid and other antibiotics is less likely to occur.

Contraindications and Precautions

The only contraindication for linezolid is hypersensitivity. Linezolid oral suspension should be used with caution in patients with phenylketonuria because the linezolid oral suspension is formulated with aspartame, which supplies roughly 20 mg of phenylalanine in each 5-mL suspension. Other linezolid products do not contain phenylalanine. Linezolid is given cautiously to patients with pre-existing blood dyscrasias because it may suppress bone marrow function. For the same reason, it should be given cautiously to patients receiving other drugs known to suppress bone marrow function. Because linezolid is a nonselective inhibitor of monoamine oxidase (MAO), it should be used with caution in patients with hypertension, untreated hyperthyroid disease, severe cardiac disease, cerebrovascular disease, or pheochromocytoma. These patients have an increased risk for poor sequelae because linezolid-induced MAO inhibition will reduce the metabolism of pressor amines, which may increase blood pressure in these individuals. Linezolid is classified as an FDA pregnancy category C drug.

Adverse Effects

Linezolid is generally well tolerated. The most common adverse effects associated with linezolid therapy are diarrhea, headache, nausea, and vomiting, usually mild to moderate in intensity and limited in duration. Serious adverse effects include thrombocytopenia, elevated hepatic enzyme levels, and pseudomembranous colitis. Hypertension is another potentially serious adverse effect in people with existing hypertension, untreated hyperthyroid disease, severe cardiac disease, cerebrovascular disease, or pheochromocytoma. As with other antibiotics, superinfections may occur during linezolid treatment.

Drug Interactions

Because linezolid is a reversible, nonselective MAO inhibitor, most potential drug interactions are related to this action of the drug. Table 39.7 presents potential drug interactions.

Food and dietary interactions with nonselective MAO inhibitors can be serious. Foods containing tyramine and beverages containing caffeine or ethanol should be avoided.

Assessment of Relevant Core Patient Variables

Health Status

Elicit a complete history from the patient focusing on pre-existing medical conditions that require cautious use of linezolid. Evaluate the patient's current medications for drugs that may interact with linezolid. Communicate positive findings to the prescriber before administering linezolid.

Review the culture and sensitivity report to establish that linezolid is an appropriate therapy. For patients requiring therapy longer than 14 days, obtain a baseline CBC and liver function tests.

Life Span and Gender

Assess the patient for potential pregnancy or breast-feeding because linezolid is a pregnancy category C drug. Linezolid is not approved for use in children.

TABLE 39.7 Agents That Interact With P Linezolid

Interactants	Effect and Significance	Nursing Management
entacapone tolcapone	Monoamine oxidase (MAO) and catechol-O-methyltransferase (COMT) are the two major enzymes involved in the metabolism of catecholamines. It is theoretically possible that the coadministration of entacapone or tolcapone with linezolid would result in inhibition of normal catecholamine metabolism.	Do not administer linezolid within 14 d of entacapone or tolcapone administration.
levodopa	Concomitant use of nonselective MAO inhibitors (MAOIs) such as linezolid with levodopa can result in hypertensive crisis.	Do not administer linezolid within 14 d of levodopa administration.
MAOIs and drugs that possess MAOI-like activity • isocarboxazid • phenelzine • tranylcypromine • selegiline • furazolidone • procarbazine	Coadministration of these drugs with linezolid may result in hypertensive crisis, convulsions, or death.	Do not administer linezolid within 14 d of these drugs.
meperidine	When meperidine is given in combination with a MAOI, accumulation of serotonin may occur and may lead to severe cardiovascular and/or neurologic adverse reactions.	Avoid administration of meperidine within 14 d of linezolid therapy. Morphine is the preferred agent in emergency situations.
selective serotonin reuptake inhibitors (SSRIs)	SSRIs potentiate the action of serotonin by inhibiting its neuronal reuptake. Because monoamine oxidase type A deaminates serotonin, administration of a nonselective MAOI concurrently with an SSRI can lead to a serious reaction known as "serotonin syndrome."	Avoid coadministration of these drugs.
serotonin-receptor agonists • naratriptan • rizatriptan • sumatriptan • zolmitriptan	The MAO type A enzyme metabolizes serotonin. Non-selective MAOIs increase the plasma concentrations of these drugs and some of their active metabolites, thus increasing levels of serotonin. This interaction could lead to "serotonin syndrome."	Do not administer linezolid within 14 d of serotonin-receptor agonists.
Sympathomimetics or psycho-stimulants with sympathomimetic actions • phenylephrine • phenylpropanolamine • pseudoephedrine • amphetamine • dexfenfluramine • dextroamphetamine • fenfluramine • methylphenidate	Linezolid has been noted to enhance the pressor response of these drugs, resulting in a rise in systolic blood pressure.	Avoid these drugs in combination if possible. Monitor blood pressure during linezolid therapy. Teach the patient to avoid OTC medications used for coughs, colds, or weight loss.
tryptophan tyrosine	When used concomitantly with tryptophan, linezolid may cause the "serotonin syndrome."	Do not coadminister these drugs.

Lifestyle, Diet, and Habits

Ask the patient about dietary intake, focusing on foods that are rich in tyramine. Evaluate the use of caffeine from coffee, tea, or carbonated beverages. Evaluate for potential alcohol abuse because alcohol consumption during therapy increases the risk for a hypertensive crisis.

Because linezolid may interact with many OTC medications, assess for self-medicating of coughs, colds, allergies, or to achieve weight loss.

Environment

Be aware of the environment in which linezolid will be administered. Parenteral linezolid should be administered in an acute hospital setting. Oral linezolid may be administered in any setting.

Nursing Diagnoses and Outcomes

- Deficient Fluid Volume related to nausea, vomiting, and diarrhea from linezolid therapy
  Desired outcome: *The patient will remain well hydrated throughout therapy.*
- Risk for Injury related to thrombocytopenia and pseudomembranous colitis
  Desired outcome: *The patient will remain free from injury and contact the health care provider immediately if any signs of bleeding or abdominal pain occur.*
- Risk for Injury related to hypertensive crisis
  Desired outcome: *The patient will remain normotensive by adhering to antihypertensive therapy and limiting foods or beverages with tyramine, caffeine, or alcohol.*

Planning and Intervention

Maximizing Therapeutic Effects

Administer linezolid at evenly spaced intervals throughout the day (Box 39.1).

Minimizing Adverse Effects

To avoid hypertensive crisis, monitor the patient's intake of food or beverages containing tyramine, caffeine, or alcohol. Serial blood pressure readings should be obtained throughout therapy.

Providing Patient and Family Education

- Explain the importance of taking linezolid exactly as prescribed for the entire course of treatment, even if the patient feels better.
- Explain the need for periodic laboratory tests if therapy is anticipated to last longer than 14 days.
- Explain dietary restrictions, focusing on food or beverages containing tyramine, caffeine, or alcohol.
- Explain the importance of not using OTC drugs that may interact with linezolid.
- Explain that linezolid may interact with many types of prescription medications. The patient should contact the prescriber before taking any other medications, even those prescribed by another health care professional.
- Teach the signs and symptoms of thrombocytopenia and pseudomembranous colitis. Advise the patient to contact the prescriber immediately if any symptoms occur.

Ongoing Assessment and Evaluation

Monitor for efficacy of treatment and the resolution of the presenting infection. Monitor for signs and symptoms of thrombocytopenia and pseudomembranous colitis and advise the prescriber if any occur. Monitor the patient's blood pressure and intake of foods or beverages containing tyramine, caffeine, or alcohol. Coordinate serial CBC and liver enzyme tests if therapy lasts more than 14 days.

When treatment ends, the initial infection should be resolved. The patient should be adequately nourished and hydrated, and any adverse drug effects should be resolved.

C STREPTOGRAMINS

Streptogramins are the newest class of antibiotics, specifically designed to eradicate "superbugs" resistant to other antibiotics. Quinupristin and dalfopristin are the only streptogramins approved for use in the United States by the FDA; they are marketed as a combination drug quinupristin/dalfopristin (Synercid).

NURSING MANAGEMENT OF THE PATIENT RECEIVING P QUINUPRISTIN/DALFOPRISTIN

Core Drug Knowledge

Pharmacotherapeutics

Quinupristin/dalfopristin is indicated for the treatment of serious or life-threatening infections associated with vancomycin-resistant *Enterococcus faecium* (VREF) bacteremia and for complicated skin and skin-structure infections caused by *Staphylococcus aureus* and *Streptococcus pyogenes*. In many hospitals, prescribing quinupristin/dalfopristin requires Infectious Diseases Committee approval to avoid inducing resistance. See the Critical Thinking Scenario: Explaining the Drug Selection Process.

Pharmacokinetics

Quinupristin/dalfopristin is administered by IV route only. Both drugs are converted to several active major metabolites and are excreted primarily through bile. The onset is rapid, duration of action is unknown, and elimination half-life is approximately 1 hour.

Pharmacodynamics

Quinupristin/dalfopristin inhibits bacterial protein synthesis by irreversibly blocking ribosome functioning. When used as single agents, these drugs are bacteriostatic. When used in combination, quinupristin/dalfopristin has up to 16 times the activity of each agent alone and is bacteriocidal against most organisms.

Contraindications and Precautions

The only contraindication to use of quinupristin/dalfopristin is hypersensitivity. It should be used cautiously in patients with decreased hepatic function.

FOCUS ON RESEARCH

Box 39.1 Decreasing the Incidence of Nosocomial MRSA

Afif, W., Huor, P., Brassard, P., et al. (2002). Compliance with methicillin-resistant *Staphylococcus aureus* precautions in a teaching hospital. *American Journal of Infection Control, 30*(7), 430–433.

The Study

This observational study was designed to determine the rate of adherence among health care providers to precautions against transmitting methicillin-resistant *Staphylococcus aureus* (MRSA) during routine patient care. The researchers anonymously observed 184 nurses, 41 physicians, 19 occupational and physical therapists, 102 unlicensed health care assistants, 28 housekeeping personnel, 65 other health care workers, and 49 visitors. Adherence to MRSA precautions was measured by observing whether participants used gowns and gloves appropriately and whether they practiced adequate hand hygiene.

Compared with nurses, occupational and physical therapists were more adherent to regulations; however, physicians, unlicensed health care assistants, housekeeping personnel, other health care workers, and visitors were less compliant. Overall, the average adherence was only 28%.

Nursing Implications

MRSA causes serious infections commonly seen in clinical settings. Health care providers have been identified as a primary route of transmission (Boyce, 2001). Current pharmacotherapy for MRSA infection includes vancomycin, linezolid, quinupristin/dalfopristin, and daptomycin. Unfortunately, these drugs are not always successful in eradicating this tenacious pathogen, and the death rate from these infections ranges from 20% to 50% (Blot, 2002). In 2003, the Centers for Disease Control developed the following guidelines to control the spread of MRSA:

Patient Considerations

- Place the patient with MRSA in a private room. When a private room is not available, the patient may be placed in a room with patients who have active infection with MRSA but no other infections (a practice called cohorting).
- Limit the movement and transport of the patient from the room for essential purposes only.
- Ensure that patient-care items, bedside equipment, and frequently touched surfaces receive daily cleaning.
- Dedicate the use of noncritical patient-care equipment and items, such as stethoscope, sphygmomanometer, bedside commode, or electronic rectal thermometer, to a single patient (or cohort) infected or colonized with MRSA and avoid sharing such items between patients.

Handwashing

- Wash hands after touching blood, body fluids, secretions, excretions, and contaminated items, whether or not gloves are worn.
- Wash hands immediately after gloves are removed, between patient contacts, and when otherwise indicated, to avoid transferring microorganisms to other patients or environments.
- Wash hands between tasks and procedures on the same patient to prevent cross-contamination of different body sites.

Gloving

- Wear gloves (clean nonsterile gloves are adequate) when touching blood, body fluids, secretions, excretions, and contaminated items.
- Put on clean gloves just before touching mucous membranes and nonintact skin.
- Remove gloves promptly after use, before touching noncontaminated items and environmental surfaces, and before going to another patient.
- Wash hands immediately after glove removal to avoid transferring microorganisms to other patients or environments.

Masking

- Wear a mask and eye protection or a face shield to protect mucous membranes of the eyes, nose, and mouth during procedures and patient-care activities that are likely to generate splashes or sprays of blood, body fluids, secretions, and excretions.

Gowning

- Wear a gown (a clean nonsterile gown is adequate) to protect skin and prevent soiling your clothes during procedures and patient-care activities that are likely to generate splashes or sprays of blood, body fluids, secretions, and excretions or otherwise soil clothing.

Appropriate Device Handling

- Handle used patient-care equipment soiled with blood, body fluids, secretions, and excretions in a manner that prevents exposure to skin and mucous membranes, contamination of clothing, and transfer of microorganisms to other patients and environments.
- Ensure that reusable equipment is not used to care for another patient until it has been appropriately cleaned and reprocessed and that single-use items are properly discarded.

Appropriate Handling of Laundry

- Handle, transport, and process used linen soiled with blood, body fluids, secretions, and excretions in a manner that prevents exposure to skin and mucous membranes, contamination of clothing, and transfer of microorganisms to other patients and environments.

MEMORY CHIP

P Linezolid

- Used for infections caused by vancomycin-resistant *Enterococcus faecium* or *E. faecalis* (VRE), methicillin-resistant *Staphylococcus aureus* (MRSA), and penicillin-susceptible *Streptococcus pneumoniae.*
- Major contraindication: hypersensitivity
- Most common adverse effects: nausea, vomiting, headache, and diarrhea.
- Most serious adverse effects: thrombocytopenia and pseudomembranous colitis.
- Maximizing therapeutic effects: Administer at evenly spaced intervals.
- Minimizing adverse effects: Monitor the patient's intake of foods and beverages containing tyramine, caffeine, or alcohol.
- Most important patient education: Teach the patient dietary restrictions and the importance of not taking any medications, including OTC medications, without the health care provider's approval.

Adverse Effects

Serious adverse effects include pseudomembranous colitis, superinfection, and hepatotoxicity. Common adverse effects include injection site reaction, injection site pain, nausea, vomiting, diarrhea, thrombophlebitis, arthralgias and myalgias, rash, pruritus, and hyperbilirubinemia.

Drug Interactions

Quinupristin/dalfopristin is a potent inhibitor of CYP3A4, a cytochrome of P-450. Serum concentrations of drugs metabolized through this pathway, such as cyclosporine, midazolam, and nifedipine, may be increased. Table 39.8 presents additional drugs metabolized through this pathway, which may therefore interact with quinupristin/dalfopristin.

Assessment of Relevant Core Patient Variables

Health Status

Elicit a complete medical history to evaluate for potential contraindications or precautions to the administration of quinupristin/dalfopristin. Be especially alert for a history of liver dysfunction. Evaluate the patient's current medications for drugs that are metabolized through the CYP3A4 enzyme system. Be sure to communicate any positive findings to the prescriber before administering this drug.

Coordinate baseline liver function and bilirubin tests on blood drawn before administration of quinupristin/dalfopristin. Coordinate liver function and bilirubin tests to be done twice weekly for the first week of therapy and once weekly thereafter.

Life Span and Gender

Evaluate the patient for pregnancy and lactation. Quinupristin/dalfopristin is an FDA pregnancy category B drug. It is unknown whether quinupristin/dalfopristin is secreted in breast milk. Consider the ratio of benefits to potential risks for the pediatric patient. Quinupristin/dalfopristin has not been approved for use in children; however, it has been administered to children in emergency situations.

Environment

Be aware of the environment in which the drug will be administered. Quinupristin/dalfopristin should be administered in an acute hospital setting. Review the policy of the parent institution and be sure that approval by the Infectious Disease Committee is documented if needed.

Nursing Diagnoses and Outcomes

- Pain related to IV administration
  Desired outcome: *The patient will inform you immediately should pain at the injection site occur.*
- Diarrhea related to potential pseudomembranous colitis
  Desired outcome: *The patient will remain well hydrated throughout therapy and report any diarrhea immediately.*
- Risk for Injury related to potential superinfection or hepatotoxicity
  Desired outcome: *The patient will remain free of injury throughout therapy.*
- Risk for Impaired Skin Integrity related to rash or pruritus.
  Desired outcome: *The patient will report itching or rash immediately to minimize potential for infection.*

Planning and Intervention

Maximizing Therapeutic Effects

Quinupristin/dalfopristin should not be administered with any other medications through a Y-site infusion unless compatibility with both the drug and diluent are established. The line should be flushed before and after administration with 5% dextrose and water (D_5W) to minimize venous irritation. *DO NOT FLUSH* the IV line with saline or heparin after administering quinupristin/dalfopristin because this procedure is not compatible with these solutions.

Minimizing Adverse Effects

Because injection site problems are very common with the administration of quinupristin/dalfopristin, these drugs should be administered in a peripherally inserted central catheter (PICC) or central line whenever possible. If administered peripherally, they should be diluted in 250 mL of D_5W and infused over 1 hour.

Providing Patient and Family Education

Because quinupristin/dalfopristin is used for serious life-threatening infections, the patient may not be able to comprehend patient teaching at the onset of therapy. When appropriate, teaching should include the following:

- Encourage the patient to report any pain during infusion.
- Teach the patient the potential adverse effects associated with quinupristin/dalfopristin such as arthralgias and myalgias, rash, or pruritus.
- Advise the patient to report cough, congestion, rash, or feeling warm because these may indicate a superinfection.
- Advise the patient to report any diarrhea immediately to avert pseudomembranous colitis, if possible.

TABLE 39.8 Agents That Interact With P Quinupristin/Dalfopristin

Interactants	Effect and Significance	Nursing Management
P-450 3A4 drugs alfentanil alosetron alprazolam aprepitant atorvastatin bortezomib buprenorphine calcium-channel blockers carbamazepine cerivastatin clarithromycin delavirdine diazepam disopyramide dofetilide donepezil erythromycin ethinyl estradiol gefitinib fexofenadine imatinib indinavir lidocaine lovastatin methylprednisolone midazolam nevirapine nifedipine norethindrone quinidine ritonavir saquinavir simvastatin sirolimus tacrolimus triazolam trimetrexate vinca alkaloids zonisamide	Quinupristin/dalfopristin inhibits cytochrome P-450 3A4 and will decrease the elimination of drugs metabolized by this pathway. This results in an increased risk for toxicity and adverse effects.	Avoid these drugs if possible. Monitor for toxicity if coadministration is unavoidable.

Ongoing Assessment and Evaluation

During infusion, monitor the IV site for signs of infiltration, edema, or phlebitis. Question the patient regarding pain at the injection site. During therapy, monitor for signs and symptoms of hyperbilirubinemia or hepatotoxicity. Monitor for diarrhea. Pseudomembranous colitis may develop from a toxin produced by *C. difficile*. Therefore, this diagnosis should be considered in any patient who complains of diarrhea after administration of quinupristin/dalfopristin.

At the end of therapy, the initial infection should be resolved. The patient will be adequately nourished and hydrated and will have normal liver function and bilirubin test results, and any adverse effects will be resolved.

C TETRACYCLINES

The tetracyclines (TCNs) were developed as semisynthetic antibiotics based on the structure of a common soil mold. They are broad-spectrum antibiotics that affect both gram-positive and gram-negative bacteria. The first syllables of their name derive from the four-ring structure common to all of these drugs. Over the years, major resistance has developed to tetracyclines, and less toxic, more effective drugs have been discovered. Still, tetracyclines are effective against certain organisms for which they remain the drug of choice. Tetracyclines include tetracycline, doxycycline, minocycline, and demeclocycline. Table 39.9 provides a summary of tetracycline antibiotics. The prototype tetracycline is tetracycline.

MEMORY CHIP

[P] Quinupristin/Dalfopristin

- Used for vancomycin-resistant *Enterococcus faecium* bacteremia and for complicated skin and skin-structure infections due to *Staphylococcus aureus*
- Major contraindication: hypersensitivity
- Most common adverse effects: injection site pain, swelling, or phlebitis
- Most serious adverse effect: hepatotoxicity
- Maximizing therapeutic effects: Do not use saline or heparin to flush the solution because they are not compatible with this drug.
- Minimizing adverse effects: Administer through PICC or central line whenever possible.
- Most important patient education: Teach the patient about the potential for injection-site adverse effects and about the importance of notifying the nurse if injection site pain occurs.

CRITICAL THINKING SCENARIO

Explaining the drug selection process

Georgia James, age 64 years, is admitted to your unit with a diagnosis of pneumonia. She has just completed her first dose of IV gentamicin when her granddaughter arrives. The granddaughter comes to the nurses' station and is very upset. She states in a very loud voice, "Why is my grandmother getting gentamicin? I saw on the Internet that there is a new type of drug for pneumonia called syner-something. Why isn't she getting the strongest kind of medication?" How would you handle this situation?

TABLE 39.9 Summary of Selected (C) Tetracycline Antibiotics

Drug (Trade) Name	Selected Indications	Route and Dosage Range	Pharmacokinetics
[P] tetracycline (Sumycin; *Canadian:* Apo-Tetra)	Various infections of varying severities (e.g., *Rickettsiae, Mycoplasma pneumoniae, Haemophilus ducreyi, Escherichia coli, Streptococcus pneumoniae, Staphylococcus aureus, Klebsiella, H. influenzae, Vibrio cholerae, Neisseria gonorrhoeae, Treponema pallidum,* and more)	*Adult:* PO, 500 mg bid or 250 mg qid *Child ≥ 8 y:* PO, 25–50 mg/kg in four equal doses	*Onset:* PO, varies *Duration:* Varies $t_{1/2}$: 6–12 h
doxycycline (Vibramycin; *Canadian:* Apo-Doxy)	Same as above and for antidiuretic hormone-secreting tumors	*Adult:* PO, 200 mg initially; maintenance, 100 mg/d; IV, 200 mg/d initially, then 100–200 mg depending on infection *Child 8 y:* PO, 4.4 mg/kg divided in two doses initially; maintenance, 2.2 mg/kg in one or two doses per day; IV, 4.4 mg/kg on first day in one or two infusions depending on infection	*Onset:* PO, varies; IV rapid *Duration:* 24–36 h $t_{1/2}$: 15–25 h
minocycline (Minocin; *Canadian:* Alti-Minocycline)	Same as tetracycline and *Neisseria meningitidis*	*Adult:* PO, 200 mg initially followed by 100 mg q12h; IV, 200 mg followed by 100 mg q12h not to exceed 400 mg/d *Child > 8 y:* PO, 4 mg/kg initially, followed with 2 mg/kg q12h; IV, 4 mg/kg followed by 2 mg/kg q12h	*Onset:* PO, varies; IV, rapid *Duration:* 24–36 h $t_{1/2}$: 11–18 h
demeclocycline (Declomycin)	Same as tetracycline	*Adult:* PO, 600 mg in four doses of 150 mg each *Child > 8 y:* PO, 6–12 mg/kg in two to four doses	*Onset:* Varies *Duration:* 18–20 h $t_{1/2}$: 12–16 h

NURSING MANAGEMENT OF THE PATIENT RECEIVING P TETRACYCLINE

Core Drug Knowledge

Pharmacotherapeutics

Oral tetracycline (Sumycin) has been in use since 1953. Initially, it was effective against most bacteria, but now it has substantial resistance patterns. It is indicated for infections caused by *Rickettsia* species, *Mycoplasma pneumoniae,* and *Chlamydia trachomatis*. It is also used to treat brucellosis, cholera, anthrax, Lyme disease, and *H. pylori* infection. Topical tetracycline is used to manage periodontal disease.

Tetracycline is also available as an ophthalmic drug to treat superficial ocular lesions due to susceptible microorganisms and as a prophylactic drug against ophthalmia neonatorum caused by *Neisseria gonorrhoeae* and *C. trachomatis*. A topical preparation is also available to treat acne vulgaris and minor skin infections.

Pharmacokinetics

Tetracycline is administered orally because it is no longer available for parenteral administration. In the fasting state, tetracycline is about 75% to 77% absorbed. Absorption takes place mainly in the stomach and upper intestine. As the dosage is increased, the percentage absorbed decreases. Absorption is decreased in the presence of food, iron preparations, and antacids containing calcium, magnesium, and aluminum salts.

Tetracycline is widely distributed into body fluids, including CSF. Tetracycline tends to concentrate in bone, liver, tumors, spleen, and teeth. It crosses the placenta and is distributed in breast milk. Tetracycline is about 65% bound to plasma protein and does not appear to undergo hepatic metabolism; however, it undergoes enterohepatic circulation and is excreted in the feces by way of the bile. The primary excretion route is the kidney. About 60% of a dose is excreted unchanged from both routes. The serum half-life of tetracycline is between 6 and 12 hours in adults with normal renal function but is greatly increased in patients with severely impaired renal function.

Tetracycline periodontal fibers are inserted into periodontal pockets. The fiber releases tetracycline in vitro at a rate of approximately 2 μg/cm per hour. Tetracycline is released at this continuous rate for 10 days at concentrations far exceeding inhibitory concentrations for most periodontal organisms.

Pharmacodynamics

The tetracyclines are bacteriostatic; they inhibit or retard the growth of bacteria but do not kill them. They retard bacterial growth by inhibiting protein synthesis in sensitive bacteria and by preventing cell division and replication. Like other antibiotics, their effect on the body is indirect.

Contraindications and Precautions

Tetracycline is contraindicated in patients with a known allergy to tetracyclines or to tartrazine (specific oral preparations contain tartrazine) and during pregnancy and lactation. Tetracycline should be used with caution in children younger than 8 years and in patients with hepatic and renal dysfunction. The ophthalmic preparation is contraindicated if the patient has a fungal, mycobacterial, or viral ocular infection.

Adverse Effects

The major adverse effects of tetracycline therapy involve the GI tract and include nausea, vomiting, diarrhea, abdominal pain, glossitis, dysphagia, damage to the teeth, and, in rare cases, hepatic toxicity and fatty liver. Like other broad-spectrum antibiotics, tetracycline has a high potential to cause superinfections.

Patients with kidney dysfunction are at risk for azotemia, especially patients with pre-existing renal dysfunction. Dermatologic effects include photosensitivity and rash. Local pain and a stinging sensation with topical or ocular application are also fairly common. Other less frequently seen effects include hemolytic anemia and suppression of bone marrow function. Hypersensitivity reactions have been reported to range from urticaria to anaphylaxis and include intracranial hypertension.

Drug Interactions

The effectiveness of penicillin G decreases if it is taken concurrently with tetracyclines. If this combination is used, the dosage of the penicillin will have to be increased. Oral contraceptives may be less effective if taken with tetracycline. Patients taking oral contraceptives should be advised to use an additional form of birth control while receiving tetracycline. For more information on drug interactions, see Table 39.10.

Assessment of Relevant Core Patient Variables

Health Status

Follow the same guidelines for evaluating health status as those for a patient receiving penicillin. Assess for known allergies to any drug with a name ending in the suffix "cycline." Additionally, closely evaluate the renal and hepatic status of patients prescribed tetracycline. Anuric patients should not receive tetracycline, and the dosage should be decreased in patients with renal insufficiency. If renal impairment exists, even usual doses may lead to excessive systemic accumulation of tetracycline, resulting in liver or kidney toxicity.

If the dermatologic preparation of tetracycline is being used, the status of the affected area should be noted and recorded carefully to allow a baseline for evaluating the drug's effects.

Life Span and Gender

Evaluate women for potential pregnancy because tetracycline is an FDA pregnancy category D drug. Because the tetracyclines bind to calcium in developing teeth and bones, women in the second and third trimesters of pregnancy should not take this drug. In babies born to mothers who take tetracyclines during pregnancy, mottled and discolored deciduous teeth may develop. To prevent damage to the developing permanent teeth, tetracycline should not be given to children younger than 8 years old.

Lifestyle, Diet, and Habits

Because many OTC drugs contain elements that may decrease the absorption of tetracycline, obtain an OTC drug history from the patient or an appropriate caregiver. Explore

TABLE 39.10 Agents That Interact With P Tetracycline

Interactants	Effect and Significance	Nursing Management
Antacids aluminum salts bismuth salts calcium salts iron salts magnesium salts zinc salts	Tetracycline forms an insoluble chelate with antacids, decreasing absorption and serum levels of either or both.	Avoid simultaneous administration. Advise patient to separate administration by 3–4 h.
Anticoagulants	Elimination of vitamin K–producing gut bacteria by tetracycline may increase the activity of anticoagulants.	Monitor anticoagulant parameter frequently. Instruct patient regarding the early signs and symptoms of bleeding.
digoxin	In some patients, digoxin is metabolized by bacteria in the GI tract. Tetracycline may reverse the process by altering GI flora, allowing more digoxin to be absorbed and increasing digoxin levels.	Monitor digoxin levels. Monitor patient for signs of digoxin toxicity.
insulin	Tetracycline may increase extrapancreatic response to insulin, resulting in hypoglycemia.	Monitor diabetic patient's blood glucose frequently.
Milk and dairy products	Foods such as milk and dairy products contain calcium, which forms poorly absorbed chelates with tetracyclines.	Administer tetracycline at least 1 h before or 2 h after meals.
methoxyflurane	Tetracycline may induce biotransformation and impairment of renal excretion of toxic metabolites of methoxyflurane, resulting in an increased risk of nephrotoxicity.	Avoid this combination.
Oral contraceptives	Tetracyclines may suppress intestinal flora, which provides an enzyme essential for enterohepatic recirculation for certain oral contraceptives. This may result in a decreased contraceptive plasma level.	Advise patients taking oral contraceptives to use an additional method of birth control while taking tetracyclines.
Penicillins	The bacteriostatic action of tetracyclines may impair the bactericidal activity of penicillins.	Avoid combination therapy.
Urinary alkalinizers	This combination may alter tubular reabsorption of tetracycline, resulting in a decreased absorption of tetracycline.	Separate administration of these drugs by 3–4 h. Monitor for efficacy of tetracycline therapy. Tetracycline dosage may need to be increased.

the dietary habits of the patient because tetracycline is not absorbed effectively if taken with food or dairy products.

Environment

Assess for the patient's potential to be outdoors while taking tetracycline. Because this drug causes photosensitivity, the patient should be taught to avoid direct sunlight, and if going outdoors is unavoidable, the patient should be encouraged to wear appropriate cover-up clothing, hat, and sunglasses, plus a sunscreen that has a sun protection factor (SPF) of at least 15.

Nursing Diagnoses and Outcomes

- Risk for Injury related to potential superinfection or allergic drug reaction
  Desired outcome: *The patient will experience no new infection and no preventable allergic reaction related to tetracycline.*
- Diarrhea related to drug-induced GI effects
  Desired outcome: *The patient will report any incidence of diarrhea and follow the prescriber's recommendation.*
- Imbalanced Nutrition: Less than Body Requirements related to adverse GI effects of nausea, vomiting, diarrhea, and altered taste
  Desired outcome: *The patient will maintain dietary intake to provide adequate nutrition.*
- Risk for Impaired Skin Integrity related to drug-induced photosensitivity
  Desired outcome: *The patient will dress appropriately and take adequate precautionary measures while outdoors to avoid unnecessary sunburn.*

Planning and Intervention

Maximizing Therapeutic Effects

To judge the efficacy of ongoing treatment, evaluate results of initial culture and sensitivity tests done on samples from the infection site. Make sure that the patient receives tetracycline

as prescribed, divided around the clock to increase effectiveness. To maximize absorption, oral preparations should be administered on an empty stomach either 1 hour before or 2 hours after any meals or other drugs. It is optimal to continue drug therapy for at least 7 to 10 days.

Minimizing Adverse Effects

Provide small, frequent meals; mouth care; and ice chips or sugarless candy to suck if stomatitis and sore mouth are problems. Monitor the patient to ensure that adequate fluids are given to replace fluid lost with diarrhea. Patients should also be reminded of the potential for photosensitivity and the need to wear protective clothing and a sunscreen with a minimum 15 SPF.

Caution patients about taking outdated tetracycline. The shelf life of tetracycline is limited, and ingestion of outdated tetracycline has been associated with the development of nausea, vomiting, and renal failure. These reactions are thought to be a result of the effects of degradation products.

Providing Patient and Family Education

- Explain that tetracycline is one drug in a class of drugs. It is important that patients understand that they should not take this drug if they have ever had a reaction to a drug with a name that ends with "cycline."
- Advise women of childbearing age that tetracycline should not be taken during pregnancy or breast-feeding.
- Explain that tetracycline is prescribed for a particular infection and should not be used to self-medicate or treat any other infection.
- Emphasize that this drug should not be given to any other person, especially a child, and that it must be kept out of the reach of children.
- Advise the patient to complete the full course of drug therapy, even if the patient feels better, and to avoid taking any outdated tetracycline because it may cause liver damage.
- Advise the patient to take tetracycline on an empty stomach, with water and not dairy products. Patients should also be instructed to take forgotten doses as soon as they remember, but not if it is almost time for the next dose.
- Instruct the patient to call the prescriber if the symptoms do not improve in 3 days.
- Explain the potential adverse effects of tetracycline and the potential remedies for these discomforts. Measures to relieve GI upset include taking small, frequent meals if the patient experiences GI distress and increasing fluid intake for diarrhea. Patients with a sore mouth or throat should be advised to suck on ice chips or hard candy.
- Teach the patient signs and symptoms of superinfection, such as discoloration of the tongue, fatigue, easy bruising, or vaginal discharge in women. Caution the patient about the potential for photosensitivity and the importance of staying out of direct sunlight and wearing sunscreen.
- Advise women who use oral contraceptives to use a backup method of contraception while taking tetracycline.

Ongoing Assessment and Evaluation

Monitor the site of infection and compare it with presenting signs and symptoms throughout the course of drug therapy. Failure to resolve these signs and symptoms may indicate a treatment failure. Also, monitor the patient to ensure that the full course of therapy is completed.

Monitor renal status to detect and prevent hepatotoxicity and to observe for any signs of superinfection. Notify the provider immediately if they occur.

At the end of therapy, the patient should be free of the initial infection. The patient will have maintained adequate nutrition and hydration, and any adverse effects will be resolved.

Drugs Closely Related to [P] Tetracycline

Doxycycline

Doxycycline (Vibramycin) is a new type of tetracycline. It has the same pharmacotherapeutics as tetracycline and is used specifically for bacterial enteritis and Lyme disease. Taken orally, it is better absorbed than tetracycline, even in the presence of food and dairy products. It is excreted mainly through feces, unlike the other tetracyclines. Because of its excretion pattern, doxycycline is useful in patients with compromised renal function. Its half-life is longer than that of tetracycline, allowing for twice-daily dosing. Contraindications, adverse effects, drug interactions, and patient management are similar to those for tetracycline.

Minocycline

Minocycline (Minocin) is another fairly new tetracycline. Like doxycycline, minocycline has a long half-life and has minimal renal clearance. In addition to sharing the utility of other tetracyclines, minocycline is also used to treat meningococcal carrier states of *Neisseria meningitidis*. Minocycline is also useful in decreasing the symptoms of rheumatoid arthritis.

Minocycline may cause vestibular toxicity with symptoms of dizziness, lightheadedness, or vertigo. Patients should be cautioned to assess for these symptoms before driving a motor vehicle or performing hazardous tasks. Contraindications, other adverse effects, drug interactions, and patient management are similar to those for tetracycline.

MEMORY CHIP

[P] Tetracycline

- Used for *Rickettsia, Mycoplasma pneumoniae,* chlamydia, and acne
- Major contraindications: pregnancy, breast-feeding, and in children younger than 8 years of age
- Most common adverse effects: discoloration of teeth, nausea, vomiting, and photosensitivity
- Most serious adverse effect: azotemia
- Maximizing therapeutic effects: Administer at evenly spaced intervals on an empty stomach.
- Minimizing adverse effects: Give frequent small meals and increase mouth care when GI distress is present.
- Most important patient education: Teach the patient to complete the entire course of medication, despite feeling better. Teach the patient to keep medication out of the reach of children.

Demeclocycline

Demeclocycline (Declomycin) is used for treating antidiuretic hormone (ADH)–secreting tumors. It inhibits ADH-induced water reabsorption in the kidneys, resulting in diuresis. For that reason, it has also been associated with the development of a nephrogenic diabetes insipidus syndrome (polyuria, polydipsia, and weakness) in patients on long-term therapy. This syndrome is dose dependent and is reversible when the drug is discontinued.

Demeclocycline is also associated with an increased risk for photosensitivity. This reaction is characterized by severe burns on sun-exposed skin. Patients at highest risk are those taking moderate to high doses of demeclocycline. Patients must be advised to remain indoors and to take precautions when outdoor activity is unavoidable. Contraindications, other adverse effects, drug interactions, and patient management are similar to those for tetracycline.

C MISCELLANEOUS ANTIBIOTICS THAT AFFECT PROTEIN SYNTHESIS

Miscellaneous antibiotics include chloramphenicol and spectinomycin. Chloramphenicol is the prototypical miscellaneous antibiotic. In 1947, chloramphenicol was isolated from *Streptomyces venezuelae* and used to treat large outbreaks of typhus. It is now available synthetically as chloramphenicol, chloramphenicol palmitate, or chloramphenicol succinate.

NURSING MANAGEMENT OF THE PATIENT RECEIVING P CHLORAMPHENICOL

Core Drug Knowledge

Pharmacotherapeutics

Chloramphenicol is a true broad-spectrum antibiotic. It is active against a wide range of gram-positive and gram-negative bacteria, many anaerobic bacteria, *Bacteroides* species, and *Salmonella* species. However, it is inactive against fungi.

Chloramphenicol is relatively toxic and so is reserved for use in serious infections against which other antibiotics have been ineffective or in patients who cannot take safer drugs because of resistance or allergies. It is the drug of choice for treating meningitis caused by *Streptococcus pneumoniae, Neisseria meningitidis,* or *Haemophilus influenzae.* It is also used in treating brain abscesses, rickettsial infections, and acute typhoid fever.

Pharmacokinetics

Chloramphenicol base is administered orally; chloramphenicol succinate is administered intravenously. For chloramphenicol succinate to be active, it must be hydrolyzed to free chloramphenicol. Free chloramphenicol is rapidly absorbed from the GI tract. Peak action occurs within 1 to 3 hours. Peak concentrations rise with repeated administration. The goal is to keep plasma concentrations below 25 μg/mL to decrease the risk for adverse hematologic effects. Plasma concentration levels of chloramphenicol are increased in patients with hepatic and renal dysfunction and in premature or newborn infants with immature systems.

Chloramphenicol is widely distributed throughout most body tissues and fluids, with highest concentrations in the liver and kidneys. Chloramphenicol can reach substantial CSF concentrations, especially in patients with inflamed meninges. In adults with adequate renal and hepatic function, the plasma half-life for chloramphenicol is 1.5 to 4.1 hours.

Following oral administration, between 5% and 15% of chloramphenicol is excreted unchanged in the urine by glomerular filtration, and the remainder is excreted by tubular secretion, mostly as inactive metabolites. Small amounts are excreted unchanged in the bile and feces.

Pharmacodynamics

Chloramphenicol is usually bacteriostatic but may be bactericidal in high concentrations or against more susceptible organisms, such as *H. influenzae* and *S. pneumoniae.* It works by inhibiting the protein synthesis of bacterial cells. Chloramphenicol also inhibits mitochondrial protein synthesis in both bacterial and human cells. In humans, the protein synthesis of rapidly proliferating cells, such as erythrocytes, may be affected. This effect may explain the mechanism of reversible depression of bone marrow function associated with chloramphenicol therapy.

Contraindications and Precautions

Chloramphenicol should not be given to patients who have had known toxic reactions to the drug because some fatal reactions have occurred. It should not be used systemically for minor infections because of the potential for serious toxicity. Chloramphenicol is also contraindicated in breast-feeding women because it can suppress bone marrow function in breast-feeding infants.

Chloramphenicol should be given with extreme caution to pregnant women, infants, and children. Other patients at high risk during chloramphenicol therapy include patients with hepatic disease, renal impairment, glucose-6-phosphate dehydrogenase (G6PD) deficiency, and acute intermittent porphyria.

Chloramphenicol should be used with caution in patients with depressed bone marrow function and in those who have received cytotoxic drug therapy or radiation therapy. Chloramphenicol can cause dose-related depression of bone marrow function and an idiosyncratic aplastic anemia.

Chloramphenicol should be used with caution in patients with dental disease. Chloramphenicol can cause myelosuppression, and risk for infection may be increased. Dental work should be performed before initiating chloramphenicol therapy or deferred until blood counts return to normal.

Ophthalmic and topical chloramphenicol should not be used continuously because such use could lead to overgrowth of nonsusceptible organisms, including fungi. The drug should be discontinued if superinfection occurs. Prolonged or repeated use of topical chloramphenicol should be avoided because the drug could be absorbed systemically, resulting in marrow hypoplasia, aplastic anemia, and possibly death.

Otic preparations of chloramphenicol should not be used in the presence of a tympanic membrane perforation. Ototoxicity may occur if chloramphenicol enters the middle ear.

Adverse Effects

A serious and potentially life-threatening adverse effect of chloramphenicol is "gray baby" syndrome. It is most common in premature infants or newborns receiving chloramphenicol, whose hepatic systems have difficulty conjugating or excreting chloramphenicol. This syndrome is characterized by failure to feed, abdominal distention, possible vomiting, progressive blue-gray skin, and vasomotor collapse. The infant may also have irregular breathing.

Other serious and potentially life-threatening adverse effects of chloramphenicol are blood dyscrasias. These include aplastic anemia, hypoplastic anemia, thrombocytopenia, pancytopenia, and granulocytopenia. These adverse effects have all occurred following short-term or long-term therapy as a result of depressed bone marrow function.

Bone marrow toxicity may or may not be dose related. Irreversible depression of bone marrow function, a type of toxicity unrelated to dose, can result in aplastic anemia, which has a high mortality rate. This type of aplasia or hypoplasia can develop months after the drug has been discontinued or from a single dose. Reversible depression of bone marrow function usually is dose related and is characterized by anemia, reticulocytopenia, leukopenia, or thrombocytopenia.

Other adverse effects, which may be dose related, are optic neuritis, which can cause blindness, and peripheral neuritis. Patients with either of these effects should discontinue the drug immediately.

Other neurotoxic effects include headache, mild depression, confusion, and delirium, but these reactions are usually mild. Patients should be monitored for other signs of peripheral neuropathy.

GI effects are usually minimal during therapy with chloramphenicol but can include nausea, vomiting, diarrhea, dysgeusia, glossitis, stomatitis, pruritus ani, or enterocolitis. Adverse GI symptoms should be reported immediately because they can indicate more severe reactions, such as superinfection.

Maculopapular rash and urticaria can occur from either systemic administration or topical application of chloramphenicol. Topical use can also cause pruritus and burning, vesicular dermatitis, or maculopapular rash. Adverse reactions require discontinuing the drug. Transient burning or itching of the eye can occur following ophthalmic application. Repeated or prolonged use of eye or topical preparations should be discouraged.

Drug Interactions

Chloramphenicol interacts with oral hypoglycemics, oral anticoagulants, hydantoins, iron salts, and vitamin B_{12}. Chloramphenicol may also interact with antibiotics, such as penicillins, cephalosporins, aminoglycosides, and erythromycin. Table 39.11 describes potential interactions.

Assessment of Relevant Core Patient Variables

Health Status

Because therapeutic benefits generally do not outweigh the risks for chloramphenicol therapy, assess the culture and sensitivity findings to evaluate the efficacy of chloramphenicol.

Evaluate the patient for risk factors that would increase the potential for severe toxicities. Such factors include recent cytotoxic or radiation therapy, anemia, depressed bone marrow function, hepatic disease, renal impairment, acute intermittent porphyria, or G6PD deficiency. Patients with recent cytotoxic or radiation therapy are at risk for blood dyscrasias. Administering chloramphenicol will increase the risk for these dyscrasias. Chloramphenicol therapy may also exacerbate acute intermittent porphyria or G6PD deficiency.

Evaluate the patient for the use of other drugs, such as oral hypoglycemics, oral anticoagulants, or antiepileptic agents, which may interact with chloramphenicol. Other drugs to consider are those with a high risk for hematologic toxicity, hepatic toxicity, or nephrotoxicity because blood, liver, or kidney problems will increase the risk for adverse effects with chloramphenicol therapy.

Before initiating therapy, evaluate baseline laboratory test results, including CBC and hepatic and renal function. Abnormal test findings should be communicated to the prescriber immediately. Perform a baseline neurologic examination because chloramphenicol may induce adverse CNS effects. For patients receiving topical chloramphenicol, perform a baseline dermatologic assessment because chloramphenicol may cause a rash or pruritus.

Life Span and Gender

Evaluate women for pregnancy. Chloramphenicol is contraindicated for pregnant women who are near term because it may depress bone marrow function or cause gray baby syndrome in the neonate. Determine whether the patient is breast-feeding. Chloramphenicol is contraindicated for use in nursing mothers. Because it is excreted into breast milk, chloramphenicol may depress bone marrow function in infants.

Assess the developmental status of infants. Premature infants and neonates may develop gray baby syndrome. This syndrome can affect children up to 2 years of age, but infants receiving chloramphenicol within the first 48 hours of life are at highest risk. Chloramphenicol should be discontinued at the first signs of gray baby syndrome because it can be fatal in a matter of a few hours.

Environment

Be aware of the environment in which the drug will be administered. Administration of chloramphenicol must occur in a setting where appropriate serum level and patient monitoring can be undertaken. Evaluate the patient daily and discontinue therapy at the first sign of adverse reactions.

Nursing Diagnoses and Outcomes

- Risk for Injury related to drug-induced adverse effects, such as blood dyscrasias, gray baby syndrome, and CNS effects, including optic or peripheral neuritis, headache, depression, confusion, or delirium
  Desired outcome: *Regular and careful monitoring will protect the patient from permanent drug-related adverse effects.*
- Risk for Impaired Skin Integrity, rash and pruritus, related to topical drug use
  Desired outcome: *The nurse and patient will observe for and report signs of unusual skin reaction and contact the prescriber.*

TABLE 39.11 Agents That Interact With P Chloramphenicol

Interactants	Effect and Significance	Nursing Management
antibiotics aminoglycosides cephalosporins penicillins	The bactericidal effects of penicillins, cephalosporins, and aminoglycosides can be affected by the bacteriostatic action of chloramphenicol.	Avoid concurrent administration of these drugs.
erythromycin	Chloramphenicol can displace erythromycin from binding sites on the 50 S subunits of bacterial ribosomes, resulting in subtherapeutic levels of erythromycin.	Concurrent use of these drugs is not recommended.
oral anticoagulants dicumarol warfarin	Chloramphenicol may interfere with hepatic metabolism of the anticoagulant and possibly the hypoprothrombinemic effect. This results in an increased risk of bleeding.	Monitor anticoagulation parameters closely. Adjust oral anticoagulant dose as needed.
oral hypoglycemic agents acetohexamide chlorpropamide glipizide glyburide tolazamide tolbutamide	Chloramphenicol may reduce hepatic clearance of oral hypoglycemics, resulting in clinical hypoglycemia.	Monitor blood glucose concentrations. Teach patient signs and symptoms of hypoglycemia.
hydantoins ethotoin mephenytoin phenytoin	Chloramphenicol alters metabolism of hydantoins, resulting in an increased risk for hydantoin toxicity.	Monitor serum concentration of hydantoins. Adjust hydantoin dosage as needed.
iron salts ferrous fumarate ferrous gluconate ferrous sulfate iron dextran iron polysaccharide	Chloramphenicol decreases iron clearance and erythropoiesis due to bone marrow toxicity. This may result in iron overload and anemia.	Choose another antibiotic if bone marrow suppression occurs. Monitor CBC. Monitor serum iron levels. Adjust iron dosage as needed.
vitamin B_{12}	Although the mechanism of action is unknown, chloramphenicol may decrease the hematologic effects of vitamin B_{12} in patients with pernicious anemia.	Monitor patient's clinical response to vitamin B_{12}. Consider alternative antibiotic therapy.

Planning and Intervention

Maximizing Therapeutic Effects

Oral chloramphenicol should be administered on an empty stomach 1 hour before or 2 hours after meals. However, for patients with GI distress, chloramphenicol may be administered with meals.

Minimizing Adverse Effects

Although adverse effects may occur when therapeutic concentrations are within normal limits, they are more likely to occur if they are high. Monitor plasma concentrations at least weekly or more often in patients with hepatic or renal impairment. Peak levels should be in the range of 10 to 20 μg/mL, whereas trough levels should be 5 to 10 μg/mL.

Avoid IM injections because they may cause bleeding, bruising, or hematomas as a result of thrombocytopenia resulting from chloramphenicol-induced depression of bone marrow function.

Providing Patient and Family Education

- Explain the importance of completing therapy.
- Point out the potential adverse effects and the need for periodic blood monitoring and daily assessment.
- Teach the patient the importance of measuring fluid intake and output accurately.
- Advise the patient to report any symptoms to the health care team immediately.

Ongoing Assessment and Evaluation

Serum concentrations and patients' responses to systemic chloramphenicol therapy are unpredictable. For patients receiving systemic therapy, coordinate serial monitoring of chloramphenicol plasma concentrations.

Assess patients receiving chloramphenicol therapy for signs of anemia and depressed bone marrow function. These signs include bleeding, easy bruising, and fatigue. Bone marrow function should be monitored with serial CBCs throughout therapy.

Monitor for signs of hepatic or renal insufficiency. For long-term or high-dose therapy or for patients with a history of hepatic or renal insufficiency, serial hepatic and renal function tests are important. In addition to increasing the risk for toxicities, impaired hepatic function has resulted in adult reactions similar to gray baby syndrome.

Other important assessments are GI and CNS effects. Although GI effects occur infrequently, they may indicate a more serious problem, such as superinfection. In the CNS, monitor for optic or peripheral neuritis, headache, depression, confusion, or delirium.

For patients receiving topical chloramphenicol, monitor for signs such as rash, itching, or burning sensation with administration.

Because most adverse effects require that therapy be discontinued, assessing the patient on a daily basis and communicating findings to the prescriber are the most important aspects of chloramphenicol therapy.

When treatment ends, the initial infection should be resolved. The patient should be adequately nourished and hydrated, and any adverse drug effects should be resolved.

Drug Significantly Different From P Chloramphenicol

Spectinomycin is related to the aminoglycosides but is somewhat different structurally. Spectinomycin is usually given as a one-time injection, followed by other antibiotic therapy, and is used to treat acute gonorrheal urethritis and prostatitis in men and acute gonorrheal cervicitis and proctitis in women. It is also a prophylactic treatment after known recent exposure to gonorrhea. Spectinomycin is active against a number of other gram-negative bacteria, although it is inferior to other antibiotics commonly used to treat these organisms. It is contraindicated in patients with a known hypersensitivity to the drug. Soreness at the injection site is the most common adverse effect. Other serious adverse effects are limited because the drug is given only once.

MEMORY CHIP

P Chloramphenicol

- Used for serious gram-positive or gram-negative infections, especially brain abscesses or meningitis
- Major contraindications: hypersensitivity and breast-feeding
- Most common adverse effects: headache, nausea, vomiting, and diarrhea
- Most serious adverse effects: blood dyscrasias, "gray-baby" syndrome
- Maximizing therapeutic effects: Administer oral preparations on an empty stomach.
- Minimizing adverse effects: Monitor peak and trough levels throughout therapy.
- Most important patient education: Teach the patient the signs and symptoms of bone marrow suppression and the importance of contacting the health care provider immediately if any symptoms occur.

CHAPTER SUMMARY

- Drugs that inhibit protein synthesis may be bacteriocidal or bacteriostatic.
- Gentamicin is the prototype for aminoglycoside agents.
- Gentamicin is used for serious infections caused by gram-negative bacilli.
- Gentamicin use is limited by its potential for adverse effects, especially nephrotoxicity, ototoxicity, and neuromuscular blockade.
- Gentamicin is generally given parenterally but may be given orally to exert a local effect on the GI tract because oral drugs are more poorly absorbed.
- Drugs similar to gentamicin include amikacin, kanamycin, netilmicin, and tobramycin.
- Clindamycin, the lincosamide prototype, is used for infections caused by gram-positive cocci and many gram-negative or gram-positive anaerobes.
- Clindamycin is reserved for treating serious infections that have not responded to less toxic antibiotics.
- Clindamycin therapy is limited by its potential for adverse effects, especially pseudomembranous colitis.
- Macrolides, such as erythromycin, are used to treat an array of infections caused by gram-positive organisms. They are less effective against gram-negative organisms.
- Erythromycin is used for patients with a hypersensitivity to penicillin.
- Erythromycin has a spectrum of activity similar to that of penicillins and cephalosporins.
- Oxazolidinones and streptogramins are the newest classes of antibiotics developed to manage "superbugs" that do not respond to vancomycin.
- The prototype oxazolidinone is linezolid (Zyvox).
- The unique mechanism of action of linezolid may reduce the emergence of resistance.
- Quinupristin/dalfopristin, the prototype streptogramin, is a combination drug that is 16 times more potent than each drug alone.
- The tetracyclines have been used for many types of infections in the past; therefore, resistance to these drugs is now a problem.
- Tetracyclines remain useful in treating infections caused by *Rickettsiae* species, *Mycoplasma pneumoniae,* and *Chlamydia* species. They are also used to treat acne.
- Chloramphenicol is used for serious gram-positive or gram-negative infections that have not responded to less toxic antibiotics.
- Chloramphenicol passes the blood–brain barrier and is useful in treating brain abscesses or meningitis.
- Chloramphenicol therapy is limited by its potential for adverse effects, especially suppression of bone marrow function.

QUESTIONS FOR STUDY AND REVIEW

1. List disadvantages of tetracycline therapy.
2. Why are aminoglycosides used only in serious infections?
3. What are the most serious adverse effects of chloramphenicol therapy?
4. After a patient receives erythromycin for 10 days for a severe skin infection, the patient develops a vaginal yeast infection. Explain why this infection occurred.
5. A patient who is taking clindamycin at home calls you to report violent, watery, and bloody diarrhea. Explain the probable cause for these symptoms. What advice would you give to this patient?
6. Describe the differences between quinupristin/dalfopristin and linezolid for managing VRE and MRSA.

? Need More Help?

Chapter 39 of the study guide for *Drug Therapy in Nursing* 2e contains NCLEX-style questions and other learning activities to reinforce your understanding of the concepts presented in this chapter. For additional information or to purchase the study guide, visit *http://connection.lww.com/go/aschenbrenner.*

REFERENCES AND BIBLIOGRAPHY

Blot, S. I., Vandewoude, K. H., Hoste, E. A., et al. (2002). Outcome and attributable mortality in critically ill patients with bacteremia involving methicillin-susceptible and methicillin-resistant *Staphylococcus aureus. Archives of Internal Medicine,* 162(19), 2229–2235.

Boyce, J. M. (2001). MRSA patients: Proven methods to treat colonization and infection. *Journal of Hospital Infection,* 48(Suppl. A), S9–S14.

Capriotti, T. (2003). Preventing nosocomial spread of MRSA is in your hands. *Dermatology Nursing,* 12(3), 193–196.

Clinical Pharmacology [Online]. Available: *http://cp.gsm.com.*

Eliopoulos, G. M. (2004). Current and new antimicrobial agents. *American Heart Journal, 147*(4), 587–592.

Facts and Comparisons. (2004). *Drug facts and comparisons.* Philadelphia: Lippincott Williams & Wilkins.

Hardman, J. G. (2001). *Goodman & Gilman's the pharmacological basis of therapeutics* (10th ed.). New York: McGraw-Hill Health Professions Division.

Kalil, A. C., Puumala, S. E., Stoner, J., et al. (2004). Unresolved questions with the use of linezolid vs vancomycin for nosocomial pneumonia. *Chest, 125*(6), 2370–2371.

Katzung, B. (2004). *Basic and clinical pharmacology* (9th ed.). New York: McGraw-Hill/Appleton & Lange.

Micromedex Healthcare Series [Online]. Available: *http://healthcare.micromedex.com.*

Muller-Serieys, C., Andrews, J., Vacheron, F., et al. (2004). Tissue kinetics of telithromycin, the first ketolide antibacterial. *Journal of Antimicrobials and Chemotherapy, 53*(2), 149–157.

Nieman, R. B., Sharma, K., Edelberg, H., et al. (2003). Telithromycin and myasthenia gravis. *Clinical Infectious Diseases, 37*(11), 1579.

Pagano, P. J., Buchanan, L. V., Dailey, C. F., et al. (2004). Effects of linezolid on staphylococcal adherence versus time of treatment. *International Journal of Antimicrobial Agents, 23*(3), 226–234.

Schito, G. C., Marchese, A., Elkharrat, D., et al. (2004). Comparative activity of telithromycin against macrolide-resistant isolates of *Streptococcus pneumoniae:* Results of two years of the PROTEKT surveillance study. *Journal of Chemotherapy, 16*(1), 13–22.

Tatro, D. S. (2004). *Drug interaction facts.* Philadelphia: Lippincott Williams & Wilkins.

Drugs That Are Miscellaneous Antibiotics

chapter 40

Learning Objectives

At the completion of this chapter the student will:

1. Identify core drug knowledge pertaining to miscellaneous antibiotic agents.
2. Identify core patient variables pertaining to miscellaneous antibiotic agents.
3. Relate the interaction of core drug knowledge to core patient variables for miscellaneous antibiotic agents.
4. Generate a nursing plan of care from the interactions between core drug knowledge and core patient variables for miscellaneous antibiotic agents.
5. Describe nursing interventions to maximize therapeutic and minimize adverse effects for miscellaneous antibiotic agents.
6. Determine key points for patient and family education for miscellaneous antibiotic agents.

KEY TERMS

arthropathy

fluoroquinolones

quinolones

FEATURED WEBLINK

http://www.cfsan.fda.gov/~mow/intro.html
Confused by the microbes that can affect humans? Log on to the "Bad Bug Book."

CONNECTION WEBLINK

Additional Weblinks are found on Connection: **http://www.connection.lww.com/go/aschenbrenner.**

Drugs That Are Miscellaneous Antibiotics

Ⓒ Quinolones/Fluoroquinolones

- [P] **ciprofloxacin**
  - First generation
    - cinoxacin
    - nalidixic acid
  - Second generation
    - lomefloxacin
    - norfloxacin
    - ofloxacin
  - Third generation
    - gatifloxacin
    - gemifloxacin
    - levofloxacin
    - moxifloxacin
    - sparfloxacin
  - Fourth generation
    - alatrofloxacin
    - trovafloxacin
- **polymyxin B**

The symbol Ⓒ indicates the **drug class.**
Drugs in **bold type** marked with the symbol [P] are prototypes.
Drugs in blue type are closely related to the prototype.
Drugs in red type are significantly different from the prototype.
Drugs in black type with no symbol are also used in drug therapy; no prototype

Miscellaneous antibiotics are those that have a mechanism of action other than disrupting the cell wall or protein synthesis of bacteria. These drugs include the fluoroquinolones, rifampin, metronidazole, and polymyxin B. This chapter discusses the fluoroquinolones, with the prototype ciprofloxacin; a drug significantly different from ciprofloxacin is polymixin B. Rifampin, the prototype for drugs affecting leprosy, is discussed in Chapter 42. Metronidazole is used most frequently to manage protozoan infections and thus is discussed in Chapter 45.

QUINOLONES/ FLUOROQUINOLONES

The **quinolones** have been used to treat infections for the past 40 years. They have undergone substantial advances in their antibiotic activity and have developed into a class of synthetic antibiotics that are effective for aerobic gram-negative and gram-positive infections. Like cephalosporins, quinolones are subdivided into four generations. The first-generation drugs are called **quinolones,** whereas subsequent generations are called **fluoroquinolones** because a fluorine atom was added to the quinolone structure of these drugs. First-generation quinolones are used only to treat uncomplicated urinary tract infections (UTIs). Second-generation fluoroquinolones have increased gram-negative and systemic activity. Third-generation fluoroquinolones have extended activity against gram-positive pathogens, but they are less active than second-generation drugs against *Pseudomonas* species. Fourth-generation fluoroquinolones share the spectrum of activity of third-generation fluoroquinolones and are also active against *Pseudomonas* species and anaerobic bacteria (Box 40.1). Table 40.1 summarizes selected fluoroquinolones. The prototype drug for the fluoroquinolone class is ciprofloxacin (Cipro).

FOCUS ON RESEARCH

Box 40.1 Efficacy of Single-Dose Fluoroquinolone Therapy for UTI

Richard, G. A., Mathew, C. P., Kirstein, J. M., et al., (2002). Single-dose fluoroquinolone therapy of acute uncomplicated urinary tract infection in women: Results from a randomized, double-blind, multicenter trial comparing single-dose to 3-day fluoroquinolone regimens. *Urology, 59*(3), 334–339.

The Study

The researchers compared the efficacy and safety of single-dose fluoroquinolone treatment with that of 3-day fluoroquinolone treatment for uncomplicated urinary tract infection (UTI). Adult women with acute uncomplicated UTI were randomized to receive either a single dose of gatifloxacin, 3 days of gatifloxacin, or 3 days of ciprofloxacin. All three regimens eradicated the most common uropathogens, including *Escherichia coli, Klebsiella pneumoniae,* and *Proteus mirabilis,* in most patients. The clinical efficacy rate for the single-dose gatifloxacin, 3-day gatifloxacin, and 3-day ciprofloxacin groups was 93%, 95%, and 93%, respectively.

Nursing Implications

UTI is the most common type of infection in adult women. Some patients have a long history of recurring infection. Historically, pharmacotherapy for uncomplicated UTI has required a 7- to 10-day course of antibiotics. However, this study showed that single-dose and 3-day gatifloxacin were equivalent, microbiologically and clinically, to 3-day ciprofloxacin for treating such infections. You must stay informed about changes in treatment methods in order to educate patients appropriately, especially women with a history of recurrent UTI. Using the newer therapeutic regimens may decrease secondary use of medical resources and improve patient adherence.

NURSING MANAGEMENT OF THE PATIENT RECEIVING P CIPROFLOXACIN

Core Drug Knowledge

Pharmacotherapeutics

Ciprofloxacin is most active against aerobic gram-negative organisms, such as *Escherichia coli, Proteus mirabilis, Klebsiella pneumoniae, Enterobacter cloacae, Proteus vulgaris, Proteus rettgeri, Morganella morganii, Citrobacter freundii, Staphylococcus aureus, Staphylococcus epidermidis,* and group D streptococci.

Ciprofloxacin also has been used extensively to treat serious gram-negative infections; however, resistance has developed in strains of *Pseudomonas aeruginosa* and *Serratia marcescens.* Ciprofloxacin is generally active against aerobic gram-positive organisms, but resistance has been noted in *S. aureus* and *Pneumococcus* species. For this reason, ciprofloxacin should be used cautiously in skin infections. Ciprofloxacin also is useful in treating sexually transmitted diseases, bacterial conjunctivitis, and otitis externa, and is used in combination with other agents against mycobacterial infections. An unlabeled use of ciprofloxacin is treatment of cystic fibrosis with pulmonary exacerbations. It is not active against anaerobic organisms.

Pharmacokinetics

Ciprofloxacin is available in oral, parenteral, and topical formulations. Topical formulations include both otic and ophthalmic preparations. Oral preparations are absorbed rapidly from the gastrointestinal (GI) tract and undergo minimal first-pass metabolism. In healthy, fasting adults, 40% to 85% is absorbed, and peak serum concentrations are reached in 0.5 to 2.3 hours. Ciprofloxacin is distributed widely into most tissues because protein binding is low. Penetration into cerebrospinal fluid is minimal when the meninges are not inflamed. Ciprofloxacin is eliminated through renal and nonrenal routes. Renal excretion accounts for 15% to 40% of unchanged drug, whereas fecal excretion accounts for 20% to 40% of the dose. Intravenous (IV) administration of ciprofloxacin has an onset of action within 10 minutes and peak effects within 30 minutes. Ciprofloxacin as a topical preparation has an onset of 5 minutes.

Pharmacodynamics

Ciprofloxacin, like other antibiotics, has no direct effect on the body but acts on the bacterial cell. Ciprofloxacin is bactericidal. It inhibits deoxyribonucleic acid (DNA) gyrase, an enzyme needed for bacterial DNA replication. Although human

TABLE 40.1 Summary of Selected (C) Fluoroquinolones

Drug (Trade) Name	Selected Indications	Route and Dosage Range	Pharmacokinetics
P ciprofloxacin (Cipro; *Canadian:* Ciloxin)	Uncomplicated UTI	*Adult:* PO, 250 mg bid × 7–14 d; IV, 200 mg q12h	*Onset:* PO, varies; IV, 10 min *Duration:* 4–5 h $t_{1/2}$: 3.5–4 h
	Complicated UTI	*Adult:* PO, 500 mg bid 10–21 d; IV, 40 mg q12h	
	Respiratory, bone, joint infections	*Adult:* PO, 500 mg q12h; IV, 400 mg q12h	
	Severe skin infections	*Adult:* PO, 750 mg q12h	
	Infectious diarrhea	*Adult:* PO, 500 mg bid 5–7 d	
	Ophthalmic	*Adult:* 1–2 gtt qd–bid	
	Otic	*Adult:* 4 gtt tid–qid *Child:* Not recommended	
First Generation			
cinoxacin (Cinobac)	Uncomplicated UTI, sexually transmitted disease (STD)	*Adult and child >12 y:* PO, 1 g/d in four divided doses 7–14 d *Child <12 y:* Not recommended	*Onset:* PO, varies *Duration:* 4–5 h $t_{1/2}$: 4–6 h
nalidixic acid (NegGram)	UTI	*Adult and child >12 y:* PO, 1 g qid 1–2 w; prolonged therapy 2 g/d *Child 3 mo–12 y:* PO, 55 mg/kg/d in four divided doses; prolonged therapy, 33 mg/k/d	*Onset:* varies *Duration:* unknown $t_{1/2}$: 1–2.5 h
Second Generation			
lomefloxacin (Maxaquin)	Lower respiratory tract infections, uncomplicated UTI	*Adult:* PO, 400 mg qd × 10 d	*Onset:* Varies *Duration:* 8–10 h $t_{1/2}$: 8 h
	Complicated UTI	*Adult:* PO, 400 mg qd × 14 d	*Onset:* Varies
	Prophylaxis	*Adult:* PO, 400 mg 2–6 h prior to surgery *Child:* Not recommended	*Duration:* Unknown $t_{1/2}$: 3–4.5 h
norfloxacin (Noroxin; *Canadian:* Apo-Norflox)	Uncomplicated UTI	*Adult:* PO, 400 mg q12h × 7–10 d	
	Complicated UTI	*Adult:* PO, 400 mg q12h × 10–21 d	
	STD	*Adult:* 800 mg single dose	
	Prostatitis	*Adult:* PO, 400 mg q12h for 28 d *Child:* Not recommended	
ofloxacin (Floxin; *Canadian:* Apo-Oflox)	Uncomplicated UTI	*Adult:* PO/IV, 200 mg bid for 3 d	*Onset:* Varies *Duration:* 9 h $t_{1/2}$: 5–10 h
	Complicated UTI, lower respiratory tract infections, skin infections	*Adult:* PO/IV, 200 mg bid for 10 d	
	Prostatitis	*Adult:* PO/IV, 300 mg bid for 6 wk	
	Uncomplicated gonorrhea	*Adult:* PO/IV, 400 mg single dose	
	Cervicitis, urethritis	*Adult:* PO/IV, 300 mg bid for 7 d *Child:* Not recommended	

(continued)

TABLE 40.1 Summary of Selected Ⓒ Fluoroquinolones (continued)

Drug (Trade) Name	Selected Indications	Route and Dosage Range	Pharmacokinetics
Third Generation			
gatifloxacin (Tequin)	Pneumonia	*Adult:* PO/IV, 400 mg qd 7–14 d	*Onset:* PO, varies; IV, rapid
	Sinusitis	*Adult:* PO/IV, 400 mg qd 10 d	*Duration:* 18–24 h
	Chronic bronchitis	*Adult:* PO/IV, 400 mg qd 7–10 d	$t_{1/2}$: 7–14 h
	Uncomplicated UTI	*Adult:* PO, 200 mg qd × 3 d; PO/IV, 400 mg single dose	
	Complicated UTI, nephritis	*Adult:* PO/IV, 400 mg qd 7–10 d *Child:* Not recommended	
gemifloxacin (Factive)	Pneumonia Chronic bronchitis	*Adult:* PO, 320 mg qd *Child:* Not recommended	*Onset:* Rapid *Duration:* 24 h $t_{1/2}$: 7 h
levofloxacin (Levaquin)	Pneumonia, skin infections	*Adult:* PO/IV, 500 mg qd for 7–14 d	*Onset:* Varies *Duration:* 3–5 h
	Sinusitis	*Adult:* PO/IV, 500 mg qd 10–14 d	$t_{1/2}$: 4–7 h
	Chronic bronchitis	*Adult:* PO/IV, 500 mg qd × 7 d	
	UTI, nephritis	*Adult:* PO/IV, 250 mg qd × 10 d *Child:* Not recommended	
moxifloxacin (Avelox)	Pneumonia, sinusitis Chronic bronchitis	*Adult:* PO, 400 mg qd × 10 d *Adult:* PO, 400 mg qd × 5 d *Child:* Not recommended	*Onset:* Varies *Duration:* unknown $t_{1/2}$: 12–13.5 h
sparfloxacin (Zagam)	Lower respiratory tract infections, sinusitis, bronchitis, skin infections	*Adult:* PO, 400 mg first day, then 200 mg qd for 7–10 d *Child:* Not recommended	*Onset:* Slow *Duration:* 8–12 h $t_{1/2}$: 16–20 h
Fourth Generation			
trovafloxacin (Trovan)	Pneumonia	*Adult:* PO/IV, 200–300 mg qd for 10–14 d	*Onset:* Rapid *Duration:* 24 h
alatrofloxacin (Trovan IV)	Sinusitis	*Adult:* PO, 200 mg qd for 10 d	$t_{1/2}$: 9–13 h
	Bronchitis	*Adult:* PO, 200 mg qd for 7–10 d	
	Complicated intra-abdominal infections, gynecologic infections	*Adult:* IV, 300 mg first day followed by 200 mg PO qd for 7–10 d	
	Skin infections	*Adult:* PO, 100 mg qd for 7–10 d	
	Complicated skin infections	*Adult:* PO/IV, 200 mg first day followed by 200 mg qd for 10–14 d	
	UTI	*Adult:* PO, 100 mg qd for 3 d	
	Chronic prostatitis	*Adult:* PO, 200 mg qd for 28 d	
	Gonorrhea	*Adult:* PO, 100 mg single dose *Child:* Not recommended	

cells contain an enzyme that functions in the same manner, this enzyme is not affected by bactericidal concentrations of ciprofloxacin. Both rapid- and slow-growing organisms are inhibited by ciprofloxacin. In addition, ciprofloxacin exhibits a prolonged postantibiotic effect; organisms may not resume growing for 2 to 6 hours after exposure to ciprofloxacin, despite undetectable drug levels. Ciprofloxacin is concentrated within human neutrophils, which may explain its effectiveness in treating mycobacterial infections.

Contraindications and Precautions

Ciprofloxacin is contraindicated in patients who are pregnant or lactating and in patients with a known allergy to any fluoroquinolone. Oral and parenteral ciprofloxacin is contraindicated for children younger than 18 years, although topical ciprofloxacin may be used in children.

Caution should be used in patients with GI disease (especially colitis), renal dysfunction, and hepatic dysfunction, and

in patients who are dehydrated. Because ciprofloxacin can stimulate the central nervous system (CNS), it should be used with caution in patients with CNS disorders (such as seizures) or cerebrovascular disease (e.g., cerebral arteriosclerosis).

Adverse Effects

Ciprofloxacin is generally well tolerated. The most clinically important adverse reaction is **arthropathy** (joint disease). This often irreversible adverse reaction tends to occur in children under 18 years old. The most common adverse reactions are GI effects, including nausea and vomiting, diarrhea, and abdominal pain. These effects occur most frequently in elderly adults or in instances of high dosages.

For the most part, CNS reactions, such as headache and restlessness, occur in only 1% to 2% of patients. Other CNS effects that occur in fewer than 1% of patients include dizziness, vertigo, insomnia, nightmares, hallucinations, confusion, agitation, drowsiness, anxiety, malaise, depression, paresthesias, and increased intracranial pressure. In predisposed patients, seizures may occur.

Cardiovascular adverse effects, such as palpitations, atrial flutter, premature ventricular contractions, syncope, angina, myocardial infarction, cardiac arrest, and cerebral thrombosis, have been reported with ciprofloxacin, but they occur infrequently.

Photosensitivity may occur with ciprofloxacin. However, this adverse effect occurs more frequently with other fluoroquinolones. Tendon rupture has been reported with ciprofloxacin therapy. Ruptures have occurred unilaterally and bilaterally and have involved the Achilles tendon, shoulder, and hands. Other adverse reactions include rash, fever, eosinophilia, and interstitial nephritis.

Adverse reactions to ophthalmic ciprofloxacin usually are associated with local effects, such as burning or discomfort. Other adverse effects of ophthalmic ciprofloxacin include lid margin crusting, crystals, scales, foreign body sensation, pruritus, conjunctival hyperemia, and a bad taste following administration.

Drug Interactions

Potential drug interactions with ciprofloxacin include those with compounds that contain various salts (e.g., aluminum, calcium, iron, magnesium, zinc). Because ciprofloxacin is bound by various cations (e.g., calcium, magnesium, iron, zinc), administration with food that contains cations can reduce bioavailability substantially. Over-the-counter (OTC) preparations of the herbal supplement St. John's wort, combined with ciprofloxacin, increase the potential for severe photosensitivity reactions. Ciprofloxacin may bind to birth control pill–receptor sites, thus increasing the risk for conception. Table 40.2 summarizes drug interactions with ciprofloxacin.

Assessment of Relevant Core Patient Variables

Health Status

Elicit a patient history to evaluate for pre-existing GI disease, renal or hepatic dysfunction, CNS disorder, pregnancy, or lactation. Any positive finding should be communicated to the prescriber. Assess for any known reactions to antibiotics.

Physical examination should include an examination of the skin for any rash or lesions, to provide a baseline for comparison if an allergic reaction is suspected or misdiagnosed. For the same reason, assess respiratory status, checking breath sounds for wheezing. Patients with pre-existing renal or hepatic disease should have baseline blood tests performed to document current functioning. Patients with pre-existing anemias or proposed long-term therapy should have a baseline complete blood count. Patients with pre-existing cardiac disorders should have a baseline electrocardiogram.

Life Span and Gender

Assess the patient for pregnancy and lactation. Because ciprofloxacin crosses the placenta and enters breast milk, pregnant or breast-feeding women should not take ciprofloxacin. As with other fluoroquinolones, the patient's age should be noted before administering ciprofloxacin. Fluoroquinolone antibiotics have caused arthropathies, such as cartilage deterioration, when administered to immature animals. Although similar consequences of therapy have not been demonstrated in humans, ciprofloxacin should not be used in patients younger than 18 years. However, ciprofloxacin ophthalmic solution is approved for use in children. Elderly patients should be monitored carefully for renal or hepatic dysfunction and receive reduced dosages of ciprofloxacin as needed.

Lifestyle, Diet, and Habits

It is important to assess the patient's typical food, caffeine, and OTC drug use. Caution the patient that food or caffeine may interrupt the action of ciprofloxacin. Patients with frequent dyspepsia should be reminded that antacids can decrease the absorption of ciprofloxacin. Some vitamins also can decrease the absorption of ciprofloxacin. The safest advice would be to take any vitamin therapy at least 2 hours before or after administration of ciprofloxacin.

Environment

Be aware of the setting in which ciprofloxacin will be administered. Ciprofloxacin may be given as an oral, parenteral, topical ophthalmic, or topic otic preparation. In acute care settings, parenteral ciprofloxacin should be administered over 60 minutes through a large vein to minimize discomfort and reduce the risk for venous irritation.

In the home, the patient should take ciprofloxacin every 12 hours on an empty stomach. Advise patients using the ophthalmic or otic solutions not to contaminate the tip of the dispenser by contact with the eye, ear, fingertips, or other surface.

Nursing Diagnoses and Outcomes

- Diarrhea related to adverse drug effects
  Desired outcome: *The patient will avoid dehydration, maintain fluid intake, and contact the prescriber if diarrhea persists.*
- Imbalanced Nutrition: More or Less than Body Requirements related to GI effects, alteration in taste, and superinfections
  Desired outcome: *The patient will maintain body weight and contact the prescriber if persistent adverse effects alter nutritional status.*

TABLE 40.2 Agents That Interact With P Ciprofloxacin

Interactants	Effect and Significance	Nursing Management
Antacids	Concurrent administration of antacids and ciprofloxacin may decrease the absorption of ciprofloxacin.	Avoid concurrent use. Administer antacids if needed 6 h before or 2 h after ciprofloxacin.
azlocillin	The clearance of ciprofloxacin may be decreased by azlocillin. This may result in increased adverse effects or toxicity.	Monitor plasma drug levels of ciprofloxacin. Monitor for signs of adverse effects or toxicity.
Caffeine	Ciprofloxacin may inhibit the hepatic metabolism of caffeine.	Monitor for excessive CNS stimulation or cardiovascular effects. Restrict caffeine intake if needed.
didanosine	The magnesium and aluminum cations in the buffers of didanosine decrease GI absorption of ciprofloxacin.	Avoid concurrent use. Administer didanosine if needed 6 h before or 2 h after ciprofloxacin.
Food	Food interferes with the absorption of ciprofloxacin.	Administer on an empty stomach. Lengthen interval between milk and ciprofloxacin as much as possible.
Hydantoins	The mechanism of action is unclear, but ciprofloxacin may reduce serum phenytoin concentrations. This may result in seizure activity.	Monitor serum phenytoin levels. Adjust phenytoin dose as needed.
Salts aluminum calcium iron magnesium zinc	GI absorption of ciprofloxacin may be decreased by the formation of iron–ciprofloxacin complex.	Avoid coadministration.
sucralfate	GI absorption of ciprofloxacin may be decreased by sucralfate.	Avoid concurrent use. Administer sucralfate if needed 6 h before or 2 h after ciprofloxacin.
Theophyllines	Ciprofloxacin inhibits the hepatic metabolism of theophyllines. This may result in theophylline toxicity.	Monitor for theophylline levels. Observe for signs of toxicity. Adjust theophylline dose as needed.

- Risk for Injury related to drug-induced dizziness, confusion, and other CNS effects
  Desired outcome: *The patient will remain free of injury and contact the prescriber about persistent CNS disturbances.*
- Risk for Impaired Tissue Integrity related to drug-induced photosensitivity
  Desired outcome: *The patient will take measures to protect his or her skin from prolonged sun exposure*

Planning and Intervention

Maximizing Therapeutic Effects

Ensure that the patient receives the full course of ciprofloxacin as prescribed, around the clock to increase effectiveness. Coordinate the administration of drugs to decrease potential drug–drug interactions.

Review culture and sensitivity reports to confirm that the causative bacteria are sensitive to ciprofloxacin.

Minimizing Adverse Effects

Institute safety measures to protect the patient if CNS effects occur. For patients with adverse GI effects, provide small, frequent meals as tolerated.

Frequent mouth care and sucking on ice chips may relieve stomatitis and sore mouth.

Providing Patient and Family Education

- One of the most important features of patient and family education is teaching the patient that ciprofloxacin is one drug within a class of drugs. Advise the patient who has ever had any type of allergic reaction to a fluoroquinolone to never take any other drug with a name that ends with "oxacin."
- Advise patients who are pregnant or breast-feeding not to take ciprofloxacin.
- It is important to explain that ciprofloxacin is prescribed for a particular infection and should not be used to self-medicate or treat any other infection or any other person, especially not a child.
- Instruct patients to call the prescriber if their symptoms do not improve within 3 days.
- It is important to instruct patients to complete the full course of drug therapy, even when they feel better.
- Advise the patient to take ciprofloxacin every 12 hours. A forgotten dose can be taken as soon as it is remembered, but not if it is almost time for the next dose.

- Teach the patient symptoms of an allergic reaction (i.e., rash, welts, itching, or shortness of breath) to ciprofloxacin and instruct the patient to stop taking the drug at once and notify the prescriber if these symptoms occur.
- Advise patients who experience GI upset to eat small, frequent meals and to increase their fluid intake, particularly if they have diarrhea. For patients with a sore mouth or throat, sucking on ice chips may provide relief.
- Caution the patient about possible photosensitivity and encourage the patient to avoid sunlight or ultraviolet light, to wear appropriate clothing, and to apply a sunscreen with a sun protection factor of at least 15 if exposure is unavoidable.
- Advise the patient of signs and symptoms of a superinfection, such as discoloration of the tongue, fatigue, easy bruising, or vaginal discharge in women. In addition, the patient needs to know that ciprofloxacin may cause CNS disturbances or cardiovascular symptoms, and that the patient should contact the prescriber immediately if these adverse reactions occur.
- Tell the patient to report any tendon pain to the prescriber immediately because of the potential for tendon rupture as an adverse effect of ciprofloxacin therapy (see the Critical Thinking Scenario: How Did That Happen?).
- Inform women who use oral contraceptives to use a backup method of contraception during ciprofloxacin therapy because their birth control pills may be less effective while they are taking ciprofloxacin.

Ongoing Assessment and Evaluation

Antibiotic therapy can result in superinfection with nonsusceptible organisms. Because overgrowth of candidal organisms can occur with ciprofloxacin therapy, monitor patients closely during treatment. In addition, patients who develop diarrhea while taking, or soon after taking, ciprofloxacin should be considered for differential diagnosis of antibiotic-associated pseudomembranous colitis.

MEMORY CHIP

P Ciprofloxacin

- Used for infections caused by aerobic gram-negative organisms
- Major contraindications: hypersensitivity, children younger than 18 years, pregnancy, or breast-feeding
- Most common adverse effects: GI
- Most serious adverse effect: arthropathy (in children younger than 18 years)
- Maximizing therapeutic effects: Complete the full course of antibiotic therapy.
- Minimizing adverse effects: Provide small, frequent meals for GI distress.
- Most important patient education: Importance of completion of therapy and, for women, use of a backup method of contraception

CRITICAL THINKING SCENARIO

How did that happen?

Keri H., age 25 years, came to your clinic after a weekend of skiing in the mountains with a complaint of chest pain, cough, and shortness of breath. She is diagnosed with pneumonia and is started on ciprofloxacin, 400 mg bid. Four days after starting the medication, Keri calls the clinic and asks, "Can I come back and get seen again? My chest pain and cough are gone but I am limping and my left heel hurts. I guess I must have done something while I was skiing, but I don't remember hurting myself." How would you respond to Keri?

Drugs Closely Related to P Ciprofloxacin

First-Generation Quinolones

NALIDIXIC ACID

Nalidixic acid (NegGram) is an oral quinolone agent that is effective against gram-negative bacteria. Gram-positive microbes are generally resistant to it. It is indicated for use only in UTIs because it concentrates in the urine and achieves only low concentrations in serum. Resistance to nalidixic acid may develop rapidly during treatment.

Nalidixic acid appears to work by interfering with DNA polymerase, thereby inhibiting bacterial DNA synthesis. It is orally administered and well absorbed; however, serum concentration levels are too low for antibacterial effects. It is metabolized by the liver into one metabolite, hydroxy nalidixic acid, which is excreted renally.

Contraindications include cerebral arteriosclerosis or seizure disorders, hepatic dysfunction, and glucose-6-phosphate dehydrogenase (G6PD) deficiency. Patients with severe cerebral arteriosclerosis or a history of seizure disorders may be at increased risk for toxicity, especially seizures. Hemolytic anemia may occur in patients with G6PD deficiency.

Nalidixic acid achieves therapeutic levels in urine in patients with moderate to severe renal impairment. However, patients with a creatine clearance of less than 10 mL/min may be at increased risk for toxicity.

Adverse effects include drowsiness, weakness, headache, dizziness, vertigo, photosensitivity, visual impairment, abdominal pain, nausea and vomiting, diarrhea, rash, pruritus, urticaria, angioedema, and arthralgia. In patients with long-term therapy, nalidixic acid may induce blood dyscrasias.

Nalidixic acid interacts with multiple drugs. It can displace anticoagulants such as warfarin from binding sites, resulting in an increased anticoagulant effect. The following agents may substantially interfere with the absorption of nalidixic acid: antacids containing magnesium, aluminum, or calcium; sucralfate or divalent or trivalent cations such as iron; multivitamins containing zinc; and didanosine chewable or buffered tablets or the pediatric powder for oral solution. These agents should not be taken within 2 hours before or 2 hours after nalidixic acid administration.

CINOXACIN

Cinoxacin (Cinobac) is another urinary tract antiseptic that works in much the same way as nalidixic acid. It is taken orally and is also used for acute or recurrent UTIs caused by

susceptible gram-negative organisms. Like nalidixic acid, cinoxacin works by interfering with DNA polymerase.

Cinoxacin is contraindicated for use in patients with severe hepatic or renal dysfunction. The adverse effect profile is the same as that of nalidixic acid; however, such effects occur less frequently.

The only important drug interaction is with probenecid. Probenecid blocks the excretion of cinoxacin, resulting in increased serum concentrations and decreased urine concentrations.

Second-Generation Fluoroquinolones

LOMEFLOXACIN

Lomefloxacin (Maxaquin) is used to treat lower respiratory tract infections, such as bronchitis, and UTIs. It also may be given as a preoperative prophylaxis to patients undergoing transurethral procedures or transrectal prostate biopsy. Lomefloxacin is a once-a-day oral preparation. Contraindications, adverse effects, and drug interactions are similar to those for ciprofloxacin. Lomefloxacin may induce serious photosensitivity reactions. It should be discontinued at the first sign of rash, redness, or burning sensation on the skin.

NORFLOXACIN

Norfloxacin (Noroxin) is used to treat UTIs, prostatitis, and urethral or endocervical gonorrhea. It is an oral agent very similar to ciprofloxacin, with the same antimicrobial spectrum. Contraindications, adverse effects, and drug interactions are the same as those listed for ciprofloxacin.

OFLOXACIN

Ofloxacin (Floxin) is available in oral, parenteral, and topical formulations. It is very similar to ciprofloxacin in antimicrobial spectrum, pharmacotherapeutics, and adverse effects. However, ofloxacin is considered to be less efficacious. Drug interactions also are similar to those of ciprofloxacin, except that ofloxacin does not affect theophylline levels.

Third-Generation Fluoroquinolones

GATIFLOXACIN

Gatifloxacin (Tequin) is a new type of fluoroquinolone. It was designed with a unique 8-methoxy structure that appears to enhance bactericidal action and decrease the rate at which resistance develops in gram-positive bacteria. Gatifloxacin is effective in treating patients with respiratory infections, such as acute exacerbation of chronic bronchitis, acute sinusitis, and community-acquired pneumonia. It also is approved for treating UTIs and gonorrhea. It is available in bioequivalent 400-mg oral and IV formulations. Oral preparations require once-a-day dosing.

Contraindications, adverse effects, and drug interactions are similar to those for ciprofloxacin. In addition, gatifloxacin may induce hyperglycemia, even in nondiabetic patients, especially in the elderly and in patients with renal insufficiency. Photosensitivity reactions occur less frequently with gatifloxacin than with other fluoroquinolones. Prolongation of the QT interval (an adverse effect of several fluoroquinolones) and torsades de pointes (associated with sparfloxacin) do not occur with gatifloxacin.

GEMIFLOXACIN

Gemifloxacin (Factive) is used to manage acute exacerbations of chronic bronchitis caused by susceptible organisms such as *Streptococcus pneumoniae, Haemophilus influenzae, Haemophilus parainfluenzae,* and *Moraxella catarrhalis.* It is also used to manage community-acquired pneumonia caused by these bacteria or by *Mycoplasma pneumoniae, Chlamydia pneumoniae,* or *Klebsiella pneumoniae.*

Gemifloxacin is a once-a-day oral drug that is well tolerated. Common adverse effects include rash, photosensitivity, and elevations in liver enzymes.

LEVOFLOXACIN

Levofloxacin (Levaquin) may be more active than other fluoroquinolones against pneumococci and certain "atypical" respiratory pathogens. It is indicated for acute maxillary sinusitis, acute bacterial exacerbation of chronic bronchitis, community-acquired pneumonia, uncomplicated skin and skin-structure infections, complicated UTIs, acute pyelonephritis, cystitis, and prostatitis; sexually transmitted diseases such as urethral and cervical gonorrhea, nongonococcal urethritis, and cervicitis; and mixed infections of the urethra and cervix. It is administered orally or parenterally. Oral preparations require once-a-day dosing.

Food has little effect on absorption; thus, levofloxacin can be taken without regard to meals.

Although levofloxacin has less affinity for cations than do many other fluoroquinolones, patients should be cautioned about taking antacids, vitamin and mineral supplements, or sucralfate 2 hours before or 2 hours after levofloxacin administration.

Important precautions include patients with CNS disorders that predispose them to seizure activity and kidney failure. Severe renal impairment requires dosage reduction. Levofloxacin is associated with QT prolongation and, like gatifloxacin, can cause photosensitization, but incidence of these adverse effects is relatively low. Interaction studies have shown that levofloxacin, unlike other fluoroquinolones, causes few or no problems with drugs such as theophylline, warfarin, digoxin, and cyclosporine.

MOXIFLOXACIN

Moxifloxacin (Avelox) is another 8-methoxy fluoroquinolone similar to gatifloxacin. It is indicated for treating acute exacerbations of chronic bronchitis, acute sinusitis, and pneumonia. It is especially efficacious in eradicating pathogens that cause exacerbations of chronic bronchitis. An important consideration for moxifloxacin is that to date, because it is a new drug, no organisms have been shown to be resistant to it. Moxifloxacin is being investigated currently for use in managing tuberculosis. Moxifloxacin is administered orally once a day for 5 to 10 days. Contraindications, adverse effects, and drug interactions are similar to those listed for ciprofloxacin. In addition, substantial prolongation of the QT segment has been reported with moxifloxacin. It should be avoided in patients who have conditions or are taking medications known to prolong the QT interval and in patients with a predisposition to arrhythmias.

SPARFLOXACIN

Sparfloxacin (Zagam) is an oral fluoroquinolone indicated for community-acquired pneumonia and acute bacterial exacerbations of chronic bronchitis. It is less active than ciprofloxacin against *Pseudomonas aeruginosa* and some other gram-negative bacilli. Because of its long half-life, sparfloxacin can be administered once daily. It is administered as two 200-mg tablets the first day, followed by one tablet daily for 9 additional days.

Sparfloxacin may cause potentially treatment-limiting photosensitivity reactions as well as QT prolongation. Torsades de pointes have been reported in patients receiving sparfloxacin who were also receiving disopyramide or amiodarone. As is the case with levofloxacin, severe renal impairment requires dosage reduction.

Fourth-Generation Fluoroquinolones

TROVAFLOXACIN AND ALATROFLOXACIN

Trovafloxacin (Trovan) and alatrofloxacin are two different names for the same active drug. Trovafloxacin is the generic name for the oral tablets, whereas alatrofloxacin is the IV prodrug, which metabolizes into trovafloxacin. Trovafloxacin is a once-a-day drug that is highly effective against resistant organisms, including anaerobic bacteria, and penetrates the CSF to a greater degree than other fluoroquinolones. Trovafloxacin is the first fluoroquinolone to be approved for oral surgery prophylaxis.

Trovafloxacin is metabolized by conjugation, which decreases the potential for cytochrome-based drug interactions and theoretically may induce fewer adverse effects than those of other fluoroquinolones. However, substantial interactions may occur with aluminum-magnesium antacids, iron, sucralfate, and IV morphine. Trovafloxacin has been associated with elevated hepatic enzymes, hepatitis, and fatal hepatotoxicity. Additionally, trovafloxacin therapy may induce acute pancreatitis.

Drug Significantly Different From Ciprofloxacin

Polymyxin B is an older antibiotic that is completely different from the fluoroquinolones. Its spectrum of activity is limited to gram-negative bacteria, with the exception of *Proteus* and *Neisseria* species. Polymyxin B binds to phospholipids in the cell membranes of gram-negative bacteria. This binding increases the permeability of the cell membrane, which results in loss of metabolites essential to bacterial existence.

Polymyxin B is administered commonly as either a topical, ophthalmic, or otic drug. It rarely is used systemically, because of its potential for causing nephrotoxicity or neurotoxicity. It frequently is used in combination with other drugs such as trimethoprim B (Polytrim) or bacitracin and neomycin (Neosporin). It also is used in combination with neomycin alone as a urinary tract irrigant.

CHAPTER SUMMARY

- Quinolone antibiotics inhibit an enzyme needed for bacterial DNA replication.
- Quinolone antibiotics, like cephalosporin antibiotics, are categorized into generations.
- First-generation quinolones are used only to treat uncomplicated UTIs.
- The second, third, and fourth generations are called fluoroquinolone antibiotics.
- Second-generation fluoroquinolones have systemic activity.
- Third-generation fluoroquinolones have extended activity against gram-positive pathogens but are less active than second-generation drugs against *Pseudomonas* species.
- Fourth-generation drugs are active against *Pseudomonas* species and anaerobic bacteria.
- Ciprofloxacin is the prototype fluoroquinolone.
- Fluoroquinolones should not be used in children, during pregnancy, or while breast-feeding because of their potential to cause arthropathies in children.
- Polymyxin B is another type of miscellaneous antibiotic.

QUESTIONS FOR STUDY AND REVIEW

1. Describe the spectrum of activity of the four generations of quinolone antibiotics.
2. How do fluoroquinolone drugs, such as ciprofloxacin, inhibit bacteria?
3. In addition to hypersensitivity, which other contraindications are associated with ciprofloxacin use?
4. Why is it important that patients take ciprofloxacin on an empty stomach?
5. Why is polymyxin B rarely used in its parenteral form?

> **Need More Help?**
>
> Chapter 40 of the study guide for *Drug Therapy in Nursing* 2e contains NCLEX-style questions and other learning activities to reinforce your understanding of the concepts presented in this chapter. For additional information or to purchase the study guide, visit *http://connection.lww.com/go/aschenbrenner.*

REFERENCES AND BIBLIOGRAPHY

Andes, D., Anon, J., Jacobs, M. R., et al. (2004). Application of pharmacokinetics and pharmacodynamics to antimicrobial therapy of respiratory tract infections. *Clinical Laboratory Medicine, 24*(2), 477–502.

Arce, F. C., Bhasin, R. S., Pasmantier, R., et al. (2004). Severe hyperglycemia during gatifloxacin therapy in patients without diabetes. *Endocrinology Practice, 10*(1), 40–44.

Clinical Pharmacology [Online]. Available: *http://cp.gsm.com.*

Cunha, B. A. (2004). Empiric therapy of community-acquired pneumonia: Guidelines for the perplexed? *Chest, 125*(5), 1913–1919.

Eliopoulos, G. M. (2004). Quinolone resistance mechanisms in pneumococci. *Clinical Infectious Diseases, 38*(Suppl. 4), S350–356.

Facts and Comparisons. (2004). *Drug facts and comparisons.* Philadelphia: Lippincott Williams & Wilkins.

Hardman, J. G. (2001). *Goodman & Gilman's the pharmacological basis of therapeutics* (10th ed.). New York: McGraw-Hill Health Professions Division.

Katzung, B. (2004). *Basic and clinical pharmacology* (9th ed.). New York: McGraw-Hill/Appleton & Lange.

Mandell, L. A., Iannini, P. B., Tillotson, G. S., et al. (2004). Respiratory fluoroquinolones: Differences in the details. *Clinical Infectious Diseases, 38*(9), 1331–1332.

Micromedex Healthcare Series [Online]. Available: *http://healthcare.micromedex.com.*

Nicolle, L. E. (2002). Urinary tract infection: Traditional pharmacologic therapies. *American Journal of Medicine, 113*(Suppl 1A), 35S–44S.

Sprandel, K. A., & Rodvold, K. A. (2003). Safety and tolerability of fluoroquinolones. *Clinical Cornerstone,* (Suppl. 3), S29–36.

Tatro, D. S. (2004). *Drug interaction facts.* Philadelphia: Lippincott Williams & Wilkins.

Yu, V. L., Greenberg, R. N., Zadeikis, N., et al. (2004). Levofloxacin efficacy in the treatment of community-acquired legionellosis. *Chest, 125*(6), 2135–2139.

Zhanel, G. G., Ennis, K., Vercaigne, L., et al. (2002). A critical review of the fluoroquinolones: Focus on respiratory infections. *Drugs, 62*(1), 13–59.

Drugs Treating Urinary Tract Infections

chapter 41

Learning Objectives

At the completion of this chapter the student will:

1 Describe the primary therapeutic uses for sulfonamides, urinary tract antiseptics, and urinary tract analgesics.
2 Identify core drug knowledge about drugs that are used for treating urinary tract infections.
3 Identify core patient variables relevant to drugs that are used for treating urinary tract infections.
4 Relate the interaction of core drug knowledge to core patient variables for drugs that are used for treating urinary tract infections.
5 Generate a nursing plan of care from the interactions between core drug knowledge and core patient variables for drugs that are used for treating urinary tract infections.
6 Describe nursing interventions to maximize therapeutic and minimize adverse effects for drugs that are used for treating urinary tract infections.
7 Determine key points for patient and family education for drugs that are used for treating urinary tract infections.

KEY TERMS

acute pyelonephritis

crystalluria

cystitis

para-aminobenzoic acid (PABA)

prostatitis

recurrent infection

reinfection

relapse

sulfonamides

urethritis

FEATURED WEBLINK

http://kidney.niddk.nih.gov/kudiseases/pubs/utiadult/
What is a urinary tract infection? Who is at risk? What are the symptoms? These questions and many others are answered at this website.

CONNECTION WEBLINK

Additional Weblinks are found on Connection:
http://www.connection.lww.com/go/aschenbrenner.

Drugs Treating Urinary Tract Infections

Ⓒ Sulfonamides

- **P SMZ-TMP**
- sulfisoxazole
- sulfasalazine
- fosfomycin

Ⓒ Urinary Tract Antiseptics

- methenamine
- nitrofurantoin

Ⓒ Urinary Tract Analgesics

- phenazopyridine

The symbol Ⓒ indicates the **drug class.**
Drugs in **bold type** marked with the symbol P are prototypes.
Drugs in blue type are closely related to the prototype.
Drugs in red type are significantly different from the prototype.
Drugs in black type with no symbol are also used in drug therapy; no prototype

A urinary tract infection (UTI) is a clinical condition caused by microorganisms infecting structures within the urinary system. It is the most common cause of infection in the United States, affecting more than 7 million individuals yearly. Females are more likely than males to have UTIs because of their short urethras and the potential for contamination of the vaginal vestibule with fecal flora. Men have protection from UTIs because of the length of their urethras and the antibacterial properties of prostatic fluid. After 50 years of age, however, men become more prone to UTIs because of prostatic hypertrophy, which can obstruct the urethra. Several disorders can be classified as UTIs. These conditions include cystitis, acute urethral syndrome, prostatitis, and acute pyelonephritis.

This chapter discusses drugs, other than fluoroquinolones (see Chapter 40), used to manage UTIs. They include sulfonamide antibiotics, urinary tract antiseptics, and urinary tract analgesics. The prototypical sulfonamide is sulfamethoxazole-trimethoprim (SMZ-TMP) (Bactrim, Septra). Drugs significantly different from SMZ-TMP include sulfasalazine, fosfomycin, and several other classes of antibiotics. Urinary tract antiseptics include methenamine (Hiprex, Urex), nitrofurantoin (Furadantin, Macrodantin, Macrobid), nalidixic acid (NegGram), and cinoxacin (Cinobac). The only urinary analgesic is phenazopyridine (Pyridium). In addition, this chapter discusses nursing management related to evaluating the patient's condition, monitoring for adverse effects, and teaching the patient and family about agents for UTI.

PHYSIOLOGY

Normally, several host defenses protect an individual from UTI. The urinary bladder is lined with a mucin layer that acts as a barrier against bacterial invasion. This layer also secretes protective substances that eventually become part of the mucin layer. Elderly and postmenopausal women produce less mucin and therefore are at a higher risk for UTI.

Another host defense is the washout phenomenon. The ureters assist the movement of urine out of the renal pelvis to the bladder by peristaltic movement. During micturition, bacteria are washed out of the ureters and bladder. Interruption of outflow, such as urethrovesicular reflux (in which urine from the urethra backs up into the bladder) or vesicoureteral reflux (in which urine from the bladder backs up into the ureters) can increase the risk for UTI by introducing bacteria into the renal system. Obstructed outflow results in stasis of urine, which under static conditions acts as a medium for microbial growth. Functional obstructions, such as neurogenic bladder, constipation, or infrequent voiding, can also increase the risk for UTIs.

Immune mechanisms provide another host defense. These mechanisms include immunoglobulin A, which provides an antibacterial defense, and phagocytic blood cells, which remove bacteria from the urinary tract. Alterations in the immune system increase the risk for UTIs.

PATHOPHYSIOLOGY

Urinary tract infections are generally classified as complicated or uncomplicated. UTIs are also divided into upper and lower UTIs. Upper UTIs are commonly associated with symptoms such as fever, nausea and vomiting, and flank or back pain. Lower UTIs are associated with symptoms such as dysuria (painful urination), hematuria (blood in urine), urgency, and frequency. It is important to use these distinctions only as general guidelines because studies have indicated that a patient may have an upper UTI while exhibiting only lower tract symptoms (Figure 41.1).

UTIs can be acute, **recurrent,** or chronic. Acute UTI is also known as the "initial infection." Recurrent UTIs are those caused by **relapse** or **reinfection.** A relapse is caused by the same organism that caused the initial infection. A reinfection is caused by a new organism. Chronic UTIs are those that need prophylactic pharmacotherapy because of the frequency of infection.

Cystitis

Cystitis is an infection of the lower urinary tract caused by introduction of a pathogen into the bladder. This infection results in redness, inflammation, irritation, and edema of the bladder mucosa, with multiple submucosal hemorrhages and sometimes pus. Symptoms may include urgency, frequency, incontinence, dysuria, hematuria, burning or a feeling of warmth on urination, bladder cramps or spasms, perineal itching, suprapubic discomfort, mild backache, or a low-grade fever. Nosocomial bladder infections, which are infections acquired in the hospital, are frequently caused by instrumentation and urinary catheterization. More commonly, bladder infections occur in the community. Factors that increase

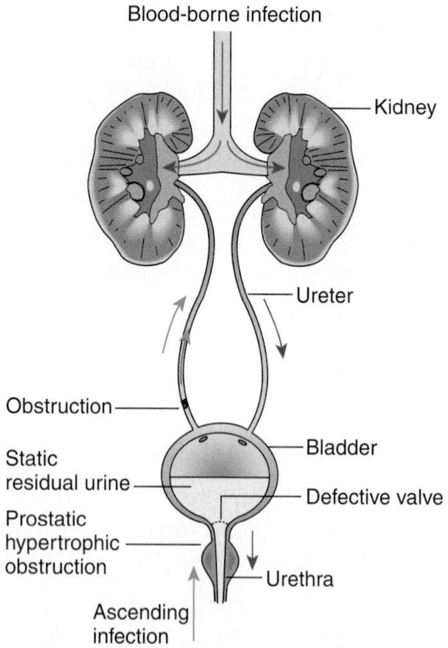

FIGURE 41.1 Urinary tract infections (UTIs) result from various causes: blood-borne infections that cycle through the renal system; ascending infection from external or other sources; stagnant urine (urinary stasis) caused by immobility or obstructions, which allows microorganisms to colonize; defective valves that may allow infected urine to flow backward; and other problems.

the risk for community-acquired UTIs include pregnancy, diaphragm with spermicide use, sexual intercourse, and delayed postcoital micturition. Complications include chronic cystitis or acute pyelonephritis.

Acute Urethral Syndrome

Acute urethral syndrome is also known as **urethritis.** It is characterized by redness, irritation, and edema of the urethral mucosa. Urethral discharge may also be evident. Common pathogens in these infections include *Ureaplasma* species, *Chlamydia* species, and *Trichomonas vaginalis.* In women, urethritis is associated with irritation by chemicals in feminine deodorants, suppositories, bubble baths, and spermicidal gels. In postmenopausal women, it is commonly caused by tissue changes related to low estrogen levels. Complications include chronic urethritis, cystitis, periurethral abscess, urethral stricture or fistula, pyelonephritis, and in men, prostatitis or epididymitis.

Prostatitis

Prostatitis is usually associated with urethritis or cystitis. Organisms can infect the prostate gland through the bloodstream or by ascending from the urethra. Symptoms include fever, chills, dysuria, urethral discharge, and a boggy, tender prostate. Diagnosis may be made by massaging the prostate, which results in a urethral discharge of prostatic secretions full of white blood cells. Complications include chronic prostatitis, epididymitis, and pyelonephritis.

Acute Pyelonephritis

Acute pyelonephritis is an infection of the kidneys and renal pelvis. Infection can occur by way of the bloodstream or ascending organisms from the bladder. Approximately 80% of cases of pyelonephritis are caused by a uropathogenic strain of *Escherichia coli* that has specific fimbriae that attach to the epithelial cells of the kidney. When microorganisms invade the kidney, an inflammatory process is initiated, resulting in local edema. As the edema subsides with treatment, fibrosis and scar tissue develop. This scarring may lead to impaired tubular reabsorption and diminished renal function.

Predisposing factors are urinary tract instrumentation, catheterization, pregnancy, vesicoureteral reflux, and neurogenic bladder. Symptoms include acute onset of chills and fever, flank pain, hematuria, general malaise or fatigue, headache, and costovertebral angle tenderness.

C SULFONAMIDES

Sulfonamides are the mainstay of treatment for UTIs. They have similar structures, functions, and therapeutic indications. Sulfonamides are categorized as short acting, intermediate acting, topical, and long acting, although the long-acting sulfonamides are not available for use in the United States because they can cause Stevens-Johnson syndrome. Sulfamethoxazole-trimethoprim is a combination of a sulfonamide and another antibacterial drug. SMZ-TMP is the prototype sulfonamide. Table 41.1 provides a summary of selected drugs used to treat UTI.

NURSING MANAGEMENT OF THE PATIENT RECEIVING P SULFAMETHOXAZOLE-TRIMETHOPRIM

Core Drug Knowledge

Pharmacotherapeutics

Sulfamethoxazole-trimethoprim (also known as cotrimoxazole) has a broad range of therapeutic uses. It is indicated for uncomplicated UTIs and systemic infections caused by susceptible organisms. SMZ-TMP is frequently used for respiratory infections caused by *Haemophilus influenzae* or *Streptococcus pneumoniae.* It is an alternative treatment for *Legionella pneumophila* pneumonia. SMZ-TMP is used for prophylaxis and treatment of *Pneumocystis carinii* pneumonia. Gastrointestinal (GI) infections treated with SMZ-TMP include shigellosis and salmonella. SMZ-TMP concentrates in prostate and vaginal fluids and thus is an effective treatment for infections at these sites. SMZ-TMP is also effective treatment for sexually transmitted diseases, such as acute gonococcal urethritis and oropharyngeal gonorrhea.

Pharmacokinetics

Sulfamethoxazole-trimethoprim is completely absorbed following oral administration. It is metabolized in the liver to inactive byproducts and excreted primarily in the urine. Peak plasma levels generally occur within 4 hours. After intravenous (IV) administration of SMZ-TMP, peak plasma levels occur in approximately 1 hour; the half-life is age dependent. SMZ-TMP is well distributed throughout the body, crosses the blood–brain barrier and the placenta, and is excreted in breast milk.

Pharmacodynamics

Sulfamethoxazole-trimethoprim inhibits microorganisms by interfering with the synthesis of folic acid (folate). Folate is necessary for the microorganism's biosynthesis of DNA, RNA, and proteins. SMZ, which is structurally similar to **para-aminobenzoic acid (PABA),** displaces PABA and blocks the synthesis of dihydrofolic acid (Figure 41.2). TMP interferes with microbial production of tetrahydrofolic acid, resulting in the formation of nonfunctional folate. SMZ-TMP is bacteriostatic: it inhibits the formation of new bacteria but has no effect on already formed bacteria. The presence of necrotic tissue, pus, or serum interferes with the action of SMZ-TMP because these materials contain PABA.

Contraindications and Precautions

Sulfamethoxazole-trimethoprim is contraindicated in patients with hypersensitivity to sulfonamides, deficiency of glucose-6-phosphate dehydrogenase (G6PD) or other folate deficiency disorders, porphyria (porphobilinogen in urine), urinary obstruction, term pregnancy, infants younger than 2 months (except for treating congenital toxoplasmosis), and lactating mothers. Patients with hypersensitivity to thiazide diuretics or sulfonylureas may have cross-sensitivity to sulfonamides because of the related sulfa structures of these drugs.

Use in pregnant women at term, in children younger than 2 months, and in mothers nursing infants younger than 2 months is contraindicated because sulfonamides may pro-

TABLE 41.1 Summary of Selected Drugs to Treat Urinary Tract Infections

Drug (Trade) Name	Selected Indications	Route and Dosage Range	Pharmacokinetics
(C) Sulfonamides			
(P) sulfamethoxazole-trimethoprim (SMZ-TMP; Bactrim) single strength (SS): 80 mgTMP/400 mg SMZ; double strength (DS): 160 mg TMP/ 800 mg SMZ; pediatric suspension: 40 mg TMP/200 mg SMZ per tsp (5 mL)	UTIs, otitis media, acute bronchitis, skin or soft tissue infections	*Adult:* 1 DS or 2 SS or 4 tsp suspension q 12 h for 10–14 d *Alternate:* 6 tablets at one time *Child >2 mo:* Up to 10 kg: 1 tsp; 11–20 kg: 2 tsp or 1 SS tab; 21–30 kg: 3 tsp or 1.5 SS tab; 31–40 kg: 4 tsp or 2 SS tab or 1 DS tab for 10–14 d	*Onset:* Varies *Duration:* 6–12 h $t_{1/2}$: 8–12 h
	Diarrhea or shigella	Same dose as above but stop after 5 days	
	PCP	*Adult and child:* 15–20 mg/kg TMP and 75–100 mg/kg SMZ in 24 h in divided doses every 6 h for 14–21 d	
	PCP prophylaxis	*Adult:* 1 DS every day *Child:* 150 mg/m2/d TMP with 750 mg/m2/d SMZ in equally divided doses 2 ×/d on 3 consecutive days per week	
sulfisoxazole (Novosoxazole; *Canadian:* Novo-Soxazole)	UTIs, chancroid trachoma, nocardiosis, meningococcal meningitis, inclusion conjunctivitis, and others	*Adult:* PO, 4–8 g/d in four to six divided doses *Child >2 y:* PO, 25–30 mg/kg am and pm	*Onset:* Varies *Duration:* Unknown $t_{1/2}$: 4.5–7.8 h
sulfasalazine (Azulfidine; *Canadian:* Alti-Sulfasalazine)	UTIs, ulcerative colitis	*Adult:* PO, 3–4 g/d in evenly divided doses; maintenance, 2 g/d (500 mg qid) *Child >2 y:* PO, 20–30 mg/kg/d in four divided doses	*Onset:* 1 h *Duration:* 6–12 h $t_{1/2}$: 5–10 h
fosfomycin (Monurol)	UTIs	*Adult and child >12 y:* PO, 3 g, one time only	*Onset:* Rapid *Duration:* Unknown $t_{1/2}$: 4–8 h
(C) Urinary Tract Antiseptics			
methenamine (Hiprex, Urex; *Canadian:* Dehydral)	UTIs	*Adult:* PO, 1 g > qid *Child 6–12 y:* PO, 500 mg qid; <6 y, PO 50 mg/kg in 3 divided doses	*Onset:* Rapid *Duration:* Unknown $t_{1/2}$: 3–6 h
nitrofurantoin (Furadantin, Macrodantin, Macrobid; *Canadian:* Apo-Nitrofurantoin)	UTIs	*Adult:* 50–100 mg qid 10–14 d; suppressive history: 50–100 mg PO hs. *Child >1 mo:* 5–7 mg/kg/d in 4 divided doses; suppressive history: 1 mg/kg/d	*Onset:* Rapid *Duration:* Unknown $t_{1/2}$: 20–60 min
(C) Urinary Tract Analgesic			
phenazopyridine (Pyridium; *Canadian:* Phenazo)	UTIs	*Adult:* PO 200 mg tid after meals *Child 6–12 y:* 12 mg/kg/d in three divided doses	*Onset:* Rapid *Duration:* Unknown $t_{1/2}$: Unknown

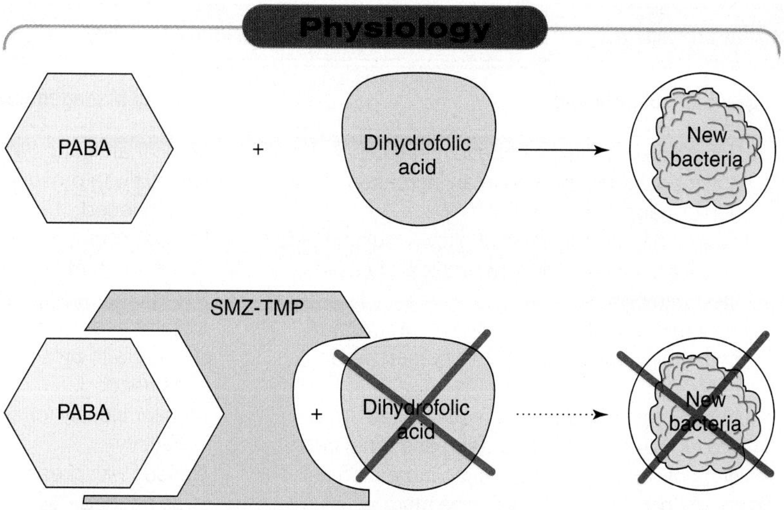

FIGURE 41.2 Simplified mechanism of action of SMZ-TMP. SMZ-TMP interferes with the formation of folic acid, which is needed to create the DNA and RNA for new microorganisms. SMZ-TMP displaces para-aminobenzoic acid (PABA) and blocks the synthesis of dihydrofolic acid. Both PABA and dihydrofolic acid are needed for new bacteria to form.

mote kernicterus (staining of certain areas of the brain by bilirubin) in the newborn by displacing bilirubin from plasma proteins.

Patients with G6PD deficiency may develop dose-related hemolytic anemia. SMZ-TMP is used cautiously in patients with hepatic or renal failure.

Adverse Effects

Sulfamethoxazole-trimethoprim is well tolerated in routine use. In immunocompromised patients, however, SMZ-TMP produces a higher incidence of adverse effects. Although nausea, vomiting, and diarrhea occur most frequently with SMZ-TMP, there are three classic potential adverse reactions to this drug: hematologic effects (such as anemia), allergic reactions, and crystalluria.

Hematologic effects are related to the direct action of SMZ-TMP on bone marrow. SMZ-TMP can induce megaloblastic anemia in patients with folate deficiency. Other blood dyscrasias, such as hemolytic anemia, agranulocytosis, leukopenia, thrombocytopenia, and aplastic anemia, may occur. Patients at high risk for folate deficiency are elderly adults, patients with long-term alcoholism, patients with malabsorption disorders, and patients with malnutrition.

Allergic reactions are common. SMZ-TMP is associated with several cutaneous reactions, including urticaria, maculopapular rashes, pruritus, contact dermatitis, and erythema nodosum. More severe reactions, such as Stevens-Johnson syndrome and exfoliative dermatitis, have been reported. Photosensitivity reactions may also occur and can continue for months after discontinuing the drug. Immunocompromised patients have a higher risk for photosensitive cutaneous eruptions. The mechanism for this increase in cutaneous eruptions is not clear.

Although the newer sulfonamides are much more soluble than older formulations, sulfonamides in general have poor solubility in water. If the urine volume and pH value drop, these drugs may crystallize in the renal tubules. This condition, called **crystalluria,** results in severe renal damage. To avoid crystalluria, patients should be instructed to maintain hydration by drinking at least 1.5 L of water every day.

Other potential adverse reactions may affect the central nervous system (CNS). Effects such as drowsiness, dizziness, and ataxia may occur. Additionally, depression and psychosis have been reported, although these effects are rare.

Drug Interactions

Certain sulfonamides are highly bound to serum proteins. When given in combination with other drugs that are also protein bound, sulfonamides may displace those drugs from their binding sites and enhance their action. This interaction occurs most frequently with drugs such as oral hypoglycemics, phenytoin, oral anticoagulants, and the antineoplastic drug methotrexate. The action of sulfonamides may be diminished when administered with local anesthetics, such as procaine, that are derived from PABA. Table 41.2 lists drugs that interact with SMZ-TMP.

Foods that can acidify the urine (such as cranberry juice) should be avoided. When the urine pH falls, the sulfonamides may precipitate and cause crystalluria.

SMZ-TMP may produce false-positive results when testing for proteinuria with sulfosalicylic acid tests. This possibility is important because SMZ-TMP actually can cause a true proteinuria, with associated nephrotoxicity. It may also give a false-positive result in tests for urine urobilinogen.

Assessment of Relevant Core Patient Variables

Health Status

Carefully assess for potential hypersensitivity to sulfonamides and other contraindications for drug therapy. Cross-sensitivity may also occur with chemically related drugs, such

TABLE 41.2 Agents That Interact With P Sulfamethoxazole-Trimethoprim (SMZ-TMP)

Interactants	Effect and Significance	Nursing Management
oral anticoagulants dicumarol warfarin	Sulfonamides inhibit the hepatic metabolism of oral anticoagulants, resulting in an increased risk for hemorrhage.	Monitor anticoagulant activity closely. Consult with prescriber about adjusting dose as needed.
cyclosporine	Although the mechanism is unknown, sulfonamides may increase the risk of nephrotoxicity associated with cyclosporine.	Monitor cyclosporine levels. Monitor serum creatinine frequently. Avoid coadministration if possible.
hydantoins	Sulfonamides inhibit the hepatic metabolism of hydantoins, resulting in an increased risk for toxicity.	Monitor hydantoin levels. Consult with prescriber about adjusting dose as needed.
methotrexate	Sulfonamides may displace methotrexate from protein binding sites and decrease renal clearance of drug. This results in an increased risk for methotrexate-induced bone marrow suppression.	Monitor closely for signs of hematologic toxicity. Consult with prescriber about adjusting dose as needed.
oral hypoglycemics	Sulfonamides inhibit the hepatic metabolism of oral hypoglycemics, resulting in hypoglycemia.	Monitor blood glucose level. Consult with prescriber about adjusting dose as needed.
zidovudine	Sulfonamides inhibit renal clearance of zidovudine, resulting in an increased effect of zidovudine in clients with impaired hepatic function.	Monitor zidovudine level. Consult with prescriber about adjusting dose as needed.

as the thiazide or loop diuretics and the oral sulfonylureas. SMZ-TMP should not be administered to patients with hepatic or renal dysfunction, porphyria, blood dyscrasias, or G6PD deficiency. Monitor patients with folate deficiency closely.

When therapy is anticipated to last more than 2 weeks, complete blood counts should be done to establish a baseline value before starting therapy.

Life Span and Gender

Evaluate the patient's pregnancy or breast-feeding status. To avoid inducing kernicterus, SMZ-TMP and the other sulfonamides should not be administered to pregnant or lactating women, nor should they be given to infants younger than 2 months.

Lifestyle, Diet, and Habits

Ask the patient about dietary intake of foods and fluids that acidify the urine because many drugs are affected by urine's pH, and acidic urine increases the risk for crystalluria. Determine whether the patient has a condition that contraindicates an increased fluid intake because increasing fluids decreases the potential for crystalluria.

Environment

Evaluate the amount of time the patient spends outdoors because photosensitivity may occur. The patient should avoid direct sunlight; if going outdoors is unavoidable, encourage the patient to wear sunscreen with a minimum skin protective factor of 15 and appropriate clothing.

Nursing Diagnoses and Outcomes

- Pain related to altered comfort level (nausea, vomiting, diarrhea, dizziness, or headache) from adverse effects of SMZ-TMP
  Desired outcome: *The patient will develop strategies to cope with pain and take the drug as directed for the full course of therapy.*
- Risk for Injury related to drug-induced hypersensitivity reactions, liver or kidney dysfunction, or blood dyscrasias
  Desired outcome: *By the end of therapy, the patient will be free from avoidable drug therapy–related injuries and infection.*
- *Risk for Impaired Tissue Integrity related to drug-induced photosensitivity*
  Desired outcome: *The patient will take measures to protect his or her skin from prolonged sun exposure.*

Planning and Intervention

Maximizing Therapeutic Effects

Administer SMZ-TMP 1 hour before or 2 hours after a meal with a full glass of water to enhance the absorption of the drug. Patients who experience adverse GI effects may take the drug with food.

Minimizing Adverse Effects

Unless contraindicated, the patient's fluid intake should increase by 1.5 L/day. Increasing fluid intake decreases the potential for crystalluria and decreases the ability of bacteria to multiply because the urine is diluted. The patient should

take precautions before exposure to the sun. When administering SMZ-TMP by the IV route, infuse the drug slowly, over 60 to 90 minutes. After completing the infusion, flush all lines to remove any residual SMZ-TMP.

Providing Patient and Family Education

- Teach the patient the optimal way to take SMZ-TMP, advising the patient to take it 1 hour before or 2 hours after a meal. However, if the patient becomes nauseated, vomits, or cannot eat, the drug may be taken with meals to minimize discomfort.
- Teach interventions to decrease the risk for adverse effects. The patient should avoid foods that may acidify the urine and drink at least 1.5 L of water a day. The patient should also wear sunscreen and protective clothing when outside. These interventions will decrease the risk for crystalluria and photosensitivity reactions, respectively.
- Explain the potential adverse effects of SMZ-TMP and advise the patient to contact the prescriber immediately if a skin rash, fever, sore throat, blood in the urine, easy bruising, or nose bleeds develop.

Ongoing Assessment and Evaluation

Monitor patients for signs of hematologic dysfunction, such as sore throat, fever, bruising, or bleeding. Also, carefully monitor fluid intake and output of hospitalized patients. Optimally, the patient should maintain an output of 1,500 mL daily. Monitor urine pH as well. Urine pH below 5.5 may potentiate crystalluria. Patients with acidic urine may need sodium bicarbonate to neutralize the urine. With prolonged therapy, monitor kidney function and perform periodic urine testing to check for crystals. For patients receiving parenteral SMZ-TMP, monitor the IV site for signs of phlebitis.

MEMORY CHIP

P Sulfamethoxazole-Trimethoprim (SMZ-TMP)

- Used for UTI, prophylaxis and treatment of Pneumocystis carinii pneumonia, and infection by *Legionella, Shigella,* or *salmonella* species, *Haemophilus influenzae,* or *Streptococcus pneumoniae*
- Major contraindications: hypersensitivity, patients with deficiencies in G6PD or other folates, porphyria, urinary obstruction, term pregnancy just ready to deliver, and infants younger than 2 months old
- Most common adverse effects: nausea, vomiting, diarrhea
- Most serious adverse effects: hematopoietic effects, crystalluria, Stevens-Johnson syndrome
- **Life span alert: to avoid inducing kernicterus, this drug should not be given to pregnant or breast-feeding women, nor to infants younger than 2 months old.**
- Maximizing therapeutic effects: Administer 1 hour before or 2 hours after a meal.
- Minimizing adverse effects: Increase fluids by 1.5 L/day to avoid crystalluria.
- Most important patient education: Teach the patient strategies to avoid photosensitivity and crystalluria.

Drug Closely Related to P Sulfamethoxazole-Trimethoprim

Of the short-acting sulfonamides, sulfisoxazole (Novo-Soxazole) is the most frequently used. Sulfisoxazole is highly water soluble, which minimizes the risk for crystalluria. Sulfisoxazole can be administered orally or parenterally. High plasma levels are possible, making sulfisoxazole appropriate for treating a variety of systemic infections, such as nocardiosis and chancroid.

Drugs Significantly Different From P Sulfamethoxazole-Trimethoprim

Sulfasalazine

Sulfasalazine (Azulfidine), another short-acting sulfonamide, is given as an enteric-coated tablet for treating ulcerative colitis. Within the colon, sulfasalazine splits into its components aminosalicylic acid and sulfapyridine, which are the active antimicrobial metabolites. Its action begins in the bowel lumen instead of systemically. Its potential adverse effects and adverse reactions are similar to those of other sulfonamides.

Drugs That Belong to Other Antibiotic Classes

Several other classes of antibiotics can also be used to manage UTIs.

Aminoglycoside drugs such as gentamicin, tobramycin, and amikacin are used for infections that originated in the urinary tract but have become systemic. This kind of infection is known as urosepsis. These drugs are all administered intravenously.

Cephalosporins may be given orally or parenterally. Oral drugs include cephalexin, cephradine, and cefadroxil. Ceftazidime and ceftriaxone may be given orally or parenterally. Although these drugs are effective, they offer no clear advantage over less expensive drugs.

The fluoroquinolones ciprofloxacin, norfloxacin, and ofloxacin are very effective for managing UTIs. Ciprofloxacin and ofloxacin may be given both orally and parenterally.

CRITICAL THINKING SCENARIO

Teaching strategies for sulfamethoxazole-trimethoprim (SMZ-TMP) therapy

Melissa Hawthorne, a 25-year-old graduate student, comes to the campus health clinic with a complaint of dysuria and urinary frequency and urgency. She is diagnosed with a UTI and given a prescription for SMZ-TMP.

1. Prepare some instructions related to drug therapy for Melissa, explaining the rationale for the instructions.
2. How would you vary the instructions if Melissa were 78 years old or had a history of congestive heart failure?

Fluoroquinolones have a broad spectrum of activity that affects most microbes that cause UTIs. Many prescribers use these drugs as first-line agents, despite their expense. Other prescribers use these drugs after treatment fails with SMZ-TMP.

The penicillin drugs ampicillin, amoxicillin, and amoxicillin-clavulanate may also be administered. Ampicillin may be given orally or parenterally. Other parenteral penicillin drugs include ticarcillin, mezlocillin, and piperacillin. Penicillins are useful against most microbes that cause UTI; however, some penicillin resistance has been reported among *Escherichia coli.*

Tetracycline drugs are most useful in managing UTI caused by *Chlamydia* species, but incidence of resistance is high among other causative microbes (Box 41.1). Both tetracycline and doxycycline are effective against sensitive organisms.

Fosfomycin

Fosfomycin (Monurol) is classified as a miscellaneous antibiotic. It works by inhibiting an enzyme, pyruvyl transferase, which is critical in the synthesis of bacterial cell walls. The drug is distributed to the kidneys, bladder wall, prostate, and seminal vesicles. Fosfomycin has been shown to cross the placenta; however, whether it enters breast milk is unknown. It is not metabolized, and excretion occurs through both urine and feces.

FOCUS ON RESEARCH

Box 41.1 UTI in Aging Women

Hu, K. K., Boyko, E. J., Scholes, D., et al. (2004). Risk factors for urinary tract infections in postmenopausal women. *Archives of Internal Medicine, 164*(9), 989–993.

The Study

Urinary tract infections (UTI), the most common type of infection in women, occur frequently in postmenopausal women. The researchers conducted a case-control study of women between 55 and 75 years of age who were enrolled in a health maintenance organization. They interviewed 899 study subjects and 911 controls about their habits, general health, and potential risk factors for UTI. Like younger women, postmenopausal women with current UTI were more likely than uninfected women to be sexually active and to have a history of UTI. The researchers found that UTI risk factors among healthy, community-dwelling, postmenopausal women reflect their overall health status. Sexual activity, history of UTI, treated diabetes, and incontinence were all associated with an elevated risk of UTI.

Nursing Implications

UTI causes substantial morbidity and even mortality, especially in elderly patients. Untreated UTI can progress to pyelonephritis or septicemia. You are in a unique position to consistently assess patients for potential UTI. Although all patients should be assessed for UTI, you should assess hospitalized postmenopausal women with diabetes, incontinence, or a history of UTI particularly carefully. Report subjective or objective signs of UTI to the patient's primary health care provider immediately to avoid unnecessary complications.

Fosfomycin is administered orally for acute UTI as a one-time dose, without regard to meals. Advise the patient to place the entire contents of a sachet containing the equivalent of 3 g of fosfomycin into 3 to 4 oz (½ cup) of water, then stir to dissolve it. It is best not to use hot water. The patient should take the medication immediately after dissolving the powder.

Fosfomycin is in FDA pregnancy category B. It is not recommended for children younger than 12 years.

The most frequent adverse effects with fosfomycin therapy are asthenia, diarrhea, dizziness, dyspepsia, headache, nausea and vomiting, rash, and vaginitis. Although rare, serious adverse effects such as angioedema, aplastic anemia, asthma exacerbation, cholestatic jaundice, hepatic necrosis, and toxic megacolon have been reported.

URINARY TRACT ANTISEPTICS

Urinary tract antiseptics are drugs that work by local action because high serum levels are not achievable. Because of their local action, few systemic effects occur. No true prototype exists; thus, each drug is discussed separately here.

Methenamine

Methenamine (Hiprex, Urex) is indicated for suppressing or eliminating bacteriuria (bacteria in urine) associated with chronic cystitis and other chronic UTIs. It is effective against both gram-positive and gram-negative organisms. In fact, the only resistance to methenamine comes from organisms such as *Proteus vulgaris* and *Pseudomonas aeruginosa,* which raise urine pH.

In acidic urine, methenamine is hydrolyzed to ammonia and formaldehyde in the bladder. Because methenamine must be hydrolyzed into its components to be effective, it does not work for upper UTIs because the time through the upper urinary tract is insufficient for this action to occur. Additionally, patients with indwelling catheters have a constant outflow of urine, again negating the time needed for hydrolization to occur. Therefore, methenamine is not useful in patients with upper UTIs and indwelling catheters.

Methenamine is contraindicated in patients with hepatic dysfunction because ammonia is also a product of its hydrolysis. Patients with hepatic dysfunction cannot eliminate ammonia, and the high ammonia levels that result can adversely affect the CNS. Methenamine should not be given concurrently with sulfonamides because the combination forms an insoluble precipitate in acidic urine.

Adverse reactions are minimal. The most common are nausea, vomiting, and anorexia. Methenamine may also cause bladder irritation, dysuria, hematuria, and crystalluria when administered as long-term prophylaxis.

Nitrofurantoin

Nitrofurantoin (Furadantin, Macrodantin, Macrobid) is another synthetic urinary tract antiseptic. Its mechanism of action is uncertain, but the drug is presumed to interfere with

several bacterial enzyme systems. Although nitrofurantoin has a broad spectrum of activity, it is not an effective systemic drug because it is rapidly excreted by the kidneys and thus does not achieve high blood levels. It is highly effective against gram-negative and gram-positive organisms in the urinary system because high concentrations are found in urine. Resistant microbes include *Enterobacter, Klebsiella, Proteus,* and *Pseudomonas* species.

Nitrofurantoin is available in two pill formulations: microcrystalline nitrofurantoin (Furadantin) and macrocrystalline nitrofurantoin (Macrodantin, Macrobid). Although both types of nitrofurantoin have equal therapeutic efficacy, macrocrystalline nitrofurantoin is absorbed more slowly and induces less GI distress.

Nitrofurantoin is contraindicated in patients with renal impairment, infants younger than 1 month, and pregnant women at term. As previously mentioned, nitrofurantoin achieves high concentrations in urine but low concentrations in blood. In the presence of kidney dysfunction, concentration in urine decreases and concentration in blood increases. This effect decreases the efficacy of treatment and increases the risk for toxic adverse effects. Nitrofurantoin is contraindicated for infants younger than 1 month because of the possibility of hemolytic anemia. It should also be used with caution in the elderly (because of their decreased renal function) and in patients with G6PD deficiency, anemia, vitamin B deficiency, diabetes mellitus, or electrolyte abnormalities.

The most common adverse reactions are anorexia, nausea, and vomiting. Other adverse reactions include abdominal pain, diarrhea, parotitis, and pancreatitis. Hepatic reactions, including hepatitis, have occurred. Nitrofurantoin may induce an asthma attack in patients with a history of asthma. As with other urinary tract antiseptics, nitrofurantoin may cause hematopoietic effects, especially in patients with folate deficiency.

Nitrofurantoin has potentially serious adverse reactions. Peripheral neuropathy is one of the most serious toxic effects; however, it is reversible if detected early. Permanent damage may result if the drug is not discontinued. Peripheral neuropathy may be enhanced in debilitating diseases, such as diabetes mellitus, anemia, and vitamin B deficiency.

Nitrofurantoin is also associated with acute and chronic pulmonary reactions. Acute reactions are manifested by sudden onset of fever, cough, chills, myalgias, and dyspnea. As with other drugs, the effects are reversible if the drug is discontinued. Subacute pulmonary reactions develop over time with many of the same symptoms; however, diffuse interstitial pulmonary fibrosis may be irreversible in some patients. Subacute pulmonary reactions occur most frequently in patients on therapy longer than 6 months.

Quinolone Antibiotics

Nalidixic acid (NegGram) and cinoxacin (Cinobac) are two additional urinary tract antiseptic drugs. Because they are first-generation quinolone drugs, they are discussed in Chapter 40.

C URINARY ANALGESIC

Phenazopyridine (Pyridium) is used frequently for UTIs but does not itself have any antibacterial activity. It is excreted in the urine, where it exerts a topical analgesic effect. It is indicated for the symptomatic relief of pain, burning, frequency, and urgency caused by the irritation that infection produces in the urinary tract mucosa. The precise mechanism of action is not known. Phenazopyridine is contraindicated for patients with known hypersensitivity or renal insufficiency. Adverse reactions include headache, rash, pruritus, and gastrointestinal disturbances. Hematologic reactions are possible with overdose. Phenazopyridine is an azo dye, which will discolor the patient's urine orange or red. It is important to inform the patient to expect this change in urine color.

CHAPTER SUMMARY

- A UTI is caused by microorganisms infecting any structure within the urinary system.
- UTI is the most frequent type of infection in the United States.
- Sulfamethoxazole-trimethoprim (SMZ-TMP) is the prototype sulfonamide, which is the drug class most commonly used to treat UTI.
- Many other drug classes may be used to treat UTI. These include aminoglycosides, cephalosporins, fluoroquinolones, penicillins, tetracyclines, and fosfomycin.
- Urinary tract antiseptics work directly in the urinary tract and have minimal systemic activity. These drugs include methenamine, nitrofurantoin, nalidixic acid, and cinoxacin.
- Phenazopyridine has no antimicrobial effects. It is used as a urinary analgesic in combination with antimicrobial drugs.

QUESTIONS FOR STUDY AND REVIEW

1. In addition to UTI, which other diseases or disorders are treated with SMZ-TMP?
2. Why are sulfonamides ineffective against organisms that do not synthesize their own folate?
3. What is the difference between antibiotics used to manage UTI and urinary tract antiseptics?
4. What is the purpose of prescribing phenazopyridine (Pyridium) for a UTI, if it has no antibacterial activity?

? Need More Help?

Chapter 41 of the study guide for *Drug Therapy in Nursing 2e* contains NCLEX-style questions and other learning activities to reinforce your understanding of the concepts presented in this chapter. For additional information or to purchase the study guide, visit *http://connection.lww.com/go/aschenbrenner.*

REFERENCES AND BIBLIOGRAPHY

Belet, N., Islek, I., Belet, U., et al. (2004). Comparison of trimethoprim-sulfamethoxazole, cephadroxil and cefprozil as prophylaxis for recurrent urinary tract infections in children. *Journal of Chemotherapy, 16*(1), 77–81.

Clinical Pharmacology [Online]. Available: *http://cp.gsm.com.*

Facts and Comparisons. (2004). *Drug facts and comparisons.* Philadelphia: Lippincott Williams & Wilkins.

Hardman, J. G. (2001). *Goodman & Gilman's the pharmacological basis of therapeutics* (10th ed.). New York: McGraw-Hill Health Professions Division.

Kahan, N. R., Chinitz, D. P., Kahan, E., et al. (2004). Longer than recommended empiric antibiotic treatment of urinary tract infection in women: An avoidable waste of money. *Journal of Clinical Pharmacology and Therapeutics, 29*(1), 59–63.

Karpman, E., & Kurzrock, E. A. (2004). Adverse reactions of nitrofurantoin, trimethoprim and sulfamethoxazole in children. *Journal of Urology, 172*(2), 448–453.

Katzung, B. (2004). *Basic and clinical pharmacology* (9th ed.). New York: McGraw-Hill/Appleton & Lange.

Micromedex Healthcare Series [Online]. Available: *http://healthcare.micromedex.com.*

McLaughlin, S. P., & Carson, C. C. (2004). Urinary tract infections in women. *Medical Clinic of North America, 88*(2), 417–429.

Tatro, D. S. (2004). *Drug interaction facts.* Philadelphia: Lippincott Williams & Wilkins.

Tempera, G., Mirabile, M., Mangiafico, A., et al. (2004). Fosfomycin tromethamine in uncomplicated urinary tract infections: An epidemiological survey. *Journal of Chemotherapeutics, 16*(2), 216–217.

Wagenlehner, F. M., & Naber, K. G. (2004). Emergence of antibiotic resistance and prudent use of antibiotic therapy in nosocomially acquired urinary tract infections. *International Journal of Antimicrobial Agents, 23*(Suppl. 1), S24–S29.

Drugs Treating Mycobacterial Infections

chapter 42

Learning Objectives

At the completion of this chapter the student will:

1. Identify core drug knowledge about drugs that are used for treating mycobacterial infections.
2. Identify core patient variables relevant to drugs that are used for treating mycobacterial infections.
3. Relate the interaction of core drug knowledge to core patient variables for drugs that are used for treating mycobacterial infections.
4. Generate a nursing plan of care from the interactions between core drug knowledge and core patient variables for drugs that are used for treating mycobacterial infections.
5. Describe nursing interventions to maximize therapeutic and minimize adverse effects for drugs that are used for treating mycobacterial infections.
6. Determine key points for patient and family education for drugs that are used for treating mycobacterial infections.

KEY TERMS

chemoprophylaxis

Ghon complex

leprosy

Hansen disease

mycobacteria

M. avium

Mycobacterium avium complex (MAC)

M. leprae

M. tuberculosis

FEATURED WEBLINK

http://www.lungusa.org/site/pp.asp?c=dvLUK9O0E&b=35778

Are you familiar with the mycobacterial diseases described in this chapter? For more information regarding tuberculosis, log on to this website.

CONNECTION WEBLINK

Additional Weblinks are found on Connection:
http://www.connection.lww.com/go/aschenbrenner.

Drugs Treating Mycobacterial Infections

Ⓒ Drugs for Treating *M. tuberculosis*

- [P] **isoniazid**
- rifampin
- ethambutol
- pyrazinamide
- streptomycin

Ⓒ Drugs for Treating *M. leprae*

- [P] **rifampin**
- rifabutin
- rifapentine
- rifaximin
- clofazimine
- dapsone

The symbol Ⓒ indicates the **drug class.**
Drugs in **bold type** marked with the symbol [P] are prototypes.
Drugs in blue type are closely related to the prototype.
Drugs in red type are significantly different from the prototype.
Drugs in black type with no symbol are also used in drug therapy; no prototype

This chapter discusses pharmacologic management of mycobacterial infections. **Mycobacteria** are slow-growing microbes that require prolonged treatment, generally with multiple medications. Many of the antimycobacterial drugs may be used for more than one type of infection. Table 42.1 presents a summary of antimycobacterial drugs.

Although many *Mycobacterium* species exist, this chapter focuses on three species: ***M. tuberculosis, M. leprae,*** and ***M. avium.*** The prototype drug for treating *M. tuberculosis* is isoniazid (INH), and the prototype for treating *M. leprae* infection is rifampin. Drugs significantly different from INH include rifampin, ethambutol, pyrazinamide, and streptomycin; leprosy drugs significantly different from rifampin include dapsone, clofazimine, and several miscellaneous antibiotics. The drugs of choice for *M. avium* are clarithromycin and azithromycin; both are macrolide drugs that are covered in Chapter 39.

PATHOPHYSIOLOGY

Tuberculosis

Tuberculosis (TB) is a mycobacterial infection that is found most frequently in the lungs; however, it may invade any organ of the body. The two types of TB are *Mycobacterium tuberculosis hominis* (human) and *Mycobacterium tuberculosis bovis* (bovine). Human TB is an airborne disease spread by tiny, invisible particles called droplet nuclei. Bovine TB is spread through the gastrointestinal (GI) system after drinking milk from infected cows. In the United States, bovine TB is very rare because dairy herds are strictly monitored, and pasteurization of milk is widespread. Symptoms of active TB include night sweats, cough, low-grade fever, fatigue, weight loss, and anorexia.

Human TB can become a devastating disease, although the bacteria themselves are not particularly virulent. The damage to the human host is a result of a hypersensitivity response evoked by the bacteria. Untreated TB may result in death, whereas inadequately treated TB may result in multidrug-resistant TB.

Human TB is subdivided into primary or reactivated TB. Primary TB occurs in a person not previously exposed to the TB bacillus. After the droplet nuclei are inhaled, the bacillus passes through the upper airways and implants in an area of rich oxygenation, such as the apices of the lungs or upper area of the lower lobes. After implantation, the bacillus is engulfed by macrophages. The combination of bacillus and macrophages becomes a gray-white granulomatous lesion called a Ghon focus. As the center of this lesion becomes necrotic, it drains into the lung lymph system and creates caseous granulomas. The combination of the primary lung lesion and lymph node granulomas is referred to as **Ghon complex.** At this stage, the patient will have a positive reaction to the screening test for TB, the purified-protein derivative (PPD). The test involves a solution that is placed intradermally on the forearm of the patient. More than 10 mm of induration at the site of injection (or 5 mm of induration for an immunocompromised patient) is a positive reaction.

The body's hypersensitive response to Ghon complex is to "wall off" the bacillus, and the patient remains asymptomatic. A small percentage of people with primary TB develop active TB and symptoms. People with the highest risk for developing active TB at this stage are those with chronic diseases or immunosuppression.

Reactivated TB results from activation of previously healed primary lesions. Reactivation may occur as the body's defenses decline as the patient ages or acquires other diseases that weaken the immune system.

The standard criterion for the diagnosis of pulmonary TB is identification of the TB bacillus in a sputum culture. Three samples are usually obtained for an acid-fast stain. Another strong indication of active TB is identification of caseation and inflammation on a chest radiograph. Multidrug therapy is used for active TB because therapy lasts long enough to create the potential for drug resistance.

Patients with primary active or reactivated TB require multidrug therapy for 6 to 12 months. Therapy is based on the susceptibility of the infecting organism and the immunocompetence of the patient. Immunocompromised patients need a longer duration of therapy because their ability to fight infections is reduced.

Treatment of TB is divided into two phases: an induction phase and a continuation phase. For most patients, four drugs are administered daily during the induction phase, with the goal of rendering the sputum noninfectious. During the continuation phase, at least two drugs are administered daily, with the goal of eliminating all intracellular bacilli. The World Health Organization advocates TB treatment with Direct Observed Treatment, Short-Course (DOTS; Box 42.1).

People who have been exposed to TB but have not developed active TB may benefit from chemoprophylaxis. **Chemoprophylaxis** should be considered for anyone younger than 35 years with a positive PPD, people who are or have been in close contact with people with active TB, people who have seroconverted from negative to positive PPD within the past 1 to 2 years, patients with a history of untreated or inadequately treated TB, patients with a chest radiograph indicating TB lesions but no evidence of active TB, and those with special risk factors. Special risk factors include diabetes mellitus, prolonged corticosteroid therapy, immunosuppression therapy, end-stage renal disease, pre-existing lung disorders, chronic malnutrition, and human immunodeficiency virus (HIV) infection or acquired immunodeficiency syndrome (AIDS). Chemoprophylaxis with isoniazid is given for 6 months, or for up to 12 months in an immunocompromised patient.

Leprosy

Leprosy (**Hansen disease**) is a chronic infectious disease caused by *M. leprae,* an acid-fast, rod-shaped bacillus. The disease mainly affects the skin, the peripheral nerves, mucosa of the upper respiratory tract, and the eyes.

The two classifications of leprosy are paucibacillary leprosy (PB) and multibacillary leprosy (MB). They can be classified on the basis of skin-smear results or clinical manifestations. In the classification based on skin smears, patients who have negative smears at all sites are grouped as having PB, whereas those who have positive smears at any site are

TABLE 42.1 Summary of Selected Antimycobacterial Drugs

Drug (Trade) Name	Selected Indications	Route and Dosage Range	Pharmacokinetics
P isoniazid (Laniazid; *Canadian:* Isotamine)	TB in conjunction with other drug therapy, prophylaxis of TB	*Adult:* PO, active TB, 5 mg/kg/d up to 300 mg in single dose; prophylaxis, 300 mg/d in single dose *Child:* PO, active TB, 10–20 mg/kg/d; prophylaxis, 10 mg/kg/d in single dose	*Onset:* Varies *Duration:* 24 h $t_{1/2}$: 1–4 h
P rifampin (Rifadin; *Canadian:* Rofact)	TB in conjunction with other drug therapy, prophylaxis of TB	*Adult:* PO or IV, 600 mg in single daily dose until improvement occurs; direct observed treatment (DOTS) 10 mg/kg 2 × wk *Child:* 10–20 mg/k not to exceed 600 mg qd	*Onset:* PO, varies; IV, rapid *Duration:* 6 h $t_{1/2}$: 3–5.1 h
	Leprosy	*Adult:* PO or IV 600 mg 1 × month for 6–24 mo *Child:* not recommended	
	Mycobacterium avium complex (MAC)	*Adult:* 600 mg PO or IV in combination with other antimycobacterials *Child:* 10–20 mg/kg PO or IV in combination with other antimycobacterials	
clofazimine (Lamprene)	Leprosy	*Adult:* 50 mg qd self-administered 300 mg q month if supervised *Child:* 1 mg/kg/d	*Onset:* 1 h *Duration:* Unknown $t_{1/2}$: Terminal 8 days, tissue 70 days
dapsone (Avlosulfon)	Leprosy	*Adult:* PO, 100 mg qd *Child:* 1–2 mg/kg/d	*Onset:* 2 h *Duration:* Unknown $t_{1/2}$: 30 h
ethambutol (Myambutol; *Canadian:* Etibi)	TB in conjunction with other drug therapy, prophylaxis of TB	*Adult:* PO, mg/kg/d as single oral dose; retreatment, 25 mg/kg/d reduced after 60 d to 15 mg/kg/d once daily *Child:* Not recommended for children younger than 13 y	*Onset:* Rapid *Duration:* 20–24 h $t_{1/2}$: 3.3 h
pyrazinamide	TB in conjunction with other drug therapy, prophylaxis of TB	*Adult:* PO, 15–30 mg/d once daily *Child:* Same	*Onset:* Rapid *Duration:* 9.5 h $t_{1/2}$: 9–10 h
rifabutin (Mycobutin)	TB, leprosy, MAC	*Adult:* 300 mg PO qd, may be given 150 mg bid to decrease GI distress *Child:* Not approved	*Onset:* 1 h *Duration:* Unknown $t_{1/2}$: 16–69 h
rifapentine (Priftin)	TB	*Adult and child >12 y:* 600 mg 2 × wk for 2 mo, then 1 × week for 4 mo *Child:* Not recommended	*Onset:* 5–6 h *Duration:* Unknown $t_{1/2}$: 13 h
rifaximin (Xifaxin)	Travelers' diarrhea	*Adult and child >12 y:* PO, 200 mg 3 x day for 3 days	*Onset:* 1 hour *Duration:* Unknown $t_{1/2}$: 5.85–5.95 h
streptomycin	TB in conjunction with other drug therapy, prophylaxis of TB	*Adult:* IM, 15 mg/kg with a maximum of 1 g/d; reduce to 25–30 mg/kg or maximum of 1.5 g two to three times a week *Child:* IM, 20–40 mg/kg/d in divided doses q6–12h to a maximum of 1 g/d; reduce to 25–30 mg/kg two to three times a week	*Onset:* Rapid *Duration:* 24 h $t_{1/2}$: 2.5 h

BOX 42.1 The Five Elements of the DOTS Strategy

- Government commitment to sustained TB control activities
- Case detection by sputum smear microscopy among symptomatic patients self-reporting to health services
- Standardized treatment regimen of 6 to 8 months for at least sputum smear–positive cases, with DOTS for at least the initial 2 months
- A regular, uninterrupted supply of all essential anti-TB drugs
- A standardized recording and reporting system that enables assessment of treatment results for each patient and the TB control program performance overall

grouped as having MB. However, in practice, most prescribers use clinical criteria for classifying the disease and deciding the appropriate treatment regimen for individual patients because skin-smear services are not always available or dependable. The clinical system of classification uses the number of skin lesions and nerves involved as the basis for grouping leprosy. Patients with fewer than five lesions are diagnosed with PB leprosy, and patients with six or more lesions are diagnosed with MB leprosy. The correct classification is important because the treatment regimens differ between the two types of leprosy. Like TB, leprosy must be treated with a multidrug regimen for a prolonged time. Drugs used to manage leprosy include rifampin, dapsone, clofazimine, ofloxacin, and minocycline.

Mycobacterium Avium Complex

***Mycobacterium avium* complex** (**MAC**) is the term used to describe an opportunistic infection caused by two similar types of bacteria named *M. avium* and *M. avium-intracellulare*. Because these bacteria are so similar, they are referred to together as a "complex." However, *M. avium* is the predominant infective organism seen in most MAC infections in people with AIDS.

M. avium and *M. intracellulare* are very common. They are found in water, soil, dust, and food, and almost everyone has them in their body. A healthy immune system will control MAC, but immunocompromised people can develop a MAC infection. MAC can be localized or disseminated (sometimes called DMAC). It often occurs in the lungs, intestines, bone marrow, liver, and spleen. Symptoms of MAC include high fevers, chills, diarrhea, weight loss, stomachaches, fatigue, and anemia. When MAC disseminates, it can cause blood infections, hepatitis, pneumonia, and other serious problems.

MAC bacteria can mutate and develop resistance to pharmacotherapy. As with other mycobacterial infections, a combination of antibacterial drugs is used to manage MAC. Immunocompromised patients are started on MAC prophylaxis when their T-cell count drops below 50. Once an immunocompromised patient develops a MAC infection, treatment must continue for life to avoid recurrence. The drugs of choice for MAC prophylaxis and treatment are azithromycin and clarithromycin. These drugs are discussed in Chapter 49. Additional drugs that may be used for MAC include rifampin, rifabutin, and clofazimine, which are described in this chapter in the sections about TB and leprosy.

C DRUGS FOR TREATING *MYCOBACTERIUM TUBERCULOSIS* INFECTION

Antitubercular drugs are divided into two major categories: first- and second-line drugs. First-line drugs are those that are effective for treatment and have manageable toxicities. First-line drugs include isoniazid, rifampin, ethambutol, pyrazinamide, and streptomycin. Because TB can easily become drug resistant, combination therapy with three to four drugs is common (Box 42.2).

Isoniazid is frequently referred to as INH, an abbreviation related to its clinical structure. Isoniazid is included in all therapeutic regimens, except in those for INH-resistant TB. For that reason, INH is the prototype for antitubercular drugs. Table 42.1 presents a summary of drugs used to treat TB.

FOCUS ON RESEARCH

Box 42.2 Successful DOTS Depends on Adherence

Van Deun, A., Salim, M. A., Das, A. P., et al. (2004). Results of a standardised regimen for multidrug-resistant tuberculosis in Bangladesh. *International Journal of Tuberculosis and Lung Disease, 8*(5), 560–567.

The Study

Researchers developed a protocol to enhance the established DOTS program in Bangladesh in order to evaluate the potential cure rate for multidrug-resistant tuberculosis (MDR-TB). As directly observed therapy, 58 patients were given a 21-month standardized regimen with kanamycin, ofloxacin, prothionamide, pyrazinamide, ethambutol, isoniazid, and clofazimine. This regimen achieved 40 cures. Three treatment failures occurred; seven patients left the study because of nonadherence; and eight patients died. The main problem identified in the study was frequent and sometimes serious adverse effects from the medications used in the study regimen. The researchers concluded that although a standardized approach can be valuable for treatment of MDR-TB, equally effective but better tolerated drug therapy must be devised.

Nursing Implications

In the United States, MDR-TB is mainly prevalent in poor socioeconomic environments or in overcrowded populations, such as prisons. However, because MDR-TB is a global problem, travelers may transfer MDR strains between states, countries, and even continents. Be diligent in assessing patients with signs or symptoms of TB. Early diagnosis and treatment are important to stop the transmission of MDR-TB. Thorough patient teaching is essential to avoid nonadherence to drug therapy. If you suspect that a patient is nonadherent, refer him or her for DOTS therapy as soon as you identify the problem.

NURSING MANAGEMENT OF THE PATIENT RECEIVING [P] ISONIAZID

Core Drug Knowledge

Pharmacotherapeutics

Isoniazid is an antibacterial drug used to treat or prevent TB and other susceptible mycobacterial infections. *Mycobacterium* organisms generally considered susceptible to INH therapy include *M. avium, M. bovis, M. intracellulare, M. kansasii, M. szulgai,* and *M. xenopi.* In unlabeled use, INH has been used to treat severe tremors associated with multiple sclerosis.

Pharmacokinetics

Isoniazid is administered orally and intramuscularly. It is absorbed rapidly from the GI tract, with peak serum levels attained within 12 hours. It is distributed into all body tissues and fluids and crosses the blood–brain barrier to achieve therapeutic levels in the cerebrospinal fluid (CSF). It also crosses the placenta and is distributed into breast milk. INH is metabolized in the liver to inactive metabolites. About 75% of the drug and its metabolites are excreted in the urine, and the rest is excreted in the feces, saliva, and sputum (see Table 42.1).

Pharmacodynamics

Isoniazid is bactericidal or bacteriostatic, depending on the drug concentration within an infected site and the susceptibility of the organism. It works by disrupting the synthesis of the bacterial cell wall. Some patients have experienced adverse effects after ingesting tyramine-containing foods. This interaction suggests that INH may inhibit plasma monoamine oxidase, although this action has not been documented. INH has no direct effect on the body.

Contraindications and Precautions

Isoniazid is contraindicated in patients with acute hepatic disease and in patients with a history of INH-induced hepatic disease. INH should be used with caution in patients with chronic hepatic disease, alcoholism, or severe renal impairment because these conditions can prolong elimination of the drug, increasing the likelihood of adverse reactions.

INH should also be given with caution to patients with diabetes mellitus, malnutrition, or alcoholism because its effects (antagonism or increased excretion) on pyridoxine (vitamin B_6) can cause peripheral neuropathy in these patients. Pyridoxine may be given concurrently with INH to decrease the risk for this adverse effect.

INH should be used with caution in patients with seizure disorders because it may cause neurotoxicity and result in seizures. It also may produce an acneiform rash or exacerbate preexisting acne.

Data conflict about INH use during pregnancy; it is classified as a United States Food and Drug Administration (FDA) pregnancy category C drug. Because INH is given as part of a multidrug regimen to combat TB, studies have not been able to elicit the exact risk that INH poses to the fetus. INH appears to be safe for use during lactation.

Adverse Effects

The major adverse effect of INH therapy is hepatitis. In addition to hepatitis, elevated hepatic enzyme levels (aspartate transaminase, alanine transaminase), bilirubinemia, and jaundice have been reported.

Another frequent adverse effect is peripheral neuropathy. This effect may present with paresthesias in the hands and feet. As previously mentioned, malnourished patients and those with diabetes and alcoholism have a higher risk for this adverse effect. Encephalopathy, convulsions, memory impairment, toxic psychosis, and optic neuritis have been reported, but these events are rare.

INH may induce endocrine changes, such as pyridoxine deficiency, pellagra, hyperglycemia, metabolic acidosis, and gynecomastia. Because it alters vitamin D metabolism, INH may cause hypocalcemia and hypophosphatemia.

Infrequently, INH may also cause adverse effects in the GI, hematologic, and integumentary systems. GI effects include diarrhea, abdominal pain, nausea, and vomiting.

Hematologic effects are agranulocytosis, hemolysis with anemia, sideroblastic anemia, aplastic anemia, pancytopenia, and thrombocytopenia. Integumentary effects include maculopapular rash, acneiform rash, or exfoliative dermatitis. Injection site reaction can be seen with intramuscular (IM) administration of INH. Rarely, INH may cause interstitial nephritis or central nervous system (CNS) toxicity, resulting in seizures.

Drug Interactions

Isoniazid interacts with a variety of drugs, including antiseizure drugs (carbamazepine and the hydantoins), alcohol, aluminum-based antacids, benzodiazepines, disulfiram, enflurane, ketoconazole, meperidine, oral anticoagulants, and rifampin. Table 42.2 lists drugs that interact with INH.

Because INH has some monoamine oxidase inhibitor activity, interactions may occur with tyramine-containing foods. INH may also interact with foods containing histamine.

Assessment of Relevant Core Patient Variables

Heath Status

Isoniazid prophylaxis is given for 6 to 12 months, whereas treatment for active TB may last 18 months. Assess for pre-existing hepatic disease or disorders such as drug or alcohol abuse, which would predispose the patient to hepatic toxic effects. Coordinate baseline liver function tests and schedule serial liver function tests throughout therapy. Some prescribers believe all patients should have these baseline tests, whereas others believe only those patients with an increased risk should be tested.

Evaluate the patient for other pre-existing disorders, such as diabetes mellitus, anemias, or seizure disorders. Patients with diabetes should have a baseline A_{1C} evaluation because INH may cause hyperglycemia. This test indicates the general glucose control for the patient over the preceding 3 months. Patients with pre-existing anemias should have a baseline complete blood count (CBC) because they are at risk for hematologic disorders. For patients with a history of seizures, perform a baseline neurologic examination. INH may cause

TABLE 42.2 Agents That Interact With P Isoniazid

Interactants	Effect and Significance	Nursing Management
alcohol	Isoniazid and alcohol may induce hepatotoxicity.	Advise the patient to limit ingestion of alcohol throughout therapy. Monitor for signs of hepatitis.
aluminum-based antacids	Aluminum salts decrease the absorption of isoniazid, decreasing serum concentrations.	Administer antacids 1 h before or 2 h after isoniazid.
oral anticoagulants	The anticoagulant activity is increased when given concurrently with isoniazid. This results in an increased risk for hemorrhage.	Monitor prothrombin time frequently. Advise patient of signs of bleeding and to report them immediately.
benzodiazepines	Isoniazid may inhibit the metabolism of benzodiazepines, resulting in enhanced action of the benzodiazepine.	Monitor patient for signs of CNS depression.
carbamazepine	Isoniazid is suspected to inhibit carbamazepine metabolism, resulting in carbamazepine toxicity. Carbamazepine may increase isoniazid degradation to hepatotoxic metabolites, resulting in an increased risk for hepatotoxicity.	Monitor carbamazepine serum concentrations. Monitor liver function test results.
disulfiram	The combination of disulfiram and isoniazid may induce excess dopaminergic activity.	Monitor patient for acute behavioral and coordination changes. Refer to health care provider immediately if any occur.
enflurane	Fast acetylation of isoniazid produces high concentrations of hydrazine, facilitating defluorination of enflurane. This may result in high-output renal failure.	Monitor renal function, especially in fast acetylators.
hydantoins	Isoniazid inhibits the metabolism of hydantoins, resulting in increased serum hydantoin concentrations and increased risk for toxicity.	Monitor serum hydantoin levels frequently.
ketoconazole	Isoniazid decreases the therapeutic benefits of ketoconazole, although the mechanism of action is unknown.	Avoid concurrent use.
meperidine	These drugs in combination may induce hypotension or CNS depression. The mechanism of action is unknown.	Use combination cautiously. Monitor blood pressure. Monitor for CNS depression.
rifampin	Hepatotoxicity may occur more frequently when combined.	Monitor liver function test results.

neurotoxicity and exacerbate seizures. Also assess baseline visual acuity.

Life Span and Gender

Isoniazid is classified as FDA pregnancy category C. Therefore, evaluate the patient's pregnancy or breast-feeding status. Although no studies have demonstrated potential fetal risk, INH use in pregnant women should be restricted to active TB therapy. Pregnant women who need INH prophylaxis should begin therapy after delivery because the risk that TB will become active increases after childbirth. Infants of nursing mothers should be assessed for signs of peripheral neuritis and hepatitis.

Determine the patient's age before therapy begins. Patients 35 years or older are three times more likely to develop drug-induced hepatitis than those younger than 35 years. INH prophylaxis for patients older than 35 years should be restricted to patients who are immunocompromised or whose PPD results indicate recent seroconversion. These patients should be closely monitored with serial liver function tests for signs of hepatotoxicity.

Lifestyle, Diet, and Habits

Ask the patient about diet and alcohol consumption. Patients should refrain from excessive intake of foods rich in tyramine, which include cheese and dairy products, beef or chicken liver, beer and ale, red wine, avocados, bananas, figs, raisins, caffeine, and chocolates. Because most people consume these food items, the diet is difficult to maintain. Although the reaction is not as severe as with patients taking monoamine oxidase inhibitors, the patient may experience hypertension.

Patients should also refrain from foods containing histamine. Foods in this category include tuna, brine, or yeast extract. The patient may experience headache, palpitations, sweating, hypotension, flushing, diarrhea, or itching.

Daily consumption of alcohol increases the risk for INH-induced hepatitis and can increase the clearance of INH.

Environment

Isoniazid therapy is routinely conducted in the home. Because of its long duration (up to 18 months), adherence to drug therapy is an issue. With the patient, explore factors in the

home environment that may affect adherence. Additionally, stress that he or she needs to have periodic follow-up examinations and laboratory testing to monitor for severe and potentially fatal adverse reactions.

Culture and Inherited Traits

Isoniazid is metabolized in the body by a process called acetylation. In some people, this process occurs more rapidly than it does in others. Fast acetylators are at higher risk for hepatic toxicity from INH therapy, whereas slow acetylators are at higher risk for high serum levels and more frequent adverse effects. Because the determination of fast acetylators or slow acetylators is genetically controlled, it is important to be aware of the patient's ethnic background. Eskimos, Asians, and about 50% of African Americans or European Americans from North America are fast acetylators. The remainder of African Americans and European Americans, Scandinavians, and people of Arab or Jewish heritage are slow acetylators.

Nursing Diagnoses and Outcomes

- Altered Protection related to drug-induced hepatitis
  Desired outcome: *The patient will call the prescriber immediately if signs or symptoms of hepatitis occur.*
- Risk for Infection related to drug-induced blood dyscrasias
  Desired outcome: *The patient will monitor for signs of infection and contact the prescriber if any occur.*
- Risk for Peripheral Neurovascular Dysfunction related to drug-induced neuropathy
  Desired outcome: *The patient will take pyridoxine throughout INH therapy to decrease potential for peripheral neuropathy.*
- Risk for Trauma related to adverse CNS effects
  Desired outcome: *The patient will encounter no injury related to CNS effects brought on by using INH.*
- Impaired Skin Integrity related to drug-induced acne
  Desired outcome: *The patient will practice careful skin care to prevent breakdown from acne resulting from drug effects.*

Planning and Intervention

Maximizing Therapeutic Effects

Administer INH to the patient with an empty stomach 1 hour before or 2 hours after meals to increase absorption. For patients with GI distress, INH may be given with meals. To avoid possible drug interactions, do not administer antacids less than 1 hour before or 2 hours after administering INH.

Minimizing Adverse Effects

The early identification of symptoms of potential adverse effects is the best way to minimize complications of INH therapy. Advise patients to report any of the prodromal symptoms of hepatitis, including fatigue, loss of appetite, and nausea and vomiting. Also advise patients to report tingling of the extremities, change in vision, or symptoms of anemia. The drug should be discontinued if clinical symptoms of hepatitis occur.

Most prescribers will discontinue the drug if liver function test results indicate elevations ranging from three to five times higher than the upper limit of normal values.

Providing Patient and Family Education

- Advise the patient to take the drug on an empty stomach every day and emphasize the importance of taking the drug daily. Patients who stop and start INH therapy repeatedly are at risk for developing drug-resistant TB. Although it is important to take the drug daily, it is more important not to double the dosage if a drug dose is forgotten.
- Explain the potential adverse effects and the importance of notifying the prescriber if any symptoms occur. Also, explain diet and alcohol restrictions to limit the risk for adverse reactions. A written list of foods that contain tyramine or histamine is most helpful to the patient.
- Explain the importance of follow-up visits, including laboratory testing and eye examinations.

Ongoing Assessment and Evaluation

Ongoing assessment is extremely important in INH therapy. Monitor for signs of adverse effects, especially hepatitis. Question the patient about symptoms such as yellow skin or eyes, anorexia, nausea, vomiting, fatigue, malaise, or weakness. Also, ask about rash, itching, or darkened urine. It is also important to question the patient regarding symmetric numbness or tingling in the extremities. Optimally, results of the patient's serial blood tests will be available for evaluation during the visit.

INH should be discontinued if signs or symptoms of hepatic damage become evident. Discontinuing INH should be considered if liver function test values exceed three to five times the upper limit of normal ranges.

At each visit, review diet and alcohol restrictions. Also, review the signs and symptoms of hepatitis and peripheral neuropathy and remind the patient to call the prescriber if any symptoms occur. You may want to arrange for the next follow-up appointment rather than wait for the patient to call.

MEMORY CHIP

P Isoniazid

- Used for prophylaxis and management of tuberculosis and for other susceptible mycobacterial infections
- Important contraindications: acute hepatic diseases
- Most common adverse effects: peripheral neuropathy, elevated liver enzyme levels
- Most serious adverse effects: hepatotoxicity, optic neuritis
- Life span alert: patients over the age of 35 years have an increased risk for isoniazid-induced hepatic dysfunction
- Maximizing therapeutic effects: Administer on an empty stomach, unless GI distress occurs.
- Minimizing adverse effects: Promptly identify signs and symptoms of potential adverse effects, especially hepatitis.
- Most important patient education: Teach patients about the role of adherence in avoiding drug resistance.

CRITICAL THINKING SCENARIO

Exposure to the tuberculosis (TB) mycobacterium

David Haversham, age 32 years works as a correctional officer in the local jail. Following policy, David goes to the clinic for his yearly TB testing. His test result last year was negative, and David does not recall having been exposed to TB. Two days later, you call David to tell him that his purified-protein derivative measured 12 mm and arrange for David to have a chest x-ray (CXR). David calls the clinic today and learns that his CXR is normal and then asks, "So, what does all this mean?"

1. How would you answer David's question?
2. What therapy, if any, would you anticipate for this patient?
3. Would this therapy change if the patient were 40 years of age?
4. What questions would you ask the patient before initiating therapy?
5. Develop a patient teaching plan for the patient.
6. How would this scenario change if David were HIV-positive?

Drugs Significantly Different From P Isoniazid

Rifampin

Rifampin (Rifadin) is another first-line drug used to manage TB. It is also the drug of choice for managing leprosy and thus will be discussed as the prototype for that disease.

Ethambutol

Ethambutol (Myambutol) appears to be more effective and less toxic than other antitubercular drugs. It is primarily bacteriostatic, although in higher doses, it also exhibits bactericidal properties. The exact mechanism is not known; however, it appears to inhibit RNA synthesis. Ethambutol is effective only against bacilli that are actively dividing.

Ethambutol is administered orally, partially metabolized in the liver, and excreted primarily in urine, with approximately 25% excreted unchanged in feces.

It is widely distributed, with high concentrations in the kidneys, lungs, and saliva. It penetrates inflamed meninges to reach therapeutic levels in the CSF. Although ethambutol crosses the placenta and is distributed into breast milk, no adverse effects on the fetus or nursing infant have been reported.

One of the main adverse effects of ethambutol is optic neuritis. Patients with preexisting ocular disease should have a baseline ophthalmologic examination and be closely monitored for changes in visual acuity and color discrimination. Ethambutol should not be used in children whose visual acuity cannot be adequately assessed. Ethambutol may also cause hyperuricemia; therefore, patients with a history of gout should be closely monitored for exacerbations.

Pyrazinamide

Like ethambutol, pyrazinamide (PZA) appears to be more effective and less toxic than other antitubercular drugs. It is indicated only for use in treating *M. tuberculosis*. PZA's exact mechanism of action is not known; however, it exhibits bacteriocidal or bacteriostatic action. Studies indicate that PZA is most effective in the initial stages of treatment.

PZA is administered orally, metabolized into active metabolites, and excreted in the urine, primarily by way of glomerular filtration. PZA is widely distributed and penetrates inflamed meninges. It is unknown whether PZA crosses the placenta, but it does enter breast milk.

Pyrazinamide should be given cautiously to pregnant patients and those with alcoholism, gout, or hepatic disease. The most severe adverse effect is hepatotoxicity. In rare instances, liver atrophy and fatalities have occurred. Common adverse effects include arthralgias, GI disturbances, and photosensitivity. Nongouty arthritis may occur because PZA inhibits urate excretion, resulting in hyperuricemia. Rarely, hematopoietic effects, such as thrombocytopenia and sideroblastic anemia, may occur.

Patients receiving pyrazinamide should have baseline laboratory tests completed before initiating treatment and periodically throughout therapy. These tests include a CBC, liver and renal function tests, and uric acid level.

Streptomycin

Streptomycin is a parenteral aminoglycoside antibiotic. Unlike other aminoglycosides, streptomycin penetrates TB cavities and caseous tissues and is therefore used in treating TB. See Chapter 39 for additional information on aminoglycoside antibiotics.

C DRUGS FOR TREATING *MYCOBACTERIUM LEPRAE* INFECTION

Leprosy was first described in 1873 by G. A. Hansen; thus, its alternate name is Hansen disease. Multidrug therapy, the standard approach for other mycobacterial infections, is also recommended for treating leprosy. Rifampin is the drug of choice for both types of leprosy (see Pathophysiology), except in cases of rifampin resistance. For that reason, rifampin is the prototype drug for treating leprosy.

NURSING MANAGEMENT OF THE PATIENT RECEIVING P RIFAMPIN

Core Drug Knowledge

Pharmacotherapeutics

In addition to treating leprosy, rifampin also is used to treat asymptomatic carriers of *Neisseria meningitidis,* as prophylaxis against infections caused by *Haemophilus influenzae* type B, and in treating Legionnaire disease, atypical mycobacterial infection, and staphylococcal infection. Rifampin is another first-line drug used in treating TB, although it should never be used as a single drug because resistance develops rapidly.

Pharmacokinetics

Rifampin may be administered orally or parenterally. It is well absorbed from the GI tract, except in the presence of food, which decreases both the rate and extent of absorption. It is widely distributed throughout the body, including the lungs, liver, bone, saliva, and peritoneal and pleural fluids. Rifampin enters CSF at concentrations approximately 10% to 20% of plasma concentration. Rifampin is metabolized in the liver to an active metabolite and undergoes enterohepatic circulation with substantial reabsorption. Rifampin is excreted primarily through biliary elimination in feces.

Pharmacodynamics

Rifampin works by inhibiting bacterial and mycobacterial RNA synthesis. It is bactericidal or bacteriostatic, depending on the concentration reached within an infected site and the susceptibility of the organism. It does not bind to RNA polymerase in human cells; thus, RNA synthesis in the host is not affected.

Contraindications and Precautions

Rifampin should not be administered to patients with known rifamycin hypersensitivity, including rifabutin, because cross-sensitivity between agents is possible. Parenteral rifampin contains sulfite sodium formaldehyde sulfoxylate. Therefore, parenteral rifampin is contraindicated in patients with sulfite hypersensitivity because it has been associated with serious or potentially fatal anaphylactoid reactions, although the incidence of such reactions is low.

Because of its potential adverse effects on the liver, rifampin is used cautiously in patients with a history of hepatic dysfunction and in patients known to have alcoholism. It is also used cautiously with patients taking other medications known to be hepatotoxic.

Adverse Effects

Rifampin may cause adverse effects similar to those of INH, especially hepatic injury. Additionally, rifampin can discolor bodily fluids, such as urine, saliva, tears, and sputum.

Wearers of soft contact lenses should be cautioned that the lenses may be permanently discolored.

Although rifampin is generally well tolerated, it may cause GI disturbances such as nausea and vomiting, anorexia, flatulence, cramps, and diarrhea. Rarely, rifampin may induce pseudomembranous colitis or pancreatitis.

High-dose therapy may induce a flu-like syndrome with fever, chills, headache, and fatigue. Other adverse effects that can be induced by high-dose therapy include leukopenia, hemolysis with anemia, shortness of breath, shock, and renal failure.

Drug Interactions

Rifampin is a potent inducer of the cytochrome P450 hepatic enzyme system and its subsets. Induction may result in reduced plasma concentrations of other drugs metabolized by the P-450 enzyme system. When these drugs are given concurrently with rifampin, their dosage may need to be increased. In some cases, the drugs are contraindicated for concurrent use. Table 42.3 lists drugs that interact with rifampin.

Assessment of Relevant Core Patient Variables

Health Status

Assess for diseases or disorders that contraindicate the use of rifampin or require strict monitoring during therapy, especially those that increase the risk for hepatotoxicity. Assess for any medications that may interact with rifampin or other drugs known to be hepatotoxic. Communicate any positive findings to the prescriber before starting therapy.

Pay special attention to patients with a diagnosis of HIV infection or AIDS. Many drugs used to treat these disorders are contraindicated for use with rifampin. Additionally, patients with HIV infection or AIDS need TB therapy for a longer duration than other patients do, increasing the problem of adherence.

Arrange for baseline laboratory tests before administering rifampin. These tests include a CBC and hepatic and renal studies.

Life Span and Gender

Rifampin is an FDA pregnancy category C drug; therefore, it is important to evaluate the patient's pregnancy status. The drug may be used in children younger than 1 month.

Lifestyle, Diet, and Habits

Assess for alcohol consumption and explain the increased risk for hepatotoxicity when alcohol consumption is combined with rifampin therapy. Because rifampin can discolor body fluids red-orange, suggest that soft contact lens wearers change to a different type of contacts or regular glasses throughout therapy. Dietary changes are not needed.

Environment

Rifampin can be given in any environment. Oral rifampin is most frequently used in the home environment; intravenous rifampin is most frequently administered in an acute care hospital. Be aware of the environment in which the drug will be administered and explore with the patient any factors in the home setting that may affect adherence with drug therapy.

Nursing Diagnoses and Outcomes

- Risk for Injury related to hepatic injury
  Desired outcome: *The patient will remain free of injury and contact the prescriber if signs such as yellow skin, itching, or fatigue occur.*
- Imbalanced Nutrition: Less than Body Requirements related to potential nausea, vomiting, anorexia, and diarrhea
  Desired outcome: *The patient will have balanced nutrition throughout therapy.*
- Ineffective Protection related to potential leukopenia or hemolysis with anemia
  Desired outcome: *The patient will remain without superinfection throughout therapy.*

Planning and Intervention

Maximizing Therapeutic Effects

Administer intravenous rifampin by slow infusion over 3 hours. Oral rifampin should be given 1 hour before or 2 hours after a meal to avoid decreasing absorption. Promote adherence to oral rifampin therapy by explaining the importance of taking the medication daily.

Minimizing Adverse Effects

Evaluate the patient for contraindications to its use and avoid administering rifampin to a patient with signs of hepatotoxicity.

Providing Patient and Family Education

- Explain the potential effect of rifampin on the liver. Patients should be advised to contact the prescriber immediately if they experience anorexia, nausea, fatigue, malaise, jaundice, cola-colored urine, or pale stools. Also, explain that

TABLE 42.3 Agents That Interact With P Rifampin

Interactants	Effect and Significance	Nursing Management
protease inhibitors, nonnucleoside reverse transcriptase inhibitors	Rifampin increases the metabolism of the antiretroviral drugs resulting in decreased plasma concentrations.	Concurrent use is not recommended.
Drugs affected by induction: • anticoagulants • beta blockers • oral contraceptives • corticosteroids • cyclosporine • digitoxin • disopyramide • doxycycline • estrogens • haloperidol • hydantoins • nifedipine • quinine derivatives • sulfonylurea agents • theophyllines • tricyclic antidepressants • zolpidem	Increased hepatic microsomal enzyme metabolism (induction) by rifampin results in decreased action of interactant drugs.	Monitor for efficacy of interactant drugs. Adjust interactant drug dosages as needed. Consult prescriber about choosing an alternate drug in place of the interactant as needed.
azole antifungal agents	Rifampin may induce the metabolism of azole antifungal drugs resulting in decreased action of azole antifungal drugs. Additionally, azole antifungal drugs interfere with the absorption of rifampin resulting in decreased serum rifampin levels.	Monitor for efficacy of azole antifungal drugs. Monitor for efficacy of rifampin. Consult with prescriber about adjusting drug dosages as needed.
benzodiazepines	The oxidative metabolism of benzodiazepines may be increased resulting in decreased pharmacologic effects.	Monitor for efficacy of benzodiazepine drugs. Consult with prescriber about adjusting benzodiazepine drug dosages as needed.
buspirone, verapamil	Rifampin induces first-pass metabolism of these drugs resulting in decreased plasma concentration.	Monitor for efficacy of interactants. Consult with prescriber about adjusting dosages of interactants as needed.
isoniazid	Rifampin may cause an alteration in the metabolism of isoniazid. Hepatotoxicity may occur at a rate higher than with either agent alone.	Monitor for signs of hepatotoxicity. Monitor liver function studies. Discontinue as needed.
macrolide antibiotics	The metabolism of rifampin may be inhibited while the metabolism of macrolide antibiotics may be increased, resulting in decreased antimicrobial effects and increased GI adverse effects.	Monitor for efficacy of macrolide antibiotics. Monitor for adverse GI effects of macrolide antibiotics. Consult with prescriber about using azithromycin or dirithromycin as alternative drugs because they do not undergo metabolism.
methadone	Rifampin stimulates the metabolism of methadone, resulting in a decreased efficacy of methadone.	Monitor the patient for signs of narcotic withdrawal.
morphine	Rifampin stimulates the metabolism of morphine resulting in a decreased efficacy of morphine.	Monitor the patient's clinical response to morphine. Administer an alternative analgesic as needed.

many drugs increase the risk for hepatic damage and that the patient should contact the prescriber before taking any new drugs, even those prescribed by another provider. Explain that alcohol consumption may also increase the risk for hepatic damage.

- Advise patients with soft contact lenses to consult their ophthalmologist for an alternate form of contacts or glasses. Assure the patient that the discoloration of body fluids is not harmful.
- Because adherence is always difficult when the medication must be taken for a prolonged time, explain the importance of taking the medication consistently, even though the patient will not feel different.
- Explain the importance of consistent follow-up visits to ensure that the mycobacteria are eradicated and to monitor for adverse effects.

Ongoing Assessment and Evaluation

Ask patients whether they have experienced any symptoms suggestive of hepatic dysfunction. Periodic testing of hematopoietic, renal, and hepatic function should also be arranged.

By the end of therapy, the mycobacteria should be eradicated, and the patient should be free from any adverse effects from rifampin therapy.

Drugs Closely Related to P Rifampin

Rifabutin

Rifabutin (Mycobutin) is an oral antimycobacterial agent that is a derivative of rifamycin. It is used for prophylaxis or treatment of TB and MAC. *M. leprae* is also considered to be susceptible to rifabutin, but leprosy is not a labeled indication. Like rifampin, rifabutin inhibits mycobacterial RNA synthesis.

Rifabutin is administered orally and is rapidly absorbed. Absorption can be slowed in the presence of a high-fat meal. The drug is metabolized in the liver. Excretion is predominantly in the urine; approximately 30% is excreted in feces, and 5% is excreted through the biliary pathway.

The most serious adverse effects of rifabutin are uveitis and blood dyscrasias. Like rifampin, rifabutin may cause discoloration of body fluids. Common adverse effects include rash, nausea, abdominal pain, and dyspepsia. Less frequently reported adverse reactions to rifabutin include seizures, taste perversion, nonspecific T-wave changes on electrocardiography, and myalgia. Rifabutin may cause hepatitis and elevated hepatic enzyme levels, but those adverse effects occur most frequently in patients with disseminated disease.

Rifabutin appears to be a less potent hepatic enzyme inducer than rifampin, although similar drug–drug interactions may still occur. Rifabutin does not interfere with the metabolism of INH. Rifabutin is contraindicated for concurrent use with nonnucleoside reverse transcriptase inhibitors, hard-gel formulation saquinavir, or ritonavir. It can be given cautiously with other antiretroviral agents, but the dosage of those agents may need to be increased.

Rifapentine

Rifapentine (Priftin) is very similar to rifampin. Although many mycobacteria are considered susceptible to rifapentine, its only approved use is in managing TB. The major difference between rifapentine and rifampin is rifapentine's extended half-life, which allows for twice-a-week dosing. Contraindications, precautions, adverse effects, and drug interactions are the same as those for rifampin.

Rifaximin

Rifaximin (Xifaxan) is a nonsystemic semisynthetic derivative of rifamycin, used specifically for travelers' diarrhea caused by noninvasive *Escherichia coli.* Rifaximin has also been evaluated for treating hepatic encephalopathy, infectious diarrhea, and diverticular disease and as antibacterial prophylaxis before colon surgery. It is currently designated as an orphan drug for use in treating hepatic encephalopathy.

Rifaximin is an oral antibiotic that works directly on the gastrointestinal tract. Less than 4% of the drug is absorbed; it is excreted primarily unchanged in feces. Because of its nonsystemic action, no important drug–drug interactions have been identified. Rifaximin is contraindicated in patients with hypersensitivity to any of the rifamycin antimicrobial agents. It is used with caution in patients with concomitant bloody stool or fever. Common adverse effects include flatulence, headache, abdominal pain, and tenesmus (a sensation of having to pass stool). Other potential adverse effects include defecation urgency or constipation, nausea or vomiting, and fever. Rifaximin should be discontinued if symptoms worsen or persist longer than 24 to 48 hours. Rifaximin is a pregnancy category C drug. Use during breast-feeding has not been approved.

Drugs Significantly Different From P Rifampin

Dapsone

Dapsone (Avlosulfon) is a synthetic sulfone that is chemically similar to sulfonamides. It is used as an antimicrobial agent for leprosy, *Pneumocystis carinii* pneumonia (PCP), and prophylaxis of malaria. It is also used as an immunosuppressive agent for systemic lupus erythematosus and as a dermatologic agent in a variety of integumentary disorders. In managing leprosy, dapsone is used in combination with other drugs such as rifampin and clofazimine (discussed later in this chapter). In the past, dapsone was the mainstay of therapy for leprosy. Now, resistance to dapsone monotherapy is common among *M. leprae.*

MEMORY CHIP

P Rifampin

- Used to manage acute TB and leprosy; also used to manage other mycobacterial infections
- Important contraindication: hypersensitivity
- Most common adverse effects: discoloration of body fluids, GI disturbances
- Most serious adverse effect: hepatotoxicity
- Maximizing therapeutic effects: Administer on an empty stomach.
- Minimizing adverse effects: Evaluate the patient for potential drug-drug interactions.
- Most important patient education: Teach patients the role of adherence in preventing resistance and the importance of contacting the prescriber if any signs of hepatic dysfunction occur.

Dapsone works by inhibiting folic acid synthesis in susceptible organisms. Although the mechanism of dapsone in integumentary disorders is unknown, it has been suggested that it may act as an immunomodulator. Dapsone is orally administered and almost completely absorbed from the GI tract. It is widely distributed throughout the body, crosses the placenta, and enters into breast milk. Dapsone is metabolized in the liver. Approximately 20% of the drug is excreted unchanged in the urine, whereas 70% to 85% is excreted as metabolites. A small amount can be detected in the feces.

Hypersensitivity is the only contraindication to the use of dapsone. Caution is used in patients with sulfonamide hypersensitivity, but no direct cross-sensitivity occurs. Dapsone is also used with caution in cases of severe anemia, glucose-6-phosphate dehydrogenase (G6PD) deficiency, or methemoglobin reductase deficiency because hemolytic anemia can occur.

Dapsone can induce serious adverse effects, including hemolytic anemia, aplastic anemia, agranulocytosis, methemoglobinemia, acute tubular necrosis, and hepatotoxicity. More common adverse effects include fever, myalgias, headache, chills, fatigue, malaise, rash, and urticaria.

Probenecid may reduce renal excretion of dapsone, resulting in an increased risk for toxicity and adverse effects. Patients receiving other hemolytic agents, such as folic acid antagonists, should be closely monitored because concurrent use increases the potential for hematopoietic adverse effects.

Clofazimine

Clofazimine (Lamprene) is used as an antimycobacterial and anti-inflammatory agent. It is bacteriocidal against *M. tuberculosis* and *M. leprae,* although its action against *M. leprae* is very slow. It is bacteriostatic against *M. avium-intracellulare.*

Clofazimine works by binding to mycobacterial DNA, thus inhibiting reproduction and growth. As an anti-inflammatory agent, it inhibits neutrophil motility and enhances the phagocytic activity of the polymorphonuclear cells and macrophages.

Clofazimine is insoluble in water and is incompletely absorbed from the GI tract. The extent of absorption varies with the individual and with the form of the drug administered. Clofazimine concentrates and can crystallize in mesenteric lymph nodes, adipose tissue, adrenals, liver, lungs, gall-bladder, bile, and spleen. It crosses the placenta and enters breast milk. Clofazimine is excreted unchanged in feces.

The only contraindication to clofazimine therapy is hypersensitivity. Precautions include pre-existing GI disease and hepatic dysfunction.

Common GI adverse effects to clofazimine include anorexia, diarrhea, nausea and vomiting, and colicky or burning abdominal pain. GI toxicity can include hepatitis (with elevated hepatic enzyme levels) or jaundice. Rare but serious adverse effects include splenic infarction, GI obstruction or ileus, and GI bleeding. Clofazimine can cause dark, black, or tarry stools that may be misinterpreted as GI hemorrhage.

Clofazimine can cause long-lasting discoloration of the skin. In white people, the skin may be bronze or dark tan. This effect may last months after clofazimine is discontinued. Like rifampin, clofazimine may discolor body fluids.

Miscellaneous Drugs

Other drugs used to manage leprosy include ofloxacin, a fluoroquinolone antibiotic, and minocycline, a tetracycline antibiotic. These drug classes are discussed in Chapters 41 and 39, respectively.

CHAPTER SUMMARY

- The most common mycobacteria are *M. tuberculosis, M. leprae, M. avium,* and *M. intracellulare.*
- INH, the prototype for antitubercular drugs, is used for both prophylaxis and treatment of acute active TB.
- Other first-line drugs for TB include rifampin, ethambutol, pyrazinamide, and streptomycin.
- Rifampin is the prototype drug for managing leprosy (Hansen disease).
- Other medications useful for leprosy include rifabutin, rifapentine, dapsone, clofazimine, ofloxacin, and minocycline.
- *M. avium* and *M. intracellulare* are the causative agents of *Mycobacterium avium* complex (MAC), a condition that frequently affects immunocompromised patients.
- Azithromycin and clarithromycin are the drugs of choice for MAC prophylaxis and treatment.
- Additional drugs used in managing MAC include rifampin, rifabutin, and clofazimine.

QUESTIONS FOR STUDY AND REVIEW

1. What type of patient has the highest risk for developing chemically induced hepatitis from INH therapy?
2. What is the difference between chemoprophylaxis and active TB therapy?
3. Why does multidrug-resistant TB occur?
4. What are the obstacles to successful drug therapy with rifampin?
5. Why is adherence an issue when treating mycobacterial infections?

Need More Help?

Chapter 42 of the study guide for *Drug Therapy in Nursing* 2e contains NCLEX-style questions and other learning activities to reinforce your understanding of the concepts presented in this chapter. For additional information or to purchase the study guide, visit *http://connection.lww.com/go/aschenbrenner.*

REFERENCES AND BIBLIOGRAPHY

Aaron, L., Saadoun, D., Calatroni, I., et al. (2004). Tuberculosis in HIV-infected patients: A comprehensive review. *Clinical Microbiology and Infection, 10*(5), 388–398.

Bastian, I., Stapledon, R., Colebunders, R., et al. (2003). Current thinking on the management of tuberculosis. *Current Opinions in Pulmonary Medicine, 9*(3), 186–192.

Clinical Pharmacology [Online]. Available: *http://cp.gsm.com.*

Facts and Comparisons. (2004). *Drug facts and comparisons.* Philadelphia: Lippincott Williams & Wilkins.

Hardman, J. G. (2001). *Goodman & Gilman's the pharmacological basis of therapeutics* (10th ed.). New York: McGraw-Hill Health Professions Division.

Katzung, B. (2004). *Basic and clinical pharmacology* (9th ed.). New York: McGraw-Hill/Appleton & Lange.

Micromedex Healthcare Series [Online]. Available: *http://healthcare.micromedex.com.*

Sheff, B. (2003). *Mycobacterium tuberculosis. Nursing, 33*(11), 75.

Stout, J. E. (2004). Safety of rifampin and pyrazinamide for the treatment of latent tuberculosis infection. *Expert Opinion on Drug Safety, 3*(3), 187–198.

Tatro, D. S. (2004). *Drug interaction facts.* Philadelphia: Lippincott Williams & Wilkins.

Drugs Treating Viral and Fungal Diseases

chapter 43

Learning Objectives

At the completion of this chapter the student will:

1. Identify core drug knowledge about drugs used to treat viral and fungal infections.
2. Identify core patient variables relevant to drugs used to treat viral and fungal infections.
3. Relate the interaction of core drug knowledge to core patient variables for drugs used to treat viral and fungal infections.
4. Generate a nursing plan of care from the interactions between core drug knowledge and core patient variables for drugs used to treat viral and fungal infections.
5. Describe nursing interventions to maximize therapeutic and minimize adverse effects for drugs used to treat viral and fungal infections.
6. Determine key points for patient and family education for drugs used to treat viral and fungal infections.

KEY TERMS

Candida

cryptococcosis

cytomegalovirus

dermatophytes

dimorphic fungi

herpes simplex virus

herpes zoster

phosphorylation

respiratory syncytial virus

tinea

FEATURED WEBLINKS

http://www.nlm.nih.gov/medlineplus/
http://www.fungal-infections.info/areas-of-intereset-en/fungal_infections-e/
Need more information regarding viral and fungal infections? For viral infections log on to the first website above, and for information regarding fungal infections, search the second site.

CONNECTION WEBLINK

Additional Weblinks are found on Connection:
http://www.connection.lww.com/go/aschenbrenner.

Drugs Treating Viral and Fungal Diseases

Ⓒ Antiviral Agents

Purine nucleoside analog drugs
- [P] **acyclovir**
- cidofovir
- famciclovir
- ganciclovir
- penciclovir
- valacyclovir
- valganciclovir
- docosanol
- foscarnet

Ophthalmic drugs
- trifluridine
- vidarabine

Drugs for influenza
- amantadine
- oseltamivir
- rimantadine
- zanamivir

Drugs for hepatitis
- adefovir dipivoxil
- interferon alpha
- interferon beta

Drugs for RSV
- palivizumab
- ribavirin
- RSV-IGIV

Ⓒ Antifungal Agents

Polyene antifungal drugs
- [P] **amphotericin B**
- azole antifungal drugs
- nystatin
- caspofungin
- flucytosine

Azole antifungal drugs
- [P] fluconazole
- itraconazole
- ketoconazole
- miconazole
- voriconazole
- butoconazole
- clotrimazole
- econazole
- oxiconazole
- sertaconazole
- sulconazole
- terconazole
- tioconazole

Miscellaneous antifungal drugs
- butenafine
- ciclopirox olamine
- griseofulvin
- naftifine
- terbinafine
- tolnaftate
- undecylenic acid

The symbol Ⓒ indicates the **drug class.**
Drugs in **bold type** marked with the symbol [P] are prototypes.
Drugs in blue type are closely related to the prototype.
Drugs in red type are significantly different from the prototype.
Drugs in black type with no symbol are also used in drug therapy; no prototype

Viral and fungal diseases affect people throughout the life span. In healthy people, these diseases may be considered an annoyance; in immunocompromised people, these diseases can be deadly.

Viruses are responsible for many infectious disorders, ranging from the common cold to life-threatening meningitis. In contrast to the number of drugs that have been developed to treat bacterial disease, few antiviral drugs have been developed. Because viruses have no metabolic enzymes of their own, they can replicate only within a living host cell by using the metabolic processes of the host. Most drugs used to eliminate a virus, therefore, may do substantial harm to the host. However, a few antiviral drugs have been developed that can target the invading virus yet leave the host intact. These drugs have a narrow spectrum of activity, and each drug has specific clinical applications.

This chapter discusses the purine nucleoside analogue drugs with the prototype acyclovir; drugs significantly different from acyclovir include docosanol, foscarnet, and the ophthalmic drugs vidarabine and trifluridine. Drugs used to manage influenza are represented by oseltamivir and drugs used in the management of hepatitis B and C are represented by interferon alfa.

Fungal infections, like viral infections, also can be life threatening in immunocompromised patients. Fungal infections can be divided into two categories:

- Systemic infections
- Superficial mycoses

Systemic infections, such as aspergillosis, cryptococcosis, blastomycosis, and histoplasmosis, can present serious medical problems. Superficial mycoses can be dermatophytic (skin related) or mucous membrane related; the most common such infections are tinea and candidiasis. The latter part of this chapter discusses two classes of antifungal drugs: polyenes (prototype, amphotericin B) and azoles (prototype, fluconazole), used to treat superficial and systemic infections. Drugs significantly different from amphotericin B are caspofungin and flucytosine; drugs significantly different from fluconazole are butoconazole, clotrimazole, econazole, oxiconazole, sulconazole, sertaconazole, terconazole, and tioconazole. This chapter also describes an additional group of drugs, the topical antimycotics, which are used to treat superficial mycoses. This arbitrary division is made to assist the student in focusing on each specific group of disorders caused by these different microbes.

PHYSIOLOGY OF VIRAL REPRODUCTION

The reproduction of viruses in humans requires five steps—adsorption, penetration, uncoating, replication, and transcription (the change of ribonucleic acid [RNA] to deoxyribonucleic acid [DNA]), all of which precede viral assembly and release. During the adsorption step, the virus attaches itself to receptor sites on the host cell surface. Once attached, the virus releases enzymes that enable the virus to penetrate the cell. After the virus enters the cell, the protein coat of the virus dissolves and releases viral genetic material. The virus then synthesizes new messenger RNA and, using host ribosomes, synthesizes viral proteins. The viral nucleic acids and proteins are assembled into mature viruses that are then released by budding off from infected cells or by lysis of the infected cell (Figure 43.1).

PATHOPHYSIOLOGY OF SELECTED VIRAL INFECTIONS

Cytomegalovirus

Cytomegalovirus (CMV) is a type of herpesvirus. CMV infection is extremely prevalent—approximately 80% of the population demonstrates evidence of infection. In most individuals, infection is asymptomatic. However, in some individuals, such as those with acquired immunodeficiency syndrome (AIDS) and bone marrow transplant recipients, CMV infection is associated with severe and usually fatal disease. CMV infection during pregnancy can be hazardous to the fetus, possibly leading to stillbirth, brain damage, and other birth defects or to neonatal illness.

Although CMV most frequently causes retinitis, it also can cause infection in the lungs, throat, brain, kidneys, gallbladder, liver, and colon. In immunocompromised patients, CMV prophylaxis is started when the $CD4^+$ T-cell count measures less than 50.

Hepatitis

In North America, the three major types of hepatitis virus are hepatitis A virus (HAV), hepatitis B virus (HBV), and hepatitis C virus (HCV). Hepatitis A infection is an acute viral syndrome spread by the oral–fecal route. It does not have the ability to become a chronic disease. Hepatitis A vaccine is the preferred method of prevention.

Hepatitis B infection is spread when blood or body fluid from an infected person enters the body of a person who is not immune. Infection may occur through having sex with an infected person, through needlesticks or sharps exposures, from an infected mother to the neonate during birth, or by sharing drugs or needles. Approximately 6% of persons infected after the age of 5 years develop chronic hepatitis B. As with HAV, vaccination is the best protection.

The hepatitis C virus is spread in the same manner as HBV, but there is no preventive vaccine. Seventy to 85% of infected individuals develop chronic hepatitis C infection, and 70% of those individuals also develop chronic liver disease.

Symptoms of hepatitis include jaundice, fatigue, abdominal pain, nausea, and anorexia. In addition, HAV hepatitis may cause diarrhea and fever; HBV hepatitis may cause joint pain, and HCV hepatitis may cause dark urine.

Herpes Simplex

Herpes simplex virus (HSV) has two types—type 1 (HSV-1) and type 2 (HSV-2). Both types cause similar infections. HSV-1 is associated generally with herpes labialis (cold sores or fever blisters), signs of which occur on or near the lips. HSV-2 may cause herpes labialis or herpes genitalis (genital lesions). Infection with either virus is characterized by the formation of painful vesicles, which rupture and form a crust.

Physiology

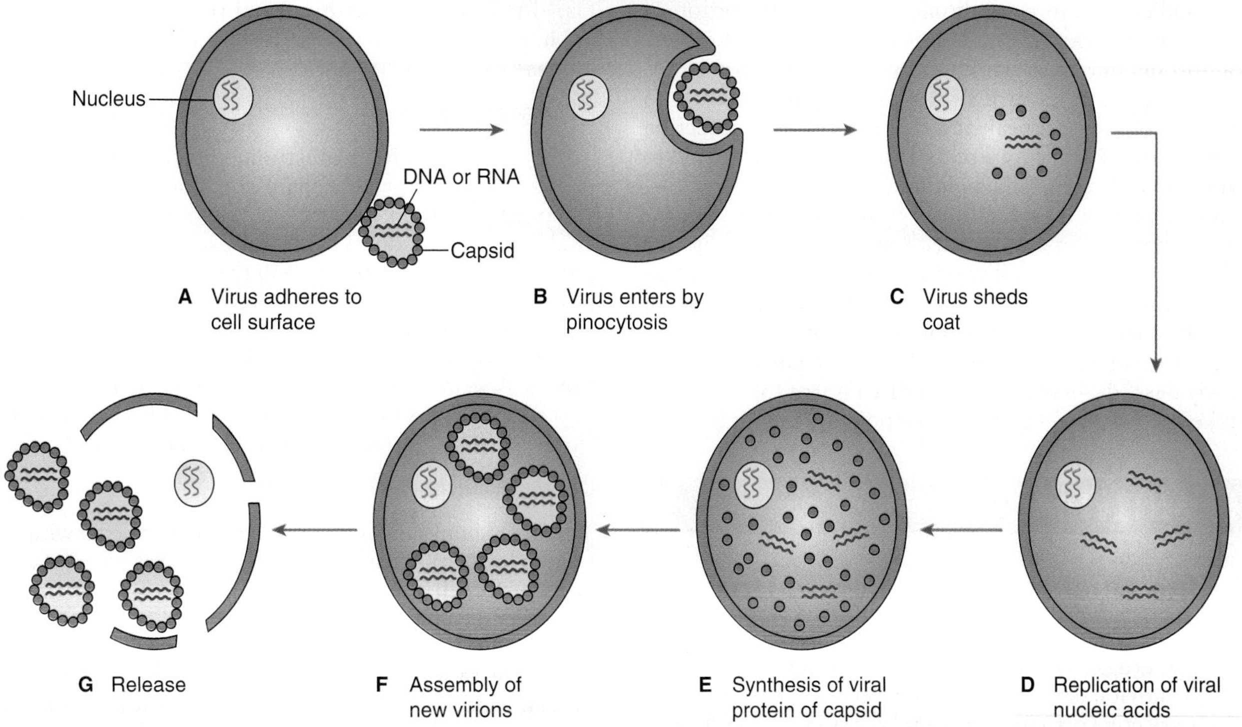

FIGURE 43.1 Viral replication. Viruses replicate in a series of steps: adsorption, penetration, uncoating, replication and transcription, and assembly and release (APURA). By adsorption (**A**), the virus adheres to receptors on the host cell surface. Then by pinocytosis promoted by enzyme activity, the virus penetrates (**B**) the cell wall. Once inside the cell, the virus uncoats (**C**), shedding its protein cover and allowing the genetic material (RNA) to be replicated (**D**) and changed to DNA. Next, new viral proteins are synthesized (**E**) and assembled (**F**) into new viruses, which are then released (**G**). Antiviral drugs interfere with the various stages of replication to limit or stop the viral disease process. (Adapted with permission from Swonger, A. K., & Matejski, M. P. [1991]. *Nursing pharmacology* [2nd ed.]. Philadelphia: J. B. Lippincott.)

when fluid from active lesions contacts parts of the body that have a break in the skin. In between outbreaks, the virus remains in a latent stage in sensory nerve ganglions. Recurrence may be triggered by other infections, sun exposure, or stress. Outbreaks are preceded by a burning or tingling sensation along the nerve and at the site of infection.

Herpes Zoster

Herpes zoster is an acute unilateral and segmental inflammation of the dorsal root ganglia caused by infection with the herpesvirus varicella zoster, which also causes chickenpox. This infection usually occurs in adults and produces localized vesicular skin lesions, confined to a dermatome, and severe neuralgic pain in peripheral areas innervated by the nerves arising in the inflamed root ganglia.

Onset of herpes zoster is characterized by fever and malaise. Within 2 to 4 days, severe deep pain, pruritus, and paresthesia or hyperesthesia develop, usually on the trunk and occasionally on the arms and legs. The pain may be continuous or intermittent and usually lasts from 1 to 4 weeks. Up to 2 weeks after the first symptoms, small, red, nodular skin lesions erupt on the painful areas.

After the initial outbreak, the virus retreats back to the dorsal root ganglia, but outbreaks may recur. Pain and neuralgia may persist after the lesions resolve, especially in elderly patients.

Influenza

Of the many types of influenza virus, influenza A and influenza B are the only types that can be affected by current antiviral agents. Influenza A and B have similar characteristics; however, infection with influenza A is more common and more severe. The virus attacks both the upper and lower respiratory tracts. It is transmitted directly by respiratory droplet or indirectly by contact with a contaminated object. Influenza virus is difficult to combat because it undergoes constant antigenic changes, which limits vaccine development and the ability of individuals to develop long-term immunity.

Influenza has a sudden, acute onset with fever and chills, marked malaise, headache, general muscle aching, sore throat, unproductive cough, and nasal congestion. It may be self-limiting or may progress to pneumonia. Elderly patients, patients with chronic diseases, and immunocompromised patients should be immunized yearly.

Respiratory Syncytial Virus

The **respiratory syncytial virus** (RSV) is a major cause of respiratory illness in all age groups. In adults, infection with

RSV tends to cause mild cold symptoms; in school-aged children, it can cause a cold and bronchial cough; and in infants and toddlers, it can cause bronchiolitis (inflammation of the smaller airways of the lungs) or pneumonia. Reinfection throughout life is common.

The highest rates of RSV illness occur in infants 2 to 6 months old, with a peak at 2 to 3 months. RSV infection is often carried home by a school-aged child and passed to a younger one, especially an infant.

RSV infection is especially dangerous in infants younger than 1 year and in children with asthma, other lung disorders, or heart disease. It is a major cause of hospitalization among children during the winter months. The symptoms of bronchiolitis include a hacking cough and wheezing on exhalation. In addition, the child typically has fever and a cloudy nasal drainage; the infant often is irritable, and oral intake decreases, sometimes to the point of dehydration.

C ANTIVIRAL AGENTS

Purine Nucleoside Analogue Drugs

The largest group of antiviral drugs is the purine nucleoside analogue drugs, initially developed as antitumor drugs but used as antiviral drugs for more than 30 years. They have relatively selective toxicity to viruses because viral DNA polymerases are more sensitive than human polymerases to inhibition by these drugs. Antiviral drugs in the nucleoside analogue subclass include acyclovir, cidofovir, famciclovir, ganciclovir, penciclovir, valacyclovir, and valganciclovir. The prototype purine nucleoside analogue antiviral drug is acyclovir (Zovirax). Table 43.1 presents a summary of purine nucleoside analogue drugs.

NURSING MANAGEMENT OF THE PATIENT RECEIVING P ACYCLOVIR

Core Drug Knowledge

Pharmacotherapeutics

Acyclovir is an oral, parenteral, and topical antiviral agent. Its antiviral spectrum is limited to the herpesviruses, including herpes simplex virus, herpes zoster virus, Epstein-Barr virus, and CMV. Acyclovir is not active against human immunodeficiency virus (HIV). Clinically, use of acyclovir is limited to treating herpes simplex, herpes genitalis, and herpes zoster infections.

Pharmacokinetics

After topical application, percutaneous absorption is minimal, and no drug is detected in the blood or urine. After oral administration, acyclovir is absorbed poorly from the gastrointestinal (GI) tract, with a bioavailability of approximately 20%. Peak serum concentrations occur in about 1.5 to 2 hours. Acyclovir distributes extensively, with the highest concentrations in the kidneys, liver, and intestines. Cerebrospinal fluid (CSF) concentrations are about 50% of plasma concentrations. Acyclovir crosses the placenta and enters breast milk. Acyclovir is metabolized minimally. Approximately 70% is eliminated by the kidneys unchanged. Half-life in patients with normal renal function is about 2.5 hours. In patients with impaired renal function, the half-life may extend to 20 hours.

Pharmacodynamics

To be active, acyclovir must undergo **phosphorylation,** a process by which a phosphate combines with an organic compound. In an infected cell, acyclovir is converted by the viral enzyme thymidine kinase. Fully active acyclovir triphosphate competes for a position in the DNA chain of the herpesvirus. Once incorporated, it terminates DNA synthesis. Uninfected cells show only minimal phosphorylation of acyclovir; thus, only a small amount of uptake into these cells occurs. Acyclovir is effective only against actively replicating viruses; it does not eliminate the latent herpesvirus. Acyclovir has only indirect effects on the body.

Contraindications and Precautions

Acyclovir should be used with caution in patients with ganciclovir hypersensitivity because acyclovir has a similar chemical structure. It also should be given with caution to women who are pregnant or breast-feeding.

Intravenous (IV) acyclovir should be used with caution in patients with renal disease and pre-existing neurologic disorders, especially seizures. Systemic acyclovir is excreted primarily by glomerular filtration and tubular secretion. Therefore, renal toxicity may occur in patients with renal disease. Patients with pre-existing neurologic disorders have an increased risk for developing tremors and myoclonus.

Adverse Effects

Acyclovir is well tolerated. Common adverse effects to acyclovir include lightheadedness, anorexia, nausea, vomiting, abdominal pain, and headache. More serious adverse effects include confusion, tremors, hallucinations, seizures, or coma. IV acyclovir may be nephrotoxic. Acyclovir nephrotoxicity appears to result from crystallization of the drug in the nephron, which can lead to renal tubular obstruction.

Drug Interactions

Acyclovir may interact with probenecid and zidovudine. The risk for nephrotoxicity increases when acyclovir is given concurrently with other drugs known to cause nephrotoxicity. Table 43.2 lists drugs that interact with acyclovir.

Assessment of Relevant Core Patient Variables

Health Status

Elicit a patient history to evaluate for pre-existing renal dysfunction, dehydration, pregnancy, or breast-feeding. Also, assess for concurrent use of any drugs known to be nephrotoxic. Any positive finding should be communicated to the prescriber. Physical examination should include a dermatologic inspection to verify that the patient has active lesions and does not have a secondary bacterial infection (acyclovir will not affect bacterial pathogens). Immunocompromised patients and patients with pre-existing renal dysfunction should have baseline renal function tests documented. For patients with pre-existing neurologic disorders, complete a baseline neurologic assessment.

TABLE 43.1 Summary of Selected Purine Nucleoside Analogue Drugs

Drug (Trade) Name	Selected Indications	Route and Dosage Range	Pharmacokinetics
P acyclovir (Zovirax; *Canadian:* Apo-Acyclovir)	Herpes simplex Herpes genitalis Herpes zoster	*Adult:* IV, 5–10 mg/kg infused over 1 h, q8h (15 mg/kg/d) for 7 d; PO (initial genital herpes), 200 mg q4h while awake (1,000 mg/d) for 10 d; PO (chronic suppressive therapy), 400 mg bid for up to 12 mo; topical, apply sufficient quantity to cover all lesions six times per day for 7 d; 1.25 cm (1/2 in) ribbon of ointment covers 2.5 cm^2 (4 in^2) surface area q3h *Child:* IV (>12 y), adult dosage; IV (<12 y), 250–500 mg/m^2 infused over 1 h, q8h (750 mg/m^2/d); PO, safety not established	*Onset:* IV, immediate; PO, varies *Duration:* IV, 8 h; PO, unknown $t_{1/2}$: 2.5–5 h
cidofovir (Vistide)	CMV retinitis in AIDS patients	*Adult:* IV, 5 mg/kg IV infused over 1 h once wk for 2 consecutive wk during induction (5 mg/kg once every 2 wk for maintenance); probenecid must be administered PO with each dose, 2 g PO 3 h before cidofovir and 1 g at 2 h and 8 h after infusion *Child:* Safety and efficacy not established for children younger than 12 y	*Onset:* Rapid *Duration:* 24 h $t_{1/2}$: 1 h
famciclovir (Famvir)	Acute herpes zoster	*Adult:* PO, 500 mg q8h for 7 d *Child:* Safety and efficacy not established	*Onset:* Varies *Duration:* 24 h $t_{1/2}$: 2 h
	Recurrent genital herpes	*Adult:* PO, 125 mg bid for 5 d	
ganciclovir (DHPG, Cytovene)	CMV infections (retinitis, colitis, esophagitis) in immunocompromised patients	*Adult:* IV, 5 mg/kg given at a constant rate over 1 h, q12h for 14–21 d (maintenance: 5 mg/kg given over 1 h once daily, 7 d/wk or 6 mg/kg/d 5d per wk; PO, 1,000 mg tid with food or 500 mg six times daily q3h with food while awake) *Child:* Safety and efficacy not established	*Onset:* IV, slow; PO, slow *Duration:* Unknown $t_{1/2}$: 2–4 h; PO, 4.8 h
	Prevention of CMV infection in transplant patients	*Adult:* IV, 5 mg/kg over 1 h q12h for 7–14 d, then 5 mg/kg/d once daily for 7 d or 6 mg/kg/d once daily for 5 d	

(continued)

TABLE 43.1 Summary of Selected Purine Nucleoside Analogue Drugs (continued)

Drug (Trade) Name	Selected Indications	Route and Dosage Range	Pharmacokinetics
penciclovir (Denavir)	Herpes labialis	*Adult:* Topical, apply thin layer to affected area q2h while awake. Therapy continues for 4 d	Not generally absorbed systemically
valacyclovir (Valtrex)	Initial or recurrent genital herpes Herpes zoster	*Adult:* PO, 500 mg bid for 5 d *Child:* Safety and efficacy not established *Adult:* PO, 1 g tid for 7 d, most effective if started within 48 h of onset of symptoms	*Onset:* Rapid *Duration:* 3 h $t_{1/2}$: 2.5–3.3 h
valganciclovir (Valcyte)	CMV retinitis Maintenance	*Adult:* PO, 900 mg 2 x/d x 21 d 900 mg/d	*Onset:* Rapid *Duration:* 12–24 h $t_{1/2}$: 4.8 h
docosanol (Abreva)	HSV	*Adult and child:* apply cream 5 times/d	*Onset:* Rapid *Duration:* Unknown $t_{1/2}$: Unknown
foscarnet (Foscarvir)	CMV retinitis in patients with AIDS	*Adult:* IV induction, 60 mg/kg q8h for 2–3 wk; maintenance, 90–120 mg/kg	*Onset:* Immediate *Duration:* Unknown $t_{1/2}$: 1.4–3 h
	Cyclovir-resistant HSV infections in immunocompromised patients	*Adult:* IV, 40 mg/kg q8–12h for 2–3 wk or until healed	

Life Span and Gender

Determine whether the patient is pregnant or breast-feeding. Acyclovir is assigned to an FDA pregnancy category C and should be used with caution during pregnancy. Breast milk concentrations of acyclovir are greater than serum concentrations; therefore, it should be given cautiously to nursing mothers.

Note the patient's age before administering acyclovir. Although acyclovir is not contraindicated for use in elderly patients, these patients should be monitored closely for the onset of nephrotoxicity because renal function diminishes with age.

Lifestyle, Diet, and Habits

Be aware of the patient's economic status. Oral acyclovir therapy is expensive. It is one of the drugs approved for reimbursement in many statewide AIDS programs. Patients may qualify for medical assistance from county, state, or federal

TABLE 43.2 Agents That Interact With P Acyclovir

Interactants	Effect and Significance	Nursing Management
probenecid	Probenecid inhibits the renal tubular secretion of acyclovir, resulting in increased acyclovir serum concentration and potential for adverse effects of acyclovir.	Monitor for adverse effects of acyclovir. Consider dosage reduction of acyclovir.
hydantoins	Serum phenytoin concentrations may be decreased, resulting in an increased risk for seizure activity.	Monitor the patient for seizure activity. Adjust the dose of phenytoin as needed.
theophylline	Acyclovir may inhibit the metabolism of theophylline, resulting in an increased risk for adverse effects to theophylline.	Monitor for adverse effects of theophylline. Adjust the dose of theophylline as needed.
valproic acid	Serum valproic acid concentrations may be decreased, resulting in an increased risk for seizure activity.	Monitor the patient for seizure activity. Adjust the dose of valproic acid as needed.
zidovudine	The mechanism of interaction is unclear; however, coadministering these drugs may induce severe drowsiness and lethargy.	Monitor for adverse effects. Consider reducing the dosage of acyclovir. Discontinue as necessary

funds or receive their drugs from local health departments. Refer patients with financial problems to the hospital or clinic's social service department.

Environment

Be aware of the environment in which acyclovir will be administered. Acyclovir is most frequently given in the outpatient community setting. Caution patients to take acyclovir only when active lesions are present to avoid inducing acyclovir-resistant virus. However, some immunocompromised patients with frequent and severe outbreaks may be placed on a prophylactic regimen. Acyclovir should be protected from light and moisture in the home environment.

Intravenous acyclovir may be administered in acute care settings to patients with a severe outbreak. Reconstituted acyclovir should be used within 12 hours. Administer the infusion over 60 minutes.

Nursing Diagnoses and Outcomes

- Disturbed Thought Processes related to drug-induced confusion, hallucinations, or seizures
  Desired outcome: *The patient will be free of thought aberrations related to drug therapy.*
- Acute Pain related to drug-induced headache
  Desired outcome: *Drug-related pain will subside after administration of acetaminophen.*
- Imbalanced Nutrition: Less than Body Requirements related to acyclovir-related anorexia, nausea and vomiting, or abdominal pain
  Desired outcome: *The patient will remain within an acceptable weight range.*
- Excess Fluid Volume related to adverse effects of drug therapy, such as nephrotoxicity
  Desired outcome: *The patient will have an adequate fluid intake and output profile.*

Planning and Intervention

Maximizing Therapeutic Effects

Administer acyclovir tablets or capsules with a full glass of water. The drug can be administered with or without food. Administering the drug at regular intervals is important.

Minimizing Adverse Effects

Oral acyclovir is well tolerated. However, for patients who report GI complaints, administer the drug with food. Advise the patient to drink at least eight 8-oz glasses of water a day.

To minimize potential nephrotoxicity, ensure that the patient is well hydrated. Administer IV acyclovir over 60 minutes. It is best to use an infusion pump to ensure that administration is timed correctly. Monitor the patient's urine output for 2 hours after the infusion and notify the prescriber if urine output is less than 500 mL/g of acyclovir administered.

Providing Patient and Family Education

- One of the most important points to stress with patients is that they should not take this drug if they have ever had a reaction to any drug with a name that ends in "vir."
- Advise patients to notify the prescriber if they are pregnant or breast-feeding.
- Explain that acyclovir is prescribed for a particular infection and should not be used to self-medicate or to treat any other infection.
- Emphasize that this drug does not prevent the transmission of infection to another person and does not cure the infection.
- Instruct patients to complete the full course of drug therapy, even if the lesions resolve. If patients are taking 200-mg tablets, advise them to take the drug five times a day. For patients who have difficulty taking pills, the drug may be taken in 400-mg doses three times a day. Consult with the prescriber, however, to be sure the alternate method is acceptable.
- It is important to advise patients to keep the drug away from light and moisture, and to instruct them to take forgotten doses as soon as they remember, but not if it is time for the next dose.
- Inform patients of the importance of remaining well hydrated while taking this drug.
- It is especially important that patients learn to recognize the symptoms of an allergic reaction to acyclovir. Patients should stop taking the drug and contact their prescriber if a rash, welts, itching, or shortness of breath occurs.
- Explain the potential adverse effects of acyclovir and the potential remedies for these discomforts. If patients experience central nervous system (CNS) effects, such as confusion, tremors, hallucinations, or coma, or if patients have signs of nephrotoxicity, such as weight gain or decreased urinary output, the prescriber should be contacted immediately.
- Because autoinoculation is possible with herpetic lesions, it is important to teach patients to wear a glove or finger cot when applying topical acyclovir. Explain the importance of washing the hands after each application, even when barriers are used. The drug should be applied to cover the lesions every 3 hours, six times a day for 7 days.
- Advise patients to contact the prescriber if the lesions turn red, become hot, or exudes purulent material, all of which are indications of a secondary bacterial infection.
- Instruct the patient to self-administer acetaminophen if headache occurs. For persistent pain, unrelieved by acetaminophen, the patient should contact the prescriber.
- Instruct the patient to consume frequent small meals if GI distress occurs. If weight loss persists, the patient should contact the prescriber.

Ongoing Assessment and Evaluation

Monitor for the effectiveness of therapy, making sure to document new lesions and assess for possible secondary bacterial infections. Also, monitor for adverse effects, such as lethargy, tremors, headache, change in mental status, and GI complaints.

For immunocompromised and elderly patients, monitoring renal function to detect early nephrotoxicity is important. Patients on long-term therapy should have periodic renal function tests. Hospitalized patients receiving IV acyclovir also should be monitored closely for developing nephrotoxicity. Measure and monitor fluid intake and output to ensure adequate hydration. Also, monitor for the development of phlebitis when administering IV acyclovir. By the completion of therapy, herpetic lesions and any adverse effects should be resolved.

MEMORY CHIP

P Acyclovir

- Used for the management of herpes simplex virus, herpes zoster virus, Epstein-Barr virus, and cytomegalovirus
- Major contraindication: hypersensitivity or cross-sensitivity to ganciclovir
- Most common adverse effects: nausea, vomiting, anorexia, lightheadedness, abdominal pain, and headache
- Most serious adverse effects: seizures and renal dysfunction
- Maximizing therapeutic effects: Administer the drug at regular intervals.
- Minimizing adverse effects: Ensure hydration to avoid nephrotoxicity.
- Most important patient education: Acyclovir treats the symptoms of the disease; it does not cure the disease or prevent its transmission to another person.

Drugs Closely Related to P Acyclovir

Cidofovir

Cidofovir (Vistide) is an IV drug indicated for treating CMV retinitis in patients with AIDS. Cidofovir gel has been effective for topical treatment of acyclovir-resistant mucocutaneous HSV infections in AIDS patients. Cidofovir may also be used in patients with ganciclovir resistance. Its major advantage is its long half-life, which allows for a once-weekly infusion.

Cidofovir use is limited by its serious potential toxic effects. Major adverse effects with cidofovir therapy include renal impairment, granulocytopenia, metabolic acidosis, uveitis, and ocular hypotony. To minimize possible nephrotoxicity, IV normal saline solution and oral probenecid must be used before and after each cidofovir dose. Renal function tests should be completed before each dose of cidofovir. Neutrophil counts also should be monitored throughout therapy. Cidofovir therapy is contraindicated in patients taking other nephrotoxic agents. Cidofovir is classified as an FDA pregnancy category C drug and should be used in pregnancy only if the benefit clearly outweighs the potential risk.

Famciclovir

Famciclovir (Famvir) is an oral antiviral agent used as an alternative to acyclovir in treating acute herpes zoster and recurrent episodes of genital herpes. In patients with chronic HBV infection, famciclovir has decreased HBV, DNA, and aminotransferase activity. Famciclovir is converted rapidly to penciclovir after oral administration.

Famciclovir's spectrum of activity is similar to that of acyclovir, but its duration of action is longer. Thus, famciclovir can be taken three times a day, unlike oral acyclovir, which requires five doses per day. Despite famciclovir's advantages of better bioavailability and longer duration of action, acyclovir possesses a higher affinity for thymidine kinase, the enzyme that promotes phosphorylation. Adverse effects and drug interactions are the same as those seen with acyclovir.

Famciclovir is classified as an FDA pregnancy category B drug; however, it should be used in pregnancy only if the benefit clearly outweighs the potential risk.

Ganciclovir

Ganciclovir (DHPG, Cytovene) is an antiviral agent used to treat CMV infections, especially retinitis, colitis, and esophagitis, in immunocompromised patients. It also is used to prevent CMV infection in transplant recipients. Its spectrum of activity also includes HSV-1 and HSV-2, herpesvirus type 6, Epstein-Barr virus, varicella zoster virus, and HBV.

Like acyclovir, ganciclovir works by terminating DNA synthesis. It is administered intravenously, orally, and by intravitreal implantation. After implantation, intravitreal ganciclovir is released at a steady rate over 5 to 8 months. After oral administration, ganciclovir is absorbed poorly from the GI tract. Bioavailability is increased when ganciclovir is administered with a high-fat meal. Following IV administration, distribution into body tissues and fluids, including the eyes, is extensive. Ganciclovir crosses the placenta and the blood–brain barrier.

Ganciclovir is not indicated for use in neonates and children and should not be taken during pregnancy and lactation. It must be used with caution in patients with depressed bone marrow function, dehydration, neutropenia, hematologic disease, thrombocytopenia, renal disease or impairment, or recent radiation therapy. Cross-sensitivity is also possible with acyclovir.

Ganciclovir can cause substantial hematologic toxicity. Granulocytopenia, neutropenia, and thrombocytopenia have all occurred during ganciclovir therapy. Ganciclovir is moderately nephrotoxic. Slight-to-moderate increases in serum creatinine and azotemia have occurred. Elevated liver function test results also may occur during therapy with ganciclovir; such changes are generally reversible. Serial laboratory tests required during therapy include complete blood count (CBC), renal function tests, and liver function tests.

Adverse effects, which occur most commonly with IV administration of ganciclovir, include diaphoresis, pruritus, pneumonia, chills, sepsis, and phlebitis. Adverse effects seen with intravitreal administration of ganciclovir may induce bacterial endophthalmitis, retinal detachment, vitreous hemorrhage, cataracts, corneal opacification, hyphema, floaters, ocular pain, posterior chamber inflammation, macular abnormalities, spikes of increased intraocular pressure, optic disc or nerve changes, and uveitis.

Ganciclovir is in FDA pregnancy category C. Based on animal studies, ganciclovir should be considered a potential teratogen in humans, with the potential to cause birth defects.

Penciclovir

Penciclovir (Denavir) is a topical antiviral agent used to treat herpes labialis. Penciclovir is the active metabolite of famciclovir. It works by inhibiting viral DNA. Penciclovir is applied every 2 waking hours.

Adverse effects associated with penciclovir use include headache, oral and pharyngeal edema, application site reactions, erythematous rash, pain, paresthesias, pruritus, skin discoloration, and urticaria.

Valacyclovir

Valacyclovir (Valtrex) is an ester of acyclovir. This oral drug was developed to improve acyclovir's oral bioavailability. Improved bioavailability means that less frequent dosing is required for valacyclovir than for acyclovir. Valacyclovir is the drug of choice in treating genital herpes, either as a first episode or as a recurrent episode. It also is the drug of choice in treating herpes zoster. Compared with acyclovir, it demonstrates earlier pain reduction or cessation of pain in treating herpes zoster.

The adverse effects and drug interactions of valacyclovir are similar to those of acyclovir. In immunocompromised patients, valacyclovir also may induce thrombotic thrombocytopenic purpura and hemolytic uremia syndrome. For that reason, it is not indicated for use in immunocompromised patients. It is used with caution in patients with renal dysfunction because accumulation of valacyclovir may induce acute renal failure or CNS toxicity. To prevent crystalluria, teach the patient to remain well hydrated to maintain a high urine volume and avoid dehydration. Valacyclovir is in FDA pregnancy category B.

Valganciclovir

Valganciclovir (Valcyte) is an ester of ganciclovir. It is an oral drug that is rapidly metabolized into its active form, ganciclovir. Pharmacotherapeutics for valganciclovir include treatment of active CMV retinitis in patients with AIDS, maintenance therapy for CMV retinitis, or secondary prophylaxis in patients with inactive CMV retinitis. It is also approved for prophylaxis against CMV following heart, kidney, or kidney-pancreas transplantation.

Oral valganciclovir has the same efficacy as intravenous ganciclovir for the management of active CMV retinitis. Adverse effects and contraindications are similar to those of ganciclovir. Serial laboratory tests required during therapy include CBC, renal function tests, and liver function tests.

Valganciclovir is classified in FDA pregnancy risk category C. In animal studies, ganciclovir was found to be mutagenic and teratogenic. Therefore, as a prodrug to ganciclovir, valganciclovir should be considered a potential teratogen in humans, with the potential to cause birth defects.

Drugs Significantly Different From P Acyclovir

Docosanol

Docosanol (Abreva) is an over-the-counter (OTC) topical cream for recurrent oral-facial herpes simplex episodes. Docosanol works by inhibiting fusion between the plasma membrane and the HSV envelope, thereby preventing viral entry into cells and subsequent viral replication. Other antivirals, such as acyclovir, work by inhibiting viral DNA replication and carry a risk for mutating the virus. Because docosanol does not act directly on the virus, it is unlikely it will produce drug-resistant mutants of HSV. Docosanol has minimal adverse effects; headache is the most common. Successful therapy occurs when the drug is applied at the earliest sign of infection.

Foscarnet

Foscarnet (Foscavir) is an IV antiviral agent that is structurally unrelated to other antiviral agents. Foscarnet currently is indicated for treating CMV retinitis in patients with AIDS. It is also being investigated for treating CMV disease, herpes simplex, and varicella zoster infection in HIV-positive patients. Its mechanism of action is similar to that of acyclovir and ganciclovir, yet it does not require phosphorylation before becoming activated.

Foscarnet therapy should be given with caution to patients with anemia, dehydration, renal impairment, and electrolyte imbalances. Patients who have cardiac disease, are receiving other drugs that influence serum electrolytes, or have a pre-existing seizure disorder or other neurologic disease require close monitoring during treatment. Foscarnet is assigned to pregnancy category C and should therefore be used with caution during pregnancy.

Foscarnet has an extensive and serious adverse reaction profile. Up to 33% of patients on foscarnet therapy acquire anemia, granulocytopenia, or leukopenia. Electrolyte imbalances, such as hypocalcemia, hypophosphatemia or hyperphosphatemia, hypomagnesemia, and hypokalemia also may occur. GI disturbances, such as anorexia, abdominal pain, nausea, and vomiting may occur in up to 30% of patients. Up to 33% of patients develop considerable renal impairment, resulting in azotemia or necrosis. Patients with renal impairment also are at high risk for developing seizures. Other CNS effects include headache, peripheral neuropathy, and anxiety.

Foscarnet should be given with caution in combination with other drugs known to be nephrotoxic, such as acyclovir, aminoglycosides, amphotericin B, cisplatin, cyclosporine, gold compounds, lithium, nonsteroidal anti-inflammatory drugs, penicillamine, pentamidine, rifampin, and vancomycin. Foscarnet, in combination with ciprofloxacin, increases the risk for seizures, whereas the combination of foscarnet and zidovudine increases the risk for anemia.

Ophthalmic Drugs

Vidarabine

Vidarabine (Vira-A) is an ophthalmic antiviral drug with activity against HSV-1 and HSV-2, varicella zoster virus, CMV, vaccinia, and HBV. Although the IV formulation of vidarabine was discontinued by the manufacturer in October 1992, the topical formulation is the most effective and least toxic of the topical nucleoside analogues.

Corticosteroids, especially ophthalmically administered steroids, should be avoided when treating herpes simplex keratitis in patients receiving ophthalmic vidarabine because corticosteroids can increase the spread of infection. In addition, vidarabine may worsen possible adverse ocular effects of the corticosteroids, such as increased intraocular pressure, glaucoma, and cataracts.

Ophthalmic doses of vidarabine are very small, and the risk for adverse systemic effects is consequently very low. Hypersensitivity reactions, such as pruritus, erythema, swelling, ocular pain or burning, or foreign body sensation, may occur. Ophthalmic administration should not be continued for longer than 21 days. Too frequent application can damage the cornea.

To administer ophthalmic vidarabine, apply 0.5 inch (1.25 cm) of ointment in the lower conjunctival sac every 3 hours up to 5 times a day while the patient is awake, until complete re-epithelialization has occurred, then 2 times a day for an additional 7 days.

Trifluridine

Trifluridine (Viroptic) is an ophthalmic antiviral preparation indicated for use in primary keratoconjunctivitis and recurrent epithelial keratitis caused by HSV-1 and HSV-2. No important interactions between trifluridine and other drugs have been reported. Adverse effects include mild transient burning or stinging on instillation, palpebral edema, epithelial keratopathy, irritation, keratitis sicca, hyperemia, and increased intraocular pressure.

To administer this drug, instill 1 drop of 1% solution into the affected eye every 2 hours during waking hours, up to a maximum daily dose of 9 drops. This therapeutic regimen should continue until the corneal ulcer has completely re-epithelialized. At this point, it is important to treat for an additional 7 days with one drop every 4 hours during waking hours up to a maximum daily dosage of 5 drops.

Drugs Used for Influenza

Amantadine

Amantadine (Symmetrel) is a synthetic antiviral agent used for the prophylactic or symptomatic treatment of influenza A virus infection, especially in high-risk patients. It also is used to relieve the symptoms of Parkinson disease.

As an antiviral, amantadine appears to block the uncoating of the virus particle and subsequent release of viral nucleic acid into the host cell. Amantadine also may interfere with penetration of the cell wall by adsorbed virus. In treating Parkinson disease, amantadine appears to potentiate CNS dopaminergic responses. It may release dopamine and norepinephrine from storage sites and inhibit the reuptake of dopamine and norepinephrine.

Amantadine is administered orally and is well absorbed from the GI tract. It crosses the blood–brain barrier and the placenta; distributes into tears, saliva, and nasal secretions; and is excreted into breast milk. About 90% of amantadine is excreted in the urine by way of glomerular filtration and tubular secretion (Table 43.3).

Amantadine should be given with caution to patients with congestive heart failure, peripheral edema, seizure disorders, eczema, and history of psychosis. These conditions may be exacerbated by amantadine therapy. Patients with renal impairment, elderly patients, and pregnant women also should be given amantadine with caution because these conditions increase the risk for adverse effects. Abrupt withdrawal of amantadine should be avoided in patients with Parkinson disease because it may precipitate symptoms of increased rigidity, confusion, urinary retention, or bulbar palsy.

Amantadine has many potential adverse effects. In the GI system, amantadine may cause nausea and vomiting, diarrhea, constipation, anorexia, and xerostomia. CNS effects include dizziness, anxiety, impaired coordination, insomnia, and nervousness. Other CNS effects that occur less commonly are headache, irritability, nightmares, depression, ataxia, confusion, somnolence and drowsiness, agitation, fatigue, and hallucinations. Patients with a history of psychosis may experience an exacerbation of symptoms, including abnormal thinking, weakness, amnesia, slurred speech, and hyperkinesia. In rare cases, amantadine has been associated with more serious effects, including increased frequency of seizures, suicidal ideation, and neuroleptic malignant syndrome. Adverse cardiovascular effects include orthostatic hypotension and peripheral edema. Livedo reticularis, a persistent purplish network-patterned discoloration of the skin, is a common adverse reaction among patients taking amantadine for Parkinson disease. This reaction is believed to be caused by abnormal capillary permeability associated with peripheral vasoconstriction, which results in decreased skin temperature and peripheral blood flow. Amantadine also may cause adverse reactions in the eyes. Diffuse, white, subendothelial corneal opacification may occur. Other ophthalmic adverse reactions include corneal edema, light sensitivity, and optic nerve palsy.

Amantadine should not be used with CNS stimulants, alcohol (ethanol), opiate agonists, hydrochlorothiazide, or triamterene. Nervousness, irritability, insomnia, seizures, or cardiac arrhythmias may occur if amantadine is taken concurrently with CNS stimulants. Ethanol use with amantadine may increase CNS effects, such as dizziness, confusion, lightheadedness, fainting, or orthostatic hypotension. Use of opiate agonists may increase the incidence of adverse effects. Hydrochlorothiazide or triamterene, used in conjunction with amantadine, can reduce renal clearance of amantadine, with subsequent increase in plasma amantadine concentrations and possible toxicity.

Rimantadine

Rimantadine (Flumadine) is an oral antiviral agent. It is indicated for prophylaxis and treatment of influenza A virus infection in adults and for prophylaxis only in children. Rimantadine is related chemically and structurally to amantadine, but it does not produce the CNS effects seen with amantadine and does not have therapeutic value in treating Parkinson disease.

Rimantadine is contraindicated for use in infants and neonates. It should be used cautiously in elderly patients and in patients with hepatic or renal dysfunction because delayed metabolism or excretion of rimantadine may increase the risk for toxic effects.

Rimantadine has a much better adverse effects profile than amantadine. The most common adverse effects reported are nausea, vomiting, insomnia, dizziness, anorexia, xerostomia, abdominal pain, headache, asthenia, nervousness, and fatigue.

Clearance of rimantadine is reduced by concurrent administration of cimetidine. Decreased serum concentration may occur if rimantadine is coadministered with acetaminophen or aspirin.

Oseltamivir

Oseltamivir phosphate (Tamiflu) is a neuraminidase inhibitor used to manage infection with influenza A or B virus. It is available as an oral capsule or as a powder for reconstitution. Influenza A and B viruses contain the viral enzyme neuraminidase on their surfaces, which facilitates the release of newly formed virus particles from infected cells. This mechanism enables infection of adjacent cells. Neuraminidase inhibitors, such as oseltamivir, appear to inhibit the release of viruses from infected cells, thus reducing spread to adjacent cells and limiting tissue damage and the duration of symptoms.

Oseltamivir is an oral agent for use in patients who have been symptomatic for no more than 2 days. The effectiveness of the drug depends on how early the treatment is initiated.

TABLE 43.3 Summary of Selected Anti-Influenza Drugs

Drug (Trade) Name	Selected Indications	Route and Dosage Range	Pharmacokinetics
amantadine (Symmetrel; *Canadian:* Gen-Amantadine)	Influenza A	*Adults <65 y and adolescents:* PO, 200 mg/d daily and continue for 24–48 h after resolution of signs/symptoms *Elderly:* PO, 100 mg/d and continue for 24–48 h after resolution of signs/symptoms *Children:* PO, 10 y and >40 kg: 100 mg 2×/d; 10 y and <40 kg: 5 mg/kg/d PO in two divided doses, not to exceed 200 mg/d; <10 y: 5 mg/kg/d (up to 150 mg/d) in 2 divided doses	*Onset:* 2 h *Duration:* 12 h $t_{1/2}$: 15–24 h
rimantadine (Flumadine)	Influenza A	*Adults and adolescents >14 y:* PO, 100 mg 2×/d for 24–48 h after resolution of signs/symptoms *Elderly:* PO, 100 mg qd for 24–48 h after resolution of signs/symptoms *Children:* PO, 10–13 y and >40 kg: 200 mg qd; 10–13 y and <40 kg: 5 mg/kg/d or 200 mg qd, whichever is less; 1–9 y: 5 mg/kg/d or 150 mg qd, whichever is less	*Onset:* Slow *Duration:* Unknown $t_{1/2}$: 25.4 h
Oseltamivir (Tamiflu)	Influenza A and B	*Adults and adolescents ≥13 y:* PO, 75 mg 2×/d for 5 d *Children:* PO, >40 kg: 75 mg (6.2 mL) 2×/d for 5 d; 24–40 kg: 60 mg (5 mL) 2×/d for 5 d; 16–23 kg: 45 mg (3.8 mL) 2×/d for 5 d; <15 kg: 30 mg (2.5 mL) 2×/d for 5 d *Infants <1 y:* Not indicated	*Onset:* Rapid *Duration:* Unknown $t_{1/2}$: 6–10 h
zanamivir (Relenza)	Influenza A and B	*Adults and children >7 y:* PO, 2 inhalations 2×/d for 5 d *Children <7 y:* Safety and efficacy have not been established	*Onset:* 1 h *Duration:* 24 h $t_{1/2}$: 2.5–5.1 h
	Influenza prophylaxis during outbreak or exposure	*Adults and children >7 y:* PO, 2 inhalations (10 mg) daily *Children ≤7 y:* Safety and efficacy have not been established	

Oseltamivir also is thought to be effective for preventing influenza; however, this use is not labeled.

Oseltamivir is a pregnancy category C drug. It is unclear whether it passes into breast milk. The most common adverse effects of oseltamivir are nausea and vomiting, bronchitis, insomnia, and vertigo. Nausea and vomiting can be reduced by administration with milk, a snack, or a meal. No important drug–drug interactions have been identified. Oseltamivir is converted extensively into oseltamivir carboxylate by the liver and then excreted renally.

Oseltamivir is not a substitute for annual influenza vaccination. It is important to encourage patients in especially at-risk populations, such as the elderly or immunocompromised patients, to receive a yearly influenza vaccine injection (Box 43.1).

Zanamivir

Zanamivir (Relenza) is the second neuraminidase inhibitor. Its mechanism of action is the same as that of oseltamivir. Zanamivir is an orally inhaled agent that is approved for use in adults and in children older than 7 years of age. It is a pregnancy category B drug. Like oseltamivir, the effectiveness of the drug is directly related to promptness with which treatment is initiated.

Zanamivir is supplied on a Rotadisk containing four blisters of a powder mixture. The Rotadisk is loaded into a Diskhaler, the blister is punctured, and the patient inhales through the mouthpiece. The actual amount of drug delivered to the respiratory tract depends on the ability of the patient to inhale adequately. Approximately 10% of zanamivir is absorbed systemically. It is excreted renally as unchanged drug.

Adverse effects with zanamivir include headache, dizziness, nausea, diarrhea, and respiratory effects such as sinusitis, bronchitis, cough, nasal symptoms, and infections. Because zanamivir is administered by oral inhalation, it is more likely to cause local adverse effects, such as bronchospasm, than systemic reactions. For this reason, zanamivir is given cautiously to patients with underlying respiratory disorders, especially asthma. Instruct the patient to have a fast-acting

FOCUS ON RESEARCH

Box 43.1 Early Oseltamivir Works Against Flu, but Vaccination is Best for Seniors

Aoki, F. Y., Macleod, M. D., Paggiaro, P., et al. (2003). Early administration of oral oseltamivir increases the benefits of influenza treatment. *Journal of Antimicrobial Chemotherapy, 51*(1), 123–129.

The Study

The researchers evaluated the benefit of early influenza treatment using oral oseltamivir (Tamiflu). They developed an open-label, international study to investigate how the overall duration of illness related to the interval from onset of illness to time of first treatment dose. The study encompassed a total of 1,426 patients (age, 12–70 years) who presented within 48 hours of the onset of influenza symptoms. Infection with influenza virus was laboratory-confirmed in 958 patients. All patients were treated with oseltamivir, 75 mg twice a day for 5 days. The study revealed that early intervention was associated with briefer illnesses. Therapy that was started within the first 12 hours after fever onset reduced the total median illness duration by 74.6 hours more than intervention at 48 hours did. Interventions started later than 12 hours but before 48 hours reduced the illness proportionately. Administration of oseltamivir within 12 hours also reduced duration of fever, severity of symptoms, and time elapsed before patients returned to baseline activity and health scores.

Nursing Implications

Influenza is a potentially life-threatening illness in the very young, the elderly, and immunocompromised patients. Although oseltamivir provides effective prophylaxis for influenza, the Centers for Disease Control and Prevention recommend that it be used only in healthy patients between the ages of 1 and 49 years. It may also be used in healthy patients 50 to 64 years of age on a case-by-case basis. Other patients should receive trivalent inactivated vaccine by subcutaneous injection.

inhaled bronchodilator, such as albuterol, available when administering zanamivir.

Like oseltamivir, zanamivir should not be substituted for yearly influenza vaccine in high-risk populations.

Table 43.3 summarizes information about drugs used to treat influenza.

Drugs Used for Hepatitis

Interferons

The interferons are a family of glycoproteins that affect many types of viral illness. They are administered parenterally, either subcutaneously or intramuscularly. Although pharmacologically similar, each is used for specific viral illnesses. The three main classes of interferons are interferon alfa, interferon beta, and interferon gamma. Interferon alpha and beta are used in the management of hepatitis (Table 43.4), whereas interferon gamma is used for other types of viral illness. The following is a brief review of the interferons, which are presented in depth in Chapter 34.

INTERFERON ALFA

Interferon alfa is an immunomodulator. The name interferon alfa actually refers to several compounds that differ slightly in their amino acid sequence:

- Interferon alfa-2a (Roferon-A)
- Interferon alfa-2b (Intron-A)
- Peginterferon alfa-2a (Pegasys)
- Peginterferon alfa-2b (PEG-Intron)
- Interferon Alfa-n3 (Alferon)
- Interferon Alfacon-1

Interferon alfa is approved for treating hairy cell leukemia, AIDS-related Kaposi sarcoma, condylomata acuminatum, chronic HBV, and chronic HCV. It also has been used investigationally for treating renal cell carcinoma, bladder carcinoma, chronic myelogenous leukemia, and lymphomas (Table 43.5).

INTERFERON BETA

Interferon beta-1a (Avonex) and Interferon beta-1b (Betaseron) are forms of native human interferon beta prepared by recombinant DNA technology. They are similar to interferon alfa and gamma in chemistry and adverse effects but differ in efficacy. They are used primarily for treating relapsing or remitting multiple sclerosis (MS) to decrease both the number and severity of attacks. They have also been tested in cutaneous T-cell lymphoma, HCV infection, HIV infection, Kaposi sarcoma, malignant melanoma, and renal cell carcinoma.

Other Drugs for Hepatitis

ADEFOVIR DIPIVOXIL

Adefovir dipivoxil (Hepsera) is a purine nucleotide analogue used in managing hepatitis B. It was initially introduced as an antiretroviral drug, but it was found to have a high incidence of nephrotoxicity at the dose needed to affect the HIV virus. Adefovir dipivoxil is a prodrug that is metabolized into the active metabolite adefovir diphosphate. As the active metabolite, adefovir replaces a nucleotide in the HBV virus, resulting in DNA chain termination. Adefovir may also stimulate endogenous interferon alfa production.

Although the prevalence of nephrotoxicity is much lower with the current recommended dosage of adefovir, it may still occur. Patients with pre-existing renal impairment have the highest risk for nephrotoxicity. Adefovir should also be given cautiously to patients with liver dysfunction.

Drug–drug interactions occur with drugs that increase the risk for renal or hepatic toxicity, such as aminoglycosides, cidofovir, nonsteroidal anti-inflammatory drugs (NSAIDs), and probenecid. Adefovir should be given cautiously in patients taking antiretroviral nonnucleoside reverse transcriptase inhibitors (NNRTIs), antiretroviral nucleoside reverse transcriptase inhibitors (NRTIs), or antiretroviral protease inhibitors (PIs) because of an increased risk for developing lactic acidosis and severe hepatomegaly with steatosis. Similarly, adefovir should be given cautiously to patients receiving metformin because both drugs have the potential to induce lactic acidosis.

Adefovir is a pregnancy category C drug. It is not known whether adefovir passes into breast milk. It is not indicated for use in adolescents or children.

Tables 43.4 and 43.5 summarize information about drugs used to treat hepatitis.

TABLE 43.4 Summary of Selected Drugs for Hepatitis

Drug (Trade) Name	Selected Indications	Route and Dosage Range	Pharmacokinetics
interferon alfa-2a (Roferon-A)	See Table 43.5	*Adult:* IM/SC, 3 million international units 3×/wk for 12 mo	*Onset:* Rapid *Duration:* Unknown $t_{1/2}$: 3.7–8.5 h
interferon alfa-2b (Intron-A)	Hepatitis B Hepatitis C	*Adult:* IM/SC, 5 million international units per day or 10 million international units 3×/wk for 16 wk 3 million international units 3×/wk for up to 18–24 mo if a positive response	*Onset:* Rapid *Duration:* Unknown $t_{1/2}$: 2–3 h
interferon alfa-2a (Pegasys)	Hepatitis B Hepatitis C	*Adult:* SC, 180 mcg once weekly for 24 wk 180 mcg once weekly for 48 wk	*Onset:* Rapid *Duration:* Unknown $t_{1/2}$: 70–90 h
interferon alfa-2b (PEG-Intron)	See Table 43.5	*Adult:* SC, 1 mcg/kg/wk	*Onset:* Rapid *Duration:* 42–72 h $t_{1/2}$: 4.6 h
interferon alfa-n3 (Alferon)	See Table 43.5	*Adult:* IM/SC, 3–6 million international units 3×/wk	*Onset:* Unknown *Duration:* Unknown $t_{1/2}$: unknown
interferon Alfacon-1 (Infergen)	See Table 43.5	*Adult:* SC, 9 mcg 3×/wk for 24 wk. At least 48 h should elapse between doses.	*Onset:* Rapid *Duration:* Unknown $t_{1/2}$: Unknown
interferon alfa-2a (SC) and ribavirin (PO) (Rebetron)	See Table 43.5	*Adults >75 kg:* Ribavirin PO 600 mg 2×/d in combination with interferon alfa-2b 3 million IU SC 3×/wk *Adults, adolescents, and children >61 kg:* Ribavirin PO 400 mg in the morning and 600 mg in the evening every day in combination with interferon alfa-2b 3 million IU SC 3×/wk *Adults, adolescents, and children 50–61 kg:* Ribavirin PO 400 mg 2×/d in combination with interferon alfa-2b 3 million IU/m2 SC 3×/wk *Adolescents and children 37–49 kg:* Ribavirin PO 200 mg in the morning and 400 mg in the evening every day in combination with interferon alfa-2b 3 million IU/m² SC 3×/wk *Adolescents and children 25–36 kg:* Ribavirin PO 200 mg 2×/d in combination with interferon alfa-2b 3 million IU/m² SC 3×/wk	*Onset:* Rapid *Duration:* Unknown $t_{1/2}$: 3.7–8.5 h
adefovir (Hepsera)	See Table 43.5	*Adult:* PO, 10 mg 1×/d	*Onset:* Unknown *Duration:* 24 h $t_{1/2}$: 7.5 h

TABLE 43.5 Drugs for Managing Hepatitis

Name	Hepatitis B Virus	Hepatitis B Infection	Hepatitis C Virus	Hepatitis C Infection
interferon alfa-2a (Roferon-A)	O		X	X
interferon alfa-2b (Intron-A)	X	X	X	X
interferon alfa-2a (Pegasys)	O	O	X	X
interferon alfa-2b (PEG-Intron)	O		X	X
interferon alfa-n3 (Alferon)	O		O	O
interferon Alfacon-1 (Infergen)	O		X	X
interferon alfa-2a and ribavirin (Rebetron)				X
adefovir (Hepsera)	X	X		

X, FDA approved; O, off-label.

Drugs Used for Respiratory Syncytial Virus

Ribavirin

Ribavirin (Virazole) is a synthetic nucleoside antiviral drug. It is used as a primary agent to treat RSV infections. Intravenous ribavirin is available from the United States Centers for Disease Control and Prevention to treat hantavirus infection and Lassa fever. Oral ribavirin is approved for treating chronic hepatitis C infection in combination with interferon alfa-2b (PEG-Intron) or interferon alfa-2b (Rebetron). The exact mechanism of antiviral activity of ribavirin is unclear; however, it is thought to increase the mutation rate of RNA viruses, leading to "error catastrophe."

Inhaled ribavirin should be administered using the SPAG-2 aerosol generator. Make sure you are thoroughly familiar with the use of this device before administering ribavirin. Solutions placed in the SPAG-2 reservoir should be discarded every 24 hours and before adding newly reconstituted solutions. Reconstituted solutions may be stored at room temperature for 24 hours.

Ribavirin is one of the few antiviral drugs that is indicated for use in children. It is contraindicated for use in children who require ventilatory support, however, because it may precipitate in the respiratory equipment.

Ribavirin is teratogenic and embryotoxic in animals; therefore, it is contraindicated for use in adults because of its potential for producing testicular lesions and teratogenic effects. It is considered a pregnancy category X drug. Pregnant health care workers should not administer aerosolized ribavirin because it can disperse into the immediate bedside area. Additionally, ribavirin should not be given concurrently with zidovudine because it blocks the action of zidovudine.

Palivizumab

Palivizumab (Synagis) is a humanized monoclonal antibody to RSV prepared by using recombinant DNA technology. As a "humanized" monoclonal antibody, the drug tends to have little immunogenicity. It is 50 to 100 times more potent than RSV-IGIV (described next) against RSV, easier to prepare, and more convenient to administer.

Palivizumab is an intramuscular injection that is given monthly during the RSV season, which is generally the beginning of fall to the end of spring. In rare circumstances, palivizumab has induced hypersensitivity reactions, including anaphylaxis. Babies who experience any type of hypersensitivity reaction should not receive additional injections. Because palivizumab is given as an intramuscular (IM) injection, it is given cautiously to babies with a history of thrombocytopenia or any coagulation disorder.

Common adverse effects include upper respiratory tract infection, otitis media, rhinitis, rash, cough, gastroenteritis, and wheezing. Rarely, babies may experience fever, diarrhea, or vomiting. Unlike RSV immune globulin (RSV-IG), palivizumab causes no risk for pulmonary edema because it is not given by infusion.

Reconstitute palivizumab powder with sterile water according to the dose of medication to be delivered. Roll the vial between the hands but do not shake the vial, then allow the solution to sit for 20 minutes before administering the injection.

Respiratory Syncytial Virus Immune Globulin

RSV-IG (RespiGam) is a polyclonal human hyperimmune globulin. It is used to prevent lower RSV disease in high-risk children younger than 24 months of age with bronchopulmonary dysplasia, chronic lung disease, or a history of premature birth. It is prepared by extracting immunoglobulin G (IgG) antibodies from the plasma of humans who have high titers of antibodies against RSV.

RSV-IG is administered intravenously over several hours. Because of the potential for infusion-related reactions and pulmonary edema resulting from fluid overload, close monitoring during the infusion is necessary.

RSV-IG administration is contraindicated in infants with cyanotic congenital heart disease and hypersensitivity to intravenous immunoglobulins. Adverse effects include infusion heart rate–related effects such as dizziness, flushing, changes in blood pressure, anxiety, palpitations, chest tightness, dyspnea, cramps, pruritus, myalgia, and arthralgia. These effects can be minimized by slowing the infusion rate. Pulmonary edema resulting from fluid overload can also occur. Because of these potential serious adverse effects, monitor the baby closely throughout the entire infusion.

PHYSIOLOGY OF FUNGAL GROWTH

Fungi can be separated into two groups—yeasts and molds. The yeasts are single-celled organisms, approximately the size of a red blood cell, that reproduce by a budding process. The buds separate from the parent cell and mature into identical daughter cells. Molds produce long, hollow, branching filaments called hyphae. The term **dimorphic fungi** describes a limited number of fungi that are capable of growing as yeasts at one temperature and as molds at another. Reproduction for most fungi may be sexual or asexual.

Fungi can produce disease in humans only if they can grow at the temperature of the infected body site. Fungi that cannot grow at core body temperature are called **dermatophytes.** Infections caused by these fungi are contained at the cutaneous level of the body. They are called superficial mycoses, as opposed to systemic mycoses, which are serious, deep-tissue fungal infections caused by organisms capable of growth at core body temperature.

The normal body has yeast colonies on the skin, mucous membranes, and GI tract. Intact immune mechanisms and competition for nutrients, provided by the body's normal bacterial flora, ordinarily keep colonizing fungi in check. Alteration of either of these components by disease states or antibiotic therapy can upset the balance, permitting fungal overgrowth and opportunistic infections.

PATHOPHYSIOLOGY OF SELECTED OPPORTUNISTIC FUNGAL INFECTIONS

Aspergillosis

Aspergillus is a fungus commonly found in soil, water, and decaying vegetation. It has been cultured from unfiltered air, ventilation systems, contaminated dust dislodged during hospital renovation and construction, horizontal surfaces, food,

and ornamental plants. It has been recognized increasingly as a cause of severe illness and mortality in highly immunocompromised patients, such as those undergoing chemotherapy, those with AIDS, or those with bone marrow or vital organ transplants.

Aspergillus infection, which is airborne, may be acquired by inhaling the fungal spores. In severely immunocompromised patients, primary *Aspergillus* pneumonia results from local lung tissue invasion. Colonization of the lower respiratory tract by *Aspergillus* in patients with pre-existing lung disease, such as chronic obstructive lung disease, cystic fibrosis, or inactive tuberculosis, can predispose patients to invasive pulmonary or disseminated infection. After pulmonary invasion, the fungus may disseminate through the bloodstream to involve multiple organs. The most reliable technique for diagnosis is a lung biopsy, although the fungus may be cultured from sputum or from specimens acquired by bronchoalveolar lavage.

Candidiasis

Candida is a yeastlike fungus that is almost always present as part of the normal population of organisms in the mouth, skin, intestinal tract, and vagina. The immune system and other organisms in the mucous membranes normally prevent it from growing in colonies. However, in immunocompromised patients, deterioration of the immune system can lead to candidal colonization; most outbreaks occur when the CD4+ T-cell count falls below 400.

HIV-infected infants and children are particularly prone to serious and extensive candidal infections. Other factors that can promote growth of *Candida* species in healthy individuals include use of broad-spectrum antibiotics (which alter the natural population of organisms in the mouth and vagina); use of topical and systemic corticosteroids; diabetes; ill-fitting dentures; drugs or conditions that alter saliva flow; radiation therapy; cancer; chemotherapy; nutritional deficiency in iron, folate, vitamin B_{12}, or zinc; oral contraceptives with a high estrogen content; pregnancy; poor oral or dental hygiene; smoking; stress; depression; and use of antihistamines.

Cryptococcosis

Cryptococcosis, which usually manifests as cryptococcal meningitis, is the most serious of the fungal infections in immunocompromised patients. Cryptococcosis rarely occurs when the CD4+ T-cell count is over 100 and is most likely when the count drops below 50. It is caused by a yeastlike organism, *Cryptococcus neoformans*. This fungus is widespread in the environment, especially in soil containing bird droppings. Exposure occurs when contaminated sources become airborne and are inhaled.

In people with intact immune systems, the fungus may form inactive fungal nodules in the lungs, which may be visible on x-ray films and can later produce active infection when the immune response decreases. As cryptococcosis progresses, either from the original infection or a later reactivation, it can take three forms (more than one of which may be present):

- CNS
- Pulmonary
- Disseminated

Meningitis, inflammation of the membranes surrounding the spinal cord or brain, is the most common manifestation of cryptococcal infection.

Mucormycosis

Mucormycosis, also known as zygomycosis, is a fungal infection of the sinuses, brain, or lungs caused by fungi such as *Mucor* or *Rhizopus*. These common fungi are found in soil and decaying vegetation. The spores are inhaled into the body through the mouth and nose. In the immunocompetent person, the spores are destroyed by phagocytosis. In the immunocompromised patient, the spores attach to the nasal or oral mucosa. The spores can then spread into the nasal cavity and maxillary sinuses. The spores can also invade the blood vessels, causing systemic spread, or a local inflammatory or thrombotic effect to the vessels.

Common syndromes associated with mucormycosis include rhinocerebral infection, pulmonary infection, or mucormycosis of the GI tract, skin, or kidneys. Symptoms associated with rhinocerebral infection include orbital and facial pain, headache, visual changes, acute sinusitis, fever, proptosis (protrusion of eye orbit), and erythema (redness) of skin overlying sinuses. Necrotic tissue may be seen on the nasal turbinates, septum, and palate. Symptoms of pulmonary involvement include cough, hemoptysis, and shortness of breath. Patients with GI involvement may have abdominal pain or vomiting.

Without treatment, mucormycosis has a mortality rate of 30% to 70%. Unlike other fungal diseases, mucormycosis requires surgical débridement of necrotic tissues in addition to pharmacotherapy to resolve the infection.

PATHOPHYSIOLOGY OF SELECTED NONOPPORTUNISTIC FUNGAL INFECTIONS

Blastomycosis

Blastomycosis is a chronic infection characterized by granulomatous and suppurative lesions. It is caused by inhaling the dimorphic fungus *Blastomyces dermatitidis*. Blastomycosis is endemic in eastern parts of the United States, but it also is seen throughout Canada and Central America.

Two basic forms of blastomycosis are recognized: pulmonary and chronic cutaneous. Most infections originate in the lungs and then disseminate to any organ, but usually to the skin and bones. In chronic cutaneous blastomycosis, the initial skin lesion presents as one or more subcutaneous nodules that eventually ulcerate. They are most common on exposed skin, such as that of the face, hands, wrist, and lower leg. Diagnosis is usually made by direct culture, agents that contain potassium hydroxide, special stains, and measurement of complement-fixing antibodies to various antigens.

Coccidioidomycosis

Coccidioidomycosis (valley fever) is primarily a disease of the lungs, which is common in the southwestern United States and northwestern Mexico. It is caused by the fungus

Coccidioides immitis, which grows in soil. The fungal spores become airborne when the soil is disturbed by wind, construction, farming, and other activities. Within the lung, the spore changes into a larger, multicellular structure called a spherule. The spherule grows and bursts, releasing endospores, which develop into other spherules. Person-to-person transmission does not occur.

Most cases of coccidioidomycosis are mild. It is thought that more than 60% of infected people have either no symptoms or experience flulike symptoms and never seek medical attention. Among patients who seek medical care, the most common symptoms are fatigue, cough, chest pain, fever, rash, headache, and joint aches. Some people develop erythema nodosum, which produces painful red bumps that gradually turn brown.

Disseminated disease occurs in less than 0.5% of patients. In patients with disseminated disease, spores may be found in lymph nodes and meningeal, spleen, liver, kidney, and adrenal tissues. Meningitis is the most common cause of death. Patients at risk for disseminated disease are immunocompromised and include patients who have undergone organ transplantation and those with lymphoma, HIV infection, adrenal corticosteroid therapy, or diabetes. Disseminated disease also occurs more frequently in men, in African Americans and Filipinos, and in pregnant women during the third trimester.

Dermatophytic Infections (Tinea, Ringworm)

Dermatophytic infections are commonly called **tinea** or ringworm. It is not a worm infection as the name suggests; rather, it is a fungal infection caused by mold-like fungi called dermatophytes. Tinea lives on the dead tissues on the skin and any structures that grow from the skin (such as hair or nails).

Tinea can affect most skin sites, depending on the specific fungal type. The descriptive terms in the following list refer to the location of the infection and not to which specific type of fungus is involved:

- Tinea pedis—athlete's foot
- Tinea cruris—ringworm of the groin
- Tinea capitis—ringworm of the scalp
- Tinea corporis—ringworm of the body
- Tinea unguium—ringworm of the nails

A slightly different type of tinea infection is known as tinea versicolor. This chronic, noninflammatory infection is characterized only by patchy, hypopigmented discoloration of the skin.

The classic features of tinea are itching, redness on the skin, and a circular patchy lesion that spreads along its borders and clears at the center. In time, it may appear as a ring or a series of rings around a clear center, hence its common name, ringworm. These particular characteristics may not always be seen in every infected person; lack of certain signs or symptoms or the presence of additional signs or symptoms depends on which site is infected and how advanced the disease is. On the palms of the hands or soles of the feet, redness may be the only sign. Sometimes there may be deep-seated blisters on the soles of the feet that, with time, dry and end up as brown crusts. There may be thick, white scales between the toes. Nails can turn thick and white and eventually crumble if untreated. On the scalp, there may be hair loss as the hairs break off at their shafts.

Histoplasmosis

Histoplasmosis is a fungus infection that affects the lungs or other organs by dissemination. The disease is acquired by inhaling fungal spores. Outbreaks may occur in groups who have been exposed to bird or bat droppings or recently disturbed contaminated soil found in chicken coops or caves. Person-to-person spread of histoplasmosis does not occur. Although anyone can get histoplasmosis, it more often infects immunocompromised patients. Infection usually results in increased resistance to further infection, although the immunity is not complete. Symptoms vary from mild to severe, ranging from flulike illness to serious lung infection.

There are four clinical forms of histoplasmosis. The most common is acute pulmonary histoplasmosis. Patients with this form of the infection experience a flulike cough, chest pains, dyspnea, fever, weight loss, and hemoptysis. The symptoms may resolve spontaneously. In children, primary histoplasmosis can lead to disseminated infection. Therefore, children who have HIV and histoplasmosis should receive suppressive therapy for life. The second form of histoplasmosis is chronic pulmonary histoplasmosis, which may develop after acute infection; this form resembles pulmonary tuberculosis. The third form is termed acute disseminated histoplasmosis. Patients with this form may develop hepatosplenomegaly, fever, and prostration. This type of histoplasmosis is usually fatal. The last form of histoplasmosis is termed chronic disseminated histoplasmosis, which may present a diagnostic problem because of the extremely varied presentation. Like the acute form, it also may be fatal.

C ANTIFUNGAL AGENTS

Antifungal drugs are generally grouped according to their pharmacotherapeutics into those used to manage systemic infections and those used to manage superficial infections, although some of the antifungal drugs may be used for both.

Polyene Antifungal Agents

Polyene antimicrobials include amphotericin B and nystatin. These drugs have high affinity for fungal infections and are therefore useful for treating systemic fungal infections. Unfortunately, the polyene antifungal drugs also have the ability to induce severe adverse effects. Amphotericin B (Fungizone) is the prototype polyene antifungal drug. Table 43.6 presents a summary of selected antifungal agents.

NURSING MANAGEMENT OF THE PATIENT RECEIVING P AMPHOTERICIN B

Core Drug Knowledge

Pharmacotherapeutics

Amphotericin B is an antifungal agent used to treat progressive and potentially fatal systemic fungal or protozoal infections. It has a wide spectrum of activity against many fungi, including *Aspergillus fumigatus, Blastomyces dermatitidis, Candida albicans, Candida guilliermondii, Candida tropicalis,*

TABLE 43.6 Summary of Selected (C) Antifungal Drugs Used for Systemic Infections

Drug (Trade) Name	Selected Indications	Route and Dosage Range	Pharmacokinetics
(C) Polyene Antifungal Drugs			
P amphotericin B (Fungizone, Fungizone, Intravenous, Abelcet [lipid complex formula])	Progressive and potentially fatal systemic fungal or protozoal infections (*Aspergillus, Blastomyces,* coccidioidomycosis, histoplasmosis, sporotrichosis, mucormycosis)	*Adult:* IV (sporotrichosis), 20 mg per injection, up to 9 mo; IV (aspergillosis), total dose of 3.6 g, treat up to 11 mo; IV (other infections in adult or child), administer over 6 h at a concentration of 0.1 mg/mL, usual dose is 0.25 mg/kg/d not to exceed 1.5 mg/kg/d	*Onset:* 20–30 min *Duration:* 20–24 h $t_{1/2}$: 24 h initially and, then 15 d; Abelcet, 173.4 h
	Aspergillosis in patients refractory to, or intolerant of, conventional therapy (Abelcet)	*Adult:* IV (Abelcet), 5 mg/kg/d given as single infusion at 2.5 mg/kg/h	
	Cutaneous and mucocutaneous mycotic infections caused by *Candida* species	*Adult:* Topical, apply liberally to candidal lesions two to four times daily, treat for 2–4 wk based on response	
nystatin (Mycostatin, Nilstat, Nystex; *Canadian:* Candistatin)	*Candida*—oropharyngeal, cutaneous, mucocutaneous, vulvovaginal, intestinal	*Adult:* PO, 500,000–1,000,000 U tid, continued for at least 48 h after clinical cure; PO suspension, 400,000–600,000 U qid (1⁄2 dose in each side of mouth, retain the drug as long as possible before swallowing); troche, dissolve 1–2 tablets in mouth four to five times daily up to 14 d; vaginal preparation, 1 tablet (100,000 U) intravaginally qd for 2 wk; topical, apply to affected area two to three times daily until healing is complete *Child:* Oral suspension (infants), 200,000 U qid (100,000 in each side of mouth); oral suspension (premature and low-birth-weight infants), 100,000 U qid	Not generally absorbed systemically
caspofungin (Cancidas)	Invasive aspergillosis	*Adult:* IV, 70 mg on day 1 then 50 mg/d *Adolescent and child:* Safety not established	*Onset:* Rapid *Duration:* Unknown $t_{1/2}$: Triphasic: alpha phase: Short beta phase: 9–11 h terminal phase: 40–50 h
	Esophageal or oropharyngeal cardidiasis	*Adult:* IV, 50 mg/d *Adolescent and child:* Safety not established	
flucytosine (5-FC, 5-fluocytosine, Ancobon)	Serious infections caused by susceptible strains of *Candida, Cryptococcus*	*Adult:* PO, 50–150 mg/kg/d q6h	*Onset:* Varies *Duration:* 10–12 h $t_{1/2}$: 2–5 h

Coccidioides immitis, Cryptococcus neoformans, Histoplasma capsulatum, Rhodotorula species, and *Sporothrix schenckii.* Certain protozoan infections also are sensitive to amphotericin B, including *Leishmania braziliensis, Leishmania donovani, Leishmania mexicana,* and *Naegleria fowleri.*

Amphotericin B is available in lipid-complex and nonlipid-complex formulations. Liposomal amphotericin B is indicated for treating invasive fungal infections in patients refractory to or intolerant of conventional amphotericin B therapy. In addition to its IV formulation, amphotericin B is also available as a topical cream, lotion, or ointment for superficial use (see Table 43.6).

Pharmacokinetics

Amphotericin B, given orally, is absorbed poorly from the GI tract. Because of its poor GI absorption, it may be given orally when GI tract sterilization is required to rid the tract of fungal colonies. Distribution of amphotericin B is limited; it crosses the placenta and may pass into breast milk. Low concentrations are achieved in aqueous humor and pleural, pericardial, peritoneal, and synovial fluids. Because CSF concentrations are approximately 3% of those in serum, amphotericin B must be given intrathecally to achieve fungistatic concentrations within the CSF.

The metabolism of amphotericin B is unknown. It is presumed that the drug enters the tissues of the body and is released slowly over time. After therapy is discontinued, amphotericin B can be detected for up to 4 weeks in blood and 4 to 8 weeks in urine. The initial half-life is approximately 24 hours, followed by a second elimination phase with a half-life of about 15 days. The drug is excreted in the urine.

Pharmacodynamics

Amphotericin B works by binding to sterols in fungal cell membranes. This binding appears to form pores or channels and results in increased cell permeability, cell leakage, and death. Because human cells also contain sterols, damage to the host's cells also may occur. At low concentrations, amphotericin B is fungistatic; higher concentrations may induce fungicidal activity.

Contraindications and Precautions

Amphotericin B can cause anemia, hypokalemia, and hypomagnesemia. Administer the drug cautiously to patients with any of these conditions because parenteral therapy with amphotericin B can cause substantial renal electrolyte loss. For patients with pre-existing renal impairment, administer amphotericin B at a lower dose and monitor the patient for signs of nephrotoxicity. Amphotericin B is assigned to pregnancy category B and should be used with caution during pregnancy and lactation.

Adverse Effects

Amphotericin B has an extensive adverse effects profile. In fact, some clinicians refer to it as "amphoterrible." Nephrotoxicity occurs in more than 80% of patients receiving IV amphotericin B. Nephrotoxicity is manifested in many forms, including renal insufficiency, azotemia, hyposthenuria, renal tubular acidosis, and frank renal failure.

Administration of IV amphotericin B may induce infusion-related reactions, such as headache, chills, fever, rigors, hypotension, bronchospasm, and nausea and vomiting. Slowing the rate of administration is not helpful. However, the severity of these symptoms usually diminishes with subsequent doses of amphotericin B.

Electrolyte abnormalities, including hypokalemia, hypomagnesemia, hypochloremia, and hypocalcemia, also may occur with amphotericin B therapy. Patients with pre-existing cardiac problems may have exacerbations of their disorders when electrolyte abnormalities occur.

A normocytic, normochromic anemia occurs in most patients receiving amphotericin B. This reaction is believed to be caused by a suppressive effect on erythropoietin production. Transfusions are not usually necessary, and the anemia resolves when therapy is discontinued. Leukopenia and thrombocytopenia also may occur.

Less common adverse effects from amphotericin B consist of ventricular fibrillation, hypertension, cardiac arrest (primarily in situations when infusion is too rapid), hypersensitivity, peripheral neuropathy, and seizures.

Intrathecal amphotericin B can cause blurred vision and, in some cases, difficulty in urination. Polyneuropathy or paresthesias can occur in some patients, resulting in numbness, tingling, pain, or weakness. Arachnoiditis, an inflammation of the arachnoid membrane, also is possible.

Drug Interactions

Amphotericin B should not be coadministered with drugs known to be nephrotoxic or hemotoxic, such as antineoplastic agents, cyclosporine, tacrolimus, or aminoglycosides. It should not be used with drugs that may be affected by electrolyte imbalances, such as corticosteroids, digitalis glycosides, and thiazide diuretics. Other drugs that interact with amphotericin B include neuromuscular blocking agents, imidazoles, and flucytosine. Table 43.7 lists agents that interact with amphotericin B.

Assessment of Relevant Core Patient Variables

Health Status

Elicit a patient history to evaluate for pre-existing renal dysfunction, cardiac disease, electrolyte imbalance, or anemia. Also, assess for use of diuretics or for any concurrent drugs known to be nephrotoxic. Communicate any positive findings to the prescriber.

Perform a complete physical examination, especially assessing the renal system. For patients with pre-existing cardiac disease, a baseline electrocardiogram should be performed. Baseline laboratory values should include CBC, complete metabolic profile, and renal function tests.

Life Span and Gender

Assess for pregnancy and lactation. Amphotericin B may be given during pregnancy. However, because of the potential adverse effects, it should be given only when absolutely needed. It should not be given to breast-feeding women because of its potential effects on the infant.

It is important to note the patient's age before administering amphotericin B. Safety of amphotericin B has not been demonstrated in children and older adults. Closely monitor patients when giving them this drug. Elderly patients are more likely to have decreased renal function, which may increase the risk for nephrotoxicity.

TABLE 43.7 Agents That Interact With P Amphotericin B

Interactants	Effect and Significance	Nursing Management
antineoplastic agents	Coadministration of antineoplastic agents and amphotericin B increases the risks for renal toxicity, bronchospasm, and hypotension.	Monitor for adverse effects. Monitor renal function tests. Adjust dosage of antineoplastic agents if needed.
corticosteroids	Concurrent use may cause potential hypokalemia.	Do not coadminister unless needed for control of adverse reactions.
digitalis glycosides	Amphotericin B may induce hypokalemia, which increases the risk for digitalis glycoside toxicity.	Monitor electrolytes. Monitor for signs of digitalis toxicity. Replace electrolytes as needed.
flucytosine	Coadministration of flucytosine and amphotericin B have a synergistic effect, which increases the risk for flucytosine toxicity.	Monitor drug levels. Monitor for flucytosine toxicity. Adjust drug dosages as needed.
hemotoxic agents	Concurrent use increases the risk for anemia, neutropenia, and thrombocytopenia.	Monitor drug levels closely. Monitor for signs of blood dyscrasias. Adjust drug dosages as needed.
imidazoles	Coadministration of imidazoles and amphotericin B has antagonistic effects, resulting in subtherapeutic levels.	Monitor for efficacy of therapy. Adjust drug dosages as needed.
nephrotoxic agents	Concurrent use increases the risk for nephrotoxicity.	Monitor drug levels closely. Monitor for signs of renal impairment. Monitor intake and output. Adjust drug dosages as needed.
neuromuscular blocking agents	Amphotericin B-induced hypokalemia may enhance the curariform effect of skeletal muscle relaxants.	Monitor electrolytes. Replace electrolytes as needed. Monitor for prolonged action of neuromuscular blocking agents. Secure airway if prolonged activity is suspected.
thiazide diuretics	Coadministration may increase electrolyte losses.	Monitor electrolytes. Replace electrolytes as needed. Adjust drug dosages as needed.
zidovudine	Coadministration increases the risk of myelosuppression and nephrotoxicity.	Monitor renal function tests. Monitor CBC. Adjust drug dosages as needed.

Lifestyle, Diet, and Habits

Assessing fluid intake in patients on amphotericin B therapy is important. Make sure that patients on amphotericin B therapy are kept well hydrated. This practice may minimize the potential for nephrotoxicity.

Environment

Note the environment in which amphotericin B will be administered. Amphotericin B should be administered in an acute care environment. Be familiar with administration of IV amphotericin B. The drug should not be reconstituted with a bacteriostatic agent in the solution because doing so may lead to precipitation. Before administration, document vital signs. Administer a test dose of amphotericin B (1 mg in 20 to 50 mL of 5% dextrose in water [D_5W] over 30 minutes) to assess for possible hypersensitivity and potential infusion reaction.

Nursing Diagnoses and Outcomes

- Risk for Injury related to infusion reaction or to electrolyte imbalance imposed by drug therapy
  Desired outcome: *The patient will remain free from injury during drug administration or respond without injury to electrolyte replacement therapy.*
- Ineffective Protection related to drug-induced leukopenia and thrombocytopenia
  Desired outcome: *The patient will remain free from opportunistic infections resulting from leukopenia and thrombocytopenia.*
- Excess Fluid Volume related to renal dysfunction resulting from drug therapy
  Desired outcome: *The patient will have an appropriate ratio of fluid intake to output.*
- Acute Pain related to infusion reaction
  Desired outcome: *The patient will have a decrease in pain after administration of analgesic drug, such as meperidine (Demerol).*
- Ineffective Breathing Patterns due to drug-induced bronchospasm
  Desired outcome: *The patient will maintain adequate oxygenation.*

- Ineffective Cardiopulmonary Tissue Perfusion related to cardiac arrest or arrhythmias resulting from drug therapy
  Desired outcome: *The patient will remain adequately perfused.*
- Disturbed Sensory Perception: Visual due to drug-related blurred vision
  Desired outcome: *The patient will regain adequate vision after therapy concludes.*
- Risk for Injury related to drug effects of numbness, tingling, or weakness
  Desired outcome: *The patient will remain injury free throughout therapy.*

Planning and Intervention

Maximizing Therapeutic Effects

Patients may desire to stop amphotericin B therapy if they have infusion reactions. Prepare the patient for the possibility of this reaction. Also, provide comfort measures, such as extra blankets, diversion therapy, or warm fluids, to offset the discomfort of this reaction.

Minimizing Adverse Effects

Be prepared for the possibility of an infusion reaction. Administering preordered drugs, such as hydrocortisone, meperidine, and ibuprofen, before starting therapy has been shown to be effective in preventing an infusion reaction. Dantrolene or meperidine can be administered if rigors occur. Coordinate the administration of amphotericin B with possible blood transfusions. Infusion-related reactions can be more severe if administration occurs shortly after platelet or granulocyte transfusions.

Administer amphotericin B in a central line, if possible, and make sure that the IV administration set has an in-line filter. The solution can be placed on an infusion pump and deliver the drug over 2 to 4 hours.

Monitor the patient carefully for signs of nephrotoxicity. In addition to accurately recording fluid input and output, monitor renal function tests and notify the prescriber immediately if the creatinine is higher than 3.5 mg/dL.

Coordinate the care of the patient when multiple prescribers are writing orders for the patient. To prevent orders for other nephrotoxic drugs, all prescribers must know that amphotericin B is being administered.

Providing Patient and Family Education

- Describe and explain the possibility of an infusion reaction and the importance of notifying staff immediately if symptoms occur.
- Explain possible adverse effects of amphotericin B and the need for serial blood tests. Because the adverse effects of amphotericin B can induce severe complications, it is important to explain the necessity of reporting any change from baseline that may occur.
- Another important area to discuss with patients and family is the importance of an accurate fluid intake and output record. It will be necessary to enlist the assistance of patients and their families to document fluid intake and output as needed.
- Inform patients using topical amphotericin B to report any skin irritation. Advise these patients to avoid occlusive dressings.
- Instruct the patient to immediately report to the prescriber any symptoms of altered protection against infection, such as easy bruising, sore throat, or fatigue.
- Instruct patients to report CNS symptoms such as numbness, tingling, or weakness to the prescriber.

Ongoing Assessment and Evaluation

During the first dose of amphotericin B, take vital signs every 15 minutes. At this time, evaluate the patient for possible infusion reactions. Should a reaction occur, stop the infusion, call for another nurse to stay with the patient, and contact the prescriber immediately. Also, monitor the IV site during administration for signs of phlebitis because amphotericin B is very irritating to tissues.

Throughout therapy, coordinate the collection of samples for laboratory tests, including a CBC, complete metabolic panel, and renal function tests. Weigh the patient daily and evaluate fluid intake and output every shift.

It is important to monitor patients with pre-existing cardiac disease for exacerbation of their symptoms. Fluid overload and electrolyte imbalances place these patients at high risk for a cardiac event.

Monitor for adverse effects that may place the patient at increased risk for injury. For patients with sensory-perceptual disturbances or numbness, tingling, and weakness, ensure that the patient understands the need for assistance to and from the bed. Keep the bed in the low position and the side rails up at all times.

Use strict aseptic technique for patients receiving amphotericin B. Most patients have anemia related to the therapy, which increases the risk for infection.

By the end of therapy, the fungal infection should be resolved. In addition, all adverse effects should be identified and appropriate intervention should be started.

Drugs Similar to P Amphotericin B

Azole Antifungal Drugs

Azole antifungal drugs can be used for both superficial mycoses and more serious systemic mycoses. Azole drugs that are used for systemic disease include fluconazole, keto-

MEMORY CHIP

P Amphotericin B

- Used for severe systemic fungal or protozoal infections
- Major contraindication: hypersensitivity
- Most common adverse effects: infusion reactions, electrolyte abnormalities, and anemia
- Most serious adverse effect: nephrotoxicity
- Maximizing therapeutic effects: Prepare the patient for the possibility of an infusion reaction so that the patient does not cease therapy.
- Minimizing adverse effects: Do not administer with other nephrotoxic drugs to minimize the potential for nephrotoxicity.
- Most important patient education: Discuss the potential for an infusion reaction and the need to monitor the hematopoietic and renal systems closely.

conazole, itraconazole, miconazole, and voriconazole. The azole family is presented in detail later in this chapter using the prototype fluconazole.

Nystatin

Nystatin (Mycostatin) is an antifungal antibiotic that is nearly identical to amphotericin B in structure. It is available in topical, vaginal, and oral formulations. Nystatin is not used for systemic fungal infections because it is poorly absorbed from the GI tract and has high potential for toxicity. It is used to treat oropharyngeal, cutaneous, mucocutaneous, and vulvovaginal candidiasis. Like amphotericin B, it may be given orally when GI tract sterilization is required to rid the GI tract of fungi.

Some formulations of nystatin, such as the oral suspension, contain methylparaben and propylparaben. Therefore, these products should be used with caution in patients with paraben hypersensitivity. In addition, some formulations of nystatin oral suspension contain sucrose, which may cause hyperglycemia, especially in the diabetic patient.

Adverse effects from nystatin are uncommon. Oral doses of nystatin can cause mild and transient nausea and vomiting, diarrhea, and abdominal pain. Topical and vaginal forms of nystatin may produce skin irritation, rash, or urticaria.

The oral suspension of nystatin is called a "swish and swallow" drug. Advise the patient to swish the solution throughout the mouth and then swallow or spit the drug as directed by the prescriber. When nystatin troches are prescribed, advise the patient to allow them to dissolve completely in the mouth and not to chew or swallow the intact troche. The troche may take up to 30 minutes to dissolve.

Drugs Significantly Different From P Amphotericin B

Caspofungin

Caspofungin (Cancidas) is a semisynthetic intravenous antifungal agent from a new class of drugs called the echinocandins. It is indicated for treating invasive aspergillosis in patients who are refractory to or intolerant of other therapies, such as amphotericin B formulations or itraconazole. Although other uses are not yet FDA approved, caspofungin is also used to manage esophageal and oropharyngeal candidiasis.

Caspofungin works by inhibiting the synthesis of a major fungal cell wall component, beta-(1,3)-D-glucan, which is not present in human cell walls. Because of its unique mechanism of action, cross-resistance with other antifungal classes of drugs is unlikely.

Caspofungin should be given cautiously to patients with pre-existing hepatic dysfunction. It is classified as a pregnancy category C drug; however, animal studies show significant embryotoxic effects. It is unclear whether caspofungin enters into breast milk. Caspofungin should be used during pregnancy and when breast-feeding only when the benefits clearly outweigh the risks. It is not approved for use in children and adolescents.

Common adverse effects associated with the use of caspofungin include abdominal pain, fever or chills, muscle cramps, pain, pain at the injection site, redness or warmth of the face, skin rash, itching, and unusual tiredness or weakness. Less common adverse effects include shortness of breath, wheezing, swelling, fluid retention, and tingling or numbness in the hands or feet. Hypersensitivity reactions, including anaphylaxis, have occurred but are rare.

Several drug–drug interactions may occur with caspofungin. When it is given concurrently with P-450 inducers, serum caspofungin levels are substantially decreased. These drugs include carbamazepine, dexamethasone, efavirenz, phenytoin, fosphenytoin, nelfinavir, nevirapine, and rifampin. When caspofungin is given concurrently with cyclosporine, caspofungin levels increase, thus increasing the risk for adverse effects, especially elevated alanine aminotransaminase (ALT) levels. When it is given concurrently with tacrolimus, serum tacrolimus levels are substantially decreased.

Flucytosine

Flucytosine (5-FC) is an oral antifungal drug. Historically, it has been used in combination with amphotericin B in treating cryptococcal meningitis. However, since the release of fluconazole in 1990, flucytosine use has declined considerably.

Flucytosine acts as an antimetabolite, interfering with pyrimidine metabolism and eventually disrupting both RNA and protein synthesis. Flucytosine is assigned to pregnancy category C and is contraindicated for use during pregnancy and breast-feeding. It is not metabolized; more than 90% is excreted by glomerular filtration as unchanged drug. Therefore, it is used cautiously in patients with pre-existing renal impairment. It also is used with caution in patients with pre-existing depression of bone marrow function, recent radiation therapy or cytotoxic drug therapy, dental disease, or a history of a hematologic disease because these patients are most susceptible to flucytosine's myelosuppressive effects. In patients with hepatic disease, flucytosine can cause hepatitis or jaundice.

Flucytosine can induce serious adverse effects. Flucytosine is toxic to rapidly proliferating tissues, such as the bone marrow and the lining of the GI tract. Therefore, common hematologic adverse effects include anemia, leukopenia, and thrombocytopenia. GI adverse effects include abdominal pain, diarrhea, nausea, vomiting, and anorexia. Other adverse effects caused by flucytosine include hepatic dysfunction, photosensitivity, and CNS effects, such as dizziness, headache, and lightheadedness. It is important to monitor patients who are concurrently taking other drugs also known to cause hematologic toxicity, nephrotoxicity, or hepatotoxicity.

Azole Antifungal Drugs

The azole antifungal drugs have two subgroups: imidazoles and triazoles. These two groups differ slightly in their chemical structures but have similar clinical applications. Azole antifungal drugs can be used for both superficial mycoses and more serious systemic mycoses. Fluconazole (Diflucan) is the prototype azole antifungal drug. Table 43.8 presents a summary of azole antifungal agents; Table 43.9 lists agents that interact with fluconazole; and Table 43.10 lists topical azole agents.

TABLE 43.8 Summary of Selected Ⓒ Azole Antifungal Agents

Drug (Trade) Name	Selected Indications	Route and Dosage Range	Pharmacokinetics
P fluconazole (Diflucan; *Canadian:* Apo-Fluconazole)	Esophageal, oropharyngeal, vulvovaginal candidiasis	*Adult:* PO/IV, 200 mg on first day, followed by 100 mg/d as indicated *Child:* PO/IV, 6 mg/kg on the first day, followed by 3 mg/kg once daily; treat for a minimum of 3 wk and at least 2 wk after resolution	*Onset:* PO, unknown; IV, immediate *Duration:* Unknown $t_{1/2}$: 20–21 h
	Systemic mycoses (cryptococcal meningitis)	*Adult:* PO/IV, 400 mg on first day, followed by 200 mg qd; 400 mg qd may be needed; continue treatment for 10–12 wk *Child:* PO/IV, 12 mg/kg on first day, followed by 6 mg/kg once daily, continue treatment for 10–12 wk	
itraconazole (Sporanox)	Blastomyces dermatitidis, histoplasma capsulatum, aspergillosis	*Adult:* PO, 200 mg qd, increase dose in 100-mg increments to a maximum 400 mg qd; give doses over 200 mg/d in divided doses; continue treatment for a minimum of 3 mo and until clinical parameters and laboratory tests indicate that the active fungal infection has subsided *Child:* Safety and efficacy not established	
	Onychomycosis	*Adult:* PO, 200 mg bid for 1 wk, followed by 3-wk rest period; repeat	
miconazole (Monistat I.V., Micatin, Monistat 3, Monistat 7, Monistat-Derm, Monistat Dual Pak)	Severe systemic fungal infections: coccidioidomycosis Candidiasis Cryptococcosis Petriellidiosis Paracoccidioldo-mycosis Vulvovaginal candidiasis	*Adult:* IV (dosage varies with organism involved), 1,800–3,600 mg for 3 to >20 wk *Adult:* 600–1,800 mg for 1–20 wk *Adult:* 1,200–2,400 mg for 3–12 wk *Adult:* 600–3,000 mg for 5–20 wk *Adult:* 200–1,200 mg for 2–16 wk *Adult:* Vaginal suppositories, insert 1 suppository intravaginally once daily hs for 3 or 7 d (depending on drug dosage regimen); repeat course as necessary	*Onset:* IV, rapid; vaginal and topical, not systemically absorbed *Duration:* IV, unknown; vaginal and topical, not systemically absorbed $t_{1/2}$: IV, 21–24 h; vaginal and topical, not systemically absorbed
	Tinea pedia, tinea cruris, tinea corporis, cutaneous candidiasis, tinea versicolor	*Adult:* Topical, apply to affected areas bid	
ketoconazole (Nizoral; *Canadian:* Apo-Ketoconazole)	Systemic fungal infections: candidiasis, chronic mucocutaneous candidiasis, oral thrush, candiduria, blastomycosis, coccidioidomycosis, histoplasmosis, chromomycosis, paracoccidioldomycosis	*Adult:* PO, 200 mg qd, up to 400 mg/d; treat from 3 wk to 6 mo, depending on infecting organism and site *Child:* PO, >2 y, 3.3–6.6 mg/kg/d as a single dose; <2 y, safety and efficacy not established	*Onset:* PO, varies; topical, slow, not appreciably systemically absorbed *Duration:* Unknown $t_{1/2}$: 8 h
	Dermatophytosis; tinea corporis, tinea cruris, tinea versicolor	*Adult:* Topical, apply daily to affected area; may be treated twice daily; continue treatment for at least 2 wk *Child:* Topical, >2 y, same as adult; <2 y, safety and efficacy not established	
voriconazole (Vefend)	Invasive aspergillosis **or** *Scedoporium* sp **or** *Fusarium* sp	*Adult and child >12 y:* IV, 6 mg/kg every 12 h day 1 followed by 3–4 mg/kg 2 ×/d *Adult and child >12 y:* PO, 400 mg every 12 h day 1 followed by 200 mg 2 ×/d	

(continued)

TABLE 43.8 Summary of Selected (C) Azole Antifungal Agents (continued)

Drug (Trade) Name	Selected Indications	Route and Dosage Range	Pharmacokinetics
	Candidiasis	*Adult and child >12 y:* IV, 6 mg/kg q12h as an IV infusion leading dose on day 1, followed by 3 mg/kg as an IV infusion q12h *Child <12 y:* Safety and efficacy have not been established *Adult and child ≥12 y (≥40 kg):* PO, 200 mg 2 ×/d for 14 d and for at least 7 d following resolution of symptoms *Adult and child ≥12 y (<40 kg):* PO, 100 mg 2×/d for 14 d and for at least 7 d following resolution of symptoms *Child <12 y:* Safety and efficacy have not been established	

TABLE 43.9 Agents That Interact With (P) Fluconazole

Interactants	Effect and Significance	Nursing Management
anticoagulants	Fluconazole may decrease the metabolism of anticoagulants such as warfarin. This may increase the anticoagulant activity and result in toxicity	Monitor prothrombin time at least every 2 d. Monitor patient for signs of bleeding. Adjust anticoagulant dosage as needed.
benzodiazepines	Metabolism of certain benzodiazepines and first-pass effect of triazolam may be decreased resulting in increased CNS depression	Monitor for CNS depression. Adjust dosage of benzodiazepines. Avoid use of itraconazole or ketoconazole.
buspirone	Inhibition of the CYP3A4 isozyme by azole antifungal agents may result in increased plasma buspirone concentrations resulting in an increased risk for adverse effects.	Avoid concurrent use if possible. Monitor for buspirone adverse effects.
cyclosporin tacrolimus	Fluconazole may inhibit cyclosporine or tacrolimus hepatic metabolism. This may induce toxicity and increase the risk for nephrotoxicity.	Monitor cyclosporine or tacrolimus levels. Monitor serum creatinine levels. Adjust cyclosporine or tacrolimus dosage as needed.
hydantoins	Fluconazole may decrease the metabolism of hydantoins, such as phenytoin. This may result in toxicity of hydantoins.	Monitor hydantoin levels. Monitor patient for sign of toxicity. Adjust hydantoin dosage as needed.
losartan	Fluconazole may inhibit the metabolism of losartan resulting in an increased antihypertensive effect and risk for adverse effects.	Monitor the blood pressure daily. Monitor the patient for adverse effects to losartan.
oral contraceptives	Concurrent use with oral contraceptives containing ethinyl estradiol/levonorgestrel may decrease serum concentration of the oral contraceptives.	Advise women taking ethinyl estradiol or levonorgestrel BCP to use another method of contraception.
rifamycins	Rifamycins may induce the metabolism of fluconazole. This may decrease plasma concentration of fluconazole and decrease antifungal activity.	Monitor for therapeutic efficacy of fluconazole. Adjust the dose of fluconazole as needed.
sulfonylureas	Although the mechanism of action is unclear, fluconazole may increase the hypoglycemic effects of sulfonylurea agents.	Monitor blood glucose levels daily. Adjust dose of sulfonylurea agent as needed.
tricyclic antidepressants	Fluconazole may inhibit the metabolism of TCA drugs resulting in an increase in therapeutic and adverse effects.	Monitor the patient's clinical response to tricyclic agents (TCA) agents. Adjust dosage of TCA as needed.
zidovudine	Coadministration of zidovudine and fluconazole increases the area under the curve (AUC) of zidovudine.	Monitor for toxic effects of zidovudine. Monitor renal function.

TABLE 43.10 Summary of Selected (C) Tropical Azole Antifungal Agents

Drug	Indications	Route and Dosage Range	Pharmacokinetics
butoconazole (Femstat-3)	Vaginal candidiasis	**Vaginal dosage (vaginal cream):** Apply 1 applicatorful of 2% cream at bedtime for 3 consecutive d (6 d if pregnant)	Not systemically absorbed
clotrimazole (Mycelex, Lotrimin)	Tinea pedis Tinea corporis Tinea cruris Candidal infections	**Topical:** *Adult and child >2 y:* Apply to affected skin and surrounding areas twice daily, morning and evening **Oral (troche) dosage:** *Adult and child >3 y:* Dissolve a 10-mg troche slowly and completely in the mouth 5×/d for 14 d **Vaginal dosage (vaginal cream):** Apply 1 applicatorful of 1% cream once daily at bedtime for 7–14 d **Vaginal dosage (tablets):** 100-mg tablet at bedtime for 7 d; or one 200-mg tablet at bedtime for 3 d; or 500-mg tablet as a single dose at bedtime	Not systemically absorbed
oxiconazole (Oxistat)	Tinea pedis Tinea corporis Tinea cruris	**Topical dosage (1% cream or lotion):** *Adult, adolescent, and child:* Apply to the affected area(s) and the immediately surrounding area(s) 1–2×/d	Not systemically absorbed
sulconazole (Exelderm)	Tinea pedis Tinea corporis Tinea cruris	**Topical dosage (cream and solution):** *Adult:* Apply 1% preparation topically to the cleansed, dry, affected area(s) once or twice daily, morning and evening, for 3 wk	Not systemically absorbed
sertaconazole (Ertaczo)	Tinea pedis	**Topical application (cream):** *Adult, adolescent, and child >12 y:* Apply a thin layer of the 2% cream to the cleansed, dry, infected area twice daily for 4 wk	Not systemically absorbed
terconazole (Terazol)	Vaginal candidiasis	**Intravaginal dosage (Terazol 7 cream):** *Adult and adolescent:* Insert 1 applicatorful intravaginally once daily at bedtime for 7 consecutive d **Intravaginal dosage (Terazol 3 cream):** *Adult and adolescent:* Insert 1 applicatorful once daily at bedtime for 3 consecutive d **Intravaginal dosage (Terazol 3 vaginal suppositories):** *Adult and adolescent:* Insert one 80-mg suppository intravaginally once daily at bedtime for 3 consecutive d	Not systemically absorbed
tioconazole (Vagistat, Monistat 1-day, Tioconastat-1)	Vaginal candidiasis	**Intravaginal dosage (cream):** *Adult and adolescent:* 1 applicatorful before bedtime as a single dose	Not systemically absorbed

NURSING MANAGEMENT OF THE PATIENT RECEIVING [P] FLUCONAZOLE

Core Drug Knowledge

Pharmacotherapeutics

Fluconazole is a triazole antifungal agent with a wide spectrum of activity. It is the drug of choice for esophageal and oropharyngeal candidiasis and is used to suppress vulvovaginal candidiasis. It is used for primary fungal prophylaxis in immunocompromised patients with a $CD4^+$ T-cell count less than 200 and as prophylaxis against coccidioidomycosis, cryptococcosis, and histoplasmosis in patients with $CD4^+$ T-cell counts below 50.

Although amphotericin B is usually the drug of choice for systemic mycoses, especially cryptococcal meningitis, fluconazole is used as an alternative drug to treat these conditions (see Table 43.8 for more information).

Pharmacokinetics

Fluconazole is administered orally and intravenously. The pharmacokinetics of both oral and IV fluconazole are similar. GI absorption is rapid and almost complete. Oral

bioavailability is more than 90% in fasting adults, and peak serum concentrations are attained within 1 to 2 hours after oral administration.

Fluconazole is distributed widely into body tissues and fluids. Saliva, sputum, nail, blister, and vaginal secretion concentrations are approximately equal to plasma concentrations. High concentrations also can be achieved in the cornea, aqueous humor, and vitreous body following IV administration. Fluconazole distributes well into the CSF and achieves CSF concentrations that are 50% to 94% of plasma concentrations, regardless of the degree of meningeal inflammation. Fluconazole crosses the placenta and enters breast milk. Elimination is mainly renal; about 60% to 80% of a dose is excreted in the urine unchanged and 11% as metabolites. Small amounts of fluconazole are excreted in the feces. Elimination of the drug can be impaired in elderly patients.

Pharmacodynamics

Fluconazole works directly by altering the fungal cell membrane. Fluconazole inhibits synthesis of ergosterol, a cytochrome P-450 enzyme that is an essential component of the fungal membrane. Inhibition of ergosterol synthesis results in increased cellular permeability, causing leakage of cellular contents. Other proposed antifungal effects of fluconazole include inhibition of endogenous respiration, interaction with membrane phospholipids, and inhibition of the transformation of yeasts to molds. It has no direct effects on the body.

Contraindications and Precautions

No absolute contraindications exist to fluconazole use. It should be used with caution during pregnancy and in patients with pre-existing hepatic and renal dysfunction.

Adverse Effects

The most common adverse effects of fluconazole are diarrhea, nausea, vomiting, abdominal pain, headache, and dizziness. Mild elevations in levels of alanine transaminase, aspartate transaminase, alkaline phosphatase, and bilirubin may occur. These abnormalities usually return to pretreatment levels after therapy is completed. Rarely, hepatotoxicity has been reported.

Other symptoms that have occurred during fluconazole therapy include alopecia and exfoliative skin disorders, such as Stevens-Johnson syndrome. These conditions occur most frequently in HIV-infected patients and in patients with a concurrent malignancy who are taking multiple drugs. A direct causative relationship has not been determined. Rarely, fluconazole therapy may induce hypokalemia, eosinophilia, and thrombocytopenia.

Drug Interactions

Many drug–drug interactions are possible with fluconazole. Fluconazole may interact with anticoagulants, benzodiazepines, hydantoins, oral contraceptives, sulfonylurea agents, tricyclic antidepressants, and zidovudine. Several drugs no longer available in the United States—astemizole, cisapride, and terfenadine—can induce fatal arrhythmias when given concurrently with fluconazole. Table 43.9 lists drugs that interact with fluconazole.

Assessment of Relevant Core Patient Variables

Health Status

Elicit a patient history to evaluate for pre-existing renal or hepatic dysfunction, pregnancy, or breast-feeding. It is important to communicate any positive findings to the prescriber. Also, assess for any known reactions to azole antifungal agents.

Perform a complete physical examination, documenting signs and symptoms of the fungal infection. For patients with pre-existing anemia, renal, or hepatic disease or patients expected to be on long-term therapy, obtain samples for baseline CBC, renal, and hepatic function tests to determine baseline organ function.

Life Span and Gender

Determine whether the patient is pregnant or breast-feeding. Fluconazole is assigned to pregnancy category C and should, therefore, be used with caution during pregnancy. It achieves high concentrations in breast milk.

Note the patient's age before administering fluconazole. Although a dosage schedule has been established for children, the safety of fluconazole has not been demonstrated in children younger than 13 years. However, drug therapy has been successful, and complications have not occurred in neonates treated with IV fluconazole in emergency treatment situations. With these concerns in mind, closely monitor children throughout therapy. Elderly patients are more likely than others to have decreased renal and hepatic function, which may increase the risk for toxicities.

Lifestyle, Diet, and Habits

Assess whether fluconazole is causing gastric distress in the patient. Fluconazole absorption and bioavailability are not affected by food or changes in gastric pH. Encourage patients who experience GI distress to take the drug with food.

Ask questions to uncover information about alcohol ingestion and other substance use (such as drugs and tobacco). Fluconazole may elevate hepatic enzymes. Caution the patient to refrain from alcohol ingestion throughout therapy because it increases the risk for hepatotoxicity. As with other drugs used as prophylaxis against opportunistic diseases in immunocompromised patients, discuss potential substance abuse (other drugs, alcohol, tobacco) with the patient. Explain how a healthy lifestyle decreases the risk for opportunistic diseases.

Determine which type of OTC pain reliever the patient generally uses. Advise the patient to use aspirin instead of acetaminophen for relief of minor discomforts because acetaminophen has the potential to damage the liver or kidneys.

Environment

Be aware of the environment in which fluconazole will be administered. Fluconazole is administered orally and intravenously. The oral preparation is used in the home environment, often as long-term prophylaxis for fungal infections in immunocompromised patients. Be sure to explain the importance of follow-up visits to assess the efficacy of therapy and to evaluate the patient for possible adverse effects.

Intravenous therapy is usually reserved for patients unable to tolerate or take fluconazole orally and is administered in

the hospital setting. Before administration, visually inspect the solution for particulate matter and discoloration. Do not administer unless the solution is clear. Fluconazole should be administered with an infusion pump at a rate not to exceed 200 mg/h.

Nursing Diagnoses and Outcomes

- Acute Pain related to fluconazole-induced headache
  Desired outcome: *The patient will self-administer aspirin to relieve headache.*
- Ineffective Protection related to adverse effects of blood dyscrasias and Stevens-Johnson syndrome
  Desired outcome: *The patient will report signs and symptoms of these adverse reactions immediately to the prescriber.*
- Disturbed Body Image from drug-related alopecia
  Desired outcome: *The patient will verbalize concerns of changes in body image to the prescriber and develop coping strategies.*
- Imbalanced Nutrition: Less than Body Requirements related to adverse effects of nausea, vomiting, and abdominal pain
  Desired outcome: *The patient will remain within acceptable weight parameters throughout therapy.*
- Risk for Injury related to elevated hepatic enzymes and hypokalemia resulting from drug therapy
  Desired outcome: *The patient will remain injury free throughout therapy.*

Planning and Intervention

Maximizing Therapeutic Effects

Administer fluconazole in evenly divided intervals throughout the day.

Minimizing Adverse Effects

Carefully screen patients for pre-existing disorders, which may increase the risk for adverse reactions. In the hospitalized patient, contact the prescriber if any drugs known to interact or increase the risk for adverse effects are added to the drug profile. Administer an antiemetic or antidiarrheal agent, if prescribed, for adverse GI effects.

Providing Patient and Family Education

- Patients must understand that they should not take this drug if they have ever had a reaction to any drug whose name includes the ending "azole."
- Advise patients to notify the prescriber if they are pregnant or breast-feeding.
- It is important to explain that fluconazole is prescribed for a particular infection and should not be used to self-medicate or treat any other infection.
- Unless such use is specified by the doctor, caution that this drug should not be used in children younger than 13 years.
- Teach the patient about the need to complete the full course of drug therapy, even if the infection resolves. Instruct patients to take forgotten doses as soon as they remember, but not if it is time for the next dose.
- Remind patients of the importance of remaining well hydrated while taking this drug.
- Explain potential adverse effects of fluconazole and potential remedies for these discomforts. It is important to advise patients to contact the prescriber immediately if they experience darkening of their urine, yellowing of the eyes or skin, unusual bruising or bleeding, skin rash (including inside the mouth), redness, blistering, peeling, or loosening of the skin. This advice is especially important for patients taking fluconazole as prophylaxis for opportunistic diseases.
- Explain that fluconazole may decrease the effectiveness of oral contraceptives and should suggest that patients use an alternative form of contraception while taking fluconazole.
- Advise patients taking sulfonylureas to monitor their blood glucose levels frequently and to notify the prescriber in the event of frequent episodes of hypoglycemia.
- Advise patients taking anticoagulants to have blood tests performed frequently to detect altered prothrombin times. Patients should contact the prescriber if they experience easy bruising or bleeding.
- It is also important to advise patients of signs and symptoms of secondary bacterial infections that may occur with superficial mycoses. Advise patients to contact the prescriber if the affected skin becomes red and hot or exudes pus.
- Ensure patients with alopecia that the condition is temporary. Patients may wish to wear a wig.

Ongoing Assessment and Evaluation

Monitor the effectiveness of therapy. When treating superficial mycoses, be sure to document new lesions and assess for possible secondary bacterial infections. In the hospital setting, monitor for hepatic or renal dysfunction. It is important to monitor fluid intake and output carefully; enlist the patient and family to document intake and output not observed by nurses.

Throughout therapy, arrange for serial blood testing to evaluate renal, hepatic, and hematopoietic function. For suspected electrolyte imbalance, reviewing complete metabolic panel test results is important.

Monitor the patient for GI distress, headache, dizziness, and exfoliative skin disorders. It is important to ensure the safety of the patient experiencing CNS effects by keeping the bed in the low position and the side rails up at all times. To avoid injury, be sure the patient understands the need to ask for ambulatory assistance if experiencing dizziness. By the end of therapy, the patient should be without symptoms of fungal infection. In addition, adverse reactions should be controlled.

MEMORY CHIP

P Fluconazole

- Used to treat candidiasis and prophylaxis for fungal diseases in immunocompromised patients
- Most common adverse effects: nausea, vomiting, diarrhea, abdominal pain, headache, and dizziness
- Most serious adverse effect: Stevens-Johnson syndrome
- Maximizing therapeutic effects: Administer adjunct medications for nausea and diarrhea.
- Minimizing adverse effects: Do not give with any drugs that increase the potential for adverse effects.
- Most important patient education: Watch for signs and symptoms of adverse effects and call the prescriber immediately if any occur.

CRITICAL THINKING SCENARIO

Fluconazole and chronic candidiasis

Janice Wind is a 40-year-old woman infected with HIV. She has been diagnosed with esophageal candidiasis, for which fluconazole therapy has been prescribed. This is her third episode of esophageal candidiasis for which she will receive prolonged therapy. Assume you are Ms. Wind's nurse.

1. Identify the assessments and evaluations you would find valuable before initiating therapy.
2. Propose or construct a patient-teaching plan. Which features would you include?
3. Develop some questions about the effects of therapy to explore with Ms. Wind when she returns to the clinic in 6 weeks for a follow-up evaluation.

Drugs Closely Related to P Fluconazole

Itraconazole

Itraconazole (Sporanox) is an oral triazole antifungal drug that is related closely to ketoconazole. Itraconazole is active against many of the same fungi as ketoconazole and fluconazole but has greater activity against *Aspergillus*. Currently, itraconazole is approved for treating *Blastomyces dermatitidis, Histoplasma capsulatum,* and onychomycosis. It is under investigation for treating dermatophytic skin infections that do not respond to topical therapy. Itraconazole also is available for IV use as an alternative to IV amphotericin B. Itraconazole's oral bioavailability may increase to as much as 100% when given with a meal or a cola beverage. Like ketoconazole, it requires an acidic environment for solubility. Itraconazole appears to have fewer adverse effects than ketoconazole. However, many drug interactions are associated with it. Concomitant administration of itraconazole and pimozide or quinidine is contraindicated. A new warning listed for this drug is that life-threatening cardiac arrhythmias, sudden death, or both have occurred in patients using quinidine, pimozide, or quinidine concomitantly with itraconazole.

Ketoconazole

Ketoconazole (Nizoral) is an imidazole antifungal agent. In addition to its antifungal activity, ketoconazole possesses actions that may make it useful in other types of conditions. For example, ketoconazole has been used successfully for treating advanced prostate cancer. When used in high doses, ketoconazole can inhibit sterol synthesis in humans, including the synthesis of aldosterone, cortisol, and testosterone. Ketoconazole also is a potent inhibitor of thromboxane synthesis and has been used clinically to prevent adult respiratory distress syndrome in patients at high risk for this syndrome.

When ketoconazole is given orally, its bioavailability is affected by the pH of the stomach. It should not be given concurrently with agents that increase gastric pH, such as food, antacids, histamine-2 blockers, and omeprazole. It also should be given with caution with other agents that induce or inhibit the P-450 isoenzymes.

Miconazole

Miconazole (Monistat I.V., Micatin) is an imidazole-type antifungal agent. When miconazole was first released, it was hoped it would replace amphotericin B as a parenteral antifungal agent. Unfortunately, it was found to be less efficacious, and it caused major toxicities. Although miconazole is still marketed in a parenteral formulation, it is used most commonly topically and intravaginally. It is the active ingredient in many OTC antifungal formulations.

Voriconazole

Voriconazole (VFEND) is another triazole antifungal agent that is structurally related to fluconazole. It is used for esophageal candidiasis, primary treatment of invasive aspergillosis, and salvage therapy for infections caused by *Scedosporium* species or *Fusarium* species in patients refractory to or intolerant of other antifungal therapy. Voriconazole can be administered by the oral or intravenous route. The mechanism of action of voriconazole is similar to that of fluconazole.

Contraindications include hypersensitivity to this drug or to any other azole antifungal agent. It is given cautiously to patients with pre-existing hepatic or renal dysfunction, especially when using the intravenous formulation. It is also given cautiously to patients with pre-existing ocular disorders because of the potential for adverse effects to vision. Voriconazole oral tablets contain lactose and should not be given to patients with the rare hereditary problems of galactose intolerance, Lapp lactase deficiency, or glucose-galactose malabsorption.

The most common adverse effect associated with the use of voriconazole is visual disturbances. Approximately 30% to 45% of patients experience visual disturbances that involve enhanced brightness, blurred vision, photophobia, or color vision changes. Voriconazole may also cause stomach upset, nausea, vomiting and anorexia, abdominal pain, diarrhea, and headache.

Serious adverse effects include hepatotoxicity and allergic reactions. Voriconazole is a pregnancy category D drug. Teratogenicity, embryotoxicity, reduced fetal weight, and multiple skeletal abnormalities were noted in animal trials.

Numerous drug–drug interactions can occur with voriconazole. Drugs that are contraindicated for concurrent use include pimozide, rifampin or rifabutin, long-acting barbiturates, quinidine, ergot alkaloids, sirolimus, and carbamazepine. Voriconazole inhibits the metabolism of cyclosporine, omeprazole, and tacrolimus, resulting in increased serum concentrations of these drugs. Phenytoin increases the metabolism of voriconazole, thereby decreasing serum drug levels of voriconazole. Patients receiving statins, benzodiazepines, vinca alkaloids, HIV protease inhibitors (other than indinavir), sulfonylureas, warfarin, and calcium channel blockers may need a reduction in their normal dose of these drugs.

Drugs Significantly Different From P Fluconazole

Butoconazole

Butoconazole (Femstat-3, Mycelex-3) is a topical imidazole antifungal agent that is effective in treating vulvovaginal candidiasis. As other azole antifungals, it exerts its anti-

fungal activity by altering cellular membranes, resulting in increased membrane permeability and growth inhibition. Approximately 5% of the vaginal preparation is systemically absorbed.

The only contraindication to the use of butoconazole is hypersensitivity. Butoconazole should be used cautiously in patients with other azole hypersensitivities because cross-sensitivity may occur. Adverse effects associated with the use of butoconazole include vaginal irritation, burning, pruritus, stinging, vaginal pain or soreness, and vaginal discharge.

Advise women using butoconazole to refrain from sexual intercourse until 72 hours after therapy is completed because butoconazole contains mineral oil, which may weaken contraceptive devices, including condoms, diaphragms, and cervical caps.

Butoconazole is available as an OTC medication. It is a pregnancy category C drug.

Clotrimazole

Clotrimazole (Mycelex, Lotrimin) is another imidazole antifungal drug. It is not orally absorbed and is too toxic for IV administration. It is marketed in various forms, including vaginal suppositories and cream, topical lotion and cream, and oral solution and lozenges. It is active against a wide variety of fungi, yeast, and dermatophytes; certain gram-positive bacteria; and superficial fungal infections. These infections include dermatophytosis, vaginal and oral candidiasis, and tinea infections. The ability of clotrimazole's formulations to reach subcutaneous tissues is poor. Therefore, clotrimazole is not indicated for treating subcutaneous mycoses.

Clotrimazole is available as an OTC medication. It is a pregnancy category C drug. Contraindications are similar to those of butoconazole. Adverse effects include skin blistering, skin irritation, burning, pruritus, and stinging.

Econazole

Econazole (Spectazole) is a topical imidazole antifungal agent used primarily to treat cutaneous candidiasis and tinea infections, including tinea versicolor. Its spectrum of activity is similar to that of clotrimazole, miconazole, or tioconazole. Econazole is not approved for ophthalmic administration or vaginal administration. It is a pregnancy category C drug and may be used in children older than 3 months of age. Contraindications and adverse effects are similar to those of clotrimazole.

Oxiconazole

Oxiconazole (Oxistat) is a topical imidazole antifungal agent used to manage tinea pedis, tinea corporis, and tinea cruris. It is available as both a cream and a lotion and is administered once daily. Oxiconazole is not approved for ophthalmic administration or vaginal administration. It is a pregnancy category B drug and may be used in children. Contraindications and adverse effects are similar to those of clotrimazole.

Sulconazole

Sulconazole (Exelderm) is a topical imidazole antifungal agent used in managing tinea pedis, tinea corporis, and tinea cruris. It has greater efficacy than clotrimazole and miconazole. Like oxiconazole, it is administered only once per day. It is not approved for ophthalmic or vaginal administration. Its contraindications and adverse effects are similar to those for oxiconazole. Topical sulconazole is classified as an FDA pregnancy risk category C drug. It is not approved for use in children.

Sertaconazole

Sertaconazole (Ertaczo) is an imidazole-type antifungal used for treating tinea pedis in immunocompetent patients. The mechanism of action of sertaconazole is the same as that of other azole antifungal agents. It is active against *Trichophyton rubrum, Trichophyton mentagrophytes,* and *Epidermophyton floccosum.*

Sertaconazole is administered as a topical cream. Systemic absorption does not occur. Antifungal hypersensitivity is the only contraindication to it use. It is a pregnancy category C drug and is generally considered safe to use while breastfeeding.

Skin irritation may occur when sertaconazole is used with other creams or lotions at the same site. Adverse effects include application site reaction, burning, and tenderness.

Terconazole

Terconazole (Terazol) is a triazole antifungal agent that is structurally related to imidazole antifungal drugs. It is available for intravaginal use only. Terconazole is as effective as clotrimazole or miconazole in managing vulvovaginal candidiasis. Contraindications and adverse effects are similar to those of butoconazole.

Tioconazole

Tioconazole (Vagistat, Monistat 1-Day, Tioconastat-1, Vagistat-1) is an imidazole antifungal agent available for intravaginal use. It is the only topical antifungal agent approved in the United States as a single-dose treatment for vulvovaginal candidiasis. It is now available as an OTC medication. Contraindications and adverse effects are similar to those of butoconazole.

C Miscellaneous Antifungal Drugs

Butenafine

Butenafine (Mentax) is an allylamine topical antifungal drug indicated for treating tinea pedis, tinea corporis, and tinea cruris. It currently is under investigation for treatment of onychomycosis. Butenafine is similar to tolnaftate (discussed later in this chapter); however, it also is effective against *Candida* species, whereas tolnaftate is not. No important drug inter-actions or adverse effects have been identified at this time.

Ciclopirox Olamine

Ciclopirox olamine (Loprox) is a miscellaneous broad-spectrum antifungal drug used to treat infections caused by dermatophytes or *Candida* species. It is used primarily for tinea pedis, tinea cruris, tinea corporis, and tinea versicolor. It works by blocking transport of amino acids into the fungal cell, thus altering the cell membrane to allow leakage of intracellular material. Ciclopirox olamine also is manufactured as a nail lacquer (Penlac) for the topical treatment of mild to moderate onychomycosis of the fingernails and toenails without lunula involvement in immunocompetent patients.

Ciclopirox olamine is absorbed deeper into the dermal layers than other topical drugs. However, little is absorbed systemically. No important drug–drug interactions are known. Potential adverse effects include irritation, pruritus at the application site, redness, pain, burning, and worsening of clinical signs or symptoms.

Griseofulvin

Griseofulvin (Grisactin, Fulvicin-U/F) is a miscellaneous antifungal drug used in treating superficial dermatophytic infections, such as ringworm and tinea. It is available in a microsize or ultramicrosize formulation. These different formulations are meant to increase the bioavailability of, and to decrease the GI intolerance to, the drug.

Griseofulvin works by disrupting the mitotic spindle structure of the fungal cell, thereby stopping cell division. It also may cause defective DNA that is unable to replicate. It is very effective for superficial mycoses because it is deposited in keratin precursor cells, creating an unfavorable environment for fungal infection. Infected skin, cells, and hair are then replaced slowly by tissue that is not infected by the dermatophyte. Griseofulvin therapy lasts until the infected area has completely regrown. This therapy may take 6 to 12 months in treating tinea unguium.

Griseofulvin is contraindicated during pregnancy and breast-feeding. It should be given with caution to patients with hepatic dysfunction, porphyria, or systemic lupus erythematosus because the drug may exacerbate these conditions.

Griseofulvin has a moderate adverse effect profile. Common adverse effects include nausea, vomiting, flatulence, and epigastric distress. CNS effects may include headache, fatigue, dizziness, insomnia, confusion, psychotic symptoms, and paresthesias of the hands and feet. Integumentary adverse effects may include maculopapular rash, urticaria, and photosensitivity. In addition, hepatitis, elevated hepatic enzymes, granulocytopenia, and leukopenia have occurred after high-dose or long-term therapy.

Griseofulvin interacts with several drugs. Most importantly, it interacts with oral contraceptives by decreasing their effectiveness. Therefore, advise women taking birth control pills to use another method of contraception during griseofulvin therapy. Griseofulvin also may decrease the effectiveness of warfarin.

Closely monitor prothrombin time if griseofulvin is either added to or discontinued from warfarin therapy. Barbiturates can decrease the antifungal activity of griseofulvin. Finally, griseofulvin may increase the adverse effects of alcohol when taken concurrently.

Naftifine

Naftifine (Naftin) is a topical allylamine antifungal drug. It is used primarily for tinea pedis, tinea cruris, and tinea corporis. Naftifine is believed to interfere with sterol biosynthesis, but by a different mechanism than azoles. No important drug interactions occur with naftifine. Adverse effects include burning, stinging, dryness, erythema, pruritus, local irritation, and rash.

TABLE 43.11 Summary of Miscellaneous Antifungal Agents

Drug (Trade) Name	Selected Indications	Route and Dosage Range	Pharmacokinetics
butenafine (Mentax)	Tinea pedis, tinea corporis, tinea cruris	*Adult:* Topical, apply to affected area once daily for 4 wk	Not generally absorbed systemically
ciclopirox olamine (Loprox)	Tinea pedis, tinea cruris, tinea corporis, tinea versicolor	*Adult:* Topical, apply to affected area as directed twice daily	Not generally absorbed systemically
griseofulvin (Fulvicin P/G, Fulvicin U/F, Grifulvin V, Gris-Peg, Grisactin, Grisactin Ultra, Grisovin-FP)	Superficial dermatophyte infections (ringworm)–tinea corporis, tinea barbae, tinea capitis, tinea ungulum Tinea pedis and tinea cruris only when unresponsive to topical therapy	*Adult:* PO, 250–500 mg bid for 2 wk, up to 18 mo	*Onset:* 4 h *Duration:* 2 d $t_{1/2}$: 9–24 h
naftifine (Naftin)	Tinea pedis, tinea cruris, tinea corporis	*Adult:* Topical, massage into area bid; do not use longer than 4 wk	Not generally absorbed systemically
terbinafine (Lamisil)	Onychomycosis	*Adult:* PO, 250 mg/d; topical, apply to area bid up to 4 wk *Child:* 20 kg, PO, 62.5 mg/d *Child:* 20–40 kg, PO, 125 mg/d	*Onset:* 24 h *Duration:* 90 d $t_{1/2}$: 100 h
tolnaftate (Aftate, Genaspor, Tinactin, Ting)	Tinea pedis, tinea cruris, tinea corporis, tinea versicolor, onychomycosis, chronic fungal scalp infections, and prophylactically for tinea pedis	*Adult:* Topical, apply bid for 2–3 wk, up to 6 wk	Not generally absorbed systemically
undecylenic acid	Tinea corporis Tinea cruris Tinea pedis	*Adult:* Apply to affected area 2 ×/d	Not generally absorbed systemically

Terbinafine

Terbinafine (Lamisil) is another allylamine antifungal drug administered either orally or topically. Its topical formulation is now available OTC. Terbinafine is pharmacologically similar to naftifine. Oral terbinafine is highly effective for treating onychomycosis because of its fungicidal activity and ability to concentrate within the nail. In fact, it has been found to be superior to griseofulvin and itraconazole for treating onychomycosis.

Oral terbinafine should be given with caution to patients with hepatic and renal insufficiency and during breast-feeding. The most common adverse effects are GI, followed by elevated hepatic enzyme levels, urticaria, pruritus, and occasionally a distorted sense of taste (dysgeusia). Rare but serious adverse effects include symptomatic idiosyncratic hepatobiliary dysfunction (including cholestatic hepatitis), serious skin reactions, severe neutropenia, and allergic reactions (including anaphylaxis).

Tolnaftate

Tolnaftate (Aftate, Genaspor, Tinactin, Ting) is a miscellaneous antifungal agent used primarily for tinea pedis, tinea cruris, tinea corporis, and tinea versicolor. Tolnaftate also is used for onychomycosis, in chronic fungal scalp infections, and prophylactically for tinea pedis. No important drug interactions occur with tolnaftate, and the only adverse reaction is mild skin irritation. It may be purchased OTC.

Undecylenic Acid

Undecylenic acid (Desenex, Cruex, Fungoid AF) is another miscellaneous antifungal agent that is available OTC. It is used primarily for athlete's foot. It is not as effective as other topical antifungal agents.

Table 43.11 presents a summary of miscellaneous antifungal agents.

CHAPTER SUMMARY

- Viral and fungal diseases range from annoying disorders to life-threatening infections.
- Antiviral drugs can be arbitrarily divided into purine nucleoside analogue drugs, ophthalmic antiviral drugs, drugs used for influenza, drugs used for hepatitis, drugs for RSV, and miscellaneous drugs.
- Few effective antiviral drugs exist because eradicating the virus also may severely damage the host.
- Acyclovir is the prototype purine nucleoside analogue drug used to treat viral infections.
- Antifungal drugs can be arbitrarily divided into those used to manage systemic infections and those used to manage superficial infections.
- The two types of fungi are yeasts and molds.
- Systemic fungal diseases are categorized by those that are opportunistic and those that occur in every population.
- Amphotericin B is the prototype polyene antifungal and is the drug of choice for most systemic fungal infections.
- Amphotericin B induces severe adverse effects, including infusion reactions.
- Fluconazole is the prototype azole antifungal drug used for both systemic and superficial mycoses.
- Superficial fungal infections are treated with both oral and topical formulations of drugs.

QUESTIONS FOR STUDY AND REVIEW

1. Why are there so few effective antiviral drugs?
2. How does acyclovir work to fight herpes infections?
3. Acyclovir should be given cautiously to patients with which types of diseases or disorders?
4. What type of antiviral agents are useful in managing hepatitis?
5. What are pharmacotherapeutic differences between amantadine (or rimantadine) and oseltamivir (or zanamivir)?
6. What special instructions should be given to immunosuppressed patients regarding oseltamivir and zanamivir?
7. Why is ribavirin not generally used in adults?
8. What are pharmacotherapeutic differences between ribavirin and palivizumab and RSV-IG?
9. List the potential adverse effects of amphotericin B.
10. What important adverse effects are associated with fluconazole therapy?
11. Which of the azole antifungal agents may be used in managing systemic fungal infections?

? Need More Help?

Chapter 43 of the study guide for *Drug Therapy in Nursing* 2e contains NCLEX-style questions and other learning activities to reinforce your understanding of the concepts presented in this chapter. For additional information or to purchase the study guide, visit *http://connection.lww.com/go/aschenbrenner.*

REFERENCES AND BIBLIOGRAPHY

Anonymous. (2004). Topical sertaconazole (Ertaczo)—another azole for tinea pedis. *Medical Letter on Drugs and Therapeutics, 46*(1185), 50–51.

Burpo, R. H. (2003). Antiviral agents in women's health: Pharmacotherapeutics of treating influenza and herpes. *Journal of Midwifery and Women's Health, 47*(3), 182–189.

Cheer, S. M., & Wagstaff, A. J. (2002). Spotlight on zanamivir in influenza. *American Journal of Respiratory Medicine, 1*(2), 147–152.

Clinical Pharmacology [Online]. Available: *http://cp.gsm.com.*

De Clercq, E. (2004). Antiviral drugs in current clinical use. *Journal of Clinical Virology, 30*(2), 115–133.

Facts and Comparisons. (2004). *Drug facts and comparisons.* Philadelphia: Lippincott Williams & Wilkins.

Gupta, A. K., & Tomas, E. (2003). New antifungal agents. *Dermatology Clinic, 21*(3), 565–576.

Hardman, J. G. (2001). *Goodman & Gilman's the pharmacological basis of therapeutics* (10th ed.). New York: McGraw-Hill Health Professions Division.

Katzung, B. (2004). *Basic and clinical pharmacology* (9th ed.). New York: McGraw-Hill/Appleton & Lange.

Luggen, A. S. (2004). Pharmacology update—managing postherpetic neuralgia. *Geriatric Nursing, 25*(2), 120–121.

Micromedex Healthcare Series [Online]. Available: *http://healthcare.micromedex.com.*

Tatro, D. S. (2004). *Drug interaction facts.* Philadelphia: Lippincott Williams & Wilkins.

Waggoner-Fountain, L. A., & Grossman, L. B. (2004). Herpes simplex virus. *Pediatric Review, 25*(3), 86–93.

Weiskittel, P. (2003). Valganciclovir hydrochloride (Valcyte): A new antiviral agent. *Nephrology Nursing Journal, 30*(1), 93–95.

Veerareddy, P. R., & Vobalaboina, V. (2004). Lipid-based formulations of amphotericin B. *Drugs Today, 40*(2), 133–145.

Yeung-Yue K. A., Brentjens, M. H., Lee, P. C. et al. (2002). Herpes simplex viruses 1 and 2. *Dermatologic Clinics, 20*(2), 249–266.

Drugs Treating HIV Infection and AIDS

chapter 44

Learning Objectives

At the completion of this chapter the student will:

1. Describe the parameters that govern the choice of antiretroviral agents.
2. Identify core drug knowledge about drugs that are used in treating human immunodeficiency virus (HIV) infection and acquired immunodeficiency syndrome (AIDS).
3. Identify core patient variables relevant to drugs that are used in treating HIV infection and AIDS.
4. Relate the interaction of core drug knowledge to core patient variables for drugs that are used in treating HIV infection and AIDS.
5. Generate a nursing plan of care from the interactions between core drug knowledge and core patient variables for drugs that are used in treating HIV infection and AIDS.
6. Describe nursing interventions to maximize therapeutic effects and minimize adverse effects for drugs that are used in treating HIV infection and AIDS.
7. Determine key points for patient and family education for drugs that are used in treating HIV infection and AIDS.

KEY TERMS

CD4+ T cells

enzyme immunoassay

enzyme-linked immunosorbent assay

fusion inhibitors

highly active antiretroviral therapy (HAART)

HIV RNA

nonnucleoside reverse transcriptase inhibitors (NNRTIs)

nucleoside reverse transcriptase inhibitors (NRTIs)

protease inhibitor (PI)

provirus

viral load

Western blot

FEATURED WEBLINK

http://www.fda.gov/oashi/aids/hiv.html

Many excellent websites give up-to-date information regarding HIV infection and AIDS. The student should evaluate the source of the information carefully to be sure that it is accurate. This FDA website offers a host of topics, from approved drugs to clinical trials.

CONNECTION WEBLINK

Additional Weblinks are found on Connection:
http://www.connection.lww.com/go/aschenbrenner.

Drugs Treating HIV Infection and AIDS

Ⓒ Nucleoside/Nucleotide Reverse Transcriptase Inhibitors

- **P** **zidovudine**
- abacavir
- didanosine
- emtricitabine
- lamivudine
- stavudine
- tenofovir
- zalcitabine

Ⓒ Non–Nucleoside Reverse Transcriptase Inhibitors

- **P** **nevirapine**
- delavirdine
- efavirenz

Ⓒ Protease Inhibitors

- **P** **saquinavir**
- amprenavir
- atazanavir
- fosamprenavir
- indinavir
- nelfinavir
- ritonavir
- lopinavir/ritonavir

Ⓒ Entry Inhibitors

- **P** **enfuvirtide**

The symbol Ⓒ indicates the **drug class.**
Drugs in **bold type** marked with the symbol **P** are prototypes.
Drugs in blue type are closely related to the prototype.
Drugs in red type are significantly different from the prototype.
Drugs in black type with no symbol are also used in drug therapy; no prototype

Human immunodeficiency virus (HIV) is a virus that disables the human immune system. The virus has many subtypes. It is transmitted from person to person through sexual contact, by blood, or perinatally. Patients infected with the HIV virus have HIV disease. The syndrome called acquired immunodeficiency syndrome (AIDS) is the late stage of HIV infection, when immunodeficiency has become profound. The Centers for Disease Control and Prevention (CDC) define AIDS as HIV infection plus a CD4+ count less than 200 cells/mm^3 or an opportunistic (AIDS-defining) illness.

Pharmacotherapy for HIV infection and AIDS has changed dramatically since AIDS was first identified in 1982, and it continues to evolve. Recommended pharmacotherapy for HIV infection and AIDS is highly individualized. However, prescribers agree that multiple drug therapy, called **highly active antiretroviral therapy (HAART)** or a "cocktail," is the only way to control the progression of the disease. Because of the staggering impact of HIV infection and AIDS-related illnesses, the Food and Drug Administration (FDA) has "fast-tracked" new drugs and new drug classes; nurses and other health care professionals are encouraged to keep abreast of rapid changes in pharmacotherapeutics for HIV infection by reviewing the most current information presented in nursing and medical journals.

This chapter presents the drug classes currently used to treat HIV infection and AIDS, which include:

- Nucleoside/nucleotide reverse transcriptase inhibitors (NRTIs; prototype, zidovudine)
- Protease inhibitors (PIs; prototype, saquinavir)
- Nonnucleoside reverse transcriptase inhibitors (NNRTIs; prototype, nevirapine)
- Fusion inhibitors (prototype, enfuvirtide)

In addition to explaining how each of these drug classes works to affect HIV infection and AIDS, this chapter addresses the core drug knowledge, core patient variables, nursing management, potential nursing diagnoses, and patient education related to the administration of antiretroviral agents. This chapter also reviews current treatment recommendations for common opportunistic diseases associated with HIV infection and AIDS.

PHYSIOLOGY

CD4+ T-Cell Function

CD4+ T cells are necessary for normal immune function. The CD4+ cell recognizes foreign antigens and infected cells and helps activate the antibody-producing B lymphocytes. CD4+ T cells also induce cell-mediated immunity, in which cytotoxic CD8+ T cells and natural killer cells directly destroy foreign antigens. Phagocytic monocytes and macrophages also are influenced by CD4+ T cells. Figure 44.1 illustrates normal CD4+ T-cell function. Chapter 34 presents a more thorough review of immune system physiology.

Human Immunodeficiency Virus

HIV is like all other viruses in structure. Its ribonucleic acid (RNA) is surrounded by core proteins, which are surrounded by a protein shell called a capsid. The capsid, in turn, is surrounded by a lipid bilayer envelope. The envelope contains glycoproteins that are used to attach to host cells. The two glycoprotein subunits, gp41 and gp120, are attached to each other and embedded in the lipid bilayer (Figure 44.2).

The HIV virus is called a retrovirus. The difference between a virus and a retrovirus is in the genetic material. Like all viruses, HIV is an obligate parasite; it cannot replicate unless it is inside a living cell. Retroviruses have positive-sense single-stranded RNA and thus must transcribe their RNA into deoxyribonucleic acid (DNA) to replicate. This process is completed by an enzyme called reverse transcriptase.

PATHOPHYSIOLOGY

HIV infection begins when gp120, a surface protein on the HIV viral envelope, binds to cells that have a CD4+ protein receptor site. These cells include CD4+ T cells, monocytes, macrophages, and certain nerve cells. Once the virus is bound to the cell, the viral envelope and the plasma membrane fuse, and HIV's genetic material enters the cell. In the cell, viral RNA is transcribed into a single strand of viral DNA with the assistance of reverse transcriptase, an enzyme made by HIV. This DNA strand replicates itself, becoming double-stranded viral DNA. At this point, viral DNA can enter the cell's nucleus and, using an enzyme called integrase, splice itself into the host cell's genome, thus becoming a permanent part of the cell's genetic structure. This action results in two major problems. First, because all genetic material is replicated during cellular division, all daughter cells from the infected host cell also will be infected. Second, because the host cell's genome now contains viral DNA, the cell's genetic codes can direct the cell to make HIV. Production of new virus then occurs by translation and transcription of the code from the integrated DNA into viral RNA. Some of this RNA is messenger RNA that codes for HIV proteins. This complex process results in long strands of **HIV RNA,** which must be cut into viable lengths. Late in replication, when the newly formed virus separates from the host cell, these HIV proteins are cleaved into small proteins by the enzyme protease. Some of these proteins become part of the HIV core, and some become part of the viral protein shell. HIV protease thus is critical for viral infectivity and replication. It has been shown that HIV **provirus** (the virus before it exits the cell) manufactured without protease is noninfectious. Figure 44.3 represents HIV replication.

The HIV virus has an affinity for CD4+ T cells. The virus destroys these important cells, responsible for normal immune function, which effectively strips the person of protection against common organisms.

Originally, researchers believed that after initial infection, HIV viral replication remained dormant until stimulated by an unknown event. Now we know that viral replication is never dormant; HIV replicates continuously from the time

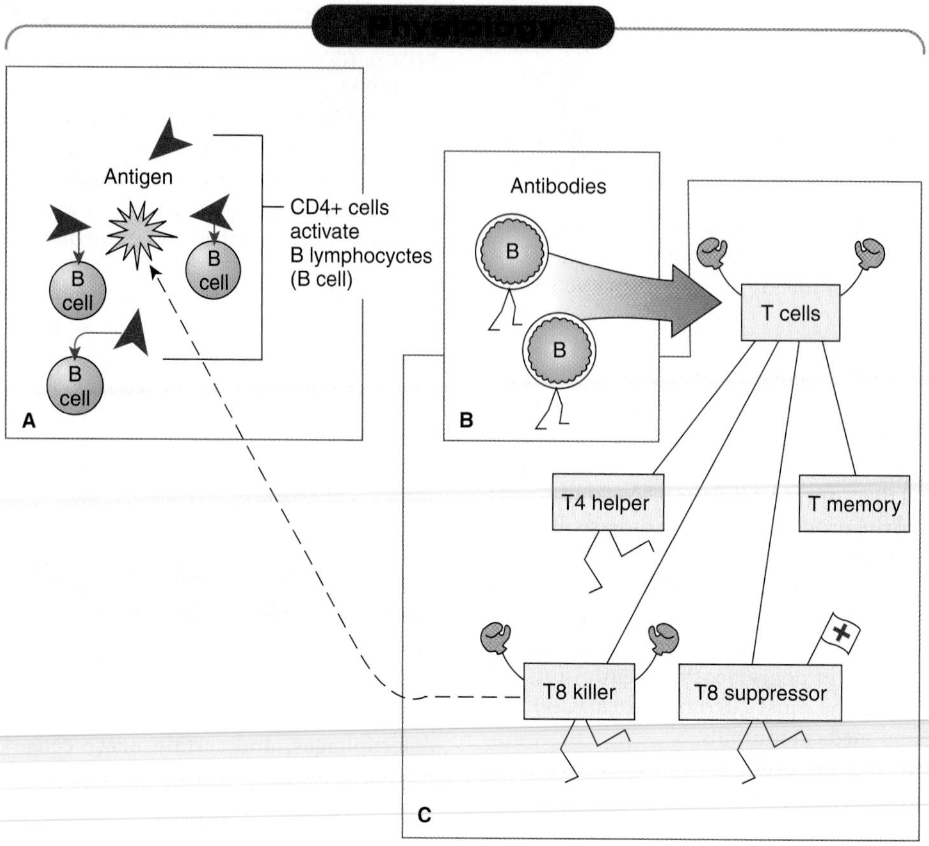

FIGURE 44.1 CD4+ cell function. CD4+ cells are the cells needed for normal immune functioning. (**A**) The CD4+ cells are the macrophages that recognize antigens (foreign substances) and signal the defenses needed to dispel them. (**B**) In beginning the defense against the antigen, the CD4+ cells activate the antibody-producing B lymphocytes, which in turn call forth the various T cells. (**C**) The T cells proliferate and differentiate to serve different functions. Cells known as T4-helper cells release lymphokines, which enhance macrophage and monocyte activity; T8 killer cells directly attack and destroy the antigen; T8 suppressor cells help to stop the immune response when appropriate; and T-memory cells are stored for future use against returning antigens.

of infection. At the initial stage of infection, the **viral load** (the amount of virus in the body) is exceptionally high. There are two reasons for this high initial viral load. First, because HIV is a new virus entering the host, the immune system is not yet sensitized to the foreign antigen, and the immune response is suboptimal. Second, because the immune system has not yet been affected by the virus, there are many CD4+ cells to invade.

During this initial stage, the patient may experience an acute retroviral syndrome that includes fever, pharyngitis, rash, myalgia or arthralgia, diarrhea, and headache. Although these symptoms are common in HIV infection, they may be dismissed initially by the patient as "the flu." After the immune system responds to the viral invasion, the viral load decreases, and the patient may become asymptomatic for a long time.

HIV infection eventually induces symptoms in every body system. In addition to those already mentioned, common symptoms associated with HIV infection include lymphadenopathy, nausea and vomiting, hepatosplenomegaly, thrush (candidiasis of the oral tissues), and weight loss. Neurologic symptoms, such as meningoencephalitis or aseptic meningitis, peripheral neuropathy, radiculopathy, facial palsy, Guillain-Barré syndrome, brachial neuritis, cognitive impairment, or psychosis, also may occur.

DIAGNOSIS OF HIV INFECTION

Diagnosis of HIV infection is initially done by a screening test followed by a confirmatory assay. Screening tests are highly sensitive, whereas confirmatory assays are highly specific. The combination use of these two types of tests produces results that are highly accurate.

The most common screening test is the **enzyme immunoassay** (EIA), or **enzyme-linked immunosorbent assay** (ELISA). The EIA detects antibodies produced in response to infection and is based on the light absorbance of antigen–antibody complexes. If the patient tests positive with the EIA test, a confirmatory **Western blot** (WB) assay test is administered. This test allows identification of antibodies specific to HIV, rather than other antibodies that can also react to the EIA test.

In addition to the EIA or WB tests, several other laboratory tests are available. They include:

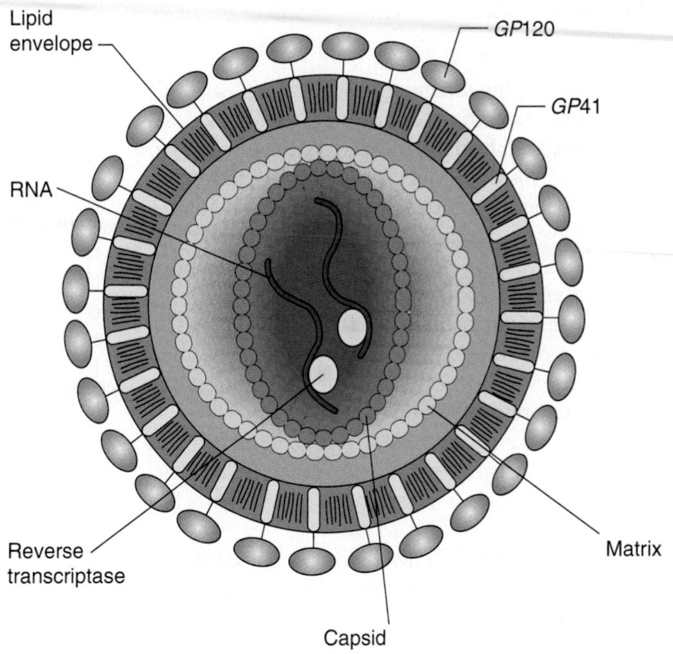

FIGURE 44.2 Structure of the HIV virus.

Physiology

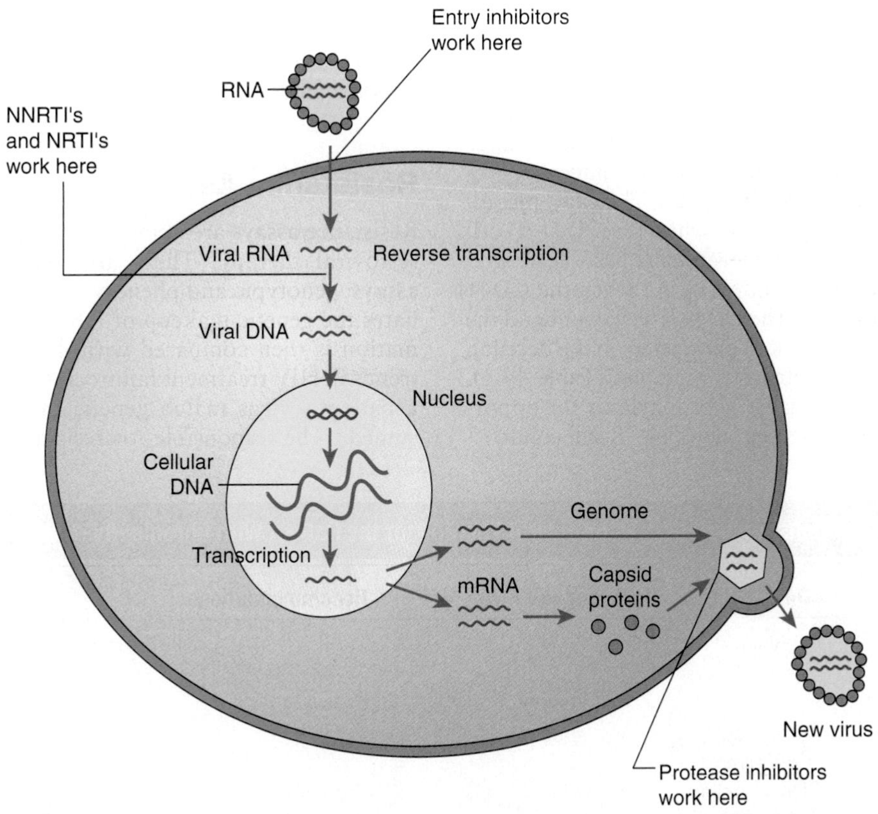

FIGURE 44.3 HIV replication. HIV enters into a CD4+ cell, sheds its protective coating, and inserts its genetic material into the cell. The genetic code of HIV, a retrovirus, is contained in single-stranded RNA instead of double-stranded DNA. In order to replicate, HIV uses the enzyme reverse transcriptase (RT) to convert its RNA to DNA. HIV DNA enters the nucleus of the CD4+ cell, uses the enzyme integrase to combine with the host cell DNA, and transmits instructions to duplicate HIV DNA. Inside the nucleus, viral DNA is transcribed into messenger RNA (mRNA), which is then translated into viral proteins. The viral RNA and viral proteins assemble at the cell membrane into a new virus. HIV proteins are processed into their functional forms by HIV protease. The newly assembled HIV leaves the cell to infect other CD4+ cells.

- *Rapid HIV testing.* This screening test produces a result within 30 minutes. As with other screening tests, any positive result requires a confirmatory assay to ensure accuracy.
- *Oral HIV testing.* This is a noninvasive screening test. Contrary to popular belief, it is not a saliva test, but instead uses a small pad to draw fluids that are derived from blood from within the mouth and gums. It also requires a confirmatory assay for a positive test result.
- *Radioimmunoprecipitation assay (RIPA).* This assay is a type of confirmatory blood test that may be used when antibody levels are very low or difficult to detect, or when Western blot assay results are uncertain.
- *Indirect fluorescent antibody assay (IFA).* This is a less commonly used confirmatory blood test used to confirm ELISA results or when Western blot test results are uncertain.
- *Polymerase chain reaction (PCR).* This specialized blood test looks for HIV genetic information. This test can detect the virus, rather than the viral antibody, even in someone only recently infected. This test is labor intensive and thus very expensive.

LABORATORY TESTS

CD4+ T-Cell Count

CD4+ T-cell counts are an indication of the current immunologic status of the patient. In the healthy patient, CD4+ range is 800 cells/mm^3 to 1,200 cells/mm^3. As HIV infection progresses, the CD4+ T-cell count decreases. The CDC recommends initiating HAART therapy when the CD4+ T-cell count falls below 200/mm^3; however, most health care prescribers offer pharmacologic intervention when the CD4+ count is less than 350/mm^3. The CD4+ T-cell count and the viral load count are the essential parameters in the decision to initiate or change antiretroviral therapies (Table 44.1). Initiation of pharmacotherapy or prophylaxis for opportunistic diseases is also based on the CD4+ T-cell count.

Viral Load (HIV RNA) Count

The HIV RNA counts are reported as copies per milliliter (mL). Viral load of HIV RNA indicates the risk for disease progression. Two tests are frequently used to measure viral load—branched-chain DNA (bDNA) and reverse transcriptase quantitative polymerase chain reaction (RT-PCR). Initially, a 2- to 2.5-fold difference existed between the results of bDNA and RT-PCR assays. Version 3.0 of the bDNA test, now in use, obtains values similar to those obtained by RT-PCR, except at the lower end of the linear range (<1,500 copies/mL).

The viral load test should be performed at the time of diagnosis and every 3 to 4 months thereafter in the asymptomatic HIV-positive patient. It should be performed immediately before starting antiretroviral therapy and again 2 to 8 weeks later. When the therapy proves effective, the patient should have repeat testing of the viral load every 3 to 4 months to evaluate the continuing efficacy of therapy. The goal is to bring the viral load to undetectable levels (i.e., <50 copies/mL) within 6 months.

When assessing the need to change antiretroviral therapy, viral load counts and CD4+ T-cell counts should be evaluated at the same time. The goal of antiretroviral therapy is to increase the CD4+ T-cell count and decrease the viral load burden. If the CD4+ T-cell count continues to decrease, or the viral load burden increases despite therapy, a change in pharmacotherapy should be considered.

Resistance Assays

Resistance assays are being used frequently to guide antiretroviral therapy. There are two types of resistance assays: genotypic and phenotypic. Genotypic testing evaluates the genetic makeup of a patient's virus. This information is then compared with data that document past trends in HIV treatment failure. If the genetic mutations in a patient's virus match genetic mutations that are presumed to be responsible for resistance to a certain drug,

TABLE 44.1 Indications for Initiating Antiretroviral Therapy for the Patient With Chronic HIV-1 Infection

Clinical Category	CD4+ Count	Plasma HIV RNA	Recommendations
Symptomatic (AIDS or severe symptoms)	Any value	Any value	Treat
Asymptomatic	CD4+ T cells <200/mm^3	Any value	Treat
Asymptomatic	CD4+ T cells 201–350 mm^3	Any value	Treatment should be offered
Asymptomatic	CD4+ T cells >350/mm^3	>100,000 copies/mL	Some clinicians recommend initiation of antiretroviral therapy; other clinicians recommend deferring therapy and monitoring the CD4+ T-cell count and HIV RNA more frequently.
Asymptomatic	CD4+ T cells >350/mm^3	<100,000 copies/mL	Most experienced clinicians recommend deferring therapy and monitoring the CD4+ T-cell count.

Adapted from U.S. Department of Health and Human Services. The DHHS Panel on Clinical Practices for Treatment of HIV Infection. (2004). *Guidelines for Use of Antiretroviral Agents in HIV-1-Infected Adults and Adolescents – October 29, 2004.* [Online]. Available: http://aidsinfo.nih.gov/guidelines/default_db2.asp?id=50.

then his or her virus is presumed to be resistant to that drug. Phenotypic testing is considered a direct way of measuring drug resistance. It places a sample of a patient's HIV in contact with antiretroviral drugs and observes how the virus reacts. Phenotypic testing is also considered quantitative because it can demonstrate how much of a drug is necessary to stop HIV from replicating.

These tests are most useful in cases of acute infection, virologic failure, suboptimal viral suppression after initiation of antiretroviral therapy, or high likelihood of exposure to resistant virus based on community prevalence or source characteristics.

PRINCIPLES OF DRUG THERAPY FOR HIV INFECTION

As researchers learn more about the HIV virus, and new drugs and drug classes are developed, the principles of drug therapy evolve. The current goals of therapy include maximal and durable suppression of viral load, restoration or preservation of immunologic function, improvement in quality of life, and reduction of HIV-related morbidity and mortality. Tools for achieving these goals include maximizing adherence to the antiretroviral regimens, sequencing drugs rationally, preserving future treatment options, and using drug-resistance testing in selected clinical settings (Department of Health and Human Services).

You have a pivotal role in maximizing adherence to the antiretroviral regimens. As a patient advocate and educator, you must be able to discuss the potential benefits and risks of HAART therapy (Box 44.1).

You are also responsible for educating the patient about self-administration of antiretroviral therapy. It is important to teach the patient how the drug works, when to take the drug, what the potential adverse effects of the drug are, which signs and symptoms to report, and ways to decrease the risk for developing resistance to the HAART regimen. Box 44.2 presents basic principles of drug therapy for HIV infection.

C NUCLEOSIDE/NUCLEOTIDE REVERSE TRANSCRIPTASE INHIBITORS

The **nucleoside reverse transcriptase inhibitors (NRTIs)** were the first class of drugs approved by the FDA to treat HIV infection and AIDS. Although more potent drug classes have emerged, nucleoside analogues continue to be crucial drugs in the pharmacologic management of HIV infection and AIDS. These drugs inhibit an enzyme critical to HIV replication (see Figure 44.3). Zidovudine was first synthesized as an antineoplastic drug in the 1960s. In 1987, it was found to inhibit the in vitro infectivity of HIV type 1 (HIV-1). Drugs within the NRTI class include abacavir, didanosine, emtricitabine, lamivudine, stavudine, zalcitabine, zidovudine, and the combination drugs lamivudine/zidovudine and abacavir/zidovudine/lamivudine. Also included in this class of drugs is tenofovir, a nucleotide reverse transcriptase inhibitor. Zidovudine (AZT, ZDV, Retrovir) is the prototype for the NRTIs. Table 44.2 presents a summary of drugs in this class.

NURSING MANAGEMENT OF THE PATIENT RECEIVING P ZIDOVUDINE

Core Drug Knowledge

Pharmacotherapeutics

Zidovudine is a synthetic nucleoside antiviral drug. Zidovudine is active against the Epstein-Barr virus and hepatitis B virus and exerts some antibacterial activity against Enterobacteriaceae, but its main indication is for treating HIV infection in adults and children and preventing transmission of HIV to the fetus in pregnant, HIV-positive women. The parameters to start antiretroviral therapy are controversial, complex, and constantly changing. Symptomatic patients

BOX 44.1 The Potential Benefits and Risks of Early and Deferred Therapy

Potential Benefits of Early Therapy
- Earlier suppression of viral replication
- Preservation of immune function
- Prolongation of disease-free survival
- Lower risk for resistance with complete viral suppression
- Possible decrease in the risk for HIV transmission

Potential Risks of Early Therapy
- Drug-related adverse effects on quality of life
- Drug-related serious toxicities
- Early development of drug resistance because of suboptimal viral suppression
- Risk for transmission of virus resistant to antiretroviral drugs (if suboptimal suppression)
- Limitation of future treatment options
- Unknown durability of current available therapy

Potential Benefits of Deferred Therapy
- Avoid negative effects of quality of life and drug-related toxicities
- More time to understand treatment demands
- Preserve future treatment options
- Delay in development of drug resistance
- Decreased total time on medication with decreased risk of treatment fatigue
- More time for the development of more potent, less toxic, and better studied combinations of drugs

Potential Risks of Deferred Therapy
- Possible risk for irreversible immune system compromise
- Possible greater difficulty in viral suppression
- Possible increased risk for HIV transmission

Adapted from U.S. Department of Health and Human Services. The DHHS Panel on Clinical Practices for Treatment of HIV Infection. (2004). *Guidelines for Use of Antiretroviral Agents in HIV-1-Infected Adults and Adolescents – October 29, 2004.* [Online]. Available: http://aidsinfo.nih.gov/guidelines/default_db2.asp?id=50.

BOX 44.2 Principles of Drug Therapy for HIV infection

When patients or patient groups ask about drug therapy for HIV, explain the following points:

- Ongoing HIV replication leads to immune system damage and progression to AIDS.*
- Plasma HIV RNA levels indicate the magnitude of HIV replication and its associated rate of CD4+ T-cell destruction; CD4+ T-cell counts indicate the extent of HIV-induced immune damage already suffered. Regular periodic measurements of plasma HIV RNA levels and CD4+ T-cell counts are necessary to determine the risk for disease progression in an HIV-infected individual and to determine when to initiate or modify antiretroviral treatment regimens.
- Because rates of disease progression differ among individuals, treatment decisions should be individualized by level of risk indicated by plasma HIV RNA levels and CD4+ T-cell counts.
- Using potent combination antiretroviral therapy to suppress HIV replication below the limits of detection of sensitive plasma HIV RNA assays narrows the potential for selection of antiretroviral-resistant HIV variants, which is the major factor limiting the ability of antiretroviral drugs to inhibit virus replication and delay disease progression. Therefore, maximum achievable suppression of HIV replication should be the goal of therapy.
- The most effective means of accomplishing durable suppression of HIV replication is to simultaneously initiate combinations of effective anti-HIV drugs with which the patient has not been treated previously and that are not cross-resistant with antiretroviral agents with which the patient has been treated previously.
- Each antiretroviral drug used in combination-therapy regimens should always be used strictly according to optimal schedules and dosages.
- The available effective antiretroviral drugs are limited in number and mechanism of action, and cross-resistance between specific drugs has been documented. Therefore, any change in antiretroviral therapy increases future therapeutic constraints.
- Women should receive optimal antiretroviral therapy, regardless of pregnancy status.
- The same principles of antiretroviral therapy apply to both HIV-infected children and adults, although the treatment of HIV-positive children and adults alike, but the treatment of HIV-positive children involves unique pharmacologic, virologic, and immunologic considerations.
- People with acute primary HIV infection should be treated with combination antiretroviral therapy to suppress virus replication to levels below the limit of detection of sensitive plasma HIV RNA assays.
- HIV-positive people, even those with viral loads below detectable limits, are infectious and should be counseled to avoid sexual and drug-use behaviors that are associated with transmission of HIV and other infectious pathogens.

*Long-term survival free from clinically important immune dysfunction has improved substantially since HAART therapy was introduced.

should begin therapy, however, regardless of laboratory values. The recommendation for initiating treatment in asymptomatic patients is a CD4+ count below 200 or plasma HIV RNA levels above 55,000 copies/mL (see Table 44.1).

Pharmacokinetics

Zidovudine is administered orally or parenterally. Following oral administration, zidovudine is absorbed rapidly from the gastrointestinal (GI) tract. The half-life of zidovudine is about 1 hour in patients with normal renal function and increases to 1.4 to 2.9 hours in patients with renal dysfunction. Hepatic dysfunction also causes a moderate prolongation of zidovudine half-life.

Zidovudine crosses the blood–brain barrier and the placenta. It is converted into its active form by intracellular conversion and its inactive metabolite by the liver. Both active drug and inactive metabolite are excreted by glomerular filtration and tubular secretion.

Pharmacodynamics

Zidovudine inhibits the synthesis of DNA by reverse transcriptase (the viral enzyme that copies viral RNA into DNA). Zidovudine, like all nucleoside analogues, bears a structural resemblance to the natural building blocks of DNA. Reverse transcriptase fails to distinguish zidovudine from its natural counterparts, and it attempts to use the drug to synthesize viral DNA. When zidovudine is incorporated into a strand of DNA being synthesized, the addition of further nucleotides is blocked, and the full-length viral DNA chain is prematurely terminated.

Contraindications and Precautions

Absolute contraindications to the use of zidovudine include hypersensitivity, breast-feeding, and existing lactic acidosis. Patients with pre-existing hepatic dysfunction, obesity, and prolonged nucleoside analogue therapy have a higher risk for developing lactic acidosis.

Zidovudine should be given with caution to patients with pre-existing depression of bone marrow function, folate deficiency, or vitamin B_{12} deficiency. Patients with these disorders are at increased risk for severe hematologic toxicity. It is also given with caution to patients who have recently received cytotoxic drugs or radiation therapy because zidovudine may induce myelosuppression. Because of the risk for myelosuppression, patients with dental disease are also given zidovudine with caution.

Zidovudine should be used with caution in patients with hepatic or renal disease. The drug is metabolized in the liver to an inactive metabolite. In patients with impaired hepatic function, zidovudine can accumulate. Both zidovudine and its inactive metabolite are excreted in the urine. Zidovudine can accumulate in patients with renal impairment, causing an increased risk for toxicity.

Adverse Effects

The most serious adverse effects of zidovudine therapy are anemia, granulocytopenia, and thrombocytopenia. These effects may indicate depressed bone marrow function. Signs of anemia can develop in 2 to 4 weeks, and signs of granulocytopenia can develop in 6 to 8 weeks. Discontinuing the drug usually resolves anemia and granulocytopenia.

Although zidovudine actually can produce an increase in platelet count, drug-induced thrombocytopenia can occur as well. Initial increases in platelet count usually occur within 1 to 2 weeks and can continue for 4 to 7 weeks of therapy.

Adverse GI effects of zidovudine therapy include nausea and vomiting, diarrhea, abdominal pain, dyspepsia, and anorexia. Esophageal ulceration also has occurred in patients

TABLE 44.2 Summary of Selected Ⓒ Nucleoside Reverse Transcriptase Inhibitors

Drug (Trade) Name	Selected Indications	Route and Dosage Range	Pharmacokinetics
zidovudine (AZT, ZDV,Retrovir)	HIV infection	*Adult and adolescent:* PO, 300 mg 2×/d or 200 mg 3×/d *Adult and adolescent:* IV, 1 mg/kg IV 5–6 times per day around the clock *Child and infant ≥90 d:* PO, 160 mg/m² every 8 h *Infant <90 d and neonate:* PO, 2 mg/kg every 6 h *Child and infant ≥90 d:* IV, 120 mg/m² every 6 h *Infant <90 d and neonate:* IV, 1.5 mg/kg every 6 h	*Onset:* Rapid *Duration:* 4 h $t_{1/2}$: 1.1 h
abacavir (ABC, Ziagen)	HIV infection	*Adult and adolescent >16 y:* PO, 300 mg 2×/d *Infant and child 3 mos–16 y:* PO, 8 mg/kg 2×/d	*Onset:* 0.7 h *Duration:* unknown $t_{1/2}$: 1.5 h
didanosine (ddI, Videx)	HIV infection	*Adult >60 kg:* PO, 400 mg qd (buffered tablets or enteric-coated capsule) or 200 mg 2×/d (buffered tablets) *Adult and adolescent <60 kg:* PO, 250 mg qd (buffered tablets or enteric-coated capsule) or 125 mg 2×/d (buffered tablets) *Child and infant ≥8 mo:* PO, 90–150 mg/m² every 12 h *Neonates <2 wk:* PO, 50 mg/m² PO every 12 h	*Onset:* Rapid *Duration:* 12 h $t_{1/2}$: 1.6 h
emtricitabine (FTC, Emtriva)	HIV infection	*Adult:* PO, 200 mg qd *Adolescent, child, and infant:* Safe and effective use has not been established.	*Onset:* Rapid *Duration:* 24 h $t_{1/2}$: 10 h
lamivudine (3TC, Epivir)	HIV infection	*Adult and adolescent >16 y & >50 kg:* PO, 300 mg qd or 150 mg 2×/d *Adult and adolescent 12–16 y and <50 kg:* PO, 2 mg/kg 2×/d *Infant >3 mo and child:* PO, 4 mg/kg 2×/d	*Onset:* Rapid *Duration:* 12 h $t_{1/2}$: 3–6 h
	Chronic hepatitis B (Epivir-HBV)	*Adult:* PO, 100 mg PO qd. If HIV+, 300 mg 2×/d for 1 y *Adolescent and child 2–17 y:* PO, 3 mg/kg qd	
stavudine (d4T, Zerit)	HIV infection	*Adult and adolescent >60 kg:* PO, 40 mg 2×/d *Adult and adolescent <60 kg:* PO, 30 mg 2×/d *Child >60 kg:* PO, 40 mg 2×/d *Child 30–60 kg:* PO, 30 mg 2×/d **Extended release capsules** *Adult and adolescent >60 kg:* PO, 100 mg qd	*Onset:* Rapid *Duration:* 12 h $t_{1/2}$: 1 h
zalcitabine (ddC, Hivid)	HIV infection	*Adult and adolescent:* PO, 0.75 mg 3×/d *Child and infant:* PO, 0.01 mg/kg every 8 h	*Onset:* Rapid *Duration:* 8 h $t_{1/2}$: 1.2 h
tenofovir (Viread)	HIV infection Chronic hepatitis B	*Adult:* PO, 300 mg PO qd *Adolescent, child, and infant:* Safe and effective dosage has not been established.	*Onset:* Rapid *Duration:* 24 h $t_{1/2}$: 17 h

treated with zidovudine. Another adverse effect is myopathy. Because myopathy also may be a component of HIV infection, it may be overlooked as an adverse effect. Discontinuation of zidovudine can provide some improvement, but rapid worsening can occur when the drug is readministered. Cardiomyopathy also has been reported.

Several central nervous system (CNS) effects have been reported during zidovudine therapy. These include headache, seizures, somnolence, paresthesias, agitation, restlessness, and insomnia. Other adverse effects that have been described include nail discoloration, rash, taste disturbance, and elevated hepatic enzymes.

As a class, NRTI drugs may induce acidosis with liver enlargement (hepatomegaly) and fatty degeneration of the liver (steatosis). Although the actual incidence of these adverse effects is low, mortality is extremely high. Patients may complain of fatigue, nausea, vomiting, abdominal pain, weight loss, or dyspnea. Evaluation shows lactic acidosis with elevated levels of creatine phosphokinase (CPK), alanine aminotransferase (ALT), lactate dehydrogenase (LDH), or all three; and abdominal computed tomography (CT) scans and liver biopsy often show steatosis. The initial clinical manifestations of lactic acidosis are variable and may include nonspecific GI symptoms without dramatic elevation of hepatic enzymes and, in some cases, dyspnea. All NRTIs have been implicated, although these adverse effects occur most frequently with stavudine and didanosine (Table 44.3).

Drug Interactions

The most important drug interaction with zidovudine is with ganciclovir, which may induce life-threatening hematologic toxicity. Other drug interactions with zidovudine include acetaminophen, interferon beta-1b, probenecid, rifampin, trimethoprim, and valproic acid.

Additionally, drugs that increase the risk for suppression of bone marrow function, such as doxorubicin (Adriamycin), dapsone, flucytosine, vincristine, and vinblastine, should be coadministered with caution. The rate and extent of zidovudine absorption may be decreased by fatty meals. Table 44.4 presents a list of drugs that interact with zidovudine.

Assessment of Relevant Core Patient Variables

Health Status

Assess the patient for hypersensitivity to zidovudine and for early pregnancy. Also assess the patient for pre-existing hepatic or renal dysfunction. Review the patient's current pharmacotherapies for drugs that are potentially myelosuppressive, nephrotoxic, or directly toxic to red blood cells. Any positive findings should be communicated to the prescriber.

Before starting therapy, perform a complete physical examination. Documenting this baseline status is important because drug therapy may be discontinued or modified based on changes from baseline. Laboratory tests should include a complete blood count (CBC), chemistry profile, liver function tests, CD4+ T-lymphocyte count, and plasma HIV RNA measurement.

Life Span and Gender

Assess the patient for pregnancy and breast-feeding. Women who are taking zidovudine and become pregnant should remain on the drug. However, if the patient is not taking zidovudine at the time of conception, it is given antenatally after 14 weeks' gestation and continued throughout pregnancy, intravenously during the intrapartum period, and to the newborn for the first 6 weeks of life. In women who have

TABLE 44.3 Potential Life-Threatening and Serious Adverse Effects of Antiretroviral Drug Classes

Class	Effects
Nucleoside/nucleotide reverse transcriptase inhibitors (NRTIs)	Bone marrow suppression Fatigue Hepatic steatosis Hepatotoxicity Lactic acidosis Muscle pain and wasting Pancreatitis Peripheral neuritis
Nonnucleoside reverse transcriptase inhibitors (NNRTIs)	Hepatotoxicity Rash Stevens-Johnson syndrome Toxic epidermal necrosis
Protease inhibitors (PIs)	Cardiovascular effects Fat maldistribution GI intolerance Hepatotoxicity Hyperlipidemia Insulin resistance/Diabetes mellitus Osteonecrosis Uncontrolled bleeding in hemophiliacs
Entry inhibitors	Injection site reactions

TABLE 44.4 Agents That Interact With P Zidovudine

Interactants	Effect and Significance	Nursing Management
acetaminophen	Enhanced nonhepatic or renal clearance of zidovudine (ZDV) may occur. This may result in subtherapeutic levels of ZDV.	Avoid coadministration if interaction is suspected. Increase dose of ZDV.
atovaquone	Atovaquone inhibits the metabolism of zidovudine, resulting in an increased zidovudine serum concentration.	Monitor for zidovudine adverse effects or toxicity.
food	The rate and extent of ZDV absorption may be decreased by fatty meals.	Administer ZDV at least 1 h before meals.
ganciclovir	Although the mechanism of action is unclear, ganciclovir in combination with ZDV may induce life-threatening hematologic toxicity.	Avoid coadministration.
interferon beta-1b	Interferon beta may inhibit the glucuronidation of ZDV. This may increase ZDV serum concentrations and induce toxic effects.	Monitor ZDV serum concentration levels. Consider decreased ZDV dose.
methadone	Concurrent use may increase zidovudine serum concentration.	Monitor for zidovudine adverse effects or toxicity.
probenecid	Probenecid appears to inhibit ZDV glucuronidation. This may increase ZDV serum concentration levels and induce toxic effects.	Monitor for systemic symptoms, such as malaise, myalgia, and fever. Consider decreased ZDV dose.
rifampin/rifabutin	Rifampin may increase hepatic metabolism of ZDV, resulting in decreased serum concentration.	Consider increasing ZDV dose if interaction is suspected.
trimethoprim	The pharmacologic effects of ZDV may be increased in patients with impaired hepatic function who receive trimethoprim.	Monitor ZDV serum concentration. Consider decreased ZDV dose.
valproic acid	First-pass glucuronide metabolism of ZDV may be decreased.	Consider ZDV dose adjustment when starting, changing, or stopping valproic acid.

not received antiretroviral therapy during pregnancy, the risk for transmitting the HIV virus to the neonate can be reduced by receiving intravenous zidovudine during labor. Box 44.3 describes considerations for the management of HIV during pregnancy.

Pregnant women taking zidovudine should be monitored closely for signs and symptoms of lactic acidosis. Pregnancy can mimic early symptoms of lactic acidosis (nausea, vomiting, fatigue, and anorexia); thus, the patient should be scheduled for periodic serum electrolyte monitoring and liver function tests, especially during the last trimester of pregnancy.

To prevent adverse effects of zidovudine in the neonate, zidovudine should not be given during lactation. In addition, HIV-positive women are advised not to breast-feed in order to avoid potential postnatal transmission to an infant who may not be infected.

Children younger than 15 months should have HIV infection (confirmed by positive PCR test result). HIV antibody test findings in infants may reflect maternal antibodies, not the infant's own antibodies.

Lifestyle, Diet, and Habits

It is important to assess the patient's understanding of HIV transmission and to explain that despite drug therapy, the patient can still transmit HIV to others. Adherence is another issue that you must assess. Even when zidovudine is taken exactly as directed, resistance may develop. However, resistance develops much more quickly when serum concentrations are suboptimal, which can be caused by imperfect adherence: either missing doses during the day or using the drug intermittently.

Assess the patient's typical dietary habits. Although zidovudine is taken without regard to meals, avoiding fatty foods is important because they decrease the drug's absorption. Outline a high-carbohydrate, moderate-protein, and low-fat diet.

It is important to investigate whether the patient has a problem or a potential problem with substance abuse. HIV infection is highly prevalent among IV drug abusers. Once the diagnosis of HIV infection is made, some patients may see no reason to change their behavior because it's already "too late." Although HIV infection had been considered unmanageable in the past, inevitably resulting in death within a few years of diagnosis, new drug classes and polytherapy now prolong life substantially. Explain the toll drug abuse takes on the body and the need for the patient to establish a healthy lifestyle.

Be aware of the patient's economic status. The cost of zidovudine is prohibitive. Many patients do not have insurance or other resources to obtain this expensive drug. Patients may qualify for medical assistance through county, state, or federal funds or receive their drugs from local health departments. Refer patients with financial problems to the hospital or clinic social worker.

Environment

Be aware of the setting in which zidovudine will be administered. Zidovudine is administered most frequently in an

BOX 44.3 **HIV Management During Pregnancy**

The goal of antiretroviral therapy during pregnancy is to preserve the health of both mother and child. In patients receiving antiretroviral therapy when conception occurs, the patient may continue HAART therapy, although certain modifications may be needed. If conception occurs when the patient is not receiving HAART therapy, the patient may consider delaying HAART therapy until after 10–12 weeks of gestation. Suggested interventions are presented below.

Perinatal Prophylaxis Throughout Pregnancy

Zidovudine Triple Therapy

Antepartum	Initiate at 14–34 weeks' gestation and continue throughout pregnancy Regimen A: zidovudine, 100 mg orally 5 times daily Regimen B: zidovudine, 200 mg orally 3 times daily *or* 300 mg 2 times daily
Intrapartum	During labor, intravenous zidovudine, 2 mg/kg of mother's body weight for 1 hour, followed by an intravenous continuous infusion of 1 mg/kg of mother's body weight until delivery
Postpartum	Zidovudine syrup, 2 mg/kg of infant's body weight every 6 h for the first 6 wk of life beginning 8–12 h after birth

Perinatal Prophylaxis in Women Without Prior Antiretroviral Therapy

Drug	Maternal Intrapartum	Infant Postpartum	Reduction (%)
Zidovudine	Intravenous zidovudine, 2 mg/kg of mother's body weight for 1 h, followed by an intravenous continuous infusion of 1 mg/kg of mother's body weight until delivery	Zidovudine syrup, 2 mg/kg of infant's body weight every 6 h for the first 6 wk of life beginning 8–12 h after birth	62
Zidovudine plus Epivir	Zidovudine, 600 mg orally at onset of labor, followed by 300 mg orally every 3 h until delivery, *and* Epivir, 150 mg orally at onset of labor, followed by 150 mg every 12 h until delivery	Zidovudine, 4 mg/kg orally every 12 h *and* Epivir, 2 mg/kg orally every 12 h for 7 d	42
Nevirapine	Single 200-mg oral dose at onset of labor	Single 2-mg/kg oral dose at age 48–72 h	47
Zidovudine plus nevirapine	Intravenous zidovudine, 2 mg/kg of mother's body weight for 1 h, followed by an intravenous continuous infusion of 1 mg/kg of mother's body weight until delivery, *and* nevirapine, single 200-mg oral dose at onset of labor	Zidovudine syrup, 2 mg/kg of infant's body weight every 6 h for the first 6 wk of life beginning 8–12 h after birth *and* single 2-mg/kg oral dose at age 48–72 h	Theoretical reduction, no data available

Adapted from U.S. Department of Health and Human Services. (2004). *Public Health Service Task Force Recommendations for Use of Antiretroviral Drugs in Pregnant HIV-1-Infected Women for Maternal Health and Interventions to Reduce Perinatal HIV-1 Transmission in the United States – June 23, 2004.* [Online]. Available: http://aidsinfo.nih.gov/guidelines/default_db2.asp?id=66.

outpatient setting. Because HIV infection is treated routinely with complicated polytherapy, assess the patient's ability to understand complex instructions. Be explicit—in both spoken and written language—concerning the instructions for taking which drug at what time of day.

Intravenous zidovudine, which can be given in any setting, is stable for 24 hours at room temperature and for 48 hours when refrigerated. The drug should be infused over 1 hour. Before infusion, examine the solution for particulate matter and discoloration. If either is present, the solution should not be administered. All preparations of zidovudine should be protected from light once prepared as well as during infusion.

Nursing Diagnoses and Outcomes

- Acute Pain related to headache from drug effects
  Desired outcome: *The patient will self-medicate with analgesics such as nonsteroidal anti-inflammatory drugs (NSAIDs).*
- Ineffective Protection related to anemia and granulocytopenia
  Desired outcome: *The patient will remain free of opportunistic diseases related to blood dyscrasias.*
- Imbalanced Nutrition: Less than Body Requirements related to GI distress
  Desired outcome: *The patient will maintain adequate weight.*
- Disturbed Sleep Pattern: Insomnia related to CNS adverse effects
  Desired outcome: *The patient will obtain adequate sleep throughout drug therapy.*
- Disturbed Thought Processes related to adverse CNS effects
  Desired outcome: *The patient will remain oriented and able to communicate effectively with others.*
- Diarrhea related to adverse drug effects
  Desired outcome: *The patient will avoid dehydration and contact the prescriber if diarrhea persists.*

- Risk for Injury related to adverse drug effects
  Desired outcome: The patient will remain injury free throughout therapy.

Planning and Intervention

Maximizing Therapeutic Effects

Administer zidovudine 1 hour before meals. Also, make sure the patient receives 600 mg/day in divided doses—200-mg tablets three times daily or 300-mg tablets twice daily. Make sure the patient is on a low-fat diet.

Minimizing Adverse Effects

Intramuscular injections should not be administered to patients receiving zidovudine; they may cause bleeding, bruising, or hematomas because of thrombocytopenia secondary to zidovudine-induced depression of bone marrow function.

Providing Patient and Family Education

- Explain the importance of adhering to the therapeutic regimen. The instructions should be clear and in writing.
- Explain the importance of periodic blood monitoring to ensure the efficacy of therapy.
- It is important to advise patients about potential adverse effects. Stress the importance of contacting the prescriber if signs of anemia or depressed bone marrow function appear, such as bleeding, easy bruising, or fatigue. Also explain that adverse effects, such as GI distress or headache, may resolve spontaneously after 3 to 4 weeks of therapy. Headaches can be treated with NSAIDs. Persistent problems should be reported to the prescriber.
- Instruct patients to advise the prescriber if any other drugs are ordered by another prescriber. Explain that many drugs may alter the way zidovudine works, and other drugs may increase the risk for adverse effects from zidovudine therapy.
- Advise the patient to postpone any dental work if myelosuppression is suspected.
- Instruct patients with sleep disturbance to attempt relaxation techniques or warm baths to facilitate sleep.
- Explain the importance of contacting the prescriber if the patient has difficulty thinking or experiences memory problems.

Ongoing Assessment and Evaluation

Perform a physical examination at each encounter with the patient. Laboratory data should be obtained every 2 to 4 weeks. Once HIV RNA levels are undetectable and the CD4+ count is stable, follow-up visits should occur every other month.

Monitor for signs and symptoms of adverse effects of lactic acidosis, anemia, depressed bone marrow function, or nephrotoxicity. Also monitor for signs of myelosuppression or myalgias. Symptoms of myalgia include proximal muscle weakness and elevations of creatinine kinase values.

Monitor for the need to change pharmacotherapy. Remember that blood analysis may be necessary to determine whether changes in therapy are needed because the patient may remain asymptomatic.

The patient should have a stable CD4+ count and a declining or undetectable HIV RNA count throughout therapy. The patient should be free of opportunistic infections and signs of anemia or depressed bone marrow function.

MEMORY CHIP

P Zidovudine

- Used for management of HIV and AIDS
- Major contraindications: hypersensitivity, first 14 weeks of pregnancy
- Most common adverse effects: nausea, headache, rash, fever, and abdominal pain
- Most serious adverse effects: anemia, granulocytopenia, and thrombocytopenia; suppression of bone marrow function; lactic acidosis; and hepatomegaly with steatosis
- Maximizing therapeutic effects: Administer 1 hour before meals.
- Minimizing adverse effects: Avoid IM injections because of thrombocytopenia.
- Most important patient education: signs and symptoms of anemia and importance of notifying the prescriber immediately

Drugs Closely Related to P Zidovudine

Abacavir

Abacavir (ABC, Ziagen) is an oral, synthetic antiretroviral agent. It may be substantially more potent than some other reverse transcriptase inhibitors. Abacavir is available in tablet and suspension formulas. It has excellent bioavailability and widespread distribution, including the cerebrospinal fluid (CSF).

Hypersensitivity is a serious and sometimes fatal adverse effect of abacavir that usually appears within 6 weeks of beginning therapy. Abacavir treatment should be discontinued if any signs of hypersensitivity occur. These signs include fever, malaise, severe nausea, diarrhea, abdominal pain, sore throat, cough, shortness of breath, and rash. Reintroduction of the drug after a hypersensitivity reaction has resulted in fatal hypotension.

Patients receiving abacavir should refrain from drinking alcohol. Alcohol increases the plasma levels of abacavir by roughly 40%, which increases the risk for adverse effects. Abacavir can be taken with or without food. Abacavir is a pregnancy category C drug. Recommendations during pregnancy are similar to those for zidovudine.

Didanosine

Didanosine (ddI, Videx) was approved in 1996 as a first-line drug for treating HIV infection. The pharmacokinetics of didanosine is similar to that of zidovudine. However, its active metabolite has a much longer half-life, which enables twice-daily dosing. Like other NRTIs, it is renally excreted, so patients with renal insufficiency should receive a reduced dose.

Didanosine is available in two formulations. In its buffered versions, didanosine decreases gastric pH, thus affecting the absorption of other drugs, such as the fluoroquinolones, dapsone, indinavir, and azole antifungals. This buffering agent also complicates the timing of administration for other antiretroviral drugs. It can be taken at the same time as other NRTIs, nevirapine, and efavirenz. Delavirdine and indinavir, however, should be taken at least 1 hour before didanosine, whereas lopinavir/ritonavir and atazanavir should be taken 2 hours before or 1 hour after didanosine. As a delayed-release capsule, didanosine is taken on an empty stomach (1 hour before or 2 hours after a meal).

The adverse effect profile of didanosine includes GI problems similar to those seen with zidovudine. Two potentially serious adverse effects associated specifically with didanosine are pancreatitis and peripheral neuropathy. Patients with prior episodes of pancreatitis, active alcohol abuse, or coadministration of other drugs that may cause pancreatitis have an even higher risk for developing pancreatitis. Didanosine should be discontinued at the first signs or symptoms of pancreatitis, such as anorexia, nausea, vomiting, and abdominal pain.

In addition, didanosine should not be given with other drugs known to cause pancreatitis, such as asparaginase, azathioprine, estrogens, ethanol, furosemide, methyldopa, nitrofurantoin, pentamidine, sulfonamides, sulindac, tetracyclines, thiazide diuretics, and valproic acid. Additionally, it should not be given with drugs known to cause peripheral neuropathy, such as chloramphenicol, cisplatin, dapsone, ethambutol, ethionamide, hydralazine, isoniazid (INH), lithium, metronidazole, nitrous oxide, phenytoin, and vincristine. Didanosine should not be given concurrently with tenofovir because this combination may increase the risk for adverse effects. Didanosine is a pregnancy category B drug. However, when taken in combination with stavudine and other antiretroviral agents, the risk for lactic acidosis is increased in pregnant women.

Emtricitabine

Emtricitabine (FTC, Emtriva) is the newest NRTI approved for managing HIV infection. Emtricitabine is structurally similar to lamivudine and has similar adverse effects and resistance patterns. The most common adverse effects associated with emtricitabine are headache, diarrhea, nausea, and rash. Hyperpigmentation on the palms, soles, or both has been observed in nonwhite patients. Emtricitabine is not indicated for treating hepatitis B virus (HBV) infection, and "flare-ups" have been reported in patients with HBV after discontinuing emtricitabine. Because emtricitabine is so similar to lamivudine, patients with virus that is resistant to lamivudine are unlikely to benefit from emtricitabine treatment. Emtricitabine is approved for patients older than 18 years. The benefit of emtricitabine is its once-daily dosing, with or without food. Because it is renally excreted, patients with renal insufficiency should receive a reduced dose. Emtricitabine is a pregnancy category B drug. Recommendations during pregnancy are similar to those for zidovudine.

Lamivudine

Lamivudine (3TC, Epivir) is a potent reverse transcriptase (RT) inhibitor. Lamivudine is approved for use in patients 3 months of age and older. Lamivudine should always be used in conjunction with other antiretroviral agents and should not be used alone to manage HIV infection. In addition to its indication for HIV infection, lamivudine is used as the drug Epivir-HBV in managing hepatitis B, but the formulation and dosage of Epivir-HBV is not sufficient to treat HIV infection.

Like stavudine, lamivudine is safe and well tolerated and has a long half-life. It is administered once or twice a day, depending on the dosage. The most common adverse effect is nausea. It is renally excreted; therefore, patients with substantial renal impairment should be given reduced doses. Exacerbations of HBV may occur in HBV/HIV coinfected patients upon discontinuation of lamivudine. Food decreases the rate but not the extent of oral absorption; therefore, lamivudine may be administered with or without food. Lamivudine is a pregnancy category C drug. Recommendations during pregnancy are similar to those for zidovudine. Additionally, lamivudine may be used in combination with zidovudine in women who did not receive zidovudine therapy throughout their pregnancy.

Stavudine

Stavudine (d4T, Zerit) was initially approved by the FDA for use in patients who cannot tolerate other antiretroviral agents. Subsequent studies have shown that stavudine induces a slower rate of disease progression than zidovudine.

Stavudine is safe and well tolerated, its absorption and serum concentrations are not affected by meals, and its half-life enables twice-daily dosing. It is excreted by the kidneys; therefore, a reduced dose should be considered for patients with decreased renal function.

A major clinical adverse effect of stavudine is peripheral neuropathy. The drug should be discontinued in patients with symptoms of neuropathy, such as tingling, burning, pain, or numbness in the distal extremities. Stavudine may induce elevations in hepatic transaminases. Therefore, baseline studies should be done for patients with a history of hepatic dysfunction or alcoholism. Stavudine may also cause pancreatitis or lactic acidosis. Although these adverse effects are rare, carefully monitor for them because they are both potentially fatal. Stavudine may be taken with or without food. It should not be combined with zidovudine or any combination product containing zidovudine. Stavudine is a pregnancy category C drug. It is important to remember that pregnant women taking stavudine in combination with didanosine and other antiretroviral agents have an increased risk for developing lactic acidosis.

Zalcitabine

Zalcitabine (ddC, Hivid) is the third agent to be approved by the FDA solely for use in treating HIV infection. It was approved for use only in conjunction with zidovudine. Zalcitabine is excreted largely unchanged by the kidneys. It should be used with caution, and dosages should be reduced, in patients with impaired renal function. Zalcitabine has a very short half-life and requires three-times-daily dosing.

As with didanosine, the major adverse effects of zalcitabine are pancreatitis and peripheral neuropathy; therefore, these drugs should not be given together. Additionally, zalcitabine may cause stomatitis. Rarely, it may induce lactic acidosis. In addition to drugs that cause pancreatitis or peripheral neuropathy, zalcitabine should not be given with aminoglycosides, amphotericin B, or foscarnet because these drugs reduce zalcitabine's renal clearance and may increase its toxicity. Zalcitabine works best when administered on an empty stomach. Zalcitabine is a pregnancy category C drug. Recommendations for use during pregnancy are similar to those for zidovudine.

Tenofovir

Tenofovir (Viread) is the only nucleotide analogue reverse transcriptase inhibitor that is approved by the FDA. Nucleotide analogues differ from nucleoside analogues because they are chemically preactivated and therefore require less processing in the body for them to become active. Tenofovir is a once-daily medication that is taken without regard to meals. Adverse effects include asthenia, headache, diarrhea, nausea, vomiting, and flatulence. Rarely, it may induce lactic acidosis. Tenofovir is also renally excreted; thus, a dosage requirement is necessary in patients with renal insufficiency.

C NONNUCLEOSIDE REVERSE TRANSCRIPTASE INHIBITORS (NNRTIs)

The **nonnucleoside reverse transcriptase inhibitors (NNRTIs)** comprise the second class of drugs used to treat HIV infection. Nevirapine, delavirdine, and efavirenz are drugs within the NNRTI class. Table 44.5 presents a summary of NNRTIs. The prototype for the NNRTI class of drugs is nevirapine (Viramune).

NURSING MANAGEMENT OF THE PATIENT RECEIVING P NEVIRAPINE

Core Drug Knowledge

Pharmacotherapeutics

Nevirapine is indicated for use in treating HIV-1 infection in combination with other antiretroviral drugs. It is not effective in HIV-2 infections. Resistant virus emerges rapidly and uniformly when nevirapine is administered as monotherapy.

Pharmacokinetics

Nevirapine is absorbed readily after oral administration. It is available as an oral tablet or oral suspension. Following administration, nevirapine has an absolute bioavailability between 91% and 93%. Nevirapine absorption is not dependent on food or fasting. Peak plasma concentrations occur within 4 hours after a single 200-mg dose. The drug is distributed widely in the body, crosses the blood–brain barrier and placenta, and enters breast milk.

Nevirapine is an inducer of hepatic cytochrome P-450 metabolic enzymes. It is biotransformed extensively in the liver into several metabolites. Nevirapine and its metabolites are eliminated mainly in the urine.

Pharmacodynamics

Nevirapine also inhibits HIV reverse transcriptase. It binds directly to reverse transcriptase, resulting in the blockage of RNA- and DNA-dependent DNA polymerase activities.

Contraindications and Precautions

Nevirapine is contraindicated for patients with hypersensitivity to any of its components. A pregnancy category C drug, it is contraindicated during pregnancy because adequate safety studies have not been completed.

Nevirapine should be given with caution to patients with hepatic or renal insufficiency. Nevirapine is metabolized by the liver; thus, patients with hepatic impairment are more likely to have increased serum concentrations of nevirapine. In addition, nevirapine is excreted through the kidneys; therefore, patients with renal insufficiency may also have an increased risk for elevated serum concentrations of nevirapine.

Adverse Effects

Severe, life-threatening hepatotoxicity, including fulminant and cholestatic hepatitis, hepatic necrosis, and hepatic failure may occur with nevirapine. Severe, life-threatening, and even fatal skin reactions, including a severe, life-threatening allergic reaction called Stevens-Johnson syndrome, toxic epidermal necrolysis, and hypersensitivity reactions characterized by rash, constitutional findings, and organ dysfunction have occurred with nevirapine treatment.

Common adverse effects of nevirapine therapy include fever, headache, nausea, vomiting, and maculopapular rash. The rash, common to all NNRTI drugs, usually consists of mild to moderate erythematous, cutaneous eruptions, with or without pruritus, and may be located on the trunk, face, and extremities.

Other adverse drug effects include abdominal pain, hepatitis, paresthesias, and ulcerative stomatitis. Antimicrobial resistance also can occur during therapy with nevirapine. Although this adverse effect develops most rapidly when nevirapine is used as monotherapy, it also may occur with polytherapy.

TABLE 44.5 Summary of Selected C Nonnucleoside Reverse Transcriptase Inhibitors

Drug (Trade) Name	Selected Indications	Route and Dosage Range	Pharmacokinetics
P nevirapine (Viramune)	HIV infection	*Adult and adolescent:* PO, 200 mg qd for 14 d, then 200 mg 2×/d *Child >8 y:* PO, 4 mg/kg qd for 14 d, then 4 mg/kg 2×/d; max: 200 mg qd *Child and infant >2 mo–8 y:* PO, 7 mg/kg qd for 14 d, then 7 mg/kg 2×/d; max: 200 mg qd	*Onset:* Rapid *Duration:* 12 h $t_{1/2}$: 25–30 h
delavirdine (Rescriptor)	HIV infection	*Adult and adolescent:* PO, 400 mg 3×/d	*Onset:* Rapid *Duration:* 8 h $t_{1/2}$: 5.8 h
efavirenz (Sustiva)	HIV infection	*Adult and adolescent >40 kg:* PO, 600 mg qd *Child 32.5–40 kg:* PO, 400 mg qd *Child 25–32.5 kg:* PO, 350 mg qd *Child 20–25 kg:* PO, 300 mg qd *Child 15–20 kg:* PO, 250 mg qd *Child 10–15 kg:* PO, 200 mg qd	*Onset:* Rapid *Duration:* 24 h $t_{1/2}$: 40–55 h

Drug Interactions

Nevirapine interacts with drugs that are metabolized by P-450 CYP3A4. It inhibits the metabolism of many drugs, resulting in elevation of their serum levels. Conversely, nevirapine induces the metabolism of some drugs, and its metabolism is induced by several drugs. Table 44.6 presents these complex drug–drug interactions.

Assessment of Relevant Core Patient Variables

Health Status

Assess the patient for hypersensitivity to nevirapine and for pregnancy or lactation. Also, assess the patient for preexisting hepatic or renal dysfunction. It is important to review the patient's current pharmacotherapies for other drugs that may react with nevirapine. Communicate positive findings to the prescriber.

Before the initiation of therapy, perform a complete physical examination. It is important to document this baseline status because drug therapy may be discontinued or modified based on changes from baseline. Laboratory tests should include CBC, chemistry profile, CD4+ T-lymphocyte count, and plasma HIV RNA measurements. For patients with preexisting hepatic or renal disorders, you may need to coordinate baseline hepatic and renal function tests.

Life Span and Gender

It is important to note the age of the patient before administering nevirapine. Nevirapine is not indicated for use in children or infants. Assess the patient for pregnancy. Nevirapine is a pregnancy category C drug and may be used during pregnancy if necessary. Recommendations for use during pregnancy are similar to those for zidovudine.

Women of childbearing age should use birth control methods other than hormonal contraceptives.

Lifestyle, Diet, and Habits

As with other anti-HIV drugs, resistance is more likely when drugs are taken inconsistently. Therefore, you need to assess the patient's understanding of the importance of taking the drug as directed. Assess for potential substance abuse by the patient and explain that a healthy lifestyle complements pharmacotherapy for HIV infection.

It is important to assess the patient's financial status. The cost of nevirapine is prohibitive, and the availability is limited. Many patients do not have insurance or other resources to obtain this expensive drug. Patients may qualify for medical assistance through county, state, or federal funds or receive their drugs from local health departments. Refer patients with financial problems to the hospital or clinic social worker.

Environment

Note the setting in which nevirapine will be administered. Nevirapine is administered most frequently in an outpatient setting. It is always administered as polytherapy. Therefore, assess the patient's ability to understand complex instructions. It is important that the instructions be explicit—both spoken and written—concerning which drug to take at which time of day. Tell the patient to store nevirapine at room temperature in a tightly closed container and to discard any unused drug after the expiration date.

Nursing Diagnoses and Outcomes

- Acute Pain related to headache from adverse drug effects
  Desired outcome: *The patient will self-medicate with analgesics such as acetaminophen.*
- Imbalanced Nutrition: Less than Body Requirements related to GI distress

TABLE 44.6 Agents That Interact With P Nevirapine

Interactants	Effect and Significance	Nursing Management
P-450 inhibitors Lipid-lowering drugs (atorvastatin, lovastatin, simvastatin)	Nevirapine may increase the serum concentration of these drugs, resulting in increased risk for adverse effects or toxicity.	Monitor for rhabdomyolysis and myopathies.
P-450 inducers carbamazepine herbal drugs (St. John's wort) phenytoin phenobarbital rifamycins	These drugs may increase the serum concentration of nevirapine, resulting in an increased risk for adverse effects or toxicity.	Monitor for adverse effects.
P-450 inducers cyclosporine estrogens methadone PIs progestins oral contraceptives warfarin	Coadministration may decrease the serum concentration level of these drugs.	Monitor for efficacy of treatment.

Desired outcome: The patient will maintain adequate weight and nutrition and notify the health care provide about persistent GI symptoms.
- Ineffective Protection related to drug-related rash
  Desired outcome: *The patient will report any rash to the prescriber.*
- Disturbed Thought Processes related to CNS adverse effects
  Desired outcome: *The patient will remain oriented and able to communicate effectively with others.*

Planning and Intervention

Maximizing Therapeutic Effects

Administer nevirapine in divided doses throughout the day. For missed doses, it is important that the patient take the drug as soon as remembered unless it is time for the next dose.

Minimizing Adverse Effects

Administer nevirapine by dose escalation (200 mg daily for 2 weeks, then 200 mg twice daily). Using dose escalation may decrease the incidence of rash. To avoid adverse effects, it is especially important never to double the dose of nevirapine.

Providing Patient and Family Education

- Explain the importance of adherence to drug therapy. Make sure the instructions are clear and in writing.
- Explain the importance of periodic blood monitoring to ensure the efficacy of therapy.
- Emphasize the need for consistent monitoring for the first 12 to 16 weeks to detect potentially life-threatening hepatotoxicity or skin reactions.
- Teach signs of potential adverse effects to patients. It is important to inform patients that the most common adverse reaction to nevirapine is rash. Also, instruct patients to monitor for signs of hepatic dysfunction, such as fatigue, jaundice, and nausea or vomiting. Tell patients to contact their prescriber immediately if signs of hepatic dysfunction or rash occur.
- Instruct patients to advise their prescriber if any other drugs are ordered by another prescriber. It is important to explain that many drugs may alter the way nevirapine works and that other drugs may increase the risk for adverse effects from nevirapine therapy.
- Instruct patients with GI distress to eat small, frequent meals. For persistent symptoms and weight loss, the patient should contact the prescriber.
- Instruct the patient to take acetaminophen for headaches but report persistent headache pain to the prescriber.
- Explain the importance of contacting the prescriber should the patient have difficulty thinking or experience memory problems.
- Explain the importance of using contraceptive measures other than hormonal contraceptives to women of childbearing age.

Ongoing Assessment and Evaluation

It is important that patients have periodic examinations and blood monitoring to assess for potential progression of the disease, treatment failure, or the emergence of resistance. CD4+ T-cell counts and HIV RNA should be assessed every 3 months. Monitor for the need to change pharmacotherapy.

Monitor for a diffuse, maculopapular, erythematous rash involving the trunk, face, and extremities, which may occur most often within the first month of dosing. A more severe integumentary reaction is Stevens-Johnson syndrome, which is characterized by aching joints and muscles; redness, blistering, peeling, or loosening of skin; and unusual tiredness or weakness accompanied by fever. Advise the prescriber immediately if these symptoms occur.

Monitor for signs of liver dysfunction. Periodic liver function tests should be evaluated. Interrupt treatment if moderate or severe liver function test abnormalities develop. Treatment may be restarted after elevated levels have returned to baseline. It is important to restart treatment at half the previous dosage, and if abnormal liver test results recur, nevirapine therapy should be discontinued permanently.

The patient should have a stable CD4+ count and a declining or undetectable HIV RNA count throughout therapy. The patient should be free of opportunistic infections and signs of rash or hepatic dysfunction.

Drugs Closely Related to P Nevirapine

Delavirdine

Delavirdine (Rescriptor) was approved by the FDA in 1997. It is indicated for combined use with NRTIs. Unlike efavirenz and nevirapine, delavirdine is a potent inhibitor of CYP3A4. As a result, concurrent administration of other CYP3A4 drugs may increase their serum drug concentrations, resulting in an increased risk for adverse effects and potential drug toxicity. Drugs that are contraindicated with delavirdine include benzodiazepines (alprazolam, midazolam, and triazolam), carbamazepine, ergot alkaloids, lipid-lowering drugs (atorvastatin, lovastatin, and simvastatin), phenobarbital, phenytoin (fosphenytoin), pimozide, rifamycins, and St. John's wort. Delavirdine should be administered at least 2 hours after antacid therapy. In patients with chronic GI disorders, proton pump inhibitors should be avoided. Histamine-2 blockers may be used if given 12 hours before or after delavirdine.

Adverse reactions associated with delavirdine include rash, increased liver enzyme levels, and headache. Delavirdine is a pregnancy category C drug; however, it is not recommended for use during pregnancy.

MEMORY CHIP

P Nevirapine

- Used for the management of HIV infection and AIDS
- Major contraindication: hypersensitivity
- Most common adverse effects: fever, headache, nausea, vomiting, and rash
- Most serious adverse effects: Stevens-Johnson syndrome and hepatotoxicity
- Maximizing therapeutic effects: Administer in equally divided doses throughout the day.
- Minimizing adverse effects: Dose escalation over a 2-week period.
- Most important patient education: Explain the symptoms of hepatotoxicity and the importance of contacting the prescriber immediately.

Efavirenz

Efavirenz (Sustiva) is the newest NNRTI. The main benefits of efavirenz are once-daily dosing and penetration into CSF. Efavirenz should be taken on an empty stomach. Taking it with food can increase the serum drug concentration of the drug, resulting in an increased risk for adverse effects or toxicity.

The major adverse effects from efavirenz affect the CNS and include dizziness, sleeplessness, intense dreams, altered mood, and anxiety. These side effects are worst during the first 2 to 4 weeks of treatment. There have been reports of severe anxiety, depression, and difficulty concentrating in people starting efavirenz therapy. To minimize the CNS effects, advise the patient to take efavirenz at bedtime. Like other NNRTI drugs, efavirenz may cause a rash. The rash is milder than that caused by other NNRTIs and usually goes away on its own. Potential drug interactions with efavirenz are similar to those with nevirapine. Efavirenz can cause a false-positive cannabinoid test. Efavirenz is a pregnancy category C drug. However, it has been found to be teratogenic in monkeys; therefore, it is not recommended during pregnancy.

C PROTEASE INHIBITORS

Protease inhibitors (PIs) are the third major class of drugs used in treating HIV infection and AIDS. Their arrival has changed the opinion of experts as to the ultimate fatality of HIV and AIDS. The PIs represent the most potent anti-HIV drugs. However, their potency and activity vary widely among individual patients. Drugs within the PI class include amprenavir, atazanavir, fosamprenavir, indinavir, nelfinavir, ritonavir, saquinavir, and the combination drug lopinavir/ritonavir. Saquinavir, the first FDA-approved PI, is the prototype for this class. Table 44.7 presents a summary of protease inhibitors.

NURSING MANAGEMENT OF THE PATIENT RECEIVING P SAQUINAVIR

Core Drug Knowledge

Pharmacotherapeutics

Saquinavir is an agent for treating HIV infection in adults. It is approved for use in combination with RT inhibitors. Combination therapy enables reduced dosage and helps to limit the incidence of adverse events. Saquinavir demonstrates activity against both HIV-1 and HIV-2 and is effective in acutely and chronically infected cells.

Pharmacokinetics

Saquinavir HGC is administered orally. It comes in two formulations—saquinavir mesylate (Invirase, HGC [hard gel capsule]) and saquinavir (Fortovase, SGC [soft gel capsule]). It is only about 4% bioavailable after dosing, because of a combination of poor absorption and extensive first-pass metabolism. A high-calorie, high-fat meal can substantially increase the bioavailability of saquinavir HGC. The bioavailability of saquinavir SGC has not been determined; however, in comparison to HGC, the relative bioavailability is estimated to be 331%.

Metabolism occurs in the liver and is affected by the P-450 enzyme system; the isozyme CYP3A4 is responsible for about 90% of the initial biotransformation of saquinavir. The metabolites of saquinavir have not been identified and appear to play little part in antiviral activity. The serum half-life of saquinavir is 1 to 2 hours. Renal elimination of saquinavir is negligible; only 1% is excreted in urine, whereas 88% is excreted in feces. It is important to remember that saquinavir HGC and SGC are not bioequivalent and cannot be used interchangeably (see Table 44.7).

Pharmacodynamics

Saquinavir is a competitive inhibitor of HIV protease, an enzyme required for HIV replication. During the later stages of the HIV growth cycle, integrated DNA is translated into polyproteins to become immature budding viral particles. Protease is responsible for packaging these polyproteins into mature virions. Virions produced without protease are immature, rendering the virus noninfectious. PIs also inhibit replication of HIV in the macrophages, which are major reservoirs of HIV.

Contraindications and Precautions

Saquinavir is contraindicated for patients with hypersensitivity to any of its components. Saquinavir is not approved for use in infants, children, or adolescents younger than 16 years.

Saquinavir should be used with caution in patients with pre-existing hepatic dysfunction because the drug is largely metabolized by the liver. It should also be used cautiously in patients with elevated triglyceride or cholesterol levels because fat redistribution and hyperlipidemia are adverse effects associated with the use of PIs. Saquinavir is also used with caution in patients with diabetes because it may induce an exacerbation requiring initiation of antidiabetic medications or a dosage change. Some patients with hemophilia A and B have experienced bleeding episodes during saquinavir therapy. Although a direct causal relation has not been established, these patients should be monitored closely.

Adverse Effects

In general, few adverse effects have been reported with saquinavir therapy. However, it is difficult to discern adverse effects thought to occur only with saquinavir because it often is given with other agents. The most common adverse effects are nausea, diarrhea, stomach discomfort, insomnia, and headache. As previously mentioned, saquinavir may induce hyperglycemia, resulting in loss of glycemic control in diabetic patients.

HIV-positive patients with hemophilia (type A or B) may be at increased risk for bleeding. Episodes of spontaneous skin hematomas and hemarthrosis, in some cases requiring additional doses of factor VIII, have been reported.

As with all other antiretroviral agents, antimicrobial resistance can develop after continued use. Combination therapy with reverse transcriptase inhibitors reduces the emergence of viral resistance.

As a class, PIs also have been associated with an unusual adverse reaction involving the deposition of fatty-

TABLE 44.7 Summary of Selected (C) Protease Inhibitors

Drug (Trade) Name	Selected Indications	Route and Dosage Range	Pharmacokinetics
P saquinavir (Invirase, Fortovase)	HIV infection	HGC, Invirase *Adult and adolescent:* PO, 1,000 mg 2×/d SGC, Fortovase *Adult and adolescent:* PO, 1,200 mg 3×/d *Child:* Safe and effective dosage has not been established.	*Onset:* Rapid *Duration:* 8 h $t_{1/2}$: 1–2 h
amprenavir (Agenerase)	HIV infection	*Adult and adolescent >16 y, or adolescent >13 y who weighs >50 kg:* PO, 1,200 mg 2×/d *Adolescent 13–16 y who weighs <50 kg:* PO, 22.5 mg/kg (1.5 mL/kg) 2×/d or 17 mg/kg (1.1 mL/kg) 3×/d *Child 4–12 y:* PO, 20 mg/kg 2×/d or 15 mg/kg 3×/d **Oral Solution** *Adult and adolescent >16 y, or adolescent >13 y who weighs >50 kg:* PO, 1,400 mg (93.3 mL) 2×/d *Child 4–12 y:* PO, 22.5 mg/kg (1.5 mL/kg) 2×/d or 17 mg/kg (1.1 mL/kg) 3×/d *Child <4 y:* Safe and effective dosage has not been established.	*Onset:* Rapid *Duration:* 8–12 h $t_{1/2}$: 7.1–10.6 h
atazanavir (Reyataz)	HIV infection	*Adult:* PO, 400 mg qd *Child:* Safe and effective dosage has not been established.	*Onset:* Rapid *Duration:* 24 h $t_{1/2}$: 7 h
fosamprenavir (Lexiva)	HIV infection	*Adult:* PO, Treatment-naive patients without ritonavir: 1,400 mg 2×/d. Treatment-naive patients with ritonavir: 1,400 mg once daily with ritonavir 200 mg qd or 700 mg 2×/d with ritonavir 100 mg 2×/d. Protease inhibitor–experienced patients: 700 mg 2×/d with ritonavir 100 mg 2×/d *Child:* Safe and effective dosage has not been established.	*Onset:* Rapid *Duration:* 12–24 h $t_{1/2}$: 7.7 h
indinavir (Crixivan)	HIV infection	*Adult and adolescent:* PO, 800 mg every 8 h; or 400 mg 2×/d plus ritonavir 400 mg 2×/d or 800 mg 2×/d *Child:* Safe and effective dosage has not been established.	*Onset:* Rapid *Duration:* 8 h $t_{1/2}$: 1.5–2 h
nelfinavir (Viracept)	HIV infection	*Adult and adolescent:* PO, 750 mg 3×/d or 1,250 mg 2×/d *Child 2–13 y:* PO, 20–30 mg/kg (max: 750 mg/dose) 3×/d	*Onset:* Rapid *Duration:* 8 h $t_{1/2}$: 3.5–5 h
ritonavir (Norvir)	HIV infection	*Adult and adolescent >16 y:* PO, 600 mg 2×/d *Adolescent and child 2–16 y:* PO, 400 mg/m^2, not to exceed 600 mg, 2×/d	*Onset:* Rapid *Duration:* 12 h $t_{1/2}$: 3–5 h
lopinavir/ritonavir (Kaletra)	HIV infection	*Adult and adolescent >45 kg:* PO, 533 lopinavir/133 mg ritonavir (4 capsules or 6.5 mL) 2×/d *Adult and adolescent >40 kg:* PO, 400 mg lopinavir/100 mg ritonavir (3 capsules or 5 mL) 2×/d	*Onset:* Rapid *Duration:* 12 h $t_{1/2}$: 5–6 h

like tissue at the base of the posterior neck ("buffalo hump") and the abdominal area ("protease paunch"). The syndrome is associated with peripheral lipodystrophy, central adiposity, female breast enlargement, hyperlipidemia, and insulin resistance. Although the long-term consequences of fat redistribution are unknown, substantial increases in triglycerides or cholesterol are of concern because of the possible association with cardiovascular events and pancreatitis.

Drug Interactions

Like nevirapine, saquinavir interacts with drugs that are metabolized by P-450 CYP3A4. Saquinavir inhibits the metabolism of many drugs, resulting in elevated serum levels of these drugs, and can be inhibited by other drugs, resulting in elevated saquinavir levels. Conversely, saquinavir induces the metabolism of some drugs, and its metabolism is induced by several drugs. Table 44.8 presents these complex drug–drug interactions.

TABLE 44.8 Agents That Interact With P Saquinavir

Interactants	Effect and Significance	Nursing Management
carbamazepine	Coadministration of these drugs may increase the serum concentration level of carbamazepine and decrease the serum concentration level of saquinavir.	Monitor for adverse effects and toxicity of carbamazepine. Monitor for decreased efficacy of saquinavir.
clarithromycin	Coadministration of these drugs may increase the serum concentration of saquinavir and decrease the serum concentration of clarithromycin.	Monitor for increased adverse effect or toxicity of saquinavir. Monitor for treatment failure of clarithromycin.
cyclosporine	Coadministration of these drugs may increase serum concentration levels of both cyclosporine and saquinavir.	Monitor for adverse effects of both drugs.
HAART therapy delavirdine indinavir nelfinavir ritonavir	Coadministration may increase the serum concentration of saquinavir.	Monitor for increased adverse effect or toxicity of saquinavir.
Rifamycins	Coadministration of these drugs may increase the serum concentration level of rifamycins and decrease the serum concentration level of saquinavir.	Monitor for adverse effects and toxicity of rifamycins. Monitor for decreased efficacy of saquinavir.
P-450 Inhibitors amiodarone benzodiazepines ergot alkaloids erectile dysfunction drugs (sildenafil, tadalafil, vardenafil) fentanyl lipid-lowering drugs (atorvastatin, lovastatin, simvastatin) pimozide risperidone tacrolimus thyroid hormones	Saquinavir may increase the serum concentration of these drugs, resulting in increased risk for adverse effects or toxicity.	Monitor for dysrhythmias, sedation, vasospasm/vasoconstriction, hypotension, respiratory depression, and rhabdomyolysis, myalgias, dysrhythmias, adverse effects, adverse effects, and hyperthyroid symptoms.
P-450 Inhibitors azole antifungals interleukin-2 grapefruit juice	Coadministration may increase the serum concentration level of saquinavir.	Monitor for adverse effects and toxicity of saquinavir.
P-450 Inducers pravastatin	Coadministration may decrease the serum concentration level of pravastatin.	Monitor for efficacy of treatment.
P-450 Inducers nevirapine phenytoin phenobarbital herbal drugs (St. John's Wort, garlic)	Coadministration may decrease the serum concentration level of saquinavir.	Monitor for efficacy of treatment.

Assessment of Relevant Core Patient Variables

Health Status

Assess the patient for hypersensitivity to saquinavir. Also, assess for pre-existing hepatic dysfunction, diabetes mellitus, or hemophilia. Patients receiving rifampin or rifabutin for tuberculosis (TB) should delay the use of saquinavir until rifampin or rifabutin has been deleted from the treatment regimen. Review the patient's current pharmacotherapies for other drugs that may react with saquinavir. It is important to communicate positive findings to the prescriber.

Before therapy begins, perform a complete physical examination. It is important to document this baseline status

because drug therapy may be discontinued or modified based on changes from baseline. Laboratory tests should include CBC, chemistry profile, lipid profile, CD4+ T-lymphocyte count, and plasma HIV RNA measurement. For patients with pre-existing hepatic disorders, liver function tests also should be performed.

Life Span and Gender

Assess the patient for pregnancy or lactation. Saquinavir is a pregnancy category B drug. In patients receiving HAART therapy when they conceive, therapy should be continued throughout the pregnancy. If a patient is not receiving therapy when the conception occurs, the patient may consider delaying HAART therapy until after 10 to 14 weeks of gestation. It is unknown whether saquinavir is excreted into breast milk. However, HIV-positive women are advised not to breast-feed to avoid potential postnatal transmission to an infant who may not be infected.

It is important to note the patient's age before administering saquinavir. Saquinavir has not been studied in patients younger than 16 years or older than 65 years.

Lifestyle, Diet, and Habits

Assess the patient's ability and willingness to adhere to drug therapy. Adherence to the saquinavir drug regimen is crucial. Viral load may increase dramatically when saquinavir is not taken as directed, and as with other anti-HIV drugs, resistance is more likely when drugs are taken inconsistently. The development of viral resistance to this PI may eliminate other drugs in this class from the patient's therapeutic strategy because cross-resistance to other PIs does occur. Vigorously discourage nonadherence and drug holidays.

Be aware of the patient's dietary and substance use habits. Administer saquinavir within 2 hours of a high-calorie, high-fat meal. Doing so can increase the low bioavailability of saquinavir by sevenfold. As with other antiretroviral agents, discuss potential substance abuse with the patient. Explain how a healthy lifestyle complements pharmacotherapy of HIV infection.

It is important to assess the patient's financial status. Many patients do not have insurance or other resources to obtain this expensive drug. Patients may qualify for medical assistance through county, state, or federal funds or receive their drugs from local health departments. Refer patients with financial problems to the hospital or clinic social worker.

Environment

It is important to be aware of the setting in which saquinavir will be administered. Saquinavir is administered most frequently in an outpatient setting. HIV infection is treated routinely with complicated polytherapy. Therefore, assess the patient's ability to understand complex instructions. It is important that the instructions be explicit—both spoken and written—concerning which drug to take at which time of the day. Saquinavir capsules should be stored at room temperature in a tightly closed bottle.

Nursing Diagnoses and Outcomes

- Acute Pain related to headache from adverse drug effect
  Desired outcome: *The patient will self-medicate with analgesics such as acetaminophen.*
- Imbalanced Nutrition: Less than Body Requirements related to GI distress
  Desired outcome: *The patient will maintain body weight and report any persistent symptoms affecting nutritional status to the prescriber.*
- Disturbed Thought Processes related to adverse CNS effects
  Desired outcome: *The patient will remain oriented and able to communicate effectively with others.*
- Diarrhea related to adverse GI effects
  Desired outcome: *The patient will avoid dehydration and report persistent diarrhea to the prescriber.*

Planning and Intervention

Maximizing Therapeutic Effects

Administer saquinavir capsules within 2 hours after eating a high-calorie, high-fat meal, three times daily in divided doses. It is important not to miss a dose because a missed dose may affect viral load.

Minimizing Adverse Effects

Give small, frequent meals when GI distress is problematic. Administer acetaminophen for complaints of headache. Encourage a regular exercise program to offset fat redistribution.

Providing Patient and Family Education

- Explain the importance of adherence to drug therapy. As previously mentioned, it is important to make sure that the instructions are clear and in writing.
- Explain the importance of periodic blood monitoring to ensure the efficacy of therapy.
- Advise patients about potential adverse effects. Also, explain that adverse effects, such as GI distress or headache, may spontaneously resolve after 3 to 4 weeks of therapy. Tell patients that persistent problems should be reported to the prescriber.
- Instruct patients to advise the prescriber if any other drugs are ordered by another prescriber. Explain that many drugs may alter the way saquinavir works and that other drugs may increase the patient's risk for adverse effects from saquinavir therapy.
- Instruct the patient to use over-the-counter (OTC) antidiarrheal agents if diarrhea occurs. If diarrhea is persistent, the patient should contact the prescriber.
- Explain the importance of contacting the prescriber if the patient has difficulty thinking or experiences memory problems.
- Instruct the patient to develop good eating habits and an exercise plan that decreases the risks associated with fat redisposition.

Ongoing Assessment and Evaluation

Patients should have periodic examinations and blood monitoring, which are important to assess for potential progression of the disease, treatment failure, or the emergence of drug resistance. CD4+ T-cell counts and HIV RNA load should be assessed every 3 months. Monitor for the need to change pharmacotherapy.

Monitor patients with hemophilia for signs of bleeding and for clinical signs, particularly those evident in laboratory

test results, if necessary. It also is important to monitor patients for hepatic dysfunction. For patients with pre-existing hepatic disorders, monitor liver function test results.

The patient should be evaluated for fat redistribution and hypertriglyceridemia or hypercholesterolemia. If these adverse effects occur, the patient should be evaluated for cardiovascular events and pancreatitis. Potential interventions include dietary modifications or discontinuation of PIs.

The patient should have a stable CD4+ count and a declining or undetectable HIV RNA load throughout therapy. The patient should have a stable lipid panel. The patient should also be free of opportunistic infections and signs of hepatic dysfunction or bleeding.

CRITICAL THINKING SCENARIO

Adding saquinavir to HAART therapy

Mark Williams is 24 years old. He was diagnosed with HIV infection 5 years ago. He is currently taking zidovudine, 300 mg bid, and lamivudine, 150 mg bid. His last visit to the clinic where you practice was 3 months ago. At that time, his CD4+ T-cell count was 375 and his viral load was 3,450 copies/mL. Today's laboratory values indicate a CD4+ T-cell count of 175 and a viral load of 15,000 copies/mL.

1. Consider what assessments should be made at this time.
2. Mark's drug therapy is changed to saquinavir (Invirase). Propose which assessments to make now, and develop a patient education checklist.
3. Discuss other therapy that you think should be initiated at this time.

Drugs Closely Related to P Saquinavir

Amprenavir

Amprenavir (Agenerase) is another drug in the PI class. Like other PIs, it works at the end of the viral replication cycle and inhibits the production of viable virions. Amprenavir is available as an oral tablet or an oral solution. The oral solution contains propylene glycol, which may induce adverse effects such as seizures, stupor, tachycardia, and various blood disorders. Because of the propylene glycol content, the oral solution should not be given to children younger than 4 years, pregnant women, patients with hepatic or renal failure, or patients being treated with disulfiram or metronidazole. It can be taken with or without food, but high-fat meals should be avoided, and antacids should be avoided within 1 hour of taking amprenavir.

Amprenavir is related structurally to sulfa. Therefore, patients with a sulfa allergy should not take this medication. Amprenavir also contains vitamin E. Because vitamin E thins the blood, patients taking anticoagulants should be monitored carefully.

The major adverse effects of amprenavir are nausea, vomiting, diarrhea, headache, stomach pains and gas, rash, and numbing sensations on the skin, particularly around the mouth. Amprenavir may induce Stevens-Johnson syndrome.

MEMORY CHIP

P Saquinavir

- Used for the management of HIV infection and AIDS
- Major contraindications: hypersensitivity, children <16 years old
- Most common adverse effects: diarrhea, abdominal discomfort, and nausea and vomiting
- Most serious adverse effects: cardiovascular events and pancreatitis resulting from fat redistribution
- Maximizing therapeutic effects: Administer within 2 hours of a high-fat, high-calorie meal.
- Minimizing adverse effects: small, frequent meals to decrease GI distress
- Most important patient education: Refrain from taking any medication that is not prescribed by the health care provider treating the patient for HIV infection.

Like other protease inhibitors, amprenavir is a P-450 CYP3A4 drug that substantially inhibits CYP3A4 hepatic enzymes. Patients taking amiodarone, lidocaine, phenobarbital, phenytoin, quinidine, tricyclic antidepressants (such as amitriptyline), and warfarin should have drug levels monitored frequently. Amprenavir should not be given with rifampin.

Amprenavir is not recommended for children younger than 3 years. Additionally, women, Asians, Native Americans, and Eskimos may be at increased risk for adverse events. It is a pregnancy category C drug; recommendations for its use during pregnancy are the same as those for saquinavir.

Atazanavir

Atazanavir (Reyataz) is a new protease inhibitor for treating HIV infection. As a new drug, it has similarities to and differences with other PIs. Like other PIs, it should be used in combination with other antiretroviral drugs. Atazanavir differs from other PIs in three ways: it is the first drug in its class to be given once daily; it does not appear to have a substantial adverse effect on lipoprotein concentrations; and it has a unique chemical structure that alters its resistance profile. If the patient's virus is resistant to other PIs, the virus may also be resistant to atazanavir. When resistance develops initially to atazanavir, however, the resistance may or may not be conferred to other PIs.

Atazanavir should be taken orally with a low-calorie, low-fat snack or meal to enhance absorption. It should not be taken within 2 hours of antacids.

The most common side effects of atazanavir are rash, nausea, diarrhea, vomiting, headache, and abdominal pain. It may also increase bilirubin levels, resulting in jaundice. Atazanavir has been associated with prolonging the PR interval, resulting in asymptomatic first-degree heart block. It should be used with caution in patients with pre-existing rhythm disturbances and in patients receiving other medications that cause PR-interval prolongation.

Like other protease inhibitors, atazanavir substantially inhibits CYP3A4 hepatic enzymes.

Drug–drug interactions are similar to those with saquinavir. Specific drug classes that should be avoided without the approval of the prescriber include proton pump inhibitors, antimigraine medications, antidysrhythmics, and antipsychotics.

Atazanavir is not approved for children younger than 16 years. It is a pregnancy category B drug, and recommendations for its use during pregnancy are the same as those for saquinavir.

Fosamprenavir

Fosamprenavir (Lexiva) is a prodrug of amprenavir. Its benefits over amprenavir include improved solubility and a smaller pill burden. Fosamprenavir is taken twice a day in combination with ritonavir by patients who have previous experience with PIs. It may be taken once daily by PI-naïve patients. Fosamprenavir may be taken with or without food. The contraindications, precautions, adverse effects, and drug–drug interactions are the same as those for amprenavir. It is not approved for children younger than 18 years. It is a pregnancy category C drug; recommendations for it use during pregnancy are the same as those for saquinavir.

Indinavir

Indinavir (Crixivan) is another oral PI indicated for treating HIV infection. When indinavir is the only PI in the HAART cocktail, it is given three times a day. It can be given twice a day if given with other PI drugs. It should be taken on an empty stomach for best absorption.

Indinavir may induce serious adverse effects such as kidney stones, elevated liver enzymes, and worsening of pre-existing thrombocytopenia. To decrease the potential for kidney stones, instruct the patient to drink at least 1 to 2 liters of water a day. Patients with pre-existing hepatic dysfunction or thrombocytopenia should be monitored closely, and appropriate laboratory testing should be scheduled regularly.

Self-limiting common adverse effects include nausea, headache, fatigue, abdominal pain, vomiting, rash, and dry skin. Other potential adverse effects include paronychia, severely dry skin, or cracked lips.

Drug–drug interactions are similar to those for saquinavir. Drugs to be avoided include rifamycins, benzodiazepines, ergotamines, and drugs for erectile dysfunction. Additionally, instruct the patient to avoid St. John's wort, garlic, and high doses of vitamin C.

Indinavir is not approved for children. It is a pregnancy category C drug; recommendations for its use during pregnancy are the same as those for saquinavir.

Nelfinavir

Nelfinavir (Viracept) is another oral PI. It is used primarily as a first-line PI because of its excellent adverse effect profile and because it is affected by cross-sensitivity to other PIs. Another benefit is that resistance that develops to nelfinavir does not always confer resistance to other PIs. Nelfinavir is taken twice daily with a large snack or meal.

The major adverse effect of nelfinavir is diarrhea, which may be controlled with loperamide or other antidiarrheals. Other interventions for nelfinavir-induced diarrhea include twice-daily calcium tablets, probiotics such as yogurt, and soluble fiber supplements. Nelfinavir also is associated with elevations in ALT, aspartate aminotransferase, and CPK levels.

Drug interactions are similar to those with saquinavir.

Nelfinavir is approved for use in children. It is a pregnancy category B drug, and recommendations for its use during pregnancy are the same as those for saquinavir.

Ritonavir

Ritonavir (RTV, Norvir) is an oral PI used to treat HIV infection. It is available as a capsule or oral suspension. Ritonavir is generally used in combination with at least two other anti-HIV drugs. Low-dose ritonavir is frequently prescribed in combination with another PI to strengthen the anti-HIV effect of the other PI. Taking ritonavir within 2 hours of a meal increases its absorption and decreases nausea.

Adverse effects are most likely to occur at the beginning of therapy and affect women more frequently than they affect men. They include headache, nausea, vomiting, diarrhea, and tingling or numbness around the mouth. Ritonavir may induce kidney failure in patients with pre-existing renal dysfunction or patients taking nephrotoxic drugs. Drug–drug interactions occur with nonsedating antihistamines, sedative hypnotics, antidysrhythmics, and ergot alkaloids.

Children are frequently given the oral solution; however, it has a very bitter taste. Ritonavir solution may be combined with chocolate milk or Ensure to mask its taste, as long as it is given within 1 hour of mixing. Ritonavir solution is kept at room temperature, but the oral capsules should be kept refrigerated.

Ritonavir is approved for use in children older than 2 years. It is a pregnancy category B drug, and recommendations for its use during pregnancy are the same as those for saquinavir.

Lopinavir/Ritonavir

Lopinavir/ritonavir (Kaletra) is a relatively new PI for adults and children. Each capsule contains 133 mg of lopinavir and 33 mg of ritonavir. The oral solution contains 42% alcohol. One of the most important attributes of lopinavir/ritonavir is its potency. Because of the addition of ritonavir, lopinavir reaches high serum levels.

Lopinavir/ritonavir is available as an oral capsule or suspension. Both formulations should be taken with meals.

Lopinavir/ritonavir is contraindicated in patients who have hypersensitivity to either component and in patients with polyoxyethylated castor oil hypersensitivity. Lopinavir/ritonavir should be given cautiously to patients with pre-existing hepatic disease because it is associated with the development of hepatic dysfunction. The most common side effects reported are diarrhea, shortness of breath, nausea, abdominal pain, headache, and vomiting.

Lopinavir/ritonavir can cause multiple drug–drug interactions, which are similar to those with saquinavir. Because ritonavir suppresses a liver enzyme used to break down dozens of drugs, it may boost the blood levels of street drugs such as Ecstasy (3,4-methylenedioxymethamphetamine, MDMA) or heroin.

Lopinavir/ritonavir is approved for use in children older than 6 months. It is a pregnancy category C drug, and recommendations for its use during pregnancy are the same as those for saquinavir.

C ENTRY INHIBITORS

Entry inhibitors are also known as **fusion inhibitors.** This class is the first new class of drugs approved for use in managing HIV infection since 1996. (For information about research regarding potential new antiretroviral agents, see Box 44.4). Before enfuvirtide's approval, anti-HIV drugs affected the HIV virus inside the infected cell. This new class

FOCUS ON RESEARCH

Box 44.4 Lessening Lipoatrophy

Valantin, M. A., Aubron-Olivier C., Ghosn, J., et al. (2003). Polylactic acid implants (New-Fill) to correct facial lipoatrophy in HIV-infected patients: Results of the open-label study VEGA. *AIDS, 17*(17), 2471–2477.

The Study

Researchers enrolled 50 patients in an open-label, single-arm, pilot study to evaluate the efficacy and safety of facial injections of poly-L-lactic acid (PLA) in HIV-positive patients with severe facial lipoatrophy. Patients received four sets of injections at the beginning of the study and then every 2 weeks for 6 weeks. Patients were evaluated by clinical examination, facial ultrasonography, and photography at baseline screening and at weeks 6, 24, 48, 72, and 96. At study entry, facial fat thickness ranged from 0.0 to 2.1 mm. At week 96, the median increase in total cutaneous thickness was 6.8 mm; 43% of patients achieved total cutaneous thickness >10 mm. Twenty-two patients (44%) developed palpable but nonvisible subcutaneous nodules; these nodules resolved spontaneously in 6 patients by week 96. This study demonstrated that PLA helps to correct facial lipoatrophy, thereby improving appearance and quality of life for HIV-positive patients. The filling material has a good efficacy and safety profile, and the injection schedule is simple.

Nursing Implications

You should be aware of this new drug and the potential benefits and drawbacks of using it. Advise the patient that poly-L-lactic acid injections may induce the appearance of small bumps under the skin in the treated area. Generally, these bumps are not visible, and they may be noticed only when pressing on the treated area. Advise the patient that other injection-related events at the site of injection, such as bleeding, tenderness, discomfort, redness, bruising, or swelling, may occur.

of drugs inhibits the HIV virus from binding to, fusing with, and entering the human cell. Enfuvirtide (Fuzeon) is the prototype for this new class of drugs.

NURSING MANAGEMENT OF THE PATIENT RECEIVING [P] ENFUVIRTIDE

Core Drug Knowledge

Pharmacotherapeutics

Enfuvirtide is approved for managing HIV infection in patients who have experienced treatment failure with drugs from each existing class of antiretrovirals or who have proved unable to tolerate previous antiretroviral regimens.

Pharmacokinetics

Enfuvirtide is a subcutaneous injection. It can be injected into the arms, upper thigh, or abdomen. It reaches peak serum concentration within 8 hours.

Pharmacodynamics

Enfuvirtide binds to the gp41 protein on the surface of HIV. This protein is considered to be the "key" used by HIV to bind onto and enter cells. By blocking gp41, enfuvirtide blocks the HIV from entering the cell.

Contraindications and Precautions

Enfuvirtide should not be used in patients with hypersensitivity to any of its components, including mannitol. Enfuvirtide is associated with the development of bacterial pneumonia; thus, it should be used with caution in patients with risk factors that predispose them to infection. Such risk factors include pre-existing pulmonary dysfunction, smoking, or use of intravenous drugs; patients with low CD4+ or high viral load counts are also predisposed to infection.

Adverse Effects

The major adverse effect of enfuvirtide is injection-site reaction. This reaction occurs in 95% of the patients using enfuvirtide. Reactions include itchy rash and red, swollen, puffy, or hardened skin. Patients using the thigh for injection are more likely than others to have cysts or nodules form.

In addition to injection site reactions, enfuvirtide may induce anorexia, nausea, weight loss, fatigue, anxiety, headache, insomnia, peripheral neuropathy, and infections such as sinusitis, herpes simplex, influenza, and conjunctivitis. Patients receiving enfuvirtide are more likely than others to acquire bacterial pneumonia and lymphadenopathy; however, a direct correlation with the drug has not yet been established.

Drug Interactions

Drug–drug interactions have not yet been identified. Patients may take rifamycins safely with enfuvirtide.

Assessment of Relevant Core Patient Variables

Health Status

Review the patient's HIV history and treatment plan carefully. Evaluate the patient's potential for adherence with self-administration of a subcutaneous medication and for the ability to follow aseptic guidelines.

Life Span and Gender

Assess the patient for pregnancy or lactation. Enfuvirtide is a pregnancy category B drug. In patients receiving HAART therapy when they conceive, therapy should be continued throughout the pregnancy. If a patient is not receiving therapy when the conception occurs, the patient may consider delaying HAART therapy until after 10 to 12 weeks of gestation. It is unknown whether enfuvirtide is excreted into breast milk. However, HIV-positive women are advised not to breast-feed to avoid potential postnatal transmission to an infant who may not be infected.

It is important to note the patient's age before administering enfuvirtide because this drug is not approved for patients younger than 6 years.

Lifestyle, Diet, and Habits

Teach the patient to avoid risk factors that predispose them to infection. Such factors include smoking and intravenous drug use. Instruct the patient to eat a healthy diet to optimize immune system function.

Be aware of the patient's economic status. The cost of enfuvirtide is prohibitive. In fact, it is so expensive that Medicaid, health maintenance organizations (HMOs), and other insurers may not add enfuvirtide to their formularies.

Environment

Enfuvirtide may be given in any clinical environment. It is most frequently self-administered by the patient. Enfuvirtide powder is stored at room temperature. Once enfuvirtide is reconstituted, it should remain in the vial, not the syringe, and should be refrigerated. Advise the patient to remove the refrigerated solution and allow it to return to room temperature before administration.

Nursing Diagnoses and Outcomes

- Pain related to injection site reactions and headache
  Desired outcome: *The patient will self-medicate with analgesics such as acetaminophen.*
- Risk for Infection related to drug action
  Desired outcome: *The patient will recognize symptoms associated with infections such as pneumonia, sinusitis, herpes simplex, influenza, and conjunctivitis and will contact the prescriber immediately for appropriate intervention.*
- Imbalanced Nutrition, Less than Body Requirements related to anorexia and nausea
  Desired outcome: *The patient will maintain optimal body weight and nutrition throughout therapy.*
- Risk for Injury related to insomnia and peripheral neuropathy
  Desired outcome: *The patient will remain injury free throughout therapy.*

Planning and Intervention

Maximizing Therapeutic Effects

Reconstitute the enfuvirtide with sterile water, and then allow the solution to sit for 10 minutes to ensure that the powder dissolves completely. When two doses of medication are prepared from the vial, the second dose should be refrigerated in the vial, not in a syringe.

Administer subcutaneous enfuvirtide at 12-hour intervals. Rotate the site of administration to optimize absorption. Avoid injecting into the umbilicus, moles, scars, bruises, or areas that could be irritated by a belt or waistband, or areas experiencing an injection-site reaction.

Minimizing Adverse Effects

Use aseptic technique when reconstituting or administering enfuvirtide. Monitor the patient for early signs of infection in areas of skin where injection-site reaction occurs. Also, monitor for signs of systemic infections, such as sinusitis or pneumonia.

Providing Patient and Family Education

- Emphasize the importance of aseptic technique when reconstituting and administering enfuvirtide.
- Teach the patient and family how to use the enfuvirtide convenience pack correctly. Be sure to explain the different types of syringes (the 3-mL syringe is used to reconstitute the powder, and the 1-mL syringe is used to administer the solution).
- Explain how to inject air into the vial in order to withdraw the solution.
- Teach the patient to accurately read the barrel of the syringe (to measure 1.1 mL of solution for administration).
- Teach the patient the correct areas of the body for subcutaneous injection of enfuvirtide (upper arms, upper thigh, and abdomen).
- Teach the patient to avoid injecting into the umbilicus, moles, scars, bruises, or areas that could be irritated by a belt or waistband, or areas of skin where an injection site reaction has occurred.
- Explain the potential for injection-site reactions and the need to rotate the injection site to ensure appropriate drug absorption.
- Teach the patient healthy lifestyle choices to decrease the potential for infections, especially the need to avoid recreational drugs and tobacco products.
- Teach the patient the signs of infection and advise him or her to contact the prescriber if such signs occur.

Ongoing Assessment and Evaluation

Assess the patient for signs of infectious disorders such as pneumonia, sinusitis, herpes simplex, influenza, and conjunctivitis. Assess for anorexia, nausea, weight loss, fatigue, anxiety, headache, insomnia, and peripheral neuropathy.

Monitor for the need to change pharmacotherapy. It is important to remember that changes in therapy may have to be based on blood analysis because the patient may remain asymptomatic.

The patient should have a stable CD4+ count and a declining or undetectable HIV RNA load throughout therapy. The patient should be free of opportunistic infections.

PROPHYLAXIS FOR OPPORTUNISTIC INFECTIONS

Patients with HIV infection are at increased risk for a multitude of opportunistic diseases. Many of these diseases must be treated on an individual basis, and routine prophylaxis is not recommended. However, several diseases do have recommendations for ongoing prophylaxis (outlined in Table 44.9). In addition to these opportunistic infections, immunocompromised patients are more vulnerable than immunocompetent patients to certain conditions of the mouth (Box 44.5).

MEMORY CHIP

P Enfuvirtide

- Used for the management of HIV infection and AIDS
- Major contraindication: hypersensitivity
- Most common adverse effects: injection-site reactions
- Most serious adverse effects: bacterial pneumonia
- Maximizing therapeutic effects: Rotate injection sites to increase absorption.
- Minimizing adverse effects: Use aseptic technique to administer subcutaneous injection.
- Most important patient education: teach to reconstitute and administer subcutaneous injections

TABLE 44.9 Recommended Preventive Regimens for Opportunistic Diseases

Infection	Indication	First Choice	Alternative
Strongly Recommended as a Standard of Care			
Pneumocystis carinii	CD4+ count <200/μL or oropharyngeal candidiasis	Sulfamethoxazole-trimethoprim (SMZ-TMP) 1 tablet daily	dapsone, 50 mg bid or 100 mg qd **or** dapsone, 50 mg daily plus pyrimethamine 50 mg weekly and leucovorin 25 mg weekly **or** dapsone, 200 mg plus pyrimethamine 75 mg plus leucovorin 25 mg weekly **or** aerosolized pentamidine 300 mg monthly **or** atovaquone, 1,500 mg daily **or** SMZ-TMP, 1 tablet 3 times per week
Mycobacterium tuberculosis (isoniazid sensitive)	Tuberculin skin test (TST) reaction >5 mm **or** contact with person with active tuberculosis, regardless of TST result	Isoniazid, 300 mg, plus pyridoxine, 50 mg daily for 9 mo **or** isoniazid, 900 mg, plus pyridoxine, 100 mg 2 times a wk for 9 mo	Rifampin 600 mg daily, or rifabutin, 300 mg for 4 mo **or** rifampin, 600 mg daily, or rifabutin 300 mg plus pyrazinamide 15–20 mg/kg of body weight for 2 mo
Mycobacterium tuberculosis (isoniazid resistant)	Same as above	Rifampin, 600 mg daily, or rifabutin, 300 mg for 4 mo	Rifampin, 600 mg daily, or rifabutin, 300 mg plus pyrazinamide 15–20 mg/kg of body weight for 2 mo
Mycobacterium tuberculosis (multiple drug resistant)	Same as above	Choice of drugs requires consultation with public health authorities; depends on susceptibility of isolate from source patient	
Toxoplasma gondii	Immunoglobin G antibody to *Toxoplasma* and CD4+ count of <100 mm³	SMZ-TMP 1 DS daily	SMZ-TMP, 1 SS daily **or** dapsone, 50 mg daily plus pyrimethamine 50 mg and leucovorin 25 mg weekly **or** dapsone, 200 mg plus pyrimethamine 75 mg and leucovorin 25 mg weekly **or** atovaquone, 1,500 mg with or without pyrimethamine 25 mg plus leucovorin 10 mg daily
Mycobacterium avium complex	CD4+ count <50/mm³	Azithromycin 1,200 mg weekly **or** clarithromycin 500 mg twice daily	Rifabutin, 300 mg daily **or** azithromycin, 1,200, plus rifabutin, 300 mg daily
Varicella-zoster virus (VZV)	Substantial exposure to chickenpox or shingles for patients who have no history of either condition or, if available, negative antibody to VZV	Varicella-zoster immune globulin (VZIG), 5 vials (1.25 mL each) IM, administered within 96 h of exposure (ideally within 48 h)	None

Adapted from Guidelines for preventing opportunistic infections among HIV-infected persons. (2002). *Morbidity and Mortality Weekly Report, 51* (RRO8), 1–46.

BOX 44.5 Oral Health Care for Immunocompromised Patients

Both immunocompetent and immunocompromised patients may have oral health problems. A few conditions are seen only in immunocompromised patients. Conditions that are seen in both populations may cause more problems in immunocompromised patients than in others. These conditions include:

- Dental caries
- Dry mouth
- Periodontal disease
- Human papillomavirus (HPV)
- Oral candidiasis (thrush)
- Aphthous stomatitis (canker sores)
- Herpes simplex virus
- Hairy leukoplakia
- Opportunistic tumors

Teach the HIV-positive patient the importance of having dental examinations twice yearly. Other suggestions may include:

- Regularly brushing and flossing the teeth and gums
- Using artificial saliva products
- Sucking on sugar-free citrus candies
- Engaging in safe oral-sex practices
- Seeking treatment for aphthous ulcers rather than allowing them to self-heal
- Not smoking
- Limiting alcohol use

Strongly Recommended as the Standard of Care

Pneumocystis Carinii Pneumonia

Pneumocystic carinii pneumonia (PCP) is a type of pneumonia that affects immunosuppressed patients. In the past, PCP was responsible for serious illness and death among patients with HIV and AIDS. Since the use of HAART began, morbidity and mortality related to PCP has dramatically decreased.

Patients should start prophylactic therapy for PCP when their CD4+ T-cell counts are less than 200 cells/mm^3 or when they have a history of oropharyngeal candidiasis. If the CD4+ count increases to at least 200 cells/mm^3, prophylaxis may be discontinued.

The drug treatment of choice is sulfamethoxazole-trimethoprim (SMZ-TMP). Patients who experience non–life-threatening adverse drug effects should continue SMZ-TMP therapy if clinically feasible. If SMZ-TMP cannot be tolerated, alternative prophylactic regimens include dapsone, dapsone plus pyrimethamine, aerosolized pentamidine, or atovaquone. Unfortunately, these alternatives are not as effective as SMZ-TMP.

For additional information on SMZ-TMP, see Chapter 41. Pentamidine is discussed in Chapter 45.

Tuberculosis

Patients with a diagnosis of HIV infection should have a baseline tuberculin skin test (TST). Depending on the progression of infection at the time of diagnosis, the TST results may be negative. Clinical evaluation for the potential of TB is needed to determine whether anergy testing should be done at this time.

All HIV-positive patients who have positive TST results (induration exceeding 5 mm) should undergo chest radiography. For patients with positive TST findings and normal chest x-ray findings, prophylaxis with INH and pyridoxine should be initiated and continued for 9 months. Alternative therapies include rifampin or rifabutin daily for 4 months, rifampin or rifabutin plus pyrazinamide daily for 2 months, or rifabutin alone for 2 months. Patients with INH-resistant or multidrug-resistant TB need alternative drug dosing.

Any HIV-positive patients who are in close contact with people who have active TB should be started on prophylaxis therapy with isoniazid regardless of their TST results. Infants of HIV-positive mothers should have a TST between 9 and 12 months. These children should be retested every 2 to 3 years. Additional information on isoniazid can be found in Chapter 42.

Toxoplasma Gondii

Patients infected with HIV should be tested for immunoglobulin G (IgG) antibody to toxoplasma soon after the diagnosis of HIV infection to detect latent infection with *Toxoplasma gondii.* Prophylaxis should be initiated for patients with IgG antibody to toxoplasma and a CD4+ T-cell count of less than 100 cells/mm^3. The drug of choice is SMZ-TMP. If unable to tolerate SMZ-TMP, the patient may receive alternative prophylaxis, including dapsone plus pyrimethamine plus leucovorin weekly, or atovaquone with or without pyrimethamine plus leucovorin daily.

Counsel patients to avoid raw or undercooked meat, particularly undercooked pork, lamb, and venison. It also is important to caution patients to wash their hands after touching raw meat, gardening, or changing a cat's litter box. Patients with cats should be advised to change the litter box daily.

Mycobacterium Avium Complex

Prophylaxis for *Mycobacterium avium* complex (MAC) should be initiated when the patient's CD4+ T-cell count falls below 50 cells/mm^3. The drugs of choice are weekly azithromycin or twice-daily clarithromycin. In addition to MAC protection, these drugs also offer protection against respiratory bacterial infections.

For patients who cannot tolerate azithromycin or clarithromycin, rifabutin is the alternative drug. It is important to remember that rifabutin interacts with almost all anti-HIV agents; therefore, it should be administered cautiously. Additional information on azithromycin and clarithromycin is located in Chapter 39.

Varicella-Zoster Virus

Prophylaxis against varicella-zoster virus (VZV) is recommended for patients who have no antibodies to VZV and for patients who have been substantially exposed to either chickenpox or shingles. In patients experiencing a VZV outbreak, treatment centers on antiviral drugs such as acyclovir, valacyclovir, or famciclovir. Information on these drugs is located in Chapter 43.

Usually Recommended Prophylaxis

Streptococcus pneumoniae

Streptococcus pneumoniae is very common in the community, and there is no effective way to limit exposure to these bacteria. For patients with a CD4+ T-cell count of at least

200 cells/mm^3, pneumococcal vaccine should be administered. For patients with a CD4+ T-cell count of less than 200 cells/mm^3, pneumococcal vaccine may be administered, but the humoral response is likely to be diminished. Additional information on pneumococcal vaccine can be found in Appendix G.

Hepatitis B

HIV-positive patients should be tested for antibodies to HBV. If the patient tests negative, the hepatitis B vaccine should be administered. This vaccine is administered in three doses, with the second dose given 1 month after the initial dose and the last dose given 6 months after the initial dose.

Hepatitis A

HIV-positive patients should be tested for antibodies to hepatitis A virus. If the patient is negative or has chronic hepatitis C, the hepatitis A vaccine should be administered. This vaccine is administered in two doses.

Influenza Virus

Every HIV-positive patient should receive annual influenza virus prophylaxis. The preferred drug is inactivated trivalent influenza virus vaccine, one dose annually. Alternate medications include oseltamivir, 75 mg daily; rimantadine, 100 mg twice daily; or amantadine, 1 mg twice daily. Additional information regarding these antiviral medications is found in Chapter 43.

Evidence for Efficacy but Not Routinely Indicated

Bacteria

Patients who are neutropenic may receive granulocyte colony-stimulating factor (G-CSF), 5 to 10 μg/kg body weight, as a subcutaneous injection daily for 2 to 4 weeks. Another frequently used drug is granulocyte-macrophage colony-stimulating factor (GM-CSF), 250 μg/mm^2 subcutaneously for 2 to 4 weeks.

Cryptococcus Neoformans

Cryptococcus neoformans causes a fungal infection. HIV-positive patients with CD4+ counts of less than 50 cells/mm^3 should begin prophylaxis with fluconazole at a dosage of 100 to 200 mg daily. An acceptable alternate drug is itraconazole capsules, 200 mg daily. See Chapter 43 for more information on these drugs.

Histoplasma Capsulatum

Histoplasma capsulatum is the organism that causes the most common fungal respiratory infections in the world. Most infections are mild; however, approximately 10% of these infections cause serious complications, including inflammation of the pericardium and fibrosis of major blood vessels (see Chapter 43). Prophylaxis is recommended for patients who live in an endemic geographic area and have a CD4+ count of less than 100 cells/mm^3. Itraconazole is the prophylactic drug of choice.

Cytomegalovirus

Cytomegalovirus (CMV) is found universally throughout all geographic locations and socioeconomic groups and infects between 50% and 85% of adults in the United States by 40 years of age. In the general population, the infection may go unnoticed; however, in the immunocompromised population, CMV may cause infection in many organs of the body, especially in the retina of the eye (see Chapter 43). Patients who are CMV antibody positive and have a CD4+ count of less than 50 cells/mm^3 should receive ganciclovir, 1 g three times daily.

CHAPTER SUMMARY

- HIV infection and AIDS are chronic diseases affecting the immune system.
- HIV infection is diagnosed by positive results on EIA, ELISA, WB, rapid HIV, oral HIV, or PCR tests.
- HIV infection is monitored by CD4+ T-cell count and HIV RNA load.
- Genotypic and phenotypic resistance assays are now available to assess patterns of resistance to HAART therapy.
- Pharmacotherapy for asymptomatic patients has benefits and risks. Patients should be informed of both before starting therapy.
- Pharmacotherapy should be considered for all symptomatic patients. For asymptomatic patients, drug therapy should be considered when the CD4+ T-cell count is less than 200 cells/mm^3 or the HIV RNA load is more than 55,000.
- Resistance develops to all classes of anti-HIV agents, especially when the therapeutic regimen is not followed.
- Absorption of individual anti-HIV agents is enhanced either by administration with food or on an empty stomach (while fasting).
- All anti-HIV drugs may produce adverse effects that decrease the patient's quality of life.
- Most anti-HIV drugs have numerous drug–drug interactions that may increase or decrease their effectiveness.
- Anti-HIV agents include NRTIs, PIs, NNRTIs, and entry inhibitors.
- Antiretroviral therapy may be given throughout pregnancy or during the intrapartum and postpartum periods.
- Opportunistic diseases develop as HIV infection progresses. Many opportunistic diseases have recommended prophylactic regimens.

QUESTIONS FOR STUDY AND REVIEW

1. How is HIV infection diagnosed?
2. Why do patients with HIV infection have an increased risk for opportunistic diseases?
3. What information is gained from CD4+ T-cell counts and viral load counts?
4. What is the rationale for highly active antiretroviral therapy (HAART)?
5. Which adverse effects of zidovudine (AZT, ZDV) therapy may indicate a need to stop therapy?
6. Before initiation of zidovudine therapy, what laboratory tests should be completed?
7. What assessments and interventions apply to lifestyle, diet, and habits for the patient taking zidovudine?
8. How do PIs inhibit HIV replication?
9. Why is adherence to drug therapy critically important with saquinavir therapy?
10. How do NNRTIs differ in action from NRTIs?
11. How does the action of the entry inhibitors affect the ability of the HIV virus to replicate?
12. Why is opportunistic disease prophylaxis necessary?

? Need More Help?

Chapter 44 of the study guide for *Drug Therapy in Nursing* 2e contains NCLEX-style questions and other learning activities to reinforce your understanding of the concepts presented in this chapter. For additional information or to purchase the study guide, visit *http://connection.lww.com/go/aschenbrenner.*

REFERENCES AND BIBLIOGRAPHY

Cahn, P. (2004). Emtricitabine: A new nucleoside analogue for once-daily antiretroviral therapy. *Expert Opinions on Investigational Drugs, 13*(1), 55–68.

Clinical Pharmacology [Online]. Available: *http://cp.gsm.com.*

Facts and Comparisons. (2004). *Drug facts and comparisons.* Philadelphia: Lippincott Williams & Wilkins.

Guidelines for preventing opportunistic infections among HIV-infected persons. (2002). *Morbidity and Mortality Weekly Report, 51* (RRO8), 1–46.

Hardman, J. G. (2001). *Goodman & Gilman's the pharmacological basis of therapeutics* (10th ed.). New York: McGraw-Hill Health Professions Division.

Hussar, D. A. (2003). New drugs of 2003. *Journal of the American Pharmacy Association, 44*(2), 168–206.

Katzung, B. (2004). *Basic and clinical pharmacology* (9th ed.). New York: McGraw-Hill/Appleton & Lange.

Maitland, D., Boffito, M., Back, D., et al. (2004). *Pharmacokinetic/pharmacodynamic considerations of once-daily dosing of antiretroviral drugs* [Online]. Available: *http://www.medscape.com/viewprogram/3193?src=search.*

McKinney, R. E., Jr., & Cunningham, C. K. (2004). Newer treatments for HIV in children. *Current Opinions in Pediatrics, 16*(1), 76–79.

Micromedex Healthcare Series [Online]. Available: *http://healthcare.micromedex.com.*

Panel on Clinical Practices for Treatment of HIV. (2002). Guidelines for using antiretroviral agents among HIV-infected adults and adolescents. *Annals of Internal Medicine, 137*(5 Pt 2), 381–433.

Saag, M. S., et al. (2004). Efficacy and safety of emtricitabine vs stavudine in combination therapy in antiretroviral-naive patients: A randomized trial. *JAMA, 292*(2), 180–189.

Sension, M. (2004). Initial therapy for human immunodeficiency virus: Broadening the options. *HIV Clinical Trials, 5*(2), 99–111.

Tatro, D. S. (2004). *Drug interaction facts.* Philadelphia: Lippincott Williams & Wilkins.

U.S. Department of Health and Human Services. (2004). *Public Health Service Task Force Recommendations for Use of Antiretroviral Drugs in Pregnant HIV-1-Infected Women for Maternal Health and Interventions to Reduce Perinatal HIV-1 Transmission in the United States – June 23, 2004.* [Online]. Available: http://aidsinfo.nih.gov/guidelines/default_db2.asp?id=66.

U.S. Department of Health and Human Services. The DHHS Panel on Clinical Practices for Treatment of HIV Infection. (2004). *Guidelines for Use of Antiretroviral Agents in HIV-1-Infected Adults and Adolescents – October 29, 2004.* [Online]. Available: http://aidsinfo.nih.gov/guidelines/default_db2.asp?id=50.

Webb, A., & Norton, M. (2004). Clinical assessment of symptom-focused health-related quality of life in HIV/AIDS. *Journal of the Association of Nurses in AIDS Care, 15*(2), 67–78.

Drugs Treating Parasitic Infections

chapter 45

Learning Objectives

At the completion of this chapter the student will:

1. Describe the guidelines that govern the choice of antiparasitic drugs.
2. Identify core drug knowledge about drugs used to treat parasitic infections.
3. Identify core patient variables relevant to drugs used to treat parasitic infections.
4. Relate the interaction of core drug knowledge and core patient variables to drugs used to treat parasitic infections.
5. Generate a nursing plan of care from the interactions between core drug knowledge and core patient variables for drugs used to treat parasitic infections.
6. Describe nursing interventions to maximize therapeutic actions and minimize adverse effects for drugs used to treat parasitic infections.
7. Determine key points for patient and family education for drugs used to treat parasitic infections.
8. Explain the hygiene measures needed to prevent parasitic reinfection.

KEY TERMS

amebiasis
arthropods
cestodes
ectoparasites
giardiasis
helminths
malaria
nematodes
parasite
Pneumocystis carinii pneumonia
protozoa
toxoplasmosis
trematodes
trichomoniasis

FEATURED WEBLINKS

Malaria: **http://www.malaria.org/**
Amebiasis: **http://www.cdc.gov/ncidod/dpd/parasites/amebiasis/default.htm**
Giardiasis: **http://www.cdc.gov/ncidod/dpd/parasites/giardiasis/default.htm**
Trichomoniasis: **http://www.cdc.gov/nchstp/dstd/TrichInfo.htm**
Toxoplasmosis: **http://www.cdc.gov/ncidod/dpd/parasites/toxoplasmosis/default.htm**
Pneumocystis carinii pneumonia: **http://www.cdc.gov/ncidod/dpd/parasites/pneumocystis/default.htm**
Helminths: **http://vetgate.ac.uk/browse/cabi/detail/896a33d6b1eb180fd524fe0b0c09cbfa.html**
Scabies: **http://www.aad.org/pamphlets/Scabies.html**
Lice: **http://www.hsph.harvard.edu/headlice.html**
Most people in the United States do not recognize parasitic diseases. Try these websites for more information concerning these diseases and disorders.

CONNECTION WEBLINK

Additional Weblinks are found on Connection: **http://www.connection.lww.com/go/aschenbrenner.**

Antiparasitic Drugs

Ⓒ Antimalarials

- **P** **chloroquine**
- hydroxychloroquine
- mefloquine
- primaquine
- pyrimethamine
- quinine sulfate

Antibacterial agents

- sulfonamides
- atovaquone/proguanil

Ⓒ Antiprotozoans

Drugs affecting amebiasis, giardiasis, trichomoniasis, and toxoplasmosis

- **P** **metronidazole**
- iodoquinol
- paromomycin
- quinacrine

Drugs affecting *Pneumocystis carinii*

- **P** **pentamidine**
- atovaquone

Ⓒ Antihelminthics

- **P** **mebendazole**
- albendazole
- thiabendazole
- diethylcarbamazine
- niclosamide
- praziquantel
- piperazine
- pyrantel
- oxamniquine

Ⓒ Antiectoparasitics

- **P** **permethrin**
- crotamiton
- lindane
- malathion
- ivermectin

The symbol Ⓒ indicates the **drug class.**
Drugs in **bold type** marked with the symbol **P** are prototypes.
Drugs in blue type are closely related to the prototype.
Drugs in red type are significantly different from the prototype.
Drugs in black type with no symbol are also used in drug therapy; no prototype

A **parasite** is an organism that must live on other organisms to survive. The parasitic diseases are commonly grouped according to the type of organism that causes them: helminths, arthropods, or unicellular organisms, such as **protozoa.** Protozoan infections include malaria, amebiasis, giardiasis, *Pneumocystis carinii* pneumonia, toxoplasmosis, and trichomoniasis. **Helminths** (worms) are grouped into three categories: **nematodes** (roundworms), **trematodes** (flukes), and **cestodes** (tapeworms). **Ectoparasites** are vectors of disease, such as ticks, mosquitoes, and biting flies, and other ectoparasites that infect external body surfaces. **Arthropods** include mites (scabies), chiggers, lice (pediculosis), and fleas.

Pharmacologic intervention for parasitic infections must be specific not only to the type of parasite but also to the appropriate stage of its life cycle. Some parasites have simple life cycles, and some have extremely complex life cycles. Thus, many parasitic diseases are treated with a combination of drugs to eradicate all stages of the parasite.

This chapter discusses the appropriate drug or drugs used to eradicate the most common parasitic diseases. Antiparasitic drugs are divided into four drug families: antimalarials, antiprotozoan drugs, anthelminthic drugs, and antiectoparasitic drugs. The antiprotozoan drugs used in treating *Pneumocystis carinii* pneumonia (PCP), a common complication of acquired immunodeficiency syndrome (AIDS), are discussed separately within the antiprotozoan drug class section.

Chloroquine is the prototype antimalarial drug; drugs also used in managing malaria that are significantly different from chloroquine include antibacterial agents, sulfonamides, and atovaquone/proguanil. Metronidazole is the prototype antiprotozoan agent; iodoquinol, paromomycin, and quinacrine are drugs significantly different from metronidazole. Another antiprotozoan drug, used for prophylaxis and treatment of PCP, is pentamidine isethionate; it is the prototype drug for this purpose. Atovaquone, a drug significantly different from pentamidine, is used to treat acute PCP infection. Mebendazole is the prototype anthelminthic; anthelminthic agents significantly different from mebendazole include pyrantel pamoate, piperazine, diethylcarbamazine, praziquantel, oxamniquine, and niclosamide. Finally, this chapter discusses antiectoparasitic agents, with permethrin as the prototype. Ivermectin (Stromectol) is an antiectoparasitic drug significantly different from permethrin. In addition to explaining how these drugs work, this chapter discusses nursing management related to evaluating the patient's condition, administering antiparasitic drugs, monitoring the patient's response, and teaching the patient and family about antiparasitic therapy.

PATHOPHYSIOLOGY

Malaria

Malaria is caused by protozoan parasites of the genus *Plasmodium.* Four species of *Plasmodium* produce disease in humans—*P. falciparum, P. vivax, P. ovale,* and *P. malariae. P. falciparum* is the most widespread and dangerous of the four. Because *P. falciparum* can destroy up to 60% of circulating red blood cells (RBCs) and induce serious adverse complications such as toxic encephalopathy, it is fatal in about 1% of all cases. That 1% accounts for more than 95% of all malaria-caused deaths worldwide.

The complex life cycle of *Plasmodium* species begins when a female *Anopheles* mosquito bites a human whose blood contains the sexual forms of the malaria parasite (gametocytes). Within the now-infected mosquito, the gametocyte completes a maturation process and becomes a sporozoite that is stored in the salivary glands. When the mosquito next feeds, it inoculates another human host with the sporozoites.

Once the sporozoites are in the human host, the asexual portion of the life cycle begins. The first stage of asexual development, the exoerythrocytic phase, occurs in the liver. During this phase, the form of the *Plasmodium* is called a tissue schizont. At the end of the phase, the *Plasmodium,* now in a form called a merozoite, is released from the liver into the bloodstream.

The second stage of asexual development, the erythrocytic phase, begins when the merozoites are released into the bloodstream. The merozoites invade the erythrocytes and develop into erythrocytic schizonts. They, in turn, develop more merozoites within the red blood cells. At the end of this phase, the RBCs rupture, releasing the merozoites and pyrogenic substances into the bloodstream, where the merozoites invade new RBCs. The release of merozoites into the bloodstream initiates malarial symptoms of fever, shivering, joint pain, and headache. With *P. vivax* and *P. ovale,* merozoites may reinvade the liver tissue and develop a dormant hepatic stage (hypnozoite), which is responsible for subsequent relapses.

The cycle of invasion, multiplication, and RBC rupture is repeated many times. After a few cycles, some of the asexual parasites develop into sexual forms (gametocytes), which remain in the bloodstream. When a mosquito bites a human with gametocytes in the blood, the cycle begins again (Figure 45.1). Because of its complex life cycle, malaria is frequently treated with combination drug therapy.

Parasitic Diseases

Amebiasis

Amebiasis is most frequently caused by the microorganism *Entamoeba histolytica,* which is passed from host to host by ingestion of fecally contaminated food or water. It also is transmitted by vectors such as flies. Amebic disease is present worldwide, but it is most common in those tropical areas where crowded living conditions and poor sanitation exist. Africa, Latin America, Southeast Asia, and India have substantial health problems associated with this disease. In the United States, amebiasis is more common among homosexual men than it is in other populations.

Ingested in its cyst form, the microorganism has thick walls that are resistant to stomach acids. In the intestine, the cysts change into a sexually active organism called a trophozoite. The trophozoite produces active amebiasis. The active disease organisms may remain in the intestine (intestinal amebiasis), or the trophozoites may penetrate the intestinal wall and produce abscesses in other tissues and organs (extraintestinal amebiasis). Symptoms may be mild or severe. Mild symptoms include mucoid diarrhea, flatulence, fatigue, weight loss, and colicky abdominal pain. Severe disease may be marked with frequent foul-smelling stools tinged with mucus and blood, fever to 105°F, tenesmus (painful but

Physiology

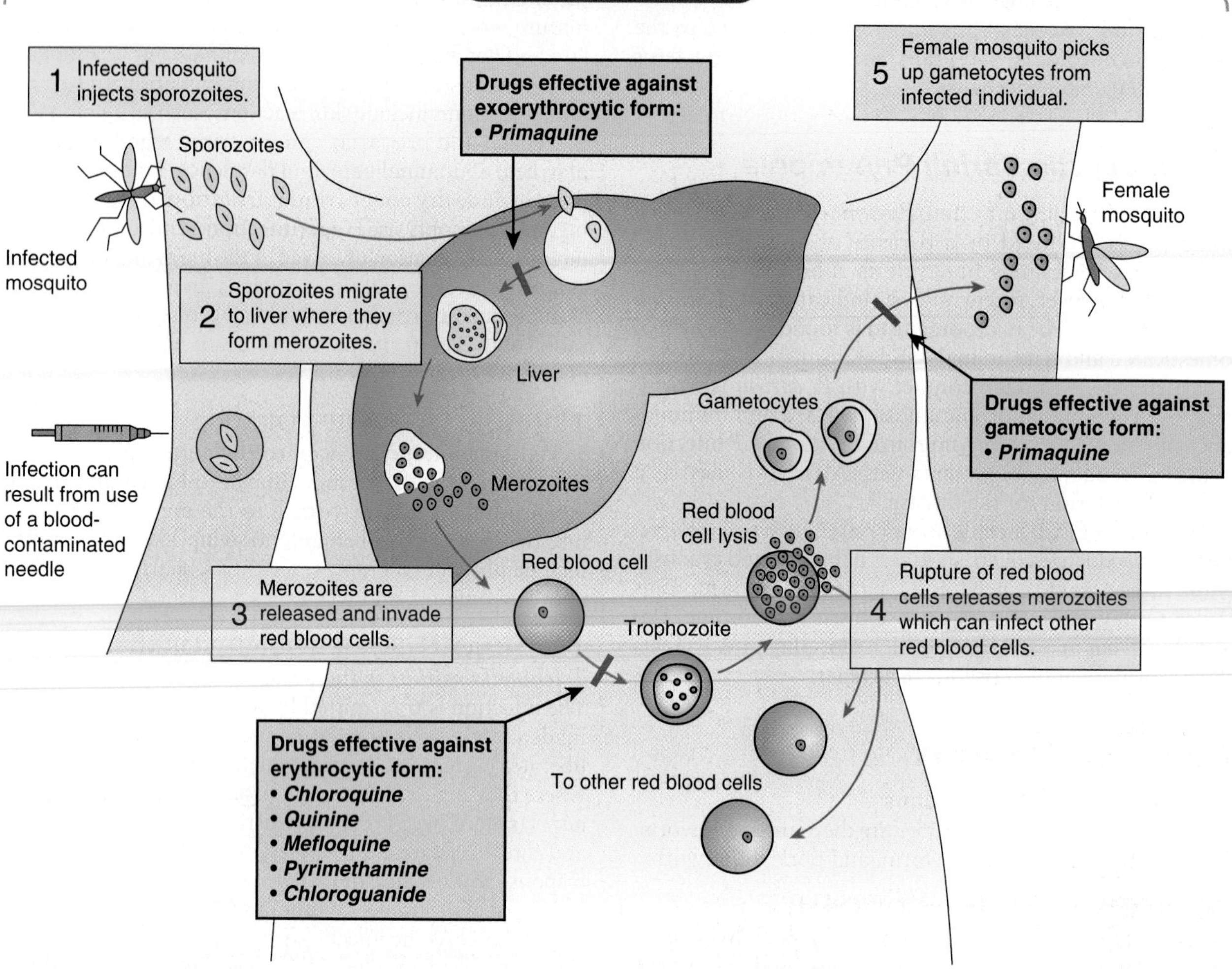

FIGURE 45.1 Life cycle of the malarial parasite and the sites of action of antimalarial drugs. (Courtesy of Mycek, M. J., Harvey, R. A., and Champe, P. C. [1997]. *Pharmacology* [2nd ed.]. Philadelphia: Lippincott-Raven.)

unsuccessful straining to defecate), generalized abdominal tenderness, and vomiting.

Giardiasis

Giardiasis is a common disease caused by a flagellated protozoan, *Giardia lamblia.* It is transmitted by fecal contamination. Hikers who drink unfiltered water or travelers to foreign countries where the water supply is impure are most susceptible. Animal reservoirs for the parasites include beavers and dogs.

Giardiasis is more prevalent in children than in adults, possibly because many individuals seem to have a lasting immunity after infection. The disease is common in children's day-care centers, especially those in which diapering is done. This disease also afflicts many homosexual men, both HIV-positive and HIV-negative individuals, presumably as a result of sexual transmission.

Giardia affects only the intestinal system, resulting in acute or chronic diarrhea and possibly malabsorption syndrome. The acute phase may last days to weeks; however, the chronic phase may last years. Symptoms include diarrheal, soft, or steatorrheal stools with mucus but without blood. Abdominal cramps, vomiting, flatulence, and weight loss also may occur.

Trichomoniasis

Trichomoniasis is an infection of the vagina caused by the parasite *Trichomonas vaginalis.* Both sexual partners are generally infected, although both may not be symptomatic. Symptoms of trichomoniasis include a thin, yellow, frothy, and malodorous discharge. The vagina may be inflamed, and the woman may also have a "strawberry" cervix, which is very friable and bleeds easily.

Toxoplasmosis

Toxoplasmosis is caused by a parasite found in a variety of animals, especially cats and birds.

Infection results from ingesting oocysts from cat feces, ingesting cysts in raw or undercooked meat, congenital transmission, or transmission during blood transfusion.

In adults, the disease is usually mild with symptoms such as fever, malaise, headache, lymphadenopathy, and sore throat. However, toxoplasmosis is very dangerous to immunocompromised patients. The infection may affect the

lungs, heart, and liver, but usually it affects the brain. Patients may succumb to meningoencephalitis.

Congenital toxoplasmosis may result in damage to the eyes (retinochoroiditis) and brain (encephalitis) of the fetus or other congenital anomalies.

Pneumocystis Carinii Pneumonia

An opportunistic lung infection, ***Pneumocystis carinii* pneumonia** (PCP) is caused by a parasite of uncertain classification. The parasite's life cycle is similar to that of a protozoan; however, recent analysis indicates that *P. carinii* may be a fungus. The microorganism is found in a variety of domesticated and wild animals, and transmission is thought to be airborne. Although contact with *P. carinii* is worldwide, only debilitated or immunosuppressed and immunodeficient patients develop symptoms. Because PCP infection occurs so frequently in patients with AIDS, it is used as a diagnostic criterion for the disease.

Symptoms of PCP include abrupt onset, high fever, tachypnea, nonproductive cough, shortness of breath, and cyanosis. As the disease rapidly progresses, patients have symptoms similar to those of adult respiratory distress syndrome. Untreated PCP has an exceptionally high mortality rate. Patients who recover are at high risk for recurrence.

Helminthic Infections

Intestinal Nematode Infections

The common intestinal nematodes are the giant roundworm, pinworm, threadworm, whipworm, and pork roundworm.

ASCARIASIS (GIANT ROUNDWORM)

Ascariasis is endemic in areas known for poor hygiene or sanitation and those where human feces are used as fertilizer. Ascariasis is transmitted by ingesting fecally contaminated foods or drinks. Once ingested, the worm eggs migrate to the small bowel, where they hatch, releasing larvae. The motile larvae migrate from the small bowel to the heart and lungs, to the esophagus, and back to the small bowel. They can survive up to 5 years and reach a length of 30 cm. Symptoms include low-grade fever, nonproductive cough, blood-tinged sputum, wheezing, dyspnea, and substernal pain.

ENTEROBIASIS (PINWORM)

Enterobius vermicularis is the most common helminthic infection in the United States. Children are infected more frequently than adults. Transmission occurs by contact with eggs in food, water, or bed linens. Adult worms inhabit the cecum and adjacent bowel areas. Female worms migrate through the anus to the perianal skin and deposit large numbers of eggs, especially at night. In a few hours, infection can be transmitted to others or remain in the host. The most common symptoms are rectal itching and vulvar itching.

STRONGYLOIDIASIS (THREADWORM)

Strongyloidiasis results from infection with *Strongyloides stercoralis*. The infection is potentially serious in adults because the worm can multiply within the host. In its filariform larvae cycle, the parasites penetrate the skin from soil, enter the bloodstream, and travel to the lungs. From the lungs, they escape the alveoli and ascend the bronchial tree to the glottis, where they are swallowed and propelled to the small intestine to mature into adult threadworms. The mature worm embeds itself in the mucosa where eggs are laid and hatched. The larvae disseminate into the lungs and most other tissues, causing local inflammation and granulomas. Symptoms include skin reactions, such as inflammation, petechiae, and urticaria, and intestinal reactions, such as diarrhea, abdominal pain, and flatulence. Pulmonary symptoms include dry cough, throat irritation, dyspnea, wheezing, and hemoptysis. Hyperinfection syndrome caused by intense dissemination of larvae to the lungs and other tissues can result in complications, such as pleural effusion, pericarditis, and myocarditis. Additional problems include perforation of the colon and peritonitis, gram-negative septicemia, and shock leading to death.

TRICHURIASIS (WHIPWORM)

Trichuriasis infection is acquired by ingesting egg-contaminated soil on hands or food. Human-to-human transmission is not possible. Worms attach to the mucosa of the large intestine by means of their anterior whip-like end. Symptoms include abdominal cramps, tenesmus, diarrhea, flatulence, nausea, vomiting, and weight loss.

TRICHINOSIS (PORK ROUNDWORM)

Trichinella spiralis is the parasite that causes trichinosis. The infection is transmitted by ingesting encysted larvae in inadequately cooked meat, especially pork. Gastric juices liberate the encysted larvae, which migrate to the intestines where they mature, mate, and produce eggs that hatch into new larvae. These larvae are distributed through the body and enter skeletal muscle tissues, producing an inflammatory response. Eventually, the larvae become re-encysted and remain within the tissues. Symptoms include diarrhea, cramps, and malaise. As the infection progresses, patients may experience muscle pain, tenderness, fever, periorbital and facial edema, and conjunctivitis.

Blood and Tissue Nematode Infections

Filarial infections are among the more serious and debilitating helminthiases associated with blood and tissue nematodes. There are two forms of filarial infections. The first form is caused by two microbes, *Wuchereria bancrofti* and *Brugia malayi*. Both microbes are transmitted by mosquitoes.

Bancroftian filariasis also is known as elephantiasis because the helminths migrate to the lymphatic system, causing lymphadenopathy and resultant edema of the extremities. Brugian filariasis also affects the lymphatic system. In this infection, microfilariae are produced and circulated in the bloodstream.

The second type of filariasis also is known as onchocerciasis or river blindness. The adult helminths reside in subcutaneous nodules and migrate to the eye, causing ocular lesions and eventual loss of vision.

Cestode Infections

Cestodes cause taeniasis infections. Tapeworm infections are transmitted in contaminated raw or improperly cooked fish (*Diphyllobothrium latum*), beef (*Taenia saginata*), and pork (*Taenia solium*). The adult tapeworm consists of a head (scolex) that attaches to the intestinal wall and segments called proglottids. The proglottids contain tapeworm eggs and are expelled in feces. Beef and fish tapeworms do not

cause serious illness. Pork tapeworms, however, produce larvae that enter the bloodstream and invade other body tissues. Symptoms include nausea, vomiting, diarrhea, fatigue, hunger, and dizziness.

Trematode Infections

Trematodes cause schistosomiasis, which is a leading cause of morbidity and mortality from parasitic diseases. The vector of schistosomiasis is a specific snail; humans acquire this parasite by drinking or contacting contaminated water. There are three major types of schistosomes. Each migrates to a specific part of the human host and produces clinical symptoms specific to each type.

Ectoparasitic Infections

Common ectoparasitic infections include scabies and pediculosis (lice).

Scabies

Scabies is a skin inflammation caused by a mite, *Sarcoptes scabiei.* The mite is barely visible with the naked eye and is transmitted by contact with an infected individual or infested bedding. Characteristic lesions consist of generalized excoriations with small pruritic vesicles, pustules, and burrows. The infestations occur on the sides of the fingers and the palms, wrists, elbows, and around the axillae. The head and neck are usually spared in adults. Diagnosis is made by identifying the parasite or its ova or feces microscopically. Treatment includes all family members and close contacts, which helps to prevent reinfestation.

Pediculosis

Pediculosis infestations occur on the scalp (pediculosis capitis), trunk (pediculosis corporis), or pubic areas (pediculosis pubis). Transmission is by direct contact with lice, particularly those on hats, combs, and body hair. Symptoms include pruritus with excoriation, nits on hair shafts, and lice on skin or clothes.

C ANTIMALARIAL DRUGS

Drug therapy for malaria has three distinct categories: suppressive therapy (prophylaxis), treatment of an acute attack (clinical cure), and prevention of a relapse (radical cure). Some drugs may be used in more than one category. All antimalarials are called schizonticides. They are further divided into tissue schizonticides or blood schizonticides. Blood schizonticides affect the erythrocytic state of the schizont replicating in the RBCs of the human host. Tissue schizonticides affect schizonts that have invaded the liver. Some antimalarial drugs, such as the prototype chloroquine, have multiple actions; it is both a blood schizonticide and a gametocytocide.

Drugs within the antimalarial class include chloroquine (Aralen), hydroxychloroquine (Plaquenil Sulfate), mefloquine (Lariam), primaquine, pyrimethamine (Daraprim), and quinine (Quinamin). Chloroquine is the prototype antimalarial drug. Table 45.1 presents a summary of selected antimalarial drugs.

NURSING MANAGEMENT OF THE PATIENT RECEIVING P CHLOROQUINE

Core Drug Knowledge

Pharmacotherapeutics

Chloroquine is indicated to suppress or treat acute attacks of malaria caused by *P. vivax, P. malariae, P. ovale,* and susceptible strains of *P. falciparum.* It does not prevent relapses because it is not effective against exoerythrocytic forms of the parasite, nor will it prevent infections caused by *P. vivax* or *P. malariae* when administered as a prophylactic. In addition to its use in treating malaria, chloroquine also is used to treat extraintestinal amebiasis, rheumatoid arthritis, and discoid lupus erythematosus.

Pharmacokinetics

Chloroquine is absorbed rapidly and completely from the gastrointestinal (GI) system. The drug concentrates in the erythrocytes (RBCs), liver, spleen, kidney, lung, melanin-containing tissues, and leukocytes (white blood cells). It penetrates the central nervous system (CNS) and crosses the placenta. Although chloroquine action peaks rapidly, its half-life is between 70 and 120 hours. About 70% of chloroquine is excreted unchanged by the kidneys. Any unabsorbed drug is excreted in feces. Small amounts of chloroquine have been detected in urine for months and even years after treatment stops.

Pharmacodynamics

Chloroquine, a 4-aminoquinoline, is classified as a blood schizonticide. In treating malaria, its direct effects are on the parasite. Chloroquine is taken up by plasmodia residing within the RBCs of the human host. Chloroquine is thought to increase blood pH and upset phospholipid metabolism in the parasite, thereby interrupting the synthesis of ribonucleic acid (RNA) and deoxyribonucleic acid (DNA). In patients with rheumatoid arthritis, chloroquine antagonizes histamine and serotonin, thereby inhibiting prostaglandin synthesis. The result is an anti-inflammatory effect. The drug's action in treating amebiasis is unknown, however.

Contraindications and Precautions

Chloroquine is contraindicated for patients with a hypersensitivity to any 4-aminoquinoline, such as hydroxychloroquine. Chloroquine also is contraindicated for patients with pre-existing eye disease because the drug can cause corneal opacities, keratopathy, or retinopathy. Retinopathy can lead to blindness and can progress even after the drug is discontinued.

Chloroquine is used with caution in patients with various pre-existing disorders. In patients with psoriasis or porphyria, chloroquine has precipitated severe attacks. Because chloroquine concentrates in the liver, it can produce toxic effects in patients with hepatic disease or alcoholism or in patients using other hepatotoxic drugs concurrently.

Chloroquine should be given with caution to patients with GI disorders, blood dyscrasias, dental disease, and neurologic disorders. Patients with these disorders may have

TABLE 45.1 Summary of Selected (C) Antimalarial Drugs

Drug (Trade) Name	Selected Indications	Route and Dosage Range	Pharmacokinetics
[P] chloroquine (Aralen)	Suppression of malaria	*Adult:* PO, 300-mg base once a week on the same day for 2 wk before exposure and continuing until 4–6 wk after exposure *Child:* PO, 5 mg base PO once a week on the same day for 2 wk before exposure and continuing until 4–6 wk after exposure	*Onset:* Rapid *Duration:* Week $t_{1/2}$: 70–120 h
	Acute malaria attack	*Adult:* PO, 600-mg base initially, then 300-mg base 6 h later and on days 2 and 3 *Child:* PO, 10-mg base/kg initially, then 5-mg base/kg 6 h later and on days 2 and 3 *Adult:* IM, 160–200 mg base initially and 6 h later if needed; not to exceed 800 mg base/d *Child:* IM, 5 mg base/kg mg base initially and 6 h later if needed	
	Amebiasis	*Adult:* PO, 1 g (600-mg base)/d for 2 d, then 500 mg (300-mg base)/d for 2–3 wk *Child:* PO, not recommended *Adult:* IM, 200–250 mg (160–200-mg base) daily for 10–12 d	
atovaquone/proguanil (Malarone)	Treatment of malaria	*Adult:* PO single dose of four tablets (total daily dose 1 g atovaquone/400 mg proguanil hydrochloride) for 3 consecutive days.	*Onset:* Rapid *Duration:* Unknown $t_{1/2}$: 3 d
	Prophylaxis	Malarone is one tablet (250 mg atovaquone/100 mg proguanil hydrochloride) per day for adults *Child:* Based on weight of child	
hydroxychloroquine (Plaquenil Sulfate)	Suppression of malaria	*Adult:* PO, 310-mg base/wk on the same day each week, beginning 2 wk before exposure and continuing for 6–8 wk after leaving the malaria area. If suppressive therapy does not begin before exposure, the initial loading dose is doubled and given in two doses 6 h apart *Child:* 5-mg base/kg/wk, then the same dosage regimen as adults	*Onset:* Rapid *Duration:* Unknown $t_{1/2}$: 50 d
	Acute malaria attack	*Adult:* PO, initial dose (day 1), 620-mg base; dose 2 (6 h after dose 1), 310 mg; dose 3 (day 2), 310 mg; dose 4 (day 3) 310 mg *Child:* PO, same as adult in the following amounts, respectively: 10 mg/kg base, 5 mg/kg, 5 mg/kg, 5 mg/kg	
mefloquine (Lariam)	Suppression of malaria	*Adult:* PO, 250 mg once weekly for 4 wk, then 250 mg every other week; CDC recommends a single dose taken weekly starting 1 wk before exposure and for 4 wk after exposure *Child:* PO, 15–19 kg 1/4 tablets; 20–30 kg 1/2 tablet; 31–45 kg 3/4 tablet; more than 45 kg 1 tablet; CDC recommends a single dose taken weekly starting 1 wk before exposure and for 4 wk after exposure	*Onset:* Delayed *Duration:* Varies $t_{1/2}$: 15–23 d
	Acute malaria attack	*Adult:* PO, 5 tablets (1,250 mg) as a single dose	

(continued)

TABLE 45.1 Summary of Selected Ⓒ Antimalarial Drugs (continued)

Drug (Trade) Name	Selected Indications	Route and Dosage Range	Pharmacokinetics
primaquine	Malaria	*Adult:* PO, begin treatment during the last week of or after a course of suppression with chloroquine or a comparable drug, then 26.3 mg (15-mg base)/d for 14 d *Child:* PO, 0.5 mg/kg/d (0.3-mg base/kg) for 14 d, maximum, 15-mg base/dose	*Onset:* Rapid *Duration:* Unknown $t_{1/2}$: 3.7–9.6 h
pyrimethamine (Daraprim)	Suppression of malaria	*Adult:* PO, 25 mg once weekly for at least 6–10 wk *Child <4 y:* PO, 6.25 mg once weekly for 6–10 wk; 4–10 y, PO, 12.5 mg once weekly for 6–10 wk	*Onset:* Unknown *Duration:* Unknown $t_{1/2}$: 56–148 h
	Acute treatment of malaria	*Adult:* PO, 25 mg/d for 2 d *Child:* PO, 4–10 y, 25 mg/d for 2 d	
	Toxoplasmosis	*Adult:* PO, initially 50–75 mg/d with 1–4 g of sulfapyridine; continue for 1–3 wk; dosage of each drug may then be decreased by half and continued for an additional 4–5 wk *Child:* PO, 1 mg/kg/d divided into two equal daily doses; after 2–4 d, reduce to half and continue for approximately 1 mo	
quinine (Quinamin)	Chloroquine-resistant malaria	*Adult:* PO, 650 mg q8h, for 5–7 d *Child:* PO, 25 mg/kg/d in divided doses q8h for 5–7 d	*Onset:* Varies *Duration:* Varies $t_{1/2}$: 4–5 h
	Chloroquine-sensitive malaria	*Adult:* PO, 600 mg q8h for 5–7 d *Child:* PO, 10 mg/kg/d in divided doses q8h for 5–7 d	

exacerbations of disease because of the actions and potential adverse effects of chloroquine. Chloroquine should be given with extreme caution to infants and children because of potentially fatal toxicities.

Adverse Effects

Potential adverse effects of chloroquine may affect the cardiovascular, GI, hematologic, integumentary, and neurologic systems. The most common adverse effects are hypotension, cardiac changes reflected on an electrocardiogram (ECG), nausea, vomiting, diarrhea, and abdominal pain.

Infrequent but important potential adverse effects include blurred vision, difficulty focusing, changes in accommodation, irreversible retinal damage, tinnitus and reduced hearing in patients with pre-existing auditory damage, headaches or psychic stimulation, convulsive seizures, and neuromyopathy.

Potential adverse hematologic effects include agranulocytosis, aplastic anemia, pancytopenia, neutropenia, and thrombocytopenia. Potential integumentary effects are pruritus, skin discoloration, skin eruption, and hair bleaching or loss.

Drug Interactions

Chloroquine may interact with cimetidine, digoxin, penicillamine, and rabies vaccine. With kaolin and magnesium-containing antacids, its absorption is decreased. Most patients will remember any prescription drugs they are taking, but they may forget to mention over-the-counter (OTC) drugs, such as cimetidine or antacids. Therefore, remember to assess the patient's use of OTC drugs as well. See Table 45.2 for more information.

Assessment of Relevant Core Patient Variables

Health Status

Before administering chloroquine, assess for anemia, porphyria, psoriasis, ocular disease, neurologic disorders, liver and kidney diseases, and other conditions that contraindicate using the drug or that require close monitoring. Next, review the patient's drug history to identify substances that may interact with chloroquine and advise the patient to consult with the prescriber before taking any OTC drugs.

Because chloroquine may affect the eyes, arrange for the patient to have a complete baseline ophthalmologic examination, including visual acuity, slit-lamp, and fundoscopic examinations. Similarly, because chloroquine may affect reflexes, muscle strength, and hearing, perform a physical examination and document baseline measurements of these factors. Additional baseline studies include laboratory results related to liver function, kidney function, and complete blood count (CBC).

Life Span and Gender

In general, chloroquine may be administered to children to prevent or treat malaria. However, careful monitoring is

TABLE 45.2 Agents That Interact With P Chloroquine

Interactants	Effect and Significance	Nursing Management
cimetidine	The metabolism of aminoquinolines may be decreased, resulting in the pharmacologic effects of aminoquinolines being increased.	Monitor for possible aminoquinoline toxicity.
digoxin	Serum levels of digoxin may be increased. The actions of digoxin may be enhanced, or toxicity may develop.	Monitor patients on combined therapy for sign and symptoms of digoxin toxicity. Monitor serum digoxin level.
kaolin magnesium antacids	Kaolin and antacids containing magnesium may decrease the absorption and therapeutic effect of aminoquinolines. The antacid activity may also be decreased.	Administer doses of chloroquine and kaolin or antacids containing magnesium at least 2 h apart.
penicillamine	Serum levels of penicillamine may be increased. This may induce hematologic, renal, or skin reactions to penicillamine.	During concurrent use of penicillamine and chloroquine, monitor patient closely for adverse effect to penicillamine. Avoid concurrent use if possible.
rabies vaccine	When the rabies vaccine is administered intradermally, chloroquine may interfere with the antibody response.	Use the IM route for rabies vaccine if concurrent use is indicated.

needed because of the drug's potential for fatal toxicity in children. Assess the adult female patient for pregnancy or lactation. Breast-feeding women need to know that chloroquine enters breast milk. Although chloroquine is assigned to pregnancy category C, most prescribers believe the benefits of chloroquine therapy outweigh the risks associated with malaria.

Lifestyle, Diet, and Habits

Determine the patient's willingness or ability to arrange activities and lifestyle to accommodate weekly therapy for suppression.

Environment

It is important to ensure that the patient understands the need for prophylactic drug therapy. People traveling to areas where malaria is endemic should begin drug prophylaxis 2 weeks before the trip begins and continue therapy for 4 to 6 weeks after returning. In addition to taking pharmacologic prophylaxis, the patient should implement activities, such as using insect repellent, protective clothing, and netting, that decrease exposure to disease-bearing mosquitoes.

Nursing Diagnoses and Outcomes

- Acute Pain related to headache and itching resulting from drug therapy
  Desired outcome: *The patient will use acetaminophen and take soothing oatmeal baths to relieve drug-related discomforts.*
- Risk for Deficient Fluid Volume related to drug-induced fluid losses from nausea, vomiting, diarrhea, and anorexia
  Desired outcome: *The patient will maintain adequate hydration despite the effects of drug therapy and minimize GI upset by taking the drug with food.*
- Ineffective Protection related to possible agranulocytosis, aplastic anemia, neutropenia, and thrombocytopenia resulting from drug therapy
  Desired outcome: *The patient will report signs and symptoms of blood abnormalities (bruising, unexplained fatigue) to the prescriber immediately.*
- Disturbed Sensory Perception, Auditory and Visual related to potential tinnitus, hearing loss, retinopathy, and blurred vision related to drug therapy
  Desired outcome: *The patient will report problems with hearing or vision to the prescriber immediately.*
- Risk for Injury: Cardiovascular Toxicity, Neuromyopathy, or Seizures related to drug therapy
  Desired outcome: *The patient will remain free of injury throughout therapy with chloroquine.*

Planning and Intervention

Maximizing Therapeutic Effects

The patient taking chloroquine on a weekly basis for prophylaxis should take the drug on the same day each week, usually by mouth. An intramuscular (IM) injection is given when the oral route is not possible. In such situations, the nurse or patient injects the drug into a large muscle mass, making sure to aspirate to avoid hitting a blood vessel. The IM route is unsuitable for children because of the risk for toxic effects. For children, the bitter-tasting tablets may be pulverized and mixed with a pleasantly flavored preparation, such as chocolate syrup or grape jam.

Minimizing Adverse Effects

The patient may take chloroquine with meals to minimize GI discomfort. After taking the drug, the patient may need to change positions slowly to minimize symptoms of dizziness or lightheadedness, which signify a hypotensive response. The patient who experiences pruritus (itching) may be soothed by an oatmeal bath because antihistamines are ineffective in such cases. To relieve a headache, the patient may take acetaminophen. Patients with blood dyscrasias or myelosuppression should postpone dental work or other procedures that increase the risk for infection. Patients with

these disorders have a higher risk for infection. Double-check pediatric doses to prevent toxicity.

Providing Patient and Family Education

- Teach the patient how to take chloroquine to prevent or treat malaria.
- Prophylactic chloroquine therapy should begin about 2 weeks before scheduled travel and should continue for about 4 to 6 weeks after the patient leaves the malarial area.
- Tell the patient to wear cover-up clothing as a barrier to mosquitoes (Box 45.1).
- Explain that if a fever develops within 2 months after a trip to a malarial area, the patient should notify the health care provider immediately.
- Point out potential adverse effects of chloroquine. For example, chloroquine use may discolor urine (red or brown). In addition, itching, nausea, vomiting, dizziness, and headaches may occur. Periodic ophthalmologic and audiometric examinations should be scheduled by patients taking prolonged therapy because the drug can cause vision and hearing problems. Instruct the patient to contact the prescriber immediately if fever, sore throat, easy bruising, unusual fatigue, or problems with hearing or eyesight develop.
- Caution the patient to avoid alcohol while taking chloroquine.
- Caution the patient to notify the prescriber if nausea, vomiting, or diarrhea is persistent.

Ongoing Assessment and Evaluation

Monitor for episodes of misty or foggy vision, difficulty reading and complaints that words tend to disappear, and visual field changes (e.g., seeing half an object, light flashes or streaks, or pigmentation changes). Evaluate the patient's gross hearing, reflexes, and muscle strength throughout therapy. Additional assessments include checking for irritability, excitability, and personality or behavioral changes and signs and symptoms of anemia and hepatic or renal dysfunction. Symptomatic patients or patients at high risk for hemolytic anemia should have periodic blood analyses, and seizure precautions should be instituted as needed.

Patients who exhibit signs of toxicity may complain of headache, drowsiness, visual disturbances, nausea, or vomiting. These symptoms may be quickly followed by cardiovascular collapse, convulsions, and respiratory or cardiac arrest. Patients suspected of experiencing toxicity should go to an emergency department.

Drugs Closely Related to P Chloroquine

Hydroxychloroquine

Hydroxychloroquine (Plaquenil Sulfate) is very similar to chloroquine but is less toxic. Although it may be used to treat malaria, it is used more commonly to treat rheumatoid arthritis and lupus erythematosus. Higher dosages are needed for treating rheumatoid arthritis.

The pharmacokinetics and pharmacodynamics of hydroxychloroquine are the same as those of chloroquine, except that it is unknown whether it enters breast milk. Because the drugs are so similar and chloroquine does enter breast milk, the safest course is to refrain from its use in patients who are breast-feeding.

Hydroxychloroquine has the same extensive adverse effects profile as chloroquine. Like chloroquine, the most common adverse effects of hydroxychloroquine affect the GI tract. Patients should take hydroxychloroquine with food to minimize these effects.

Mefloquine

Mefloquine (Lariam), a 4-quinolinemethanol derivative, is related chemically to quinine. Mefloquine is the drug of choice for chloroquine-resistant and multidrug-resistant *P. falciparum*. Because it is the only drug available for treating these parasites, it is reserved for these conditions, to avoid inducing resistance. As a blood schizonticide, it prevents erythrocytic parasites from replicating but has no action on exoerythrocytic parasites. Its mechanism of action is unknown, but it may work by raising intravascular pH in parasite acid vesicles, causing death.

Mefloquine is given orally, despite its variable absorption, because it is irritating to tissues. It is distributed widely, crosses the placenta, and may enter breast milk. It is highly bound to plasma proteins and concentrates in blood erythrocytes.

COMMUNITY-BASED CONCERNS

Box 45.1 Stop Malaria Before It Starts!

In addition to prophylactic pharmacotherapy instructions, include the following when educating the patient about malaria:

- Be sure to use mosquito netting. Check for holes in the net.
- Always sleep in screened areas. Spray the area with permethrin-containing insecticide before the sun sets.
- Wear protective clothing. Use 30-mL DEET (N,N-diethyl meta-toluamide) in 250 mL of water to impregnate cotton garments.
- Minimize nocturnal exposure; long-sleeved clothing and long pants should be worn outdoors after sunset.
- DEET insect repellents should be applied to exposed skin. Refined lemon eucalyptus oil also may be used on the skin but is not as effective.

MEMORY CHIP

P Chloroquine

- Used primarily for malaria; secondarily for amebiasis, rheumatoid arthritis, and lupus
- Major contraindications: pre-existing eye diseases
- Most common adverse effects: hypotension, nausea, vomiting, diarrhea, and abdominal pain
- Most serious adverse effects: retinopathy and aplastic anemia
- Maximizing therapeutic effects: Administer medication on the same day each week.
- Minimizing adverse effects: Administer with meals to decrease potential GI effects.
- Most important patient education: Begin prophylaxis 2 weeks before entering any area where malaria is endemic and continue for 4 to 6 weeks after leaving the area.

Mefloquine is contraindicated in persons with known hypersensitivity. In cases of overwhelming acute *P. falciparum* infections, the patient should receive an intravenous (IV) antimalarial treatment initially, followed by oral mefloquine. Mefloquine is contraindicated for use in patients with seizure disorders or psychiatric disturbances. It also is contraindicated during pregnancy because it is potentially teratogenic and embryotoxic.

The most common adverse effects of mefloquine when used in suppressive therapy are vomiting, dizziness, syncope, and extrasystoles. When it is used for acute malaria, the most common symptoms are similar to those of the disease itself, including nausea, vomiting, fever, headache, myalgias, and chills. Additional adverse effects include diarrhea, skin rash, abdominal pain, fatigue, loss of appetite, tinnitus, alopecia, sinus bradycardia, and ECG changes. Neuropsychiatric adverse effects include vertigo, visual disturbances, and psychotic manifestations such as hallucinations, nightmares, confusion, anxiety, severe mood swings, and depression.

Several important drug–drug interactions can occur with mefloquine. Concurrent use of beta blockers or quinine can result in ECG abnormalities or cardiac arrest. Coadministration with chloroquine or quinine increases the risk for seizure activity. Concurrent use with valproic acid may decrease valproic acid concentrations, resulting in loss of seizure control.

Primaquine

Primaquine is an 8-aminoquinoline. It is classified as a tissue schizonticide. The exact mechanism of action is uncertain, although it is believed to interfere with the function of plasmodial DNA. Primaquine is the only tissue schizonticide available for the radical cure of *P. vivax* and *P. ovale*. In addition to destroying exoerythrocytic (tissue) forms, primaquine prevents the development of erythrocytic (blood) forms, which cause relapses in *P. vivax*. Primaquine also is gametocidal for all four *Plasmodium* species.

Because of its potential toxicity, primaquine is not used as a first-line drug, except in cases of chloroquine-resistant malaria. Toxicity may occur when primaquine is given concurrently with other antimalarial drugs, such as quinacrine.

Primaquine is contraindicated for patients with known sensitivity. Patients with iodoquinol hypersensitivity may have cross-sensitivity to primaquine. It is administered cautiously to black Americans and ethnic groups of the Eastern Mediterranean region, in whom glucose-6-phosphate dehydrogenase (G6PD) deficiency is highly prevalent, because of its association with hematologic effects. Patients with pre-existing hematologic conditions secondary to G6PD deficiency are at risk for developing hemolytic anemia and methemoglobinemia.

Symptoms such as dark urine, anorexia, pallor, unusual tiredness or weakness, and back, leg, or abdominal pain may indicate that the patient is developing hemolytic anemia. Bluish fingernails, lips, or skin; dizziness; breathing difficulty; or unusual tiredness or weakness may indicate methemoglobinemia. This adverse effect occurs most frequently with high-dose therapy. If any of these adverse reactions occur, primaquine treatment must be discontinued immediately.

Pyrimethamine

Pyrimethamine (Daraprim) is a folic acid antagonist that blocks the protozoal enzyme dihydrofolic reductase, thereby blocking the parasite's folic acid metabolism. Like chloroquine and hydroxychloroquine, pyrimethamine is a blood schizonticide and has some tissue schizonticidal activity. However, its blood schizonticidal activity is slower than that of the 4-aminoquinoline compounds.

Pyrimethamine is used for to prevent malaria caused by susceptible strains of plasmodia. It may be used concurrently with fast-acting antimalarials, such as chloroquine, for transmission control and suppressive care but should not be used alone for an acute attack. In combination with antibiotics, it may be used for acute malaria. In combination with a sulfonamide or clindamycin, it also may be used for toxoplasmosis.

Pyrimethamine is administered orally. Distribution is mainly into kidneys, lungs, liver, and spleen, with concentrations in blood erythrocytes. It crosses the placenta and enters breast milk. Metabolism produces several unidentified metabolites that all are excreted in the urine. Urine excretion of this agent can persist for up to 30 days.

Pyrimethamine should be used cautiously in patients with anemia, folate deficiency, and suppressed bone marrow function. It is used cautiously in patients with pre-existing anemia because folic acid antagonism can potentiate anemias, especially megaloblastic anemia. Suppression of bone marrow function may result in myelosuppression, leading to leukopenia, agranulocytosis, or thrombocytopenia. Some clinicians routinely prescribe folic acid when treating toxoplasmosis because higher doses of pyrimethamine are necessary. Routine CBCs are also prudent. High doses of pyrimethamine may precipitate seizures.

Pyrimethamine should be used with extreme caution during the first 14 to 16 weeks of pregnancy. Possible interference with folic acid metabolism could cause birth defects. If its use cannot be avoided, concurrent use of folinic acid is recommended. Use during breast-feeding should be avoided because the drug may interfere with the infant's folic acid metabolism.

Common GI complaints with pyrimethamine include anorexia, nausea, vomiting, abdominal pain, and diarrhea. As with other antimalarials, taking the medication with food may decrease these symptoms.

Potential dermatologic reactions include urticaria, toxic epidermal necrolysis, exfoliative dermatitis, and Stevens-Johnson syndrome. Pyrimethamine should be discontinued at the first sign of rash.

CNS effects related to pyrimethamine therapy include weakness, ataxia, tremor, and, rarely, respiratory failure. In patients with pre-existing seizure disorders, pyrimethamine may precipitate seizures, especially in those on high-dose therapy.

Drug–drug interactions include the potential for the development of blood dyscrasias if pyrimethamine is used with other bone marrow depressants or folate antagonists. Bone marrow function may be more likely to be depressed with sulfonamide combination therapy. Other drugs that can interact with pyrimethamine in this manner include carbamazepine, clozapine, chloramphenicol, phenothiazines, procainamide, antiretroviral agents, antineoplastic agents, or antithyroid agents. Folic acid (vitamin B_9) can interfere with the action of pyrimethamine and therefore should not be used concomitantly with pyrimethamine.

Quinine Sulfate

Quinine sulfate has been used to treat malaria for more than 170 years. Quinine is substantially more toxic than chloroquine. It is active against the asexual erythrocytic forms of *Plasmodium*. It does not provide a radical cure for malaria

because it is not effective against exoerythrocytic forms of malaria.

Although the exact mechanism of action is unknown, quinine elevates the pH of parasitic acid vesicles and may upset molecular transport and phospholipase activity. Quinine is administered orally and distributes widely into liver, lungs, kidneys, and spleen, with some distribution into the cerebrospinal fluid (CSF). Although it crosses the placenta and enters breast milk, the American Academy of Pediatrics considers quinine compatible with breast-feeding.

Quinine should not be used for patients with a known allergy to quinidine. Patients with quinidine hypersensitivity may have cross-sensitivity to quinine. Quinine is a pregnancy category X drug. Quinine can cause congenital malformation and has been associated with stillbirths. In addition to the potential effects on the fetus, quinine stimulates the release of insulin and may induce hypoglycemia in pregnant women.

Quinine should not be used for patients with optic neuritis or tinnitus because it can exacerbate these conditions. Even at therapeutic dosages, quinine may cause cinchonism (tinnitus, headache, nausea, vertigo, and vision impairment).

Quinine should be used cautiously for patients with G6PD deficiency, myasthenia gravis, or cardiac arrhythmias. Patients with G6PD deficiency have a higher than usual risk for developing hemolytic anemia. Quinine produces neuromuscular blockade and can exacerbate muscular weakness and cause respiratory distress and dysphagia in myasthenic patients. Patients with cardiac arrhythmias may be at risk for developing quinine-induced dysrhythmias. Patients treated with quinine have shown prolonged Q-T intervals.

Quinine can cause several important drug–drug interactions. High doses of quinine can affect the clearance of digitalis glycosides and require dosage adjustment to avoid digoxin toxicity.

Alkalinization of the urine by acetazolamide can decrease the renal clearance of quinine, resulting in an increased risk for toxicity. Conversely, rifampin has been shown to substantially accelerate quinine clearance and reduce its half-life. Higher doses of quinine may be required in patients who are receiving rifampin.

Quinine can increase the hypoprothrombinemic (anticoagulant) effects of warfarin. The patient should be closely monitored for signs and symptoms of bleeding. Additionally, the possibility of cinchonism is increased if quinine and quinidine are administered concomitantly.

Finally, quinine should not be used concomitantly with mefloquine because additive cardiac effects can produce arrhythmias and seizures.

Drugs Significantly Different From [P] Chloroquine

Antibacterials

Antibacterial drugs, which belong to different drug classes altogether, are used in conjunction with antimalarial drugs to treat malaria. Tetracycline and doxycycline are used to eradicate *Plasmodium* in the erythrocytic stage. They are not considered first-line drugs because they work very slowly. Tetracycline is used in conjunction with quinine in treating *P. falciparum*. Doxycycline is an alternative regimen for *P. falciparum* prophylaxis in patients who cannot tolerate mefloquine. This antibacterial drug is not used to treat acute malaria. Clindamycin also is used to eradicate *Plasmodium* in the erythrocytic stage. Like tetracycline, it is used in conjunction with quinine to treat of *P. falciparum*. These three drugs are discussed in Chapter 39.

Sulfonamides

Sulfonamides also are used in managing malaria. They are generally combined with pyrimethamine. The most common drug combination is pyrimethamine and sulfadoxine (Fansidar). Fansidar is given concurrently with quinine to treat chloroquine-resistant *P. falciparum*. Sulfonamides are discussed in Chapter 40.

Atovaquone/Proguanil

Malarone is the trade name for a combination of atovaquone and proguanil hydrochloride. Atovaquone is currently marketed in the United States under the trade name Mepron as a treatment for PCP. Proguanil was approved in the United States in 1948 for use in malaria. Because it was not widely used in this country, it ceased to be marketed here in the 1970s. The advantage of Malarone is that it is effective in regions where resistance to other antimalarial drugs has developed. Another unique feature of Malarone is that it is not metabolized. It is eliminated by biliary excretion.

Malarone therapy should be started 1 or 2 days before entering a malaria-endemic area and continued daily during the stay and for 7 days after return. It should be taken at the same time each day with food or milk to increase its bioavailability. In the event of vomiting, a repeat dose should be taken within 1 hour of dosing.

Among adults who receive Malarone for malaria, the side effects can include abdominal pain, nausea, vomiting, and headache. Among pediatric patients, vomiting and itching have been reported. When Malarone is used to prevent malaria, the most common side effects are headache and abdominal pain.

C ANTIPROTOZOAN DRUGS

Antiprotozoan drugs are used to treat many human infections, including amebiasis, giardiasis, trichomoniasis, toxoplasmosis, and opportunistic infections such as PCP. The most frequently used drugs are metronidazole, iodoquinol, quinacrine hydrochloride, pentamidine, and atovaquone. Some drugs are effective for many types of infections, whereas others are effective for only one or two types of infections (Box 45.2). Because of an increase in the past decade in

BOX 45.2 Drugs Used for Protozoan Infections

Amebiasis: metronidazole, iodoquinol, paromomycin, diloxanide furoate, chloroquine
Giardiasis: metronidazole, quinacrine
Pneumocytosis: pentamidine, atovaquone, sulfamethoxazole-trimethoprim
Schistosomiasis: praziquantel, oxamniquine, metrifonate
Toxoplasmosis: metronidazole, pyrimethamine with sulfonamides
Trichomoniasis: metronidazole

protozoan infections in the United States, many new antiprotozoan drugs are being developed. Investigational drugs such as albendazole, diloxaride furoate, and dehydroemetine are obtainable only from the Centers for Disease Control and Prevention (CDC) in Atlanta, Georgia.

Drugs Affecting Amebiasis, Giardiasis, Trichomoniasis, and Toxoplasmosis

Metronidazole is the prototype antiprotozoan drug for treating amebiasis, giardiasis, and trichomoniasis. In addition to its antiprotozoan effects, metronidazole has antibacterial effects and is extremely effective against the anaerobic bacteria that cause intra-abdominal infections and *Helicobacter pylori,* which is a cause of peptic ulcer disease. For a summary of selected antiprotozoan drugs, see Table 45.3.

NURSING MANAGEMENT OF THE PATIENT RECEIVING [P] METRONIDAZOLE

Core Drug Knowledge

Pharmacotherapeutics

Metronidazole (Flagyl) is a synthetic antibacterial and antiprotozoan drug. As an antiprotozoan drug, it is used in treating *T. vaginalis,* amebiasis, and giardiasis. As an antibacterial drug, it is extremely effective against anaerobic infections. It also is useful in treating Crohn disease, antibiotic-associated diarrhea, and rosacea.

Pharmacokinetics

Metronidazole can be administered orally, intravenously, and topically. About 90% of metronidazole is absorbed orally, with food delaying but not interfering with absorption. Minimal amounts of metronidazole are absorbed systemically when it is used as an intravaginal drug. Both IV and oral metronidazole are distributed widely into most body tissues and fluids, including CSF. Metronidazole is metabolized in the liver. It crosses the placenta and enters breast milk.

Pharmacodynamics

Metronidazole has no direct effects on the human body. It is taken up readily by anaerobic organisms and cells. Its selectivity for anaerobic bacteria results from the ability of these organisms to reduce metronidazole to its active form intracellularly because the electron transport proteins necessary for this reaction are found only in anaerobic bacteria. Metronidazole acts against anaerobic bacteria by inhibiting DNA synthesis, which causes bacterial cell death.

Contraindications and Precautions

Major precautions are taken when using metronidazole in patients who are alcohol dependent or pregnant. Metronidazole enters fetal circulation rapidly. A theoretical risk remains for the fetus. Most prescribers prefer to postpone using metronidazole during pregnancy until after the first trimester.

Because of the capacity for a disulfiram-like interaction (i.e., nausea, vomiting, headache, and chest pain), ingestion of metronidazole and alcohol should be separated by at least 1 day. Patients with hepatic dysfunction should be monitored for toxicity resulting from decreased clearance and possible accumulation of metronidazole. Dosage reduction may be necessary for patients with severe hepatic dysfunction. Because metronidazole can cause leukopenia, the drug should be used with caution in patients with active or previous depression of bone marrow function.

Adverse Effects

The most common adverse effects of metronidazole are nausea and vomiting, dry mouth (xerostomia), altered sense of taste (dysgeusia), anorexia, and abdominal pain. Other consequences of xerostomia include periodontal disease and dental caries. Some patients report discolored (reddish brown) urine while taking metronidazole.

Intravenous metronidazole contains 28 mEq of sodium per gram of metronidazole, which may promote water retention and exacerbate pre-existing congestive heart failure (CHF) or peripheral edema. Oral preparations of metronidazole do not contain this large amount of sodium and can be used without jeopardy.

Other common adverse effects include CNS effects, such as dizziness, lightheadedness, and headache. CNS toxicity has occurred and is exhibited as ataxia, mood changes, encephalopathy, or clumsiness. High dosages and prolonged use of metronidazole are associated with peripheral neuropathy and seizures.

As noted previously, patients receiving metronidazole who drink alcoholic beverages may experience disulfiram-like adverse effects. The flavor of alcoholic beverages also may be altered as well.

Vaginal candidiasis occurs in some women because metronidazole can suppress natural bacteria, leading to an overgrowth of *Candida* organisms. Candidal overgrowth may also occur in the mouth. Symptoms include glossitis, stomatitis, and furry tongue.

Thrombophlebitis can occur from administration of IV metronidazole and is characterized as pain, redness, and swelling at the injection site. The potential for this adverse effect can be minimized by avoiding prolonged use of indwelling IV catheters.

Less common potential adverse effects include visual impairment, photophobia, and ocular motility disorders. Rare reports of optic neuritis have occurred. Additionally, using metronidazole may lead to blood dyscrasias and leukopenia. Pancreatitis is another serious, but rare, adverse reaction.

Drug Interactions

Metronidazole interferes with the metabolism of ethanol (alcohol), resulting in disulfiram-like effects, such as nausea, vomiting, and abdominal cramps. Patients taking disulfiram have reported psychotic reactions with concomitant use of metronidazole. Metronidazole may interact with barbiturates, anticoagulants, ethanol, and disulfiram (Table 45.4).

TABLE 45.3 Summary of Selected (C) Antiprotozoan Drugs

Drug (Trade) Name	Selected Indications	Route and Dosage Range	Pharmacokinetics
P metronidazole (Flagyl; *Canadian:* Apo-Metronidazole)	Anaerobic bacterial infection	*Adult:* IV, 15 mg/kg infused over 1 h, then 7.5 mg/kg infused over 1 h every 6 h for 7–10 d; not to exceed 4 g/d *Child:* IV, not recommended	*Onset:* PO, varies; IV, rapid *Duration:* Variable $t_{1/2}$: 6–8 h
	Amebiasis	*Adult:* PO, 750 mg tid for 5–10 d *Child:* PO, 35–50 mg/kg in three divided doses for 10 d	
	Trichomoniasis	*Adult:* PO, 2 g at one time for 250 mg tid for 7–10 d	
	Bacterial prophylaxis	*Adult:* IV, 15 mg/kg infused over 30–60 min and completed about 1 h before surgery, then 7.5 mg/kg infused over 30–60 min at 6 to 12-h intervals after initial dose during the day of surgery	
	Gardnerella vaginalis	*Adult:* PO, 500 mg bid for 7 d	
	Antibiotic-associated pseudomembranous colitis	*Adult:* PO, 1–2 g/d for 7–10 d	
	Inflammatory papules, pustules, and erythema of rosacea	*Adult:* Topical, apply and rub in a thin film twice daily, morning and evening, to entire affected areas after washing	
		Adult and child: IM/IV, 4 mg/kg once a day for 14 d by deep IM injection or IV infusion over 60 min *Adult and child:* Inhalational, 300 mg once every 4 wk administered by nebulizer (e.g., Respirgard II)	
P pentamidine (NebuPent, Pentam 300; *Canadian:* Pentacarinate)	PCP	*Adult and child:* Inhalational, 300 mg once every 4 wk with Respirgard nebulizer; IM/IV 4 mg/kg once daily for 14 d by deep IM injection or IV infusion over 60 min	*Onset:* Inhalation, rapid; IM, slow *Duration:* 6–8 wk $t_{1/2}$: 6.5–9.5 h
atovaquone (Mepron)	PCP	*Adult:* PO, 750 mg, tid for 21 d	*Onset:* Varies *Duration:* 3–5 d $t_{1/2}$: 2–3 d
iodoquinol (Yodoxin; *Canadian:* Diodoxaquin)	Amebiasis	*Adult:* PO, 650 mg tid before meals for 20 d *Child:* PO, 40 mg/kg/d in three divided doses before meals for 20 d, not to exceed 1.95 g/d	*Onset:* Minimal absorption *Duration:* Unknown $t_{1/2}$: Unknown
quinacrine (Atabrine)	Malaria	*Adult and child >8 y:* PO, 200 mg with 1 g sodium bicarbonate every 6 h for 5 doses; then 100 mg every 8 h for 6 d. The maximum dose is 2.8 g in 7 d *Child 4–8 y:* PO, 200 mg every 8 h; then 100 mg every 12 h for 6 d *Child 1–4 y:* PO, 100 mg every 8 h; then 100 mg daily for 6 d	*Onset:* Unknown *Duration:* 4–6 wk $t_{1/2}$: 5 d
	Giardiasis	*Adult:* PO, 100 mg tid for 5–7 d *Child:* PO, 7 mg/kg/d in 3 divided doses for 5 d	
quinacrine	Cestodiasis	*Adults and child >14 y:* PO, 4 doses of 200 mg given 10 min apart with 600 mg of sodium bicarbonate given with each dose *Child 11–14 y:* PO, 600 mg in 3–4 divided doses given 10 min apart with 300 mg of sodium bicarbonate given with each dose *Child 5–10 y:* PO, 400 mg in 3–4 divided doses given 10 min apart with 300 mg of sodium bicarbonate given with each dose	

TABLE 45.4 Agents That Interact With P Metronidazole

Interactants	Effect and Significance	Nursing Management
anticoagulants	Hepatic metabolism of anticoagulants may be decreased by metronidazole, resulting in enhanced effects of the anticoagulant. This may induce hemorrhage.	Monitor patients more frequently, and teach them to recognize signs and symptoms of bleeding. Notify the prescriber who may need to prescribe a lower dose of anticoagulant.
barbiturates	Barbiturates may induce a faster elimination of metronidazole, resulting in therapeutic failure of metronidazole.	Observe for treatment failure in patients receiving a barbiturate concurrently with metronidazole. If necessary, the metronidazole dose may need to be increased accordingly. Alternatively, the prescriber may order a higher initial metronidazole dose.
disulfiram	The coadministration of disulfiram and metronidazole may result in an acute psychosis or confusional state. The mechanism of the interaction is unclear.	Monitor patients closely for signs of confusion. Discontinue both agents if symptoms occur. Avoid coadministration.
ethanol	Metronidazole can inhibit alcohol dehydrogenase and other alcohol-metabolizing enzymes. This can lead to an accumulation of drug in the blood and the development of disulfiram-like side effects.	Caution patient to avoid ethanol during therapy and 1–2 d after therapy stops.

Assessment of Relevant Core Patient Variables

Health Status

Before administering metronidazole, assess the patient for potential medical conditions that contraindicate use or require close monitoring, such as alcoholism, cardiac disease, dental disease, hepatic disease, seizure disorders, and depressed bone marrow function.

Perform a baseline neurologic assessment because metronidazole may cause CNS toxicity or exacerbate peripheral neuropathy and seizure disorders. In addition, a baseline visual acuity assessment may be needed. Other important assessments include liver function tests, because metronidazole is metabolized in the liver, and a CBC, particularly for patients with a history of depressed bone marrow function or severe anemia. The patient's drug history must be reviewed to identify drugs that may interact with metronidazole.

Life Span and Gender

Assess women for possible pregnancy because metronidazole is not recommended in the first trimester. Metronidazole enters breast milk and is not recommended for use in children or infants.

Lifestyle, Diet, and Habits

Determining the patient's typical intake of alcohol is important. Caution patients to refrain from alcohol ingestion for 48 hours after completing metronidazole therapy. They should also be reminded that many OTC products contain alcohol, so that they should avoid taking OTC drugs without consulting their health care providers.

Environment

Be aware of the setting in which metronidazole will be administered. Hospitalized patients usually receive metronidazole by IV infusion. Monitor the patient's cardiovascular and respiratory status frequently because IV metronidazole may promote fluid retention, leading to an exacerbation of CHF or peripheral edema. Also, monitor the IV site frequently for signs of thrombophlebitis.

Nursing Diagnoses and Outcomes

- Risk for Deficient Fluid Volume: Anorexia, nausea, vomiting, and diarrhea related to drug administration
  Desired outcome: *The patient will maintain adequate hydration throughout therapy.*
- Risk for Disturbed Sensory Perception: Drug-induced dizziness, vertigo, syncope, and ataxia
  Desired outcome: *The patient will compensate for sensory-perceptual disturbances by moving slowly and carefully to prevent accidents and asking for help with ambulation as needed.*
- Disturbed Thought Processes: Acute confusional state related to potential disulfiram-like interaction
  Desired outcome: *The patient will refrain from alcohol consumption for 48 hours after completing drug therapy.*
- Risk for Injury: Potential teratogenic effects related to drug administration
  Desired outcome: *The patient will act to prevent conception while taking metronidazole.*

Planning and Intervention

Maximizing Therapeutic Effects

To avoid reinfection, patients taking metronidazole for *Trichomonas* infection need to understand that their sexual partners must be treated at the same time. To avoid early cessation of therapy, advise the patient that the drug may discolor the urine and reassure the patient that this discoloration is harmless.

Minimizing Adverse Effects

Because some patients will downplay their intake of ethanol or neglect to mention they take disulfiram because of the social stigma attached to alcoholism, emphasize the importance of potential adverse effects resulting from the interaction of ethanol and metronidazole.

To minimize possible GI irritation, metronidazole may be administered with meals. Patients who experience dry mouth can use sugar-free hard candies or ice chips to moisten the mouth. Sugar-containing products tend to promote dental caries in dry mouth, an environment that is already friendly to decay-causing organisms. IV metronidazole must be infused slowly over 1 hour.

Providing Patient and Family Education

- Create teaching plans that focus on explaining the potential adverse effects (such as, GI upset, altered taste, discolored urine), adapting to adverse effects (taking drug with meals to relieve GI upset), and identifying which effects to report to the prescriber. For example, candidal overgrowth, ataxia, easy bruising, or bleeding may represent adverse effects that require immediate intervention.
- Discuss the importance of refraining from ethanol or disulfiram use during metronidazole therapy.
- For patients taking metronidazole for giardiasis, stress the importance of treating sex partners simultaneously for trichomonal infections and of having follow-up stool examinations.
- Emphasize the need for birth control measures for women taking metronidazole long-term.

Ongoing Assessment and Evaluation

When administering intravenous metronidazole, monitor for thrombophlebitis and signs of edema or CHF. When administering oral metronidazole, monitor all patients for signs of oral candidiasis (white spots in the mouth) and women for symptoms of vaginal candidiasis.

Additional evaluative assessments include monitoring for signs and symptoms of peripheral neuropathy (numbness and tingling of the extremities) and CNS toxicity (mood changes and irritability).

For patients on prolonged therapy, arrange for periodic CBCs and liver function tests as well as tests for visual acuity. Remind the patient to schedule frequent dental checkups.

For patients with giardiasis, arrange testing of three stool specimens, taken several days apart. Three negative stool test results indicate successful metronidazole therapy.

MEMORY CHIP

P Metronidazole

- Used for *Trichomonas vaginalis*, amebiasis, giardiasis, and anaerobic infections
- Major contraindications: alcohol dependency and pregnancy
- Most common adverse effects: nausea, vomiting, xerostomia, and dysgeusia
- Most serious adverse effect: blood dyscrasias
- Maximizing therapeutic effects: Treat both partners at the same time.
- Minimizing adverse effects: Assess alcohol intake closely.
- Most important patient education: reinforce the need to refrain from alcohol intake during therapy.

Drugs Significantly Different From P Metronidazole

Iodoquinol

Iodoquinol (Yodoxin) is an oral antiprotozoan agent used to treat intestinal amebiasis. It exerts its action directly in the large intestine, although the exact mechanism of this action is unknown. Iodoquinol is active against both the trophozoite and encysted forms of the parasite. It can be used alone in mild cases or in asymptomatic carriers. In more severe cases, it should be used in combination with other amebicidal drugs.

Adverse effects associated with iodoquinol include mild GI disturbances, skin disorders, discoloration of hair and nails, thyroid enlargement, fever, chills, headache, vertigo, and malaise. Neurotoxicity from iodoquinol may induce optic neuritis, optic atrophy, and peripheral neuropathy.

Protein-bound serum iodine levels may increase during iodoquinol treatment, and therapy may therefore interfere with certain thyroid function tests. These effects may persist for up to 6 months after therapy discontinues.

Paromomycin

Paromomycin (Humatin) is not an antiprotozoan drug; it is an oral aminoglycoside antibiotic with broad-spectrum antibacterial and amebicidal activity. Paromomycin is used for extraintestinal amebiasis and tapeworm infestation. It is absorbed poorly from the GI tract and thus is used only for intestinal forms of amebiasis and helminths.

Adverse GI effects of paromomycin include anorexia, nausea, vomiting, gastric burning and pain, abdominal cramps, and diarrhea. The only important drug–drug interaction with paromomycin occurs with succinylcholine. When given in combination, paromomycin may potentiate the neuromuscular effects of succinylcholine.

Quinacrine

Quinacrine (Atabrine) is an oral antiprotozoan agent used most commonly to treat giardiasis. It also has been used to treat malaria and cestodiasis, although more efficacious drugs are currently used for those disorders. Quinacrine is absorbed readily from the GI tract and concentrates primarily in the liver. Quinacrine is metabolized and excreted slowly. It may be detected in the urine up to 2 months after therapy has been discontinued.

Because quinacrine achieves high concentrations in the liver, it should be used with caution in patients with hepatic disease, other hepatotoxic drugs, or alcoholism. Quinacrine should be used with caution in patients with psoriasis and porphyria because it can exacerbate these conditions. Quinacrine should be administered with caution to infants (younger than 1 year) and to patients with renal disease and severe renal impairment, cardiac disease, or G6PD deficiency. Quinacrine should be used with caution in patients with a history of psychosis and in patients older than 60 years because the drug can

cause a transient psychosis in these patients. Other potential neuropsychiatric disturbances include nightmares, restlessness, confusion, anxiety, irritability, euphoria, aggressive behavior, nervousness, and emotional changes.

When small doses of quinacrine are taken, potential adverse effects include mild headache, dizziness, and GI disturbances. Large doses of quinacrine can produce adverse effects such as severe headache and GI disturbances, including nausea and vomiting, abdominal pain or cramps, and mild diarrhea. Other adverse side effects during therapy with quinacrine include blood dyscrasias, hepatitis (and elevated hepatic enzymes), aplastic anemia, pancytopenia, fainting, seizures, and retinopathy.

Quinacrine may induce integumentary adverse effects such as urticaria, black and blue skin and nail discoloration, exfoliative dermatitis, and contact dermatitis. It temporarily imparts a yellow color to the urine and skin.

Quinacrine may potentiate the toxicity of aminoquinolines such as primaquine and chloroquine. Quinacrine is metabolized extensively in the liver. Therefore, it should be given cautiously with other drugs that may induce hepatotoxicity, such as acetaminophen.

Drugs Affecting *Pneumocystis Carinii* Pneumonia

Drugs used to treat PCP include pentamidine isethionate, atovaquone, and sulfamethoxazole-trimethoprim (SMZ-TMP). SMZ-TMP is not an antiprotozoan drug but an antibiotic (see Chapter 41). Patients at high risk for PCP (low T-cell count or high viral load count) and those unable to take SMZ-TMP (also known as cotrimoxazole) should be maintained on a prophylactic dosage of pentamidine. The prototype antiprotozoan drug for prophylaxis and treatment of PCP is pentamidine isethionate.

NURSING MANAGEMENT OF THE PATIENT RECEIVING P PENTAMIDINE ISETHIONATE

Core Drug Knowledge

Pharmacotherapeutics

Historically, pentamidine (Pentam 300) was used only for trypanosomiasis (African sleeping sickness) and leishmaniasis. Currently, pentamidine is an important therapeutic drug for prophylaxis and treatment of PCP.

Pharmacokinetics

Pentamidine is absorbed readily and binds to body tissues. It is sequestered in the liver and kidney and eliminated unchanged by the kidneys. Pentamidine can be detected in the urine up to 8 weeks after therapy has ended.

Pharmacodynamics

Pentamidine is administered by inhalation or parenterally. Its mechanism of action is unclear, but it appears to interfere with nucleotide, phospholipid, and protein synthesis of the parasite. It causes local tissue damage when given intramuscularly and is therefore usually given intravenously. For prophylaxis, pentamidine is delivered by inhalation through an aerosol device to the alveoli where *P. carinii* lodges.

Contraindications and Precautions

Pentamidine is contraindicated for use in patients with a history of an anaphylactic reaction to it. However, once the diagnosis of PCP is established, no absolute contraindications apply. The drug is given with caution to patients with asthma; hematologic disorders; cardiac, hepatic, and renal diseases; and diabetes mellitus.

Adverse Effects

Sudden severe effects may develop after a single dose of pentamidine. Patients should be lying down and monitored closely during administration. Equipment for emergency resuscitation should be readily available.

The most frequent adverse effects from pentamidine are cough and bronchospasm, especially in patients with asthma. Another frequent adverse reaction to pentamidine is a sudden, severe hypotension.

Thrombocytopenia, leukopenia, and anemia are potential hematologic problems; arrhythmias, tachycardia, torsades de pointes, or other adverse cardiac effects may occur as well. Pentamidine is toxic to pancreatic cells. When receiving IV pentamidine, patients with diabetes mellitus can become acutely hypoglycemic immediately after the infusion. Additionally, pentamidine may precipitate pancreatitis. Pentamidine also can cause elevations in aspartate transaminase (AST), alanine transaminase (ALT), bilirubin, and alkaline phosphatase. Patients with pre-existing hepatic diseases are more vulnerable to these effects. Pentamidine can cause azotemia and acute renal insufficiency as well.

Drug Interactions

Concomitant use of other drugs associated with suppression of bone marrow function, electrolyte imbalance, pancreatitis, or nephrotoxicity may cause additive effects. Pentamidine also may interact with drugs that have similar adverse effects (Table 45.5).

Assessment of Relevant Core Patient Variables

Health Status

Assess for concurrent drug use that is potentially nephrotoxic. Obtain and review baseline measurements. These measurements include vital signs (especially blood pressure), CBC, hepatic and renal function values, and glucose and amylase levels.

Closely monitor administration of aerosolized pentamidine to patients with a history of asthma because the drug may induce bronchospasm and acute asthma.

Lifestyle, Diet, and Habits

It is important to assess lifestyle because patients at risk for PCP and diseases associated with compromised immune function include IV drug abusers, men who have sex with men, and people with multiple sex partners. Immunocompromised patients may be taking multiple drugs, placing them at risk for potential hematologic, renal, and hepatic

TABLE 45.5 Agents That Interact With P Pentamidine

Interactants	Effect and Significance	Nursing Management
Bone Marrow Suppressants		
antineoplastic agents azathioprine carbamazepine clozapine cotrimoxazole phenothiazines zidovudine	Concomitant use of bone marrow suppressants and pentamidine has the potential to cause additive hemotoxicity.	Monitor for sore throat, easy bruising, or bleeding. Monitor CBC and platelet counts.
Diuretics		
loop diuretics thiazide diuretics	Diuretics and pentamidine can produce similar toxicities.	Monitor for hypokalemia, hypomagnesemia, and pancreatitis. Monitor serum electrolyte and amylase levels.
Drugs That May Cause Nephrotoxicity		
aminoglycosides amphotericin B cyclosporine vancomycin	Drugs associated with nephrotoxicity and pentamidine have the potential for causing additive renal toxicity.	Monitor for nephrotoxicity, hypokalemia, hypomagnesemia, and bone marrow depression.
Drugs That May Cause Pancreatitis		
azathioprine didanosine estrogens furosemide tetracycline valproic acid	Drugs associated with pancreatitis and pentamidine have the potential for causing additive pancreatic toxicity.	Monitor for signs of pancreatitis. Monitor amylase levels.

toxicities. Because pentamidine also may affect these systems, monitor patients closely for adverse effects.

Environment

Note the environment in which pentamidine will be administered. Many patients receive IV or aerosolized pentamidine therapy at home.

Nursing Diagnoses and Outcomes

- Ineffective Protection: Risk for drug-induced leukopenia, thrombocytopenia, and anemia
  Desired outcome: *The patient will report any signs and symptoms of blood abnormalities (i.e., unusual fatigue, fever and infection, and bruising).*
- Risk for Deficient Fluid Volume related to drug-induced nausea, vomiting, and anorexia
  Desired outcome: *The patient will remain adequately hydrated throughout therapy.*
- Risk for Injury: Hypoglycemia, hyperglycemia, or acute renal failure related to drug therapy and bronchospasm, cough, hypotension, or cardiovascular complications related to drug administration
  Desired outcome: *The patient will remain free of injury or complications related to pentamidine administration.*

Planning and Intervention

Maximizing Therapeutic Effects

Intravenous pentamidine should be protected from the light and used within 24 hours of preparation. It should not be mixed with other drugs, because of incompatibilities; nor should it be mixed with saline solutions because a precipitate will form. When pentamidine is administered by inhalation, a bronchodilator can be given before treatment to reduce bronchospasm and increase drug effectiveness.

Minimizing Adverse Effects

Administer pentamidine with the patient lying down. Baseline vital signs are obtained initially and monitored continuously during the infusion, and then every 2 hours after the infusion until blood pressure stabilizes. Patients receiving pentamidine should not receive IM injections because they may cause bleeding, bruising, or hematomas as a result of thrombocytopenia secondary to pentamidine-induced depression of bone marrow function. Pentamidine should not be administered at bedtime because hypoglycemia may occur at a time when the patient cannot respond to the symptoms.

Appropriate respiratory precautions must be taken to protect health care staff from contact with organisms, such as *Mycobacteria,* that may be aerosolized if the patient coughs.

Providing Patient and Family Education

- Make sure that the patient and family understand the therapeutic and adverse effects of pentamidine and the importance of monthly treatments for PCP prophylaxis. In addition, they need to realize that PCP infection is still possible despite pentamidine prophylaxis.
- Urge the patient to contact the prescriber if fever or respiratory difficulties occur. Other conditions for which the patient should contact the prescriber include nausea, vomiting, or diarrhea that does not subside; persistent urinary frequency, inability to void, continual hunger and thirst, or unexplained weight loss; and abdominal pain, leg cramps, fever, sore throat, unexplained bruising, or extreme fatigue.
- Emphasize the need for small, frequent meals despite the patient's anorexia.

Ongoing Assessment and Evaluation

Care of hospitalized patients includes monitoring blood urea nitrogen, serum creatinine, serum calcium, and blood glucose levels; CBC and platelet counts; and liver function test results (including bilirubin, alkaline phosphatase, AST, and ALT levels) on a daily basis. ECGs should be scheduled at regular intervals throughout therapy. It is important to measure daily fluid intake and output.

Drug Significantly Different From P Pentamidine

Oral atovaquone is indicated for the acute treatment of mild to moderate *P. carinii* in patients who are intolerant to SMZ-TMP (cotrimoxazole). Atovaquone is roughly equivalent to IV pentamidine, but less effective than cotrimoxazole, for treating PCP.

Atovaquone is unique among agents used to manage PCP because it can kill *Pneumocystis* organisms rather than merely inhibiting their growth. Besides *Pneumocystis,* atovaquone is active against other protozoans including *Plasmodium* species, *Toxoplasma gondii, Entamoeba histolytica, Trichomonas vaginalis, Leishmania* species, and microsporidia. The antiprotozoan activity of atovaquone is probably related to its ability to selectively inhibit mitochondrial electron transport, leading to inhibition of pyrimidine synthesis.

Atovaquone is absorbed poorly from the GI tract. It is a highly lipophilic compound; thus, administering it with a fatty meal will improve its absorption. Because many patients who are treated with atovaquone have advanced human immunodeficiency virus (HIV) infection, distinguishing adverse effects caused by atovaquone from those caused by underlying medical conditions is often difficult. No life-threatening effects have yet been attributed to atovaquone.

MEMORY CHIP

P Pentamidine

- Used for prophylaxis and management of PCP
- Major contraindication: previous anaphylactic reactions to the drug
- Most common adverse effects: cough and bronchospasm
- Most serious adverse effects: cardiac abnormalities, renal failure, and suppressions of bone marrow function
- Maximizing therapeutic effects: Protect from light and administer within 24 hours of preparation.
- Minimizing adverse effects: Monitor blood pressure throughout administration.
- Most important patient education: Contact the health care provider if fever or respiratory difficulties occur; PCP may occur despite prophylactic treatment.

C ANTHELMINTHIC DRUGS

As discussed previously, helminthic infections result from cestodes, nematodes, and trematodes. The most commonly used anthelminthic drugs are mebendazole, thiabendazole, niclosamide, pyrantel pamoate, diethylcarbamazine, oxamniquine, and praziquantel. Box 45.3 summarizes which drugs are used to treat the various types of helminths.

Of all the drugs in the class, the prototype for treating most helminths is mebendazole (Vermox). Mebendazole is indicated to treat infection with cestodes and nematodes, such as pinworm, whipworm, common roundworm, common hookworm, and American hookworm. It also is used to treat enterobiasis. Mebendazole is usually the drug of choice in helminthic infections because mixed infections are common. Table 45.6 presents a summary of selected anthelminthic drugs.

NURSING MANAGEMENT OF THE PATIENT RECEIVING P MEBENDAZOLE

Core Drug Knowledge

Pharmacotherapeutics

Mebendazole is an oral, broad-spectrum, synthetic anthelminthic drug. It is particularly effective against susceptible GI nematodes, such as whipworms, pinworms, and hookworms. Mebendazole, like pyrantel pamoate, is considered a drug of choice for treating infections caused by these nematodes.

BOX 45.3 Which Drug for Which Worm?

Most antihelminthic agents are effective against many types of helminths; only a few have limited application. The following helminths are controlled by the following drugs:

- Intestinal nematodes: mebendazole, thiabendazole, albendazole, ivermectin, pyrantel
- Blood and tissue nematodes: diethylcarbamazine, ivermectin
- Trematodes: praziquantel, oxamniquine
- Cestodes: praziquantel, niclosamide

TABLE 45.6 Summary of Selected (C) Anthelminthic Drugs

Drug (Trade) Name	Selected Indications	Route and Dosage Range	Pharmacokinetics
[P] mebendazole (Vermox)	Trichuriasis, ascariasis, hookworm infections	*Adult:* PO, 100 mg bid for 3 consecutive d *Child >2 y:* same as adults; *<2 y,* safety and efficacy not established	*Onset:* Under 2 h *Duration:* 48 h $t_{1/2}$: 3–9 h
	Enterobiasis	*Adult:* PO, 100 mg once; if not cured in 3 wk, a second dose may be given	
diethylcarbamazine (Hetrazan)	Ascariasis	*Adult:* PO, 13 mg/kg/d for 7–10 d *Child:* PO, 6–10 mg/kg tid for 7–10 d	*Onset:* 1 h *Duration:* Variable
	Filariasis	*Adult:* PO, 6–10 mg/kg tid pc for 3–4 weeks	$t_{1/2}$: 8 h
niclosamide (Niclocide)	Beef or fish tapeworm	*Adult:* PO, 2 g as a single dose *Child 11–34 kg:* PO, 1 g as a single dose; *> 34 kg,* 1.5 g as a single dose	*Onset:* Minimal absorption *Duration:* Unknown $t_{1/2}$: Unknown
	Dwarf tapeworm	*Adult:* PO, 2 g daily for 7 d *Child 11–34 kg:* PO, 1 g as a single dose; *>34 kg,* 1.5 g on day 1, then 1 g for the next 6 d	
oxamniquine (Vancil)	Strains of *S. mansoni*	*Adult:* PO, 12–15 mg/kg as a single dose *Child 30–40 kg:* PO, 500 mg; *41–60 kg,* 750 mg; *61–80 kg,* 1,000 mg; *81–100 kg,* 1,250 mg	*Onset:* Rapid *Duration:* 24 h $t_{1/2}$: 1–2.5 h
praziquantell (Biltricide)	Schistosomiasis	*Adult:* PO, 60 mg/kg in three equally divided doses as a 1-day treatment with 4–6 h between doses *Child:* Safety and efficacy not established	*Onset:* Rapid *Duration:* Unknown $t_{1/2}$: 0.8–1.5 h
	Clonorchiasis and opisthorchiasis	*Adult:* PO, 75 mg/kg in three equally divided doses as a 1-day treatment *Child:* Safety and efficacy not established	
pyrantel pamoate (Antiminth; *Canadian:* Combantrin)	Pinworm and roundworm infections	*Adult:* PO, 11 mg/kg as a single dose; maximum dose of 1 g *Child >2 y:* PO, same as adults; *<2 y,* safety and efficacy not established	*Onset:* Poorly absorbed *Duration:* Unknown $t_{1/2}$: Unknown
thiabendazole (Mintezol)	Enterobiasis	*Adult <150 lb and child >30 lb:* PO, 10 mg/kg per dose, *>150 lb,* PO, 1.5 g/dose; maximum daily dose, 3 g two doses/day for 1 d; repeat in 7 d to reduce risk of reinfection	*Onset:* Rapid *Duration:* 24 h $t_{1/2}$: 1.2 h

Pharmacokinetics

Mebendazole is absorbed minimally from the GI tract because of substantial first-pass metabolism. It is metabolized to an inactive metabolite. Approximately 10% of the drug is excreted unchanged in the urine, and the remainder is excreted in the feces.

Pharmacodynamics

Direct pharmacodynamics occurs in the parasite. Mebendazole is a broad-spectrum anthelminthic, available in chewable tablets. It selectively damages cytoplasmic microtubules in the absorptive and intestinal cells of the helminth but not in those of the host. This microtubular deterioration is irreversible and leads to disruption of absorptive and secretory functions of the cells that are essential to the helminth's survival. Efficacy varies, depending on pre-existing diarrhea and GI transit time, degree of infection, and helminth strains.

Contraindications and Precautions

Mebendazole is contraindicated in patients with hypersensitivity to the drug, and it is used with caution in patients with inflammatory bowel disease or hepatic disease and during pregnancy, especially during the first trimester. In patients with Crohn disease or ulcerative colitis, drug absorption, and therefore the risk for toxicity, is increased. Mebendazole is metabolized primarily by the liver and can accumulate in patients with hepatic impairment, increasing the risk for adverse effects. Because it is not known whether mebendazole is excreted in breast milk, the drug is used with caution in breast-feeding mothers. It has not been evaluated for use in children younger than 2 years old.

Adverse Effects

Because of its poor absorption, mebendazole rarely causes systemic toxicity, except in patients with diseases that increase absorption of drugs from the bowel. Transient abdominal

pain, diarrhea, dizziness, headache, and fever are common. However, these symptoms may result from expulsion of worms rather from the drug. Other reported adverse effects include blood abnormalities, such as leukopenia, thrombocytopenia, and eosinophilia. Integumentary effects include pruritus, rash, and flushing. In the renal system, hematuria and crystalluria are possible. In addition, mebendazole may elevate liver enzyme levels.

Drug Interactions

Mebendazole may interact with anticonvulsant drugs, such as carbamazepine and the hydantoins. Although the mechanism of interaction is unknown, mebendazole's pharmacologic effects may be decreased, resulting in failure to eradicate the helminth. However, no special precautions appear necessary. If an interaction is suspected, dosage may have to be increased.

Assessment of Relevant Core Patient Variables

Health Status

Assess the patient for medical conditions that contraindicate or require close monitoring during therapy. Additional assessments should be made to prepare for potential drug interactions. Helminth specimens should be collected to ensure that mebendazole will be therapeutic. A baseline CBC is needed because mebendazole may cause blood abnormalities.

Patients with a history of Crohn disease or ulcerative colitis should be monitored closely. Patients in whom the bowel lumen is no longer intact may absorb mebendazole in toxic quantities.

Life Span and Gender

Assess for pregnancy and lactation, and determine the age of the patient, before administering mebendazole. Laboratory studies show that even one dose of mebendazole is teratogenic and embryotoxic. Therefore, it should not be given during pregnancy. Because it has not been adequately tested in children younger than 2 years of age, it should not be given to them or to breast-feeding women.

Environment

Evaluate the patient's close contacts because helminthic infections are highly contagious. Ideally, all family members are treated simultaneously, and care is taken to disinfect clothing and bedding.

Nursing Diagnoses and Outcomes

- Acute Pain related to headache, abdominal discomfort, rash, and perianal itching from drug therapy
  Desired outcome: *The patient will adopt measures to help tolerate therapy, including taking acetaminophen for headache, taking with food if GI distress occurs, and applying cream if indicated to sooth perianal itching.*
- Risk for Deficient Fluid Volume related to drug-induced diarrhea
  Desired outcome: *Unless contraindicated, the patient will maintain fluid intake to prevent dehydration.*

Planning and Intervention

Maximizing Therapeutic Effects

Anthelminthic tablets may be crushed and mixed with applesauce or other food. Chewing the drug offers the greatest effectiveness, as does taking the drug with fatty foods, such as milk, cheese, or ice cream. All family members and close patient contacts should be treated at the same time to avoid reinfection.

Minimizing Adverse Effects

Mebendazole may be given with small, frequent meals if GI distress occurs. Recommend soothing oatmeal baths to relieve pruritus or rash because antihistamines are not effective. Relaxation techniques or acetaminophen may be used to manage headaches or constant GI distress. Unless contraindicated, fluid intake may be increased to at least eight 8-oz glasses of fluid daily to minimize the potential for crystalluria.

Providing Patient and Family Education

- Provide information about potential adverse drug effects, such as anemia and other blood problems signaled by sore throat, fever, and fatigue. In addition, stress the importance of contacting the prescriber if serious adverse effects occur. Explain that minor adverse effects, such as itching, may be relieved with oatmeal baths.
- Urge the patient to follow the instructions of the prescriber; printed directions may be given if appropriate.
- To prevent treatment failure, encourage the patient to complete the full course of drug therapy.
- To prevent future infections, urge the patient to wear shoes and wash all fruits and vegetables well before eating. Moreover, it is important to teach the patient about hygiene (such as laundering infested bedclothes and undergarments daily) and other measures that help to prevent reinfection.

Ongoing Assessment and Evaluation

Evaluation of nursing care includes monitoring to ensure that the helminth has been eradicated and for complications of therapy, such as dehydration in instances of severe nausea and vomiting; sore throat, fever, and easy bruising; and hematuria or crystalluria. Periodic CBC counts and liver function tests should be performed for patients at risk for hematologic or hepatic effects and for patients on long-term therapy.

MEMORY CHIP

P Mebendazole

- Used for management of helminthic infections
- Major contraindication: hypersensitivity
- Most common adverse effects: abdominal pain, diarrhea, dizziness, and headache
- Most serious adverse effect: blood dyscrasias
- Maximizing therapeutic effects: Treat all family members at the same time.
- Minimizing adverse effects: small, frequent meals to decrease GI effects
- Most important patient education: Wash all clothing and bed linens at the same time the whole family is being treated.

Drugs Closely Related to P Mebendazole

Albendazole

Albendazole (Albenza), an oral agent, is not available routinely in the United States and is not approved by the FDA. However, it can be obtained from the CDC in Atlanta. It is well absorbed from the GI tract and relatively free of adverse effects. Like mebendazole, it is teratogenic and has not been tested for use in children. In most clinical trials, it has been shown to be more efficacious than mebendazole in treating intestinal and systemic nematodes. In limited trials, it has been effective against systemic cestode infections, which have been historically refractory to chemotherapy.

Thiabendazole

Thiabendazole (Mintezol) is a vermicidal drug related structurally to mebendazole. It has more limited usefulness than mebendazole because of its potential toxicity. The precise mechanism of action is not clear. It inhibits specific enzymes in the helminth and is used to treat pinworm, roundworm, threadworm, and hookworm infections. It is the drug of choice for strongyloidiasis.

Because thiabendazole is better absorbed than mebendazole from the bowel, adverse effects are more common than with mebendazole. It is used with caution in children weighing less than 15 kg, in patients with hepatic or renal dysfunction, and in patients with severe dehydration, malnutrition, or anemia.

Drugs Significantly Different From P Mebendazole

Pyrantel Pamoate

Like mebendazole, pyrantel pamoate (Antiminth) is used to treat pinworm and roundworm infections. Unlike mebendazole, pyrantel pamoate exhibits a selective depolarizing neuromuscular blocking action that causes spastic paralysis of worms.

Pyrantel is administered as an oral suspension that is absorbed poorly from the GI tract. Because of its poor absorption, it is well tolerated by patients older than 2 years. It is metabolized in the liver and excreted mainly in feces and secondarily in urine.

Pyrantel is used with caution in patients who have liver dysfunction, anemia, or both and in patients who are malnourished or dehydrated. Its safety has not been proved during pregnancy or for children younger than 2 years of age. Pyrantel and piperazine are mutually antagonistic and should not be given together because each blocks the other's activity.

Piperazine

Another drug used in treating roundworms and pinworms is piperazine. It differs from mebendazole in its mechanism of action: it works by hyperpolarizing the parasite's membranes, which produces flaccid paralysis. The parasites are not killed by the drug but are expelled from the host by normal peristalsis.

Also unlike mebendazole, piperazine may be used during pregnancy. However, it has the potential for producing neurotoxicity and is contraindicated in patients who have seizures. It is an antagonist to pyrantel.

Diethylcarbamazine

Diethylcarbamazine (Hetrazan) is the only drug currently used for suppressing and curing bancroftian and brugian filariasis. It works in two ways. First, it decreases muscular activity in the microfilariae and eventually paralyzes them. It also causes changes in the microfilarial surface that make the parasite more susceptible to the host's immune responses.

Common adverse effects include nausea and vomiting, anorexia, and headache. Another type of reaction, caused by the dying microfilariae, is called the Mazzotti reaction. This reaction is characterized by severe itching, papular rash, tachycardia, and an intense headache. Rapid drug-induced death of *Onchocerca volvulus* microfilariae in the eye can result in permanent loss of vision.

Praziquantel

Praziquantel (Biltricide) is used in treating infection with schistosomes: flukes and tapeworms. It increases the helminths' permeability to calcium, thereby causing contracture and paralysis of the helminth.

Adverse effects are minimal; the most common include malaise, headache, dizziness, and abdominal discomfort. Patients should be warned not to drive a car or operate machinery on the day of treatment and the day after. Praziquantel did not exhibit mutagenicity, carcinogenicity, or teratogenicity in animal trials. However, prescribers advise breastfeeding women to refrain from nursing on the day of treatment and for 72 hours thereafter.

Oxamniquine

Oxamniquine (Vansil) is a tetrahydroquinoline derivative that is effective against *Schistosoma mansoni* infections, although it is ineffective against other helminths. This selectivity restricts its use. It is thought to act through a reaction that affects the macromolecules of the parasite.

Administered orally, oxamniquine is absorbed readily from the GI tract. Absorption is slowed by the presence of food, yet the drug is better tolerated after a meal. The major adverse effects are dizziness, drowsiness, nausea, and diarrhea. Oxamniquine should be given with caution to patients with pre-existing seizure disorders because its use has been associated with convulsions. It is contraindicated in pregnancy.

Niclosamide

Niclosamide (Niclocide) differs from mebendazole both in its therapeutic effects and mechanism of action. Used to treat cestodes, it inhibits oxidative phosphorylation in the cestodal mitochondria. Contact with the drug kills the tapeworm's scolex and proximal segments. The scolex of the tapeworm, loosened from the gut wall, may be digested in the intestine and may not be identified in the feces, even after extensive purging. Niclosamide affects intestinal cestodes only. It has no effect on encysted larvae in subcutaneous, muscle, or CNS tissues (cysticercosis). Niclosamide is indicated for treating dwarf tapeworms and those ingested with beef and fish.

A laxative is given before administration to purge the bowel of all dead cestode segments. If the segments remain in the bowel, digestion may liberate the eggs and lead to cysticercosis. The most common adverse effects of niclosamide treatment are abdominal distress, anorexia, nausea, and vomiting.

C ANTIECTOPARASITIC DRUGS

Antiectoparasitic drugs include permethrin, lindane, crotamiton, and malathion. These are topical drugs with local action. Although they can eradicate the parasite, they have minimal effect on the pruritus that frequently accompanies ectoparasitic infections. Permethrin, designated the drug of choice by the American Academy of Pediatrics (AAP website, 2004), is the prototype drug for antiectoparasitic drugs. Table 45.7 presents a summary of selected antiectoparasitic drugs.

NURSING MANAGEMENT OF THE PATIENT RECEIVING P PERMETHRIN

Core Drug Knowledge

Pharmacotherapeutics

Permethrin is a topical scabicide and pediculicide. For lice, it is available OTC as a 1% cream (Nix). Scabies should be treated with the 5% prescription cream (Elimite).

Pharmacokinetics

Permethrin is applied topically. A small amount may be systemically absorbed, especially from abraded or denuded skin. It is excreted as inactive metabolites through the kidneys.

Pharmacodynamics

Direct effects of permethrin occur in the parasite. Permethrin disrupts the parasite's nerve cell membrane, resulting in paralysis and death. Permethrin also exhibits residual ovicidal activity for approximately 2 weeks.

Contraindications and Precautions

Permethrin should not be used in patients who have had previous hypersensitivity reactions to household insecticides because it contains similar substances.

Adverse Effects

Common adverse effects include burning, itching, numbness, rash, redness, stinging, swelling, or tingling of the scalp. Pruritus, edema, and erythema caused by the parasite can be exacerbated during therapy. Inhaling substantial quantities of permethrin can aggravate bronchial asthma.

Drug Interactions

No drug–drug interactions are known to occur with permethrin.

TABLE 45.7 Summary of Selected C Antiectoparasitic Drugs

Drug (Trade) Name	Selected Indications	Route and Dosage Range	Pharmacokinetics
P permethrin (Elimite, Nix)	Scabies	*Adult and child:* Topical cream, apply cream to clean, dry skin from the neck to the toes and rub in well; leave on skin for 8–12 h; wash skin well	*Onset:* 10 min *Duration:* Unknown $t_{1/2}$: 16 h
	Pediculosis	*Adult and child:* Topical lotion, apply the lotion to the head and leave for 10 minutes; rinse thoroughly	
crotamiton (Eurax)	Scabies	*Adult:* Apply 10% preparation to the affected skin. Massage gently into skin until completely absorbed. Repeat as needed	*Onset:* Unknown *Duration:* Unknown $t_{1/2}$: Unknown
ivermectin (Stromectol)	Onchocerciasis Strongyloidiasis Scabies	*Adult and child >15 kg:* PO, 150 μg/kg 1 h after breakfast *Adult and child >15 kg:* PO, 200 μg/kg 1 h after breakfast *Adult and child >15 kg:* PO, 150–200 μg/kg	*Onset:* Well absorbed *Duration:* Unknown $t_{1/2}$: 16–35 h
lindane (Kwell, Scabene)	Scabies and pediculosis	*Adult and child:* Topical cream, apply cream to clean, dry skin from the neck to the toes and rub in well; leave on skin for 8–12 h; wash skin well *Adult and child:* Topical shampoo, wash and dry the hair and allow to cool; apply shampoo to dry hair and rub into the scalp; allow shampoo to remain in place for 4 min; use enough water to work up a good lather; rinse thoroughly and towel dry; use a fine-toothed comb when hair is thoroughly dry	*Onset:* Rapid *Duration:* 3 h $t_{1/2}$: 18 h
malathion (Ovide)	Scabies and pediculosis	*Adult and child >6 y:* Apply approximately 30 mL and leave in place for 8–12 h. Rinse thoroughly	*Onset:* Rapid *Duration:* 2 d–2 wk $t_{1/2}$: 8–48 h

Assessment of Relevant Core Patient Variables

Health Status

Evaluate the extent of infection. Lice that are visible in the eyebrows or eyelashes should not be treated by the patient at home.

Life Span and Gender

Permethrin is not approved for use in children younger than 2 years of age. It is a pregnancy category B drug. Whether permethrin enters breast milk is unknown; however, the American Academy of Pediatrics recommends discontinuing breast-feeding during therapy (AAP website, 2004).

Lifestyle, Diet, and Habits

Determine the patient's use of creams, ointments, or oils. The patient should be cautioned not to use them during permethrin therapy.

Environment

Because permethrin is routinely used at home, the patient needs to clearly understand how to use the drug properly. Explain that the infection may take up to 2 weeks to resolve.

Nursing Diagnoses and Outcomes

- Risk for Impaired Skin Integrity: Rash and pruritus related to drug therapy
  Desired outcome: *The patient will self-medicate with OTC diphenhydramine.*

Planning and Intervention

Maximizing Therapeutic Effects

Permethrin is for external use only, and the patient should be encouraged to use it exactly according to directions. When treating pubic lice, a second application of permethrin may be required.

Minimizing Adverse Effects

The patient needs to follow the directions for using permethrin carefully to avoid potential adverse effects. The drug must be kept out of the reach of children, who may ingest it accidentally.

Providing Patient and Family Education

- Emphasize the potential adverse effects of permethrin and the importance of contacting the provider should any such effects occur.
- Provide directions for using permethrin correctly. It is important to cover the following teaching points for use with scabies:
  - Thoroughly wash and dry the skin.
  - Massage the cream into the skin from the head to the soles of the feet, paying special attention to creases in the skin, hands, feet, underarms, and groin, and between fingers and toes.
  - Scabies rarely infests the scalp of adults, although the hairline, neck, side of the head, and forehead may be infested in older people and in infants. Treat infants on the scalp, side of the head, and forehead.
  - Leave the permethrin cream on the skin for 8 to 14 hours.
  - Wash off by taking a shower or bath.
  - Change into clean clothes.
- It is important to cover the following teaching points for use with lice:
  - Shampoo the hair and scalp using regular shampoo.
  - Rinse thoroughly and towel-dry the hair and scalp.
  - Allow hair to air dry for a few minutes.
  - Shake the permethrin lotion well before applying.
  - Wet the hair and scalp thoroughly with the permethrin lotion. Be sure to cover the areas behind the ears and on the back of the neck also. Allow the lotion to remain in place for 10 minutes.
  - Rinse the hair and scalp thoroughly and dry with a clean towel.
  - Remove nits only after the hair is completely dry.
- Instruct the patient how to eliminate nits (tiny, white, oval-shaped eggs of the adult louse, which lodge on hair close to the scalp):
  - Buy a good metal lice or nit comb.
  - Choose a well-lit area in your home for your lice-picking station.
  - Comb through the hair a section at a time, using metal clips to divide sections—and a magnifying glass if you have one handy.
  - Remove lice and nits from the comb with a tissue after each stroke, or rinse the comb in sudsy hot water between strokes.
  - Continue combing for at least 30 strokes or until the scalp and hair are nit-free. Hand-pick any remaining nits.
  - Repeat the procedure every 2 days for 2 weeks
- Additional information to reduce the potential for reinfection includes:
  - Machine-wash all clothing (including hats, scarves, and coats), bedding, towels, and washcloths in very hot water and dry them by using the hot cycle of a dryer for at least 20 minutes. Clothing or bedding that cannot be washed should be dry-cleaned or sealed in an airtight plastic bag for 2 weeks.
  - Shampoo all wigs and hairpieces.
  - Wash all hairbrushes and combs in very hot soapy water (above 130°F) for 5 to 10 minutes and do not share them with other people.
  - Clean the house or room by thoroughly vacuuming upholstered furniture, rugs, and floors.
  - Wash all toys in very hot soapy water (above 130°F) for 5 to 10 minutes.
  - Place all stuffed animals in sealed plastic bags for about a month. (Lice live only about 25 days.)

Ongoing Assessment and Evaluation

After-treatment evaluations consist of monitoring for signs of successful treatment (eradication) or failure (reinfection).

MEMORY CHIP

P Permethrin

- Used for scabies and pediculosis
- Major contraindications: hypersensitivity to household insecticides
- Most common adverse effects: skin irritation and pruritus
- Maximizing therapeutic effects: Apply only as directed.
- Minimizing adverse effects: Keep out of reach of children.
- Most important patient education: To minimize the risk for systemic absorption, do not leave on the scalp or body for longer than the recommended time.

Drugs Closely Related to P Permethrin

Crotamiton

Crotamiton (Eurax) is a scabicidal and antipruritic drug used for treating *S. scabiei* (scabies) and relieving pruritus. The drug can be used with caution during pregnancy, and the only contraindication to its use is hypersensitivity. Pediatric safety has not been established. Crotamiton should not be applied in the eyes or around the mouth because it may cause irritation. It should not be applied to acutely inflamed skin or raw or weeping surfaces until the acute inflammation resolves. The only potential adverse reaction is rash.

Crotamiton should be applied from the chin to the toes after taking a routine bath or shower. A second application is advisable 24 hours later. A cleansing bath should be taken 48 hours after the last application. Clothing and bed linens should be changed the second day. Contaminated clothing and bed linen may be dry cleaned or washed in very hot water.

Lindane

Lindane (Kwell) is another topical drug used to treat *S. scabiei* (scabies and its eggs), pediculosis capitis, pediculosis corporis, and *Phthirus pubis* (crab louse). Its use is highly controversial. In fact, many states have banned it as a pharmaceutical.

Lindane is absorbed slowly and incompletely through intact skin, through the GI tract when ingested, and through mucous membranes when inhaled. Following topical administration, some lindane is absorbed systemically. In the parasite, lindane is absorbed through the exoskeleton and causes excessive CNS stimulation that results in convulsion and death. If absorbed systemically, lindane is a CNS stimulant, producing adverse effects similar to those of dichlorodiphenyltrichloroethane (DDT), a potent insecticide.

In March 2003, the FDA approved a "black box" warning stating that lindane be used only in patients who cannot tolerate first-line treatment with safer medications to treat lice or scabies infestation or in whom such treatment has failed. Lindane is contraindicated for patients with known seizure disorders and for individuals with known hypersensitivity. CNS toxicity may precipitate seizures. Lindane should not be used where skin rash, abrasion, or inflammation exists because such use can enhance systemic absorption and increase the possibility of CNS toxicity. Lindane also is contraindicated for children younger than 2 years of age, who have more permeable skin than adults do, and may therefore be at high risk for systemic absorption. Caution should be used with this drug in children between 2 and 10 years of age because the risk for toxicity is greater in this age group than in others. Lindane is a pregnancy category C drug. It is not recommended for use while breast-feeding because it is secreted into breast milk. An alternative form of infant feeding should be used for at least 2 days after using lindane.

Malathion

Malathion (Ovide) is an organophosphate insecticide commonly known to the public as an aerosolized insecticide that is sprayed over vegetation. It was originally approved by the FDA in 1989, then removed from the market, and then reintroduced in 1999. It is used to manage human lice infections that are resistant to permethrin.

Malathion works by enabling acetylcholine to overstimulate cholinergic receptor sites, which leads to rapid insect death. It is not recommended for children under the age of 6 years and is contraindicated for use in infants because their scalp is more permeable and allows more absorption. The topical formulation contains isopropyl alcohol, making it flammable. For that reason, it should not be used in proximity to any heat source, such as electric rollers, curling irons, and especially cigarettes, pipes, lighters, matches, and other smoking-related items.

If ingested, malathion is a poison. The most serious symptom of organophosphate poisoning is respiratory distress, including potential respiratory arrest. Other respiratory symptoms include rhinorrhea, chest tightness, and wheezing. In addition to affecting the respiratory system, organophosphate poisoning can induce gastrointestinal peristalsis, diarrhea or fecal incontinence, and abdominal pain or cramps. It can also cause miosis, loss of ocular accommodation, blurred vision, and ocular pain. In the cardiovascular system, potential symptoms include bradycardia or hypotension. CNS symptoms include confusion, drowsiness or lethargy, and seizures. The patient may also experience weakness or muscle paralysis. Atropine and pralidoxime are the antidotes to organophosphate poisoning.

Malathion is a pregnancy category B drug; whether it is excreted into breast milk is unknown.

CRITICAL THINKING SCENARIO

Home care concerns in antiectoparasitic therapy

After treatment and recovery from status epilepticus, your patient, J. Colone, is discharged home on phenytoin (Dilantin) therapy. One of your assignments as a student nurse is to accompany the visiting nurse who will visit with Mr. Colone to assess his progress. When you arrive, you are surprised to learn that the whole family is being treated for head lice. Examine your concerns about Mr. Colone's current situation. In addition to teaching him about drug therapy, what other points will you emphasize in the teaching plan? What is especially important for Mr. Colone to know?

Drug Significantly Different From P Permethrin

Ivermectin (Stromectol) is an oral drug used in managing onchocerciasis or strongyloidiasis. It is an anthelminthic drug that also is used as an antiectoparasitic drug. Although it is not FDA approved to treat scabies, ivermectin has been

used successfully to treat this condition. Ivermectin is used only when treatment with topical agents fails.

Ivermectin should not be used during pregnancy or by women who breast-feed. It should be given cautiously to patients with severe illness such as hepatic, cardiovascular, renal, or pulmonary diseases.

CHAPTER SUMMARY

- Parasites include protozoa, helminths, and arthropods.
- Helminths include cestodes, nematodes, and trematodes.
- Arthropods include ectoparasites, such as scabies and lice.
- Pharmacologic intervention for parasites must be specific not only to the type of parasite but also to the stage of its life cycle.
- Chloroquine is the prototypical antimalarial drug. Additional drugs used in treating malaria include hydroxychloroquine, mefloquine, primaquine, pyrimethamine, and quinine.
- Metronidazole is the prototypical antiparasitic drug. Additional antiprotozoan drugs include iodoquinol, paromomycin, and quinacrine.
- PCP occurs most often in immunocompromised patients. Drug treatment for PCP includes pentamidine, atovaquone, and SMZ-TMP.
- Mebendazole is the prototypical anthelminthic drug. The choice of anthelminthic therapy, however, depends on the type of helminth. Other anthelminthic drugs include albendazole (in clinical trial), thiabendazole, pyrantel pamoate, piperazine, diethylcarbamazine, praziquantel, oxamniquine, and niclosamide.
- Permethrin is the prototypical antiectoparasitic drug. Drugs closely related to permethrin include crotamiton, lindane, and malathion.

QUESTIONS FOR STUDY AND REVIEW

1. Why should patients with chloroquine therapy continue to have their eyes examined after completing therapy?
2. Why is chloroquine used cautiously in children?
3. What baseline evaluations should be done for a patient on long-term antimalarial therapy?
4. Why would a patient with alcoholism need to be monitored closely during antiparasitic therapy?
5. Why should you take respiratory protective measures during the administration of inhaled pentamidine?
6. How can you intervene to minimize potential severe adverse effects from the administration of pentamidine?
7. What are the major causes of treatment failure with lindane?

> **Need More Help?**
>
> Chapter 45 of the study guide for *Drug Therapy in Nursing* 2e contains NCLEX-style questions and other learning activities to reinforce your understanding of the concepts presented in this chapter. For additional information or to purchase the study guide, visit *http://connection.lww.com/go/aschenbrenner.*

REFERENCES AND BIBLIOGRAPHY

American Academy of Pediatrics [Online]. Available: *http://www.aap.org.*

Bagheri, H., Simiand, E., Montastruc, J. L., et al. (2004). Adverse drug reactions to anthelmintics. *Annals of Pharmacotherapeutics, 38*(3), 383–388.

Cayley, W. E. (2004). Mefloquine for preventing malaria in nonimmune adult travelers. *American Family Physician, 69*(3), 521–522.

Clinical Pharmacology [Online]. Available: *http://cp.gsm.com.*

Facts and Comparisons. (2004). *Drug facts and comparisons.* Philadelphia: Lippincott Williams & Wilkins.

Hardman, J. G. (2001). *Goodman & Gilman's the pharmacological basis of therapeutics* (10th ed.). New York: McGraw-Hill Health Professions Division.

Jones, K. N., & English, J. C. (2003). Review of common therapeutic options in the United States for the treatment of pediculosis capitis. *Clinical Infectious Diseases, 36*(11), 1355–1361.

Katzung, B. (2004). *Basic and clinical pharmacology* (9th ed.). New York: McGraw-Hill/Appleton & Lange.

Kremsner, P. G., & Krishna, S. (2004). Antimalarial combinations. *Lancet, 364*(9430), 285–294.

Kucik, C. J., Martin G. L., Sortor, B. V., et al. (2004). Common intestinal parasites. *American Family Physician, 69*(5), 1161–1168.

Montoya, J. G., & Liesenfeld, O. (2004). Toxoplasmosis. *Lancet, 363*(9425), 1965–1976.

Micromedex Healthcare Series [Online]. Available: *http://healthcare.micromedex.com.*

Petri, W. A., Jr. (2003). Therapy of intestinal protozoa. *Trends in Parasitology 19*(11):523–526.

Schlagenhauf, P. (2004). Malaria: From prehistory to present. *Infectious Disease Clinics of North America, 18*(2), 189–205.

Sheff, B. (2004). Microbe of the month: *Giardia lamblia. Nursing, 34*(4), 76.

Tatro, D. S. (2004). *Drug interaction facts.* Philadelphia: Lippincott Williams & Wilkins.

Taylor, W. R., & White, N. J. (2004). Antimalarial drug toxicity: A review. *Drug Safety, 27*(1), 25–61.

Wright, J. M., Dunn, L. A., Upcroft, P., et al. (2003). Efficacy of antigiardial drugs. *Expert Opinions on Drug Safety, 2*(6), 529–541.

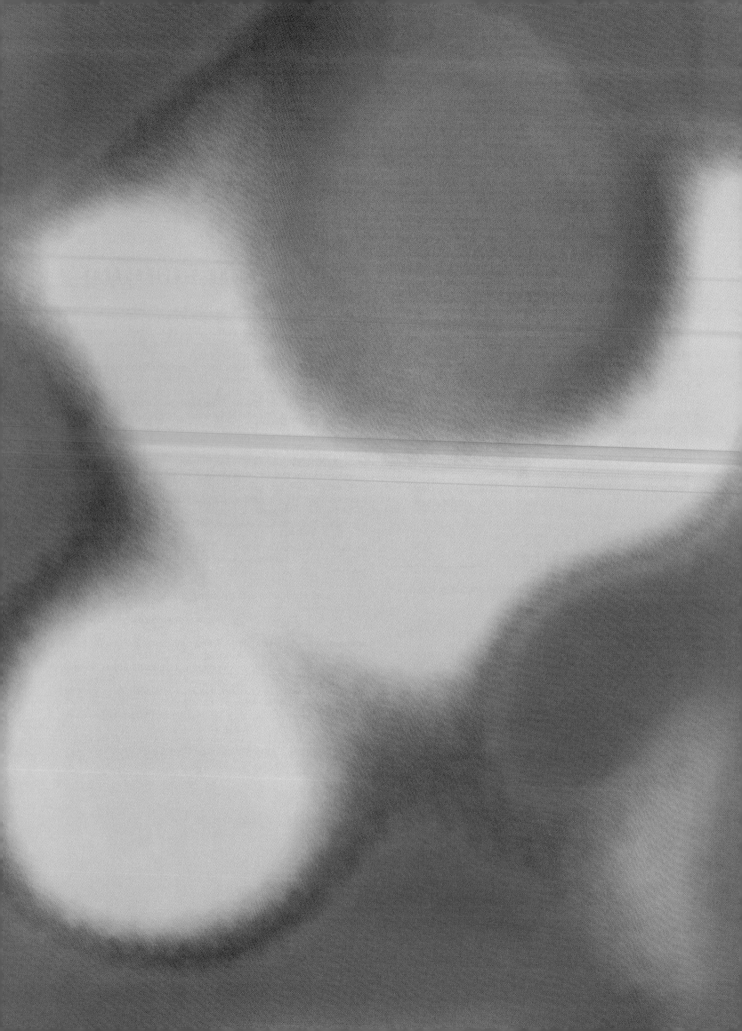

Respiratory System Drugs

unit 11

Drugs Affecting the Upper Respiratory System

chapter 46

Learning Objectives

At the completion of this chapter the student will:

1. Describe the anatomy and physiology of the upper respiratory system.
2. Identify core drug knowledge pertaining to drugs that affect the upper respiratory system.
3. Identify core patient variables pertaining to drugs that affect the upper respiratory system.
4. Relate the interaction of core drug knowledge to core patient variables for drugs that affect the upper respiratory system.
5. Generate a nursing plan of care from the interactions between core drug knowledge and core patient variables for drugs that affect the upper respiratory system.
6. Describe nursing interventions to maximize therapeutic effects and minimize adverse effects for drugs that affect the upper respiratory system.
7. Determine key points for patient and family education for drugs that affect the upper respiratory system.

FEATURED WEBLINK

http://www.aaaai.org/patients/allergic_conditions/rhinitis.stm
Got allergies? Visit the Professionals Center at the website of the American Academy of Allergy Asthma and Immunology.

CONNECTION WEBLINK

Additional Weblinks are found on Connection:
http://www.connection.lww.com/go/aschenbrenner.

KEY TERMS

antihistamines
antitussives
cilia
common cold
decongestants
expectorants
histamine
influenza
laryngitis
pharyngitis
rebound congestion
rhinitis
sinuses
sinusitis

Drugs Affecting the Upper Respiratory System

Ⓒ Antitussives

[P] dextromethorphan
codeine
hydrocodone bitartrate
benzonatate

Ⓒ Decongestants

[P] pseudoephedrine
phenylephrine

Topical decongestants
ephedrine
naphazoline
oxymetazoline
tetrahydrozoline
xylometazoline

Ⓒ Antihistamines

[P] fexofenadine
azelastine
cetirizine
desloratadine
loratadine
brompheniramine
chlorpheniramine
diphenhydramine
inhaled steroids
inhaled mast cell stabilizers

Ⓒ Expectorants

[P] guaifenesin
terpin hydrate
iodine preparations

The symbol Ⓒ indicates the **drug class.**
Drugs in **bold type** marked with the symbol [P] are prototypes.
Drugs in blue type are closely related to the prototype.
Drugs in red type are significantly different from the prototype.
Drugs in black type with no symbol are also used in drug therapy; no prototype

This chapter discusses drugs that affect the upper respiratory system. The upper respiratory system is essential for bringing oxygen into the body and body tissues. The classes of drugs that affect the upper respiratory system work to keep the airways open. The following drug classes are discussed in this chapter:

- **Antitussives**—drugs that block the cough reflex
- **Decongestants**—drugs that decrease the blood flow to an area and thus decrease overproduction of secretions
- **Antihistamines**—drugs that block the release or action of **histamine,** a chemical released during inflammation, which increases secretions and narrows airways
- **Expectorants**—drugs that increase productive cough to clear the airways

PHYSIOLOGY

The respiratory system is composed of the upper and lower respiratory systems. The upper respiratory system, or conducting airway, is composed of the nose, mouth, pharynx, larynx, trachea, and the bronchial tree (Figure 46.1). Air moves from the nasal cavity through the pharynx and into the larynx. The larynx contains the vocal chords and the epiglottis, the latter of which closes during swallowing to protect the lower respiratory tract from any foreign particles. From the larynx, air proceeds to the trachea, the main conducting airway into the lungs.

Air Filtration

Air usually moves into the nasal cavity through the nose. Nasal hairs catch and filter foreign substances, and the air is warmed and humidified as it passes by blood vessels close to the surface of the epithelial lining in the nasal passage. This epithelial lining contains goblet cells that produce mucus, which traps dust, microorganisms, pollen, and other foreign substances. These actions help to purify the air and increase the efficiency of gas diffusion when the air reaches the lower respiratory tract.

The cells of the epithelial lining also contain **cilia,** microscopic hair-like projections of the cell membrane. The cilia are in constant motion, moving the mucus and any trapped substances toward the throat, where they will be swallowed and destroyed. Three pairs of **sinuses** (air-filled passages through the skull) open into the nasal passage. The epithelial lining of the nose is continuous with the lining of the sinuses, and the mucus produced in the sinuses drains into the nasal cavity. The mucus drains into the throat, is swallowed, and proceeds to the gastrointestinal (GI) tract, where foreign materials are destroyed by the stomach acids.

Other Air-Purifying Mechanisms

The walls of the nasal cavity are sensitive to irritation. When receptors in these walls are stimulated, a central nervous system (CNS) reflex is initiated, and a sneeze results. The sneeze causes air to push through the nasal cavity under tremendous pressure, cleaning out any foreign irritant and opening the passages for more efficient flow of air. Throughout the airways, many macrophage scavengers are free to move throughout the epithelium and destroy invaders. Mast cells are present in abundance and release histamine, serotonin, adenosine triphosphate, and other chemicals to ensure a rapid and intense inflammatory reaction to any cell injury.

PATHOPHYSIOLOGY

The most common conditions that affect the upper respiratory system can be classified as inflammatory responses. For example, the rhinovirus and adenovirus are two types of common cold viruses that invade the tissues of the upper respiratory tract, initiating the release of histamine and prostaglandins and causing an inflammatory response.

Common Cold

The **common cold** is a viral infection that starts in the upper respiratory tract, sometimes spreads to the lower structures, and may contribute to secondary infections in the eyes or middle ears. The main differences between the common cold and other respiratory infections are the absence of fever and the relative mildness of the symptoms. Cold symptoms vary from person to person. Manifestations may include sneezing, headaches, fatigue, chills, sore throat, inflammation of the

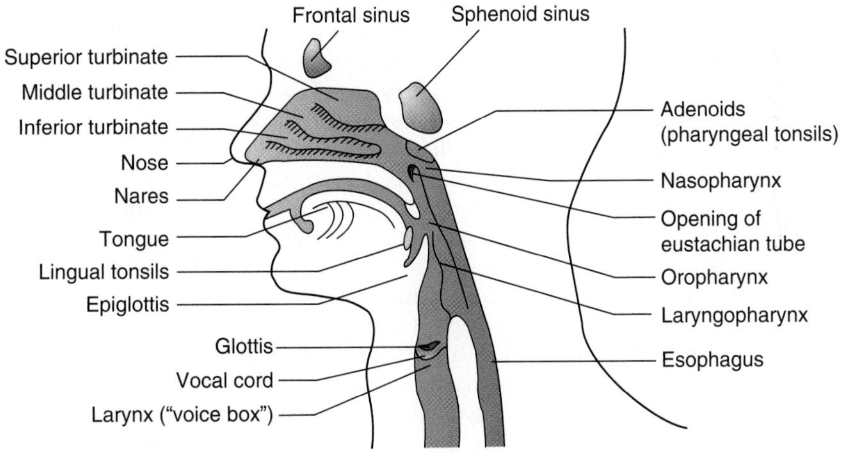

FIGURE 46.1 Structures of the upper airway.

nose (**rhinitis**), and nasal discharge. Usually, there is no fever. The secretions are generally watery and clear. Pathologic changes occurring in the mucous membrane that lines the nose, the nasal sinuses, the nasopharynx, and other upper respiratory passages may include tissue swelling, congestion of blood, and oozing of fluids.

Allergic or Seasonal Rhinitis

A condition similar to the common cold that afflicts many people is called allergic or seasonal rhinitis. This inflammation of the nasal cavity also is commonly called hay fever. It occurs when the upper airways respond to a specific allergen (e.g., pollen, mold, or dust) with a vigorous inflammatory response, resulting in nasal congestion, sneezing, stuffiness, and watery eyes. Other areas of the upper respiratory tract can become irritated or infected, resulting in inflammation.

Sinusitis

Sinusitis occurs when the epithelial lining of the sinus cavities becomes inflamed. It can be caused by bacteria or viruses. The resultant swelling often causes severe pain because the bony cavity cannot stretch and the swollen tissue pushes against the bone and blocks the sinus passages. The danger of a sinus infection is that if it is untreated, the causative microorganisms can move up the sinus passages and into brain tissue.

Pharyngitis

Pharyngitis is an inflammation or infection of the pharynx (throat) caused by bacteria or viruses. The symptoms of pharyngitis caused by bacteria are generally redness and swelling of the throat, a pustulant fluid on the tonsils or discharged from the mouth, extreme soreness of the throat that is felt during swallowing, swelling of lymph nodes, and a slight fever. Viral pharyngitis infections produce raised whitish to yellow lesions in the pharynx that are surrounded by reddened tissue. They also cause fever, headache, and sore throat that last for 4 to 14 days. Lymphatic tissue in the pharynx also may become involved.

Laryngitis

Laryngitis is an inflammation of the larynx or voice box, caused by chemical or mechanical irritation, viral infections, or bacterial infections. Simple laryngitis usually is associated with the common cold or similar infections. Usually, the mucous membrane lining the larynx is the primary site of infection; it becomes swollen and filled with blood, secretes a thick mucous substance, and contains many inflammatory cells.

When the epiglottis, which closes the larynx during swallowing, becomes swollen and infected by influenza viruses, the larynx can become obstructed, and suffocation may result. Excessive smoking, alcoholism, or overuse of the vocal cords may cause chronic laryngitis. The mucous membrane becomes dry and covered with polyps, small lumps of tissue that project from the surface. In addition, the wall of the larynx may thicken and become inflamed. Additional causes of laryngitis include diphtheria, tuberculosis, and syphilis—serious infections that require aggressive treatment.

Influenza

Influenza is an infection caused by any of several strains of myxoviruses, categorized as types A, B, and C. Influenza is transmitted from person to person through the respiratory tract by inhalation of infected droplets ejected by coughing and sneezing. As the virus particles gain entrance to the body, they selectively attack and destroy the ciliated epithelial cells that line the upper respiratory tract, bronchial tubes, and trachea. The onset of symptoms is abrupt, with sudden and distinct chills, fatigue, and high temperature. A diffuse headache and severe muscular aches throughout the body are experienced and often are accompanied by irritation or a sense of rawness in the throat. Symptoms associated with other respiratory tract infections, such as coughing and nasal discharge, also may occur.

C ANTITUSSIVE DRUGS

Antitussives are drugs that suppress the cough reflex. Many disorders of the upper and lower respiratory tracts, including the common cold, sinusitis, pharyngitis, and pneumonia, are accompanied by an uncomfortable, nonproductive cough. Coughing normally is a protective mechanism that forces foreign irritants out of the respiratory system, opening it for more efficient flow of air. However, persistent coughing can be exhausting, cause muscle strain, and further irritate the respiratory tract. A cough that occurs without an active disease process or that persists after treatment may be a symptom of another disease process and should be investigated before any drug is given to alleviate it. Antitussive drugs include dextromethorphan, codeine, and hydrocodone bitartrate. Dextromethorphan (Benylin) is selected as the prototype of the antitussives. Table 46.1 presents a summary of antitussive drugs.

NURSING MANAGEMENT OF THE PATIENT RECEIVING P DEXTROMETHORPHAN

Core Drug Knowledge

Pharmacotherapeutics

Dextromethorphan is used in treating chronic, nonproductive cough. It is available widely in a variety of nonprescription forms, such as capsules, lozenges, syrups, extended-release oral suspension, and chewable tablets.

Pharmacokinetics

Dextromethorphan is absorbed rapidly from the GI tract, with antitussive activity occurring within 15 to 30 minutes (see Table 46.1). It undergoes extensive hepatic metabolism. Excretion is mainly renal, with some drug eliminated unchanged, but most eliminated as metabolites.

Pharmacodynamics

Dextromethorphan is related chemically to the opiate agonists and can suppress coughing as effectively as narcotics. Cough suppression occurs by several mechanisms, but mainly

TABLE 46.1 Summary of Selected Ⓒ Antitussives

Drug (Trade) Name	Selected Indications	Route and Dosage Range	Pharmacokinetics
P dextromethorphan (Benylin, Delsym, Robitussin Maximum Strength Cough, Robitussin Cough Calmers, Sucrets Cough Control Formula, Vicks 44 Cough; *Canadian:* Balminil DM, Calmyline #1, Robidex, Koffer)	Cough suppression	*Adult and adolescent:* PO, Regular-release formulation: 10–20 mg PO every 4 h; or 30 mg every 6–8 h; Max: 120 mg/day *Child 6–11 y:* PO, 5–10 mg every 4 h; or 15 mg every 6–8 h; Max: 60 mg/day *Child 2–5 y:* 2.5–5 mg every 4 h; or 7.5 mg every 6–8 h; Max: 30 mg/day *Child <2 y:* Safe and effective usage is not established. Extended-release formulation: *Adult and adolescent:* 10 mL every 12 h; Max: 20 mL/day *Child 6–11 y:* 5 mL every 12 h; Max: 10 mL/day *Child 2–5 y:* 2.5 mL every 12 h; Max: 5 mL/day. *Child <2 y:* Safe and effective usage is not established.	*Onset:* 15–30 min *Duration:* 5–6 h $t_{1/2}$: 11 h
benzonatate (Tessalon Perles)	Cough suppression	*Adult and child >10 y:* PO, 100 mg 3×/d or every 4 h; Max: 600 mg/day *Child <10 y:* Safe and effective usage is not established.	*Onset:* 15–20 min *Duration:* 3–8 h $t_{1/2}$: Unknown
codeine (*Canadian:* Paveral)	Cough suppression	*Adult:* PO, 10–20 mg every 4–6 h; Max: 120 mg/24 h *Elderly:* May require reduced doses *Child 6–12 y:* 5–10 mg every 4–6 h; Max: 60 mg/day *Child 2–5 y:* 2.5–5 mg every 4–6 h; Max: 30 mg/day *Child and infant <2 y:* Safe dosage has not been established.	*Onset:* 15–20 min *Duration:* 4–6 h $t_{1/2}$: 1.5–4 h
hydrocodone bitartrate (Hycodan, Hydromet, Hydropane, Mycodone, Tussigon; *Canadian:* Robidon)	Cough suppression	*Adult:* PO, 5–10 mg every 4–6 h Maximum single adult dose: 15 mg *Adolescent >12 y:* PO, 0.6 mg/kg/day in 3–4 divided doses. Maximum single dose: 10 mg *Child 2–11 y:* 0.6 mg/kg/day in 3–4 divided doses. Maximum single dose: 5 mg	*Onset:* 10–20 min *Duration:* 3–6 h $t_{1/2}$: 3–8 h

the drug directly affects the cough center in the medulla. Therapeutic doses do not affect ciliary activity.

Contraindications and Precautions

Dextromethorphan is contraindicated for treating chronic coughs resulting from emphysema and asthma. Because of its extensive hepatic metabolism, dextromethorphan is used with caution in patients with hepatic impairment. It also is used with caution during pregnancy. Although teratogenic effects have not been demonstrated, dextromethorphan is rated FDA pregnancy category C.

Adverse Effects

Although adverse effects are generally rare, dextromethorphan toxicity can occur and is characterized by nausea and vomiting, drowsiness, dizziness, irritability, and restlessness.

Drug Interactions

Dextromethorphan may potentiate sedation when used with other CNS depressants. It may interact with monoamine oxidase inhibitors (MAOIs), resulting in serotonin syndrome, a dangerous condition that consists of nausea, hypotension,

excitation, hyperpyrexia, and possible coma. It also may interact with fluoxetine, quinidine, and sibutramine. Table 46.2 lists drugs that interact with dextromethorphan.

Assessment of Relevant Core Patient Variables

Health Status

Before administering dextromethorphan, review the patient's record to determine whether dextromethorphan may be administered safely. This drug is contraindicated for patients with emphysema or asthma. If coughing is suppressed in these patients, they may retain secretions that will exacerbate their disease.

Review the patient's record for drugs that may interact with dextromethorphan, especially antidepressants. Finally, evaluate the patient for a history of hepatic insufficiency because dextromethorphan is processed by the liver.

Perform a baseline evaluation of the head, eyes, ears, nose, and throat (HEENT) in addition to a complete lung assessment.

Life Span and Gender

Determine whether the patient is pregnant. Dextromethorphan, a pregnancy category C drug, should be used with caution during pregnancy. It also is important to be aware of the patient's age before administering dextromethorphan because it is not indicated for use in children younger than 6 years old.

Lifestyle, Diet, and Habits

Investigate the patient's need to drive or operate potentially dangerous equipment and advise the patient to refrain from these activities until the sedative effects of dextromethorphan use are known. It is important to assess the patient's typical intake of alcohol. Caution the patient about the potentially additive effects of dextromethorphan when used with alcohol because both are CNS depressants. Find out how frequently the patient drinks grapefruit or orange juice, because these juices can substantially increase the concentration of dextromethorphan.

Environment

Be aware of the environment in which dextromethorphan will be administered. Dextromethorphan is used commonly in over-the-counter (OTC) cough and cold preparations, and prescribed dextromethorphan is just as commonly self-administered by patients at home. Therefore, caution patients to read labels of all drugs they are taking to avoid a possible overdose.

Nursing Diagnoses and Outcomes

- Risk for Injury related to sensory-perceptual alteration from drug-induced drowsiness and sedation
  Desired outcome: *The patient will remain free from injury related to sedation and drowsiness.*
- Risk for Ineffective Airway Clearance related to suppression of cough reflex
  Desired outcome: *The patient will maintain his or her baseline respiratory function.*

Planning and Intervention

Maximizing Therapeutic Effects

In acute or long-term care settings, administer dextromethorphan at evenly spaced intervals to maintain blood levels of the drug at steady state. Provide environmental controls, including appropriate lighting, reduced noise, and comfortable temperature, to ease sensory-perceptual alteration and aid relaxation.

Minimizing Adverse Effects

During therapy, ensure that safety precautions are used, such as side rails and ambulation assistance. It also is important to

TABLE 46.2 Agents That Interact With P Dextromethorphan

Interactants	Effect and Significance	Nursing Management
fluoxetine	Fluoxetine interferes with the metabolism of dextromethorphan, resulting in hallucination or a serotonin syndrome–like reaction.	Avoid coadministration if possible. Monitor for adverse effects.
juice grapefruit orange	Grapefruit and orange juice inhibit the metabolism and intestinal efflux of dextromethorphan, resulting in increased risk for pharmacologic and adverse effects that last for several days.	Avoid administration of dextromethorphan with grapefruit or orange juice. Monitor for adverse effects.
monoamine oxidase inhibitors	Dextromethorphan can block neuronal uptake of serotonin and may produce serotonin syndrome.	Maintain an interval of at least 2 weeks between administration of these drugs.
quinidine	Quinidine may inhibit the hepatic metabolism of dextromethorphan, resulting in an increased risk for adverse effects and toxicity.	Monitor for adverse effects.
sibutramine	Coadministration of these agents may have additive serotonergic effects.	Avoid coadministration if possible. Monitor for adverse effects. Monitor for serotonin syndrome.

monitor respiratory status and movement of air periodically during drug use. Refrain from administering dextromethorphan with grapefruit or orange juice.

Providing Patient and Family Education

- Explain to patients and their families that taking dextromethorphan will help to quiet a cough.
- Emphasize that sedation, drowsiness, and impaired orientation can occur. Because it can be sedating, it is important to tell patients to take dextromethorphan only as directed and not to drive or perform other tasks that require alertness. Some patients may require assistance walking if they react strongly to dextromethorphan.
- It is important to explain to patients that they should not take dextromethorphan if they have ever had a reaction to it, are pregnant or breast-feeding, or have a history of liver problems.
- Caution patients who are taking certain antidepressants or drugs for irregular heartbeat or obesity about the potential for serious drug–drug interactions.
- Alert patients not to take any OTC drugs or consume alcohol while taking dextromethorphan because doing so could increase sedation.
- Caution patients to keep dextromethorphan out of the reach of children.
- It is important to tell patients to report immediately any chest tightness, difficulty breathing, noisy breathing, or shortness of breath. These symptoms may indicate that the drug is not working, or that the patient is having a reaction to the drug.

Ongoing Assessment and Evaluation

Monitor the effect of dextromethorphan on the patient's motor control, sedation, and respiratory status. By the end of therapy, the patient should remain free of injury related to sedation and have cough relief.

MEMORY CHIP

P Dextromethorphan

- Used to manage nonproductive cough
- Major contraindication: cough resulting from emphysema or asthma
- Most common adverse effects: nausea, vomiting, and irritability
- Most serious adverse effects: drowsiness and dizziness
- Maximizing therapeutic effects: Administer at evenly spaced intervals throughout the day.
- Minimizing adverse effects: Institute precautions to ensure safety during potential drowsiness or dizziness.
- Most important patient education: Advise the patient to seek medical attention if cough does not resolve.

Drugs Closely Related to P Dextromethorphan

Codeine

Codeine is a controlled substance used in treating cough. Like dextromethorphan, it works directly on the medullary center to suppress the cough reflex. Codeine is more sedating than dextromethorphan and also may induce respiratory depression. Codeine is contraindicated for patients who must cough to maintain a patent airway (e.g., postoperative patients). Codeine is used with caution in patients who are pregnant or breast-feeding and in patients with head injuries. It also is used cautiously in patients with chronic cough (e.g., that caused by emphysema or asthma) or in patients with a history of drug addiction. Adverse effects include sedation, dry mouth, nausea, vomiting, and constipation. Codeine also is discussed in Chapter 23.

Hydrocodone Bitartrate

Hydrocodone bitartrate (Hycodan), also a controlled substance, is a derivative of codeine and acts directly on the cough reflex center in the medulla. It is somewhat more sedating than codeine and has the same properties, contraindications, and adverse effects.

Drug Significantly Different From P Dextromethorphan

Benzonatate

Benzonatate (Tessalon, Tessalon Perles) is an oral non-narcotic antitussive agent that is rarely used because it is not as effective as other antitussives. Benzonatate works by anesthetizing the stretch receptors in the respiratory tract, lung tissue, and pleura, interfering with their activity, and thereby reducing the cough reflex. At normal doses, it does not affect the respiratory center.

Benzonatate is used to coat the oropharynx to depress the gag reflex before intubation or endoscopy. The "Perles" are also topically applied to discrete areas of the body, such as a defined lesion or abnormality, before magnetic resonance imaging (MRI), because they show up as "markers" for more accurate mapping and measurement. Of course, neither of these uses is approved by the FDA.

C DECONGESTANT DRUGS

Decongestants are drugs taken to decrease nasal congestion related to the common cold, sinusitis, and allergic rhinitis, a condition that is caused by an inflammatory response in the upper respiratory tract. Nasal decongestants work by constricting the nasal arterioles, thereby decreasing the swelling of the nasal membrane. These drugs can be administered orally or topically. When decongestants are taken orally, they are absorbed in the body, thus increasing the chance of adverse effects. When used topically, the drug has the same therapeutic effects; however, the potential for adverse effects is diminished.

Drugs within the decongestant class include pseudoephedrine, phenylpropanolamine, ephedrine, oxymetazoline, and phenylephrine. The intranasal steroid dexamethasone sodium phosphate is not in the decongestant drug class, but

it is used for its anti-inflammatory effect on nasal conditions. The prototype decongestant is pseudoephedrine (Sudafed), an orally administered decongestant. Table 46.3 presents a summary of decongestant drugs.

NURSING MANAGEMENT OF THE PATIENT RECEIVING P PSEUDOEPHEDRINE

Core Drug Knowledge

Pharmacotherapeutics

Pseudoephedrine can reduce the volume of nasal mucus and is recommended for the temporary relief of nasal congestion related to the common cold, allergic rhinitis, and sinusitis. It also is used to relieve the pressure of otitis media by promoting drainage of the eustachian tubes.

Pharmacokinetics

Pseudoephedrine is an oral drug readily absorbed from the GI tract, with onset of activity occurring within 30 minutes. Duration of action ranges from 4 to 6 hours in regular formulations, to 8 to 12 hours in extended-release preparations (see Table 46.3). Pseudoephedrine is metabolized by the liver and excreted in the urine. This drug also crosses the placenta and is secreted in breast milk.

Pharmacodynamics

Pseudoephedrine mimics the actions of the sympathetic nervous system and achieves its nasal decongestant effects by causing vasoconstriction in the nasal mucous membranes. This shrinkage decreases membrane size and promotes sinus drainage and improved airflow. Stimulation of other sympathetic receptors while the patient is taking pseudoephedrine can result in cardiovascular stimulation, constriction of renal arterioles, and anxiety.

Contraindications and Precautions

Pseudoephedrine is categorized in pregnancy category C and should be used with caution during pregnancy or lactation because of its possible effects on the fetus and neonate. This drug should not be used by patients with severe hypertension and coronary artery disease because it produces sympathomimetic effects such as increased heart rate and blood pressure. Special caution should be used in patients with diabetes, thyrotoxicosis, coronary artery disease, benign prostatic hypertrophy, and increased intraocular pressure because of the risk for sympathomimetic adverse effects, which could aggravate these conditions.

Adverse Effects

Adverse effects related to pseudoephedrine use are related primarily to its sympathomimetic effects on the CNS and cardiovascular system. They will occur almost immediately

TABLE 46.3 Summary of Selected C Decongestants

Drug (Trade) Name	Selected Indications	Route and Dosage Range	Pharmacokinetics
Oral Decongestants			
P pseudoephedrine (Sudafed, Dimetapp, Pedia Care, Triaminic, Contac; *Canadian:* Balmiminil Decongestant, Drixoril, Robidrine)	Nasal decongestion	*Adult and child >12 y:* PO, 60 mg every 4–6 h *Child >6 y:* PO, 30 mg every 4–6 h *Child <6 y:* PO, 15 mg every 4–6 h Sustained release: *Adult and child >12 y:* PO, 120 mg every 12 h *Child <12 y:* not recommended Controlled release: *Adult and child >12 y:* PO, 240 mg every 24 h *Child <12 y:* not recommended	*Onset:* 30 min *Duration:* 4–6 h $t_{1/2}$: 7 h
Phenylephrine (AH-Chew D; *Canadian*: Dionephrine)	Nasal decongestion	*Adult and child >12 y:* PO, 10–20 mg every 4 h *Child >6 y:* PO, 10 mg every 4 h	*Onset:* 5–10 min *Duration:* 3–4 h $t_{1/2}$: Unknown
Topical Decongestants			
ephedrine (Pretz-D)	Nasal decongestion	*Adult and child >12 y:* Nasal spray, 2–3 sprays 0.025% every 4 h *Adult and child >6 y:* Nasal spray, 1–2 sprays 0.025% every 4 h	Minimal systemic absorption
naphazoline (Privine, Vasocon, Naphcon Forte, Nafazair, All Clear, VasoClear)	Nasal decongestion	Intranasal dosage (0.05% nasal spray): *Adult:* 1–2 sprays in each nostril every 4–6 h as needed	Minimal systemic absorption

(continued)

TABLE 46.3 Summary of Selected Decongestants (continued)

Drug (Trade) Name	Selected Indications	Route and Dosage Range	Pharmacokinetics
		Intranasal dosage (0.05% nasal drops): *Adult:* 1–2 drops in each nostril every 3 h as needed	
	Ocular decongestion	Ophthalmic dosage (0.012, 0.03% and 0.1% ocular solutions): *Adult and child >6 y:* Topical, 1–2 drops in the affected eye(s) up to 4 times per day	
oxymetazoline (Afrin, Allerest 12 Hour Nasal, Dristan 12 Hr Nasal, Visine, Ocu-Clear)	Nasal decongestion	Nasal dosage: *Adult and child >6 y:* Use 1–2 drops or sprays of 0.05% solution in each nostril 2× day or as required, but no more frequently than every 6 h *Child 2–5 y:* 2–3 drops or spray of the 0.025% solution in each nostril 2× day.	Minimal systemic absorption
	Ocular decongestion	Ophthalmic dosage: *Adult and child:* Instill 1–2 drops of 0.025% solution in the affected eye(s) 2–4×/d, but no more frequently than every 6 h	
phenylephrine (Neo-Synephrine)	Nasal decongestion	*Adult and child >12 y:* Apply 2–3 drops or 1–2 sprays of 0.25%–0.5% solution in each nostril or a small quantity of 0.5% nasal jelly applied into each nostril every 4 h as needed *Child 6–12 y:* 2–3 drops of 0.25% solution in each nostril every 4 h as needed *Child <6 y:* Apply 2–3 drops or sprays of 0.125% or 0.16% solution in each nostril every 4 h as needed *Infants >6 mo:* 1–2 drops of 0.16% solution in each nostril every 3 h	Minimal systemic absorption
tetrahydrozoline (Tyzine, Visine)	Nasal decongestion	Nasal dosage: *Adult and child ≥6 y:* 2–4 drops or 3–4 sprays of 0.1% nasal solution in each nostril every 3–4 h as necessary, never more often than every 3 h *Child 2–6 y:* 2–3 drops of 0.05% pediatric nasal drops in each nostril as needed, never more often than every 3 h	Minimal systemic absorption
	Ocular decongestion	Ophthalmic dosage: *Adult:* Instill 1–2 drops of 0.05% ophthalmic solution into the eye(s) up to 4× day	
xylometazoline (Otrivin, Natru-Vent)	Nasal decongestion	*Adult and adolescent ≥12 y:* 1 spray of 0.1% solution in each nostril every 8–10 h as needed	Minimal systemic absorption

and include feelings of tension, anxiety, restlessness, tremor, insomnia, and weakness. Severe CNS reactions have included hallucinations, delusions, and convulsions. Adverse cardiovascular effects include palpitations, tachycardia, hypertension, and arrhythmias. Allergic reactions that have been reported with pseudoephedrine use include skin rashes and urticaria. Extreme dryness of the mucous membranes, resulting in pain and irritation, has been reported in some cases.

When sympathomimetic adverse effects occur, patients with diabetes, thyrotoxicosis, coronary artery disease, hypertension, benign prostatic hypertrophy, or increased intraocular pressure should discontinue using pseudoephedrine; patients without concurrent disease may continue taking the drug.

Drug Interactions

Increased hypertension may occur if pseudoephedrine is taken concurrently with MAOIs, guanethidine, methyldopa, or furazolidone. Instruct the patient to avoid such combinations. The duration of pseudoephedrine's effect may increase if it is taken with any urinary alkalinizer (e.g., potassium citrate, sodium citrate, sodium lactate, tromethamine, sodium acetate, and sodium bicarbonate) because the drug cannot be excreted into alkaline urine. An increased dose of pseudoephedrine may be necessary when giving it with urinary acidifiers, such as ammonium chloride, potassium phosphate, or sodium acid phosphate. Table 46.4 lists drugs that interact with pseudoephedrine.

Assessment of Relevant Core Patient Variables

Health Status

Review the patient's health history and perform a physical examination to determine any contraindications to the use of this drug. Contraindications include hypersensitivity to the drug, thyrotoxicosis, diabetes, hypertension, benign prostatic hypertrophy, cardiovascular disorders, pregnancy, and lactation.

It is especially important to assess patient orientation, affect, respiratory rate and sounds, blood pressure, and pulse. In addition, monitor cardiovascular effects carefully to prevent serious complications and arrange for dosage adjustment as appropriate.

Life Span and Gender

Be aware of the patient's age before administering pseudoephedrine. Pseudoephedrine must be given cautiously to elderly patients because they may experience more serious adverse effects than other patients do. Avoid sustained-release preparations and use short-duration preparations. Assess female patients for pregnancy. Pseudoephedrine is ranked in pregnancy category C; it should be avoided by pregnant women unless the benefits outweigh the potential risks.

Lifestyle, Diet, and Habits

Assess the use of over-the-counter medications. Pseudoephedrine is used in combination with many other agents, including antihistamines. Teach the patient to read ingredient labels carefully.

Environment

Pseudoephedrine is generally taken in the outpatient setting. Because it is an over-the-counter medication and patients have easy access to the drug, caution the patient about overuse of pseudoephedrine and other decongestants. Frequent, long-term, or excessive use of decongestants will induce rebound congestion. **Rebound congestion** occurs when the nasal passages become congested as the drug effect wears off and the body compensates by vasodilating the same nasal arterioles

TABLE 46.4 Agents That Interact With P Pseudoephedrine

Interactants	Effect and Significance	Nursing Management
furazolidone	May increase the pressor sensitivity to mixed and indirect-acting sympathomimetics, such as pseudoephedrine, resulting in hypertension	Avoid coadministration. If used concurrently, monitor for hypertension. If hypertensive crisis results, consider the use of phentolamine.
guanethidine	Depletes norepinephrine stores, resulting in hypertension	Use an alternative antihypertensive therapy.
monoamine oxidase inhibitors	Increase the amount of norepinephrine available for release by pseudoephedrine, resulting in severe headache, hypertension, and hyperpyrexia; hypertensive crisis possible	Avoid coadministration. If these are used together and hypertension develops, administer phentolamine.
methyldopa	Coadministration of methyldopa and pseudoephedrine may result in an increased pressor response, resulting in hypertension	Monitor the blood pressure during coadministration. Discontinue pseudoephedrine if hypertension occurs.
urinary acidifiers	Tubular reabsorption of pseudoephedrine possibly decreased due to a decreased urinary pH by urinary acidifiers	Monitor possible need for an increased dose of pseudoephedrine to achieve desired results. Acidification of the urine may be useful in the treatment of sympathomimetic intoxication.
urinary alkalinizers	Tubular reabsorption of pseudoephedrine possibly increased due to an increased urinary pH by urinary alkalinizers	Decrease the dose of pseudoephedrine during coadministration of a urinary alkalinizer.

that the drug constricted. When rebound occurs, patients tend to use more of the drug to decrease the congestion, and a vicious cycle of congestion–drug use–congestion develops.

Nursing Diagnoses and Outcomes

- Risk for Injury caused by visual sensory-perceptual alterations (hallucinations) related to drug-induced CNS effects
  Desired outcome: *The patient will be protected from injury related to drug use and will demonstrate safety procedures to use if these effects occur.*
- Ineffective Tissue Perfusion: Cerebral or Cardiopulmonary related to sympathomimetic effects
  Desired outcome: *The patient will be monitored and dosage adjusted to minimize potential perfusion deficits or CNS effects.*

Planning and Intervention

Maximizing Therapeutic Effects

In conjunction with pseudoephedrine therapy, the patient should use a humidifier, drink plenty of fluids, and avoid smoke-filled rooms because dry air, dry mucous membranes, and airborne irritants may render the drug less effective.

Minimizing Adverse Effects

Provide the patient with appropriate safety measures, such as side rails, adequate lighting, and assistance with movement to avoid injury if CNS effects are experienced.

Providing Patient and Family Education

- Explain to patients that the purpose of pseudoephedrine is to promote breathing and relieve congestion.
- Tell patients not to take pseudoephedrine if they have ever had a reaction to it, have high blood pressure, or are breast-feeding. In addition, instruct patients to take the drug exactly as prescribed. Higher doses may cause nervousness, dizziness, chest pain, or sleeplessness.
- Tell patients not to take pseudoephedrine for more than 4 days. They should contact their health care providers to schedule an appointment if respiratory symptoms do not subside after 4 days.
- Caution patients to avoid using other OTC drugs, many of which also contain pseudoephedrine, because a serious overdose could occur.
- To avoid rebound congestion, teach patients strategies for decreasing the discomfort of nasal congestion and explain why excessive drug use should be avoided.
- Outline safety measures that may be necessary if CNS effects occur, such as getting assistance with ambulation, using adequate lighting, and avoiding driving or other tasks that require alertness.
- Urge patients to report excessive dizziness, weakness, palpitations, and sleeplessness, and to keep pseudoephedrine out of the reach of children.

Ongoing Assessment and Evaluation

Monitor for rebound congestion, sedation, dizziness, weakness, tremor, and urinary retention. By the end of therapy, the patient will be free from nasal congestion and free from potential CNS or cardiovascular adverse effects.

MEMORY CHIP

P Pseudoephedrine

- Used to relieve nasal congestion
- Major contraindications: severe hypertension, severe cardiac disorders
- Most common adverse effects: tachycardia, palpitations, and nervousness
- Most serious adverse effects: dysrhythmias, hypertension, and coronary vasospasm
- Maximizing therapeutic effects: Use humidifier and increase fluid intake.
- Minimizing adverse effects: Adhere to safety precautions.
- Most important patient education: Take pseudoephedrine exactly as prescribed to avoid rebound congestion.

Drugs Closely Related to P Pseudoephedrine

Phenylephrine

Phenylephrine (AH-Chew D) is a powerful alpha-adrenergic stimulant that decreases nasal congestion. It is available in oral, spray, and drop formulations. Special caution must be taken to avoid use in abraded nasal membranes, because systemic absorption of this drug can result in severe cardiac, CNS, and urinary effects. As with other decongestants, continuous use may induce rebound congestion.

Topical Decongestant Drugs

Topical decongestants stimulate alpha-adrenergic receptors in the nasal passages, causing constriction in the nasal arterioles. As a result, the nasal membrane is reduced in size, swelling is limited, and the size of the nostril is increased, allowing for more efficient airflow. Although topical decongestants have the same potential adverse effects as pseudoephedrine, the risks are diminished because their action is localized rather than systemic. In very young children, the vascularity of the nasal membranes, developing nasal passages, and eustachian tubes increases the risk for systemic absorption and adverse effects.

Use of topical decongestants for longer than 5 continuous days can lead to rebound congestion. Instruct the patient to stop using the drug if rebound congestion occurs.

CRITICAL THINKING SCENARIO

Prolonged use of nasal decongestants

Noah Rightman, age 16 years, comes to the clinic for a recheck of his allergic rhinitis. He uses a nasal decongestant daily. Lately, he has needed to use his nasal decongestant "10 times a day," and asks, "What's wrong with this drug? I want something stronger." Understanding the sympathetic nervous system, how would you respond to Noah?

C ANTIHISTAMINES

Antihistamines are used to relieve symptoms of allergies. These drugs, which block the action of histamine as it is released during the inflammatory response to an antigen, are very effective for allergic rhinitis. Their action restores normal airflow through the upper respiratory system. Because of their OTC availability, these drugs are often misused to treat colds and influenza. Drugs within the antihistamine class can be separated into first generation and second generation. First-generation antihistamines include diphenhydramine, brompheniramine, and chlorpheniramine. Second-generation antihistamines include fexofenadine, loratadine, and cetirizine. Fexofenadine (Allegra) is the prototype for antihistamines. Table 46.5 presents a summary of antihistamine drugs.

NURSING MANAGEMENT OF THE PATIENT RECEIVING [P] FEXOFENADINE

Core Drug Knowledge

Pharmacotherapeutics

Fexofenadine is used to relieve symptoms associated with seasonal and perennial allergic rhinitis, allergic conjunctivitis, uncomplicated urticaria, and angioedema. It is most effective if used before the onset of symptoms.

Pharmacokinetics

Fexofenadine is taken orally and is absorbed rapidly. The peak drug effect is seen within 2 to 6 hours. Fexofenadine is only slightly (5%) metabolized in the liver and is excreted in the feces (80%) and urine (11%). This drug is assigned to pregnancy category C. This drug crosses the placenta and enters breast milk; therefore, it should be avoided or used with caution by pregnant and lactating women.

Pharmacodynamics

Fexofenadine selectively blocks the effects of histamine at H_1-receptor sites, decreasing the allergic response. Fexofenadine also has anticholinergic and antipruritic effects. However, fexofenadine, a second-generation antihistamine, has less of an anticholinergic effect than the first-generation antihistamines because it binds to lung receptors substantially more than it binds to cerebellar receptors, resulting in a reduced sedative potential.

Contraindications and Precautions

Fexofenadine should not be used in a patient with hypersensitivity to fexofenadine or terfenadine or any of their components, in children younger than 12 years old, or in pregnant or lactating women. Fexofenadine also should be used with caution in patients with renal impairment because the drug's half-life will be prolonged in these patients. In addition, peak plasma levels in patients with renal impairment are increased.

Adverse Effects

The most common adverse reactions associated with fexofenadine therapy include viral infection (e.g., colds and flu), nausea and vomiting, dysmenorrhea, drowsiness, dyspepsia, and fatigue. Fexofenadine is a metabolite of terfenadine. Terfenadine has been associated with QT-interval prolongation and ventricular tachycardias and is no longer manufactured. Fexofenadine has not induced QT-interval prolongation, but patients should still be monitored for this adverse effect.

Drug Interactions

Only a few drug interactions are associated with fexofenadine. They are presented in Table 46.6.

Assessment of Relevant Core Patient Variables

Health Status

Assess the patient's history for allergy to any antihistamine and for pregnancy, lactation, or renal impairment. Before beginning therapy, assess the patient's respiratory system, orientation and affect, and skin condition. If long-term therapy is anticipated, renal function should be assessed as well.

Life Span and Gender

Note the age of the patient before administering fexofenadine. Use special precautions in elderly patients, who are more likely than others to experience dizziness, sedation, and syncope. The drug should not be used by children younger than 12 years old. Determine whether the patient is pregnant because fexofenadine should not be used during pregnancy.

Lifestyle, Diet, and Habits

Evaluate how often the patient drinks apple, grapefruit, or orange juice because these juices decrease the absorption of fexofenadine. Teach the patient to avoid these juices for 1 hour before and 2 hours after taking fexofenadine.

Caution patients taking fexofenadine to assess the level of sedation caused by the drug before driving a vehicle or performing tasks that require concentration.

Environment

Be aware of the environment in which fexofenadine will be administered. Fexofenadine usually is administered at home and in the community setting. Caution patients taking fexofenadine to read the labels of nonprescription products to be sure that they are not taking another product that also contains an antihistamine, which could potentiate the effects of both drugs.

Nursing Diagnosis and Outcome

- Risk for Injury caused by drowsiness and fatigue related to drug-induced CNS effects
  Desired outcome: *Safety precautions will prevent injury related to drug-induced CNS effects.*

Planning and Intervention

Maximizing Therapeutic Effects

Institute measures to prevent dangers associated with thickening of respiratory secretions. Examples of appropriate measures include use of a humidifier, forcing fluids as appropriate,

(*text continues on page 858*)

TABLE 46.5 Summary of Selected (C) Antihistamines

Drug (Trade) Name	Selected Indications	Route and Dosage Range	Pharmacokinetics
Second-Generation Antihistamines			
[P] fexofenadine (Allegra; *Canadian:* Allegra 12 hr)	Allergy relief	*Adult and child >12 y:* PO, 60 mg 2×/d or 180 mg daily *Child 6–11 y:* PO, 30 mg 2×/d	*Onset:* 1–2 h *Duration:* 12 h $t_{1/2}$: 14 h
cetirizine (Zyrtec)	Allergy relief	Tablets, chewable tablets, or oral syrup: PO, *Adult and child >6 y:* 5–10 mg daily *Child 2–5 y:* 2.5 mg (½ teaspoonful or 2.5 mL of oral syrup) daily or 5-mg chewable tablet daily *Child 1–2 y:* PO, 2.5 mg (½ teaspoonful or 2.5 mL) every 12 h *Child 6–11 mo:* PO, 2.5 mg (½ teaspoonful or 2.5 mL) daily	*Onset:* 30 min *Duration:* 24 h $t_{1/2}$: 8–11 h
desloratadine (Clarinex)	Allergy relief	*Adult and child >12 y:* PO, 5 mg daily	*Onset:* 1 h *Duration:* 24 h $t_{1/2}$: 27 h
loratadine (Alavert, Claritin)	Allergy relief	*Adult and child >6 y:* PO, 10 mg daily *Child 2–5 y:* PO, 5 mg (5 mL oral syrup) daily *Child <2 y:* Safe and effective use has not been established.	*Onset:* 1–3 h *Duration:* 24 h $t_{1/2}$: 8.4 h
Inhaled Antihistamine			
azelastine (Astelin)	Allergy relief	*Adult and child >12 y:* 2 sprays per nostril twice daily *Child 5–11 y:* 1 spray per nostril twice daily	Minimal systemic absorption
First-Generation Antihistamines			
brompheniramine (Dimetane, Dimetapp)	Allergy relief	*Adult and child >12:* 4–8 mg PO q6–8 h *Child 6–11:* 2–4 mg q6–8 h *Child 2–5:* 1 mg PO q4–6 h (in children 2–5 y, consult health care provider before administering)	*Onset:* 1 h *Duration:* 9–24 h $t_{1/2}$: 12–34 h
chlorpheniramine (Chlor-Trimeton; *Canadian:* Chlor-Tripalan)	Allergy relief	*Adult and child >12:* 4 mg PO q4–6 h max. 24/mg/d Exten release 8–12 mg q8–12h *Child 6–11:* 2 mg PO q4–6h max 12/mg/d *Child 2–5:* 1 mg PO q4–6 h max 4/mg/d *Adult:* SC, IM, IV; 5–40 mg single dose max. 40 mg/d *Child:* SC (only), 87.5 µg/kg q6h	*Onset:* 15–30 min *Duration:* 4–12 h $t_{1/2}$: 20–24 h
diphenhydramine (Benadryl; *Canadian:* Allerdryl)	Allergy relief	*Adult:* PO, 25–50 mg qid; IV/IM, 10–50 mg to maximum of 400 mg *Child:* PO, 5 mg/kg/d to maximum of 300 mg daily; IV/IM, same	*Onset:* 15–30 min *Duration:* 4–8 h $t_{1/2}$: 2.5–7 h

(continued)

TABLE 46.5 Summary of Selected Ⓒ Antihistamines (continued)

Drug (Trade) Name	Selected Indications	Route and Dosage Range	Pharmacokinetics
Combination Drugs			
acrivastine and pseudo-ephedrine (Semprex-D)	Allergy and congestion relief	*Adult and child >12 y:* PO, 1 capsule (acrivastine 8 mg and pseudo-ephedrine 60 mg) every 4–6 h	See individual components
chlorpheniramine and pseudoephedrine (Sudafed Cold and Allergy)	Allergy and congestion relief	*Adult and child >12 y:* PO, 1 tablet PO every 4–6 h, not to exceed 4 doses in 24 h *Child 6–12 y:* PO, ½ tablet every 4–6 h, not to exceed 4 doses in 24 h	See individual components
loratadine and pseudo-ephedrine (Claritin-D)	Allergy and congestion relief	12-h extended-release tablets: *Adult and child >12 y:* PO, 1 tablet every 12 h 24-h extended-release tablet: *Adult and child >12 y:* PO, 1 tablet every 24 h *Child <12 y:* Safe and effective use has not been established.	See individual components
fexofenadine and pseudo-ephedrine (Allegra-D)	Allergy and congestion relief	*Adult and adolescent:* PO, 1 tablet 2×/d *Child:* Safe and effective use has not been established.	See individual components
triprolidine and pseudo-ephedrine (Actifed Cold and Allergy)	Allergy and congestion relief	*Adult and child >12 y:* PO, 1 tablet or capsule every 4–6 h, not to exceed 4 doses per 24 h *Child 6–12 y:* PO (tablets only), ½ tablet every 4–6 h, not to exceed 4 doses per day Syrup PO: *Adult:* 10 mL PO every 4–6 h Max: 40 mL/day. *Child 6–12 y:* 5 mL PO 3–4 times per day *Child 4–6 y:* 3.75 mL PO 3–4 times per day *Child 2–4 y:* 2.5 mL PO 3–4 times per day *Child 4 mos–2 y:* 1.25 mL PO 3–4 times per day	See individual components
Inhaled Nasal Steroids			
beclomethasone (Beconase, Vancenase)	Allergy and congestion relief	**Metered-dose inhalers (42 µg/spray)** *Adult and child >12 y:* 1 spray into each nostril 2–4 ×/d *Child 6–12 y:* 1 spray into each nostril 3×/d. **AQ pump nasal sprays (42 µg/spray)** *Adult and child >6 y:* 1–2 sprays into each nostril 2×/d **AQ double-strength pump nasal spray (84 µg/spray)**	Minimal systemic absorption

(continued)

TABLE 46.5 Summary of Selected Antihistamines (continued)

Drug (Trade) Name	Selected Indications	Route and Dosage Range	Pharmacokinetics
		Adult and child >6 y: 1–2 sprays into each nostril once daily in the morning Children <6 y: not recommended	
budesonide (Rhinocort)	Allergy and congestion relief	**Metered-dose inhaler (32 µg/spray)** *Adult and child >6 y:* 2 sprays in each nostril in the morning and in the evening, or 4 sprays in each nostril in the morning **AQ pump nasal sprays (32 µg/spray)** *Adult and adolescent:* 1 spray in each nostril once daily in the morning Max: 256 µg/d *Child >6 y:* 1 spray in each nostril once daily in the morning Max: 128 µg/d	Minimal systemic absorption
flunisolide (Nasalide)	Allergy and congestion relief	**AQ pump nasal sprays (25 µg/spray)** *Adult and child >14 y:* 2 sprays in each nostril 2×/d. Max: 200 µg per nostril per day *Child 6–14 y:* 1 spray in each nostril 3×/d, or 2 sprays in each nostril 2×/d Max: 100 µg per nostril per day *Child <6 y:* Safe and effective use has not been established.	Minimal systemic absorption
fluticasone (Flonase)	Allergy and congestion relief	**AQ pump nasal sprays (50 µg/spray)** *Adult >18 y:* 2 sprays per nostril once daily or 1 spray per nostril twice daily Max: 200 µg/d *Child 4–17 y:* 1 spray per nostril once daily *Child <4 y:* Safe and effective dosage has not been established.	Minimal systemic absorption
mometasone (Nasonex)	Allergy and congestion relief	**AQ pump nasal sprays (50 µg/spray)** *Adult and child >11 y:* 2 sprays in each nostril once daily (total daily dose of 200 µg) *Child 2–11 y:* 1 spray in each nostril once daily (total daily dose of 100 µg) *Child <2 y:* Safe and effective use has not been established.	Minimal systemic absorption
triamcinolone (Nasacort)	Allergy and congestion relief	**Metered-dose inhaler (55 µg/pump)** *Adult and adolescent >12 y:* 2 sprays into each nostril once per day Max: 440 µg/d	Minimal systemic absorption

(continued)

TABLE 46.5 Summary of Selected C Antihistamines (continued)

Drug (Trade) Name	Selected Indications	Route and Dosage Range	Pharmacokinetics
		Child 6–11 y: 2 sprays into each nostril once per day Max: 220 μg/d **AQ pump nasal sprays (55 μg/spray)** *Adult and child >12 y:* 2 sprays into each nostril once per day (total dose of 220 μg) *Child 6–11 y:* 1–2 sprays into each nostril once per day	
Inhaled Mast Cell Stabilizer			
cromolyn sodium (NasalCrom)	Allergy and congestion relief	**Metered-dose inhaler (5.2 mg/spray)** *Adult and child >2 y:* 1 spray in each nostril 3–4 times per day	Minimal systemic absorption

and encouraging the patient to avoid dry or smoke-filled areas.

Minimizing Adverse Effects

Refrain from giving the patient apple, grapefruit, or orange juice with fexofenadine because these juices decrease its absorption.

Provide safety measures, such as side rails, and assistance with ambulation if CNS effects occur.

Providing Patient and Family Education

- Explain that fexofenadine is formulated to relieve allergy symptoms.
- Caution patients not to take fexofenadine if they have ever had a reaction to it, are pregnant, or are breast-feeding. In addition, if patients miss a dose, they should take it as soon as they remember, unless it is almost time for the next dose; two doses should not be taken at the same time.
- Tell patients to avoid the use of other OTC drugs, many of which contain similar antihistamines that could cause serious adverse effects if taken concurrently with fexofenadine. Inform patients to avoid alcohol while taking fexofenadine and not to drive or perform tasks that require alertness until the drug's effect has been determined.
- Tell patients to take fexofenadine with food if GI upset occurs and to suck on sugarless lozenges if dry mouth is a problem.
- Teach patients to take fexofenadine with a glass of water. Explain why apple, grapefruit, and orange juices should not be taken at the same time as fexofenadine.
- Warn patients to report difficulty breathing, tremors, hallucinations, and palpitations; teach patients and their families about safety measures that may be needed if these CNS effects occur. Caution patients to keep fexofenadine out of the reach of children.
- Encourage patients to use a humidifier, drink fluids, and avoid overly dry spaces and smoke-filled areas to help decrease the problems associated with the drying effects of antihistamines.

Ongoing Assessment and Evaluation

After several days taking this drug, the patient should experience little discomfort associated with the drug's adverse effects. The patient should be free of injury related to the CNS effects of fexofenadine. The patient should not experience respiratory difficulty related to the anticholinergic effects of the drug.

TABLE 46.6 Agents That Interact With P Fexofenadine

Interactants	Effect and Significance	Nursing Management
juices Apple Grapefruit Orange	Apple, grapefruit, and orange juice decrease the absorption of fexofenadine.	Monitor for continued allergy symptoms. May require increased dose of fexofenadine.
rifampin	Rifampin reduces the absorption of fexofenadine.	Monitor for continued allergy symptoms.
St. John's wort	St. John's wort may induce the metabolism of fexofenadine, resulting in decreased serum concentration of fexofenadine.	Monitor for continued allergy symptoms. May require increased dose of fexofenadine.

MEMORY CHIP

P Fexofenadine

- Used for allergic disorders
- Major contraindication: use in children younger than 12 years old
- Most common adverse effects: flu-like symptoms, nausea and vomiting, dysmenorrhea, and drowsiness
- Most serious adverse effect: potential for QT interval prolongation
- Maximizing therapeutic effects: Use a humidifier and increase fluid intake.
- Minimizing adverse effects: Adhere to safety precautions.
- Most important patient education: Use for symptoms related to allergic disorders; do **not** use for symptoms related to common viral illness, such as colds and flu.

Drugs Closely Related to P Fexofenadine

Azelastine

Azelastine (Astelin) is a second-generation H_1-receptor antagonist that is administered as a nasal spray. It is approved to treat the symptoms of seasonal allergic rhinitis and vasomotor rhinitis such as rhinorrhea, nasal congestion, sneezing, nasal pruritus, and postnasal drip. It acts by locally antagonizing the effects of histamine at the H_1-receptor sites but does not bind to or inactivate histamine. Adverse effects include drowsiness, dizziness, epistaxis, nasal burning, sneezing, dry mouth, and a bitter taste. An FDA pregnancy category C drug, it is approved for use in children older than 5 years.

Cetirizine

Cetirizine (Zyrtec) is the active metabolite of hydroxyzine; it differs from the parent compound by having greater affinity for the H_1 receptor. Cetirizine is effective in treating chronic idiopathic urticaria, perennial allergic rhinitis, and seasonal allergic rhinitis. It causes more sedation than other second-generation antihistamines such as desloratadine, loratadine, and fexofenadine but much less sedation than first-generation antihistamines. Cetirizine is approved for use in children as young as 6 months of age.

Cetirizine is classified as a pregnancy category B drug. It is excreted in human breast milk; because the concentration of drug in breast milk has not been quantified, the manufacturer recommends against using cetirizine during breast-feeding.

Desloratadine

Desloratadine (Clarinex) is the active metabolite of loratadine. It is a potent, long-acting antihistamine. Because it penetrates poorly into the CNS and has low affinity for CNS H_1 receptors, it does not cause intense drowsiness. It is available as regular or rapidly disintegrating tablets. It is approved for use in children older than 12 years.

Desloratadine is a pregnancy category C drug. It enters breast milk and reaches a concentration equal to that in maternal serum. Potential adverse effects in the infant include irritability, disturbed sleeping patterns, drowsiness, hyperexcitability, and excessive crying.

Loratadine

Loratadine (Claritin), like fexofenadine, is a second-generation antihistamine. It has fewer CNS effects than other H_1 receptor blockers and can be administered once a day. It is not indicated for children younger than 2 years old. Loratadine should be given cautiously to patients with pre-existing hepatic dysfunction. To minimize the risk for hepatotoxicity, these patients should take loratadine on an every-other-day regimen. Loratadine is most effective when taken on an empty stomach.

Loratadine is a pregnancy category C drug. Like desloratadine, it enters breast milk in a concentration equal to that in maternal serum.

Drugs Significantly Different From P Fexofenadine

Brompheniramine and Chlorpheniramine

Brompheniramine (Dimetane) and chlorpheniramine (Chlor-Trimeton) are OTC antihistamines, which also may be used in conjunction with decongestants. They are nonselective H_1 blockers (first-generation antihistamines) and thus have sedative effects. Brompheniramine causes less sedation than other first-generation antihistamine agents. These drugs are given to treat allergies such as hay fever, allergic conjunctivitis, urticaria (hives), and angioedema (allergic swelling). They reduce sneezing, runny noses, and itching eyes in hay fever. In addition, they have a mild anticholinergic action that suppresses mucus secretion. Their advantage is that they are relatively inexpensive. The major detriment is that they must be taken every 4 to 6 hours.

Brompheniramine is a pregnancy category C drug. It is contraindicated during the first trimester of pregnancy and should be avoided during the following trimesters. If brompheniramine must be used during pregnancy, extended-release products should be avoided to limit fetal exposure. Chlorpheniramine is a pregnancy category B drug, although it also should be avoided during pregnancy. Both drugs enter breast milk and may induce adverse effects in the breast-feeding infant.

Diphenhydramine

Diphenhydramine (Benadryl) is a first-generation antihistamine known as an ethanolamine. Other ethanolamine antihistamines are carbinoxamine, clemastine, dimenhydrinate, doxylamine, and phenyltoloxamine. Ethanolamine antihistamines have substantial antimuscarinic activity and produce marked sedation in most patients. In general, GI effects are minimal. In addition to treating allergic symptoms, diphenhydramine is effective in relieving nausea, vomiting, and vertigo associated with motion sickness. It also is used commonly to treat drug-induced extrapyramidal symptoms and mild cases of Parkinson disease.

Diphendydramine is a pregnancy category B drug. Although the use of H_1 antagonists is discouraged during pregnancy, diphenhydramine is the parenteral antihistamine of choice for managing acute or severe allergic reactions in pregnant patients. First-generation H_1 antagonists are not used during breast-feeding because they may inhibit lactation. In addition, they may induce paradoxical CNS stimulation in neonates or seizures in premature infants.

Inhaled Nasal Steroids

Inhaled nasal steroidal preparations are used to treat seasonal or perennial allergic rhinitis. In fact, studies have shown that they are superior to oral antihistamines for alleviating nasal, eye, and global allergy symptoms.

Two types of inhaled nasal steroids are available: aqueous sprays that spray a liquid from a bottle through a nozzle fixed at the top of the unit, and metered dose nasal inhalers that deliver the drug from a pressurized canister through a nozzle on the side near the bottom of the unit. Aqueous sprays are less irritating than those delivered by metered dose inhaler.

Common adverse effects of inhaled nasal steroids include a burning or itching sensation and a drying effect on the nasal mucosa. By delivering steroids directly to the nasal passage, inhaled nasal steroids maximize the beneficial therapeutic effects of corticosteroids while minimizing their potential systemic adverse effects, although systemic adverse effects may still occur during long-term or high-dose therapy. Despite these drugs' reduced risk for systemic adverse effects, children receiving inhaled nasal steroids should be evaluated routinely for possible growth retardation, although the risk is extremely small.

The available inhaled nasal steroids are presented in Table 46.5. Discussion of oral steroids is presented in Chapter 51.

Inhaled Mast Cell Stabilizer

Cromolyn sodium (NasalCrom Nasal Spray) is the only treatment indicated for nasal allergy symptoms that is available OTC. Cromolyn sodium provides a protective layer that shields mast cells lining the nasal passage and prevents them from breaking down and releasing histamines. Common adverse effects include irritation inside of the nose, flushing, and an increase in sneezing. Cromolyn sodium has been approved for adults and children older than 2 years. For best results, cromolyn sodium should be taken for 1 full week before coming in contact with allergens and should then be taken three to four times daily.

(C) EXPECTORANT DRUGS

Expectorants are drugs that liquefy lower respiratory tract secretions. This effect decreases the viscosity of the secretions (which makes it easier for the patient to cough them up) and improves airflow. Expectorants are available in many OTC preparations, making them widely available to the patient without advice from a health care provider. Drugs within the expectorant class include guaifenesin and terpin hydrate. Although not within the expectorant class, iodine preparations have actions very similar to drugs within this class. Guaifenesin (Robitussin) is the prototype expectorant drug. Table 46.7 presents a summary of selected expectorant drugs.

NURSING MANAGEMENT OF THE PATIENT RECEIVING [P] GUAIFENESIN

Core Drug Knowledge

Pharmacotherapeutics

Guaifenesin is used to relieve the symptoms of respiratory conditions characterized by a dry, nonproductive cough. These disorders include the common cold, acute bronchitis, and influenza. Guaifenesin is often found in combination with antihistamines and decongestants (see Table 46.6).

Pharmacokinetics

Guaifenesin is taken orally and is absorbed readily from the GI tract, with an onset of action of 30 minutes. The duration of action is 4 to 6 hours.

Pharmacodynamics

Guaifenesin enhances the output of respiratory tract fluids by reducing the adhesiveness and surface tension of the flu-

TABLE 46.7 Summary of Selected (C) Expectorants

Drug (Trade) Name	Selected Indications	Route and Dosage Range	Pharmacokinetics
[P] guaifenesin (Robitussin, Scot-Tussin, Mytussin, Fenesin, and many more)	Relief of conditions characterized by dry, nonproductive cough Presence of mucus in the respiratory tract	*Adult:* PO, 100–400 mg q4h, not to exceed 2.4 g/d *Child >12 y:* PO, adult dosage *6–12 y:* PO, 100–200 mg q4h, not to exceed 1.2 g/d *2–6 y:* PO, 50–100 mg q4h, not to exceed 600 mg/d	*Onset:* 30 min *Duration:* 4–6 h $t_{1/2}$: Unknown
terpin hydrate (various)	Symptomatic relief of dry, nonproductive cough	*Adult:* PO, 85–170 mg tid–qid *Child:* Do not give unless prescribed *10–12 y:* 85 mg tid–qid *5–9 y:* 40 mg tid–qid *1–4 y:* 20 mg tid–qid	*Onset:* 30–60 min *Duration:* Unknown $t_{1/2}$: Unknown
iodine preparations (SSKI, Potassium Iodide)	Symptomatic treatment of COPD diseases in which tenacious mucus complicates the problem	*Adult:* PO, 300–1000 mg after meals bid–tid *Child:* PO, 150–500 mg after meals bid–tid	*Onset:* 30 min *Duration:* Unknown $t_{1/2}$: Unknown

ids, thus allowing easier movement of the less viscous secretions. Thinned secretions result in a more productive cough. With a more productive cough, the frequency of coughing should decrease.

Contraindications and Precautions

The only known contraindication to guaifenesin is a known allergy to the drug. The drug is assigned to pregnancy category C and therefore should be used with caution in patients who are pregnant or lactating. The most important consideration in the use of this drug is discovering the cause of the underlying cough. Prolonged use of the OTC preparation could result in masking important symptoms of a serious underlying disorder. The drug should not be used for more than a week; if the cough persists, encourage the patient to visit the prescriber.

Adverse Effects

The most common adverse effects of guaifenesin use are GI symptoms, including nausea, vomiting, and anorexia. Some patients experience headache or dizziness, and an occasional person will develop a mild rash.

Drug Interactions

Guaifenesin has no important drug–drug interactions. However, it may interfere with colorimetric tests and give false results with urinary catecholamine determinations.

Assessment of Relevant Core Patient Variables

Health Status

Assess the patient for any past hypersensitivity to guaifenesin; history of persistent cough for more than 1 week; cough caused by smoking, asthma, or emphysema; or a very productive cough. In addition, perform a physical assessment, which should include an examination of the patient's skin condition (as a baseline if a rash develops), temperature (to monitor for underlying problems), respiratory status, and adventitious breath sounds.

Life Span and Gender

Determine whether the patient is pregnant. Guaifenesin is a pregnancy category C drug and so should be used very cautiously by pregnant patients.

Lifestyle, Diet, and Habits

It is important to assess the patient's smoking habits and typical alcohol intake. Smokers will not benefit from the action of guaifenesin because the etiology of their cough is irritation. When using guaifenesin, the patient should take care not to drink alcohol or use other drugs containing alcohol. Although guaifenesin and alcohol do not interact, both cause drowsiness; therefore, they should not be taken together.

Nursing Diagnoses and Outcomes

- Imbalanced Nutrition: Less than Body Requirements related to GI symptoms of nausea and vomiting
  Desired outcome: *The patient will maintain baseline weight and nutritional status.*
- Ineffective Airway Clearance related to increased viscosity of secretions
  Desired outcome: *The patient will demonstrate effective coughing technique and make use of several methods to increase airway clearance.*

Planning and Intervention

Maximizing Therapeutic Effects

Teach the patient about good pulmonary hygiene, which includes coughing, deep breathing, drinking plenty of fluids, and using a humidifier. Show the patient how to perform effective coughing technique. Family members may assist with percussion and postural drainage as appropriate.

Minimizing Adverse Effects

Suggest that the patient eat small, frequent meals to alleviate GI upset. Additionally, give the drug with meals if symptoms become intolerable.

Providing Patient and Family Education

- Explain to patients that guaifenesin will help make it easier to cough up secretions from the lungs.
- Warn patients not to take guaifenesin if they have ever had a reaction to it, if their cough is caused by smoking, or if their cough is chronic (unless use of the drug is approved by their provider).
- Tell patients not to use guaifenesin for longer than 1 week, and that if the cough persists after that time, or if fever or rash develops, they should consult with their prescriber.
- Caution patients taking guaifenesin not to take any other drugs without their provider's approval and not to drink alcohol while taking this drug.
- Tell patients that if a dose is missed, it should be taken as soon as remembered unless it is time for the next dose. Two doses should never be taken at the same time.
- Teach patients ways to augment guaifenesin therapy, such as drinking a glass of water with each dose. Lots of water will help the body thin the secretions in the lungs and will help guaifenesin work more efficiently. Other ways to augment drug therapy include use of a humidifier, deep breathing, chest percussion, and positional drainage if needed. In addition, teach patients good coughing technique and encourage patients to use the technique regularly.

Ongoing Assessment and Evaluation

Monitor the patient's reaction to the drug carefully; fever, rash, or persistent cough may indicate a more serious underlying medical problem, and appropriate follow-up should be arranged. The patient will tolerate drug adverse effects through use of small, frequent meals and proper timing of dosage. Within 1 week, the patient will exhibit an increasingly productive cough and good movement of respiratory secretions, as demonstrated by productive cough and clearing breath sounds.

MEMORY CHIP

P Guaifenesin

- Used to manage dry cough
- Major contraindication: hypersensitivity
- Most common adverse effects: nausea, vomiting, and anorexia
- Maximizing therapeutic effects: good pulmonary hygiene
- Minimizing adverse effects: small, frequent meals to decrease GI distress
- Most important patient education: Seek medical attention if cough does not resolve.

Drugs Closely Related to P Guaifenesin

Terpin Hydrate

Terpin hydrate stimulates the glands of the respiratory tract to increase the amount of fluid secreted. Actions and management related to this drug are very similar to those for guaifenesin. However, terpin hydrate contains about 42% alcohol, which crosses the placenta and may result in congenital abnormalities. The alcohol in terpin hydrate also is excreted in breast milk and can be harmful to infants.

Iodine Preparations

These drugs have been used for many years to stimulate an increase in the fluid produced by the lungs. They are used in treating chronic obstructive pulmonary disease and as adjunctive treatment in respiratory tract conditions, such as cystic fibrosis and chronic sinusitis, and after surgery to prevent atelectasis. These drugs tend to have a bitter flavor, which limits their popularity. They must be used with caution in many conditions because of the effect of iodine on the thyroid gland. Iodine preparations are assigned to pregnancy category X because of potential damage to the fetal thyroid.

CHAPTER SUMMARY

- The upper respiratory system is composed of upper or conducting airways, including the nares, nasal sinus, pharynx, larynx, and trachea.
- Disorders of the upper respiratory system include inflammation and irritation of the upper airways.
- Antitussives, such as dextromethorphan, are drugs used to suppress the cough reflex when dry, nonproductive coughing is tiring and irritating to the respiratory system.
- Decongestants, such as pseudoephedrine, are drugs used to decrease the swelling and blood flow to the mucosa of the respiratory tract. Oral decongestants have greater potential than topical decongestants, which are applied directly to the mucosa, to cause systemic adverse effects. However, the topical decongestants are more likely to cause rebound congestion if used longer than 5 consecutive days.
- Antihistamines are classified as first- or second-generation drugs. First-generation antihistamines are more sedating than second-generation drugs.
- Antihistamines, such as fexofenadine, are used to block the action of histamine as it is released in response to an inflammatory reaction. These drugs block the swelling and congestion that follow histamine release.
- Antihistamines may be taken orally, or by nasal or topical administration.
- Inhaled nasal steroids are also used to manage allergic rhinitis and vasomotor rhinitis.
- Expectorants, such as guaifenesin, are drugs used to increase the viscosity and volume of the respiratory tract secretions, which helps patients to clear the lower respiratory tract of tenacious secretions.

QUESTIONS FOR STUDY AND REVIEW

1. What is the difference between dextromethorphan and narcotic antitussive agents?
2. Why are antihistamines inappropriate for treating the common viral cold?
3. What property of fexofenadine makes it an excellent antihistamine?
4. What are the advantages of inhaled antihistamine or steroid drugs over oral formulations?
5. How does guaifenesin assist in controlling cough?

Need More Help?

Chapter 46 of the study guide for *Drug Therapy in Nursing* 2e contains NCLEX-style questions and other learning activities to reinforce your understanding of the concepts presented in this chapter. For additional information or to purchase the study guide, visit *http://connection.lww.com/go/aschenbrenner.*

REFERENCES AND BIBLIOGRAPHY

Clinical Pharmacology [Online]. Available: *http://cp.gsm.com.*

Facts and Comparisons. (2004). *Drug facts and comparisons.* Philadelphia: Lippincott Williams & Wilkins.

Hardman, J. G. (2001). *Goodman & Gilman's the pharmacological basis of therapeutics* (10th ed.). New York: McGraw-Hill Health Professions Division.

Katzung, B. (2004). *Basic and clinical pharmacology* (9th ed.). New York: McGraw-Hill/Appleton & Lange.

Micromedex Healthcare Series [Online]. Available: *http://healthcare.micromedex.com.*

Tatro, D. S. (2004). *Drug interaction facts.* Philadelphia: Lippincott Williams & Wilkins..

Drugs Affecting the Lower Respiratory System

chapter 47

KEY TERMS

bronchodilators

bronchospasm

chemoreceptors

chronic airway limitation (CAL)

chronic obstructive pulmonary disease (COPD)

mucolytics

perfusion

respiration

ventilation

Learning Objectives

At the completion of this chapter the student will:

1. Describe the anatomy and physiology of the lower respiratory system.
2. Identify core drug knowledge pertaining to drugs that affect the lower respiratory system.
3. Identify core patient variables pertaining to drugs that affect the lower respiratory system.
4. Relate the interaction of core drug knowledge to core patient variables for drugs that affect the lower respiratory system.
5. Generate a nursing plan of care from the interactions between core drug knowledge and core patient variables for drugs that affect the lower respiratory system.
6. Describe nursing interventions to maximize therapeutic and minimize adverse effects for drugs that affect the lower respiratory system.
7. Determine key points for patient and family education for drugs that affect the lower respiratory system.
8. Compare and contrast drugs used for maintenance treatment of lower respiratory disorders with those used to manage acute exacerbations of lower respiratory disorders.

FEATURED WEBLINK

http://www.lungusa.org
Asthma, bronchitis, emphysema—how do you know what is happening to your patient? Log on to this site for information concerning these chronic lung disorders.

CONNECTION WEBLINK

Additional Weblinks are found on Connection:
http://www.connection.lww.com/go/aschenbrenner.

Drugs Affecting the Lower Respiratory System

© Mucolytics

- [P] **acetylcysteine**
- dornase alfa

© Bronchodilators

© Beta agonists
- [P] **albuterol**
- epinephrine
- formoterol
- isoproterenol
- levalbuterol
- metaproterenol
- pirbuterol
- salmeterol
- terbutaline

© Anticholinergics
- [P] **ipratropium bromide**
- tiotropium

© Xanthine derivatives
- [P] **theophylline**
- aminophylline
- dyphylline
- caffeine

© Anti-Inflammatory Agents

© Inhaled glucocorticoid steroids
- [P] **flunisolide**
- beclomethasone
- budesonide
- fluticasone
- triamcinolone

© Mast cell stabilizers
- [P] **cromolyn sodium**
- nedocromil
- **omalizumab**

© Leukotriene receptor antagonists
- [P] **zafirlukast**
- montelukast
- zileuton

The symbol © indicates the **drug class.**
Drugs in **bold type** marked with the symbol [P] are prototypes.
Drugs in blue type are closely related to the prototype.
Drugs in **red type** are significantly different from the prototype.
Drugs in black type with no symbol are also used in drug therapy; no prototype

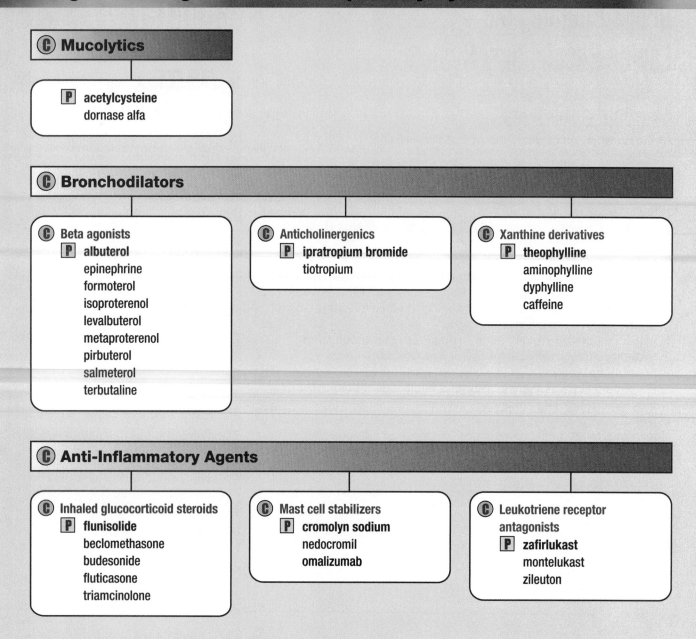

This chapter discusses drugs that affect the lower respiratory system. The lower respiratory system is affected by many serious conditions, which all, to some extent, affect the ability to move air in and out of the lungs. Examples of these conditions include pneumonia, bronchitis, chronic obstructive pulmonary diseases, and cystic fibrosis.

Drugs used to manage lower respiratory system disorders include mucolytics such as acetylcysteine; bronchodilators, which include several subclasses, such as sympathomimetics (respiratory beta agonists), anticholinergics, and xanthines; and anti-inflammatory drugs, which also have several subclasses, including glucocorticoids, mast cell stabilizers, monoclonal antibodies, and leukotriene receptor antagonists.

PHYSIOLOGY

The lower respiratory tract is virtually sterile because of the various defense mechanisms in the upper respiratory system. The lower respiratory system, or the respiratory airway, begins at the trachea. The trachea bifurcates, or divides, into two main bronchi, which further divide into smaller and smaller branches, forming the bronchial tree. The bronchial tree flows into the lungs, a pair of organs composed of a network of blood vessels and small bronchi and alveoli: the functional units of the lungs (Figure 47.1).

Protective Mechanisms

The bronchial tubes have three layers: cartilage, muscle, and epithelial cells. The cartilage keeps the tube open and becomes progressively less abundant as the bronchi divide and get smaller. The muscles also help to keep the bronchi open, and they too become smaller and less abundant, with only a few muscle fibers remaining in the terminal bronchi and alveoli.

All the tubes in the lower airway contain goblet cells, which secrete mucus to entrap any particles that may have escaped the upper airway protective mechanisms. In addition, during the passage through the bronchi, microorganisms and other foreign bodies are removed from the air by tiny hair-like structures called cilia, which project from the cells that line the bronchial wall. With a wave-like motion, these cilia sweep the foreign material and mucus upward toward the trachea and larynx. The walls of the trachea and the conducting bronchi are very sensitive to irritation. Foreign material and mucus stimulate nerve endings in the bronchial wall and initiate the cough reflex. Coughing completes the expulsion of the foreign material and mucus from the bronchial tree.

Gas Exchange, Perfusion, and Respiration

Lung tissue receives its blood supply from the bronchial artery, which branches directly off the thoracic aorta. The alveoli receive unoxygenated blood from the right ventricle

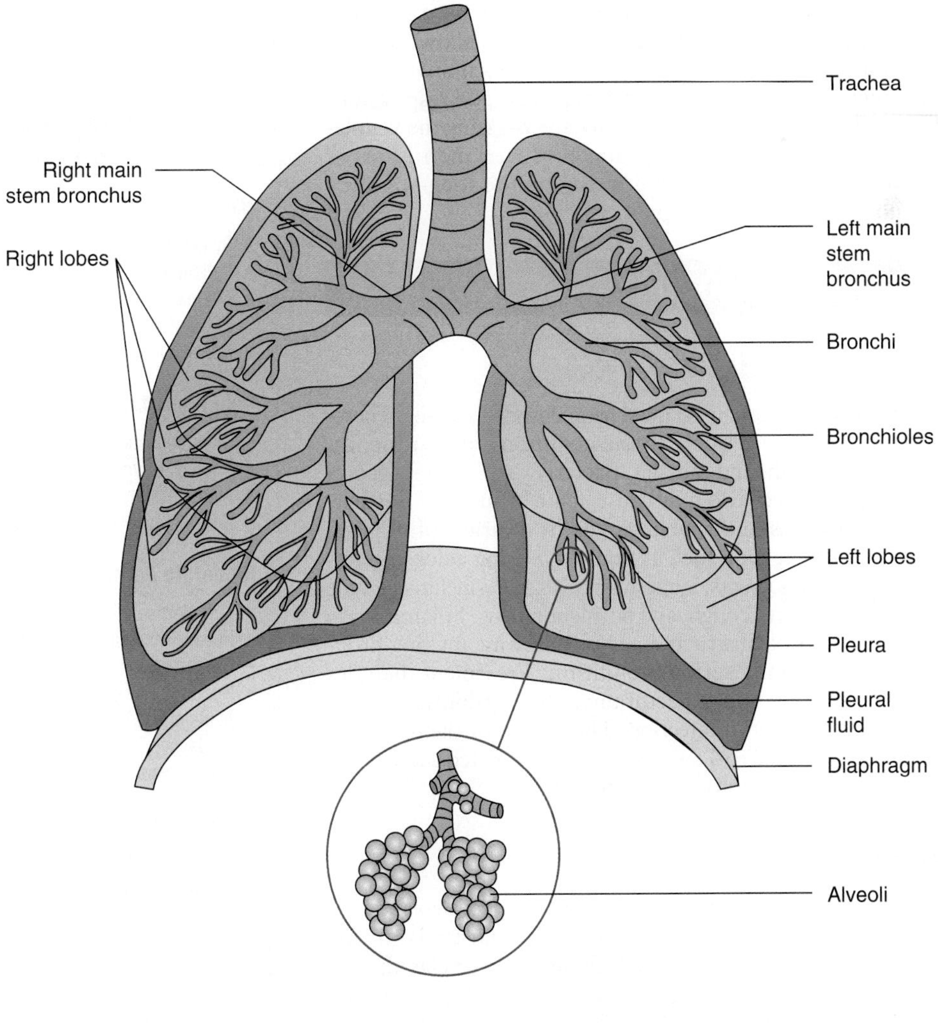

FIGURE 47.1 Lower respiratory system.

by way of the pulmonary artery. Blood delivery to the alveoli is referred to as **perfusion.** In the alveoli, gas exchange occurs; carbon dioxide is removed from the blood, while oxygen from inhaled air diffuses into the blood. This exchange of gases at the alveolar level is called **respiration.** The alveolar sac stays open even during exhalation because the nitrogen and oxygen gases it contains exert outward pressure and because the lungs produce a lipoprotein surfactant that decreases the surface tension of the alveolar walls, preventing alveolar collapse. Oxygenated blood is returned from the lungs to the left atrium through the pulmonary veins. From there, it is pumped throughout the body to deliver oxygen and pick up waste products.

Ventilation

Ventilation, or the act of breathing, is controlled by the central nervous system (CNS). The inspiratory muscles (the diaphragm and the external intercostal and abdominal muscles) are stimulated to contract by the respiratory center in the medulla. The medulla receives input from **chemoreceptors** (neuroreceptors in the medulla, aorta, and carotid arteries that are sensitive to carbon dioxide and acid levels) and increases the rate or depth of respiration to maintain homeostasis in the body. The vagus nerve, a predominantly parasympathetic nerve, plays a key role in stimulating the diaphragm to contract, causing inspiration. Vagal stimulation also leads to bronchoconstriction (tightening of the bronchi). The sympathetic system also innervates the respiratory system. Stimulation of the sympathetic system leads to increased rate and depth of respiration and dilates the bronchi to allow freer airflow through the system. During a physical examination, you document vital signs as temperature, pulse, and respirations (TPR). To be accurate, you actually are assessing the ventilatory rate, not the respiratory rate. However, the authors of this text do not recommend changing the long-standing method of charting vital signs.

PATHOPHYSIOLOGY

Acute Bronchitis

Acute bronchitis is caused most frequently by viruses. Therefore, it may be a sequela to the common cold, influenza, whooping cough, and measles. Bacteria such as streptococci and staphylococci also may cause acute bronchitis. Furthermore, bronchitis can be precipitated by a variety of physical and chemical agents, such as fumes of strong acids, ammonia, or organic solvents. Symptoms of acute bronchitis include fever, a productive cough, and purulent mucus. Inflammation often narrows or obstructs a person's airway, making bronchitis a potentially serious condition. Treatment includes bronchodilators and expectorants, plus antibiotic therapy if there is a bacterial infection. The course of the disease is commonly short: 2 to 4 days. However, untreated acute bronchitis may develop into chronic bronchitis.

Asthma

Asthma is a disorder characterized by recurrent episodes of **bronchospasm,** bronchial muscle spasm that leads to narrowed or obstructed airways. Asthma has been classified as either intrinsic or extrinsic. Intrinsic asthma has no identifiable cause but has been associated with exercise and emotional stress. Extrinsic asthma occurs as a result of an allergic reaction to an environmental allergen. Exposure to the antigen causes a rapid and intense inflammatory reaction with the release of histamine, serotonin, and leukotrienes. These chemicals cause severe bronchoconstriction and increased mucus production. In addition, as airway obstruction increases pressure in the respiratory system, fluid moves into the tissues and results in further obstruction. This reaction usually occurs within 5 to 30 minutes after exposure to the allergen. Classifications of asthma are shown in Box 47.1. An extreme type of asthma is called status asthmaticus. This is a life-threatening bronchospasm, which occludes airflow into the lungs and requires emergency treatment. Pharmacotherapy for asthma is dependent on the current classification because the patient may fluctuate between classes, depending on their response to medication as well as environmental, psychological, and physical stressors (Table 47.1). Figure 47.2 shows where various asthma drugs exert their effects.

Chronic Obstructive Pulmonary Diseases

Chronic airway limitation (CAL) is a new term for **chronic obstructive pulmonary disease** (COPD). CAL is an umbrella term that describes gradually progressive, degenerative diseases, such as chronic bronchitis, emphysema, or repeated, severe asthma attacks. In CAL, the bronchioles become thick and edematous, the upper respiratory defense mechanisms are

BOX 47.1 Classifications of Asthma

Mild Intermittent

- Symptoms occur two or fewer times per week
- Patient asymptomatic and normal peak flow between exacerbations
- Acute exacerbations tend to be brief but may range from moderate to severe
- Normal peak flow is greater than 80% of predicted value

Mild Persistent

- Symptoms occur more than twice per week but not daily
- Nocturnal symptoms occur more than twice per month
- Acute exacerbations interfere with daily activities
- Normal peak flow is greater than 80% of predicted value

Moderate Persistent

- Symptoms occur daily
- Rescue medication used daily
- Exacerbations affect activity
- Nocturnal symptoms occur more than once per week
- Acute exacerbations occur two or more times per week and may last for days
- Normal peak flow is 60% to 80% of predicted value

Severe Persistent

- Continued symptoms that limit physical activity
- Frequent acute exacerbations
- Frequent nocturnal symptoms
- Normal peak flow is less than 60% of predicted value

TABLE 47.1 A Systematic Approach to Asthma: National Education and Prevention

Asthma Classification	Daily Medications	Rescue Drugs
Step 1: mild intermittent	No daily medications	Short-acting, inhaled beta-2 agonist*
Step 2: mild persistent	Inhaled anti-inflammatory: glucocorticoid (low dose) **or** cromolyn sodium **or** nedocromil **or** zafirlukast for patient >12 years of age **or** Sustained release theophylline may be used but not preferred	Short-acting, inhaled beta-2 agonist*
Step 3: moderate persistent	Inhaled glucocorticoid (moderate dose) **or** Inhaled glucocorticoid (low-medium) dose **plus** long acting bronchodilator: • inhaled salmeterol • sustained-release theophylline • long-acting beta-2-agonist tablets	Short-acting, inhaled beta-2 agonist*
Step 4: severe persistent	Daily combined use of a high-dose inhaled corticosteroid **and** long-acting bronchodilator: • inhaled salmeterol • sustained-release theophylline • long-acting beta-2-agonist tablets **and** Systemic steroids (tablets or syrup) as needed (make every attempt to control with high dose inhaled steroids rather than systemic steroids)	Short-acting, inhaled beta-2 agonist*

*Use of short-acting inhaled beta-2 agonists on a daily basis, or increasing use, indicates the need for additional long-term control therapy.

destroyed, and constant irritation and inflammation of the lower respiratory tract are present. With time, the fragile alveoli enlarge and collapse or fuse. Air is trapped in the lungs as the elastic fibers are lost, and increasing amounts of energy are required to try to move the air through the narrowed bronchial tubes. The lungs overinflate and the efficiency of gas exchange is lost. The person suffering from CAL complains of dyspnea and shortness of breath. A barrel chest develops as the lungs overinflate. The person is fatigued from the poor oxygenation of the blood and from the increased expenditure of energy required for breathing.

Chronic Bronchitis

Chronic bronchitis is long-standing, largely irreversible inflammation of the bronchial tree. The continuous inflammatory injury to the lining of the bronchial tree has destroyed many of the cells, the cilia are absent, and the defense mechanism against invading foreign material is lost. The bronchial tubes are narrow, rigid, and distorted. Viscous mucous materials are hypersecreted, resulting in a chronic, deep, and productive cough. The cough is difficult to suppress and in fact should not be, because the abundant secretions must be eliminated to avoid the danger of severe superimposed infection.

Excessive and prolonged tobacco smoking can cause chronic bronchitis and is certainly one of its most aggravating factors. Infections of the sinus cavities also provide a reservoir of microorganisms that can continually reinfect the lungs. Damaged bronchi are ideal sites for harboring infections and for accumulation of excess fluids and secreted mucus. Episodes of acute bronchitis and pneumonia are frequent because the respiratory tract is more susceptible to invasion by pathogenic microorganisms.

Emphysema

Emphysema is an abnormal distention of the lungs with air characterized by loss or degeneration of elastic tissue, disappearance of capillary walls, and breakdown of the alveolar walls. The alveoli first stretch and then tend to disintegrate. The lungs become filled with large pools of air, and loss of elastic support around small airways, or loss of the small airways themselves, severely interferes with expiration. As with chronic bronchitis, smoking is the main cause of emphysema. Symptoms include severe breathlessness on exertion, weight loss, and swelling in the extremities. The skin takes on a bluish color from lack of sufficient gas exchange, there is tightness in the chest, and the affected person wheezes.

Bullous emphysema is a variety of emphysema in which the distended alveoli form large air cysts on one or both of the lungs and occasionally rupture, causing lung collapse.

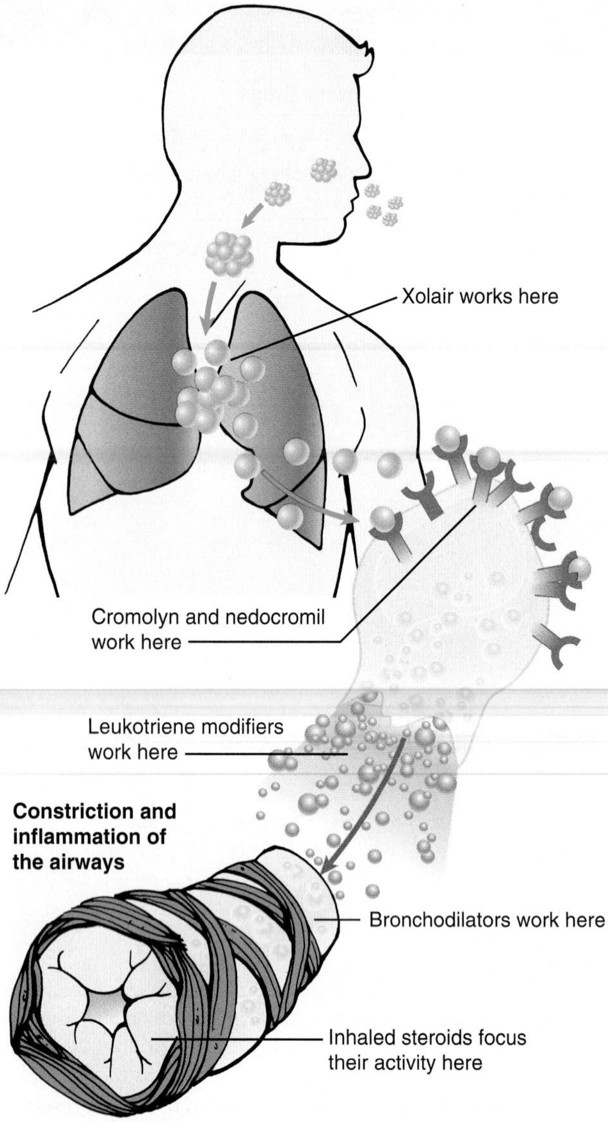

FIGURE 47.2 Drugs used in the management of asthma.

FOCUS ON RESEARCH

Box 47.2 Identifying Respiratory Pathogens Using an Electronic "Nose"

Lai, S. Y., Deffenderfer, O. F., Hanson, W., et al. (2002). Identification of upper respiratory bacterial pathogens with the electronic nose. *Laryngoscope, 112*(6), 975–979.

The Study

The sense of smell has been an important diagnostic tool since ancient times. An electronic nose (Cyranose 320), initially created by the California Institute of Technology (Caltech) with a grant funded by NASA's Jet Propulsion Laboratory (JPL) for quality-control purposes in the food and chemical industries, has been further developed and incorporated into a unit that monitors closed human habitats such as the Space Shuttle, where air must be recycled. The Cyranose 320 is now available for commercial uses. These researchers developed a study to evaluate its ability to identify common upper respiratory bacterial pathogens. The researchers programed the electronic nose to identify the odor of six types of common bacteria. The electronic nose was able to distinguish between control swabs and bacterial samples. Using a complex mathematical equation, researchers were able to determine that the electronic nose could differentiate among various common bacterial pathogens of the upper respiratory tract, including *Staphylococcus aureus, Streptococcus pneumoniae, Haemophilus influenzae,* and *Pseudomonas aeruginosa.* The researchers concluded that the electronic nose could provide a rapid means to identify organisms causing upper respiratory infections. Subsequent research determined that the electronic device was 70% to 92% accurate in diagnosing lower airway infections such as pneumonia (Sniffing out pneumonia, 2004).

Nursing Implications

Nurses use a variety of biomedical equipment. Although this device is not yet FDA approved, many hospitals may be involved in clinical trials using this device. The implication for this new device is that serious infections such as pneumonia and sinusitis may be identified early in the disease process, enabling the health care team to coordinate timely initiation of appropriate medications such as bronchodilators, antibiotics, and oral and nasal inhalers.

Pneumonia

Pneumonia is an inflammation of the lungs. It can be caused by bacterial or viral invasion of the tissue or by aspiration of foreign substances into the lower respiratory tract. The lung tissue progresses through an inflammatory reaction that produces symptoms of difficulty breathing, fever, productive cough, shortness of breath, and sometimes chest pain. Pneumonia is more frequently seen when a person's immune system is compromised or when the person has an upper respiratory disorder that causes the normal protective mechanisms to be inefficient. Its etiology can be challenging to pinpoint. Box 47.2 describes a novel approach to identifying respiratory pathogens.

Cystic Fibrosis

Cystic fibrosis is a hereditary disease that affects the functioning of the body's exocrine glands: the mucus-secreting and sweat glands. In persons with this disease, a protein is produced that lacks the amino acid phenylalanine. This flawed protein distorts the movement of salt and water across the membranes that line the lungs and gut, resulting in dehydration of the mucus that normally coats these surfaces. Thus, the normal mucous secretions in the respiratory and digestive systems become abnormally thick, sticky, and concentrated. The thick, sticky mucus accumulates in the lungs, plugging the bronchi and making breathing difficult. This condition results in chronic respiratory infections, often bacterial. Chronic cough, recurrent pneumonia, and the progressive loss of lung function are the major manifestations of this disease. The goals of treatment are to keep the secretions fluid and moving and to maintain airway patency as much as possible. Because the disease increases tenacious mucus secretions, acetylcysteine (Mucomyst), a mucolytic drug, is the drug of choice.

Ⓒ MUCOLYTIC DRUGS

Mucolytics break down mucus and help the high-risk respiratory patient cough up thick, tenacious secretions to improve breathing and airflow. The drugs can be administered by a nebulizer or by direct instillation into the trachea through an endotracheal tube or tracheostomy. Mucolytics usually are reserved for patients who have major difficulty mobilizing and coughing up secretions. Mucolytic drugs include acetylcysteine and dornase alfa. Acetylcysteine is the prototypical mucolytic agent. Table 47.2 presents a summary of selected mucolytic agents.

NURSING MANAGEMENT OF THE PATIENT RECEIVING P ACETYLCYSTEINE

Core Drug Knowledge

Pharmacotherapeutics

Acetylcysteine is used to liquefy the thick, tenacious secretions of patients whose respiratory disorders make it difficult to mobilize and cough up these secretions. These disorders include CAL, cystic fibrosis, pneumonia, and tuberculosis. Acetylcysteine also is indicated for patients who develop atelectasis (collapse of the alveoli) because of thick mucus secretions. It can be used during diagnostic bronchoscopy to clear the airway, to facilitate the removal of secretions postoperatively, and to facilitate airway clearance and suctioning in patients with tracheostomies. Other uses for acetylcysteine include treating acetaminophen overdose, hepatorenal syndrome, and toxic renal effects caused by cisplatin therapy. It is also used to prevent contrast-induced renal complications in patients receiving contrast agents for diagnostic imaging tests.

Pharmacokinetics

Acetylcysteine is delivered directly to the respiratory system by nebulizer (inhalation) or direct instillation. Onset of effect occurs within 1 minute, with a peak effect occurring within 5 to 10 minutes. The drug is metabolized in the liver and is excreted in the urine (see Table 47.2).

Pharmacodynamics

Acetylcysteine affects the mucoproteins in the respiratory secretions. It splits disulfide bonds that are responsible for holding the mucous material together. The result is a decrease in the tenacity and viscosity of the secretions. This drug also protects liver cells from being damaged during episodes of acetaminophen toxicity. It has this effect because it normalizes hepatic glutathione levels and binds with a reactive hepatotoxic metabolite of acetaminophen. In its role in preventing contrast-induced nephrotoxicity, acetylcysteine acts as an antioxidant. Antioxidants prevent oxygen free radicals from bonding with other unbound radicals and thus reduce cell damage.

TABLE 47.2 Summary of Selected Ⓒ Mucolytics

Drug (Trade) Name	Selected Indications	Route and Dosage Range	Pharmacokinetics
P acetylcysteine (Mucomyst; *Canadian:* Parvolex)	Mucolytic adjuvant therapy for abnormal or viscous mucous secretions in acute and chronic bronchopulmonary disease Diagnostic bronchial studies Acetaminophen antidote	Nebulization with face mask, mouthpiece, tracheostomy 1–10 mL of 20% solution or 2–20 mL of 10% solution q2–6h Nebulization with tent, croupette: up to 300 mL per treatment Instillation: Direct or by tracheostomy 1–2 mL of a 10%–20% solution q1–4h Diagnostic bronchogram: Before the procedure, give two to three administrations of 1–2 mL of a 20% solution or 2–4 mL of a 10% solution by nebulization or intratracheal instillation Acetaminophen antidote: PO, 140 mg/kg loading dose followed by 17 maintenance doses of 70 mg/kg starting 4 h after the loading dose	*Onset:* Instillation and inhalation, 1 min *Duration:* 2–3 h $t_{1/2}$: 6–25 h
dornase alfa (Pulmozyme)	Management of respiratory symptoms associated with cystic fibrosis	*Adult:* Inhaled, 2.5 mg qid through nebulizer *Child >5 y:* Inhaled, adult dosage	*Onset:* Slow *Duration:* 1 wk $t_{1/2}$: Unknown

Contraindications and Precautions

Acetylcysteine is contraindicated in patients who are hypersensitive to the drug. It should be used with caution in patients with a history of respiratory compromise. For example, acetylcysteine should be used with caution in any condition that compromises the patient's ability to cough because the increased volume of secretions can compromise the airway if it is not cleared. It should also be used with caution in patients who have asthma because bronchospasm can occur.

Intravenous (IV) acetylcysteine is used with caution in patients with serious hepatic disease because these patients may have higher serum concentrations of acetylcysteine than other patients do. Oral acetylcysteine may induce vomiting; thus, it should be given cautiously to patients with esophageal varices or peptic ulcer disease because vomiting can result in acute bleeding.

Adverse Effects

Inhaled acetylcysteine may induce bronchospasm, bronchoconstriction, chest tightness, a burning feeling in the upper airway, and rhinorrhea. Some patients report stomatitis as well. Less common adverse effects are fever, chills, drowsiness, and clammy skin.

IV acetylcysteine may induce anaphylactoid reactions such as angioedema, chest tightness, rash, hypotension, and tachycardia. Both IV and oral acetylcysteine may cause nausea and vomiting.

Drug Interactions

No important drug interactions have been reported for acetylcysteine.

Assessment of Relevant Core Patient Variables

Health Status

Before initiating therapy, perform a physical examination to establish baselines. This examination should include temperature, skin evaluation, respiratory evaluation (including adventitious sounds and ability to cough), and an abdominal assessment for potential hepatomegaly.

Life Span and Gender

Determine whether the patient is pregnant or breast-feeding because acetylcysteine should be avoided during pregnancy and lactation unless the benefit to the mother outweighs the potential risk to the fetus or child.

Environment

Note the environment in which acetylcysteine will be administered. Inhaled acetylcysteine usually is administered under the supervision of a respiratory therapist or specially trained nurse, although some patients or caregivers trained to administer it may give it at home.

Patients receiving acetylcysteine for contrast-induced nephrotoxicity or acetaminophen overdose must be closely monitored; thus, acetylcysteine given for these purposes is administered in the acute care hospital.

Nursing Diagnoses and Outcomes

- Ineffective Airway Clearance related to drug effect or bronchospasm
  Desired outcome: *The patient's airway will be maintained without increased difficulty breathing.*
- Disturbed Sensory Perception, Olfactory, related to odor of drug and route of administration
  Desired outcome: *The patient will remain comfortable and able to tolerate drug therapy.*
- Imbalanced Nutrition: Less than Body Requirements, related to nausea and vomiting.
  Desired outcome: *The patient will maintain nutritional balance throughout therapy.*
- Risk for Injury related to anaphylactoid reaction
  Desired outcome: *Potential anaphylactoid reactions will be recognized and treated appropriately.*

Planning and Intervention

Maximizing Therapeutic Effects

Administer an inhaled beta agonist before administering acetylcysteine, to dilate the bronchial tree and enable the drug to permeate the entire tree. Read the instructions for using the inhalation mask before administering inhaled acetylcysteine. Monitor the nebulizer for any buildup of the drug in the mask from evaporation. Dilute oral acetylcysteine in order to mask the taste.

Minimizing Adverse Effects

Inform the patient that nebulization may produce an initially disagreeable odor, but that this odor is transient. Remove residual drug from the patient's face after administration by face mask; the drug may irritate the face and will make it feel sticky and uncomfortable. Establish a routine for pulmonary hygiene to eliminate secretions as efficiently as possible; keep suction equipment available.

Carefully monitor the patient receiving IV acetylcysteine for signs of anaphylactoid reaction. If the patient's face becomes flushed, slow the administration of acetylcysteine and administer diphenhydramine as ordered.

Providing Patient and Family Education

- Explain the rationale for receiving acetylcysteine.
- Instruct patients to report all adverse effects, including difficulty breathing, severe nausea, and dizziness.
- Explain to patients that inhaled acetylcysteine will help to get rid of mucus in the lungs.
- Inform the patient that she or he must not take this drug without the assistance of a respiratory therapist or other health care provider unless the patient has been taught how to prepare the drug and how to use the nebulizer for administration.
- Warn patients not to take any other drugs without their provider's approval and not to drink alcohol while taking this drug.
- Teach patients and their family members all aspects of pulmonary hygiene, including drainage, cupping, coughing, and deep-breathing exercises. Encourage other methods of keeping secretions loose: drinking plenty of fluids, using a humidifier, and avoiding dry or smoke-filled areas.

- Inform the patient that nebulization may produce a disagreeable odor, but that this odor is transient. In addition, explain the need to wipe the face with water to remove residual drug after administration by face mask because the drug may irritate the face and will make it feel uncomfortable. These patient education tips will help to increase adherence to drug therapy.

Ongoing Assessment and Evaluation

For the patient receiving acetylcysteine for acetaminophen overdose, monitor for anaphylactoid reactions and schedule serial liver function tests. For the patient receiving acetylcysteine to prevent contrast-induced nephrotoxicity, monitor kidney function tests, urinalysis, and intake and output of food and fluids. For the patient receiving acetylcysteine for its mucolytic effects, assess the patient for proper techniques of pulmonary hygiene.

Determinants of successful therapy depend on the pharmacotherapeutic use of acetylcysteine. In managing acetaminophen overdose, the patient will recover without permanent hepatic dysfunction. The patient receiving acetylcysteine before contrast imaging will have normal renal function. The patient receiving acetylcysteine for its respiratory effects will have had no incidents of difficulty breathing and will be tolerating and continuing with drug therapy. There will be evidence, by history and breath sounds, that secretions are loosening and the patient is having success coughing and moving secretions out.

Drug Closely Related to P Acetylcysteine

Dornase alfa (Pulmozyme) is a mucolytic agent prepared by techniques that use recombinant deoxyribonucleic acid (DNA). The mucus of people with cystic fibrosis contains excess DNA. The drug selectively breaks down respiratory tract mucus by separating this extracellular DNA from proteins. This drug is used as adjunctive therapy to relieve the buildup of secretions in cystic fibrosis. It does not replace any other therapy for cystic fibrosis, but it does help to keep the airways open and functioning longer. Caution must be used in anyone with a history of hypersensitivity to hamster protein because the drug is manufactured using Chinese hamster ovary cells. It is not yet approved for use in children younger than 5 years old. Adverse effects can include hoarseness and sore throat related to nebulizer use, skin rash, and conjunctivitis.

MEMORY CHIP

P Acetylcysteine

- Used to liquefy thick tenacious secretions
- Major contraindication: hypersensitivity
- Most common adverse effects: nausea, vomiting, and rhinorrhea
- Most serious adverse effects: bronchospasm and bronchoconstriction
- Maximizing therapeutic effects: Refrigerate the solution and use it within 96 hours.
- Minimizing adverse effects: Keep suction equipment close by.
- Most important patient education: correct use of special equipment

C BRONCHODILATORS

Bronchodilators are drugs used to facilitate respiration by dilating the airways. Sympathomimetics (beta-2 adrenergic agonists), such as albuterol; anticholinergics, such as ipratropium bromide; and xanthine derivatives, such as theophylline, are bronchodilators commonly used to treat respiratory diseases. Table 47.3 presents a summary of selected bronchodilators.

C Beta Agonists (Sympathomimetics)

As discussed in Chapter 14, sympathomimetics are drugs that mimic the effects of the sympathetic nervous system. As a quick review, the body has two subtypes of beta receptors: beta-1 and beta-2. Drugs that stimulate these receptors may be nonspecific or selective to either beta-1 or beta-2 receptors. Beta-2 receptors are more predominant in the lungs, whereas beta-1 receptors are more predominant in the heart. One of the actions of beta stimulation in the sympathetic nervous system is dilation of the bronchi and increased rate and depth of respiration. For respiratory disorders, the drugs of choice would be those that are beta-2 selective. Albuterol (Proventil, Ventolin) is the prototypical beta-agonist agent.

NURSING MANAGEMENT OF THE PATIENT RECEIVING P ALBUTEROL

Core Drug Knowledge

Pharmacotherapeutics

Albuterol is used as a bronchodilator in managing CAL and asthma (see Table 47.3).

Pharmacokinetics

Albuterol may be administered orally in tablet or liquid form and by inhalation. Oral inhalation is by metered dose inhaler (MDI) or by nebulizer (Box 47.3). Following oral inhalation, bronchodilation occurs in 5 to 15 minutes, after which albuterol is absorbed over several hours from the respiratory tract. The kidneys excrete 80% to 100% of a dose within 72 hours, whereas 10% may be eliminated in feces.

When albuterol is administered orally in tablet or liquid form, bronchodilation occurs within 30 minutes. The kidneys excrete 75% of a dose within 72 hours as metabolites, and 4% may be found in feces.

Pharmacodynamics

Albuterol is a moderately selective beta-2 agonist. It selectively stimulates receptors of smooth muscle in the lungs, the uterus, and the vasculature that supplies skeletal muscle. The main result of albuterol binding to beta-2 receptors in the lungs is

TABLE 47.3 Summary of Selected (C) Bronchodilators

Drug (Trade) Name	Selected Indications	Route and Dosage Range	Pharmacokinetics
(C) Beta-Agonists			
(P) albuterol (Proventil, Ventolin, Salbutamol; *Canadian:* Gen-Salbutamol, Novo-Salmol) 2 mg, 4 mg; 2/5 mL	Asthma, bronchospasm	*Adult and child >12 y:* PO, 2–4 mg 3–4×/d Max: 32 mg/d *Child 6–11 y:* PO, 2 mg 4×/d Max: 24 mg/d *Child 2–6 y:* PO, 0.1 mg/kg 3×/d Max: 12 mg/d	*Onset:* 30 min *Duration:* 4–8 h $t_{1/2}$: 2–4 h
albuterol, inhaled (Proventil, Ventolin) 90 µg/spray MDI; 2.5/3 mL, 5/mL NEB	Asthma, bronchospasm	*Adult and child >12 y:* MDI, 2 puffs every 4–6 h Max: 12 puffs/d Exercise induced: 2 puffs 15 min before exercise *Adult and child >12 y:* Nebulizer, 2.5 mg 3–4×/d Max: 10 mg/d *Child 6–11 y:* MDI, 1–2 puffs every 4–6 h Max: 12 puffs/d *Child 6–11 y:* Nebulizer, 2.5 mg every 4–6 h *Child 2–5 y:* Nebulizer, 0.1–0.15 mg/kg/dose every 4–6 h	*Onset:* 5 min *Duration:* 3–8 h $t_{1/2}$: 2–4 h
	Acute bronchospasm	*Adult and child >12 y:* MDI, 4–8 puffs every 1–4 h Start: 4–8 puffs INH q20 min for 4 h *Adult and child >12 y:* Nebulizer, 2.5–5 mg every 20 min ×3, then 2.5–10 mg NEB q1–4h or 10–15 mg/h continuous NEB *Child <12 y:* Nebulizer, 0.15 mg/kg every 20 min ×3, then 0.15–0.3 mg/kg every 1–4 h or 0.5 mg/kg/h by continuous NEB	
albuterol (AccuNeb) 0.63/3 mL or 1.25/3 mL NEB	Asthma, bronchospasm	*Child 11–12 y:* Nebulizer, 1.25 mg 3–4×/d *Child 2–11 y:* Nebulizer, 0.63–1.25 mg 3–4×/d	*Onset:* 5 min *Duration:* 3–8 h $t_{1/2}$: 2–4 h
epinephrine 10 mg/mL NEB	Bronchospasm	*Adult and child >4 y:* Nebulizer, 0.5 mL up to every 3 h Max: 0.5 mL q3h	*Onset:* SC 5–10 min; IM, 5–10 min; inhalation, 1–5 min *Duration:* SC, 20–30 min; IM, 20–30 min; inhalation, 1–3 h $t_{1/2}$: SC, 5–6 h; IM, 5–6 h; inhalation, 5–6 h
formoterol (Foradil) 12 µg/powder cap INH	Asthma, prophylaxis COPD	*Adult and child >5 y:* INH, 12 µg (contents of one capsule) every 12 h using the aerolizer Max: 24 µg/d *Child <5 y:* Safety not established	*Onset:* 1–3 h *Duration:* Unknown $t_{1/2}$: 10 h
	Asthma, exercise induced	*Adult and child >12 y:* 12 µg formoterol (contents of one capsule) via aerolizer at least 15 min before exercise	

(continued)

TABLE 47.3 Summary of Selected (C) Bronchodilators (continued)

Drug (Trade) Name	Selected Indications	Route and Dosage Range	Pharmacokinetics
isoproterenol (Isuprel Mistometer) 103 μg/spray INH	Bronchospasm	*Adult:* INH, 1 puff every 4 h as needed Max: 5 doses/d *Child:* Safety not established	*Onset:* Inhalation, rapid; IV, immediate; SL, rapid *Duration:* Inhalation, 50–60 min; IV, 1–2 min; SL, 2 h $t_{1/2}$: Unknown
metaproterenol (Alupent) 10, 20, 10/5 mL sol; MDI; NEB	Bronchospasm	*Adult:* PO, 20 mg 3–4×/d *Adult:* MDI, 2–3 puffs every 3–4 h Max: 12 puffs/d *Adult:* Nebulizer, 0.2–0.3 mL 5% sol every 4 h	*Onset:* PO, 15 min; inhalation, 1–4 min *Duration:* PO, 4 h; inhalation, 3–4 h $t_{1/2}$: Unknown
levalbuterol (Xopenex) 0.31/3 mL, 0.63/3 mL, 1.25/3 mL NEB	Bronchospasm	*Adult:* Nebulizer, 0.63–1.25 mg every 6–8 h *Child >11 y:* Nebulizer, 0.63 mg 3×/d Max: 1.25 mg 3×/d *Child 6–11 y:* Nebulizer, 0.31 mg 3×/d Max: 0.63 mg 3×/d	*Onset:* Rapid *Duration:* 5–6 h $t_{1/2}$: 3.3–4 h
pirbuterol (Maxair) 0.2 mg/spray	Bronchospasm	*Adult and child >12 y:* INH, 1–2 puffs every 4–6 h Max: 12 puffs/d	*Onset:* Rapid *Duration:* 6 h $t_{1/2}$: 2–3 h
salmeterol (Serevent Diskus)	Asthma, COPD Asthma, exercise induced	*Adult and child >4 y:* DPI, 50 μg every 12 h *Adult and child >4 y:* DPI, 50 μg 1× 30–60 min before exercise Max: 50 μg every 12 h	*Onset:* 5–20 min *Duration:* 12 h $t_{1/2}$: 3–4 h
terbutaline	Asthma	*Adult and child >15 y:* PO, 5 mg 3×/d Max: 15 mg/d *Adult and child >15 y:* SC, 0.5 mg every 4 h *Child 12–15 y:* PO, 2.5–5 mg 3×/d Max: 7.5 mg/d *Child 12–15 y:* SC, 0.5 mg every 4 h SC *Child 6–12 y:* PO, 0.05 mg/kg 3×/d Max: 0.15 mg/kg/dose or 5 mg/d *Child 6–12 y:* SC, 0.005–0.01 mg/kg SC q15–30 min ×2 Max: 0.4 mg/d	*Onset:* PO, 30 min; SC, 30 min; inhalation, 5–30 min *Duration:* PO, 4–8 h; SC, 1.5–4 h; inhalation, 3–4 h $t_{1/2}$: PO, 3–4 h; SC, 3–4 h; inhalation, 3–4 h
(C) Anticholinergic Agents			
(P) ipratropium (Atrovent) 18 μg/spray MDI; 500 μg NEB	Bronchospasm	*Adult:* MDI, 2–3 puffs 3–4×/day Max: 12 puffs/d *Adult:* Nebulizer, 500 μg every 6–8 h *Child >12 y:* MDI, 2–3 puffs 3–4×/d Max: 12 puffs/d *Child >12 y:* Nebulizer, 250–500 μg every 6–8 h *Child <12 y:* MDI, 1–2 puffs 3–4×/d Max: 8 puffs/d *Child <12 y:* Nebulizer, 250 μg every 6–8 h	*Onset:* 15 min *Duration:* 3–4 h $t_{1/2}$: 2–3 h
tiotropium (Spiriva) 18 μg/inhalation DPI	Bronchospasm	*Adult:* DPI, 1 inhalation every day *Child:* Safety not established	*Onset:* 5 min *Duration:* 24 h $t_{1/2}$: 5–6 d

(continued)

TABLE 47.3 Summary of Selected Ⓒ Bronchodilators (continued)

Drug (Trade) Name	Selected Indications	Route and Dosage Range	Pharmacokinetics
Combination Inhalers			
albuterol/ipratropium (Combivent Duo-Neb) 120/21 μg/spray MDI 3/0.5/3 mL NEB	COPD	*Adult:* INH, 1–2 puffs 4×/d Max: 12 puffs/d *Adult:* NEB, 3 mL 4×/d Max: 6 doses/d *Child:* Safety not established.	See individual drugs
fluticasone/salmeterol (Advair Diskus) 100/50, 250/50, 500/50 μg/spray DPI	Asthma	*Adult and child >12 y:* INH, 100/50 μg INH 2×/d if not on inhaled steroid, 100/50–500/50 μg INH bid if on other inhaled steroid *Child 4–11 y:* INH, 100/50 μg 2×/d (off-label in this age group)	See individual drugs
	Bronchitis	250/50 μg INH 2×/d	
Ⓒ Xanthine Derivatives			
Ⓟ theophylline (Slo-Phyllin; *Canadian:* Acet-Amp)	Acute asthma symptoms	*Adult 16–60 y:* PO/IV, 300 mg/d in divided doses; titrate to maximum of 600 mg/d in divided doses; maintenance, up to 600 mg/d *Child 1–15 y:* PO/IV, 12–14 mg/kg/d to maximum of 600 mg daily in divided doses; maintenance, up to 400 mg daily *Infant <53 wk:* 0.2 mg × age in weeks; maintenance, 16 m	*Onset:* PO, varies; Peak: 2 h *Duration:* 2–3 d $t_{1/2}$: 3–5 h nonsmoker; 4–5 h smoker
	Methotrexate toxicity	*Adult and child >3 y:* IV, 2.5 mg/kg	
	Neonatal apnea	Premature to 24 d: 1 mg/kg q12h 24 d+: 1.5 mg/kg q12h	
	Sleep apnea	*Adult only:* 3.3 mg/kg bid	
aminophylline (Truphylline)	Acute asthma (child)	*Adult and child >12 y:* IV 0.7 mg/kg IV 0.5 mg/kg	*Onset:* PO 15–60/m IV rapid *Duration:* 6–8/h $t_{1/2}$: Variable
	Neonatal apnea	0–24 d: 2 mg/kg/d divided dose q12h	
	Maintenance	*Adult:* PO, 3 mg/kg q8h *Child 9–12 y:* 3 mg/kg q6h *Child 6–9 y:* 4 mg/kg q6h	
dyphylline (Dilor, Lufyllin)		*Adult:* 15/mg/kg qid PO 250–500 mg q6h IM *Child:* Safety not established	*Onset:* Unknown *Duration:* Unknown $t_{1/2}$: Unknown

relaxation of bronchial smooth muscles. This relaxation of bronchial smooth muscle relieves bronchospasm, reduces airway resistance, facilitates mucous drainage, and increases vital capacity.

Contraindications and Precautions

The only absolute contraindication to albuterol is hypersensitivity to the drug or any components of the delivery system, such as fluorocarbons.

Precautions include hypertension, cardiac disease, cardiac arrhythmias, ischemic heart disease, hyperthyroidism, diabetes mellitus, and seizures. Selectivity is relative; therefore, potential beta-1 stimulation may exacerbate these conditions. Another precaution is pregnancy because beta-2 agonists may interfere with uterine contractility.

Adverse Effects

Adverse effects to albuterol are related to its sympathomimetic action. Adverse effects occur more frequently when albuterol is administered orally than when it is inhaled. The most common adverse effects of inhaled albuterol include throat irritation, palpitations, sinus tachycardia, anxiety,

BOX 47.3 Types of Inhalation Devices

Metered-dose inhaler (MDI)

- A small, hand-held device that delivers a set amount of drug with each activation
- Requires coordination to inhale medication correctly
- Optimally approximately 10% of drug reaches the lung
- Important to wait at least 1 minute between puffs
- May be used with a "spacer" to increase amount of drug delivered to the lungs
- Environmental hazard because it uses chlorofluorocarbon propellant that can damage the ozone layer

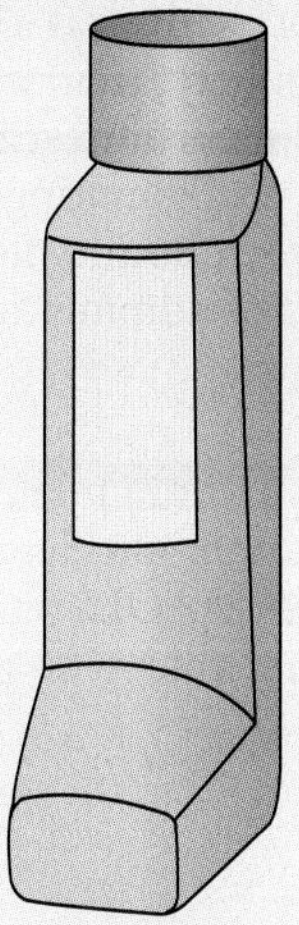

MDI

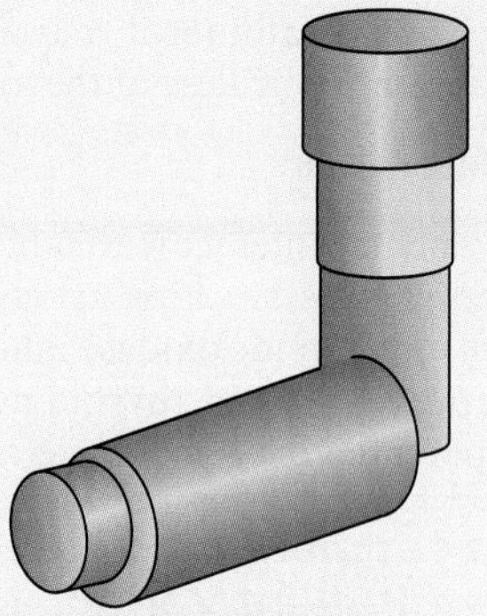

MDI with spacer

Dry-powder inhaler (DPI)

- A small, hand-held device that delivers a dry micronized powder with each inhalation
- Does not require coordination
- Optimally approximately 20% of drug reaches the lung
- Important to wait at least 1 minute between inhalations
- No environmental concerns because no propellant is used

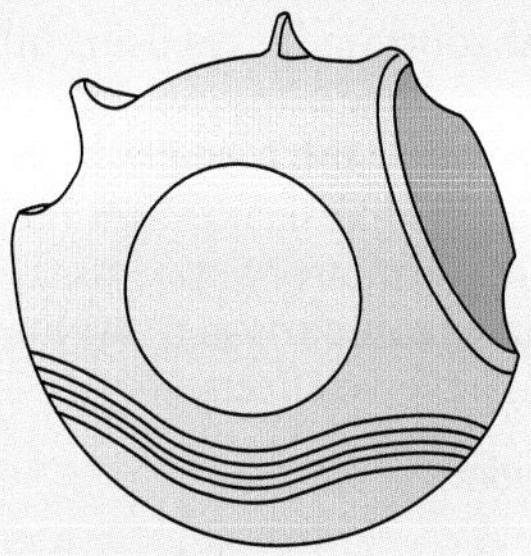

Dry powder inhaler

Nebulizer

- A small machine that delivers misted droplets of drug into the lungs
- Delivered through a mouthpiece or mask
- Takes longer time to deliver medication to the lungs than MDIs or DPIs
- More effective for some patients than MDIs or DPIs

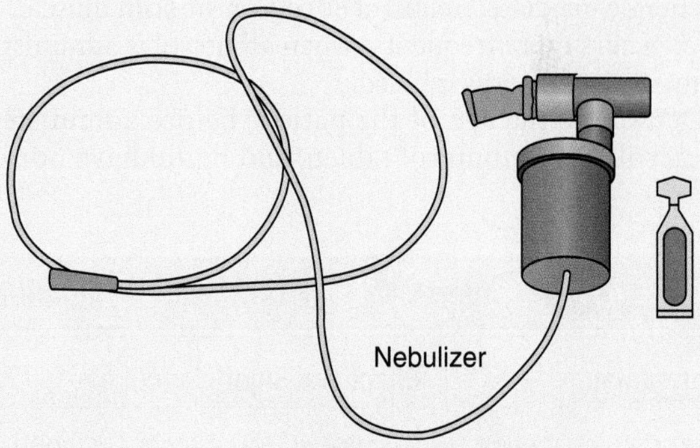

Nebulizer

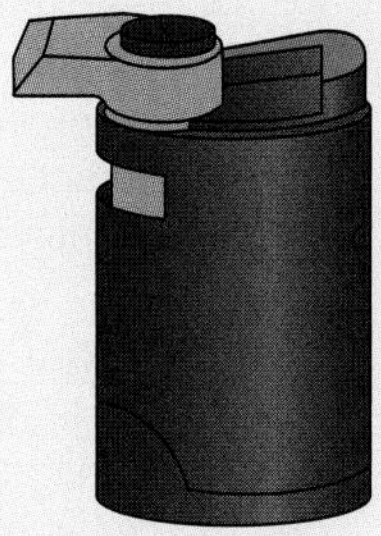

Portable nebulizer

tremor, and increased blood pressure. Rarely, serious adverse effects such as bronchospasm, urticaria, or angioedema may occur.

Frequent adverse effects associated with oral albuterol include tachycardia or palpitations, anxiety, tremors, headache, insomnia, muscle cramps, and gastrointestinal (GI) symptoms such as dyspepsia, nausea, and vomiting.

Overuse of albuterol may induce rebound bronchoconstriction, regardless of the method of administration.

Drug Interactions

Albuterol may interact with other sympathomimetic agents, beta-adrenergic blocking agents, digoxin, antidepressants such as monoamine oxidase inhibitors (MAOIs) or tricyclic antidepressants, and thyroid agents. Table 47.4 presents these potential drug–drug interactions.

Assessment of Relevant Core Patient Variables

Health Status

Evaluate the patient for potential medical conditions or other drug therapy that contraindicates using albuterol or requires close patient monitoring. Any positive findings should be communicated to the health care provider.

Perform a baseline physical examination, concentrating on the cardiac and respiratory systems. Document the baseline findings for later comparison to evaluate efficacy of treatment or potential adverse effects.

Life Span and Gender

Evaluate the pregnancy status of the patient, as needed. Albuterol is classified as a pregnancy class C drug because it can interfere with uterine contractility as a result of its beta-adrenergic–mediated relaxant effects on smooth muscle. This effect occurs more frequently when albuterol is administered orally than when it is inhaled.

Determine the age of the patient before administering albuterol. Oral albuterol tablets and liquid have not been established as safe for children younger than 2 years. Extended-release tablets have not been approved for children younger than 12 years.

Lifestyle, Diet, and Habits

Assess the patient's intake of caffeine, including coffee, tea, soda, cocoa, candy, and chocolate. Caffeine has sympathomimetic effects that may increase the risk for adverse effects. Also, assess for use of over-the-counter (OTC) medications such as pain relievers, appetite suppressants, and cold medicines because they frequently contain caffeine.

Environment

Note the environment in which the drug will be administered. Patients who self-administer albuterol may use their MDIs more frequently than recommended. This practice can result in rebound bronchoconstriction, which may motivate the patient to increase MDI use, stimulating the cycle of rebound.

Nursing Diagnoses and Outcomes

- Anxiety related to sympathomimetic effects of albuterol administration
  Desired outcome: *The patient will engage in interventions that decrease anxiety.*
- Ineffective Tissue Perfusion: Cardiopulmonary related to rebound bronchoconstriction caused by overuse of albuterol
  Desired outcome: *The patient will use albuterol as prescribed by the health care provider and contact that person if symptoms do not abate.*

Planning and Intervention

Maximizing Therapeutic Effects

Because albuterol is most commonly administered by inhalation, it is important to supervise the patient's ability to use the MDI or nebulizer appropriately (Box 47.4).

TABLE 47.4 Agents That Interact With P Albuterol

Interactants	Effect and Significance	Nursing Management
sympathomimetics	Additive effects may occur when albuterol is administered in combination with other sympathomimetic drugs. This increases the risk for cardiovascular adverse effects.	Monitor vital signs frequently. Avoid concurrent use if possible.
beta-adrenergic blocking agents	Albuterol has the exact opposite effect on the body as beta-adrenergic blocking agents. Coadministration will counteract each agent when given concomitantly.	Do not give concurrently.
digoxin	Albuterol may decrease serum digoxin levels.	Monitor for therapeutic effects of digoxin. Monitor serum digoxin levels. Adjust digoxin dose as needed.
MAOI or tricyclic antidepressants	MAOI and tricyclic antidepressants potentiate albuterol's effect on the peripheral vasculature. This may result in severe hypotension.	Monitor the patient's blood pressure. Avoid coadministration, if possible.
thyroid agents	Concomitant use of albuterol and thyroid hormones can enhance the effects of either drug on the cardiovascular system. Combined use of these agents may further increase this risk for coronary insufficiency.	Avoid coadministration, if possible. Monitor for signs of cardiac insufficiency.

COMMUNITY-BASED CONCERNS

Box 47.4 How to Use a Metered-Dose Inhaler

When a patient is first diagnosed with asthma and prescribed inhalation therapy, he or she may need to learn how to use the inhaler that will deliver drug therapy. The nurse may be the health care provider who supplies instructions such as these:

1. Hold the device upright and shake it.
2. Tilt the head back slightly.
3. Exhale and open mouth.
4. Position the inhaler in one of three ways:
   - Held 1–2 inches from the mouth (this is preferred)
   - Using a spacer
   - With the inhaler between the lips
   - When using dry powder inhalers, always place the mouthpiece between the lips.
5. Start to inhale slowly and press down on the inhaler to release the medication.
6. Breathe in for 3 to 5 seconds.
7. Hold your breath for 10 seconds to allow the drug to reach deep into the lungs.
8. Repeat for the ordered number of puffs, allowing 1 minute between each puff.

Spacers are recommended for children, older adults and anyone who has difficulty using a nebulizer alone. Spacers are indicated when using inhaled steroids.

Use the prescribed bronchodilator first to open air passages, and then use other prescribed medications.

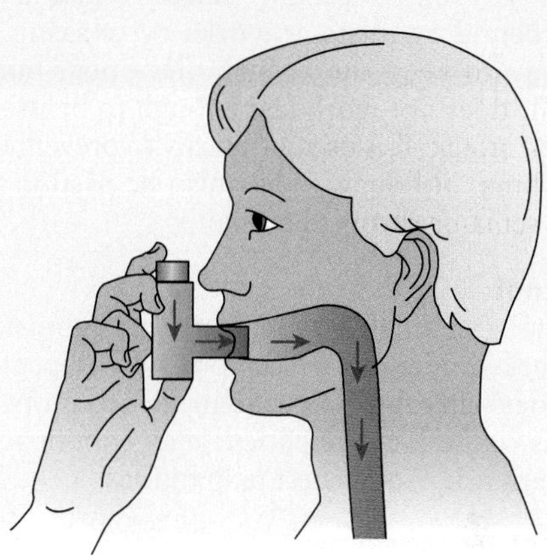

Minimizing Adverse Effects

Explain the need to adhere to the recommended frequency of administration. The patient should be encouraged to contact the health care provider to obtain adjunctive medications if symptoms persist, rather than increase the frequency of albuterol use.

Providing Patient and Family Education

- Teach the patient that inhaled albuterol is called a "rescue drug" and should be the *first drug* to use when symptoms of an acute attack occur.
- Teach the patient how to use an MDI. Include the correct procedure for administering medication, methods of keeping the equipment clean, and how to assess when to change the canister (Box 47.5).
- Explain the importance of using the drug as prescribed and encourage the patient to communicate with the health care provider if the symptoms do not abate with the recommended therapy.
- Explain the importance of limiting caffeine intake.
- Explain the importance of refraining from use of OTC drugs without the health care provider's knowledge.

COMMUNITY-BASED CONCERNS

Box 47.5 How to Care for Your Inhaler

Keep the inhaler clean. Once a week, remove the medication canister from the plastic casing and wash the casing in warm, soapy water. When the casing is dry, replace the medication canister and place the cap on the mouthpiece. Ensure that the hole is clear. Check the expiration date. Keep a log of doses used to know when medication should be replaced.

Ongoing Assessment and Evaluation

Evaluate for abatement of the symptoms of asthma or CAL. Evaluate for CNS symptoms, such as anxiety, tremors, insomnia, or CNS disturbances. Determine the frequency of use and refer the patient to the health care provider if albuterol is needed more frequently than prescribed.

Drugs Closely Related to P Albuterol

Several other beta-agonist agents are used as bronchodilators. The pharmacodynamics and pharmacokinetics of all of these drugs are very similar; slight variations or different vehicles make them the drugs of choice for different patients. A patient may need to try several of these before finding the one that works most effectively. In addition, combination inhalers, with beta agonists combined with either anticholinergic drugs or inhaled steroids, are available (see Table 47.3).

MEMORY CHIP

P Albuterol

- Used for acute and chronic management of CAL and asthma
- Major contraindication: hypersensitivity
- Most common adverse effects: throat irritation, palpitations, tachycardia, anxiety, tremors, and increased blood pressure
- Most serious adverse effects: bronchospasm, urticaria, and angioedema
- Maximizing therapeutic effects: Ensure correct use of inhalation device.
- Minimizing adverse effects: Do not use more than prescribed.
- Most important patient education: This rescue drug should be used first for all acute symptoms of shortness of breath or wheezing.

Epinephrine

Epinephrine is the active ingredient in OTC inhalers such as Primatene Mist. It is a nonselective adrenergic agonist; therefore, it stimulates alpha-1, alpha-2, beta-1, and beta-2. For that reason, it is prone to induce multiple adverse reactions, especially tachycardia, hypertension, chest palpitations, and anxiety.

Formoterol

Formoterol (Foradil) is a highly selective beta-2 agonist. Like other beta-2 agonists, it works by relaxing muscles in the airway to keep the bronchioles open, but its onset is slow. It does not work fast enough to be used for an acute asthma attack. It is used primarily to prevent exercise-induced asthma, although it may also be used in patients with emphysema or chronic bronchitis.

Isoproterenol

Isoproterenol (Medihaler-Iso) is a potent agonist of both beta-1 and beta-2 adrenergic receptors. At therapeutic doses, it has little to no effect on alpha-adrenergic receptors. Because of its effects on beta-1, the patient may experience tachycardia, hypertension, and chest palpitations.

Levalbuterol

Levalbuterol (Xopenex) is a moderately selective beta-2 agonist. It is the R-isomer of albuterol and has approximately 2-fold greater binding affinity than racemic albuterol and approximately 100-fold greater binding affinity than the S-isomer of albuterol. It is available as a solution for nebulization, although approval as an MDI is anticipated in the near future.

Metaproterenol

Metaproterenol (Alupent) is another of the beta-2 selective agonists. It has more selectivity for beta-2 than isoproterenol, but less than albuterol. It is not as frequently used as albuterol or salmeterol because of its ability to induce cardiac adverse events.

Pirbuterol

Pirbuterol (Maxair) is structurally very similar to albuterol. It is used to interrupt an acute asthmatic event or to prevent bronchospasm associated with asthma, exercise-induced bronchospasm, bronchitis, emphysema, and bronchiectasis.

Salmeterol

Salmeterol (Serevent Diskus) is another highly selective beta-2 agonist used for asthma, bronchospasm, and emphysema. Like formoterol, it has a slow onset, which makes it useful for the prevention of attacks, but not for an acute attack. In 1996, the FDA requested a black box warning placed on salmeterol because of preliminary results of the Salmeterol Multi-center Asthma Research Trial (SMART). Early data showed a small but significant increase in asthma-related deaths in patients receiving salmeterol versus those on placebo (13 versus 4). Subsequent subgroup analyses suggest the risk may be greater in African American patients compared with Caucasians (FDA Talk Paper, 2003).

Terbutaline

Terbutaline (Brethine) is another beta-2 selective adrenergic agonist. It is longer acting than isoproterenol and metaproterenol but shorter acting than albuterol or salmeterol. Its main pharmacotherapeutic use is the prevention of bronchospasm, but it is also used clinically to abort premature labor.

(C) Respiratory Anticholinergic Agents

Inhaled anticholinergic drugs are considered first-line treatment for patients with CAL whose symptoms have become persistent. Anticholinergic agents diminish the effect of acetylcholine, the terminal neurotransmitter in the parasympathetic nervous system. In the respiratory system, use of inhaled anticholinergic drugs stops the bronchoconstriction that is caused by stimulation of the parasympathetic nervous system. Ipratropium bromide (Atrovent) is the prototypical respiratory anticholinergic agent.

NURSING MANAGEMENT OF THE PATIENT RECEIVING [P] IPRATROPIUM BROMIDE

Core Drug Knowledge

Pharmacotherapeutics

Ipratropium bromide is used for maintenance treatment of bronchospasm associated with asthma, bronchitis, pulmonary emphysema, or CAL.

Pharmacokinetics

Ipratropium bromide is administered by oral inhalation or intranasal spray. Following oral inhalation, onset occurs between 15 to 30 minutes, peaks in 1 to 2 hours, and lasts 4 to 5 hours. Ipratropium bromide is not readily absorbed into the systemic circulation after inhalation either from the surface of the lung or from the GI tract. Approximately 50% of the absorbed drug is excreted unchanged in the urine. After intranasal dosing, less than 20% of an ipratropium dose is absorbed from the nasal mucosa into the systemic circulation. The metabolism of intranasal ipratropium bromide is the same as that of the inhaled drug.

Pharmacodynamics

Ipratropium antagonizes the action of acetylcholine by blocking muscarinic cholinergic receptors. Blockade of these cholinergic receptors decreases the formation of cyclic guanosine monophosphate (cGMP), resulting in decreased contractility of smooth muscle and thereby reducing bronchospasm.

Contraindications and Precautions

Ipratropium aerosol inhalation is contraindicated in patients who have soya lecithin hypersensitivity, including those patients with a history of peanut oil hypersensitivity or hypersensitivity to related foods and legumes such as soybeans and peanuts. Ipratropium should also not be used in patients with hypersensitivity to atropine or atropine derivatives, those with bromide hypersensitivity, or patients with hypersensitivity to propellant fluorocarbons.

Because of its anticholinergic effects, ipratropium should be used with caution in patients with bladder obstruction, prostatic hypertrophy, or closed-angle glaucoma. Ipratropium

may precipitate urinary retention in patients with pre-existing bladder obstruction or prostatic hypertrophy. It may increase intraocular pressure and aqueous outflow resistance in patients with closed-angle glaucoma, especially if the medication gets into the eyes.

Adverse Effects

Ipratropium aerosols can produce a paradoxic acute bronchospasm that can be life threatening in some patients. This rare problem, when it occurs, is usually seen with the first inhalation from a newly opened MDI. The patient should "test-spray" three times before using a new MDI for the first time. Another serious, but rare, adverse effect is an anaphylactoid reaction. Symptoms include urticaria; angioedema of tongue, lips, and face; maculopapular rash; bronchospasm; laryngospasm; pruritus; and oropharyngeal edema. This reaction may occur when a patient has an unknown allergy to soybeans, legumes, or soya lecithin.

More commonly, ipratropium may induce cough, hoarseness, throat irritation, or dysgeusia. The classic anticholinergic adverse effects—dry mouth, constipation, urinary retention, and blurred vision—may also occur, but not as frequently or intensely as with systemic anticholinergic drugs.

Nasal administration of ipratropium may induce epistaxis, headache, rhinitis, nasal congestion, rhinorrhea, and general nasal irritation.

Temporary ocular irritation, ocular pain, mydriasis, cycloplegia, blurred vision, conjunctivitis, or visual impairment may result from spraying ipratropium products inadvertently into the eyes.

Drug Interactions

No serious drug–drug interactions are associated with ipratropium. Ipratropium inhalation solution forms a precipitate with cromolyn sodium inhalation solution if they are mixed together in a nebulizer. Theoretically, potential exists for ipratropium to have additive anticholinergic effects when administered with other antimuscarinics.

Assessment of Relevant Core Patient Variables

Health Status

Assess the patient for potential medical conditions or other drug therapy that contraindicates using ipratropium or requires close patient monitoring. Perform a baseline respiratory examination and document the findings. This baseline assessment will be used to evaluate the efficacy of treatment.

Life Span and Gender

Evaluate the pregnancy status of the patient, as needed. Ipratropium is classified as an FDA pregnancy category B drug. However, human studies have not been done. Therefore, ipratropium should be used during pregnancy only when the benefits to the mother outweigh the possible risk to the fetus. Minimal amounts of inhaled ipratropium reaches breast milk; therefore, the potential risk to the breast-feeding infant is negligible. Safety and effectiveness of ipratropium have not been established in infants or in children younger than 5 years.

Lifestyle, Diet, and Habits

Determine whether the patient smokes. Smoking causes vasoconstriction, the opposite of the action of ipratropium.

Environment

Note the environment in which the drug will be administered. If ipratropium will be self-administered, assist the patient to identify the correct MDI to use for acute symptoms. Although beta-agonist drugs, such as albuterol, are the drugs of choice for acute symptoms, ipratropium may still be delivered during exacerbations of asthma.

Nursing Diagnoses and Outcomes

- Risk for Injury (bronchospasm) related to use of new canister of ipratropium
  Desired outcome: *The patient will "test-spray" a new canister three times before inhaling the medication.*
- Risk for Injury (anaphylactoid reactions) related to allergies to soybeans, legumes, or soya lecithin.
  Desired outcome: *The patient will review past allergic responses to assess whether any of the causative foods may have been responsible.*

Planning and Intervention

Maximizing Therapeutic Effects

Explain the importance of taking ipratropium daily, despite the absence of symptoms. Watch the patient demonstrate the use of the MDI to assess correct use (see Box 47.4).

Minimizing Adverse Effects

Explain the importance of using the inhaler as prescribed to avoid systemic absorption that will lead to an increased risk for adverse effects.

Providing Patient and Family Education

- Advise the patient that ipratropium is used prophylactically to reduce the frequency and severity of future asthma attacks. It will not abort an asthma attack in progress.
- Advise patients to avoid using ipratropium if they have a history of allergy to soybeans, legumes, or soya lecithin.
- Remind the patient that ipratropium must be taken daily, despite the absence of symptoms of asthma.
- Remind the patient that overuse of ipratropium may induce adverse effects or increase their intensity.
- Teach the patient to use an MDI. Include the correct procedure for administering the medication, keeping the equipment clean, and assessing when to change the canister (see Box 47.5).

Ongoing Assessment and Evaluation

Assess the patient's need for beta-agonist drugs in addition to ipratropium. If the patient continues to need beta agonists more than twice a week, refer the patient to the health care provider for additional assessment.

Drugs Closely Related to P Ipratropium Bromide

Tiotropium

Tiotropium (Spiriva) is structurally close to ipratropium but pharmacodynamically different. It is selective for muscarinic

MEMORY CHIP

P Ipratropium Bromide

- Used for maintenance therapy of CAL or asthma
- Major contraindications: hypersensitivity to fluorocarbons or legumes, such as soybeans or peanuts
- Most common adverse effects: cough, hoarseness, throat irritation, dysgeusia, and anticholinergic effects
- Most serious adverse effects: bronchospasm and anaphylaxis
- Maximizing therapeutic effects: Administer the medication daily, despite the absence of symptoms.
- Minimizing adverse effects: Use only as directed to decrease potential systemic absorption.
- Most important patient education: This drug will not abort an acute asthma attack.

receptors 1 to 3; however, it dissociates from them much slower than ipratropium does. This slow dissociation gives tiotropium a long duration of action and enables once-daily dosing. Another advantage is that tiotropium is minimally absorbed, which decreases the risk for systemic adverse effects.

Tiotropium should be used with caution in the elderly because they may experience anticholinergic effects such as blurred vision, constipation, urinary retention, and dry mouth despite the drug's minimal systemic absorption. It should also be used with caution in women who are pregnant. Tiotropium is a pregnancy category C drug; whether it crosses into breast milk is unknown.

As with ipratropium, there is potential for additive anticholinergic effects when tiotropium is administered with other antimuscarinics.

C Xanthine Derivatives

The xanthine derivatives, including theophylline, aminophylline, diphylline, and caffeine, come from a variety of naturally occurring sources. They are excellent bronchodilators but do not work as quickly as beta-adrenergic agonist drugs. Theophylline is the prototype xanthine derivative bronchodilator.

NURSING MANAGEMENT OF THE PATIENT RECEIVING P THEOPHYLLINE

Core Drug Knowledge

Pharmacotherapeutics

Theophylline is indicated for the symptomatic relief or prevention of bronchial asthma and reversal of bronchospasm associated with CAL. An unlabeled use is to treat apnea and bradycardia in premature infants.

Pharmacokinetics

Theophylline is well absorbed when given orally. Its peak effects occur in 2 hours, with a duration of effect from 4 to 8 hours. The drug is metabolized in the liver and excreted in the urine. It crosses the placenta and may enter breast milk (see Table 47.3).

Pharmacodynamics

Theophylline has a direct effect on the smooth muscles of the respiratory tract, both those in the bronchi and those in the blood vessels. The exact mechanism of action is not known. One theory suggests that theophylline works by directly affecting the mobilization of calcium within the cell. Theophylline stimulates two prostaglandins, which results in smooth muscle relaxation. This effect increases the respiratory capacity that has been impaired by bronchospasm or air trapping. Theophylline also inhibits the release of slow-reacting substance of anaphylaxis (SRS-A) and of histamine, decreasing the bronchial swelling and narrowing that occur resulting the presence of these two chemicals.

Contraindications and Precautions

Theophylline is contraindicated in patients with hypersensitivity to any xanthines, in association with status asthmaticus, or in patients with a peptic ulcer. It has been assigned to pregnancy category C and therefore is contraindicated or used with caution during pregnancy. Use caution with any patient with a cardiac problem, such as arrhythmia, coronary artery disease, congestive heart failure, or hypertension, because of the drug's stimulatory effects. Caution also should be used in patients with renal or hepatic disease because the drug is metabolized in the liver and excreted through the kidneys. Also, it is not known whether theophylline enters into breast milk, but there is a possibility that the drug has a stimulatory effect on the infant. Therefore, the drug should be used with caution during lactation.

Adverse Effects

Adverse effects related to theophylline use are related directly to serum levels of the drug. If serum levels of theophylline are less than 20 μg/mL, adverse effects are uncommon. At serum levels from 20 to 25 μg/mL, the most common adverse effects are GI symptoms of nausea, vomiting, and diarrhea and CNS effects of headache, insomnia, and irritability. When serum levels exceed 30 μg/mL, adverse effects such as hyperglycemia, hypotension, arrhythmias, seizures, brain damage, and even death may occur. Even at therapeutic doses, theophylline may cause CNS effects, such as irritability (especially in children), restlessness, and muscle twitching. It also may cause GI effects, such as loss of appetite, hematemesis, and gastroesophageal reflux. Potential cardiovascular effects include palpitations, tachycardia, and circulatory failure. In the respiratory system, theophylline may cause tachypnea. Possible genitourinary effects include urinary retention in men with prostate enlargement and diuresis. Generalized effects, such as fever, flushing, rash, and elevated liver enzymes, also have occurred.

Drug Interactions

Theophylline levels and effects are influenced by a large number of other drugs. Increased effects and potential toxicity occur if the drug is taken concurrently with histamine-2 antagonists, such as cimetidine or ranitidine; macrolide antibiotics, such as erythromycin and troleandomycin; quinolone anti-

- Explain the importance of tak prescribed and instruct patie that can interfere with their dr OTC drugs, and smoking). M their families are aware of pr and know when to contact the change their diets, use OTC d ing habits.
- Teach patients never to chew or they should be swallowed who capsules should always be tal 1 hour before or 2 hours after a solution, it should be shaken the patient to take immediate- tions of the drug with food if
- Caution the patient not to ch out consulting the health care regular checkups or blood tes evaluated.
- Instruct patients to take the d dose is missed, it should be tal bered unless it is almost time f two doses should never be tak
- Instruct patients to avoid con caffeine-containing foods (e.g. (e.g., coffee, cola, and tea) wh to contact their health care pr consumption substantially. In check the ingredients of any O using it.
- Advise the patient to ingest s distress occurs.
- Advise a quiet environment or tion or insomnia from theoph
- Caution against using theoph attack because its onset is not acute attack.
- Urge the patient to report such a insomnia, restlessness, muscle t severe GI pain, palpitation, and

Ongoing Assessment a

Monitor the patient for potentia adverse effects. The patient's seru be maintained between 10 and 2 peutic effects and minimal advers on theophylline, the patient shoul imal discomfort from adverse effe to the therapy prescribed.

Drugs Closely Related to P Theophylline

Aminophylline

Aminophylline (Truphylline), a th cologically identical to theophylli theophylline; thus, it is preferred needed. It is important to adminis rate not to exceed 25 mg/minute. A

biotics, such as ciprofloxacin, norfloxacin, and ofloxacin; oral contraceptives; and rifampin.

Theophylline also may have substantial interactions with halothane, barbiturates, charcoal, benzodiazepines, nondepolarizing neuromuscular blockers, and beta blockers. It also may interact with thyroid hormones, hydantoins, adenosine, disulfiram, mexiletine, and thiabendazole (Table 47.5).

Assessment of Relevant Core Patient Variables

Health Status

When taking the patient history before starting theophylline therapy, screen the patient for any hypersensitivity to xanthines and for peptic ulcer, active gastritis, status asthmaticus,

TABLE 47.5 Agents That Interact With P Theophylline

Interactants	Effect and Significance	Nursing Management
activated charcoal	Can reduce absorption of theophylline and remove it from the systemic circulation, resulting in subtherapeutic levels of theophylline	Monitor for increased symptoms of respiratory distress if activated charcoal must be administered.
adenosine	Mechanism of action unclear; theophylline may decrease effectiveness of adenosine	Administer higher dose of adenosine.
barbiturates	May induce cytochrome P450, stimulating theophylline metabolism and increasing clearance, resulting in subtherapeutic levels of theophylline	Assess for need of increased theophylline dosage with coadministration of barbiturates.
benzodiazepines	Possible antagonistic action by competitive binding to intracerebral adenosine receptors, resulting in decreased sedative effects of benzodiazepines	Assess the clinical status of the patient, and tailor the dosage of benzodiazepines as needed.
beta blockers	May reduce the n-demethylation of theophylline, resulting in a decreased effect of one or both agents	Monitor patient for clinical changes. Monitor plasma theophylline levels when a beta blocker is added or deleted from a regimen. Beta-selective agents are preferred.
disulfiram	Inhibits the hydroxylation and demethylation pathways of theophylline metabolism, resulting in potential theophylline toxicity	Monitor theophylline levels closely when coadministered with disulfiram. Adjust theophylline dose as needed.
halothane	Catecholamine-induced arrhythmias possible when halothane is administered after theophylline	Do not administer halothane to patient taking theophylline.
histamine-2 antagonists	Inhibition of the hepatic metabolism of theophylline, resulting in potential toxicity	Monitor theophylline levels; 20%–40% reduction in dosage of theophylline may be necessary.
hydantoins	Phenytoin and theophylline metabolism increased, resulting in subtherapeutic levels of both drugs	Monitor plasma levels of both drugs and adjust as necessary.
macrolide antibiotics	Inhibit the metabolism of theophylline, and theophylline reduces the bioavailability and increases renal clearance of oral erythromycin, resulting in theophylline toxicity and macrolide ineffectivity	Monitor drug levels and adjust dosages as needed, with addition or deletion of macrolides.
mexiletine	Inhibits the cytochrome P450 oxidase system, resulting in theophylline toxicity	Monitor theophylline levels and adjust dose as needed.
nondepolarizing muscle relaxants	Antagonistic activity between theophylline and nondepolarizing muscle relaxants—nontherapeutic effects of muscle relaxants	Assess the need for higher dosage of muscle relaxants.
oral contraceptives	Decrease the oxidative degradation of theophylline by cytochrome P448, resulting in theophylline toxicity	Monitor theophylline levels and adjust dose as needed.
quinolone antibiotics	Inhibition of the hepatic metabolism of theophylline resulting in potential theophylline toxicity	Monitor theophylline levels and adjust dose as needed.
rifampin	Appears to induce the hepatic metabolism of theophylline, resulting in subtherapeutic levels	Monitor theophylline levels and adjust dose as needed if rifampin is added or deleted.
thiabendazole	Possible metabolic inhibition of theophylline , resulting in theophylline toxicity	Monitor theophylline levels and adjust dose as needed
thyroid hormones and preparations	Direct correlation between plasma thyroid hormones/preparations and theophylline clearance; hypothyroid or hyperthyroid patients, alteration in theophylline clearance	Adjust dose according to plasma theophylline levels. Achieving a euthyroid state is critical in controlling theophylline clearance.

coronary disease, hyperthyroi
pregnancy, and lactation.
Patients with cardiac disea
during theophylline therapy
cardiovascular effects, such a
elevated blood pressure.
Perform a baseline physic
color, texture, and lesions; re
and heart rate. Assess the re
rate, adventitious sounds, and
volume in 1 second (FEV_1) (Bo
obtain baseline thyroid, liver,

Life Span and Gender

Assess the patient for pregnar
phylline is contraindicated d
mothers who used theophyll
iness, and withdrawal apnea.
possible enlarged prostate glar
should be taken when admir
patients: they should be mon
changes.

Lifestyle, Diet, and Habits

Determine whether the patier
may decrease serum theophyll
who smoke require an incre
up to 50%. Monitor patient
in smoking habits. It also is i
patients taking theophylline
increased by a low-carbohyd
charcoal-broiled beef. Theoph
by a high-carbohydrate, low-p
phylline can be increased by fo

COMMUNITY-BASED

Box 47.6 Using a Peak F

Patients receiving inhaled bronchod
effectiveness of drug therapy and lu
meter to monitor peak expiratory flo
inexpensive and may be available fr
prescription from the pharmacist.
Peak flow values are a way to q
tion. Daily monitoring helps to det
lung function, sometimes even bef
toms. Daily monitoring also permit
before the patient experiences a se
gency care.
The peak flow meter consists of a
measuring device. The patient inhale
places the mouthpiece in the mouth,
patient blows out as hard and as fast
pels an indicator up a scale to a num
of air per minute, represents the peal
the provider, the patient can determi
patient can then keep a record of the
in PEFR to the health care provider.

Drugs Affecting the Upper Gastrointestinal Tract

Drug Therapy for *Helicobacter pylori*

- amoxicillin (see Chapter 38)
- bismuth
- clarithromycin (see Chapter 39)
- metronidazole (see Chapter 45)
- tetracycline (see Chapter 39)

(C) Proton Pump Inhibitors

- (P) **omeprazole**
- sucralfate

(C) GI Stimulants

- (P) **metoclopramide**
- dexpanthenol

(C) Lipase Inhibitors

- (P) **orlistat**
- sibutramine

(C) H_2 Receptor Antagonists

- (P) **ranitidine**
- cimetidine
- famotidine
- nizatidine
- misoprostol

(C) Digestive Enzymes

- (P) **pancrelipase**
- pancreatin

(C) Antiemetics

- (P) **ondansetron**

(C) Antacids

- (P) **aluminum hydroxide with magnesium hydroxide**
- aluminum compounds
- magnesium compounds
- calcium carbonate
- sodium bicarbonate

(C) Gallstone Solubilizing Agents

The symbol (C) indicates the **drug class.**
Drugs in **bold type** marked with the symbol (P) are prototypes.
Drugs in blue type are closely related to the prototype.
Drugs in red type are significantly different from the prototype.
Drugs in black type with no symbol are also used in drug therapy; no prototype

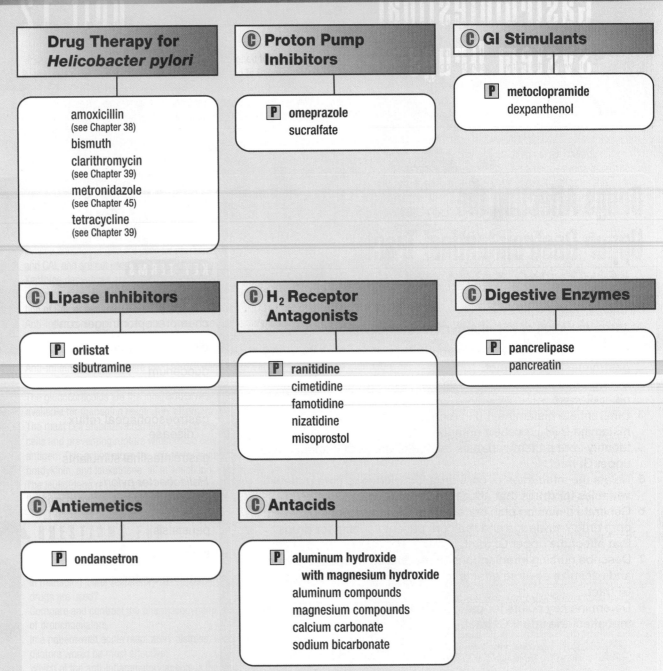

Numerous prescription drugs and over-the-counter (OTC) preparations are used to treat or prevent disorders of the upper gastrointestinal (GI) tract, such as gastroesophageal reflux disease, hiatal hernia, peptic ulcer disease, digestive problems, nausea, and vomiting. These problems may be caused by innate physiologic problems, such as poor organ functioning or excessive acid production, or they may be secondary to therapeutic treatment, such as surgery or other drug therapy.

Many of these drugs have a local effect in the GI tract and can interfere with the absorption of other drugs that are administered orally. Other GI drugs act systemically and can produce interactions with other drugs. Because many of the drugs used to treat these disorders are available OTC, the potential for self-diagnosis and self-medication is great. Patients might not consider OTC drugs to be part of their drug therapy and therefore might not mention using these agents unless questioned directly.

This chapter discusses the most common drug classes used to treat disorders of the upper GI tract, including:

- Drugs to treat *Helicobacter pylori* infection
- Proton pump inhibitors
- Histamine-2 (H_2) receptor antagonists
- Antacids
- GI stimulants
- Digestive enzymes
- Lipase inhibitors
- Antiemetics
- Gallstone-solubilizing agents. These drugs are mentioned briefly in this chapter, but no prototype is presented.

PHYSIOLOGY

The upper GI tract consists of the mouth, oropharynx, esophagus, stomach, and duodenum (small intestine). The **duodenum,** which is responsible for most digestive functions, is composed of four layers—the mucosa, submucosa, muscularis externa, and serosa. The mucosa is a mucous membrane covering the entire inner surface of the GI tract. In the duodenum, where some of the glands necessary for digestion and absorption are located, the mucosa forms folds and projections that increase the surface area of the intestine. The submucosa is composed of loose connective tissue containing blood, lymphatic vessels, and nerves. The blood vessels provide nutrients and oxygen to the tissues and remove the products of digestion. The muscularis externa is composed of two layers of smooth muscle. One layer encircles and constricts the tract; the other layer consists of longitudinal muscle fibers that contract to decrease the length of the tract. The serosa, which covers the outside of the GI tract, contains secretory cells that keep the outer surface of the tract moist and lubricated.

Digestion begins in the mouth, where food is chewed into fine particles, and salivary glands secrete substances that begin breaking down the food. The salivary glands consist of two types of secretory cells—serous and mucous. The serous cells contain amylase, an enzyme that splits the starch and glycogen contained in carbohydrates into disaccharides. This process is the first step of digestion. The mucous cells secrete mucus, which binds the food and facilitates swallowing. The tongue mixes food with the salivary gland secretions and moves the food toward the pharynx for swallowing.

Swallowing is a complex reflex that requires coordination of several muscle groups. After the bolus of food is moved toward the pharynx by the tongue, stimulated sensory nerves in the pharyngeal area trigger the swallowing reflex. Swallowing begins when the soft palate rises, preventing food from entering the nasal cavity. The epiglottis moves down over the trachea, preventing food from entering the lungs. Next, muscles in the lower pharynx relax, enabling food to move into the esophagus. **Peristalsis,** a rhythmic movement of contraction and expansion of the smooth muscle, propels the food toward the stomach.

The esophagus, a long, hollow tube that connects the mouth to the stomach, passes through the diaphragm and joins the stomach in the abdomen. The lower esophageal sphincter contains circular muscle fibers that contract to prevent regurgitation of gastric contents into the esophagus. Peristalsis causes these muscles to relax and allows food to enter the esophagus.

The stomach, which is situated between the esophagus and the duodenum, is a temporary storage and mixing site for food undergoing digestion. Three types of cells—mucous, chief, and parietal—secrete fluids commonly referred to as gastric juice. Chief cells in the stomach release pepsinogen, which is activated to the digestive enzyme pepsin by hydrochloric acid (secreted from parietal cells). Pepsin begins the process of protein digestion. The mucus secreted by mucous cells in the stomach protects against pepsin and hydrochloric acid, which can help form or aggravate peptic ulcers (Figure 48.1).

Gastric secretions are regulated primarily by the parasympathetic nervous system. The sight, smell, or thought of food stimulates parasympathetic nerve impulses that trigger the release of the hormone gastrin, which stimulates production of gastric juice. The movement of food mixed with gastric juice, a substance called chyme, into the duodenum inhibits further secretion of gastric juice. Fat-rich, acid chyme entering the duodenum triggers the release of cholecystokinin, a hormone produced in the intestinal wall that decreases gastric motility.

The acid in chyme also triggers release of secretin, another hormone. Secretin and cholecystokinin stimulate the release of pancreatic juice that contains bicarbonate, which buffers the effects of gastric acid, and **digestive enzymes.** The digestive enzymes, which break down chyme into nutrients the body can absorb, are secreted by the pancreas in inactive forms and changed to their active forms in the duodenum. The duodenum also produces some digestive enzymes. The pancreatic enzymes include amylase (which splits starch and glycogen into disaccharides), lipase (which hydrolyzes fats to fatty acids), and trypsin, chymotrypsin, and carboxypeptidase (which split proteins into amino acids).

Vomiting of GI contents is controlled by the **vomiting center** (VC) in the medulla of the brain. The GI tract contains sensory receptors that send nerve impulses to the brain in response to abdominal distention or irritation. Inflammation, spasms, and ischemia can also irritate nerve endings and activate the VC. These impulses are transmitted to the VC, which returns impulses that trigger abdominal contractions and reverse peristalsis, thereby inducing vomiting. The VC can also be directly stimulated through the cortical

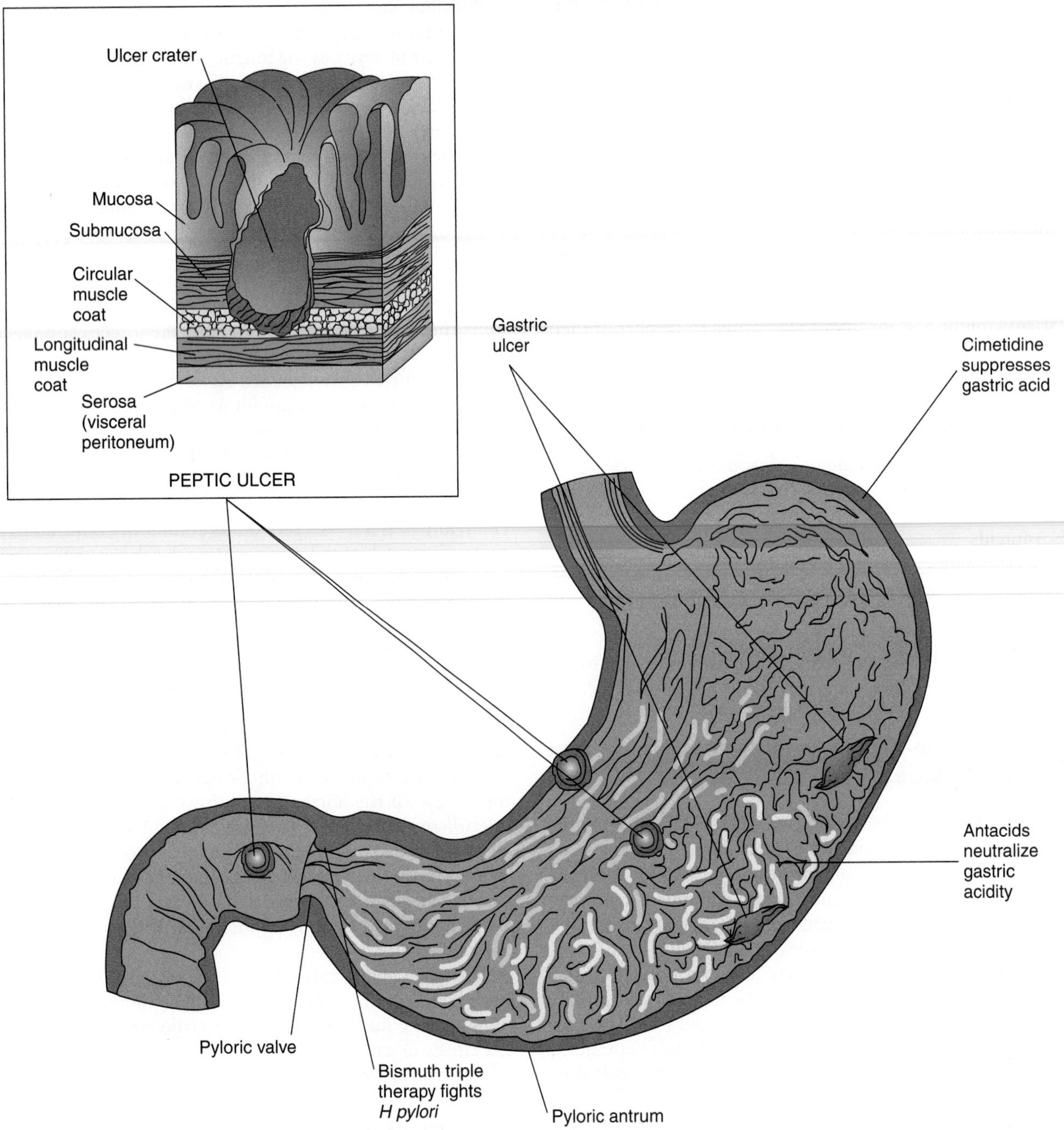

FIGURE 48.1 Drugs used in treating peptic ulcer disease need to retard further ulceration and promote healing. Lesions known as peptic ulcers are those that affect the mucosa of the stomach (gastric ulcer) or the duodenum (duodenal ulcer). With an advanced duodenal ulcer, gastric acid burrows through the gastric mucosa, submucosa, and muscle layers and perforates the peritoneum. As the illustration indicates, antacids neutralize excess acidity, H_2 receptor antagonists suppress gastric acid production; and bismuth triple therapy treats ulcers caused by *Helicobacter pylori.*

pathway by unpleasant olfactory and visual stimuli, pain, emotional factors, increased intracranial pressure, migraine headaches, or vestibular (inner ear) disturbances.

Additionally, the VC can be stimulated when the **chemoreceptor trigger zone** (CTZ) is stimulated. Located near the VC, the CTZ is stimulated by drugs, chemicals, toxins, radiation, hormonal changes, some disease states, and altered metabolic states. It also is stimulated by vestibular mechanisms. When the CTZ is stimulated, it acts on the VC to maintain a state of excitability to other incoming vestibular impulses.

PATHOPHYSIOLOGY

Gastroesophageal Reflux Disease

The esophagus normally is not exposed to much gastric acid because the lower esophageal sphincter prevents reflux (upward movement of gastric juices into the esophagus). When reflux occurs frequently and in larger amounts than normal, chronic symptoms of heartburn and dyspepsia occur, and ulceration of the mucosal lining may result. This condition is known as **gastroesophageal reflux disease** (GERD). Although GERD may sometimes occur alone, it often results from a hiatal hernia, a condition in which the cardiac portion of the stomach moves up through an opening in a weakened diaphragm. The movement of the stomach through the diaphragm decreases the pressure of the lower esophageal sphincter, so that the acid easily moves into the esophagus. Because cancer of the esophagus has the same symptoms as a hiatal hernia, cancer must be ruled out before drug therapy starts.

Ulcers

A **peptic ulcer** exists when all layers of the wall of the stomach or duodenum have been eroded. Untreated, a peptic ulcer can erode through the serosa and result in perforation. Peptic ulcers can occur in any part of the upper GI tract that is in contact with gastric hydrochloric acid and pepsin. The symptoms depend on the location of the ulcer. Gastric ulcer pain usually occurs 1 to 2 hours after eating, whereas duodenal ulcer pain begins 2 to 4 hours after eating and often results in night pain. Both types of ulcer can be complicated by perforation, hemorrhage, or obstruction. A **stress ulcer** is a peptic ulcer that is caused by acute or chronic stress. Stress ulcers occur frequently in critically ill patients. Clinically important complications of stress ulcers (bleeding that requires transfusion, bleeding associated with hemodynamic instability) are substantial sources of morbidity and mortality in the intensive care setting (Sung, 2003).

Helicobacter Pylori Infection

Helicobacter pylori is a gram-negative, spiral bacterium that colonizes the gastric mucosa. *H. pylori* infection, the most common chronic bacterial infection worldwide, is found in more than half of the human population. The natural history of *H. pylori* infection is still unknown. Person-to-person contact may be responsible for transmission. Infection persists unless treated. Research has shown an etiologic association between *H. pylori* infection and a number of important diseases, including chronic active gastritis, peptic ulcer disease, mucosa-associated lymphoid tissue lymphoma, gastric polyps, and gastric cancer. *H. pylori* infection has been identified in 90% to 95% of patients with duodenal ulcers, 50% to 80% of gastric ulcer patients, and in almost 100% of patients with chronic active gastritis. *H. pylori* plays a causative role in chronic gastritis and peptic ulcer disease and is associated with the development of gastric cancer (Zheng & Jones, 2003). Chronic *H. pylori* infection, particularly that acquired in early childhood, increases the risk for developing gastric cancer. The World Health Organization has classified *H. pylori* as a type 1 human carcinogen because of this finding (Chelimsky & Czinn, 2000). Studies have indicated that recurrent abdominal pain in children might be associated with gastritis induced by *H. pylori*, but the implications for therapy remain unclear. There also have been suggestions in the literature that *H. pylori* may be involved in diseases outside the upper GI tract.

Historically, stress, caffeine intake, and smoking were considered contributors to excessive acid production, which led to ulcer formation. This theory has been abandoned since the link between *H. pylori* and peptic ulcers was found. Excess acid alone does not produce gastric ulcers. Still, 80% of people infected with *H. pylori* never develop an ulcer. Other factors in the person's internal environment play a role in creating peptic ulcers when *H. pylori* is present. These factors are not known yet, but diet may be one of them. A review of the literature from 1966 to 1999 showed that soluble fiber from fruits and vegetables seems to protect against developing duodenal ulcers, whereas a diet with large amounts of refined sugars appears to be a risk factor for developing duodenal ulcers (Misciagna et al., 2000). Smokers do have a higher rate of peptic ulcer disease than nonsmokers, most likely because of the detrimental effects of smoking on the gastric mucosa. Surface-active phospholipids, which are surfactants in the gastric mucus, are believed to play a key role in protecting the gastric mucosa. Both *H. pylori* and smoking alter the concentrations of some of the phospholipid subclasses. This alteration makes the mucosa more vulnerable to damage from the gastric acid present in the stomach (Wenner et al., 2000). *H. pylori* infection that persists after treatment has been shown to be the only independent predictor of recurrent duodenal ulcer bleeding (Lai et al., 2000).

Pancreatitis

The pancreas contributes pancreatic juice and vital digestive enzymes to digestion. Production of these enzymes is reduced or no longer occurs in patients who have chronic pancreatitis or in those who have undergone a pancreatic resection or removal. In pancreatitis, digestive enzymes that normally are maintained in the pancreas in their inactive form become activated, destroying parts of the gland. With time, destruction of the pancreas decreases the amount of enzymes produced because the cells that produce the enzymes have been lost. Chronic pancreatitis occurs following repeated attacks of acute pancreatitis. The digestive enzyme pancrelipase is used to treat pancreatitis and other pancreatic deficiency states.

Obesity

The incidence of overweight and obesity is increasing at an alarming rate, both in the United States and worldwide. It has been estimated that 61% of American adults are now overweight or obese (Wyatt, 2003). Obesity and overweight reflect the extent to which a patient's body mass index (BMI) exceeds the normal range. The BMI is calculated as weight in kilograms divided by the square of height in meters. Normal BMI is 18.5 kg/m^2 to 24.9 kg/m^2. The term overweight is used if the patient's BMI is 25 to 29.9 kg/m^2, whereas the term obesity is used if the BMI exceeds 29.9 kg/m^2. Overweight and obesity are the result of a mismatch between energy consumed in calories and energy expended in activities. The

lifestyle in industrialized countries is increasingly sedentary. The energy expenditure of the average American worker at the beginning of the 21st century is estimated to be about half of that of the American worker at the start of the 20th century. Additionally, a high-fat diet, common in these countries, also contributes to obesity (Jeffrey & Utter, 2003). High blood pressure, type 2 diabetes, coronary heart disease, elevated blood cholesterol, gallbladder disease, and osteoarthritis are associated with overweight and obesity. High blood pressure is the most common overweight- and obesity-related health condition, and its incidence increases as weight increases (Bray, 2003). Type 2 diabetes, gallbladder disease, and osteoarthritis also are more prevalent as weight increases. The risk for coronary heart disease, somewhat higher than normal in overweight patients, is substantially elevated if the patient is obese. Elevated blood cholesterol levels are found at all levels of overweight and obesity. Preventing and treating obesity are important to control these lifelong morbidities and the mortality that accompanies them.

Nausea and Vomiting

Disorders of the upper GI tract are often accompanied by nausea and vomiting. Increased activity of neurotransmitters—for example, dopamine in the CTZ and acetylcholine in the VC—appears to play an important role in inducing vomiting. Serotonin also has a role in vomiting, and special serotonin receptors are located in the CTZ. The CTZ is stimulated through peripheral and central pathways. Peripheral stimulation happens when chemotherapy causes damage to the gastrointestinal mucosa, activating afferent input through the vagus nerve. Serotonin is the neurotransmitter for peripheral stimulation. The neurotransmitter substance P, found in the gut and the central nervous system, is capable of mediating emesis and is responsible for central pathway stimulation. Substance P exerts its antiemetic effect by binding to the tachykinin neurokinin (NK1) receptor, found throughout the central and peripheral systems and in the gut. The release of serotonin from the small intestine during chemotherapy stimulates these receptors and therefore stimulates vomiting. Major breakthroughs in combating emesis have occurred since the discovery of serotonin antagonists and more recently NK1 receptor antagonists.

DRUGS USED TO TREAT *HELICOBACTER PYLORI* INFECTION

Eliminating *H. pylori* from the GI tract improves healing and decreases the recurrence of ulcers. Once the infection has been eradicated, reinfection rates are less than 0.5% per year; ulcer recurrence rates also are reduced dramatically. The cure rate from the various treatment options ranges from about 70% to 90% or higher. Eradication therapy is the standard of care for patients with active or inactive peptic ulcers, including patients who use nonsteroidal anti-inflammatory drugs (NSAIDs). No routine antimicrobial treatment is recommended for patients with *H. pylori* infection who do not have ulcers. In addition, using antibiotics to eradicate *H. pylori* in an attempt to prevent gastric cancer is not recommended because research has not been done (NIH Guidelines, 1998). Strong indications for treating *H. pylori* infections include mucosa-associated lymphoid tissue lymphoma, hyperplastic polyps, hyperplastic gastropathy, postendoscopic resection for gastric cancer, and acute *H. pylori* gastritis. Currently, no single treatment is recognized as the standard, or best, treatment option. The FDA has approved six different options for treating *H. pylori* infections (Table 48.1). Other variations of combination drug therapy have been used in practice and in clinical trials.

Use of a single antibiotic is not recommended because of the potential for developing resistance to that antibiotic. Prior exposure to antibiotics also increases the risk for drug resistance (see Chapter 37). Antibiotic resistance has been reported with metronidazole and clarithromycin but not with bismuth, amoxicillin, or tetracycline. Resistance to metronidazole often can be overcome if the dose and the duration of therapy are increased. Clarithromycin resistance cannot be overcome by increasing the dose or the duration.

Using a single antibiotic with a proton pump inhibitor has been shown to be effective in curing *H. pylori* infection,

TABLE 48.1 Therapies Approved by the Food and Drug Administration for *H. Pylori* Infection

Drug Therapy	Dose and Duration of Therapy
*lansoprazole +	30 mg bid for 10–14 d
clarithromycin +	500 mg bid for 10–14 d
amoxicillin	1 g bid for day to 14 d
omeprazole +	20 mg bid for 10 d
clarithromycin +	500 mg bid for 10 d
amoxicillin	1 g bid for 10 d
ranitidine bismuth citrate +	400 mg bid for 14 d
clarithromycin	500 mg tid for 14 d
followed by ranitidine bismuth citrate	400 mg bid for additional 14 d
bismuth subsalicylate +	525 mg qid for 14 d
metronidazole +	250 mg qid for 14 d
tetracycline +	500 mg qid for 14 d
H_2 receptor antagonist	per individual drug dosing for 28 d
†omeprazole +	40 mg qd for 10 d
clarithromycin	500 mg tid for 14 d
followed by additional omeprazole	20 mg once/daily for additional 14 d
†lansoprazole +	30 mg tid for 14 d
amoxicillin	1 g tid for 14 d

*This combination therapy has ≥90% or higher eradication rate of *H. pylori* infection.

†Practice guidelines from the American College of Gastroenterology do not recommend a single antibiotic combined with a proton pump inhibitor because cure rate is <70%.

but only 30% to 70% of the time, so it is not recommended. Double antibiotic therapy with the addition of an antisecretory drug (one that prevents the secretion of gastric acid) is very effective and is the most preferred therapy. Triple and quadruple therapy regimens also are effective in curing *H. pylori* infection. They include bismuth subsalicylate (Pepto-Bismol), antibiotics, and an antisecretory agent. These therapies carry more risk for adverse effects than simpler therapies. Adherence also is a limiting factor for these therapies, because of the number of drugs that must be taken every day.

Studies have concluded that curing *H. pylori* infection significantly reduces the risk for recurring ulcer disease. Thus, maintenance therapy with antisecretory agents is not needed for patients with a history of uncomplicated ulcer disease once *H. pylori* has been eradicated. For patients who have had complicated ulcer disease, the decision about whether they should continue taking antisecretory drugs must be made on an individual basis. Factors that should be considered and may lead to a decision to continue with therapy are presence of comorbid disease; use of medications, such as NSAIDs and anticoagulants, that increase risk for recurrence or complications; and the severity of the previous ulcer-related complications.

Ulcers that are refractory, or unresponsive, to therapy for *H. pylori* infection often indicate failure to eradicate the organism. Resistance to the therapy, patients' nonadherence to therapy, and concurrent use of NSAIDs also may be involved in refractory ulcers. Retreatment regimens following treatment failure should not include antibiotics to which the patient's organisms might have acquired resistance. With antibiotic-resistant *H. pylori* infections, higher doses and longer durations of treatment usually result in better cure rates. When multiple treatment regimens fail, salvage therapy with quadruple therapy may be used. Furazolidone, another antibiotic for serious infections, may be substituted for the metronidazole (Roghani et al., 2003). Further discussion of the antimicrobials used to treat *H. pylori* is found in Chapters 39 and 45.

Prophylactic and therapeutic vaccines have been developed against *H. pylori* in animals. Research toward developing vaccines against *H. pylori* for use in humans is now under way (Sutton & Doidge, 2003).

C PROTON PUMP INHIBITORS

The secretion of gastric acid can be suppressed by inhibiting the H^+/K^+ adenosine triphosphatase (ATPase) enzyme system at the secretory surface of the gastric parietal cell. Because this enzyme system is the "acid pump," also known as the "proton pump," within the gastric mucosa, drugs that inhibit this system are known as proton pump inhibitors. These drugs block the final step of gastric acid production. Their effect is dose related; they inhibit acid secretion regardless of the stimulus producing the acid. The prototype drug is omeprazole. Other drugs in this class are lansoprazole, pantoprazole, and rabeprazole. A drug significantly different from omeprazole is sucralfate. Table 48.2 presents a summary of antisecretory drugs.

NURSING MANAGEMENT OF THE PATIENT RECEIVING P OMEPRAZOLE

Core Drug Knowledge

Pharmacotherapeutics

Omeprazole is used for symptomatic treatment of heartburn and other symptoms of GERD. It also is used to treat duodenal ulcers associated with *H. pylori* infection. It is sometimes used for short-term treatment (4–8 weeks) of active duodenal and gastric ulcer when *H. pylori* is not present and is also used as short-term treatment for erosive esophagitis, diagnosed by endoscopy, to maintain healing. It can be used long term in chronic hypersecretory conditions, such as Zollinger-Ellison syndrome, multiple endocrine adenomas, and systemic mastocytosis. Unlabeled uses are treatment of posterior laryngitis, and adjunctive treatment to enhance the efficacy of pancreatin in treating steatorrhea (large quantities of fat in stool) in cystic fibrosis.

Pharmacokinetics

Omeprazole, like other proton pump inhibitors, is acid labile. Therefore, it is formulated as enteric-coated granules delivered in a capsule. The drug is absorbed rapidly after leaving the stomach. Omeprazole is metabolized extensively by the cytochrome P-450 system in the liver, and several metabolites are formed. These metabolites do not have an antisecretory function, except perhaps minimally. The antisecretory effect of omeprazole is long lasting and is not related closely to elimination half-life: its half-life in plasma is less than 2 hours, whereas the antisecretory effect lasts longer than 24 hours. This extended effect is attributed to prolonged binding of the drug to the parietal H^+/K^+ ATPase enzyme. When the drug is discontinued, normal secretory activity returns within 3 to 5 days. Little of the drug is excreted unchanged. The metabolites are excreted mostly in the urine, although about one fourth of them are eliminated in the feces. Duration of action is longer in Asians than in whites. Therefore, dose adjustments may be necessary.

Pharmacodynamics

Omeprazole suppresses the last phase of gastric acid production by suppressing the H^+/K^+ ATPase enzyme system. Intragastric pH is therefore elevated, and as a result, blood flow in the antrum, pylorus, and duodenal bulb is decreased. Omeprazole increases serum pepsinogen levels and decreases pepsin activity. The increases in gastric pH are associated with increased numbers of nitrate-reducing bacteria and elevated nitrate concentrations in gastric juice in patients with gastric ulcers. Serum gastrin levels increase as acid secretion is inhibited. Continued treatment does not provoke serum gastrin levels to rise continually; however; they reach a certain degree of elevation and remain there.

Contraindications and Precautions

Omeprazole is contraindicated for patients who are hypersensitive to the drug or any of its components. Omeprazole is an FDA pregnancy category C drug.

TABLE 48.2 Summary of Selected Antisecretory Drugs and Other Drugs Used in Peptic Ulcer Disease

Drug (Trade) Name	Selected Indications	Route and Dosage Range	Pharmacokinetics
(C) Proton Pump Inhibitors			
(P) omeprazole (Prilosec)	Active duodenal ulcer Gastric ulcer GERD Hypersecretory conditions *Helicobacter pylori*	20 mg/d PO × 4–8 wk 40 mg/day PO × 4–8 wk 20 mg/day × 4–8 wk 60 mg once daily PO initially 20 mg bid PO (in combination with other therapy)	*Onset:* Within 1 h *Duration:* 72 h $t_{1/2}$: 30–60 min
lansoprazole (Prevacid)	Active duodenal ulcer Erosive esophagitis, GERD Hypersecretory conditions *H. pylori*	15 mg/d PO × 4 wk 15–30 mg/day PO × 8 wk 60 mg/d 30 mg/d × 2 wk (in combination with other drug therapy)	*Onset:* Unknown *Duration:* 24 h $t_{1/2}$: 1.5 h
(C) H_2 Receptor Antagonists			
(P) ranitidine (Zantac, Zantac 75, GELdose)	Duodenal and gastric ulcers	PO, 150 mg bid, or 300 mg at bedtime (duodenal) short-term use for active ulcers; maintenance dose, 150 mg at bedtime; parenteral (any use), IM, 50 mg (2 mL premixed) q6–8h; IV push, 50 mg (2 mL) diluted with 0.09% NaCl solution (normal saline) to make 20 mL, over 5 min or more; intermittent IV, 50 mg diluted in 100 mL dextrose 5% in water (D5W) or other compatible solution, run over 15–20 min, q6–8h, not to exceed 400 mg/d	*Onset:* PO, varies; IV, rapid *Duration:* 8–12 h $t_{1/2}$: 2–3 h
	GERD	PO, 150 mg bid	
	Pathologic hyper-secretory conditions (i.e., Zollinger-Ellison syndrome)	PO, 150 mg bid, may give up to 6 g/d; continuous IV infusion (dilute in compatible solution to no more than 2.5 mg/mL); run at 1 mg/kg/h, after 4 h may be adjusted upward in 0.5 mg/kg/h increments up to 2.5 mg/kg/h	
	Erosive esophagitis	PO, 150 mg qid; maintenance 150 mg bid	
cimetidine (Tagamet, Tagamet HB)	Duodenal and gastric ulcers	PO, 800 mg at bedtime, or 300 mg qid with meals and at bedtime for 4–6 wk (duodenal) or 8 wk (gastric); IV or IM, 300 mg q 6–8 h, not to exceed 2,400 mg/d	*Onset:* PO, varies; IV, rapid *Duration:* 4–13 h (depending on dose and regimen) $t_{1/2}$: 2 h
	Prevention of upper GI bleeding	IV, infusion at 50 mg/h	
	Erosive GERD	PO, 1,600 mg/d divided into 2 or 4 doses for 12 wk; IV or IM, dosing and regimen not established	
	Pathologic hypersecretory conditions	PO, 300 mg qid with meals and at bed-time not to exceed 240 mg/d, given as long as clinically needed.	
	Heartburn/acid indigestion	PO OTC, 200 mg twice daily; continuous IV infusion, 300 mg q 6–8 h	

(continued)

TABLE 48.2 Summary of Selected Antisecretory Drugs and Other Drugs Used in Peptic Ulcer Disease (continued)

Drug (Trade) Name	Selected Indications	Route and Dosage Range	Pharmacokinetics
famotidine (Pepcid, Pepcid AC)	Same as ranitidine, for ulcers and related conditions	PO (acute duodenal ulcer), 40 mg/d at bedtime or 20 mg bid for 6–8 wk; maintenance, 20 mg/d at bedtime; (acute benign gastric ulcer), 40 mg/d at bedtime; IV (patient NPO), 20 mg q12h (dilute 2 mL, or 20 mg, in 5 or 10 mL normal saline or other) compatible solution, and inject over at least 2 min; intermittent IV, 20 mg (dilute in 100 mL D5W or other compatible solution, infuse over 15–30 min)	*Onset:* PO, ≤1 h; IV, rapid *Duration:* 10–12 h $t_{1/2}$: 2.5–3.5 h
	Hypersecretory conditions	PO (individualize), 20 mg q6h to start, up to 160 mg q6h; continue as long as needed	
	GERD	PO, 20 mg bid up to 6 wk	
	Esophagitis due to GERD	PO, 20 or 40 mg bid for up to 12 wk	
	Heartburn, acid indigestion	PO (OTC), 10 mg (1 tablet); prevention 1 h before eating a meal expected to cause GI distress; up to 2 tablets in 24 h	
nizatidine (Axid AR)	Duodenal ulcer, benign active gastric ulcer	PO (active ulcer), 300 mg once daily at bedtime or 150 mg bid (less for patients with renal insufficiency); maintenance 150 mg once daily at bedtime	*Onset:* Varies *Duration:* 3–10 h $t_{1/2}$: 1–2 h
	GERD	Adult: PO, 150 mg bid	
(C) Miscellaneous			
misoprostol (Cytotec)	Prevention of NSAID-induced gastric ulcers	PO, 200 µg qid with food; if not well tolerated, may use 100 µg per dose	*Onset:* Rapid *Duration:* 3 h $t_{1/2}$: 20–40 min
sucralfate (Carafate)	Duodenal ulcer	1 g PO qid 1 h before meals and at bedtime for 4–8 wk	*Onset:* 30 min *Duration:* 5 h $t_{1/2}$: 6–20 h

Adverse Effects

Omeprazole is generally well tolerated. The most common adverse effects are headache and diarrhea. However, during clinical trials, these effects also were found in patients receiving placebo. Other adverse effects reported in clinical trials include central nervous system (CNS) effects of dizziness and asthenia; GI effects of constipation, abdominal pain, nausea, and vomiting; and miscellaneous effects of upper respiratory infection, cough, rash, and back pain.

Rare adverse effects (which occurred in fewer than 1% of patients in clinical studies) are numerous and diverse. They include confusion, drowsiness, blurred vision, tachycardia, diaphoresis, flushing, dry mouth, severe generalized skin reactions, elevated liver enzyme levels, and overt hepatic disease.

Overdosage with omeprazole has been reported rarely, and no serious outcomes have been reported from overdosage. In patients who received 16 to 45 times the usual dose, symptoms were transient and included confusion, drowsiness, blurred vision, tachycardia, nausea, diaphoresis, flushing, headache, and dry mouth.

Drug Interactions

Omeprazole can interact with other drugs that also are metabolized through the cytochrome P-450 pathway. Examples of these drugs include cyclosporine, disulfiram, and the benzodiazepines. Such interactions can produce elevated levels of these other drugs because their metabolism is decreased. Because omeprazole causes prolonged and substantial decreases in gastric acidity, drugs that depend on an acid environment for absorption may not be absorbed optimally. Table 48.3 lists drugs that interact with omeprazole.

Assessment of Relevant Core Patient Variables

Health Status

Determine that the patient has a clinical indication for the use of omeprazole. Hepatic and renal diseases do not require a decreased dosage.

TABLE 48.3 Agents That Interact With P Omeprazole

Interactants	Effect and Significance	Nursing Management
clarithromycin	Increases the plasma levels of both clarithromycin and omeprazole. This may be beneficial because the two are given as cotherapy to treat *Helicobacter pylori.*	Give as ordered. Assess for possible adverse effects.
sucralfate	Delayed absorption and reduced bioavailability of omeprazole by about 17% when the two are given at the same time. This decreases desired therapeutic effect.	Give omeprazole ≥30 min before sucralfate.
benzodiazepines (diazepam, flurazepam, triazolam)	Large increases (130%) in the half-life of the benzodiazepines, most likely due to decreased metabolism of the benzodiazepines. Plasma levels also increased and total clearance decreased.	Decreased dose of benzodiazepines may be indicated. Monitor for adverse effects.
phenytoin	Reduced plasma clearance of phenytoin and increased half-life, most likely caused by inhibition of its metabolism.	Decreased dose of phenytoin may be indicated. Monitor for adverse effects. Monitor blood levels of phenytoin.
warfarin	Prolong the elimination of warfarin due to inhibition of its metabolism.	Monitor for adverse effects. Assess protime carefully. Adjust dose if warranted.

Life Span and Gender

Assess female patients for pregnancy or breast-feeding. Omeprazole is a pregnancy category C drug; no adequate or well-controlled studies of the drug have been done in pregnant women. Omeprazole should be used during pregnancy only if the potential benefit to the mother justifies the potential risk to the fetus. It is not known whether omeprazole is secreted in breast milk. Animal studies showed decreased weight gain from nursing when the mother received large doses (35–345 times the human dose) of omeprazole. Therefore, use in breast-feeding is not recommended. Note the patient's age. Omeprazole's efficacy and safety in children have not been established. Although bioavailability of the drug may be increased in older adults, no dosage adjustment is needed.

Lifestyle, Diet, and Habits

Assess the patient's diet and smoking habits. Highly acidic foods, such as tomato juice, and highly spiced foods may worsen the symptoms of GERD or peptic ulcer disease until the ulcer heals. Omeprazole should be taken before eating. Smoking also may aggravate the symptoms of peptic ulcer disease.

Environment

Omeprazole may be given in any environment.

Culture and Inherited Traits

Assess the patient's culture and genetic background before administering omeprazole. Asians can experience elevated serum levels (up to fourfold higher) than whites and thus might need a decreased dose.

Nursing Diagnoses and Outcomes

- Altered Comfort related to symptoms of GERD, peptic ulcer disease, or chronically elevated acid production
  Desired outcome: *Drug therapy will relieve the symptoms from the GI disorder.*
- Imbalanced Nutrition: Less than Body Requirements related to symptoms of GERD, peptic ulcer disease, or chronically elevated acid production
  Desired outcome: *Drug therapy will allow adequate dietary intake.*
- Collaborative Problem: *H. pylori* infection
  Desired outcome: *Treatment regimen to eradicate* H. pylori *will be effective, with minimal adverse effects.*

Planning and Intervention

Maximizing Therapeutic Effects

Make sure that omeprazole is administered for the recommended time, based on the clinical indication for therapy, usually between 2 and 8 weeks. For chronic pathologic hypersecretory conditions, administer daily for as long as needed. Some patients are known to have received omeprazole for 5 years or longer.

Minimizing Adverse Effects

Daily dosages larger than 80 mg should be given in divided doses. Because the drug is enteric coated, it cannot be crushed before use.

Providing Patient and Family Education

- Teach the patient to take omeprazole before meals and to continue therapy for the duration prescribed.
- Emphasize that the drug should not be crushed or chewed because doing so alters absorption and effectiveness.
- Explain that antacids can be used while taking omeprazole if symptoms require additional management.

Ongoing Assessment and Evaluation

Therapy is effective when the symptoms of GERD, peptic ulcer disease, or hypersecretory conditions are controlled or the duodenal ulcer is healed.

MEMORY CHIP

P Omeprazole

- Used to treat peptic ulcers resulting from *H. pylori*, GERD, erosive esophagitis, and chronic hypersecretory conditions (e.g., Zollinger-Ellison syndrome)
- May interact with other drugs metabolized by CYP 450
- Most common adverse effects: headache and diarrhea
- **Life span alert: use not recommended during breast feeding**
- Most important patient education: Take omeprazole before meals; do not crush or chew drug.

Drug Significantly Different From P Omeprazole

Sucralfate (Carafate), like omeprazole, is used to treat duodenal ulcers (see Table 48.2). Unlabeled uses of sucralfate include accelerating the healing of gastric ulcers and long-term management of gastric ulcers. Other unlabeled uses include treating reflux ulcers, reflux and peptic esophagitis, and NSAID-induced GI symptoms (including those caused by aspirin), and preventing stress ulcers and GI bleeding in critically ill patients. Sucralfate suspension also has been used to treat oral and esophageal ulcers caused by radiation, chemotherapy, and sclerotherapy.

Unlike omeprazole, sucralfate is not a proton pump inhibitor and does not prevent the secretion of gastric acid. Sucralfate is an aluminum salt of sulfated sucrose, a polysaccharide with antipeptic activity. In the acidic medium of gastric fluid, the aluminum ion splits off, leaving a highly polar anion. An essentially nonabsorbent paste forms and adheres to the ulcer lesion, protecting the lesion from acid, pepsin, and bile salts. This protection allows the ulcer to heal. The drug also has minimal antacid effects, but these effects do not contribute to ulcer healing.

Sucralfate should be used cautiously during pregnancy (pregnancy category B) and breast-feeding because it is not known whether the drug is secreted in breast milk. Safety and efficacy in children have not been established. In dialysis patients and others with chronic renal failure, sucralfate given concurrently with aluminum antacids increases the risk for aluminum toxicity because small amounts of aluminum, given off by sucralfate, are absorbed from the GI tract. This toxicity is not a potential problem for patients with normal renal function.

Adverse effects from sucralfate are usually mild. The drug rarely had to be discontinued during clinical trials. The most common adverse effect was constipation, which occurred in only 2% of patients. Sucralfate may decrease the effectiveness of anticoagulants, digoxin, hydantoins, ketoconazole, quinidine, and the quinolones.

Teach the patient to take sucralfate at least 1 hour before meals and at bedtime to maximize the therapeutic effect. Sucralfate may block the absorption of other drugs; therefore, it should be taken 1 hour before or after other drugs are administered. Antacids should be taken 30 minutes before or after sucralfate.

C THE HISTAMINE-2 RECEPTOR ANTAGONISTS

Various terms are used to describe the H_2 receptor antagonists, including histamine-2 receptor antagonists, H_2 receptor blockers, H_2 antagonists, H_2 blockers, and histamine blockers. H_2 receptor antagonists block the effect of histamine at H_2 receptors, particularly those in the parietal cells of the stomach. Antihistamines that block histamine-1 (H_1) receptors, the most frequent site of action for antihistamines, do not affect H_2 receptor sites, and H_2 receptor antagonists do not block H_1 sites; they also are not anticholinergic.

By blocking histamine at the parietal cells, these drugs inhibit gastric acid secretion in all phases, and other secretions caused by histamine, muscarinic agonists, and gastrin are also inhibited. H_2 receptor antagonists also inhibit the fasting secretions that occur during the night, as well as secretions stimulated by food, insulin, caffeine, pentagastrin, and betazole. These drugs also reduce the volume of, and the hydrogen ion concentration in, gastric secretions. H_2 receptor antagonists include ranitidine (Zantac), cimetidine (Tagamet), famotidine (Pepcid), and nizatidine (Axid AR). A drug significantly different from ranitidine is misoprostol. Although cimetidine was the first drug in this class, it is not used as frequently now because of its numerous drug interactions; these interactions are not found with other H_2 receptor antagonists. Ranitidine is the prototype drug for this class.

NURSING MANAGEMENT OF THE PATIENT RECEIVING P RANITIDINE

Core Drug Knowledge

Pharmacotherapeutics

Ranitidine (Zantac) is used to treat patients with active duodenal or benign gastric ulcers and (at reduced dosage) in maintenance therapy after acute ulcers have healed. It is also used to treat pathologic hypersecretory conditions, such as Zollinger-Ellison syndrome. It is used to treat GERD and endoscopically diagnosed erosive esophagitis and as maintenance therapy to promote healing of erosive esophagitis.

Pharmacokinetics

Ranitidine is a competitive, reversible inhibitor of the action of histamine at the H_2 receptors, including receptors on the gastric cells. Zantac is 50% absorbed after oral administration. It is metabolized by the liver to N-oxide, S-oxide, and desmethyl ranitidine.

The drug's principal route of excretion is in the urine, with approximately 30% of the orally administered dose collected in the urine as unchanged drug in 24 hours. The elimination half-life is 2.5 to 3 hours.

Pharmacodynamics

Ranitidine inhibits both daytime and nocturnal basal gastric acid secretions as well as gastric acid secretion stimulated by food, betazole, and pentagastrin. Ranitidine does not affect pepsin secretion. It has little or no effect on fasting or

postprandial serum gastrin secretion. It has no effect on prolactin levels, gonadotropins, thyroid-stimulating hormone, growth hormone, cortisol, aldosterone, androgen or estrogen levels, or sperm count.

Contraindications and Precautions

Ranitidine is contraindicated in patients who are hypersensitive to the drug. It is a pregnancy category B drug; no adequate, well-controlled studies of this drug have been performed in pregnant women. It also is not recommended for use by nursing mothers because it has been found in breast milk. The safety and effectiveness of ranitidine have been established in patients 1 month to 16 years of age.

Ranitidine should be used cautiously in patients with hepatic or renal impairment because the drug is metabolized by the liver and excreted by the kidneys. Patients with gastric ulcers should be monitored closely when using ranitidine because the drug can mask symptoms of GI cancer temporarily. Such patients should be evaluated thoroughly to rule out cancer. In geriatric populations, as compared with younger subjects, no overall differences in safety or effectiveness have been observed. However, greater sensitivity of some older individuals to the drug cannot be ruled out.

Adverse Effects

Ranitidine generally is well tolerated. Headache, sometimes severe, seems to be related to administration of ranitidine. Blood count changes (leukopenia, granulocytopenia, and thrombocytopenia) have occurred. These effects were usually reversible. Rash has been reported. GI effects include constipation, diarrhea, nausea and vomiting, and abdominal discomfort or pain; pancreatitis has also been reported, but rarely. Hepatocellular, cholestatic, or mixed hepatitis, with or without jaundice, has occasionally been reported. CNS, cardiovascular, musculoskeletal, integumentary, and other effects such as hypersensitivity are rare.

Drug Interactions

Ranitidine does not inhibit the cytochrome P-450 system, whereas cimetidine does. Cimetidine decreases hepatic metabolism and increases the potential for interaction with many other drugs. For this reason, cimetidine use is decreasing, and ranitidine, famotidine, and others are being used as drugs of first choice.

Assessment of Relevant Core Patient Variables

Health Status

Before administering ranitidine, assess the patient for epigastric, abdominal, and esophageal pain, commonly described as heartburn or a burning sensation that occurs after eating. Also, explore complaints of dyspepsia; nausea and vomiting; dark, tarry stools; hepatic dysfunction; and renal impairment. If the patient has a nasogastric tube in place, inspect for frank or occult bleeding.

The drug history should include the prescription and OTC drugs the patient is taking currently because many drugs, including aspirin, other NSAIDs, and corticosteroids, can cause gastric irritation. Additional drug history involves determining whether the patient is taking any OTC H_2 receptor antagonists and asking how long and why the patient has been using these drugs.

Life Span and Gender

Assess whether the patient is pregnant or breast-feeding because pregnant and breast-feeding patients should take ranitidine only if necessary. Determine the patient's age. Elderly patients should be assessed carefully for decreased renal and hepatic function.

Lifestyle, Diet, and Habits

Assess the patient's diet and smoking habits. Caffeine, alcohol, and spicy foods may aggravate gastric symptoms from GERD, peptic ulcer disease, and hypersecretory conditions. Smoking reverses the drug-induced inhibition of nocturnal gastric acid production and hinders ulcer healing. Cigarette smoking also is related closely to ulcer recurrence.

Environment

Ranitidine can be administered in any setting. The oral form is self-administered easily. Administration through the intravenous (IV) or intramuscular (IM) route is done most commonly in an inpatient setting.

Culture and Inherited Traits

Cultural influences on dietary patterns must be considered if the patient normally eats a diet consisting of highly spiced foods, such as jalapeño peppers, Thai curries, or Szechwan cuisine.

Nursing Diagnoses and Outcomes

- Chronic Pain related to alteration in the gastric mucosa, ulceration, or irritation
  Desired outcome: *The patient will report decreased pain while receiving drug therapy.*
- Acute Pain related to adverse drug effects, such as headache
  Desired outcome: *The patient will not experience adverse effects while taking ranitidine.*
- Risk for Injury related to drug-induced somnolence, dizziness, confusion, or hallucinations
  Desired outcome: *The patient will not suffer injury from adverse effects of drug therapy.*
- Diarrhea related to adverse effects of drug therapy
  Desired outcome: *The patient's elimination patterns will remain within normal parameters.*

Planning and Intervention

Maximizing Therapeutic Effects

If both ranitidine and antacids are prescribed, give them at least 2 hours apart to prevent decreased absorption of ranitidine.

Minimizing Adverse Effects

Monitor serum trough levels in patients with renal or hepatic impairment because CNS effects are more likely to occur when serum levels are elevated above the therapeutic level. Drug therapy may have to be discontinued if serious adverse effects occur.

Administer intravenous ranitidine therapy slowly to prevent hypotension and cardiac arrhythmias. It is important

to administer single IV push doses, diluted in 20 mL of normal saline or other compatible solution, over at least 2 minutes. Intermittent IV infusions of 300 mg in at least 50 mL of D_5W or other compatible solution should be administered over at least 15 minutes or 20 minutes. Give a continuous IV infusion at a rate of 37.5 mg/h.

Providing Patient and Family Education

- Instruct the patient to take the drug exactly as directed for the entire course of therapy, even if symptoms disappear (it usually takes 4–6 weeks for an ulcer to heal but less time for the symptoms to subside).
- Caution the patient not to take a double dose if a dose is missed.
- Counsel the patient on smoking cessation. OTC or prescription smoking cessation aids may be recommended, if appropriate.
- Explain that alcohol, caffeine, spicy foods, products containing aspirin or ibuprofen, and smoking all contribute to gastric irritation and slow healing of the ulcer.
- Caution the patient not to drive until the effects of ranitidine on the patient are known.
- Urge the patient to report immediately any tarry, black stools or coffee ground–like emesis, which are signs of gastric bleeding that must be treated.
- Caution the patient not to substitute OTC ranitidine for prescribed ranitidine because these products have different potencies (Box 48.1).
- Teach the patient to stagger ranitidine and antacid dosing schedules to allow at least 2 hours between doses.

Ongoing Assessment and Evaluation

During long-term therapy, the patient's blood counts should be monitored to detect changes from baseline. Drug therapy is effective when epigastric pain decreases, peptic ulcers heal, hypersecretion of gastric acid declines, or GI bleeding is prevented without adverse effects.

Drug Significantly Different From P Ranitidine

Misoprostol (Cytotec), unlike ranitidine, is not an H_2 antagonist. It is a synthetic form of prostaglandin E and is used to prevent NSAID-induced gastric ulcers in high-risk patients, such as older adults, patients with other debilitating diseases, and patients with a history of gastric ulcers (see Table 48.2). An unlabeled use is treating duodenal ulcers. Misoprostol may be useful in treating duodenal ulcers refractory to treatment with H_2 receptor antagonists. While misoprostol does not prevent duodenal ulcers, it is effective in decreasing the incidence of gastric ulcers associated with the use of PSI drugs.

NSAIDs inhibit prostaglandin synthesis, causing diminished bicarbonate and mucus secretion in the gastric mucosa. Misoprostol binds at the prostaglandin receptors and can increase bicarbonate and mucus secretion, thereby protecting the stomach lining. This action results in decreased peptic ulcer formation in patients taking NSAIDs. Misoprostol decreases pepsin concentration moderately during basal conditions but not during histamine stimulation. It has no significant effect on gastrin levels, either before or after meals. Misoprostol does decrease normal daytime and nocturnal gastric acid secretion. It also decreases the gastric acid that is produced in response to stimuli, including meals, histamine, pentagastrin, and coffee. Activity of the drug begins within 30 minutes of administration and lasts for 3 hours or more.

Misoprostol is classified as a pregnancy category X drug because it has abortifacient properties. The drug causes uterine contractions and miscarriage. Women of childbearing potential must receive written and oral warnings about the hazards of misoprostol, be able to adhere to effective contra-

COMMUNITY-BASED CONCERNS

Box 48.1 Using Over-the-Counter (OTC) Gastrointestinal Drugs Responsibly

Various antacids, such as Maalox and Mylantin, and histamine-2 (H_2) receptor antagonists (also called H_2 blockers), such as cimetidine (Tagamet HB), ranitidine (Zantac HB), and famotidine (Pepcid AC), are available currently OTC. Nurses who provide home care or who treat patients on an outpatient basis need to be aware that many patients self-medicate with these preparations. They may use them alone, as an adjunct to prescribed therapy, or in place of their prescribed drug. The following guidelines may help nurses help such patients use these drugs responsibly:

- Assess specifically for OTC antacid and H_2-blocker use. The patient may not think of OTC products as "real drugs" and so fail to identify them during the drug history.
- Advise the patient taking a prescribed H_2 blocker to take only that drug and not to substitute any OTC preparation for it. Explain that the dosages and drug formulations may be different.
- Caution the patient not to take any OTC H_2-blocker in addition to the prescribed drug. In such cases, "more is not better."
- If a particular antacid has been prescribed for a patient, warn the patient not to switch brands or type of antacid without consulting the prescriber. Some forms of antacids are contraindicated in certain medical conditions (e.g., congestive heart failure and hypertension).
- Urge patient to consult own health care provider before taking antacids in conjunction with an H_2-blocker.

MEMORY CHIP

P Ranitidine

- Blocks histamine competitively at histamine-2 (H_2) receptors in the gastric parietal cells; these receptors are not affected by H_1 antagonists.
- Inhibits all phases of gastric acid secretion
- Used for gastroesophageal reflux disease, duodenal ulcer, gastric ulcer, pathologic hypersecretory conditions; to prevent upper GI bleeding; and for heartburn and acid indigestion (OTC strength only)
- Interacts with numerous other drugs, many by decreasing their hepatic metabolism
- Most serious adverse effects (all rare): neutropenia, agranulocytosis, thrombocytopenia, autoimmune hemolytic or aplastic anemia
- Maximizing therapeutic effects: Give ranitidine at least 2 hours apart from antacids.
- Most important patient education: Do not substitute OTC drug for prescription drug nor add OTC drug to prescribed drug therapy.

ceptive measures, and have had a negative serum pregnancy test result in the 2 weeks before beginning therapy. Therapy should be started on the second or third day of the next normal menstrual cycle. It is not known whether the drug enters breast milk; thus, its use by nursing mothers is not recommended. Efficacy and safe use in children have not been established. Additionally, elderly patients may not be able to tolerate the usual dose. Cautious use is recommended for patients with renal failure. However, a dosage reduction is not normally necessary. Other uses of misoprostol are discussed in Chapters 24, 54 and 55.

The most common adverse effect of misoprostol therapy is diarrhea; the next most common is abdominal pain. Other adverse effects are nausea and vomiting, dyspepsia, flatulence, constipation, and headache. Possible gynecologic problems include spotting, cramps, and menstrual disorders.

When antacids are administered with misoprostol, the availability of misoprostol is reduced, but this effect does not appear to be important clinically. Although food decreases plasma concentrations of misoprostol, the specific receptors for misoprostol in the GI tract are still activated, and a therapeutic response is evident. The effect of misoprostol is topical, rather than systemic. Patients should take misoprostol with food. If diarrhea is a problem, it can be diminished if the drug is taken after the meal.

C ANTACIDS

Antacids are drugs that increase the gastric pH, thereby neutralizing gastric acidity. These preparations are used for various upper GI disorders, including symptoms of GERD (heartburn, indigestion, and upset stomach), esophagitis, hiatal hernia, gastritis, and peptic ulcer disease. Antacids are composed of inorganic salts of aluminum, magnesium, calcium, or sodium used alone or in various combinations. Antacids include aluminum hydroxide with magnesium hydroxide, aluminum, magnesium, calcium, and sodium bicarbonate. The prototype antacid is aluminum hydroxide with magnesium hydroxide (Maalox, Mylanta). Table 48.4 presents a summary of antacid drugs.

NURSING MANAGEMENT OF THE PATIENT RECEIVING P ALUMINUM HYDROXIDE WITH MAGNESIUM HYDROXIDE

Core Drug Knowledge

Pharmacotherapeutics

The combination drug aluminum hydroxide with magnesium hydroxide is used in conditions of hypersensitivity to relieve the symptoms of upset stomach, heartburn, gastric reflux, and sour stomach associated with GERD, and the discomfort from peptic ulcers (Table 48.5). Unlabeled uses include treatment and maintenance therapy for duodenal ulcer.

Pharmacokinetics

A single oral dose of an aluminum- and magnesium-based antacid typically results in minimal absorption from the GI tract. Patients taking this type of drug for a prolonged period may absorb between 5% and 20% of the magnesium and very little of the aluminum. The small amounts of magnesium and aluminum that are absorbed are distributed widely throughout the body. Small amounts of the drugs are found in breast milk. Aluminum hydroxide with magnesium hydroxide is eliminated in the feces.

The onset of action is rapid. Duration of action varies according to when the drug was taken in relation to meals. If it is taken on an empty stomach, the duration is 20 to 60 minutes; if it is taken following a meal, the duration is 3 hours.

Pharmacodynamics

Antacids do not coat the lining of the stomach, despite what is commonly believed. Aluminum hydroxide with magnesium hydroxide raises the gastric pH in the stomach and duodenal bulb above 4, which inhibits pepsin's proteolytic activity and increases the tone of the lower esophageal sphincter. Antacids, in general, may have a local astringent effect. The aluminum in this drug, and in other aluminum antacids, inhibits gastric emptying by inhibiting contraction of the smooth muscle of the stomach. The aluminum in the drug binds with phosphate in the GI tract and can lower phosphate levels effectively.

Antacids have different acid-neutralizing capacities (ANCs). The ANC is expressed as mEq/mL. The definition is the milliequivalent (mEq) of HCl required to keep the antacid suspension at a pH of 3.5 for 10 minutes, in vitro (in the laboratory). To be an antacid, a substance must neutralize 5 mEq/dose or more. Antacids with high ANCs are usually more effective in vivo (in the patient). Of the various forms of antacids available, suspensions have the greatest neutralizing capacity.

Contraindications and Precautions

Aluminum hydroxide with magnesium hydroxide may cause hypophosphatemia, especially if dietary intake of phosphorus is inadequate. Patients with renal insufficiency should use magnesium-containing antacids with caution because a small amount of magnesium is absorbed systemically, and hypermagnesemia is possible, especially if the patient takes more than 50 mEq daily. Pregnant or breast-feeding patients should consult the prescriber before taking aluminum hydroxide with magnesium hydroxide.

Aluminum hydroxide with magnesium hydroxide should be used cautiously in patients who have recently experienced massive upper GI bleeding.

Adverse Effects

Antacids that contain aluminum alone can cause constipation, whereas antacids that contain magnesium alone can cause diarrhea. Aluminum and magnesium are combined to balance the constipating effects of aluminum with the diarrheal effects of magnesium. Other possible adverse effects include hypermagnesemia (in patients with renal failure) and hypophosphatemia. Less common adverse effects are accumulation of aluminum in serum, bone, and the CNS (with large doses); osteomalacia; and encephalopathy. Acid rebound may occur, although this effect may not be important clinically because the buffers in the antacid may neutralize any elevation in acidity.

TABLE 48.4 Summary of Selected (C) Antacids

Drug (Trade) Name	Selected Indications	Route and Dosage Range	Pharmacokinetics
[P] aluminum hydroxide with magnesium hydroxide (Maalox)	Hyperacidity; prevention of stress ulcer bleeding; treatment and maintenance of duodenal and gastric ulcers; initially for gastroesophageal reflux disease (GERD)	PO, 15–30 mL up to 4 × d	*Onset:* Immediate *Duration:* 20–40 min on empty stomach, 3 h if 1 h after meals $t_{1/2}$: Not systemically absorbed
magnesium hydroxide (Milk of Magnesia)	Hyperacidity; bleeding; treatment and maintenance of duodenal and gastric ulcers; initially for GERD	PO, liquid, 5–15 mL up to four times a day; liquid concentrate, 2.5–7.5 mL up to 4 × d; tablets, 622–1,244 mg up to 4 × d	*Onset:* Immediate *Duration:* 20–40 min on empty stomach, 3 h if 1 h after meals $t_{1/2}$: Not systemically absorbed
aluminum hydroxide (Amphojel)	Hyperacidity; prevention of stress ulcer bleeding; treatment and maintenance of duodenal and gastric ulcers; initially for GERD; reduction of phosphate absorption in hyperphosphatemia in chronic renal failure	PO, suspension, 5–30 mL as needed after meals and at bedtime; tablets/capsules, 500–1,500 mg three to six times a day between meals and at bedtime	*Onset:* Immediate *Duration:* 20–40 min on empty stomach, 3 h if 1 h after meals $t_{1/2}$: Not systemically absorbed
aluminum carbonate (Basaljel)	Hyperacidity; treatment, control, management of hyperphosphatemia; use with a low-phosphate diet to prevent formation of phosphate urinary stones	PO, suspension, 10 mL in water or juice up to every 2 h; tablets/capsules, 2 up to every 2 h	*Onset:* Immediate *Duration:* 20–40 min on empty stomach, 3 h if 1 h after meals $t_{1/2}$: Not systemically absorbed
calcium carbonate (Tums)	Hyperacidity (occasional use); calcium replacement	PO, tablets, 0.5–1.5 g as needed	*Onset:* Immediate *Duration:* 20–40 min on empty stomach, 3 h if 1 h after meals $t_{1/2}$: Unknown
magnesium oxide (Mag-ox)	Hyperacidity; magnesium replacement	PO, capsules, 140 mg tid–qid; tablets 400–800 mg/d	*Onset:* Immediate *Duration:* 20–40 min on empty stomach, 3 h if 1 h after meals $t_{1/2}$: Not systemically absorbed
magaldrate (Riopan)	Hyperacidity; treatment and maintenance of duodenal and gastric ulcers; initially for GERD	PO, suspension liquid, 5–10 mL between meals and at bedtime	*Onset:* Immediate *Duration:* 20–40 min on empty stomach, 3 h if 1 h after meals $t_{1/2}$: Not systemically absorbed
sodium bicarbonate (Bell/Ans)	Hyperacidity (occasional use)	PO, tablets, 0.3–2 g up to qid	*Onset:* Immediate *Duration:* 20–40 min on empty stomach, 3 h if 1 h after meals $t_{1/2}$: Unknown
sodium citrate (citra pH)	Hyperacidity (occasional use)	PO, liquid, 30 mL daily	*Onset:* Immediate *Duration:* 20–40 min on empty stomach, 3 h if 1 h after meals $t_{1/2}$: Unknown

No specific recommendations for a child's dose.

TABLE 48.5 Agents That Interact With (C) Antacids

Interactants	Effect and Significance	Nursing Management
allopurinol	Decreased effect with aluminum salts	Monitor for drug effectiveness. Alert prescriber to need for possible dosage adjustment. Do not administer both drugs at same time if significant interactions occur.
amphetamines	Increased effect with sodium bicarbonate	Same as above.
benzodiazepines	Increased effect with aluminum salts; decreased effect with magnesium salts, sodium bicarbonate, and magnesium/aluminum combination	Same as above.
captopril	Decreased effect with magnesium/aluminum combinations	Same as above.
chloroquine	Decreased effect with aluminum and magnesium salts	Same as above.
corticosteroids	Decreased effect with aluminum, magnesium, and magnesium/aluminum combinations	Same as above.
dicumarol	Increased effect with magnesium salts	Same as above.
diflunisal	Decreased effect with aluminum salts	Same as above.
digoxin	Decreased effect with aluminum and magnesium salts	Same as above.
ethambutol	Decreased effect with aluminum salts	Same as above.
flecainide	Increased absorption with sodium bicarbonate	Same as above.
fluoroquinolones	Decreased effect with calcium salts and magnesium/aluminum combinations	Same as above.
H_2 receptor antagonists	Decreased effect with aluminum salts, magnesium salts, and magnesium/aluminum combinations	Same as above.
hydantoins	Decreased effect with calcium salts, magnesium salts, and magnesium/aluminum combinations	Same as above.
iron salts	Decreased effect with all antacids	Same as above.
isoniazid	Decreased effect with aluminum salts	Same as above.
ketoconazole	Decreased effect with sodium bicarbonate and magnesium/aluminum combinations	Same as above.
levodopa	Increased effect with magnesium/aluminum combinations	Same as above.
lithium	Decreased effect with sodium bicarbonate	Same as above.
methenamine	Decreased effect with sodium bicarbonate	Same as above.
methotrexate	Decreased effect with sodium bicarbonate	Same as above.
nitrofurantoin	Decreased effect with magnesium salts	Same as above.
penicillamine	Decreased effect with aluminum salts and magnesium salts	Same as above.
phenothiazines	Decreased effect with aluminum salts, magnesium salts, and magnesium/aluminum combinations	Same as above.
quinidine	Increased effect with calcium salts, magnesium salts, sodium bicarbonate, and magnesium/aluminum combinations	Same as above.
salicylates	Decreased effect with calcium salts, sodium bicarbonate, and magnesium/aluminum combinations	Same as above.
sodium polystyrene sulfonate	Concurrent use, possible metabolic alkalosis in patients with renal impairment	Same as above.
sulfonylurease	Increased effect with magnesium salts and magnesium/aluminum combinations; decreased effect with sodium bicarbonate	Same as above.
sympathomimetics	Increased effect with sodium bicarbonate	Same as above.
tetracycline	Decreased effect with all antacids	Same as above.
thyroid hormones	Decreased effect with aluminum salts	Same as above.
ticlopidine	Decreased effect with aluminum salts, magnesium salts, and magnesium/aluminum combinations	Same as above.
valproic acid	Increased effect with magnesium/aluminum combinations	Same as above.

Drug Interactions

Magnesium and aluminum affect the action of many orally administered drugs (see Table 48.5). This interaction may stem from decreased acidity of gastric juices, which affects absorption; absorption or binding by the magnesium and aluminum to the surface of drugs, which decreases their bioavailability; or increased urine alkalinity, which changes the rate of drug elimination (slowing the excretion of basic drugs and speeding the elimination of acidic drugs).

Assessment of Relevant Core Patient Variables

Health Status

Determine whether the patient has symptoms that warrant the use of aluminum hydroxide with magnesium hydroxide. Assess for GI bleeding; coffee grounds–like emesis indicates GI bleeding, as do dark, tarry stools in a patient who is not taking iron supplements. Patients who have had massive upper GI bleeding should use caution when taking products that contain aluminum. Also assess for renal insufficiency. Patients with a history of renal insufficiency should not receive aluminum hydroxide with magnesium hydroxide. Although antacids that are solely aluminum based are used to decrease elevated phosphate levels found in renal failure, aluminum in combination with magnesium hydroxide should be avoided because these patients do not excrete magnesium at the normal rate. The additional magnesium that can be absorbed from this product and all magnesium-containing antacids may be sufficient to cause hypermagnesemia in the patient with renal failure. Also, determine the patient's serum phosphate level because aluminum binds with phosphate.

Ask the patient about use of OTC drugs because the patient may not consider these agents important to mention during the drug history. Assess which type of drugs the patient uses and determine why they are being used, to detect possible drug interactions.

Lifestyle, Diet, and Habits

Evaluate the patient's normal dietary, alcohol, and smoking habits. Caffeine, alcohol, spicy food, and smoking may contribute to the severity of symptoms experienced.

Environment

Aluminum hydroxide with magnesium hydroxide is easily self-administered. It may be used in any care setting, including the home. (see Box 48.1).

Nursing Diagnoses and Outcomes

- Chronic Pain related to alteration in the gastric mucosa, ulceration, or irritation
  Desired outcome: *The patient will report that pain has decreased while on drug therapy.*
- Potential Complication: Electrolyte Imbalance related to hypophosphatemia, hypermagnesemia, or hyperalbuminemia secondary to drug therapy
  Desired outcome: *The patient's electrolyte levels will remain within normal limits.*
- Diarrhea or Constipation secondary to drug therapy
  Desired outcome: *The patient's elimination patterns will remain within normal parameters.*

Planning and Intervention

Maximizing Therapeutic Effects

Liquid preparations are usually preferred, because of their rapid action. Shake suspensions well before use to disperse the drug evenly. If tablets are used, they must be chewed thoroughly before swallowing and followed with a glass of water. Tablets should be administered 1 to 3 hours after meals and at bedtime for the best therapeutic effects.

Minimizing Adverse Effects

Administer or teach the patient to administer aluminum hydroxide and magnesium hydroxide 2 hours after other drugs to prevent drug interactions. Assess for use of antacids and other OTC preparations during drug history; patients might not consider these to be drugs and might fail to mention them unless asked.

Monitor for signs of acid rebound, such as increased GI pain and complaints of acid reflux. Monitor serum phosphorus and magnesium levels in patients receiving high doses of aluminum hydroxide and magnesium hydroxide (the maximum dosage for more than 2 weeks) or in patients on long-term therapy or with renal impairment. Monitor for signs of aluminum deposits in serum, bone, and CNS and for dialysis encephalopathy and osteomalacia syndromes when high doses are given to patients with renal failure.

Providing Patient and Family Education

- Teach the patient to take the antacid 2 hours after other drugs and 1 hour after meals and at bedtime.
- Caution the patient not to take the maximum dose for longer than 2 weeks unless directed by the prescriber.
- Instruct the patient not to substitute this drug for prescription drugs to treat peptic ulcer disease.
- Urge the patient to contact the prescriber if diarrhea or constipation occurs, if abdominal pain does not diminish, or if black, tarry stools or coffee grounds–like emesis is seen.
- Teach the patient to shake liquid forms well and measure the proper dose; the patient should not just drink some undetermined amount.
- Instruct the patient to chew the tablet form thoroughly and then drink water.

Ongoing Assessment and Evaluation

Drug therapy is considered effective if the patient's pain is decreased or eliminated, electrolytes remain at normal levels, and elimination patterns remain normal.

Drugs Closely Related to P Aluminum Hydroxide With Magnesium Hydroxide

All antacid preparations are related closely and are used in various combinations to produce the desired results. In addition to the prototype aluminum hydroxide with magnesium hydroxide, aluminum preparations and magnesium preparations may be used individually. Additionally, sodium bicarbonate and calcium carbonate are used as antacids, either alone or in combination with other antacids. Various combinations of aluminum salts, magnesium salts, calcium

MEMORY CHIP

P Aluminum Hydroxide With Magnesium Hydroxide

- Treats hyperacidity and its symptoms in GERD and peptic ulcers; prevents stress ulcer bleeding
- Interacts with many other drugs by increasing the pH (i.e., increasing alkalinity), which alters absorption, adsorption, or binding with drugs; or by increasing urinary pH (i.e., affecting drug elimination rate)
- Major contraindication: avoid use in chronic renal failure (multiple doses)
- Most common adverse effects: constipation (aluminum antacids) and diarrhea (magnesium antacids); combination usually negates the adverse effect of each, although either may occur
- Most serious adverse effect: potential electrolyte imbalance
- Minimizing adverse effects: Administer 2 h after other drugs to prevent drug interactions.
- Most important patient education: Do not substitute this drug for prescription drugs to treat peptic ulcer disease.

carbonate, and sodium bicarbonate are useful. The aluminum salts used in antacids include aluminum carbonate, aluminum hydroxide, aluminum phosphate, and dihydroxyaluminum aminoacetate. The magnesium salts include magnesium carbonate, magnesium hydroxide, magnesium oxide, and magnesium trisilicate. The calcium salt calcium carbonate is often given with simethicone (an antiflatulent), magnesium carbonate, magnesium hydroxide, or aluminum hydroxide. However, it can be used alone.

The pharmacotherapeutics of the antacids vary. Unlike aluminum or magnesium preparations, neither calcium carbonate nor sodium bicarbonate is recommended for long-term use, such as in treating peptic ulcer disease. Aluminum hydroxide is used to treat hyperphosphatemia associated with chronic renal failure. Aluminum carbonate can be used to treat, control, or manage hyperphosphatemia. It can also be used with low-phosphate diets to prevent phosphate-based renal calculi (kidney stones) from developing. Calcium carbonate is used in treating hypocalcemia. Magnesium sulfate is used to treat hypomagnesemia.

The pharmacokinetics of the antacids varies slightly because sodium bicarbonate and calcium carbonate undergo much more systemic absorption than the aluminum or magnesium preparations.

The main variation in pharmacodynamics is in the acid-neutralizing capacity of the antacids.

Sodium bicarbonate and calcium carbonate have the greatest acid-neutralizing capacity. Suspension forms of antacids have greater acid-neutralizing capacity than tablets. Box 48.2 lists selected antacids by their acid-neutralizing ability.

Sodium bicarbonate and calcium carbonate can cause metabolic alkalosis and acid rebound because of their systemic absorption, especially with large doses and frequent use. When given together in large doses, they may cause milk alkali syndrome. Milk alkali syndrome can be acute (with symptoms of weakness, headache, nausea, and irritability) or chronic (with alkalosis, hypercalcemia, and possible renal impairment).

BOX 48.2 Antacids' Acid-Neutralizing Capacity

The antacids listed below appear in descending order of their acid-neutralizing capacity (e.g., sodium bicarbonate most effective). Aluminum phosphate has the lowest acid-neutralizing effect.

- sodium bicarbonate
- calcium carbonate
- magnesium hydroxide
- magnesium and aluminum hydroxide mixtures
- magaldrate
- magnesium trisilate
- aluminum hydroxide
- aluminum phosphate

The major core patient variable that must be considered for the different forms of antacids is health status. Aluminum hydroxide may be used therapeutically in patients with renal failure, whereas multiple doses of magnesium oxide are avoided in renal failure because of the risk for magnesium toxicity. Because of its high sodium content, sodium bicarbonate should not be given to people on low-sodium diets or those who have underlying pathologies that make sodium restrictions necessary, such as hypertension, congestive heart failure, or renal failure. Neither sodium bicarbonate nor calcium carbonate is recommended for peptic ulcer disease.

C GASTROINTESTINAL STIMULANTS

The **gastrointestinal stimulants** increase the effect of acetylcholine on the GI system. Acetylcholine is responsible for normal GI function. GI stimulants increase peristalsis and gastric emptying. Drugs in the GI stimulant class include metoclopramide (Reglan), dexpanthenol (Ilopan), and cisapride (Propulsid). The prototype GI stimulant is metoclopramide (Reglan). Table 48.6 presents a summary of selected gastrointestinal stimulants.

NURSING MANAGEMENT OF THE PATIENT RECEIVING P METOCLOPRAMIDE

Core Drug Knowledge

Pharmacotherapeutics

Metoclopramide is used to relieve symptoms of diabetic gastroparesis, also known as diabetic gastric stasis. Symptoms of this disorder include nausea, vomiting, heartburn, persistent fullness after meals, and anorexia. Metoclopramide also is used short term to treat GERD in patients who do not respond to usual therapy. It also can be used parenterally to prevent nausea and vomiting associated with postoperative states (if nasogastric suctioning is not desirable) or chemotherapy. It may be administered as a single dose before small

TABLE 48.6 Summary of Selected (C) GI Stimulants

Drug (Trade) Name	Selected Indications	Route and Dosage Range	Pharmacokinetics
P metoclopramide (Reglan, Octamide)	Diabetic gastroparesis, gastroesophageal reflux disease (GERD), prevention of postoperative nausea and vomiting, prevention of chemotherapy-induced vomiting	*Adult:* PO, 10 mg 30 min before each meal and at bedtime for 2–8 wk; IM, 10–20 mg near end of surgery; IV, infuse over at least 15 min, 30 min before chemotherapy, repeat every 2 h for two doses, then every 3 h for three doses; for highly emetogenic drugs, such as cisplatin and decarbazine, give 2 mg/kg for first two doses; for less emetogenic drugs, give 1 mg/kg	*Onset:* PO, 30–60 min; IM, 10–15 min; IV, 1–3 min *Duration:* PO, IM, IV 1–2 h $t_{1/2}$: PO, IM, IV, 5–6 h

bowel intubation, especially in instances in which the tube does not pass through the pylorus easily. It may be used to promote the transit of barium through the GI tract after a diagnostic procedure if the delayed passage of barium interferes with further radiographic diagnostic procedures in the stomach and small intestine.

Unlabeled uses of metoclopramide include improving lactation (it can increase milk production by elevating serum prolactin levels); minimizing nausea and vomiting in a variety of conditions, including during pregnancy and labor; treating gastric ulcers and anorexia nervosa; improving response to ergotamine, analgesics, and sedatives used in migraine headache; treating postoperative gastric bezoars (boluses of food that have hardened and remain in the stomach); treating diabetic atonic bladder; and treating esophageal variceal bleeding.

Pharmacokinetics

Metoclopramide is given orally and is absorbed readily from the GI tract. The drug is distributed widely throughout the body; it crosses the blood–brain barrier and placenta and is found in breast milk. The drug is not highly protein bound (30%).

A small amount of the drug is metabolized by the liver, and most is excreted in the urine. Patients with renal insufficiency may require a dosage reduction.

Pharmacodynamics

Metoclopramide's mechanism of action is unclear. However, it appears to sensitize tissues to the effect of acetylcholine. It has the cholinergic-like effect on the upper GI tract of stimulating motility but does not stimulate gastric, pancreatic, or gallbladder secretions. Metoclopramide increases peristalsis of the duodenum and jejunum, thus shortening the transit time through the stomach and small intestine. It also increases the tone of the lower esophageal sphincter, increases gastric contractions, and relaxes the pyloric sphincter.

Dopamine produces nausea and vomiting by stimulating the medullary CTZ. Metoclopramide is a dopamine receptor antagonist that exerts antiemetic effects directly on the CTZ. It is believed to lessen the sensitivity of visceral nerves to stimuli that induce nausea and vomiting.

Contraindications and Precautions

Metoclopramide is contraindicated when stimulation of GI motility may be dangerous, as in GI hemorrhage, perforation, or mechanical obstruction. Other contraindications include hypersensitivity to the drug; pheochromocytoma (the drug may cause a hypertensive crisis that probably results from a release of catecholamines from the tumor); history of seizure disorders (seizure activity may increase with this drug); and concomitant use of drugs that produce extrapyramidal effects (because these effects may increase).

Depression, from mild to severe, including suicidal ideation, has occurred in patients with and without a history of depression. Use caution in giving metoclopramide to patients with a history of depression; it should be given only if the benefits of the drug outweigh the potential risks from depression. Metoclopramide should be given very cautiously, if at all, to patients with Parkinson disease because they may experience an exacerbation of symptoms. Use caution if giving this drug to patients with hypertension. Theoretically, metoclopramide may increase the pressure on a suture line following a gut anastomosis or closure. Although this effect has not been reported in the literature, use some caution when giving this drug to postoperative patients. Elevated prolactin levels will persist during chronic administration of metoclopramide. One third of human breast cancers are prolactin dependent in vitro. Therefore, use caution if the patient has previously detected breast cancer. Studies have not, however, shown a definite link between elevated prolactin levels and breast cancer in animals or in humans. Metoclopramide is classified as a pregnancy category B drug.

Adverse Effects

Approximately 20% to 30% of patients receiving metoclopramide experience adverse effects of the drug. The adverse effects are usually mild, transient, and reversible after discontinuing the drug. Incidence correlates with dose and duration of therapy. The possible adverse reactions are many.

Effects on the CNS are common and include restlessness, drowsiness, fatigue, insomnia, headache, dizziness, confusion, anxiety, dystonia, mental depression (even in patients who had never experienced clinical depression before) with suicidal ideation and suicide, convulsive seizures, and hallucinations. Extrapyramidal symptoms, Parkinson-like reactions, tardive dyskinesia, and akathisia also may occur. Extrapyramidal symptoms are manifested primarily as acute dystonic reactions. They occur more commonly in children and young adults during the first 24 to 48 hours of treatment. They occur even more frequently when metoclopramide is used in high doses to control vomiting caused by chemotherapy. Tardive dyskinesia, potentially irreversible, occurs most often in the elderly, particularly older women. Additional adverse effects are nausea, diarrhea, and transient hypertension.

Drug Interactions

Metoclopramide interacts with several drugs because it increases gastric motility, thereby altering absorption. The most important drug interactions are with levodopa, anticholinergics, and narcotics. Levodopa and metoclopramide have opposite effects on dopamine receptors. Metoclopramide's effects on GI motility are antagonized by anticholinergics and narcotics. Table 48.7 presents agents that interact with metoclopramide.

Assessment of Relevant Core Patient Variables

Health Status

Before beginning therapy with metoclopramide, assess the patient indications for metoclopramide use, such as diabetic gastroparesis, GERD, cancer that requires chemotherapy, or postoperative status. Also assess for depression, Parkinson disease, seizures, or hypertension because these conditions are precautions to its use. Also, assess the patient's drug history; it should not include current use of levodopa, anticholinergics, or narcotics. Any renal or hepatic impairment should be noted because the dosage may need to be adjusted.

Life Span and Gender

Determine whether the patient is pregnant. Several case reports show no adverse effects on the fetus with the use of metoclopramide; however, no adequate and well-controlled studies exist. Although metoclopramide is excreted into breast milk, the levels are well below the maximum therapeutic infant dose. Therefore, there appears to be no contraindication to breast-feeding if the mother receives no more than 45 mg/day of metoclopramide. Note the patient's age and gender because older adults, especially older women, are more likely than others to develop the adverse effect of tardive dyskinesia.

Environment

Note the environment in which metoclopramide will be administered. Oral metoclopramide can be given in any setting and can be self-administered. IV administration of metoclopramide is performed in an acute care setting or an outpatient center.

Nursing Diagnoses and Outcomes

- Risk for Self-Directed Violence secondary to adverse effects of drug therapy
  Desired outcome: *The patient will do no self-harm related to depression from drug therapy.*

TABLE 48.7 Agents That Interact With [P] Metoclopramide

Interactants	Effect and Significance	Nursing Management
alcohol	Increases the rate of absorption, raising blood levels more quickly	Teach patient to avoid alcohol while on drug therapy.
cimetidine	Decreases absorption so bioavailability may be reduced	Monitor for effectiveness of cimetidine.
cyclosporine	Faster gastric emptying, which may allow for increased absorption, possibly increasing immunosuppression and adverse effects from cyclosporine	Monitor white blood cell counts and watch for other adverse effects, such as tremor, hypertension, and renal dysfunction.
digoxin	Absorption, plasma levels, and therapeutic response may be decreased; capsule, elixir, and tablets with a high dissolution rate least affected	Monitor drug levels and therapeutic response. Consult with the prescriber regarding dosage or preparation change if therapeutic response declines significantly.
levodopa	Has the opposite effect on the dopamine receptors; bioavailability of levodopa may be increased; may decrease effect of metoclopramide on gastric emptying and lower esophageal pressure	Monitor for therapeutic and adverse effect of both. Administration of metoclopramide to patients with Parkinson's disease is relatively contraindicated.
monoamine oxidase inhibitors	Metoclopramide releases catecholamines in patients with essential hypertension; MAO inhibitors also have a sympathomimetic effect, blood pressure may be elevated	Use cautiously in hypertensive patients. Monitor blood pressure closely throughout therapy.
succinylcholine	Metoclopramide inhibits plasma cholinesterase, may increase the neuromuscular blocking effects of succinylcholine	Monitor respiratory function.
anticholinergics	Antagonize the effects of metoclopramide on GI motility	Monitor for therapeutic effects.

- Powerlessness related to extrapyramidal effects, Parkinson-like symptoms, or tardive dyskinesia secondary to adverse effect of drug therapy
  Desired outcome: *The patient will make decisions regarding own care, treatment, and future (when possible) while on drug therapy.*
- Risk for Injury related to drowsiness, fatigue, insomnia, confusion, and hallucination secondary to adverse effects of drug therapy
  Desired outcome: *The patient will not suffer injury while on drug therapy.*

Planning and Intervention

Maximizing Therapeutic Effects

Give oral doses 30 minutes before each meal to allow for onset of action and give an IM injection near the end of surgery to prevent postoperative nausea and vomiting. Administer IV metoclopramide over at least 15 minutes, 30 minutes before the start of chemotherapy to prevent chemotherapy-induced vomiting. Repeat every 2 hours for two doses, then every 3 hours for three doses. Do not administer metoclopramide concurrently with anticholinergic or narcotic drugs.

Minimizing Adverse Effects

Monitor for evidence of depression and report positive findings to the prescriber. Institute interventions to protect the patient if he or she expresses suicidal ideas. If extrapyramidal symptoms (e.g., involuntary movements of the limbs, facial grimacing, and rhythmic protrusion of the tongue) occur, especially during the first 48 hours of therapy, withhold the metoclopramide dose, notify the prescriber, and seek orders for diphenhydramine (Benadryl), 50 mg IM, or benztropine (Cogentin), 1 to 2 mg IM. Either of these drugs usually reverses the symptoms.

Withhold the dose and notify the prescriber if Parkinson-like symptoms (e.g., bradykinesia, tremor, cog-wheel motions, and mask-like faces) occur, particularly in the first 6 months of therapy. Effects usually subside gradually within 2 to 3 months after drug discontinuation. Contact the prescriber regarding discontinuing the drug if signs of tardive dyskinesia (involuntary movements of face, tongue, mouth, or jaw and sometimes involuntary movements of trunk or extremities) occur because tardive dyskinesia may be irreversible.

Providing Patient and Family Education

- Tell the patient to take metoclopramide 30 minutes before meals.
- Caution the patient to prevent injury by avoiding activities that require mental alertness, coordination, or physical dexterity (e.g., operating motor vehicles or other heavy machinery) until the effects of the drug are known.
- Caution the patient to avoid alcoholic beverages, sedatives, and other CNS depressants during metoclopramide therapy because these substances may cause additive sedation.
- Explain to the patient how to recognize any involuntary movements of the eyes, face, or limbs, such as tremors or cogwheel motion of the arms; depression; or serious diarrhea, and report these to the prescriber at once. In such cases, the patient should not take any more of the drug without discussing these signs and symptoms with the prescriber.

Ongoing Assessment and Evaluation

With careful monitoring and follow-up assessments, nursing care and drug therapy can be considered successful if the patient's GI complaints diminish or subside and the patient does not experience depression or other adverse effects, such as nausea or Parkinson-like symptoms.

Drug Closely Related to [P] Metoclopramide

Dexpanthenol (Ilopan) is used prophylactically after major abdominal surgery to minimize the possibility of paralytic ileus. It also is used to treat paralytic ileus, intestinal atony that causes abdominal distention, postoperative or postpartum retention of flatus, and postoperative delay in resuming intestinal motility. Dexpanthenol contributes to the final step of acetylcholine production. Acetylcholine, the neurohumoral transmitter in the parasympathetic system, maintains normal intestinal function. Decreased acetylcholine results in decreased peristalsis. Dexpanthenol is the alcohol analogue of D-pantothenic acid. Pantothenic acid is a precursor of coenzyme A, which is a cofactor for enzyme-catalyzed reactions involving the transfer of acetyl groups. The final step in acetylcholine synthesis is the choline acetylase transfer of an acetyl group from acetylcoenzyme A to choline. Thus, dexpanthenol contributes to the production of acetylcholine and promotes peristalsis.

Dexpanthenol is contraindicated in hemophilia and in paralytic ileus caused by mechanical obstruction. It is a pregnancy category C drug. Dexpanthenol causes intestinal colic (30 minutes after administration), vomiting, and a slight drop in blood pressure. Other adverse effects include itching, tingling, difficulty breathing, red patches of skin, generalized dermatitis, and urticaria. Unlike metoclopramide, dexpanthenol does not cause extrapyramidal symptoms, parkinsonism, or tardive dyskinesia.

MEMORY CHIP

[P] Metoclopramide

- Used as a GI stimulant in diabetic gastric stasis, and GERD; as an antiemetic postsurgery and with chemotherapy for cancer
- Major contraindication: when stimulation of GI motility might be dangerous
- Most common adverse effects: CNS complaints
- Most serious adverse effects: tardive dyskinesia and severe depression
- **Life span alert: Older women are more likely to experience tardive dyskinesia as an adverse effect.**
- Maximizing therapeutic effects: Give metoclopramide 30 min before meals or chemotherapy.
- Minimizing adverse effects: Monitor for depression, Parkinson-like symptoms, extrapyramidal effects, and tardive dyskinesia; holding further drug administration and contact the prescriber if noted.
- Most important patient education: Teach patient to recognize signs of serious adverse effects; to call prescriber at once when noted.

Ⓒ DIGESTIVE ENZYMES

Digestive enzymes are responsible for breaking down food into forms that can be absorbed easily in the GI tract. The digestive process normally begins in the mouth with digestive enzymes in salivary secretions and then continues in the stomach with the action of gastric acid and pepsin. It is completed in the duodenum with the release of the pancreatic enzymes that change protein, carbohydrate, and fat into absorbable forms.

Replacement of many of these enzymes is not necessary or truly useful because rarely does a deficiency of endogenous enzymes actually cause GI problems. Many of the drug preparations of digestive enzymes are combinations of various enzymes, frequently paired with anticholinergics, barbiturates, or antacids (Table 48.8). In those few situations in which an endogenous deficit does exist, it is nearly impossible to correct the deficit adequately with these combinations. In addition, combination therapy increases the risk for adverse effects from the other drug entities in the compound.

Pancreatic enzymes comprise one group of digestive enzymes that is an exception. Deficiencies of pancreatic enzymes do occur on a fairly frequent basis, usually in pancreatitis, duct obstruction, and following pancreatectomy. Replacement of these enzymes is indicated and therapeutic. Pancreatic digestive enzymes include pancrelipase (Pancrease, Cotazym, Ku-Zyme, Viokase, Ilozyme, Zymase, and Ultrase) and pancreatin (Dizymes, Entozyme, Donnazyme, Pancreazyme, Hi-Vegi-Lip, and Creon). The prototype for pancreatic digestive enzymes is pancrelipase.

NURSING MANAGEMENT OF THE PATIENT RECEIVING Ⓟ PANCRELIPASE

Core Drug Knowledge

Pharmacotherapeutics

Pancrelipase is enzymatic replacement therapy for patients with deficient exocrine pancreatic secretions; cystic fibrosis; chronic pancreatitis; ductal obstructions caused by cancer of the pancreas or common bile duct; pancreatic insufficiency; or steatorrhea from malabsorption syndrome; and after pancreatectomy, gastrectomy, or post-GI surgery, such as Billroth II gastroenterostomy. Table 48.8 describes these uses. Pancrelipase also can be used as a presumptive test to evaluate pancreatic function. Pancrelipase is administered orally.

TABLE 48.8 Summary of Selected Ⓒ Digestive Enzymes and Drugs Preventing Digestion

Drug (Trade) Name	Selected Indications	Route and Dosage Range	Pharmacokinetics
Ⓟ pancrelipase (Pancrease, Ku-Zyme, Viokase, Ilozyme, Zymase, Ultrase; *Canadian:* Creon)	Deficient exocrine pancreatic secretions	Adjust dosage until steatorrhea minimizes and good nutritional status is maintained	Unknown
	Pancreatic insufficiency, steatorrhea from malabsorption syndrome and post-gastrectomy, or post-GI surgery, Billroth II gastroenterostomy	*Adult:* PO, 4,000 to 48,000 U with each meal and with snacks; severe deficiencies, increase to 64,000–88,000 units with each meal or increase hourly if tolerated *Child <6 mo:* PO, dose not established; 6–12 mo, 2,000 U with each meal; 1–6 y, 4,000–8,000 U with each meal and 4,000 U with each snack; 7–12 y, 4,000–12,000 U with each meal and snack	
	Postpancreatectomy, ductal obstructions caused by cancer of the pancreas or common bile duct	*Adult:* PO, 8,000–16,000 U at 2 h intervals, or as prescribed	
	Cystic fibrosis	Use powder form: 0.7 g with meals	
pancreatin (Dizymes, Entozyme, Donnazyme, Hi-Vegi-Lip, Creon)	Same as above	*Adult:* PO, 1 or 2 tablets with meals and snacks; adjust according to individual meals *Child:* Dosage not established	Unknown
Ⓟ orlistat (Xenical)	Management of obesity	120 mg tid with meals that contain fat	*Onset:* Immediate *Duration:* Unknown $t_{1/2}$: Not absorbed
sibutramine (Meridia)	Management of obesity	10 mg/d PO; after 4 wk may titrate to 15 mg/d	*Onset:* Unknown *Duration:* To 24 h $t_{1/2}$: Unknown

Pharmacokinetics

Absorption, distribution, metabolism, and excretion of this drug are unknown. The onset, peak, and duration are also unknown. Because pancrelipase is affected by gastric acid, the drug is enteric coated. This formulation may decrease absorption in the duodenum, however. The site of metabolism and route of elimination from the body are unknown.

Pharmacodynamics

Pancrelipase contains the enzymes lipase, protease, and amylase, which are responsible for the final phase of digestion. During this phase, fats are hydrolyzed to fatty acids, proteins to proteoses and derived substances, and starches to sugars and dextrins so that they can be absorbed in the small intestine. Pancreatic enzymes normally exert their effects in the duodenum and in the first part of the jejunum.

Contraindications and Precautions

Pancrelipase is contraindicated in patients who are hypersensitive to pork protein or enzymes because the drug is derived from pork. It should not be used by patients with acute pancreatitis or acute exacerbations of chronic pancreatitis. Pancrelipase is a pregnancy category C drug and should be used only if necessary. It is not known whether it crosses into breast milk; therefore, it should be administered with caution to nursing mothers.

Caution must be used not to spill the powder on one's hands because it may irritate the skin. Inhaling the powder irritates the nasal mucosa and the respiratory tract, triggering an asthma attack in those susceptible.

Adverse Effects

Caution must be used with large doses because they may cause nausea, abdominal cramps, and diarrhea. Hyperuricosuria and hyperuricemia have occurred with extremely high doses. Less often, allergic reactions have occurred.

Drug Interactions

The antacids calcium carbonate and magnesium hydroxide can interfere with the beneficial effects of pancrelipase. Serum iron response to oral iron supplements may be decreased by concurrent dosing of pancrelipase. Table 48.9 lists agents that interact with pancrelipase.

Assessment of Relevant Core Patient Variables

Health Status

Assess the patient's health history for chronic pancreatitis, cystic fibrosis, ductal obstructions from cancer, pancreatic insufficiency, pancreatectomy, gastrectomy, or other GI surgery. Results of laboratory studies to review include serum amylase and lipase levels to determine pancreatic functioning and findings of steatorrhea. Foul-smelling, frothy stools are a sign of steatorrhea. Assess the patient's nutritional status because deficiency of pancreatic enzymes prevents the absorption of fats, proteins, and starches and may leave the patient malnourished. Also, determine whether the patient is allergic to pork because pancrelipase is derived from pork.

Life Span and Gender

Determine whether the patient is pregnant or breast-feeding. Because pancrelipase is in pregnancy category C, it should be given only if clearly necessary. Caution should be used when administering pancrelipase to a breast-feeding woman. Note the patient's age. The drug can be given to children, but the dosage for children younger than 6 months old has not been established.

Environment

Pancrelipase can be administered in any setting, including the home.

Culture and Inherited Traits

Consider the religious affiliation of patients taking pancrelipase. Some religious groups, such as Muslims and Orthodox Jews, forbid the consumption of pork products in any form, and pancrelipase is pork based. Therefore, these patients may not accept this drug therapy.

Nursing Diagnoses and Outcomes

- Imbalanced Nutrition: Less than Body Requirements related to impaired digestion secondary to insufficient pancreatic enzymes
  Desired outcome: *The patient's nutrient absorption will be adequate to meet body needs while on drug therapy.*
- Risk for Pain, acute abdominal, secondary to adverse effects of drug therapy
  Desired outcome: *The patient will not develop pain as an adverse effect of drug therapy.*

Planning and Intervention

Maximizing Therapeutic Effects

Brands of pancrelipase should not be changed without consulting the prescriber because the brands do not have equal bioavailability. Administer antacids or H_2 receptor antagonists, if prescribed, to maintain the patient's gastric pH within an alkaline range. An alkaline pH prevents pancrelipase tablets from dissolving in the stomach and becoming inactivated.

TABLE 48.9 Agents That Interact With (C) Digestive Enzymes

Interactants	Effect and Significance	Nursing Management
calcium carbonate, magnesium hydroxide	May negate effect of enzymes	Administer 2 h apart. Monitor for therapeutic effect.
iron	Serum levels may not increase as expected with oral supplements	Monitor blood iron levels. Seek order to adjust dose if iron levels are significantly affected

Minimizing Adverse Effects

Be sure to administer or make sure the patient is administering pancrelipase exactly as prescribed to prevent excessive dosing.

Providing Patient and Family Education

- Explain to the patient and family the need to learn about the role of the digestive enzyme in digesting and absorbing food. Insufficient amounts of enzyme result in weight loss and steatorrhea (foul-smelling and frothy stools). Although it is not usually possible to dose pancrelipase to eradicate steatorrhea completely, pancrelipase should greatly decrease steatorrhea.
- Tell the patient to take the drug every time she or he eats, either before or with meals and snacks.
- Caution the patient not to crush or chew pancrelipase because doing so will destroy the enzyme by exposing it to gastric acid.
- Urge the patient to notify the prescriber of any abdominal pain, diarrhea, nausea, or return of steatorrhea.
- If the form of pancrelipase is a capsule that is to be opened and mixed with food, caution the patient to avoid getting the powder on the hands or sniffing the powder contained in the capsules. Asthma attacks can occur in susceptible patients who inhale pancrelipase powder.

Ongoing Assessment and Evaluation

Assess the patient for decreased steatorrhea, weight gain, and improved nutritional status. Drug therapy is successful if digestion and nutritional status improve without the occurrence of adverse effects.

Drug Closely Related to P Pancrelipase

Pancreatin is a digestive enzyme that has the same action and indication for use as pancrelipase (see Table 48.8). The difference between the two is that pancreatin is not as concentrated as pancrelipase and therefore may not control steatorrhea as well. Pancreatin may be from beef or pork sources.

MEMORY CHIP

P Pancrelipase

- Used as enzyme replacement therapy for patients deficient in this pancreatic enzyme
- Most common adverse effects: nausea, abdominal cramps, and diarrhea at large doses
- Most important patient education: Do not crush or chew tablets; take before or with meals, avoid breathing powder and skin contact.

C LIPASE INHIBITORS

A drug that inhibits the digestive enzyme lipase is orlistat (Xenical), which is used to manage obesity. A drug significantly different from orlistat is the reuptake inhibitor sibutramine (Meridia).

NURSING MANAGEMENT OF THE PATIENT RECEIVING P ORLISTAT

Core Drug Knowledge

Pharmacotherapeutics

Orlistat (Xenical) is used to manage obesity by promoting weight loss and weight maintenance (see Table 48.9). It is to be used in conjunction with a weight-loss diet. Orlistat also is used to reduce the risk for regaining weight after weight loss and for obese patients with an initial BMI of 30 kg/m^2 or more or a BMI of 27 kg/m^2 of more in those who have other cardiovascular risk factors (e.g., hypertension, diabetes, or dyslipidemia).

Pharmacokinetics

Very little orlistat is absorbed into the systemic circulation after oral administration; most of its effect is from its local action in the GI tract. In laboratory studies, orlistat was more than 99% protein bound. Metabolism appears to occur predominantly within the GI wall. Two metabolites are formed, but they do not seem to be pharmacologically important. Fecal excretion is the main route of elimination.

Pharmacodynamics

Orlistat is a reversible lipase inhibitor. By inhibiting the action of lipase, it decreases the absorption of dietary fats. Its therapeutic effect occurs in the lumen of the stomach and small intestine, where it prevents the formation of active gastric and pancreatic lipases. The inactivated enzymes are unable to hydrolyze dietary fat, in the form of triglycerides, into absorbable free fatty acids and monoglycerides. Undigested triglycerides are not absorbed, and therefore fewer calories are absorbed. This reduced caloric intake enables weight loss. At the recommended therapeutic dose of 120 mg three times a day, orlistat inhibits dietary fat absorption by about 30%.

In clinical trials, weight loss was observed within the first 2 weeks of starting therapy with orlistat. For the first year of use, the overall mean weight loss was between 12.4 and 13.4 pounds for people receiving orlistat, compared with 5.8 to 6.2 pounds for those receiving placebo. At the end of 1 year, 57% of the orlistat-treated patients (compared with 31% on placebo) had lost at least 5% of their baseline body weight. The percentage of weight lost was similar for the two groups after 2 years of therapy as well. In studies, patients taking placebo regained between 52% and 63% of the weight lost, whereas orlistat patients regained only 26% to 35%.

Contraindications and Precautions

Orlistat is contraindicated if the patient has chronic malabsorption syndrome or cholestasis. It also is contraindicated

if the patient is hypersensitive to the drug or any of its elements. Organic causes of obesity, such as hypothyroidism, should be ruled out before prescribing orlistat.

Some patients may develop increased levels of urinary oxalate following treatment. Caution should be used if the patient has a history of hyperoxaluria or calcium oxalate nephrolithiasis. The weight loss brought about by orlistat use may improve metabolic control in diabetic patients. They may require a reduced dose of oral hypoglycemic medication or insulin. Orlistat is a pregnancy category B drug.

Adverse Effects

GI symptoms, the most common adverse effects, are related to the pharmacodynamics of the drug. These adverse effects are generally mild and transient, although for some patients, they may last for 6 months or longer and be severe enough to warrant discontinuing the drug. These GI symptoms are oily spotting, flatus with discharge of stool, fecal urgency, fatty or oily stool, oily evacuation, increased defecation, and fecal incontinence.

Other adverse effects that can occur, but are not common, include:

- CNS: anxiety, depression, dizziness, and headache
- Dermatologic: dry skin and rash
- GI: abdominal pain, gingival disorder, infectious diarrhea, nausea, rectal pain or discomfort, tooth disorders, and vomiting
- Musculoskeletal: arthritis, back pain, joint disorders, myalgia, tendonitis, and pain in the lower extremities
- Reproductive, female: menstrual irregularity and vaginitis
- Respiratory: ear, nose, and throat symptoms, influenza, lower respiratory tract infection, and upper respiratory tract infection
- Miscellaneous: fatigue, otitis, pedal edema, sleep disorder, and urinary tract infection

No adverse effects related to overdose are known to have occurred. If necessary, stop the drug and observe the patient for 24 hours. The systemic effects attributable to lipase inhibition should be rapidly reversible.

Drug Interactions

Because orlistat impairs fat absorption, the absorption of fat-soluble vitamins (A, D, E, beta-carotene) will decrease. A few other known drug interactions are listed in Table 48.10.

Assessment of Relevant Core Patient Variables

Health Status

Verify that the patient does not have a physiologic cause for obesity before starting orlistat.

Life Span and Gender

Determine whether the patient is pregnant or breast-feeding. Because no adequate and well-controlled studies of orlistat have been done in pregnant women, it is not recommended during pregnancy. It is not known whether orlistat is excreted in breast milk, and therefore, its use is not recommended during breast-feeding. Determine the patient's age because safety and efficacy have not been established in children.

Lifestyle, Diet, and Habits

Take a dietary history to determine how many calories in the patient's diet, and what percentage of the calories, come from fat. The patient should be eating a nutritionally balanced, reduced-calorie diet; no more than 30% of the patient's caloric intake should come from fat while he or she receives orlistat.

Environment

Know the setting in which orlistat will be administered. Orlistat is normally self-administered in the patient's home.

Nursing Diagnoses and Outcomes

- Imbalanced Nutrition: More than Body Requirements
  Desired outcome: *The patient will lose weight during drug therapy.*

TABLE 48.10 Agents That Interact With P Orlistat

Interactants	Effect and Significance	Nursing Management
cyclosporine	Exact clinical effect is unknown. Changes in cyclosporine absorption have been reported with variations in dietary intake.	Monitor for clinical effectiveness of cyclosporine.
fat-soluble vitamins	Decreased absorption rate of fat-soluble vitamins; 30% decrease in beta carotene and about 60% reduction in vitamin E absorption have been shown. Decrease in other vitamin levels not known exactly. Vitamin deficiency may result.	Teach patient to take a multivitamin that includes fat-soluble vitamins to prevent deficiencies.
pravastatin	Additive lipid lowering effect of pravastatin. Increases pravastatin serum levels about 30%. May possibly be a helpful adjunct therapy in hypercholesterolemia (not shown yet by research)	Monitor patient's HDL and LDL serum levels
warfarin	Possible decrease in Vitamin K absorption. No known effect on pharmacokinetics or pharmacodynamics of warfarin currently.	Monitor for changes in coagulation, increased effect of warfarin.

- Risk for Imbalanced Nutrition: Less than Body Requirements related to impaired absorption of fat-soluble vitamins during drug therapy
  Desired outcome: *The patient will not have serious vitamin deficiencies while taking drug therapy.*
- Risk for Bowel Incontinence related to adverse effects of drug therapy
  Desired outcome: *Bowel incontinence will not occur or will be minimal and transient.*
- Risk for Diarrhea related to adverse effects of drug therapy
  Desired outcome: *Diarrhea will not occur or will be minimal and transient.*

Planning and Intervention

Maximizing Therapeutic Effects

Ensure that the patient takes orlistat with all meals that contain fat and that he or she limits dietary fat to 30% of calories. The patient should also be encouraged to participate in exercise while on drug therapy.

Minimizing Adverse Effects

Advise the patient to take a multivitamin that contains fat-soluble vitamins to prevent imbalances from drug therapy. GI symptoms need to be tolerated; no specific action is known to minimize them.

Providing Patient and Family Education

- Teach the patient to limit dietary fat. Calories from fat should be no more than 30% of daily calories. This percentage promotes weight loss and prevents and minimizes GI adverse effects.
- Instruct the patient to divide daily fat intake equally between meals and to take the drug with each meal containing fat (during or up to 1 hour after eating). The patient should skip a dose if the meal has no fat or if the meal is missed.
- Encourage the patient to take a vitamin supplement that includes fat-soluble vitamins.

Ongoing Assessment and Evaluation

Orlistat therapy is effective if weight loss occurs without major GI adverse effects or vitamin deficiency occurring.

CRITICAL THINKING SCENARIO

Adverse effects from orlistat

Ms. Benson has been taking orlistat, a lipase inhibitor, to promote weight loss for 1 month. She returns to the clinic for follow up. You, the nurse, ask her how she is tolerating the medication. She tells you that initially she only had some problems with "needing to go to the bathroom a couple of times a day." However, she says that in the last few days she has been bothered by "real oily poop." She tells you that she has to run to the bathroom "like mad, 'cause I can't hold it. Sometimes I can't get there fast enough and spot my panties with that stuff."

What questions should you ask Ms. Benson to assess her problem thoroughly?

MEMORY CHIP

P Orlistat

- Used to promote weight loss in obesity; prevents absorption of dietary fat
- Major contraindication: chronic malabsorption syndrome or cholestasis
- Most common adverse effects: GI (oily spotting, flatus with stool, and fecal urgency)
- Most important patient education: Take with all meals containing fat; limit dietary fat to 30% of calories; take a multivitamin with fat-soluble vitamins.

Drug Significantly Different From P Orlistat

Sibutramine (Meridia), like orlistat, is used to manage obesity, including weight loss and weight loss maintenance. Sibutramine works in a very different manner than orlistat does, however. Sibutramine inhibits the reuptake of norepinephrine, serotonin, and dopamine. Norepinephrine levels are increased most, and dopamine levels are increased least. The changes in neurotransmitter levels bring about appetite suppression; thus, sibutramine is an anorexiant. It does not alter fat absorption or digestion, as orlistat does. A full discussion of sibutramine is found in Chapter 13.

Other anorexiants in use today include diethylpropion, benzphetamine, phendimetrazine, and phentermine.

C ANTIEMETICS

Antiemetics, which suppress stimulation of the CTZ and the VC, are used to treat nausea and vomiting. Antiemetic drugs are primarily from three main drug classifications—selective serotonin receptor antagonists, antidopaminergics, and anticholinergics.

The antidopaminergic drugs (also referred to as phenothiazides) block the action of dopamine, a neurotransmitter found in both the GI tract and the CTZ; they also have sedative properties. These drugs also are considered antipsychotics. The prototype for phenothiazides, chlorpromazine (Thorazine), is discussed in Chapter 17. Other drugs in this class used as antiemetics include prochlorperazine (Compazine), triflupromazine (Stelazine), perphenazine (Trilafon), promethazine (Phenergan), thiethylperazine (Torecan), and metoclopramide (Reglan).

The anticholinergic antiemetics, such as meclizine, block the action of acetylcholine in the VC. They affect motion sickness by reducing the sensitivity of the labyrinthine apparatus. This reduced sensitivity inhibits vestibular input to the CNS, reducing stimulation of the CTZ and the VC. The anticholinergics are used to treat nausea, vomiting, and motion sickness, and some anticholinergics, such as meclizine (Antivert), are used to treat vertigo. Anticholinergic drugs, such as the prototype atropine, are discussed in Chapter 14. Atropine is not used as an antiemetic. Other drugs in this class that are used as antiemetics include scopolamine (Transderm-Scop), cyclizine (Marazine), buclizine (Buculadin-S Softabs), diphen-

hydramine (Benadryl), and trimethobenzamide (Tigan) (see also Appendix H: Antiemetic Drugs).

A different drug class altogether, the **emetics**, includes drugs that induce vomiting. Historically, they have been used in cases of accidental ingestion of a noncorrosive agent. Ipecac, a product that is available OTC to inducing vomiting, is no longer recommended for use in cases of accidental poisonings in children because no data are available to show that it prevents the poison from entering the bloodstream, even though it induces vomiting.

C SELECTIVE SEROTONIN RECEPTOR ANTAGONISTS

The selective serotonin receptor antagonists, also known as the 5-HT_3 receptor antagonists (to specify which of the serotonin receptors are blocked), prevent the stimulation of special serotonin receptors in the CTZ. Selective serotonin receptor antagonists include ondansetron (Zofran), dolasetron (Anzemet), and granisetron (Kytril). The prototype selective serotonin receptor antagonist is ondansetron.

NURSING MANAGEMENT OF THE PATIENT RECEIVING P ONDANSETRON

Core Drug Knowledge

Pharmacotherapeutics

Ondansetron (Zofran) is used to prevent nausea and vomiting associated with cancer chemotherapy and radiotherapy, and in postoperative states when expectation is high that nausea or vomiting will occur or when nausea and vomiting must be avoided (Box 48.3).

Unlabeled uses of ondansetron include treating nausea and vomiting associated with acetaminophen poisoning; treating acute levodopa-induced psychosis (visual hallucinations); treating nausea and vomiting caused by prostacyclin therapy; reducing bulimic episodes in patients with bulimia nervosa; and treating spinal or epidural morphine–induced pruritus. It also may have potential benefit in patients with social anxiety disorder.

New research is indicating that alcoholism that occurs relatively early in life is associated with serotonergic abnormality and antisocial behaviors. Patients with early-onset alcoholism who received ondansetron in a clinical trial had fewer drinks per day, and more days without any drinking, than patients who received placebo. Ondansetron appears to be effective treatment for these patients, presumably by relieving an underlying abnormality in serotonin stimulation (Johnson et al., 2000). More studies are needed in this area to confirm this finding.

Pharmacokinetics

Ondansetron is metabolized by the liver. It is moderately protein bound (about 75%). It crosses the placenta, may enter breast milk, and is excreted in the urine.

FOCUS ON RESEARCH

Box 48.3 Control of Postoperative Nausea and Vomiting

Loewen, P. S., Marra, C. A., & Zed, P. J. (2000). 5–HT_3 receptor antagonists versus traditional agents for the prophylaxis of postoperative nausea and vomiting. *Canadian Journal of Anaesthesia, 47*(10), 1008–1018.

The Study

A review of the literature that was published in English between 1966 and 1999 was conducted; it focused on studies that examined the control of postoperative nausea and vomiting. The effectiveness of "traditional" antiemetic therapy (i.e., metoclopramide, perphenazine, prochlorperazine, cyclizine, and droperidol [an off-label use of this anesthetic not approved by the Food and Drug Administration]) was compared to the effectiveness of 5–HT_3 receptor antagonists (selective serotonin receptor antagonists), which include ondansetron, dolasetron, granisetron, and tropisetron. The review showed that the group of selective serotonin receptor antagonists was superior statistically to other drug treatments in the prevention of postoperative nausea and vomiting.

Nursing Implications

Nurses should be aware that the selective serotonin receptor antagonists are superior in their efficacy to other antiemetics for postoperative nausea and vomiting. This knowledge allows nurses to better meet the needs of patients who are at increased risk for postoperative nausea and vomiting, or who are having severe postoperative nausea and vomiting not controlled by other methods. Severe nausea and vomiting are also undesirable in certain postoperative patients because of strain on surgical incision and internal sutures. Nurses should seek orders for selective serotonin receptor antagonist antiemetics from physicians and other prescribers when the patient's situation warrants this drug therapy.

Pharmacodynamics

Serotonin receptors of the 5-HT_3 type are located peripherally on the vagal nerve terminal and centrally in the CTZ. During chemotherapy, special mucosal cells in the small intestine release serotonin, which stimulates these receptors. Ondansetron blocks these receptor sites, thus preventing nausea and vomiting.

Contraindications and Precautions

Ondansetron is contraindicated in patients with hypersensitivity to the drug or its components. Ondansetron is a pregnancy category B drug.

Adverse Effects

The most common adverse effects of ondansetron are headache, constipation, and malaise. Potentially serious adverse effects are arrhythmias, hypotension, and extrapyramidal effects (e.g., Parkinson-like symptoms). Other adverse effects that can occur include:

- Cardiovascular: hypertension
- CNS: anxiety, dizziness, drowsiness, and chills or shivering
- GI: abdominal pain, diarrhea, and xerostomia
- Miscellaneous: wound problems, musculoskeletal pain, cold sensation, fever, gynecologic disorders, hypoxia, injection-site reaction, paresthesia, pruritus, urinary retention, weakness, increases in aspartate transaminase and alanine aminotransferase, and pain.

Drug Interactions

Because ondansetron is metabolized by the cytochrome P-450 enzymes, drug interactions may occur with other drugs that are metabolized by these enzymes or those that inhibit P-450 metabolism. However, no dosage adjustment has been recommended based on available data regarding this finding.

Assessment of Relevant Core Patient Variables

Health Status

Verify that the patient has clinical indications for receiving ondansetron and is not known to have a hypersensitivity to it.

Life Span and Gender

Assess whether the patient is pregnant. Ondansetron is a pregnancy category B drug. Therefore, it should be used only if the potential benefit to the mother justifies potential risks to the fetus. Determine the patient's age. Ondansetron is used to prevent nausea and vomiting associated with cancer chemotherapy in children. However, dosage information for children 3 years of age or younger is limited. Dosage adjustment is not needed in older adults.

Environment

Note the setting in which ondansetron will be administered. Ondansetron normally is administered in the hospital.

Nursing Diagnoses and Outcomes

- Imbalanced Nutrition: Less than Body Requirements related to severe nausea and vomiting
  Desired outcome: *Nutritional needs will be met, and ondansetron therapy will prevent severe nausea and vomiting.*
- Risk for Altered Comfort related to severe nausea and vomiting
  Desired outcome: *Comfort will be maintained, and ondansetron therapy will prevent severe nausea and vomiting.*
- Potential Complication: Altered Cardiac Output related to adverse effects of ondansetron
  Desired outcome: *Cardiac output will not be affected adversely by possible hypotension and arrhythmias from ondansetron.*

Planning and Intervention

Maximizing Therapeutic Effects

Administer ondansetron 30 minutes before the start of chemotherapy. Infusions should be given over 15 minutes. Additional doses are used after chemotherapy. When used for postoperative nausea and vomiting, ondansetron should be given immediately before induction into anesthesia. If ondansetron is used with radiation therapy, the dose should be given orally, 1 to 2 hours before treatment. Oral disintegrating tablets should be removed from the pack by peeling back the foil, not by pushing the drug tablet through the foil. Place ondansetron on the patient's tongue and have the patient swallow it. The drug does not have to be administered with a fluid.

Providing Patient and Family Education

- Explain the purpose of the drug.
- Teach the patient to report any tremor, gait problems, or other Parkinson-like symptoms.

Ongoing Assessment and Evaluation

Ondansetron therapy is considered effective if nausea and vomiting are controlled and adverse effects do not occur.

Drugs Significantly Different From [P] Ondansetron

A new drug, aprepitant (Emend), is a substance P/NK1 receptor antagonist that has been approved for preventing delayed emesis from chemotherapy. It has little or no affinity for serotonin (5-HT), dopamine, and corticosteroid receptors, the targets for other antiemetics. Aprepitant is highly protein bound at 95%. The drug is extensively metabolized by the P-450 system, primarily by CYP3A4. Aprepitant is also a moderate inhibitor of CYP3A4. Minor metabolism occurs through CYP1A2 and CYP2C19. Metabolism is the route of elimination; aprepitant is not renally excreted. The half-life is 9 to 13 hours. No clinically statistical pharmacokinetic differences in aprepitant use exist among men and women, older and younger adults, and Hispanics, blacks, and whites. No dosage adjustments are indicated for any of these groups. Aprepitant has not been studied in children younger than 18 years.

Studies show that, given orally once a day for 3 days (the day of therapy, and then 2 days afterward) 1 hour before administration of chemotherapy, this drug decreased delayed emesis by 30% over placebo. Aprepitant is used in combination with ondansetron and dexamethasone as a standardized regimen. It is not used alone. The aprepitant regimen prevents acute and delayed nausea and vomiting associated with highly emetogenic drugs, including high doses of cisplatin. Aprepitant is not effective in treating current conditions of nausea.

A major difference between aprepitant and odansetron is the potential for drug interactions. Aprepitant must be used with extreme caution in patients who also receive other drugs that are primarily metabolized through CYP3A4, and elevations of their plasma levels are likely to occur. It should not

MEMORY CHIP

[P] Ondansetron

- Used to prevent nausea and vomiting associated with cancer chemotherapy, radiation, and certain postoperative states
- Most common adverse effects: headache, constipation, and malaise
- Most serious adverse effects: arrhythmias, hypotension, and extrapyramidal effects
- Maximizing therapeutic effects: Administer 30 min before treatment.
- Most important patient education: Notify the nurse if any adverse effects occur.

be used at all concurrently with pimozide, cisapride, terfenadine, or astemizole because inhibition of CYP3A4 in these drugs and the elevated plasma concentrations of these drugs can potentially cause serious or life-threatening reactions. Several chemotherapy drugs are metabolized by CYP3A4 and include docetaxel, paclitaxel, etoposide, vinblastine, vincristine, irinotecan, ifosfamide, and imatinib. During clinical trials aprepitant was commonly coadministered with etoposide, vinorelbine, or paclitaxel. These drugs did not require dosage adjustments. Use of the other chemotherapeutic CYP3A4 substrates has not been studied, and they may require downward dosage adjustments if coadministered with the aprepitant regimen. Aprepitant also interacts substantially with warfarin, which may result in a clinically significant decrease in the INR, leading to a risk for clotting. Patients need to have their INR monitored for 14 days, especially between days 7 and 10, following initiation of the 3-day aprepitant regimen. The efficacy of oral contraceptives may also be reduced by aprepitant. A backup method of contraception should be used. Aprepitant is generally well tolerated and in clinical trials had a similar adverse effect pattern as placebo. The most common adverse effects were tiredness, hiccups, constipation, diarrhea, and loss of appetite.

C GALLSTONE-SOLUBILIZING AGENTS

Gallstone-solubilizing agents, including ursodiol (Actigall) and monoctanoin (Moctanin), work to dissolve gallstones. They are used only under specific circumstances and are summarized in Table 48.11.

CHAPTER SUMMARY

- Drug therapy for the upper GI tract is related to problems from bacterial infection, acid production, digestion, and nausea and vomiting.
- Dietary factors can influence symptoms experienced from the disease process; can contribute to the effectiveness of the therapy; and can contribute to adverse effects from therapy. Current dietary habits should be explored, and additional dietary teaching provided as indicated, with all patients requiring drug therapy for upper GI problems.
- *Helicobacter pylori* causes a bacterial infection that is a causative factor in peptic ulcers. When *H. pylori* is eradicated, an ulcer rarely reoccurs. Treatment involves various drug choices but optimally includes the combination of antibiotics (usually two) and a proton pump inhibitor. A bismuth salicylate may be added as well. H_2 receptor antagonists sometimes are used instead of a proton pump inhibitor.
- Proton pump inhibitors, such as omeprazole, decrease gastric acid production. They are used to manage the symptoms of GERD and peptic ulcers and to treat hypersecretory conditions.
- H_2 receptor antagonists, such as ranitidine, block histamine at parietal cells, thus reducing the hydrogen ion concentration and the volume of gastric acid. Common uses of H_2 receptor antagonists include treating peptic ulcer disease, gastric esophageal reflux disease, and hypersecretory conditions and preventing stress ulcers. OTC ranitidine is used for heartburn and indigestion.
- Antacids are basic salts that increase the gastric pH, thereby neutralizing gastric acidity. These preparations are used for upper GI disorders such as gastroesophageal reflux esophagitis, hiatal hernia, gastritis, and peptic ulcer disease. Antacids do not cure these conditions but help to manage the symptoms and discomfort associated

TABLE 48.11 Summary of Selected C Gallstone-Solubilizing Agents

Drug (Trade) Name	Selected Indications	Contraindications and Precautions	Adverse Effects	Route and Dosage Range
ursodiol (Actigall)	Dissolution of radiolucent, noncalcified, smaller than 20-mm gallstones in patients who are not candidates for surgery due to age, disease states, or idiosyncratic reactions to anesthesia	Will not dissolve calcified, radiopaque, or radiolucent bile pigment stones in patients with compelling needs for cholecystectomy	Nausea, vomiting, dyspepsia	*Adult:* PO, 8–20 mg/kg/d in two to three doses, for 1 y or more (if partial or full dissolution does not occur in 1 y, likelihood of success is reduced)
monoctanoin (Moctanin)	Dissolution of radiolucent gallstones retained in biliary tract after cholecystectomy when other means have failed or cannot be used	Impaired hepatic function, significant biliary tract infection, recent history of duodenal ulcer or duodenitis, portosystemic shunting, acute pancreatitis, or any life-threatening problem that would be complicated by biliary tract infusion	Abdominal pain, nausea, vomiting, diarrhea, anorexia, indigestion, fever	*Adult* (direct infusion into biliary tract only after a catheter has been placed endoscopically as close to the stones as possible): Dilute 120-mL vial with 13 mL of sterile water; perfuse stone 3–5 mL/h for 2–10 d

with them. All antacids are closely related and are used in various combinations to produce the desired effects and to minimize adverse effects.

- Two antacids are absorbed systemically: sodium bicarbonate and calcium carbonate. In large doses, they can cause metabolic alkalosis. Sodium bicarbonate contains large quantities of sodium. It should not be given to patients who have pathologies that require salt restriction.
- Magnesium antacids should not be given to patients with chronic renal failure because these drugs increase the risk for developing magnesium toxicity in such patients. Aluminum carbonate is used in patients with chronic renal failure because it binds with phosphorus, reducing serum phosphate levels.
- Sucralfate, although an aluminum salt, is not an antacid. When it dissolves in the stomach, it forms a sticky paste that adheres to ulcerated areas, preventing gastric acids from touching the ulcer and allowing healing to occur.
- The GI stimulants, such as metoclopramide, are used in diabetic gastroparesis and with symptomatic gastroesophageal reflux. They increase GI motility, apparently by sensitizing the tissues to acetylcholine. Metoclopramide, because of its dopamine antagonist characteristics, also is used as an antiemetic postoperatively and during chemotherapy.
- Digestive enzymes are a replacement for the body's intrinsic enzymes when the body does not produce enough to meet the needs for digestion. The enzymes that are replaced most frequently and with the greatest therapeutic effects are the pancreatic enzymes. They should be taken with meals and with snacks.
- Orlistat, a lipase inhibitor, prevents the absorption of dietary fat. It is used in obesity to promote and maintain weight loss.
- Antiemetics prevent nausea and vomiting; they prevent stimulation of the CTZ and the VC by interfering with neurotransmitter receptors. They are primarily selective serotonin receptor antagonists, antidopaminergics, or anticholinergics.
- Selective serotonin receptor antagonists, such as ondansetron, are used to prevent the nausea and vomiting associated with cancer chemotherapy and radiation therapy, and after some types of surgery.

QUESTIONS FOR STUDY AND REVIEW

1. If a patient is treated for active peptic ulcer disease solely with an antisecretory drug, such as the proton pump inhibitor omeprazole or an H_2 receptor antagonist such as ranitidine, is it likely that the ulcer will recur?
2. Your patient is receiving the proton pump inhibitor omeprazole for GERD. Explain how dietary factors may interact with the therapeutic action of omeprazole.
3. Why is it important to assess the pharmacokinetics of other drugs that a patient is receiving when you plan to start the patient on omeprazole therapy?
4. How do H_1 receptor antagonists differ from H_2 receptor antagonists?
5. What is the advantage of combining aluminum hydroxide with magnesium hydroxide as an antacid?
6. Why are aluminum antacids given to patients with chronic renal failure?
7. What are the main adverse effects of orlistat, a lipase inhibitor used in treating obesity?
8. Why is ondansetron especially helpful in preventing nausea and vomiting caused by cancer chemotherapy?

Need More Help?

Chapter 48 of the study guide for *Drug Therapy in Nursing* 2e contains NCLEX-style questions and other learning activities to reinforce your understanding of the concepts presented in this chapter. For additional information or to purchase the study guide, visit *http://connection.lww.com/go/aschenbrenner.*

REFERENCES AND BIBLIOGRAPHY

Axon, A. T. (2000). Treatment of *Helicobacter pylori:* An overview. *Alimentary Pharmacology and Therapeutics, 14*(Suppl. 3), 1–6.

Bray, G. A. (2000). A concise review on the therapeutics of obesity. *Nutrition, 16*(10), 953–960.

Candelli, M., Carloni, E., Armuzzi, A., et al. (2000). Role of sucralfate in gastrointestinal diseases. *Panminerva Medicine, 42*(1), 55–59.

Centers for Disease Control and Prevention. (2001). *Helicobacter pylori* and peptic ulcer disease. [Online]. Available: *http://www.cdc.gov/ulcer.md.htm.*

Chelimsky, G., & Czinn, S. J. (2000). *Helicobacter pylori* infection in children: Update. *Current Opinion in Pediatrics, 12*(5), 460–462.

Ernst, P. B., & Pappo, J. (2000). Preventive and therapeutic vaccines against *Helicobacter pylori:* Current status and future challenges. *Current Pharmaceutical Design, 6*(15), 1557–1573.

Facts and Comparisons. (2004). *Drug facts and comparisons.* Philadelphia: Lippincott Williams & Wilkins.

Flake, Z., Scalle, R., & Bailey, A. (2004). Practical selection of antiemetics. *American Family Physician, 69*(5), 1169–1174, 1176.

GlaxoSmithKline. (2002). Zantac prescribing information. Research Triangle Park, NC.

Gomollon, F., Sicilia, B., Ducons, J. A., et al. (2000). Third line treatment for *Helicobacter pylori:* A prospective, culture-guided study in peptic ulcer patients. *Alimentary Pharmacology and Therapeutics, 14*(10), 1335–1338.

Graham, D. Y., & Qureshi, W. A. (2000). Antibiotic-resistant *H. pylori* infection and its treatment. *Current Pharmaceutical Design, 6*(15), 1537–1544.

Hawkins, C., & Hanks, G. W. (2000). The gastroduodenal toxicity of nonsteroidal anti-inflammatory drugs: A review of the literature. *Journal of Pain and Symptom Management, 20*(2), 140–151.

Healthnotes. (2002). Safetychecker antacids/acid blockers. [Online]. Available: *http://www.mcustompak.com/healthNotes/Drug/Antacids.htm.*

Jeffrey R. W., & Utter J. (2003). The changing environment and population obesity in the United States. *Obesity Research, 11*(Suppl), 12S–22S.

Johnson, B. A., Roache, J. D., Javors, M. A., et al. (2000). Ondansetron for reduction of drinking among biologically predisposed alcoholic patients: A randomized controlled trial. *Journal of the American Medical Association, 284*(8), 963–971.

Kandel, G. (2000). *Helicobacter* and disease: Still more questions than answers. *Canadian Journal of Surgery, 43*(5), 339–346.

Lai, K. C., Hui, W. M., Wong, W. M., et al. (2000). Treatment of *Helicobacter pylori* in patients with duodenal ulcer hemorrhage—a long-term randomized, controlled study. *American Journal of Gastroenterology, 95*(9), 2225–2232.

Macleo, A. D. (2000). Ondansetron in multiple sclerosis. *Journal of Pain and Symptom Management, 20*(5), 388–391.

McManus, T. J. (2000). *Helicobacter pylori:* An emerging infectious disease. *Nurse Practitioner, 25*(8), 40, 43–44.

Misciagna, G., Cisternino, A. M., & Freudenheim, J. (2000). Diet and duodenal ulcer. *Digest for Liver Disease, 32*(6), 468–472.

Nakajima, S., Graham, D. Y., Hattori, T., et al. (2000). Strategy for treatment of *Helicobacter pylori* infection in adults. Updated indications for test and eradication therapy suggested in 2000. *Current Pharmaceutical Design, 6*(15), 1503–1514.

National Digestive Diseases Information Clearinghouse. (2002). *H. pylori* and peptic ulcer [Online]. Available: *http://digestive.niddk.nih.gov/ddiseases/pubs/hpylori.*

National Institutes of Health. (1998). *Helicobacter pylori* in peptic ulcer disease. Guidelines [On-line]. Available: *http://www./summary.asp?guideline=000428&summary_type=brief_summary&view=brief_summary&sSe.*

Powell, R. M., & Buggy, D. J. (2000). Ondansetron given before induction of anesthesia reduces shivering after general anesthesia. *Anesthesia and Analgesia 90*(6), 1423–1427.

Roghani, H. S., Massarrat S., Shirekhoda, M., et al. (2003). Effect of different doses of furazolidone with amoxicillin and omeprazole on eradication of *Helicobacter pylori. Journal of Gastroenterology and Hepatology, 18*(7), 778–782.

Sung, J. J. (2003). The role of acid suppression in the management and prevention of gastrointestinal hemorrhage associated with gastroduodenal ulcers. *Gastroenterology Clinics of North America, 32*(3 Suppl), S11–23.

Sutton, P., & Doidge, C. (2003). *Helicobacter pylori* vaccines spiral into the new millennium. *Digestive and Liver Diseases, 35*(10), 675–687.

Trepanier, E. F. (2000). Intravenous pantoprazole: A new tool for acutely ill patients who require acid suppression. *Canadian Journal of Gastroenterology, 14*(Suppl. D), 11D–20D.

Vanderhoff, M. T., & Rundsarah, M. (2002). Proton pump inhibitors: An update. *American Family Physician, 66,* 273–280.

Wadden, T. A., Berkowitz, R. I., Womble, L. G., et al. (2000). Effects of sibutramine plus orlistat in obese women following 1 year of treatment by sibutramine alone: A placebo-controlled trial. *Obesity Research, 8*(6), 431–437.

Weiss, D. (2000). How to help your patients lose weight: Current therapy for obesity. *Cleveland Clinic Journal of Medicine, 67*(10), 739, 743–746.

Wenner, J., Gunnarsson, T., Graffner, H., et al. (2000). Influence of smoking and *Helicobacter pylori* on gastric phospholipids. *Digestive Diseases and Science, 45*(8), 1648–1652.

Wyatt, H. R. (2003). The prevalence of obesity. *Primary Care, 30*(2), 267–279.

Zheng, P. Y. & Jones, N. L. (2003). Recent advances in *Helicobacter pylori* infection in children: From the petri dish to the playground. *Canadian Journal of Gastroenterology, 17*(7), 448–454.

Drugs Affecting the Lower Gastrointestinal Tract

chapter 49

Learning Objectives

At the completion of this chapter the student will:

1 Identify core drug knowledge about drugs that affect the lower gastrointestinal (GI) tract.
2 Identify core patient variables related to drugs that affect the lower GI tract.
3 Relate the interaction of core drug knowledge to core patient variables for drugs that affect the lower GI tract.
4 Generate a nursing plan of care from the interactions between core drug knowledge and core patient variables for drugs that affect the lower GI tract.
5 Describe nursing interventions to maximize therapeutic effects and minimize adverse effects for drugs that affect the lower GI tract.
6 Determine key points for patient and family education for drugs that affect the lower GI tract.

KEY TERMS

constipation
Crohn disease
diarrhea
fecal impaction
flatus
inflammatory bowel disease (IBD)
irritable bowel syndrome (IBS)
peristalsis
ulcerative colitis

FEATURED WEBLINK

http://www.mayoclinic.com/invoke.cfm?id=DS00104
This site from the Mayo Clinic provides complete information about inflammatory bowel disease and its treatments.

CONNECTION WEBLINK

Additional Weblinks are found on Connection:
http://www.connection.lww.com/go/aschenbrenner.

Drugs Affecting the Lower Gastrointestinal Tract

(C) Antiflatulents

- (P) **simethicone**
- charcoal

(C) Antidiarrheals

- (P) **diphenoxylate HCl with atropine sulfate**
- difenoxin
- loperamide
- bismuth subsalicylate
- kaolin and pectin

(C) Drugs Used to Treat Irritable Bowel Syndrome

- (P) **alosetron**
- dicyclomine
- hyoscyamine
- tegaserod

(C) Drugs Used to Treat Inflammatory Bowel Disease

- balsalazide
- mesalamine
- olsalazine
- sulfasalazine

(C) Laxatives

(C) Saline laxatives

- (P) **magnesium hydroxide**
- magnesium sulfate
- magnesium citrate
- sodium phosphate

(C) Hyperosmotic laxatives

- glycerin
- lactulose
- polyethylene glycol electrolyte solution

(C) Stimulant laxatives

- bisacodyl
- calcium salts of sennosides A and B
- cascara sagrada
- castor oil
- phenolphthalein
- senna

(C) Bulk-forming laxatives

- polycarbophil
- psyllium

(C) Stool softener

- docusate sodium

(C) Lubricant laxative

- mineral oil

The symbol (C) indicates the **drug class**.
Drugs in **bold type** marked with the symbol (P) are prototypes.
Drugs in blue type are closely related to the prototype.
Drugs in red type are significantly different from the prototype.
Drugs in black type with no symbol are also used in drug therapy; no prototype

This chapter discusses drugs used to treat the most common alterations of the lower gastrointestinal (GI) tract, including flatus (gas), diarrhea, constipation, irritable bowel syndrome, and irritable bowel disease. All are digestive disorders. Their occurrence may be mild and episodic or severe, debilitating, and chronic. Patients may self-treat these problems with over-the-counter (OTC) medications, or they may seek medical attention. These problems may be related to other drug therapy, diet, emotions, or changes in activity. The drug classes used to treat flatus, diarrhea, and constipation are called antiflatulents, antidiarrheals, and laxatives, respectively. In addition, drugs used to treat irritable bowel syndrome and inflammatory bowel disease (including ulcerative colitis and Crohn disease) are presented.

Some drugs begin acting in the lower GI tract. However, their therapeutic uses are for alterations of other systems. These drugs include potassium-removing resins, such as sodium polystyrene sulfonate (Kayexalate), and a lipid-lowering agent, such as cholestyramine (Questran). These drugs are discussed in Chapters 26 and 30, respectively.

PHYSIOLOGY

The large intestine is approximately 5 feet long (1.5 m) and 2.5 inches (6.5 cm) in diameter. The longitudinal muscle fibers on the outer surface of the large intestine are in three layers and do not cover the entire colon uniformly. This arrangement of the muscle exerts a tension on the wall of the intestine, drawing it up and giving it a puckered appearance.

The large intestine is composed of the cecum, colon, rectum, and anal canal. The cecum, located on the right side of the abdomen, is a small pouch-like structure. The appendix is a blind tube of lymphoid tissue attached to the cecum. The colon has four sections—ascending, transverse, descending, and sigmoid. The area immediately after the sigmoid colon is the rectum, which is followed by the anal canal. The anal canal has two sphincters—the internal and the external.

The contents from the small intestine enter the cecum through the ileocecal valve. **Peristalsis,** wave-like muscular contractions and squeezing of the intestines, moves the contents through the small and large intestines. The movement of fecal material into the rectum triggers defecation. The distended rectum activates the defecation reflex, relaxing both the internal and external anal sphincters. As peristaltic action increases, the diaphragm lowers, and the abdominal muscles contract, forcing the feces out of the body through the anus. Defecation is controlled in the healthy person by maintaining a contracted external anal sphincter. The normally brown color of fecal material is caused by the breakdown of bilirubin. The normal content of fecal matter includes dead bacteria, fat, inorganic matter, protein, dried digestive juices, and indigestible components of food.

Large amounts of mucus are secreted by goblet cells in the epithelial layer of the large intestine. This mucus protects the epithelial surface from abrasive fecal material and aids in holding the fecal material together. Certain bacteria normally present in the large intestine produce some needed vitamins, including vitamin K, vitamin B_{12}, riboflavin, and thiamine. The bacteria produce gases that contribute to the formation of flatus.

During the movement of stomach contents through the large intestine, water and some electrolytes are reabsorbed. Absorption of fluid and electrolytes occurs primarily in the proximal colon. The longer the contents remain in the large intestine, the greater the amount of water that is reabsorbed (Figure 49.1).

PATHOPHYSIOLOGY

Flatus

Flatus is a normal byproduct of digestion. Flatus becomes problematic, causing discomfort or pain from excessive production (caused by ingesting gas-producing foods) or from an inability to pass it through the large intestine (a disruption of peristalsis, such as occurs temporarily after surgery).

Diarrhea

When peristalsis occurs too rapidly and stomach contents move more quickly than normal through the large intestine, diarrhea results. **Diarrhea** occurs when frequency of stools increases and the content of the stools becomes loose and

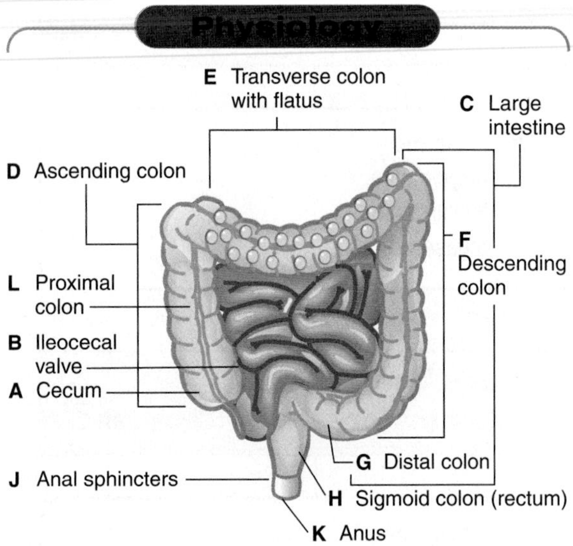

FIGURE 49.1 Moving through the lower gastrointestinal tract. Once the contents of the small intestine enter the cecum (**A**) through the ileocecal valve (**B**), they are transported through the large intestine (**C**) by peristalsis (wave-like propulsion of gastric contents). The three segments of the large intestine are termed the ascending colon (**D**), the transverse colon (**E**) and the descending colon (**F**). When the contents leave the distal colon (**G**) and enter the sigmoid colon (**H**) (rectum), the distended rectum activates the defecation reflex, which causes the internal and external anal sphincters (**J**) to relax. As peristaltic activity increases, the diaphragm lowers and the abdominal muscles contract, forcing the feces out of the body through the anus (**K**). Certain bacteria normally present in the intestine produce gases that are commonly known as flatus. Absorption of fluid and electrolytes occurs primarily in the proximal colon (**L**), although some absorption occurs throughout the length of the large intestine. The longer the contents remain in the large intestine, the more water is absorbed.

watery. Nutrients cannot be absorbed normally under these conditions.

The causes of diarrhea may include malabsorption syndrome, bacterial or viral infections, irritable bowel syndrome, ulcerative colitis, lactose intolerance, cancer, and laxative abuse. The cause of the diarrhea should be determined before instituting treatment. If the cause is an infection, drug therapy may not be recommended.

Diarrhea may be acute or chronic. Acute diarrhea is most often the result of bacterial infection, food poisoning, viral infection, or drug toxicity. It is usually self-limiting and responds to treatment within 48 hours. Chronic diarrhea is most often secondary to a disease process, such as irritable colon, ulcerative colitis, diverticulitis, or cancer, or secondary to removal of some of the bowel through surgery. Treatment of the disease usually eliminates the diarrhea. When diarrhea becomes chronic, antidiarrheal drug therapy may be needed for an extended time.

Constipation and Fecal Impaction

Constipation is infrequent or incomplete passage of hard stools that results from a decrease in peristaltic activity and slow movement of fecal material through the colon. This slow movement through the colon allows more water to be absorbed from the feces, resulting in hard, dry stools. The hard, dry fecal material is more difficult to pass and can cause painful defecation. Prolonged constipation may lead to **fecal impaction,** in which the patient is unable to pass the hardened mass of feces. The many causes of constipation include the following:

- Inadequate fiber in the diet
- Not defecating when the urge is felt
- Inactivity
- Decreased fluid intake
- Irritable bowel syndrome
- Weakened abdominal muscles caused by aging or disease
- Inability to perform the Valsalva maneuver effectively
- Hemorrhoids
- Cancer
- Hypothyroidism
- Adverse effects from drug therapy

Patients' definitions of constipation reflect what their normal patterns are. For this reason, an individual's definition may or may not reflect the actual slowed movement through the colon with resultant dry, hard stools.

Irritable Bowel Syndrome

Irritable bowel syndrome (IBS) is a common disorder of the intestines characterized by abnormal movement through the lower GI tract (either too quickly or too slowly) and abnormal sensations (abdominal discomfort or pain). It affects an estimated one in five adult Americans and up to three times as many women as men. IBS is the most common GI diagnosis among gastroenterology practices in the United States. American and European cultures have similar frequencies of IBS, and these rates generally cross the racial and ethnic groups in these cultures. Within the United States, however, some research indicates a lower prevalence of IBS in Hispanics living in Texas and Asians living in California (Lehrer & Lichentenstein, 2003). Onset of IBS usually occurs at a young age, with half of the people diagnosed with IBS reporting the onset of symptoms before age 35 years, and many reporting that the symptoms began in childhood.

IBS is a problem with colonic motility that has no known cause. It is called a functional disorder because no evidence of disease is seen when the colon is examined. IBS does not lead to any serious, organic diseases. IBS has not been linked to inflammatory bowel diseases such as Crohn disease or ulcerative colitis and it does not cause cancer of the bowel. However, IBS is a chronic disorder that can be very painful, limiting the ability of a person to fully participate in life, diminishing quality of life, and incurring substantial cost. A review of the literature on the yearly direct costs per individual for management of IBS reported figures of UK £90, Canadian $259, and U.S. $619 per patient (Inadomi et al., 2003).

Although the exact cause of IBS is not known, research has shown that neurotransmitters affect the nervous system of the enteric, or GI, tract. Stimulation by neurotransmitters at these sites produces localized effects in the lower GI tract, such as GI motility and sensations (Gershon, 2003; Chey, 2003). Serotonin (also called 5–HT for 5-hydroxytryptamine) is a primary neurotransmitter affecting the enteric tract, and it plays a role in visceral sensation and the normal functioning of the tract, including secretion and motility. Abnormalities in motility and visceral sensation correspond to the pathology of many of the symptoms of IBS (Chey, 2003). Although seven serotonin receptor sites have been identified, 5-HT_3 and 5 HT_4 receptors are the most important sites in IBS.

IBS is a complex syndrome whose presentation varies. Some people primarily have problems with diarrhea, some with constipation, and others alternate between diarrhea and constipation. No definitive test exists for IBS; thus, it has been difficult to clearly diagnose patients. A consensus panel of gastroenterologists created a set of conditions for the diagnosis of IBS known as the Rome Criteria. To be diagnosed with IBS, a patient must have symptoms that are continuous or recurrent over at least 3 months. The symptoms must include abdominal pain or discomfort that is characterized by being relieved by defecation, associated with a change in stool frequency, and associated with a change in stool consistency. In addition, two or more of the following symptoms must be present at least 25% of the time for at least 3 months: altered stool frequency, altered stool form, altered stool passage, mucorrhea (large amounts of mucus in the stool), and abdominal bloating or subjective distention.

In IBS, the bowel is hypersensitive and overreacts to mild stimulation. The normal distention of the bowel that can occur with food intake, gas, or a high-fiber diet can be enough to trigger IBS. Thus, IBS patients exhibit pain and discomfort at lower volumes of gastric distention than occur in patients who do not have IBS. The symptoms of IBS are painful diarrhea or constipation, or diarrhea that alternates with constipation. Other symptoms are crampy abdominal pain, bloating, gas pain, excessive flatulence, increased belching, mucus in the stool, small stools ("rabbit-like pellets"), or flat "ribbon" stools. Bleeding, fever, weight loss, and persistent severe pain are *not* symptoms of IBS and may indicate other problems. IBS symptoms have been found to affect general health, vitality, social functioning, bodily pain, diet, sexual function, and sleep negatively. IBS symptoms also contribute to time lost from work.

For those with IBS, the symptoms of spastic contractions may be triggered by stress because the bowel is controlled partly by the nervous system. IBS, however, is *not* related to a personality disorder; it is a disorder of digestion. Stress management or use of stress-reduction techniques may help relieve some of the symptoms or make them less severe. Diet also can trigger flares of IBS. An increase in peristalsis is normal after eating. For people with IBS, strong contractions of the colon may come sooner after eating than usual, accompanied by cramps and diarrhea. Because fat is a strong stimulus for colonic contractions, eating a high-fat meal will bring on contractions in some people that may be stronger or more violent than usual. Large meals also can cause cramping and diarrhea in people with IBS. Lack of fiber may potentiate constipation in IBS. Finally, women with IBS experience more symptoms when they have their menstrual period, which is hypothesized to be related to female sex hormones increasing the susceptibility of the colon to spasm. Research has not shown, however, that stress reduction or dietary modification is helpful or effective in all patients with IBS. Even in patients who experience a positive effect, these lifestyle modifications may not replace the need for drug therapy.

Inflammatory Bowel Disease

Inflammatory bowel disease (IBD) is a general term that includes both ulcerative colitis and Crohn disease. IBD has no known cause but is characterized by inflammation of the large or small intestine. **Ulcerative colitis** is an inflammatory disease of the large intestine in which ulcers form in the mucosa of the colon or rectum. Diarrhea, blood, and pus may result. **Crohn disease** is an inflammation extending into the deeper layers of the intestinal wall. It is most often found in the ileum and the cecum. However, Crohn disease can develop anywhere along the intestines. It may cause ulcers along the entire colon, form a string of ulcers in one part of the colon, or cause multiple scattered clusters of ulcers in the colon. The main symptom of IBD is diarrhea, which may, especially in ulcerative colitis, contain blood. Constipation also may develop during active flare-ups. Cramps and intestinal pain may occur. Fever, fatigue, loss of appetite, and weight loss also may occur.

Approximately 1 to 2 million Americans have IBD (the wide variation is because of the difficulty of diagnosing IBD and because people may have long remissions and not be identified as having IBD). Men and women seem to be affected equally. IBD most often is diagnosed between 15 and 40 years of age. Jewish Americans of European descent have a risk for IBD that is five times that of the general population. IBD is more common among city dwellers than country dwellers and is more prevalent in developed countries.

Although the exact cause is not known, genetic factors have been implicated. Up to 25% of people with IBD have family members with the disease. Genetic abnormalities linked to the two disorders may share locations on chromosomes 1, 3, 4, 7, 12, and 16. Some researchers believe that the disease develops in people who have a genetic susceptibility that allows an agent, such as a virus or bacterium, to trigger an abnormal immune response. When an organism injures the lining of the intestine in a normal, healthy person, the immune system reduces the inflammation and injury by producing suppressor T cells. In people with IBD, however, when an organism injures the lining of the intestine, the immune system produces helper T cells. Helper T cells produce a protein called a cytokine. Cytokines cause intestinal inflammation and damage, which attract even more helper T cells to the area. Because IBD is more prevalent in industrialized countries, environmental factors, such as diet, are believed to also play a role in producing IBD. No clear insight into this phenomenon is yet available from research.

C ANTIFLATULENTS

Antiflatulents decrease gas production, coalesce gas bubbles, and facilitate the passage of gas through belching and expelling flatus. Antiflatulents include simethicone and charcoal (Table 49.1). The prototype antiflatulent is simethicone (Mylicon). It is available alone or combined with antacids and digestants (see Chapter 48).

NURSING MANAGEMENT OF THE PATIENT RECEIVING P SIMETHICONE

Core Drug Knowledge

Pharmacotherapeutics

Antiflatulents are drugs used to relieve the discomfort of excess gas in the GI tract caused by swallowing air, postoperative gas distention, peptic ulcer, spastic or irritable colon, or diverticulitis. These drugs relieve pain and discomfort by promoting belching and the passing of flatus.

Pharmacokinetics

Simethicone is inert and is not absorbed from the GI tract. Because the drug is inactive, it is excreted unchanged in feces and does not interfere with absorption of water or nutrients or the secretion of mucus in the GI tract. Simethicone is not distributed systemically in the body and is excreted unchanged in the feces. It begins to act immediately in the GI tract and has a duration of approximately 3 hours. Its peak and half-life are unknown.

Pharmacodynamics

Simethicone has a defoaming action that alters the surface tension of gas bubbles. As the surface tension is changed, gas bubbles unite, forming larger gas bubbles that are eliminated more easily by belching or expulsion as flatus. It also is combined with antacids to decrease flatulence, but it has no antacid properties. An unlabeled use is treating the symptoms of infant colic.

Contraindications and Precautions

Simethicone has no contraindications or precautions.

Adverse Effects

No substantial adverse reactions have been reported with the use of simethicone.

Drug Interactions

No drug interactions with simethicone are known.

TABLE 49.1 Summary of Selected (C) Antiflatulent and (C) Antidiarrheal Drugs

Drug (Trade) Name	Selected Indications	Route and Dosage Range	Pharmacokinetics
(C) Antiflatulents			
[P] simethicone (Mylanta Gas, Gas Relief, Gas-X, Major-Con, Phazyme, Flatulex, Mylicon)	Relief of symptoms and pressure from excess gas in the intestinal tract	*Adult:* PO, 125-mg capsules qid with meals; 40–125-mg tablets qid with meals; 40–80-mg drops qid up to 500 mg/d *Child <2 y:* PO, 20 mg qid up to 240 mg/d; 2–12 y, 40 mg qid	*Onset:* Not absorbed systemically *Duration:* None $t_{1/2}$: None
(C) Antidiarrheals			
[P] diphenoxylate HCl with atropine sulfate (Lomotil, Logen, Lonox, Lomanate)	Diarrhea	*Adult:* PO, 5 mg qid *Child (2–12 y):* 0.3–0.4 mg/kg/d in 4 doses	*Onset:* Unknown *Duration:* Unknown $t_{1/2}$: 12–14 h
loperamide (Imodium, Kaopectate II Caplets, Pepto Diarrhea Control)	By prescription: control of acute nonspecific diarrhea or chronic diarrhea associated with inflammatory bowel disease	*Adult* (acute): PO, 4 mg initially, then 2 mg after each loose stool, not to exceed 16 mg/d; chronic, 4 mg initially, then 2 mg after each loose stool until diarrhea controlled *Child* (acute): PO, first day, 13–20 kg weight, 1 mg tid; 20–30 kg weight, 2 mg bid; >30 kg weight, 2 mg tid; after first day, 1 mg/10 kg after loose stools (not to exceed first day recommended doses); chronic, not established	*Onset:* Unknown *Duration:* Unknown $t_{1/2}$: 9.1–14.4 h
	OTC: traveler's diarrhea (acute diarrhea)	*Adult:* PO, 4 mg initially, then 2 mg after each loose stool, no more than 8 mg/d for no more than 2 d *Child 9–11 y:* PO, 2 mg initially then 1 mg after each loose stool up to 6 mg/d for no more than 2 d; (6–8 y): 1 mg initially and after each loose stool up to 4 mg/d for up to 2 d	
bismuth subsalicylate (Pepto-Bismol, Bismatrol, Pink Bismuth)	Indigestion, nausea, diarrhea (including traveler's diarrhea), abdominal cramps	*Adult:* PO, 2 tablets or 30 mL every 30 min to 1 h as needed, up to 8 doses in 24 h *Child 9–12 y:* PO, 1 tablet or 15 mL; 6–9 y: 2/3 tablet or 10 mL; 3–6 y: 1/3 tablet or 5 mL, same dosing schedule as adults	*Onset:* Bismuth, unknown; salicylate, rapid *Duration:* Bismuth, unknown; salicylate, 3–6 h $t_{1/2}$: Bismuth, unknown; salicylate, 2–3 h

Assessment of Relevant Core Patient Variables

Health Status

Before administering simethicone, assess for abdominal pain, distention, and bowel sounds.

Lifestyle, Diet, and Habits

Assess the patient's dietary choices for gas-producing foods such as cucumbers, cabbage, onions, beans, and radishes.

Environment

Note the setting in which simethicone will be administered. Simethicone is easily self-administered and can be given in any setting. Some preparations are available OTC.

Nursing Diagnosis and Outcome

- Acute Pain related to the presence of flatus
  Desired outcome: *Within 2 to 3 hours of using simethicone, the patient will experience a decrease in abdominal pain and distention.*

Planning and Intervention

Maximizing Therapeutic Effects

Simethicone should be given after meals and at bedtime to increase its effectiveness. Have the patient chew tablets thoroughly or allow them to dissolve in the mouth to promote dispersion. The suspension form of the drug must be shaken to ensure that the active ingredients are well dispersed.

To ensure accuracy of dosing liquid forms of the drug, use or teach the patient to use a calibrated dropper. When administering to infants, simethicone should be mixed with 30 mL of a suitable liquid, preferably formula or cool water.

Providing Patient and Family Education

- Teach the patient to take simethicone after each meal and at bedtime, to chew tablets thoroughly before swallowing, and to shake the liquid suspension form well before measuring a dose.
- Tell the patient to expect to pass gas and have increased belching after taking this drug.
- The patient must be cautioned not to increase the dosage unless instructed to do so by the prescriber.
- Instruct the patient to avoid gas-producing foods. A high-fiber diet will increase peristalsis, and a low-fat diet will decrease production of carbon dioxide gas.

Ongoing Assessment and Evaluation

Assess abdominal pain and distention periodically throughout therapy to monitor the effectiveness of the drug. Simethicone is effective if abdominal distention is decreased and the patient reports feeling more comfortable. If effectiveness is not observed, the dose may need to be increased. Verify that the patient does not have any increase in abdominal pain, nausea, vomiting, or fever because these findings are not symptoms of excessive flatus and may indicate that the patient requires medical attention.

MEMORY CHIP

P Simethicone

- Relieves the pain of excess gas in the GI tract; antifoaming action changes surface tension of gas bubbles, causing them to coalesce and pass more easily
- Most important patient education: Chew tablets to promote effectiveness; take after meals and at bedtime.

Drug Closely Related to P Simethicone

Charcoal is an absorbing, detoxifying, and soothing agent. The drug relieves gas and cramping by absorbing toxins and gas on the surfaces of its carbon particles. Like simethicone, it is useful for the relief of gas, diarrhea, and GI distress associated with indigestion and cramping.

Unlike simethicone, charcoal is used as an antidote in poisonings from drug overdose because it reduces absorption of certain drugs and chemicals and can actually remove them from the systemic circulation. Charcoal also is used for preventing nonspecific pruritus associated with kidney dialysis. It should not be given to children younger than 3 years of age. Charcoal can be combined with simethicone to treat gas pains; the charcoal decreases the amount of gas produced, and the simethicone promotes elimination of gas.

C ANTIDIARRHEALS

Antidiarrheals slow intestinal motility, allowing time for fluid reabsorption and better stool formation. The most effective antidiarrheal drugs include opiate derivatives, the opiates themselves, and loperamide, a drug related to the antipsychotic drug haloperidol. These drugs act systemically to reduce intestinal motility and slow peristalsis. Several locally acting drugs are available OTC and are effective in mild cases of diarrhea.

The drugs discussed in the following sections include diphenoxylate HCl, difenoxin, loperamide, and the locally acting agents bismuth subsalicylate, kaolin, and pectin. The prototype antidiarrheal drug is diphenoxylate HCl with atropine sulfate.

NURSING MANAGEMENT OF THE PATIENT RECEIVING P DIPHENOXYLATE HCL WITH ATROPINE SULFATE

Core Drug Knowledge

Pharmacotherapeutics

Diphenoxylate HCl with atropine sulfate (Lomotil, Lomanate, Lonox, Logen) is used as an adjunct in treating diarrhea (see Table 49.1).

Pharmacokinetics

Diphenoxylate HCl with atropine sulfate is absorbed readily in the GI tract. When the tablet form is used instead of the solution, bioavailability is decreased by approximately 10%. Diphenoxylate HCl with atropine sulfate is found in breast milk; however, the distribution is unknown. The drug is metabolized in the liver to difenoxin, which is an active metabolite that produces the desired therapeutic effects. It leaves the liver as bile and is excreted in feces. A tiny amount is excreted unchanged in the urine.

Pharmacodynamics

This drug is a synthetic narcotic similar in structure to meperidine. The dosage used in treating diarrhea is not high enough to provide pain relief. The drug acts on the smooth muscle of the intestine to slow intestinal motility and prolong intestinal transit time, allowing for the reabsorption of fluid. A small amount of atropine sulfate is combined with diphenoxylate to discourage deliberate abuse. When excessive dosages are taken, the adverse reactions of atropine sulfate, which include dry mouth and tachycardia, are particularly unpleasant. This preparation is very effective in treating diarrhea.

Contraindications and Precautions

Hypersensitivity to the drug or to atropine sulfate is a contraindication. Treatment using diphenoxylate HCl with atropine sulfate is contraindicated for diarrhea caused by GI organisms that penetrate the gastric mucosa (e.g., *Shigella, Salmonella,* and some toxic strains of *Escherichia coli*) because the drug slows peristalsis and may aggravate and prolong the diarrhea. The drug is contraindicated in patients with pseudomembranous colitis that occurs with broad-spectrum antibiotic therapy because it may worsen and prolong diarrhea. It also is contraindicated in patients with obstructive jaundice caused by hepatic impairment. Diphenoxylate HCl with atropine sulfate is contraindicated in children younger than 2 years of age. The drug is an FDA pregnancy category C drug.

Caution is used when administering the drug to patients with advanced hepatic and renal disease because of the risk for hepatic coma, to those with ulcerative colitis because of the risk for inducing toxic megacolon, and to patients with severe dehydration because it may cause variability of drug response that may predispose the patient to delayed diphenoxylate intoxication. Caution should be used in lactating women and in children because adverse effects from the atropine sulfate are more likely to occur in these patients. Children with Down syndrome are at special risk for atropine sulfate toxicity when taking diphenoxylate, even if it is taken in recommended doses. Although diphenoxylate HCl with atropine sulfate does not produce morphine-like effects or addiction in recommended dosages, at high doses, addiction can occur.

Adverse Effects

The most common adverse effects of diphenoxylate HCl with atropine sulfate are drowsiness and dizziness related to the drug's chemical similarity to meperidine, an opioid. Dry mouth and other anticholinergic effects (e.g., flushing, tachycardia, hyperthermia, and urinary retention) from the atropine in the drug are not common in adults receiving normal, therapeutic doses of diphenoxylate HCl, although children are at greater risk for these effects. Diphenoxylate HCl with atropine sulfate also may have the following adverse effects:

- GI: nausea, vomiting, abdominal discomfort, paralytic ileus, toxic megacolon, and pancreatitis
- Central nervous system (CNS): sedation, headache, malaise, lethargy, restlessness, euphoria, depression, and numbness of extremities
- Allergic: pruritus, swelling of gums, angioneurotic edema, urticaria, and anaphylaxis

Drug Interactions

When diphenoxylate HCl with atropine sulfate is given to patients taking monoamine oxidase inhibitors (MAOIs), the combination of the two drugs could precipitate a hypertensive crisis because diphenoxylate is similar chemically to meperidine. Diphenoxylate HCl with atropine sulfate may potentiate the depressive effects of alcohol, barbiturates, and tranquilizers. Table 49.2 lists drugs that interact with diphenoxylate HCl with atropine sulfate.

Assessment of Relevant Core Patient Variables

Health Status

Before administering diphenoxylate HCl with atropine sulfate, assess the patient for abdominal pain and distention to have a baseline for monitoring therapy. Auscultate bowel sounds. Patients with diarrhea will usually have frequent, high-pitched bowel sounds. Determine whether the patient has a diagnosis of hepatic impairment, obstructive jaundice, pseudomembranous colitis, or ulcerative colitis. Pertinent information about stools that should be assessed and documented includes frequency, color, consistency, and odor. Examine laboratory reports of stool specimens and do not administer diphenoxylate HCl with atropine sulfate if stool

TABLE 49.2 Agents That Interact With P Diphenoxylate HCl With Atropine Sulfate

Interactants	Effect and Significance	Nursing Management
monoamine oxidase inhibitors	Chemical structure of diphenoxylate similar to meperidine—hypertensive crisis possible	Administer together cautiously. Monitor BP while on both drugs.
barbiturates, tranquilizers, and alcohol	Depressant effect on central nervous system may be potentiated, leading to respiratory depression or sedation	Closely observe patient when patient is receiving both drugs. Monitor level of consciousness and respirations.

cultures are positive for *E. coli, Salmonella, Shigella,* or *Clostridium difficile*. While taking a drug history, determine whether the patient is receiving MAOIs and check the condition of mucous membranes and the skin for signs of dehydration. If the patient is a child, observe for Down syndrome.

Life Span and Gender

Determine whether the patient is pregnant or breast-feeding, and if the patient is a child, verify that he or she is older than 2 years of age.

Lifestyle, Diet, and Habits

Determine whether the patient has a history of substance abuse because it may make the patient more likely to use diphenoxylate HCl with atropine sulfate inappropriately.

Environment

Be aware of the setting in which diphenoxylate HCl with atropine sulfate will be administered. Although diphenoxylate HCl with atropine sulfate requires a prescription, oral doses are easily self-administered and can be given in any setting.

Culture and Inherited Traits

Cultural and social variations exist regarding how regular bowel movements and diarrhea are defined. Determine the patient's perception of normal elimination and diarrhea.

Nursing Diagnoses and Outcomes

- Diarrhea related to the causative factor (if identified)
  Desired outcome: *Diarrhea will be controlled through use of diphenoxylate HCl with atropine sulfate.*
- Risk for Injury related to drowsiness and dizziness secondary to drug therapy
  Desired outcome: *The patient will not sustain injury from drug therapy.*

Planning and Intervention

Maximizing Therapeutic Effects

To maximize the therapeutic effect, administer diphenoxylate HCl with atropine sulfate as ordered, four times daily, to obtain therapeutic results. Use the dropper provided when administering liquid preparations to ensure the correct dose.

Minimizing Adverse Effects

Decrease the dosage of diphenoxylate HCl with atropine sulfate when the number of stools decreases. The recommended dosage should not be exceeded. If the patient's condition does not improve with the maximum daily dose for 10 days, diarrhea symptoms are unlikely to be controlled with further use of this drug. In such cases, assess for adverse effects. Assess for toxic megacolon (abdominal distention and pain are possible indications). Because the massive dilation and atony of the colon from toxic megacolon can result in serious complications, signs of abdominal distention should be reported immediately.

Assess for and report signs of atropine sulfate toxicity (e.g., dry mouth, flushing, hypothermia, tachycardia, and urinary retention) because this condition requires immediate treatment. Children must be assessed very carefully because they are especially susceptible to atropine sulfate toxicity.

Providing Patient and Family Education

- Teach the patient not to exceed the prescribed dosage and to lower the dosage as instructed as soon as symptoms of diarrhea are controlled. Furthermore, if a dose is missed, instruct the patient not to take two doses.
- Instruct the patient to notify the prescriber if diarrhea persists for more than 10 days.
- Encourage the patient to avoid alcohol and other CNS depressants and not to drive or perform tasks that require mental alertness until the effects of diphenoxylate HCl with atropine sulfate on the individual are known.
- Caution the patient to maintain adequate fluid intake during periods of diarrhea to prevent dehydration and electrolyte imbalance.
- Caution the patient to store diphenoxylate HCl with atropine sulfate out of the reach of children.
- For liquid forms of diphenoxylate HCl with atropine sulfate, tell the patient not to use a household teaspoon to measure doses but rather a specially marked dropper or measuring spoon.
- If dry mouth occurs, recommend that the patient suck on hard candy or sip water.

Ongoing Assessment and Evaluation

It is important to assess skin turgor and mucous membranes for loss of moisture because these signs indicate dehydration. Monitoring electrolyte laboratory reports for electrolyte imbalance that may occur with the loss of fluid through diarrhea is also a priority. Weakness, muscular cramping, or dizziness should be reported because they are subjective symptoms of electrolyte imbalance. Any change in amount, color, consistency, or odor of stools should be noted. Drug therapy is effective when diarrhea is controlled without any adverse effects.

CRITICAL THINKING SCENARIO

Diphenoxylate in antidiarrheal therapy

Mr. Rothberg is 46 years old. He enters the emergency clinic with complaints of acute diarrhea for the last 36 hours. He also complains of abdominal pain and cramping. "Every time I eat," he says, "I have to run to the bathroom. I can't seem to keep anything in."

1. What questions you would ask when assessing Mr. Rothberg's condition?
2. After assessment is completed, Mr. Rothberg is diagnosed as having diarrhea secondary to an acute viral illness of the GI tract. He is given a prescription for diphenoxylate HCl with atropine sulfate. What additional core patient variables need to be assessed to provide patient education geared to Mr. Rothberg's personal learning needs?

MEMORY CHIP

[P] Diphenoxylate HCL With Atropine Sulfate

- Used to treat diarrhea not responsive to symptomatic and supportive treatment
- This drug is related chemically to meperidine, an opioid, but lacks any analgesic effect. Atropine is added to discourage abuse.
- Major contraindications: diarrhea associated with organisms that penetrate intestinal mucosa; pseudomembranous enterocolitis
- Most common adverse effects: drowsiness, dizziness, and dry mouth
- Most serious adverse effects: atropine overdose and toxic megacolon
- **Life span alert: Children are more likely to have adverse effects from atropine, especially if they have Down syndrome; variable response in children; avoid use if patient is <2 years old.**
- Minimizing adverse effects: Decrease the dose when diarrhea becomes less frequent; monitor for signs of atropine overdose (in children) and toxic megacolon.
- Most important patient education: Do not exceed the prescribed dose.

Drugs Closely Related to [P] Diphenoxylate HCl With Atropine Sulfate

Difenoxin (Motofen) is the principal active metabolite of diphenoxylate and is effective at one fifth the dose of diphenoxylate. It is metabolized to an inactive form. Loperamide (Imodium) is chemically similar to haloperidol, an antipsychotic drug. Unlike diphenoxylate, loperamide may be used for chronic and acute diarrhea. Loperamide comes in prescription and OTC strengths. Because loperamide does not contain the anticholinergic drug atropine sulfate, the contraindications and adverse reactions related to atropine sulfate are not applicable. For this reason, it may also be better tolerated than diphenoxylate HCl with atropine sulfate.

Drugs Significantly Different From [P] Diphenoxylate HCl With Atropine Sulfate

Bismuth Subsalicylate

Bismuth subsalicylate (Pepto-Bismol, Bismatrol, Pink Bismuth), a locally acting antidiarrheal, is available without a prescription and is used widely as an antidiarrheal agent. The salicylate component of this drug seems to have an antisecretory effect, whereas the bismuth component has a direct antimicrobial effect against bacteria and viral pathogens in the GI tract. Bismuth subsalicylate is used to treat diarrhea, indigestion, nausea, and abdominal cramps. Unlabeled uses include treating chronic infantile diarrhea and the symptoms of Norwalk virus–induced gastroenteritis, as well as preventing traveler's diarrhea. Bismuth subsalicylate is not given to children or adolescents with viral diseases because of the possibility that the salicylate component may cause Reye syndrome.

Kaolin and Pectin

Kaolin and pectin (Kaopectate) are locally acting antidiarrheals frequently used in combination. These drugs are used widely to treat mild diarrhea, even though clinical studies have not firmly established their effectiveness. Kaolin and pectin are different from the prototype diphenoxylate. These drugs act as absorbents; that is, toxins, bacteria, and other irritants in the GI tract bind to them. Commercial products usually contain two or more adsorbents. For example, Kaopectate is a combination of kaolin and pectin. The adsorptive action is not selective and therefore can interfere with normal GI absorption, particularly absorption of other drugs.

(C) LAXATIVES

Drugs used to treat constipation are referred to as laxatives. Laxatives are drugs that act directly on the intestine to promote peristalsis and evacuation of the bowel. Laxatives are classified as saline laxatives, hyperosmotics, stimulants, and bulk-forming laxatives. Table 49.3 presents a summary of laxative drugs. Stool softeners (surfactants) and lubricants are also used to promote easy passage of stool, but they are not technically laxatives.

(C) Saline Laxatives

Saline laxatives include magnesium hydroxide, magnesium sulfate, magnesium citrate, and sodium phosphate. The prototype saline laxative is magnesium hydroxide (Milk of Magnesia).

NURSING MANAGEMENT OF THE PATIENT RECEIVING [P] MAGNESIUM HYDROXIDE

Core Drug Knowledge

Pharmacotherapeutics

Magnesium hydroxide is used for acute or chronic constipation, preoperatively to prepare the bowel for surgery, and to clear the lower bowel tract before or after radiologic and other diagnostic studies (see Table 49.3). Magnesium hydroxide also is used as an antacid (see Chapter 48).

Pharmacokinetics

Magnesium hydroxide has a local effect in the lower GI tract and is absorbed poorly. Approximately 15% to 30% of the magnesium in magnesium hydroxide is absorbed in the small intestine. Onset of action is 30 minutes to 3 hours after administration. A bowel movement usually occurs within 6 hours of administration. Excretion occurs in the kidneys and the GI tract.

Pharmacodynamics

Magnesium hydroxide is a salt. It works in the small intestine and large intestine by attracting and retaining water in the intestinal lumen, thereby increasing pressure within the

TABLE 49.3 Summary of Selected (C) Laxatives

Drug (Trade) Name	Selected Indications	Route and Dosage Range	Pharmacokinetics
(C) Saline Laxatives			
[P] magnesium hydroxide (Milk of Magnesia)	Constipation, preparation for diagnostic tests of lower GI tract, post-GI diagnostic tests	*Adult:* PO, 30–60 mL/d; 15–30 mL/d (if concentrated) *Child 2–5 y:* PO, 5–15 mL/d *Child 6–11:* PO, 15–30 mL	*Onset:* 0.5–3 h *Duration:* Unknown $t_{1/2}$: None
magnesium sulfate (epsom salts)	Same as above	*Adult:* PO, 10–15 g in glass of water *Child:* PO, 5–10 g in glass of water	*Onset:* 0.5–3 h *Duration:* Unknown $t_{1/2}$: None
magnesium citrate (Citrate of Magnesia, Citro-Nesia)	Same as above	*Adult:* PO, 240 mL *Child:* PO, 120 mL	*Onset:* 0.5–3 h *Duration:* Unknown $t_{1/2}$: None
sodium phosphate (Phospho-Soda, sodium phosphates)	Same as above	*Adult:* PO, 20–45 mL mixed in half glass cool water *Child (5–11 y):* PO, 5–20 mL mixed in half glass cool water	*Onset:* 0.5–3 h *Duration:* Unknown $t_{1/2}$: None
(C) Hyperosmotic Laxatives			
polyethylene glycol-electrolyte solution (PEG-ES) (Colovage, CoLyte, Golytely, OCL)	Induce diarrhea to cleanse bowel tract before GI examination	*Adult:* PO, 240 mL every 10 min until 4 L consumed or effluent is clear; may be given through nasogastric tube 20–30 mL/min	*Onset:* 30–60 min *Duration:* About 4 h $t_{1/2}$: None
lactulose (Cephulac, Cholac, Chronulac, Constilac, Constulose, Duphalac, Enulose)	Constipation	*Adult:* PO, 15–30 mL/d up to 60 mL/d if needed *Child (infant):* PO, 2.5–10 mL in divided doses; older children and adolescents, 40–90 mL	*Onset:* 24–48 h *Duration:* Unknown $t_{1/2}$: None
	Prevention and treatment of portal-systemic encephalopathy, including hepatic precoma and coma	*Adult:* PO, 30–45 mL tid or qid; adjust dose every day or two to produce two or three soft but formed stools; may give hourly doses to induce rapid effect initially *Adult:* rectal, 300 mL in 700 mL water or normal saline solution, retain for 30–60 min; repeat every 4–6 h until patient is awake enough to take oral form	
glycerin (Sani-Supp, Fleet Babylax)	Constipation	*Adult and child:* Rectal, 1 suppository, retain 15 min (sized for adults and children)	*Onset:* 0.25–0.5 h *Duration:* Unknown $t_{1/2}$: None
(C) Stimulant Laxatives			
cascara sagrada (cascara sagrada fluid extract aromatic)	Constipation	*Adult:* PO, 325 mg tablet at bedtime or 5 mL *Child (<12 y):* No recommended dosage	*Onset:* 6–10 h *Duration:* Unknown $t_{1/2}$: None

(continued)

TABLE 49.3 Summary of Selected (C) Laxatives (continued)

Drug (Trade) Name	Selected Indications	Route and Dosage Range	Pharmacokinetics
senna (Senokot, Senexon, Senolax, Senna-Gen, Senokotxtra, Black Draught, Gentlax, Dr. Caldwell Senna Laxative, Fletcher's Castoria)	Same as above	*Adult:* PO, 1 or 2 tablets once or twice/d (depending on brand) *Child 6–12 y:* PO, 1 tablet once or twice/d	*Onset:* 6–10 h *Duration:* Unknown $t_{1/2}$: None
castor oil (Fleet flavored Castor Oil, Purge, Emulsoil)	Same as above	*Adult:* PO, 15–60 mL, depending on the product *Child 2–12 y:* PO, 5–15 mL, depending on product	*Onset:* 2–6 h *Duration:* Unknown $t_{1/2}$: None
bisacodyl (Dulcagen, Dulcolax, Fleet laxative, Bisco-Lax)	Same as above, pre- and postdiagnostic studies of lower GI tract	*Adult:* PO, 10–15 mg/d up to 30 mg/d prediagnostic study *Child 6–12 y:* PO, 5 mg/d *Adult:* Rectal, suppository form of 10 mg/d *Child 6–12 y:* rectal, suppository form of 5 mg/d	*Onset:* 0.25–1 h *Duration:* Unknown $t_{1/2}$: None
(C) Bulk-Forming Laxatives			
polycarbophil (Fibercon, Equalactin, Mitrolan, Fiber-Lax, Fiberall)	Constipation or diarrhea associated with conditions such as irritable bowel syndrome and diverticulitis; acute nonspecific diarrhea	*Adult:* PO, 1 g/d to qid not to exceed 4 g/d; severe diarrhea, repeat every 30 min not to exceed maximum dose *Child 6–12 y:* PO, 500 mg no more than qid not to exceed 2 g/d	*Onset:* 12–24 h *Duration:* Unknown $t_{1/2}$: None
psyllium (Fiberall, Hydrocil Instant, Konsyl, Metamucil, natural vegetable powder, Reguloid, Serutan, Syllact, Konsyl-D, Modane Bulk, V-Lax)	Constipation, promotion of regularity	*Adult:* PO, 1 rounded teaspoon in 8 oz water one to three times daily	*Onset:* 12–24 h *Duration:* Unknown $t_{1/2}$: None
(C) Stool Softener			
docusate sodium (Colace, Regutol, Disonate, DOK, DOS Softgel, D-S-S, Modane Soft, Pro-Sof, Regular SS, Dioeze, Surfak Liquigels, DC Softgels, Pro-Cal-Sof, Sulfalax Calcium, Diolose, Diocto-K, Kasof)	Softens stool to prevent constipation and straining in defecation	*Adult:* PO, 50–300 mg/d *Child 6–12 y:* PO, 50–150 mg/d (depending on product)	*Onset:* 24–72 h *Duration:* Unknown $t_{1/2}$: None
(C) Lubricant Laxative			
mineral oil (Neo-Cultol, Milkinol, Agoral Plain, Kondremul Plain)	Constipation	*Adult:* PO, 15–45 mL/d *Child (6–12 y):* PO, 5–15 mL/d	*Onset:* 6–8 h *Duration:* Unknown $t_{1/2}$: None

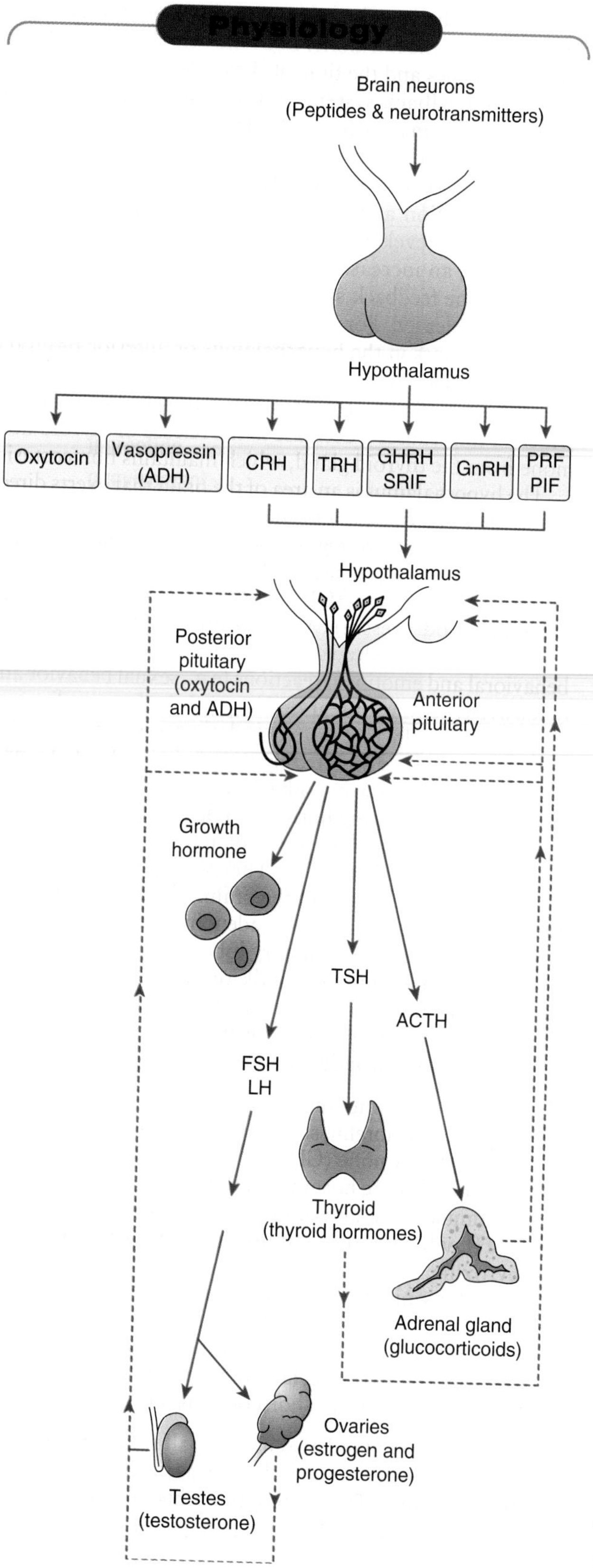

FIGURE 50.1 Control of hormone production by hypothalamic-pituitary-target cell feedback mechanism. Hormone levels from the target glands regulate the release of hormones from the anterior pituitary by means of a negative feedback system. The *dashed line* represents feedback control.

levels (ACTH), body growth and metabolism (GH), function of the thyroid gland (TSH), gonadal function (FSH and LH), and milk production and breast growth (prolactin). The hypothalamus is now recognized as the master controller in the body because it stimulates the pituitary gland to either release or not release a specific hormone. The first five hormones listed are **tropic hormones,** which means that they stimulate other organs or glands to secrete substances that are hormonally active. Secretion varies with physiologic activity (such as exercise) or with the time of day, and these substances are released into the bloodstream in a pulsatile manner. Various drugs, the central nervous system (CNS), hypothalamic hormones, some diseases, and hormones of the peripheral endocrine system affect their synthesis and release. Prolactin acts directly on breast tissue to stimulate milk production.

GH does not have a specific target gland. In children, it stimulates linear body growth. It regulates cellular metabolism, increases protein synthesis, enhances amino acid transport across cell membranes (which stimulates an anabolic effect), decreases the rate of carbohydrate use in cells, increases the rate of fatty acids for food use, and maintains or increases blood glucose levels in both children and adults. Many of the effects of GH depend on the production of insulin-like growth factor-1 (IGF-1), which is produced mainly in the liver.

GH is the most apparent of the pituitary hormones. Its secretion is regulated by two hypothalamic hormones: GHRH (GH-releasing hormone), which increases the release of GH; and somatostatin, which inhibits GH release. GH secretion fluctuates over a 24-hour period, with peak levels occurring during sleep stages 3 and 4 (1–4 hours after the onset of sleep). GH is also released during periods of hypoglycemia, stress, exercise, and excitement, and in response to levodopa and arginine.

Posterior Lobe of the Pituitary Gland

The posterior pituitary stores and secretes two **effector hormones** (hormones that produce an effect when stimulated): oxytocin and vasopressin (also known as antidiuretic hormone [ADH]). Both are synthesized in the hypothalamus and transported to the posterior lobe for future use.

Oxytocin stimulates uterine smooth muscle contraction in the later part of pregnancy and causes the milk let-down reflex in lactating women. Vasopressin controls the concentration of body fluids. It is released in response to decreases in blood volume, hypotension, or increases in plasma osmolarity (concentration). Vasopressin release can also be stimulated by stress, pain, trauma, nausea, use of tranquilizers or morphine, a positive-pressure apparatus, and some anesthetics. Vasopressin alters the permeability of the distal renal tubules and collecting ducts in the kidneys to conserve water.

Thyroid Gland Function

The bilobar thyroid gland is a shield-shaped gland located in the anterior middle portion of the neck, between the larynx and the trachea. The gland is composed of a series of circular follicles containing a material called colloid in the center. The colloid consists largely of thyroglobulin, which is a glycoprotein–iodine complex. It is synthesized in the thyroid cells and secreted into the follicle, where the thyroid hormone is stored. In making thyroid hormone, the thyroid gland is

very efficient in its use of iodide, which it receives from food, water, or medications.

A daily dietary absorption of 100 to 200 μg of iodide is adequate for the thyroid gland to make normal quantities of thyroid hormone. Iodide is pumped into the follicular cells against a concentration gradient in the process of removing it from the blood for storage. Because of this mechanism, the concentration of iodide in the normal thyroid gland is much higher than in the blood.

Once the iodide is in the follicle, it is oxidized by an enzyme called peroxidase in a reaction with a tyrosine molecule to form monoiodotyrosine and diiodotyrosine. Thyroxine (T_4) is formed when two diiodotyrosine residues are coupled. Triiodothyronine (T_3) is formed when a monoiodotyrosine and a diiodotyrosine are coupled. Collectively, these two hormones are referred to as thyroid hormone. When thyroid hormone is needed, T_4 and T_3 are released into the bloodstream. Once in the bloodstream, T_3 and T_4 are more than 99% bound to thyroid-binding globulin and other plasma proteins for transport. The three major thyroid-binding proteins are thyroid hormone-binding globulin (TBG), thyroxine-binding prealbumin (TBPA), and albumin. Some medications (e.g., corticosteroids, phenytoins, salicylates, and diazepam), systemic diseases, and congenital diseases can affect either the amount of binding protein in the blood or the binding ability of the hormone.

The hypothalamic-pituitary-thyroid feedback system regulates secretion of thyroid hormone. The hypothalamus produces TRH, which controls the release of TSH from the anterior pituitary gland. TSH increases the release of thyroid hormone from the follicles into the bloodstream and thyroglobulin breakdown, which increases thyroid activity. This increased activity activates the iodide pump, which increases the oxidation of iodide and increases the size and number of follicle cells. The increase in thyroid hormone levels sends a message to the hypothalamus to decrease TRH release and to the pituitary to decrease TSH. The decrease in TRH levels causes a decrease in TSH levels, which in turn causes the thyroid hormone levels to drop. The drop in thyroid hormone is sensed by the hypothalamus and pituitary, which respond by once again increasing TRH and TSH release (Figure 50.2).

Thyroid hormones control cellular metabolism and promote normal growth and development. They regulate heat and energy production, blood volume, cardiac output, oxygen consumption, and metabolism of fats, carbohydrates, and proteins (Table 50.1). All major organs are affected by disorders of the thyroid gland.

The thyroid gland also produces calcitonin, which maintains the serum calcium level by preventing release of calcium from the bone.

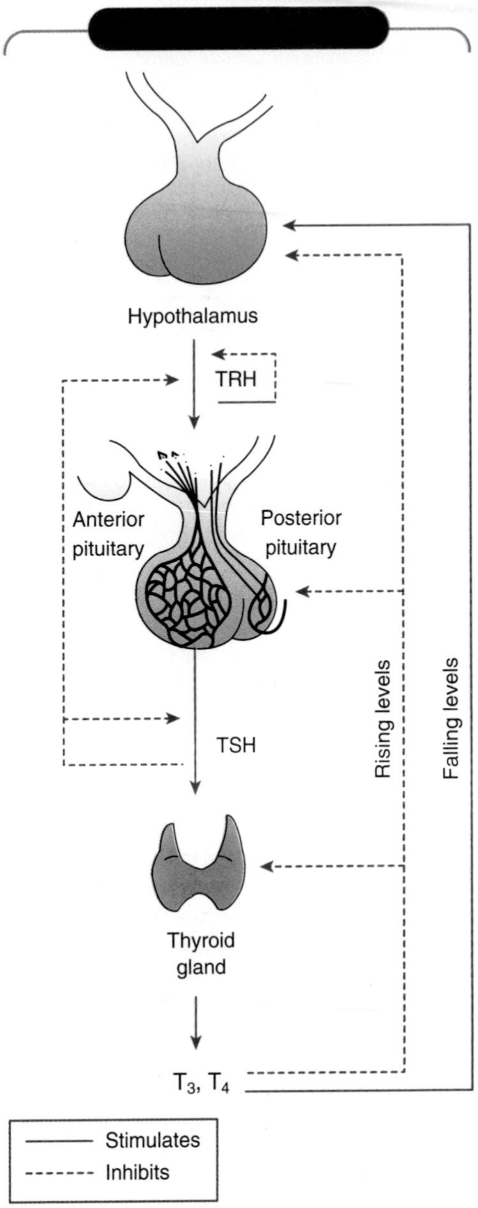

FIGURE 50.2 Thyroid-releasing hormone (TRH) from the hypothalamus stimulates the anterior pituitary to release thyroid-stimulating hormone (TSH). It also inhibits the hypothalamus from releasing TRH. TSH stimulates the thyroid gland to releases T_3 and T_4. It also inhibits the hypothalamus from releasing TRH and the anterior pituitary from releasing more TSH. The release of T_3 and T_4 from the thyroid gland inhibits TRH release from the hypothalamus, TSH release from the pituitary, and further T_3 and T_4 release from the thyroid gland. Falling T_3 and T_4 levels will stimulate the hypothalamus to release TRH, and the process repeatedly continues to maintain effective hormone levels.

Parathyroid Gland Function

The four tiny, highly vascular parathyroid glands work together as a single gland to produce PTH, which helps to regulate serum calcium and phosphate. These glands are located on the dorsal surface of the thyroid. In the healthy individual, plasma calcium concentration is maintained within narrow limits.

PTH affects three target organs: bone, kidneys, and GI tract. The primary storage site for calcium is in the bone. The major controlling factor for PTH secretion is serum calcium.

TABLE 50.1 Effects of Thyroid Hormone

Target Physiologic Process or Body System	Primary Effects
Carbohydrate metabolism	Increases cellular glucose uptake Increases gluconeogenesis and glycolysis Increases GI carbohydrate absorption Increases insulin secretion
Cardiovascular system	Increases heart rate, cardiac output, arterial pressure
Central nervous system	Increases mental processes Increases activity in spinal cord areas controlling muscle tone
Fat metabolism	Increases fat metabolism, including lipid mobilization from fat tissues and free fatty acid oxidation
GI function	Increases appetite, food absorption, digestive enzyme secretions, GI motility
Growth metabolism	Accelerates growth (in children) Accelerates food use for energy, speeds protein synthesis and catabolism, excites mental processes Increases other endocrine gland functions

When serum calcium levels are low, the parathyroid gland stimulates the release of PTH. Release of this hormone promotes increased bone resorption, which increases the serum calcium level. PTH also activates vitamin D in the kidney, which boosts absorption of phosphate and calcium from the GI tract. When serum calcium levels are elevated, PTH secretion decreases. Magnesium and phosphate levels also affect PTH secretion.

PATHOPHYSIOLOGY

Pituitary Gland Dysfunction

Pituitary dysfunction may occur from many causes, such as congenital defects, developmental abnormalities, acute or chronic inflammation, invasive tumors, circulatory disturbances (infarction or hemorrhage), surgery, radiation therapy, injury (head trauma), or infection. These conditions may cause either a decrease or increase in hormonal secretions. A single hormone or multiple hormones may be affected.

Anterior Pituitary Gland Dysfunction

Conditions of anterior pituitary dysfunction include growth hormone deficiency and excess.

GROWTH HORMONE DEFICIENCY

Several forms of GH deficiency can occur in children, including idiopathic and congenital. Idiopathic is the most common. Children with idiopathic GH deficiency have adequate somatotropes but inadequate GHRH (GH-releasing hormone), leading to short stature or dwarfism.

Adults with GH deficiency also fit into two categories: those who manifest GH deficiency as children, and those who develop GH deficiency in adulthood secondary to a pituitary tumor or its treatment. Aging can cause decreases in GH levels; the effects of decreasing GH levels in the elderly is being investigated. Metabolic disorders that affect mobility, energy levels and socialization, and cardiovascular mortality are all associated with GH deficiency in adults.

GROWTH HORMONE EXCESS

When GH excess occurs before puberty and the fusion of the epiphysis of the long bones, linear skeletal growth is accentuated and causes **gigantism.** Gigantism is an uncommon condition, caused by excessive secretion of GH by somatotrope adenomas. These children have normal body proportions but grow to be 7 feet or taller.

Acromegaly is the term used to describe excessive GH secretion that occurs in adulthood, after puberty and the closure of the epiphyseal plate. The most common cause of acromegaly is also somatotrope adenoma, but it can also be caused by hypothalamic or some nonendocrine tumors. Because the epiphysis of the long bones has closed, these people cannot grow taller, but soft tissues continue to grow. As a result, small bones of the feet and hands and membranous bones of the skull and face enlarge. This enlargement causes the hands and feet to grow and gives the face coarse features, such as a broadening nose, slanting forehead, and protruding jaw. All body organs are affected, leading to an enlarged heart, hypertension, accelerated atherosclerosis, peripheral neuropathies, and muscle weakness.

Posterior Pituitary Gland Dysfunction

Two major disorders that arise from posterior pituitary gland dysfunction are **diabetes insipidus** (DI) and **syndrome of inappropriate antidiuretic hormone** (SIADH). DI is caused by a deficiency in antidiuretic hormone (ADH), and SIADH is caused from excessive ADH. Most disorders of the posterior pituitary gland are secondary to lymphoma, metastatic cancer, septicemia, or disseminated intravascular coagulation (DIC).

DIABETES INSIPIDUS

Increases in plasma osmolarity or decreases in blood volume stimulate the release of ADH. ADH is produced in the kidney, causing areas of the collecting duct to become more permeable to water and allowing water reabsorption to increase. Increased water reabsorption will increase both plasma osmolarity and blood volume.

DI occurs with either a decreased response to, or a deficiency of, ADH. As a result, the person is unable to concentrate urine. This disorder is characterized by excretion of very large amounts of urine (as much as 3–20 L/day). As long as the thirst mechanism is normal and fluids are replenished, fluid levels are not altered. However, if the person with DI is unable to communicate a need for water or does not have access to fluids, hypertonic dehydration and increased serum osmolality occur. Causes of DI include head injury or surgery,

defects in the synthesis or release of ADH, or electrolyte disturbances such as hypercalcemia or hypokalemia. DI can be an acute or chronic problem.

SYNDROME OF INAPPROPRIATE ANTIDIURETIC HORMONE

Syndrome of inappropriate antidiuretic hormone (SIADH) is a condition in which ADH secretion continues, regardless of decreased serum osmolarity, which causes dilutional hyponatremia and marked water retention. It results from a failure of the negative feedback system that regulates the release and inhibition of ADH. SIADH may be chronic (secondary to tumors or CNS disorders) or acute (secondary to stress, pain, or surgery). A variety of drugs can also cause SIADH (Box 50.1). Clinical manifestations seen in SIADH (as a result of the dilutional hyponatremia) include lethargy, anorexia, muscle cramps, nausea, vomiting, seizure, coma, and death.

Thyroid Gland Dysfunction

Thyroid function alterations can occur from a hyperfunctioning or hypofunctioning gland, misfunctions that may be caused by either a congenital defect or by a problem that occurs later in life. Dramatic changes in patterns of growth and development, and in functions of the cardiovascular, respiratory, GI, neuromuscular, skeletal, and reproductive systems, can result.

An increase in the size of the thyroid gland (goiter) can occur in hyperthyroid, euthyroid, and hypothyroid states. Goiters may be toxic or nontoxic. Toxic goiters cause signs of extreme hyperthyroidism or thyrotoxicosis, described later in this section.

Hypothyroidism

Congenital **hypothyroidism** is present at birth, and acquired hypothyroidism occurs later in life as a result of either a primary or secondary disorder of the hypothalamus or pituitary gland.

Untreated congenital hypothyroidism can have devastating effects, such as mental retardation and impaired physical growth. Congenital hypothyroidism occurs from abnormal biosynthesis of thyroid hormone, deficient TSH hormone, or an absence of the thyroid gland. **Cretinism**, the term used for the condition of untreated hypothyroidism, does not apply to the normally developing infant, born with hypothyroidism, who receives thyroid hormone replacement therapy soon after birth. Fortunately, a very effective screening test for hypothyroidism is readily available. A drop of blood is taken from the infant's heel and analyzed for T_4 and TSH, and treatment can be instituted immediately if hypothyroidism is detected.

Hypothyroidism that is evident in older children and adults occurs as a result of either dysfunction or destruction of the thyroid gland (primary hypothyroidism) or of impaired hypothalamic or pituitary function (secondary hypothyroidism). Primary hypothyroidism may result from surgical removal of the thyroid gland (thyroidectomy) or from radiation, which ablates the gland. Certain drugs (e.g., lithium carbonate, used for manic depression, and propylthiouracil and methimazole, which are antithyroid drugs) can block hormone synthesis and cause hypothyroidism with a goiter. Thyroid hormone production can be blocked by drugs containing iodine (e.g., kelp tablets, radiographic contrast media, and cough syrups containing iodide). Thyroid problems are also being reported from the use of the antiarrhythmic medication amiodarone, because of its high iodine content. In the United States, the use of iodized salt and other dietary iodide sources has decreased the incidence of iodine deficiency, which causes hypothyroidism and goiter. The major cause of goiter and hypothyroidism in children and young adults is Hashimoto thyroiditis, an autoimmune disorder that damages the thyroid.

Clinical manifestations of hypothyroidism can vary widely. Subclinical hypothyroidism can cause nonspecific complaints. Overt manifestations of hypothyroidism occur as a result of decreased cellular metabolism secondary to thyroid hormone deficiency and myxedematous involvement of the body tissues. These manifestations include lethargy, hypoactive reflexes, weight gain, anxiety, impaired memory, constipation, hypotension, bradycardia, intolerance to cold, loss of hair, decreased sexual function, menstrual irregularities, infertility, edema of the hands, feet, and face, pale and rough skin, thickened tongue, and husky voice. The signs and symptoms of hypothyroidism are summarized in Table 50.2.

Hyperthyroidism

An excessive amount of thyroid hormone in the peripheral tissues results in **hyperthyroidism,** or **thyrotoxicosis.** Patients with hyperthyroidism exhibit signs and symptoms of overactive cellular metabolism of all body systems; tachycardia, palpitations, hypertension, increased body temperature, heat intolerance, weight loss, amenorrhea, and goiter. These manifestations result from increased oxygen consumption and increased sympathetic nervous system activity. Graves disease, the most common cause of hyperthyroidism, is accompanied by goiter and exophthalmos (bulging of the eyeballs). Other causes of hyperthyroidism include thyroid gland adenoma, multinodular goiter, and ingestion of excessive thyroid hormone.

Graves disease is an autoimmune disorder that arises from sustained overactivity of the thyroid gland, caused by thyroid-stimulating antibodies and growth of the entire thyroid gland (goiter). Infiltrative ophthalmopathy (exophthalmos) occurs in as many as 50% of all patients with Graves disease, and skin lesions (dermopathy) are also common.

BOX 50.1 Drugs That May Cause Syndrome of Inappropriate Antidiuretic Hormone Secretion (SIADH)

- carbamazepine (Tegretol)
- chlorpropamide (Diabinese)
- clofibrate (Atromid S)
- cyclophosphamide (Cytoxan)
- isoproterenol (Isuprel)
- morphine
- oxytocin (Pitocin)
- phenothiazines
- prostaglandins
- thiazide diuretics
- tricyclic antidepressants
- vasopressin
- vincristine (Oncovin)

TABLE 50.2 Clinical Comparison of Hypothyroidism and Hyperthyroidism

Body System	Clinical Picture of Hypothyroidism	Clinical Picture of Hyperthyroidism
Central nervous system	General slowing of mental processes Lethargy Neuropathies	Emotional lability Hyperkinesia Nervousness
Cardiovascular system	Decreased peripheral vascular resistance, heart rate, stroke volume, cardiac output, pulse pressure ECG changes: bradycardia, increased PR interval, flat T wave, low voltage Low-output congestive heart failure Pericardial effusion	Increased peripheral vascular resistance, heart rate, stroke volume, cardiac output, pulse pressure High-output congestive heart failure Increased inotropic and chronotropic effects Angina Arrhythmias
EENT	Enlarged tongue Eyelid drooping Periorbital edema Puffy, nonpitting face	Diplopia (Graves disease) Exophthalmos (Graves disease) Periorbital edema Retraction of upper lid with wide stare
Gastrointestinal system	Decreased appetite Decreased frequency of bowel movements Ascites	Increased appetite Increased frequency of bowel movements Hypoproteinemia
Hematopoietic system	Decreased erythropoiesis Anemia	Increased erythropoiesis Anemia
Metabolic system	Decreased basal metabolic rate with slight positive nitrogen balance Delayed degradation of insulin with increased insulin sensitivity Increased cholesterol and triglycerides Decreased hormone degradation Decreased requirements for fat- and water-soluble vitamins Decreased drug detoxification	Increased basal metabolic rate with negative nitrogen balance Hyperglycemia Increased free fatty acids Decreased cholesterol and triglycerides Increased hormone degradation Increased requirements for fat- and water-soluble vitamins Increased drug detoxification
Musculoskeletal system	Stiffness and muscle fatigue Decreased deep tendon reflexes Increased alkaline phosphatase, LDH, AST	Weakness and muscle fatigue Increased deep tendon reflexes Hypercalcemia Osteoporosis
Renal system	Impaired water excretion Decreased renal blood flow Decreased glomerular filtration rate	Mild polyuria Increased renal blood flow Increased glomerular filtration rate
Reproductive system	Hypermenorrhea infertility* decreased libido* Men: impotency, oligospermia decreased gonadal steroid metabolism*	Women: menstrual irregularities decreased fertility, decreased gonadal steroid metabolism*
Respiratory	Pleural effusions Hypoventilation Hypercarbia	Dyspnea Decreased vital capacity
Skin	Pale, cool, puffy skin (myxedema) Dry, brittle hair Brittle nails Cold intolerance	Warm, moist, diaphoretic skin Fine, thin hair Heat intolerance

*Both men and women

Patients with exophthalmos appear to have protruding eyes. Even with treatment, once exophthalmos exists, it remains essentially unchanged. Vision loss (secondary to involvement of the optic nerve) and corneal ulceration (secondary to the eyelids not closing tightly) also occur.

An extreme, life-threatening form of thyrotoxicosis is called **thyroid crisis** (also known as thyroid storm). It is seen in patients who are not adequately treated for their hyperthyroidism or who are undiagnosed. Thyroid crisis is frequently precipitated by infection (usually respiratory), diabetic ketoacidosis, stress, manipulation of a hyperactive thyroid gland during thyroidectomy, or emotional or physical trauma. Manifestations of thyroid crisis include severe CNS effects (e.g., restlessness, agitation, or delir-

ium), extreme cardiovascular effects (e.g., angina, heart failure, or tachycardia), and high fever. Treatment must be implemented immediately; it includes administration of methimazole (MMI), beta blockers, corticosteroids, fluids and electrolytes, measures to control hyperthermia, and oxygen.

Parathyroid Gland Dysfunction

PTH is secreted by the parathyroid glands. This hormone is a major regulator of serum calcium and phosphate. A decrease in serum calcium concentration is the dominant regulator of PTH, with a response rate of just a few seconds. A decrease in phosphate causes an indirect effect on PTH by combining with calcium and decreasing serum calcium concentrations. Magnesium also affects the secretion, synthesis, and action of PTH; severe and prolonged hypomagnesemia can have a marked effect on the inhibition of PTH levels. Hypocalcemia can cause tetany, convulsions, muscle spasm, and neuromuscular excitability. Hypercalcemia has been associated with life-threatening cardiac dysrhythmias, CNS abnormalities, renal damage, and soft tissue calcification. For these reasons, maintaining calcium at the desired level is important. Table 50.3 summarizes disorders of bone and calcium metabolism.

Hypoparathyroidism

Hypoparathyroidism (inadequate PTH levels) can be either inherited or acquired. This condition is characterized by hypocalcemia and frequently by hypophosphatemia. As stated previously, hypocalcemia can cause tetany, convulsions, muscle spasm, and neuromuscular excitability. Acquired hypoparathyroidism occurs most commonly as a result of surgery in the neck, but this adverse outcome has become less common with the advent of improved surgical techniques and the increased use of nonsurgical therapy. Lack of PTH can cause vitamin D deficiency, leading to osteomalacia in adults and rickets in children.

Hyperparathyroidism

Hypersecretion of PTH leads to hyperparathyroidism. Primary hyperparathyroidism is most common in women older than 50 years and is caused by an adenoma, a carcinoma of the parathyroid gland, or hyperplasia. Hyperparathyroidism causes excessive levels of calcium in both serum (hypercalcemia) and urine (hypercalciuria). Urine phosphate levels are also high, and serum phosphate levels are normal to low. Potential complications of these imbalances include nervous system complaints, pancreatitis, peptic ulcers, kidney stones, severe osteoporosis and osteopenia, and pathologic bone fractures. These complications can be remembered by the rhyme, "moans, groans, stones, and bones." Secondary hyperparathyroidism occurs primarily in persons with renal failure, but it can also occur with multiple myeloma, bone metastasis, and Paget disease. Regardless of the cause, hyperparathyroidism is characterized by deposits of calcium salts in body tissues and bone decalcification. In primary hyperparathyroidism, the severity of hypercalcemia reflects the quantity of hyperfunctioning tissue. Excessive quantities of PTH stimulate transport of calcium into the serum from the kidneys, bones, and intestines. Nephrolithiasis (formation of kidney stones) can occur secondary to calcium deposits in the soft tissues of the kidney.

The influence of PTH on the cells of the bones is very strong and causes them to release calcium into the serum. Under normal conditions, the amount of calcium in the bones remains at a constant level, but in the presence of too much PTH, the bones release their calcium into the bloodstream at a high rate, resulting in osteopenia and osteoporosis (Figure 50.3). PTH also influences the lining of the intestine to absorb more calcium from the diet (Table 50.4).

Secondary hyperparathyroidism is caused most often by corticotropin-releasing factor and hyperphosphatemia. There is an inverse relationship between the glomerular filtration rate and serum phosphate levels: as the glomerular filtration rate decreases, serum phosphate levels increase. In turn, this increase decreases serum calcium levels, and this drop then stimulates secretion of PTH.

TABLE 50.3 Disorders of Bone and Calcium Metabolism

Disorder	Examples	Management
Hypocalcemia	• Inadequate dietary intake of Ca++ and/or vitamin D • Malabsorption caused by vitamin D lack or end-organ resistance • Hypoparathyroidism, pseudohypoparathyroidism • Renal failure	• Treatment with calcium and vitamin D compounds
Hypercalcemia	• Hyperparathyroidism • Hypervitaminosis D • Neoplasia • Hyperthyroidism • Immobilization	• Treatment with fluids, low calcium diet, calcitonin, bisphosphonates, glucocorticoids, loop diuretics
Impaired bone remodeling	• Osteoporosis	• Treatment with bisphosphonates, calcitonin, calcium, estrogen (female)

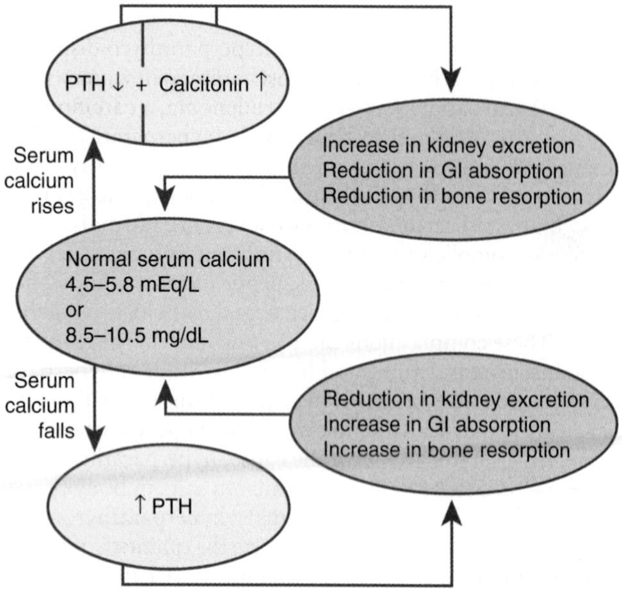

FIGURE 50.3 Regulation of serum calcium. Parathyroid hormone (PTH) and calcitonin regulate normal serum calcium. As serum calcium rises, PTH is inhibited by calcitonin. The kidney then excretes more calcium, the GI system absorbs less, and a reduction in bone resorption occurs. As serum calcium falls, PTH is secreted and raises the calcium level by decreasing the amount of calcium lost in the kidney, increasing the amount absorbed in the GI tract, and increasing bone resorption.

As the serum calcium level rises, neuromuscular irritability decreases, because of the sedative effect of serum calcium on the body. Hypercalcemia is commonly associated with hyperparathyroidism, but it can also occur secondary to neoplastic disease or immobilization, during which movement of calcium out of the bones increases. Renal failure also decreases renal excretion of calcium and thus also leads to hypercalcemia.

Ⓒ PITUITARY DRUGS

The primary effects of drugs used to affect pituitary function are to either mimic or antagonize the pituitary hormone. GH, somatostatin, ADH, and oxytocin are the most frequently used drugs. Table 50.5 presents a summary of selected pituitary drugs.

Ⓒ Growth Hormones

Growth hormone deficiency, leading to short stature, was initially treated with GH injections that were extracted from the pituitary glands of cadavers. Because cadavers were the only source, the availability of the treatment was limited. Additionally, several cases of Creutzfeldt-Jakob disease (a neurologic disturbance that progresses to coma and death, caused by encephalopathy) secondary to an infectious agent in the GH put an end to this practice. Presently, synthetic human GH (rhGH), produced from recombinant DNA, is available. Although rhGH therapy is very expensive, it has been shown to be effective in treating children and adolescents with GH deficiencies. Somatropin (Humatrope) is the prototype rGH discussed in this chapter.

NURSING MANAGEMENT OF THE PATIENT RECEIVING [P] SOMATROPIN

Core Drug Knowledge

Pharmacotherapeutics

Somatropin is a recombinant DNA formulation of GH (rGH) that has an amino acid sequence identical to that of pituitary-derived GH. It is used as long-term replacement therapy for children who have a growth failure because of inadequate endogenous GH secretion and for those with short stature

TABLE 50.4 Actions of Parathyroid Hormone (PTH) and Vitamin D

	PTH	Vitamin D (and metabolites)
Bone	• High doses—calcium and phosphate resorption increased • Low doses—may increase bone formation	• Increased calcium and phosphate resorption by calcitriol • Increased bone formation
Kidney	• Decreased calcium excretion • Increased phosphate excretion	• Calcium and phosphate excretion may be decreased by calciferol and calcitriol
Intestine	• Increased calcium and phosphate absorption by increased calcitriol production	• Increased calcium and phosphate absorption by calcitriol
Effect on serum levels	Serum calcium is increased and serum phosphate is decreased	Serum calcium and serum phosphate are both increased

TABLE 50.5 Summary of Selected (C) Pituitary Drugs

Drug (Trade) Name	Selected Indications	Route and Dosage Range
(C) Growth Hormones		
[P] somatropin (Genotropin)	Treatment of growth failure from growth-hormone deficiency or chronic renal failure (prior to transplant)	SC, 0.16 to 0.24 mg/kg/wk 6–7 × /wk
Humatrope,		*Child:* SC or IM, 0.18 mg/kg/wk 3 or 6 × /wk
Norditropin,		SC, 0.024–0.034 mg/kg 6–7 × /wk
Saizen		SC or IM, 0.06 mg/kg 3 × /wk
Nutropin	Turner syndrome	SC, ≤ 0.375 mg/kg/wk
Serostim	AIDS wasting syndrome	SC, ≈ 0.1 mg/kg/d
somatrem (Protropin)	Treatment (long-term) of growth failure in children	*Child:* IM, up to 0.1 mg/kg 3qwk Dosage is based on individual response
	Short stature of Turner's syndrome (orphan use)	*Child:* IM, <0.1 mg/kg 3 ×/wk
Growth Hormone Antagonists		
octreotide acetate (Sandostatin)	Acromegaly (reduce growth hormone levels) Severe diarrhea	*Adult:* SC, 50–600 µg bid–qid *Child:* safety and efficacy not established
bromocriptine mesylate (Parlodel)	Acromegaly	*Adult:* PO, 1.25–30 mg/d
	Parkinson disease (idiopathic)	*Adult:* PO, 2.5–100 mg/d; efficacy for >2 yr not established
	Suppression of physiologic lactation following parturition	*Adult:* PO, 2.5 mg bid × 14–21 d
	Hyperprolactinemia	*Adult:* PO, 5–10 mg/d
(C) Posterior Pituitary Hormone Regulators		
[P] desmopressin (DDAVP, Stimate*)	Neurogenic diabetes insipidus	*Adult:* Intranasal, 0.1–0.4 mL/d qd or bid; 1 spray (300 mg)/nostril; SC, IV—0.5–1.0 mL/d bid PO—0.05 mg bid *Child 3 mo-12 y:* Intranasal—0.05–0.3 mL/d qd or bid; 1 spray (300 mg)/nostril; SC, IV—0.5–1.0 ml/d bid; PO—0.05 mg bid (*Dosage adjusted according to water turnover pattern*)
	Primary nocturnal enuresis	*Adult and child >6 y:* Intranasal 20–40 µg hs:
	Hemophilia A (with factor VIII >5%) von Willebrand's disease	*Adult and child:* IV, 0.3 µg/kg (*Repeated administration based on patient response*)
vasopressin (Pitressin)	Neurogenic diabetes insipidus	*Adult:* IM, SC, intranasal; 5–10 U repeated bid to tid
	Abdominal distention	*Adult:* IM, 5–10 U repeated q3–4 H intervals
	Antiflatulent effect for abdominal roentgenography	*Adult:* IM, SC, 10 U at 2 h and 10 U at ½ hr before procedure *Child:* decrease dosage proportionately
lypressin (Diapid)	Neurogenic diabetes insipidus	*Adult:* Intranasal, 1–2 sprays qid in one or both nostrils (*Dosage dependent on urination or significant thirst*)

*Used for hematological effects only

caused by Turner syndrome. Somatropin stimulates linear growth in patients who lack adequate endogenous growth hormone, resulting in an increase in skeletal growth.

Pharmacokinetics

Somatropin is well absorbed and distributed. The absolute bioavailability of somatropin is 75% and 63% after subcutaneous (SC) and intramuscular (IM) administration, respectively. GH localizes to the liver and kidney. It is filtered by the glomerulus in the kidney, reabsorbed in the proximal tubule, and broken down within renal cells into amino acids. A portion of the breakdown products is returned to the systemic circulation. Intravenous (IV) somatropin has a mean half-life of 0.36 hours, whereas SC- and IM-administered somatropin doses have mean half-lives of 3.8 and 4.9 hours, respectively. The longer half-life of SC and IM administration is attribut-

able to slower absorption from the injection site. The liver and kidney are the major elimination organs for exogenously administered GH. Caution must be used in administering somatropin to patients with severe hepatic and renal function because reduced clearance will occur.

Pharmacodynamics

Treatment with GH has powerful effects on growth and metabolism. It stimulates cell growth and cellular mitosis, facilitates cellular uptake of amino acids for protein synthesis, and promotes use of fatty acids for energy. These effects are caused indirectly by an increase in insulin-like growth factor-1 (IGF-1), an intermediary peptide. In vitro and clinical testing has demonstrated that somatropin is equivalent therapeutically to GH of pituitary origin in adults.

Contraindications and Precautions

Somatropin should not be used to promote growth in children with closed epiphyses. Pediatric patients with endocrine disorders, including growth hormone deficiency, are more likely to develop slipped-capital epiphysis. For this reason, if a pediatric patient taking GH begins to limp, the limp must be evaluated. Patients with a history of scoliosis who are being treated with GH are at elevated risk for developing more severe scoliosis, which occurs more frequently if rapid growth occurs. Patients with Turner syndrome have an increased risk for otitis media or hearing disorders. They are also at a greater risk for developing cardiovascular disorders (aortic aneurysm, stroke, and hypertension). Somatropin is in FDA pregnancy category C. It should be given only when clearly needed because it is not known whether it can cause fetal harm or is excreted in breast milk. It also is contraindicated in patients who have evidence of intracranial tumors because tumor growth rate may increase. Cautious use also is advised in diabetic patients because insulin resistance resulting in hyperglycemia may develop. Some product formulations contain diluent preservatives that may cause hypersensitivity.

Adverse Effects

Adverse effects with high-dose somatropin include headache, hypertension, joint and back pain, peripheral edema, muscle aches, and rhinitis. Many of these adverse effects occur initially and then resolve spontaneously or in response to dosage adjustments. Others include hypothyroidism, hyperglycemia, glycosuria, and pain at the injection site. Recurrent growth of intracranial tumor also may occur. Leukemia has occurred in a small number of children receiving somatropin or somatrem, but its relation to therapy is uncertain.

A small percentage of patients (approximately 2%) may develop antibodies to the rGH protein molecule. However, GH antibody–binding capacities (2 mg/L) have not been associated with any growth reduction.

Drug Interactions

GH reduces the activity of hepatic mixed-function oxidases. This reduction may alter drug metabolism. Glucocorticoid or other corticosteroid therapy may inhibit the growth-promoting effect of rGH. Patients with coexisting ACTH deficiency may need their glucocorticoid replacement dosages adjusted carefully to avoid an inhibitory effect on growth. Therefore, patients should be monitored closely if this combination must be used. Use of somatropin with anabolic steroids, androgens, estrogens, or thyroid hormones may accelerate epiphyseal maturation.

Assessment of Relevant Core Patient Variables

Health Status

Before administering somatropin, review the patient's record to determine whether it can be administered safely. A physical assessment will establish baseline data from which to monitor the effects of the drug. This assessment should include height and weight measurements, bone age determinations, thyroid function tests, glucose tolerance tests, and levels of GH. These data must be monitored and reviewed periodically during treatment. If the growth rate does not meet or exceed the pretreatment rate by at least 2 cm per year, nonadherence to therapy, antibody formation, malnutrition, or hypothyroidism must be considered as possible causes. X-rays of the hip and funduscopic examination are recommended before starting and periodically during the course of GH therapy.

Patients with diabetes or glucose intolerance should be observed closely during somatropin therapy. Individuals with GH deficiency secondary to an intracranial lesion should be evaluated regularly for progression or recurrence of the underlying disease process. Individuals should be assessed routinely for any malignant transformation of skin lesions. Those with growth failure secondary to chronic renal insufficiency should be monitored regularly for progression of renal osteodystrophy progression because slipped-capital femoral epiphysis or avascular necrosis of the femoral head may be seen in children with advanced renal osteodystrophy. Whether these problems are affected by GH therapy is uncertain. Examine the injection site for pain and swelling.

Life Span and Gender

It is important to assess whether the patient is pregnant or breast-feeding. Somatropin is classified in pregnancy category C and should only be given to a pregnant or lactating woman if use is clearly indicated. It is not known whether somatropin is excreted in breast milk. Available data suggest that rGH clearances are similar in adults and children. Treatment with GH requires a long-term regimen. Children receiving this drug will need continual monitoring, and once therapy has begun, the patient's height and weight should be measured and recorded at regular intervals.

Lifestyle, Diet, and Habits

Adherence to the drug regimen is imperative; therefore, evaluating the patient's ability and willingness to adhere is important. Actual somatropin dosage is individualized to each patient. SC injections each evening are most effective because nightly injections mimic the natural hormone surge that occurs after sleep. Stimulation of growth is most effective when treatment begins early and injections are continued until the epiphyses close. Response to treatment tends to decrease with time.

Environment

It is important to assess the setting in which somatropin will be administered, the ability of the patient or caregiver to administer the drug properly, and the patient's and family's financial situation. Most often, the patient or caregiver is

instructed in the proper way to reconstitute and administer the medication according to the manufacturer's instructions because it is frequently given in the home. They also need to be instructed to refrigerate the drug following reconstitution. The drug is very expensive, and some insurance companies resist covering the cost of treatment. In such cases, sources of financial support may have to be solicited. Health care visits are decreased if parents or caregivers administer the injections, but regular visits to the physician must still occur to monitor blood and urine samples, make bone age determinations, and track growth rate. Regular follow-up health care is necessary.

Nursing Diagnoses and Outcomes

- Delayed Growth and Development related to deficiency of GH secretion
  Desired outcome: *The patient will demonstrate an increase in linear growth.*
- Imbalanced Nutrition: More (or Less) than Body Requirements related to endocrine changes and rapid changes in height and weight
  Desired outcome: *The patient will receive adequate nutrition for growth appropriate to age and need.*
- Impaired Tissue Integrity related to pain and swelling at injection site
  Desired outcome: *The patient will not experience pain and swelling at the injection site.*
- Altered Comfort related to headache, joint, and muscle discomfort secondary to somatropin effects
  Desired outcome: *The patient will describe measures to improve comfort.*

Planning and Intervention

Maximizing Therapeutic Effects

Hypothyroidism may develop during somatropin therapy and, if untreated, may prevent an optimal response. For this reason, periodic thyroid function tests must be performed, and thyroid hormone replacement therapy should be initiated if indicated. Glucocorticoid replacement dosage must be carefully adjusted in patients with coexisting ACTH deficiency to avoid an inhibitory effect on growth. Patients taking somatropin who require dialysis in a daytime ambulatory setting should take their doses before bedtime. Patients who require chronic cycling peritoneal dialysis should receive their doses of somatropin in the morning, after the dialysis is completed.

Minimizing Adverse Effects

GH therapy may induce insulin resistance; thus, monitoring the patient closely for glucose intolerance is important. Children being treated with rGH for growth failure secondary to chronic renal insufficiency may develop problems of renal osteodystrophy (generalized bone changes resembling osteomalacia and rickets). Slipped-capital femoral epiphyses or avascular necrosis of the femoral head can also occur in these patients. Although it is uncertain whether these problems are a direct result of GH therapy, x-rays of the hip should be obtained before initiating GH therapy. Health care providers and parents should be alert for the development of a limp or complaints of hip or knee pain. Slipped-capital femoral epiphysis may occur more frequently in patients with endocrine disorders or in patients undergoing rapid growth. Pain and discomfort related to headache, bone, and muscle discomfort can be treated with appropriate analgesics and environmental controls.

Sudden growth spurts and changes in growth and development, coupled with potential thyroid changes and insulin resistance, may cause nutritional imbalance that can complicate the desired effect of the GH. Consider nutritional assessment and appropriate replacement of necessary nutrients.

Providing Patient and Family Education

- Explain that this drug is replacing an important hormone (GH) that is necessary for normal growth and development.
- Explain to patients and their families that the drug can be given only by injection. Teach patients, family members, or caregivers how to reconstitute and administer the drug. Review injection site rotation to maximize therapeutic effect and avoid problems of lipodystrophy. Periodic review of injection technique is important to ensure effectiveness and decrease adverse effects.
- Instruct patients to refrigerate the reconstituted solution. Vials are stable for up to 14 days if reconstituted with diluent or bacteriostatic water for injection. If sterile water is used, only one dose of somatropin can be used, and the unused portion must be discarded.
- Diabetic patients must be alerted to the fact that insulin resistance may develop. Instruct these patients to monitor blood sugar closely and to report variations to their health care team.
- Instruct patients or their families to report any adverse drug effects and emphasize the importance of reporting a limp or any hip or knee pain as soon as possible. Slipped-capital femoral epiphysis may occur more frequently in patients with endocrine disorders or in patients undergoing rapid growth.

Ongoing Assessment and Evaluation

Evaluate thyroid function at regular intervals because hypothyroidism will compromise rGH drug effects. Additionally, it is important to be alert for signs of glucose intolerance because insulin resistance may develop and disrupt diabetes control. As with all protein pharmaceuticals, a small percentage of patients may develop antibodies to the protein. Evaluate adherence to the prescribed treatment program, assess thyroid status, and test for GH antibodies in any patient who fails to respond to therapy. Stress the importance of follow-up appointments and periodic analysis of thyroid function, glucose tolerance, and GH levels to evaluate the effectiveness of the drug and possible development of adverse effects. Therapy is considered effective when anticipated growth occurs. The patient and family should demonstrate appropriate drug administration technique, acknowledge the importance of monitoring for adverse effects, and show understanding of when to report findings to the health care team (Box 50.2).

Drugs Closely Related to P Somatropin

Commercially available drug preparations of somatropin include Genotropin, Humatrope, Norditropin, Nutropin, Saizen, and Serostim. All are powders that need reconstitu-

COMMUNITY-BASED CONCERNS

Box 50.2 Children Receiving Growth Hormone (somatropin)

As a nurse educating patients and families about the use of growth hormone (GH) therapy, you should include the following information:

- GH is indicated for children with inadequate endogenous GH secretion and for those with short stature caused by Turner syndrome.
- GH is not clearly indicated for children who are born to a short family but whose parents want them to be taller.
- GH is not indicated for children with closed epiphyses.
- GH therapy requires long-term commitment from the patient; treatment generally lasts 3 to 9 years.
- Although GH may be covered in part by insurance, the cost of treatment can be as much as $50,000 annually.
- GH is given as a daily SC injection, usually in the evening, because this timing mimics the natural hormone surge that occurs after sleep.
- Parents or other caregivers are taught how to administer the injections, but regular physician visits are mandatory during treatment to monitor bone age determinations, growth rate, and blood and urine samples.
- Insulin resistance may develop in a diabetic patient taking GH; therefore, blood sugar in these patients must be closely monitored.

tion, with the exception of Nutropin AQ. They differ in the amounts of rGH IU (international units) contained in the vial, whether vials are single or multiple dose, and what diluents are used (some diluents are preservative free).

Humatrope's new indication for short stature (FDA approved in 2003) is the first indication in children that specifies a height restriction. The American Association of Clinical Endocrinologists and Growth Hormone Research Society define short stature as height more than 2 standard deviations (SD) below the mean for sex and age. The indication for this medication is for those more than 2.25 SD below the mean for sex and age. To ensure appropriate use of this medication, marketing of this product for this new pediatric use is limited to pediatric endocrinologists.

Nutropin is indicated for long-term treatment of growth failure stemming from inadequate endogenous GH secretion, for growth failure associated with renal insufficiency (until renal transplant), and for short stature related to the chromosomal disorder, Turner syndrome. This syndrome exclusively affects females and is characterized in part by short stature and incomplete sexual development.

Serostim is indicated for concomitant use with antiviral therapy for human immunodeficiency virus (HIV)-associated cachexia (wasting syndrome), to increase lean muscle mass and body weight. Serostim is in FDA pregnancy category B.

Somatrem (Protropin) is an artificial human GH with therapeutic effects very similar to those of somatropin. Its chemical structure differs from that of somatropin by one additional amino acid. Approximately 30% to 40% of all somatrem-treated individuals develop persistent antibodies to GH. Other adverse effects include decrease in thyroid function and insulin resistance.

MEMORY CHIP

P Somatropin

- Genetically engineered (recombinant DNA) human growth hormone used for long-term treatment of children with deficient endogenous growth hormone
- Major contraindications: closed epiphyses and cranial lesions
- Most common adverse effects: joint and muscle pain
- Most serious adverse effects: development of antibodies to growth hormone, hypothyroidism, and insulin resistance
- Maximizing therapeutic effects: Reconstitute drug according to manufacturer's directions.
- Minimizing adverse effects: periodic testing of glucose tolerance, thyroid function, and presence of growth hormone antibodies
- Most important patient education: proper preparation and storage of medication; proper SC or IM injection technique

Drugs Significantly Different From P Somatropin

Growth hormone antagonists decrease GH secretion. Almost all conditions of GH hypersecretion are caused by pituitary tumors and are usually treated by radiation therapy or surgery. Pharmacotherapy for GH excess includes two groups of drugs: the somatostatin analogues (octreotide acetate) and the dopamine agonists (bromocriptine) (see Table 50.5). Hypothalamic somatostatin (from the hypothalamus) is an effective GH inhibitor, but it is rarely used because of its short initial half-life (1 to 3 minutes) and its multiple effects on many secretory systems (e.g., it inhibits the release of gastrin, glucagon, insulin).

Octreotide Acetate

Octreotide acetate (Sandostatin) is a more potent inhibitor than somatostatin of growth hormone, insulin, and glucagon. It also suppresses LH (luteinizing hormone) response to GnRH (gonadotropin-releasing factor) and secretion of TSH (thyroid-stimulating hormone). Sandostatin is highly effective in treating both children and adults with excess GH, and it has replaced bromocriptine as the most commonly used agent for acromegaly. It is indicated to reduce growth hormone blood levels and IGF-1 (somatomedin C) levels in patients with acromegaly, who either cannot be treated surgically or who have an inadequate response to surgery or irradiation of the pituitary.

Other indications include treating symptoms associated with metastatic carcinoid tumors (diarrhea and flushing) and vasoactive intestinal peptide (VIP) secreting adenomas (watery diarrhea) as well as esophageal varices. In single doses, Sandostatin has been shown to decrease bile secretion and to inhibit gallbladder contractility.

Off-label uses include acquired immunodeficiency syndrome (AIDS)-associated diarrhea, breast cancer, insulinomas, small bowel fistulas, Cushing syndrome, dumping syndrome after gastrectomy, and graft-versus-host disease (GVHD)-induced diarrhea.

The elimination of octreotide from the plasma has a half-life of 1.7 hours, with approximately 32% of the dose

excreted unchanged in the urine. Because of a significant increase in the half-life of the drug (46%) and a significant decrease in clearance (26%) during clinical trials in elderly patients, dose adjustment may be necessary in these patients. In patients with severe renal failure requiring dialysis, octreotide half-life is increased, which also necessitates adjusting the maintenance dose.

Individuals with acromegaly may experience either hypoglycemia (3%) or hyperglycemia (16%) during therapy. This effect may result in overt diabetes mellitus or require dosage changes for insulin or other hypoglycemic agents.

Side effects of GI discomfort (diarrhea, loose stools, abdominal discomfort, and nausea), headache, sinus bradycardia or other cardiac arrhythmias, and decreased glucose tolerance may also occur. Octreotide therapy may cause acute cholecystitis, cholestatic jaundice, biliary tract obstruction, or pancreatitis. More frequently, it causes cholelithiasis in patients requiring therapy for 12 months or more. Dietary fat absorption may be altered in some patients. Periodic fecal fat and serum carotene determinations should be performed to help assess possible drug-induced fat malabsorption. It is important to stress the importance of reporting icterus (jaundice), dark urine, or clay-colored stools to the health care team immediately, as well as any abdominal pain, edema, chest pain, shortness of breath, or fainting.

When octreotide is administered concomitantly with cyclosporine, it may decrease blood levels of cyclosporine and cause rejection of transplanted organs. Octreotide is associated with alterations in nutrient absorption and may have an effect on oral medications. Drug and food interactions include altered absorption of dietary fats, decreased vitamin B_{12} levels, and abnormal Schilling test results. (The Schilling test is done to diagnose pernicious anemia).

For prolonged storage, unused drug should be protected from light and stored in the refrigerator. If refrigerated, the solution should be allowed to warm to room temperature before administration. At room temperature, octreotide is stable for 14 days if protected from light. Octreotide is usually administered subcutaneously but can also be delivered through a continuous subcutaneous infusion. Because it is most often given subcutaneously, teach the patient and family details of sterile technique, injection-site rotation, and signs of infection for which to watch. The patient receiving octreotide therapy will require long-term follow-up and regular evaluation for signs of acromegaly and other endocrine dysfunction (e.g., thyroid or insulin resistance), which may require dosage adjustment. Emphasize the importance of regular follow-up visits with the health care provider. Responsiveness to octreotide therapy may be evaluated by assessing GH and IGF-1 serum levels (Box 50.3).

FOCUS ON RESEARCH

Box 50.3 Octreotide for Acromegaly

National Institute of Diabetes and Digestive and Kidney Diseases (NIDDK). Sandostatin LAR Depot vs. Surgery for Treating Acromegaly.

The Study

The purpose of this study was to compare the efficacy of Sandostatin LAR Depot (octreotide) to transsphenoidal surgery in previously untreated acromegalic patients with macroadenomas. The primary goal was to normalize insulin-like growth factor-1 (IGF-1) levels. Secondary goals were to compare the effectiveness of Sandostatin LAR Depot treatment and transsphenoidal surgery in suppressing growth hormone (GH) levels to 2.5 ng/mL or less, relieving the clinical signs and symptoms of acromegaly, reducing the size of the macroadenomas, and producing few side effects. The researchers also assessed the prognostic value of baseline pituitary adenoma size, extension, and baseline growth hormone level on posttreatment growth hormone and IGF-1 levels, and assessed the resource use of each treatment type.

More information about the study can be obtained at *http://clinicalstudies.info.nih.gov.*

Nursing Implications

1. The goal of treatment in acromegaly is to reduce GH and IGF-I levels to normal.
2. Sandostatin LAR Depot can be used in patients for whom surgical resection is not an option.
3. In patients with acromegaly, octreotide reduces GH to within normal ranges in 50% of patients and reduces IGF-I to within normal ranges in 50% to 60% of patients. Because the effects of pituitary irradiation may not become maximal for several years, adjunctive therapy with octreotide to reduce blood levels of growth hormone and IGF-I offers potential benefit before the effects of irradiation are manifested.
4. Octreotide suppresses secretion of thyroid-stimulating hormone; patients may develop a hypothyroid state. Baseline and periodic assessment of thyroid function (TSH total or free T4) is recommended during chronic therapy.
5. Octreotide inhibits gallbladder contractility and decreases bile secretion; the incidence of gallstone or biliary sludge formation is markedly increased.

Bromocriptine Mesylate

Bromocriptine mesylate (Parlodel) is a semisynthetic ergot alkaloid that inhibits prolactin secretion. In acromegaly, it also lowers elevated blood levels of GH, with varying efficacy. It can be used alone or as an adjunct to irradiation. In some children, bromocriptine and octreotide used in combination have proved successful. Bromocriptine, a dopamine agonist, is also used to treat Parkinson disease. Dopamine agonists inhibit GH secretion in some patients with acromegaly, although the opposite effect occurs in healthy individuals. Dopamine increases somatostatin release from the hypothalamus. This effect may explain the GH-inhibiting properties of bromocriptine. Off-label uses for bromocriptine include treating hyperprolactinemia associated with pituitary adenomas, neuroleptic malignant syndrome, cocaine addiction, and cyclical mastalgia (pain in the breast). Bromocriptine is administered orally. It has a substantial hepatic first-pass effect; 28% of an oral dose is absorbed from the GI tract. Bromocriptine undergoes first-pass metabolism, and only a small percentage (6%) of the absorbed dose reaches the systemic circulation unchanged. Plasma half-life is 6 to 8 hours. Bromocriptine is highly bound (90%–96%) to serum albumin and is metabolized in the liver before being excreted in the feces and urine. Contraindications for bromocriptine include sensitivity to ergot alkaloids, severe ischemic heart disease, or peripheral vascular disease. Safe use of bromocriptine has not been

demonstrated in pregnancy, and use in pregnancy is contraindicated. If pregnancy occurs, treatment should be discontinued immediately.

Lanreotide and Pegvisomant

Two new agents recently approved for treating acromegaly include lanreotide and pegvisomant. Lanreotide is a sustained-release formulation of a somatostatin analogue. It is administered intramuscularly every 2 weeks and is both safe and effective in treating adults with acromegaly. Preliminary evidence suggests it is also effective for use in children, but it has not yet been approved for this use. Pegvisomant is a genetically engineered GH receptor antagonist that has selective affinity for the GH receptor. It reduces IGF-1 levels and improves the clinical symptoms of GH excess. It is given as a subcutaneous injection once a day.

(C) Posterior Pituitary Hormone Regulators

The posterior pituitary stores two hormones that are produced in the hypothalamus: vasopressin (also known as ADH), which controls the concentration of body fluids; and oxytocin, which stimulates uterine contractions and causes the milk let-down reflex.

Desmopressin, vasopressin, lypressin, and terlipressin are synthetic analogues of the naturally occurring posterior pituitary hormone, vasopressin, that are used to treat DI (diabetes insipidus). In pharmacologic doses, oxytocin can be used to induce or improve uterine contractions during labor. The prototype posterior pituitary hormone is desmopressin acetate. It is the preferred treatment for most individuals with chronic DI because it has a longer duration of action, a more specific antidiuretic action, and an antidiuretic-to-pressor ratio significantly greater than that of vasopressin.

NURSING MANAGEMENT OF THE PATIENT RECEIVING [P] DESMOPRESSIN

Core Drug Knowledge

Pharmacotherapeutics

Desmopressin (DDAVP, Stimate) may be administered intranasally, orally, or parenterally (IV or SC) to manage central DI. Primary nocturnal enuresis and episodes of spontaneous or trauma-induced bleeding are also effectively managed with intranasal desmopressin. Parenteral desmopressin maintains homeostasis in hemophilia A and von Willebrand disease (type I) during the intraoperative and postoperative periods when administered 2 hours before the procedure (see Table 50.5). It is ineffective for treating nephrogenic DI.

An off-label use for intranasal desmopressin is treating chronic autonomic failure characterized by nocturnal polyuria, morning postural hypotension, and overnight weight loss. Individualized dosage is necessary to maintain normal urine volume.

Pharmacokinetics

Desmopressin provides prompt onset of antidiuretic action with a long duration after administration because it has a biphasic half-life of 7.8 and 75.5 minutes for the fast and slow phases, respectively. The injectable form has an antidiuretic effect 10 times that of an equivalent dose of intranasal desmopressin. The half-life of the nasal spray is approximately 3.5 hours. Plasma concentrations of the nasal spray are highest 40 to 45 minutes after dosing. Desmopressin is metabolized rapidly by the liver and excreted by the kidneys.

Pharmacodynamics

The naturally occurring posterior pituitary hormone, vasopressin (ADH), and its synthetic analogues (desmopressin, lypressin) interact with V1 and V2 receptors. V1 receptors have a pressor response, whereas V2 receptors have both an antidiuretic and hemostatic response. General vasoconstriction by smooth muscle contraction of most blood vessels occurs with the binding of the V1 receptors. At higher concentrations, ADH interacts with these receptors. This vasoconstriction is marked in the portal vessels, somewhat less in cerebral, coronary, peripheral, and pulmonary vessels, and slightly in intrahepatic vessels. GI motility and tone are also enhanced. V2 receptors are found on renal tubule cells. They mediate antidiuresis by stimulating the increase of water permeability and resorption in the renal collecting tubules. Release of and increase in circulating levels of factor VIII and von Willebrand factor occurs with the binding of the V2 receptors. These proteins are involved in blood coagulation.

Contraindications and Precautions

The only contraindication to desmopressin use is hypersensitivity. Intranasal delivery may be inappropriate if the patient has an impaired level of consciousness. Use with caution in patients with coronary artery insufficiency or those who are hypertensive because high intranasal doses of desmopressin may elevate the blood pressure slightly. Caution should also be used in patients who are predisposed to thrombus formation, because of reports of thrombotic events, such as thrombosis, acute cerebrovascular thrombosis, or myocardial infarction, although such reports are rare. Use with caution in patients with conditions associated with fluid and electrolyte imbalance, such as cystic fibrosis, because these patients are especially prone to hyponatremia.

Adverse Effects

Most adverse effects of desmopressin are mediated through the V1 receptor acting on vascular and GI smooth muscle. Adverse reactions are mild and infrequent and are often resolved with dosage reduction. Possible reactions for intranasal or parenteral administration include mild abdominal pain and cramps, transient headache, nasal congestion, nausea, rhinitis, and facial flushing. Injection of desmopressin is associated with local erythema, burning, pain, or swelling. Changes in blood pressure (either a slight elevation or a transient fall) with a compensatory heart rate increase have also been reported infrequently. Oral administration of tablets for 12 to 44 months has shown a transient increase in AST;

however, the elevated AST returned to normal range despite continued use of the medication. The major V2 receptor-mediated adverse effect is water intoxication. Rare severe allergic reactions have been reported with desmopressin.

Drug Interactions

Although desmopressin pressor activity is very low, large intranasal or parenteral doses (>0.3 μg/kg) should be used cautiously with other pressor agents because of the potential for additive or synergistic effects. Carbamazepine, chlorpromazine, and nonsteroidal anti-inflammatory drugs (NSAIDs) enhance the antidiuretic response to vasopressin; thus, these drugs may potentiate the effects of desmopressin.

Assessment of Relevant Core Patient Variables

Health Status

Assess for pre-existing health conditions that require cautious use of desmopressin. A baseline assessment, including measurements of weight, serum and urine osmolality, and serum sodium must be established to determine effectiveness of the drug. Careful monitoring for cardiac reactions during desmopressin treatment is also important. Posterior pituitary agonists should be used with caution in patients with vascular disease, especially coronary artery disease, because changes in blood pressure can occur. Desmopressin should also be used cautiously in patients with conditions associated with fluid and electrolyte imbalances, such as cystic fibrosis, because these patients are prone to hyponatremia and water intoxication while taking this drug. Early signs include confusion, drowsiness, listlessness, and headache.

Life Span and Gender

Determine whether the patient is pregnant or breast-feeding. Desmopressin is a pregnancy category B medication. Although there are several publications describing the use of desmopressin to manage diabetes insipidus during pregnancy, no adequate and well-controlled studies have determined its safety and efficacy for use during pregnancy and lactation. Thus, use in pregnancy and lactation should occur only when the potential benefits outweigh the potential hazards to the fetus.

Clinical trials have demonstrated that desmopressin is an effective agent in both adults and children and has few side effects. Safety and efficacy of parenteral desmopressin in children (<12 years of age) or intranasal desmopressin in infants (<3 months of age) have not been established. Infants and children require careful fluid intake restriction to prevent possible hyponatremia and water intoxication, which can cause seizures.

Lifestyle, Diet, and Habits and Environment

Assess the patient's lifestyle in terms of work, rest patterns, leisure activities, and use of social or recreational drugs. Decreased plasma volume, pain, stress, sleep, exercise, and use of certain drugs (e.g., barbiturates, nicotine, morphine, and vincristine) are all factors that stimulate the secretion of ADH.

Nursing Diagnoses and Outcomes

- Risk for Fluid Volume Excess related to administration of desmopressin, secondary to diabetes insipidus
  Desired outcome: *The patient will not demonstrate signs and symptoms of water intoxication and will maintain urine specific gravity within a normal range.*
- Risk for Ineffective Therapeutic Regimen Management related to lack of knowledge of diabetes insipidus, disease management, and signs and symptoms of complications
  Desired outcome: *The patient will describe the disease process, causes, and factors contributing to symptoms and the regimen for disease or symptom control, relate intent to practice health behaviors needed or desired to control disease and prevent complications, and report less anxiety from fear of the unknown and loss of control.*

Planning and Intervention

Maximizing Therapeutic Effects

Establish baseline values for weight, blood pressure, electrolytes, and urine specific gravity. Individualize the dosage of desmopressin according to the diurnal pattern of water elimination, control of nocturia, and adequate duration of sleep. During long-term therapy, periodically assess the condition of nasal passages. Inappropriate administration may lead to nasal ulceration and, as a consequence, subsequent administered doses may be inadequate.

ADH solutions must be protected from agitation and temperature extremes (excessive heat or freezing). To maintain potency, it is important to refrigerate nasal and parenteral solutions of desmopressin.

Minimizing Adverse Effects

Assess the patient for pre-existing cardiovascular disorders and monitor patients carefully for cardiac reactions from desmopressin. The very young and elderly require careful fluid intake restriction to prevent possible water intoxication and hyponatremia. Instruct patients to drink one to two glasses of water with each dose of desmopressin to help reduce the GI effects of the drug.

When administering the drug by IV infusion, ensure patency of venous access, preferably in a large vein, and use an infusion-control device. This precaution will decrease the chance of extravasation.

Providing Patient and Family Education

- Information about antidiuretic drugs, including action, use, adverse effects, and drug interactions that may occur, should be provided. It is important to emphasize to the patient and family that sudden changes in weight, pulse rate, and blood pressure may indicate serious fluid imbalance.
- Alcohol can alter the therapeutic response to desmopressin. Caution the patient against consuming alcohol during therapy. Many over-the-counter (OTC) products contain alcohol, so it is important to discuss the need to read drug labels before taking any OTC medications. Also, advise the patient to carry appropriate medical identification to alert medical personnel in case of an emergency.
- Review with the patient and family or caregiver the proper administration technique for nasally administered dosage forms. Intranasal preparations are administered through a flexible nasal catheter that measures the appropriate dose. After the drug is drawn into the catheter, one end is placed in the patient's mouth and the other end in the nose.

The patient should then blow into the catheter to deposit the drug into the nasal passageways. Proper technique will lessen nasal irritation that may occur. Nasal congestion may impair absorption when desmopressin is administered intranasally.
- Stress the importance of taking desmopressin as directed and to consult the health care provider before discontinuing its use.

Ongoing Assessment and Evaluation

The patient should be instructed to monitor urine specific gravity and intake and output as well as to weigh himself or herself daily to determine drug efficacy. Decreased urine output and thirst are signs of therapeutic drug response. If desmopressin is being used for abdominal distention, it is important to assess bowel sounds and the presence or absence of flatus. During prolonged therapy, electrocardiographic (ECG) studies should be monitored as well as fluid and electrolyte status.

Drugs Closely Related to P Desmopressin

Vasopressin

Synthetic vasopressin (Pitressin) is effective for treating diabetes insipidus resulting from a partial or complete deficiency in production and secretion of posterior pituitary ADH. It also may be used to prevent or treat postoperative abdominal distention and to facilitate abdominal radiography (see Table 50.5).

An off-label use of vasopressin is managing bleeding esophageal varices. Following SC, IM, or IV injection, synthetic vasopressin aqueous solution has a plasma half-life of 10 to 20 minutes. The duration of antidiuretic activity is 2 to 8 hours. Vasopressin is metabolized rapidly by the liver and is excreted by the kidneys.

Use of vasopressin is contraindicated in patients with hypersensitivity or chronic nephritis with increased levels of blood urea nitrogen (BUN). Vasopressin is in pregnancy category C. Its effect on lactation is unknown. The literature reports that vasopressin, when used during pregnancy in doses sufficient for an antidiuretic effect, is not likely to produce tonic uterine contractions that could be harmful to the fetus or threaten the continuation of the pregnancy.

Lypressin

Lypressin (Diapid) is a synthetic derivative of vasopressin. It acts principally as an ADH and is used to treat DI (see Table 50.5). Lypressin has little pressor or oxytocic activity. When administered as a short-acting nasal spray in therapeutic doses, it has a prompt onset of action, duration of activity of 3 to 8 hours, and minimal cardiovascular pressor effects. Large doses may cause coronary artery constriction. The safety of lypressin use during pregnancy and lactation has not been established.

The effectiveness of lypressin may be decreased during nasal congestion, allergic rhinitis, or upper respiratory tract infections because of decreased absorption by the nasal mucosa. In these situations, larger doses may be required. Infrequent and mild adverse effects include localized cases of rhinorrhea, nasal congestion and irritation, and pruritus. Systemic effects include headache, conjunctivitis, and heartburn secondary to excessive intranasal use.

Terlipressin

Terlipressin (Glypressin), a synthetic analogue of vasopressin, has orphan-drug status for treating bleeding esophageal varices. It can be administered as intermittent injections instead of continuous intravenous infusion, and it has a safer adverse reactions profile than vasopressin.

MEMORY CHIP

P Desmopressin

- Synthetic analogue of human ADH; for treatment of neurogenic diabetes insipidus
- Major contraindications: presence of hemophilia A with factor VIII levels 5% or less
- Most common adverse effects: localized erythema with intranasal administration; burning pain with parenteral injection
- **Life span alert: Infants, children, and the elderly require careful fluid intake restriction to prevent possible hyponatremia and water intoxication.**
- Maximizing therapeutic effects: Keep solutions (nasal, parenteral) refrigerated.
- Minimizing adverse effects: Monitor urine volume/osmolality, plasma osmolality; patients with conditions associated with fluid/electrolyte imbalances are prone to hyponatremia.
- Most important patient education: Inform patients that medication bottle accurately delivers 25 to 50 doses and any solution remaining after 25 to 50 doses should be discarded because the amount delivered thereafter may be substantially less than prescribed. The remaining solution should not be transferred to another bottle.

THYROID DRUGS

Thyroid hormones influence essentially every organ system in the body. They have numerous biological effects, including stimulation of the basal metabolic rate, which affects protein, carbohydrate, and lipid metabolism. Thyroid hormones are essential for normal growth and development throughout the entire life cycle. Like most endocrine glands, the thyroid glands can secrete too much hormone (hyperthyroidism) or too little hormone (hypothyroidism).

Thyroid disorders involve an alteration in the quantity of thyroid hormone secretion, enlargement of the thyroid gland (goiter), or both and are classified as either hyperthyroidism or hypothyroidism.

The prevalence of hyperthyroidism (thyrotoxicosis) and hypothyroidism are similar—approximately 2% of women and 0.2% of men are affected. Increasing age is associated with an increase in the incidence of hypothyroidism. Six percent of women and 2.5% of men older than 60 years have TSH levels greater than twice the upper limit of normal. Hypothyroidism may be mistaken for the normal aging process.

(C) Thyroid Hormones

The only treatment for hypothyroidism is lifelong replacement of thyroid hormones that are adequate to meet the individual's metabolic needs. A number of pharmacologic preparations of endogenous thyroid hormone, including levothyroxine, desiccated thyroid, liothyronine sodium, and liotrix can completely correct hypothyroidism. The preferred treatment, and prototype drug, for hypothyroidism is levothyroxine (T_4; Levothroid, Synthroid), and it is used almost universally. Table 50.6 presents a summary of selected thyroid hormones.

NURSING MANAGEMENT OF THE PATIENT RECEIVING [P] LEVOTHYROXINE

Core Drug Knowledge

Pharmacotherapeutics

Levothyroxine (T_4) is used as replacement therapy in hypothyroidism of any etiology, except transient hypothyroidism during the acute phase of subacute thyroiditis. It also can be used for pituitary suppression of TSH in treating and preventing euthyroid goiter, in managing hypothyroidism secondary to thyroid cancer, and in treating **myxedema coma.** T_4 also may used in conjunction with antithyroid drugs to treat thyrotoxicosis and to prevent goiter formation, hypothyroidism, and thyrotoxicosis during pregnancy (see Table 50.6).

Pharmacokinetics

The absorption of levothyroxine (T_4) from the GI tract varies from 48% to 79% of the administered dose. Absorption is increased during fasting states. Excessive fecal loss has been found with malabsorption syndromes. T_4 must be converted to triiodothyronine (T_3) for its clinical effects. When the drug is taken orally, the onset of effect occurs very slowly, with the peak effect occurring in 1 to 3 weeks. When the drug is administered intravenously to treat myxedema, the onset of effect is 6 to 8 hours, with a peak effect in 24 to 48 hours. T_4 has a half-life of 6 to 7 days. Levothyroxine is metabolized in the liver and excreted in the bile. It crosses the placenta and enters breast milk.

Pharmacodynamics

Levothyroxine acts as replacement for natural thyroid hormone. Increased oxygen consumption, respiration, heart rate, growth and maturation, and speed of fat, protein, and carbohydrate metabolism occur secondary to increases in the basal metabolic rate.

Contraindications and Precautions

Levothyroxine is an FDA pregnancy category A drug. It is safe for maintaining and regulating thyroid function during pregnancy but should be used with caution in lactating women because it crosses into breast milk and can affect the infant's thyroid-pituitary balance. Levothyroxine should also be used with caution in patients with coronary artery disease or coronary insufficiency because the resulting increase in basal metabolic rate may aggravate angina pectoris caused by the increased myocardial oxygen demand. Use of T_4 in cardiovascular disease should be initiated at a low dosage and titrated upward gradually. Use of levothyroxine for patients with concomitant DI, diabetes mellitus, or adrenal insufficiency (Addison disease) will exacerbate the intensity of their symptoms. An appropriate adjustment in therapy for these concomitant diseases is necessary. For those with myxedema, it is necessary to begin treatment with low doses with gradual increases because they are particularly sensitive to thyroid preparations.

TABLE 50.6 Summary of Selected (C) Thyroid Hormones

Drug (Trade) Name	Selected Indications	Route and Dosage Range	Pharmacokinetics
[P] levothyroxine (L-thyroxine; Synthroid, Levothroid)	Replacement therapy for hypothyroidism, including cretinism	*Adult:* PO, 50–200 µg/d *Child:* PO, 0–6 mo, 8–10 µg/kg/d; 6–12 mo, 6–8 µg/kg/d; 1–5 y, 5–6 µg/kg/d; 6–12 y, 4–5 µg/kg/d; over 12 y, 2–3 µg/kg/d	*Onset:* Slow *Duration:* 3 wk $t_{1/2}$: 2–7 d
	Emergency treatment of myxedema coma	*Adult:* IV, 400 µg initially	
thyroid dessicated (T_3 and T_4; Armour Thyroid)	Same as above	*Adult:* PO, 300 mg/d initially, increase by 15 mg q 2–3 wk; maintenance 60–120 mg/d *Child:* PO, 1.2–6 mg/kg/d, depending on age	*Onset:* Slow *Duration:* 3 wk $t_{1/2}$: 2–7 d
liothyronine (T_3; Cytomel, Triostat)	Same as above	*Adult:* PO, 25 µg/d increase every 1–2 wk by 12.5–25 µg; maintenance, 25–75 µg/d *Child (and elderly adult):* PO, 5–50 µg/d	*Onset:* Varies *Duration:* 3–4 d $t_{1/2}$: 1–2 d
liotrix (T_4 and T_3; Thyrolar)	Same as above	*Adult:* PO, 15–30 mg/d increase every 2 wk to a maximum of 60–120 mg/d	*Onset:* Slow *Duration:* 3 wk $t_{1/2}$: 2–7 d

Contraindications include hypersensitivity, thyrotoxicosis uncomplicated by hypothyroidism, and acute myocardial infarction (MI) complicated by hypothyroidism. The metabolic stimulating effects of T_4 could worsen the MI, cause arrhythmias, and lead to further complications.

Adverse Effects

Adverse effects observed with the use of thyroxine are related to therapeutic overdosage. These include hypertension, tachycardia, arrhythmias, anxiety, headache, nervousness, GI irritation, sweating, and heat intolerance. Patients with sensitivity to lactose may show intolerance because lactose is used in the manufacture of this product. There is no well-documented evidence of allergic reactions to thyroid hormones. In children, partial hair loss may occur in the first few months of therapy.

Drug Interactions

Risk for bleeding is increased if T_4 is given with anticoagulants (e.g., warfarin). The dose of the anticoagulant should be reduced by one third before beginning levothyroxine therapy. Bleeding times (e.g., international normalized ratio [INR], prothrombin time [PT], and partial thromboplastin time [PTT]) should be monitored closely. Digitalis levels and therapeutic effects may be reduced when digitalis is given concurrently with T_4. If this combination of drugs is used, monitor the serum digoxin levels closely and make appropriate dosage adjustments. Effects of beta-adrenergic blockers and theophylline may be altered as the individual returns to a euthyroid state. If these drugs are given in combination with T_4, monitor the patient closely, and adjust the dosage of theophylline or beta blockers as needed (Table 50.7). Patients with diabetes, who also take thyroid supplements, may need to increase their doses of insulin or oral hypoglycemic agents. Conversely, a decrease in the thyroid hormone dose may necessitate a decrease in their antidiabetic agents. Medicinal or dietary iodine interferes with all in vivo tests of radioactive iodine uptake. This interference produces low uptakes that may not reflect a true decrease in hormone synthesis.

Some drugs may interfere with thyroid hormone absorption or metabolism. Antilipemic agents (e.g., cholestyramine and lovastatin), aluminum-containing antacids, ferrous sulfate, and sucralfate may inhibit absorption. Administration of these drugs should be separated from the administration of T_4 by a 4- or 5-hour interval. Some antiepileptic drugs (phenytoin, carbamazepine), amiodarone, or rifampin may require an adjustment in T_4 dosage because these agents can affect T_4 metabolism. Dosages of oral anticoagulants, insulin, oral hypoglycemic agents, cardiac glycosides, tricyclic antidepressants, catecholamines, and sympathomimetic agents may require adjustment when a patient starts thyroid replacement therapy or when the dosage is changed to avoid serious adverse consequences. Table 50.7 lists agents that interact with T_4.

Assessment of Relevant Core Patient Variables

Health Status

Before administering T_4, review the patient's record to determine whether the drug can be administered safely. Perform a baseline physical examination to monitor the effects of the drug. Skin color, temperature, texture, and presence of any lesions should be noted to monitor for any reactions and to assess thyroid hormone effectiveness. Note muscle tone, weight, temperature, blood pressure, pulse, and respirations to assess for the desired therapeutic effects of T_4 and to monitor for toxic or adverse effects. Thyroid function tests, ECGs, and serum laboratory analyses must be completed to monitor appropriate dosage and response to the drug.

Individuals with known cardiac problems should begin drug therapy with smaller doses of thyroid hormone replacement, because of the cardiac stimulant effect of T_4. Carefully monitor the individual for angina and cardiac arrhythmias.

Life Span and Gender

Determine the patient's age before administering T_4. Geriatric patients should start with a low dosage of thyroid hormone replacement. Gradual increases will prevent serious cardiovascular and neurologic adverse effects. If the pulse rate is greater than 100 bpm, withhold the T_4 dose. Closely monitor elderly patients who are also receiving beta blockers or digitalis glycosides, because of the increased risk for toxic effects. In both premenopausal and postmenopausal women, long-term T_4 therapy has been associated with decreased bone density in the spine and hip. A basal bone density measurement and monitoring for osteoporosis would be beneficial.

Monitor children maintained on T_4 for growth and development and for toxic effects. Additionally, adjust the dosage as the child grows.

Because pregnant patients who are receiving thyroid hormone replacement may require a dosage increase during pregnancy, assess the patient for pregnancy. Thyroid hormone deficiency may have an adverse effect on fetal nervous system development and on the outcome of the pregnancy.

Lifestyle, Diet, and Habits

Assess the patient's ability to adapt to a long-term drug regimen. Patients maintained on T_4 most often take the drug for life. T_4 is best taken as a single daily dose before break-

CRITICAL THINKING SCENARIO

Levothyroxine and weight control

A woman comes to the clinic and asks for a prescription for thyroid hormone. She has tried multiple diets without success and is convinced that she must have a "glandular" problem. She tells you that she read that thyroid hormone is an effective way to lose weight because it increases your metabolism, and she wants to try it. After obtaining thyroid function tests, it is determined that this patient has normal thyroid function.

1. Think about the problems that could occur if thyroid replacement hormone is given to a euthyroid patient. Outline the normal controls of thyroid activity, and predict what could happen.
2. Develop a patient education tool to explain this situation to the patient, and propose other ways of dealing with her weight problem.

TABLE 50.7 Agents That Interact With P Levothyroxine

Interactants	Effect and Significance	Nursing Management
cholestyramine and colestipol	Loss of efficacy of thyroid hormone; potential for hypothyroidism	Monitor thyroid hormone levels closely; administer drugs 4–6 h apart.
anticoagulants	Increased effect of anticoagulant; bleeding problems possible	Monitor INR, PT, PTT tests closely; assess patient for signs of overt or occult bleeding Anticoagulant dose may need adjustment.
beta-adrenergic blockers	Actions of beta blockers possibly blocked as patient returns to euthyroid state	Assess for decreased beta blocking action; consider alternative therapy or increased beta blocker dose.
digitalis glycosides	Reduced serum levels of digitalis and decreased therapeutic effects	Evaluate serum digoxin levels; adjust dose as needed for therapeutic effects.
theophylline	Increased theophylline levels as patient reaches euthyroid state and normal theophylline clearance	Monitor serum theophylline levels closely; increase dose as needed to maintain therapeutic levels.

fast. Assist the patient to establish a routine for taking the medication.

Caution the patient to avoid changing from one brand of this drug to another without first consulting the pharmacist or prescriber. Products manufactured by different companies may not be equally effective, and bioavailability differences have occurred with different preparations of T_4.

Environment

Know the environment where the drug will be administered. Most often, T_4 is taken at home as oral drug. IV T_4 is administered only for myxedema coma. It is used for short-term therapy until the patient is able to take the oral drug.

Nursing Diagnoses and Outcomes

- Imbalanced Nutrition: More than Body Requirements related to dietary intake in excess of metabolic demands secondary to hypothyroidism
  Desired outcome: *The patient will maintain normal body weight, describe reasons why weight gain may occur, discuss nutritional needs related to age, lifestyle, and diagnosis, and discuss the effects of exercise and diet on weight control.*
- Risk for Injury related to adverse drug reactions
  Desired outcome: *The patient will not experience adverse reactions to thyroid hormone replacement.*
- Risk for Injury related to pre-existing health status that requires cautious use of a thyroid agent
  Desired outcome: *The patient will not experience complications of pre-existing health conditions linked to the prescribed thyroid hormone replacement therapy. Such complications include coronary artery disease, angina, myocardial infarction, and hypertension secondary to increased metabolic demands on the heart, and acute adrenal crisis secondary to increased tissue demand for adrenal hormones.*
- Knowledge Deficit related to thyroid dysfunction and the necessity for thyroid hormone replacement
  Desired outcome: *The patient and family will express an accurate understanding of the teaching regarding the disease process and the prescribed thyroid hormone replacement therapy. An example includes avoidance of myxedema coma from interrupted drug therapy.*

Planning and Intervention

Maximizing Therapeutic Effects

Replacement therapy is a lifelong occurrence. T_4 is absorbed best when taken once a day on an empty stomach, preferably before breakfast. During drug therapy, monitor cardiovascular response and serum thyroid function to determine the appropriate dosage and response to T_4. Monitor children regularly to assess the need to change dosage to allow for appropriate growth and development. If the patient is on other medications, it is important to monitor the response to these drugs and to T_4, especially as the patient achieves a euthyroid state. Offer support and encouragement to deal with the need for lifelong therapy.

Minimizing Adverse Effects

Young adults without evidence of coronary artery disease can begin a full replacement dose of T_4. Older individuals and those with (or at risk for) coronary artery disease, atrial arrhythmias, or both should begin with a low dose (e.g., 25 to 50 μg/day), which can be slowly titrated to the target dosage.

Check adrenal function in hypothyroid patients because some of these individuals also have adrenal insufficiency. Without appropriate glucocorticoid replacement, thyroid administration in these individuals can precipitate an acute adrenal crisis because thyroid agents increase tissue demand for adrenal hormones.

Thyroid agents may potentiate the hypo-prothrombinemic effect of oral anticoagulants by increasing the catabolism of vitamin K. Administering thyroid agents to diabetic patients may increase the dosage requirement of insulin or oral agent.

Providing Patient and Family Education

- Explain to patients and their families that this drug is a hormone that is being used to replace the thyroid hor-

mone that their body is not able to produce. Tell them that this hormone is responsible for regulating the body's metabolism. Explain to patients that they will most likely need to take levothyroxine for life and that it should be taken every day, preferably in the morning before breakfast.
- Explain that although this drug causes few adverse effects, patients should report any increase in the symptoms of thyroid dysfunction, such as weight changes, nervousness, skin changes, lethargy, and sleeplessness, or any skin rash or lesions.
- Advise patients to avoid OTC drugs and to check with the prescriber if they feel that an OTC medication is needed. Many OTC drugs contain ingredients that interfere with thyroid function, and patients may want to obtain a medical identification tag or card so that people taking care of them in an emergency are aware that they are taking a thyroid replacement drug.
- Educate patients to keep this drug out of the reach of children.
- Stress the importance of notifying the health care provider if manifestations of hyperthyroidism (e.g., headache, nervousness, chest pain, palpitations, increased pulse rate, diarrhea, diaphoresis, or heat intolerance) occur.

Ongoing Assessment and Evaluation

Monitor serum thyroid hormone levels periodically. As a patient reaches a euthyroid state, reassess the potential for drug interactions and the need to adjust the dosage of other drugs appropriately. It is important to monitor pulse rate and rhythm as well as respiratory rate to assess the effect of the thyroid hormone on these systems and the possible need for dosage adjustment. Medications are administered to the patient with hypothyroidism very cautiously because of altered metabolism and excretion and depressed metabolic rate and respiratory status.

Long-term use of T_4 may decrease hip and spine bone density in women. Measure bone density before beginning T_4 therapy to establish a baseline and then monitor it routinely.

Thyroid hormones may increase blood glucose levels, necessitating adjustment in doses of insulin or oral hypoglycemic agents for diabetic patients. Patients with hypothyroidism have an increased susceptibility to all hypnotic and sedative agents, analgesics, and anesthetics. These drugs, even in small doses, may induce profound somnolence lasting far longer than anticipated. Respiratory depression is likely as a result of the decreased respiratory reserve and alveolar hypoventilation that occurs with hypothyroidism.

As the patient moves from a hypothyroid to a euthyroid state, the body's response to many drugs may be altered. Closely monitor patients taking multiple drugs as they return to a euthyroid state and adjust dosages of the other drugs as needed. For example, the actions of some beta-adrenergic blockers may be impaired. Serum digitalis levels may be reduced, reducing the therapeutic effect of digitalis glycosides. Theophylline clearance will be altered. Nursing management of drug therapy is considered effective if the patient adheres successfully to drug therapy, can recognize various signs and symptoms of hypothyroidism, and seeks appropriate attention from the health care team.

MEMORY CHIP

[P] Levothyroxine

- Synthetic thyroid hormone replacement
- Major contraindications: acute myocardial infarction, thyrotoxicosis; use cautiously in hypoadrenalism
- Most common adverse effects: symptoms of hyperthyroidism, alopecia with initial therapy (particularly in children)
- Maximizing therapeutic effects: Monitor drug response carefully at the start of therapy; administer oral drug as a single daily dose before breakfast.
- Minimizing adverse effects: Monitor cardiac response as increased basal metabolic rate may exacerbate angina pectoris.
- Most important patient education: Have patient wear medical ID (tag or bracelet) to alert emergency medical personnel of drug therapy.

Drugs Closely Related to [P] Levothyroxine

Desiccated Thyroid

Desiccated thyroid (Armour Thyroid) is composed of desiccated animal thyroid glands. It is much less pure, stable, and predictable than synthetic preparations of thyroid hormone. The active thyroid hormones (T_4 and T_3) are available in their natural states and at their natural ratios. Although these preparations are the least expensive, their standardization by iodine content or bioassay is inexact. Optimal dosage is determined by the patient's clinical response and laboratory findings. Therapy is instituted using low doses, with increments that depend on cardiovascular status. The usual starting dose is 30 mg, with increments of 15 mg every 2 to 3 weeks. Patients with long-standing myxedema are started at a lower dose (15 mg/day), particularly if cardiovascular impairment is suspected. The drug dosage should be reduced if angina occurs.

Liothyronine Sodium

Liothyronine sodium (Cytomel [oral form]; Triostat [parenteral form]) is a synthetic form of the natural thyroid hormone T_3. It has the pharmacologic activities of the natural hormone. Its short duration of activity enables quick dosage adjustment and facilitates control of overdosage. Patients who are allergic to thyroid extract derived from pork or beef can be safely treated with this medication. Liothyronine injection is for IV use only and should be stored between 2° and 8°C (36° to 46°F).

Liotrix

Liotrix (Thyrolar) is a uniform mixture of synthetic T_4 and T_3 in a 4:1 ratio by weight. Optimal dosage is determined by patient's clinical response and laboratory findings.

(C) Antithyroid Compounds

The antithyroid agents used clinically to manage hyperthyroidism include methimazole, propylthiouracil, iodide or iodine solutions (Lugol solution), radioactive iodine (I-131), and propranolol. Methimazole (MMI) is the prototype antithyroid compound. Table 50.8 presents a summary of selected antithyroid agents.

TABLE 50.8 Summary of Selected (C) Antithyroid Drugs

Drug (Trade) Name	Selected Indications	Route and Dosage Range	Pharmacokinetics
[P] methimazole (Tapazole)	Treatment of hyperthyroidism Amelioration of hyperthyroidism before thyroidectomy, radioactive iodine	*Adult:* PO, 15 mg/d for mild hyperthyroidism; 30–40 mg/d for moderate hyperthyroidism; 60 mg/d for severe hypothyroidism *Child:* PO, 0.4 mg/kg/d; maintenance, ½ initial dose	*Onset:* 1 wk *Duration:* Weeks $t_{1/2}$: 5–13 h
propylthiouracil (PTU)	Treatment of hyperthyroidism Attain euthyroid state before thyroidectomy, radioactive iodine therapy	*Adult:* Initial dose, PO, 300–900 mg/d maintenance; PO, 100–150 mg/d *Child:* PO, 6–10 y, 50–150 mg/d; ≥ 10 y, 150–300 mg/d; maintenance, based on response	*Onset:* 10–21 d *Duration:* Weeks $t_{1/2}$: 1–2 h
sodium iodide I-131 (Iodotope, Sodium iodide I-131 [therapeutic])	Treatment of hyperthyroidism, thyroid cancer	*Adult:* PO, hyperthyroidism, 4–10 mCi; thyroid cancer, 50 mCi; then 100–150 mCi as needed	*Onset:* Rapid *Duration:* Unknown $t_{1/2}$: 7.61 d
strong iodine solution (Lugol solution, Thyro-Block)	Treatment of hyperthyroidism	*Adult:* PO, 2–6 drops tid for 10 d before surgery	*Onset:* 24–48 h *Duration:* 6 wk $t_{1/2}$: Unknown

NURSING MANAGEMENT OF THE PATIENT RECEIVING [P] METHIMAZOLE (MMI)

Core Drug Knowledge

Pharmacotherapeutics

Thyroid-hormone antagonist drugs, surgery, or radioactive iodine is used to treat hyperthyroidism. The purpose of treatment is to reduce the amount of functional thyroid tissue. Antithyroid drugs are used for palliative treatment of hyperthyroidism, as adjunct in preparation for surgery (thyroidectomy) or radioactive iodine therapy, or to manage thyrotoxic crises. Additionally, if thyroidectomy is contraindicated or otherwise not advised, MMI is the drug of choice (see Table 50.8).

Pharmacokinetics

MMI is readily absorbed from the GI tract. Onset of action is slow, and it requires an average of 5.8 weeks to lower T_4 levels to normal. The half-life of MMI is 5 to 13 hours. It is metabolized in the liver and excreted in the urine. MMI is usually preferred over propylthiouracil (PTU), another thionamide, because it reverses hyperthyroidism more quickly and has fewer side effects. MMI can be administered in single or divided doses, whereas PTU must be given in three equal doses at approximately 8-hour intervals.

Pharmacodynamics

MMI inhibits the synthesis of thyroid hormones (T_4 and T_3); hence, new T_3 and T_4 are not produced. It does not inactivate existing thyroxine and triiodothyronine that are stored in the thyroid, nor does it interfere with the effectiveness of thyroid hormones given as tablets or by injection. Some clinical evidence suggests that the thionamide drugs have immunosuppressant effects. Thus, they are beneficial for suppressing the immune-mediated hyperthyroidism of Graves disease.

Contraindications and Precautions

Methimazole is contraindicated with any known hypersensitivity to antithyroid drugs. It is also contraindicated during pregnancy and nursing because the drug crosses the placenta and is excreted in breast milk.

Adverse Effects

Most adverse effects are minor, but some major side effects can occur. Up to 15% of people taking an antithyroid drug experience minor side effects. Both MMI and PTU can cause hives, itching, rash, fever, arthralgia, joint swelling, vertigo, drowsiness, nausea and vomiting, and altered taste sensation. The nausea and vomiting may depend on the amount of the drug ingested with each dose. For this reason, spreading large total daily doses out over the day may reduce these side effects. If adverse effects occur with one drug, frequently the same effects will occur if the patient switches to the other drug.

Major side effects include agranulocytosis, which affects only 0.2% to 0.5% of all people taking antithyroid medication. If this adverse effect occurs, it usually does so within the first 3 months of treatment. Agranulocytosis resolves within a few days when treatment is discontinued. Liver damage, aplastic anemia, and vasculitis are other rare complications. Most people recover fully when the drug is stopped.

Drug Interactions

Increased toxicity has been reported when MMI is administered along with iodinated glycerol, lithium, and potassium iodide. The anticoagulant effect of warfarin may be increased if it is given with MMI. Dosage of some drugs (including beta blockers, theophylline, and digoxin) requires adjustment during the treatment of hyperthyroidism.

Assessment of Relevant Core Patient Variables

Health Status

Before administering MMI, review the patient's record to determine whether the drug can be administered safely. Antithyroid agents are in pregnancy category D. They readily cross the placenta and can induce goiter and cretinism in the developing fetus. Fortunately, in many pregnant women, thyroid dysfunction decreases as the pregnancy proceeds. This decrease enables reduction of the thionamide dose. If thionamide therapy is necessary during pregnancy, PTU is preferred because it crosses the placenta to a lesser extent than MMI does.

Perform a physical examination before starting drug therapy to establish a baseline for monitoring the drug's effects. Note skin color, temperature, texture, and presence of any lesions to assess for allergic reactions and thyroid hormone effectiveness. It also is important to review liver and renal function tests because the drug is metabolized in the liver and excreted in the urine. Perform a complete blood count (CBC) with differential as a baseline for potential hematologic changes that can occur during therapy. In addition, perform thyroid function tests to monitor the effect of the drug on thyroid function.

Life Span and Gender

Determine whether the patient is pregnant or breast-feeding. Counsel women of childbearing age to avoid pregnancy while using this drug because serious fetal effects can occur. Patients receiving antithyroid preparations during the postpartum period should use formula preparations to feed their babies.

Note the patient's age before administering MMI. Hepatotoxicity has occurred in some pediatric patients. Monitor children closely to ensure that thyroid function is maintained and that growth and development proceed normally. Dosage adjustment may be required with prolonged use.

Lifestyle, Diet, and Habits

Assess the patient's ability to adapt to a long-term drug regimen because patients taking MMI may require prolonged therapy to achieve the full effect. The drug can be taken once daily or in divided doses every 8 hours around the clock. Help the patient establish a schedule that will cause the least interference with the patient's sleep pattern. Drowsiness and vertigo are potential adverse effects of this drug. Therefore, caution the patient to avoid driving or performing tasks that require precision and alertness if these effects occur.

Environment

This drug is usually given in the home. It is necessary to teach the patients the importance of taking the drug as prescribed and the necessity of making special arrangements in their schedules and routines to facilitate this need.

Nursing Diagnoses and Outcomes

- Imbalanced Nutrition: Less than Body Requirements related to increased metabolic demands secondary to hypothyroidism
  Desired outcome: *The patient will describe reasons why weight loss may occur and discuss nutritional needs related to age, lifestyle, and diagnosis.*
- Risk for Injury related to blood dyscrasias (e.g., granulocytosis) or to drowsiness and vertigo secondary to adverse reactions of PTU
  Desired outcome: *The patient will demonstrate no adverse hematologic reactions to thyroid therapy (e.g., hypoprothrombinemia or bleeding), identify factors that increase the risk from injury (e.g., from CNS side effects), and relate intentions to practice and use safety measures to prevent injury.*
- Nonadherence related to long-term use of the antithyroid agent and need to take the prescribed medication frequently
  Desired outcome: *The patient will describe the reasons for the therapeutic regimen, identify barriers to adherence, and identify the behaviors that must change to facilitate adherence.*

Planning and Intervention

Maximizing Therapeutic Effects

Ensure that the drug is being administered appropriately (three equal doses at 8-hour intervals) to maintain serum concentration. Encourage fluid intake of 3 to 4 L/day unless contraindicated. MMI can be given with meals to minimize GI irritation.

Minimizing Adverse Effects

During drug therapy, arrange for periodic blood tests to monitor for hematologic and thyroid functions. Also, encourage frequent, small meals to alleviate GI symptoms and to help maintain nutrition while the patient is taking MMI. Encourage the patient to avoid driving or performing hazardous tasks if drowsiness or vertigo occurs. Monitor the patient's bone marrow function. It is important to obtain a baseline assessment of the CBC with a differential. Emphasize the importance of regular follow-up care and monitoring of bone marrow, CBC, and thyroid functions at intervals determined by the physician.

Providing Patient and Family Education

- Explain to patients and their families that this agent is an antithyroid drug that blocks the production and activity of the thyroid hormone responsible for regulating the body's metabolism, that is, the speed with which the body's cells burn energy. This drug will most likely have to be taken for a prolonged time to achieve the desired effect.
- If the drug is taken in divided doses, instruct the patient to take them every 8 hours around the clock. Work with patients and the family to establish a schedule that will cause the least interference with sleep.
- Adverse effects of this drug include vertigo and drowsiness. Advise the patient to avoid driving or performing hazardous tasks while taking this drug and to take extra precautions to prevent falls and injuries.
- Other adverse effects include nausea, vomiting, and epigastric distress. Encourage the patient to eat small, frequent meals to maintain nutrition and alleviate some of the discomfort associated with these adverse effects.

- Advise the patient that he or she will have periodic blood tests while taking this drug to monitor its effectiveness and possible adverse effects. Stress the need to report fever, sore throat, unusual bleeding or bruising, and headache to the health care team.
- As with all medications, instruct patients to keep this drug out of the reach of children.

Ongoing Assessment and Evaluation

Monitor serum thyroid hormone levels periodically to evaluate the effectiveness of the drug and to assess the need for replacement thyroid hormone because the thyroid gland is suppressed. With continued antithyroid therapy, an insidious goitrogenic hypothyroidism may appear. Alert the patient to watch for signs of this adverse effect, such as decreased cardiac rate, intolerance to cold, and weight gain. Thyroid function tests, used to evaluate drug therapy, should be measured routinely (every 4–6 weeks). It is important to review periodically the signs of hypothyroidism and hyperthyroidism with the patient and significant others. As the patient reaches a euthyroid state, assess the need for dosage adjustment with drugs affected by metabolic rate and activity. Therapy is considered successful when normal thyroid status is maintained, and the patient can explain and demonstrate self-monitoring techniques.

Drug Closely Related to P Methimazole

Propylthiouracil (PTU) is a thionamide with similar characteristics to those of MMI. Adverse effects are also similar and include pruritus, rash, urticaria, arthritis, fever, abnormal taste, nausea, and vomiting. Serious complications, such as agranulocytosis, are dose dependent. Serum aminotransferase concentrations increase transiently in up to one third of patients taking PTU. Well-documented hepatotoxicity is equally divided between PTU and MMI.

MEMORY CHIP

P Methimazole (MMI)

- Inhibits the synthesis of thyroid hormones; antithyroid agent
- Major contraindications: sensitivity to the drug; nursing mothers, because the drug is excreted in breast milk
- Most common adverse effects: GI (nausea, vomiting, epigastric pain), itching, rash, hives, and arthralgia
- Most serious adverse effects: agranulocytosis, liver damage, aplastic anemia, and vasculitis. Most adverse effects resolve spontaneously with discontinuation of the drug.
- Maximizing therapeutic effects: Administer drug around the clock at 8-hour intervals, although it can be given in a single daily dose.
- Minimizing adverse effects: periodic blood tests to assess bone marrow function and bleeding tendencies
- Most important patient education: Drug must be taken for a prolonged period (months) to achieve the desired effects; report fever, sore throat, unusual bleeding or bruising, and malaise.

Drugs Significantly Different From P Methimazole

Iodide or Iodine Solutions (Lugol Solution, Thyro-Block [tablets])

Iodine is the oldest of the antithyroid drugs. Low doses of iodine are needed in the body to form thyroid hormone. High doses, however, tend to inhibit thyroid function. A hyperfunctioning thyroid gland responds to iodine by promptly inhibiting the release of hormone. Iodine helps to firm the thyroid gland by reducing its size and vascularity. This effect helps prevent postoperative hemorrhage and the surgical complication of thyroid storm.

Potassium iodide, or occasionally strong iodine solution, is used preoperatively to reduce the vascularity of the gland before thyroidectomy and, alone or in combination with the beta blocker, propranolol, to manage thyrotoxic crisis (thyroid storm), usually in conjunction with other antithyroid agents (e.g., MMI). When used preoperatively, potassium iodide is administered 10 to 14 days before surgery.

Chronic toxicity may occur when potassium iodide is given in large doses or over a long duration. Chronic toxicity is usually dose dependent and is manifested as a metallic taste, burning in the mouth and throat, sore teeth and gums, increased salivation, and eye irritation with swollen eyelids. Gastric irritation is common, and diarrhea may occur. When the drug is discontinued, the clinical manifestations of toxicity generally subside spontaneously within a few days.

Hypersensitivity reactions to iodides may cause angioedema, cutaneous and mucosal hemorrhage, and clinical signs (e.g., fever, arthralgia, lymphadenopathy, and eosinophilia) resembling serum sickness.

Prolonged use or excessive doses of iodides may result in thyroid gland hyperplasia, thyroid adenoma, goiter, and severe hypothyroidism.

Concomitant use of lithium salts, other iodides, or antithyroid agents and potassium iodide may result in an additive or synergistic hypothyroid effect. If these drugs are used together, the patient should be monitored closely for signs and symptoms of hypothyroidism. Simultaneous use of potassium iodide and potassium-containing drugs or potassium-sparing diuretics may result in hyperkalemia.

Cautious initial administration of potassium iodide is recommended because some individuals are markedly sensitive to iodides. Persons at highest risk are those with goiter or autoimmune thyroid disease (Hashimoto thyroiditis). Some commercially available formulations of potassium iodide contain sodium bisulfite, a sulfite that may cause allergic-type reactions, including anaphylaxis and life-threatening asthmatic episodes, in susceptible individuals. Question the patient carefully about the presence of goiter, autoimmune thyroid disease, or asthma because this sensitivity occurs more frequently in asthmatic individuals.

Iodine-131

I-131 (radioactive iodine) is used to treat hyperthyroidism and well-differentiated thyroid carcinoma. While destroying thyroid tissue, it exposes only the thyroid tissue to the altering radiation, eliminates the problems of surgery, and enables outpatient treatment. Most patients treated with radioactive iodine become euthyroid and then require lifelong replacement therapy with thyroid hormones.

respond to the increased ACTH by increasing their production of adrenal androgens. Consequently, testosterone levels are abnormally high, which results in masculinization.

Hyperaldosteronism

Hyperaldosteronism is another abnormality of adrenal hormone production. Certain tumors of the adrenal cortex produce excessive amounts of aldosterone (or occasionally another mineralocorticoid). Two problems occur as a result of hyperaldosteronism: hypertension secondary to sodium and water retention and hypokalemia-induced muscle weakness. Both problems represent excessive aldosterone actions on the distal renal tubule. Treatment ultimately involves surgical removal of the tumor.

C STEROID HORMONE AGONISTS

C Glucocorticoids

The primary endogenous glucocorticoids produced by the adrenal gland are cortisol (hydrocortisone) and cortisone. Cortisol and cortisone are used for replacement therapy in patients with adrenal insufficiency. They have no role in any systemic anti-inflammatory therapeutic regimen because of their high mineralocorticoid activity relative to their anti-inflammatory activity.

All natural and synthetic glucocorticoids act by binding to a specific cytoplasmic glucocorticoid receptor. Currently, glucocorticoids are available in numerous formulations, including oral, topical, ophthalmic solutions and ointments, oral inhalers, nasal formulations, parenteral, and rectal preparations. The main therapeutic uses of glucocorticoids include anti-inflammatory agent, immunosuppressive agent, replacement therapy for individuals with adrenal insufficiency, and adjunctive treatment in selected malignant disorders. Synthetic glucocorticoids include prednisone, methylprednisolone, dexamethasone, and betamethasone (Figure 51.2). Table 51.1 presents a summary of selected glucocorticoids.

A common adverse effect of synthetic glucocorticoids administered in high doses for anti-inflammatory and immunosuppressant effects (combined or separately) is suppression of the HPA axis. This effect appears within days of beginning glucocorticoid therapy. The time needed for the HPA axis to recover depends on the type of glucocorticoid given, the dose and frequency of administration (daily dosing or alternate-day dosing), and the duration of treatment. Occasionally, the patient's hypothalamic-pituitary-adrenal (HPA) axis remains permanently suppressed by glucocorticoid anti-inflammatory therapy. Consequently, the corticosteroid therapy reverts to replacement therapy.

Abrupt discontinuation of a glucocorticoid following a prolonged administration time may result in acute adrenal insufficiency because of a lack of both exogenous and endogenous glucocorticoids. Acute adrenal insufficiency is characterized by increased morbidity and mortality. To prevent acute adrenal insufficiency, exogenously administered glucocorticoids must be withdrawn gradually (tapered) so that the HPA axis can resume secretion of cortisol at a normal level and rate.

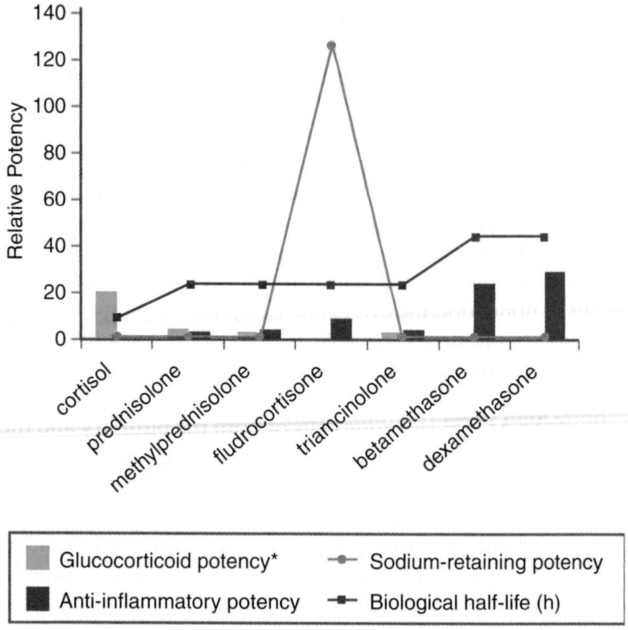

*Glucocorticoid activity signifies the stimulation of glucose formation, a reduction in its utilization, and the promotion of its storage as glycogen.

FIGURE 51.2 Comparison of glucocorticoids.

Prednisone, a synthetic analogue of cortisone, is the prototype glucocorticoid. It is four times more potent than naturally occurring cortisol; thus, its results are longer acting and have a more potent anti-inflammatory effect. Prednisone and its derivatives are the most commonly used glucocorticoids for the treatment of inflammatory conditions and a variety of autoimmune diseases.

NURSING MANAGEMENT OF THE PATIENT RECEIVING P PREDNISONE

Core Drug Knowledge

Pharmacotherapeutics

Therapeutic uses of prednisone include anti-inflammatory treatment for conditions such as asthma, rheumatoid arthritis, and ulcerative colitis. They also include immunosuppressive treatment for a variety of chronic conditions, such as scleroderma and post-transplantation rejection; and as replacement therapy for adrenal deficiency states.

Prednisone may be used as either short- or long-term therapy. Short-term therapies include during acute allergic reactions, during periods of acute exacerbation of chronic diseases such as chronic obstructive pulmonary disease, and at the beginning of treatment for a chronic condition to manage symptoms until other drugs become effective. Long-term high-dose or low-dose therapy may be indicated depending on the underlying condition (e.g., transplantation) or disease (e.g., rheumatoid arthritis) being treated (see Table 51.1).

is adrenal hypofunction, the treatment includes immediate replacement of adrenocortical hormone (e.g., intravenous [IV] hydrocortisone [Solu-Cortef]), salt, and fluids to restore normal blood volume and blood pressure.

In secondary adrenal insufficiency, the deficiency of cortisol secretion is secondary to insufficient secretion of ACTH by the anterior pituitary. Little or no alteration in aldosterone secretion occurs. Thus, glucocorticoid insufficiency occurs without affecting mineralocorticoid levels. The most common cause of secondary adrenal insufficiency is long-term treatment of nonendocrine disorders with pharmacologic doses of glucocorticoid drugs. Because it bypasses the negative feedback loop, this treatment results in gradual loss of adrenal and pituitary hormonal reserves and some degree of atrophy of the ACTH-secreting cells of both the pituitary and the adrenal cortex. Sudden withdrawal of the glucocorticoid drug may result in secondary adrenal insufficiency, manifested clinically by acute adrenal insufficiency. HPA axis suppression resulting from glucocorticoid therapy may last for as long as 1 year after drug therapy has been discontinued.

A patient receiving pharmacologic doses of glucocorticoids for more than 2 weeks may have some degree of HPA axis suppression. Prevention of secondary adrenal insufficiency following prolonged administration of glucocorticoid drugs can be avoided by "weaning" the patient from the drug over weeks or months.

Cushing Syndrome

Cushing syndrome is a rare disorder resulting from increased adrenocortical secretion of cortisol, resulting in chronic elevation in glucocorticoid and adrenal androgen hormones. Mineralocorticoid hormone levels are usually not affected because increased adrenocorticotropic hormone (ACTH) production is usually the causative agent. Cushing syndrome may be caused by any one of the following sources:

- ACTH-dependent adrenocortical hyperplasia
- Tumor
- ACTH-secreting tumor
- Long-term administration of large doses of any steroid that is a potent glucocorticoid (iatrogenic Cushing syndrome)

The term *cushingoid* refers to the variable number of the physiologic changes associated with Cushing syndrome (Box 51.2).

Salt-Losing Adrenogenital Syndrome

Salt-losing adrenogenital syndrome, a congenital condition, is characterized by an inherited enzymatic interference with the normal biosynthesis of glucocorticoids and mineralocorticoids. The resulting low levels of these corticosteroids stimulate the body's feedback mechanism to produce large amounts of corticotropin (ACTH). The adrenal glands are only able to

BOX 51.2 Cushingoid Characteristics

Some cardinal signs of Cushing syndrome include:
Moon face
Glaucoma and cataract formation
Hirsutism and masculinization
Cervicodorsal fat (buffalo hump)
Extremity thinning and atrophy
Abdominal striae (purplish)
Protuberant abdomen
Truncal obesity
Swelling (fluid retention and edema)
Brittle bones (osteoporosis)

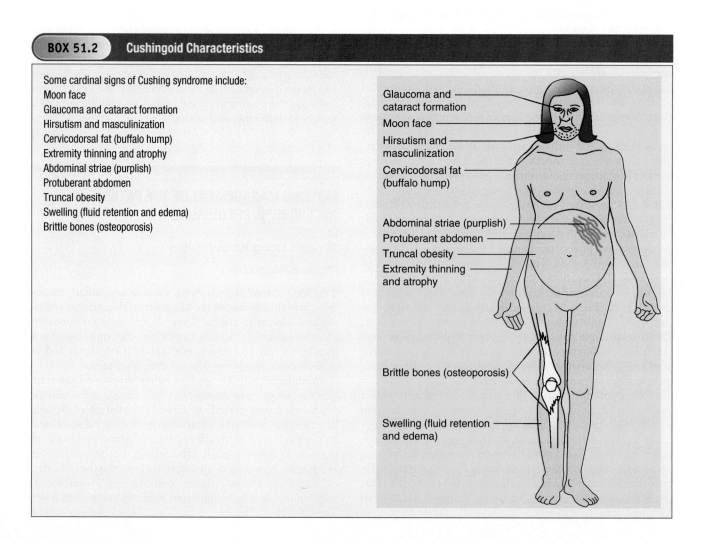

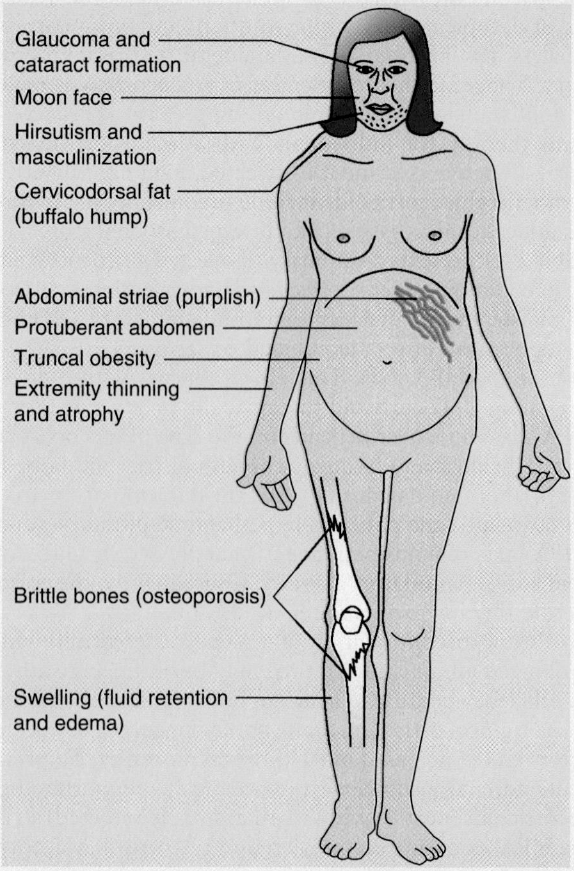

Hypothalamic corticotropin-releasing factor (CRF) stimulates the release of pituitary adrenocorticotropic hormone (ACTH). The hypothalamic-pituitary-adrenal (HPA) axis regulates and stimulates cortisol synthesis release by the adrenal cortex. Each of these substances is regulated by a complex feedback loop because the production of each substance is regulated by the plasma concentrations of the other two. Glucocorticoid, androgen, and estrogen secretion depend on adrenocortical stimulation by ACTH from the anterior pituitary. CRF controls ACTH release into the bloodstream (Figure 51.1).

Three factors are important in regulating ACTH secretion:

- Circulating cortisol levels
- Stress levels
- Circadian (diurnal) rhythms

Pituitary production of ACTH is very sensitive to suppression by exogenous glucocorticoids. Long-term or chronic administration may result in adrenocortical atrophy and subsequent reduction in the ability to produce these hormones.

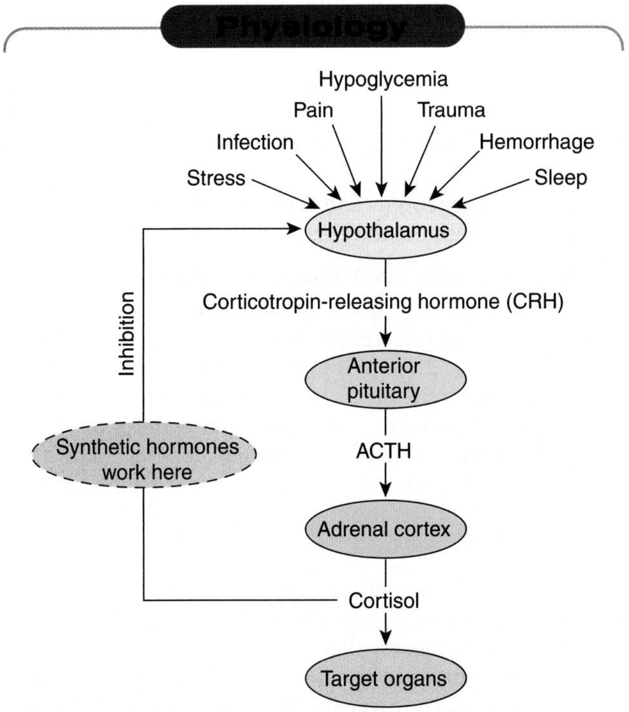

FIGURE 51.1 The hypothalamic-pituitary-adrenal (HPA) feedback system regulates and stimulates cortisol synthesis and release by the adrenal cortex. Each hormone in the HPA axis is influenced by a complex feedback loop because synthesis of one substance is regulated by plasma concentrations of the others. For instance, secretion of glucocorticoid, androgen, and estrogen depends on adrenocortical stimulation by adrenocorticotropic hormone (ACTH) from the anterior pituitary. Corticotropin-releasing factor, produced by the hypothalamus, controls ACTH release into the bloodstream. Circulating cortisol levels, stress, and circadian rhythms are also important in regulating ACTH secretion. ACTH in turn regulates cortisol release. The objectives of replacement and pharmacologic drug therapy involve maintaining balance in the HPA feedback system.

Mineralocorticoids

The mineralocorticoids (**aldosterone** is the most prevalent naturally occurring mineralocorticoid) exert a major influence on regulating potassium, sodium, and water balance. Mineralocorticoids are produced in the outer layer of cells of the adrenal cortex (zona glomerulosa). Numerous systemic factors affect the synthesis and secretion of aldosterone. Angiotensin II is the most potent of these factors. In the distal renal tubules, aldosterone promotes the reabsorption of sodium into the blood in exchange for potassium secreted into the renal tubules for urinary excretion.

Several mechanisms control aldosterone levels:

- Extracellular sodium and potassium levels—when serum sodium levels are low or potassium levels are high, aldosterone levels rise.
- Renal renin release—a reduction in renal blood flow increases aldosterone levels by the renin-angiotensin-aldosterone system.
- Pituitary adrenocorticotropic hormone (ACTH)—the glucocorticoid hormones produced in the adrenal cortex have mineralocorticoid effects.

Sex Steroids

The adrenal cortex produces small amounts of sex steroids (e.g., testosterone and estrogens) and some weak anabolic androgens (e.g., dehydroepiandrosterone and androstenedione). These hormones are produced by the adrenal glands in males and females. The amounts, however, are usually insignificant compared with the hormone amounts secreted by the gonads. However, under certain conditions (e.g., tumors, cushingoid effects), their excess may cause a substantial endocrine imbalance. These gonadal hormones are discussed in depth in Chapters 53 and 54.

PATHOPHYSIOLOGY

Adrenal Insufficiency

There are two forms of **adrenal insufficiency**—primary and secondary. Primary adrenal insufficiency (**Addison disease**) results from the destruction of the adrenal cortex caused by infection or hemorrhage, which results in hyposecretion of all adrenocortical hormones—most importantly the glucocorticoid, cortisol and the mineralocorticoid, aldosterone. Characteristics of Addison disease include those related to glucocorticoid deficiency, such as hypoglycemia, anorexia, nausea, vomiting, flatulence, diarrhea, hyperpigmentation of skin, anxiety, depression, and loss of mental acuity; and those related to mineralocorticoid deficiency, such as fluid and electrolyte imbalance, orthostatic hypotension, hyponatremia, hyperkalemia, general malaise, muscle weakness, muscle pain, and cardiac arrhythmias.

The major complication of Addison disease is a sudden, life-threatening exacerbation called **addisonian crisis** (adrenal crisis). The patient experiences severe hypotension, hyponatremia, dehydration, hyperkalemia, and hyperthermia in the absence of another cause. A stressor is often the trigger for an addisonian crisis. These physiologic responses are initially treated with standard resuscitative therapy (e.g., vasopressors, plasma expanders). When the source of these symptoms

Corticosteroids are used for replacement therapy to maintain adequate levels of hormones in patients with inadequate adrenal function. Corticosteroids are also used for their anti-inflammatory, antiallergenic, and immunosuppressive effects (Box 51.1).

The benefits derived from chronic use of corticosteroids are often accompanied by a number of risks (adverse effects). Corticosteroid complications vary from mild to life threatening and are a function of the dosage, route of administration, and duration of therapy.

PHYSIOLOGY

The hormones of the endocrine system are important messengers in the communication between cells. The nervous system, adrenal glands, and other endocrine glands contribute to homeostasis, thus allowing physical and emotional adaptation to internal and external changes.

Two adrenal glands are located one at the top of each kidney. Each gland is composed of two distinct parts—the medulla and the cortex.

The medulla and cortex are crucial to metabolism, the body's stress response, and fluid and electrolyte balances. The adrenal medulla synthesizes and secretes catecholamines—epinephrine and norepinephrine. These hormones are important in counteracting short-term stress.

BOX 51.1 Therapeutic Uses for the Corticosteroids

Glucocorticoid and Mineralocorticoid Effects at Physiologic Doses

Adrenocortical insufficiency
Adrenogenital syndrome (salt-losing)

Glucocorticoid Effects at Supraphysiologic Doses

Acute allergic conditions (e.g., bronchial asthma, serum sickness)
Acute spinal injury
Cerebral edema
Collagen diseases, rheumatic disorders (e.g., systemic lupus erythematosus, acute rheumatic carditis)
Dermatologic diseases (e.g., seborrheic dermatitis, severe psoriasis)
Gastrointestinal diseases (e.g., Crohn disease, intractable sprue, ulcerative colitis)
Hematologic disorders (e.g., autoimmune hemolytic anemia, thrombocytopenia)
Hepatic diseases (e.g., liver cirrhosis with ascites)
Joint inflammation (e.g., bursitis)
Meningitis
Neoplastic diseases (e.g., leukemias, lymphomas)
Nephrotic syndrome
Ocular disorders (e.g., allergic conjunctivitis, chorioretinitis, iritis, keratitis)
Organ transplantations
Respiratory diseases (e.g., interstitial pulmonary fibrosis, pulmonary emphysema with bronchial edema)
Thyroiditis

The adrenal cortex is involved primarily in the synthesis and secretion of **glucocorticoids** and **mineralocorticoids** (collectively referred to as the corticosteroids) from plasma-derived, low-density lipoproteins and high-density lipoproteins (cholesterol). Corticosteroids are characterized by mineralocorticoid and glucocorticoid effects, depending on the predominant pharmacologic action of the agent. Adrenal corticosteroids exert effects on almost every organ in the body. Their pharmacologic actions are generally an extension of their physiologic effects. Their primary actions include carbohydrate, protein, and fat metabolism; electrolyte and water metabolism; cardiovascular functions; and immune effects. The zona reticularis region of the adrenal cortex produces and secretes other steroid hormones, including adrenal androgens, progesterone, and the estrogens.

Glucocorticoids

The glucocorticoids acquired their name from their role in glucose metabolism; they increase blood glucose concentrations by:

- Stimulating gluconeogenesis and glucose secretion by the liver
- Increasing the hepatic sensitivity to the gluconeogenic actions of glucagon and catecholamines
- Decreasing glucose uptake and utilization by peripheral tissue
- Increasing proteolysis and decreasing protein synthesis in muscles to support the gluconeogenesis activities

Glucocorticoids exert potent and diverse actions on glucose, protein, and bone metabolism and possess anti-inflammatory, antiallergenic, and immunosuppressant actions. Metabolic effects of glucocorticoids include gluconeogenesis, mobilization of amino acids from protein in striated muscle, protein catabolism, fat synthesis and lipolysis, and hepatic enzymatic activities that convert amino acids to glucose, with most of the excess glucose stored in the liver as glycogen. The metabolic effects of the glucocorticoids result in the following:

- An increase in circulating amino acid levels
- An overall depletion of muscle protein
- A negative nitrogen balance
- A mobilization of fatty acids, converting cell metabolism from using glucose for energy to using fatty acids for energy

Other physiologic effects of the glucocorticoids include:

- An antagonistic effect on antidiuretic hormones to maintain water balance
- A lowering of the threshold for electrical excitation in the brain
- A reduction in the amount of new bone synthesis

In addition, glucocorticoids have actions that allow the body to cope effectively with physiologic or psychological stress (e.g., overwhelming illness or trauma). For example, the glucocorticoid **cortisol** sensitizes the arterioles to norepinephrine for vasopressor effects and allows epinephrine and glucagon to activate gluconeogenesis and glycogenolysis.

(C) Glucocorticoids

- **[P] prednisone**
  - betamethasone
  - dexamethasone
  - hydrocortisone
  - methylprednisolone
- Inhaled glucocorticoids
  - beclomethasone dipropionate
  - budesonide
  - flunisolide
  - fluticasone
  - triamcinolone
- Topical glucocorticoids
  - betamethasone
  - dexamethasone
  - hydrocortisone
  - methylprednisolone
  - triamcinolone

(C) Mineralocorticoids

- **[P] fludrocortisone**

(C) Steroid Hormone Antagonists

- **[P] aminoglutethimide**
  - corticosterone and desoxycorticosterone
  - cyproheptadine
  - ketoconazole
  - mifepristone
  - mitotane

The symbol (C) indicates the **drug class.**
Drugs in **bold type** marked with the symbol [P] are prototypes.
Drugs in blue type are closely related to the prototype.
Drugs in red type are significantly different from the prototype.
Drugs in black type with no symbol are also used in drug therapy; no prototype

chapter 51

Drugs Affecting Corticosteroid Levels

Learning Objectives

At the completion of this chapter the student will:

1. Describe the physiologic effects of and clinical indications for mineralocorticoids and glucocorticoids.
2. Discuss complications associated with glucocorticoids.
3. Discuss nursing interventions to maximize therapeutic and minimize adverse effects for drugs that affect corticosteroid hormone levels and have anti-inflammatory action.
4. Describe the most frequently encountered adverse effects associated with the glucocorticoids and mineralocorticoids.
5. Identify dosing strategies that may minimize glucocorticoid-related adverse effects.
6. Determine key points for patient and family education for drugs that affect corticosteroid hormone levels and have anti-inflammatory action.
7. Discuss the clinical indications of drugs referred to as steroid hormone antagonists.

KEY TERMS

Addison disease

addisonian crisis

adrenal insufficiency

aldosterone

cortisol

Cushing syndrome

glucocorticoid

hyperaldosteronism

mineralocorticoid

salt-losing adrenogenital syndrome

steroid hormone inhibitors

FEATURED WEBLINK

http://www.niddk.nih.gov/health/endo/endo.htm
Confused about endocrine disorders? Log on to this website for help with understanding these complex disorders.

CONNECTION WEBLINK

Additional Weblinks are found on Connection:
http://www.connection.lww.com/go/aschenbrenner.

CHAPTER SUMMARY

- A combination of neural and endocrine systems, originating in the hypothalamus, regulates CNS, autonomic nervous system, and endocrine functions.
- The hypothalamus produces two hormones—oxytocin and vasopressin—that are stored in and released from the posterior lobe of the pituitary gland. The hypothalamus releases a series of stimulating and inhibiting factors to promote the release of stimulating hormones from the anterior pituitary gland. These stimulating hormones affect several other endocrine glands.
- The anterior lobe of the pituitary gland produces growth hormone (GH), a hormone important for the regulation of growth and development. Release of GH is determined by inhibiting and releasing factors and by chemical signals for growing tissue.
- The thyroid gland is a bilobar gland located in the neck around the trachea. This vascular gland uses dietary iodine to produce two thyroid hormones (T_3 and T_4). These hormones affect the way many body cells utilize energy and maintain metabolism. These hormones are regulated by a balance between TRH, TSH, and the thyroid hormone levels.
- The parathyroid glands are four very small groups of tissue located on the back of the thyroid gland. These cells produce PTH (parathyroid hormone), the most important regulator of serum calcium levels in the body. PTH stimulates osteoclasts to release calcium from the bone, increases intestinal absorption of calcium, and increases calcium resorption from the kidneys. It also stimulates cells in the kidney to produce calcitriol, the active form of vitamin D, which stimulates intestinal transport of calcium into the blood. Calcium is a vital anion that is used in many of the body's metabolic processes, including membrane transport processes, conduction of nerve impulses, muscle contraction, and blood clotting. To be effective, the serum levels of calcium must be maintained between 9 and 11 mg/dL.
- The GH somatropin is an example of a drug used to replace a pituitary hormone. It is given by injection to children with GH deficiency, to some adults with GH deficiency, and to girls with Turner syndrome.
- Release of GH is blocked by octreotide, bromocriptine, and GH-inhibiting factor (somatostatin). These drugs can be used to treat acromegaly and must be given by injection.
- Vasopressin (or ADH) is administered by injection or intranasally in order to regulate water loss when levels of ADH are low or absent. Vasopressin blocks the release of water in the nephron and increases vascular volume while decreasing osmolarity. The dosage of this drug is determined by patient response and water balance.
- Thyroid hormone is given to replace low levels of thyroid hormone resulting from surgery, radiation, autoimmune disorders, inadequate iodine in the diet, malignancies, or pituitary-hypothalamic disorders. Levothyroxine (T_4) is the most commonly used thyroid hormone because of its predictability and reliability.
- Patients treated with thyroid hormone need lifelong therapy. They should be monitored for nutritional balance related to changes in metabolism and should be evaluated periodically for the effectiveness of other maintenance drugs as the patient reaches normal thyroid function and metabolism changes.
- Drugs used to block thyroid function include the thionamides—methimazole (MMI) and propylthiouracil (PTU)—and iodine preparations. The thionamides block the coupling of iodine to the thyroid hormone, whereas the iodine preparations prevent formation of thyroid hormone by blocking iodine uptake. I-131 is used in diagnostic imaging to isolate areas of increased thyroid gland activity or in one large dose to cause thyroid gland destruction by beta ray emission. Patients effectively treated with antithyroid drugs will need to be monitored for hypothyroidism and the need for thyroid hormone replacement.
- Hypercalcemia is treated with calcitonin (a thyroid hormone that counters the action of PTH), the bisphosphonates, and gallium. These drugs are used to treat any condition characterized by increased calcium levels or bone resorption, such as postmenopausal osteoporosis, Paget disease, and hypercalcemia associated with malignancy.
- Hypocalcemia is treated with vitamin D derivatives. Vitamin D compounds regulate the following processes: absorption of calcium and phosphate from the small intestine, mineral resorption in bone, and reabsorption of phosphate from the renal tubules. Working with PTH and calcitonin to regulate calcium homeostasis, vitamin D actually functions as a hormone. Patients receiving vitamin D products need to be cautioned about using OTC multiple-vitamin preparations and should be encouraged to increase dietary intake of calcium.

QUESTIONS FOR STUDY AND REVIEW

1. What is the importance of calcium balance, and how is it maintained in the body?
2. How do the hypothalamus and pituitary glands interact to help maintain homeostasis in the body?
3. What are the special educational needs of the patient and family when somatropin is used to replace deficient GH?
4. List the signs and symptoms of hypothyroidism.
5. A patient with malignancy-induced severe hypercalcemia is admitted with a serum calcium level of 18. The patient is given IV gallium as an emergency treatment. What special precautions need to be observed with the use of this drug?
6. An order is written for calcitonin, salmon to treat hypercalcemia. Before administering the drug, the patient assessment reveals a history of allergy to animal products. What steps should you take before administering the drug?

? Need More Help?

Chapter 50 of the study guide for *Drug Therapy in Nursing* 2e contains NCLEX-style questions and other learning activities to reinforce your understanding of the concepts presented in this chapter. For additional information or to purchase the study guide, visit *http://connection.lww.com/go/aschenbrenner.*

REFERENCES AND BIBLIOGRAPHY

Bilezikian, J. P., & Silverberg, S. J. (2000). Clinical spectrum of primary hyperparathyroidism. *Endocrine and Metabolic Disorders, 1*(4), 237–245.

Gutierrez, K., & Queener, S. F. (2003). *Pharmacology for nursing practice*. St. Louis: Mosby.

Marcus, R. (2000). Diagnosis and treatment of hyperparathyroidism. *Endocrine and Metabolic Disorders, 1*(4), 247–252.

Porth, C. M. (2004). *Essentials of pathophysiology: Concepts of altered health states* (7th ed.). Philadelphia: Lippincott Williams & Wilkins.

Rogol, A. D. (2003). Causes of short stature. In: Rose, B. D. (Ed.), *UpToDate*. Wellesley, MA: UpToDate.

Ross, D. S. (2003a). Patient information: Antithyroid drugs. In B. D. Rose (Ed.), *UpToDate*. Wellesley, MA: UpToDate.

Ross, D. S. (2003b). Pharmacology and toxicology of thionamides. In B. D. Rose (Ed.), *UpToDate*. Wellesley, MA: UpToDate.

Sherman, S. I. (2003). Radioiodine treatment of differential thyroid cancer. In B. D. Rose (Ed.), *UpToDate*. Wellesley, MA: UpToDate.

Snyder, P. J. (2003). Treatment of hypopituitarism. In B. D. Rose (Ed.), *UpToDate*. Wellesley, MA: UpToDate.

Providing Patient and Family Education

- Explain to patients and their families that this drug is a form of vitamin D and that it is being used to increase the patient's low calcium levels. Calcium is needed for many of the body's activities, and it is important to keep calcium levels in the blood in an effective range.
- Discuss the possible adverse effects of the drug, including GI upset with nausea, vomiting, and epigastric upset. Advise patients to eat small, frequent meals to maintain nutrition and decrease some of the unpleasant side effects of the drug.
- Advise patients to monitor noise, temperature, and light and to take prescribed analgesics as needed to decrease discomfort of the headache, muscle ache, and irritability that are common adverse effects of the drug.
- Instruct patients to report lethargy, weight loss, severe bone pain, excessive urine output, or constipation.
- Instruct patient that, as with all medications, this drug should be kept out of the reach of children.

Ongoing Assessment and Evaluation

Dosage adjustment is required as soon as clinical improvement occurs. Therapy should be started at the lowest possible dose, with increases made after careful monitoring of the serum calcium. It is important to estimate daily dietary calcium intake and adjust the intake when indicated. Patients with normal renal function taking calcitriol should avoid dehydration by maintaining adequate fluid intake. The range between therapeutic and toxic doses is narrow. When high therapeutic doses are used, it is especially important to chart the progress with frequent determinations of urinary calcium, phosphate, and BUN and to chart serum calcium, phosphate, magnesium, and alkaline phosphatase levels. Twenty-four hour urinary calcium and phosphate levels should also be monitored. These laboratory determinations are especially important in hypoparathyroid and dialysis patients. Serum calcium levels should be maintained between 9 and 10 mg/dL.

Nursing management in drug therapy is considered effective when calcium levels are maintained within a normal range and when the patient recognizes and expresses the importance of self-monitoring for adverse effects and takes responsibility for reporting significant adverse effects to the health care provider.

MEMORY CHIP

P Calcitriol

- Vitamin D; management of hypocalcemia and resultant bone disease in patients undergoing chronic renal dialysis
- Major contraindications: hypercalcemia, hypervitaminosis D, malabsorption syndrome, and decreased renal function
- Most common adverse effects: weakness, headache, somnolence, nausea, vomiting, dry mouth, constipation, muscle or bone pain, and metallic taste
- Most serious adverse effect: chronic hypercalcemia can lead to generalized vascular calcification, nephrocalcinosis, and other soft tissue calcification
- **Life span alert: Use caution in elderly patients, especially those with coronary disease, renal function impairment, and arteriosclerosis.**
- Maximizing therapeutic effects: Patients with normal renal function taking calcitriol should maintain adequate fluid intake and avoid dehydration; periodically monitor serum calcium, phosphate, magnesium, alkaline phosphatase, and 24-hour urinary calcium and phosphate, especially in hypoparathyroid and dialysis patients.
- Minimizing adverse effects: Maintain serum calcium levels between 9 and 10 mg/dL.
- Most important patient education: Adequate dietary calcium is necessary for a clinical response to vitamin D therapy; compliance with dosage instructions, diet, phosphate-binder use, and calcium supplementation is essential; avoid use of nonprescription drugs, including magnesium-containing antacids.

Drugs Closely Related to P Calcitriol

Dihydrotachysterol

Dihydrotachysterol (DHT) is a vitamin D derivative that is indicated for treating postoperative tetany (acute, chronic, and latent), idiopathic tetany, and hypothyroidism. Off-label, it is used for familial hypophosphatemia and renal osteodystrophy. DHT mobilizes bone calcium and stimulates intestinal calcium absorption in the absence of PTH. It also increases the excretion of phosphate from the kidneys. It exerts a slow but persistent effect and can be used for long periods. The beginning dose is 0.8 to 2.4 mg/day for several days, followed by a maintenance dose of 0.2 to 1.0 mg/day to maintain normal serum calcium levels. It can be supplemented with 10 to 15 mg of calcium gluconate or calcium lactate PO daily if needed. Toxicity is manifested by symptoms of hypercalcemia. It is important to carefully monitor standard hypercalcemia-related metabolic parameters (e.g., serum levels of calcium, phosphate, magnesium, and potassium).

Doxercalciferol

Doxercalciferol (Hectorol), a vitamin D analogue, is indicated to treat hyperparathyroidism secondary to renal failure. It can be administered intravenously or orally and has a mean half-life of 32 to 37 hours. Doxercalciferol is a prohormone of vitamin D that undergoes hepatic conversion to active vitamin D. Hyperphosphatemia lessens its effectiveness. Decreased absorption may occur when it is combined with agents known to interfere with the absorption of fat-soluble vitamins (e.g., cholestyramine and mineral oil). Adverse effects include edema, headache, dizziness, malaise, nausea, and vomiting.

Paricalcitol

Paricalcitol (Zemplar) is a parenterally administered synthetic vitamin D analogue used for hyperparathyroidism secondary to renal failure. It has a mean half-life of 15 hours. Paricalcitol suppresses PTH levels in patients with CRF. It may also reduce serum total alkaline phosphatase levels. Effective therapy with paricalcitol requires a dietary regimen of calcium supplementation and phosphorus restriction. Phosphate-binding compounds may be needed. Excessive use of aluminum-containing compounds should be avoided.

TABLE 50.11 Agents That Interact With P Calcitriol

Interactants	Effect and Significance	Nursing Management
Cholestyramine, ketoconazole, mineral oil, phenytoin, phenobarbital, thiazide diuretics	Decreased pharmacologic effects of vitamin D Intestinal absorption of vitamin D may be reduced Ketoconazole may inhibit both synthetic and catabolic enzymes of calcitriol Absorption of vitamin D is reduced with prolonged use of mineral oil Hypoparathyroid patients on vitamin D may develop hypercalcemia due to thiazide diuretics Endogenous synthesis of calcitriol will be inhibited; higher doses of calcitriol may be necessary with concurrent administration of phenytoin and phenobarbital	Appraise the patient for management of concurrent disease states. Assess the patient for evidence of therapeutic effects of interacting drugs. Check for therapeutic serum levels (if applicable) of interacting drugs.
Mg^{++}-containing antacids, digitalis glycosides, verapamil	Increased pharmacologic effects from interaction with vitamin D Hypermagnesemia may develop in patients on chronic renal dialysis Hypercalcemia in patients on digitalis may precipitate cardiac arrhythmias.	Assess the patient for control of concurrent disease states. Evaluate patient for evidence of therapeutic effects of interacting drugs. Measure therapeutic serum levels (if applicable) of interacting drugs. Monitor cardiac rhythm and function.

Lifestyle, Diet, and Habits

Calcitriol is generally given in the home setting. IV doses can be given following dialysis to increase calcium levels. Evaluate vitamin D ingested in fortified foods, dietary supplements, and other concomitantly administered drugs. It may be necessary to limit dietary vitamin D and its derivatives during treatment.

Patients receiving calcitriol are likely to experience multiple GI effects. Small, frequent meals may help alleviate some of these symptoms. A bowel-training program may be needed if constipation is a problem. Closely monitor nutritional status.

Nursing Diagnoses and Outcomes

- Imbalanced Nutrition: Less than Body Requirements related to reduced absorption of fat-soluble vitamins, including calcitriol, in the presence of very low-fat diet
  Desired outcome: *The patient will ingest a nutritionally balanced diet to allow for normal absorption of fat-soluble vitamins.*
- Imbalanced Nutrition: More than Body Requirements related to drug–vitamin interaction of vitamin D and calcium supplements
  Desired outcome: *The patient will identify sources of dietary vitamin D and calcium, consume these foods in moderation, and refrain from consuming vitamin or dietary supplements containing vitamin D and calcium.*
- Acute Pain related to headache and general discomfort secondary to drug effects
  Desired outcome: *The patient will not experience undue pain and discomfort as a result of drug therapy.*

Planning and Intervention

Maximizing Therapeutic Effects

Calcitriol capsules should be swallowed whole, rather than crushed or chewed. Eating a balanced diet and getting exposure to sunlight usually satisfies normal vitamin D requirements. Caution the patient and family to avoid using vitamin supplements as a substitute for a balanced diet. Monitor serum calcium levels before and during drug therapy because adequate dietary calcium is necessary for a clinical response to vitamin D therapy. Begin therapy at the lowest possible dose, with dosage increases made only after careful analysis of the serum calcium. Adjust the dosage as soon as clinical improvement is seen. It is essential to estimate the daily dietary calcium intake and adjust that intake as indicated. Patients with normal renal function taking calcitriol should maintain an adequate fluid intake to avoid dehydration because the range between therapeutic and toxic doses is narrow. When high therapeutic doses are used, frequent serum and urinary calcium, phosphate, and BUN determinations are necessary.

Monitor serum calcium, phosphate, magnesium, and alkaline phosphatase levels routinely. Serum calcium levels should be maintained between 9 and 10 mg/dL.

Minimizing Adverse Effects

Avoid use of mineral oil. Chronic dialysis patients should avoid magnesium-containing antacids while taking these drugs. Arrange for small, frequent meals to alleviate GI discomfort and to provide adequate nutrition. Monitor bowel function and begin a bowel-training program as appropriate. Provide analgesics as appropriate to decrease discomfort and pain related to drug effects.

supplies of vitamin D depend on UV light for conversion of 7-dehydrocholesterol to vitamin D_3 or ergosterol to vitamin D_2. Following exposure to UV light, vitamin D_3 is converted to the active form of vitamin D, calcitriol, in the liver and kidneys. Calcitriol is believed to be the most active form of vitamin D_3. It stimulates intestinal calcium and phosphate transport. Calcitriol is a fat-soluble vitamin that helps to regulate calcium homeostasis, bone growth, and maintenance. It increases calcium absorption from the intestine, thereby increasing serum calcium levels. It decreases alkaline phosphatase and possible PTH levels.

Biologically active vitamin D metabolites control the intestinal absorption of dietary calcium, the tubular reabsorption of calcium by the kidney, and, in conjunction with PTH, the mobilization of calcium from the skeleton. They act directly on bone cells (osteoblasts) to stimulate skeletal growth and on the parathyroid glands to suppress PTH synthesis and secretion. Vitamin D also is involved in magnesium metabolism.

Contraindications and Precautions

Excessive doses of calcitriol can cause hypercalcemia and hypercalciuria. For these reasons, it is important to monitor serum calcium twice a week during initial dosing. In dialysis patients, decreased serum alkaline phosphatase levels often precede hypercalcemia. An abrupt increase in calcium intake, usually from dietary sources, may trigger hypercalcemia. If hypercalcemia develops, it is necessary to discontinue calcitriol immediately. During periods of hypercalcemia, daily serum calcium and phosphate levels must be determined. When calcium levels return to normal, calcitriol can be readministered at a daily dose 0.25 μg lower than initially used. Patients on digitalis therapy are at an increased risk for cardiac arrhythmias; thus, calcitriol must be given cautiously. Chronic hypercalcemia can lead to generalized vascular calcification, nephrocalcinosis, and other soft tissue calcification. Chronic hypercalcemia may be associated with a transient increase in serum creatinine levels in patients with normal renal function. It is important for these patients to pay careful attention to factors that may lead to hypercalcemia. Patients with end-stage renal disease are unable to adequately synthesize calcitriol, the active hormone formed from the precursor vitamin D. Resultant hypocalcemia and secondary hyperparathyroidism are major causes of the metabolic bone disease of renal failure.

Some vitamin D products contain tartrazine, which may cause allergic-type reactions (including bronchial asthma) in susceptible individuals. Although the incidence of this sensitivity is low, it is frequently seen in patients with aspirin hypersensitivity. Products containing tartrazine are identified in product listings on the label.

Calcitriol therapy should always be started at the lowest possible dose and increased only with careful monitoring of serum calcium levels. During periods when the medication is adjusted, serum calcium levels should be monitored twice a week. Once the optimal dose is determined, serum calcium levels require monthly monitoring.

Adverse Effects

Adverse effects are similar to those encountered with vitamin D excess. Early signs include weakness, headache, nausea and vomiting, dry mouth, constipation, and bone pain. Late signs include polyuria, polydipsia, weight loss; elevated BUN, serum glutamic-oxaloacetic transaminase (SGOT), and serum glutamate pyruvate transaminase (SGPT); cardiac arrhythmias, hypertension, and dehydration.

Drug Interactions

Hypermagnesemia is a risk if calcitriol is taken with magnesium-containing antacids. If both drugs must be taken, they should be spaced 2 to 4 hours apart. Patients on chronic renal dialysis should not take both types of medications. Reduced absorption of calcitriol occurs if it is taken with cholestyramine or mineral oil. This combination also should be avoided or spaced 2 to 4 hours apart. A possible risk for hypercalcemia occurs in some patients when thiazide diuretics and calcitriol are combined. Table 50.11 lists drugs that interact with calcitriol.

Assessment of Relevant Core Patient Variables

Health Status

A thorough health history is necessary to identify any factors that relate to the cause of hypoparathyroidism. Calcitriol should be used with caution in elderly patients, especially those with coronary disease, renal function impairment, and arteriosclerosis. Before administering calcitriol, review the patient's record to determine whether calcitriol can be safely administered. Caution should be used when administering the drug to patients with renal stones.

Before beginning drug therapy, perform a physical examination including skin color, temperature, orientation, and status of mucous membranes to establish a baseline from which to monitor the effects of the drug. Determine serum levels of calcium, phosphorus, magnesium, alkaline phosphatase, and renal and liver function to establish a baseline from which to measure drug activity and adverse effects.

Life Span and Gender

Assess the patient for pregnancy or breast-feeding. Calcitriol is in pregnancy category C. No adequate, well-controlled studies have been performed in pregnant women. It should be used during pregnancy only if the potential benefits outweigh the potential hazards to the fetus. Vitamin D may be excreted in breast milk; therefore, breast-feeding should be avoided when taking calcitriol. Safety of vitamin D in amounts over 400 IU/day is not established.

Safety and efficacy of calcitriol given to pediatric patients undergoing dialysis have not been studied but are based on adult patients. Dosing guidelines have not been established for patients with hypoparathyroidism who are younger than 1 year or for those younger than 6 years with pseudohypoparathyroidism. Long-term calcitriol therapy is well tolerated by pediatric patients who are not undergoing dialysis. Pediatric doses should be individualized and monitored closely.

Sufficient numbers of subjects older than 65 years have not been studied to determine whether or not they respond differently from younger adults. Dosage for elderly patients should start at the low end of the dosing range, because of their greater risk for decreased renal, hepatic, or cardiac function.

TABLE 50.10 Summary of Selected (C) Antihypocalcemic Drugs

Drug (Trade) Name	Selected Indications	Route and Dosage Range	Pharmacokinetics
P calcitriol (Calcijex, Rocaltrol)	Management of hypocalcemia in chronic renal dialysis Hypoparathyroidism Predialysis	*Adult:* 0.25 μg/d. May increase *by 0.25 μg/d at 4–8 wk intervals* *Hypoparathyroidism:* 0.25 μg/d. Children ≥ 6 y and adults usually respond to 0.5–2 μg/d. *<6 y:* 0.25–0.75 μg *Adult and child >3 y:* 0.25 μg/d	*Onset:* 2–6 h *Duration:* 3–5 d $t_{1/2}$: 3–6 h
dihydrotachysterol (DHT, Hytakerol)	Treatment of hypoparathyroidism Postoperative or idiopathic tetany	*Adult:* PO, 0.75–2.5 mg/d initially; maintenance, PO, 0.2–1.75 mg/d to maintain serum calcium levels	*Onset:* 10–24 h *Duration:* 3–5 d $t_{1/2}$: 16 d
doxercalciferol (Hectorol)	Reduction of elevated parathyroid hormone levels in the management of secondary hyperparathyroidism in patients undergoing chronic renal dialysis	10 μg administered three times a week at dialysis; initial dose adjusted as needed to lower blood PTH into 15- to 300-pg/mL range. Increase dosage at 8-week intervals by 2.5 μg. The maximum recommended dose is 20 μg administered three times a week at dialysis for a total of 60 μg/week.	*Onset:* 10–24 h *Duration:* 3–5 d $t_{1/2}$: 32–37 h
paricalcitol (Zemplar)	Prevention and treatment of secondary hyperparathyroidism associated with chronic renal failure	Initial dose is 0.04 to 0.1 μg/kg (2.8 to 7 μg); dose may be increased by 2–4 μg at 2–4 wk intervals to maximum of 0.24 μg/kg (16.8 μg) administered as a bolus dose every other day during dialysis.	*Onset:* 10–24 h *Duration:* 16 d $t_{1/2}$: 15 h

Hypoparathyroidism is treated primarily with vitamin D. If necessary, dietary supplements of calcium are also given. Patients with hypoparathyroidism have deficient levels of PTH, which result in hypocalcemia. Vitamin D stimulates calcium absorption from the intestine and restores the serum calcium to a normal level. It is a fat-soluble vitamin derived from natural sources (fish liver oils) or from conversion of provitamins. In humans, natural supplies of vitamin D depend on ultraviolet (UV) light for conversion to vitamin D_3 or vitamin D_2. Following exposure to UV light, vitamin D_3 must then be converted to its active forms by the liver and kidneys. Vitamin D is hydroxylated by the hepatic microsomal enzymes to calcifediol. It is further hydroxylated in the kidney to calcitriol and doxercalciferol. Calcitriol (Rocaltrol [capsules, solution]; Calcijex [parenteral]) is believed to be the most active form of vitamin D in stimulating intestinal calcium and phosphate transport.

Pharmacotherapeutics

Clinical indications for calcitriol include management of hypocalcemia and resulting bone disease in patients on chronic renal dialysis; management of secondary hyperparathyroidism and metabolic bone disease in predialysis patients with moderate to severe chronic renal failure (creatinine clearance, 15–55 mL/min); and management of hypocalcemia and its clinical manifestations in patients with hypoparathyroidism (postsurgical, idiopathic, or pseudohypoparathyroidism). Off-label uses for calcitriol (oral) include increasing bone mass and preventing fractures in patients with osteoporosis, and (topical) decreasing severity of psoriatic lesions (see Table 50.10).

Pharmacokinetics

Calcitriol can be administered orally or intravenously. It is rapidly absorbed from the small intestine, with a peak effect occurring in 3 to 6 hours. Absorption is reduced with liver or biliary disease because bile is essential for adequate absorption. Vitamin D is chiefly stored in the liver but is also found in fat, muscle, skin, and bones. Calcitriol is 99% bound in blood. It is transported in blood by an alpha-globulin vitamin D–binding protein. Vitamin D is converted to calcifediol in the liver and then to doxercalciferol in the kidney. The half-life of calcitriol is 5 to 8 hours. Its pharmacologic activity persists for 3 to 5 days. The half-life increases at least twofold in patients with chronic renal failure and in hemodialysis patients. The primary route of vitamin D excretion is in the bile, but a small percentage is found in the urine.

Pharmacodynamics

Vitamin D is a fat-soluble vitamin derived from natural sources (fish liver oils) or from conversion of provitamins, 7-dehydrocholesterol, and ergosterol. In humans, natural

6 to 8 ounces of plain water 2 hours before or after other medications or meals. It should be given only for a 3-month period. Beverages other than plain water (including mineral water), food, and some medications (e.g., indomethacin) are likely to reduce the absorption of tiludronate. Following therapy, an interval of 3 months should be allowed to assess response. The effectiveness of this drug beyond 3 months is not known. The tablets should not be removed from the foil strip packaging until they are to be used.

Plicamycin

Plicamycin (Mithracin) is an antineoplastic, antihypercalcemic agent that is indicated for hypercalcemia secondary to neoplasms. It has been reported to be effective in treating Paget disease; however, it has not been approved by the FDA for this use. This medication is for IV administration only, and it is highly recommended that it be given only under the supervision of a qualified physician experienced in the use of chemotherapeutic agents. The patient must be hospitalized during administration, because of the possibility of severe reactions.

When plicamycin is used for Paget disease, the dose should be about 10% of that used for cancer treatment. Adverse effects are much less common with this use, because of the lower dose. The dosage is based on body weight; ideal body weight should be used if the individual has abnormal fluid retention. Extravasation may cause local irritation and cellulitis at injection sites. Plicamycin blocks the hypercalcemic action of pharmacologic doses of vitamin D, acts on osteoclasts, and blocks the action of PTH. Plicamycin inhibition of DNA-dependent RNA synthesis renders osteoclasts unable to respond fully to PTH with the biosynthesis necessary for osteolysis. Decreases in serum phosphate levels and urinary calcium excretion accompany the lowering of serum calcium concentrations. The drug is cleared rapidly from blood within the first 2 hours; excretion also is rapid (90% in the first 24 hours after injection). Contraindications to use are thrombocytopenia, coagulation disorders, impaired bone marrow function, and pregnancy (plicamycin is in FDA pregnancy category X). Most common adverse effects include GI symptoms (anorexia, nausea, vomiting, diarrhea, and stomatitis). Electrolyte disturbances and depression of serum calcium, phosphorus, and potassium levels may occur. Calcium supplements are sometimes needed during plicamycin therapy.

Drugs Significantly Different From [P] Calcitonin, Salmon

Furosemide

Furosemide (Lasix) is a loop diuretic that promotes renal excretion of calcium. Dosage of up to 100 mg IV may be given. Adverse effects include dehydration, hypokalemia, hyperuricemia, hypomagnesemia, and hypochloremic alkalosis. Fluid balance, blood pressure, pulse, and serum electrolytes must be carefully monitored when furosemide is administered. Furosemide is discussed in depth in Chapter 32.

Gallium

Gallium (Ganite) inhibits calcium resorption from bone and reduces bone turnover, effects that result in a lowered serum calcium level. Gallium is indicated for treating cancer-related hypercalcemia. It is administered intravenously over a 5-day period for patients that are symptomatic and do not respond to conventional treatment. This drug carries a substantial risk for severe renal insufficiency, especially if it is administered concomitantly with other nephrotoxic agents (e.g., amphotericin B or aminoglycosides). Renal function tests must be monitored closely for any sign of renal toxicity. It is crucial to maintain adequate hydration in patients receiving gallium and to monitor serum electrolytes closely.

Cinacalcet

Cinacalcet (Sensipar), an oral calcimetric agent, is the first approved agent in this drug class. It is indicated to treat patients with secondary hyperparathyroidism caused by chronic kidney disease and patients with hypercalcemia associated with parathyroid carcinoma. Cinacalcet directly reduces PTH levels, while lowering calcium and phosphorus levels. This action is consistent with the National Kidney Foundation Disease Outcomes Quality Initiative clinical practice guidelines for bone metabolism and disease in chronic kidney disease. In a clinical trial reported by the manufacturer, cinacalcet was shown to reduce high serum calcium levels in patients with parathyroid carcinoma. With nearly 500 patients developing this rare condition annually, cinacalcet was granted orphan designation by the FDA.

(C) Antihypocalcemic Drugs

Blood calcium and phosphate levels are usually adequately regulated by using replacement therapy with vitamin D compounds combined with calcium salts and a high dietary intake. Calcitriol (1,25-dihydroxy-vitamin D3) (Rocaltrol [capsules]; Calcijex [parenteral]) is the active form of vitamin D and the prototype antihypocalcemic. Table 50.10 presents a summary of selected antihypocalcemic drugs.

NURSING MANAGEMENT OF THE PATIENT RECEIVING [P] CALCITRIOL

Core Drug Knowledge

Vitamin D compounds regulate absorption of calcium and phosphate from the small intestine, reabsorption of phosphate from the renal tubules, and mineral resorption in bone. Vitamin D is considered a hormone, although it is not a natural human hormone. The commonly used term "vitamin D" refers to both ergocalciferol (D_2) and cholecalciferol (D_3). Vitamin D_2, a plant vitamin, is predominantly used to fortify milk and cereals, and it can substitute for D_3.

Vitamin D metabolites control intestinal absorption of dietary calcium, tubular reabsorption of calcium by the kidney, and mobilization of calcium from the skeleton, in conjunction with PTH. They act directly on bone cells (osteoblasts) to stimulate skeletal growth and on the parathyroid glands to suppress PTH synthesis and secretion. Vitamin D is also involved in magnesium metabolism.

Vitamin D works together with PTH and calcitonin to regulate calcium homeostasis. It functions as a hormone.

bodies may form after several months of therapy, causing resistance to the drug and decreased therapeutic effects. Monitor the hormone status and clinical response in those receiving long-term therapy.

Nursing management of drug therapy is judged effective when calcium levels are maintained within a normal range. The patient should express the importance of self-monitoring for adverse effects and of reporting significant effects to the prescriber.

Drugs Closely Related to P Calcitonin, Salmon

Bisphosphonates

The bisphosphonates are calcium-regulator drugs closely related to calcitonin. The major pharmacologic action of this class of drugs is to inhibit normal and abnormal bone resorption. Reduction of abnormal bone resorption is responsible for therapeutic benefit in hypercalcemia. Bisphosphonate drugs are recommended for long-term management of hypercalcemia to increase bone resorption of calcium, in treating and preventing osteoporosis in postmenopausal women, and in managing Paget disease.

Caution patients taking bisphosphonates that the expected benefits of the drug are obtained only when each tablet is taken upon arising in the morning with a full glass of plain water (6–8 oz) and at least 30 minutes before ingesting any other medications, food, or beverages. Taking bisphosphonates with juice or coffee markedly reduces absorption (especially of alendronate). After taking the drug, the patient must stay in an upright position for 30 minutes to facilitate drug delivery to the stomach and prevent esophageal irritations. Patients must be instructed not to take this medication at bedtime or before arising for the day. Sucking on or chewing these medications can cause oropharyngeal ulceration. Supplemental calcium and vitamin D must also be administered for the bisphosphonates to be effective. Weight-bearing exercise and modifying certain behavioral factors (e.g., cigarette smoking and alcohol consumption) may aid in diminishing bone resorption. Bisphosphonates are very effective when given as a once-a-week medication. If a dose is missed, the patient should be instructed to take a tablet on the morning after they remember, then resume taking the medication on the regularly chosen day.

ALENDRONATE

Alendronate sodium (Fosamax) is a bisphosphonate that inhibits osteoclast-mediated bone resorption. It is indicated to treat or prevent osteoporosis in postmenopausal women (see Chapter 54), to increase bone mass in men with osteoporosis, to treat glucocorticoid-induced osteoporosis in men and women, and for Paget disease. It is likely that calcium supplements, some oral medications, and antacids will interfere with the absorption of alendronate. The patient should be instructed not to take any other medication for at least 30 minutes after taking alendronate.

ETIDRONATE

Etidronate (Didronel) has a similar action to that of alendronate. It lowers serum calcium levels by blocking calcium removal from bone. Etidronate is indicated for managing Paget disease, hypercalcemia related to malignancy, and heterotropic ossification that can occur after total hip replacement or spinal cord injury. Off-label, it is used for postmenopausal or steroid-induced osteoporosis. Etidronate is excreted unchanged in the urine and has a serum half-life of 6 hours and a bone half-life of 90 days. It crosses the placenta and may enter breast milk.

Etidronate should be used cautiously in patients with renal dysfunction or upper GI tract disease. The most common adverse effects of etidronate are GI complaints, such as metallic taste sensation, nausea, and diarrhea. Giving the medication in two divided doses helps to alleviate GI effects. Initiation of drug therapy can exacerbate the pain of Paget disease, but pain usually resolves as therapeutic levels are reached. Hypersensitivity reactions are rare but have included angioedema, urticaria, rash, and pruritus.

RISEDRONATE

Risedronate (Actonel) modulates bone metabolism and inhibits osteoclast-mediated bone resorption. It has an initial half-life of about 1.5 hours and a terminal half-life of 480 hours. Supplemental calcium and vitamin D should be ingested concurrently, if dietary intake is inadequate. Agents containing calcium, aluminum, or magnesium should be taken at a different time of the day to prevent interference with risedronate absorption. Risedronate is not recommended for use in patients with severe renal impairment (creatinine clearance, <30 mL/min). No dosage adjustment is necessary for the elderly. Risedronate has not been studied in patients younger than 18 years.

TILUDRONATE

Tiludronate (Skelid) is similar in action to risedronate. It is indicated to treat Paget disease in patients who also have serum alkaline phosphatase (SAP) levels twice the normal upper limit, are at risk for future complications of their disease, and are symptomatic. As with the other medications discussed, patients should receive supplemental calcium and vitamin D if dietary intake is inadequate. Tiludronate should be given as a single daily oral dose of 400 mg, taken with

MEMORY CHIP

P Calcitonin, Salmon

- Calcium regulator used to treat postmenopausal osteoporosis, Paget disease, hypercalcemia
- Major contraindications: hypersensitivity to fish products
- Most common adverse effects: nausea, vomiting, and diarrhea
- **Life span alert: *Children*—safety and efficacy not established.**
- Maximizing therapeutic effects: Store unopened bottle (nasal drug formulation) in the refrigerator between 36° and 43°F; once the pump has been activated, store at room temperature.
- Minimizing adverse effects: Periodically examine urine sediments of patients on chronic therapy; coarse granular casts and renal tubular epithelial cell casts result from therapy and may cause renal calculi.
- Most important patient education: With intranasal dosing, alternate nostrils daily; notify health care provider if significant nasal irritation occurs.

Include the family history because primary hyperparathyroidism occurs in a number of familial syndromes. Use caution when administering calcitriol to patients with renal dysfunction or upper GI disease. Perform a nasal examination before nasal calcitonin administration and repeat it if the patient experiences nasal complaints.

Life Span and Gender

Calcitonin is in FDA pregnancy C. Assess for pregnancy and lactation. Whether calcitonin is excreted in human milk is unknown. For this reason, nursing is not recommended while the patient is on this drug. No studies have been conducted with pregnant women, but in animal studies, decreased fetal birth weights have been shown.

Lifestyle, Diet, and Habits and Environment

Long-term treatment with calcitonin occurs in the home or community. Monitor the patient's responses to detect adverse effects or previously unrecognized effects of the drug. Abnormal serum calcium levels and signs of allergy may occur.

Take a thorough health history to identify factors relating to the cause of hyperparathyroidism, such as vitamin D intoxication, hyperphosphatemia, and osteolytic bone metastases. Obtain a broad database about the patient for comparison during therapy; for example, record dietary practices, visible bone deformities that may or may not interfere with activities, allergic tendencies, emotional lability, and lethargy.

Nursing Diagnoses and Outcomes

- Imbalanced Nutrition: Less than Body Requirements related to GI effects of drug therapy
  Desired outcome: *The patient will relate the importance of good nutrition and ingest daily nutritional requirements in accordance with activity level and metabolic needs.*
- Pain, Acute or Chronic related to complications of calcium or phosphate imbalances (e.g., renal stones, pathologic fractures, and osteoporosis)
  Desired outcome: *The patient will practice pain relief measures to avoid or manage the pain.*

Planning and Intervention

Maximizing Therapeutic Effects

The recommended intranasal dose of calcitonin for postmenopausal osteoporosis is 200 IU intranasally, alternating nostrils each day. This practice will decrease nasal irritation. An adequate diet and supplemental calcium carbonate (1.5 g daily), plus vitamin D intake (400 units daily), is essential. SC and IM injections of 100 IU/day are also available.

For Paget disease, the drug must be given by injection. The recommended starting dose is 100 IU/day SC (preferred for outpatient administration) or IM. Serum alkaline phosphatase and 24-hour urinary hydroxyproline should be periodically measured in order to measure drug effect. Decrease in bone pain and normalization of biochemical abnormalities usually occur within the first few months of treatment, if it is going to occur. When normalization does occur, 50 IU/day or every other day is often sufficient to maintain clinical and biochemical improvement.

The recommended starting dose for hypercalcemia is 4 IU/kg every 12 hours, SC or IM. If adequate response does not occur within 2 days, an increase to 8 IU/kg every 12 hours is expected. If this dosage is inadequate, it can be further increased to 8 IU/kg every 6 hours. If the volume is greater than 2 mL, IM injection is preferred.

Minimizing Adverse Effects

Nausea is the most common adverse effect with SC or IM administration. It is most evident at the initiation of treatment and tends to decrease or disappear with continued administration. Local inflammatory reactions from SC and IM injections can be minimized by rotating injection sites. Rhinitis, nasal crusts, and dryness are the most common adverse effects of nasal calcitonin. Alternating nostrils daily is recommended.

Providing Patient and Family Education

- Instruct the patient or family members in sterile SC and IM injection technique.
- For nasal forms of the drug, teach patients how to activate the pump and instruct them to evaluate the mucous membranes daily.
- This drug is designed to decrease the level of calcium in the blood. Calcium is needed for many of the body's activities, and it is important to keep the blood calcium levels in an effective range.
- Explain that adverse effects are usually mild but may include GI upset with nausea, vomiting, and epigastric discomfort or local inflammation. The drug should be taken once a day at the same time each day. If GI upset occurs, suggest small, frequent meals to maintain nutrition and decrease the unpleasant effects of the drug. Explaining that these adverse effects usually decrease with continued use may promote adherence.
- Starting therapy may exacerbate Paget disease bone pain. It is important to assure patients that such exacerbation is usually transient. Teach the patient the following ways to manage bone pain associated with Paget disease:
- Non-narcotic analgesics (e.g., NSAIDs, cytochrome-C-oxidase-2 [COX-2] inhibitors)
- Applications of heat
- Massage
- Bracing
- Guided imagery
- Relaxation techniques
- Biofeedback
- Meditation
- The patient should be instructed to report twitching, muscle pain, severe diarrhea, or dark urine.
- As with all medications, this drug should be kept out of the reach of children.
- Alert the patient and family that skeletal deformities (e.g., bowed tibia or femur, kyphosis, or barrel-shaped chest) are not corrected by treatment. You can teach the patient to camouflage deformities using clothing (e.g., slacks for women, tunic-style tops, and loosely fitted apparel).

Ongoing Assessment and Evaluation

Calcitonin can cause the serum calcium level to drop, resulting in tetany and cardiac arrhythmias. In addition, anti-

NURSING MANAGEMENT OF THE PATIENT RECEIVING P CALCITONIN, SALMON

Core Drug Knowledge

Pharmacotherapeutics

Calcitonin, salmon (Miacalcin) is indicated to treat symptomatic Paget disease of the bone (osteitis deformans), postmenopausal osteoporosis, and hypercalcemia. **Paget disease** is an idiopathic disease characterized by chronic bone inflammation that results in thickening, softening, and bowing of the affected bones. Many people with Paget disease are not symptomatic because only small areas of the bones are involved. Those with symptomatic disease experience bone pain and deformity, fractures, spinal cord compression, or cranial and spinal cord entrapment. Because vascularity of the bone is increased, high-output congestive heart failure may be evident. When a large mass of bone is involved, urinary hydroxyproline excretion may increase secondary to the breakdown of the collagen-containing bone matrix. Serum alkaline phosphatase also increases, secondary to increased bone formation. Calcitonin, salmon decreases the rate of bone turnover, with a resultant decrease in both urinary hydroxyproline excretion and serum alkaline phosphatase. It can be administered by the SC, IM (for all three conditions), or intranasal (for postmenopausal osteoporosis) route. There is a risk for allergic reaction to the salmon antigens in calcitonin, salmon. For this reason, if a person is suspected to have sensitivity to Miacalcin, skin testing is recommended. The skin test consists of administering 0.1 mL of a 10-IU/mL solution subcutaneously on the inner aspect of the forearm. The appearance of a wheal or mild erythema, usually within 15 minutes, indicates a positive reaction (see Table 50.9).

Calcitonin, human (Cibacalcin) is a synthetic form of the hormone produced by the human thyroid gland. Calcitonin, human is used to treat Paget disease. It must be administered subcutaneously up to three times a week. It should be discontinued once symptoms are relieved.

Calcitonin, salmon is a synthetic polypeptide of 32 amino acids that has actions very similar to those of the hormone secreted by the parafollicular cells of the thyroid gland, but with a greater (about 50.fold) potency per milligram and longer duration of action. It inhibits **bone resorption** (pathologic or physiologic loss or destruction of bone tissue, which can occur as a result of neoplasm, hyperparathyroidism, osteoporosis, or prolonged immobility). Calcitonin also increases the excretion of calcium, sodium, and phosphorus by the kidney, thereby lowering serum calcium levels. Intranasal calcitonin increases spinal bone mass in postmenopausal women with established osteoporosis, but has not been shown to be effective early in menopause.

Pharmacokinetics

Calcitonin is rapidly metabolized, primarily in the kidneys, by conversion to smaller inactivated fragments. A small amount of unchanged hormone and its inactive metabolites are excreted in the urine. Half-life is 1.2 hours. Calcitonin does not cross the placenta. Whether it passes to breast milk and cerebrospinal fluid has not been determined.

Pharmacodynamics

In mammals, calcitonin is a polypeptide hormone that is secreted by the parafollicular cells of the thyroid gland. Calcitonin, salmon is a synthetic polypeptide with essentially the same actions as calcitonin. It plays a role in the regulation of calcium and bone metabolism and has direct renal effects and actions on the GI tract. Single injections of calcitonin cause a transient but marked inhibition of bone resorption. With prolonged use, a persistent, smaller decrease occurs in the rate of bone resorption. This decrease is associated with a decreased number of osteoclasts and a reduction in their resorptive activity. Endogenous calcitonin, in conjunction with PTH, has been shown to regulate blood calcium in animal studies. High blood calcium levels increase secretion of calcitonin, which inhibits bone resorption. This effect returns the blood calcium to normal.

Contraindications and Precautions

Rare but serious allergic-type reactions, such as anaphylaxis, have been reported with injectable calcitonin, salmon. Because of this possibility, the major contraindication to the use of calcitonin, salmon is allergy. People who are allergic to fish products are at a greater risk for anaphylaxis. Patients with multiple allergies should undergo skin testing before receiving calcitonin treatment. No serious allergic-type reactions have been reported with the nasal spray.

Adverse Effects

Adverse effects are generally infrequent and mild. GI disturbances are most evident at the start of treatment and tend to decrease with continued use. Other adverse effects include dermatologic effects of skin rash and flushing of the face and hands, nasal irritation or rhinitis (if using the nasal spray), and localized inflammatory reactions at the injection site.

Drug Interactions

If calcitonin, salmon is taken with calcium supplements, antacids, or vitamin D, there is a risk for hypercalcemia, and therapeutic effect is decreased. Advise patients against using OTC vitamin and mineral preparations and antacids because many of these products contain calcium. Concurrent administration of theophylline may increase bone resorption. Formal studies to evaluate drug interactions with the nasal spray have not been done.

Assessment of Relevant Core Patient Variables

Health Status

Before administering calcitonin, review the patient's record to determine whether calcitonin can be administered safely. Perform a physical examination to establish a baseline from which to monitor the drug's effects. It is important to evaluate bone pain, muscle tone, bowel sounds, renal function tests, and serum calcium levels. While collecting a thorough health history, ask about bone disease, endocrine disorders, kidney stones, or ulcer diseases. Also, obtain a complete drug history, including use of prescription and OTC drugs. Thiazide diuretics and excessive ingestion of vitamin D can cause hypercalcemia.

drugs used to treat PTH excess or high levels of serum calcium. These drugs do not directly affect the parathyroid gland or PTH, but rather inhibit bone resorption of calcium. Calcitonin is a polypeptide hormone secreted by the thyroid gland. Commercially available calcitonin drugs are calcitonin, salmon and calcitonin, human. Both are derived synthetically and are used when the hypercalcemia is related to hyperparathyroidism. The prototype calcium-regulator drug is calcitonin, salmon. Table 50.9 presents a summary of selected antihypercalcemic drugs.

TABLE 50.9 Summary of Selected (C) Antihypercalcemic Drugs

Drug (Trade) Name	Selected Indications	Route and Dosage Range	Pharmacokinetics
P calcitonin, salmon (Calcimar, Miacalcin Nasal Spray, Miacalcin; *Canadian:* Caltine)	Treatment of Paget disease Postmenopausal osteoporosis with calcium and vitamin D Emergency treatment of hypercalcemia	*Adult:* Paget disease, initial dose, SC or IM, 100 IU/d; maintenance, 50 IU/d or qod; postmenopausal osteoporosis, SC or IM, 100 IU/d; hypercalcemia, SC or IM, 4 IU/kg q12h, may increase to 8 IU/dg q6h *Child:* Safety and efficacy not established	*Onset:* 15 min *Duration:* 8–24 h $t_{1/2}$: 1.2 h
cinacalcet (Sensipar)	Secondary hypertension in patients on renal dialysis Parathyroid cancer	*Adult:* PO, 30 mg/d, increase gradually to maximum 180 mg/d *Adult:* PO, 30 mg bid up to 90 mg qid	*Onset:* Unknown *Duration:* Unknown $t_{1/2}$: 30–40 h
alendronate (Fosamax)	Treatment of Paget disease in patients at risk for complications	*Adult:* Osteoporosis, PO, 70 mg/wk or 10 mg/d; Paget disease, PO, 40 mg/d for 6 mo *Child:* Safety and efficacy not established	*Onset:* Slow *Duration:* Days $t_{1/2}$: Unknown
etidronate (Didronel)	Treatment of Paget disease Heterotopic ossification Hypercalcemia resulting from malignancy	*Adult:* Paget disease, PO, 5–10 mg/kg/d up to 6 mo or 11–20 mg/kg/d not to exceed 3 mo; Heterotropic ossification, PO, 20 mg/kg/d, total; treatment not to exceed 4 mo; Hypercalcemia, IV, 7.5 mg/kg/d x 3 days. May repeat with at least 7-day interval between course of tx. Follow with oral dose of 20 mg/kg/d not to exceed 3 mo.	*Onset:* Slow *Duration:* 6 h; 6 h (serum) $t_{1/2}$: 90 d
furosemide (Lasix; *Canadian:* Apo-Furosemide)	Promotes renal excretion of calcium	Up to 100 mg IV	*Onset:* 5 min *Duration:* 2 h $t_{1/2}$: 2 h
gallium nitrate (Ganite)	Treatment of malignancy-related hypercalcemia	*Adult:* IV, 200 mg/m²/d for 5 consecutive d *Child:* Safety and efficacy not established	*Onset:* Slow *Duration:* 3–4 d $t_{1/2}$: Unknown
pamidronate (Aredia)	Treatment of hypercalcemia resulting from malignancy Paget disease Osteolytic bone lesions Postmenopausal osteoporosis	*Adult:* Hypercalcemia, IV, 60–90 mg over 24h; Paget disease, IV 30 mg/d over 4 h for 3 d; osteolytic bone lesions, IV, 90 mg over 4 h each month *Child:* Safety and efficacy not established	*Onset:* Rapid *Duration:* 72 h $t_{1/2}$: 1.6 h, then 27.3 h
plicamycin (Mithracin)	Hypercalcemia and hypercalciuria in symptomatic patients associated with advanced neoplasms	Base dose on body weight. Use ideal weight if patient has abnormal fluid retention. 25 µg/kg/d for 3 or 4 d; may repeat at intervals of ≥1 wk to maintain serum and urinary calcium excretion at normal levels.	*Onset:* Rapid *Duration:* Unknown $t_{1/2}$: Unknown
risedronate (Actonel)	Treatment of Paget disease Prevention of bone loss in postmenopausal women	*Adult:* PO, 30 mg/d for 2 mo *Adult:* PO, 5 mg/d or 35 mg/wk	*Onset:* Rapid *Duration:* Unknown $t_{1/2}$: 480 h
tiludronate (Skelid)	Treatment of Paget disease	*Adult:* PO, 400 mg/d for 3 mo *Child:* Safety and efficacy not established	*Onset:* 2 h *Duration:* Days $t_{1/2}$: 150 h

The total amount of I-131 needed to achieve clinical remission of hyperthyroidism without destroying the entire gland varies widely. The usual dosage range to treat hyperthyroidism is 4 to 10 millicuries (mCi). The usual dosage for ablation of normal thyroid tissue (in thyroid carcinoma) is 50 mCi, with subsequent therapeutic doses of 100 to 150 mCi.

The exposure level around a patient treated with I-131 depends on the administered dose, the time elapsed following treatment, and the amount absorbed by thyroid tissue. Hospital radiation-safety protocols (based on the U.S. Nuclear Regulatory Commission [NRC] regulations for radiopharmaceutical therapy) must be strictly followed during the hospitalization. Radioactive iodine therapy is considered safe. Some individuals, particularly the elderly, may be treated with antithyroid drugs before I-131 therapy to minimize the risk for exacerbating the hyperthyroidism.

I-131 has orphan-drug status for detection of hepatocellular carcinoma, hepatoblastoma, and alpha-fetoprotein–producing germ-cell tumors; detection of tumors that produce human chorionic gonadotropin; adrenal cortical imaging; and B-cell lymphomas and leukemias. It also has orphan-drug status as a diagnostic adjunct in pheochromocytoma.

I-131 is absorbed readily from the GI tract and distributed primarily within the extracellular fluid of the body. It is trapped and rapidly converted by the thyroid to protein-bound iodine. It is then concentrated by the stomach and salivary glands and excreted within several days by the kidney. The physical half-life of I-131 is 8.04 days.

I-131 is in FDA pregnancy category X. It is contraindicated for women who are or may become pregnant because it crosses the placenta and can cause permanent damage to the fetus' thyroid gland. It is also contraindicated for lactating women because iodine is excreted in breast milk. Another contraindication to therapy is pre-existing vomiting because if the patient vomits during the first few hours after therapy, the vomitus will be highly radioactive. I-131 is seldom used in patients younger than 30 years unless circumstances preclude other treatment.

The immediate adverse reactions following I-131 treatment for hyperthyroidism are usually mild. More severe reactions occur following larger doses, such as those used in thyroid carcinoma. Severe reactions include depression of the hematopoietic system (acute leukemia, depressed bone marrow function, anemia, leukopenia, and thrombocytopenia). Signs of radiation sickness may also occur. Manifestations may include nausea and vomiting, tachycardia, chest pain, itching skin, hives, rash, chromosomal abnormalities, acute thyroid crisis, and death. Tenderness and swelling around the neck area, pain on swallowing, sore throat, and cough may occur 72 hours after treatment. These manifestations usually respond to treatment with analgesics.

The uptake of I-131 will be affected by recent intake of iodine in any form and by thyroid and antithyroid agents. Antithyroid therapy (e.g., methimazole) of a severely hyperthyroid patient is usually discontinued 3 to 4 days before I-131 is administered.

Fears of radiation-induced genetic damage, leukemia, and neoplasia have shaped this practice, although these fears have not been realized during several decades of clinical experience. Studies indicate that the risk for infertility and birth defects following I-131 treatment is not increased if pregnancy is avoided for at least 1 year following treatment.

Patients with Graves disease may be given an antithyroid drug, such as MMI, for several months preceding radiotherapy in order to establish a euthyroid state. I-131 dosing is then based on the ability of the abnormal thyroid tissue to absorb and eliminate I-131.

Question the patient regarding previous medication and procedures involving radiographic contrast media because the uptake of I-131 will be affected by recent intake of these agents. Reassure patients that they will not be isolated from other household members. Instead, caution them to avoid prolonged, close contact with others, particularly children and pregnant women, for about 1 week following therapy with I-131.

Household contamination is not a great risk, but saliva and urine may be contaminated for several days following treatment. Provide the patient and family with both verbal and written instructions specific to their living situations. Instruct the patient to sleep alone, to avoid close personal contact with family members, and to drink liberal amounts of fluids for 2 days after treatment. Eating utensils should be washed thoroughly with soap and water after every meal. Emphasize the importance of hand washing. Typically, the toilet is the most contaminated item because most of the I-131 dosage is excreted in the urine. The NRC recommends an annual radiation dose limit of 100 mrem for the general public. This limit excludes exposure to family members of outpatients receiving radiation, however. Hyperthyroid patients treated with I-131 typically emit only low levels of radiation beyond a 1-meter distance (approximately 3.3 feet). Make certain household members understand that they can minimize their exposure by staying 1 meter or more away from the patient for a the first few days. Anxious household members should understand that exposure from diagnostic x-rays (typically, 10–2,000 mrem) is considerably greater than exposure that results from minimal contact with the patient.

Advise the patient that temporary thinning of the hair may occur 2 to 3 months after treatment. Educate the patient and family about the signs and symptoms of hypothyroidism, which may occur following I-131 therapy.

Propranolol

Propranolol (Inderal), a beta-adrenergic blocker, is commonly used intravenously in treating thyroid storm to minimize the excessive cardiac stimulation that results from the catecholamine activity. Therefore, it controls the symptoms but does not alter the disease. Propranolol is discussed in depth in Chapter 13.

PARATHYROID DRUGS

C Antihypercalcemic, Calcium-Regulator Drugs

Calcitonin (human and salmon) and the bisphosphonates (alendronate, etidronate, risedronate, tiludronate, plicamycin, pamidronate, furosemide, and gallium) are calcium-regulator

- Advise the patient that he or she will have periodic blood tests while taking this drug to monitor its effectiveness and possible adverse effects. Stress the need to report fever, sore throat, unusual bleeding or bruising, and headache to the health care team.
- As with all medications, instruct patients to keep this drug out of the reach of children.

Ongoing Assessment and Evaluation

Monitor serum thyroid hormone levels periodically to evaluate the effectiveness of the drug and to assess the need for replacement thyroid hormone because the thyroid gland is suppressed. With continued antithyroid therapy, an insidious goitrogenic hypothyroidism may appear. Alert the patient to watch for signs of this adverse effect, such as decreased cardiac rate, intolerance to cold, and weight gain. Thyroid function tests, used to evaluate drug therapy, should be measured routinely (every 4–6 weeks). It is important to review periodically the signs of hypothyroidism and hyperthyroidism with the patient and significant others. As the patient reaches a euthyroid state, assess the need for dosage adjustment with drugs affected by metabolic rate and activity. Therapy is considered successful when normal thyroid status is maintained, and the patient can explain and demonstrate self-monitoring techniques.

Drug Closely Related to P Methimazole

Propylthiouracil (PTU) is a thionamide with similar characteristics to those of MMI. Adverse effects are also similar and include pruritus, rash, urticaria, arthritis, fever, abnormal taste, nausea, and vomiting. Serious complications, such as agranulocytosis, are dose dependent. Serum aminotransferase concentrations increase transiently in up to one third of patients taking PTU. Well-documented hepatotoxicity is equally divided between PTU and MMI.

MEMORY CHIP

P Methimazole (MMI)

- Inhibits the synthesis of thyroid hormones; antithyroid agent
- Major contraindications: sensitivity to the drug; nursing mothers, because the drug is excreted in breast milk
- Most common adverse effects: GI (nausea, vomiting, epigastric pain), itching, rash, hives, and arthralgia
- Most serious adverse effects: agranulocytosis, liver damage, aplastic anemia, and vasculitis. Most adverse effects resolve spontaneously with discontinuation of the drug.
- Maximizing therapeutic effects: Administer drug around the clock at 8-hour intervals, although it can be given in a single daily dose.
- Minimizing adverse effects: periodic blood tests to assess bone marrow function and bleeding tendencies
- Most important patient education: Drug must be taken for a prolonged period (months) to achieve the desired effects; report fever, sore throat, unusual bleeding or bruising, and malaise.

Drugs Significantly Different From P Methimazole

Iodide or Iodine Solutions (Lugol Solution, Thyro-Block [tablets])

Iodine is the oldest of the antithyroid drugs. Low doses of iodine are needed in the body to form thyroid hormone. High doses, however, tend to inhibit thyroid function. A hyperfunctioning thyroid gland responds to iodine by promptly inhibiting the release of hormone. Iodine helps to firm the thyroid gland by reducing its size and vascularity. This effect helps prevent postoperative hemorrhage and the surgical complication of thyroid storm.

Potassium iodide, or occasionally strong iodine solution, is used preoperatively to reduce the vascularity of the gland before thyroidectomy and, alone or in combination with the beta blocker, propranolol, to manage thyrotoxic crisis (thyroid storm), usually in conjunction with other antithyroid agents (e.g., MMI). When used preoperatively, potassium iodide is administered 10 to 14 days before surgery.

Chronic toxicity may occur when potassium iodide is given in large doses or over a long duration. Chronic toxicity is usually dose dependent and is manifested as a metallic taste, burning in the mouth and throat, sore teeth and gums, increased salivation, and eye irritation with swollen eyelids. Gastric irritation is common, and diarrhea may occur. When the drug is discontinued, the clinical manifestations of toxicity generally subside spontaneously within a few days.

Hypersensitivity reactions to iodides may cause angioedema, cutaneous and mucosal hemorrhage, and clinical signs (e.g., fever, arthralgia, lymphadenopathy, and eosinophilia) resembling serum sickness.

Prolonged use or excessive doses of iodides may result in thyroid gland hyperplasia, thyroid adenoma, goiter, and severe hypothyroidism.

Concomitant use of lithium salts, other iodides, or antithyroid agents and potassium iodide may result in an additive or synergistic hypothyroid effect. If these drugs are used together, the patient should be monitored closely for signs and symptoms of hypothyroidism. Simultaneous use of potassium iodide and potassium-containing drugs or potassium-sparing diuretics may result in hyperkalemia.

Cautious initial administration of potassium iodide is recommended because some individuals are markedly sensitive to iodides. Persons at highest risk are those with goiter or autoimmune thyroid disease (Hashimoto thyroiditis). Some commercially available formulations of potassium iodide contain sodium bisulfite, a sulfite that may cause allergic-type reactions, including anaphylaxis and life-threatening asthmatic episodes, in susceptible individuals. Question the patient carefully about the presence of goiter, autoimmune thyroid disease, or asthma because this sensitivity occurs more frequently in asthmatic individuals.

Iodine-131

I-131 (radioactive iodine) is used to treat hyperthyroidism and well-differentiated thyroid carcinoma. While destroying thyroid tissue, it exposes only the thyroid tissue to the altering radiation, eliminates the problems of surgery, and enables outpatient treatment. Most patients treated with radioactive iodine become euthyroid and then require lifelong replacement therapy with thyroid hormones.

TABLE 51.1 Summary of Selected (C) Glucocorticoids

Drug (Trade) Name	Selected Indications	Route and Dosage Range	Pharmacokinetics
(P) prednisone (Deltasone, Prednisone; *Canadian:* Apo-Prednisone) or prednisolone (Delta-Cortef; *Canadian:* Novo-Prednisolone)	Rheumatic disorders Collagen disorders Dermatologic disorders Allergic states Ophthalmic disorders Respiratory diseases Hematologic disorders Neoplastic diseases GI diseases	*Adult:* PO, 5–60 mg/d	*Onset and duration:* Vary with administration and dosage preparation Plasma $t_{1/2}$: (for prototype glucocorticoid prednisone): 60 min Biologic $t_{1/2}$: 18–36 h
betamethasone (Celestone)	Anti-inflammatory and immunosuppressant effects (similar to those of prednisone)	*Adult:* PO, 0.6–7.2 mg/d	*Onset and duration:* Vary with administration and dosage preparation
betamethasone dipropionate† (Alphatrex; *Canadian:* Taro-Sone)	Localized anti-inflammatory effects	Topical	
betamethasone sodium phosphate* (Cel-U-Jec, Selestoject; *Canadian:* Betnesol)	Anti-inflammatory and immunosuppressant effects (similar to prednisone)	*Adult:* IM, IV, up to 9 mg/d	Plasma $t_{1/2}$ (for betamethasone): 300+ min
betamethasone sodium phosphate† betamethasone acetate* (Celestone Soluspan)	Localized anti-inflammatory effects	*IL, 0.5–2 mL (1 mL = 3 mg each compound)	Biologic $t_{1/2}$: 36–54 h
betamethasone valerate+ (Valisone)	Localized anti-inflammatory effects	Topical	
cortisone acetate (Cortone Acetate)	Glucocorticoid replacement therapy for adrenocortical insufficiency	*Adult:* PO, 25–300 mg/d	
dexamethasone*† (Decadron; *Canadian:* Dexasone)	Anti-inflammatory and immunosuppressant effects (similar to prednisone) Cerebral edema Chemotherapeutic antiemetic Diagnostic aid for Cushing syndrome and major (endogenous) depression	*Adult:* PO, 0.75–9 mg/d	*Onset and duration:* Vary with administration and dosage preparation Plasma $t_{1/2}$ (for dexamethasone): 110–210 min
dexamethasone acetate (Decadron-LA) or	Anti-inflammatory and immunosuppressant effects (similar to those of prednisone)	*Adult:* IM, 8–16 mg; *IL, 00.8–16 mg	Biologic $t_{1/2}$: 36–54 h
dexamethasone sodium phosphate† (Decadron Phosphate, Hexadrol)	Localized anti-inflammatory effects	*Adult:* IV, 0.5–9 mg/d *IL, 0.4–4 mg	*Duration:* 2–3 d (PO, IM, or IV)
flunisolide (AeroBid; *Canadian:* Bronalide)	Localized anti-inflammatory effects Bronchial asthma	Aerosol	*Onset:* Slow *Duration:* 4–6 h
fluocinolone acetonide	Localized anti-inflammatory effects	Topical	Plasma $t_{1/2}$: 1–2 h
fluticasone propionate (aerosol, Flonase; topical, Cutivate)	Localized anti-inflammatory effects	Aerosol, topical	Biologic $t_{1/2}$: wk

(continued)

TABLE 51.1 Summary of Selected Glucocorticoids (continued)

Drug (Trade) Name	Selected Indications	Route and Dosage Range	Pharmacokinetics
cortisone/hydrocortisone† (Cortef)	Primary or secondary adrenal cortical insufficiency (hydrocortisone or cortisone is drug of choice; synthetic analogues, however, may be used in conjunction with mineralocorticoids)	*Adult:* PO, 20–240 mg/d	*Onset and duration:* Vary with administration and dosage preparation Plasma t½ (for hydrocortisone): 80–120 min Biologic $t_{1/2}$: 8–12 h
hydrocortisone sodium phosphate (Hydrocortisone Phosphate) or hydrocortisone sodium succinate (Solu-Cortef)	Localized anti-inflammatory effects	*Adult:* IM, IV, SC, 15–240 mg/d *Adult:* IM, IV, 100–500 mg at 2-, 4-, or 6-h intervals; *IL; 12.5–75 mg	
hydrocortisone acetate*†	Localized anti-inflammatory effects		
methylprednisolone (Medrol; *Canadian:* Meprolone)	Anti-inflammatory and immunosuppressant effects (similar to those of prednisone)	*Adult:* PO, 4–48 mg/d	*Onset and duration:* Vary with administration and dosage preparation
methylprednisolone acetate*† (Depo-Medrol; *Canadian:* Medrol Veriderm)		*Adult:* IM, 40–120 mg/wk	
methylprednisolone sodium succinate (Solu-Medrol)		*Adult:* IM, IV, 10–40 mg; high-dose therapy, 30 mg/kg	Plasma $t_{1/2}$: (for methylprednisolone): 78–188 min Biologic $t_{1/2}$:18–36 h
prednisolone acetate (Prednisolone Acetate, Predcor) or	Anti-inflammatory and immunosuppressant effects (similar to those of prednisone)	*Adult:* IM, IV, 4–60 mg/d *IL, 4–100 mg	*Onset and duration:* Vary with administration and dosage preparation
prednisolone sodium phosphate (IV-Predate, IM-Hydeltrasol)	Localized anti-inflammatory effects	*Adult:* IM, IV, 4–60 mg/d *IL, 5–20 mg/d	
prednisolone tebutate (Prednisolone Tebutate, Hydeltra-T.B.A.)	Localized anti-inflammatory effects	*Adult:* *IL, 4–30 mg *Child:* Individualize dosage depending on severity of condition and patient's response	
triamcinolone (Aristocort, Kenacort; *Canadian:* Oracort)	Anti-inflammatory and immunosuppressant effects (similar to those of prednisone)	*Adult:* PO, 4–48 mg (in divided doses depending on the disease)	*Onset:* Varies with administration and dosage preparation Plasma $t_{1/2}$: 200† min Biologic $t_{1/2}$: 18–36 h
triamcinolone diacetate (Aristocort)	Localized anti-inflammatory effects	*Adult:* IM, Up to 40 mg/wk *IL, 5–48 mg	
triamcinolone hexacetonide (Aristospan Intralesional, Aristospan Intraarticular)	Localized anti-inflammatory effects	*IL, 2–20 mg	

*May be administered for localized effects (e.g., intra-articular, intrabursal, intradermal, intralesional, intrasynovial, or soft tissue [IL]). Dosage varies according to size of treatment area and desired local effects.

†May be administered topically (e.g., dermatologic, inhalation, or ophthalmic).

Pharmacokinetics

Prednisone, like other glucocorticoids, is absorbed readily from the gastrointestinal (GI) tract because of its lipophilic nature. Glucocorticoids also are absorbed at a moderate rate from the synovial and the conjunctival spaces and very slowly through the skin. Consequently, topical administration is used for a localized action. Excessive and prolonged local application of certain drugs may result in enough absorption to cause systemic effects. In contrast to oral dosage forms, injectable preparations (e.g., esters, suspensions) have greatly altered onsets and durations of action; they are, however, absorbed slowly and completely. Prednisone—inactive on its own—must be metabolized in the liver into pharmacologically active prednisolone. Prednisolone is excreted in the urine, crosses the placenta, and enters the breast milk.

Metabolic factors can increase or decrease the levels of prednisone in the blood. The liver and kidney are the major sites of glucocorticoid inactivation. Drugs that are cyproheptadine (CYP) inducers (e.g., phenobarbital, phenytoin,

rifampin) may accelerate the hepatic biotransformation of glucocorticoids. Conditions such as hypothyroidism may cause the hepatic metabolism to be decreased.

Pharmacodynamics

Prednisone has primarily glucocorticoid activity, although some mineralocorticoid activity is present and more apparent when the drug is administered in high doses (see Figure 51.2). Prednisone may cause salt and water retention, resulting in edema and hypertension. Prednisone affects virtually all body cells but not in the same way. Anti-inflammatory effects include retardation of the migratory polymorphonuclear leukocytes, suppression of tissue repair and granulation, reduction in the erythrocyte sedimentation rate, decrease in fibrinogenesis, and diminished C-reactive protein. Prednisone does not, however, affect antigen-antibody reactions or immediate hypersensitivity reactions.

Its immunosuppressant effects are attributable to suppression of phagocytosis, decrease in the number of circulating eosinophils and lymphocytes, suppression of delayed hypersensitivity reactions, decrease in antigen–antibody tissue reactions, and a decrease in plasma immunoglobulins.

Glucocorticoid effects on carbohydrate, fat, and protein metabolism are responsible for both the beneficial and adverse effects. The normal physiologic action of systemic glucocorticoids, including prednisone, is increased gluconeogenesis and decreased glucose use. These actions provide for glucose production (and energy) during periods of stress or decreased carbohydrate intake (Box 51.3).

Contraindications and Precautions

Contraindications to prednisone use are a hypersensitivity to the drug and systemic fungal infections. Precautions include closely monitored use for individuals with sensitivity to additives such as tartrazine or sulfites because they may develop severe allergic or anaphylactic reactions to some preparations.

Avoid abrupt withdrawal of systemic prednisone for replacement with an inhaled glucocorticoid. A corticosteroid withdrawal syndrome (e.g., malaise, myalgia, nausea, headache, and low-grade fever) and asthma relapse are problems encountered when systemic glucocorticoids are withdrawn too quickly after beginning inhalation therapy. Withdrawal syndrome is more likely if prednisone is being given for adrenal insufficiency.

BOX 51.3 Pharmacodynamic Effects of Glucocorticoids

Metabolic
- Increased glycogenolysis and gluconeogenesis
- Increased protein catabolism and decreased protein synthesis
- Decreased gastrointestinal absorption of calcium
- Decreased secretion of thyroid-stimulating hormone (TSH)
- Decreased activity and formation of osteoblasts

Anti-inflammatory (systemic and local effects)
- Decreased production of prostaglandins, cytokines, and interleukins
- Decreased proliferation and migration of lymphocytes and macrophages

Adverse Effects

Treatment with prednisone may produce adverse effects. These effects include central nervous system (CNS) complaints of stimulation, anxiety, mood swings, insomnia, and headache. GI complaints include nausea, vomiting, increased appetite, weight gain, and dyspepsia. Endocrine changes of menstrual irregularities, hyperglycemia, and suppression of pituitary ACTH release (after 2–3 days) are common with continued prednisone use. In addition, dermatologic and integumentary adverse effects include acne, suppression of skin test reactions, and delayed healing of wounds. Other effects of continued prednisone use include muscle weakness, increased susceptibility to infections (especially herpes virus, varicella virus, *Candida* and *Mycobacterium* species), suppression of physiologic responses to infection, sodium and fluid retention, fatigue, and malaise.

Administration of prednisone produces a negative feedback effect on the HPA axis; this effect results in the suppression of endogenous cortisol production. Suppression of ACTH release and cortisol secretion has been shown to occur with 50 mg/day of oral prednisone for as few as 5 days. Although long believed to be important, high doses and long-term use of glucocorticoids are no longer thought to be reliable predictors of a probable HPA axis deficiency. There appears to be considerable patient variability in responses to dosages and duration of therapy. Acute adrenal insufficiency caused by HPA axis suppression following drug withdrawal is one of the most serious complications of prednisone therapy (Box 51.4).

Adverse reactions occur with long-term administration of supraphysiologic (pharmacologic) doses of prednisone. Cushingoid characteristics include redistribution of fat deposits (e.g., buffalo hump, moon face, and truncal obesity). Signs of protein catabolism, such as loss of muscle mass and thinning of the extremities, muscle aches, and weakness may also develop. Visual acuity may be affected by the development of cataracts and glaucoma. Hyperlipidemia and thrombus formation also may occur. Other adverse effects from long-term therapy (doses above 5 mg/day) include undesired dermatologic responses of acne, hirsutism, delayed wound healing, skin atrophy, tearing, and striae. Women and the elderly of both genders are more prone to these effects.

A clinically important adverse effect of long-term prednisone therapy is osteoporosis, which is often considered to be a major limitation of long-term prednisone therapy. Long-term prednisone therapy (doses over 7.5 mg/day) enhances calcium loss, and increases parathyroid hormone levels. Calcium loss from bones decreases bone mineral density, thereby promoting an osteoporotic condition that increases the risk for hip, pelvic, rib, or vertebral fractures.

Substantial bone effects (e.g., suppression of bone growth) may occur when these drugs are used in long-term and intermittent treatment of a variety of diseases. The bones most often affected are the vertebrae, ribs, and long bones, although all bones are at risk. A high incidence of vertebral compression fractures exists in both male and female patients who receive extended prednisone treatment.

There appears to be a direct correlation between the extent of bone loss and the duration of prednisone therapy; research suggests that the majority of bone loss occurs within the

BOX 51.4 Complications of Prednisone (and Other Glucocorticoid Therapy)

Central Nervous System Problems
- Emotional lability
- Anxiety
- Paresthesias
- Seizures
- Increased intracranial pressure with papilledema
- Insomnia
- Psychosis
- Paradoxical suicidal depression
- Aggravation of preexisting psychiatric disorders

Endocrine/Metabolic Problems
- Antagonistic effects on insulin, parathyroid, and thyroid hormones
- Glucose intolerance
- Hirsutism
- Suppression of HPA axis
- Hyperglycemia
- Hyperlipidemia
- Iatrogenic diabetes
- Obesity
- Increased serum lipids
- Increased serum triglycerides (in transplant and asthmatic patients and those with organ transplantation treated with >5 mg/d of prednisone)
- Protein wasting
- Amenorrhea
- Postmenopausal bleeding

Cardiovascular Problems
- Thromboembolism (fat embolism)
- Arrhythmias secondary to K+ alterations
- Hypertension
- CHF

Gastrointestinal Problems
- Fatty liver infiltrates
- Pancreatitis
- Increased appetite (which leads to weight gain)
- Ulcerative esophagitis
- Nausea and vomiting
- Peptic ulceration with perforation or hemorrhage

Fluid and Electrolyte Problems
- Fluid retention
- K+ loss (hypokalemia)
- Na+ retention (hypernatremia)
- Ca++ loss (hypocalcemia)

Hematologic and Immunologic Problems
- Altered inflammatory response
- Eosinopenia
- Leukocytosis
- Opportunistic infections
- Leukopenia

Musculoskeletal Problems
- Aseptic necrosis (femur, humerus head)
- Growth failure
- Myopathy
- Osteopenia
- Osteoporosis

Ophthalmic Problems
- Increased intraocular pressure
- Cataracts
- Glaucoma
- Exophthalmos

Integumentary Problems
- Acne
- Ecchymoses
- Petechiae
- Skin atrophy
- Striae purpura
- Subcutaneous fat atrophy

General Problems
- Cushingoid characteristics
- Withdrawal syndrome

first 3 to 12 months, with a slowing of bone loss thereafter. Although alternate-day therapy has been shown to delay some of the adverse effects of long-term prednisone therapy, it does not appear to decrease the risk for development of osteoporosis. The prevalence of osteoporosis is difficult to assess when corticosteroids are used in diseases in which the risk for osteoporosis is already increased (e.g., rheumatoid arthritis and renal disease).

Finally, glucose tolerance is affected by prednisone. This reaction occurs in as many as 15% of individuals on long-term therapy. The risk for iatrogenic diabetes mellitus increases with age, obesity, a previous history of glucose intolerance, and a family history of diabetes. Even low-dose therapy can impair glucose tolerance in patients with type 1 and 2 diabetes. Patients with diabetes may need changes in diet or hypoglycemic therapy (e.g., insulin, oral drugs) to maintain control of blood sugar.

Drug Interactions

Major interactions may occur between prednisone and a variety of drugs. Prednisone also causes some interactions with laboratory measurements. Urine glucose and serum cholesterol levels may be increased. Serum levels of K^+ may be decreased. Triiodothyronine (T_3), thyroxine (T_4), thyroid iodine-131 (I-131) uptake, and protein-bound iodine concentrations may be decreased, making it difficult to monitor the therapeutic response of patients receiving the drugs for thyroiditis or assessing patients for thyroid dysfunction. Prednisone also may produce a false-positive result in some tests for systemic bacterial infections. In addition, reactions to skin tests may be suppressed. Prednisone alters glucose tolerance tests. Diabetic patients should be monitored closely and adjustments in dosage of insulin or oral antidiabetic drugs made accordingly. Table 51.2 lists drugs that interact with prednisone.

Assessment of Relevant Core Patient Variables

Health Status

Before administering prednisone, review the patient's drug history for use of prescription, over-the-counter (OTC), and herbal medications and recreational drugs. In addition, it is important to review the patient's medical history for GI prob-

TABLE 51.2 Agents That Interact With P Prednisone

Interactants	Effect and Significance	Nursing Management
Anticholinesterases • ambenonium • edrophonium • neostigmine • pyridostigmine	Corticosteroids antagonize the effects of anticholinesterases in patients with myasthenia gravis, resulting in profound muscle depression.	Monitor patient's muscle strength.
Azole antifungal agents • fluconazole • itraconazole • ketoconazole • miconazole • voriconazole	Prednisone clearance possibly decreased	Observe for adverse effects to prednisone.
Barbiturates	Barbiturates induce hepatic metabolism of prednisone, resulting in subtherapeutic serum concentrations of prednisone.	Observe for subtherapeutic effects of prednisone. Dosage may require adjustment.
Hydantoins	Hydantoins induce hepatic metabolism of prednisone, resulting in subtherapeutic serum concentrations of prednisone.	Observe for subtherapeutic effects of prednisone. Dosage may require adjustment.
Oral anticoagulants	Anticoagulant dose requirements possibly reduced; conversely, prednisone may oppose the anticoagulant action.	Monitor prothrombin time and coagulation tests.
Oral contraceptives	Possible increased prednisone half-life and concentration and decreased clearance	Evaluate for excess effects of prednisone. Dosage may require adjustment.
Potassium-depleting agents (diuretics)	May increase the depletion of potassium	Observe patients for muscular and systemic effects of hypokalemia.
Rifamycins	Rifamycins induce hepatic metabolism of prednisone, resulting in subtherapeutic serum concentrations of prednisone.	Avoid coadministration if possible. Observe for subtherapeutic effects of prednisone. Dosage may require adjustment.
Salicylates	Prednisone stimulates the metabolism of salicylates, resulting in decreased serum salicylate levels, and may decrease their effectiveness.	Evaluate for subtherapeutic effects of salicylate. Dosage may require adjustment.
Somatrem	Growth-promoting effect of somatrem possibly inhibited	Increased dosage of somatrem may be necessary. Monitor closely for pharmacologic side effects.
Theophylline	Alterations in the pharmacologic activity of either agent possible	Observe for subtherapeutic effects of either drug. Dosage adjustments may be necessary.

lems. Assess the patient's nutritional status, weight control, and disease or trauma history. Perform a complete physical examination and review current laboratory data. In addition, muscle strength and body proportions should be observed, as should patterns of hair growth and distribution. Depending on the findings, further testing (e.g., hepatic and renal function studies) may be indicated. Throughout therapy, continue to assess the patient for signs of adrenal insufficiency.

Life Span and Gender

Prednisone is an FDA pregnancy category C drug. It is secreted in breast milk and may suppress growth or cause other adverse effects in nursing infants. Growth suppression can occur in children receiving prolonged prednisone therapy. Growth suppression is proportional to the duration, dose, and frequency of prednisone administered. Divided daily doses are more growth inhibiting than a single daily dose.

Elderly patients are more prone to adrenal suppression from prolonged prednisone administration. Elderly patients may require lower doses because of physiologic changes resulting from aging, such as decreased muscle mass and plasma volume or impairment of hepatic or renal functions. Blood pressure and blood glucose and electrolyte levels should be monitored regularly.

Lifestyle, Diet, and Habits

Assess the patient's typical diet. The patient's diet plan should include low sodium and high potassium. A diet that controls carbohydrate and calorie intake is important (unless contraindicated) because of the increased gluconeogenesis, decreased glucose use, increased appetite, and weight gain effects of pharmacologic glucocorticoid therapy. Encourage increased protein intake to decrease the risk for protein deficiency.

It also is important to assess the patient's typical daily activities and fall risk. The weak muscles and easily fatigued state characteristic of glucocorticoid excess predispose the patient to accidents. Osteoporosis and vertebral-compression effects of excessive glucocorticoid therapy may make bone fractures more likely. Passive and active range-of-motion exercises to offset the tendency toward muscle weakness and atrophy are important. Physical or occupational therapy referrals may be necessary.

Nursing Diagnoses and Outcomes

- Excess Fluid Volume related to sodium and water retention secondary to corticosteroid therapy
  Desired outcome: *The patient will relate causative factors and methods of preventing edema and exhibit decreased peripheral and sacral edema.*
- Risk for Infection or Risk for Injury related to anti-inflammatory, immunosuppressive, dermatologic, and metabolic effects of chronic corticosteroid therapy
  Desired outcome: *The patient will demonstrate knowledge of risk factors associated with potential for infection or injury and will practice appropriate precautions for prevention.*
- Imbalanced Nutrition: More than Body Requirements related to increased appetite secondary to corticosteroid medications
  Desired outcome: *The patient will maintain a healthy weight, discuss current nutritional needs, and discuss the effects of exercise on weight control.*
- Altered Body Image related to cushingoid characteristics or physical changes secondary to glucocorticoid therapy
  Desired outcome: *The patient will verbalize and demonstrate acceptance of appearance (grooming, dress, posture, presentation of self), verbalize and demonstrate increased positive feelings, and demonstrate healthy adaptation and coping skills.*

Planning and Intervention

Maximizing Therapeutic Effects

Hormone production by the adrenal gland is influenced by many factors. Normal cortisol production follows a diurnal cycle. Levels peak in the early morning hours (6 AM to 8 AM) and decline throughout the day with a second, lower peak in the late afternoon (4 PM to 6 PM). Cortisol secretion increases in response to stress (physical or emotional) and low endogenous glucocorticoid levels. Thus, the most opportune time for administration of daily doses or alternate day doses of glucocorticoids is early in the morning.

When prednisone is prescribed for replacement therapy, teach the patient:

- Signs and symptoms of glucocorticoid imbalances
- Monitoring the response to therapy
- Drug schedule
- Identifying factors that increase adrenal stress (e.g., physical illness, injury, trauma, or emotional upset)
- Stress management
- Dosage changes during periods of stress or illness
- Prevention of injury and infection
- Drug interactions

Alert the patient that following intra-articular injection, the injected joint should not be overused. Weight-bearing joints, such as the knee, should be rested 24 to 48 hours after the injection.

Minimizing Adverse Effects

Emphasize the importance of adherence to the drug regimen, especially the adverse consequences of stopping therapy abruptly, such as the danger of adrenal insufficiency. Like other anti-inflammatory drugs, prednisone administration can lead to peptic ulcer disease. Therefore, teach the patient to reduce gastric irritation from prednisone use by consuming milk (unless contraindicated), food, or nonsystemic antacids (e.g., Al^+, Ca^{2+}, or Mg^+ salts), or by using adjunct antiulcer drug therapy (for instance H_2-receptor antagonists, proton pump inhibitors) when taking the medication. Caffeine, alcohol, and products containing aspirin interact with prednisone, increasing the secretion of gastric acid irritating the gastric mucosa and leading to an increased risk for GI bleeding.

Altered growth and development is a risk with systemic glucocorticoid therapy. Inhaled glucocorticoids may cause hoarseness, fungal infections, throat irritation, and dry mouth. Teach the patient to rinse the mouth or brush the teeth following use of the inhaled steroids to minimize the risk for oral, laryngeal, or pharyngeal fungal infections.

Alternate-day administration (glucocorticoids given every other day instead of daily) of long-term, systemic glucocorticoids has been used to lessen the suppression of the hypothalamus, the anterior pituitary, and the rate of bone loss. However, alternate-day dosing does not minimize the risk for osteoporosis or cataract formation. Intermediate-acting glucocorticoids, such as prednisone, are most appropriate for alternate-day therapy. Ensure that the change from daily to alternate-day administration does not occur abruptly because this abrupt change may cause signs and symptoms of adrenal insufficiency (e.g., fatigue, nausea, vomiting, and hypotension) on the days between doses.

When a patient receiving ongoing corticosteroid therapy requires surgery, review the preoperative orders to ensure a dose of a rapid-acting corticosteroid has been added to the patient's daily dose of corticosteroid. If not, obtain the order from the prescriber. To promote recovery after the stress of surgery, an increased dose of steroid should be continued postoperatively in decreasing doses over several days, returning to the patient's baseline dose of corticosteroid.

Providing Patient and Family Education

- Discuss taking the drug exactly as prescribed.
- Discuss not stopping the drug abruptly because of the risk for acute adrenal insufficiency.
- Discuss dealing with missed doses and the dosing strategy (Box 51.5).
- Discuss the purpose of the medication therapy and the need for maintaining therapy.
- Teach that prednisone replacement therapy is used to treat the chronic, lifelong conditions of adrenal cortical insufficiency.
- Provide emotional support and assistance in the grieving process over loss of health and loss of control as needed (PRN).
- Advise the patient to wear a medical identification device with the diagnosis and drug therapy clearly indicated.

COMMUNITY-BASED CONCERNS

Box 51.5 Home Dosing Strategies

One Dose Every Other Day

If a dose is missed, take the missed dose as soon as possible. If the medication is remembered the same morning, take it and then go back to the regular dosing schedule.

If the dose is remembered several hours late, then wait and take it the following morning. Skip the next day and start the regular dosing schedule the day after.

One Dose Every Day

If a dose is missed, take the missed dose as soon as possible, then go back to the regular schedule.

If the missed dose is not remembered until the next day, skip it and do not double the next dose.

Several Doses Every Day

If a dose is missed, it is important to take the missed dose as soon as possible, then go back to the regular schedule.

If the missed dose is not remembered until the next dose is due, double the next dose.

Periods of Stress, Illness, Injury, or Surgery

Make sure that the directions for dosage adjustment are clearly indicated on the drug label.

- Emphasize the importance of the patient's notifying all health care providers about glucocorticoid therapy when seeking medical treatment.
- Discuss the adverse effects of drug therapy and identify symptoms that should be reported to the prescriber.
- Discuss alterations in appearance that may cause disturbances in self-concept from long-term therapy.
- Discuss strategies to deal with the changes that occur (e.g., truncal obesity, thinning of extremities, or "buffalo hump" may be camouflaged with loosely fitted clothing).
- Discuss bone health (supplemental daily intake of 1,500 mg of oral calcium and 510 IU of vitamin D is recommended).
- Teach how to identify signs and symptoms of acute adrenal insufficiency, including symptoms of anorexia, hypoglycemia, lethargy, malaise, nausea, psychological despondency, restlessness, and weakness, and to report symptoms to the prescriber.
- Discuss the importance of rest, sleep, and health-maintenance behaviors.
- Teach ways to avoid infection and how to recognize signs of infection.
- Discuss self-medication for minor illnesses handled at home (e.g., flu with vomiting and diarrhea) that may require dosage adjustments, medical intervention, or hospitalization.
- Provide patients and their caregivers with written instructions on what to do on sick days.
- Discuss safety issues and fall preventions. Emphasize the possible occurrence of osteoporosis and encourage the patient and caregiver to report all bone pain.
- Evaluate the safety of the home environment. Stress the importance of reporting bone pain because aseptic necrosis or pathologic fractures may occur spontaneously.

Ongoing Assessment and Evaluation

During prednisone therapy, the patient must be monitored for therapeutic drug response, adverse drug reactions, and indications of drug toxicity. Monitor for periods of stress (e.g., trauma, surgery, or severe illness) in order to coordinate medication adjustment of prednisone dosage to avoid drug-induced adrenal insufficiency. Assess for appropriate healing of all wounds and infections during and after hospitalizations or minor surgery because prednisone delays wound healing and increases the risk for infection. Common indicators of infection (including temperature elevation, erythema, and leukocytosis) are repressed because corticosteroids block the inflammatory responses. Also, assess for changes in energy level, activity level, and appetite as indicators of infection.

Glucocorticoids cause an increase in gluconeogenesis and a decrease in glucose utilization, causing hyperglycemia to occur. Monitor patients for the development of iatrogenic diabetes mellitus. Patients with existing diabetes may require an adjustment in therapy to maintain glucose control. Prophylactic antitubercular drug therapy may be required in infected persons because high glucocorticoid levels are likely to reactivate encapsulated tuberculosis.

Maintain vigilance in assessing patients receiving long-term prednisone (and other glucocorticoids) therapy. Adrenal suppression may occur, whereas effects of endogenous glucocorticoid hormones on the body may be exaggerated. Indications of adrenal suppression include anorexia, diarrhea, fluid and electrolyte imbalances (especially decreased Na^+, decreased glucose, and increased K^+), fatigue, nausea, vomiting, and weight loss. If fluid volume deficit occurs, it is important to assess for hypotension, pyrexia, tachycardia and tachypnea, dry skin, and dry mucous membranes. Also, assess for adverse reactions from prednisone (and other glucocorticoids), such as changes in mood or affect (e.g., agitation, depression, euphoria, and insomnia), edema, muscle weakness, nausea, vomiting, and weight gain.

While caring for a patient on glucocorticoid therapy, monitor specific laboratory tests. Actual serum levels of cortisol and ACTH may be determined by a 24-hour urine collection. Electrolytes are measured with a metabolic panel. Lymphocyte levels (primarily T_4) should decrease when glucocorticoids are being used for immunosuppressive effects. In addition, monitor patients receiving digoxin or other digitalis-based drugs for toxicity.

Evaluate for the effectiveness of the therapy and assess signs and symptoms that precipitated the use of glucocorticoid drugs. When prednisone is used as replacement therapy, the patient should report an increased state of health (e.g., absence of fatigue, hypoglycemia, hypovolemia, and weakness) and a feeling of well-being. When prednisone is used for chronic inflammatory conditions (e.g., rheumatoid arthritis), the patient should experience less pain and discomfort and increased joint mobility.

Drugs Closely Related to P Prednisone

Among the glucocorticoids closely related to prednisone are hydrocortisone, methylprednisolone, dexamethasone, betamethasone, inhaled glucocorticoids, and topical glucocorticoids.

MEMORY CHIP

P Prednisone

- Anti-inflammatory or immunosuppressive therapy
- Hepatic dysfunction may impair prednisone conversion into active prednisolone
- Prednisone use may cause HPA axis suppression if given for more than 2 weeks and is then withdrawn too abruptly, placing the patient at risk for acute adrenal insufficiency
- Major contraindications: hypersensitivity to prednisone; systemic fungal infections
- Most common adverse effects: CNS complaints of euphoria, headache, and vertigo; GI complaints of nausea, vomiting, increased appetite, weight gain, and dyspepsia
- Most serious adverse effect: acute adrenal insufficiency due to HPA axis suppression following prednisone withdrawal
- Maximizing therapeutic effects: Administer prednisone according to established schedule (preferably one that follows the normal diurnal pattern of cortisol secretion); increase the dosage in times of stress to prevent drug-induced adrenal insufficiency.
- Minimizing adverse effects: give prednisone with meals and/or antacids.
- Most important patient education: Advise the patient to wear medical identification so that any emergency medical personnel will know about this drug therapy

Hydrocortisone

Hydrocortisone is bound reversibly to corticosteroid-binding albumin and globulin. Hydrocortisone is metabolized by the liver and excreted in the urine. Hydrocortisone is absorbed partially following rectal administration. Rectal preparations of hydrocortisone (e.g., retention enema, intrarectal foam) are absorbed as much as 50% and used as adjunctive therapy in patients with ulcerative colitis and other steroid-responsive conditions. Contraindications to rectal hydrocortisone use are systemic fungal infections, recent ileocolostomy or intestinal anastomoses, abscess, obstruction, peritonitis, and perforation.

Methylprednisolone

Methylprednisolone (Medrol) and its derivatives, methylprednisolone sodium succinate (Solu-Medrol), such as betamethasone, dexamethasone, and triamcinolone, are synthetic glucocorticoids characterized by potent anti-inflammatory and immunosuppressive effects. These drugs have little mineralocorticoid activity and usually are not used to manage adrenal insufficiency unless a more potent mineralocorticoid is administered concomitantly. Pharmacokinetics, pharmacodynamics, contraindications, and adverse effects are similar to those associated with prednisone.

Methylprednisolone is used for the following conditions:

- Short-term management of inflammatory and allergic disorders, such as rheumatoid arthritis
- Collagen diseases, such as systemic lupus erythematosus, and skin diseases
- Status asthmaticus
- Autoimmune disorders
- Cancer-related hypercalcemia
- Ulcerative colitis
- Acute exacerbations of multiple sclerosis
- Palliative therapy in some leukemias and lymphomas
- Blood disorders, such as thrombocytopenia purpura
- Severe spinal cord injury, if used within 8 hours, to improve neurologic function (approved use in Canada)

Methylprednisolone is metabolized by the liver, crosses the placenta, and is secreted in breast milk. It is excreted in the urine. Dosages are individualized according to patient and dosage form. Methylprednisolone is administered orally, whereas methylprednisolone sodium succinate may be given by intramuscular (IM) or IV injection. Methylprednisolone acetate may be administered by IM, intra-articular, intralesional, or soft-tissue injection. As in prednisone therapy, systemic methylprednisolone must be discontinued gradually or changed to an oral form of a glucocorticoid to prevent acute adrenal insufficiency. Adverse reactions include vertigo, headache, weight gain and increased appetite, sodium and fluid retention, immunosuppression, and impaired wound healing.

Teach patients:

- To avoid people with known infections
- To avoid receiving live virus vaccines while taking methylprednisolone
- To report adverse effects, such as unusual weight gain, edema, muscle weakness, black or tarry stools, and prolonged cold-like infections

Dexamethasone

Dexamethasone exhibits essentially no mineralocorticoid activity and maximal anti-inflammatory activity with a prolonged plasma half-life (see Figure 51.2). It is used almost exclusively in short-term situations requiring maximum anti-inflammatory activity (e.g., cerebral edema and septic shock). Diagnostic testing for Cushing disease (idiopathic adrenocortical hyperfunction) may include dexamethasone administration and a 24-hour urine sample.

CRITICAL THINKING SCENARIO

Concerns raised by methylprednisolone and other glucocorticoids

Mr. Vito, 62 years old, is admitted to the emergency department with acute respiratory distress related to chronic obstructive pulmonary disease. Emergency treatment consists of respiratory inhalation therapy and IV methylprednisolone sodium succinate (Solu-Medrol), after which Mr. Vito is transferred to the telemetry unit. The nursing history that accompanies him discloses that he has type 2 diabetes that is controlled by diet and oral antidiabetic drugs.

1. Discuss assessment data needed to ensure safe administration of methylprednisolone to Mr. Vito, identifying any condition that represents a need for particularly cautious drug administration.
2. Define any concerns related to respiratory therapy and diabetes control. As Mr. Vito recovers, plans are made for him to begin long-term, anti-inflammatory corticosteroid therapy. At discharge, he will be on a tapering dose of oral prednisone and a beclomethasone (Vanceril) inhaler as needed.
3. Identify any important assessments that should be done to ensure safe administration of prednisone. In addition, propose important points to include in a patient education program.

Betamethasone

Betamethasone binds to intracellular corticosteroid receptors to produce anti-inflammatory and immunosuppressive effects. Clinical uses and adverse effects for betamethasone are similar to those for dexamethasone and methylprednisolone.

Figure 51.2 presents a comparison of glucocorticoids.

Inhaled Glucocorticoids

Beclomethasone, budesonide, flunisolide, fluticasone, and triamcinolone acetonide constitute a class of pulmonary and intranasal steroids, possessing enhanced topical anti-inflammatory activity and low systemic potency. Inhaled glucocorticoids are metabolized in the lung before they are absorbed, thereby reducing their systemic effects. These drugs are relatively equal in potency and clinical effectiveness and are thought to have variable systemic activity and complications. The intranasal and inhaled glucocorticoids are covered in depth in Chapters 46 and 47.

Topical Glucocorticoids

Topical steroids are effective therapy for a variety of inflammatory skin conditions. They are ranked according to their potency from super-high potency to lowest potency (Table 51.3). Available formulations include lotions, creams, ointments, or foams. Ointments are often preferred because they facilitate steroid absorption and penetration by trapping the moisture in the epidermis.

The primary therapeutic effects of the topical corticosteroids are their nonspecific anti-inflammatory activity acting on most causes of inflammation, including chemical, immunologic, mechanical, and microbiologic etiologies. When the glucocorticoids are applied to inflamed skin, they inhibit the migration of macrophages and leukocytes into the area by reversing the vascular dilation and permeability. The clinical result is a decrease in edema, erythema, and pruritus.

Topical application of corticosteroids rarely produces systemic effects. Topical steroids may be absorbed systemically if applied to the nasal mucosa or large areas of abraded skin, inhaled excessively for prolonged periods, or used in large doses. Optic and otic steroid preparations are not absorbed systemically.

Adverse effects with topical application are usually milder and more transient than those seen after systemically administered steroids. However, adrenal function may be suppressed when potent topical agents are used in large amounts for long periods, especially when the skin surface is denuded or when occlusive dressings are used. Occlusive dressings substantially increase percutaneous absorption, increasing the risk for local adverse effects (e.g., skin atrophy) and systemic adverse effects. Increased skin temperature, hydration, and application to skin with a thin surface layer also enhance absorption.

Intra-articularly Injected Glucocorticoids

Intra-articular injection produces localized effects for symptomatic relief of joint pain and increase joint mobility. Patients receiving this form of the drug need to be cautioned to allow time for the treated area to heal. The pain-induced limitation may be eliminated, but overusing the joint may still aggravate the active inflammatory process. Frequent intra-articular injections may damage joint tissues.

C Mineralocorticoids

Aldosterone, the naturally occurring mineralocorticoid, is expensive and requires parenteral administration. Therefore, fludrocortisone (Florinef Acetate) is the prototype exogenous mineralocorticoid. This adrenal corticosteroid has both high mineralocorticoid and glucocorticoid activity (its glucocorticoid potency is 15 times greater than that of

TABLE 51.3 Comparative Potency of Topical Glucocorticosteroids

Very High Potency	High Potency	Medium Potency	Low Potency
Betamethasone dipropionate (augmented)	Amcinonide	Beclomethasone	Alclometasone
Clobetasol	Betamethasone dipropionate	Betamethasone benzoate	Clocortolone
Diflorasone diacetate ointment	Desoximetasone gel or ointment, or cream ≥0.25%	Betamethasone valerate	Desonide
Halobetasol	Diflorasone diacetate cream	Clobetasone	Dexamethasone
	Fluocinolone cream ≥0.2%	Desoximetasone cream <0.25%	Flumethasone
	Fluocinonide	Diflucortolone	Flurandrenolide <0.025%
	Halcinonide	Fluocinolone ointment or topical solution or cream <0.2%	Hydrocortisone base
	Triamcinolone ≥0.5%	Flurandrenolide ≥0.025%	Hydrocortisone acetate
		Fluticasone	
		Hydrocortisone butyrate	
		Hydrocortisone valerate	
		Mometasone	
		Triamcinolone <0.5%	

hydrocortisone). However, when used as replacement therapy in adrenocortical deficiency, its therapeutic effect is the mineralocorticoid activity.

NURSING MANAGEMENT OF THE PATIENT RECEIVING P FLUDROCORTISONE

Core Drug Knowledge

Pharmacotherapeutics

Fludrocortisone is used for partial replacement therapy for primary adrenocortical insufficiency and for treating salt-losing adrenogenital syndrome.

Pharmacokinetics

Orally administered, fludrocortisone is absorbed readily from the GI tract, with peak concentration in 1.7 hours. It is metabolized in the liver and excreted by the kidney. Plasma half-life is approximately 3.5 hours, but biological half-life ranges from 18 to 36 hours. Fludrocortisone crosses the placenta and is secreted in breast milk. The usual adult dosage is 0.1 mg/day (range, 0.1 mg three times a week up to 0.2 mg/day).

Pharmacodynamics

Fludrocortisone acts on the distal renal tubule to enhance the reabsorption of sodium and to increase the urinary excretion of both potassium and hydrogen ions. In small oral doses, the mineralocorticoid effects of fludrocortisone predominate: urinary excretion of potassium, marked sodium retention, and a rise in blood pressure as a result of the physiologic effects of these electrolyte levels. Larger doses of fludrocortisone result in predominance of glucocorticoid effects.

Contraindications and Precautions

Fludrocortisone hypersensitivity and conditions not requiring intense mineralocorticoid activity are contraindications to use. Fludrocortisone's glucocorticoid activity places patients at risk for infection and is contraindicated in systemic fungal infections. The drug should be used cautiously during lactation because it is secreted into breast milk, and safety and efficacy are not established in children. It should also be used cautiously in patients with cardiovascular disease because it can elevate sodium and fluid levels.

Adverse Effects

In small oral doses, fludrocortisone produces marked sodium retention and increased urinary potassium excretion causing a rise in blood pressure. In larger doses, fludrocortisone inhibits endogenous adrenal cortical secretion and pituitary corticotropin excretion. It promotes the deposition of liver glycogen. It induces negative nitrogen balance when protein intake is inadequate. Adverse effects usually occur when the dosage is too high or when the drug is withdrawn too rapidly. Cardiovascular adverse effects may include edema, hypertension, congestive heart failure, and cardiomegaly. Dermatologic adverse effects may include bruising, diaphoresis, urticaria, or allergic skin rash. Hypokalemic alkalosis may occur. Additionally, fludrocortisone may cause adverse effects similar to those seen with the glucocorticoids.

Drug Interactions

Fludrocortisone interacts with many of the same drugs as prednisone because of its high glucocorticoid activity. The drugs with which fludrocortisone interacts include barbiturates, hydantoins, rifampin, anticholinesterases, and salicylates Table 51.4 lists agents that interact with fludrocortisone.

TABLE 51.4 Agents That Interact With P Fludrocortisone

Interactants	Effect and Significance	Nursing Management
Anticholinesterases • ambenonium • edrophonium • neostigmine • pyridostigmine	Corticosteroids antagonize the effects of anticholinesterases in patients with myasthenia gravis, resulting in profound muscle depression.	Monitor patient's muscle strength.
Barbiturates	Barbiturates induce hepatic metabolism of prednisone, resulting in subtherapeutic serum concentrations of prednisone.	Observe for subtherapeutic effects of prednisone. Dosage may require adjustment.
Hydantoins	Hydantoins induce hepatic metabolism of prednisone, resulting in subtherapeutic serum concentrations of prednisone.	Observe for subtherapeutic effects of prednisone. Dosage may require adjustment.
Oral anticoagulants	Anticoagulant dose requirements possibly reduced; conversely, prednisone may oppose the anticoagulant action.	Monitor prothrombin time and coagulation tests.
Rifamycins	Rifamycins induce hepatic metabolism of prednisone, resulting in subtherapeutic serum concentrations of prednisone.	Avoid coadministration if possible. Observe for subtherapeutic effects of prednisone. Dosage may require adjustment.
Salicylates	Prednisone stimulates the metabolism of salicylates, resulting in decreased serum salicylate levels, and may decrease their effectiveness.	Evaluate for subtherapeutic effects of salicylate. Dosage may require adjustment.

Assessment of Relevant Core Patient Variables

Health Status

Review the patient's history for pre-existing conditions that require cautious use of fludrocortisone (e.g., diabetes mellitus, hypertension, osteoporosis, or impaired renal function).

Report any positive findings to the health care provider. Before administering fludrocortisone, assess the patient's fluid and electrolyte balance, nutritional status, and weight control history. In small doses, fludrocortisone produces marked sodium retention, increased urinary excretion of potassium, and elevated blood pressure. In larger doses, the glucocorticoid effects of fludrocortisone promote the deposition of liver glycogen and induce a negative nitrogen balance unless enough protein is consumed. Depending on the patient's condition before drug administration, assess appropriate laboratory or diagnostic tests to manage the adverse events associated with fluid and electrolytes (particularly hypertension).

Life Span and Gender

Fludrocortisone is an FDA pregnancy category C drug, which means that safety for use during pregnancy has not been established. If fludrocortisone is given during pregnancy, observe the newborn for signs of adrenocortical insufficiency because of adrenal suppression. Fludrocortisone is secreted in breast milk. Therefore, use caution when giving it to lactating women. It is important to note the patient's age before administering fludrocortisone. Monitor growth and development of infants and children on long-term therapy.

Lifestyle, Diet, and Habits

Assess the patient's diet because fludrocortisone-mediated sodium retention and potassium loss are affected by food choices.

Environment

Fludrocortisone may be given in any setting, including the home environment.

Culture and Inherited Traits

Traditional foods and herbal and home remedies consumed by patients of various ethnic or cultural groups may be high in sodium. For example, Chinese foods are traditionally prepared with high-sodium soy sauce and monosodium glutamate (MSG). Many other preserved and fermented foods are high in sodium. Take a complete dietary history, including usual dietary intake, food preferences and intolerances, and use of home remedies. This information allows you to assess the patient's risk for weight gain or edema and will also provide the knowledge to use when teaching the patient, family, and caregivers.

Nursing Diagnoses and Outcomes

- Excess Fluid Volume related to mineralocorticoid-induced sodium and water retention
  Desired outcome: *The patient will relate causative factors and methods of preventing fluid retention and exhibit decreased peripheral and sacral edema.*
- Risk for Injury related to adrenocortical insufficiency
  Desired outcome: *The patient will demonstrate knowledge of risk factors associated with potential for injury and will practice appropriate precautions for prevention.*

Planning and Intervention

Maximizing Therapeutic Effects

Assess for drugs that may interact with fludrocortisone and decrease its efficacy. These drugs include barbiturates, cholestyramine, oral contraceptives, and salicylates. As with prednisone, evaluate the need for an increased dose of fludrocortisone during times of injury, stress, or infection, or surgery.

Minimizing Adverse Effects

Monitor blood pressure, fluid balance, and electrolyte status. Patients with a history of renal or cardiovascular dysfunction are at risk for adverse effects from fludrocortisone. Review the importance of following a diet high in potassium-rich foods in order to prevent potassium loss and moderate sodium intake to reduce the risk for hypertension, weight gain, and edema.

Providing Patient and Family Education

- Instruct patients to adhere to drug therapy as prescribed, stressing the importance of regular follow-up visits with the prescriber.
- Encourage the patient to wear a medical identification bracelet that states the patient's medical condition and the specific drug therapy.
- Teach patients to report unusual weight gain, lower extremity edema, muscle weakness, and severe or continuing headache.
- Teach the patient to monitor blood pressure.
- Schedule follow-up appointments to monitor serum electrolytes (including calcium) regularly to prevent fludrocortisone overdosage.
- Help the patient develop a low-sodium and high-potassium dietary plan.
- Teach the patient to weigh herself or himself daily; any sudden increase indicates fluid retention.
- Teach signs and symptoms for self-monitoring for adverse effects to drug therapy.

Ongoing Assessment and Evaluation

Monitor for edema, weight gain, hypertension, cardiac arrhythmias, or muscular weakness that may develop because of the drug's sodium-retaining effects. Potassium supplementation may be necessary related to potassium loss. Periods of stress (e.g., those related to trauma, surgery, or severe illness) may require medication adjustment of mineralocorticoid and glucocorticoid dosage to avoid drug-induced adrenal insufficiency.

Assess the patient for adverse reactions to fludrocortisone including fluid retention (e.g., increased blood pressure, sudden weight gain), ankle edema, and respiratory crackles. Additionally, monitor for acute adrenal insufficiency or characteristic adverse glucocorticoid reactions. Fludrocortisone replacement therapy is effective when the patient exhibits a normal blood pressure, and fluid and electrolyte balance is

within normal limits. The patient should be able to explain the importance of self-monitoring for adverse effects.

C STEROID HORMONE ANTAGONISTS

Steroid hormone antagonists, otherwise known as adrenal **steroid hormone inhibitors,** act to inhibit or suppress the adrenal cortex, thus controlling the symptoms of Cushing syndrome. Drugs within this class include aminoglutethimide, cyproheptadine, ketoconazole, mifepristone, and mitotane. Aminoglutethimide (Cytadren) suppresses adrenal cortical function and is the prototype steroid hormone antagonist.

NURSING MANAGEMENT OF THE PATIENT RECEIVING P AMINOGLUTETHIMIDE

Core Drug Knowledge

Pharmacotherapeutics

Aminoglutethimide is used to treat hypercortisolism (Cushing syndrome). It does not affect the underlying pathology of the hypercortisolism and is used for a short period (less than 3 months) until more definitive therapy (e.g., surgery or pituitary radiation) can be initiated.

Pharmacokinetics

Aminoglutethimide is well absorbed orally and is bound minimally to plasma proteins. Its plasma half-life of 5 to 9 hours (initially, 11–16 hours) decreases following 1 to 2 weeks of therapy because of its action as a hepatic enzyme inducer. Aminoglutethimide crosses the placenta and is secreted in breast milk. It is excreted in the urine. The usual adult dosage for Cushing syndrome is 250 mg every 6 hours up to a maximum of 2 g/day.

MEMORY CHIP

P Fludrocortisone

- Fludrocortisone is given for adrenal insufficiency (Addison disease)
- Fludrocortisone may cause HRA axis suppression if given for more than 2 weeks and withdrawn too abruptly; abrupt withdrawal places the patient at risk for acute adrenal insufficiency
- Major contraindications: hypersensitivity to fludrocortisone; conditions not requiring intense mineralocorticoid activity
- Most common adverse effects: sodium retention and increased urinary potassium excretion
- Most serious adverse effects: congestive heart failure, cardiomegaly, and hypokalemic alkalosis
- Maximizing therapeutic effects: Increase the dosage in times of stress to prevent drug-induced adrenal insufficiency.
- Minimizing adverse effects: Monitor fluid balance.
- Most important patient education: Eat potassium-rich foods and moderate sodium intake.

Pharmacodynamics

Aminoglutethimide blocks the first step in steroid syntheses and reduces the synthesis of all hormonally active steroids.

Contraindications and Precautions

Hypersensitivity to glutethimide (a nonbarbiturate sedative-hypnotic) or aminoglutethimide is a contraindication for use. Under conditions of stress, aminoglutethimide may cause cortical hypofunction. Glucocorticoid (hydrocortisone) and mineralocorticoid supplements may be needed.

Adverse Effects

Adverse reactions include drowsiness, skin rash, nausea, headache, myalgia, and anorexia. These effects usually disappear spontaneously within 1 to 2 weeks of therapy. Because hypothyroidism may occur, baseline thyroid function should be established, and supplemental thyroid hormone may be necessary. Monitor the complete blood count (CBC) for hematologic abnormalities. Elevations in levels of aspartate aminotransferase (AST), alkaline phosphatase, and bilirubin have been reported.

Orthostatic hypotension and tachycardia may occur. Adverse effects of the CNS are headache and dizziness, possibly caused by decreased vascular resistance. Rash and cholestatic jaundice are considered to be allergic or hypersensitivity reactions. Masculinization and hirsutism in females and precocious sex development in males have been reported.

Drug Interactions

Drug interactions with aminoglutethimide occur because of its action as an enzyme inducer. Aminoglutethimide interacts with coumarin, warfarin, other oral anticoagulants, theophylline, digoxin, medroxyprogesterone, and dexamethasone. Table 51.5 lists agents that interact with aminoglutethimide.

Assessment of Relevant Core Patient Variables

Health Status

Review current laboratory data because hypothyroidism and hematologic abnormalities (e.g., agranulocytosis, anemia, leukopenia, neutropenia, and thrombocytopenia) have occurred with aminoglutethimide use. These tests include a CBC, serum electrolyte levels, thyroid function studies, kidney and liver function, glucose tolerance test results, electrocardiogram, x-ray films of spine and chest, and tuberculin skin test results. Assess the patient's history of prescription, OTC, recreational, or illicit drug use; GI upset; ulcers; or epigastric pain. Also assess nutritional status, weight control, concurrent disease, and trauma history. Include orthostatic vital signs in the physical assessment. Observe muscle strength and body proportions as well as hair growth and distribution patterns. Throughout therapy, continue to assess for signs of adrenal insufficiency.

Life Span and Gender

Aminoglutethimide is a pregnancy category D drug and should be avoided during pregnancy. It is unknown whether it is secreted in breast milk; safety in lactation and safety and efficacy in children have not been established. It is impor-

TABLE 51.5 Agents That Interact With P Aminoglutethimide

Interactants	Effect and Significance	Nursing Management
oral anticoagulants	Aminoglutethimide increases warfarin metabolic clearance, reducing the action of warfarin.	Monitor PT when adding or stopping aminoglutethimide. Dosage change may be required.
dexamethasone	Aminoglutethimide may induce loss of dexamethasone induced adrenal suppression, resulting in an unsuccessful chemical adrenalectomy.	Doses of dexamethasone higher than usually required may be necessary. Consider substituting hydrocortisone for dexamethasone.
theophyllines	Aminoglutethimide is a potent inducer of hepatic enzymes responsible for the metabolism of theophylline.	Monitor serum theophylline levels. Dosage change may be required.

tant to note the patient's physical condition and age before administering aminoglutethimide. Geriatric patients may have increased sensitivity to CNS effects and may become lethargic.

Lifestyle, Diet, and Habits

Assess the patient's typical daily activities. Dizziness and drowsiness may occur with aminoglutethimide use, and caution when performing activities requiring alertness and concentration is necessary until drug effects are known. It also is important to determine the patient's alcohol intake because alcohol potentiates aminoglutethimide's effect.

Environment

Aminoglutethimide may be given in any setting, including the home environment.

Nursing Diagnoses and Outcomes

- Risk for Injury related to CNS effects of hypotension and sedation, endocrine effects of hypothyroidism, or hematologic effects of agranulocytosis, leukopenia, and thrombocytopenia
  Desired outcome: *The patient will remain injury free during aminoglutethimide therapy.*
- Imbalanced Nutrition: Less than Body Requirements related to adverse effects of anorexia and nausea
  Desired outcome: *There will be no change or an improved nutritional status.*
- Disturbed Body Image related to hirsutism and masculinization (in females)
  Desired outcome: *The patient will identify and incorporate methods for camouflaging the adverse hormonal effects of aminoglutethimide therapy.*

Planning and Intervention

Maximizing Therapeutic Effects

Advise the patient to carry medical identification and to inform health care professionals that aminoglutethimide is being taken. It is important to remind the patient that an injury, infection, or illness may cause adrenocortical insufficiency, and the patient may require a medication dose adjustment.

Minimizing Adverse Effects

Suppression of aldosterone production may cause orthostatic or persistent hypotension. Teach the patient to change positions slowly and to avoid situations or environments that enhance hypotension (e.g., consumption of alcohol, overheated areas) to decrease the risk for accidental injury from postural hypotension.

Providing Patient and Family Education

- Discuss the adverse reactions of aminoglutethimide, including dizziness or drowsiness, nausea, anorexia, headache, orthostatic hypotension, and hirsutism.
- Caution patients about driving or performing other tasks that requires alertness, coordination, or physical dexterity until the effects of the drug are known.
- Teach the patient that small, frequent meals of bland foods may reduce the symptoms of nausea.
- Teach the patient to change positions slowly to reduce fall risk caused by orthostatic hypotension.
- Teach the patient to report skin rash, severe drowsiness or dizziness, headache, or severe nausea.
- Teach the patient to avoid pregnancy, alcohol consumption, and overheated environments while taking this drug.

Ongoing Assessment and Evaluation

Continuously assess for adrenal insufficiency because medication adjustment may be necessary. Monitor blood pressure and assess for hematologic abnormalities and physical and mental changes associated with hypothyroidism. Thyroid hormone replacement may be necessary.

Nursing management of aminoglutethimide therapy is considered successful when the patient sustains a reduced plasma cortisol level. The patient should be able to state the importance of self-monitoring for adverse effects and of reporting symptoms to the prescriber.

Drugs Significantly Different From P Aminoglutethimide

Corticosterone and Desoxycorticosterone

Corticosterone and desoxycorticosterone (Metyrapone) are potent inhibitors of endogenous adrenal corticosteroid

MEMORY CHIP

P Aminoglutethimide

- Used to treat adrenocortical hormone excess (Cushing syndrome); it suppresses adrenal cortical function
- Major contraindication: hypersensitivity to glutethimide
- Most common adverse effects: drowsiness, skin rash, nausea, headache, myalgia, and anorexia
- Most serious adverse effects: orthostatic hypotension and tachycardia
- Maximizing therapeutic effects: Provide supplemental doses of steroids during times of injury, infection, or illness.
- Minimizing adverse effects: Help the patient change positions slowly to decrease the risk of injury related to orthostatic hypotension.
- Most important patient education: Take the drug with small, frequent meals to lessen GI effects; do not drive or perform other tasks that require alertness, coordination, or physical dexterity until the effects of the drug are known.

synthesis and are used as diagnostic drugs for testing hypothalamic-pituitary ACTH function.

Cyproheptadine

Cyproheptadine (Periactin) is a potent serotonin and cholinergic antagonist that inhibits secretion of adrenocorticotropic hormone (ACTH) from pituitary microadenoma cells. It is used for treatment of ACTH hypersecretion and Cushing syndrome secondary to pituitary disorders. Remission of Cushing syndrome usually occurs 1 to 3 months after beginning therapy.

Ketoconazole

Ketoconazole (Nizoral) is an antifungal that strongly inhibits all gonadal and adrenal steroid hormone synthesis. It is used in conjunction with surgery or radiation to inhibit glucocorticoid synthesis.

Mifepristone

Mifepristone (RU-486) is a synthetic progesterone and glucocorticosteroid receptor antagonist. It also weakly binds to the androgen receptor. Its antagonistic activity at the glucocorticoid receptor disrupts the negative pituitary feedback resulting from the normal morning rise in cortisol levels. Mifepristone is absorbed rapidly following oral administration, with peak plasma levels occurring 1 to 3 hours after administration. The antiglucocorticoid action of mifepristone (dosages of 20 mg/kg per day) is useful in some patients for the treatment of Cushing syndrome. Common adverse effects include abdominal pain, mild to moderate nausea and vomiting, headache, and diarrhea. These adverse effects can usually be controlled with mild analgesic and antiemetic agents.

RU-486 has been used to treat endometriosis and breast cancer. It can be used as a contraceptive drug that acts by inhibiting follicle maturation, ovulation, and egg implantation. It also is used to interrupt pregnancy through the release of prostaglandins and increased uterine contractions.

Mitotane

Mitotane (Lysodren) is an adrenal cytotoxic agent, although it can cause adrenal inhibition without cellular destruction. It is used for palliative treatment of inoperable adrenal cortical carcinoma. Its biochemical action is unknown, but it reduces production of adrenal steroids and is thought to modify the peripheral metabolism of steroids and directly suppress the adrenal cortex. Approximately 51% of oral mitotane is absorbed; it is primarily stored in fat and undergoes hepatic metabolism. It is excreted in the urine (10%–25%) and feces (up to 60%). Its blood levels, detectable for up to 10 weeks after discontinuation of therapy because of the drug's lipophilic nature, do not appear to be related to therapeutic or toxic effects.

Mitotane is assigned to FDA pregnancy category C. Reliable contraceptive measures are recommended during therapy. Precautions include concomitant drug therapy, hepatic enzyme induction, and the possibility that adrenal insufficiency may develop. Adverse reactions include GI distress, lethargy and somnolence, and transient skin rashes.

CHAPTER SUMMARY

- Corticosteroids affect every body system and have the potential to cause severe adverse effects. Prolonged high-dose corticosteroid therapy increases the incidence of disabling and lethal effects.
- Glucocorticoids occupy an important role in the pharmacologic management of various inflammatory diseases despite the numerous complications that may occur from therapy. Uses for the corticosteroids include replacement, anti-inflammatory, and immunosuppressive therapies. Glucocorticoids are used as replacement therapy in Addison disease, as pharmacologic anti-inflammatory drugs for serious inflammatory disorders and autoimmune diseases, and for a chemotherapeutic effect in certain malignant neoplasms.
- Glucocorticoids are potentially useful in many situations when used with caution. To prevent or manage adverse effects, you, the patient, and the family need a clear understanding of the drugs' actions and uses.
- Glucocorticoids used therapeutically are usually synthetic analogues of the naturally occurring adrenal corticosteroid cortisol, also known as cortisone. The prototype glucocorticoid is prednisone.
- Some patients are at high risk for the serious adverse or toxic effects of the glucocorticoids. Use precautions to avoid viral infections and live virus vaccines. Use with caution in children, pregnant or lactating women, and patients with diseases and disorders, such as cardiovascular disease, renal impairment, peptic ulcer disease, diabetes mellitus, osteoporosis, and treatment-resistant infections.
- Adverse effects, also known as cushingoid effects or characteristics, may be debilitating and life threatening. Cushingoid effects occur with long-term high dosages of systemic glucocorticoids.
- Acute adrenal insufficiency (addisonian crisis) may occur after abrupt withdrawal of pharmacologic dosages of glucocorticoids. A patient experiencing acute adrenal insufficiency is in a potentially life-threatening situation because of the multiple body systems involved.
- During steroid therapy, the underlying disease or condition and its extent will suggest the therapeutic goals that direct the nursing care. Patient and family education is fundamental to nursing management.
- Mineralocorticoids are essential for fluid, sodium, and potassium homeostasis.
- Fludrocortisone is the prototype mineralocorticoid. It is used therapeutically with a glucocorticoid for treating patients with adrenocortical insufficiency (Addison disease).
- Episodes of acute stress (e.g., surgery or trauma) may require an adjustment of the mineralocorticoid dosage to prevent acute adrenal insufficiency.

- Aminoglutethimide, an adrenal steroid inhibitor, suppresses adrenal cortical function. It is used for disorders chiefly characterized by adrenocortical hormone excess (Cushing syndrome).

QUESTIONS FOR STUDY AND REVIEW

1. What are the main effects of glucocorticoids on metabolism?
2. What are the physiologic changes that occur as a result of untreated acute and chronic adrenal insufficiency (Addison disease)?
3. What is Cushing syndrome? What is the physiologic effect of chronic pharmacologic dosage of glucocorticoids? How is Cushing syndrome different from "cushingoid" characteristics?
4. What are the three major actions of the adrenal steroids?
5. What are the two major clinical uses of adrenal steroids?
6. Why should glucocorticoid therapy never be stopped suddenly in a patient who has been receiving long-term therapy?
7. What are the advantages and disadvantages of glucocorticoid alternate-day therapy?
8. What drug interactions commonly occur with glucocorticoids?
9. What is the major clinical use of fludrocortisone? What steroid characteristics does it possess?
10. What patient teaching should be done with patients taking fludrocortisone?
11. What is the major clinical indication for use of the adrenal steroid inhibitors? Name the prototype adrenal steroid inhibitor. Explain its function.

Need More Help?

Chapter 51 of the study guide for *Drug Therapy in Nursing* 2e contains NCLEX-style questions and other learning activities to reinforce your understanding of the concepts presented in this chapter. For additional information or to purchase the study guide, visit *http://connection.lww.com/go/aschenbrenner.*

REFERENCES AND BIBLIOGRAPHY

Clinical Pharmacology [Online]. Available: *http://cp.gsm.com.*

Facts and Comparisons. (2004). *Drug facts and comparisons.* Philadelphia: Lippincott Williams & Wilkins.

Hardman, J. G. (2001). *Goodman & Gilman's the pharmacological basis of therapeutics* (10th ed.). New York: McGraw-Hill Health Professions Division.

Katzung, B. (2004). *Basic and clinical pharmacology* (9th ed.). New York: McGraw-Hill/Appleton & Lange.

Micromedex Healthcare Series [Online]. Available: *http://healthcare.micromedex.com.*

Tatro, D. S. (2004) *Drug interaction facts.* Philadelphia: Lippincott Williams & Wilkins.

Drugs Affecting Blood Glucose Levels

chapter 52

Learning Objectives

At the completion of this chapter the student will:

1. Discuss the importance of diabetes in terms of prevalence and costs.
2. Compare the characteristics of type 1, type 2, and gestational diabetes; describe their pathophysiologic processes.
3. Explain the principles and practices of insulin therapy, including measures to prevent and treat hypoglycemia.
4. Identify core drug knowledge and core patient variables for the oral antidiabetic drugs.
5. Generate a nursing plan of care from the interactions between core drug knowledge and core patient variables for drugs that affect blood glucose.
6. Describe nursing interventions to maximize therapeutic effects and minimize adverse effects for the drugs that lower blood glucose.
7. Identify the peak action time for the four types of insulin and determine when a hypoglycemic episode is most likely to occur with the use of each type.
8. Determine key points for patient and family education for insulin and the oral antidiabetic drugs that affect blood glucose levels.

KEY TERMS

basal insulin
dawn phenomenon
diabetes mellitus
diabetic ketoacidosis
gestational diabetes mellitus
gluconeogenesis
glycogenolysis
glycosylated hemoglobin
hyperglycemia
hypoglycemia
insulin
islets of Langerhans
lipodystrophy
metabolic syndrome
nonketotic hyperglycemia
prandial insulin
Somogyi effect
type 1 diabetes
type 2 diabetes

FEATURED WEBLINK

www.niddk.nih.gov
The website of the National Institute of Diabetes and Digestive and Kidney Diseases (NIDDK) has information about clinical research trials, ongoing laboratory research projects, and current congressional reports and plans. Diabetes information for patients is available in both English and Spanish.

CONNECTION WEBLINK

Additional Weblinks are found on Connection:
http://www.connection.lww.com/go/aschenbrenner.

Drugs Affecting Blood Glucose Levels

(C) Insulins

- [P] **regular**
- aspart
- lispro
- regular concentrated iletin II
- NPH
- lente
- glargine

(C) Oral Antidiabetics

(C) Sulfonylureas

- [P] **glyburide**
- **First-generation sulfonylureas**
  - acetohexamine
  - chlorpropamide
  - tolazamide
  - tolbutamide
- **Second-generation sulfonylureas**
  - glimepiride
  - glipizide

(C) Meglitonides

- repaglinide
- nateglinide

Nonsulfonylureas

- (C) **Biguanides**
  - [P] **metformin**
- (C) **Thiazolidinediones**
  - rosiglitazone
  - pioglitazone
- (C) **Alpha-glucosidase inhibitors**
  - acarbose
  - miglitol
- **Antidiabetic combination agents**
  - glucovance
  - metaglip

(C) Glucose-elevating agents

- [P] **glucagon**
- diazoxide
- glucose

The symbol (C) indicates the **drug class**.
Drugs in **bold type** marked with the symbol [P] are prototypes.
Drugs in blue type are closely related to the prototype.
Drugs in red type are significantly different from the prototype.
Drugs in black type with no symbol are also used in drug therapy; no prototype

The fifth leading cause of death by disease in the United States, **diabetes mellitus** is a common chronic disease that affects 18.2 million people, or 6.2% of the population (American Diabetes Association [ADA], 2004a). An estimated 13 million people are diagnosed with diabetes, yet 5.2 million are unaware they have the disease (ADA, 2004a). Approximately 5% to 10% of Americans diagnosed with diabetes have type 1 (lack of endogenous insulin), whereas 90% to 95% have type 2 (diminished insulin effectiveness). People with diabetes are at increased risk for cardiovascular disease, kidney failure, blindness, and extremity amputations.

These morbidities add to the cost of care for diabetes. In 2002, the total annual economic cost of diabetes was estimated to be $132 billion, or 1 of every 10 health care dollars spent in the United States (ADA, 2004b). Diabetes has serious consequences that require patient self-management education and continuing medical care provided by an interdisciplinary team of health care professionals. Although research is exploring how to correct the pathologies in the pancreas that produce diabetes (e.g., transplantation of islets of Langerhans cells), at this time, diabetes is normally controlled by drug therapy and cannot be cured.

Exogenous insulins (manufactured versions of the protein hormone that helps regulate the use of sugar and other carbohydrates) are used to replace deficient intrinsic insulins. Regular insulin is the prototype drug; drugs similar to regular insulin are the analogues aspart and lispro. Drugs significantly different from regular insulin are the analogues NPH (a suspension of isophane), lente (a zinc suspension), and glargine. Combinations of some of these drugs also exist.

Oral antidiabetic drugs are also used to control diabetes. These agents belong to two groups: sulfonylureas and nonsulfonylureas (also known as antiglycemics or antihyperglycemics). The prototype for the sulfonylureas is glyburide; drugs similar to glyburide are acetohexamide, chloropropamide, tolazamide, tolbutamide, glimepride, and glipizide. Drugs significantly different from glyburide are repaglinide and nateglinide. The prototype for the nonsulfonylureas is metformin. Drugs similar to the prototype are rosiglitazone and pioglitazone. Acarbose and miglitol are significantly different from the prototype metformin.

PHYSIOLOGY

Glucose is made available to the body from food that is ingested and from the production of glucose by the liver. Unable to store or synthesize glucose, the brain depends on a steady supply of glucose from the circulation and extracts its energy on a nearly continuous basis.

Three body systems are involved in the regulation and use of glucose—the liver, pancreas, and skeletal muscle tissue. The liver synthesizes its own glucose supply (a process called **gluconeogenesis**) in addition to storing and releasing glucose that has been ingested from the diet. Normally, the liver releases some of its stored or synthesized glucose when blood levels are low and stops producing and releasing glucose when blood levels are high.

The pancreas is both an exocrine and endocrine gland. Its exocrine pancreatic function is to produce digestive enzymes. Its endocrine function is to synthesize and secrete peptide hormones—insulin, glucagon, and somatostatin—by the **islets of Langerhans.** The islets of Langerhans are cellular structures that lie in the interstitial tissue of the pancreas and are richly innervated by adrenergic and cholinergic nerves. Insulin, glucagon, and somatostatin play an important role in regulating the metabolic activities of the body as well as in regulating and maintaining the homeostasis of blood glucose. The islets of Langerhans contain the following types of cells:

- Beta cells, which secrete the hypoglycemic hormone insulin
- Alpha cells, which secrete the hyperglycemic hormone glucagon
- Delta cells, which release somatostatin, a hormone that inhibits both glucagon and insulin secretion
- F cells, which synthesize and secrete pancreatic polypeptides used in digestion

The muscle tissue is the target organ for the action of insulin; it contains the majority of insulin receptor sites. When insulin binds with receptor sites on the skeletal muscle, glucose is able to cross over the membrane and enter the cell. When muscle tissue has fewer available receptor sites than are needed by the cells for glucose entry, a condition called insulin resistance occurs. Insulin resistance plays a major role in the development of type 2 diabetes.

Insulin

Insulin is a small protein, consisting of two polypeptide chains, which is synthesized as a precursor protein (proinsulin) that then undergoes enzymatic splitting to form insulin and peptide C—both of which are secreted by the pancreatic beta cells. Measurement of circulating C peptide provides an index of insulin levels.

Insulin secretion is regulated tightly by a coordinated interaction of blood glucose levels, gastrointestinal (GI) and pancreatic hormones, and autonomic neurotransmitters. Insulin secretion is most commonly triggered by high blood glucose. Glucose is one of the body's most important energy sources, and some tissues—especially those in the brain—are highly dependent on glucose for energy, particularly the glucose extracted from the blood. Therefore, careful regulation of blood glucose levels and cellular uptake is essential.

Numerous hormones are involved in regulating blood glucose levels. However, two hormones—insulin and glucagon, secreted by the pancreas—exert the most direct influence.

Functions of Insulin

Insulin has a number of important actions. Primarily, it regulates carbohydrate metabolism, but it also plays an important role in metabolizing fats and proteins. Insulin and its analogues lower blood glucose levels by stimulating peripheral glucose uptake, especially by skeletal muscle and fat. Insulin resistance leads to an inappropriately elevated hepatic glucose output and impaired glucose uptake by the muscle tissue. In the liver, insulin has several functions; it promotes the uptake and storage of glucose in the form of glycogen, promotes the conversion of excess glucose into fat, and suppresses hepatic gluconeogenesis (production of glucose) and **glycogenolysis** (breakdown of glycogen to glucose). Most tissues in the body need insulin so that glucose can enter their cells (Figure 52.1). However, the tissues of the brain, nerves, intestine, liver, retina, erythrocytes, and renal tubules do not.

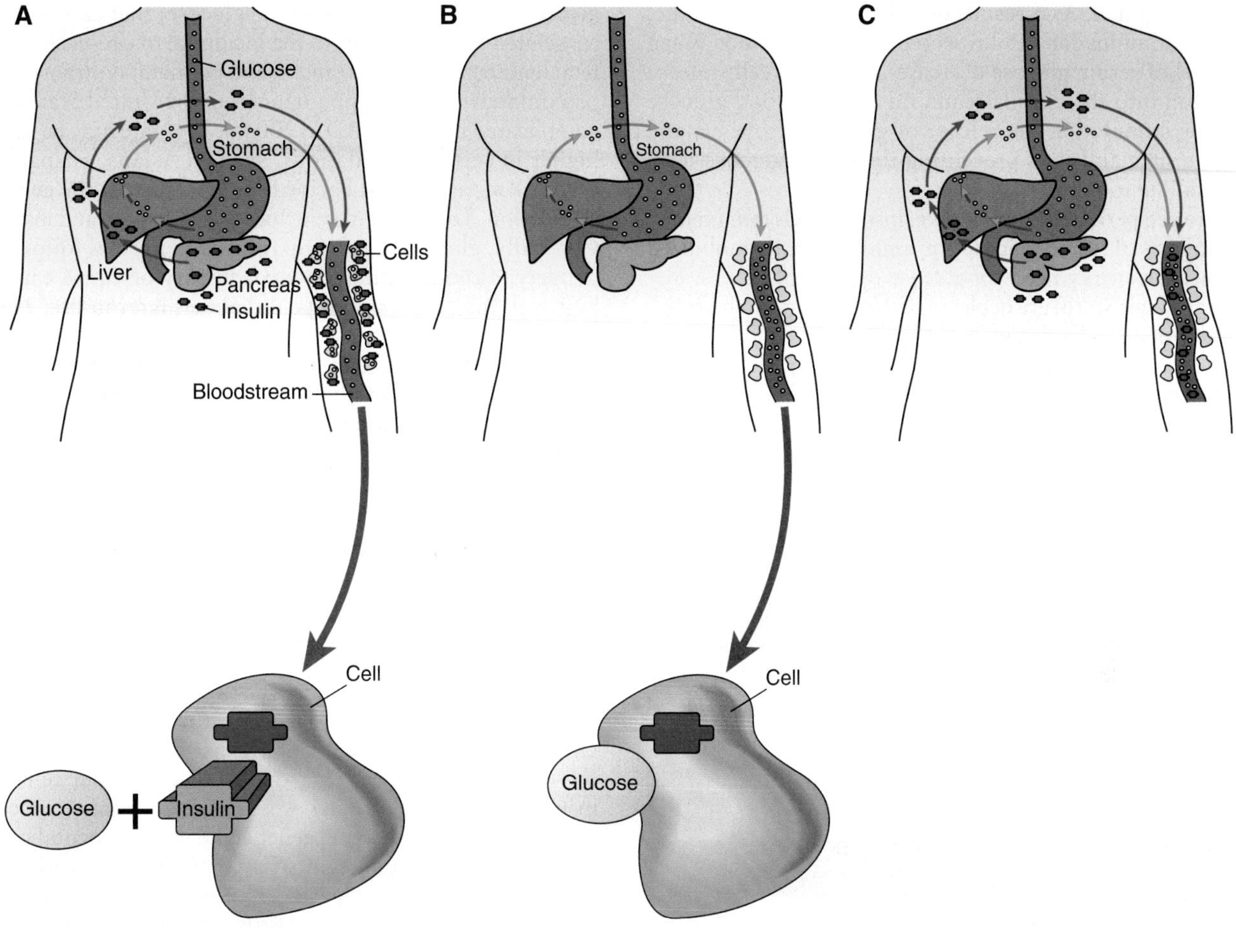

FIGURE 52.1 (**A**) Normally, glucose is made available to the body from the food that is ingested and from glucose production by the liver. Insulin secreted by beta cells in the pancreas binds to the skeletal muscle cells, allowing glucose to cross the plasma membrane and enter the cell. As depicted in the enlargement, insulin provides the key that unlocks the cellular membrane to allow glucose to enter. (**B**) In type 1 diabetes, the pancreas does not produce insulin, so glucose cannot refuel the cells. Without insulin (the key), glucose is unable to enter the cell. (**C**) In type 2 diabetes, insulin is produced by the pancreas but it does not work properly and the glucose is not absorbed by the cell. Both types of diabetes have the same result: failure of glucose to be absorbed into the cells, leading to hyperglycemia.

Insulin Synthesis and Release

The plasma glucose level is the single most important factor in controlling the rate of insulin synthesis and release. Other factors that directly or indirectly influence insulin release or its action include blood levels of sugars (fructose, sucrose, and others), levels of free fatty acids, growth hormone, thyroid-stimulating hormone, glucagon, sympathetic and parasympathetic stimulation, adrenocorticotropic hormone, and cortisol.

Stimulated by plasma glucose levels, insulin secretion occurs in two phases. During the first phase, insulin secretion peaks after 1 to 2 minutes and is short lived. Delayed onset and a longer duration of action characterize the second phase. The exact mechanism by which glucose stimulates insulin release is not fully understood.

Blood glucose levels may be influenced by several factors other than insulin secretion. Any of the following can cause changes in blood glucose levels:

- Stress or illness
- Secretion of insulin-antagonistic hormones (counter-regulatory hormones) that affect glucose metabolism (e.g., cortisol, epinephrine, growth hormone, glucagon, and somatostatin)
- Rates of hepatic synthesis of glucose (gluconeogenesis) or conversion of glycogen to yield glucose (glycogenolysis)
- Presence and levels of insulin antibodies
- Use of glucose by peripheral cells or tissues
- Number of cellular insulin receptors

In response to postprandial elevations of blood glucose levels (those that occur after a meal), insulin is released into the bloodstream by the beta cells. A prompt increase in insulin release occurs so that absorbed carbohydrates are transported rapidly to the liver and other tissues where carbohydrates are stored or used, preventing the serum glucose level from

rising too much. As a result, blood glucose levels decline, and the stimulus for insulin secretion is suppressed. When the level of serum glucose decreases, the alpha cells release glucagon into the bloodstream, raising the blood glucose level by stimulating the release of glycogen from hepatic storage sites and thus preventing the serum glucose level from falling too low.

Between periods of food intake, insulin levels remain low, and sources of stored glucose and amino acids are mobilized to meet the energy needs of glucose-dependent tissues. Hepatic glycogen stores are depleted within 6 hours after a meal. If additional food is not ingested by this time, muscles begin to release amino acids that are converted to glucose. Lipolysis occurs in adipose tissue, and serum levels of free fatty acids rise. Free fatty acids are used for energy by muscle and liver cells, thus conserving glucose for use by the brain.

Glucagon

Glucagon also plays a role in regulating the blood glucose level. Glucagon is a small protein hormone, and declining blood glucose levels stimulate its release from pancreatic islet alpha cells. Sympathetic nerve impulses, exercise, infection, and trauma also stimulate its release. In the liver, glucagon stimulates glycogenolysis and gluconeogenesis, resulting in a release of glucose into the blood.

PATHOPHYSIOLOGY

Diabetes mellitus is a serious chronic disease that affects people of all ages and ethnic groups. Type 2 diabetes appears in a disproportionately higher prevalence in some groups in the United States, including African Americans, Hispanic Americans, and Native Americans. A different type of diabetes, termed diabetes insipidus, is a metabolic disorder in which high amounts of dilute urine are formed because of deficient production of antidiuretic hormone (ADH) or inability of the kidney tubules to concentrate urine (see Chapter 50). This type of diabetes does not alter blood glucose levels and is not treated by insulin or oral antidiabetic drugs. For simplicity, this text will use the term "diabetes" to refer to diabetes mellitus.

Types of Diabetes

Most cases of diabetes fall into two broad categories—type 1 and type 2. In 1997, the American Diabetes Association issued the new classifications in an attempt to classify diabetes according to differences in etiology rather than the age of onset or the treatment type, both of which were imprecise methods of classifying the pathophysiology. Another type of diabetes, **gestational diabetes mellitus** (GDM), is a condition characterized by glucose intolerance with onset during pregnancy. It occurs when a woman's pancreatic function is not sufficient to overcome the insulin resistance created by the anti-insulin hormones secreted by the placenta (e.g., estrogen, prolactin, cortisol, and progesterone) and the increased fuel consumption needed for the mother and the fetus. Diagnosis and treatment are essential because the severe **hyperglycemia** (abnormally high blood glucose) that can result is associated with increases in the incidence of pre-eclampsia, fetal macrosomia, birth trauma, and perinatal mortality. Approximately 4% of all pregnancies in the United States are complicated by GDM (ADA, 2004c). This rate may be much higher in certain populations, such as Asians, Hispanics, Native Americans, and Pacific Islanders, than in the general population. Treatment may include diet, exercise, and insulin. Generally, glucose regulation returns to normal following delivery, although women with a history of GDM carry a high risk for developing type 2 diabetes later in life, as do their offspring.

Other pathologies can induce a diabetes-like state with hyperglycemia, including diseases such as carcinomas, pancreatitis, and infections; hormonal abnormalities such as acromegaly and Cushing syndrome; drugs such as corticosteroids; and genetic defects of the beta cell.

Type 1 Diabetes Mellitus

Type 1 diabetes is an autoimmune disorder characterized by the destruction of the insulin-secreting beta cells in the pancreas, leading to absolute insulin deficiency (see Figure 52.1). The body's reserve of insulin is depleted, resulting in hyperglycemia and ketoacidosis. By the time the signs and symptoms of type 1 diabetes appear, most pancreatic beta cells have been destroyed. Although the pathogenesis is unclear, considerable evidence (e.g., the presence of islet cell and insulin autoantibodies) suggests that the destructive process is autoimmune, with some genetic and environmental components. The autoimmune destruction of the pancreatic beta cells may occur over a period of months to several years before the onset of clinical disease is observed. The final result of type 1 diabetes is an extensive and selective loss of pancreatic beta cells and a state of absolute insulin deficiency (insulinopenia). Therefore, insulin therapy is indicated in all cases of type 1 diabetes. Insulin is used as replacement therapy by supplementing the deficient endogenous levels and temporarily restoring the ability of the body to use carbohydrates, fats, and proteins properly.

The onset of type 1 diabetes commonly occurs during childhood or puberty; however, it can develop at any age. In fact, another small peak of onset is seen during midlife.

Type 2 Diabetes Mellitus

Type 2 diabetes is the result of insulin resistance by the tissues and usually a decrease in insulin production (see Figure 52.1). Abnormalities of carbohydrate, fat, and protein metabolism occur in type 2 diabetes. Type 2 diabetes is linked closely to obesity, sedentary lifestyle, and lack of physical activity; scientific experts declare that the dramatic rise in the number of patients with this type of diabetes is attributable, in great part, to America's weight problem. More than 60% of the U.S. adult population is either overweight or obese.

Type 2 diabetes historically was rare in children, adolescents, and young adults. This is no longer the case, however, because type 2 diabetes is increasing in these younger age groups as the childhood population becomes increasingly overweight. Type 2 diabetes is now seen as an emerging epidemic in the pediatric population. Obesity and diabetes are also risk factors for cardiovascular disease, and as incidence of diabetes increases in the pediatric population so does the risk for cardiovascular disease.

Insulin resistance can be considered the primary defect in type 2 diabetes. An insulin-resistance syndrome known as **metabolic syndrome** (or Syndrome X) is a precursor to the development of type 2 diabetes. This syndrome is a combination of conditions, namely: insulin resistance with a compensatory hyperinsulinemia to maintain glucose homeostasis; obesity (especially abdominal or visceral obesity); dyslipidemia characterized by high triglycerides, low high-density lipoproteins, or both; and hypertension. The focus of these signs and symptoms is an increasing inability to use insulin.

No appreciable loss of pancreatic beta cells or cellular activity from the islets occurs in type 2 diabetes. Plasma concentrations of insulin are essentially normal or may even be increased because the pancreas tries to overcome the resistance by producing more insulin; because the peripheral tissue is resistant to insulin, the insulin does not enter the cells but stays in the bloodstream.

Undiagnosed type 2 diabetes is common in the United States, with estimates that approximately 5.2 million individuals are undiagnosed. Hyperlipidemia linked to insulin abnormalities leads to atherosclerotic plaques in the vessels. Thus, patients with undiagnosed type 2 diabetes are at greatly increased risk for coronary heart disease, stroke, and peripheral vascular disease.

In many cases, type 2 diabetes can be controlled with weight reduction, age-appropriate physical activity, dietary modifications, and oral drug therapy or injections of insulin.

Table 52.1 compares type 1 and type 2 diabetes.

Criteria for Diabetes Mellitus Diagnosis

Three criteria are used to diagnose diabetes:

1. Symptoms of diabetes and plasma glucose ≥200 mg/dL at any time of day regardless of time since last meal, *or*
2. Plasma glucose ≥126 mg/dL after fasting for 8 hours, *or*
3. Plasma glucose ≥200 mg/dL during an oral glucose tolerance test (OGTT) in which 75 g of glucose dissolved in water is ingested (ADA, 2003a).

A finding of any of these three criteria must be confirmed on a subsequent day for the diagnosis to be valid.

TABLE 52.1 Comparison of Type 1 and Type 2 Diabetes Mellitus

Patient Characteristics	Type 1 (Absolute Insulin Deficiency)	Type 2 (Relative Insulin Deficiency)
Age at onset	Usually before 20 y; onset sudden	Usually after 40 y with incidence increasing as age and weight increase; gradual onset; may occur in youth
Incidence	5%–10%	90%–95%
Body weight	Usually thin/underweight or normal weight	Usually overweight/obese
Endogenous insulin production/activity	Significantly decreased/absent	Slightly decreased; normal or may be increased; insulin effects reduced by inadequate tissue (receptor) response.
Insulin receptors/ resistance	Normal receptors/no resistance	Decreased or defective receptors/definite insulin resistance
Dietary modifications	Necessary	Beneficial for blood glucose and weight control
Exogenous insulin requirement	Required for all patients with type 1 diabetes	May be necessary for patients with type 2 diabetes
Clinical signs/symptoms	Hyperglycemia, significant polyphagia/ polydipsia/polyuria, weight loss	Hyperglycemia, fatigue, weakness, mild polyphagia/polydipsia/polyuria, fungal infections (especially skin, vaginal), blurred vision
Complications		
Acute - ketoacidosis	Likely	Unlikely; may occur in the presence of severe illness/stress
Chronic - microvascular and macrovascular disorders	Frequent	Frequent
Etiology/genetic susceptibility	Not fully known; related to human leukocyte antigen (HLA-DR3, HLA-DR4), proposed beta-cell destruction by viral infection or autoimmune process	Not fully known; strong familial component
Clinical management	Insulin injections, dietary controls, exercise regimen	Weight reduction, dietary controls, exercise regimen, oral drug therapy, insulin

The preferred screening and diagnostic test is measuring the fasting plasma glucose (FPG) because it is less expensive and easier to perform than the other methods. The OGTT is more sensitive and more specific than the FPG, yet it is poorly reproducible and rarely used in clinical practice. A random screening is more likely to vary because of dietary intake and is not conclusive by itself. If a random screening is unexplainably elevated, a fasting specimen is ordered to confirm or disprove the diagnosis of diabetes.

Prediabetes is a condition in which a patient's blood glucose levels are higher than normal but do not meet the criteria for diabetes. Under new guidelines established by the ADA, an FPG of less than 100 mg/dL is normal, and 100 to 125 mg/dL is considered prediabetes. An estimated 16 million people in the United States have prediabetes, which is almost always a precursor to type 2 diabetes (ADA, 2004d).

Complications of Diabetes

The consequences of uncontrolled diabetes are serious and can result in acute or chronic complications.

Acute Complications

Hyperglycemia is an abnormally high concentration of glucose in the circulating blood. According to the 2003 ADA guidelines, hyperglycemia is a fasting plasma glucose value of more than 126 mg/dL (ADA, 2003b). The classic signs of hyperglycemia include excessive urination (polyuria) and excessive thirst (polydipsia) caused by the osmotic pull of glucose. Other symptoms include fatigue, dry or itchy skin, poor wound healing, and vision changes (often blurred vision).

Diabetic ketoacidosis (DKA) and **nonketotic hyperglycemia** (NKH), also known as hyperosmolar hyperglycemic nonketotic syndrome (HHNS), are two serious acute complications of diabetes that greatly contribute to the morbidity and mortality among patients with diabetes. These disorders are extreme manifestations of impaired carbohydrate regulation that can occur in diabetes.

Diabetic ketoacidosis occurs primarily in type 1 diabetes. It occurs when ketone production by the liver outpaces ketone loss through the kidneys. Lack of insulin is usually the cause of the ketone imbalance. The onset of diabetic ketoacidosis is slow and gradual. The major metabolic imbalances present in diabetic ketoacidosis are hyperglycemia, ketosis, and metabolic acidosis. Glucose levels are more than 250 mg/dL and can potentially be more than 1,000 mg/dL. These elevated glucose levels can cause loss of consciousness. Other symptoms that may occur include osmotic diuresis, dehydration, electrolyte imbalance, tachycardia, acetone smell to the breath (sometimes referred to as a fruity breath), and hypotension. Treatment for diabetic ketoacidosis is regular insulin administered by intravenous (IV) infusion and IV replacement of fluids and electrolytes.

Nonketotic hyperglycemia also has a slow, gradual onset, but unlike diabetic ketoacidosis, it occurs primarily in type 2 diabetes. In NKH, insulin is present, but it is not as effective as it should be. This circulating insulin prevents the formation of ketones, yet is ineffective in moving the glucose from the blood into the cells. The two primary factors that contribute to NKH are the body's increased resistance to insulin and high dietary carbohydrate consumption. The symptoms of NKH are severe hyperglycemia (glucose level, >600 mg/dL), hyperosmolarity of the blood (≥310 mOsm/L), and dehydration. The severe hyperosmolarity pulls water out of cells, including brain cells, causing neurologic changes such as altered reflexes (presence of Babinski sign), grand mal seizures, aphasia, hyperthermia, visual hallucinations, and hemiparesis. NKH may initially be misdiagnosed as stroke because of the overlap of some of the neurologic changes. Treatment involves careful rehydration and drug therapy to lower blood glucose.

Two types of fasting hyperglycemia can occur in diabetics receiving insulin treatment: the **dawn phenomenon** and the **Somogyi effect** (Figure 52.2). In the dawn phenomenon, blood glucose levels are at their highest between 5 AM and 6 AM. The release of growth hormone overnight is believed to produce this increase in blood glucose. Dawn phenomenon is treated by providing larger doses of intermediate-acting insulin at bedtime to prevent early morning elevations of glucose. The Somogyi effect also produces early-morning hyperglycemia, but the precipitating factor is actually a hypoglycemic event sometime after midnight. The body compensates for the low blood glucose by using counter-regulatory hormone release, directing the liver to release glucose to restore the glucose level to normal. When the body overcompensates, rebound hyperglycemia occurs. The Somogyi effect is treated by lowering the insulin dose, increasing dietary intake at bedtime, or both. The patient's exercise habits should also be evaluated to determine the appropriate balance between calorie intake and insulin needs.

Chronic Complications

The chronic complications of diabetes are usually classified as microvascular or macrovascular, according to the type of blood vessel damage that underlies the problem. Among the macrovascular chronic complications are atherosclerotic vascular disease, myocardial infarction (MI), and cerebral vas-

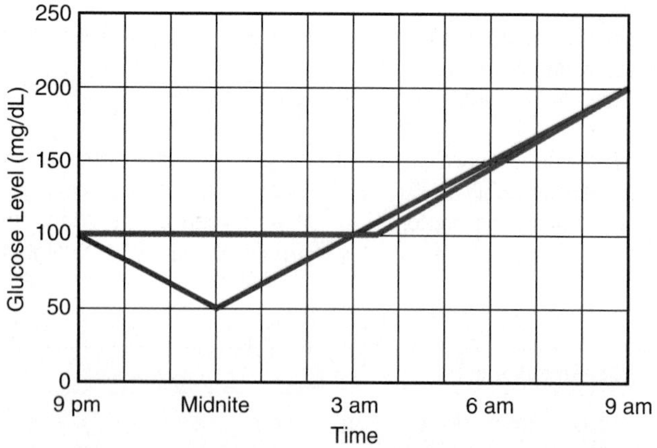

FIGURE 52.2 Blood glucose levels characteristic of unusual phenomena: the Somogyi effect (*red line*) and the dawn phenomenon (*blue line*). In the Somogyi effect, the blood glucose dips around midnight but rises significantly in the morning before breakfast. In the common problem known as the dawn phenomenon, the blood glucose level is stable until about 3 AM but begins rising after dawn. These kinds of problems illustrate why diabetic drug dosages are tailored to meet the individual patient's needs. They present the health care practitioner with challenges and opportunities to mix insulins and adjust dosage regimens to benefit the patient.

cular accident. Among the microvascular complications are cataracts, glaucoma and blindness from retinopathy, lower-extremity infections and gangrene, foot ulcers and Charcot joints resulting in amputation, renal failure from nephropathy and gastroparesis, and sexual dysfunction as a result of autonomic neuropathy.

Landmark Diabetic Clinical Trials

The Diabetic Control and Complications Trial (DCCT) was an early landmark study conducted from 1983 to 1993 by the National Institute of Diabetes and Digestive and Kidney Diseases. This study demonstrated conclusively that the onset and progression of chronic complications of diabetes (e.g., retinopathy, nephropathy, and neuropathy) are slowed by keeping blood sugar levels as close to normal as possible—about 70 to 100 mg/dL (ADA, 2003c). The study also showed that any sustained lowering of the blood glucose level helps, even in patients with a history of poor control.

Although the DCCT studied patients with type 1 diabetes exclusively, the findings have been clinically extrapolated to patients with type 2 diabetes. Another large study, The United Kingdom Prospective Diabetes Study conducted between 1977 and 1991, focused on patients with type 2 diabetes and provided substantial direct evidence of the link between glycemic control and diabetic complications. Results of this study demonstrated that hemoglobin A_{1C} levels (a lab measurement of long-term glucose levels), risk for microvascular complications, and progression of retinopathy were significantly lower with intensive treatment (ADA, 2003d). In addition, no significant effects of lowering blood glucose on cardiovascular complications were observed (ADA, 2003c).

These two trials have had major therapeutic implications for health care providers and their patients. A treatment goal for type 1 diabetes should be a mean glucose of 120 mg/dL and hemoglobin A_{1c} of less than 7.0%. These parameters are similar to those followed in the intensively treated cohort in the DCCT. To achieve this tight control, patients required three or more daily insulin injections or the use of an insulin pump.

The danger of keeping tight control of blood glucose levels is **hypoglycemia,** a condition in which blood glucose levels are abnormally low. Severe hypoglycemia can result in altered consciousness or coma. The risk for hypoglycemia can be reduced by frequent blood glucose monitoring, adjusting the insulin regimen, and altering the time, frequency, and content of the patient's meals. Recent research suggests that achieving appropriate glycemic control can be particularly challenging when patients have limited access to health care (Box 52.1).

FOCUS ON RESEARCH

Box 52.1 Diabetes Case Management Among Low-Income Ethnic Minority Populations

Jovanovic, L., Wollitzer, A. O., Gorke, K., et al. (The California Med-Cal Type 2 Diabetes Study Group). (2004). Closing the gap: Effect of diabetes case management on glycemic control among low-income ethnic minority populations. *Diabetes Care, 27*(1), 95–103.

The Study

A primary objective of diabetes management is to improve glycemic control. When normal glycemic control can be achieved in patients with diabetes, microvascular and macrovascular complications are reduced. Therefore, it is cost effective to monitor glycemic control by measuring hemoglobin A_{1c} levels periodically and by self-monitoring blood glucose daily. However, research indicates that many patients with diabetes have poor glycemic control. In particular, disparities exist among low-income ethnic minority populations relative to other groups. Barriers to care include high cost of glucose monitoring strips and medications, lack of English language skills, and poor cultural sensitivity of health care providers.

In this study, 362 participants were randomized into two groups: a control group that continued to receive usual care from their primary care provider, and an intervention group that received individualized education from registered nurses and dietitians. The intervention group was assessed for diet, exercise, and self-care behaviors, and strategies to improve self-care education and management were used throughout the study in this group. The strategies considered the patient's level of education, literacy, and functional understanding and also his or her treatment goals, general health status, cultural beliefs, and support network. All interactions occurred in a clinic setting or by telephone; appointments were monitored and were rescheduled if missed. Transportation issues were also addressed to ensure visits were completed. Both groups had similar mean hemoglobin A_{1c} levels at baseline. During the 2 years of study, a progressive reduction in hemoglobin A_{1c} levels was seen in both groups; however, the reduction in the intervention group was significantly greater at each time ($p < 0.01$). By the end of the study, the mean difference from baseline in hemoglobin A_{1c} levels in the intervention group was 0.87 greater than that in the control group. The authors conclude that diabetes case management, added to primary care, substantially improves glycemic control.

Nursing Implications

Registered nurses play a vital role in patient education and diabetic management for people with diabetes. Diabetes management can help reduce disparities among low-income ethnic populations but also can improve diabetic health status in all populations. You need a clear understanding of drug therapies and management strategies for diabetes to ensure that patients receive high-quality, accurate patient education that will lead to better control of their diabetes.

Diabetic Therapy

The treatment for type 1 diabetes includes two different insulin regimens. The nonphysiologic regimen does not mimic normal beta-cell secretion and is ideal for those newly diagnosed patients who still produce some endogenous insulin and have not progressed to complete beta-cell failure. This regimen includes one or two daily injections of long-acting insulin. The physiologic regimen attempts to mimic normal insulin secretion, consisting of basal and prandial insulin. **Basal insulin** is the continuous secretion that maintains glucose homeostasis, that is, the body's baseline level of insulin. **Prandial insulin** is the insulin secretion stimulated in response to meals. A regimen that meets both basal and prandial needs combines quick-onset, short-duration insulin with slower-onset, longer-duration insulin. Typically, this mixed basal and prandial regimen includes giving a mixture of NPH (intermediate-acting) and regular (short-acting) insulin before breakfast, regular insulin before dinner, and NPH at bedtime. Meal timing and consistency are very important to avoid hypoglycemic episodes. The physiologic regimen has several variations, which use a combination of rapid-acting insulin (prandial insulin) and intermediate-acting insulin (basal

insulin). Overall, the main goal of this therapy is to avoid hypoglycemic episodes and improve hemoglobin A_{1C} levels, yet maintain a simple regimen to which the patient can adhere.

The first line of treatment for type 2 diabetes consists of oral antidiabetic agents in addition to weight reduction and dietary modification. Starting insulin therapy is recommended if hemoglobin A_{1c} approaches 8% despite optimal oral therapy. The best regimen uses bedtime basal insulin (NPH or glargine) while continuing one or two daytime oral anti-diabetic medications. Metformin combined with insulin may be the best regimen for most type 2 diabetes patients because this combination has resulted in fewer hypoglycemic episodes, lower insulin doses, and less weight gain than other regimens that combine sulfonylureas and insulin. Because of the insulin resistance associated with type 2 diabetes, the patient may require large doses of exogenous insulin; therefore, the goal of therapy is to lower the hemoglobin A_{1c} level, not the insulin dose. Patients with type 2 diabetes require insulin if they become pregnant, have major surgery, or experience severe trauma, infections (including gangrene), fever, hepatic or renal dysfunction, and hyperthyroidism or other endocrine dysfunction.

Table 52.2 presents a summary of selected antidiabetic drugs.

INSULINS

Synthetic insulin (exogenous; i.e., not produced within a person's body) acts in the same manner as endogenously produced insulin. Sources for exogenous insulin include pork pancreas and recombinant DNA technology or genetic engineering to create human-like insulin. Modifying the amino acid sequence of the human insulin molecule has resulted in new, rapid-acting insulin analogues, such as aspart or lispro (produced by rDNA technology). Human-sourced insulin is considered the standard therapy, and almost all patients who are now started on insulin will receive a recombinant DNA form. Some patients who have been on insulin for many years may still use pork-derived insulin. Animal-derived insulins are slower acting than human insulin, however, and produce more allergic responses than human insulin.

Insulin is available as rapid-, short- (also known as "regular"), intermediate- and long-acting types. Type usually refers to the action time of a particular product, which includes the onset, peak, and duration of effects. Some insulins are injected separately, whereas others may be mixed together in a syringe. Other insulins are available premixed in standard concentrations in one vial.

The potency of insulin is expressed in United States Pharmacopeia (USP) units. Most types of insulin are prepared in solutions of 100 units per milliliter. The numbers after the "U" indicate the number of units per milliliter (for example, U-100). Insulin is available commercially in concentrations of 100 or 500 U/mL, (U-100 or U-500). In the United States, U-100 is the standard insulin preparation; U-500 is used only in rare cases of insulin resistance when the patient requires extremely large doses. The syringe that is used to administer the insulin should be calibrated to provide the same concentration per unit as the insulin (e.g., a U-100 syringe should be used with U-100 insulin). U-500 and rapid-acting rDNA insulins (aspart, lispro) require a prescription, whereas the other insulins do not. Different types and species sources (porcine, rDNA) of insulin have different pharmacologic properties. Consequently, the properties of insulin concentration, type, and species source—as well as injection technique, presence of insulin antibodies, site of injection, and individual patient response differences—can all affect the onset, peak, degree, and duration of insulin activity.

Short-acting regular insulin is the prototype insulin.

NURSING MANAGEMENT OF THE PATIENT RECEIVING [P] REGULAR INSULIN

Core Drug Knowledge

Pharmacotherapeutics

Insulin therapy is indicated for all patients with type 1 diabetes and for those patients with type 2 diabetes whose hyperglycemia cannot be controlled properly by diet, exercise, weight reduction, oral antidiabetic drugs, or a combination of these interventions. Regular insulin is also indicated for patients with hyperkalemia because an infusion of glucose and insulin produces a shift of potassium into cells and lowers serum potassium levels. Regular insulin, like all insulins, is administered subcutaneously. Regular insulin is the only insulin that can be administered intravenously. Regular insulin can also be administered through an implantable insulin pump.

Subcutaneous insulin therapy for type 1 diabetes frequently consists of daily injections of mixtures of short-acting regular insulin with intermediate-acting insulins; multiple doses of regular insulin before each meal in association with one or two daily doses of long-acting insulin may also be used. Combining the two types of insulin allows for rapid adjustment to elevated glucose levels as well as for prolonged control, such as all day or overnight. Some premixed combinations are also available.

Regular insulin may be used on a "sliding scale," whereby the dose is based on blood glucose levels, according to guidelines provided in a specific medication order. Sliding scale insulin may be used before meals and at bedtime or every 4 to 6 hours if a patient is receiving continuous total parenteral nutrition (TPN). A sliding scale is ordered frequently for hospitalized diabetic patients when insulin needs may be greatest, for example, with fever, infection, internal stress, or after surgery or trauma.

Pharmacokinetics

Regular insulin, like all insulins, is destroyed by gastric acids and must be given parenterally. The subcutaneous route usually produces slow, steady absorption. The rate of absorption is affected by the site of administration. The most rapid absorption occurs when administration is into the abdominal subcutaneous layer (as much as 50% faster than other routes). The next most rapid is into the arm, followed by the thigh, and finally the buttocks.

When regular insulin is given by IV infusion, some of the drug—usually between 20% and 30%—is absorbed into the plastic tubing set. Up to 80% loss has occasionally been reported. Close monitoring of the therapeutic effect is necessary because it is not possible to determine the exact amount that will be lost and never received by the patient.

TABLE 52.2 Summary of Selected Antidiabetic Drugs

Drug (Trade) Name	Selected Indications	Route and Dosage Range	Pharmacokinetics
(C) Insulins			
Short Acting			
(P) Regular insulin (Humulin R, Novolin R, Regular Iletin I; *Canadian:* Novolin ge Toronto)	**All insulin preparations,** types 1 and 2 diabetes mellitus	*Adult and child:* SC, dosages determined and adjusted depending on plasma glucose, diet, activity, and health status	*Onset:* 0.5–1 h *Duration:* 8–12 h $t_{1/2}$: Varies with preparation
Rapid Acting			
insulin lispro (Humalog)			*Onset:* 0.25 h *Duration:* 6–8 h $t_{1/2}$: 1 h
insulin aspart (Novolog)			*Onset:* 5–10 min *Duration:* 3–5 h $t_{1/2}$: 1.5 h
Intermediate Acting			
isophane insulin suspension, NPH (Humulin N, NPH Iletin I, *Canadian:* Novolin ge)			*Onset:* 1–1.5 h *Duration:* 18–24 h $t_{1/2}$: Unknown
insulin zinc suspension, Lente (Humulin L, Lente Iletin I, Lente L, Novolin L)			*Onset:* 1–2.5 h *Duration:* 24 h $t_{1/2}$: Unknown
Long Acting			
glargine (Lantus)			*Onset:* 1 h *Duration:* 24 h $t_{1/2}$: Unknown
Combination			
Isophane insulin suspension (NPH) and insulin injection (70% NPH and 30% regular insulin) (Novolin 70/30)			*Onset:* 30 min *Duration:* 24 h $t_{1/2}$: Unknown
(C) Oral Antidiabetics			
(C) Sulfonylureas			
(P) glyburide (Diabeta; *Canadian:* Albert Glyburide)	**All oral antidiabetics,** type 2 diabetes mellitus	*Adult:* PO, initially 2.5–5 mg with breakfast; maintenance, 1.25–20 mg/d *Child:* Safety and efficacy not determined	*Onset:* 1–2 h *Duration:* 16–24 h $t_{1/2}$: 10 h
glipizide (Glucotrol)		*Adult:* PO, initial, 5 mg before breakfast; then increase in increments of 2.5–5 mg not to exceed 15 mg/d *Child:* Safety and efficacy not determined	*Onset:* 1–3 h *Duration:* 10–24 h $t_{1/2}$: 2–4 h
chlorpropamide (Diabenese; *Canadian:* Apo-Chlorpropamide)		*Adult:* PO, 200–500 mg/d; maximum dose is 750 mg/d	*Onset:* 1 h *Duration:* 24–60 h $t_{1/2}$: 36 h
tolazamide (Tolinase)		*Adult:* PO, maintenance 100–1,000 mg/d	*Onset:* 4–6 h *Duration:* 12–24 h $t_{1/2}$: 7 h
tolbutamide (Orinase; *Canadian:* Apo-Tolbutamide)		*Adult:* PO, 0.25–3 g/d in single or divided doses maintenance *Child:* Safety and efficacy not determined	*Onset:* 1 h *Duration:* 6–12 h $t_{1/2}$: 7 h

(continued)

TABLE 52.2 Summary of Selected Antidiabetic Drugs (continued)

Drug (Trade) Name	Selected Indications	Route and Dosage Range	Pharmacokinetics
acetohexamide (Dymelor; *Canadian:* Dimelor)		*Adult:* PO, 250 mg–1.5 g /d initially *Child:* Safety and efficacy not determined	*Onset:* 1 h *Duration:* 12–24 h $t_{1/2}$: 6–8 h
Meglitinides			
repaglinide (Prandin)		*Adult and child:* PO, 0.5–4 mg before meals; maximum dose is 16 mg/d	*Onset:* Rapid *Duration:* Unknown $t_{1/2}$: 1 h
nateglinide (Starlix)		*Adult and child:* PO, 120 mg tid (60 mg tid if Hb A_{1C} is near therapeutic goal), 1–30 min before meals	*Onset:* Rapid *Duration:* Unknown $t_{1/2}$: 1.5 h
(C) **Biguanides**			
[P] metformin (Glucophage)		*Adult:* 500–2,000 mg/d in divided doses *Child:* Safety and efficacy not determined	*Onset:* 2–2.5 h *Duration:* 10–16 h $t_{1/2}$: 1.5–6.2 h
(C) **Alpha-Glucosidase Inhibitors**			
[P] acarbose (Precose; *Canadian:* Prandase)		*Adult:* PO, 50–100 mg tid with the first bite of each main meal *Child:* Safety and efficacy not determined	*Onset:* <30 min *Duration:* 4–6 h $t_{1/2}$: 2 h
miglitol (Glyset)		*Adult and child:* PO, initial dose of 25 mg tid at first bite of meal; may start at 25 mg/d if GI effects are severe. Maintenance dose of 50 mg/tid; maximum dose of 100 mg tid	*Onset:* Rapid *Duration:* Unknown $t_{1/2}$: 2 h
(C) **Thiazolidinediones**			
[P] rosiglitazone (Avandia)		*Adult and child:* PO, 4 mg/d as single dose or divided into two doses; may increase to maximum of 8 mg/d after 8 wks	*Onset:* Rapid *Duration:* Unknown $t_{1/2}$: 3–4 h
pioglitazone (Actos)		*Adult and child:* PO, 15–30 mg/d as single dose; may increase to maximum of 45 mg/d	*Onset:* Rapid *Duration:* Unknown $t_{1/2}$: 3–7 h
(C) **Glucose-Elevating Agents**			
[P] glucagon	Reverse severe hypoglycemia resulting from insulin overdosage	*Adult and child (<20 kg):* SC, IM, IV, 1.0 mg; dose may be repeated once or twice *Child (≤20 kg):* 0.5 mg	*Onset:* IM, 8–10 min; IV, 1 min *Duration:* IM, 19–32 min; IV, 9–20 min $t_{1/2}$: 3–10 min

Regular insulin has a quick onset and a short duration of action; therefore, it can be administered to a patient several times a day. In comparison to regular insulin, other forms of insulin have slower onsets but longer durations of action (see Table 52.2). Insulin deteriorates if exposed to excessive heat or light. Regular insulin is stable at room temperature for 1 month. For longer storage, place insulin in the refrigerator.

Insulin is filtered at the glomerulus, with most of the dose (98%) reabsorbed in the proximal renal tubule. Slightly more than half of the reabsorbed insulin is metabolized and excreted; the remaining insulin is returned to the venous blood. Renal function impairment occurs commonly in diabetic patients because of vascular insufficiency. Renal function impairment reduces the amount of insulin excreted, thus reducing the amount of insulin required.

Pharmacodynamics

Insulin is the principal hormone required for proper glucose use in normal metabolic processes. Most of the body's cells require insulin to facilitate entry of glucose. Insulin's effects are tissue specific; it facilitates membrane transport of

glucose (and some other amino acids and ions) into muscle, adipose, and connective tissue cells and into leukocytes. Nerve tissues, erythrocytes, kidney epithelium (tubules), and cells of the brain, intestines, liver, and retina do not require insulin to absorb glucose.

Injected insulin mimics the effect of endogenous insulin. Serum glucose level is regulated by insulin control over the metabolism of carbohydrates, fats, and proteins. At the cellular level, insulin increases the cell membrane permeability to glucose, amino aids, and fatty acids and maintains a constant glucose level by changing glycogen into glucose. In addition, insulin converts excess glucose into glycogen and promotes the storage of fat by combining alpha-glycerophosphate (a product of glucose metabolism) with fatty acids to form triglycerides. Consequently, one effect of insulin on metabolism is weight gain.

Contraindications and Precautions

Regular insulin is contraindicated in times of hypoglycemia or if the patient has any sensitivity to any of its components. When changing the type of insulin (e.g., from rapid acting to intermediate acting, or vice versa), caution should be used and the patient monitored carefully for hypoglycemia or hyperglycemia, either of which may occur as the body adjusts to the different pharmacokinetics of the preparation.

Adverse Effects

Hypoglycemia, the most common adverse effect of insulin therapy, may result from an excessive insulin dose or from increased physical activity without eating. Hypoglycemia is a substantial drop in blood glucose level (to <60 mg/dL) that may result from excessive insulin entering the bloodstream or from insufficient glucose levels to meet tissue demands. The earliest signs of hypoglycemia are neurologic in nature because the brain uses only glucose for fuel. They include fatigue and malaise, trembling, irritability, headache, nausea, numbness, paresthesias, muscle weakness, blurred vision, confusion, and ultimately convulsions, stupor, coma, and death. Hypoglycemia may cause increased sympathetic activity and manifest as hunger, tachycardia, sweating, and nervousness.

Subcutaneous fat may also break down because of repeated insulin injections into the same site. This adverse effect, known as **lipodystrophy** (also called lipoatrophy), causes a depression in the skin and may delay insulin absorption, adversely affecting pharmacotherapeutics.

Drug Interactions

Table 52.3 lists important drug interactions with insulin.

Assessment of Relevant Core Patient Variables

Health Status

Assess patients for allergies and for immunocompromised states and determine whether the patient has been receiving daily insulin, either as a lifelong therapy or short-duration therapy (such as that needed during acute infections). When the patient has been receiving regular insulin at home, determine the type, amount, usual time of administration, who administers it, and what sites are used. Also, determine the frequency of hypoglycemic reactions and how the patient or family handles these reactions. This information helps the health care team to assess knowledge, usual practices, and teaching needs.

Complete a thorough history and physical assessment from which to establish a baseline. Solicit current drug history, including information on all prescription and over-the-counter (OTC) drugs, from the patient or family. A careful review of this information may identify drugs that can alter the action of insulin. Drugs taken for other disorders (e.g., thiazide diuretics, corticosteroids, and estrogens) may cause hyperglycemia, which complicates diabetic control and requires higher dosages of an antidiabetic medication or insulin.

Assess for complications related to diabetes, such as neuropathy, nephropathy, or retinopathy, and for the patient's ability to perform psychomotor skills such as self-monitoring of blood glucose or self-injection of insulin.

Assess the integumentary system and inquire into the patient's general health practices, especially in regard to the

TABLE 52.3 Agents That Interact With P Regular Insulin

Interactants	Effect and Significance	Nursing Management
acetazolamide, AIDS antivirals, calcitonin, corticosteroids, diazoxide, diltiazem, thiazide diuretics, dobutamine, epinephrine, estrogens (including oral contraceptives), isoniazid, lithium carbonate, morphine sulfate, niacin, phenothiazines, phenytoin, nicotine, thyroid hormones	Decreased hypoglycemic effect of insulin	Monitor plasma glucose and A_{1C} levels. Observe for hyperglycemic complications
ACE inhibitors, alcohol, beta blockers, calcium, chloroquine, clofibrate, guanethidine, lithium carbonate, MAO inhibitors, mebendazole, octreotide, pentamidine, phenylbutazone, pyridoxine, salicylates, sulfinpyrazone, sulfonamides, tetracyclines	Increased hypoglycemic effect of insulin	Monitor blood glucose level. Observe for hypoglycemic complications.

skin. For example, you should assess for lipoatrophy or lipodystrophy at injection sites, color and temperature of the lower extremities, presence of calluses and ulcers on feet, delayed healing of wounds, and signs of peripheral neuropathy.

It is important to obtain baseline and periodic assessments of blood glucose levels, blood cell counts, electrolytes (especially potassium), blood lipid levels (e.g., cholesterol and triglycerides), and hemoglobin A_{1C} levels. Assess the patient's knowledge of diabetes and basics of self-care.

Life Span and Gender

Assess the patient for pregnancy. Human insulin is preferred for use during gestation (both in gestational diabetes and in women who have diabetes before becoming pregnant). Human insulin is also recommended for women with diabetes who are considering pregnancy. Insulin is ranked in FDA pregnancy category B. Inquire about breast-feeding status. Although the hormone does not pass into breast milk, lactation may decrease insulin requirements despite the increase in caloric intake necessitated by it.

Adjust care to meet the patient's chronologic and developmental age. Infants and toddlers must be assessed carefully to avoid hypoglycemic episodes, which could have harmful effects on the developing brain and spinal column. With adolescents, the nursing assessment includes monitoring growth spurts, which can cause a substantial increase in insulin requirements. Also, assess the adolescent's acceptance of and actual adherence to therapy. Adolescents with type 1 or 2 diabetes may resist medication, especially insulin injections. They may delay or omit their insulin dosages to fit in socially or to control their weight.

Assess the older adult for changes in the management and control of diabetes and glucose levels. Changes in the diet and activity level of the elderly patient pose challenges to control of blood glucose levels. Examples of these changes include ill-fitting dentures, difficulty chewing and swallowing, decreased ability and interest in cooking, age-related changes in taste perception, reluctance to change long-established eating patterns, limited finances, and reliance on others for meals. Furthermore, decreased motor coordination and visual acuity may impair the patient's ability to perform self-monitoring of blood glucose levels and self-injection of insulin. Older adults may have impaired vision, decreased motor coordination, or other health problems that affect their ability to perform tasks needed for diabetic control, such as fingersticks, self-administration of insulin, and managing diet and exercise.

Lifestyle, Diet, and Habits

An assessment of psychosocial aspects of diabetes, such as role changes and presence of financial concerns, may help to ascertain the patient's ability to cope with a chronic illness that involves major changes in lifestyle.

Exercise increases the permeability of the cell membrane to glucose, decreasing the need for insulin to transport glucose into the cell. Therefore, you must determine the activity and exercise patterns of the patient, which can be accomplished by asking about the patient's usual activity level, occupation, amount and type of recreational activities, and daily exercise patterns. Also, assess the patient's typical eating habits because they also alter the individual response to regular insulin.

The patient's typical alcohol intake is also a factor because consuming alcohol may cause hypoglycemia or hyperglycemia. Alcohol has no nutritional value, although if consumed, it must be included in the fat allowances of the diabetic diet plan. Patients taking insulin and consuming alcohol may need to adjust the insulin dosage because alcohol potentiates the hypoglycemic effect of insulin. Also, assess for the use of dietary supplements and herbal products because they may alter glucose production or storage or interact with insulin.

Environment

Note the environment in which regular insulin will be administered. Insulin is most commonly self-administered by the patient in the home. Proper needle disposal is a growing concern because of the large number of patients administering medications with syringes in the home care setting. Current Environmental Protection Agency (EPA) guidelines recommend that syringes, lancets, and other sharp objects be placed in a hard plastic or metal container with a screw-on or other tight-fitting lid. Patients should check local regulations regarding sharps disposal. For information on methods of insulin administration other than subcutaneous injections see Box 52.2.

Culture and Inherited Traits

Before administering insulin, note the patient's ethnic background. Human regular insulin is preferred in patients whose religion forbids pork products.

Nursing Diagnoses and Outcomes

- Deficient Knowledge related to insulin pharmacotherapeutics
  Desired outcome: *The patient (or family) will state brand, type, onset, peak, duration, and dose of insulin.*
- Risk for Nonadherence to Self-Care related to the complexity and chronic nature of the insulin regimen.
  Desired outcome: *The patient will adhere to the treatment regimen and communicate an understanding of the insulin regimen and its importance (i.e., demonstrate techniques for administering insulin and verbalize recommendations for site rotation, storage of insulin, and disposal of syringes).*
- Potential Complication: Hypoglycemia related to administration of too much insulin.
  Desired outcome: *The patient will assess for and report signs and symptoms of hypoglycemia and if an episode should occur will implement the appropriate treatment.*
- Pain related to insulin injections and self-monitoring blood glucose testing via fingerstick.
  Desired outcome: *The patient will state two nonpharmacologic methods used to control pain and will demonstrate proper subcutaneous injection and fingerstick techniques to minimize pain.*

Planning and Intervention

Maximizing Therapeutic Effects

Store opened vials of regular insulin at room temperature. Extra supplies are stored in the refrigerator, but not the freezer. Extreme temperatures (<2°C or >30°C) should be avoided to prevent loss of maximum function.

COMMUNITY-BASED CONCERNS

Box 52.2 Insulin Delivery Devices

Insulin Infusion Pump

An insulin pump is a small (2- × 3-in) precise computerized device that consists of a reservoir filled with insulin. The reservoir is connected by an infusion set (a thin plastic tube) to a subcutaneous SC catheter or needle. The catheter is changed every 2 to 3 days. An insulin pump can be programmed to deliver a basal infusion of insulin (microdoses; about 0.1 U) 24 hours a day. Continuous delivery of insulin helps maintain blood glucose concentrations between meals and overnight. Insulin dosing adjustments require little or no patient effort. When the patient eats, a predetermined bolus dose of insulin is delivered that is matched to the estimated caloric intake. The bolus mode requires the patient to determine the dose and push a button to administer insulin before or after each meal. Pump devices help patients achieve tighter blood glucose control, thus minimizing potential complications. The pumps have an alarm system that alerts the patient if insulin delivery is interrupted. Some patients may find the pump complicated to use. The individual needs to be very motivated and adherent to therapy. The pump is not automatic; the user must decide how much insulin to give. Some combinations of pumps and glucose monitors are available. See below.

Jet Injectors

Jet injectors deliver insulin transcutaneously without a needle. A fine stream of insulin directed at high speed and pressure penetrates the skin. The dose of insulin is controlled by a dial-a-dose mechanism similar to that used in insulin pens. An advantage to this method is a more rapid absorption of regular human insulin. Their use is limited, however, by size (about 8 oz) and expense. Other limitations include pain or bruising at the injection site and the potential for a decreased amount of absorbed insulin.

Insulin Pens

Pen devices are unique because they combine the insulin container and the syringe into a single modular unit. Although insulin pens are available in a variety of types and styles (e.g., prefilled or reusable) generally, they have a characteristic design—the patient must attach a needle, prime the pen, dial the dose, and depress a plunger to deliver the dose. The convenient insulin delivery can add lifestyle flexibility (because pens are pocket sized and easy to carry) and may lead to improved glycemic control.

Insulin Dosers

The Innovo by Novo-Nordisk Pharmaceuticals is a new insulin-delivery device. It is the size of a pager, advertised as a "doser" rather than an injectable pen. The top half of the device is a miniature screen that displays the dose amount and elapsed time since the last dose. All doses can be dialed in 1-U increments up to 70 U. The device includes a compartment for an insulin-syringe cartridge.

Future Insulin Delivery Devices

In the future, insulin may be delivered by intranasal, transdermal, inhalation, or oral systems. The intranasal route of insulin administration has been demonstrated to be effective in clinical trials. However, some concerns over this method include low intranasal insulin bioavailability (8%), nasal irritation, loss of olfactory sense, and the effects of nasal congestion on insulin absorption. Transdermal insulin appears to be effective (70% absorbed into bloodstream) but slow.

Inhaled Therapeutic System and Pfizer, Inc., are developing a device for inhaled insulin to treat both type 1 and type 2 diabetes. This portable aerosol delivery system—about the size of a flashlight—is similar to an asthma inhaler. It delivers a dose of insulin in a dry powder through the mouth, directly into the lungs, where it enters the blood to act as a rapid-acting insulin. Two multicenter clinical trials—one for type 1 patients and one for type 2 patients—have demonstrated that the inhaled insulin worked as well as injected insulin in achieving overall blood glucose control as measured by the hemoglobin A_{1c}. Aventis and Pfizer together have developed the inhaled insulin, Exubera, which is currently in Phase 3 clinical trials.

Generex Biotechnology Corporation has announced that it has completed an important series of short-term clinical trials of Oralgen (Canada-Oralin), its proprietary insulin formulation that is administered to the oral cavity using a lightweight, handheld spray device. Oralgen is continuing clinical testing in long-term trials.

GlaxoSmithKline is developing an oral insulin pill that can be taken approximately 15 minutes before a meal to provide adequate glucose metabolism. The pill has a polymer coating that allows the insulin to be absorbed in the intestine and not broken down earlier in digestion. Early research suggests the pill can obtain insulin levels that are comparable to that achieved through insulin injections.

Blood Glucose Monitoring Devices

Newer blood glucose meters may offer alternate sites for testing such as blood drawn from the thigh, forearm, or upper arm using a lancet (e.g., One-Touch Ultra, FreeStyle) or an all-inclusive system that incorporates the meter and sampler into a single unit (such as At-Last).

The GlucoWatch G2 Biographer is a wristwatch-like device for patients with diabetes (>7 years old) that automatically, and painlessly, checks blood sugar levels every 10 minutes by sending tiny electric currents through the skin. The device works by having the patient slide a thin plastic sensor onto the watch back each time it is strapped on; small electric currents then extract fluid from the skin and measure its glucose content. This measurement occurs every 10 minutes for 13 hours. GlucoWatch supplements rather than replaces the routine finger (or arm or thigh in newer blood glucose meters) sticks because it sometimes gives false readings. An alarm sounds if blood sugar reaches dangerous levels—either too high or too low—even when the patient is asleep.

Combinations of Glucose Monitoring Devices and Insulin Administration Devices

The InDuo by Novo-Nordisk Pharmaceuticals is a combined blood glucose monitoring and insulin dosing system. This compact device tests glucose levels from the patient's arm and automatically stores results in the memory and calculates 14- and 30-day averages. The insulin delivery system is similar to that of the insulin pen.

A combination of a glucose meter and an insulin pump with a dose calculator is available by Medtronic MiniMed Inc. and Becton Dickinson. The combination of these two products allows for better interchange of data between the two. Glucose values are automatically sent to the insulin pump, thus preventing possible errors that can result when the patient inputs the glucose data manually into the pump. The software that accompanies this glucose monitor/insulin pump also allows for transfer of data to a personal computer fitted with the appropriate software program.

Administer regular insulin with an insulin syringe into an appropriate subcutaneous site. Regular insulin is administered about 30 to 60 minutes before eating. To promote regular absorption, one anatomic area should be selected for regular insulin injections (e.g., the abdomen). Serial locations within that anatomic area are chosen to rotate the exact injection site. This practice is sometimes called intrasite rotation. Do *not* rotate injection sites by using the arm one day, the stomach the next day, and the thigh the next day because this practice will substantially change the absorption of the insulin and the blood glucose levels of the patient. If the patient routinely receives regular insulin in the morning and in the evening, one anatomic area may be selected for each time of day (e.g., use the abdomen for all morning injections and the thighs for all evening injections).

Frequent monitoring of blood glucose by fingersticks and periodic determinations of hemoglobin A_{1c} levels helps determine the therapeutic effect of insulin and overall consistency of diabetic control and provide the necessary data to change the insulin regimen (if necessary) so that maximal effects are achieved.

When a patient receives regular insulin intravenously, carefully monitor blood sugar levels to account for varying absorption of the drug into the plastic tubing.

Minimizing Adverse Effects

Avoid administering cold insulin to help limit local irritation (e.g., lipodystrophy) at the injection site. Injection-site rotation also helps prevent lipodystrophy. Prevention is especially important in infants and children.

Assess the current blood sugar level of the patient before administering regular insulin. Caution is necessary if the blood glucose level is below 70 mg/dL before administration. Usually, the dose is withheld until the blood sugar level has risen to normal levels. Consult with the physician or nurse practitioner before administering regular insulin if the blood sugar is low.

The patient should be monitored closely for hypoglycemic reactions, especially near the peak action time of the insulin (see Table 52.2). Reassess the patient's blood glucose level if signs or symptoms of hypoglycemia occur. If the regular insulin dose is too low for the patient's current metabolic needs, hyperglycemia may occur. Monitor the patient for signs and symptoms of hyperglycemia and re-evaluate blood glucose levels as appropriate.

When you draw up insulin, the dose should always be double-checked by another nurse to prevent accidental overdosage because insulins are very potent. A small dose creates a big effect and could cause serious and even life-threatening consequences to the patient.

Special consideration is needed when caring for infants and toddlers with type 1 diabetes. Infants and toddlers require low dosages of insulin to maintain a goal serum glucose level of 100 to 200 mg/dL. Hypoglycemia may occur because of unpredictable food intake and activity levels in preschool-aged children. The brain and spinal column do not develop normally without an adequate and available source of glucose. Therefore, hypoglycemia must be avoided in infants and young children because it can have potentially damaging effects on growth and development.

Providing Patient and Family Education

In addition to the information provided within this section, which is specific to insulin therapy, see Box 52.3.

Discussing Diet

- Emphasize the importance of eating the prescribed diet after insulin dosing. Warn the patient that hypoglycemia might occur from omission of a meal or from altered absorption of food if a meal is postponed.
- Counsel the patient not to take any nonprescription or OTC preparations, including herbs or alcohol, without first consulting the prescriber, because these substances may interact with regular insulin and alter its effectiveness.

Understanding Activity and Rest

Emphasize that changing the daily exercise or activity pattern will vary the hypoglycemic effect from insulin. If the patient is more active than usual, he or she will use more glucose, thus lowering the available glucose for insulin to act on. The molecules of insulin administered in the patient's ordered dose each have the pharmacodynamic ability to move a certain number of molecules of glucose. If less glucose is available in the bloodstream than is usual for that patient, when insulin moves the set number of glucose molecules into the cells, hypoglycemia will result. Therefore, the patient may need to eat more to offset the glucose burned

BOX 52.3 Patient and Family Education Common to Diabetic Drug Therapy

In addition to receiving routine medical care provided by health care professionals, patients and their families need to be educated on important topics of self-management and drug therapy for diabetes if their management is going to be successful. People with diabetes need to understand:

- What diabetes is and why treatment is necessary
- How to administer and store insulin
- How and when to test their blood glucose
- How and when to take oral medications if they have type 2 diabetes

Emphasize that drug therapy is not a substitute for diet control, exercise, and weight loss. The patient must understand the balance among exercise, diet, and drug therapy, realizing that changes in dietary intake and exercise will result in a change drug therapy.

Caution the patient against consuming alcohol because of its hypoglycemic or hyperglycemic effects with insulin and other antidiabetic drugs, and because of the possibility of a disulfiram-like reaction when alcohol is combined with some sulfonylureas.

Teach the patient to recognize and report symptoms of hypoglycemia (e.g., fatigue, excessive hunger, diaphoresis, and numbness or tingling of extremities), or hyperglycemia (e.g., excessive thirst or urination, urinary glucose, or ketones) to the health care team.

Teach the patient to notify the prescriber when his or her blood sugar is consistently outside of the set parameters (too high or too low), so that changes in the drug regimen can be made.

Encourage the patient to carry some type of medical identification (e.g., a Medic Alert bracelet) and to inform all health care providers of current drug therapy.

by exercising. If the increase in exercising is a permanent change, the insulin dose may need to be adjusted.

Recognizing the Role of Stress

- Teach the patient and family that stress, both physiologic (e.g., from illness, surgery, and trauma) and psychological (e.g., from death in the family, divorce, and job changes), might change insulin requirements because the hormones released in stressful situations are antagonistic to insulin.
- In cases of stress, urge the patient to consult the prescriber to see whether a change is needed in the insulin dosage or regimen.

Monitoring the Blood Glucose Level

- Most diabetic patients learn to test their own blood to measure the level of circulating glucose. Various kits and devices are commercially available for this task.
- Typically, blood is monitored periodically (e.g., before meals and bedtime), and regular insulin is given according to the degree of glucose detected.

Administering Insulin

- Most patients with type 1 diabetes administer their own insulin with disposable needle and syringe injection devices (see Box 52.2). Teach the patient to perform aseptic technique, select the appropriate type of insulin, mix insulin properly (if necessary), administer insulin correctly by subcutaneous injection (see Chapter 3 on injection technique), rotate sites serially in an anatomic location (intrasite rotation), and store insulin carefully (Box 52.4). If an acute infection is present or resistance to infection is impaired, the needles should not be reused.
- Manufacturers of disposable syringes recommend a single use. Some patients, however, prefer to reuse a syringe until its needle becomes dull, usually up to three or four times. Reuse reduces the cost of injections, which may be important for patients with limited financial resources. Most insulin preparations have bacteriostatic additives that inhibit growth of bacteria commonly found on the skin. If reuse is planned, the needle must be carefully recapped by the patient after each use. Aseptic technique should be followed. The patient who reuses a syringe should be taught to inspect the skin around the injection sites for unusual redness or signs of infection.
- Teach the patient thoroughly about safe insulin administration. Needles or syringes should never be shared with anyone else because this practice may cause transmission of blood-borne infections (e.g., hepatitis B or C, or human immunodeficiency virus [HIV] infection).
- Nearly as important as learning about injection techniques is learning about safe and proper disposal of insulin injection equipment. The EPA recommends that insulin needles and lancets be discarded whole in opaque, puncture-resistant containers to avoid the hazards of

BOX 52.4 Insulin Administration

ADA Guidelines for Preparing and Administering a Subcutaneous Dose of Insulin

- Check the type of insulin and the expiration date
- Inspect the solution for visible changes (e.g., solid clumps) that indicate deterioration of the drug.
- If possible, verify Dose, Expiration date, Concentration, Type, Species source (DECTS) with another individual (nurse if in health care setting).
- Wash hands.
- Cleanse injection site and insulin vial by wiping with alcohol.
- If using suspension (cloudy solution), roll gently between palms of hand to resuspend the insulin.
- Inject an amount of air into the vial (each vial if using two) that is equal to the dose of insulin.
- When mixing two types of insulin in one syringe, the short-acting clear insulin should be drawn into the syringe first; do not mix insulins if 1) they are from a different species source (e.g., human, porcine), or 2) their purity level is different, or 3) they are produced by different manufacturers.
- Eliminate air bubbles from the syringe to ensure an accurate dose.
- Injection sites—in their order of rapidity of absorption—include the 1) abdomen (excluding 2 in around the umbilicus), 2) subcutaneous tissue of the upper arm, 3) anterior and lateral aspects of the thigh, and 4) buttocks.*
- Insulin injections are made into SC tissue so it is not necessary to aspirate for blood routinely before injecting the insulin.
- The needle angle during the injection (45 to 90 degrees) should be individualized to avoid IM injection; the needle length is usually ⅝ in. Gently pinch a skin fold to determine the angle that will deliver an SC injection.

Other Considerations

- Insulin vials in current use may be stored at room temperature; avoid exposure to direct sunlight and high temperatures. Some potency of product may be lost after 30 days.
- Spare insulin vials should be stored in the refrigerator. No potency is lost when stored in the refrigerator.
- Prefilled syringes:
  Are stable up to 30 days when stored in the refrigerator.
  Filled with an insulin suspension (cloudy solution) should preferably be stored with the needle pointed up (vertical position) to avoid clumping of suspended insulin molecules in the needle.
  Insulin combinations inappropriate for pre-filling and storage:
  aspart insulin with crystalline zinc preparations
  regular insulin mixed with lente or ultralente insulins
  glargine insulin mixed with any other type of insulin
- Adaptive equipment—several products are available for patients with diabetes who are visually or functionally impaired. Some of the commonly-used assistive devices include:
  Syringe magnifiers to enlarge the measurements on the syringe barrel.
  Needle guides to help direct the needle into the vial stopper.
  Vial stabilizers mounted on a surface to hold the vial in place during needle insertion.
  Insertion aids add bulk to the syringe for patients unable to hold a small syringe.
  Dose-measuring devices assist the visually impaired patient to draw up the recommended insulin dosage into a syringe.
  "Talking" blood glucose meters produce audible test results with tactile guides for test strip insertion.

*Site selection influences absorption; it is recommended that rotation of insulin injection sites take place within the same anatomic area.

exposed or broken needles and that the lid be taped on tightly before putting the container in the trash. For example, a plastic milk container or a coffee can is preferable to a glass jar, which can break.

Explaining Other Safety Measures

- Encourage patients to wear diabetic identification, such as a Medic Alert bracelet, so that appropriate treatment can be given if complications, such as diabetic coma, occur away from home.
- Also, caution the patient that changing the kind of insulin normally used may affect blood glucose control and should be done only under the supervision of the health care professional.
- Advise the patient always to carry a spare vial of each type of insulin used and to pay attention to the expiration date stamped on the vial.

Ongoing Assessment and Evaluation

It is important to evaluate the technical skills (e.g., insulin injection) that will be used by the patient for self-care at home. Specific assessment and evaluation criteria may include the patient's stated willingness to adhere to recommended drug therapy and management techniques for diabetes and may also include blood glucose levels that remain within normal limits as specified by the prescriber.

Fasting blood glucose and hemoglobin A_{1C} levels are valuable in monitoring the patient's response to therapy.

Nursing management of drug therapy is considered successful if the patient experiences few episodes of hypoglycemia or hyperglycemia, demonstrates the ability to correctly perform the technical tasks necessary for managing diabetes at home, follows the ADA diet and incorporates it into his or her lifestyle, incorporates an exercise regimen to attain or maintain normal body weight, and recognizes situations in which knowledge deficit may require the guidance of a diabetes health care professional for additional information or follow-up care.

MEMORY CHIP

P Regular Insulin

- Used primarily to treat type 1 diabetes mellitus; only type of insulin used for intravenous administration, in external insulin pumps, and for "sliding scale" coverage for hypoglycemia
- Most common adverse effect: hypoglycemia
- Most serious adverse effects: anaphylaxis and hypersensitivity
- Maximizing therapeutic effects: Protect insulin from excessive heat and light to avoid deterioration.
- Minimizing adverse effects: Use the same type and brand of syringe to avoid dosage errors; rotate injection sites to prevent tissue damage.
- Most important patient education: thorough patient teaching regarding dosage, administration techniques for subcutaneous injection, delivery devices, diet and exercise, and capillary blood glucose testing; wear medical alert tag identifying diabetic condition treated with insulin to alert emergency medical personnel

Drugs Closely Related to P Regular Insulin

Rapid-acting Insulins: Aspart and Lispro

Compared with regular insulin, the pharmacodynamically rapid-acting (rDNA) insulins aspart (NovoLog) and lispro (Humalog) have a faster onset of glucose-lowering activity (15 minutes), an earlier peak glucose-lowering effect (0.5–1.5 hours), and a shorter duration of action (6–8 hours) after subcutaneous (SC) administration. The rapid onset of action allows patients more flexibility in taking insulin and preparing and consuming meals. Both aspart and lispro are well suited for use in implantable pumps because its short duration of action mimics endogenous insulin more closely than regular insulin.

Although the pharmacologic actions of these analogues are quite similar, their chemical characteristics differ, in that insulin lispro contains zinc. Lispro and aspart are normally used in regimens along with an intermediate- or long-acting insulin. In patients with type 1 diabetes, insulin lispro is used in regimens that include a longer-acting insulin. In patients with type 2 diabetes, however, insulin lispro may be used without a longer-acting insulin when used in combination therapy with sulfonylureas. It may also be used with sulfonylureas in adults and children. Unlike regular insulin, these rapid-acting insulins should be administered closer to the time a meal is started because of their onset of action. Lispro is to be administered 10 to 15 minutes before a meal; aspart is to be administered just before starting a meal, no more than 5 minutes. Adverse effects and patient education are similar to those for regular insulin. To compare pharmacokinetics of various insulins, see Table 52.4.

Regular [Concentrated] Iletin II

Regular [concentrated] Iletin II, like regular insulin, has no additives to prolong onset or duration of action. Unlike regular insulin, its higher concentration (500 U/mL) extends its duration of action to 24 hours. This insulin is indicated for diabetic patients who have developed insulin resistance because a large dose may be administered in a reasonable volume. It is administered subcutaneously only and usually once a day. However, some patients require doses two or three times a day. Hypoglycemia may occur 18 to 24 hours after an injection. Unlike regular insulin, the only available form of Iletin II is pork based. Concentrated insulin is a pregnancy category C drug.

Drugs Significantly Different From P Regular Insulin

Insulin is available in a variety of forms, with the different forms made by adding zinc or isophane with a buffer. These modifications delay the absorption of the insulin from a subcutaneous site, resulting in a later onset of action, peak action, and an extended duration of action. Thus, insulin preparations may be rapid-, short-, intermediate-, or long-acting. NPH, lente, and glargine differ from regular insulin primarily in terms of duration of action. NPH and lente are considered intermediate acting. They are cloudy in appearance, administered subcutaneously once or twice daily, and never used for sliding-scale coverage or in implantable pumps. Because these insulins are suspensions and tend to

TABLE 52.4 Pharmacokinetics of Injectable Insulins

Insulin	*Onset* (h)	*Peak* (h)	*Duration* (h)
Regular (short-acting)	0.5–1	2–3	8–12
Lispro (rapid-acting)	0.25	0.5–1.5	6–8
NPH (intermediate-acting)	1–1.5	4–12	18–24
Glargine (long-acting)	1	—	24

separate inside the vial, they must be mixed by rolling the vial between the palms of both hands before withdrawing the mixture into the insulin syringe. Excessive agitation should be avoided to prevent damaging the additive used to create a long-term drug action. Glargine is a long-acting insulin, and it is clear in appearance.

NPH and Lente

NPH and lente insulins are intermediate-acting insulins that contain protamine and zinc to prolong their duration of action. Onset of action is 1 to 1.5 hours, peak action occurs in 4 to 12 hours, and duration of action is up to 24 hours. These insulins are mixed frequently with regular insulin and given twice daily.

NPH (isophane insulin suspension) insulin is the most widely used intermediate-acting insulin. It contains protamine and a small amount of zinc. Occasionally, a white precipitate (flocculus) may appear as frosting that adheres to the vial. This effect, called flocculation, occurs for unknown reasons, although vigorous mixing of the vial is thought to contribute. Flocculation decreases the potency of the insulin; if it is present, the insulin should be discarded. NPH insulin may be mixed with regular insulin; premixed solutions of NPH and regular insulin are available in ratios of 70:30 and 50:50 (i.e., for every 100 units of insulin, there are 70 of NPH and 30 of regular insulin, or 50 of NPH and 50 of regular insulin). Use of premixed insulin is especially useful for patients who are visually impaired or have difficulty with fine motor skills and may reduce the number of errors that might occur using the standard mixing technique. A limitation of the premixed solutions is that the patient's insulin requirements must match the fixed ratio of the premixed preparations.

Lente insulin is an intermediate-acting preparation of insulin that is a zinc suspension. Lente insulin may not be mixed with nonlente insulins.

Nursing interventions specific for intermediate-acting insulins include observing patients for adequate nutritional intake and monitoring for hypoglycemia during mid to late afternoon (after an early morning dose) because the lengthy peak action time produces additional risks for hypoglycemic reactions. The onset of hypoglycemia with the intermediate-acting insulins is insidious and more prolonged. Adverse effects, nursing actions, and patient education are also similar to those for regular insulin (see Table 52.4).

Glargine

Insulin glargine (rDNA) is characterized by a chemical structure that regulates its release from the SC tissue into the circulation, providing a relatively constant glucose-lowering effect with no pronounced peak of action over a 24-hour period. Glargine, unlike NPH, is a clear insulin, similar to regular insulin in its appearance. Extreme caution must be used not to confuse glargine for regular insulin because serious adverse effects, including hypoglycemia, can occur. Glargine must not be diluted or mixed with any other insulin or solution because its onset of action may be delayed, and the solution will become cloudy. Insulin glargine is administered subcutaneously once daily at bedtime. This timing of administration is unique for glargine. Patients who have previously received twice-daily injections of NPH insulin may be switched over to glargine's once-daily regimen under medical supervision. The initial dose of glargine is usually 20% less than the previous NPH dose. Taking one injection daily instead of two may be viewed as an improvement in quality of life for some patients. Adverse effects, administration techniques, and patient education are similar to those for regular insulin (see Table 52.4).

ORAL ANTIDIABETIC MEDICATIONS

Five chemical classes of oral antidiabetic agents are available for treating type 2 diabetes. They are grouped here based on chemical composition into sulfonylureas and nonsulfonylureas.

(C) Sulfonylureas

The sulfonylureas consist of first- and second-generation drugs. The terms first generation and second generation are applied to groups of drugs that are in the same class but are developed at different times and have some different characteristics. The first-generation drugs are the original group of drugs in the class, and the second-generation drugs are those that are developed to overcome recognized limitations of the first generation. For example, second-generation sulfonylurea drugs have fewer drug interactions than those in the first generation. The first-generation sulfonylureas—acetohexamide, chlorpropamide, tolazamide, and tolbutamide—are rarely used today. Until the mid-1990s, the sulfonylureas were the only class of oral antidiabetic agents available to manage type 2 diabetes. Glyburide, a second-generation drug, is the prototype sulfonylurea.

A group of drugs that are significantly different from the prototype glyburide are the meglitinides, consisting of repaglinide and nateglinide. These drugs act in a way similar to the sulfonylurea drugs but have a different chemical structure.

NURSING MANAGEMENT OF THE PATIENT RECEIVING P GLYBURIDE

Core Drug Knowledge

Pharmacotherapeutics

Glyburide is a potent second-generation oral sulfonylurea that is indicated as an adjunctive treatment to lower blood glucose levels in patients with type 2 diabetes in whom hyperglycemia cannot be controlled by diet and exercise alone (see Table 51.2).

Combination administration of a sulfonylurea and insulin has been used with some success in patients with type 2 diabetes whose disease is difficult to control with diet and sulfonylurea therapy alone. One such method is the "BIDS" system—*B*edtime *I*nsulin (usually NPH) in combination with a *D*aytime (morning only or morning and evening) *S*ulfonylurea. Temporary use of insulin in addition to glyburide may be necessary during periods of physiologic stress (e.g., from systemic infection, trauma, surgery, or fever); stress can induce alterations in glucose regulation that can be controlled only with exogenously administered insulin.

Pharmacokinetics

Administered orally, glyburide is absorbed rapidly and completely from the GI tract. The onset of action occurs within 2 hours, with a maximal decrease in serum glucose occurring within 3 to 4 hours. Like other second-generation sulfonylureas, glyburide is highly protein bound by nonionic binding, which differs from the ionic protein binding observed with first-generation sulfonylureas. Therefore, first-generation sulfonylureas are more likely to be displaced by drugs that competitively bind to proteins (e.g., warfarin), resulting in greater hypoglycemic response.

Glyburide is metabolized completely in the liver by the CYP3A3/4 isoenzyme to two metabolites, both of which are only weakly active. Both unchanged drug and metabolites are excreted equally in the urine and feces. The elimination half-life of the drug is 10 hours, and the duration of action is 24 hours in patients with normal renal function.

There are two forms of glyburide—micronized and nonmicronized. The two forms differ in absorption, onset of action, and delivery system, and consequently also differ in their bioavailability. Patients transferring to micronized glyburide from conventional glyburide or other oral antidiabetic agents should have their dosages adjusted.

Pharmacodynamics

The hypoglycemic action of glyburide results from the stimulation of pancreatic beta cells, leading to increased insulin secretion. Glyburide, like other sulfonylureas, is ineffective in type 1 diabetes, in which no endogenous release of insulin occurs, and in severe cases of type 2 diabetes, in which the release of insulin is severely impaired. Glyburide also reduces the glucose output from the liver by decreasing liver glycogenolysis (breakdown of glycogen stored in liver into glucose) and gluconeogenesis (formation of glycogen from fatty acids and proteins rather than from carbohydrates). Glyburide also increases insulin sensitivity at cellular sites. These mechanisms lower blood glucose levels.

Contraindications and Precautions

Glyburide is contraindicated in patients with a known hypersensitivity to sulfa drugs because the sulfonylureas are related chemically to the antimicrobial sulfonamides (although they do not demonstrate any antimicrobial activity). Glyburide should not be used in type 1 diabetes and should be used cautiously in individuals with renal or hepatic disease.

Adverse Effects

Glyburide and other sulfonylureas are generally well tolerated. The primary adverse effect associated with glyburide (and the other sulfonylureas) is hypoglycemia. Renal or hepatic insufficiency may elevate drug blood levels, and hepatic insufficiency may also diminish gluconeogenic capacity. Both effects increase the risk for serious hypoglycemic reactions. In addition to excessive dosage, other factors that result in hypoglycemia include altered hepatic metabolism and renal excretion, improper diet, excessive physical activity, ingestion of alcohol (more of a problem with first-generation sulfonylureas), or concomitant use of more than one glucose-lowering drug. The hypoglycemia induced by glyburide and other sulfonylureas, although typically mild, may occasionally be severe and require immediate re-evaluation and adjustment of the drug dosage and the patient's lifestyle (e.g., diet and activity). GI effects may include anorexia, nausea, vomiting, heartburn, and a metallic taste in the mouth. Elderly, debilitated, or malnourished patients and those with adrenal or pituitary insufficiency are particularly susceptible to the hypoglycemic action of glucose-lowering drugs. Signs of allergic reactions to glyburide therapy can include maculopapular rash, urticaria, pruritus, and erythema. These reactions are usually mild, but if they persist or become severe, the drug should be discontinued. Photosensitivity reactions also may occur with sulfonylureas. Rarely, blood dyscrasias occur (e.g., leukopenia, thrombocytopenia, pancytopenia, agranulocytosis, aplastic anemia, hemolysis) that may lead to hemolytic anemia. These effects typically subside once the drug is stopped, assuming the condition is detected early after its onset; if undetected and untreated, these conditions may progress and be fatal.

Hyponatremia and the syndrome of inappropriate secretion of antidiuretic hormone (SIADH) have occurred in patients receiving sulfonylureas. As the medication stimulates ADH release, the normal feedback mechanism that controls ADH release is overridden, making the kidneys more permeable to water. This effect results in an increased plasma volume and dilutional hyponatremia. Signs and symptoms of SIADH include water intoxication characterized by mental confusion, nausea, anorexia, dizziness, decreased sodium concentration, increased urinary osmolality, and decreased serum osmolality.

Research performed in the 1970s demonstrated a higher rate of cardiovascular death in patients who received a first-generation sulfonylurea than patients treated with placebo or diet plus insulin. Although the question has always lingered concerning second-generation sulfonylurea drugs, a recent review of the literature indicates that glyburide or other second generation sulfonylureas cause no cardiovascular effects of any clinical consequence (Riveline et al., 2003).

CRITICAL THINKING SCENARIO

Unexpected hypoglycemia

At the beginning of your 7 AM shift, Mr. B, an 81-year-old African American male, arrives unresponsive to the emergency department by ambulance. He is accompanied by his wife. She states she was unable to wake him up this morning. Mr. B is found to have a serum glucose level of 8. One amp of D_{50} (50% dextrose) is administered, and his glucose level increases to 40 and is closely monitored. He becomes responsive, alert and oriented. Mr. B has a past medical history of hypertension (HTN), congestive heart failure (CHF), and end-stage renal disease (ESRD), for which he undergoes hemodialysis three times a week. He does not have diabetes, and there is no family history of diabetes, although his wife has type 2 diabetes. He and his wife are able to care for one another and live in their own home. Throughout your 12-hour shift, you continue to administer amps of D_{50} after checking his blood glucose every hour. His blood sugar continues to fluctuate and remains low, never getting above 60. Mr. B's head computed tomography scan is negative, and his cardiac enzymes are also negative, indicating there has been no heart damage. After all of the fluid is administered, you notice crackles in the bases of his lung, leading to fluid overload and exacerbation of his CHF. By the end of your shift, you start a continuous infusion of D_{50} at 75 mL/h while continuing to check his blood glucose levels every hour. Without the D_{50}, Mr. B's blood glucose will drop.

1. After analyzing all of this information, how do you account for Mr. B's symptoms?
2. What further information might be helpful to fully assess Mr. B's condition?

Drug Interactions

As with other first- and second-generation sulfonylureas, a synergistic drug interaction occurs between glyburide (which stimulates insulin release) and the "insulin sensitizers" metformin and rosiglitazone (which improve tissue use of insulin). Hypoglycemia may occur. A disulfiram-like reaction (see Chapter 5) may occur when glyburide or other sulfonylureas are administered with alcohol. This disulfiram-like reaction is characterized by facial flushing and occasional breathlessness but without the nausea, vomiting, and hypotension seen with a true alcohol–disulfiram reaction. A number of drug interactions are possible because these drugs are metabolized by the CYP3A3/4 system. Table 52.5 lists drugs that interact with glyburide.

Concomitant use of some alternative therapies (e.g., juniper berries, ginseng, garlic, fenugreek, coriander, dandelion root, or celery) increases the risk for hypoglycemia.

Assessment of Relevant Core Patient Variables

Health Status

Assessments to be made before therapy with glyburide are similar to those necessary with insulin. Because glyburide undergoes hepatic metabolism and renal excretion, impairment in these functions can result in elevated serum concentrations of glyburide and increase the risk for hypoglycemia. Therefore, assess renal and hepatic function. To detect or prevent possible adverse drug interactions, additional assessments should include a review of all other drugs—prescription and OTC, including herbal products and dietary supplements—used by the patient. If hypoglycemic reactions occur, it is important to determine their frequency and how the patient or family handles these reactions. This information helps to assess knowledge, usual practices, and teaching needs.

Life Span and Gender

Assess the patient for pregnancy or lactation. Glyburide is in FDA pregnancy category B. Animal reproduction studies have shown adverse fetal effects with glyburide; thus, insulin is recommended instead to maintain blood glucose levels

TABLE 52.5 Agents That Interact With [P] Glyburide

Interactants	Effect and Significance	Nursing Management
antacids (MG+ salts)	Increased glyburide serum levels due to increased glyburide absorption	Monitor blood glucose level for hypoglycemia.
sulfonamides, chloramphenicol, phenylbutazone, salicylates, clofibrate, anticoagulants, fluconazole, H_2-antagonists (e.g., cimetidine), MAOIs, probenecid, sulfonamides, tricyclic antidepressants	Increased risk for hypoglycemia	Monitor blood glucose level for hypoglycemia. Teach patient to recognize signs of hypoglycemia, and to carry food with sugar to eat if necessary.
diazoxide, beta blockers, cholestyramine, hydantoins, thiazide diuretics, rifampin	Decreased hypoglycemic effect	Monitor blood glucose level for hyperglycemia. Monitor A_{1C} levels.
digitalis	Increased serum digitalis levels	Monitor serum digitalis levels and heart rate and rhythm. Observe for symptoms of digitalis toxicity.
alcohol	Disulfiram-like reaction with some sulfonylureas. May cause hypoglycemia or hyperglycemia	Avoid concomitant use.

during pregnancy. Prolonged severe neonatal hypoglycemia may occur if glyburide is administered near the time of delivery. Whether glyburide is excreted in breast milk is unknown; however, some first-generation sulfonylureas are excreted in breast milk. Because of the possibility of hypoglycemia in breast-fed infants, lactating women should avoid use of glyburide.

Note the age of the patient before administering glyburide. The drug's safety and efficacy have not been established in children. Although the FDA has not approved any of the oral antidiabetic drugs for use in children with type 2 diabetes, they are frequently prescribed by physicians who treat this population. Elderly patients may be more susceptible to the hypoglycemic effects of glyburide because of age-related decline in renal function that slows down the drug excretion. Rapid and prolonged hypoglycemia (<12 hours), despite hypertonic glucose injections, has been reported. Hypoglycemic reactions may be more difficult to recognize in elderly individuals because they may be obscured by other pathologies or drug therapies.

Lifestyle, Diet, and Habits

It is a good idea to assess the patient's willingness or ability to adhere to strict drug therapy. Patients should take their pills daily and at the same time each day. Note the patient's weight and typical alcohol consumption before therapy is initiated. Obese patients (those more than 20% over ideal body weight) may not respond to glyburide. Concomitant alcohol use increases the rate of glyburide metabolism and may cause a disulfiram-like reaction. Also, assess for use of herbs that might interact with glyburide.

Environment

Be aware of the environment in which glyburide will be administered. Glyburide is most commonly self-administered by the patient in the home setting.

Nursing Diagnoses and Outcomes

- Ineffective Health Maintenance related to glyburide-induced nausea, vomiting, abdominal pain, and disulfiram-like reaction secondary to alcohol ingestion
  Desired outcome: *The patient will follow ADA dietary guidelines and avoid consuming alcohol.*
- Imbalanced Nutrition: More than Body Requirements related to weight gain secondary to glyburide/sulfonylurea therapy
  Desired outcome: *The patient will follow ADA dietary guidelines and not experience a weight gain.*
- Ineffective Protection related to leukopenia secondary to bone marrow depression associated with glyburide use
  Desired outcome: *The patient will be free from infection while taking glyburide.*

Planning and Intervention

Maximizing Therapeutic Effects

Administer glyburide before breakfast or the first main meal of the day in order to stimulate insulin production. In addition, glyburide should be stored in a tightly capped container at room temperature.

Minimizing Adverse Effects

Monitor the patient's blood glucose levels periodically throughout therapy to detect hypoglycemia. Blood glucose levels should be assessed most closely at the start of therapy and whenever the dose is increased. Because older adults are more sensitive to the hypoglycemic effects of glyburide, administer the drug cautiously at a reduced dosage until the effects on the patient are known. More frequent monitoring of blood glucose levels may be required with older adults.

Monitor patients with renal and hepatic impairment for signs of adverse effects. General blood work should also be monitored periodically throughout therapy to detect blood dyscrasias.

Providing Patient and Family Education

In addition to general teaching on diabetes and diabetic management (see Box 52.3), you must teach specific information about glyburide.

- Teach the patient and family the signs and symptoms of hypoglycemia (irritability, confusion, nervousness, weakness, hunger), which is a common adverse effect of glyburide. The patient and family should know to treat hypoglycemia with a small amount of quickly absorbed carbohydrate, such as a hard candy, orange juice, or a teaspoon of sugar.
- Alert the patient and family to the signs and symptoms of out-of -control diabetes, such as hyperglycemia, polydipsia, polyphagia, and polyuria. Persistent hyperglycemia may indicate a need to adjust the glyburide dose or some other aspect of the therapeutic regimen, such as diet.
- Teach the patient to avoid alcohol while using glyburide.
- It is important to caution the patient to avoid OTC medications and herbal or dietary supplements without first consulting the prescriber. Drug interactions may occur; for example, cough syrups containing alcohol and sugar may cause an unintended effect.
- Provide the patient with oral and written information amount and timing of the doses to be taken.

Also see Box 52.3.

Ongoing Assessment and Evaluation

Interview the patient and family and observe for therapeutic and adverse responses to glyburide and adherence to prescribed treatments. When assessing the success of nursing management, be alert for adverse drug effects (especially hypoglycemia) and appropriately refer the patient to the prescriber for re-evaluation of pharmacotherapy if pertinent symptoms are identified. Blood tests monitoring glucose levels (e.g., fasting, 2-hour postprandial, and hemoglobin A_{1C}) are as important as they are for patients taking exogenous insulin. Review the patient's hepatic and renal function periodically, particularly if he or she has preexisting liver or kidney impairment. Drug therapy with glyburide is considered effective if blood glucose levels are controlled and the patient does not experience appreciable adverse effects.

MEMORY CHIP

P Glyburide

- Oral hypoglycemic that stimulates insulin release and increases peripheral tissue sensitivity to insulin effects; used as adjunct with dietary restrictions to treat type 2 diabetes mellitus. Is available commercially combined with metformin to manage type 2 diabetes (e.g., Glucovance).
- Major contraindications: severe hepatic or renal impairment; allergy to sulfa drugs
- Most common adverse effects: nausea, epigastric fullness, heartburn
- Most serious adverse effect: hypoglycemia
- **Life span alert: Older adults may be at greater risk for hypoglycemia related to drug accumulation from age-related decline in hepatic and renal functions.**
- Maximizing therapeutic effects: Daily dosage of >10 mg should be divided into two doses and taken 30 minutes before the meal.
- Minimizing adverse effects: Avoid taking glyburide with certain alternative dietary therapies, supplements, or herbs because of increased risk for hypoglycemia.
- Most important patient education: signs and symptoms of out-of-control diabetes, such as hyperglycemia, polydipsia, polyphagia, and polyuria; dietary restrictions for serum glucose control and weight loss

Drugs Significantly Different From P Glyburide

Repaglinide

Repaglinide (Prandin), which belongs to the meglitinide class, is an oral hypoglycemic agent. This class shares many of the pharmacologic actions and adverse effects of the sulfonylureas. In lowering blood glucose levels, repaglinide has a mechanism of action much like that of the sulfonylureas. It stimulates the secretion of insulin from the pancreatic beta cells by binding to the beta cell sites. In contrast to the sulfonylureas, this agent is absorbed rapidly and undergoes minimal renal excretion, making it suitable for elderly patients or others with decreased kidney function. Peak action occurs within 1 hour of ingestion; the drug is metabolized completely in 3 to 4 hours. Administered orally before each meal, repaglinide is effective in lowering postprandial glucose levels as the amount of insulin released from the pancreas increases during and just after a meal, mimicking the normal blood glucose response to eating. Because of its rapid elimination in contrast to the sulfonylureas, repaglinide does not cause the beta cells to continuously release insulin for long periods of time. Therefore, insulin levels return to normal before the next meal. The number of meals eaten is equivalent to the number of doses taken; for example, if a meal is missed, the corresponding dose of medication also is skipped. Conversely, a dose is added when an extra meal or large snack is taken.

Nateglinide

Nateglinide (Starlix) is a meglitinide that may be used alone or in combination therapy with metformin. It lowers blood glucose by stimulating insulin secretion from the pancreas within 20 minutes following oral administration; the extent of pancreatic insulin release is glucose dependent and diminishes at low glucose levels. Used before meals, it causes a rapid rise in plasma insulin with peak levels occurring within 1 hour and a fall to baseline by 4 hours. Nateglinide is metabolized predominantly by the CYP450 system and is rapidly and completely eliminated renally. Nateglinide is a category C drug and is contraindicated in pregnancy and lactation. It should be used with caution in chronic hepatic disease, and its safety and efficacy in children is not established. Although hypoglycemia occurs infrequently, it is the most common adverse reaction. Drug interactions that potentiate the hypoglycemic effect of nateglinide include nonsteroidal anti-inflammatory drugs (NSAIDs), salicylates, and nonselective beta-adrenergic blockers. Drug interactions that reduce the hypoglycemic effect of nateglinide include thiazides, corticosteroids, thyroid products, and sympathomimetics.

Nonsulfonylureas

The nonsulfonylurea antidiabetics comprise three different classes grouped by their chemical structure: biguanides, thiazolidinediones, and alpha-glucosidase inhibitors. More commonly, however, these drugs are considered by their mode of action, which is either improving insulin action or delaying the digestion of carbohydrates; thus, the terms antiglycemic or antihyperglycemic may also be used. Metformin, a biguanide, works by improving insulin action and is the prototype drug. Drugs closely related to metformin are the thiazolidinediones, including rosiglitazone and pioglitazone. These drugs also enhance the effectiveness of insulin. Drugs significantly different from the prototype metformin are the alpha-glucosidase inhibitors acarbose and miglitol. These drugs reduce the absorption of oral carbohydrates.

C Biguanides

NURSING MANAGEMENT OF THE PATIENT RECEIVING P METFORMIN

Core Drug Knowledge

Pharmacotherapeutics

Metformin is used as an adjunct to diet and exercise to lower blood glucose in type 2 diabetes (see Table 52.2). Metformin is not a hypoglycemic agent because it does not stimulate insulin secretion; rather, it is an antihyperglycemic or "insulin sensitizer" agent. Metformin works by suppressing hepatic glucose production (reducing glyconeogenolysis) while enhancing insulin sensitivity in adipose and skeletal muscle tissue, increasing glucose uptake into those cells. As a result, insulin resistance is lessened. Metformin is ineffective if patients are without some residual functioning pancreatic islet cells.

In addition, metformin lowers triglyceride levels and total and low-density lipoprotein (LDL) cholesterol levels, and promotes weight loss. Metformin may be used with a sulfonylurea or with insulin to control glucose levels in type 2 diabetes.

Pharmacokinetics

Administered in oral tablet form, metformin is absorbed slowly but incompletely from the GI tract; this incomplete absorption results in a bioavailability of only 50% to 60%. Food slightly delays and decreases the extent of its absorption. The absorbed drug is distributed rapidly into peripheral body tissues and fluids, and peak serum levels are achieved in 2 to 3 hours after administration. Metformin does not bind to plasma proteins and does not undergo hepatic metabolism. Metformin is excreted mostly unchanged by the kidneys; 90% of the absorbed drug is eliminated renally within the first 24 hours, with a plasma elimination half-life of 6.2 hours. Half-life is longer in patients with impaired renal function.

Pharmacodynamics

Metformin decreases hepatic glucose production, decreases intestinal absorption of glucose, and improves insulin sensitivity by increasing peripheral glucose uptake and use in skeletal muscle and adipose tissue through increased transport of glucose across the cell membrane.

Unlike the sulfonylureas, metformin rarely causes hypoglycemia when used alone because it does not stimulate insulin secretion. In fact, insulin secretion remains unchanged, whereas fasting insulin levels and daylong plasma insulin response may actually decrease. In addition, metformin lowers triglyceride levels and promotes weight loss. Metformin lowers fasting and postprandial hyperglycemia. Full therapeutic effect from a given dose takes up to 2 weeks to occur; thus, when the dose is being titrated upward, increases should occur no more frequently than every 1 to 2 weeks.

Contraindications and Precautions

Metformin is contraindicated in patients with hepatic disease, alcoholism, acute or chronic metabolic acidosis, congestive heart failure, clinical situations that predispose to hypoxemia, and renal impairment (creatinine clearance, <40 mL/minute) because these conditions may predispose the patient to developing lactic acidosis.

Adverse Effects

Minor but common side effects of metformin include GI disturbances such as anorexia, nausea and vomiting, weight loss, abdominal discomfort, dyspepsia, flatulence, diarrhea, and a metallic taste sensation. These adverse effects tend to decline with continued use and can be minimized by initiating therapy with lower doses of metformin. Hypoglycemia can occur if metformin is combined with a sulfonylurea drug or with insulin.

Serious adverse effects are rare and usually occur in individuals with impaired renal or hepatic function. Lactic acidosis, although very rare, is the most serious adverse effect and carries a mortality rate of nearly 50%. Lactic acidosis is a metabolic complication characterized by an increased anion gap, elevated blood lactate levels, decreased blood pH, and electrolyte disturbances. Lactic acidosis onset is often subtle and presents with nonspecific symptoms such as malaise, myalgias, respiratory distress, increasing somnolence, and nonspecific abdominal distress. Hypothermia, hypotension, and bradyarrhythmias may be present with more marked acidosis. When metformin is implicated as the cause of lactic acidosis, plasma levels generally exceed 5 µg/mL. Hemodialysis is recommended to correct lactic acidosis caused by metformin accumulation because metformin is dialyzable and its removal results in the reversal of symptoms and recovery. Other rare, serious adverse effects associated with metformin include blood dyscrasias such as aplastic anemia, agranulocytosis, and thrombocytopenia.

Drug Interactions

Metformin, which improves insulin use, interacts synergistically with the sulfonylureas, which stimulate insulin production. This interaction causes hypoglycemic adverse effects. Metformin may react with contrast media used for radiographic procedures. Table 52.6 lists drugs that interact with metformin.

Assessment of Relevant Core Patient Variables

Health Status

Assessments to be made before therapy with metformin are similar to those necessary with insulin. Assessment of current health status should include diet, activity, medication, any adverse effects from medications, and methods used for monitoring blood glucose. The patient receiving metformin should have periodic renal and hepatic function tests. Metformin's half-life is prolonged and its excretion is decreased in patients with impaired renal function, especially those with decreased creatinine clearance. Hepatic function impairment may increase the risk for lactic acidosis. The patient also should have periodic blood tests because blood dyscrasias are rare but possible. Assess the patient's weight during therapy because weight loss—a beneficial side effect for overweight type 2 diabetics—may occur. The patient should also have lipid levels monitored because metformin decreases LDL cholesterol; again, this result is usually a positive effect for the diabetic patient.

TABLE 52.6 Agents That Interact With P Metformin

Interactants	Effect and Significance	Nursing Management
cimetidine	Increased risk for hypoglycemia	Monitor blood glucose levels.
sulfonylureas	Synergistic reaction between metformin and sulfonylurea that improves insulin use; may increase risk for hypoglycemia	Monitor blood glucose levels. Observe for hypoglycemic complications.
glucocorticoids, alcohol	Increased risk of lactic acidosis	Monitor serum lactate levels.

Life Span and Gender

Assess whether the patient is pregnant or breast-feeding. Metformin is in FDA pregnancy risk category B. Animal studies demonstrate metformin excretion into breast milk, but studies in lactating women have not been performed. It is important to determine the age of the patient before administering metformin. Safety and efficacy in children have not been established. Age-related changes in renal function account for altered pharmacokinetics; metformin should be used cautiously in elderly patients because of the prevalence of decreased renal function in this age group. In general, elderly patients are better able to tolerate lower doses of metformin.

Lifestyle, Diet, and Habits

Ask patients about their typical diet and exercise habits and about alcohol intake. Hypoglycemia is more common when metformin is administered concomitantly with other oral hypoglycemic agents, if caloric intake is deficient, or if the patient exercises strenuously. Caution patients against excessive alcohol intake while taking metformin because alcohol use increases the risk for lactic acidosis. Concurrent use with chromium, garlic, gymnema, or alcohol may increase the risk for hypoglycemia.

Environment

Note the environment in which metformin will be administered. Metformin is an oral drug that is easily self-administered in the home setting.

Culture and Inherited Traits

In controlled clinical studies of metformin in individuals with type 2 diabetes, the antihyperglycemic effect was comparable among whites, African Americans, and Hispanics.

Nursing Diagnosis and Outcome

- Risk for Imbalanced Nutrition: Less than Body Requirements related to anorexia secondary to adverse GI effects of weight loss, diarrhea, and anorexia from metformin
  Desired outcome: *The patient will ingest daily nutritional requirements in accordance with activity level and metabolic needs and relate the importance of good nutrition.*

Planning and Intervention

Maximizing Therapeutic Effects

Administer metformin twice a day with the morning and evening meal. The dosage is individualized on the basis of both effectiveness and tolerance. Fasting plasma glucose and hemoglobin A_{1C} (**glycosylated hemoglobin**) are used to identify the minimum effective dose of metformin, when used either as monotherapy or in combination with a sulfonylurea or insulin. Adherence with the recommended diabetic diet and daily exercise will assist in the control of type 2 diabetes, when used in conjuncture with metformin.

Minimizing Adverse Effects

Adverse GI effects during initiation of metformin therapy appear to be dose related. Taking the drug at mealtimes and using gradual dosage increments will minimize these effects. Because it is excreted renally, metformin should be withheld temporarily when patients undergo any procedure using iodinated contrast dye, which is also excreted renally. Lower doses are usually indicated in older adults to prevent adverse effects.

Providing Patient and Family Education

- Teach the patient to take metformin with meals, morning and evening.
- Emphasize that the patient should not use alcohol while taking metformin.
- Advise the patient not to take any OTC preparations, including dietary and herbal supplements, without first consulting the prescriber.
- For general teaching, see Box 52.3.

Ongoing Assessment and Evaluation

Monitor blood glucose levels (fasting and hemoglobin A_{1C}) throughout therapy. Periodic screening for hematologic changes is recommended during therapy with metformin because blood dyscrasias may occur. Metformin therapy is effective when glucose levels are controlled and the patient does not experience any important adverse effects (see also the "Ongoing Assessment and Evaluation" section within the "Insulin" discussion).

Drugs Closely Related to P Metformin

C Thiazolidinediones: Rosiglitazone and Pioglitazone

The actions of the thiazolidinedione oral antihyperglycemic drugs are similar to those of the biguanides; they are antihyperglycemics and "insulin sensitizers." However, thiazolidinedione drugs do not lower triglyceride levels, decrease

MEMORY CHIP

P Metformin

- Oral antihyperglycemic that increases peripheral tissue sensitivity to the effects of insulin and decreases hepatic glucose production. Is available commercially combined with glyburide to manage type 2 diabetes (e.g., Glucovance)
- Major contraindications: serious hepatic or renal function impairment
- Most common adverse effects: nausea, diarrhea, abdominal bloating, flatulence, and anorexia; GI adverse effects appear to be dose related
- Most serious adverse effects: lactic acidosis and hypoglycemia
- **Life span alert: Older adults may be at greater risk for lactic acidosis from age-related decline in renal function.**
- Maximizing therapeutic effects: Individualize the dosage on the basis of both the effect and tolerance while not exceeding the maximum recommended daily dose.
- Minimizing adverse effects: Daily dosage of >2 g should be divided into three doses taken at each meal; the drug should be taken with food to decrease adverse GI effects.
- Most important patient education: dietary restrictions for serum glucose control and weight loss

total and LDL cholesterol levels, or promote weight loss. Thiazolidinedione antidiabetic drugs include rosiglitazone (Avandia) and pioglitazone (Actos). Rosiglitazone and pioglitazone are both indicated as an adjunct to diet and exercise to lower blood glucose in patients with type 2 diabetes. They are prescribed for monotherapy or in combination with a sulfonylurea, metformin, or insulin when adequate glycemic control is not achieved (see Table 52.2). Both drugs are absorbed rapidly after oral administration. They are both highly protein bound and undergo hepatic metabolism through the P-450 system, although they are metabolized by different isoenzymes. These drugs are excreted in the urine and feces. Rosiglitazone and pioglitazone should not be given to patients exhibiting clinical evidence of active liver disease or increased serum transaminase or aminotransferase levels (ALT or AST more than 2.5 times the upper limits of normal). Patients treated with these drugs should undergo periodic monitoring of liver enzymes. Hepatic enzymes should be measured before therapy begins. In patients with normal baseline liver enzymes, liver enzymes should be monitored every 2 months for the first 12 months and periodically thereafter. Rosiglitazone and pioglitazone therapy are well tolerated with few adverse effects that include fluid retention, headache, and weight gain. Plasma volume expansion may occur with rosiglitazone therapy. As a result, small decreases in hemoglobin, hematocrit, and neutrophil counts (within the normal range) have occurred.

In vitro drug metabolism studies suggest that rosiglitazone does not inhibit any of the major P-450 enzymes at clinically relevant concentrations; therefore, drug interactions are minimal. Specific data on pioglitazone and other drugs metabolized by the same isoenzyme (P-3A4) have not been documented; however, potential drug interactions are possible through this pathway. Drugs that are metabolized by CYP3A4, such as erythromycin, calcium channel blockers, cortical steroids, cyclosporine, the statins, tacrolimus, triazolam, and trimetrexate, may have their metabolism impaired, and caution should be used. Drugs that inhibit CYPP3A4, such as ketoconazole, appear to increase the metabolism of pioglitazone.

The assessment of current health status is the same as the assessment for metformin. Particular attentions to hepatic function blood tests are needed because rosiglitazone and pioglitazone can cause hepatotoxicity. It is necessary to emphasize the importance of follow-up blood work and to teach patients to report signs of early liver impairment (e.g., nausea, vomiting, malaise, and dark urine). Premenopausal, anovulatory diabetic women taking either rosiglitazone or pioglitazone are at risk for resuming ovulation with this drug therapy and so are at risk for pregnancy. Female patients should be counseled to consider an alternative method of contraception or be referred to their prescribers to discuss a dosage increase in the oral contraceptive.

Drugs Significantly Different from P Metformin

C Alpha-Glucosidase Inhibitors: Acarbose and Miglitol

Alpha-glucosidase inhibitors provide yet a different mechanism of action for patients with type 2 diabetes. These medications do not enhance insulin secretion, nor are they insulin sensitizers like metformin. Rather, the antihyperglycemic activity results from a substantial reduction in postprandial glucose levels. Alpha-glucosidase inhibitors are an ideal alternative therapy for patients with type 2 diabetes who have mild to moderate hyperglycemia and who are at risk for hypoglycemia or lactic acidosis (see Table 52.2). Acarbose and miglitol are the two alpha-glucosidase inhibitors.

Acarbose (Precose) and miglitol (Glyset) effectively lower postprandial serum glucose when administered alone or in combination with insulin, metformin, or a sulfonylurea. Administered orally with the first bite of food, acarbose undergoes exclusive metabolism within the GI tract—principally by intestinal bacteria but also by digestive enzymes. An active metabolite is created that produces the therapeutic effects of acarbose. Little of the active metabolite is absorbed; only about 35% of the dose is converted and then absorbed. Plasma half-life of acarbose is about 2 hours. The absorbed drug is eliminated through the kidneys. Unlike acarbose, miglitol is not metabolized and is eliminated by renal excretion as unchanged drug. The half-life of miglitol is similar to that of acarbose, about 2 hours.

Acarbose differs from metformin in that it inhibits enzymes needed to digest carbohydrates; specifically, it inhibits alpha-glucosidase enzymes in the brush border of the small intestine and inhibits pancreatic alpha-amylase. Pancreatic alpha-amylase hydrolyzes complex starches to oligosaccharides in the lumen of the small intestine, whereas the membrane-bound intestinal alpha-glucosidases hydrolyze oligosaccharides, trisaccharides, and disaccharides to glucose and other monosaccharides in the small intestine. Inhibition of these enzyme systems reduces the rate of digestion of complex carbohydrate. Less glucose is absorbed because the carbohydrates are not broken down into glucose molecules. In diabetic patients, the short-term effect of these drug therapies is to decrease current blood glucose levels; the long-term effect is a small reduction in the hemoglobin A_{1C} level.

Acarbose and miglitol are contraindicated in patients with diseases of the bowel (e.g., inflammatory bowel disease, absorptive disorders, colonic ulceration, and history of bowel obstruction). They should be used cautiously in patients with hiatal hernia or other conditions that might be exacerbated by increased formation of gas, which is a side effect of acarbose. The drugs are also contraindicated in patients with chronic liver diseases and substantial renal impairment (serum creatinine, >2 mg/dL). Acarbose and miglitol are in FDA pregnancy risk category B. They are excreted into breast milk and should not be given to lactating women.

Adverse effects of acarbose and miglitol are primarily GI in nature and include flatulence, diarrhea, and abdominal distention. These effects occur because the delay in carbohydrate absorption increases fermentation and formation of intestinal gases.

Assessments to be made before starting therapy with the alpha-glucosidase inhibitors are similar to those necessary with insulin. In addition, 1-hour postprandial blood glucose and serum transaminase levels should be obtained as baseline data.

Stress the importance of notifying the health care team if unusual fatigue or muscle pain, difficulty breathing, GI distress, dizziness, lightheadedness, or irregular heartbeat occurs because these symptoms may indicate the onset of lactic acidosis, which is often insidious.

When first educating the patient, tell the patient that acarbose and miglitol inhibit the absorption of regular cane sugar

(such as in candy or orange juice). The most important difference between these drugs and insulin or metformin therapy is that if a hypoglycemic reaction occurs, the patient must not use cane or table sugar products because the sugar will not be absorbed. Emphasize that he or she should use oral glucose tablets instead to increase blood glucose levels. See Box 52.3.

Antidiabetic Combination Agents: Glucovance and Metaglip

Glucovance and Metaglip are both combination antidiabetic agents consisting of a sulfonylurea and a biguanide. Glucovance is a combination of glyburide and metformin, and Metaglip is a combination of glipizide and metformin. Both are indicated as an adjunct to diet and exercise to improve glycemic control. They are also indicated as a second-line therapy when initial treatment with a sulfonylurea or metformin does not result in adequate glycemic control in type 2 diabetes. For patients taking Glucovance who require additional therapy, a thiazolidinedione can be added. Both medications are administered once or twice daily with meals to avoid hypoglycemia (largely because of glyburide or glipizide) and to reduce GI side effects (largely because of metformin). These agents are not recommended for use during pregnancy or in children. Careful consideration is needed in the elderly population and those with renal function impairment. One of the advantages of a combined drug is that it helps to promote adherence to drug therapy because the patient has to take fewer pills daily. For other information, please refer to the individual prototype drugs (see Table 52.2).

C GLUCOSE-ELEVATING AGENTS

Glucagon is a hyperglycemic polypeptide hormone produced by the alpha cells of the pancreatic islets of Langerhans. Its physiologic effect is generally the opposite of that of insulin. Glucagon is the body's first line of defense against hypoglycemia. Whether endogenous or exogenous, it reduces the effectiveness of insulin and some commonly used drugs.

The main stimulus to glucagon secretion is a decrease in intracellular glucose concentrations that usually occurs as a result of a drop in serum blood sugar. Diabetic patients have been shown to have high levels of glucagon, although the cause-and-effect relationship is uncertain. Theoretically, glucagon imbalances could contribute to many of the diabetic patient's problems with glucose metabolism.

NURSING MANAGEMENT OF THE PATIENT RECEIVING P GLUCAGON

Core Drug Knowledge

Pharmacotherapeutics

Most commonly, glucagon is used in unconscious diabetic patients to reverse the severe hypoglycemia resulting from insulin overdosage. Glucagon is effective in hypoglycemia only if liver glycogen is available. It is administered by the intramuscular (IM), IV, or SC route. Glucagon also is used to induce intestinal relaxation before radiographic examinations. Unlabeled uses for glucagon include as treatment for propranolol (beta-adrenergic antagonist) overdose and cardiovascular emergencies.

Pharmacokinetics

Glucagon has a plasma half-life of 3 to 10 minutes (see Table 52.2). The hormone undergoes hepatic metabolism and is excreted in urine and bile.

Pharmacodynamics

Glucagon increases blood glucose levels by stimulating glycogenolysis in the peripheral tissues, exerts a positive inotropic and chronotropic effect on the heart (increasing heart contraction and heart rate, respectively) by increasing cyclic adenosine monophosphate, and relaxes the GI smooth muscle. After parenteral injection of glucagon, the maximum hyperglycemic effect occurs within 30 minutes. The duration of action is about 1 to 2 hours. GI smooth muscle relaxation occurs within 15 minutes and lasts for approximately 30 minutes. The mechanism by which glucagon relaxes GI smooth muscle is not known.

Contraindications and Precautions

A hypersensitivity to glucagon contraindicates its use. Glucagon causes insulin release and is contraindicated when insulin levels are high. It causes catecholamine release and is contraindicated in pheochromocytoma. It should be used cautiously in pregnancy and lactation.

Adverse Effects

Glucagon may cause hypotension, respiratory distress, nausea and vomiting, hypersensitivity reactions of urticaria, and hypokalemia in overdosage.

Drug Interactions

Glucagon increases the hypoprothrombinemic effect of oral anticoagulants and may cause bleeding. The interaction appears to be dose related.

Assessment of Relevant Core Patient Variables

Health Status

Assess the patient's blood sugar levels and level of consciousness. After emergency use of glucagon, assess the patient's level of adherence to the therapeutic regimen and the patient's level of understanding of the disease and its treatment.

Life Span and Gender

Note whether the patient is pregnant or breast-feeding. Glucagon crosses the placental barrier and enters breast milk. Emergency use would over shadow concerns regarding breast feeding, however.

Lifestyle, Diet, and Habits

Review the patient's adherence to the diabetic treatment plan. It is important to assess whether the patient is administering the insulin and monitoring blood glucose correctly,

and whether he or she is adhering to the prescribed dietary and exercise regimens. Adherence to the treatment plan will help to prevent episodes of hypoglycemia.

Environment

Be aware of the environment in which glucagon will be administered. Glucagon is usually administered as an emergency treatment. Although it most frequently is administered in an acute care setting, it might be administered in extended care settings or in the home. Home use would be limited to patients at high risk for experiencing severe hypoglycemia when a family member or caregiver can be taught how to assess for hypoglycemia and administer the drug.

Nursing Diagnosis and Outcome

- Risk for Injury related to hypotension from the adverse effects of glucagons
  Desired outcome: *Substantial hypotension will not result from glucagon treatment.*

Planning and Intervention

Maximizing Therapeutic Effects

Glucagon is administered by the IM, SC, or IV route. The drug is dispensed in a powder form and must be reconstituted to a concentration of 1 mg/mL using the diluent supplied by the manufacturer. Reconstituted glucagon should be used immediately, although refrigerated solution may be kept for 48 hours. The solution should be clear after dilution; otherwise, it should be discarded. A dose of 0.5 to 1.0 mg is usually effective. Doses exceeding 2 mg should be reconstituted with sterile water and used immediately. An additional dose may be administered if the patient's response is inadequate or incomplete after 20 minutes.

Minimizing Adverse Effects

Supplemental carbohydrates should be administered as soon as possible once consciousness has been achieved to restore liver glycogen and prevent secondary hypoglycemia.

Providing Patient and Family Education

- Emphasize to patients and family members measures to prevent hypoglycemic reactions from insulin (reasonable uniformity from day to day with regard to diet, insulin, and exercise; routine blood glucose self-monitoring; and carrying sugar, candy, or other readily absorbable carbohydrate so that it may be taken at the first warning of hypoglycemia).
- Teach family members the importance of quick intervention if severe hypoglycemia occurs to prevent CNS damage.
- Instruct the family in the proper technique for emergency administration of glucagon, if appropriate.

Ongoing Assessment and Evaluation

Blood glucose levels should be monitored before, during, and after glucagon administration, and the patient's emergency supply of glucagon should be restored (if appropriate) as soon as possible. Survival and return to normal function are signs of effective nursing management.

MEMORY CHIP

[P] Glucagon

- Glucose-elevating agent that accelerates hepatic glyconeogenesis, increasing blood glucose levels
- Major contraindications: insulinoma and pheochromocytoma
- Most common adverse effects: nausea, vomiting, generalized allergic reactions, including urticaria, respiratory distress, and hypotension
- Most serious adverse effect: hypokalemia
- Maximizing therapeutic effects: Use the diluent provided in preparation of glucagons for parenteral injection (SC, IM, or IV). Reconstituted glucagons should be clear, watery, and used immediately. Any unused portion should be discarded. Provide supplemental carbohydrates as soon as possible after drug injection to restore liver glycogen and prevent secondary hypoglycemia.
- Minimizing adverse effects: Teach the patient and family members preparation and administration techniques for glucagons before an emergency arises
- Most important patient education: Teach the patient and family members measures to prevent hypoglycemic reactions due to insulin; convey importance of early recognition and treatment of hypoglycemic episodes.

Drugs Significantly Different From [P] Glucagon

Diazoxide

Administered orally, diazoxide (Proglycem) produces a prompt, dose-related increase in blood glucose levels. Its hyperglycemic effects occur because it inhibits insulin release from the pancreas and has an extrapancreatic effect. Its clinical indications are hyperinsulinism caused by an inoperable islet cell cancer, islet cell hyperplasia, or an extrapancreatic cancer. Diazoxide administered intravenously will quickly lower blood pressure in a hypertensive emergency. See Chapter 27 for a discussion of this use of the drug.

Diazoxide is absorbed rapidly. Onset of action occurs within 1 hour. It is highly protein bound (more than 90%), has an 8-hour duration of effect, and has a half-life that ranges from 24 to 36 hours. Diazoxide undergoes hepatic metabolism and renal elimination. Diazoxide is in FDA pregnancy risk category C.

The most common adverse effects from oral dosing are sodium and fluid retention, hyperglycemia, and glycosuria. In some patients, congestive heart failure may develop secondary to sodium and fluid retention.

Other adverse effects can include dizziness and weakness, GI discomfort (e.g., nausea, vomiting, anorexia, abdominal pain, and constipation), and taste alterations.

The usual dosage of diazoxide (adult or child) is 3 to 8 mg/kg per day divided into two or three doses every 8 or 12 hours. Infants and newborns may be given 8 to 15 mg/kg per day every 8 to 12 hours. The total daily dose is divided equally, and administration times also are evenly spaced within the 24-hour day.

Glucose

Glucose, a monosaccharide, is absorbed directly from the intestine, resulting in a rapidly increased blood glucose concentration. It is indicated for managing hypoglycemia. The

dosage is 10 to 20 g orally, repeated in 10 minutes if necessary. An occasional adverse effect is nausea. Glucose is not absorbed from the buccal mucosa. It must be swallowed to be effective. It should be used with caution in children younger than 2 years of age. Intravenous glucose (dextrose) is also used to treat hypoglycemia. Solutions with a concentration of 25% dextrose are used in neonates and infants, and solutions of 50% dextrose are used in other age groups.

CHAPTER SUMMARY

- Diabetes is primarily a disorder of carbohydrate metabolism, although it is associated with derangements of protein and fat metabolism and a series of vascular disorders.
- The patient with type 1 diabetes has an absolute insulin deficiency, cannot maintain a normal blood glucose level, and depends on exogenous insulin for survival. Combinations of short- and longer-acting insulins may be administered to fully manage and control glucose levels.
- The patient with type 2 diabetes has a developed insulin resistance. Although insulin is produced, it is not effective in moving glucose into the cells. Oral antidiabetic agents are used to improve glucose control. Occasionally, this patient may need insulin to achieve glucose balance during times of stress, such as illness, or to achieve maximum control of blood sugar.
- All insulins manage hyperglycemia by promoting cellular glucose uptake and metabolism. Insulins vary in peak, onset, and duration of action; they are similar in absorption, distribution, metabolism, and excretion.
- Hypoglycemia is the most common adverse effect of insulin therapy. Severe hypoglycemia may produce loss of consciousness and is termed insulin shock.
- Regular insulin has a quick onset and peak, and a short duration of therapy. Because of these pharmacokinetic features, it can be used multiple times a day, usually before meals and at bedtime. The dose of regular insulin is often variable and based on the current blood glucose reading. This approach is known as sliding-scale insulin.
- Rapid-acting insulins, such as lispro and aspart, have a more rapid onset of action than regular insulin. When administered subcutaneously, they are administered closer to the time of a meal than regular insulin. These insulins can also be administered by an insulin pump.
- Intermediate-acting insulins, such as NPH, have a slower onset with a peak effect occurring later than with regular insulin. Their effects also last longer than those of regular insulin. These longer-acting insulins are normally assigned a standard daily dosage that the patient takes once or twice a day. Intermediate-acting insulins may be combined with regular insulin to meet both the current and long-term glucose levels of the patient. Intermediate or long-acting insulins are not administered by IV route or used in sliding-scale regimens. These insulins are suspensions and appear cloudy.
- Long-acting glargine does not create the peak and trough in blood insulin levels that NPH does. It has a more flat, sustained effect, which lasts for 24 hours. It is taken subcutaneously once daily at bedtime. Unlike NPH, it is a clear solution.
- Insulins are very potent (a small dose creates a big effect). When drawing up insulin, the dose should always be double-checked by another nurse to prevent accidental overdosage, which could cause serious, even life-threatening, consequences to the patient.
- Nursing care of the patient receiving insulin therapy calls for balancing diet, exercise, and insulin requirements; preventing and monitoring for complications of therapy; and teaching the patient how to do the same.
- Glyburide is the prototype oral antidiabetic sulfonylurea drug. It is used to treat type 2 diabetes. It works by stimulating insulin release from the beta cells of the pancreas and by reducing glucose output from the liver. It also increases the sensitivity of the peripheral cells to insulin. The patient must make some endogenous insulin for glyburide to work. The most common adverse effect is hypoglycemia.
- Other antidiabetic drugs work in different ways than the sulfonylureas. Metformin is the prototype for these drugs. Metformin decreases intestinal absorption of glucose and improves insulin sensitivity. It rarely causes hypoglycemia when used alone.
- Glucagon is a protein made by the pancreas that is used for emergency treatment of severe hypoglycemia. It regulates the rate of glucose production through glycogenolysis, gluconeogenesis, and lipolysis.

QUESTIONS FOR STUDY AND REVIEW

1. What effect does insulin have on blood glucose levels?
2. What effect does glucagon have on glucose metabolism? What effect does it have on the effect of insulin?
3. How do the characteristics of type 1 and type 2 diabetes compare?
4. Why must insulin be injected?
5. What effect would be expected from too much insulin? How would this effect be recognized?
6. Why is regular insulin often combined with NPH insulin?
7. Which insulins are used to provide sliding-scale coverage (insulin dose based on current blood glucose level)?
8. What is the difference between NPH and glargine insulins
9. What is the most common adverse effect of glyburide, a sulfonylurea oral antidiabetic drug?
10. How does acarbose produce its therapeutic effect?
11. What patient and family education should be given if the patient is prescribed glucagons for emergency home use?

? Need More Help?

Chapter 52 of the study guide for *Drug Therapy in Nursing* 2e contains NCLEX-style questions and other learning activities to reinforce your understanding of the concepts presented in this chapter. For additional information or to purchase the study guide, visit *http://connection.lww.com/go/aschenbrenner.*

REFERENCES AND BIBLIOGRAPHY

American Diabetes Association. (2003a). Standards of medical care for patients with diabetes mellitus. *Diabetes Care, 26*(Suppl. 1), S33–S47.

American Diabetes Association. (2003b). Report of the expert committee on the diagnosis and classification of diabetes mellitus. *Diabetes Care, 26*(Suppl. 1), S5–S20.

American Diabetes Association. (2003c). Implications of the diabetes control and complications trial. *Diabetes Care, 26*(Suppl. 1), S25–S27.

American Diabetes Association. (2003d). Implications of the United Kingdom prospective diabetes study. *Diabetes Care, 26*(Suppl. 1), S28–S32.

American Diabetes Association Website. (2004a). [Online]. Available: *www.diabetes.org/diabetes-statistics/national-diabetes-fact-sheet.jsp.*

American Diabetes Association Website. (2004b). [Online]. Available: *www.diabetes.org/diabetes-statistics/cost-of-diabetes-in-us.jsp.*

American Diabetes Association Website. (2004c). [Online]. Available: *www.diabetes.org/gestational-diabetes.jsp.*

American Diabetes Association Website. (2004d). [Online]. *www.diabetes.org/for-media/diabetes-care/10-24-03.jsp.*

Riveline, J. P., Danchin, N., Ledru, F., et al. (2003). Sulfonylureas and cardiovascular effects: from experimental data to clinical use. Available data in humans and clinical applications. *Diabetes Metabolism, 29*(3), 207–222.

Drugs Affecting Men's Health and Sexuality

chapter 53

Learning Objectives

At the completion of this chapter the student will:

1 Identify common health problems of men that are treated with drug therapy.
2 Identify core drug knowledge about drugs that affect men's health and sexuality.
3 Identify core patient variables relevant to drugs that affect men's health and sexuality.
4 Relate the interaction of core drug knowledge and core patient variables for drugs that affect men's health and sexuality.
5 Generate a nursing plan of care from the interactions between core drug knowledge and core patient variables for drugs that affect men's health and sexuality.
6 Describe nursing interventions to maximize therapeutic and minimize adverse effects of drugs that affect men's health and sexuality.
7 Determine key points for patient and family education related to drugs that affect men's health and sexuality.

KEY TERMS

androgens

benign prostatic hypertrophy

erectile dysfunction

follicle-stimulating hormone

luteinizing hormone

male pattern baldness

FEATURED WEBLINK

www.pslgroup.com/enlargprost.htm
This website includes medical news, alerts, and various other articles related to benign prostatic hypertrophy (BPH) as well as links to other genitourinary disorders.

CONNECTION WEBLINK

Additional Weblinks are found on Connection:
http://www.connection.lww.com/go/aschenbrenner.

Drugs Affecting Men's Health and Sexuality

(C) Androgens

(P) testosterone
(short-acting, long-acting, transdermal system, methyltestosterone, fluoxymesterone)

Anabolic steroids
- oxymetholone
- stanozolol
- oxandrolone
- nandrolone phenpropionate
- nandrolone decanoate

(C) Drugs to Treat Erectile Dysfunction

(P) sildenafil
- tadalafil
- vardenafil
- alprostadil
- yohimbine

(C) Drugs to Treat BHP

(P) finasteride

Alpha-1 blockers
- prazosin
- terazosin
- doxazosin
- tamsulosin

(C) Drugs to Treat Male Pattern Baldness

(P) minoxidil
- finasteride

The symbol (C) indicates the **drug class.**
Drugs in **bold type** marked with the symbol (P) are prototypes.
Drugs in blue type are closely related to the prototype.
Drugs in red type are significantly different from the prototype.
Drugs in black type with no symbol are also used in drug therapy; no prototype

Men's health and sexuality differ from women's. Men, over their lifetime, experience unique health problems. Some problems may be directly related to deficiencies of the male sex hormone testosterone; others may be indirectly related to changing hormone levels. Additionally, changes in the cardiovascular (e.g., peripheral vascular disease, ischemic heart disease), neurologic (e.g., neuropathies), and endocrine (e.g., diabetes mellitus) systems are responsible for other health problems in men.

This chapter discusses drug therapy used to treat insufficient testosterone, erectile dysfunction, benign prostatic hypertrophy (BPH), and male pattern baldness. It discusses the prototype male sex hormone testosterone. The prototype for treating erectile dysfunction is sildenafil (Viagra). The prototype drug for treating BPH is finasteride (Proscar, Propecia). The prototype drug for treating male pattern baldness is minoxidil (Rogaine, Minoxidil for Men).

In addition, this chapter briefly discusses prostatic cancer. Chapters 35 and 36 present a fuller discussion of the drugs used to treat prostate cancer.

PHYSIOLOGY

Hormones

Androgens are naturally occurring or synthetic steroidal compounds that produce the masculinizing and tissue-building properties of testosterone, the main male sex hormone. Other androgens include dihydrotestosterone, androstenedione, and dehydroepiandrosterone. During puberty, the pituitary gland secretes large volumes of **follicle-stimulating hormone** (FSH) and **luteinizing hormone** (LH). The predominant effect of FSH is forming sperm cells. LH in males stimulates the interstitial cells of the testes, which produce approximately 95% of the body's testosterone. Interstitial cell development is also influenced by interstitial cell-stimulating hormone (ICSH). Therefore, increased production of ICSH stimulates production of testosterone.

Testosterone is responsible for the normal growth and development of the male sex organs. Testosterone is also responsible for development and maintenance of the male secondary sexual characteristics: hair distribution (beard, pubic area, chest, and axillae); all hair related to secondary sex characteristics; hair texture and color (more deeply pigmented, heavier, and sometimes more curly); laryngeal enlargement and vocal cord thickening (resulting in voice deepening); and alterations in body musculature and fat distribution.

Testosterone causes retention of sodium, potassium, and phosphorus as well as decreased urinary excretion of calcium. Sodium retention may lead to fluid retention. Testosterone also has multiple effects on bone. It stimulates the growth of skeletal muscle tissue and enhances the growth of long bones in prepubescent boys—the growth spurt of adolescence. The ossification (hardening) of the epiphyseal growth plates, which stops the growth of the long bones, occurs with prolonged elevation of testosterone levels. Testosterone also is reported to stimulate the production of red blood cells by enhancing the production of erythropoietin-stimulating factor.

The adult male produces approximately 7 to 8 mg of testosterone daily. In women, the adrenal cortex and the ovaries secrete androgens, including testosterone, although in much smaller amounts than are found in men.

Penis

The male penis has a dermal layer of smooth muscle, under which is loose connective tissue. This pliable connective tissue allows the skin of the penis to move without distorting the underlying structures. This important characteristic enables the penis to become erect. Beneath the connective tissue is a dense network of elastic fibers that encircle the internal structures of the penis. Most of the shaft of the penis is composed of three cylindrical columns of erectile tissue, each of which consists of a maze of vascular channels incompletely separated by partitions of elastic connective tissue and smooth muscle fibers. In the nonaroused state, the arterial branches are constricted, and the muscular partitions are tense, so that blood flow into the erectile tissue is restricted.

The parasympathetic system innervates the penile arteries. Normal erection involves the release of nitric oxide, secondary to sexual stimulation, in the erectile tissue of the penis. The nitric oxide activates an intermediary enzyme that boosts cyclic guanosine monophosphate (cGMP), a substance that mediates the action of certain hormones. By some unknown mechanism, cGMP stimulates smooth muscle, producing relaxation and an inflow of blood into the erectile tissue.

Urethra and Prostate

Passing through the penis is the urethra, which in men transports both urine and semen. The prostate gland is a small, muscular, rounded organ that encircles the proximal portion of the urethra as it leaves the urinary bladder (Figure 53.1). The ejaculatory duct joins the urethra in the prostate. The prostate gland is very small until puberty, when it begins to grow as a result of hormonal changes. The growth of the prostate gland slows after age 20 years but continues throughout the rest of a man's life. The primary hormone in prostate cells that affects growth of the prostate is dihydrotestosterone (DHT). A special enzyme, 5-alpha reductase, converts testosterone to DHT.

PATHOPHYSIOLOGY

Hormonal Problems

If a male is deficient in endogenous sex hormones, he will not experience normal sexual development. The primary sex organs will not mature, secondary sexual characteristics will not develop, reproduction will not be possible, and the normal growth spurt of adolescence will not happen. If the level of endogenous hormones drops after puberty has occurred and the sexual organs and reproductive system have matured, secondary sexual characteristics may diminish. Ability to reproduce, despite developed organs, will be diminished,

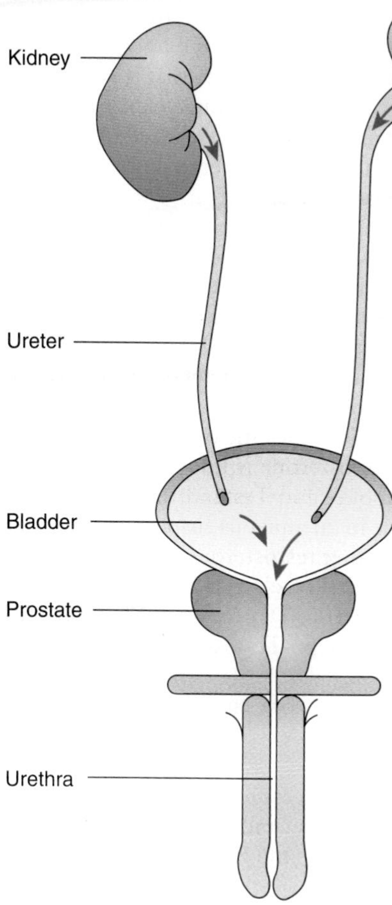

FIGURE 53.1 Normal urine flow.

and the man may not create enough sperm to impregnate a woman.

Erectile Dysfunction

Erectile dysfunction is the inability to achieve or maintain an erection in at least every three of four attempts at intercourse. Erectile dysfunction affects more than 30 million men in the United States and more than 150 million men worldwide and accounts for half a million visits in the United States to health care providers every year (Gaines, 2004). It may be a temporary or chronic problem. Erectile dysfunction may be caused by certain drug therapies, alcohol use, trauma, or illness that affects either the autonomic nervous system or the central nervous system (CNS). Physiologic causes such as vascular or neural changes may also cause erectile dysfunction, as can emotions. Severe stress, emotional problems, depression, anxiety, or fear of impaired performance may all result in sexual dysfunction. Almost 90% of men older than age 50 years have an organic cause for their erectile dysfunction; in younger men, most cases of erectile dysfunction are psychogenic. Vascular disease is the most common physical cause of erectile dysfunction, and atherosclerosis of the penile artery is the primary cause in more than half of men older than age 50 years. Men with diabetes have a high risk for erectile dysfunction because of a combination of vascular disease and neuropathy.

Benign Prostatic Hypertrophy

Prostatic enlargement that is not caused by cancer is called **benign prostatic hypertrophy or hyperplasia** (BPH). BPH occurs spontaneously in men as they age, and incidence rises after age 40 years. By age 80 years, almost 80% of men will have BPH. The exact cause of BPH is not well understood. Although testosterone levels fall with aging, DHT (the primary hormone in the prostate) levels remain fairly constant. DHT is the hormone primarily responsible for prostate growth. Additionally, the small amount of estrogen in the man may also affect prostate growth because decreasing testosterone levels no longer offset the effects of estrogen.

BPH first affects the urethra as the enlarged prostate tightens around it. The pressure of the gland against the urethra is like a clamp on a garden hose, making passage of fluid more difficult (Figure 53.2). The man has difficulty initiating a stream or stopping the flow of urine (dribbling). This pressure on the urethra from the prostate causes the man's bladder to thicken. Initially, the bladder is irritable and contracts even when it contains only a small amount of urine, resulting in frequent urination and nocturia. As the prostate continues to place pressure on the bladder, the bladder weakens, resulting in poor contraction during urination. Eventually, the bladder can no longer empty completely, causing urinary retention. Urinary tract infections may result. Complete inability to void may also occur.

Male Pattern Baldness

The adult has two major types of hair: vellus hair and terminal hair. *Vellus hair* is the fine "peach fuzz" located over much of the body surface. *Terminal hair* is heavy, more deeply pigmented, and sometimes curly. It is located mostly on the head. Hair follicles may alter the structure of the hair on the body in response to circulating hormones. In men, decreasing levels of sex hormones can affect the scalp, causing a shift from terminal hair to vellus hair production beginning at the temples and the crown of the head. Changes in the

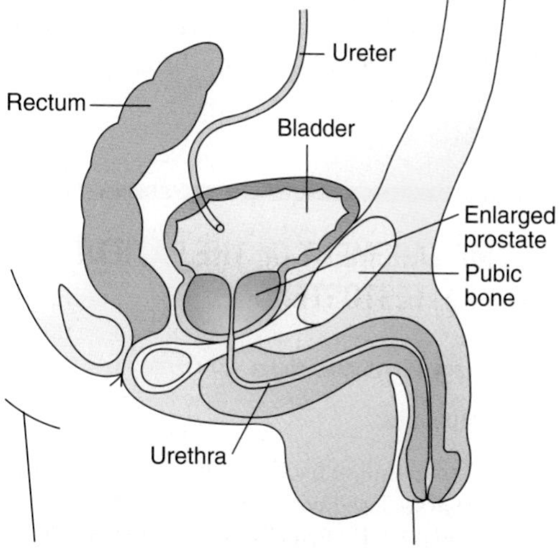

FIGURE 53.2 Urine flow with benign prostatic hypertrophy.

receptors for testosterone and other male sex hormones may also induce hair loss.

Male pattern baldness, also called androgenetic alopecia, is baldness of the vertex of the scalp. Women may also have hair loss related to decreased sex hormone levels, but it differs from hair loss in men in that the loss is diffuse or may involve thinning of the frontoparietal areas.

Prostate Cancer

Prostate cancer is a malignant metastasizing cancer and the second most common cause of cancer death in men. One in 5 men in the United States will develop prostate cancer. Prostate cancer is not caused by BPH. It usually originates in one of the secretory glands. As the cancer grows, it produces a nodular lump on the surface of the prostate. During a digital examination, this lump can be palpated through the rectal wall. If diagnosis is not made until after the cancer has metastasized, the prognosis for survival decreases because metastasis can rapidly involve the lymphatic system, lungs, bone marrow, liver, or adrenal glands.

Prostate cancer treatment varies for each affected man. Treatment options include surgical intervention, radiation therapy, cryotherapy, and hormonal therapy (antiandrogen antineoplastics and gonadotropin-releasing hormone analogues). Drugs used to treat prostate cancer are discussed in Chapters 35 and 36.

C ANDROGENS

The prototype male sex hormone is testosterone. When testosterone is administered exogenously as a drug, it may be given in different forms. These differences may relate to the onset or duration of action or to the route of administration (oral, buccal, parenteral, topical, and subdermal implants). Drugs similar to testosterone are the anabolic steroids, which include oxymetholone (Anadrol-5), stanozolol (Winstrol), oxandrolone (Oxandrin), nandrolone phenpropionate (Durabolin, Hybolin Improved), and nandrolone decanoate (Deca-Durabolin, Hybolin Decanoate-50, Hybolin Decanoate-100, Neo-Durabolic, and Androlone-D 200).

Table 53.1 provides a summary of selected drugs used to treat men's health problems.

NURSING MANAGEMENT OF THE PATIENT RECEIVING P TESTOSTERONE

● Core Drug Knowledge

Pharmacotherapeutics

In males, testosterone is used as replacement therapy for hypogonadism associated with low or no endogenous testosterone (see Table 53.1). Boys with low or no testosterone before puberty need testosterone treatment to develop secondary sexual characteristics and must continue it after puberty to maintain them. Men who develop a deficiency of testosterone after puberty require testosterone to maintain sexual characteristics. Testosterone may also be given to males with delayed puberty (puberty that is expected to occur but much later than normal) to stimulate the onset of puberty. These patients must be carefully selected and have a clear familial pattern of delayed puberty that is not secondary to a pathologic disorder. Brief treatment with conservative doses may be justified if these patients are having serious emotional problems as a result of delayed puberty. Testosterone is also used in treating erectile dysfunction and male climacteric symptoms when these conditions are secondary to androgen deficiency.

In women 1 to 5 years after menopause, testosterone may be used as secondary treatment to slow the growth of advanced, inoperable metastatic breast cancer.

Short-acting testosterone is known by the trade names Histerone, Tesamone, and Testandro. Short-acting testosterone is available in an aqueous suspension or in an oil for injection. Long-acting testosterone is known by the trade names Andro L.A. 200, Delatestryl, Durathate-200, Everone 200, depAndro100, DepAndro 200, Andropository-200, Depotest 100, Depo-Testosterone, Duratest-100, and Duratest-200.

Implantable testosterone pellets have the trade name Testopel. Transdermal patches of testosterone have the trade names Testoderm and Androderm. Oral forms of testosterone are methyltestosterone and fluoxymesterone. Trade names for these drugs are Android-10, Android-25, Oreton Methyl, Testred, Virilon, and Halotestin.

Pharmacokinetics

Natural testosterone undergoes a high first-pass effect and is not used orally. The form of testosterone that is used orally is a synthetic androgen that is less extensively metabolized and has a longer half-life than natural testosterones. The synthetic androgens are also available as buccal tablets. They are absorbed directly into the bloodstream, bypassing the gastrointestinal (GI) tract and the first-pass effect. These buccal androgens have approximately twice the potency of oral androgens. Peak serum level from buccal administration occurs in 1 hour, compared with 2 hours for oral administration. Testosterone esters are less polar than free testosterone. Testosterone esters in oil are given intramuscularly. These testosterone esters will be slowly absorbed, allowing for dosing intervals of 2 to 4 weeks.

In the plasma, testosterone is about 98% bound to a specific testosterone-estradiol–binding globulin. The amount of binding globulin in the plasma determines the relative percentages of free and bound testosterone. The concentration of free testosterone determines half-life. Inactivation of testosterone occurs mostly in the liver. The conjugates and metabolites of testosterone are eliminated in the urine and feces. Testosterone crosses the placenta and enters the breast milk.

Pharmacodynamics

The effects of exogenous testosterone on males are the same as the effects of endogenous testosterone. In females, the drug causes masculinization. In addition, increased testosterone levels in women slow the growth of advanced breast cancers, which are estrogen dependent.

TABLE 53.1 Summary of Selected Drugs Used to Treat Men's Health Problems

Drug (Trade) Name	Selected Indications	Route and Dosage Range	Pharmacokinetics
C Androgens			
P testosterone			
testosterone (short-acting; Histerone, Tesamone)	*Males:* replacement therapy in hypogonadism, delayed puberty, impotence secondary to androgen deficiency	Male hypogonadism (initiation of puberty), IM 40–50 mg/m²/dose/mo or 50–400 mg/dose q 2–4 wk; androgen replacement, IM, 25–50 mg two to three times per week	*Onset:* Slow *Duration:* 1–3 d $t_{1/2}$: 10–100 min
testosterone (long-acting; Delatest, Everone, Andronate, Depo, Duratest; Canadian: Scheinpharm Testone - CYP)	*Males:* replacement therapy in hypogonadism, delayed puberty *Females:* palliation of inoperable breast cancer	*Adult:* hypogonadism (initiation of puberty), IM, 50–200 mg q 2–4 wk; androgen replacement, IM, 50–400 mg q 2–4 wk *Females:* IM, 200–400 mg q 2–4 wk	*Onset:* Slow *Duration:* 2–4 wk $t_{1/2}$: Up to 8 d
testosterone, transdermal (Testoderm, Androderm)	*Males:* primary hypogonadism, hypogonadotropic hypogonadism	*Adult:* Patch, 4–6 mg/d applied to scrotal skin (Testoderm); 5 mg/d applied to nonscrotal skin (Androderm)	*Onset:* Rapid *Duration:* 24 h $t_{1/2}$: 10–100 min
Drugs to Treat Erectile Dysfunction			
P sildenafil (Viagra)	Erectile dysfunction	PO: usual dose 50 mg once/d, may use 25–100 mg based on effectiveness and tolerance	*Onset:* <30 minutes *Duration:* up to 4 hours $t_{1/2}$: 4 h
alprostadil (Caverject, Edex, Muse)	Erectile dysfunction	Intracavernosal injection: initial dose 2.5 µg; titrate upward by first another 2.5 µg, then by 5–10 µg until desired effect achieved; give no more than 3 times/week. Intraurethral: 125–1000 µg; use smallest effective dose; no more than 2 doses in 24 hours	*Onset:* Intracavernosal—rapid Intraurethral—5–10 min *Duration:* Intracavernosal— up to 1 h Intraurethral—30–60 min $t_{1/2}$: Unknown
vardenafil (Levitra)	Erectile dysfunction	PO, 2.5–20 mg once/day with recommended starting dose of 10 mg	*Onset:* 15–30 min *Duration:* Up to 4 h
tadalafil (Cialis)	Erectile dysfunction	PO, 10 mg or 20 mg once/day	*Onset:* <30 min *Duration:* Up to 36 h
Drugs to Treat Benign Prostatic Hypertrophy (BPH)			
P finasteride (Propecia, Proscar)	BPH Male pattern baldness	PO: 5 mg/d PO: 1 mg/d	*Onset:* <2 h *Duration:* 24 h $t_{1/2}$: 6 h
C Alpha-1 Blockers			
P tamsulosin (Flomax)	BPH	PO: 0.4 mg/d about 30 min after the same meal daily	*Onset:* Varies *Duration:* 24 h $t_{1/2}$: 9–13 h
Drugs to Treat Male Pattern Baldness			
P minoxidil (Rogaine, Minoxidil for Men)	Male pattern baldness	Topically to affected area of scalp—1 mL bid	*Onset:* ≥4 mo *Duration:* 3–4 mo after discontinuing effective dosing $t_{1/2}$: Unknown

Contraindications and Precautions

Testosterone is contraindicated for patients with serious cardiac, hepatic, or renal disease because edema with or without congestive heart failure (CHF) may be a complication in these patients. It is also contraindicated in those people hypersensitive to the drug and in men with carcinomas of the breast or prostate. Testosterone is not normally used in premenopausal women, but it is nonetheless designated as an FDA pregnancy category X drug because it causes masculinization of the genitalia in the female fetus.

Caution must be used when administering testosterone to the following patients:

- Young males with delayed puberty, because of testosterone's adverse effect on bone maturation
- Males with pre-existing gynecomastia (breast enlargement) because testosterone may compound the problem
- Elderly men because they may be at increased risk for BPH and prostate cancer
- Patients with BPH because they may develop acute urethral obstruction
- Patients with acute intermittent porphyria (a group of disorders that result from a disturbance in the metabolism of porphyrins, nitrogen-containing organic compounds in protoplasm) because androgens have precipitated attacks of this condition
- Patients with a history of myocardial infarction (MI) or coronary artery disease (CAD) because testosterone may promote hypercholesterolemia

Adverse Effects

Most adverse effects are related to high doses of the drug. In males, the most common adverse effects include gynecomastia, excessive frequency and duration of penile erections, decreased ejaculatory volumes, and oligospermia (low sperm count).

In females, the most common adverse effects are androgenic and include amenorrhea and other menstrual irregularities (if given before menopause), inhibition of gonadotropin secretion, and virilization, including deepening of the voice and clitoral enlargement. Clitoral enlargement is not reversible after therapy ends.

Other effects related to the actions of testosterone on the body may occur. They include hypercalcemia, particularly in immobile patients and patients with metastatic breast cancer; retention of sodium, chloride, water, potassium, calcium, and inorganic phosphates; hypercholesterolemia; and edema. In addition, rash, acne, seborrhea, and hirsutism may occur. Prostatic hypertrophy, prostatic cancer, and urethral obstruction are also possibilities. Other potential adverse effects include hepatitis (which can be life threatening), hepatocellular carcinoma (with prolonged use of high doses), premature closing of the long bones, dizziness, headache, sleep disorders, fatigue, changes in libido, and polycythemia (excess of red blood cells).

Drug Interactions

No important drug interactions are associated with natural testosterone. With the synthetic forms, anticoagulation effect is increased if anticoagulants are given with either fluoxymesterone or methyltestosterone. Coadministering methyltestosterone and imipramine may result in paranoia-like symptoms.

Assessment of Relevant Core Patient Variables

Health Status

Assess for existing serious heart, kidney, or liver disease, which are contraindications for therapy, and screen for established hypersensitivity to testosterone. Determine whether male patients have carcinoma of the breast or prostate, which is a contraindication, or whether they have gynecomastia or BPH, because these conditions require precautions. Assessing for a history of MI, CAD, or acute intermittent porphyria is important because all these factors require caution in use of testosterone. Because of testosterone's effects on bone growth, only people with expert training and knowledge of the drug and its effects on bone growth should prescribe it.

Life Span and Gender

Carefully consider age-related assessment data for problems possibly related to the use of testosterone. When testosterone is used in prepubescent boys to treat hypogonadism or delayed onset of puberty, premature closure of the long bones may lead to stunted growth. Caution also is necessary when testosterone is used in elderly men. Testosterone is not normally used in premenopausal females because it is likely to produce masculinization. If a woman is prescribed testosterone, assess the patient for pregnancy. Testosterone will cause masculinization of the female fetus, as characterized by clitoromegaly, abnormal vaginal development, and fusion of the genital folds to form a scrotum-like structure. These effects are most likely to occur if testosterone is given during the first trimester. If large amounts of the drug are given to a male fetus, adverse effects also are possible. It is not known whether testosterone crosses into breast milk, but testosterone is rarely used in young women.

Lifestyle, Diet, and Habits

Although anabolic steroids are abused more frequently to enhance athletic performance, testosterone has also been abused for this purpose. This use is not a safe and effective one for this drug. Verify that the patient is not abusing testosterone (Box 53.1).

Environment

Testosterone may be administered in any setting.

COMMUNITY-BASED CONCERNS

Box 53.1 Athletes and Testosterone

Nurses perform a significant service when they teach patients or community groups about pitfalls of unorthodox drug use:

- Athletes have used and abused testosterone and anabolic steroids in an effort to increase muscle mass. These drugs have not been shown to be effective for this purpose.
- Serious potential adverse effects include early closure of epiphyseal growth plates, which stunts normal growth; edema (with or without CHF); and male gynecomastia.
- Increase in weight and muscle size is partially the result of water retention.

Nursing Diagnoses and Outcomes

- Delayed Growth and Development related to potential for early epiphyseal closure secondary to drug therapy
  Desired outcome: *The patient will attain normal height while receiving drug therapy.*
- Ineffective Sexuality Patterns related to effect of drug therapy
  Desired outcome: *The male patient will develop normal male sexual organs and characteristics. The female patient will not experience excessive masculinization during therapy.*
- Excess Fluid Volume related to potential effects of drug therapy
  Desired outcome: *The patient will not experience enough increase in fluid volume to become edematous during drug therapy.*
- Potential Complication: Hypercalcemia related to drug therapy, immobility, breast cancer
  Desired outcome: *The patient will not develop hypercalcemia.*

Planning and Intervention

Maximizing Therapeutic Effects

Administer the drug at regular intervals to maintain therapeutic testosterone levels. He or she adjusts the dose upward when giving testosterone to treat hypogonadism and induce puberty. At the end of the growth spurt, the patient should remain on a maintenance dose.

Some nursing actions specific to the route of administration can maximize the therapeutic effect of testosterone. When administering testosterone as Testoderm transdermal patches, place the patches on clean, dry scrotal skin that has been dry shaved for optimal skin contact. Chemical depilatories must not be used for this purpose. The patient should wear these transdermal patches for 22 to 24 hours before replacing them.

Do not place Testoderm TTS patches on the scrotum. Rather, place them on clean, dry skin on the arm, back, or upper buttocks. The skin area should not be oily, damaged, or irritated. The patient wears these patches for 24 hours and then replaces them.

Place Androderm transdermal patches on the back, abdomen, upper arms, or thighs. Avoid placing them on the scrotum or over bony areas such as the shoulder and hip. These patches stay in place for 7 days before replacement.

Either the nurse or the patient places buccal tablets between the gum and the cheek. The tablets should be allowed to dissolve; they should never be swallowed.

For suspensions, agitate the vial to mix the drug thoroughly before drawing it into a syringe and administering it intramuscularly.

Minimizing Adverse Effects

When prepubescent boys undergo testosterone therapy, radiographs should be taken every 6 months to assess bone age. Radiographs help to document bone maturation and the effect of testosterone on the epiphyseal centers.

Some nursing actions can minimize the adverse effects of testosterone. Monitor serum cholesterol levels and liver function periodically. Check hemoglobin and hematocrit levels periodically for polycythemia during treatment with high doses. Monitor serum and urine calcium levels in women receiving testosterone for disseminated breast cancer. In women receiving testosterone for palliative treatment of metastasized breast cancer, monitor the disease progression closely because occasionally the drug may accelerate the disease process.

When administering testosterone by intramuscular (IM) injection, inject deep into the gluteal muscle to prevent inflammation and pain at the administration site. Never administer the drug intravenously.

Discard used transdermal patches by folding them and putting them into trash in an appropriate manner or flush them down the toilet. Active drug remains after use, so accidental application or ingestion of patches by children would be dangerous.

Assess for signs of adverse effects and contact the prescriber if adverse effects are noted, especially severe masculinization in women or edema or jaundice in either sex. Dosage adjustments or cessation of therapy may be indicated.

Providing Patient and Family Education

- Teach the patient and family the rationale for use of the drug, including therapeutic effects and potential adverse effects.
- Instruct the patient and family about proper administration technique. If drug administration is IM, teach the patient how to safely dispose of needles and syringes. If the patient will be using transdermal patches, teach him or her how to dispose of used patches.
- Review the importance of scheduling and keeping follow-up appointments for radiographs and blood tests.
- Teach patients taking buccal tablets to place the tablet between gum and cheek and not to swallow it. Remind these patients not to eat, drink, or smoke while the tablet is in place because doing so will alter absorption of the drug.
- Alert patients to notify the prescriber if swelling of the extremities (edema), jaundice, or prolonged painful erection develops. Women should notify the prescriber if they develop hoarseness, deepening of the voice, menstrual irregularities, acne, or facial hair growth.

Ongoing Assessment and Evaluation

Monitoring for adverse effects throughout therapy is necessary, as is regular monitoring of blood test results and bone growth, as noted previously. Therapy is considered effective if development of male sex organs and male sexual characteristics occurs normally or if males maintain secondary male sexual characteristics without adverse effects. If given to women with breast cancer, testosterone therapy is considered effective if discomfort from the malignant tumor is minimized and the disease advances no further.

Drugs Closely Related to [P] Testosterone

The anabolic steroids include oxymetholone, stanozolol, oxandrolone, nandrolone phenpropionate, and nandrolone decanoate. They are derived from testosterone and, like

MEMORY CHIP

P Testosterone

- Used as hormone replacement therapy in male hypogonadism that is associated with low or absent endogenous testosterone
- Major contraindication: serious cardiac, hepatic, or renal disease because edema with or without CHF may be a complication
- Most common adverse effects: gynecomastia, excessive frequency and duration of penile erections, decreased ejaculatory volumes, and oligospermia; masculinization in females
- Most serious adverse effect: life-threatening hepatitis
- **Life span alert: Pregnancy category X drug; prepubescent boys may have premature closing of long bones.**
- Maximizing therapeutic effects: Administer at regular intervals; place transdermal patches appropriately on skin (varies by trade preparation).
- Minimizing adverse effects: radiographs every 6 months to determine bone maturation and the effect on the epiphyseal growth centers when treating prepubescent boys; safe disposal of used transdermal patches
- Most important patient education: Notify health care provider if swelling of the extremities (edema), jaundice, or painful, continued erection develop.

testosterone, have both anabolic and androgenic effects. Unlike testosterone, these drugs have anabolic effects that are much stronger than their androgenic effects. In fact, their two major actions are to promote body tissue-building processes and reverse catabolic or tissue-depleting processes. Anabolic steroids are indicated for treating certain anemias because they stimulate erythropoiesis. They are also used prophylactically to decrease the frequency and severity of attacks of hereditary angioedema (characterized by episodic edema of the abdominal viscera, extremities, face, and airway). Anabolic steroids are also used to control metastatic breast cancer in women.

An abuse or addiction syndrome has been recognized with the chronic use of anabolic steroids to improve athletic performance (see Box 53.1). The use of these drugs to improve athletic performance is questionable because of the possibility of serious adverse effects, which may be irreversible. Serious adverse effects include peliosis hepatitis (in which blood-filled cysts replace normal liver cells and sometimes spleen cells, a condition that can be associated with liver failure), liver tumors (possibly malignant), and blood lipid changes associated with an increased risk for atherosclerosis (resulting from decreased high-density lipoprotein and sometimes increased low-density lipoprotein). In females, masculinization effects similar to those effects produced by (short-acting) testosterone occur with use of anabolic steroids. Like testosterone, anabolic steroids are in pregnancy category X because of the possibility of fetal masculinization.

DRUGS USED TO TREAT ERECTILE DYSFUNCTION

Agents to treat erectile dysfunction work to mimic the body's natural methods of achieving an erection. The prototype is sildenafil (Viagra). Two FDA-approved drugs, which are represented by the prototype sildenafil, are vardenafil (Levitra) and tadalafil (Cialis). Both drugs are cGMP specific phosphodiesterase type 5 (PDE5) inhibitors. Tadalafil has a longer duration of action and is effective for up to 36 hours in most cases. Both drugs are administered orally; both drugs produce adverse effects and have contraindications similar to the adverse effects and contraindications for sildenafil. As with sildenafil, tadalafil was initially developed as a treatment for cardiovascular disease, whereas vardenafil was developed specifically as an erectogenic (Rosen & McKenna, 2002).

A drug closely related to sildenafil is alprostadil (Caverject, Edex, Muse). A drug significantly different from sildenafil is yohimbine (Aphrodyne, Dayto Himbin, Yocon, Yohimex).

NURSING MANAGEMENT OF THE PATIENT RECEIVING P SILDENAFIL

Core Drug Knowledge

Pharmacotherapeutics

Sildenafil is used to treat erectile dysfunction. It is administered orally, usually 1 hour before sexual activity. Sildenafil is effective only with accompanying sexual stimulation. It is effective in erectile dysfunction after a radical prostatectomy, but only if either a bilateral or unilateral nerve-sparing procedure has been performed. Sildenafil may be effective in men younger than 55 years of age if one nerve is not cut (unilateral sparing) (Zagaja et al., 2000).

Pharmacokinetics

Sildenafil is rapidly absorbed. Maximum plasma concentrations are reached within 30 to 120 minutes of oral dosing when taken on an empty stomach (the most frequent peak time is 60 minutes). When taken with a high-fat meal, absorption is delayed, so that approximately 60 extra minutes are needed to reach peak plasma levels. A high-fat meal also reduces peak serum concentrations by 29%.

Sildenafil is metabolized by two hepatic microsomal isoenzymes. The primary isoenzyme involved in metabolism is CYP3A4. A second isoenzyme, with a more minor effect on metabolism, is CYP2C9. Through these pathways, sildenafil is converted into an active metabolite that is further metabolized. The metabolite has pharmacologic properties similar to the parent drug and accounts for about 20% of sildenafil's pharmacologic effect. The metabolite of sildenafil is excreted primarily in the stool and to a small extent in the urine. Men older than 65 years have a reduced sildenafil clearance and elevated free plasma concentrations that are about 40% greater than in younger men.

Pharmacodynamics

Sildenafil inhibits PDE type 5, the isoenzyme that metabolizes cGMP. The decreased metabolism of cGMP allows it to remain active longer, increasing smooth muscle relaxation and inflow of blood. These circumstances allow for an improved and more sustained erection. Because sildenafil works at the end of a cascade of events that produce erection, starting with sexual stimulation releasing nitric oxide,

sildenafil is not effective in normal doses without sexual stimulation. Men must continue sildenafil treatment to maintain improvement in erectile function.

Contraindications and Precautions

Sildenafil is contraindicated if the patient is currently using nitrates because its vasodilating effects potentiate the hypotensive effects of nitrates. Sildenafil is also contraindicated if the patient has hypersensitivity to any component of the tablet.

The American College of Cardiology and the American Heart Association recommend caution when sildenafil is prescribed to patients who have coronary ischemia, CHF, or hypotension, or to those patients with a history of MI, cerebrovascular accident (stroke), or life-threatening arrhythmias within the past 6 months. These professional groups also recommend that any patients with strong cardiac risk factors or known cardiac disease should undergo an exercise stress test before beginning any treatment for erectile dysfunction.

Adverse Effects

Adverse effects from sildenafil are generally transient and mild to moderate in nature. The most common adverse effects are facial flushing, headache, nasal congestion, and heartburn. Other adverse effects are diarrhea, urinary tract infections, blue-tinged vision and light sensitivity, blurred vision, dizziness, and rash.

Although some cardiovascular system–related deaths have been reported in patients taking sildenafil since the drug has been on the market, research and statistical analysis have found that sildenafil is not responsible for causing an excessive number of cardiovascular deaths. The anecdotal reports of deaths are believed to be caused by pre-existing cardiac risk factors (e.g., hypertension, diabetes mellitus, smoking, and depression) and the cardiovascular "work" or effort involved in sexual intercourse. Based on these incidents, however, precautions must be used with patients who have known cardiovascular problems because they may have greater risk for cardiovascular adverse effects from sildenafil (see Contraindications and Precautions, above).

Overdosing produces adverse effects similar to those effects associated with normal dosing but at an increased rate of incidence. Standard supportive measures for drug overdose should be used. Renal dialysis is not helpful because little of the drug is excreted renally.

Drug Interactions

The CYP3A4 isoenzyme and, to a lesser degree, the CYP2C9 isoenzyme mediate sildenafil metabolism. Any drug that inhibits these systems may produce a drug interaction with sildenafil and decrease its clearance, raising plasma levels as a result. Strong CYP3A4 inhibitors (e.g., ketoconazole, itraconazole, erythromycin, and cimetidine) have been shown to increase the plasma levels of sildenafil as much as 200%. Any drug that induces CYP3A4, such as rifampin, will therefore probably increase the metabolism of sildenafil and subsequently decrease plasma levels of sildenafil. However, this association has not been definitively proved. As previously discussed, nitrates interact with sildenafil, increasing both vasodilation and hypotension. Table 53.2 lists drugs that interact with sildenafil.

A drug–food interaction occurs when a patient takes sildenafil with a high-fat meal, delaying the rate of absorption and reducing peak serum levels.

Assessment of Relevant Core Patient Variables

Health Status

Review the patient's medication history to determine whether the patient is taking nitrates because nitrate use is a contraindication for use of sildenafil. Assess for any of the cardiovascular problems that require cautious use of sildenafil:

TABLE 53.2 Agents That Interact With P Sildenafil

Interactants	Effect and Significance	Nursing Management
nitrates	Sildenafil potentiates the vasodilating effect of nitric oxide from nitrates, resulting in a significant and potentially fatal decrease in blood pressure (BP).	Teach patient that he should not use any nitrate while taking sildenafil.
amlodipine	In hypertensive patients, produces mean additional BP reduction of 7–8 mg.	Monitor the patient's BP. In most cases, this drop is not clinically significant.
beta blockers, nonspecific	Beta blockers increase the level of sildenafil's active metabolite; this is not believed to be clinically significant.	None
cimetidine	Coadministration increases the plasma concentrations of sildenafil by more than 50%.	Monitor for adverse effects; a decreased dose may be indicated; consider starting dose of 25 mg.
diuretics	Diuretics increase the level of sildenafil's active metabolite; this is not believed to be clinically significant.	None
erythromycin	A single dose of 100 mg of sildenafil administered with erythromycin at steady state (500 mg bid for 5 days) resulted in a 182% increase in sildenafil's peak concentration.	Monitor for adverse effects; a decreased dose may be indicated; consider starting dose of 25 mg.

coronary ischemia, CHF, or hypotension; or a history of MI, cerebrovascular accident, or life-threatening arrhythmias within the past 6 months. Verify that the patient is not allergic to any component of sildenafil. Assess also for hepatic cirrhosis, which decreases metabolism of sildenafil and increases blood level of active sildenafil. Such patients may need a decreased dose. Although only a small portion of sildenafil is excreted renally, severe renal impairment does increase the maximum blood concentration of the drug. A decreased dose may also be indicated in this situation.

Life Span and Gender

Inquire about the patient's age. Men aged 65 years or older show increased circulating levels of sildenafil, which is most likely the result of decreased metabolism from normal age-related changes in the liver. These patients may require a decreased dose. Sildenafil is not approved for use in women.

Lifestyle, Diet, and Habits

A high-fat meal eaten before the use of sildenafil will decrease the rate of absorption and reduce the maximum blood level achieved by drug therapy by about 29%. If the patient states that the drug is not always effective, assess his dietary intake. Decreasing dietary fat may increase the effectiveness of the drug therapy without a need for an increased dose.

Environment

Sildenafil is self-administered in the home.

Culture and Inherited Traits

Although most research on sildenafil has been performed on white men, it has also been studied in Asian men and found to be effective and well tolerated in this population (Tan et al., 2000).

Nursing Diagnoses and Outcomes

- Sexual Dysfunction related to erection dysfunction
  Desired outcome: *Use of sildenafil will allow the patient to experience normal expression of sexuality.*
- Risk for Injury related to adverse effects of drug therapy
  Desired outcome: *The patient will not experience adverse effects from sildenafil, or effects will be mild, transient, and well tolerated.*

Planning and Intervention

Maximizing Therapeutic Effects and Minimizing Adverse Effects

Nursing strategies to maximize the therapeutic effects and minimize the adverse effects of sildenafil are related to the patient education that is provided.

Providing Patient and Family Education

- Sildenafil is not effective without sexual stimulation and arousal.
- The patient should take sildenafil about 1 hour before sexual activity.
- The patient should not take nitrates (e.g., nitroglycerin, isosorbide) while taking sildenafil.
- Sexual activity increases the risk for cardiovascular problems, including MI, for people with known cardiovascular risks. If a patient experiences any symptoms of cardiovascular problems during sexual intercourse (e.g., angina, dizziness, nausea), he must stop the sexual activity. He should discuss any such problems with the prescriber.
- The patient must avoid high-fat meals before using sildenafil.

Drugs Closely Related to P Sildenafil

Vardenafil

Vardenafil treats erectile dysfunction similarly to sildenafil. Like sildenafil, it is taken orally 1 hour before intercourse for best results. Vardenafil is metabolized by the P-450 system, primarily CYP3A4 and CYP2C isoforms. Patients who take other drugs that inhibit CYP3A4, such as ritonavir, may have elevated blood levels of vardenafil, although no specific recommendations to decrease the dose of vardenafil exist. Coadministering vardenafil with alpha blockers can produce severe hypotension and is contraindicated. Nitrate use is also contraindicated for vardenafil, as it is for sildenafil. Adverse effects for vardenafil are similar to sildenafil. The incidence of visual disturbances is somewhat less with vardenafil than with sildenafil.

Tadalafil

The third cGMP drug for treating erectile dysfunction is tadalafil (Cialis). Like the other two drugs in this class, sildenafil and vardenafil, tadalafil works by blocking the degradation of cyclic guanosine monophosphate. Like the other drugs, tadalafil should not be taken within 48 hours of taking nitrates, such as nitroglycerine, because substantially lower blood pressure and possibly death may result. Nitroglycerine use is a contraindication for taking tadalafil. Additionally, tadalafil should not be taken with alpha blockers, other than Flomax, because the same drug interaction may occur. Adverse effects are similar to the other drugs in the class. The major advantage of tadalafil is that it has a longer duration of action than the other two drugs used to treat erectile dysfunction. Improved ability to achieve and sustain an erection can occur as soon as 30 minutes after taking tadalafil and up to 36 hours after taking the drug, compared with about 4 hours after taking sildenafil. This

CRITICAL THINKING SCENARIO

Effectiveness of sildenafil

Joe Rosenbaum is 64 years old and takes sildenafil for erectile dysfunction. He returns to the clinic for follow-up. On assessment, you learn that the drug therapy appears to be effective and that Mr. Rosenbaum is tolerating it well without apparent adverse effects. You ask whether he has any other concerns or questions. He hesitates, and then laughingly says, "The only thing is, this pill doesn't seem to be as helpful if we've gone out to a restaurant for dinner. I guess it likes my wife's cooking better." What questions might you ask Mr. Rosenbaum to help determine a possible cause of this variation in sildenafil's effectiveness?

MEMORY CHIP

[P] Sildenafil

- Used to treat erectile dysfunction in men
- Major contraindication: current use of nitrates
- Most common adverse effects: facial flushing, headache, nasal congestion, and heartburn
- Most serious adverse effect: may increase risk of cardiovascular death in patients with current cardiovascular problems
- Most important patient education: Sexual stimulation and arousal are needed for drug effectiveness; take 1 hour before engaging in sexual activity.

longer duration may be an advantage for those patients who felt that the need to take the drug within 60 minutes of desired sexual activity produced emotional anxiety or interrupted sexual activity.

Alprostadil

A drug closely related to sildenafil is alprostadil, which is also used to treat erectile dysfunction. Unlike sildenafil, which is administered orally, alprostadil is administered by injection into the dorsal lateral aspect of the proximal third of the penis, or by intraurethral pellets. Alprostadil produces various pharmacologic effects; the most important are relaxation of smooth muscle, vasodilation of the arteries in the erectile tissue, and inhibition of platelet aggregation. Erection is achieved by the combination of relaxation of smooth muscles in the penis and vasodilation. An erection should occur within 5 to 20 minutes after administration. Unlike sildenafil, sexual arousal is not a prerequisite to the effectiveness of alprostadil.

Alprostadil is also given intravenously as palliative treatment for infants with patent ductus arteriosus until surgery can be performed. Unlabeled uses of alprostadil include activity in the performance of diagnostic peripheral arteriography and in treating atherosclerosis, gangrene, and pain related to peripheral vascular disease. In a recent study, about 40% of the men who used intracavernous injection to treat erectile dysfunction and later used sildenafil considered the sildenafil response (as indicated by quality of erection) inferior. Some men preferred to continue with intracavernous alprostadil in addition to sildenafil or to use it as an alternative to sildenafil (McMahon et al., 2000).

Absorption of alprostadil occurs from the urethra with both forms of administration. With the intraurethral technique, urination should precede drug administration. The residual urine then disperses the medicated pellet, allowing absorption through the urethral mucosa. Little alprostadil enters the general circulation. Alprostadil is rapidly converted to compounds that are further metabolized before excretion. Metabolism occurs in the first pass through the lung by way of enzymatic oxidation, and almost all the drug is metabolized. This finding accounts for the very low systemic concentration of alprostadil. Excretion of the metabolites occurs primarily through the kidneys.

Contraindications to alprostadil use are those conditions that might predispose the patient to priapism (erection lasting more than 6 hours), including sickle cell anemia or trait, multiple myeloma, and leukemia. Alprostadil is also contraindicated in patients with anatomic deformations of the penis (e.g., angulation, cavernosal fibrosis) or penile implants (intracavernosal placement), if sexual activity is inadvisable or contraindicated for the man, and for sexual intercourse with a pregnant woman unless a condom is used vasodilation from the drug's action may be harmful to the fetus. The most common adverse effect for both routes of administration is penile pain, which is usually mild or moderate. The most common adverse effects that are solely related to intraurethral administration are urethral pain and burning. Vaginal burning, itching, or both can occur in the female partner of the man using intraurethral alprostadil. Other adverse effects that may occur with intracavernosal administration are penile fibrosis, hematoma at the injection site, prolonged erection, and penile rash or edema. Priapism may occur, although it is not common. The pharmacodynamics of alprostadil may lead to hemodynamic changes, such as decreased blood pressure and increased heart rate, although these changes are not clinically important.

Patient education on the administration technique is important. Assess the patient's technique before the patient uses the drug on his own at home.

Drugs Significantly Different From [P] Sildenafil

Yohimbine

Yohimbine, although recognized as a drug by the FDA, has no FDA-approved indications. However, it is prescribed for unlabeled uses as a sympatholytic and mydriatic. It may also have activity as an aphrodisiac. It has been used successfully in treating erectile dysfunction with vascular or diabetic origins, but related data are scant. Yohimbine may be helpful in improving sexual function and desire in some men whose sexual dysfunction is related to the use of selective serotonin reuptake inhibitors.

Yohimbine is taken orally, three times a day. It is an alkaloid with chemical similarities to the drug reserpine. Yohimbine is believed to have properties similar to *Rauwolfia* alkaloids. It is primarily an alpha-2 adrenergic blocker of presynaptic alpha-2 receptors, which causes release of norepinephrine. It affects the peripheral autonomic nervous system by increasing parasympathetic (cholinergic) activity and by decreasing sympathetic (adrenergic) activity, thus producing erection. Yohimbine has a stimulating effect on mood and may increase anxiety, although mostly at high doses. Yohimbine is contraindicated in renal disease. All major adverse effects occur in the CNS (e.g., nervousness, irritability, tremor, dizziness, headache, and skin flushing). Reportedly, the drug exerts no appreciable influence on cardiac stimulation. Its exact effect on blood pressure is not known.

Apomorphine

Another drug that is significantly different from sildenafil is apomorphine SL (Uprima). Although this drug has been available in Europe since 2000, it is not yet approved by the FDA. It is the first centrally acting drug for erectile dysfunction in that it acts on dopamine receptors in the hypothalamus that are essential to erection. Unlike sildenafil, which has been known to cause cardiovascular changes such as decreased blood pressure, apomorphine SL has been shown to have very

little effect on the cardiovascular system. It interacts minimally with nitrates (Heaton et al., 2002).

DRUGS TO TREAT BENIGN PROSTATIC HYPERTROPHY

As discussed earlier, 5-alpha reductase (specifically type II) converts testosterone into the androgen 5-alpha dihydrotestosterone (DHT). Because the prostate gland depends on DHT for growth, interference with this process is helpful in treating BPH. Surgical intervention is another option. Transurethral resection of the prostate (TURP) is the most common surgical intervention, although a prostatectomy or radical prostatectomy may be performed.

The prototype drug for treating BPH is finasteride (Proscar). Drugs significantly different from finasteride are the alpha-1 blockers, which include prazosin (Minipress), terazosin (Hytrin), doxazosin (Cardura), and tamsulosin (Flomax).

NURSING MANAGEMENT OF THE PATIENT RECEIVING [P] FINASTERIDE

Core Drug Knowledge

Pharmacotherapeutics

Finasteride is used to treat BPH and androgenetic alopecia (male pattern baldness); the dose used for male hair loss is much smaller than that used for BPH. Two separate trade names are used to differentiate these preparations. Proscar is the trade name of finasteride used in BPH. Propecia is the trade name of finasteride used for male pattern baldness. The therapeutic effect for BPH is seen within 6 to 12 months of treatment, although it sometimes occurs earlier. Daily usage for more than 3 months is needed to see therapeutic effects when treating baldness. The therapeutic effects are reversed for both BPH and hair loss if the patient stops drug therapy.

Pharmacokinetics

Finasteride is well absorbed after oral administration. Food does not affect its absorption. Finasteride is highly protein bound, at a rate of about 90%. It is extensively metabolized in the liver through oxidative pathways. The inactive metabolites are excreted in the bile and feces (see Table 53.1).

Pharmacodynamics

Finasteride specifically inhibits the steroid 5-alpha reductase and consequently blocks the peripheral conversion of testosterone to DHT. The results are substantial decreases in serum and tissue DHT concentrations, and a complementary increase in testosterone level. Finasteride reduces prostatic DHT by as much as 90% and circulating levels of DHT by between 60% and 80%. Finasteride also decreases DHT prostate-specific antigen (PSA) levels by between 41% and 71%. These changes improve BPH-related symptoms, increase maximum urinary flow rates, and decrease prostate size.

In men with male pattern hair loss, DHT is found in increased amounts in the scalp. Finasteride decreases scalp and serum DHT concentrations in these men. Finasteride does not appear to affect body hair.

Contraindications and Precautions

Finasteride is contraindicated in women and children. It is a pregnancy category X drug because it causes abnormalities of the external genitalia in the male fetus. Because of these risks, pregnant women or women who may become pregnant should not handle crushed or broken finasteride tablets. Finasteride is also contraindicated if hypersensitivity to the drug or any of its components exists. Caution should be used if the patient has impaired liver function because finasteride is metabolized extensively in the liver.

Adverse Effects

Finasteride is generally well tolerated; adverse effects are usually mild and transient. Adverse effects, which occur in less than 4% of patients taking finasteride, include erectile dysfunction, decreased libido, and decreased volume of ejaculate. Sexual adverse effects resolved with continued treatment in more than 60% of patients who reported these effects. Overdose of finasteride has not been associated with adverse effects.

Drug Interactions

Finasteride decreases PSA levels by about 50%. A decrease in PSA level occurs even if the patient has prostate cancer. This reduction does not suggest a beneficial effect of finasteride on prostate cancer but rather an effect of the drug.

Assessment of Relevant Core Patient Variables

Health Status

Before administering the drug, verify that the patient has the clinical indications for receiving finasteride. Assess patients with BPH for prostate cancer before beginning therapy and periodically throughout therapy.

Life Span and Gender

Finasteride is not given to women or children.

Lifestyle, Diet, and Habits

Assess the patient for use of alternative medications, such as herbs (Box 53.2).

Environment

Be aware of the environment in which the medication will be administered. Finasteride may be administered in any environment but is most frequently self-administered in the home.

Nursing Diagnoses and Outcomes

- Risk for Sexual Dysfunction related to drug therapy
  Desired outcome: *If the patient experiences sexual dysfunction, it will resolve with continued drug therapy.*
- Impaired Urinary Elimination related to BPH
  Desired outcome: *Following drug therapy with finasteride, the patient will have no or fewer lower urinary tract symptoms from BPH.*

FOCUS ON RESEARCH

Box 53.2 Saw Palmetto and Benign Prostatic Hypertrophy (BPH)

Gerber, G. S. (2000). Saw palmetto for the treatment of men with lower urinary tract symptoms. *Journal of Urology, 163*(5), 1408–1412.
Gordon, A. E., & Shaughness, A. F. (2003). Saw palmetto for prostate disorders. *American Family Physician, 67*(6), 1281–1283.
Marks, L. S., Partin, A. W., Epstein, J. I., et al. (2000). Effects of a saw palmetto herbal blend in men with symptomatic benign prostatic hyperplasia. *Journal of Urology, 163*(5), 1451–1456.
Wilt, T., Ishani, A., Stark, G., et al. (2000). *Serenoa repens* for benign prostatic hyperplasia. *Cochrane Database System Review, 2,* CD001423.

The Studies

Saw palmetto, also known as *Serenoa repens,* is an herb sold over the counter with claims that it improves a man's prostate health and decreases the urinary symptoms of BPH. Several studies have been done to determine whether saw palmetto is indeed a safe and effective therapy for BPH. Two reviews of the literature (Gerber, 2000; Wilt et al., 2000) were conducted with the aim of determining mechanisms of action and effectiveness of saw palmetto. An additional small clinical study also examined the effects of this herb.

Clinical studies reported in the literature suggest that saw palmetto does positively affect urinary flow rates and lower urinary tract symptoms in men with mild to moderate BPH when compared with placebo. The literature also suggests that saw palmetto produces similar improvements in urinary symptoms and flow rate when compared with finasteride. Saw palmetto appears to be safe and have few or no adverse effects. Long-term efficacy, safety, and ability to prevent BPH complications, however, have not been determined. There has been concern that saw palmetto could mask the presence of prostate cancer by lowering prostate-specific antigen (PSA) levels. A study of 1,000 patients did not support this concern, although it did show a decrease in the PSA level with finasteride therapy (Gordon & Shaughness, 2003).

Research studies have demonstrated various potential mechanisms of action of saw palmetto. These mechanisms include 5-alpha reductase inhibition, adrenergic receptor antagonism, intraprostatic androgen receptor blockade, and prostate epithelial contraction.

Nursing Implications

Americans are widely using alternative medicines and complementary therapies. People are self-treating with herbs for various problems. Frequently, people do not tell their doctors or nurses that they are using herbs. Be aware that male patients may be using saw palmetto to treat symptoms of BPH. When obtaining a drug history, ask whether the patient uses saw palmetto, so that the drug history is complete. Patients may seek information from nurses on the safety and efficacy of this herb. Although you would not prescribe saw palmetto (unless you are a nurse practitioner), patient teaching can include that this herb appears to be safe and effective if the patient has mild to moderate symptoms of BPH. Caution patients that more research needs to be done in a large controlled clinical drug study to fully determine the long-term effects and safety of saw palmetto. Teach patients not to randomly substitute this herb for any prescribed medication. Encourage patients seeking assistance for symptoms of BPH to discuss the use of saw palmetto as one treatment option with the prescriber.

Planning and Intervention

Maximizing Therapeutic Effects

No specific actions maximize the therapeutic effects of finasteride.

Minimizing Adverse Effects

Adverse effects are a concern for the female nurse as well as the patient. The drug is in pregnancy category X. If you are female, and pregnant or in the childbearing years, you should not handle crushed or broken finasteride tablets because absorption is more likely to occur in these circumstances.

When the drug is given at home, teach the patient and family how to handle the drug to minimize risks.

Providing Patient and Family Education

Teach the patient the following information:

- Rationale for drug use
- Possible adverse effects of the drug (impotence and decreased libido) and that these effects are usually transient
- That volume of ejaculate may decrease with the use of finasteride but that this effect does not interfere with normal sexual function
- That female family members who are pregnant or capable of having children must not handle broken or crushed finasteride

Ongoing Assessment and Evaluation

Monitor the patient for improvement in BPH-related symptoms and increased ease of urination. If finasteride is used for male pattern baldness, increased hair growth and decreased hair loss indicate effectiveness. Throughout therapy, monitor men with BPH for prostate cancer. PSA levels require monitoring throughout therapy. Carefully evaluate any man on finasteride whose PSA levels increase; this development may be related to nonadherence to the drug regimen or to prostate cancer.

MEMORY CHIP

P Finasteride

- Used to treat BPH and male pattern baldness
- Major contraindication: use in women and children
- Most common adverse effects: altered sexual function (effects are mild and transient)
- **Life span alert: pregnancy category X**
- Most important patient education: Women should not handle crushed or broken tablets.

Drugs Significantly Different From P Finasteride

The alpha-1 blockers include prazosin (Minipress), terazosin (Hytrin), doxazosin (Cardura), tamsulosin (Flomax), and alfuzosin hydrochloride (Uroxatral). These drugs benefit patients with BPH by relaxing prostatic smooth muscle and relieving the lower urinary tract symptoms of BPH. Although a review of clinical drug trials shows that all the alpha-adrenergic receptor antagonists are similar in their efficacy for symptom relief and urodynamic improvement, the FDA has approved only terazosin, doxazosin, tamsulosin, and alfuzosin for this use. One recent study suggests that tamsulosin may be safer than the other alpha-1 blockers for older men and patients with hypertension who have impaired blood pressure regulation. This study also suggests that terazosin may be more effective in improving lower urinary tract symptoms than the other alpha-1 blockers (Tsujii, 2000), although other studies have not supported this possibility.

Alfuzosin hydrochloride (Uroxatral) is known outside of the United States as Oxatral OD. It works by selectively blocking the alpha-1 adrenergic receptors in the smooth muscle of the bladder neck and prostate, which results in improved urine flow. It has a low incidence of possible adverse effects such as postural hypotension, syncope, and sexual side effects. This medication is dosed as a once-daily extended release formula (Benign prostatic hypertrophy, 2003).

Alpha-1 blockers have a rapid onset of action, producing a therapeutic response within weeks (regardless of the presence of prostatic enlargement or bladder outlet obstruction). In contrast, finasteride takes longer to achieve therapeutic effects and alleviates only those symptoms associated with a large prostate. Except for tamsulosin, alpha-1 blockers are also used to treat hypertension (see Chapter 27 for more information). Tamsulosin is similar to finasteride in that neither drug lowers blood pressure and therefore neither is associated with the cardiovascular adverse effects (e.g., dizziness, postural hypotension) that are linked with the other alpha blockers. Both are associated, however, with an increased risk for sexual dysfunction; tamsulosin is associated with ejaculatory dysfunction, and finasteride is associated with decreased libido and erectile dysfunction.

DRUGS TO TREAT MALE PATTERN BALDNESS

Male pattern baldness may respond to drug therapy with topical minoxidil (Rogaine, Minoxidil for Men), which is the prototype drug. A drug significantly different from minoxidil is finasteride (Propecia), as previously discussed.

NURSING MANAGEMENT OF THE PATIENT RECEIVING P MINOXIDIL

Core Drug Knowledge

Pharmacotherapeutics

Minoxidil is used topically to treat androgenetic alopecia. Although men primarily use minoxidil, women also may use it. Minoxidil is effective in male pattern baldness of the vertex and in women with diffuse hair loss or thinning of the frontoparietal areas. It is not effective in patients who have predominantly frontal hair loss. Topical minoxidil is available as an over-the-counter (OTC) medication.

Pharmacokinetics

Topical minoxidil is poorly absorbed from normal intact scalp. Decreased integrity of the epidermal barrier from conditions such as inflammation, excoriations of the scalp, scalp psoriasis, or severe sunburn may increase systemic absorption. These abnormal scalp conditions may increase absorption enough to pose a risk for increased adverse effects.

Pharmacodynamics

The exact mode of action for topical minoxidil is unknown. Oral minoxidil was originally developed as a peripheral vasodilator used in treating hypertension, and hair growth was considered an adverse effect of the drug (see Chapter 27 for more information on peripheral vasodilators used in hypertension). Topical applications require at least 4 months of twice-daily application before the patient can expect evidence of hair growth. About 60% of patients who use minoxidil experience hair growth. Patients who respond to drug therapy need to continue the drug to maintain therapeutic effects. Reports indicate that the balding process resumes 3 to 4 months after drug therapy is stopped.

Contraindications and Precautions

The only contraindication to topical minoxidil is hypersensitivity to any component of the drug. Topical minoxidil is classified as a pregnancy category C drug because no adequate and well-controlled studies in pregnant women have been conducted. Thus, women must avoid using it during pregnancy. Safety and efficacy in children younger than 18 years have not been established.

Adverse Effects

The most common adverse effects of topical minoxidil are irritant dermatitis and allergic contact dermatitis. Other dermatologic effects are eczema, local erythema, pruritus, dry skin and scalp flaking, and exacerbated hair loss. Systemic absorption can cause the adverse effects associated with orally administered minoxidil, including edema, chest pain, increased or decreased blood pressure, and increased or decreased pulse.

Topical minoxidil contains alcohol. Burning or irritation may develop if the drug gets into the eyes, mouth, or mucous membranes or onto sensitive skin. Overdose has not been reported with topical applications of minoxidil.

Drug Interactions

Topical minoxidil should not be used with other topical agents (e.g., corticosteroids, retinoids, petrolatum) known to enhance cutaneous drug absorption.

Assessment of Relevant Core Patient Variables

Health Status

Verify that the patient has male pattern baldness and does not have predominantly frontal hair loss because topical

minoxidil is not effective for frontal hair loss. If the drug is given to women, the hair loss must be diffuse or identified as thinning of the frontoparietal area for therapy to be effective. Ensure that the patient has a normal, healthy scalp before and throughout therapy. A nonintact scalp promotes systemic absorption, and adverse effects may be more prominent, especially in patients with a history of heart disease. Monitor these patients closely for any problems with tachycardia or fluid retention.

Life Span and Gender

Topical minoxidil is used primarily in men, although it may be used in women. In female patients, assess for pregnancy and intention to become pregnant because use of minoxidil in pregnancy is to be avoided. Ensure that the patient is older than 18 years of age because the drug's safety in children has not been established.

Environment

Be aware of the environment in which minoxidil will be administered. Topical minoxidil is self-administered in the patient's home.

Nursing Diagnoses and Outcomes

- Situational Low Self-Esteem related to hair loss
  Desired outcome: *The patient's self-esteem will improve related to hair growth from drug therapy.*
- Risk for Injury related to adverse effects of drug therapy
  Desired outcome: *The patient will not experience adverse effects of drug therapy.*

Planning and Intervention

Maximizing Therapeutic Effects

Nursing actions to maximize the therapeutic effect are related to patient education.

Minimizing Adverse Effects

Nursing actions to minimize the adverse effects are related to patient education.

Providing Patient and Family Education

- Teach the patient receiving topical minoxidil the purpose and possible adverse effects of the drug.
- Teach the patient to administer the drug using this technique:
  1. Dry the hair and scalp before application.
  2. Apply 1 mL to the total affected area of the scalp twice daily, once in the morning and once at night.
  3. Wash hands after applying the drug.
- Advise the patient not to use minoxidil with other topical medications on the scalp.
- Caution the patient not to apply minoxidil if the scalp is irritated or sunburned because these conditions may increase the risk for adverse effects.
- Advise the patient not try to make up for any missed doses but to simply resume the normal administration schedule instead.
- Teach the patient not use more than the prescribed amount twice a day.
- Advise the patient that twice-daily use for 4 months or longer may be needed to see results. Fine, soft, colorless hair that is barely visible may be the first hair to grow. Over time, the new hair will become the same color and thickness as the other hair on the scalp.
- Keep medication out of the eyes and mouth; avoid applying it to sensitive skin on the face. If accidental exposure occurs, flush the area with large amounts of cool tap water. Consult with the prescriber if irritation continues.
- If no response to treatment occurs in 4 months or more, consult with the physician about the appropriateness of continuing therapy.

Ongoing Assessment and Evaluation

Assess the patient's scalp periodically to determine whether irritation has developed. The patient will usually check his own scalp during therapy. Topical minoxidil treatment is effective when hair growth has occurred with no adverse effects.

CHAPTER SUMMARY

- Testosterone is the main male sex hormone. Insufficient testosterone will prevent the growth spurt of adolescence and the development of secondary male sex characteristics. Lack of testosterone after development of secondary sex characteristics will cause those characteristics to diminish.
- Exogenous testosterone is used when endogenous levels are low. Exogenous testosterone will cause the same effects on the body as endogenous testosterone.
- One problem affecting male sexuality is erectile dysfunction. This problem may result from multiple factors, such as stress, adverse effects of drug therapy, and cardiovascular or neurologic impairments.
- When erectile dysfunction is a recurring problem, drug therapy may be used. Drug therapy used in erectile dysfunction includes sildenafil, alprostadil, and occasionally yohimbine. Sildenafil has the advantage of being an oral drug that is very effective; however, it is effective only in conjunction with sexual stimulation.
- A common problem of the older man is BPH. The exact cause of BPH is unknown, although excessive growth of the prostate is believed to be caused primarily by elevated levels of DHT (the primary hormone in the prostate cells). Overgrowth of the prostate places pressure on the urethra and the bladder, causing lower urinary tract symptoms.
- Drug therapy is one type of treatment for BPH. Drug therapy for BPH includes finasteride, which decreases the size of the prostate over time, and alpha-1 blockers, which relax the smooth muscle of the bladder and decrease difficulties in voiding.

MEMORY CHIP

P Minoxidil (topical)

- Used topically to promote growth of hair in male pattern baldness
- Use for 4 months or more required to see effect
- Is an over-the-counter drug
- Most common adverse effects: irritation and dermatitis at application site
- Most serious adverse effects: edema and tachycardia
- Most important patient education: Use bid; do not increase dosage or frequency; do not use if scalp is irritated or sunburned.

- Male pattern baldness is another men's health issue. This problem may be related to changing testosterone levels or alterations in the male sex hormone receptors.
- Topical minoxidil can be effective in promoting hair growth for male pattern baldness. This drug is available OTC. Women may also use minoxidil.

▲ QUESTIONS FOR STUDY AND REVIEW

1. What effects does testosterone have on the male?
2. What is the main risk when administering testosterone to induce the growth spurt of puberty?
3. How does sildenafil act to help the man achieve an erection?
4. Why should women not handle broken or crushed finasteride?
5. Topical minoxidil is poorly absorbed into the systemic circulation. What is the advantage of this factor?

? Need More Help?

Chapter 53 of the study guide for *Drug Therapy in Nursing* 2e contains NCLEX-style questions and other learning activities to reinforce your understanding of the concepts presented in this chapter. For additional information or to purchase the study guide, visit *http://connection.lww.com/go/aschenbrenner.*

■ REFERENCES AND BIBLIOGRAPHY

Benign prostatic hypertrophy drug available in U.S. (2003). *Health and Medicine Week, 83.*

Gaines, K. (2004). Tadalafil (Cialis) and vardenafil (Levitra) recently approved drugs for erectile dysfunction. *Urologic Nursing, 24*(1), 46–48.

Heaton, J. P. W., Dean, J., & Sleep, D. J. (2002). Rapid communication sequential administration enhances the effect of apomorphine sl in men with erectile dysfunction. *International Journal of Impotence Research, 14,* 61–64.

McMahon, C. G., Samali, R., & Johnson, H. (2000). Efficacy, safety and patient acceptance of sildenafil citrate as treatment for erectile dysfunction. *Journal of Urology, 164*(4), 1192–1196.

Rosen, R. C., & McKenna, K. E. (2002). PDE-5 inhibition and sexual response: Pharmacological mechanisms and clinical outcomes. *Annual Review of Sex Research, 13,* 36–80.

Tan, H. M., Moh, C. L., Mendoza, J. B., et al. (2000). Asian sildenafil efficacy and safety study (ASSESS-1): A double-blind, placebo-controlled, flexible-dose study of oral sildenafil in Malaysian, Singaporean, and Filipino men with erectile dysfunction. *Urology, 56*(4), 635–640.

Tsujii, T. (2000). Comparison of prazosin, terazosin and tamsulosin in the treatment of symptomatic benign prostatic hyperplasia: A short-term open, randomized multicenter study. BPH Medical Therapy Study Group. Benign prostatic hyperplasia. *International Journal of Urology, 7*(6), 199–205.

Zagaja, G. P., Mhoon, D. A., Aikens, J. E., et al. (2000). Sildenafil in the treatment of erectile dysfunction after radical prostatectomy. *Urology, 56*(4), 631–634.

chapter 54

Drugs Affecting Women's Health and Sexuality

Learning Objectives

At the completion of this chapter the student will:

1. Identify core drug knowledge about drugs that affect women's health and sexuality.
2. Identify core patient variables relevant to drugs that affect women's health and sexuality.
3. Relate the interaction of core drug knowledge to core patient variables for drugs that affect women's health and sexuality.
4. Compare the risks and benefits of hormone replacement therapy in postmenopausal women.
5. Generate a nursing plan of care from the interactions between core drug knowledge and core patient variables for drugs that affect women's health and sexuality.
6. Describe nursing interventions to maximize therapeutic effects and minimize adverse effects of drugs that affect women's health and sexuality.
7. Determine key points for patient and family education for drugs that affect women's health and sexuality.

KEY TERMS

estrogen
follicle-stimulating hormone
gonadotropin-releasing hormone
luteinizing hormone
menopause
osteoporosis
Paget disease
progestin
proliferative phase
secretory phase

FEATURED WEBSITE

http://www.fda.gov/womens/menopause/default.htm
This site, hosted by the U.S. Food and Drug Administration, has links to updates on hormonal therapy for postmenopausal women, labeling changes for estrogen and progestin, and other information about hormonal drug therapy.

CONNECTION WEBLINK

Additional Weblinks are found on Connection:
http://www.connection.lww.com/go/aschenbrenner.

Drugs Affecting Women's Health and Sexuality

Ⓒ Estrogens

- [P] **conjugated estrogen**
- synthetic conjugated estrogens, A
- contraceptives
- **clomiphene**
- **gonadotropins**
- **menotropins**
- **human chorionic gonadotropin**
- **gonadotropin-releasing hormones and agonists**
- androgen-estrogen combinations
- synthetic androgens

Ⓒ Progestins

- [P] **progesterone**
- levonorgestrel implants
- intrauterine progesterone contraceptive system
- contraceptives
- **megestrol acetate**
- **mifepristone**

Ⓒ Bisphosphonates

- [P] **alendronate**
- etidronate
- tiludronate
- pamidronate
- risedronate
- **raloxifene**

Ⓒ Contraceptives

- Ⓒ oral contraceptives
- Ⓒ emergency oral contraceptives
- Ⓒ combination hormone contraceptives
- norelgestromin/ethinyl estradiol transdermal system
- etonogestrel/ethinyl estradiol vaginal ring

The symbol Ⓒ indicates the **drug class.**
Drugs in **bold type** marked with the symbol [P] are prototypes.
Drugs in blue type are closely related to the prototype.
Drugs in red type are significantly different from the prototype.
Drugs in black type with no symbol are also used in drug therapy; no prototype

The female sex hormones are responsible for the normal development and maintenance of adult female sexual characteristics. If endogenous hormone levels are insufficient, sexual characteristics fail to develop. If endogenous levels are low after female sexual characteristics develop, the woman may be unable to become pregnant or maintain a pregnancy. If levels of sex hormones become low enough, masculinization may occur. Additionally, research has shown that low levels of female sex hormones contribute to some common women's health problems. This chapter presents the use of female sex hormones as replacement drug therapy when endogenous levels are absent or insufficient. It discusses two classes of female sex hormones: estrogens and progestins. The prototype estrogen is conjugated estrogen (Premarin), and the prototype progestin is progesterone (Prometrium, Progesterone).

This chapter also presents drug therapy used in treating osteoporosis, a common health problem in postmenopausal women. The prototype drug is alendronate (Fosamax).

PHYSIOLOGY

The female sex hormones are responsible for producing female sexual characteristics, developing the female reproductive system, and maintaining pregnancy. The two types of female sex hormones are **estrogen** and **progestin.** Both are steroidal compounds that the ovaries begin to secrete at puberty and that the placenta secretes during pregnancy. The adrenal cortex also secretes estrogen and progestin, but in much smaller amounts.

Estrogen

The female body produces six different estrogens but only three in substantial amounts: estradiol, estrone, and estriol. Estradiol is the most potent and the major estrogen secreted by the ovaries. In addition to promoting and maintaining female organs and secondary sexual characteristics (e.g., distribution of body hair, high-pitched voice), estrogen affects the release of pituitary gonadotropins, causes capillary dilation, and promotes fluid retention. It also enhances protein anabolism, promotes thinning of cervical mucus, inhibits or facilitates ovulation, and prevents postpartum breast pain. Estrogen also maintains the tone and elasticity of the urogenital structures and stimulates growth of axillary and pubic hair and pigmentation of the nipples and genitals.

Estrogen promotes growth during the adolescent growth spurt; continued elevated levels of estrogen terminate growth by stimulating closure of the epiphyses of the long bones. Closure occurs because estrogen stimulates the osteoblasts in the bone to produce bone faster than the epiphyseal cartilage can expand. Because estrogens cause a faster epiphyseal closure than androgens, women are generally shorter than men by adulthood. Estrogen indirectly contributes to strengthening the skeleton by conserving calcium and phosphorus and encouraging bone formation. After puberty, estrogen is important in maintaining normal bone density and composition. The organic and mineral components of bone are continuously being recycled and renewed throughout life; this process is called bone remodeling.

Progestin

Progestins, which include progesterone and its derivatives, are the other female sex hormones. Progesterone is the primary endogenous progestin. The progestins change the proliferative endometrium into a secretory endometrium. Through positive feedback, they also inhibit or facilitate secretion of pituitary gonadotropins. Doing so either prevents follicular maturation and ovulation or promotes maturation for the primed follicle. Progestins also inhibit spontaneous uterine contractions and contractions of other smooth muscles throughout the body. They may also demonstrate some anabolic or androgenic activity.

Menstrual Cycle

Much secretion of the female sex hormones is cyclic, and these cyclic changes constitute the menstrual cycle. **Gonadotropin-releasing hormone** (GRH), which is secreted by the hypothalamus and then perfused throughout the anterior pituitary, stimulates the release of **follicle-stimulating hormone** (FSH) and **luteinizing hormone** (LH). During puberty, the pituitary gland secretes large volumes of FSH and LH to initiate and establish the menstrual cycle. These hormones stimulate the development of the ovarian follicles and the release of the ovum from the mature follicle (Figure 54.1). As the follicles grow, they produce estrogen. Estrogen increases the vascularity of the uterine lining, preparing it for implantation of a fertilized egg. This phase of the menstrual cycle is termed the **proliferative phase.** The rapidly rising estrogen levels further stimulate GRH, encouraging further release of LH. The high levels of LH trigger the rupture of the mature follicle, and ovulation occurs.

After ovulation, the follicle is transformed into the corpus luteum, which secretes progesterone and estrogen. This phase is known as the **secretory phase** of the menstrual cycle. In response to the rising levels of estrogen and progesterone, the endometrial glands continue to grow, the arteries of the endometrium become spiraled, and the endometrium prepares for implantation of a fertilized egg. When estrogen and progesterone have reached critical levels, they create negative feedback, directly preventing further release of GRH and indirectly preventing the release of FSH and LH. If fertilization does not occur, the corpus luteum disintegrates, estrogen and progesterone levels fall, and the endometrial tissue sloughs off in the menses. As the levels of estrogen and progesterone continue to decline, GRH is again secreted, reinitiating the process. If fertilization occurs, the corpus luteum remains and continues to secrete estrogen and progesterone for the first month of pregnancy. By the second month, the placenta has developed, and it becomes the major source of estrogen and progesterone to maintain the pregnancy.

PATHOPHYSIOLOGY

If a woman is deficient in endogenous sex hormones, she will not experience normal sexual development. The primary sex organs will not mature, secondary sexual characteristics will not develop, reproduction will not be possible, and the normal growth spurt of adolescence will not happen. If levels of endogenous hormones drop after puberty

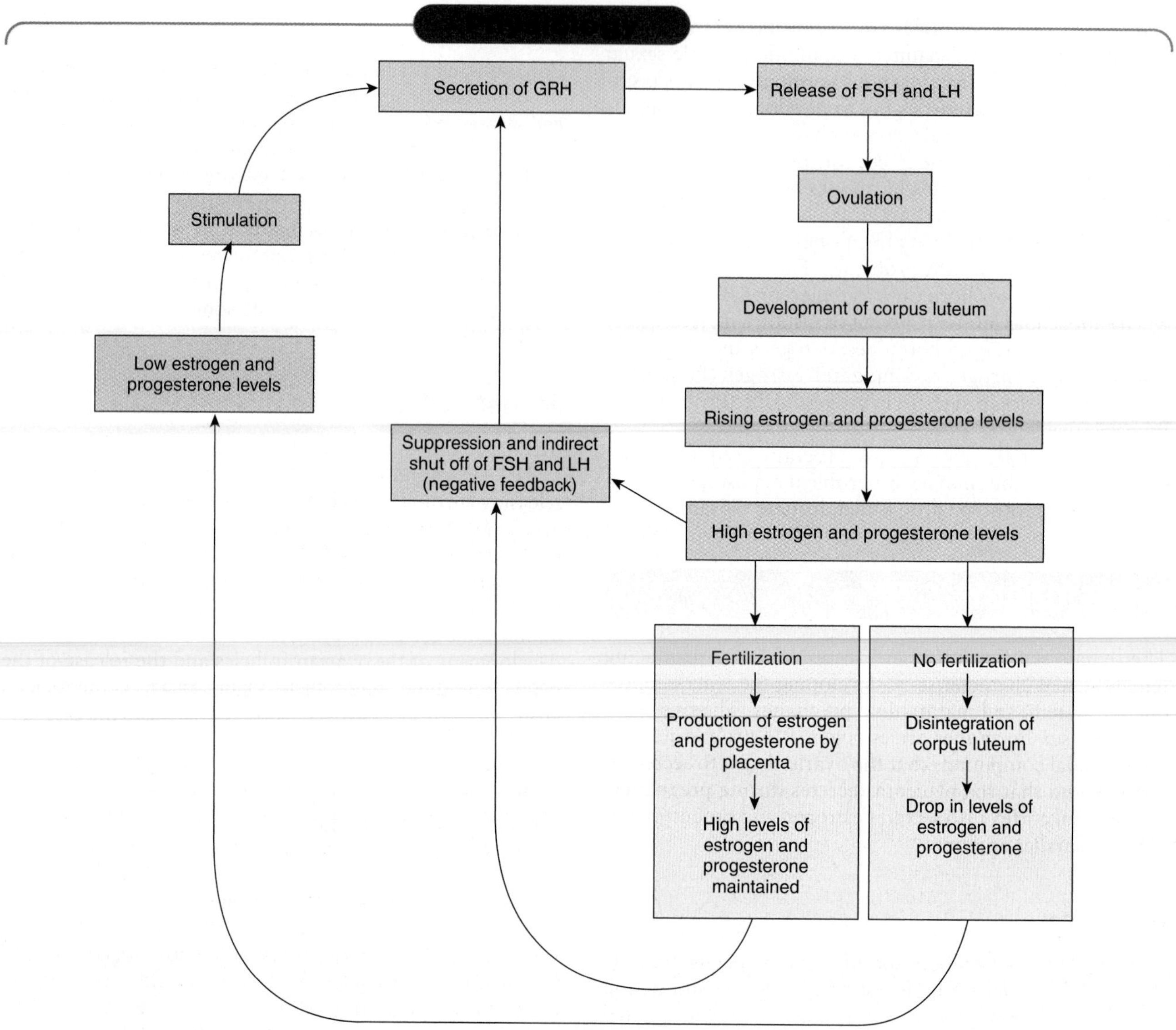

FIGURE 54.1 Menstrual cycle and fertility. In the *proliferative phase* of the menstrual cycle gonadotropin-releasing hormone (GRH) is secreted by the hypothalamus and perfused through the anterior pituitary, which stimulates release of both follicle-stimulating hormone (FSH) and luteinizing hormone (LH). In response, estrogen production is stimulated in preparation for implantation of a fertilized egg. Then the *secretory phase* of the menstrual cycle begins, during which rising estrogen levels stimulate GRH, which stimulates release of more LH, which in turn prompts ovulation and the formation of the corpus luteum. Estrogen and progesterone levels continue to rise in preparation for implantation of a fertilized egg. When estrogen and progesterone levels peak, they halt additional release of GRH and indirectly, FSH and LH. When fertilization does not occur, the corpus luteum is sloughed off, and estrogen and progesterone levels fall. GRH is again secreted to continue the cycle. When fertilization occurs, the corpus luteum remains to provide estrogen and progesterone until the second month of pregnancy when the placenta is developed and becomes the major source of estrogen and progesterone to maintain the pregnancy.

has occurred and the sexual organs and reproductive system have matured, secondary sexual characteristics may diminish. The ability to reproduce will be diminished, despite the presence of developed organs, and the woman may be unable to carry a pregnancy to term.

When a woman's estrogen levels drop during **menopause,** the ending of the monthly ovarian cycles, she experiences several changes. A vasomotor response is typical. The woman will experience periods of hot flashes not related to physical exertion and perfuse periodic sweating, even at night, which may awaken the woman from sleep. Menstrual periods become irregular because the frequency and quality of ovulation decrease. In addition, vaginal secretions diminish, so that the drier vagina may be uncomfortable, and intercourse may become uncomfortable or painful.

For some as yet unknown reason, postmenopausal women are at increased risk for cardiovascular disease and myocardial infarction (MI). For example, the risk for coronary artery disease (CAD) increases twofold after menopause, and heart disease is the primary cause of death for postmenopausal

women. The possible causes of this effect on the cardiovascular system are still being researched.

In postmenopausal women, the loss of estrogen and its positive effects on bone remodeling contribute to the development of osteoporosis. **Osteoporosis,** characterized by low bone mineral density, is a loss in bone mass sufficient to compromise normal function. Osteoporosis occurs when the body fails to form enough new bone, reabsorbs too much of the old bone, or both. Approximately 20% of women older than 50 years in the United States have osteoporosis, and about 50% have low bone density that may deteriorate into osteoporosis. Deficiency of sex hormones is the leading cause of osteoporosis. Approximately 80% of people with osteoporosis are women because decreases in estrogen levels occur sooner and are more substantial in women than decreases of testosterone in men.

Osteoporosis produces weak bones and leads to an increased risk for fractures. Fractures can have serious complications, including pain, loss of mobility, complications related to immobility, and death. Bone changes in postmenopausal women may also be related to decreased physical activity. Heavily stressed bones, such as those that develop with regular weight-bearing exercise (e.g., walking, running), are stronger and thicker than bones not subjected to these ordinary stresses, which become thin and brittle. Moderate physical activity and weight bearing are essential for bone remodeling. Osteoporosis may be caused by corticosteroid excess (e.g., in Cushing disease), hyperthyroidism, hyperparathyroidism, immobilization, bone malignancies, and genetic disorders. Risk factors for osteoporosis include Asian or white race, family history of osteoporosis, smoking, eating disorders, excessive alcohol intake, low dietary calcium, eating disorders, and use of steroid medications.

C ESTROGENS

The many different types of exogenous estrogen differ by indications, route of administration, and pharmacokinetics. Most of these estrogens are used for hormone replacement therapy (HRT). Conjugated estrogen (Premarin) is the prototype. Other estrogens are categorized as follows:

- Estradiol (Estrace, FemPatch, Vivelle, Vivelle-Dot, Climara, Alora, Estraderm, Delestrogen, Gynogen, Valergen); formulations include oral preparations, transdermal patch, in oil for IM injection, vaginal cream, and vaginal ring
- Estrone (Kestrone), given as an intramuscular (IM) injection
- Esterified estrogens (Estratab, Menest), estropipate (Ortho-Est, Ogen, estropipate), ethinyl estradiol (Estinyl), all of which are taken orally; estradiol hemihydrate (Vagifem), available as vaginal tablets; and estradiol cypionate (dep-Gynogen, Depo-Estradiol Dypionate, DepoGen), which is given by IM injection

Drugs closely related to conjugated estrogen are oral contraceptives and synthetic conjugated estrogens, A (Cenestin). Table 54.1 provides a summary of selected estrogens.

Several drugs that affect female sexuality are significantly different from conjugated estrogen. These drugs are clomiphene (Clomid, Milophene, Serophene), the gonadotropins (follitropin alfa [Gonal-F], follitropin beta [Follistim], urofollitropin [Fertinex]) and menotropins (which are purified preparations of gonadatropins) [Pergonal, Humegon, Repronex], human chorionic gonadotropin (HCG) (A.P.L., Chorex-5, Profasi, Choron 10, Gonic, Pregnyl), gonad-releasing hormones (gonadorelin acetate [Lutrepulse], nafarelin acetate [Synarel], and histrelin acetate [Supprelin]), androgen-estrogen combination drugs (DepAndrogyn, Depo-Testadiol, Dura-Estrin, Valertest No. 1, Premarin with Methyltestosterone, Estratest), and synthetic androgens (danazol) (Danocrine).

NURSING MANAGEMENT OF THE PATIENT RECEIVING P CONJUGATED ESTROGEN

Core Drug Knowledge

Pharmacotherapeutics

Conjugated estrogen is used primarily as HRT in female hypogonadism, female castration, and primary ovarian failure. Estrogen replacement therapy is also used in menopausal women to treat moderate to severe vasomotor responses (hot flashes). Other uses in menopause include treating atrophic vaginitis, vaginal dryness, painful intercourse, mood swings, and loss of tone in genitourinary muscles. Menopausal symptoms should be treated with as small a dose as possible for as short a time as possible. It should not be considered life-long therapy. Although estrogen is approved for use in postmenopausal women who have evidence of bone loss (osteoporosis) and has been shown to reduce further bone loss and to improve bone density, it is *not* currently recommended as a first-line treatment for this condition because of complications arising from estrogen use. Other drugs to help promote bone density are safer and should be used first. (See the discussion of alendronate later in this chapter; also Table 54.3). Conjugated estrogen is also used to treat abnormal uterine bleeding resulting from hormonal imbalance with no organic pathology. Additionally, conjugated estrogen is used as palliative therapy in advanced prostatic cancer, in men with metastatic breast cancer, and in selected women with breast cancer who do not have an estrogen-dependent tumor. Estrogen replacement therapy should *not* be used in postmenopausal women in an attempt to prevent cardiovascular disease or complications.

Pharmacokinetics

Absorption from the gastrointestinal (GI) tract is complete. Estrogen binds to specific receptor proteins in tissues that are responsive to estrogen (female genital organs, breasts, hypothalamus, pituitary). Metabolism occurs primarily in the liver. While circulating through the liver, estrogen is degraded to less active estrogenic compounds. Some estrogens are excreted into the bile and then reabsorbed from the intestines and returned to the liver. The estrogen conjugates are water soluble and are excreted through the kidneys, with minimal resorption. Conjugated estrogen crosses the placenta and enters breast milk.

TABLE 54.1 Summary of Selected (C) Estrogens

Drug (Trade) Name	Selected Indications	Route and Dosage Range	Pharmacokinetics
P conjugated estrogen (Premarin; *Canadian:* Congest)	Hormone replacement therapy	*Adult:* PO, 0.3–.625 mg/d cyclically (3 wk on, 1 wk off)	*Onset:* Slow *Duration:* 24 h $t_{1/2}$: Unknown
estradiol, transdermal (Vivelle, Estraderm, Climara)	Female hypogonadism Vasomotor symptoms associated with menopause Hormone replacement therapy	*Adult:* .025–.05 mg applied to skin once or twice weekly (brand dependent)	*Onset:* Slow *Duration:* 3–7 d $t_{1/2}$: Unknown
estradiol, oral (Estrace)	Hormone replacement therapy Inoperable breast cancer	*Adult:* PO, 1–2 mg/d *Adult:* 10 mg tid; prostatic cancer 1–2 mg tid	*Onset:* Slow *Duration:* Unknown $t_{1/2}$: Unknown
estradiol valerate in oil (Gynogen, Delestrogen, Estra-L, Valergen, Dioval)	Hormone replacement therapy Prostate cancer	*Adult:* IM, 10–20 mg q4wk *Adult:* IM, 30 mg q1–2wk	*Onset:* Slow *Duration:* 4 wk $t_{1/2}$: Unknown
diethylstilbestrol (DES; *Canadian:* Honvol)	Female breast cancer (inoperable) Prostate cancer	*Adult:* PO, 15 mg/d *Adult:* PO, 1–3 mg/d	*Onset:* Rapid *Duration:* 24 h $t_{1/2}$: Unknown
(C) Selected Non-estrogens			
P clomiphene (Clomid, Milophene)	Ovulatory failure	*Adult:* PO, 50–100 mg/d for 5 d	*Onset:* 5–8 d *Duration:* 6 wk $t_{1/2}$: 5 d
menotropins (Pergonal, Humegon)	Ovulation stimulation Spermatogenesis stimulation	*Adult:* IM, 75 IU/d for 7–12 d, follow with hCG *Adult:* IM, 75–150 IU three times a week, pretreat and cotreat with human chorionic gonadotropin	*Onset:* Slow *Duration:* Months t½: Unknown
chorionic gonadotropins (Choron, Pregnyl)	Hypogonadotropic Hypogonadism (males) Ovulation stimulation Spermatogenesis stimulation	*Adult:* 500–4,000 USP three times a week *Adult:* 5,000–10,000 USP 1 d after last menotropin dose *Adult:* Pretreatment, IM, 5,000 IU three times a week for 4–6 mo; cotreatment, 2,000 IU two times a week with menotropins	*Onset:* Unknown *Duration:* Unknown $t_{1/2}$: Unknown after pretreatment with menotropins

Pharmacodynamics

Estrogen given to females with insufficient endogenous estrogen (hypogonadism) stimulates the development of the female sex organs and secondary female sexual characteristics. Estrogen also stimulates the long-bone growth spurt of adolescence; when circulating estrogen reaches a certain level, it triggers closure of the epiphyseal plates to stop growth. Other actions of estrogen include facilitating or inhibiting ovulation (depending on dose), increasing fluid retention, facilitating protein anabolism, conserving calcium and phosphorus, stimulating bone formation, and maintaining tone and elasticity of urogenital structures.

When given during and after menopause, conjugated estrogen reduces hot flashes. It also increases vaginal secretions, improves urogenital tone, and reduces irritability and emotional lability. When given to postmenopausal women for treating or preventing osteoporosis, estrogen substantially increases spinal bone mineral density. The risks accompanying therapy are greater than this benefit, however, and estrogen should not be used routinely to treat osteoporosis. The Women's Health Initiative (WHI), a large clinical trial, found that menopausal women who had moderate to severe vasomotor symptoms at the start of the study experienced a small benefit in their sleep quality with 3 years of estrogen-progestin therapy. However, therapy provided no benefit for other health-related quality-of-life measures, such as general health, vitality, mental health, relief from depressive symptoms, or sexual satisfaction (Hays et al., 2003). Additionally, the WHI study found that estrogen-progestin combinations created deleterious effects in the cardiovascular system (see Adverse Effects, below) and slightly increased the risk for cognitive decline and probable dementia in women older than 65 years (Rapp et al., 2003; Shumaker et al., 2003).

Contraindications and Precautions

Based on the findings from the Women's Health Initiative and the Women's Health Initiative Memory Study, the FDA

asked all manufacturers of estrogen products to carry a warning in their labels that the drug increases the risk for cardiovascular events, including stroke; memory loss; and dementia.

Estrogen is contraindicated in patients with breast cancer because it stimulates the growth of breast cancer cells. However, it may be used in appropriately selected patients receiving treatment for metastatic disease. For a discussion of the role of hormones in cancer, see Chapter 36. Estrogen is also contraindicated in the following conditions:

- Estrogen-dependent neoplastic diseases
- Undiagnosed abnormal genital bleeding
- Active thrombophlebitis or thromboembolic disorders
- History of thrombophlebitis, thrombosis, or thromboembolic disorders associated with previous estrogen use (except when used in treating breast or prostatic malignancy)
- Known or suspected pregnancy (estrogen is an FDA pregnancy category X drug because of known adverse effects on the developing fetus)

Conjugated estrogen should be administered with caution to breast-feeding women because estrogen has been shown to decrease the quantity and quality of breast milk and may be excreted into it. Its safety and efficacy in children have not been established. Cautious use must be observed in patients with incomplete bone growth because of the epiphyseal closure that accompanies estrogen use. Caution also is necessary in patients for whom some degree of fluid retention may cause complications, such as those with epilepsy, migraine headaches, cardiac dysfunction, or renal dysfunction. Caution should also be used in patients with renal insufficiency or metabolic bone diseases associated with hypercalcemia.

Adverse Effects

Postmenopausal estrogen use has been associated with some serious and important adverse effects. Although postmenopausal women are more at risk for cardiovascular disease and MI than premenopausal women, recent landmark research from the Women's Health Initiative trial indicates that estrogen given to postmenopausal women in combination with progestin significantly increases the risk for stroke and coronary heart disease in all subgroups examined (Box 54.1).

Findings from the Women's Health Initiative also indicate that estrogen-progestin combinations increase the incidence of breast cancers, and that when cancer is detected, it is at a more advanced stage than if the woman were not taking HRT. Additionally, it is more likely that a woman receiving estrogen-progestin will have an abnormal mammogram. Estrogen with progestin, therefore, may stimulate breast cancer growth and hinder breast cancer diagnosis (Chlebowski et al., 2003). Findings from the WHI study also indicate that estrogen with progestin appears to increase the risk for ovarian cancer, although it does not have this effect on endometrial cancer (Anderson et al., 2003). Estrogen given alone is known to increase the risk for endometrial cancer. The progestin in combination therapy has a positive effect on the endometrium, offsetting any increase in risk for endometrial cancer from estrogen.

The branch of the WHI study that examined the use of estrogen alone continued until March 2004, when it was stopped a year early. Early data analysis shows that, like combination HRT, estrogen replacement appears to increase the risk for stroke and probably for dementia or mild cognitive impairment but decreases the risk for hip fracture. Unlike combination HRT, estrogen alone did not appear to have any effect (positive or negative) on heart disease and did not increase the risk for breast cancer (National Institutes of Health, 2004).

The use of estrogen during early pregnancy may have teratogenic effects on the fetus. Use of conjugated estrogen in patients with breast cancer and bone metastases may cause severe hypercalcemia. Estrogen use increases the risk for thrombosis formation (thrombophlebitis and thromboembolism) in all women receiving the drug, regardless of age.

Most adverse effects of estrogen therapy are related to the effect of estrogen on the body and may be dose related. Common adverse effects include breakthrough bleeding, changes in menstrual flow, dysmenorrhea, premenstrual-like syndrome, headache, nausea, vomiting, bloating, abdominal cramps, chloasma (dark, patchy pigmentation to skin), and photosensitivity. Other adverse effects include cholestatic jaundice, colitis, acute pancreatitis, steepened corneal curvature, intolerance to contact lenses, migraine headaches, dizziness, mental depression, pain at injection site, edema, changes in libido, and breast tenderness, enlargement, or secretion.

Drug Interactions

No important drug interactions are associated with conjugated estrogen.

Assessment of Relevant Core Patient Variables

Health Status

Before the patient begins estrogen therapy, assess his or her blood pressure (for hypertension) and breasts (for masses). The patient should also undergo a pelvic examination and a Papanicolaou test to rule out cervical cancer. It is important to determine whether the patient has breast cancer, undiagnosed genital bleeding, active thrombophlebitis or thromboembolic disorders, or a history of thrombophlebitis, thrombosis, or thromboembolic disorders associated with previous estrogen use (except in the palliative treatment of breast or prostate cancer). These conditions are contraindications to use of conjugated estrogen.

Other assessment data to look for in the patient are a personal or family history of breast cancer, a history of benign breast tumors, early menarche, a first pregnancy late in life, or never having been pregnant. These factors are thought to increase the risk for breast cancer with estrogen replacement therapy.

It is also important to determine whether the patient has a metabolic bone disease associated with hypercalcemia or renal insufficiency because these conditions mandate cautious use of estrogen. Determine whether the patient has a condition that might be adversely affected by fluid retention, such as epilepsy, migraine headaches, cardiac dysfunction, or renal insufficiency.

Life Span and Gender

Check the patient's age. The use of parenteral conjugated estrogen in premature infants has been associated with the development of a fatal "gasping syndrome" because of the

FOCUS ON RESEARCH

Box 54.1 Summary of Findings from the Women's Health Initiative

Anderson, G. L., Judd, H. L., Kaunitz, A. M., et al., Women's Health Initiative Investigators. (2003). Effects of estrogen plus progestin on gynecologic cancers and associated diagnostic procedures: The Women's Health Initiative randomized trial. *Journal of the American Medical Association, 290*(13), 1739–1748.
Chlebowski, R. T., Hendrix, S. L., Langer, R. D., et al., Women's Health Initiative Investigators. (2003). Influence of estrogen plus progestin on breast cancer and mammography in healthy postmenopausal women: The Women's Health Initiative Randomized Trial. *Journal of the American Medical Association, 289*(24), 3243–3253.
Manson, J. E., Hsia, J., Johnson, K. C., et al., Women's Health Initiative Investigators. (2003). Estrogen plus progestin and the risk of coronary heart disease. *New England Journal of Medicine, 349*(6), 523–534.
Shumaker, S. A., Legault, C., Rapp, S. R., et al., Women's Health Initiative Memory Study Investigators. (2003). Estrogen plus progestin and the incidence of dementia and mild cognitive impairment in postmenopausal women. The Women's Health Initiative Memory Study: A randomized controlled trial. *Journal of the American Medical Association, 289*(20), 2651–2662.
Wassertheil-Smoller, S., Hendrix, S. L., Limacher, M., et al., Women's Health Initiative Investigators. (2003). Effect of estrogen plus progestin on stroke in postmenopausal women. The Women's Health Initiative: A randomized trial. *Journal of the American Medical Association, 289*(20), 2673–2684.

The Study

The Women's Health Initiative was a large, multicenter, randomized clinical trial of 16,608 postmenopausal women between the ages of 50 and 79 years. The goal of the trial was to determine whether estrogen-progestin hormone replacement therapy was cardioprotective for postmenopausal women. The chief outcome criterion was the incidence of coronary heart disease (nonfatal myocardial infarction or death caused by CHD). The study was designed to follow the women for 8.5 years. However, after participants had received treatment for an average of 5.2 years, the study was prematurely stopped because the data indicated that the overall risks of continuing the study exceeded any benefits that could be obtained. The study found that estrogen plus progestin does not provide cardiac protection and may increase the risk for CHD in generally healthy postmenopausal women. The risk appeared highest during the first year of hormone use.

A subgroup of the women in the study was also assessed to determine the effect of estrogen plus progestin on the risk for stroke. This part of the study showed that HRT also increased the risk for stroke in all subgroups with baseline stroke risk (e.g., the presence of hypertension or smoking). From the main study, 4,532 of the women were also recruited to participate in a study (Women's Health Initiative Memory Study) to evaluate the effect of HRT on memory and cognitive processes. The findings from these women showed that, contrary to previous thinking, HRT increased the risk for dementia, including Alzheimer disease, and did not prevent mild cognitive impairment.

Data were also collected from the Women's Health Initiative to determine the effect of HRT on postmenopausal women who still had a uterus. HRT appears to increase the risk for ovarian cancer but not endometrial cancer. Data were also examined to determine whether HRT had an effect on breast cancer, and the incidence of breast cancer was found to be increased for women taking HRT. Additionally, the stage at which breast cancer was diagnosed was more advanced if the woman had been on HRT. This finding suggests that HRT not only stimulates breast cancer growth but may make its diagnosis more difficult.

All of these findings caused the researchers to conclude that postmenopausal estrogen plus progestin conferred greater risks than benefits and that this therapy should generally be avoided.

Nursing Implications

The results of the Women's Health Initiative study dramatically changed the thinking in the medical community about the use of HRT in postmenopausal women. Although postmenopausal women are known to be at a substantially higher risk for coronary heart disease, and estrogen is known to reduce (low-density lipoprotein (LDL) cholesterol, a cardiovascular risk factor), exogenous hormone therapy with estrogen and progestin is obviously not the answer, as was previously thought. Couple this information with the knowledge that HRT increases the risk for Alzheimer disease, breast cancer, and ovarian cancer, and the therapy now appears to pose too great a risk compared to its known benefits (e.g., increasing postmenopausal bone density and slightly improving sleep). How is it possible that the scientific thinking could switch from encouraging women to use HRT to avoiding its use as much as possible?

First, you need to understand that science and the state of knowledge on any topic are constantly evolving. As more is learned through research, different recommendations about therapy may be indicated. Second, the Women's Health Initiative was an exceedingly large study, much larger than any previous studies, some of which had a few thousand participants. The larger the number of participants in a clinical drug study, the more likely adverse effects of drug therapy will be identified. Similarly, the larger the trial, the more likely that findings regarding drug efficacy (whether the drug is found effective or not) are valid and can be applied to a larger population. Here, although the study was initially intended to prove a positive effect, the data pool was large enough to show there was too much risk for any small benefit that could be achieved.

It is important that you understand how clinical trials are conducted and how their results modify practice. Patients will often hear of an outcome from a trial reported in the general media. The report may or may not accurately or completely represent the facts from the clinical trial. Patients can become fearful, angry, or confused as to why medical advice regarding a particular drug therapy may change. You need to be able to discuss the facts of these studies with patients to help them sort out and understand the findings in relation to their own health.

benzyl alcohol in the preparation. Assess whether long-bone growth has been completed. If the patient is prepubescent, monitor growth throughout therapy to prevent premature closing of the epiphyses.

Assess for pregnancy, which is a contraindication for therapy. Use of conjugated estrogen during pregnancy may promote congenital defects, including heart and limb-reduction defects. Male fetuses exposed to conjugated estrogen through maternal use may develop genitourinary structural problems and, later, abnormal semen. Use of estrogen to treat threatened or habitual miscarriage has not been proved effective. Also, assess the patient's menopausal or postmenopausal status. If the patient is menopausal, assess for severity of symptoms.

Environment

Conjugated estrogen may produce photosensitivity. Patients who are outdoors frequently need to take precautions against the sun's ultraviolet rays until tolerance to the drug is determined. Be aware of the environment in which estrogen will be administered. Oral conjugated estrogen may be administered in any setting, including in the home by the patient. Parenteral conjugated estrogen (IM or intravenous [IV]) is administered in a hospital setting.

Nursing Diagnoses and Outcomes

- Ineffective Sexuality Patterns related to therapy for female hypogonadism or lack of intrinsic estrogen
  Desired outcome: *The patient will develop normal sex organs and secondary sexual characteristics while using estrogen drug therapy.*
- Risk for Delayed Growth and Development related to intrinsic estrogen deficiency and early hypophysis closing from estrogen replacement therapy
  Desired outcome: *The patient will achieve normal growth and development while using drug therapy.*
- Decisional Conflict related to comparison of risks and benefits of postmenopausal estrogen replacement therapy
  Desired outcome: *The patient will make an informed decision about estrogen replacement therapy after comparing personal risks and benefits.*

Planning and Intervention

Maximizing Therapeutic Effects

Several nursing actions are geared toward maximizing the therapeutic effects of estrogen. Conjugated estrogens are administered cyclically (3 weeks of daily administration followed by 1 week off) to simulate the normal cycling of endogenous estrogen (except when given for carcinomas or postpartum breast engorgement). The drug should stay refrigerated before reconstitution (IV or IM use); after reconstitution, the solution can remain refrigerated for up to 60 days. The solution should not be used if it darkens or if precipitation occurs.

Minimizing Adverse Effects

To minimize adverse effects of estrogen therapy, monitor for signs of thrombophlebitis and thromboembolus. The estrogen dosage should remain as low as possible to minimize the chances for development of endometrial cancer (if given without progestin), ovarian cancer, or breast cancer, but still achieve the desired therapeutic effects. HRT should be limited to treating only those menopausal women who have substantial menopausal symptoms. The dose and the duration of therapy should be minimized in menopausal women to decrease the risk for cancer, stroke, and coronary heart disease. Applying estrogen topically to urogenital structures may decrease the risk for systemic adverse effects, compared with risk of oral preparations, when it is used to treat the symptoms of menopause. Do not administer IV conjugated estrogen with other agents. (An exception is in emergencies in which a separate drug infusion has already been started. In such cases, inject the drug into the IV tubing as close to the angiocatheter insertion site as possible.) Protect the patient from ultraviolet light until it is determined whether the patient will experience photosensitivity.

Providing Patient and Family Education

- Teach patients and their families about the therapeutic purpose of estrogen. Provide and clarify information on risks and benefits of postmenopausal therapy, so that the patient can make an informed choice regarding drug therapy.
- Provide instruction on how to take estrogen cyclically, unless the patient is taking it for palliative cancer treatment or postpartum breast engorgement.
- Instruct the patient on the signs and symptoms of thrombophlebitis and thromboembolism (pain in groin or calves, sharp chest pain or sudden shortness of breath, sudden severe headache, dizziness or fainting, vision or speech disturbance, weakness or numbness in arm or leg). Urge the patient to notify the physician or nurse practitioner at once if these signs or symptoms occur.
- Teach the patient to notify the physician or nurse practitioner if any of the following signs or symptoms occurs: abnormal vaginal bleeding, missed menstrual period or suspected pregnancy, lumps in the breast, severe abdominal pain, yellowing of the skin or eyes, or severe depression.
- Teach the patient to avoid prolonged exposure to the sun and to use sunblock and appropriate clothing in the sun because photosensitivity may occur.
- In addition, emphasize to the patient the importance of returning for follow-up care and physical examinations while receiving estrogen therapy.

Ongoing Assessment and Evaluation

If the patient is a prepubescent girl, evaluate for normal sexual development with therapy and monitor the patient's growth as appropriate. Checking for evidence of early epiphyseal closure is essential. Monitor the postmenopausal woman for development of endometrial cancer (when estrogen is used alone) and ovarian or breast cancer (when estrogen is used in combination with progestin), as well as for cardiovascular complications. Therapy is considered effective when normal growth and sexual development occur, the symptoms of menopause are controlled, and the patient does not show any serious adverse effects from the drug therapy.

Drugs Closely Related to P Conjugated Estrogen

Contraceptives are combinations of estrogen and progesterone and are discussed later in the chapter. Synthetic conjugated estrogens (Cenestin) are very similar to conjugated estrogen. The major difference is that Cenestin is made of nine synthetic estrogen components obtained from plant material, whereas conjugated estrogen is derived from the urine of a pregnant mare. Cenestin is approved only for short-term use in treating vasomotor symptoms of menopause.

Drugs Significantly Different From P Conjugated Estrogen

Clomiphene

Clomiphene is an ovulation stimulant. This nonsteroidal agent promotes ovulation by indirectly increasing the output of the pituitary gonadotropins. Clomiphene binds to

CRITICAL THINKING SCENARIO

Individual decisions about hormone replacement therapy

Sue Rosario is 46 years old and is undergoing menopause. She reports that she hasn't slept well in the past 3 months because she awakens two or three times a night with such severe episodes of sweating that she has to get up and change her night clothes because they are soaked in perspiration. She states she is having trouble focusing at work, where she is a computer software engineer, because she is fatigued. Additionally, she often has severe hot flashes and episodes of sweating at work, which further impairs her ability to be productive. Her physician has ordered her a course of HRT to treat the menopausal symptoms. She discusses with you her concerns about taking HRT. She says, "I heard these drugs cause you to have a heart attack. Isn't this drug too dangerous to take?"

1. How will HRT be helpful to Sue at this time?
2. What points will you include in your patient education to help Sue understand the risks and benefits of HRT in her situation? Include what precautions should be used to minimize any risk she might incur.

MEMORY CHIP

P Conjugated Estrogen

- Used as hormone replacement when premenopausal endogenous levels of estrogen are low
- Used in combination with progesterone in oral contraceptives
- Used to treat moderate to severe symptoms of menopause (small dose, short duration of therapy)
- Major contraindications: most breast cancers, estrogen-dependent cancers, thrombophlebitis or thromboembolic disorders (active or history of), undiagnosed abnormal genital bleeding
- Most common adverse effects: menstrual cycle problems (breakthrough bleeding, changes in menstrual flow, dysmenorrheal, premenstrual-like syndrome, headache, nausea, vomiting, bloating, abdominal cramps, chloasma, and photosensitivity)
- Most serious adverse effects (when used alone): thromboembolic events, increased risk for stroke, increased risk for dementia or mild cognitive impairment, increased risk for endometrial cancer
- Most serious adverse effects (when used with progestin): increased risk for stroke, increased risk for coronary heart disease, increased risk for breast and ovarian cancers
- **Life span alert: pregnancy category X drug**
- Maximizing therapeutic effects: Administer cyclically.
- Minimizing adverse effects: Monitor for thrombophlebitis or thromboembolism; minimize dose and duration of therapy (in postmenopausal women); monitor bone growth for early epiphyseal growth plate closure (in prepubescent girls).
- Most important patient education: Report signs and symptoms of thrombophlebitis or thromboembolism at once; benefits and risks of postmenopausal HRT.

estrogenic receptors, preventing estrogen from binding. The hypothalamus and pituitary gland interpret this development as indicative of low estrogen levels and respond by increasing secretion of LH, FSH, and gonadotropins, thus stimulating ovulation. Clomiphene is used in treating ovulatory failure in patients who want to become pregnant and have a fertile partner. Use of clomiphene increases the chance of multiple pregnancy, although most births are single births. Clomiphene therapy is not effective in primary pituitary or ovarian failure. Clomiphene is administered orally. Hot flashes are the most common adverse effect; they are usually not severe and disappear after treatment stops.

Gonadotropins and Menotropins

The gonadotropins are preparations of FSH. Follitropin alpha and follitropin beta are human FSH preparations made using recombinant DNA technology. Urofollitropin is an FSH preparation extracted from the urine of postmenopausal women. Menotropins, purified preparations also made from the urine of postmenopausal women, are biologically standardized for FSH and LH activity. All of these drugs stimulate ovarian follicular growth in women who do not have primary ovarian failure yet do not experience an endogenous surge in LH level. They must be administered in conjunction with, but slightly before, HCG to induce ovulation (see below for discussion of HCG). HCG is administered after it has been determined by laboratory analysis that sufficient follicular development has occurred. The gonadotropins are also used in follicle stimulation for women being treated with assisted reproduction technologies, such as in vitro fertilization. Urofollitropin is used to induce ovulation in women with polycystic ovary disease who are unresponsive to clomiphene therapy. Menotropins with HCG are also given to men with primary or secondary hypogonadism to stimulate spermatogenesis.

Overstimulation of the ovary occurs in approximately 20% of women receiving therapy with gonadotropins, resulting in mild to moderate uncomplicated ovarian enlargement with or without abdominal distention or pain. A more severe condition, ovarian hyperstimulation syndrome, may occur and result in severe ovarian enlargement, abdominal pain and distention, nausea, vomiting, diarrhea, dyspnea, and oliguria. Ascites, pleural effusion, hypovolemia, electrolyte imbalance, hemoperitoneum, and thromboembolic events may also occur.

Use of follitropins is associated with multiple births, including triplets, quadruplets, and quintuplets. The incidence of multiple births is about 12% with follitropin alpha, 8% with follitropin beta, and 21% with urofollitropin. Singleton births still outnumber multiple births, however. Follitropin alpha and urofollitropin are administered by subcutaneous (SC) injection, follitropin beta is administered by SC or IM injection, and menotropins are administered by IM injection. All gonadotropins are in pregnancy category X. Adverse effects include vascular and pulmonary complications, ovarian enlargement, ovarian cysts, nausea, headaches, and sensitivity reactions.

Human Chorionic Gonadotropin

Human chorionic gonadotropin is a polypeptide hormone that stimulates the interstitial cells to produce androgens in male patients. In women, it can substitute for LH to trigger

ovulation. It is used to induce ovulation in females after pretreatment with follitropins or menotropins. It is also used to treat prepubertal cryptorchidism not resulting from anatomic obstruction and to treat hypogonadism in males. HCG is administered by IM injection. It is a pregnancy category X drug. Adverse effects include headache, irritability, edema, precocious puberty, and ovarian hyperstimulation syndrome.

Gonadotropin-Releasing Hormones

Gonadorelin acetate is a synthetic GRH used to induce ovulation in women with primary hypothalamic amenorrhea. The hypothalamus releases endogenous GRH in a pulsating manner. As discussed in the Physiology section of this chapter, GRH also helps to synthesize and promote the release of FSH and LH. FSH and LH stimulate the gonads to produce steroids necessary for reproductive processes. Gonadorelin acetate works similarly. It is administered by a special pump, a Lutrepulse pump, through an IV line. Gonadorelin acetate may cause multiple pregnancy, ovarian hyperstimulation syndrome, and anaphylaxis.

Nafarelin acetate is a potent agonistic analogue of GRH and stimulates the release of FSH and LH from the pituitary. Repeated dosing abolishes the stimulatory effect on the pituitary gland and leads to decreased secretion of FSH and LH. Therefore, tissues and body functions that depend on gonadal steroids for their maintenance become inactive. Nafarelin acetate is used to treat endometriosis and central precocious puberty of children of both sexes. When used in children with precocious puberty, nafarelin causes the LH and sex steroid hormone levels to remain at prepubertal levels. This effect arrests development of secondary sexual characteristics and slows linear growth and skeletal maturation. Nafarelin acetate is a pregnancy category X drug. It is administered as a nasal spray. Adverse effects are hypoestrogenic (hot flashes, decreased libido, vaginal dryness) and androgenic (acne, myalgia, reduced breast size, edema) effects. An additional adverse effect is nasal irritation.

Histrelin acetate is a synthetic nonapeptide agonist of naturally occurring GRH and is more potent than GRH. Histrelin acetate acts similarly to nafarelin acetate in initially stimulating and then suppressing release of FSH and LH. Like nafarelin, histrelin is used to control central precocious puberty in boys and girls. Common adverse effects are vasodilation, headache, dermatologic reactions at the medication site, vaginal dryness, and dyspepsia.

Gonadotropin-Releasing Hormone Antagonist

Ganirelix inhibits the premature LH surges in women undergoing controlled ovarian hyperstimulation as part of treatment for infertility. It suppresses natural gonadotropin secretion. When gonadotropin is suppressed, LH and FSH secretion by the pituitary are suppressed—LH more so than FSH. After starting FSH therapy on day 2 or 3 of the menstrual cycle, begin daily SC injections of ganirelix. Continue with therapy until the day that HCG is to be administered, as determined by follicular development. Ganirelix is packaged in a container with a natural rubber stopper and should not be given to patients with latex allergies. It is a pregnancy category X drug and will cause resorption of fetal contents if administered to a pregnant woman. Confirm that the patient is not pregnant before administering this drug.

Androgen-Estrogen Combination Drugs and Synthetic Androgens

Androgen-estrogen combination drugs are indicated for treating moderate to severe vasomotor symptoms associated with menopause (e.g., hot flashes) if estrogen use alone has been ineffective. Effects are similar to those of each hormone individually. See Chapter 53 for a discussion of the effects of testosterone.

Danazol (Danocrine) is a synthetic androgen with weak, dose-related androgenic effects. Its similarities to testosterone are limited. Danazol suppresses pituitary ovarian response by inhibiting pituitary gonadotropins. It is used to treat endometriosis because it inactivates and atrophies the normal and ectopic endometrial tissue. It is also used in treating fibrocystic breast disease when pain and tenderness are severe enough to warrant suppression of ovarian function. Danazol is also used prophylactically for hereditary angioedema. Three unlabeled uses include treatment of precocious puberty, gynecomastia, and menorrhagia.

Adverse effects are mostly androgenic and hypoestrogenic (flushing, sweating, vaginitis, nervousness, emotional lability); they also include hepatic dysfunction. Like testosterone, danazol can cause masculinization in the female fetus.

C PROGESTINS

Progestins consist of progesterone and its derivatives. Through stimulation or inhibition, they regulate secretion of pituitary gonadotropins, which in turn regulates development of the ovarian follicle. Progestins also inhibit spontaneous uterine contractions.

The prototype progestin is progesterone (Prometrium, Crinone). Other drugs in this class are medroxyprogesterone (Cycrin, Provera, Amen, Curretab), hydroxyprogesterone (Hylutin), and norethindrone acetate (Aygestin). Closely related drugs are levonorgestrel (Norplant), intrauterine progesterone (Progestasert), and contraceptives including oral contraceptives, emergency oral contraceptives, and other combination hormone contraceptives. Drugs significantly different from progesterone are megestrol acetate (Megace) and mifepristone (Mifeprex). Table 54.2 provides a summary of selected progestins.

NURSING MANAGEMENT OF THE PATIENT RECEIVING P PROGESTERONE

Core Drug Knowledge

Pharmacotherapeutics

Progesterone helps produce normal menstrual cycles in patients with amenorrhea and stops dysfunctional uterine bleeding. These seemingly opposite uses are possible because of the timing of drug administration and the drug's pharmacodynamics (see Table 54.2). Progesterone is also added to postmenopausal HRT to decrease the risk for endometrial cancer from estrogen therapy. It may be added cyclically (i.e., for so many days in every cycle) or daily. The exact dose and the preferred number of days the drug is given in a month

TABLE 54.2 Summary of Selected (C) Progestins

Drug (Trade) Name	Selected Indications	Route and Dosage Range	Pharmacokinetics
(P) progesterone (Gesterol)	Amenorrhea Abnormal uterine bleeding	*Adult:* IM, 5–10 mg/d for 6–8 d	*Onset:* Varies *Duration:* Unknown $t_{1/2}$: Unknown
medroxyprogesterone (Provera, Depo-Provera [IM])	Amenorrhea Abnormal uterine bleeding Contraception Inoperable recurrent endometrial or renal cell cancer	*Adult:* PO, 5–10 mg/d for 5–10 d *Adult:* IM, 150 mg q 3 months *Adult:* IM, 400 mg–1g q week	*Onset:* Unknown *Duration:* Unknown $t_{1/2}$: Unknown
megestrol (Megace)	Breast cancer, palliative Endometrial cancer, palliative Appetite enhancement in AIDS patients	*Adult:* PO, 400–800 mg/d	*Onset:* Unknown *Duration:* Unknown $t_{1/2}$: Unknown
levonorgestrel implants (Norplant)	Prevention of pregnancy	*Adult:* Insertion of six capsules, each containing 36 mg levonorgestrel	*Onset:* Slow *Duration:* Up to 5 y $t_{1/2}$: Unknown
intrauterine progesterone (Progestasert)	Prevention of pregnancy	*Adult:* Insertion of a single system into the uterine cavity; contains 38 mg progesterone	*Onset:* Unknown *Duration:* 1 y $t_{1/2}$: None

(if dosing is cyclic) are still unknown, and research continues in this area.

Pharmacokinetics

Progesterone is absorbed rapidly, whether administration is oral or by IM injection. Hepatic transformation is rapid; metabolites are present in the bloodstream for several days. Nonmetabolized progesterone and the metabolites of progesterone are excreted in the urine. Progesterone crosses the placenta and enters breast milk.

Pharmacodynamics

Exogenous progesterone will affect the body in ways similar to endogenous progesterone. When the ovarian follicle creates the corpus luteum, progesterone is produced. Progesterone changes the endometrium from its proliferative phase into its secretory stage. When levels of progesterone (in combination with estrogen) are high enough, a signal is sent to the pituitary gonadotropins to stop producing FSH and LH, thus preventing further ovulation. Progesterone is necessary to increase endometrial receptivity for implantation of an embryo. Once the embryo is implanted, progesterone helps maintain the pregnancy. If pregnancy does not occur, the corpus luteum will disintegrate, progesterone levels will fall, the pituitary gonadotropins will be stimulated, and more FSH and LH will be produced, causing ovulation again. Progesterone also inhibits spontaneous uterine contractions and contractions of other smooth muscles in the body, but because of its potential teratogenic effects, its use to prevent spontaneous abortion (miscarriage) is not recommended. Progesterone has some anabolic or androgenic activity, although it is minor.

Progesterone decreases the risk for endometrial cancer in postmenopausal women receiving estrogen. Progesterone, when combined with estrogen, increases bone mineral density and reduces the risk for fracture (Cauley et al., 2003). However, the risks of therapy outweigh these benefits in treating osteoporosis.

Contraindications and Precautions

Progesterone is contraindicated in patients with hypersensitivity to progestins. It is also contraindicated for patients with thrombophlebitis, thromboembolic disorder, cerebral hemorrhage, or a history of any of these conditions. Further contraindications include impaired liver function or disease, carcinoma of the breast or genital organs, undiagnosed vaginal bleeding, or missed abortion. Progesterone is a pregnancy category D drug, and its use during pregnancy has led to fetal abnormalities, including masculinization of the female fetus. It passes into breast milk, although the effect on the infant remains undetermined.

Caution should be used in patients with pathologies that may be adversely affected by fluid retention (epilepsy, migraine headaches, asthma, cardiac dysfunction, or renal dysfunction). Patients who have a history of depression should be observed carefully for signs of this disorder while taking progesterone. Photosensitivity may occur with use of this drug. The benzyl alcohol that some of these products contain may produce a fatal gasping syndrome if given to premature infants.

Adverse Effects

Recent research from the Women's Health Initiative indicates that progesterone may increase the risk for breast and ovarian cancer when given in combination with estrogen to postmenopausal women (Chlebowski et al., 2003; Anderson et al., 2003).

Common adverse effects include breakthrough bleeding, spotting, change in menstrual flow, amenorrhea, changes in cervical secretions, breast tenderness, changes in weight, and nausea. Uncommon but serious adverse effects include sudden partial or complete loss of eyesight, thrombophlebitis, mental depression, and cholestatic jaundice. Progesterone is irritating at the injection site; the aqueous form is especially painful.

Drug Interactions

No known drug interactions are associated with progesterone. Progesterone, however, may affect results of the following laboratory tests: hepatic function, coagulation (decrease in prothrombin and factors VII, VIII, IX, and X), thyroid, metyrapone, and endocrine function.

Assessment of Relevant Core Patient Variables

Health Status

Assess for conditions that contraindicate use of progesterone: a history of or current thrombophlebitis, thromboembolic disorder, and cerebral hemorrhage; impaired liver function or disease; depression; and undiagnosed vaginal bleeding. Before progesterone treatment, a complete physical examination is required, including assessment of the breasts and pelvic organs. A Papanicolaou test should be performed. Assess the patient's menstrual cycles for irregularities. All vaginal bleeding should be diagnosed carefully before therapy starts.

Life Span and Gender

Assess the patient for pregnancy or intention to become pregnant because progesterone is associated with genital and congenital abnormalities when exposure occurs in the first 4 gestational months. Genital abnormalities include masculinization of the genital organs in the female fetus and hypospadias in the male fetus. Congenital abnormalities include congenital heart defects and limb reduction defects. If the patient is in the later stages of pregnancy, progesterone might be used to halt premature labor. Assess whether the patient is breast-feeding because progesterone's effects on the infant are unknown. Progesterone may be added to postmenopausal HRT.

Environment

Caution patients about exposure to ultraviolet light. Be aware of the environment in which progesterone will be administered. Progesterone may be administered in any environment, including the home, if the patient or family member has learned to administer an IM injection correctly.

Nursing Diagnoses and Outcomes

- Disturbed Body Image related to potential breakthrough bleeding, spotting, changes in menstrual flow, weight gain, or breast tenderness secondary to adverse effects of drug therapy
  Desired outcome: *The patient will not experience substantial adverse effects from drug therapy to alter body image.*
- Risk for Injury related to loss of vision, onset of thrombotic disorders, and depression secondary to adverse effects of drug therapy
  Desired outcome: *The patient will not suffer an injury related to adverse effects of drug therapy.*

Planning and Intervention

Maximizing Therapeutic Effects

The dosing schedule varies depending on the clinical indication for using progesterone. In treating amenorrhea, the drug should be administered for 6 to 8 consecutive days. For treating dysfunctional uterine bleeding, the drug should be administered daily for 6 days. The best dosing schedule when progesterone is used in HRT is currently unknown.

Minimizing Adverse Effects

You can take steps to minimize the adverse effects of progesterone therapy. To avoid risk for injury to the fetus, do not administer the drug to any woman who is in the first 4 months of pregnancy. Postmenopausal dosage should be the minimum effective dose to decrease risk for endometrial cancer while limiting any increased risk for breast or ovarian cancer. Assessment throughout therapy for signs and symptoms of breast or ovarian cancer is essential. Do not give progesterone to patients with a history of or active thrombophlebitis, thromboembolic disorders, breast cancer, ovarian cancer, or cerebral hemorrhage because these conditions are possible adverse effects of therapy. Therapy must be discontinued at the first sign of any of these conditions. Carefully monitor patients who may be adversely affected by fluid retention. Therapy also must be discontinued if excessive fluid retention places patients at risk in their primary disease or disorder.

Providing Patient and Family Education

- Instruct patients and their families on the therapeutic and adverse effects of progesterone.
- Teach patients how to perform breast self-examination.
- Teach patients to notify the prescriber if they suspect that they are pregnant or if sudden loss of vision, severe headache, or numbness in an arm or leg occurs.
- Inform the patient who is using the vaginal gel form of progesterone that it is the only intravaginal therapy she should be using. If she requires other intravaginal therapy, administration should be at least 6 hours before or after progesterone gel. If indicated, discuss with the patient how to time self-administration of intravaginal therapies.

Ongoing Assessment and Evaluation

Monitor premenopausal women for return of normal menstrual flow and cessation of abnormal bleeding. If amenorrhea or dysfunctional uterine bleeding is corrected without adverse effects, the drug therapy has been effective. Assess postmenopausal women throughout therapy for signs or symptoms of breast or ovarian cancer. Combination therapies of estrogen and a progestin (e.g., progesterone) are effective in the postmenopausal woman if they relieve symptoms while avoiding serious adverse effects.

Drugs Closely Related to P Progesterone

Levonorgestrel implants (Norplant system) and intrauterine progesterone systems (Progestasert, Mirena) are unique forms of progesterone. Their main effects on the body and reproductive system are the same as those of other forms of progesterone. Like progesterone in combined estrogen-progestin oral contraceptives, these drugs are used solely to prevent

MEMORY CHIP

P Progesterone

- Used to treat amenorrhea to help produce normal menstrual cycles, to stop dysfunctional uterine bleeding, or as part of postmenopausal HRT to decrease risk for endometrial cancer
- Used in combination with estrogen in oral contraceptives
- Major contraindications: thrombophlebitis, thromboembolic disorder, cerebral hemorrhage (current or history of), breast or genital organ cancer, undiagnosed vaginal bleeding, and missed abortion
- Most common adverse effects: menstrual irregularities (breakthrough bleeding, spotting, change in menstrual flow, amenorrhea, changes in cervical secretions, breast tenderness, changes in weight, and nausea)
- Most serious adverse effects (when used alone): thrombophlebitis, thromboembolism
- Most serious adverse effects (when used with progestin): increased risk for stroke, increased risk for coronary heart disease, increased risk for breast and ovarian cancers
- **Life span alert: pregnancy category D drug**
- Maximizing therapeutic effects: Dosing schedule will vary based on clinical indication for drug.
- Minimizing adverse effects: Minimize dose and duration of therapy in postmenopausal women.
- Most important patient education: In premenopausal women, report serious adverse effects at once; in postmenopausal women, perform breast self-examination.

pregnancy. The major difference is in their route of administration and length of effectiveness. The oral contraceptives—estrogen-progestin combination drugs—also are closely related to progesterone and are discussed fully in the section on estrogen-progestin combination drugs.

Levonorgestrel Implant

Levonorgestrel implants consist of six flexible closed capsules made of a synthetic material (Silastic). Each capsule contains 36 mg of levonorgestrel. The capsules are implanted subdermally in the midportion of the upper arm, about 8 to 10 cm above the antecubital space, in a fan-like pattern. Diffusion of levonorgestrel through the capsules provides continuous, slow release of progesterone to prevent pregnancy for up to 5 years. The capsules may be removed at any time to reverse the contraceptive effect. A new set of capsules may be placed after the initial 5 years if the woman desires continued contraceptive protection.

Intrauterine Progesterone Systems

Intrauterine progesterone inserts (Progestaserts) are T-shaped units filled with progesterone. They are placed in the uterine cavity for 1 year by a health care provider; the system must be replaced 1 year after insertion. Its exact mechanism of action is unknown. The progesterone is thought to inhibit the survival of sperm or alter the uterine environment to prevent implantation. Suppression of endometrial tissue proliferation is one known progestational influence of the insert on the endometrium.

Adverse effects of the intrauterine progesterone inserts are unique to the administration route and may be severe. They include increased risk for septic abortion or congenital anomalies if pregnancy does occur, increased risk for pelvic inflammatory disease, device embedment in the endometrium, perforation of the uterine wall or cervix by the device, endometritis, vaginitis, midcycle spotting, increased menstrual flow, pain, cramping, and amenorrhea.

The levonorgestrel-releasing intrauterine system (Mirena) is also placed in the uterine cavity by a health care provider. It provides birth control for up to 5 years. Adverse effects are similar to the intrauterine inserts left in place for 1 year.

Drugs Significantly Different From P Progesterone

Megestrol

Megestrol (Megace) is a progestin-like progesterone and shares many of progesterone's qualities and characteristics. The two drugs differ mostly in their pharmacotherapeutic effects. Unlike progesterone, megestrol is used as palliative treatment for patients with advanced breast or endometrial cancer (tablet form) or to increase appetite in patients with acquired immunodeficiency syndrome (AIDS) (suspension form). Exactly how megestrol increases appetite in patients with AIDS who have anorexia and cachexia is unknown. The resulting weight gain is not related to water retention. Megestrol is not used as part of HRT in postmenopausal women. Its contraindications are similar to those of progesterone. Safety and efficacy of megestrol acetate therapy in children have not been established.

Mifepristone

Mifepristone (Mifeprex) is used to end an early pregnancy (defined as 49 days or less from the start of the last menstrual period). It competes with progesterone for binding at the progesterone-receptor sites and is a progesterone antagonist. Mifepristone inhibits the activity of endogenous and exogenous progesterone, resulting in termination of pregnancy. Mifepristone also has antiglucocorticoid and weak antiandrogenic effects. Compensatory elevation of adrenocorticotropic hormone (ACTH) and cortisol levels have been observed in some patients. Animal studies have indicated some antiandrogenic effects with large doses, but no studies have been done on this effect in humans. Mifepristone is rapidly absorbed. It is highly protein bound and is metabolized by the CYP3A4 pathway in the liver. Most mifepristone is excreted in the feces.

Mifepristone, although effective for most women who use it, may result in an incomplete medical abortion, necessitating surgical intervention. Mifepristone may also fail to initiate an abortion or produce substantial vaginal bleeding; either of these events may also require a surgical procedure. Between 1% and 5% of women will require a surgical procedure related to one of these problems. For this reason, the FDA has established very specific and unique requirements in the United States for the use of mifepristone. Although it is a prescription drug, mifepristone is not available in pharmacies. Instead, it is distributed directly to physicians, who can determine the duration of a patient's pregnancy through menstrual history and clinical examination and are able to detect an ectopic pregnancy. Ultrasonographic scanning should be used if the duration of pregnancy is uncertain or if ectopic pregnancy is suspected. Physicians must be able to

provide surgical intervention in cases of incomplete abortion or severe bleeding, or they must have pre-established plans for providing such care through others. Some states allow nurse practitioners or nurse midwives who work closely with physicians to be authorized prescribers of mifepristone.

Drug therapy with mifepristone should not be used if the patient cannot return or is unwilling to return to the physician's office for two follow-up visits. It also should not be administered to patients who do not have adequate access in the following 2 weeks to medical facilities equipped for emergency treatment of incomplete abortion, blood transfusion, and emergency resuscitation. The prescriber must give the patient the FDA Written Medication Guide for mifepristone and discuss the information thoroughly. The Medication Guide contains FDA-approved information written especially for patients. Medication Guides accompany drugs that the FDA has determined to pose a serious risk; appropriate patient education reduces the risk. The patient must sign an agreement before receiving treatment.

After the patient meets all the baseline requirements, she swallows three tablets of mifepristone in the physician's or other provider's office. This visit is considered Day 1. At Day 3, the woman returns to the provider's office to determine whether she is still pregnant. If medical abortion is incomplete, the woman takes two tablets of misoprostol. (Misoprostol is a different drug, a synthetic prostaglandin E_1 analogue. Although it is used to prevent gastric ulcers resulting from the use of nonsteroidal anti-inflammatory drugs [NSAIDs], it also is known to have abortifacient properties, by producing uterine contractions. See Chapter 48 for more information on the antiulcer properties of misoprostol.) In clinical trials, about 44% of women who took misoprostol following mifepristone expelled the products of conception within 4 hours; approximately 63% expelled them within 24 hours after the misoprostol dose. The patient returns to the provider's office at Day 14 to verify complete ending of the pregnancy. Although bleeding itself is not proof that the pregnancy has been terminated, lack of bleeding indicates that the therapy was ineffective in causing a medical abortion. If the pregnancy has not been completely terminated, surgical intervention to end the pregnancy is recommended. Pregnancies that are carried to term after use of mifepristone may result in fetal deformities.

Contraindications for using mifepristone are a pregnancy that has lasted longer than 49 days since the start of the last menstrual period; confirmed or suspected ectopic pregnancy; intrauterine device (IUD) in place (which must be removed before drug therapy begins); chronic adrenal failure; concurrent long-term corticosteroid therapy; bleeding disorders or use of anticoagulant drugs; allergy to mifepristone, misoprostol, or other prostaglandins; and inherited porphyrias (rare inherited disturbances in porphyrin metabolism that may cause hemolytic anemia and splenomegaly).

The most common adverse effects of mifepristone are heavy vaginal bleeding, abdominal pain, and uterine cramping. Most women will have vaginal bleeding or spotting for 9 to 16 days after ending the pregnancy; some women will bleed for 30 days or more. Vaginal bleeding may be severe enough to warrant blood transfusion, treatment with vasoconstrictor or uterotonic drugs, surgical intervention, or IV fluids. Other common adverse effects include nausea, vomiting, and diarrhea. Pelvic pain, fainting, headache, dizziness, and muscle weakness may also occur, but they are rare. Reported adverse effects decrease after day 3 and are rare by day 14, except for complaints of bleeding and spotting.

Specific drug or food interactions with mifepristone have not been studied; however, because as the CYP3A4 pathway metabolizes this drug, other drugs that are metabolized by or inhibit metabolism from this pathway may produce a drug interaction.

Mifepristone does not prevent subsequent pregnancies. The patient should resume contraception after verifying that the pregnancy has been completely eliminated or before resuming sexual activity.

CONTRACEPTIVES

Contraceptives are forms of estrogen and progesterone, usually in combination. They are administered orally and through a number of different other routes (Box 54.2).

(C) Oral Contraceptives

The oral contraceptives are closely related to both estrogen and progestin because they contain varying amounts of these drugs in combination. A very few oral contraceptives contain progestins only. Oral contraceptives are given to prevent pregnancy; the patient's cultural beliefs may affect their use because some cultures and religions do not support interference with reproduction. Combination oral contraceptives inhibit ovulation by suppressing the gonadotropins FSH and LH. In addition, oral contraceptives alter the quality of cervical and other mucus in the female genital tract (inhibiting sperm penetration) and change the characteristics of the endometrium (reducing the likelihood of implantation). These drug effects may also assist in preventing pregnancy.

Oral contraceptives differ in the type and relative strength (potency) of their components and the relative dominance of estrogen or progesterone activity. Their ultimate effect is

COMMUNITY-BASED CONCERNS

Box 54.2 Contraceptives and Sexually Transmitted Diseases

Women who use any of the hormonal contraceptives are protected against pregnancy. Pregnancy can also be prevented with over-the-counter preparations that are spermicides, although they are not as effective in preventing pregnancy as the hormonal contraceptives are. None of these contraceptives protect women from sexually transmitted diseases, such as syphilis, gonorrhea, chlamydia, or HIV. Barrier protection from a condom is needed to prevent the transmission of the bacteria or viruses that cause these diseases. Condoms may be used with any of the other contraceptives. After ejaculation, care must be taken not to allow the semen to spill out of the condom during withdrawal of the penis from the vagina.

related to combined activity. Progestin-only oral contraceptives prevent pregnancy in a way that is not clearly understood. They are known to alter the cervical mucus and exert a progestational effect on the endometrium, which apparently produces cellular changes that render the endometrium hostile to implantation of a fertilized egg. In some patients, the effects of progestin also prevent ovulation.

The three types of combination oral contraceptives are as follows:

- Monophasic: the dose of estrogen and progestin remains the same throughout the entire cycle.
- Biphasic: the amount of estrogen remains the same, but the amount of progestin rises in the second half of the cycle.
- Triphasic: estrogen amounts remain the same or may vary throughout the cycle, whereas progestin varies throughout the cycle.

Some serious adverse effects may occur with oral contraceptive use. These effects are usually related to high doses of estrogen in the drug. Oral contraceptives should be prescribed with the smallest effective dose of estrogen possible; thus, high-dose estrogen formulations are prescribed infrequently, usually only when a lower dose has been ineffective. Dose-related serious adverse effects include thromboembolism, stroke, MI, hepatic lesions, and gallbladder disease. The risk for cardiovascular and cerebrovascular effects is substantially increased in women age 35 years or older with other risk factors (e.g., smoking, uncontrolled hypertension, hypercholesterolemia, elevated low-density lipoprotein (LDL) cholesterol, obesity, and diabetes). Mortality rates associated with circulatory disease have been shown to increase substantially in smokers older than 35 years and in nonsmokers older than 40 years.

In addition, a decrease in glucose tolerance has been observed in a small percentage of patients on estrogen-progestin combination drugs; the mechanism appears to be related to estrogen dose. Elevated blood pressure may be related to the use of oral contraceptives and is believed to result from estrogen and progesterone effects. Other adverse effects are related to the dosage of estrogen and progestin and reflect the individual adverse effects of these drugs. Lower doses minimize these effects, which include breakthrough bleeding (transitory), spotting, amenorrhea during and after treatment, breast tenderness, nausea and vomiting (usually transitory), steepening of the corneal curvature, contact lens intolerance, weight gain or loss, edema, migraine, elevated triglyceride levels, and depression.

Oral contraceptives are known to interact with the penicillins and the tetracyclines (both classes of antimicrobials). This drug interaction decreases the level of circulating hormones, and contraceptive failure may result. Although the interaction is well documented with these classes of antimicrobials, it can potentially occur with other antimicrobials as well. Women should be cautioned about this potential lack of effectiveness and encouraged to use another form of birth control while they are taking a penicillin or a tetracycline. A small recent study showed a drug interaction between oral contraceptives and St. John's wort, an over-the-counter (OTC) herb used as an antidepressant (Hall et al., 2003). St. John's wort induces the P-450 system, specifically the CYP3A isoenzymes. It was found to substantially increase the clearance rate of the oral contraceptive used in the study, suggesting that the effectiveness of oral contraceptives is likely to be diminished with concurrent use of St. John's wort. Patients should be cautioned that they may experience some breakthrough bleeding if they use this combination. They should also be counseled to use a second form of birth control if they use St. John's wort while taking oral contraceptives.

For greatest effectiveness, the woman should take the oral contraceptive every day at the same time, such as with a particular meal or at bedtime. Packets have either 21 or 28 pills. The last 7 pills in the 28-day pack are inert and do not contain hormones. If the woman is using a 21-pill pack, she takes one pill daily for 21 days and then no pill for 7 days. If she is using the 28-day pack, she takes one pill every day. Patients may follow one of several regimens for beginning a cycle. The patient should refer to the package insert with each preparation. If the woman misses one dose, she should take the next dose as soon thereafter as possible; a woman may take two tablets on the same day. If a woman misses two doses, she should make up two missed pills over 2 days. If she misses three consecutive pills, she may not have adequate birth control protection. At that point, she has two choices for how to proceed. She can either begin a new cycle pack as soon as she realizes that she has missed 3 days' worth of pills, or she can wait until it has been 7 days since she last took a pill and then begin a new cycle pack. She should use another form of birth control as a backup for at least the first 7 consecutive days after starting a new cycle pack and preferably for the entire new cycle.

A new form of combination oral contraceptive is taken daily for 84 days followed by 7 days of no pills. The menstrual period therefore occurs only once every 3 months, or 4 times a year. The trade name for this form of oral contraceptive is Seasonale.

If a woman misses a menstrual period while on any form of oral contraceptive, she should be evaluated for pregnancy. Oral contraceptives should be withheld until pregnancy is ruled out because of possible damage to the fetus if the woman takes the drug during early pregnancy.

Mothers who do not breast-feed may begin use of oral contraceptives 4 to 6 weeks after delivery even if they have not resumed spontaneous menstrual periods. Oral contraceptives are not recommended in breast-feeding women, although they may be used carefully if absolutely necessary.

A new choice of oral contraceptive is now available for women. Ovcon 35 is the first chewable oral contraceptive. It is spearmint flavored and is chewed and then swallowed. To guarantee that the entire dose reaches the stomach, it should be followed with a glass of water after chewing the tablet. It can also be swallowed whole. Like other oral contraceptives, Ovcon 35 contains a progestin (norethindrone) and an estrogen (ethinyl estradiol) and therefore has the same risks for adverse effects. Ovcon 35 comes in 28-day packs with 21 white active pills and 7 green inert pills.

Emergency Oral Contraceptives

Emergency oral contraceptives are available as either a progestin-only product (Plan B) or a combination of progestin and estrogen (Preven). The drug is used to prevent pregnancy

after unprotected sexual intercourse or a known or suspected contraceptive failure. The first dose should be taken as soon as possible after intercourse; the drug is most effective if taken within 24 hours of unprotected sex but may be taken up to 72 hours after the event. The second dose is taken 12 hours after the first. The two forms of emergency contraception are equally effective in preventing pregnancy when taken as directed. Emergency contraceptive pills are not used for routine contraception. Some debate exists as to whether this form of contraception should be available as an OTC medication.

Other Combination Hormone Contraceptives

Norelgestromin/Ethinyl Estradiol Transdermal System

The norelgestromin/ethinyl estradiol transdermal system is similar to oral contraceptives in that it is a combination of a progestin and an estrogen. Unlike oral contraceptives, the combination of hormones is administered topically from a patch that releases the drugs. Efficacy in preventing pregnancy and adverse effects is similar to oral contraceptives. Like 21-day cycle packs of oral contraceptives, the transdermal system is designed to be used for 3 weeks and then not used for 1 week, creating a 4-week cycle. A new patch is applied weekly on the same day of the week for three consecutive weeks. During the fourth week, no patch is applied. Menstruation will begin during this week, when the woman is not wearing a patch.

The first time a woman uses the norelgestromin/ethinyl estradiol transdermal system, she should start it after her menstrual period begins. She can choose to apply the first patch either the day her period starts or the following Sunday. If she chooses the Sunday after the start of her period, she needs to use backup contraception for the first week of her first cycle (unless there is no delay in starting the method because the start of the menstrual period is on a Sunday). Directions for applying the patch are as follows:

- Choose a site to apply the patch on clean, dry, intact, healthy skin on the buttocks, abdomen, upper outer arm, or upper torso. Do not place on the breasts. The patch should be placed so that it will not be rubbed by tight clothing.
- Avoid using makeup, creams, lotions, powders, or other topical products on the site where the patch will be placed.
- Peel apart the foil pouch that contains the patch and open flat. Grasp a corner of the patch and gently remove it from the pouch.
- Using a fingernail, lift one corner of the patch, removing both the patch and the plastic liner from the foil liner.
- Peel away half of the clear plastic protective liner. Care should be taken to avoid touching the sticky surface of the patch.
- Apply the sticky surface of the patch to the skin and then remove the other half of the backing.
- Press down on the patch with the palm for 10 seconds to guarantee that the edges stick well to the skin.
- Change the patch weekly, using a new location for each patch. Before discarding the used patch, fold it in half so that it sticks to itself and seals in any active hormone remaining in the patch.

If the patch comes off and remains off for less than 24 hours, it can be reapplied if still sticky, or it can be replaced with a new patch. If the patch has been off for more than 24 hours, a new 4-week cycle must be started immediately and the "Day 1" patch from a new packet applied. Backup contraception should be used for the first week of the new cycle. If a woman forgets to replace a patch at the start of a new cycle (the end of week 4), she should apply the new week "Day 1" patch as soon as she remembers and use backup contraception for the first week. Birth control is not guaranteed if more than 7 days elapse without wearing a patch. In that case, backup birth control is needed.

If the woman forgets to change the patch for up to 48 hours at the end of week 1 or 2, she should change the patch as soon as she remembers. No backup contraception is needed in this situation. If more than 48 hours have elapsed, she should stop the current cycle and start a new 4-week cycle. Backup contraception should be used for the first week. If she forgets to remove the patch at the end of the third week, she should remove it as soon as possible. The first patch of the next cycle should be applied on the usual patch change day.

Etonogestrel/Ethinyl Estradiol Vaginal Ring

The etonogestrel/ethinyl estradiol vaginal ring (NuvaRing) is another combination of progestin and estrogen used for contraception. It has actions and adverse effects similar to those of the norelgestromin/ethinyl estradiol transdermal system. It is inserted into the vagina by the woman, left in place for 3 weeks, and then removed for 1 week. The drug is absorbed through the mucous membranes of the vagina and into the vascular system. Exact placement of the ring inside the vagina is not critical for effective birth control. The ring is removed by hooking the index finger under the forward rim of the ring or by grasping the rim between the index and middle finger and pulling it out. Removed rings should be wrapped in the foil pouch and discarded in the trash; they should not be flushed down the toilet. Menstruation will follow after the ring is removed, usually 2 or 3 days later.

C BISPHOSPHONATES

The bisphosphonate drug class affects normal and abnormal bone resorption. The prototype is alendronate (Fosamax). Drugs closely related to alendronate are risedronate, tiludronate, etidronate, and pamidronate. A significantly different drug is raloxifene. Table 54.3 provides a summary of selected drugs used to treat bone resorption.

TABLE 54.3 Summary of Selected C Drugs Used to Treat Bone Resorption

Drug (Trade) Name	Selected Indications	Route and Dosage Range	Pharmacokinetics
P alendronate (Fosamax)	Treat/prevent postmenopausal osteoporosis	PO, 10 mg/d	*Onset:* Slow *Duration:* Days $t_{1/2}$: Unknown
	Paget disease	PO, 40 mg/d for 6 mo	
etidronate (Didronel)	Paget disease	PO, 5–10 mg/kg/d not to exceed 6 months	*Onset:* Slow for PO, rapid for IV *Duration:* Days $t_{1/2}$: 6 h in plasma; >90 d in bone
	Hypercalcemia of malignancy	IV, 7.5 mg/kg/d for 3 successive d diluted in at least 250 mL sterile normal saline	
pamidronate (Aredia)	Paget disease	IV, 30 mg diluted in 500 mL normal saline or 0.45% saline, infuse over 4 h for 3 consecutive d	*Onset:* Rapid *Duration:* Days $t_{1/2}$: biphasic in plasma 1.6 h, then 27.3 h
	Hypercalcemia of malignancy	IV, 60–90 mg as a single-dose infusion diluted in 1 L normal saline, 0.45% saline, or 5% dextrose. Infuse 60 mg over 4 h, 90 mg over 24 h	From bone up to 300 d
	Breast cancer with bone metastases	IV, 90 mg over 4 h every 3 to 4 wk in at least 500 mL	
risedronate (Actonel)	Paget disease	PO, 30 mg/d for 2 mo	*Onset:* Rapid *Duration:* Days $t_{1/2}$: Multiphasic, 1.5 to 220 h
tiludronate (Skelid)	Paget disease	PO: 400 mg active tiludronate/d (comes in 240 mg tablets each with 200 mg active drug) for 2 mo	*Onset:* Rapid *Duration:* Unknown $t_{1/2}$: Unknown

NURSING MANAGEMENT OF THE PATIENT RECEIVING P ALENDRONATE

Core Drug Knowledge

Pharmacotherapeutics

Alendronate is used to treat and prevent osteoporosis in postmenopausal women. Alendronate is also approved to treat men who have osteoporosis. Other uses (described in Chapter 50) are treating glucocorticoid-induced osteoporosis (in men and women) and treating patients with **Paget disease.** Paget disease is an idiopathic bone disease characterized by chronic, focal areas of bone destruction complicated by concurrent excessive bone repair. The result is thick but weak bones that may fracture or bend under stress.

Pharmacokinetics

Alendronate is absorbed orally. Food and beverages other than plain water can decrease its absorption and bioavailability by about 40%. After absorption, alendronate is stored in the skeleton and does not appear to be metabolized. It is excreted in the urine as it is slowly released from the skeleton.

Pharmacodynamics

The major action of alendronate is to inhibit both normal and abnormal bone resorption. Alendronate is a highly selective and potent inhibitor of bone resorption, which occurs following recruitment, activation, and polarization of osteoclasts. The exact mechanism of antiresorptive action is not fully understood but may be related to the inhibition of hydroxyapatite crystal dissolution or the drug's action on bone-resorbing cells. Reduction of abnormal bone resorption is responsible for reductions in serum calcium and phosphate concentrations. Alendronate greatly increases bone-mineral density (BMD) in patients with osteoporosis. Evidence of increased BMD is seen after 3 months of use and continues throughout therapy. Alendronate thus appears to reverse the progression of osteoporosis.

Contraindications and Precautions

Alendronate is contraindicated if the patient is hypocalcemic or hypersensitive to the drug or any of its components. It is also contraindicated if the patient has any abnormalities of the esophagus that delay esophageal emptying, such as stricture or inability of the esophagus to relax. Alendronate should not be used if the patient is unable to stand or sit upright for at least 30 minutes. Alendronate is not recommended for patients with severe renal insufficiency, which can cause increased accumulation of alendronate in the bone. Alendronate is a pregnancy category C drug. Animal studies show increases in maternal and fetal hypocalcemia and deaths; no studies have been done on pregnant women.

Alendronate is used in pregnancy only if benefits outweigh risks. Although it is unknown whether alendronate enters breast milk, based on the fetal risks determined from results of animal studies, the drug should not be given to breast-feeding mothers. Its safety and efficacy in children have not been established.

Recently, spontaneous osteonecrosis of the jaw has been reported in cancer patients who have received bisphosphonates as a component of their therapy. A dental examination with appropriate preventive dentistry should be considered before treatment with bisphosphonates in patients with concomitant risk factors (e.g., cancer, chemotherapy, corticosteroid therapy, or poor oral hygiene).

Adverse Effects

When given to treat osteoporosis, the most common adverse effect of alendronate is abdominal pain; musculoskeletal pain is also fairly common. Other adverse effects are flatulence, acid regurgitation, esophageal ulcer, abdominal distention, gastritis, headache, rash, and erythema (rare). GI irritation is more likely to occur if the patient does not take the drug with a full glass of water, or if the patient lies down after taking the drug. When given to treat Paget disease, alendronate increases the risk for upper GI symptoms; otherwise, the adverse effects are similar to use for osteoporosis.

Overdose of alendronate produces hypocalcemia, hypophosphatemia, and upper GI adverse effects. Administering milk or antacids to bind with the alendronate may be helpful in counteracting the effects of overdose, but dialysis is not beneficial. Otherwise, care is directed at treating the symptoms of overdosage.

Drug Interactions

Drug interactions are known to occur between alendronate and some other drugs. Because of potential interactions, the patient is recommended to wait at least 30 minutes after taking alendronate before taking any other drug. Table 54.4 lists drugs that interact with alendronate.

Assessment of Relevant Core Patient Variables

Health Status

Assess whether the patient has hypocalcemia or other disturbances in mineral metabolism, such as phosphate or vitamin D deficiency. These imbalances must be corrected before starting drug therapy with alendronate because alendronate may cause additional slight decreases in serum calcium and phosphate levels. Verify that the patient has a clinical indication for use of alendronate (e.g., treating or preventing osteoporosis or Paget disease) before beginning therapy. Also, assess for a family history of osteoporosis, which increases a woman's risk for developing osteoporosis. Assess for severe renal insufficiency as well because this condition may necessitate a dose reduction.

Life Span and Gender

Alendronate is used in postmenopausal women to treat or prevent osteoporosis; it may be used as treatment for all patients with Paget disease. Assess the patient for pregnancy or intention to become pregnant because alendronate is a pregnancy category C drug. Also, assess the patient's lactation status because administration to breast-feeding mothers must be avoided. Use of this drug in children requires caution because safety and efficacy have not been established. Older adults require no precautions or dosage adjustments.

Lifestyle, Diet, and Habits

Review the patient's normal eating habits because food and beverages (e.g., coffee, orange juice, and mineral water) will decrease absorption of alendronate. Verify that the patient's diet contains adequate intake of calcium and vitamin D. Patients who have a history of eating disorders, such as excessive dieting, have an increased risk for osteoporosis. Assess for normal weight-bearing exercise, which helps prevent osteoporosis. Also, ask the patient about smoking and alcohol consumption because these factors increase the risk for osteoporosis.

Environment

Be aware of the setting in which alendronate will be administered. Alendronate is normally self-administered in the home, although it could be given in any setting.

Culture and Inherited Traits

Asian and white women are at increased risk for osteoporosis.

Nursing Diagnoses and Outcomes

- Risk for Injury related to fractures from osteoporosis or Paget disease
  Desired outcome: *The patient using drug therapy will have no fractures.*

TABLE 54-4 Agents That Interact With [P] Alendronate

Interactants	Effect and Significance	Nursing Management
ranitidine	IV ranitidine doubles alendronate's bioavailability. Clinical significance is unknown.	Monitor for therapeutic and adverse effects.
calcium supplements, antacids	Products with calcium and other multivalent ions interfere with absorption of alendronate.	Separate doses of alendronate and calcium or antacids by 2 h.
aspirin	Coadministration increases risk of adverse effects in upper gastrointestinal system.	Monitor for adverse effects. If severe adverse effects develop, discontinue aspirin.

- Potential Complication: Electrolyte Imbalance related to drug therapy with alendronate
  Desired outcome: *The patient will not experience electrolyte imbalance.*
- Potential Complication: Altered GI Function related to adverse effects of drug therapy with alendronate
  Desired outcome: *The patient will experience either no or minimal adverse effects.*

Planning and Intervention

Maximizing Therapeutic Effects

Nursing actions to maximize therapeutic effects are related to patient education.

Minimizing Adverse Effects

To minimize adverse effects from hypocalcemia, take measures to correct pre-existing hypocalcemia before treatment. Monitor electrolyte levels throughout therapy as indicated. Other actions to minimize adverse effects are related to patient education.

Providing Patient and Family Education

- Teach the patient to take alendronate at least 30 minutes before eating, drinking any beverage other than plain water, or taking any other medication. The patient should swallow the medicine with 6 to 8 ounces (180–240 mL) of plain water, which improves absorption of the drug.
- Instruct the patient not to lie down for at least 30 minutes after swallowing alendronate, to decrease adverse GI effects.
- Encourage the patient to take supplemental calcium and vitamin D if dietary intake is inadequate to meet the needs of the bones. Calcium or vitamin D will decrease absorption of alendronate, however, if either is taken at the same time as alendronate. Instruct the patient to take alendronate at least 1 hour before taking calcium or vitamin D.
- Encourage the patient to make lifestyle changes that will benefit bone health, such as engaging in weight-bearing exercise (including walking as tolerated and permitted by the patient's physical condition), limiting or stopping cigarette smoking, and limiting or stopping alcohol use.

Ongoing Assessment and Evaluation

Verify throughout therapy that the patient is not experiencing hypocalcemia or other adverse effects from drug therapy. Therapy is effective when adverse effects are absent or minimal, bone mass density increases, and bone resorption and bone formation decrease.

MEMORY CHIP

P Alendronate

- Used to treat or prevent osteoporosis in postmenopausal women; also used to treat Paget disease
- Prevents bone resorption
- Major contraindication: hypocalcemia
- Most common adverse effects: GI problems
- Most serious adverse effect: hypocalcemia (uncommon)
- **Life span alert: used in postmenopausal women**
- Most important patient education: Take medication at least 30 minutes before eating, drinking, or taking other medication; take with plain water only.

Drugs Closely Related to P Alendronate

The other bisphosphonates are etidronate (Didronel), tiludronate (Skelid), pamidronate (Aredia), and risedronate (Actonel). They all act primarily on bone to prevent bone resorption. Unlike alendronate, they are not used to treat or prevent osteoporosis; their therapeutic indication is for treatment of Paget disease. Like alendronate, tiludronate and risedronate are used for patients with Paget disease who have alkaline phosphatase levels at least two times greater than the upper limit of normal or who are symptomatic or at risk for future complications. Oral etidronate is used to treat symptomatic Paget disease, and pamidronate is used to treat moderate to severe Paget disease.

Additional therapeutic uses for these drugs are treating and preventing heterotopic ossification (formation of bone in an abnormal location) after total hip replacement or spine injury (oral etidronate); treating moderate to severe hypercalcemia of malignancy, with or without bone metastasis (pamidronate, parenteral etidronate); and treating breast cancer or multiple myeloma in conjunction with standard chemotherapy (pamidronate). Unlabeled uses include treating postmenopausal osteoporosis (etidronate, pamidronate, risedronate) and hyperparathyroidism (pamidronate); preventing glucocorticoid-induced osteoporosis (pamidronate); reducing bone pain in patients with prostate cancer (pamidronate); and treating hypercalcemia caused by immobilization (pamidronate).

Pharmacokinetics, pharmacodynamics, and adverse effects for all of these drugs are similar to those of alendronate.

Drug Significantly Different From P Alendronate

Like alendronate, raloxifene (Evista) is prescribed to prevent osteoporosis in postmenopausal women. It reduces resorption of bone and decreases overall bone turnover. Unlike alendronate, however, raloxifene works as a selective estrogen-receptor modulator. Raloxifene is actually an estrogen antagonist at some sites because it blocks estrogen from attaching itself to the estrogen-receptor sites. At other estrogen-receptor sites, it produces estrogen-like effects. These effects include increasing bone-mass density and decreasing levels of total and LDL cholesterol. Raloxifene does not share estrogen's effects on the uterus or the breasts because it is an antagonist at these receptor sites.

Raloxifene is rapidly absorbed after oral dosing. It has extensive first-pass metabolism, although the P-450 pathways do not appear to metabolize it. The metabolites that are formed have a long half-life. The drug is highly protein bound. Raloxifene is excreted in the feces. It may cause fetal harm if given to pregnant women. It is a pregnancy category X drug, and its use is therefore contraindicated in pregnant women. Raloxifene is also contraindicated if the woman has a history of or active venous thromboembolic events (deep vein thrombosis, pulmonary embolism, retinal vein thrombosis). Caution should be used if raloxifene is coadministered with other highly protein-bound drugs, such as lidocaine, diazoxide, or diazepam. Raloxifene may decrease the binding of these drugs, which results in more free and active drug. Lab studies have not shown that raloxifene displaces the binding of warfarin, phenytoin, or tamoxifen. Ampicillin and cholestyramine both greatly decrease the absorption of raloxifene; these drugs should not be administered with raloxifene.

Common adverse effects of raloxifene are hot flashes and leg cramps. Raloxifene increases the risk for venous thromboembolic events, especially during the first 4 months of treatment. To minimize this risk, patients should discontinue use of raloxifene at least 72 hours before an expected prolonged immobilization (e.g., a planned surgical event requiring immobilization or bed rest). Raloxifene also should be discontinued throughout periods of prolonged immobilization and bed rest. Patients should resume raloxifene therapy only when fully ambulatory. If patients are traveling, advise them to avoid prolonged sitting in the same position.

Teach patients to take supplemental calcium and vitamin D if their dietary intake is inadequate. As with alendronate, encourage the patient to do weight-bearing exercises and to decrease alcohol consumption and cigarette smoking to promote bone density.

CHAPTER SUMMARY

- Women need adequate levels of sex hormones to develop and maintain the sexual and reproductive organs, create and maintain the secondary sexual characteristics, induce and stop the growth spurt of adolescence, and achieve and maintain pregnancy.
- Estrogen and progestin are the primary female sex hormones.
- Estrogen causes capillary dilation, promotes fluid retention, enhances protein anabolism, contributes to strengthening the skeleton, and maintains normal bone density and composition.
- Progestins are composed of progesterone and its derivatives. They regulate, through stimulation or inhibition, the secretion of pituitary gonadotropins. This secretion, in turn, regulates the development of the ovarian follicle. Progestins also inhibit spontaneous uterine contractions.
- Decreased levels of female sex hormones (primarily estrogen) that result from menopause increase the risk for cardiovascular disease and osteoporosis. Cardiovascular disease is the primary cause of death for postmenopausal women. Osteoporosis affects women more than men because levels of male sex hormones (testosterone) fall more gradually and at a later age than the decline of estrogen occurs in women.
- Postmenopausal hormone replacement therapy (HRT) carries substantial risks. Research has found that the risk for coronary artery disease and stroke increases substantially with the use of postmenopausal hormones. An adverse effect on cognition and a greater risk for Alzheimer disease also exist.
- Use of HRT should be limited to menopausal women who have considerable vasomotor symptoms. The dose and the length of time therapy is administered should be kept to a minimum.
- Most contraceptives are combinations of estrogen and progestin, although some contain progestin only. They may have serious adverse effects, but these effects are usually related to higher doses of estrogen in the drugs. Contraceptives should be prescribed with the smallest effective dose of estrogen possible.

QUESTIONS FOR STUDY AND REVIEW

1. Explain why progesterone can be used to treat amenorrhea and abnormal uterine bleeding.
2. What are the serious adverse effects that may result from estrogen therapy?
3. What is the benefit of using the selective estrogen receptor modulator raloxifene instead of conjugated estrogen to treat postmenopausal osteoporosis?
4. What teaching points regarding missed pills would you review with a patient who is starting oral contraceptives?
5. What unique instructions about drug administration do you need to give to a patient who is to receive alendronate for osteoporosis?

Need More Help?

Chapter 54 of the study guide for *Drug Therapy in Nursing* 2e contains NCLEX-style questions and other learning activities to reinforce your understanding of the concepts presented in this chapter. For additional information or to purchase the study guide, visit *http://connection.lww.com/go/aschenbrenner.*

REFERENCES AND BIBLIOGRAPHY

Anderson, G. L., Judd, H. L., Kaunitz, A. M., et al., Women's Health Initiative Investigators. (2003). Effects of estrogen plus progestin on gynecologic cancers and associated diagnostic procedures: The Women's Health Initiative randomized trial. *Journal of the American Medical Association, 290*(13), 1739–1748.

Cauley, J. A., Robbins, J., Chen, Z., et al., Women's Health Initiative Investigators. (2003). Effects of estrogen plus progestin on risk of fracture and bone mineral density. The Women's Health Initiative randomized trial. *Journal of American Medical Association, 290*(13), 1729–1738.

Chlebowski, R. T., Hendrix, S. L., Langer, R. D., et al., Women's Health Initiative Investigators. (2003). Influence of estrogen plus progestin on breast cancer and mammography in healthy postmenopausal women: the Women's Health Initiative Randomized Trial. *Journal of the American Medical Association, 289*(24), 3243–3253.

Hall, S. D., Wang, Z., Huang, S. M., et al. (2003). The interaction between St. John's wort and an oral contraceptive. *Clinical Pharmacology and Therapeutics, 74*(6), 525–535.

Hays, J., Ockene, J. K., Brunner, R. L., et al., Women's Health Initiative Investigators. (2003). Effects of estrogen plus progestin on health-related quality of life. *New England Journal of Medicine, 348*(19), 1839–1854.

Manson, J. E., Hsia, J., Johnson, K. C., et al., Women's Health Initiative Investigators. (2003). Estrogen plus progestin and the risk of coronary heart disease. *New England Journal of Medicine, 349*(6), 523–534.

National Institutes of Health. (2004). NIH asks participants in Women's Health Initiative estrogen-alone study to stop study pills, begin follow-up phase. *NIH News,* March 2. [Online]. Available: *http://www.nhlbi.nih.gov/new/press/04-03-02.htm.*

Rapp, S. R., Espeland, M. A., Shumaker, S. A., et al., WHIMS Investigators. (2003). Effect of estrogen plus progestin on global cognitive function in postmenopausal women. The Women's Health Initiative Memory Study: A randomized controlled trial. *Journal of the American Medical Association, 289*(20), 2663–2672.

Shumaker, S. A., Legault, C., Rapp, S. R., et al., WHIMS Investigators. (2003). Estrogen plus progestin and the incidence of dementia and mild cognitive impairment in postmenopausal women. The Women's Health Initiative Memory Study: A randomized controlled trial. *Journal of the American Medical Association, 289*(20), 2651–2662.

Wassertheil-Smoller, S., Hendrix, S. L., Limacher, M., et al., Women's Health Initiative Investigators. (2003). Effect of estrogen plus progestin on stroke in postmenopausal women. The Women's Health Initiative: A randomized trial. *Journal of the American Medical Association, 289*(20), 2673–2684.

Drugs Affecting Uterine Motility

chapter 55

Learning Objectives

At the completion of this chapter the student will:

1. Identify core drug knowledge about drugs that affect uterine motility.
2. Identify core patient variables relevant to drugs that affect uterine motility.
3. Relate the interaction of core drug knowledge to core patient variables for drugs that affect uterine contraction.
4. Generate a nursing plan of care from the interactions between core drug knowledge and core patient variables for drugs that affect uterine motility.
5. Describe nursing interventions to maximize therapeutic effects and minimize adverse effects for drugs that affect uterine motility.
6. Determine key points for patient and family education for drugs that affect uterine motility.

KEY TERMS

antepartum

intrapartum

oxytocics

postpartum

tocolytics

uterine tetany

FEATURED WEBLINK

http://www.awhonn.org

The site for the Association of Women's Health, Obstetric, and Neonatal Nurses has many links related to education and practice for nurses. These links include clinical updates, continuing education, a practice resource center, a fetal heart monitoring program, a section on cardiovascular health, competence-assessment tools, evidence-based clinical practice standards and guidelines (which are available for purchase), and a prematurity resource center. Other links go to news and events, publications and research, and legislation and health policy.

CONNECTION WEBLINK

Additional Weblinks are found on Connection:
http://www.connection.lww.com/go/aschenbrenner.

Drugs Affecting Uterine Motility

Ⓒ Oxytocics

- **P** **oxytocin**
- ergonovine maleate
- methylergonovine
- carboprost
- dinoprostone
- misoprostol

Ⓒ Tocolytics

- **P** **terbutaline**
- ritodrine
- magnesium sulfate
- indomethacin

The symbol Ⓒ indicates the **drug class.**
Drugs in **bold type** marked with the symbol **P** are prototypes.
Drugs in blue type are closely related to the prototype.
Drugs in red type are significantly different from the prototype.
Drugs in black type with no symbol are also used in drug therapy; no prototype

For labor and delivery of the fetus, normal uterine function is necessary. Normal uterine function consists of labor contractions beginning between 38 and 42 weeks of gestation. The contractions must be regular and strong enough to facilitate delivery of the fetus. At times, labor occurs prematurely, and stopping the uterine contractions is desirable. This chapter examines two classes of drugs that are used when the uterus does not function normally:

- **Oxytocics:** uterine stimulants used to initiate or augment a contractile pattern of labor
- **Tocolytics:** uterine relaxants used to stop labor contractions that occur before completion of the 37th week of gestation

Oxytocin (Pitocin, Syntocin) is the prototype oxytocic drug. Drugs significantly different from the prototype are ergonovine maleate, methylergonovine maleate, and misoprostol. The prototype tocolytic drug is terbutaline. A drug represented by the prototype is ritodrine. A drug significantly different is magnesium sulfate.

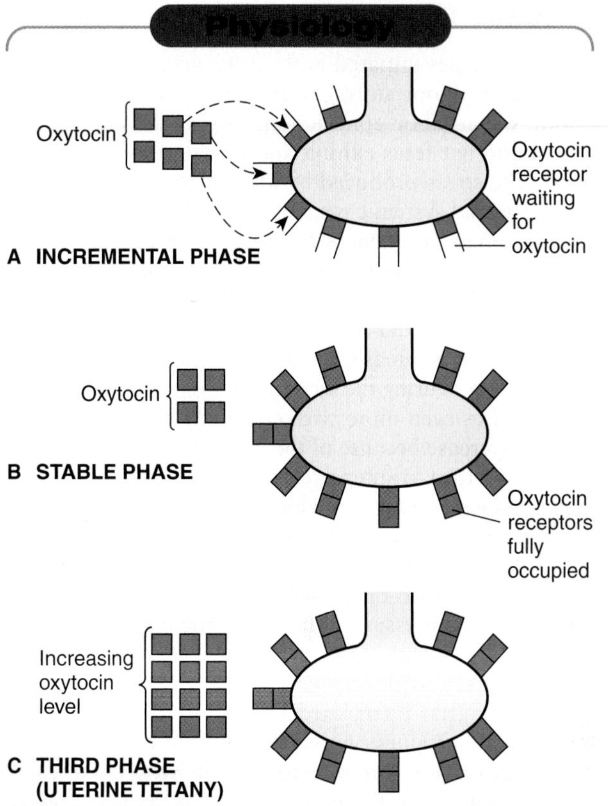

FIGURE 55.1 Phases of oxytocin activity. Oxytocic drug therapy is usually initiated to mimic the role of natural oxytocin in prompting or augmenting labor. Oxytocin undergoes three phases of activity. (**A**) In the incremental phase, oxytocin levels rise, and oxytocin receptors are stimulated, producing increased intensity and frequency of uterine contractions. (**B**) In the stable phase, receptor sites are occupied with oxytocin, so no further oxytocin effects occur until a receptor site opens again. (**C**) In the third phase—uterine tetany—oxytocin levels continually rise. Uterine contractions increase in number while the force of the contractions decreases. In such instances, the uterus experiences hyperstimulation.

PHYSIOLOGY

Contractions and Related Changes

Most women progress through pregnancy with contractions beginning between 38 and 42 gestational weeks. The onset of labor begins the **intrapartum** period of pregnancy, which concludes with delivery. The induction of labor is related to oxytocin, a hormone that is produced in the hypothalamus, stored in the posterior pituitary, and released into the circulatory system. Once the pituitary releases oxytocin, oxytocin binds to cell membrane receptors on target tissues, primarily the uterine myometrium (muscle cells) and the mammary epithelium. The fetus may also secrete some oxytocin during labor. Oxytocin receptors are also located in the decidua, which is the endometrium (or lining) of the uterus. Although the exact mechanism of oxytocin in labor is unknown, endogenous oxytocin stimulates the myometrial cells of the uterus, initiating uterine contractions (Figure 55.1). The myometrial cells increase in sensitivity as pregnancy progresses because the number of oxytocin receptors doubles just before labor. Estrogen may have a role in the creation of additional oxytocin receptors. The oxytocin receptors that are located in the endometrium increase during labor and reach peak levels at birth. If the number of oxytocin receptors is limited, the response of the uterus to oxytocin will be diminished. Oxytocinase, produced by the placenta, rapidly degrades oxytocin, which allows circulating oxytocin to restimulate the oxytocin receptors.

Endogenous oxytocin also has some vasopressive effects (causing vascular constriction) and antidiuretic effects (causing increased water resorption from the glomerular filtrate). Oxytocin is also necessary for the let-down of breast milk. Additionally, oxytocin is believed to have an intricate role in the creation and maintenance of maternal behavior (e.g., bonding with and caring for the infant).

In addition to the necessary number of oxytocin receptors and the amount of available oxytocin, contraction of uterine muscle also depends on oxygenation and glucose. Oxygen and glucose are required to provide the energy needed for muscle contraction. If these two elements are inadequate, the uterine contractions will be too weak or too few to advance labor and progress to delivery. For example, if the woman in labor has pathophysiology that impairs her respiratory status (e.g., a chronic respiratory disease), she may be unable to fully oxygenate the uterus. Or, if the woman has had a prolonged labor, she may have exhausted her glucose reserves.

Prostaglandins also have a role in preparing the uterus for labor and delivery. Prostaglandin E_2 (PGE_2) leads to sensitization of the myometrium to oxytocin. PGE_2 primarily plays a role in assisting with cervical ripening (by which the cervix becomes softened, yielding, and dilated to allow for the passage of the fetus in vaginal delivery) without affecting uterine contractions. PGE_2, however, is capable of initiating uterine contractions and may interact with oxytocin to increase uterine contractility.

Systemic Changes in Labor

Systemic changes initiated in the **antepartum** period (pregnancy before labor starts) continue into the intrapartum period. When labor contractions begin, the childbearing woman and her fetus exhibit additional physiologic alterations. The stress produced by uterine contractions affects many maternal systemic responses.

The woman experiences cardiovascular system changes. Blood pressure remains close to the antepartal baseline, except during uterine contractions. With contractions during the first stage of labor, the systolic pressure may increase by 35 mm Hg, whereas the diastolic pressure may increase by 25 mm Hg. During the second stage of labor, blood pressure increases even more with efforts to bear down. Pulse rate may increase because of the pain of labor contractions but should return to antepartal baselines. The bearing-down efforts of the second stage (which involve pushing against a closed glottis) also increase intrathoracic pressure, which interrupts venous return from the lower extremities. This interruption in turn decreases cardiac output, pulse pressure, and blood pressure. When the patient breathes again, the intrathoracic pressure decreases, helping cardiac output, pulse pressure, and blood pressure return to baseline values. Immediately after birth, cardiac output increases to 80% above prelabor values; within the first hour after delivery, cardiac output slowly returns to normal. Most childbearing women can adapt to these cardiovascular changes successfully without requiring drug therapy.

During the intrapartum period, the woman experiences respiratory system changes because oxygen demand and consumption increase. Uterine contractions cause the respiratory rate to increases above pregnancy rates. This hyperventilation causes the level of $PaCO_2$ to fall; consequently, respiratory alkalosis develops.

As labor progresses, the contracting uterus increases muscular activity and oxygen requirements, which produces a mild metabolic acidosis. This mild metabolic acidosis continues, so that during the second stage of labor and by the time of birth, the acid-base balance remains because metabolic acidosis is uncompensated by respiratory alkalosis. The acid-base imbalances created by labor are quickly reversed after delivery because respiratory rates return to prepregnancy values and lactic acid production decreases. By 24 hours after birth, acid-base status is similar to prepregnancy levels.

The major labor adaptation in the hemopoietic system is the development of leukocytosis above pregnancy levels. The childbearing patient's white blood cell count may be between 25,000 and 30,000 mm^3. Although an elevated white blood cell count is normally considered a sign of infection, laboratory assessment that shows an elevation of the white blood cells in the woman who has just delivered must not routinely be considered a sign of infection. This leukocytosis most likely results from labor stress, heavy exertion, and healing of the opened placental site.

Profuse perspiration and hyperventilation alter fluid and electrolyte balance during labor. Most women are not permitted to eat or drink as labor progresses to prevent nausea, vomiting, and possible aspiration. Generally, healthy women having uncomplicated vaginal deliveries do not require intravenous (IV) fluids during labor but merely do not have any food or drink during this period. If labor is long, the woman may experience dehydration and electrolyte imbalance. She may require hydration with IV fluids.

The renal system compensates for this decreased oral intake and increased water loss in part by excreting urine that is more concentrated. Also, the increasing uterine muscular activity leads to a breakdown of proteins and the presence of a trace of protein in the urine. As the fetal head descends in the pelvis, it extends pressure against the bladder walls and the urethra. The woman may not be sensitive to bladder filling.

The gastrointestinal (GI) system experiences a reduction or cessation of gastric motility and absorption of solid foods as labor begins. Gastric emptying time is prolonged, and more than 25 mL of gastric contents remains in the stomach regardless of when the woman consumed her last meal. Gastric acidity increases, and more than 50% of laboring women have a gastric pH below 2.5. Most circulating blood shifts away from the GI system to more vital maternal organs during labor.

The healthy fetus can progress through a normal labor and delivery with no adverse effects. The labor process produces a stressful physiologic state in the fetus with each contraction, but fetal compensatory mechanisms generally allow the fetus to respond successfully to those events.

Fetal acid-base status in labor depends on the maternal contractile pattern and the fetus's ability to compensate for contraction-produced decreases in oxygen. Oxygen/carbon dioxide exchange between the mother and the fetus occurs primarily between contractions when the blood flow is not impeded. In women who are laboring efficiently, the contractions occur at intervals that allow the intervillous spaces in the placenta to refill with oxygenated blood between contractions; this refilling maintains an adequate oxygen supply to the fetus. The healthy fetus thus maintains a pH above 7.25. The two main indicators of fetal well-being and adequate fetal compensation during labor are a stable fetal heart rate (FHR) and the presence of fetal movements. The mature FHR ranges within a baseline of 120 to 160 bpm.

PATHOPHYSIOLOGY

Occasionally, uterine function proceeds abnormally, causing failure of labor to occur or failure of labor to progress. The two main categories of obstetric situations that require drug administration to initiate the onset of contractions include labor that does not begin at term and a pregnancy that is detrimental to the patient or her fetus.

Stimulation of uterine contractions using drugs before spontaneous labor has started is called induction of labor. Specific maternal and fetal conditions that may require induction of labor include the following:

- Diabetes
- Preeclampsia
- Premature rupture of the membranes
- Fetal demise
- Renal disease
- Post-term pregnancy
- Chorioamnionitis (inflammation of the membrane covering the fetus)
- Isoimmunization (response of an Rh-negative mother when exposed to Rh-positive blood from her infant)

- Intrauterine fetal growth retardation
- Mild abruptio placentae with no fetal distress

Before induction is initiated, the patient's cervix is assessed using the Bishop scoring system, and the fetus is assessed for evidence of maturity. The Bishop scale is a prelabor scoring system used to assist in predicting patient success if labor is induced. The system consists of five assessment parameters:

1. Cervical dilation
2. Cervical effacement
3. Fetal station
4. Cervical consistency
5. Cervical position

Each parameter is scored on a scale of 0 to 3. The higher the score, the greater is the likelihood that induction will lead to a vaginal delivery. The favorable cervix is described as one that is anterior, soft, at least 50% effaced and 2 cm dilated, with the fetal station at +1 or lower. These findings are equal to a Bishop score of 9.

Drugs may be administered to increase uterine contractions if labor is spontaneous but its patterns are dysfunctional, particularly when labor patterns are not strong or rhythmic enough to spur delivery. This type of labor needs augmentation with drug therapy that increases uterine contractions.

Another obstetric event usually requiring drug therapy is premature labor. The parturitional (child-birthing) process is now known to begin long before clinically detected preterm labor. Increases in gap junctions, oxytocin receptors, and enhanced uterine contractility accompany the parturitional process. If labor begins before completion of the 37th gestational week, drug therapy may be used (in addition to conservative methods of bed rest in side-lying position, hydration, and sedation) to stop the uterine contractions and prolong the pregnancy. None of the currently used drug therapies appear to alter the fundamental process of parturition. The goal of tocolytic drug therapy, covered later in this chapter, is to secure some additional time before delivery to administer drugs to the mother. Delaying delivery allows other drugs, which help to promote fetal respiratory function, to be administered and to allow time to transfer the mother, if necessary, to a hospital capable of providing acute medical care to the mother and neonatal intensive care to the newborn. During this short but crucial interval, corticosteroids are administered to improve neonatal outcomes. Corticosteroid administration significantly reduces the risk for neonatal death, respiratory distress syndrome (RDS), and intraventricular hemorrhage (IVH), a risk factor for cerebral palsy. These effects of corticosteroids are greatest if the pregnancy is prolonged for at least 24 hours; the benefits continue for at least 7 days. (See Chapter 51 for a complete discussion of corticosteroids.)

C OXYTOCICS

Oxytocic drugs are synthetic forms of the endogenous posterior pituitary hormone oxytocin. They produce uterine contractions and milk ejection for breast-feeding. The prototype oxytocic drug is oxytocin (Pitocin, Syntocin). Drugs closely related to oxytocin are ergonovine maleate (Ergotrate Maleate) and methylergonovine (Methergine). Drugs significantly different from oxytocin are carboprost (Hemabate), dinoprostone (Prepidil, Cervidil), and misoprostol (Cytotec). Table 55.1 provides a summary of selected uterine motility drugs.

NURSING MANAGEMENT OF THE PATIENT RECEIVING P OXYTOCIN

Core Drug Knowledge

Pharmacotherapeutics

Oxytocin is given by IV drip infusion to initiate or augment (improve) labor contractions when important fetal or maternal reasons to do so exist. Examples of such reasons include Rh problems, maternal diabetes, preeclampsia near term, premature rupture of placental membranes, or uterine inertia. IV oxytocin may also be used to treat incomplete or inevitable spontaneous abortion during the second trimester. IV infusion or intramuscular (IM) injection of oxytocin is used to control bleeding or hemorrhage that occurs **postpartum,** that is, after delivery of the fetus. Oxytocin should be dosed to mimic the release of endogenous oxytocin, which is about 2 to 3 mU/min in spontaneous labor. The proper dose of oxytocin is one that achieves adequate uterine contractility while minimizing maternal and fetal adverse effects. The dose should be low initially, no more than 0.5 to 1 mU/min. Determining the appropriate dose of oxytocin requires slow upward titration in increments of 1 to 2 mU/min. Most women with cervical ripening develop adequate labor patterns with 6 mU/min or less of oxytocin (Arias, 2002; Simpson & Knox, 2003). The dosage necessary to achieve adequate labor is generally lower if labor is being augmented than if it is not. The desired contractile pattern consists of one contraction every 2 to 3 minutes, with durations of 40 to 90 seconds per contraction and an intensity of 40 to 90 mm Hg for internal uterine monitoring, or firm to palpation for external monitoring. In some other established protocols, called high-dose active management protocols, oxytocin is initiated at a higher rate and titrated with higher doses of the drug; dose changes may be as frequent as every 15 minutes. The use of these high-dose protocols is controversial (Clayworth, 2000). These protocols were designed for use in the nulliparous woman in spontaneous active labor. All aspects of the protocol must be followed, not just the sections related to oxytocin dosing (Simpson & Knox, 2003).

An unusual use of oxytocin is currently being researched: the use of oxytocin infusion as a treatment for autism or Asperger syndrome. The reasoning behind this research is that oxytocin has been found to play a role in social and repetitive behaviors, and alterations in these behaviors are found in autism (Hollander et al., 2003).

No labeled use of oxytocin exists in children or in men.

Pharmacokinetics

Onset of action occurs almost immediately after IV administration. Steady-state plasma levels are reached in approximately 40 minutes with continuous IV infusion, during which maximum uterine contraction occurs. Physiologic steady state

TABLE 55.1 Summary of Selected Ⓒ Uterine Motility Drugs

Drug (Trade) Name	Selected Indications	Route and Dosage Range	Pharmacokinetics
Ⓒ Oxytocics			
P oxytocin (Pitocin, Syntocinon; nasal spray, Syntocinon)	Antepartum: to induce or augment uterine contractions Postpartum: to control postpartum bleeding or hemorrhage (parenteral)	*Adult:* IV (induction or augmentation of labor), 1–2 mU/min, through infusion pump, and should be increased by this amount at 30–60 or 40–60 min intervals; do not exceed 20 mU/min; IV (treatment of incomplete or spontaneous abortion), infusion of 10-U oxytocin with 500-mL physiologic saline solution or 5% dextrose in physiologic saline infused at a rate of 10–20 mU/min; (control of postpartum uterine bleeding), IV drip, add 10–40 U to 1,000 mL of a nonhydrating diluent: run at a rate to control uterine atony; IM, 10 U after delivery of placenta; (initial milk letdown)	*Onset:* IV, immediate; IM, 3–5 min; nasal, varies *Duration:* IV, 60 min; IM, 2–3 h; nasal, 20 min $t_{1/2}$: 1–6 min
ergonovine maleate (Ergotrate Maleate)	Prevention and treatment of postpartum and postabortal hemorrhage due to uterine atony	*Adult:* IM, 0.2 mg, severe bleeding may require repeat dosing q2–4 h; IV, 0.2 mg in emergency situations	*Onset:* IM, 7–8 min; IV, immediate *Duration:* IM, 3 h; IV, 45 min $t_{1/2}$: 0.5–2 h
methylergonovine (Methergine)	Routine management after delivery of the placenta Treatment of postpartum atony and hemorrhage; subinvolution of the uterus	*Adult:* IM, 0.2 mg after delivery of the placenta, after delivery of the anterior shoulder, or during puerperium; may be repeated q2–4 h; IV, same dosage as IM, infuse slowly over at least 60 seconds, monitor BP very carefully because severe hypertensive reaction can occur; oral, 0.2 mg tid or qid daily in the puerperium for up to 1 wk	*Onset:* IM, 2–5 min; IV, immediate; oral, 5–10 min *Duration:* IM, 3 h; IV, 1–3 h; oral, 3 h $t_{1/2}$: 30 min
Ⓒ Tocolytics			
P terbutaline sulfate (Brethaire, Brethine, Bricanyl)	Unlabeled use: inhibition of premature labor	*Adult:* IV, initially 10 mg/min; titrate upward to a maximum of 80 mg/min; maintain at minimum effective dosage for 4 h; oral, 2.5 mg q4–6 h daily as maintenance therapy	*Onset:* IV, unknown oral, 30 min *Duration:* IV, unknown oral, 4–8 h $t_{1/2}$: Unknown
ritodrine (Yutopar)	Management of preterm labor in selected patients ≥ 20 wk gestation	*Adult:* IV, 0.05 mg/min initially; gradually increase by 0.05 mg/min q10min until desired result is attained; usual effective dosage between 0.15 and 0.35 mg/min continued for at least 12 h after uterine contractions cease	*Onset:* Rapid *Duration:* Unknown $t_{1/2}$: 1.7–2.6 h
Others			
carboprost (Hemabate)	Termination of pregnancy 13–20 wk Evacuation of the uterus in instance of missed abortion or intra-uterine fetal death in the second trimester	*Adult:* (Abortion) IM, 250 μg at 1½ to 3½ h intervals; may be increased to 500 μg; do not exceed 12 mg total dose or continuous administration over 2 d; (postpartum hemorrhage) IM, 250 μg as one dose; multiple doses at 15–90 min intervals may be used; do not exceed a total dose of 2 mg	*Onset:* 15 min *Duration:* Unknown $t_{1/2}$: 8 h

(continued)

TABLE 55.1 Summary of Selected C Uterine Motility Drugs (continued)

Drug (Trade) Name	Selected Indications	Route and Dosage Range	Pharmacokinetics
	Postpartum hemorrhage due to uterine atony that does not respond to conventional methods		
dinoprostone (Prostaglandin E_2)	Termination of pregnancy 12–20 wk Evacuation of the uterus in missed abortion or intrauterine fetal death up to 28 wk gestational age Management of non-metastatic gestational trophoblastic disease (benign hydatidiform mole) Initiation of cervical ripening before induction of labor	*Adult:* (Abortion) Intravaginal, one suppository (10 mg); additional suppositories may be given at 3–5 h intervals; (cervical ripening) intravaginal gel, 0.5 mg dose; repeat dose may be given if no response in 6 h	*Onset:* 10 min *Duration:* 2–3 h $t_{1/2}$: 2.5–5 min
magnesium sulfate	Unlabeled use: inhibition of premature labor; seizure prevention and control in preeclampsia and eclampsia	*Adult:* IM, 4–5 g of a 50% solution q4h as necessary; IV, 4 g of a 10%–20% solution; do not exceed 1.5 mL/min of a 10% solution; IV infusion, 4–5 g in 250-mL 5% dextrose; do not exceed 3 mL/min	*Onset:* IV, immediate; IM, 60 min *Duration:* IV, 30 min; IM, 3–4 h $t_{1/2}$: Unknown

is achieved when no further uterine response to increased oxytocin infusion occurs because the receptor sites are already bound with oxytocin and are temporarily unavailable. Elimination is through the liver, kidneys, and mammary glands and by the enzyme oxytocinase (see Table 55.1).

Pharmacodynamics

Synthetic, exogenous oxytocin has the same effects on the body as natural, endogenous oxytocin. It stimulates uterine contractions and milk let-down for breast-feeding. Although the endogenous hormone has a known effect on milk production, exogenous oxytocin is not administered for this purpose.

Response to oxytocin therapy has three phases (see Figure 55.1):

1. Incremental phase: uterine activity increases evenly as the dose of oxytocin increases.
2. Stable phase: uterine activity remains constant even if the oxytocin dose increases because the myometrial receptor sites are already fully bound with oxytocin. Because the sites are full, they cannot be receptive to more effects from the oxytocin. As half-life and elimination of oxytocin occur, the uterus again has open receptors and is responsive to increases in oxytocin levels. The uterus shifts periodically between the incremental and stable phases.
3. Hyperstimulation: if this third phase of uterine response to oxytocin occurs, it indicates adverse effects from the drug. If the dose continually increases, the frequency of contractions will increase, but the uterine pressure will decrease so that the contractions are less effective. The result is hyperstimulation of the uterus, with uterine fibrillation and prolonged contraction. This condition is known as **uterine tetany.** Uterine tetany is generally recognized as a persistent pattern of more than 5 contractions in 10 minutes, contractions lasting 2 minutes or more, or contractions of normal duration occurring within 1 minute of each other (Simpson & Knox, 2003; American College of Obstetricians and Gynecologists [ACOG], 1999a; ACOG, 1995).

Oxytocin therapy also has vasopressive and antidiuretic effects. Oxytocin affects the cardiovascular system by initially decreasing blood pressure. With prolonged oxytocin administration, baseline blood pressure may increase by 30%. Cardiac output and stroke volume also increase. Oxytocin doses of 20 mU/min or above have antidiuretic effects when administered over a prolonged period. Although these antidiuretic effects are weak, fatal water intoxication has occurred with the use of oxytocin. Additionally, oxytocin increases the water permeability of the nephron, which causes more water retention than sodium reabsorption and in turn leads to water intoxication and dilutional hyponatremia. Symptoms of water intoxication affect primarily the CNS and musculoskeletal systems. CNS effects range from headache, fatigue, nausea, and anorexia to lethargy, confusion, disorientation, agitation, vomiting, seizures, and coma. Musculoskeletal symptoms may include cramps and weakness. Cardiovascular effects, such as tachycardia and hypotension, can also occur.

Oxytocin and vasopressin are known to play a role in social and repetitive behaviors. A small study of adults with autism or Asperger disorder who were administered oxytocin infusions showed a significant reduction in repetitive behaviors after the infusion, compared with placebo (Hollander et al., 2003).

Contraindications and Precautions

Oxytocin is contraindicated in cephalopelvic disproportion (fetal head relative to maternal pelvis) and with unfavorable fetal positions or presentations that must be converted before delivery (such as transverse lie). It is also contraindicated in the following conditions:

- Obstetric emergencies in which the benefit-to-risk ratio for either mother or fetus favors cesarean section
- Fetal distress without signs of imminent delivery
- Prolonged use in uterine inertia or severe toxemia
- Hypertonic or hyperactive uterine patterns
- Failure of uterine activity to achieve satisfactory progress
- Contraindication to vaginal delivery (e.g., invasive cervical carcinoma, active genital herpes, cord presentation or prolapse, total placenta previa, vas previa)
- Hypersensitivity to the drug

Oxytocin must be administered very cautiously if cyclopropane anesthesia is used because maternal sinus bradycardia with abnormal atrioventricular rhythms and hypotension may result. Water intoxication is possible with oxytocin use and should be considered if oral fluids are given in addition to oxytocin infusion. Overstimulation of the uterus, which may be hazardous to the mother or fetus, can occur with oxytocin administration, even with proper administration and supervision.

Adverse Effects

Adverse effects of oxytocin are dose related and take two forms: maternal and fetal. The most common maternal adverse effects are nausea, vomiting, uterine hypertonicity, and cardiac arrhythmias. Less common but potentially fatal is severe water intoxication and hyponatremia. Other maternal adverse effects are spasm and rupture of the uterus (usually from excessive doses or hypersensitivity to the drug), postpartum hemorrhage, subarachnoid hemorrhage, and pelvic hematoma. The most common fetal adverse effect is bradycardia. Other adverse fetal effects are premature ventricular contractions and other arrhythmias, impaired fetal oxygenation, permanent brain or central nervous system (CNS) damage and death (from excessive uterine motility), low Apgar scores 5 minutes after birth, neonatal jaundice, and retinal hemorrhage.

When administered intrapartally for induction or augmentation of labor, oxytocin does not cause fetal structural defects or congenital anomalies but may be responsible for fetal CNS depression. Such CNS depression severely compromises the neonate's ability to successfully adapt to the extrauterine environment.

Overdosage depends on uterine hyperactivity. Hyperstimulation with hypertonic or tetanic contractions or a resting tone of 15 to 20 mm Hg or more between contractions can cause tumultuous labor, uterine rupture, cervical and vaginal lacerations, postpartum hemorrhage, uteroplacental hypoperfusion, deceleration of FHR, fetal hypoxia, fetal hypercapnia, or fetal demise. These effects occur because uterine hyperstimulation, or a resting tone above 20 mm Hg, can produce uteroplacental hypofusion, a state in which the placenta does not have time to recover and be refilled with oxygenated blood. The lack of oxygenated blood creates a state of fetal hypoxia. The greatest drop in fetal oxygen saturation occurs 90 seconds after a contraction, and the fetus needs an additional 90 seconds to recover. In women who are laboring efficiently, intervals occur between the contractions that allow the fetus to be reoxygenated. In hyperstimulation from oxytocin therapy, no rest between contractions exists. Recovery of the fetus from oxytocin-induced hypoxia therefore requires cessation of oxytocin administration. A normal, healthy fetus with sufficient metabolic reserve can tolerate hyperstimulation for a short time, but if hyperstimulation continues, the ability of the fetus to buffer the byproducts of anaerobic metabolism will eventually be depleted. Consequently, the fetus will begin to show signs of compromise (Clayworth, 2000).

Water intoxication with convulsions may occur if large doses of oxytocin (40–50 mL/min) are given for a long time. Treatment consists of discontinuing the drug, restricting fluid intake, initiating diuresis, administering IV hypertonic saline solutions, correcting electrolyte imbalance, controlling convulsions cautiously with barbiturates, and following general nursing measures to care for an unconscious patient.

Drug Interactions

If oxytocin is given at the same time as sympathomimetic drugs (those drugs that stimulate the sympathetic nervous system), the vasopressor effect may be increased. A possible consequence is postpartum hypertension.

Assessment of Relevant Core Patient Variables

Health Status

Assess, or verify that the physician or nurse midwife has assessed, the patient's pelvic adequacy before beginning oxytocin therapy. You must determine or confirm with the physician or nurse midwife that the fetal position is favorable for vaginal delivery. Assess for fetal distress and for conditions that would contraindicate vaginal delivery (e.g., invasive cervical carcinoma, active genital herpes, cord presentation or prolapse, total placenta previa, vas previa). Assess contractions for hypertonic or hyperactive patterns or for contractions that should be successful in advancing labor but are not. Evaluating whether uterine inertia has been prolonged or if severe toxemia is present is important because these factors are contraindications for oxytocin therapy.

Assess whether the patient's cervix is favorable for induction (Bishop score of 5 or better). Before and throughout therapy, assess maternal vital signs, length of contractions, time between contractions, FHR, fetal movement, and fluid status. Many institutions monitor FHRs over 20 minutes to produce a 20-minute FHR tracing. The tracing is evaluated with nonstress testing criteria to determine fetal well-being. Nonstress testing criteria for a reactive FHR tracing include two fetal movements with FHR accelerations 15 bpm above baseline for 15 seconds in a 10-minute period. These movements with accelerations are reassuring signs of fetal well-being.

Life Span and Gender

Before oxytocin is administered, assess the duration of the pregnancy. Oxytocin is not used during the first trimester except in cases of spontaneous or induced abortion.

Lifestyle, Diet, and Habits

Consider the patient's risk for water intoxication if the patient is receiving oral fluids and oxytocin by IV drip.

Environment

Be aware of the environment in which oxytocin will be administered. Oxytocin is administered in a hospital labor and delivery suite where the patient and fetus can be continually monitored.

Nursing Diagnoses and Outcomes

- Risk for Fetal or Maternal Injury related to uterine hypertonicity secondary to oxytocin therapy
  Desired outcome: *The mother and fetus will progress through labor and delivery without injury while on oxytocin therapy.*
- Excess Fluid Volume related to drug-induced water intoxication and altered electrolyte levels
  Desired outcome: *The patient's fluid status will remain normal while on oxytocin therapy.*

Planning and Intervention

Maximizing Therapeutic Effects

Assess cervical ripening using the Bishop scoring system before oxytocin therapy starts. If the cervix is not ripe, PGE_2 gel may need to be instilled or vaginal doses of misoprostol given at least 4 hours before administering oxytocin. (For further discussion of these drugs, see the section on Drugs Significantly Different From Oxytocin.) Specific orders from the prescriber are required for administering either of these drugs. A protocol may also be required.

Use an infusion pump for precise administration of oxytocin. Add 1 mL (10 U) per 1,000 mL of a physiologic electrolyte solution, such as 0.9% sodium chloride, to make a solution of 10 mU/mL (0.01 U/mL). Use of normal saline is preferred over 5% dextrose because it helps to prevent the hyponatremia that can occur with oxytocin infusion (Box 55.1). Start the infusion at 0.5 to 1 mU/min and increase the dose by 1 to 2 mU/min every 40 to 60 minutes until the desired contractile pattern is achieved. Titrate the oxytocin based on the frequency of contractions, the progress of labor, and fetal tolerance, regardless of which induction/augmentation protocol you are following (Clayworth, 2000). If labor is progressing at 1 cm/hour, oxytocin dosage does not need to be increased (Simpson & Knox, 2003; Crane & Young, 1998; Simpson, 1998).

Minimizing Adverse Effects

Piggyback the diluted oxytocin solution into a primary IV line, which also supplies a physiologic electrolyte solution. Doing so enables you to discontinue the solution immediately if adverse maternal or fetal effects occur. An infusion pump is continuously used throughout therapy to prevent overdosage.

FOCUS ON RESEARCH

Box 55.1 Current Practices in Oxytocin Dilution

Ruchala, P. L., Metheny, N., Essenpreis, H., et al. (2002). Current practice in oxytocin dilution and fluid administration for induction of labor. *Journal of Obstetric, Gynecologic, and Neonatal Nursing, 31*(5), 545–550.

The Study

Nurse managers of obstetric units, randomly recruited from eligible hospitals in the American Hospital Association (AHA) guide (1998), responded to questionnaires, of which 256 were analyzed to determine which intravenous fluids were being used to dilute oxytocin for infusion and for mainline fluid in women receiving oxytocin induction. Ninety-eight percent of those surveyed responded that they followed current guidelines and used physiologic electrolyte solutions for both purposes. However, 2% reported using 5% dextrose in water, which does not follow the current guidelines. The use of 5% dextrose in water does not prevent the hyponatremia that can occur with oxytocin infusion.

Nursing Implications

You need to understand that your institution's protocols for administering a particular drug (oxytocin in this case) may not reflect the research on best practices or current clinical guidelines or recommendations. Be as active as possible in helping to write hospital policy that reflects accurate and current knowledge of drug pharmacokinetics and pharmacodynamics, as well as current clinical guidelines published by professional nursing organizations. In cases of poor maternal or fetal outcome after oxytocin infusion, you will be held to nationally accepted standards. If legal action is taken against you or the hospital, the fact that you followed institutional policy, if that policy does not reflect the current beliefs in the field, may not be considered an acceptable defense.

Use of drugs that stimulate uterine activity requires close monitoring of the patient and fetus throughout administration of the drug. Assess maternal vital signs, FHR, and contractile pattern before each increase in the oxytocin infusion rate. If maternal vital signs show hypertension or substantial changes, if the FHR decreases, or if fetal movement stops, notify the prescriber immediately.

The FHR monitor continuously records the patient's uterine contraction pattern. If the dose of oxytocin remains unchanged, assess FHR and uterine activity every 15 minutes during the active phase of stage one labor and every 5 minutes during the second stage of labor. Maternal vital signs should be checked at least every 4 hours during induction (Simpson & Knox, 2003; American Academy of Pediatrics [AAP]/ACOG, 2002; Association of Women's Health, Obstetric and Neonatal Nursing [AWHONN], 1998).

Assess for evidence of hyperstimulation. Hyperstimulation occurs when contractions are more frequent than every 2 minutes, last longer than 90 seconds, have a resting tone exceeding 15 mm Hg pressure, or have a normal pattern but occur within 1 minute of each other. If a hypercontractile labor pattern develops from the oxytocin infusion, stop the oxytocin infusion immediately and notify the physician or nurse midwife at once. Ideally, you will notice the hyperstimulation soon after it begins and stop the oxytocin before fetal demise can occur. Other interventions include placing the woman in a left-lateral position, increasing IV fluids, and administering oxygen by tight face mask at a rate of 10 to 12 L/min.

The appropriate dose for restarting oxytocin after hyperstimulation is unknown. Based on the physiology of contractions and the pharmacokinetics of oxytocin, it has been suggested that the infusion of oxytocin may be restarted after 5 to 10 minutes if the fetal status is reassuring and the contractions no longer meet the definition of hyperstimulation. It may be necessary to restart at a lower dose and increase the interval between dosage increases. However, if oxytocin has been discontinued for more than 40 minutes, essentially all the circulating oxytocin has been metabolized. Consequently, the patient should be considered similar to a patient who has not received any exogenous oxytocin, and the infusion of oxytocin should resume from the initial dose, with dose increases occurring less frequently. If, on reassessment, the woman still has a pattern of hyperstimulation after the oxytocin infusion is stopped, the infusion should not be resumed (Clayworth, 2000).

Making these assessments in the intrapartum period is challenging and raises issues of nursing conduct and patient safety. If you have a professional difference of opinion with the physician about whether the patient is experiencing hyperstimulation or whether the oxytocin should be slowed or stopped, use the appropriate chain of command in the institution to seek appropriate assistance for the patient. Failure to continue to seek care for a patient when necessary may legally be considered negligence on your part if the patient or fetus has an adverse outcome from oxytocin therapy (Simpson & Knox, 2003).

Assess the patient's fluid intake and urinary output and urge the patient to urinate at least every 2 hours throughout oxytocin therapy. Assess for signs of water intoxication, including anorexia, nausea, vomiting, headache, confusion, muscle cramps, hypotension, and tachycardia.

Providing Patient and Family Education

- Educating the patient and family about the rationale for oxytocin use, the desired effects, and the potential adverse effects of oxytocin therapy is important.
- Explain that the patient and fetus will be monitored closely to determine the effectiveness of the therapy and to detect any early signs of adverse effects.

Ongoing Assessment and Evaluation

Throughout induction, monitor continually for evidence of adverse maternal or fetal effects. Oxytocin drug therapy is considered effective when labor progresses predictably, no maternal or fetal adverse effects occur, vaginal delivery happens without complications, and the postpartum period is uneventful.

MEMORY CHIP

P Oxytocin

- Used to induce labor or to augment labor
- Works similarly to endogenous oxytocin by attaching to oxytocin receptors and stimulating them
- Major contraindications: conditions that require cesarean section; hypermotility of the uterus
- Most common adverse effects: maternal—nausea, vomiting, uterine hypertonicity, and cardiac arrhythmias; fetal—bradycardia
- Most serious adverse effects: maternal—uterine rupture, water intoxication (uncommon); fetal—fetal demise, hypoxia, permanent brain damage, death
- **Life span alert: used in third trimester of pregnancy**
- Maximizing therapeutic effects: Administer when the cervix has ripened; titrate the dose upward slowly based on the frequency of contractions and uterine response.
- Minimizing adverse effects: Assess mother and fetus carefully throughout therapy for adverse effects and poor fetal tolerance; stop the infusion if hypertonicity or fetal compromise occurs.
- Most important patient education: purpose of drug; rationale for frequent assessment

Drugs Closely Related to P Oxytocin

Ergonovine maleate (Ergotrate Maleate) and methylergonovine (Methergine), ergot derivatives, are two additional oxytocic drugs. Unlike oxytocin, they are primarily used to prevent postpartum or postabortal hemorrhage.

Ergonovine Maleate

Ergonovine maleate, when used after placental delivery, increases the strength, duration, and frequency of uterine contractions and decreases uterine bleeding. Ergonovine maleate exerts its effects by acting as a partial agonist or antagonist at the alpha-adrenergic, dopaminergic, and tryptaminergic receptors. Ergonovine maleate may also be used to treat migraine headache (an unlabeled use of this drug), although it is less effective for this condition than the drug ergotamine.

Onset of action is rapid, although it varies by route of administration. IM injection is the preferred method. IV injection is confined to emergencies, such as excessive uterine bleeding, because of the higher incidence of adverse effects that accompany IV administration. Uterine contractions will continue for 3 or more hours after IM injection. Ergonovine maleate promotes a higher uterine tone than oxytocin and therefore is not recommended for routine use before the delivery of the placenta. As with oxytocin, hypertension and headache may occur with use of ergonovine maleate. The principal manifestations of serious overdosage of ergonovine maleate are convulsions (acute overdosage) and gangrene of the fingers and toes (chronic overdosage). Other symptoms of overdosage include nausea, vomiting, diarrhea, hypertension or hypotension, weak pulse, dyspnea, loss of consciousness, numbness and coldness of extremities, tingling, chest pain, hypercoagulability, confusion, excitement, delirium, hallucinations, and coma.

Methylergonovine

Methylergonovine also has substantial effects on uterine tone. It acts directly on the smooth muscle of the uterus and induces a rapid and sustained tetanic uterotonic effect, which shortens the third stage of labor and reduces blood loss. Excretion is rapid and appears to be both renal and hepatic. IM use of methylergonovine is considered routine management after delivery of the placenta, although it may also be administered after the delivery of the anterior shoulder if full obstetric supervision is available. It is given orally three or four times a day immediately postpartum for a maximum of

1 week. Hypertension, sometimes with seizures or headache, is the most common adverse effect. Other adverse effects are hypotension, nausea, vomiting, dizziness, tinnitus, transient chest pain, hematuria, thrombophlebitis, water intoxication, hallucinations, leg cramps, nasal congestion, diarrhea, diaphoresis, palpitations, and dyspnea. Signs of acute overdosage include nausea, vomiting, abdominal pain, numbness, tingling of the extremities, and increase in blood pressure.

Drugs Significantly Different From P Oxytocin

Carboprost

Carboprost (Hemabate) is a prostaglandin used to induce abortion in pregnancies of 13 to 20 weeks' duration. Prostaglandins stimulate the myometrium of the pregnant uterus to contract in a manner similar to that of labor. The exact mechanisms of action of carboprost are unknown. Carboprost may also be used to control postpartum hemorrhage resulting from uterine atony that has not responded to oxytocin and IM ergot preparations. Carboprost is contraindicated in the following conditions: acute pelvic inflammatory disease; active cardiac, pulmonary, renal, or hepatic disease; and hypersensitivity to the agents. Carboprost is administered intramuscularly.

Carboprost also stimulates the smooth muscle of the GI tract, which may be responsible for the nausea, vomiting, and diarrhea that sometimes accompany its use. Nausea is the most common adverse effect. Other possible adverse effects are cardiovascular (arrhythmia, chest pain), CNS related (headache, flushing, anxiety, hot flashes, paresthesia, dizziness, weakness), genitourinary (endometritis, uterine rupture, uterine or vaginal pain), and respiratory (coughing, dyspnea). Other miscellaneous adverse effects include chills and shivering, backache, blurred vision, breast tenderness, diaphoresis, eye pain, muscle cramps, fever, rash, and leg cramps.

Dinoprostone

Dinoprostone (Prepidil, Cervidil) has two major uses. Dinoprostone given as a vaginal suppository (Prostin E2) is used to terminate pregnancies of 12 to 20 weeks. It is usually reserved for evacuating the uterus in managing incomplete spontaneous abortion or intrauterine fetal death up to 28 weeks. It is also used in managing nonmetastatic gestational trophoblastic disease (benign hydatidiform mole).

Dinoprostone in a gel form (PGE_2 gel; Prepidil) or a vaginal insert (Cervidil) is used as an agent for cervical ripening at term when induction of labor is indicated. In most patients, treatment with dinoprostone will change the consistency, dilation, and effacement of the cervix.

The liver appears to be the primary site of metabolism for dinoprostone. Metabolites are excreted renally.

Misoprostol

Misoprostol (Cytotec) is a synthetic PGE_1 analogue. It produces uterine contractions. It also has antisecretory and mucosal protective properties. Although the only approved use of misoprostol is to prevent gastric ulcers induced by therapy with nonsteroidal anti-inflammatory drugs (NSAIDs), many research studies have demonstrated that misoprostol is safe and effective in producing cervical ripening and initiating labor. This off-label use is widespread in clinical practice but is considered controversial by some authorities, including the Food and Drug Administration (FDA). The agency has not approved the drug for this use, and the manufacturer of the drug has placed a warning on the label not to use misoprostol for labor induction.

Multiple studies have indicated that misoprostol is more effective than PGE_2 in achieving vaginal deliveries within 24 hours of administration, decreases the need for a cesarean section (Goldberg & Wing, 2003), and reduces the need and the total amount of oxytocin required for augmentation of labor (Hofmeyr & Gulmezoglu, 2000). Research studies have not found a difference in the frequency of serious maternal adverse effects or neonatal outcomes with low-dose misoprostol therapy when compared with oxytocin or PGE_2 (Goldberg & Wing, 2003). Women at term who experienced prelabor rupture of their amniotic membranes were found to have less need for epidural analgesia and fetal heart monitoring when labor was induced with prostaglandins rather than with oxytocin. The risk for chorioamnionitis and neonatal infections between these two groups, however, was similar (Tan & Hannah, 2000). Numerous research studies have shown that hyperstimulation and meconium-stained amniotic fluid is possible, although relatively rare, with misoprostol; these adverse effects appear to be related to high doses (greater than 25 μg). The ACOG has concluded that intravaginal misoprostol tablets are effective in inducing labor in pregnant women who have unfavorable cervices and wrote to the FDA to emphasize its conclusions (ACOG, 1999b). To limit the risk for adverse fetal and maternal effects, the following standards of clinical practices should accompany the use of misoprostol (Simpson & Knox, 2003; ACOG, 1999b):

- The initial dose should be small, one fourth of a 100-μg tablet (i.e., approximately 25 μg). The pharmacy should prepare the doses because the tablets are not scored.
- Doses should not be administered more frequently than every 3 to 6 hours.
- Oxytocin should not be administered any sooner than 4 hours after the last dose of misoprostol.
- Misoprostol should not be used in patients with a previous cesarean delivery or prior major uterine surgery to prevent uterine rupture.

Some research has examined the role of oral misoprostol in inducing labor when premature rupture of membranes at term occurs. Although oral misoprostol does not seem to induce labor more rapidly than IV oxytocin, it is possible that it decreases the rate of hyperstimulation. This finding is inconclusive, however, and requires more research to substantiate it (Mozurkewich et al., 2003, Crane et al., 2003). Oral misoprostol appears to be less likely than oxytocin to produce postpartum hemorrhage, but this finding also is inconclusive and requires more research (Mozurkewich et al., 2003). See Chapter 48 for more information on the antiulcer properties of misoprostol and Chapter 54 for a discussion of its use as an abortifacient.

C TOCOLYTICS

Drugs that inhibit uterine activity are classified as tocolytics. Preterm labor is the medical complication requiring the administration of tocolytics. Tocolytics are used when true labor begins after 20 weeks' gestation and usually

before completion of the 34th gestational week. During the last 2 weeks of the preterm period (from 35 to 37 weeks), most fetuses are producing sufficient amounts of surfactant so that viability is not threatened by respiratory distress, and labor is thus not interrupted with a tocolytic but allowed to proceed. Although the use of tocolytic drugs can stop preterm labor, they have not been found to have an effect on perinatal or neonatal outcomes. The use of tocolytics stops labor for 24 to 48 hours, which affords additional time before delivery for the mother to receive corticosteroids. During that interval, the corticosteroids can exert a therapeutic effect on the fetal lungs so that they are prepared for life outside the uterus. If necessary, the mother can also be transferred to another facility during that time.

Currently, several drugs are used for their tocolytic properties, including beta-adrenergic agents, such as terbutaline and ritodrine, and magnesium sulfate. A new drug class, the oxytocin antagonists, is under investigation for use in treating preterm labor. Atosiban, the first drug in this class, has not been approved for use in the United States. Indomethacin, an NSAID, has been used as a tocolytic, but such use is rare because indomethacin poses substantial risks to the fetus. (Indomethacin is discussed in greater detail later in the chapter.) Thus far, the FDA has approved only ritodrine for use as a tocolytic. However, despite its approval and proven short-term effectiveness, this drug is seldom used to treat preterm labor because it causes many maternal adverse effects. Discontinuation rates because of adverse effects have been reported as high as 38%, contributing to the obstetric community's lack of confidence in ritodrine and a general view that ritodrine therapy is unsafe. A drug that acts similarly is terbutaline. Although using terbutaline to control preterm labor is an off-label use, the drug is widely used for this purpose. It is perceived to have fewer adverse effects than ritodrine, although some clinical studies dispute this conclusion. Because of its widespread use, terbutaline is the prototype tocolytic for this chapter.

Research on tocolytics has produced mixed results, with some studies showing that all of the tocolytics are equally effective in stopping preterm labor, some showing that a particular drug is better than other drugs, and some studies indicating that none of the drugs are very effective. Thus, the efficacy of all tocolytic drugs remains unclear, which is one reason for the continued controversy surrounding their use.

NURSING MANAGEMENT OF THE PATIENT RECEIVING [P] TERBUTALINE

Core Drug Knowledge

Pharmacotherapeutics

Terbutaline is used off-label to control preterm labor in pregnancies of 20 weeks to 34 weeks. Some disagreement exists as to what the earliest gestational age to use terbutaline should be, and some authorities believe drug therapy should be started later than 20 weeks. Using terbutaline to control preterm labor, although widespread, is still considered controversial by many experts who feel that the effectiveness of the drug for this use has never been clearly demonstrated.

Intervention should begin as soon as a diagnosis of preterm labor is established and contraindications are ruled out. Conservative therapy (e.g., bed rest and lying on the left side) may be tried first and may also be used simultaneously with drug therapy. Terbutaline has also been used to prevent further preterm labor after an episode of preterm labor has been stopped. This use is also considered controversial, and many experts feel that the drug's effectiveness has never been demonstrated by positive perinatal or neonatal outcomes. Despite the controversy about the effectiveness of terbutaline and of other drugs used as tocolytics, terbutaline is still commonly used for controlling preterm labor and preventing additional episodes of preterm labor. It should be used concomitantly with corticosteroids, which are effective in preventing respiratory complications in the premature newborns. Terbutaline therapy prolongs delivery long enough for the corticosteroids to take effect.

Because terbutaline increases fetal heart rate, it has occasionally been given orally to mothers in an attempt to treat fetal heart block. Although these few small studies and case reports indicate that terbutaline increases the heart rate in some fetuses, evidence to demonstrate a prolonged effect or improved fetal or neonatal outcomes is insufficient. This use of terbutaline is off-label and experimental (Kulier & Hofmeyr, 2000; Robinson et al., 2001; Yoshida et al., 2001). Other, labeled uses of terbutaline include treatment of asthma and bronchospasm (see Chapter 47, Table 47.2 for more information on this use). Terbutaline is administered orally, subcutaneously, or intravenously.

Pharmacokinetics

Terbutaline is well absorbed orally. Its onset of action is quicker when administered subcutaneously, but its duration of action is shorter. Other aspects of pharmacokinetics are not well known.

Pharmacodynamics

Terbutaline is a beta-receptor agonist (stimulant) that selectively prefers the beta-2 receptors over beta-1 receptors. Stimulation of these receptors inhibits contractility of uterine smooth muscle and provides bronchial dilation, vasodilation, and hepatic glycogenolysis and gluconeogenesis, among other effects (for a full discussion of the effects from beta-2 receptor stimulation, see Chapter 13). Although terbutaline prolongs pregnancy, it has not been found to decrease the incidence of premature births or have any effect on perinatal or neonatal outcomes.

Contraindications and Precautions

Terbutaline is contraindicated before the 20th week of pregnancy because the impetus for a spontaneous abortion may be related to genetic fetal defects. Terbutaline is also contraindicated in the following conditions, in which continuing the pregnancy is hazardous to the mother or fetus:

- Antepartum hemorrhage that requires immediate delivery
- Eclampsia and severe preeclampsia
- Intrauterine fetal death
- Chorioamnionitis (inflammation of the amniotic membranes)
- Maternal cardiac disease

- Pulmonary hypertension
- Maternal hyperthyroidism
- Uncontrolled maternal diabetes mellitus

Additional contraindications include pre-existing maternal medical conditions that would be seriously affected by the pharmacologic properties of a beta-agonist such as terbutaline. Examples include hypovolemia, cardiac arrhythmias associated with tachycardia or digitalis toxicity, uncontrolled hypertension, and pheochromocytoma (a hypertension-producing tumor of the adrenal glands). Hypersensitivity to any component of the drug is also a contraindication. Precautions that apply to the use of terbutaline include controlled diabetes, controlled hypertension, and bronchial asthma already being treated with beta agonists. Terbutaline is an FDA pregnancy category B drug.

Adverse Effects

Terbutaline is a potent drug that may produce serious, even fatal, adverse effects in the woman and the fetus. The adverse effects are related to the other effects of beta stimulants on the body, including beta-1 stimulation effects, because although terbutaline is relatively selective for beta-2 receptors, some stimulation of beta-1 receptors still occurs. These maternal adverse effects include tachycardia, palpitations, hypotension, cardiac arrhythmias, electrocardiographic changes, dyspnea, nervousness, tremor, transient hyperglycemia, hypokalemia (occurring possibly through intracellular shunting), pulmonary edema, cerebral and myocardial ischemia, nausea, and vomiting. Fetal and neonatal effects include increased fetal heart rate and neonatal hypoglycemia. Of these adverse effects, tachycardia (maternal and fetal), cardiac arrhythmias, palpitations, and tremor (maternal) are probably the most common, and pulmonary edema and cerebral and myocardial ischemia are the most serious. Cardiac arrhythmias are also potentially serious.

In instances of overdose, the drug should be discontinued, and an appropriate beta blocker, such as propranolol, should be given as an antidote.

Drug Interactions

Additive effects may occur if terbutaline is administered with other beta stimulants. Coadministration of terbutaline and beta blockers decreases the effectiveness of terbutaline. Table 55.2 lists drugs that interact with terbutaline.

Assessment of Relevant Core Patient Variables

Health Status

Determine whether the patient has any conditions that contraindicate therapy or require cautious use of terbutaline. These conditions may include cardiac arrhythmias associated with tachycardia, uncontrolled hypertension, pheochromocytoma, diabetes, or bronchial asthma already being treated with beta agonists. Assess the patient's pulse rate and blood pressure. A baseline electrocardiogram (ECG) should be performed to rule out undiagnosed maternal heart disease before beginning terbutaline infusion. Determine whether the patient is taking beta blockers.

Life Span and Gender

Ask whether the woman's pregnancy is 20 weeks' gestation or more because pregnancy of less than 20 weeks is a contraindication.

Environment

Be aware of the environment required to administer terbutaline. Terbutaline given to control a current episode of preterm labor must be given in a hospital labor and delivery suite where the mother and fetus can be monitored while the IV solution or the continuous subcutaneous (SC) solution is infused. Oral terbutaline given to prevent future episodes of preterm labor may be administered in any setting.

Nursing Diagnoses and Outcomes

- Risk for Injury to mother from adverse effects of drug therapy
  Desired outcome: *No adverse effects will occur from drug therapy.*
- Risk for Injury to infant stemming from premature delivery or adverse effects from drug therapy
  Desired outcome: *Drug therapy will prevent premature delivery of infant and will not cause adverse effects to the newborn.*
- Excess Fluid Volume, pulmonary edema, related to potential adverse effects of drug therapy
  Desired outcome: *The patient's fluid volume will remain within normal limits.*

TABLE 55.2 Agents That Interact With [P] Terbutaline

Interactants	Effect and Significance	Nursing Management
Beta blockers	Will compete with terbutaline for the same receptors, thereby preventing terbutaline from having its effect	Give as antidote if overdosage of terbutaline; otherwise, not recommended to be coadministered.
Beta-2 agonists; other sympathomimetic drugs	Increased effects at other beta receptors; may significantly increase blood pressure	Avoid coadministration if possible; monitor patient's BP carefully if coadministration is essential.
Halothane, cyclopropane (halogenated hydrocarbon anesthetics)	Increases the risk for cardiac arrhythmias	Monitor patient carefully if this combination must be used.

Planning and Intervention

Maximizing Therapeutic Effects

Begin drug therapy as soon as possible after preterm labor is diagnosed and the order to start therapy has been received. Terbutaline therapy is usually given by the IV route initially and can be switched to an oral route if use is expected to continue longer than 24 hours.

Minimizing Adverse Effects

Monitor the patient's pulse rate and blood pressure closely throughout therapy. Have the patient lie on her left side during infusion to help minimize the risk for hypotension and promote circulation to the fetus. Closely monitor the patient's fluid status and avoid fluid overload. Related measures include monitoring intake and output of fluids, assessing peripheries for edema, and auscultating breath sounds for rales and rhonchi every hour. If pulmonary edema develops, discontinue drug administration and notify the prescriber or nurse midwife immediately. Seek orders to manage the edema by diuretic therapy.

If the patient demonstrates signs of adverse effects, such as palpitations, tachycardia, hypotension, or nervousness, the dosage of terbutaline should be decreased. Ensure that a beta blocker such as propranolol is available as an antidote in case of overdosage. If the patient is diabetic or receives potassium-depleting diuretics, monitor the serum glucose and potassium levels carefully. Administer terbutaline infusions through an IV infusion controller or pump to keep the dosage rate accurate. Because of the risk for pulmonary edema, avoid diluting terbutaline with saline (0.9% sodium chloride solution or lactated Ringer solution) and Hartmann solution; use a dextrose solution instead.

Providing Patient and Family Education

- Educate the patient and family about the therapeutic and adverse effects of the drug.
- Explain to the patient the rationale for lying on her left side.
- Instruct the patient to notify you or another health care provider immediately if she experiences swelling in her hands or feet, shortness of breath, palpitations, or chest pain.

For more on patient and family education, see Box 55.2.

Ongoing Assessment and Evaluation

Monitor the maternal heart rate, FHR, and maternal blood pressure and fluid status throughout therapy. Terbutaline drug therapy is considered effective when the premature contractions decrease in intensity and frequency, the woman and fetus do not experience adverse effects, and premature birth is avoided for at least 24 hours so that administered corticosteroids can exert their beneficial effects.

CRITICAL THINKING SCENARIO

Maternal monitoring and terbutaline

Susan Hartmann, who is 30 weeks pregnant, has diabetes that is well controlled with glyburide, an oral antidiabetic agent. She begins preterm labor, and terbutaline is ordered for her.

1. Discuss which laboratory values you would monitor most closely if you were her nurse.
2. Explain the rationale for your choices.

COMMUNITY-BASED CONCERNS

Box 55.2 Teaching About Drugs That Affect Uterine Function

Prenatal teaching should include the following:

- Signs of preterm labor
- Rationale for not giving ritodrine to stop preterm labor before 20-weeks' gestation (spontaneous abortion may be related to fetal defects; ritodrine's effects on fetus less than 20 weeks are unknown)
- Rationale regarding use of oxytocin (these should focus on medical indications, not convenience of delivery)

Drugs Significantly Different From P Terbutaline

Magnesium Sulfate

Magnesium is a trace mineral involved in many chemical reactions in the body. Therefore, the pharmacotherapeutics of magnesium sulfate are diverse, and more potential therapeutic uses are under consideration. Oral magnesium sulfate preparations are used in laxatives and antacids (see Chapters 48 and 49). Oral and IV forms of magnesium sulfate are often given to correct electrolyte imbalances (hypomagnesemia). IV magnesium effectively suppresses ventricular ectopy and is a first-line therapy for torsades de pointes, a variation on ven-

MEMORY CHIP

P Terbutaline

- Used off-label to control preterm labor after 20 weeks' and up to 34 weeks' gestation; allows time for administered corticosteroids to be effective in newborn
- Beta-2 receptor agonist (stimulant); antidote: beta blockers
- Major contraindications: before the 20th week of pregnancy; when continuing the pregnancy is hazardous to the woman or fetus; pre-existing maternal medical conditions that would be seriously affected by the pharmacologic properties of a beta agonist
- Most common adverse effects: maternal and fetal tachycardia; maternal palpitations, cardiac arrhythmias, tremor
- Most serious adverse effects: maternal—pulmonary edema, cerebral and myocardial ischemia, some cardiac arrhythmias
- Maximizing therapeutic effects: Administer as soon as preterm labor is diagnosed and order is written for drug therapy.
- Minimizing adverse effects: Monitor maternal pulse rate, blood pressure, fluid status, and fetal heart rate; decrease infusion rate if adverse effects (excessive beta stimulation) are present.
- Most important patient education: Drugs to control preterm labor help buy time for other drug therapy to have an effect in preventing complications in the newborn.

tricular tachycardia that can progress to fibrillation and be fatal. It may also be useful in treating patients with congestive heart failure or acute myocardial infarction. Magnesium sulfate is used to control hypertension, encephalopathy, and convulsions in children with acute nephritis. IV magnesium may be useful in treating asthma and chronic lung disease that have been unresponsive to conventional therapy with beta agonists.

Magnesium sulfate is the drug of choice for treating or preventing seizures associated with preeclampsia, eclampsia, and pregnancy-induced hypertension. Its effectiveness in preventing seizures in eclampsia is well accepted and documented. A review of research trials shows that magnesium sulfate decreases the risk from eclampsia by more than half, and probably reduces the risk for maternal death.

When used in eclampsia, magnesium sulfate does not appear to improve the short-term outcomes for the baby, although it does not increase the risk for poor outcomes either (Duley et al., 2003). One recent study on its use in mild preeclampsia showed that it did not have a major impact on disease progression, meaning that it did not significantly prevent the preeclampsia from worsening or developing into eclampsia. Nonetheless, using magnesium sulfate in mild preeclampsia did not in itself produce negative outcomes for the mother or baby because it did not increase the need for cesarean delivery, the occurrence of infectious diseases, the incidence of postpartum hemorrhage, or the incidence of low Apgar scores in the newborn (Livingston et al., 2003). Magnesium sulfate has some effectiveness as a tocolytic. As with terbutaline, its use as a tocolytic is unlabeled, and the research showing magnesium sulfate's effectiveness is likewise mixed. Some research demonstrates that it is as effective as terbutaline, others that it is more effective. The effectiveness of magnesium sulfate as a tocolytic remains controversial, although it is widely used for this purpose. It appears to inhibit myometrial contractility but does not prolong pregnancy much. It can help prevent labor long enough to allow corticosteroids to be administered to the mother to protect the infant's lungs. Short-term neonatal outcomes from magnesium sulfate may not ultimately improve early neonatal outcomes (Jazayeri et al., 2003), but long term it may reduce the risk for cerebral palsy or death in very preterm infants without causing negative effects (Crowther et al., 2003). Research on the possible benefits of using magnesium sulfate to control preterm labor continues.

Magnesium sulfate's mechanism of action makes it particularly suitable for use in complications of pregnancy. Magnesium sulfate acts as a CNS and muscular depressant, producing peripheral neuromuscular blockade. It prevents or controls convulsions by blocking neuromuscular transmission and by decreasing the amount of acetylcholine freed at the end plate by the motor nerve impulse. Secondarily, magnesium sulfate relaxes smooth muscle, decreasing uterine contractions and blood pressure. This effect may be related to its antagonistic effect on calcium, which prevents calcium influx into the cells for cellular contraction.

Although magnesium sulfate is a pregnancy category A drug (which means that it does not cause fetal structural defects), its use still carries some risk to the fetus because the drug may cause other adverse effects. Magnesium sulfate may also cause adverse effects in the mother. Adverse effects are related to how the drug works and are usually associated with elevated serum levels or magnesium intoxication (Table 55.3). A serum level of 10 to 12 mg/dL is associated with toxicity (normal levels without any infusion of magnesium sulfate are 1.8–3). The most common maternal adverse effects are the following:

- Headache
- Hyporeflexia
- Weakness
- Thirst
- Flushing
- Burning at infusion site

The most life-threatening maternal adverse effects are:

- Circulatory collapse
- Respiratory depression
- Pulmonary edema

The most common fetal and neonatal adverse effects are:

- Heart rate changes
- Neonatal hypotonia
- Neonatal respiratory depression (possibly serious)

Other maternal adverse effects from magnesium toxicity are sweating, hypotension, flaccid paralysis, hypothermia, and cardiac depression. IV infusion, especially for prolonged periods (more than 24 hours), may produce hypermagnesemia in the newborn, including neuromuscular or respiratory depression. Overdosage produces a sharp drop in the blood pressure, respiratory paralysis, and ECG changes (increased PR interval, increased QRS complex, and prolonged QT interval). Heart block and asystole may also occur. Serum levels need to be monitored closely when the patient is receiving magnesium sulfate to prevent overdosage and adverse effects from therapy. Calcium gluconate antagonizes the effects of magnesium toxicity and is the antidote for overdose.

Magnesium sulfate may be administered by the IM or IV route or by IV infusion (see Table 55.1). An IV pump should be used to regulate the flow of magnesium sulfate infusion. Dosing is accomplished with a loading dose followed by a maintenance dose. The IV route is preferred for initial stabilization; after that, an oral dose may be used for maintenance.

TABLE 55.3 Correlation of Serum Levels and Effects of Magnesium Sulfate

Serum Level (mEq/L)	Effect
1.5–3	Normal level
4–7	Therapeutic level for preeclampsia/eclampsia/convulsions
7–10	Loss of deep tendon reflexes, hypotension, loss of consciousness
13–15	Respiratory paralysis
16–25	Cardiac conduction altered (lengthened PR interval, QRS widening, prolonged QT interval arrhythmias)
25	Cardiac arrest

The goal is to maintain a therapeutic serum level without causing adverse effects. The therapeutic level varies, depending on the clinical indication for the therapy. It is 5 to 8 mg/dL in preterm labor and 4 to 8 mg/dL in pregnancy-induced hypertension. These levels are higher than would normally be found in the serum but are the elevations required to produce a therapeutic effect.

In addition to using an IV pump, several other nursing actions can minimize adverse effects. Assess for signs of magnesium toxicity by monitoring the serum magnesium levels and the patient's clinical response to drug administration. Use continuous maternal cardiac monitoring and continuous fetal monitoring while the patient is receiving IV magnesium sulfate. Place the patient on bed rest in the left lateral recumbent position to prevent hypotension and to maximize blood flow to the fetus. The patient must receive nothing orally to eat or drink (i.e., remain NPO) during stabilization to help prevent nausea and vomiting. Document uterine activity, cervical changes, and maternal-fetal responses with each change in dose. Implement safety measures or seizure precautions if the drug is used to prevent or treat seizures associated with pregnancy-induced hypertension. Finally, always keep calcium gluconate at the bedside to use as an antidote if magnesium toxicity occurs.

Indomethacin

Indomethacin is an NSAID that suppresses uterine activity by inhibiting prostaglandin synthesis. It is effective in stopping premature labor, but its use as a tocolytic is very limited because of concerns over fetal safety. Indomethacin appears to increase the risk for necrotizing enterocolitis, intercranial hemorrhage, and patent ductus arteriosus. These serious effects severely limit the use of this and other prostaglandin inhibitors in treating preterm labor. Use of the drug for treating preterm labor is not recommended. For information about the other uses of indomethacin, see Chapter 24.

CHAPTER SUMMARY

- Drug therapy may be used when labor does not occur at term, does not bring about delivery effectively, or begins preterm.
- Oxytocin is given by IV drip infusion to initiate or augment (improve) labor contractions when important fetal or maternal reasons to do so exist. It is also used to control postpartum bleeding or hemorrhage.
- Response to oxytocin therapy has three phases: the incremental phase, the stable phase, and hyperstimulation. The hyperstimulation phase is undesirable and indicates that administration of oxytocin has been excessive.
- Adverse effects of oxytocin are dose related.
- You need an accurate understanding of the physiology involved in producing contractions, the core drug knowledge (most specifically the pharmacokinetics, pharmacodynamics, and adverse effects of oxytocin), and the relevant core patient variables to be able to make sound professional judgments in managing patients receiving oxytocin therapy.
- You are responsible for determining the maternal and fetal response to oxytocin therapy (frequency of contractions, progress of labor, and fetal tolerance) and for titrating the dose, per the physician's or nurse midwife's orders, based on this assessment.
- You must stop the infusion of oxytocin if hyperstimulation of the uterus occurs.
- Tocolytic drugs are used to stop preterm labor. Although they are effective for short-term use, they have not decreased the number of preterm births, neonatal morbidity, or neonatal mortality. Tocolytic drugs do help prolong labor long enough to allow administration of corticosteroids and to transfer the mother (if necessary) to an institution that has facilities for premature infants.
- Terbutaline is a beta-receptor agonist (stimulant) that attaches to receptors in the uterine smooth muscle. Stimulation of these receptors inhibits contractility of uterine smooth muscle. Infusing terbutaline decreases the intensity and frequency of uterine contractions. Beta-blocking compounds stop the effects of terbutaline.
- Dose-related maternal and fetal tachycardia and changes in maternal blood pressure can occur in patients receiving terbutaline. Adverse effects reflect stimulation of the beta receptors.
- Magnesium sulfate infusions depress the CNS and cause muscle relaxation. Magnesium sulfate is the drug of choice to treat preeclampsia and seizures in eclampsia and is used off-label to stop preterm labor. Excessive loss of tone and reflexes can occur as an adverse effect. Adverse effects are related to high levels of the drug in the blood.
- Drugs that alter uterine motility are potentially dangerous to the woman and fetus. Infusions of these drugs should be regulated with IV controllers or pumps. These patients need close monitoring for signs of adverse effects throughout therapy.

QUESTIONS FOR STUDY AND REVIEW

1. Why should you titrate oxytocin slowly upward with dosage adjustments every 40 to 60 minutes?
2. Define the three phases of oxytocin response.
3. Which adverse effect of oxytocin is most dangerous to the pregnant woman?
4. What nursing assessments should be made to minimize adverse effects from oxytocin?
5. How does terbutaline stop preterm labor?
6. If the patient develops tachycardia, palpitations, and nervousness while on terbutaline infusion, what action should you take?
7. List the reasons that magnesium sulfate may be prescribed during pregnancy.
8. State the antidote to magnesium sulfate overdosage.
9. What are the most common maternal, fetal, and neonatal adverse effects from infusion of magnesium sulfate?

Need More Help?

Chapter 55 of the study guide for *Drug Therapy in Nursing* 2e contains NCLEX-style questions and other learning activities to reinforce your understanding of the concepts presented in this chapter. For additional information or to purchase the study guide, visit *http://connection.lww.com/go/aschenbrenner.*

REFERENCES AND BIBLIOGRAPHY

American Academy of Pediatrics and American College of Obstetricians and Gynecologists. (2002). *Guidelines for perinatal care* (5th ed.). Elk Grove Village, IL: Author.

American College of Obstetricians and Gynecologists. (1995). *Dystocia and the augmentation of labor.* (Technical Bulletin Number 217). Washington, DC: Author.

American College of Obstetricians and Gynecologists. (1999a). *Induction of labor.* (Practice Bulletin Number 10). Washington, DC: Author.

American College of Obstetricians and Gynecologists. (1999b). *Induction of labor with misoprostol.* (Committee Opinion No. 228). Washington, DC: Author.

Arias E. (2002). Pharmacology of oxytocin and prostaglandins. *Clinical Obstetrics and Gynecology, 43,* 455–468.

Association of Women's Health, Obstetric and Neonatal Nurses. (1998). *Standards and guidelines for professional nursing practice in the care of women and newborns* (5th ed.). Washington, DC: Author.

Clayworth, S. (2000). The nurse's role during oxytocin administration. *MCN American Journal of Maternal Child Nursing, 25*(2), 80–85.

Crane, J. M., Delaney, T., & Hutchens, D. (2003). Oral misoprostol for premature rupture of membranes at term. *American Journal of Obstetrics and Gynecology, 189*(3), 720–724.

Crane, J. M., & Young, D. C. (1998). Meta-analysis of low dose versus high dose oxytocin for labour induction. *Journal of the Society of Obstetrics and Gynaecology in Canada, 20,* 1215–1223.

Crowther, C. A., Hiller, J. E., Doyle, L. W., et al., Australasian Collaborative Trial of Magnesium Sulphate (ACTOMgSO4) Collaborative Group. (2003). Effect of magnesium sulfate given for neuroprotection before preterm birth: A randomized controlled trial. *Journal of the American Medical Association, 290*(20), 2730–2732.

Duley, L., Gulmezoglu, A. M., & Henderson-Smart, D. J. (2003). Magnesium sulphate and other anticonvulsants for women with preeclampsia. *Cochrane Database Systematic Reviews, 2,* CD000025.

Goldberg, A. B., & Wing, D. A. (2003). Induction of labor: The misoprostol controversy. *Journal of Midwifery and Women's Health, 48*(4), 244–248.

Hofmeyr, G. J., & Gulmezoglu, A. M. (2000). Vaginal misoprostol for cervical ripening and labour induction in late pregnancy. *Cochrane Database Systematic Reviews,* (2), CD000941.

Hollander, E., Novotny, S., Hanratty, M., et al. (2003). Oxytocin infusion reduces repetitive behaviors in adults with autistic and Asperger's disorders. *Neuropsychopharmacology, 28*(1), 193–198.

Jazayeri, A., Jazayeri, M. K., & Sutkin, G. (2003). Tocolysis does not improve neonatal outcomes in patients with preterm rupture of membranes. *American Journal of Perinatology, 20*(4), 189–193.

Kulier, R., & Hofmeyr, G. J. (2000). Tocolytics for suspected intrapartum fetal distress. *Cochrane Database Systematic Reviews, 2,* CD000035.

Livingston, J. C., Livingston, L. W., Ramsey, R., et al. (2003). Magnesium sulfate in women with mild preeclampsia: A randomized controlled trial. *Obstetrics and Gynecology, 101*(2), 217–220.

Mozurkewich, E., Horrocks, J., Daley, S., et al., the MisoPROM Study. (2003). The MisoPROM Study: A multicenter randomized comparison of oral misoprostol and oxytocin for premature rupture of membranes at term. *American Journal of Obstetrics and Gynecology, 189*(4), 1026–1030.

Robinson, B. V., Ettedgui, J. A., & Sherman, F. S. (2001). Use of terbutaline in the treatment of complete heart block in the fetus. *Cardiology in the Young, 11*(6), 683–686.

Simpson, K. R. (1998). *Cervical ripening and induction and augmentation of labor.* (Practice monograph). Washington, DC: Association of Women's Health, Obstetric, and Neonatal Nurses.

Simpson, K. R., & Knox, G. E. (2003). Common areas of litigation related to care during labor and birth: Recommendations to promote patient safety and decrease risk exposure. *Journal of Perinatal and Neonatal Nursing, 17*(2), 110–125.

Tan, B. P., & Hannah, M. E. (2000). Prostaglandins versus oxytocin for prelabour rupture of membranes at term. *Cochrane Database Systematic Reviews,* (2), CD000159.

Yoshida, H., Iwamoto, M., Sakakibara, H., et al. (2001). Treatment of fetal congenital complete heart block with maternal administration of beta-sympathomimetics (terbutaline): A case report. *Gynecologic and Obstetric Investigation, 52*(2), 142–144.

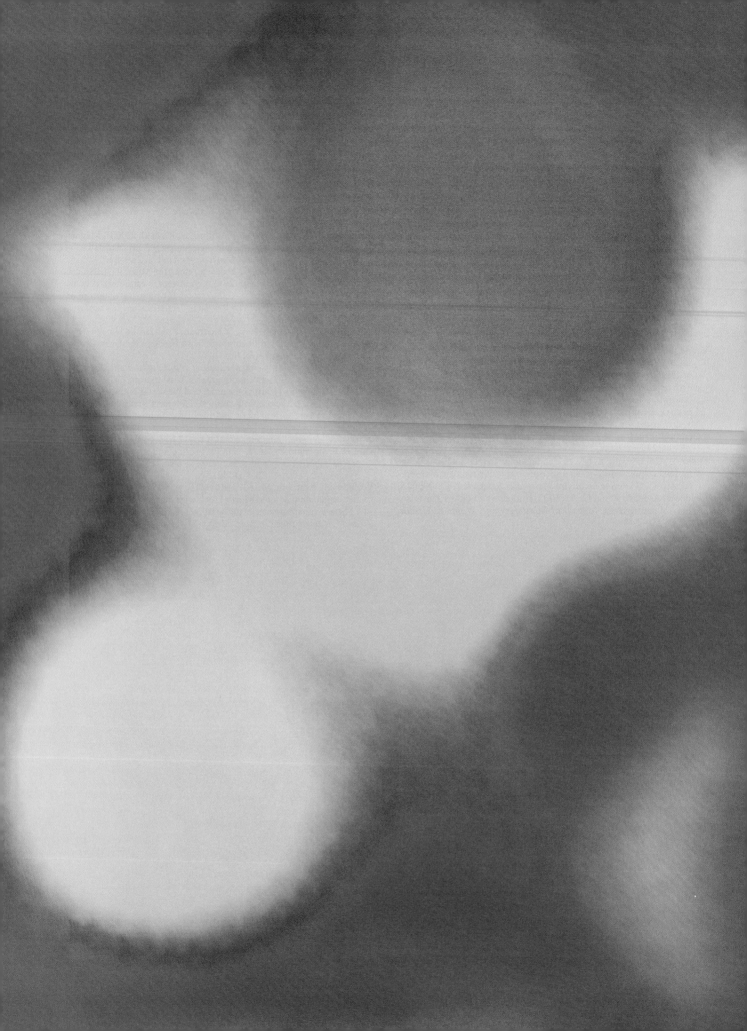

appendix A

Supplemental Canadian Drug Information

NARCOTICS, CONTROLLED DRUGS, BENZODIAZEPINES, AND OTHER TARGETED SUBSTANCES

Table 1 summarizes the requirements for prescribing, dispensing, and record keeping for narcotics, controlled drugs, benzodiazepines, and other targeted substances. This information does not present a comprehensive review; additional and confirmatory information can be found in the Controlled Drugs and Substances Act, Narcotic Control Regulations, Controlled Drugs Regulations, and the Benzodiazepines and Other Targeted Substances Regulations. (Reviewed 2004 by the Office of Controlled Substances, Health Canada.)

TABLE 1 Narcotic, Controlled Drugs, Benzodiazepines and Other Targeted Substances Summary

Classification and Description	Legal Requirements
Narcotic Drugs*	
• 1 narcotic (e.g., cocaine, codeine, hydromorphone, morphine) • 1 narcotic + 1 active non-narcotic ingredient (e.g., Cophylac, Empracet-30, Novahletex DH, Tylenol No. 4) • All narcotics for parenteral use (e.g., fentanyl, pethidine) • All products containing diamorphine (hospitals only), hydrocodone, oxycodone, methadone or pentazocine • Dextropropoxyphene, propoxyphene (straight) (e.g., Darvon-N, 642)	• Written prescription required. • Verbal prescriptions not permitted. • Refills not permitted. • Written prescription may be prescribed to be dispensed in divided portions (part-fills). • For part-fills, copies of prescriptions should be made in reference to the original prescription. Indicate on the original prescription: the new prescription number, the date of the part-fill, the quantity dispensed and the pharmacist's initials. • Transfers not permitted. • Record and retain all documents pertaining to all transactions for a period of at least 2 years, in a manner that permits an audit. • Sales reports required except for dextropropoxyphene, propoxyphene. • Report any loss or theft of narcotic drugs as well as forged prescriptions within 10 days to the Office of Controlled Substances at the address indicated on the forms.
Narcotic Preparations*	
• Verbal prescription narcotics: 1 narcotic + 2 or more active non-narcotic ingredients in a recognized therapeutic dose (e.g., Fiorinal with Codeine, Robitussin AC 692, 282, 292, Tylenol No. 2 and No. 3) • Exempted codeine compounds: contain codeine up to 8 mg/solid dosage form or 20 mg/30 mL liquid + 2 or more active non-narcotic ingredients (e.g., Atasol-8, Robitussin with Codeine).	• Written or verbal prescriptions permitted. • Refills not permitted. • Written or verbal prescriptions may be prescribed to be dispensed in divided portions (part-fills). • For part-fills, copies of prescriptions should be made in reference to the original prescription. Indicate on the original prescription: the new prescription number, the date of the part-fill, the quantity dispensed and the pharmacist's initials. • Transfers not permitted. • Exempted codeine compounds when dispensed pursuant to a prescription follow the same regulations as for verbal prescription narcotics. • Record and retain all documents pertaining to all transactions for a period of at least 2 years, in a manner that permits an audit. • Sales reports not required. • Report any loss or theft of narcotic drugs as well as forged prescriptions within 10 days to the Office of Controlled Substances at the address indicated on the forms.
Controlled Drugs*	
• Part I e.g., amphetamines (Dexedrine) methylphenidate (Ritalin) pentobarbital (Nembutal) secobarbital (Seconal, Tuinal)	• Written or verbal prescriptions permitted. • Refills not permitted for verbal prescriptions. • Refills permitted for written prescriptions if the prescriber has indicated in writing the number of refills and dates for, or intervals between, refills.

(continued)

TABLE 1 Narcotic, Controlled Drugs, Benzodiazepines and Other Targeted Substances Summary (continued)

Classification and Description	Legal Requirements
preparations: 1 controlled drug + 1 or more active noncontrolled drug(s) (Cafergot-PB)	• Written or verbal prescriptions may be prescribed to be dispensed in divided portions (part-fills). • For refills and part-fills, copies of prescriptions should be made in reference to the original prescription. Indicate on the original prescription: the new prescription number, the date of the repeat or part-fill, the quantity dispensed and the pharmacist's initials. • Transfers not permitted. • Record and retain all documents pertaining to all transactions for a period of at least 2 years, in a manner that permits an audit. • Sales reports required except for controlled drug preparations. • Report any loss or theft of controlled drugs as well as forged prescriptions within 10 days to the Office of Controlled Substances at the address indicated on the forms.
• Part II e.g., barbiturates (amobarbital, phenobarbital) butorphanol (Stadol NS) diethylpropion (Tenuate) nalbuphine (Nubain) phentermine (Ionamin) preparations: 1 controlled drug + 1 or more active noncontrolled ingredient(s) (Fiorinal, Neo-Pause, Tecnal) • Part III e.g., anabolic steroids (methyltestosterone, nandrolone decanoate)	• Written or verbal prescriptions permitted. • Refills permitted for written or verbal prescriptions if the prescriber has authorized in writing or verbally (at the time of issuance) the number of refills and dates for, or intervals between, refills. • Written or verbal prescriptions may be prescribed to be dispensed in divided portions (part-fills). • For refills and part-fills, copies of prescriptions should be made in reference to the original prescription. Indicate on the original prescription: the new prescription number, the date of the repeat or part-fill, the quantity dispensed and the pharmacist's initials. • Transfers not permitted. • Record and retain all documents pertaining to all transactions for a period of at least 2 years, in a manner that permits an audit. • Sales reports not required. • Report the loss or theft of controlled drugs as well as forged prescriptions within 10 days to the Office of Controlled Substances at the address indicated on the forms.
Benzodiazepines and Other Targeted Substances*	
e.g., alprazolam (Xanax) bromazepam (Lectopam) chlordiazepoxide (Librium) clobazam (Frisium) ethchlorvynol lorazepam (Ativan) mazindol meprobarnate oxazepam (Serax)	• Written and verbal prescriptions permitted. • Refills for written or verbal prescriptions permitted if indicated by prescriber. • Part-fills permitted as per prescriber's instructions. • For refills or part-fills of prescriptions, the following information should be recorded: date of the repeat or part-fill, prescription number, quantity dispensed and the pharmacist's initials. • Transfer of prescriptions permitted except a prescription that has been already transferred. • Sales reports not required. • Report any loss or theft of benzodiazepines and other targeted substances within 10 days to the Office of Controlled Substances at the address indicated on the forms.

*The products noted are examples only.

Reprinted with permission from *Compendium of Pharmaceuticals and Specialties,* 39th ed., Canadian Pharmacists Association, Ottawa, 2004.

IMMUNIZATION SCHEDULES FOR INFANTS AND CHILDREN

TABLE 2 Routine Immunization Schedules

Age at Vaccination	DTaP[1]	IPV	Hib[2]	MMR	Td[2] or dTap[10]	Hep B[4] (3 doses)	V	PC	MC
Birth									
2 months	X	X	X					X[8]	X[9]
4 months	X	X	X			Infancy		X	X
6 months	X	(X)[5]	X			or		X	X
12 months				X		preadolescence	X[7]	X	
18 months	X	X	X	(X)[5] or		(9–13 years)			or
4–6 years	X	X		(X)[4]					
14–16 years					X[10]				X[9]

DTaP, diphtheria, tetanus, pertussis (acellular) vaccine; IPV, inactivated poliovirus vaccine; Hib, *Haemophillus influenzae* type b conjugate vaccine; MMR, measles, mumps and rubella vaccine; Td, tetanus and diphtheria toxoid, adult type with reduced diphtheria toxoid; dTap, tetanus and diphtheria toxoid, acellular pertussis, adolescent/adult type with reduced diphtheria and pertussis components; Hep B, hepatitis B vaccine; V, varicella; PC, Pneumococcal conjugate vaccine; MC, meningococcal C conjugate vaccine.

TABLE 3 Routine Immunization Schedule for Children <7 Years of Age Not Immunized in Early Infancy

Timing	DTaP[1]	IPV	Hib	MMR	Td[2] or dTap[10]	Hep B[4] (3 doses)	V	P	M
First visit	X	X	X[11]	X[12]		X	X[7]	X[8]	X[9]
2 months later	X	X	X	(X)[6]		X		(X)	(X)
2 months later	X	(X)[5]						(X)	
6–12 months later	X	X	(X)[11]			X			
4–6 years of age[12]	X	X							
14–16 years of age					X				

P, pneumococcal vaccine; M, meningococcal vaccine.

TABLE 4 Routine Immunization Schedule for Children >7 Years of Age Not Immunized in Early Infancy

Timing	dTap[10]	IPV	MMR	Hep B[4] (3 doses)	V	M
First visit	X	X	X	X	X	X[9]
2 months later	X	X	X[6]	X	(X)[7]	
6–12 months later	X	X		X		
10 years later	X					

M, meningococcal vaccine.

Notes

1. DTaP (diphtheria, tetanus, acellular or component pertussis) vaccine is the preferred vaccine for all doses in the vaccination series, including completion of the series in children who have received >1 dose of DPT (whole cell) vaccine.
2. Hib schedule shown is for PRP-T or HbOC vaccine. If PRP-OMP is used, give at 2, 4, and 12 months of age.
3. Td (tetanus and diphtheria toxoid), a combined adsorbed "adult type" preparation for use in people >7 years of age, contains less diphtheria toxoid than preparations given to younger children and is less likely to cause reactions in older people.
4. Hepatitis B vaccine can be routinely given to infants or preadolescents, depending on the provincial/territorial policy; three doses at 0-, 1-, and 6-month intervals are preferred. The second dose should be administered at least 1 month after the first dose, and the third at least 2 months after the second dose. A two-dose schedule for adolescents is also possible.
5. This dose is not needed routinely, but can be included for convenience.
6. A second dose of MMR is recommended, at least 1 month after the first dose, for the purpose of better measles protection. For convenience, options include giving it with the next scheduled vaccination at 18 months of age or with school entry (4–6 years) vaccinations (depending on the provincial/territorial policy), or at any intervening age that is practicable. The need for a second dose of mumps and rubella vaccine is not established but may be beneficial (given for convenience as MMR). The second dose of MMR should be given at the same visit as DTaP IPV (+ Hib) to ensure high uptake rates.
7. Children aged 12 months to 12 years should receive one dose of varicella vaccine. Individuals >13 years of age should receive two doses at least 28 days apart.
8. Recommended schedule, number of doses, and subsequent use of 23 valent polysaccharide pneumococcal vaccine depend on the age of the child when vaccination is begun (see page 177 in the *6th Edition 2002 Canadian Immunization Guide* for specific recommendations).
9. Recommended schedule and number of doses of meningococcal vaccine depends on the age of the child (see page 151 in the *6th Edition 2002 Canadian Immunization Guide* for specific recommendations).
10. dTap adult formulation with reduced diphtheria toxoid and pertussis component.
11. Recommended schedule and number of doses depend on the product used and age of the child when vaccination is begun (see page 87 in the *6th Edition 2002 Canadian Immunization Guide* for specific recommendations). Not required past age 5.
12. Delay until subsequent visit if child is <12 months of age.
13. Omit these doses if the previous doses of DTaP and polio were given after the fourth birthday.

REFERENCES

Health Canada [Online]. Available: *http://www.hc-sc.gc.ca/pphb-dgspsp/dird-dimr/is-cv.*

National Advisory Committee on Immunization. (2002). *Canadian immunization guide* (6th ed.). Ottawa, ON: Health Canada.

appendix B

Diagnostic Imaging Agents

New medical test procedures continue to rely on diagnostic imaging agents. Common imaging agents include radiopaque contrast agents, such as barium sulfate; ionic iodinated imaging agents, such as diatrizoate meglumine; nonionized iodinated imaging agents, such as metrizamide; oral cystographic compounds, such as iocetamic acid; provocative agents, such as arginine; and skin testing agents, such as coccidioidin.

Radiopaque contrast agents highlight and provide contrast among internal structures. Iodinated imaging agents and cystographic compounds are composed of iodine compounds with radiopaque properties. Provocative agents provoke measurable responses that indicate disease or its absence. Skin testing agents help to identify allergic responses and other disorders.

As technology advances, more patients will undergo testing procedures with these agents. Nurses must be prepared to administer and monitor some of these agents and provide care for patients receiving them. Like therapeutic drugs, these diagnostic agents require special administration methods, produce adverse effects, and call for careful patient education. Such education of course requires a firm understanding of the interrelationship between *core drug knowledge* related to diagnostic drugs and *core patient variables* specific to the testing procedures. A summary of various pharmacologic test agents follows.

Drug (Trade) Name	Indications	Nursing Management
Imaging Agent		
barium sulfate suspensions (Baro-CAT, Prepcat, Entrobar) concentrated suspensions (Tomocat) powder (Baroflave) powder for suspension (Barosperse, Anatrast, Tonopaque)	GI diagnostics	Do not administer if obstruction of GI tract is suspected. Keep the patient fasting (NPO) for 8 h for oral, administration. Provide mouth care for NPO patients. Administer cathartic or enema posttest as ordered. Assess GI status posttest; document passage of stool. Keep patient well hydrated to expel barium. Monitor for constipation, intestinal cramping, distention, diarrhea, and bowel obstruction.
Ionic Iodinated Imaging Agents		
diatrizoate meglumine (Gastrografin) diatrizoate sodium (Hypaque Sodium)	GI diagnostics, discography, urography, angiography, angiocardiography, arteriography, aortography, ventriculography, venography, venacavography, computed tomography (CT)	Assess for allergy to iodine, iodine compounds, foods that contain iodine, or dye allergy. Assess patient history of: bronchial asthma; renal, hepatic, or thyroid diseases; sickle cell disease. Notify the provider of any positive allergy or history before administering the drug. Monitor fluid and electrolyte status. Have emergency equipment available for possible allergic reactions. Monitor extravasation from injection site.
ethiodized oil (Ethiodol)	Hysterosalpingography	Same as diatrizoate meglumine. When injected into lymph nodes, monitor for compromised pulmonary function. Monitor for infection in the insertion site and delayed wound healing.
iodamide meglumine (Renovue-Dip, Renovue-65)	Urography, pyelography, CT	Same as diatrizoate meglumine.
iodipamide meglumine (Cholografin Meglumine)	Cholecystography, cholangiography	Same as diatrizoate meglumine.
iophendylate	Lumbar, thoracic, and total columnar myelography	Same as diatrizoate meglumine. Keep patient in a flat position for 24 h after test procedure. Monitor for signs of meningeal irritation or subarachnoid bleeding.

(continued)

Continued

Drug (Trade) Name	Indications	Nursing Management
iothalamate meglumine iothalamate sodium (Conray)	Cholangiography, urography, pyelography, cystourethrography, arthrography, angiography, angiocardiography, arteriography, aortography, CT, cholangiopancreatography, cystography	Same as diatrizoate meglumine.
Nonionized Iodinated Imaging Agents		
metrizamide (Amipaque)	Myelography, angiocardiography, arteriography, ventriculography, CT, cisternography	Assess for history of iodine sensitivity. Assess for the following: seizure disorder, local or systemic infection, pheochromocytoma, multiple sclerosis, sickle cell anemia, severe cardiovascular disease, impaired hepatic function, active alcoholism. Notify the provider of any positive history prior to administering the drug. Assess pretest and posttest fluid and electrolyte balance. Monitor for CNS effects after test.
iopamidol (Isovue)	Urography, angiography, angiocardiography, arteriography, aortography, ventriculography, venography	Same as for metrizamide.
iohexol (Omnipaque)	Urography, myelography, angiography, angiocardiography, arteriography, aortography, ventriculography, venography, CT	Same as for metrizamide. After intrathecal administration, elevate the head of the bed 45 degrees.
ioversol (Optiray)	Urography, angiography, arteriography, aortography, ventriculography, venography, CT	Same as for metrizamide.
ioxaglate meglumine (Hexabrix)	Urography, arthrography, angiography, angiocardiography, arteriography, aortography, ventriculography, venography, hysterosalpingography, CT	Same as for metrizamide.
Oral Cholecystographic Compounds		
iocetamic acid (Cholebrine)	Cholecystography	Assess for allergy to iodine, iodine compounds, or foods that contain iodine. Assess for allergy to dyes (FD&C yellow dye No. 5). Assess for the following: bronchial asthma, hyperuricemia, renal disease, hepatic impairment, GI absorption diseases, cardiovascular disease, and thyroid diseases. Administer high-fat diet the day before the test. Administer the contrast medium as ordered. Keep the patient NPO, except for water, after administration of contrast medium. Administer laxative or enema as ordered. Keep patients well hydrated, especially those with hyperuricemia.
iopanoic acid (Telepaque)	Cholecystography, cholangiography	Same as iocetamic acid.
ipodate calcium (Oragrafin calcium)	Cholecystography, cholangiography	Same as iocetamic acid.

(continued)

Continued

Drug (Trade) Name	Indications	Nursing Management
ipodate sodium (Oragrafin sodium, Bilivist) tyropanoate sodium (Bilopaque)	Cholecystography, cholangiography	Same as iocetamic acid.
Provocative Drugs		
arginine	Evaluate pituitary growth hormone reserve	Assess for allergy or hypersensitivity reactions. Assess for sickle cell anemia and renal disease. Notify the provider of any positive history before administration of the test. Administer through an indwelling catheter to prevent extravasation. Draw blood sample at 30 min before and again immediately before the test. Draw blood sample at the initiation of the injection and at 30-min intervals for 2½ h thereafter.
corticotropin (ACTH)	Evaluate adrenal function	Assess for porcine protein sensitivity. Notify provider of positive allergic response prior to administration of the drug. Advise low-carbohydrate diet for 48 h prior to day of testing. Keep patient NPO 12 h before test. Restrict patient's activity 12 h before test. Withhold the following medications: amphetamines, calcium gluconate, corticosteroids, estrogens, lithium, and spironolactone.
cosyntropin	Assist in diagnosing adrenocortical insufficiency	Assess for allergy to corticotropin or cosyntropin. Notify the provider of any positive allergy history before administration of the drug. The following drugs may interfere with test results: cortisone, hydrocortisone, estrogens, and spironolactone. Draw blood specimen 30–60 min after administration of cosyntropin.
edrophonium (Tensilon)	Assist in the diagnosis of myasthenia gravis Differentiate between cholinergic crisis and myasthenic crisis Evaluate therapy	Withhold the following medications: anticholinergics, muscle relaxants, prednisone, procainamide, and quinidine. Have 1-mg atropine available to reverse possible severe cholinergic reactions. Interpretation timing: myasthenia gravis diagnosis 45 s after administration; differentiation between cholinergic crisis and myasthenic crisis—1 min after administration; and evaluation of treatment—1 min after administration.
gonadorelin (Factrel)	Evaluate anterior pituitary function	Withhold the following medications: androgens, estrogens, gonadotrophins, and glucocorticoids. Avoid interacting drugs: digoxin, dopamine antagonists, levodopa, phenothiazines, and spironolactone. Draw blood sample every 15 min for the first hour, then at 2 h postadministration.
histamine phosphate	Evaluate production of hydrochloric acid	Ensure NPO status for 12 h before test. Allow no smoking for 8 h before test.

(continued)

Continued

Drug (Trade) Name	Indications	Nursing Management
	Assist in diagnosing pheochromocytoma	Withhold the following medications: adrenaline blockers, alcohol, antacids, anticholinergics, cimetidine, corticosteroids, and reserpine. Have epinephrine available for severe hypotension. Monitor blood pressure and pulse rate closely.
metyrapone	Evaluate hypothalamic-pituitary function	Same as gonadorelin.
pentagastrin (Peptavlon)	Evaluate gastric acid secretion Assist in diagnosing Zollinger-Ellison syndrome	Assess for the following: allergies, pancreatic disease, biliary disease, and hepatic disease. Notify the provider of any positive history before administration of the test. Do not use in patients with acute bleeding or penetrating ulcers. Place a nasogastric tube for the procedure. Obtain gastric acid specimen 60 min after administration of pentagastrin.
secretin	Assist in diagnosing pancreatic exocrine disorders and gastrinoma	Assess for the following: allergies, asthma, anticholinergic therapy, inflammatory bowel disease, and vagotomy. Notify the provider of any positive history before administration of the test. Assist in the insertion of a double-lumen catheter. Administer test dose if the patient has a history of asthma or allergies; continue test if no reaction after 1 min. For pancreatic disorders: obtain gastrin and duodenal secretion samples taken during the first 60 min after secretin injection. For gastrinoma: draw blood sample during the first 30 min after secretin injection.
thyrotropin	Assist in diagnosing low thyroid reserve and subclinical hypothyroidism Differentiate between primary and secondary hypothyroidism Detect thyroid cancer Evaluate treatment	Assess for a history of: angina pectoris, cardiac failure, hypopituitarism, adrenal cortical suppression, corticosteroid therapy, coronary thrombosis, untreated Addison disease, and hypersensitivity to thyrotropin. Notify the provider of any positive history before administration of the test. Monitor for signs of hypersensitivity reaction. Monitor for nausea, vomiting, headache, fever, tachycardia, and ventricular fibrillation.
tolbutamide sodium	Assist in diagnosing diabetes mellitus, insulinoma, pancreatic carcinoma, acute pancreatitis	Assess for a history of hypersensitivity to tolbutamide or other sulfonylureas, and identify current drug therapy that may enhance the hypoglycemic effect of tolbutamide. Notify the provider of any positive history before administration of the test. Monitor for signs and symptoms of hypoglycemia. Have IV glucose on hand for severe hypoglycemia. Draw blood for baseline glucose level and serial glucose levels as ordered after administration.
xylose	Assist in diagnosing malabsorptive conditions	Assess for a history of impaired renal function, thyroid dysfunction, pernicious anemia, and iron-deficiency anemia.

(continued)

Continued

Drug (Trade) Name	Indications	Nursing Management
		Notify the provider of any positive history before administration of the test. To avoid inaccurate results, assess for vomiting or diarrhea, gastric stasis, bacterial infections, and cardiovascular dysfunction. Encourage fluid intake before and after procedure.
Skin Testing Drugs		
coccidioidin	Assist in the diagnosis of coccidiomycosis Evaluate cell-mediated immune status	Assess for diagnosis of coccidioidal erythema nodosum or allergy to mercury. Notify the provider of any positive history before administration of the test. Assess for an allergy to mercury. Administer by intradermal injection being sure to produce a wheal. Repeat the test in another location (at least 5 cm away) if no wheal appears. Assess for induration at the injection site 24 h later. False-positive results may be reported if assessed after 48 h. A positive test result is an area of induration.
histoplasmin	Assist in diagnosing histoplasmosis	Assess for a history of histoplasmosis or previous positive test results. Notify the provider of any positive history before administration of the test. Do not use more than 0.1 mL for testing because larger doses may cause necrosis and ulceration. Have epinephrine available in case of severe reaction. Administer by intradermal injection being sure to produce a wheal. Repeat the test in another location (at least 5 cm away) if no wheal appears. Assess for induration at the injection site 48–72 h later.
penicilloylopolylysine (PPL)	Assist in assessing risk for hypersensitivity reaction with the administration of penicillin	Assess for a history of penicillin or cephalosporin allergy. Monitor these patients closely. Notify the provider of any positive history before administration of the test. Administer the scratch test first. If no reaction, or questionable reaction to the scratch test, administer the intradermal test. A positive result will be itching or increased size of the wheal within 15 min.
mumps	Assess cell-mediated immunity	Assess for previous hypersensitivity to the test. Assess for allergy to avian protein or to thimerosal because these patients have a higher risk for an anaphylactic reaction to the test. Notify the provider of any positive history before administration of the test. Administer by intradermal injection, being sure to produce a wheal. Repeat the test in another location (at least 5 cm away) if no wheal appears.

(continued)

Continued

Drug (Trade) Name	Indications	Nursing Management
		Assess for induration at the injection site 48–72 h later. In immunocompromised patients, a positive test result is any amount of induration. In immunocompetent patients, a positive test result is 5 mm or more of induration.
tuberculin	Assist in diagnosing tuberculosis Evaluate cell-mediated immune status	Assess for previous positive test results. Notify the provider of any positive history before administration of the test. Administer by intradermal injection, being sure to produce a wheal. Repeat the test in another location (at least 5 cm away) if no wheal appears. To avoid false-positive results, do not administer in an area of atopic dermatitis, sun-damaged skin, or ultraviolet treatment. Assess for induration at the injection site 48–72 h later. In immunocompromised patients, a positive test result is 5 mm or more of induration. In immunocompetent patients, a positive test result is 10 mm or more of induration.

appendix C

Enzyme or Débridement Therapy

Enzymes and débridement agents are composed of proteins and similar substances. Having catalytic action, they are used to slow or speed organic processes, replace or supplement deficient enzymes, break down proteins (such as blood clots), and débride wounds.

The nurse administering enzyme or débridement therapy is responsible for understanding the drug's action and effects (core drug knowledge); assessing the patient's health history and physical condition (core patient variables); and planning and implementing associated patient education.

Drug (Trade) Name	Indications	Nursing Management
Enzymes		
agalsidase beta (Fabrazyme)	Treatment of Fabry disease	Assess for mannitol hypersensitivity. If positive, advise health care provider before administering drug. Monitor for signs of allergic reactions such as difficulty breathing, closing of the throat, hives, rash, and itching. Monitor for signs of infusion reaction such as fever, shaking, chest tightness, high or low blood pressure, fast heartbeats, muscle pain, stomach pain, nausea or vomiting, dizziness, numbness or tingling, and headache. Administer pretreatment medications to minimize infusion reactions as ordered.
alglucerase (Ceredase)	Replacement of glucosylceramidase in patients with Gaucher disease (a congenital disorder of lipid metabolism)	Assess the patient's health history for an immune-deficiency disease, unusual or allergic reaction to alglucerase, other drugs, foods, dyes, or preservatives. Determine whether the patient is pregnant, trying to get pregnant, or breast-feeding. Monitor for fever, chills, or stomach discomfort; nausea, vomiting; pain, burning, swelling, or irritation at the injection site.
chymopapain (Chymodiactin)	Decreases intradisk pressure and relieves compressive symptoms in patients with vertebral disk herniation	Use in the lumbar region only. Assess the patient for papaya sensitivity, spondylolisthesis, spinal stenosis, progressive paralysis, spinal cord tumor, and previous injection of chymopapain. Administer pretreatment with H_1 and H_2 blockers to reduce the severity of possible anaphylactic reaction. Monitor for anaphylaxis, erythema, pilomotor erection, urticaria, conjunctivitis, vasomotor rhinitis, angioedema, back pain/spasm, and transverse myelitis/myelopathy.
desoxyribonuclease and fibrinolysin (Elase)	Attacks protein (DNA) component of purulent exudates Attacks fibrin of blood clots and fibrinous exudates	Replenish at least once daily because significant activity is lost after 24 h.
hyaluronidase (Wydase)	Adjunct therapy to increase the absorption and dispersion of other injected drugs or during urography to improve reabsorption of radiopaque agents Antidote for extravasation	Change needle after each injection when used for extravasation. Monitor for urticaria and anaphylactic-like reactions.
imiglucerase (Cerezyme)	DNA recumbent enzyme used for Gaucher disease	Assess the patient's health history for an unusual or allergic reaction to imiglucerase and other drugs, foods, dyes, or preservatives; pregnancy or plans for pregnancy; breast-feeding.

(continued)

Continued

Drug (Trade) Name	Indications	Nursing Management
		Monitor for fever, chills, or stomach discomfort; nausea; vomiting.
pancreatin (Donnazyme)	Used as a pancreatic enzyme supplement for conditions in which pancreatic enzymes are deficient or absent, such as cystic fibrosis, chronic pancreatitis, pancreatectomy, gastrointestinal bypass surgery, and ductal obstruction from neoplasm	Administer PO with meals. Advise the patient to refrain from keeping drug in the mouth prior to swallowing because it may cause mucosal irritation and stomatitis. Do not give concurrently with antacids or iron salts. Give with caution during pregnancy, breast-feeding, or in porcine hypersensitivity. Monitor for maculopapular rash (sign of porcine hypersensitivity).
pancrelipase (Cotazym, Creon, Ilozyme, Pancrease, Viokase)	Same as pancreatin Has 12 times the lipolytic activity, 4 times the proteolytic activity, and 4 times the amylolytic activity of pancreatin	Administer pancrelipase orally. Products are not interchangeable. Administer delayed-release capsules containing enteric-coated spheres, microspheres, or microtablets by opening and mixing the contents with liquids or soft food. Advise patient not to chew or crush to avoid destruction of enteric coating. The enteric coating will dissolve if in contact with food with a pH greater than 6. Powder drug form may be administered with liquids or mixed with food. Avoid inhaling the powder.
pegademase bovine (Adagen)	Replacement in patients with adenosine deaminase (ADA) deficiency	Give with caution in patients with thrombocytopenia or coagulopathy. Monitor for headache; also monitor injection site. Do not coadminister with vidarabine.
thrombin (Thrombinar, Thrombostat)	Used during surgery to control incisional or surgical bleeding	Avoid parenteral administration because intravascular clots may be fatal. Do not administer to pregnant patients or to patients with bovine hypersensitivity. Before applying, sponge away blood from the surface to which thrombin is to be applied. Apply as a dry powder, spray, or with a saturated absorbable gelatin sponge. Prepare spray and saturated absorbable gelatin sponge as directed by the manufacturer. To avoid disturbing the clot after applying thrombin, do not sponge the area.
Débridement Agents		
collagenase (Santyl)	Chemical débridement of acute or chronic dermal ulcers and severely burned areas associated with necrotic material.	Assess need for pain medication prior to treatment. Gently wash the site with normal saline, using sterile gauze. It is not necessary to remove previously applied collagenase. Apply the ointment within the boundaries of the wound. Do not let the tip of the tube touch anything.
dextranomer (Debrisan)	Cleansing of exudative wounds. Treatment of decubitus or leg ulcers.	Assess need for pain medication prior to treatment.

(continued)

Continued

Drug (Trade) Name	Indications	Nursing Management
		Débride and cleanse wound by irrigation before applying three times per day. Paste is easier to apply than beads. Apply dressing and seal on all four sides.
papain and urea (Accuzyme)	Enzymatic débridement agent for wounds such as diabetic or decubitus ulcers, burns, postoperative wounds, and traumatic or infected wounds.	Assess need for pain medication prior to treatment. Gently wash the site with normal saline with sterile gauze. Do not use hydrogen peroxide solution, because it may inactivate papain. Apply the ointment within the boundaries of the wound. Do not let the tip of the tube touch anything.

appendix D

Enteral and Nutritional Supplements

Vitamins and minerals are substances that the body requires for essential metabolic reactions. The body cannot synthesize enough of these components to meet all of its needs. Therefore, vitamins and minerals must be obtained from animal and vegetable sources ingested as food. In a well-balanced diet, humans take in all they need. Only small amounts of vitamins and minerals are needed because they function as coenzymes that activate the protein portion of enzymes, which catalyze a great deal of biochemical activity.

Vitamins are either water soluble and excreted in the urine or fat soluble and capable of being stored in adipose tissue. Additional *core drug knowledge* includes specific uses of enteral nutrition. Enteral nutrition treats vitamin or mineral deficiencies, supplements the diet when needed, and provides specific therapeutic effects related to vitamin or mineral activity.

Enteral nutrients are classified in pregnancy category C and are contraindicated in cases of allergy to components of the vitamin or mineral, such as colorants, additives, or preservatives. Adverse effects to anticipate from enteral nutrition include nausea, diarrhea, and sometimes toxic reactions, particularly in instances of overdose.

Core patient variables should be assessed. The health history should disclose any condition that would contraindicate using enteral nutrition. The physical examination should include a skin evaluation, respiratory status, pulse rate, and blood pressure. Each enteral drug should be checked for special administration needs. The patient or family should be cautioned to avoid additional supplements in OTC products because overdose can occur. Patients also should be cautioned to avoid using mineral oil if they are taking fat-soluble vitamins.

Nutritional Component	Purpose	Nursing Management
Fat-Soluble Vitamins		
vitamin A (Aquasol A, Del-Vi-A) Preformed vitamin A is retinol. Provitamin A carotenoids are beta-carotene and alpha-carotene.	Treats vitamin A deficiency Necessary for growth and repair of body tissues Helps maintain integrity of skin and mucous membranes of the mouth, nose, throat, and lungs Assists in adaptation to light Aids in bone and teeth formation	Administer PO or IM. Protect IM vial from light. Teratogenic with excessive dosage. Watch for hypervitaminosis A: nausea, vomiting, hepatomegaly, splenomegaly, jaundice, CNS symptoms including increased intracranial pressure.
vitamin D ergocalciferol (vitamin D_2 Calciferol)	Used to manage hypophosphatemia, hypoparathyroidism, and resistant rickets	Administer as prescribed. Encourage balanced diet and exposure to sunlight. Do not use with mineral oil.
cholecalciferol (vitamin D_3, Delta-D)	Treats vitamin D deficiency	Monitor calcium levels before administration and periodically during therapy.
calcifediol (25-Hydroxy-D_3, Calderol)	Used to manage hypocalcemia and potential bone disease in patients receiving chronic renal dialysis	Discontinue if patient does not respond or if hypercalcemia occurs.
vitamin E (Aquasol E, Vita-Plus E, Softgels)	Reduces toxic effects of oxygen on the lung and retina in certain premature infants Treats severe vitamin E deficiency Maintains adequate levels of vitamin E during periods of stress and growth	Do not administer IV. Instruct patient to report fatigue, weakness, nausea, headache, blurred vision, diarrhea. If above adverse effects occur, stop vitamin therapy immediately.
vitamin K phytonadione (Mephyton, AquaMEPHYTON)	Treats hypoprothrombinemia due to vitamin K deficiency, overdose of anticoagulants or hemorrhagic disease of the newborn Given as prophylaxis for vitamin K deficiency in newborns	Administer Mephyton orally. Administer AquaMEPHYTON SC or IM. IV administration is possible, but only if the benefits outweigh the risks. If given IV, monitor for potential shock or respiratory or cardiac arrest. Monitor prothrombin time (PT) prior to and throughout therapy.
Water-Soluble Vitamins		
vitamin C (ascorbic acid) (Cebid, Vita-C, Cevalin, N'ice Vitamin C Drops)	Treats severe vitamin C deficiency (scurvy) Enhances wound and burn healing	Monitor combination and OTC products for vitamin C content. Be forewarned: many patients receive more than the recommended dose.

(continued)

Continued

Nutritional Component	Purpose	Nursing Management
		Administer PO and, if necessary, IM, slow IV, or SC, depending on patient's condition. Keep in mind that dose may decrease effectiveness of anticoagulant therapy and increase adverse effects of oral contraceptives.
vitamin B_{12} (cyanocobalamin) (Ener-B)	Treats severe vitamin B_{12} deficiency, which may present as megaloblastic anemia, neuronal damage, or oral ulcerations and GI disturbances Used to prevent anencephaly, spina bifida, and neural tube defects in the developing fetus Used to prevent colorectal cancer Used to reduce plasma homocysteine levels	Administer PO, SC, or IM. Patients without intrinsic factor must receive drug IM. Monitor patient for mouth sores or skin breakdown. Monitor plasma vitamin B_{12} levels every 3–6 months. Monitor potassium levels for patients on long-term therapy.
vitamin B_3 (niacin) (Nicotinic Acid)	Prevents and treats pellagra, niacin deficiency, and hyperlipidemia in patients not responsive to diet therapy	Advise patient that he or she may feel sensation of warmth and flushing on administration, but sensation usually subsides within 24 h. Monitor serum lipid levels in patients being treated for hyperlipidemia. Encourage proper diet and exercise. Advise patient that adverse effects of nausea, abdominal pain, and diarrhea may occur and that taking vitamin with meals may relieve these problems.
vitamin B_6 (pyridoxine) (Nestrex, Beesix)	Treats severe vitamin B_6 deficiency Prevents peripheral neuropathy with isoniazid therapy	Avoid administering to patients taking levodopa, because serious toxic interaction may result. Monitor for adverse effects, such as sensory neuropathic syndrome, marked by unsteady gait and somnolence. Provide safety measures if this effect occurs.
vitamin B_2 (riboflavin)	Treats severe B_2 deficiencies Maintains adequate B_2 levels during periods of stress or growth	Monitor patient for response to treatment. Warn patient that this drug may discolor urine yellow-orange; explain that the discoloration will subside when therapy discontinues.
vitamin B_1 (thiamine) (Thiamilate, Biamine)	Treats severe B_1 deficiencies (e.g., beriberi) Prevents Wernicke-Korsakoff syndrome in alcoholics	Do not mix in alkaline solutions. Advise patient that this vitamin changes composition of sweat and body odor. Warn patient that a warm and flushing sensation may accompany administration, but sensation will subside quickly.
Minerals		
calcium (Calciday, Chooz, Dicarbosil, Oystercal, Tums)	Treats severe calcium deficiency Maintains calcium levels Reduces gastric acid levels Helps cardiac contraction during cardiac arrest	Administer with meals to decrease GI effects. Avoid combination with digoxin, thiazide, oral contraceptives (toxicity may occur). Keep in mind that calcium may decrease absorption of atenolol, iron, quinolones, tetracyclines. Avoid combining with high-fiber diets, oxalate, or zinc, because these combinations may decrease absorption. Combining with milk or dairy products may increase the risk of hypercalcemia.

(continued)

Continued

Nutritional Component	Purpose	Nursing Management
		Monitor calcium levels in acute situations; also monitor for signs of hypercalcemia, hypophosphatemia. Caution patient to avoid OTC multiple-combination products that may increase risk of hypercalcemia.
iron (ferrous fumarate, gluconate, and sulfate) (Feostat, Feosol, Fer-in-sol)	Treats severe iron deficiency Treats iron deficiency anemia Supplements epoetin alfa therapy	Avoid administering iron with tetracycline (decreases absorption of both), antacids, cimetidine, vitamin C, chloramphenicol (decreases iron absorption). If appropriate, tell patient that absorption of levodopa, methyldopa, penicillamine, and quinolones is decreased if these drugs are taken with iron. Administer with food to relieve GI upset. Other adverse effects may include anorexia, vomiting, constipation, green or dark stools. Dilute liquid form and have patient drink it through a straw to decrease dental staining. Keep out of reach of children. Serious toxicity can occur if accidentally ingested.
magnesium, citrate and hydroxide (Citrate of Magnesia, Milk of Magnesia)	Decreases gastric acidity when used as antacid Relieves mild constipation Evacuates colon when used before rectal/bowel examinations	Caution patients to read labels of OTC products carefully to avoid magnesium overdose. Forewarn patients that diarrhea may occur. When administering magnesium, recognize that combination with the following drugs will decrease their absorption: digoxin, penicillamine, amino quinolones, nitrofurantoin, and tetracyclines. Administer these drugs at least 2 h apart.
phosphorus (Neutra-Phos)	Dietary supplement for periods of growth or stress	Avoid using phosphorus if patient is on a sodium- or potassium-restricted diet. Reconstitute powdered drug form before administering. Monitor potassium level if patient is receiving potassium or using potassium-sparing diuretics. Caution patient that antacids and calcium vitamin D products may decrease phosphorus levels. Explain that adverse effects may include GI upset, diarrhea, dizziness, seizures, confusion, muscle cramps. Advise patient to stop taking drug and report excessive diarrhea if it occurs.
zinc (Orazinc, Verazinc, Zincate)	Supplements diet to treat or prevent zinc deficiency Speeds healing Treats rheumatoid arthritis, Wilson's disease, and common cold	Administer with food if GI upset occurs. Avoid high-fiber diets, calcium, and phosphates in combination; administer at least 2 h apart. Encourage patients to check OTC products to avoid zinc overdose. Caution patients that adverse effects may include nausea, vomiting, and diarrhea.

(continued)

Continued

Nutritional Component	Purpose	Nursing Management
Enteral Supplements		
Contain: amino acids carbohydrates fats electrolytes vitamins trace elements	Supplements intake for anorectic patients, those with impaired swallowing, or those with digestive or absorptive disorders	Check placement of feeding tube prior to administration. Check order for continuous or intermittent administration. Check for residual per institution's protocol. Monitor for signs of aspiration. Check glucose. Monitor for signs of electrolyte imbalance.

appendix E

Parenteral Nutrition

Parenteral nutrition (PN) is administration through a central or other IV line of essential proteins, amino acids, carbohydrates, vitamins, minerals, trace elements, lipids, and fluid. PN is used to improve or stabilize the nutritional status of cachetic or debilitated patients who cannot take or absorb oral nutrition to maintain their nutritional status. The exact composition of the PN solution is determined after a nutritional assessment and takes into account *core drug knowledge* related to the parenteral solution and *core patient variables* of the patient's current health status, age, and metabolic needs.

PN is contraindicated in anyone with known allergies to any of the solution's components. Many multiple combination products are available and a solution that is suitable for any patient can be given. Adverse effects that may accompany PN include mechanical problems (related to the IV line, such as pneumothorax, infections, air emboli, or emboli related to protein or lipid aggregations), infections related to the nutrient-rich solution and invasive administration, metabolic imbalances related to the composition of the solution, gallstone development (especially in children), and nausea (associated with administering lipids).

Before PN begins, a nutritional assessment should be performed with additional assessments made periodically during therapy. Core patient variables to include in the assessment are the patient's height, weight, dietary and medical histories, current illness, and current drug therapy regimens. Daily assessments include daily weights, fractional urine analyses, blood glucose levels every 6 to 8 hours, vital signs, strict intake and output, condition of the infusion pump and insertion site (checked at every shift), neurologic status, and blood chemistry values (to evaluate the effectiveness of therapy).

Parenteral solutions should be refrigerated until ready to be administered. Just before administration, the solution's components should be checked against the prescribed components. Then, the solution should be inspected for abnormalities, such as precipitates, cloudiness, or color changes. The solution should not hang for more than 24 hours, after which it should be replaced. In most cases, inline filters are recommended to decrease the opportunity for bacteria or aggregates to be infused with the solution.

PN is used during pregnancy in patients whose conditions limit nutritional intake. Elderly patients should be assessed carefully when receiving PN because they may not tolerate the increased volume or concentrated glucose solutions. Extreme caution must be used when giving intralipids to premature infants in whom hepatic clearance is decreased. PN should be discontinued slowly by gradually reducing the infusion rate over several hours. PN should not be discontinued, however, until an alternate source of nutrition has been established.

Patient and family education materials should focus on why PN is being given, the need for monitoring both the patient and the infusion equipment (pump and line) regularly, signs and symptoms to report to the health care provider—particularly chest pain, difficulty breathing, pain at the injection site, fever, and flulike symptoms. Many patients now receive PN at home and must deliver their own infusions. These patients need special instructions in maintaining sterile technique and recognizing warning signs of infection or emboli to be reported immediately. Information about typical PN formulas follows.

PN Component*	Purpose	Nursing Management
Typical Central PN Solution (1L)		
Provides 1,350 total nonprotein calories in 1,250-mL volume of solution with 25% dextrose concentration, 5% amino acid concentration, and osmolarity of 1900 mOsm/L Actual concentration and components of any PN solution are determined by the patient's current status and nutritional needs.		
10% amino acids	Provides 50 g protein for growth and healing	*Dosage:* 500 mL Monitor blood pressure, cardiac output, blood chemistries, urine analyses to determine effect of intravascular protein pull.
50% dextrose	Provides 850 kcal for energy	*Dosage:* 500 mL Monitor blood glucose level. Evaluate injection site for signs of infection or irritation.
20% fat emulsion	Provides 500 fat calories, ready energy	*Dosage:* 250 mL Monitor for emboli; signs include shortness of breath, chest pain, deep leg pain, neurologic changes. Monitor for signs of increased vascular workload, especially in very young and very old patients.
sodium chloride	Provides sodium and chloride needed for various chemical reactions within the body	*Dosage:* 40 mEq Monitor cardiac rhythm and serum electrolyte levels.

(continued)

Continued

PN Component*	Purpose	Nursing Management
calcium gluconate	Provides essential calcium for muscle contraction, blood clotting, and numerous chemical reactions	*Dosage:* 4.8 mEq Monitor cardiac rhythm, muscle strength, and serum electrolyte levels.
magnesium sulfate	Provides magnesium for various chemical reactions within the body	*Dosage:* 8 mEq Monitor blood pressure and serum electrolyte levels.
potassium phosphate	Provides needed potassium for nerve functioning and muscle contraction	*Dosage:* 9 mMol Monitor blood pressure, cardiac rhythm, muscle function, and serum electrolyte levels.
multivitamins	Provides essential vitamins to maintain cell integrity and promote healing	*Dosage:*10 mL Monitor for signs of vitamin deficiency or toxicity.
trace elements zinc 3 mg copper 1.2 mg manganese 0.3 mg chromium 12 μg selenium 20 μg	Provides small amounts of elements essential for various chemical reactions in the body and maintenance of cell integrity and healing	Periodically monitor blood chemistry findings to determine adequacy of elemental replacement.
Typical Peripheral Parental Nutrition Solution (1L)		
Provides 840 total nonprotein calories in 1,250-mL volume of solution with 10% dextrose concentration, 4.25% amino acid concentration, and osmolarity of 900 mOsm/L Actual concentration and components of any PN solution are determined by the patient's current status and nutritional needs.		
8.5% amino acids	Provides 41 g protein for growth and healing	*Dosage:* 500 mL Monitor blood pressure, cardiac output, blood chemistries, urine analyses to determine effect of intravascular protein pull.
20% dextrose	Provides 340 calories for energy	*Dosage:* 500 mL Monitor blood glucose level. Evaluate injection site for signs of infection or irritation.
20% fat emulsion	Provides 500 fat calories, ready energy	*Dosage:* 250 mL Monitor for emboli; signs include shortness of breath, chest pain, deep leg pain, neurologic changes. Monitor for signs of increased vascular workload, especially in very young and very old patients.
sodium chloride	Provides sodium and chloride needed for various chemical reactions within the body	*Dosage:* 40 mEq Monitor cardiac rhythm and serum electrolyte levels.
calcium gluconate	Provides essential calcium for muscle contraction, blood clotting, and numerous chemical reactions	*Dosage:* 4.8 mEq Monitor cardiac rhythm, muscle strength, and serum electrolyte levels.
magnesium sulfate	Provides magnesium for various chemical reactions within the body	*Dosage:* 8 mEq Monitor blood pressure and serum electrolyte levels.
potassium phosphate	Provides needed potassium for nerve functioning and muscle contraction	*Dosage:* 9 mMol Monitor blood pressure, cardiac rhythm, muscle function, and serum electrolyte levels.
multivitamins	Provides a combination of essential vitamins to maintain cell integrity and promote healing	*Dosage:* 10 mL Monitor for signs of vitamin deficiency or toxicity.

(continued)

Continued

PN Component*	Purpose	Nursing Management
trace elements zinc 3 mg copper 1.2 mg manganese 0.3 mg chromium 12 μg selenium 20 μg	Provides small amounts of elements essential for various chemical reactions in the body and maintenance of cell integrity and healing	Periodically monitor blood chemistry findings to determine adequacy of replacement.

*Multiple combination preparations are available commercially. Each preparation varies in the concentration of one or more components and should be checked carefully before administering.

appendix F

Antidotes

Antidotes are usually given in emergency situations for which the nurse must be prepared with sufficient knowledge (*core drug knowledge*) of their uses and administration. Specific antidotes react chemically with or block the receptor sites of specific toxins. This decreases the toxic effect or, in many cases, reverses the effect of the poison. There are generally no contraindications for using antidotes, although they are appropriate only in potentially serious or life-threatening situations when their benefits clearly outweigh the risk of their use. Antidotes are drugs and, as such, produce adverse effects, which vary with the antidote.

Before an antidote is administered, the nursing assessment should focus on *core patient variables* and include a careful history of the time and amount of exposure to the toxin. In many situations, timing is crucial to treatment. The physical assessment should include vital signs, orientation, and blood chemistries appropriate to the toxin and the antidote. Supportive measures should be readily available, including life support, IV fluids to counteract shock, ventilating devices, and so forth. Patient and family education, which may occur after the situation stabilizes, should cover reasons for the antidote, adverse effects to expect, and drugs and other products to avoid after receiving the antidote. In cases of accidental overdose, the nurse should help the patient and family determine ways to prevent accidents in the future.

Antidote (Trade) Name	Poison	Nursing Management
acetylcysteine (Mucomyst, Mucosil, Mucomyst 10 IV)	*acetaminophen:* Prevents or minimizes hepatic injury after acetaminophen overdose	Administer 140 mg/kg PO as a loading dose followed by 70 mg/kg q4h starting 4 h after loading dose. IV dose is available if oral route is not. Begin treatment within 24 h of overdose. Empty stomach by gastric lavage, and use activated charcoal if feasible to decrease absorption of acetaminophen. Obtain blood chemistries and measure acetaminophen levels before antidote administration and daily until blood chemistry returns to nontoxic levels. Provide supportive care for electrolyte imbalances, hypoglycemia, and clotting problems related to hepatic injury.
aminocaproic acid (Amicar)	Management of acute bleeding syndromes resulting from fibrinolysis	Dilute drug per manufacturer's recommendation. Use cautiously in patients with cardiac, renal, or hepatic disease. Monitor fibrinogen levels.
atropine	*anticholinesterases* (organophosphorus insecticides) and *muscarine/mushroom* poisoning	Administer 2–3 mg IM or IV, and repeat until signs of atropine toxicity disappear. Provide ventilatory support and cardiac massage as needed. Monitor vital signs continually until they stabilize.
calcium chloride, calcium gluconate	*calcium channel blocker:* overdose	Administer 4.6–16 mEq IV. Monitor vital signs continually. Monitor serum calcium levels. Be prepared to provide life support and to counteract hypotension and bradycardia as appropriate.
activated charcoal (Antidose-Aqua, CharcoAid, LiquiChar)	*various poisons:* (including chemicals and drugs, such as acetaminophen, benzodiazepines, and others)	Administer 30–100 g or 1 g/kg PO (5–10 times the amount of toxin ingested) as an emergency treatment to absorb toxic substances from the GI tract and inhibit GI absorption. Administer as soon as possible after ingestion. Induce emesis before giving to conscious patient only. Have life-support equipment on standby. Give only to conscious patients.
deferoxamine (Desferal)	*iron:* acute or chronic toxicity	Adult: Administer 1 g IM followed by 0.5 g IM q4h; then 0.5 IM q4–12 h based on patient's response.

(continued)

Continued

Antidote (Trade) Name	Poison	Nursing Management
		Child: Administer 50 mg/kg IM or IV q6h. Monitor neurologic status periodically. Anticipate common adverse effects: skin rash and pain at injection site. Stop drug administration and reevaluate if patient reports impaired vision.
dexrazoxane (Zinecard)	*doxorubicin:* reduces incidence and severity of cardiotoxicity associated with chemotherapy with doxorubicin	Administer IV as prescribed; dexrazoxane: doxorubicin ratio should be 10;1. Administer by slow IV push or rapid IV drip. Do not mix with other drugs. Use special caution when handling and disposing of dexrazoxane.
digoxin immune fab (Digibind)	digoxin: overdose or toxicity (life threatening)	Administer in an amount determined by serum digoxin level or amount of digoxin ingested. If this information is unobtainable, give 800 mg IV (20 vials). Monitor serum digoxin levels before and periodically during therapy. Monitor cardiac response continually. Keep life-support equipment on hand at all times. Do not redigitalize patient until digoxin has cleared the system (several days to 1 week). Teach patient to report palpitations, dizziness, muscle cramps.
dimercaprol (BAL in oil)	acute and chronic *mercury* poisoning; *arsenic* and *gold* poisoning; *lead* poisoning in combination with edetate disodium	Administer 2.5–5 mg/kg q4–6 h IM; continue for up to 10 d. Administer this chelating agent by deep IM injection only. Monitor for severe nausea and vomiting because medication may be needed. Advise patient to report severe headache or weakness and tingling in the hands and feet.
edetate calcium disodium (Calcium Disodium Versenate) edetate disodium (Disotate, Endrate)	*lead* poisoning, *calcium* overdose, *digitalis* toxicity	*Adult (lead):* Administer 5 mL IV undiluted bid for up to 5 d or 35 mg/kg IM bid; (calcium or digitalis) 50 mg/kg/d IV for 5 consecutive d, then 2 free d followed by another antidote series. *Child (lead):* Administer 35 mg/kg IM bid for 3–5 d followed by a 2-d rest before repeating antidote therapy; (calcium or digitalis) 40 mg/kg/d IV. Prepare a schedule of drug administration days and rest days. Monitor electrolytes and BUN before and periodically during therapy. Monitor cardiac rhythm if treating digitalis overdose. Instruct patient to report pain at injection site or difficulty voiding.
flumazenil (Romazicon)	*benzodiazepine* (to reverse serious adverse effects completely or partially)	Administer 0.2 mg IV; wait 45 s and repeat at 60-s intervals until effect is apparent. Administer 0.2 mg IV and give repeated doses of 0.3 mg IV to a maximum of 3 mg for acute overdose. Inject into running IV line. Monitor clinical response and sedation carefully.

(continued)

Continued

Antidote (Trade) Name	Poison	Nursing Management
		Have life-support equipment on standby. Teach patient to avoid OTC drugs and alcohol for at least 18–24 h after receiving this drug.
glucagon	*insulin* overdose/shock (counteracts hypoglycemia)	Administer 0.5–1.0 mg SC, IV, or IM; repeat 1 to 2 times until response is apparent. Monitor skin, color, orientation, and vital signs. Evaluate blood glucose levels and adjust dosage accordingly. Teach diabetic patients, family members, and caregivers how to recognize signs of hypoglycemia and how to administer glucagon by injection.
leucovorin calcium (Wellcovorin)	*methotrexate*	Administer 12–15 g/m^2 PO, IM, or IV followed by 10 mg/m^2 PO q6h for 72 h as rescue drug to reverse toxic effects of high-dose methotrexate therapy on normal cells. Begin rescue within 24 h of methotrexate administration. Arrange for fluid loading and urine alkylinization to decrease methotrexate toxicity. Give drug orally if possible. Be sure to have life-support equipment on standby.
mesna (Mesnex)	*ifosfamide* (reacts chemically with urotoxic ifosfamide and used prophylactically to prevent hemorrhagic cystitis from ifosfamide therapy)	Administer mesna at 20% of the ifosfamide dose as a single IV dose at the time of each ifosfamide injection; repeat at 4 h and 8 h. Prepare within 6 h of use. Discard any unused portion. Record times of injection to ensure accurate timing of dose. Monitor patient for signs of hemorrhagic cystitis.
methylene blue (Urolene Blue)	*cyanide* or *nitrite* poisoning (converts ferrous iron of reduced hemoglobin to the ferric form, producing methemoglobin)	Inject 1–2 mg/kg IV slowly over several minutes; avoid SC injection. Monitor blood chemistries. Keep life-support equipment on standby.
nalmefene (Revex) naloxone (Narcan) naltrexone (Re Via)	*opioid* overdose (to block opioid receptors and displace the opioid from the receptor)	Administer nalmefene 0.5 mg/70 kg IV, then 0.5 mg/70 kg IV 2–5 min later (maximum dose 1.5 mg/70 kg). Administer naloxone 0.4–2.0 mg IV; repeat at 2- to 3-min intervals (maximum dose 10 mg). Administer naltrexone 50 mg/24 h PO (maintenance program for narcotic withdrawal). Keep life-support equipment on standby. Monitor patient continually. Anticipate common adverse effects of dizziness and drowsiness. Advise patient to avoid opiate-containing drugs, including analgesics and cough and cold medicines, for several weeks after receiving this drug.
neostigmine (Prostigmin)	*nondepolarizing neuromuscular junction blockers*	Administer atropine sulfate 0.6–1.2 mg IV before giving neostigmine. Administer neostigmine 0.5–2.0 mg IV by slow injection; repeat as needed (maximum dose 5 mg).

(continued)

Continued

Antidote (Trade) Name	Poison	Nursing Management
		Monitor patient continually. Keep life-support equipment on standby.
penicillamine (Cuprimine Depen)	*copper* (chelating agent that forms inactive complex with copper, leading to rapid urinary excretion)	Administer 1 g/d PO in divided doses qid (up to two doses may be needed). Monitor patient for potentially lethal myasthenic syndrome and bone marrow depression. Arrange for blood chemistries prior to and at least every 2 wk during therapy. Administer antidote on an empty stomach at least 30–60 min before meals and at least 2 h after evening meal.
physostigmine (Antilirium)	*anticholinergics,* including *tricyclic antidepressants* and *diazepam* overdoses	Administer 2 mg IM or IV slowly 1 mg/min or less. Keep atropine on standby in case of cholinergic crisis. Monitor patient response carefully.
pralidoxime chloride (Protopam Chloride)	*organophosphate pesticides* and *chemicals with anticholinesterase activity*	Administer 1–2 g IV as a 15–30-min infusion; repeat in 1 h; give additional doses as needed. Administer 2–4 mg atropine IV concomitantly with pralidoxime. Give antidote as soon as possible after exposure to poison. Maintain airway and have life-support equipment on standby.
protamine sulfate	*heparin* (heparin antagonist that treats heparin overdose)	Administer in amount determined by heparin dose; 1 mg IV neutralizes 90 USP U heparin from lung sources or 115 USP U heparin from intestinal sources. Monitor coagulation studies to adjust dosage and to detect heparin rebound response to protamine sulfate. Have life-support equipment on standby.
pyridoxine (Nestrex, Beesix)	*isoniazid* (competitively blocks isoniazid effects in cases of toxicity)	Administer 4 g IV followed by 1 g IM every 30 min. Monitor injection sites for signs of irritation. Have life-support equipment on standby.
succimer (Chemet)	*lead* (chelates lead in the system)	Administer 10 mg/kg PO q8h for 5 d then 10 mg/kg PO q12h for 2 wk. Obtain serum lead levels before therapy. Ensure adequate hydration during therapy. Also ensure that patient completes full 19-d course of therapy.
vitamin K (Mephyton, AquaMEPHYTON)	*oral anticoagulant* (overdosages) (treats prothrombin deficiency)	Administer 2.5–10 mg IM, SC, or PO; repeat in 12–48 h if needed. Because adequate coagulation will take time, protect patient from injury or invasive procedures. Monitor coagulation studies. Have plasma or whole blood on standby if patient does not respond as anticipated.

appendix G

Immunizations

People develop immunity to disease either naturally or by receiving biologic drugs, such as vaccines. These formulations provide preformed antibodies to specific antigens, which provide passive immunity, or they stimulate the body to produce antibodies to an injected antigen, which provide active immunity. Passive immunity does not provide long-term protection and must be repeated as needed. Active immunity provides long-term protection against various antigens.

The nurse who is administering a biologic product should have an understanding of *core drug knowledge* related to these preparations. For example, most must be injected and are metabolized within the RES system. If at all possible, they should not be used during pregnancy or given when the patient has an acute infection. Specific formulations may be associated with allergies to other drugs and should not be used if the patient has these allergies. In addition, biologic drugs should be used with caution in instances of immunosuppression and chronic illness, after blood transfusions, and in combination with other biologic drugs. Adverse effects associated with these drugs include pain and swelling at the injection site, fever, flulike symptoms, lethargy, and fatigue.

Before administering a biologic formulation, the nurse should review *core patient variables*—for example, the patient's health and medical history—for any condition that contraindicates using the vaccine or for any condition suggesting the need for extra caution. Physical assessment should include temperature, respiratory status, pulse rate, and blood pressure. The biologic drug should be injected using sterile technique into the site recommended by the manufacturer. The patient or caregivers should receive information on comfort measures (analgesics and antipyretics, warm compresses to the injection site), a written record of the drug/vaccine given, and the dates on which to return for repeated immunizations.

Product (Trade) Name	Action and Purpose	Nursing Management
Immunoglobulins		
cytomegalovirus immune globulin (CytoGam)	Attenuation of CMV associated with kidney transplantation	Administer 150 mg/kg IV within 72 h; then 100 mg/kg at 2, 4, 5, and 8 wk after transplantation; then 50 mg/kg at 12 and 16 wk. Give to seronegative recipient of seropositive kidney. Do not give during acute infection. Give injection in deltoid muscle and provide comfort measures (e.g., analgesics, warm compresses). Provide written record of immunization and dates for booster follow-up.
hepatitis B vaccine (Energix-B, Recombivax-HB)	Active immunity to infection caused by all subtypes of hepatitis B	*Adult:* Administer 1 mL IM followed by 1 mL IM at 1 mo and 6 mo after initial dose. *Child:* Energix-B, give 0.5 mL IM followed by 0.5 mL at 1 mo and 6 mo; Recombivax-HB, give 0.25 mL IM followed by 0.25 mL IM at 1 mo and 6 mo. Avoid immunization during any active infection and use caution with compromised patients. Shake container well before withdrawing solution. Inject deltoid muscle in adults, anterolateral thigh muscle in children. Provide comfort measures for pain and reactions. Provide written record of immunization and dates for booster follow-up.
influenza virus vaccine (Fluogen, Fluzone, Flu-Shield)	Stimulates active immunity to influenza virus antigens in people at high risk for developing complications from influenza	Administer according to patient's age: 6–35 mo, 0.25 mL IM repeated in 4 wk; 3–6 y, 0.5 mL IM repeated in 4 wk, older than 6 y, 0.5 mL IM. Do not give to anyone allergic to chicken eggs, feathers, chicken dander. Do not administer with other vaccines or to patients with acute respiratory infections. Monitor for toxicity if combined with theophylline or warfarin. Provide comfort measures and written record of immunization.

(continued)

Continued

Product (Trade) Name	Action and Purpose	Nursing Management
Intranasal influenza vaccine (FluMist)	Stimulates the production of antibodies to prevent influenza A and B.	Administer in October or November each year. Be sure you are using the current year's vaccine. Use for patients between 5 and 49 years of age. Do not administer to patients with immune disorders, because the vaccine contains live, attenuated influenza viruses that may cause serious infections in immunocompromised patients. Do not administer to patients with underlying chronic disorders such as diabetes mellitus, renal failure, or sickle cell disease, because these conditions predispose the patient to serious infections. Do not administer to patients with reactive airway diseases such as chronic obstructive pulmonary disease (COPD) or asthma, because bronchospasm may occur. Advise the patient to report any possible adverse effects to their health care provider, because the provider should report vaccine adverse effects to the Vaccine Adverse Event Reporting System (VAERS).
measles (rubeola) virus vaccine (Attenuvax)	Stimulates active immunity in those never infected with measles	Administer 0.5 mL SC in the upper, outer arm, and repeat if first given before age 15 mo. Do not give to patients with acute infection or anaphylactic reaction to neomycin. Use caution in patients allergic to chicken products. Do not administer within 1 mo of any live virus vaccine. Refrigerate vaccine and protect it from light. Provide comfort measures. Provide written record of immunization.
mumps virus vaccine, live (Mumpsvax)	Stimulates active immunity to mumps virus in patients older than 12 y	Administer 0.5 mL SC in the upper, outer arm. Do not give to patients with acute infection or anaphylactic reaction to neomycin. Use caution in patients allergic to chicken products. Do not administer within 1 mo of any live virus vaccine. Refrigerate vaccine and protect it from light. Provide comfort measures. Provide written record of immunization.
palivizumab (Synagis)	Monoclonal antibody that interferes with the ability of respiratory syncytial virus (RSV) to replicate in and infect cells. Prevents RSV infection in high-risk pediatric patients.	Administer 15 mg/kg IM once monthly during RSV season (November through April) to high-risk children less than 24 months of age. Do not administer to patients with known murine protein hypersensitivity or to patients with anaphylactic reactions to murine proteins. Monitor closely for allergic reactions. Have epinephrine available.

(continued)

Continued

Product (Trade) Name	Action and Purpose	Nursing Management
poliovirus vaccine, live, oral, trivalent—OPV, TOPV, Sabin (Orimune)	Stimulates active immunity to prevent poliomyelitis caused by poliovirus types 1, 2, and 3	Administer 0.5 mL PO at 2, 4, and 18 mo of age; older children: two doses of 0.5 mL PO given 8 wk apart and a third dose 6–12 mo later. *Adults:* follow dose schedule for older children if necessary. Do not administer to patients sensitive to streptomycin or neomycin or to patients with persistent vomiting or diarrhea or with immunosuppression. Refrigerate or freeze vaccine; thaw before use. Caution unimmunized adults about risk of exposure to children receiving TOPV. Provide comfort measures. Provide written record of immunization.
poliovirus vaccine inactivated—IPV, Salk (Ipol)	Stimulates active immunity; given to patients unwilling or unable to take oral vaccine	*Child:* Administer 0.5 mL SC at 2, 4, and 18 mo with booster at time of entry to elementary school. *Adult:* Seldom administered but if needed, inject 0.5 mL SC, two doses given at 1–2 mo intervals and a third dose given 6–12 mo later. See other management measures for live vaccine above.
rabies vaccine (HDCV, Imovax Rabies)	Preexposure rabies immunization for patients at high risk Postexposure antirabies regimen given with rabies immunoglobulin	*Preexposure:* Administer 1 mL IM on d 0, 7, 21, and 28. *Postexposure:* Give 1 mL IM on d 0, 3, 7, 21, 28. Refrigerate vaccine. If titer values are low, booster may be needed.
Respiratory syncytial virus immune globulin (RS-VIG, RespiGam)	A polyclonal human hyperimmune globulin that relies on passive transfer of antibodies from healthy adults with especially high levels of antibodies directed against RSV.	Administer 750 mg/kg IV once monthly during RSV season (November through April) to high-risk children less than 24 months of age. Monitor for allergic reaction, symptoms of aseptic meningitis, and fluid overload. Monitor for infusion-related symptoms such as dizziness, flushing, changes in blood pressure, anxiety, palpitations, chest tightness, dyspnea, abdominal pain, pruritus, myalgia, or arthralgia. Slow the infusion rate should any occur.
rubella virus vaccine, live (Meruvax II)	Stimulates active immunity against the rubella virus	Inject total contents of reconstituted vial SC in the upper outer aspect of arm. Do not give to pregnant patients or those with allergy to neomycin or immune deficiency. Defer vaccine in cases of acute infection. Do not administer within 1 mo of other live vaccines or 3 mo of blood transfusion. Refrigerate and protect vaccine vials from light. Provide comfort measures. Provide written record of immunization.
varicella virus vaccine, live (Varivax)	Stimulates active immunity against the chickenpox virus	Administer 0.5 mL SC as a single dose in children 1–12 y; inject 0.5 mL SC in the deltoid area to children 13 y and older. Avoid in patients with allergy to neomycin or gelatin. Do not give salicylates for up to 6 wk after vaccine.

(continued)

Continued

Product (Trade) Name	Action and Purpose	Nursing Management
		Do not administer while child has acute infection. Provide comfort measures and record of immunization.
yellow fever vaccine (YF-Vax)	Immunity for travelers to areas where yellow fever is endemic	Administer 0.5 mL SC and booster dose every 10 y. Administer with caution in patients allergic to chicken or egg products.
diphtheria and tetanus toxoids, combined, adsorbed (DT, Td)	Active immunity of patients older than 7 y against diphtheria and tetanus	Administer 2 doses of 0.5 mL IM at 4–8-wk intervals, then 0.5 mL IM at 6–12 mo and booster every 10 y. Do not give to treat acute tetanus or diphtheria or during acute infection. Administer IM only. Provide comfort measures and record of immunization with dates for follow-up immunizations.
diphtheria and tetanus toxoids and whole cell pertussis vaccine, adsorbed—DTwP (Tri-Immunol)	Active immunity in children 6 wk to 7 y against diphtheria, tetanus, pertussis	Administer 0.5 mL IM on three occasions at 4–8-wk intervals, then booster 1 y after third injection and booster needed in 4–6 y. Do not give to treat acute tetanus, diphtheria, or whooping cough. Do not administer to anyone older than 7 y. Use with caution if patient has history of adverse reaction to early injections. Provide comfort measures and record of immunization with dates for follow-up immunizations.
diphtheria and tetanus toxoids and acellular pertussis vaccine, adsorbed—DTwP (Acel-Imune, Infanrix, Tripedia)	Stimulates active immunity against diphtheria, tetanus, and pertussis (fourth and fifth doses in a series of immunizations)	Administer as fourth dose in series: 0.5 mL IM at 18 mo or 6 mo after last dose of DTwP; then administer fifth dose in series: 0.5 mL IM at 4–6 y. Do not give to treat acute tetanus, diphtheria, or whooping cough. Do not administer to anyone older than 7 y. Use with caution if patient has history of adverse reaction to early injections. Provide comfort measures. Provide written record of immunization and dates for follow-up immunizations.
diphtheria and tetanus toxoids and whole cell pertussis vaccine with *H. influenzae B* conjugate vaccine—DTwp-HIB (Tetramune)	Stimulates active immunity against diphtheria, tetanus, pertussis, and *H. influenzae B* in children 2 mo–5 y	Administer in three doses of 0.5 mL IM at 2-mo intervals with a fourth dose at 15 mo. Do not give to treat acute tetanus, diphtheria, *H. influenzae B,* or whooping cough. Do not administer to patient older than 5 y. Use with caution if patient has history of adverse reaction to early injections. Provide comfort measures, record of immunization, and dates for follow-up immunizations.
H. influenzae B conjugated vaccine hepatitis B surface antigen (Comax)	Stimulates active immunity to *H. influenzae B* and hepatitis B	Administer only to children of HBsAg-negative mothers. Do not give to adults or to children with febrile illnesses. Administer IM only. Provide comfort measures. Provide written record of immunization and dates for follow-up immunizations.

(continued)

Continued

Product (Trade) Name	Action and Purpose	Nursing Management
H. influenza B conjugated vaccine tetanus toxoid (ActHIB, OmniHIB)	Stimulates active immunity to *H. influenzae B* and tetanus in children at 2 mo–5 y	Administer 0.5 mL IM at 2, 4, and 6 mo and then at 12–15 mo. Do not give to treat acute *H. influenzae B* infection. Do not give to children older than 5 y. Administer IM only. Provide comfort measures, record of immunization, and dates for follow-up immunizations.
measles, mumps, rubella vaccine, live (MMR-II)	Stimulates active immunity to measles, mumps, and rubella in children older than 15 mo	Administer 0.5 mL SC in the upper outer aspect of the arm. Provide booster immunization at entry into school (5–6 y) and at entry into junior high school (12–13 y). Do not give to pregnant patients or those with allergy to neomycin or immunosuppression. Give cautiously to patient with allergy to eggs, chickens, or chicken feathers. Do not give within 1 mo of other live vaccines or 3 mo of blood transfusion. Refrigerate and protect vaccine from light. Provide comfort measures, record of immunization, and dates for follow-up immunizations.

Recommended Childhood and Adolescent Immunization Schedule—United States, January—June 2004

range of recommended ages | catch-up vaccination | preadolescent assessment

Vaccine ▼ / Age ▶	Birth	1 mo	2 mos	4 mos	6 mos	12 mos	15 mos	18 mos	24 mos	4-6 yrs	11-12 yrs	13-18 yrs
Hepatitis B[1]	HepB #1	only if mother HBsAg (-)							HepB series			
		HepB #2			HepB #3							
Diphtheria, Tetanus, Pertussis[2]			DTaP	DTaP	DTaP		DTaP			DTaP	Td	
Haemophilus influenzae Type b[3]			Hib	Hib	Hib	Hib						
Inactivated Polio			IPV	IPV	IPV					IPV		
Measles, Mumps, Rubella[4]						MMR #1				MMR #2	MMR #2	
Varicella[5]						Varicella			Varicella			
Pneumococcal[6]			PCV	PCV	PCV	PCV			PCV	PPV		
Vaccines below this line are for selected populations												
Hepatitis A[7]									Hepatitis A series			
Influenza[8]					Influenza (yearly)							

This schedule indicates the recommended ages for routine administration of currently licensed childhood vaccines, as of December 1, 2002, for children through age 18 years. Any dose not given at the recommended age should be given at any subsequent visit when indicated and feasible. ▓ Indicates age groups that warrant special effort to administer those vaccines not previously given. Additional vaccines may be licensed and recommended during the year. Licensed combination vaccines may be used whenever any components of the combination are indicated and the vaccine's other components are not contraindicated. Providers should consult the manufacturers' package inserts for detailed recommendations.

1. Hepatitis B vaccine (HepB). All infants should receive the first dose of hepatitis B vaccine soon after birth and before hospital discharge; the first dose may also be given by age 2 months if the infant's mother is HBsAg-negative. Only monovalent HepB can be used for the birth dose. Monovalent or combination vaccine containing HepB may be used to complete the series. Four doses of vaccine may be administered when a birth dose is given. The second dose should be given at least 4 weeks after the first dose, except for combination vaccines which cannot be administered before age 6 weeks. The third dose should be given at least 16 weeks after the first dose and at least 8 weeks after the second dose. The last dose in the vaccination series (third or fourth dose) should not be administered before age 6 months.

Infants born to HBsAg-positive mothers should receive HepB and 0.5 mL Hepatitis B Immune Globulin (HBIG) within 12 hours of birth at separate sites. The second dose is recommended at age 1-2 months. The last dose in the vaccination series should not be administered before age 6 months. These infants should be tested for HBsAg and anti-HBs at 9-15 months of age.

Infants born to mothers whose HBsAg status is unknown should receive the first dose of the HepB series within 12 hours of birth. Maternal blood should be drawn as soon as possible to determine the mother's HBsAg status; if the HBsAg test is positive, the infant should receive HBIG as soon as possible (no later than age 1 week). The second dose is recommended at age 1-2 months. The last dose in the vaccination series should not be administered before age 6 months.

2. Diphtheria and tetanus toxoids and acellular pertussis vaccine (DTaP). The fourth dose of DTaP may be administered as early as age 12 months, provided 6 months have elapsed since the third dose and the child is unlikely to return at age 15-18 months. **Tetanus and diphtheria toxoids (Td)** is recommended at age 11-12 years if at least 5 years have elapsed since the last dose of tetanus and diphtheria toxoid-containing vaccine. Subsequent routine Td boosters are recommended every 10 years.

3. *Haemophilus influenzae* type b (Hib) conjugate vaccine. Three Hib conjugate vaccines are licensed for infant use. If PRP-OMP (PedvaxHIB® or ComVax® [Merck]) is administered at ages 2 and 4 months, a dose at age 6 months is not required. DTaP/Hib combination products should not be used for primary immunization in infants at ages 2, 4 or 6 months, but can be used as boosters following any Hib vaccine.

4. Measles, mumps, and rubella vaccine (MMR). The second dose of MMR is recommended routinely at age 4-6 years but may be administered during any visit, provided at least 4 weeks have elapsed since the first dose and that both doses are administered beginning at or after age 12 months. Those who have not previously received the second dose should complete the schedule by the 11-12 year old visit.

5. Varicella vaccine. Varicella vaccine is recommended at any visit at or after age 12 months for susceptible children, i.e. those who lack a reliable history of chickenpox. Susceptible persons aged ≥13 years should receive two doses, given at least 4 weeks apart.

6. Pneumococcal vaccine. The heptavalent **pneumococcal conjugate vaccine (PCV)** is recommended for all children age 2-23 months. It is also recommended for certain children age 24-59 months. **Pneumococcal polysaccharide vaccine (PPV)** is recommended in addition to PCV for certain high-risk groups. See *MMWR* 2000;49(RR-9);1-38.

7. Hepatitis A vaccine. Hepatitis A vaccine is recommended for children and adolescents in selected states and regions, and for certain high-risk groups; consult your local public health authority. Children and adolescents in these states, regions, and high risk groups who have not been immunized against hepatitis A can begin the hepatitis A vaccination series during any visit. The two doses in the series should be administered at least 6 months apart. See *MMWR* 1999;48(RR-12);1-37.

8. Influenza vaccine. Influenza vaccine is recommended annually for children age ≥6 months with certain risk factors (including but not limited to asthma, cardiac disease, sickle cell disease, HIV, diabetes, and household members of persons in groups at high risk; see *MMWR* 2002;51(RR-3);1-31), and can be administered to all others wishing to obtain immunity. In addition, healthy children age 6-23 months are encouraged to receive influenza vaccine if feasible because children in this age group are at substantially increased risk for influenza-related hospitalizations. Children aged ≤12 years should receive vaccine in a dosage appropriate for their age (0.25 mL if age 6-35 months or 0.5 mL if aged ≥3 years). Children aged ≤8 years who are receiving influenza vaccine for the first time should receive two doses separated by at least 4 weeks.

For additional information about vaccines, including precautions and contraindications for immunization and vaccine shortages, please visit the National Immunization Program Website at www.cdc.gov/nip or call the National Immunization Information Hotline at 800-232-2522 (English) or 800-232-0233 (Spanish).

Approved by the Advisory Committee on Immunization Practices (www.cdc.gov/nip/acip), the American Academy of Pediatrics (www.aap.org), and the American Academy of Family Physicians (www.aafp.org).

appendix H

Antiemetic Drugs

Stimulation of the chemoreceptor trigger zone (CTZ) in the brain stimulates the vomiting center (VC). When the VC is stimulated, vomiting occurs. The VC may also be directly stimulated by conditions such as GI irritation, motion sickness, and vestibular neuritis. Increased activity of neurotransmitters, for example, dopamine in the CTZ and acetylcholine in the VC, appears to have an important role in inducing vomiting. Serotonin also has a role in vomiting, and special serotonin receptors are located in the CTZ. The release of serotonin from the small intestine during chemotherapy stimulates these receptors and therefore stimulates vomiting. Nurses administering antiemetic drugs need an understanding of *core drug knowledge* related to these drugs.

The nurse should be knowledgeable regarding why the drug is prescribed and how it works prior to administering it. The nurse should also determine whether the pharmacokinetics of the drug may be altered by any disease processes, or whether the drug has contraindications or precautions relevant to administration. Assess for drug interactions with other current medications while administering antiemetics. Appropriate dosage should be determined for each drug relevant to the patient's age and weight.

The nurse needs to determine core patient variables relevant to antiemetic drug therapy. Assess the patient's health status and life span to determine whether there are conditions that may prohibit the use of the drug. Determine whether the patient's lifestyle, diet, or habits are contributing to the nausea and vomiting. It may be helpful to place the patient on clear liquids or only ice chips to promote the antiemetic effect and minimize additional nausea and vomiting. If vomiting is severe and prolonged, the patient may need to be NPO and receive IV fluids during antiemetic drug therapy. A quiet environment with dimmed lighting is often helpful as an adjunct therapy to control nausea and vomiting.

To maximize the therapeutic effects of antiemetics, administer through an appropriate route on a regular basis. When severe nausea is anticipated as a result of a procedure or drug therapy, such as antineoplastic therapy, the prophylactic use of antiemetics is often recommended.

Drug (Trade) Name	Indications	Nursing Management
Antidopaminergics		
chlorpromazine (Thorazine) perphenazine (Trilafon) prochlorperazine (Compazine) promethazine (Phenergan) thiethylperazine (Torecan) metoclopramide (Reglan)	Nausea and vomiting Chlorpromazine and perphenazine are also used for relieving intractable hiccups	Limit use in children with prolonged vomiting of known etiology due to possible adverse effects. Anticipate drowsiness and caution patients not to drive or perform activities requiring mental alertness until effects of the antiemetic drug are known. Teach patients to avoid alcohol and other CNS depressants due to possible additive effects. Administer by whichever route is recommended, depending on the drug.
Anticholinergics		
cyclizine (Marezine) meclizine (Antivert) buclizine (Buculadin-S Softabs) dimenhydrinate (Dramamine) diphenhydramine (Benadryl) trimethobenzamide (Tigan) scopolamine (Transderm-Scop)	Nausea and vomiting Diphenhydramine and scopolamine only indicated for motion sickness Meclizine and dimenhydrinate also used for vertigo	Use with caution in patients with glaucoma, obstructive disease of the GI or GU tract, and elderly men with possible prostatic hypertrophy. Caution patients about additive effects with alcohol and other CNS depressants. Teach patients to wash hands after handling scopolamine transdermal disks because temporary dilation of the pupil and blurred vision are possible if drug comes in accidental contact with the eyes. Safety and efficacy in children have not been established.

(continued)

Continued

Drug (Trade) Name	Indications	Nursing Management
Selective Serotonin Receptor Antagonists		
ondansetron (Zofran) granisetron (Kytril)	Nausea and vomiting associated with initial and repeated courses of chemotherapy and radiation therapy. Ondansetron also used to prevent postoperative nausea and vomiting, also an unlabeled use for granisetron	Little is known about the dosing of ondansetron in children 3 y or younger. Dosage recommendations are available for children 4–18 y. Safety and efficacy for children younger than 2 y have not been established for granisetron. Dosage recommendations are available for children 2–16 y. These drugs may be administered PO or by IV infusion. Stable under normal lighting conditions for storage, protect from excessive light.
dolasetron (Anzemet)	Dolasetron is used to prevent nausea and vomiting associated with chemotherapy	Administer orally (100 mg) before chemotherapy. It can be mixed in juice for children. It is given with caution to patients with potential cardiac problems from electrolyte imbalances and patients taking antiarrhythmic drugs.
Miscellaneous		
diphenidol (Vontrol)	Nausea and vomiting related to postoperative status, malignant neoplasms, or labyrinthine disorders	Because drug has weak peripheral anticholinergic effect, use with care in patients sensitive to these effects. Administer orally.
benzquinamide (no other names)	Nausea and vomiting associated with surgery and anesthesia Prophylactic use reserved for patients in whom emesis would cause harm or endanger outcome of surgery	Administer preferably by IM route because IV route may cause sudden increases in blood pressure and transient arrhythmias. Safety and efficacy in pregnancy and children have not been established.
hydroxyzine (Vistaril)	Nausea and vomiting (unlabeled use)	Administer by deep IM into a large muscle. The Z-tract method is often recommended to minimize tissue irritation.
phosphorated carbohydrate solution (Emetrol)	Nausea associated with flu, pregnancy, food indiscretions, and emotional upsets	Do not administer to patient with fructose intolerance. Safe for children with flu or fever. Administer 10–20 mL g15min until distress subsides but no more than 5 doses. Do not dilute because the optimal pH for functioning may be destroyed.
Cannabinoids		
dronabinol (Marinol) nabilone (Cescamet)	Treatment of nausea and vomiting associated with cancer chemotherapy	Administer 1–3 h before chemotherapy begins with last dose 1 h after chemotherapy is completed. Monitor for tachycardia, hypotension, and dysphoria.
Glucocorticoids		
dexamethasone (Decadron) methylprednisolone (Solu-Medrol)	Treatment of nausea and vomiting associated with cancer chemotherapy	Administer intravenously just prior to chemotherapy. Adverse effects are rare due to short duration of treatment.

appendix I

Therapeutic and Toxic Levels of Selected Drugs

In evaluating the effects of drug therapy, nurses always need to keep an eye on the drug concentration in the patient's blood or serum. The following table identifies therapeutic and toxic concentrations commonly established for adults. These ranges are presented in conventional measures and SI units.

The Systeme Internationale (SI) is helpful to understand because, as with the metric system, it has been adopted by most countries in an effort to standardize clinical data in the world community and across all disciplines. The SI is structured on biologic substances reacting in the human body on a molar basis. Like the conventional system, the SI uses the kilogram as a measure of mass or weight and the meter as a measure of length. Unlike the conventional system, the SI uses the mole as a measure of volume.

A mole is the amount of a chemical compound whose weight in grams equals its molecular weight. Thus, the concentration of a solution is expressed in moles, millimoles, or micromoles per liter (mol/L, mmol/L, mmol/L, respectively) instead of in grams or milligrams per milliliter (mL) or deciliter (dL). Although a few laboratory values are the same in conventional and SI units, many differ dramatically, and normal values in both systems vary depending on laboratory methods, equipment calibrations, and other reference sources.

Quantifying the amount of drug in blood plasma or serum is helpful to health care professionals because it informs drug dosages and dosage adjustments, identifies inadequate and therapeutic responses, and diagnoses drug toxicity.

Drug	Blood Component*	Conventional Units	SI Units
acetaminophen	P		
therapeutic		0.2–0.6 mg/dL	13–40 μmol/L
toxic		>5.0 mg/dL	>300 μmol/L
barbiturate, therapeutic: see *phenobarbital*	S		
bromide, toxic	S		
as bromide ion		>20 mg/dL	>15 mmol/L
as sodium bromide		>150 mg/dL	>15 mmol/L
		>15 mEq/L	>15 mmol/L
carbamazepine, therapeutic	P	4.0–10.0 mEq/L	17–42 μmol/L
chlordiazepoxide	P		
therapeutic		0.5–5.0 mg/L	2–17 μmol/L
toxic		>10.0 mg/L	>33 μmol/L
chlorpropamide, therapeutic	P	76–250 mg/L	270–900 μmol/L
citrate (as citric acid)	B	1.2–3.0 mg/dL	60–160 μmol/L
corticotropin (ACTH)	P	20–100 pg/mL	4–22 pmol/L
cyanocobalamin (vit. B_{12})	S	200–1000 pg/mL	150–750 pmol/L
desipramine, therapeutic	P	50–200 ng/mL	170–700 nmol/L
diazepam	P		
therapeutic		0.1–0.25 mg/L	350–900 nmol/L
toxic		>1.0 mg/L	>3510 nmol/L
digoxin, therapeutic	P	0.5–2.2 ng/mL	0.6–2.8 nmol/L
		0.5–2.2 μg/L	0.6–2.8 nmol/L
diphenylhydantoin, therapeutic	P	10–20 mg/L	40–80 μmol/L
doxepin, therapeutic	P	50–200 ng/mL	180–720 nmol/L
epinephrine (radioenzymatic procedure)	P	31–95 pg/mL	170–520 pmol/L
estrogens (as estradiol)	S		
female		20–300 pg/mL	70–1100 pmol/L
peak production		200–800 pg/mL	750–2900 pmol/L
male		<50 pg/mL	<180 pmol/L
ethchlorvynol, therapeutic	P	>40 mg/L	>280 μmol/L
ethosuximide, therapeutic	P	40–110 mg/L	280–780 μmol/L
folate (as pteroylglutamic acid)	S	2–10 ng/mL	4–22 nmol/L
fructose	P	≤10 mg/dL	≤0.55 mmol/L
glucagon	S	50–100 pg/mL	50–100 ng/L
glucose	P	70–110 mg/dL	3.9–6.1 mmol/L
glutethimide	P		
therapeutic		<10 mg/L	<46 μmol/L
toxic		>20 mg/L	>92 μmol/L

(continued)

Continued

Drug	Blood Component*	Conventional Units	SI Units
gold	S	300–800 µg/dL	15.0–40.0 µmol/L
imipramine, therapeutic	P	50–200 ng/mL	180–710 nmol/L
insulin	P, S	5–20 µU/mL	35–145 pmol/L
		5–20 mU/L	35–145 pmol/L
		0.20–0.84 µg/L	35–145 pmol/L
iron	S		
male		80–180 µg/dL	14–32 µmol/L
female		60–160 µg/dL	11–29 µmol/L
isoniazid	P		
therapeutic		<2.0 mg/L	<15 µmol/L
toxic		>3.0 mg/L	>22 µmol/L
lithium, therapeutic	S	0.50–1.50 mEq/L	0.50–1.50 mmol/L
magnesium	S	1.8–3.0 mg/dL	0.80–1.20 mmol/L
		1.6–2.4 mEq/L	0.80–1.20 mmol/L
meprobamate	P		
therapeutic		<20 mg/L	<90 µmol/L
toxic		>40 mg/L	>180 µmol/L
methsuximide, therapeutic	P	10–40 mg/L	50–210 µmol/L
norepinephrine (radioenzymatic procedure)	P	215–475 pg/mL (at rest for 15 min)	1.27–2.81 nmol/L
phenobarbital, therapeutic	P	2–5 mg/dL	85–215 µmol/L
phenylbutazone, therapeutic	P	<100 mg/L	<320 µmol/L
potassium	S	3.5–5.0 mEq/L	3.5–5.0 mmol/L
primidone	P		
therapeutic		6–10 mg/L	25–45 µmol/L
toxic		>10 mg/L	>46 µmol/L
procainamide	P		
therapeutic		4.0–8.0 mg/L	17–34 µmol/L
toxic		>12 mg/L	>50 µmol/L
propoxyphene, toxic	P	>20 mg/L	>5.9 µmol/L
propranolol hydrochloride (inderal), therapeutic	P	50–200 ng/mL	190–770 nmol/L
pyruvate (as pyruvic acid)	B	0.3–0.9 mg/dL	35–100 µmol/L
quinidine	P		
therapeutic		1.5–3.0 mg/L	4.6–9.2 µmol/L
toxic		>6.0 mg/L	>18.5 µmol/L
salicylate (salicylic acid)	S	Toxic >20 mg/dL	>1.45 mmol/L
sulfonamides, all as sulfanilamide, therapeutic	B	10.0–15.0 mg/dL	580–870 µmol/L
theophylline, therapeutic	P	10.0–20.0 mg/L	55–110 mmol/L
thiocyanate (nitroprusside toxicity)	P	10 mg/dL	1.75 mmol/L
thyroxine (T_4)	S	4–11 µg/dL	51–142 nmol/L
trimethadione, therapeutic	P	<50 mg/L	<350 µmol/L
trimipramine, therapeutic	P	50–200 ng/ml	170–680 nmol/L
vitamin B_2 (riboflavin)	S	2.6–3.7 µg/dL	70–100 nmol/L
vitamin B_6 (pyridoxal)	B	20–90 ng/mL	120–540 nmol/L
vitamin B_{12} (cyanocobalamin)	P, S	200–1000 pg/mL	150–750 pmol/L
vitamin E (alpha-tocopherol)	P, S	0.78–1.25 mg/dL	18–29 µmol/L

*P, plasma; B, blood; S, serum.

appendix J

Drugs That May Cause Photosensitivity

PHARMACIST'S LETTER
PRESCRIBER'S LETTER

Detail-Document #200509

– This Detail-Document accompanies the related article published in–

PHARMACIST'S LETTER / PRESCRIBER'S LETTER

May 2004 ~ Volume 20 ~ Number 200509

Drug-Induced Photosensitivity

Lead author: Kelly M. Shields, Pharm.D.

Drugs Reported to Cause Photosensitivity Reactions [1-11]

Therapeutic Class	Drugs	Comments
Antihistamines	cetirizine (*Zyrtec*), cyproheptadine (*Periactin*), diphenhydramine (*Benadryl*), loratadine (*Claritin*), promethazine (*Phenergan*)	Reactions have been seen both with topical and systemic administration of antihistamines.
Anti-infectives	Fluoroquinolones: ciprofloxacin (*Cipro*), gemifloxacin (*Factive*), levofloxacin (*Levaquin*), lomefloxacin (*Maxaquin*), moxifloxacin (*Avelox*), norfloxacin (*Noroxin*), ofloxacin (*Floxin*) Tetracyclines: demeclocycline (*Declomycin*), doxycycline (*Vibramycin*), minocycline (*Minocin*), oxytetracycline (*Terramycin*), tetracycline (*Achromycin*) Others: azithromycin (*Zithromax*), capreomycin (*Capastat*), ceftazidime (*Fortaz*), cefazolin (*Ancef*), cycloserine (*Seromycin*), dapsone, ethionamide (*Trecator-SC*), isoniazid (*Nydrazid*), metronidazole (*Flagyl*), nalidixic acid (*NegGram*), pyrazinamide, sulfamethoxazole/trimethoprim (*Bactrim*), sulfasalazine (*Azulfidine*), sulfisoxazole (*Gantrisin*)	Lomefloxacin has higher incidence than other quinolones, no reports with gatifloxacin. Tetracyclines- reactions seen most often with demeclocycline. Cefazolin reaction was noted in one case report with concurrent gentamicin use.
Antifungals	flucytosine (*Ancobon*), griseofulvin (*Fulvicin, Gris-PEG*), terconazole (*Terazol*) voriconazole (*VFEND*)	
Antiretroviral	ritonavir (*Norvir*), saquinavir (*Fortovase, Invirase*), zalcitabine (*Hivid*)	Reactions seen in less than 2% of patients.
Antimalarial	chloroquine (*Aralen*), hydroxychloroquine (*Plaquenil*), pyrimethamine (*Daraprim*), pyrimethamine/sulfadoxine (*Fansidar*), quinine	Limited reports of reactions exist.
Antivirals	amantadine (*Symmetrel),* acyclovir (*Zovirax*)	About 1% incidence.
Antineoplastics	bexarotene (*Targretin*), capecitabine (*Xeloda*), dacarbazine (*DTIC*), epirubicin (*Ellence*), fluorouracil (*5-FU*), interferon alfa (*Intron A, Alferon-N*), methotrexate (*Mexate*), pentostatin (*Nipent*), procarbazine (*Matulane*), tretinoin, oral (*Vesanoid*), vinblastine (*Velban, Velbe*)	Incidence varies from 1% to 5% by agent.
Antiplatelet	clopidogrel (*Plavix*)	Only one case report.

More. . .

Therapeutic Class	Drugs	Comments
Cardiovascular	Thiazide diuretics: bendroflumethiazide (*Corzide*), chlorthalidone (*Thalitone*), hydrochlorothiazide (*Microzide*), hydroflumethiazide (*Diucardin*), indapamide (*Lozol*), methyclothiazide (*Enduron*), metolazone (*Zaroxolyn*), polythiazide (*Renese*) Diuretics, Other: furosemide (*Lasix*), triamterene (*Dyrenium*) Antihypertensives: captopril (*Capoten*), diltiazem (*Cardizem, Tiazac*), enalapril (*Vasotec*), nifedipine (*Procardia*), sotalol (*Betapace*) Statins: fluvastatin (*Lescol*), lovastatin (*Mevacor*), pravastatin (*Pravachol*), simvastatin (*Zocor*) Other: amiodarone (*Cordarone, Pacerone*), fenofibrate (*Tricor*), quinidine	Any combination product with hydrochlorothiazide has a risk of photosensitivity. Incidence of photosensitivity with amiodarone is about 10%.
Anticonvulsants	carbamazepine (*Tegretol*), felbamate (*Felbatol*), gabapentin (*Neurontin*), lamotrigine (*Lamictal*), oxcarbazepine (*Trileptal*), topiramate (*Topamax*), valproic acid (*Depakene*)	Incidence is generally low ranging from 0.1% to 1%.
Antipsychotics	Antipsychotics,Phenothiazines: chlorpromazine (*Thorazine*), fluphenazine (*Prolixin*), perphenazine (*Trilafon*), prochlorperazine (*Compazine*), thioridazine (*Mellaril*), trifluoperazine (*Stelazine*) Antipsychotics, Other: clozapine (*Clozaril*), haloperidol (*Haldol*), loxapine (*Loxitane*), olanzapine (*Zyprexa*), quetiapine (*Seroquel*), risperidone (*Risperdal*), thiothixene (*Navane*), ziprasidone (*Geodon*)	Phenothiazines-reactions most common with chlorpromazine (incidence of 2% to 3%).
Antidepressants	Tricyclic Antidepressants: amitriptyline (*Elavil*), amoxapine (*Asendin*), clomipramine (*Anafranil*), desipramine (*Norpramin*), doxepin (*Sinequan*), imipramine (*Tofranil*), maprotiline (*Ludiomil*), nortriptyline (*Pamelor*), protriptyline (*Vivactil*), trimipramine (*Surmontil*) Selective serotonin reuptake inhibitors: citalopram (*Celexa*), escitalopram (*Lexapro*), fluoxetine (*Prozac*, *Sarafem*), fluvoxamine (*Luvox*), paroxetine (*Paxil*), sertraline (*Zoloft*) Antidepressant, Other: bupropion (*Wellbutrin*), mirtazapine (*Remeron*), nefazodone (*Serzone*), trazodone (*Desyre*l), venlafaxine (*Effexor*)	In the case of most of these drugs, incidence of photosensitivity has not been definitely attributed to the antidepressant. No reports noted with escitalopram, but included because structurally related to citalopram.
Sedative/Hypnotics	alprazolam (*Xanax*), chlordiazepoxide (*Librium*), zaleplon (*Sonata*), zolpidem (*Ambien*)	Incidence ranges from 0.1% to 1%.

More. . .

Therapeutic Class	Drugs	Comments
Analgesic Agents	NSAIDs: celecoxib (*Celebrex*), diclofenac (*Voltaren, Cataflam*), diflunisal (*Dolobid*), etodolac (*Lodine*), ibuprofen (*Motrin*), ketoprofen (*Orudis*), mefenamic acid (*Ponstel*), meloxicam (*Mobic*), nabumetone (*Relafen*), naproxen (*Anaprox*), oxaprozin (*Daypro*), piroxicam (*Feldene*), rofecoxib (*Vioxx*), sulindac (*Clinoril*), valdecoxib (*Bextra*) Other: cyclobenzaprine (*Flexeril*), dantrolene (*Dantrium*), sumatriptan (*Imitrex*)	
Hormones	Oral contraceptives, corticosteroids	
Antidiabetic Agents	Sulfonylureas: acetohexamide (*Dymelor*), chlorpropamide (*Diabinese*), glimepiride (*Amaryl*), glipizide (*Glucotrol*), glyburide (*DiaBeta, Micronase*), tolazamide (*Tolinase*), tolbutamide (*Orinase*)	
Skin Agents	benzocaine (*Americaine*), coal tar, hexachlorophene (*PHisoHex*), isotretinoin (*Accutane*), methoxsalen (*Uvadex, Oxsoralen*), minoxidil (*Rogaine*), tacrolimus (*Prograf, Protopic*), tazarotene (*Tazorac*), tretinoin, topical (*Renova, Retin-A*) Sunscreen agents: PABA, cinnamates, benzyphenones	Isotretinoin incidence is 5% to 10%.
Miscellaneous	chlorhexidine (*Peridex, Hibiclens*), gold salts, selegiline (*Eldepryl*), thalidomide (*Thalomid*)	
Vitamins	pyridoxine (Vitamin B6), Vitamin A	Based on case reports.
Dietary Supplements	bitter orange, chlorella, dong quai, gossypol, gotu kola, St. John's wort	Limited reporting of adverse reactions with dietary supplements makes this listing incomplete.

Many of the drugs listed in the proceeding table were labeled as photosensitizing based on unclear data. Unclear and incomplete reporting of adverse drug reactions lead to this confusion. Chemicals that are planar, tricyclic, or polycyclic absorb ultraviolet light, which lead them to be classified as photosensitizer drugs.[10]

Types of Photosensitivity

Drug-induced photosensitivity may present in a variety of ways. Most reactions are generally classified as either phototoxic or photoallergic. Photoallergy is a relatively rare, immunological response, which is not dose-related. The allergy develops after multiple days of continuous exposure. It occurs when light causes a drug to act as a hapten, triggering a hypersensitivity response. The reaction usually manifests as pruritic and eczematous.[10-13]

Phototoxic reactions are chemically-induced reactions when the drug absorbs UVA light and causes cellular damage. This reaction can be seen with initial exposure to a drug, may be dose-related, and doesn't demonstrate cross-sensitivity. It usually has rapid onset and manifests as an exaggerated sunburn. This reaction will be seen only on skin areas exposed to the sun.[10-13]

Management of Photosensitivity

Prevention of photosensitivity reactions is based on patient education. Patients should be educated to minimize sun exposure. Use of UVA-protective sunscreens and physical barriers such as clothing can provide additional light protection.

More. . .

Sunscreens that provide UVA coverage include: avobenzone, dioxybenzone, oxybenzone, titanium dioxide, zinc oxide. Remind patients of the need to frequently reapply while in the sun. Patients should definitely be counseled to avoid sources of high-intensity light such as tanning beds. Additionally, as some reactions may be dose-related, a decrease in dose may be considered to help minimize the reaction or possibly selection of an alternative agent.

An acute attack may be managed in a number of different ways based on severity. A mild reaction may be handled similarly to a sunburn, with skin protectants and topical or systemic analgesics.[12] Patients may also benefit from application of cooling creams or gels. If patients have blisters that are broken, antibacterial creams may be necessary to prevent infection.[10] Severe reactions may be handled by oral or topic corticosteroids.[13] Antihistamines may also alleviate pruritus associated with reactions.

Users of this document are cautioned to use their own professional judgment and consult any other necessary or appropriate sources prior to making clinical judgments based on the content of this document. Our editors have researched the information with input from experts, government agencies, and national organizations. Information and Internet links in this article were current as of the date of publication.

References

1. Anderson PO, Knoben JE, Troutman WG. Handbook of clinical drug data. 10th ed. New York: McGraw-Hill; 2002.
2. Dukes MNG, Aronson JK. Meyler's side effects of drugs. 14th ed. Amsterdam: Elsevier; 2000.
3. Cohen HE. Red Book. 2003 ed. Montvale (NJ): Thomson Medical Economics; 2003.
4. Warnock JK, Morris DW. Adverse cutaneous reactions to mood stabilizers. *Am J Clin Dermatol* 2003;4:21-30.
5. Warnock JK, Morris DW. Adverse cutaneous reactions to antipsychotics. *Am J Clin Dermatol* 2002;3:629-36.
6. Arana GW. An overview of side effects caused by typical antipsychotics. *J Clin Psychiatry* 2000;61(supp 8):5-11.
7. Dogra S, Kanwar AJ. Clopidogrel bisulphate-induced photosensitivity lichenoid eruption. *Br J Dermatol* 2003;148:609-10.
8. McEvoy GK. AHFS Drug Information 2004 [database on the Internet]. Bethesda(MD): American Society of Health System Pharmacy. C2004 [updated 2004 Jan 1; cited 2004 April 19]. Available from: http://www.statref.com.
9. Jellin JM, Gregory PJ, Batz F, et al. Therapeutic Research Faculty. *Natural Medicines Comprehensive Database*. http://www.naturaldatabase.com. (Accessed April 17, 2004).
10. Moore DE. Drug-induced cutaneous photosensitivity. *Drug Saf* 2002;25:345-72.
11. Allen JE. Drug-induced photosensitivity. *Clin Pharm* 1993;12:580-7.
12. Berbardi RR. Handbook of nonprescription drugs. 14th ed. Washington DC: American Pharmacists Association; 2004.
13. Morison WL. Photosensitivity. *N Engl J Med* 2001;350;1111-7.

Answers to Questions for Study and Review

Unit 1: Foundation for Drug Therapy in Nursing

CHAPTER 1: NURSING MANAGEMENT IN DRUG THERAPY

1-1. Core drug variables are assessed in several ways: the patient interview, the physical assessment, and the medical record. Data on some of the variables can be obtained from more than one source.

1-2. Core drug knowledge contains basic pharmacologic facts about the drug. The nurse needs to know this information to administer drugs safely, to determine interactions with core patient variables, to devise strategies, to maximize therapeutic effects and minimize adverse effects, and to educate patients and their families.

1-3. Learning about a prototype drug gives the nurse information about a group of drugs instead of just one drug, which simplifies learning and helps the nurse organize drug information logically.

1-4. Core patient variables may affect the form the patient education should take (i.e., written, visual with pictures, or spoken), who in the family should be included in the teaching, and what content is most important to include in the teaching.

CHAPTER 2: PHARMACEUTICALS: DEVELOPMENT, SAFEGUARDS, AND DELIVERY

2-1. The *United States Pharmacopeia* (USP) and the *National Formulary* (NF) are compendia of drugs available in the United States. The drugs are listed by their official names.

2-2. Drugs are named to describe their organic structure (chemical structure), their chemical composition (chemical name), their general properties derived from their chemical components (generic name), and their desired effect as intended by the manufacturer (trade name).

2-3. Drugs are classified according to chemical composition, physiologic effect, or therapeutic use. Organizing a multitude of drugs into family groups—drug classes—with similar characteristics facilitates learning about an individual drug within the group. A general characteristic of the drug class is likely to apply to a single drug within the class.

2-4. The 1938 Food, Drug, and Cosmetic Act prohibited the marketing of new drugs before they had been properly tested for safety. It further stipulated that pharmaceutical companies had to submit an investigational new drug application to the government for review of a drug's safety before it could sell the product. The Durham-Humphrey Amendment provided further safeguards. This amendment distinguished between legend drugs (requiring a prescription) and over-the-counter drugs (not requiring a prescription) and required that labels of legend drugs carry the legend: "Caution—Federal law prohibits dispensing without a prescription." It further specified certain drugs that could not be refilled without a new prescription from the health care provider. The Canadian Narcotics Council Act (1961) regulated possession, sale, manufacture, production, and distribution of narcotics.

2-5. Clinical trials proceed after extensive animal testing provides initial evidence of the safety and efficacy of a new drug. Clinical trials have four phases. Phase I establishes optimal dosage range and pharmacokinetics. Phase II closely monitors study participants for the drug's effectiveness and adverse effects. Phase III begins if no serious adverse effects have been identified in phase II. Beginning in this phase, double-blind studies (in which neither the investigator nor the study subject knows whether the drug being administered is a placebo or the new drug being studied) establish the drug's clinical effectiveness, safety, and dosage range. Phase IV consists of postmarketing studies. Some drugs make it through all phases of clinical trials without problems, only to have severe adverse effects show up after they are used more widely in the general population. Examples of this phenomenon are the links uncovered between felbamate and aplastic anemia and between troglitazone and hepatic failure.

2-6. Controlled substances are drugs defined and categorized according to their abuse potential and dependence-producing liability. The 1970 Controlled Substance Act requires an accounting of all controlled drugs on a special record and an accounting of all discarded or wasted medication. Another licensed nurse must countersign the special record filled out by a first. Furthermore, all controlled substances must be kept under double lock. Only authorized people have access to the keys.

2-7. All patients should be taught not to share drugs with anyone else, to follow directions for use that appear on the drug label, to avoid drinking alcohol with any prescription or over-the-counter drug, and not to take a drug after its expiration date.

2-8. The patient teaching plan for drug therapy should include the drug name and reason for use; the dosage (amount, frequency, duration of therapy, what to do about a missed dose or a double dose); administration route; special directions or procedures (for drug administration, drug stability, storage, disposal); minor adverse effects and reportable serious adverse effects; drug interactions (among drugs and foods); effects of other disease states on drug therapy; and self-monitoring techniques.

CHAPTER 3: DRUG ADMINISTRATION

3-1. The most frequently used drug administration route is the enteral route for oral drugs.

3-2. An enteric coating prevents the drug from breaking down in the stomach and thus prevents GI irritation and inactivation of the drug by stomach acid. Sustained release may also occur with enteric coating.

3-3. The parenteral route may be recommended for a patient who is unable to swallow, is confused and uncooperative with oral medications, is unconscious, or has a physiologic need to keep the GI tract empty (e.g., in preparation for a diagnostic test or surgery, or to rest the tract). The parenteral route may be used when the drug has a high first-pass effect when administered orally, which eliminates most of the active drug, or when the drug will be inactivated by gastric acid.

3-4. The greatest risk for rapid drug toxicity is the intravenous route, especially in cases of continuous intravenous infusion.

Unit 2: Core Drug Knowledge

CHAPTER 4: PHARMACOTHERAPEUTICS, PHARMACOKINETICS, AND PHARMACODYNAMICS

4-1. Pharmacokinetics is what happens to the drug as it moves through the body (i.e., the body's effect on the drug). Pharmacodynamics is the manner in which the drug produces its action in the body (i.e., the drug's effect on the body).

4-2. Lipophilic drugs are soluble in lipid, or fats. Because the cell membrane is composed primarily of lipids, being lipophilic allows a drug to pass through the cell membrane easily.

4-3. Hydrophilic drugs or particles are water soluble. Water solubility promotes excretion in the urine, which is water based.

4-4. Drugs attach to specialized receptors on the cell. Attachment to the receptor either turns on the receptor's specialized action or blocks other substances from attaching to the receptor.

4-5. One hundred percent of drugs that are given orally present to the liver first after absorption. If the drug is extensively metabolized, most of the drug dose will be lost before it enters the systemic circulation. Giving the drug by another route (such as the intravenous route or the sublingual route) bypasses the liver initially, allowing 100% of the drug dose to enter the systemic circulation.

4-6. In a person with renal insufficiency or hepatic dysfunction, the dose given may be lower than the typical dose given to other patients because improperly functioning kidneys cannot excrete drugs at the rate that is normally expected and a poorly functioning liver cannot metabolize drugs as rapidly. Both of these impairments increase the amount of circulating drug and prolong the effect from a drug dose. An increase in the amount of the circulating drug increases the therapeutic effects of the drug, but it also increases the risk for adverse effects.

4-7. A patient with decreased albumin levels who is receiving a drug that is known to be highly protein bound is at higher risk for adverse drug effects than a patient with normal albumin levels because drug that is bound to protein is not active. Only free drug is active and can create an effect. Because the protein, albumin, is low, there is no place for the drug to bind, and more drug than would normally be expected is free, active, and able to cause therapeutic and adverse effects.

CHAPTER 5: ADVERSE EFFECTS AND DRUG INTERACTIONS

5-1. Rash, hives, redness, itching, swelling of the eyes or another body part, and difficulty swallowing or breathing (laryngeal edema) are all signs of allergic reactions to drug therapy. Complaints such as nausea or vomiting would more likely indicate adverse effects.

5-2. Changes in hearing and balance may naturally occur with aging, but they are also signs of ototoxicity. Thus, adverse effects could be misconstrued as age-related changes.

5-3. The circulating blood level of Drug A will be decreased. When Drug B stimulates the hepatic pathway, more of the isoenzyme CYP3A4 will be active, thus creating more metabolism of Drug A. As Drug A is metabolized at a faster than normal rate, the circulating level will decrease.

5-4. No, the circulating blood levels of the drug will differ. The effect of grapefruit juice on metabolism varies greatly among people because people have different amounts of CYP3A4 in their GI tract.

5-5. Owing to normal circulatory patterns, all the dose of the oral drug is presented initially to the liver, where damage may occur. When the drug is administered parenterally, the drug molecules first go to the heart, and then only about 25% of the molecules are sent to the liver. Because fewer drug molecules are present in the liver at any given time, less damage may occur.

5-6. The combination of these drugs will result in an additive CNS depressive effect, greatly increasing the risk for CNS toxicity.

5-7. As the nurse, you consider the possibility that Drug A and Drug B have had an interaction, producing decreased therapeutic response from Drug A. Look up both drugs and determine whether this is an accurate assessment.

Unit 3: Core Patient Variables

CHAPTER 6: LIFE SPAN: CHILDREN

6-1. In the infant and especially the neonate, immature liver function affects drug distribution. The neonate's immature liver produces fewer plasma proteins, especially albumin; many drugs bind strongly to albumin. The pharmacologic effects of drugs result from unbound, or free, drug. In the neonate and infant, more free drug is available because less drug is bound to plasma protein. This state results in increased blood levels of drugs and, in turn, more side effects and toxicity.

6-2. Body surface area is the external surface of the body expressed in square meters. The ratio of body surface area to weight is inversely proportional to length.

6-3. An increased dose of some drugs may be given to the infant because the drug is diluted by the infant's higher body water content.

6-4. No. Some drugs have adverse effects only in children and are contraindicated in them. Other drugs are not supported by enough clinical study to determine what effect they would have on a child. Extreme caution must be used if these drugs are administered.

6-5. Vastus lateralis or rectus femoris.

6-6. If past experiences were unpleasant, the child would more likely be fearful and anxious about this interaction or drug therapy. Because parents and sometimes other family members are normally responsible for seeing that the child receives the appropriate drug therapy at home, including them in the planning and education relevant to drug therapy is crucial. Children also need to be involved, at an age-appropriate level, in their drug therapy.

CHAPTER 7: LIFE SPAN: PREGNANT OR BREAST-FEEDING WOMEN

7-1. A drug assigned to FDA pregnancy category X should not be used because it is almost sure to harm the fetus. The benefits of drug therapy cannot compensate for the risk to the fetus.

7-2. Drugs that have low molecular weight and are lipophilic and not bound to protein pass through the placenta's lipid membrane easily.

7-3. Gestational weeks 3 through 8 mark the period of organogenesis, which is when all major fetal organ systems are developing. Teratogenic exposure during this period may cause major malformations that are usually recognized at birth.

7-4. Physiologic changes in the renal system that increase drug excretion rates include renal blood flow increases of 40% to 50%, which increase filtration through the glomerulus about 50% and contribute to increased excretion rates.

7-5. Lipophilic (fat-soluble) drugs pass into breast milk because of the high fat content in breast milk.

CHAPTER 8: LIFE SPAN: OLDER ADULTS

8-1. Liver function and metabolism are impaired because of decreased liver mass, decreased hepatic blood flow and hepatic tissue perfusion, and changes in the phases of metabolism.

8-2. Normal renal function decreases with aging. Drugs that depend on renal elimination are not excreted as quickly in the older adult. This decrease in function leads to elevated circulating active drug levels, which places the patient at risk for adverse effects or drug toxicity.

8-3. Polypharmacy is the simultaneous use of multiple prescription and over-the-counter (OTC) drugs by one person, and it puts the person at increased risk for drug interactions, adverse effects, and nonadherence to drug therapy. Polypharmacy occurs frequently in older adults because they often experience multiple health problems related to organ and body system deterioration with advanced age.

8-4. Adverse drug effects often mimic cognitive and functional changes that occur naturally with advanced age.

8-5. Activity will affect absorption and distribution of some drugs. Dietary habits will indicate whether a patient will be able to swallow oral tablets or pills. Quality of life may be impaired from adverse effects of drug therapy. The patient may have strict habits related to administration of drug therapy; following the patient's normal routine may reduce stress. The patient's economic status, including drug insurance coverage, may affect whether the patient obtains prescribed drugs regularly.

CHAPTER 9: LIFESTYLE: SUBSTANCE ABUSE

9-1. Alcohol is a CNS depressant. In combination with other CNS depressants, alcohol can produce additive pharmacologic effects of CNS depression.

9-2. Drug abuse is the excessive self-administration of a drug (often dependence producing) for other than therapeutic purposes. Drug misuse is the inadvertent incorrect use of a drug, often because the individual lacks knowledge of the drug. Addiction is physical dependence on a drug, which leads to serious physical and behavioral problems. Without the drug, physical symptoms of withdrawal begin to occur. Withdrawal is marked by a variety of physical effects, including nausea, muscle cramping, dysphoria, and convulsions. Characteristics of addiction include compulsive drug use, drug craving, and drug seeking. Psychological dependence (habituation) is an intense desire or craving for the drug when it is not available.

9-3. Disulfiram is used as an adjunct to behavioral therapy in treating alcohol abuse. It causes a severe intolerance reaction when alcohol is ingested. This reaction is manifested by flushing, throbbing headache, respiratory difficulty, palpitations, and confusion.

9-4. Factors that place an individual at risk for substance abuse include chronic pain; struggles with self-esteem issues and peer pressure; poverty and illiteracy among the socioeconomically underprivileged; wealth and influence among the very privileged; profession (health care providers); history of child abuse or sexual assault; and family history of substance abuse, including alcoholism.

9-5. Methadone is an opioid with a dependence-producing liability. During therapy, patients develop a dependence on methadone. Oral methadone dosing suppresses opioid withdrawal symptoms, and the drug has a long duration of action (24 hours), which are advantages of methadone therapy.

9-6. Hallucinogenic drugs distort perceptions and reality. Nursing interventions for a "bad trip" rely on decreasing sensory stimuli and providing for safety and support.

9-7. Two major substances that are abused are alcohol and nicotine (cigarettes). Categories of additional drugs of abuse include CNS depressants (alcohol, marijuana, opioids, sedatives and hypnotics, antipsychotics, and antianxiety drugs), CNS stimulants (cocaine, amphetamines, caffeine), and mind-altering or psychedelic drugs (LSD, mescaline, MDMA). Some individuals use drugs to alter thoughts and feelings.

CHAPTER 10: LIFESTYLE, DIET, AND HABITS: NUTRITION AND COMPLEMENTARY MEDICATIONS

10-1. Adverse drug–nutrient interactions are most likely to occur if medications are taken over long periods, if several medications are taken, or if nutrition status is poor or deteriorating.

10-2. Drugs and nutrients can interact and alter metabolism by acting as structural analogues, competing with each other for metabolic enzyme systems, altering enzyme activity, and contributing pharmacologically active substances.

10-3. Foods can alter drug absorption by changing the acidity of the digestive tract, stimulating secretion of digestive enzymes, altering rate of absorption, binding to drugs, or competing for absorption sites in the intestines.

10-4. Patients may not consider these substances to be potentially harmful or capable of interacting with prescribed drug therapy and therefore may not volunteer this information unless directly questioned.

CHAPTER 11: ENVIRONMENT: INFLUENCES ON DRUG THERAPY

11-1. The nurse assesses for exposure to chemicals in the workplace, home, and community. Exposure to these chemicals is thought to be responsible for alteration of the hepatic drug-metabolizing enzymes resulting in decreased drug efficacy, prolonged pharmacologic effects, or increased toxicity.

11-2. Alcohol, tobacco, or exposure to chemicals (e.g., industrial chemicals, pesticides) may adversely affect the pharmacokinetics of certain drugs by altering hepatic drug-metabolizing enzymes and altering drug responses, which increases the patient's risk for drug reactions.

11-3. The nurse inquires about the patient's home and workplace environment because they may have a bearing on drug therapy. The nurse also obtains a complete patient history that also documents lifestyle habits, which may affect drug therapy (e.g., ethanol, tobacco) as well as exposure to workplace chemicals; these factors all influence the hepatic drug-metabolizing enzymes. This information is important and will help the nurse determine whether the desired effect of drug therapy is achieved.

CHAPTER 12: CULTURE AND INHERITED TRAITS: CONSIDERATIONS IN DRUG THERAPY

12-1. A culture is a background of customs and traditions, values, institutions, art, history, and folklore that is shared by a people. An ethnic group has a common heritage linked by race, nationality, or language.

12-2. An awareness of cultural differences alerts the nurse to assess for factors that might have an effect on drug therapy, such as current health status, genetic variations in pharmacokinetics, self-medication (with traditional or alternative medicines), and dietary practices. This awareness also assists the nurse in forming a therapeutic relationship, in communicating effectively with the patient and family, and in providing appropriate and effective teaching.

12-3. Obtain an interpreter or translator. Speak to the patient. Speak slowly. Do not shout or exaggerate your mouth movements. Allow time for the patient to think and respond. Use as few words as possible. Use as many words in the patient's language as possible. Use nonverbal language.

12-4. If the patient is present oriented, explain problems that may occur now, if medicine is not taken as directed. If patient is future oriented, she or he will be more receptive to learning that the medication will prevent future problems if taken as directed.

12-5. The genetic background of Mexican Americans is quite varied. Their bodies may or may not handle drugs in the same way that they are handled in the bodies of Hispanics in general. Drug information that is related to findings for Hispanic people can be generalized only tentatively to Mexican Americans.

Unit 4: Peripheral Nervous System Drugs

CHAPTER 13: DRUGS AFFECTING ADRENERGIC FUNCTION

13-1. Predrug therapy assessments include ensuring that there is no known hypersensitivity to beta-adrenergic antagonists (beta blockers) and that the patient does not have contraindications to drug therapy such as bronchial asthma or chronic obstructive lung disease, severe sinus bradycardia, right ventricular hypertrophy or failure secondary to pulmonary hypertension, second- and third-degree atrioventricular block, overt cardiac failure, or cardiogenic shock. Additional assessments include detecting any disorder requiring precautions with beta blockers, such as peripheral vascular disease, allergies, asthma, chronic obstructive lung disease or bronchospastic disease, congestive heart failure, hepatic disease, diabetes mellitus, hyperthyroidism, and cerebrovascular insufficiency.

13-2. When monitoring therapeutic effects of beta-blocker therapy for angina, the nurse monitors for reduced use of nitroglycerin and reduced frequency, severity, onset, and duration of angina-related pain. The heart rate is monitored as well.

13-3. Impending propranolol toxicity is recognized by bradycardia, severe hypotension, depression, confusion, hallucinations, and bronchospasm.

13-4. If the patient shows cardiotoxic effects, the nurse should withhold the next drug dose and notify the prescriber immediately.

13-5. Dopamine increases renal perfusion. As the kidney becomes adequately perfused, it will resume its normal functioning and produce urine at a normal rate. Monitoring urinary output indicates whether the dose of dopamine is sufficient to perfuse the kidneys adequately. The systolic blood pressure should rise from dopamine administration. If the diastolic pressure rises greatly or disproportionately, it indicates that the alpha-2 effects of dopamine are overriding the beta-2 and dopaminergic effects. Such an increase in diastolic pressure means that the drug dosage must be decreased.

13-6. The use of radiocontrast dye may induce nephropathy and resultant acute renal failure in patients with preexisting renal insufficiency. Activation of peripheral dopamine-1 receptors produces vasodilation to the coronary, renal, mesenteric, and peripheral arteries, thus reducing the potential for renal adverse effects from contrast dye.

13-7. Prazosin may induce "first-dose syncope." Patients should be advised to sit or lie down after taking the first dose to minimize postural hypotension.

CHAPTER 14: DRUGS AFFECTING CHOLINERGIC FUNCTION

14-1. In the absence of bowel sounds or with hypoactive bowel sounds, bethanechol is given to increase gastrointestinal motility. Its effectiveness would be gauged by the assessment of active bowel sounds, passage of flatus, or production of stool. Shortness of breath would be assessed by listening to breath sounds and measuring respiratory rate. Shortness of breath indicates cholinergic toxicity and should be treated immediately with the antidote atropine. To ease the work of respiration, the head of the bed can be raised. The patient should be checked every 15 minutes after atropine administration and observed until stable.

14-2. Headache, decreasing blood pressure, and decreased pulse rate are due to the stimulation of muscarinic receptors in the cardiovascular system. These signs may indicate impending toxicity or adverse effects.

14-3. A cholinergic crisis results from overstimulation of cholinergic receptors following the inhibition of cholinesterase or overdosing with a cholinergic agent. It is treated by administering an anticholinergic to block the muscarinic receptors and a sympathomimetic to increase peripheral resistance and restore blood pressure; if the crisis is caused by the use of an irreversible inhibitor, such as an insecticide, then an oxime, such as pralidoxime, is needed to regenerate the postsynaptic cholinesterase enzyme.

14-4. Parasympathetic nerves innervate the salivary glands and some sweat glands. Stimulation of these nerves causes the production of large amounts of saliva and sweat. Inhibition of parasympathetic stimulation by anticholinergic drugs prevents the secretion of saliva and sweat, causing dry mouth and skin.

Unit 5: Central Nervous System Drugs

CHAPTER 15: DRUGS PRODUCING ANESTHESIA AND NEUROMUSCULAR BLOCKING

15-1. Producing general anesthesia with a single agent is not always desirable because too deep a level of unconsciousness may ensue. To overcome this limitation, a process called balanced anesthesia is employed. Balanced anesthesia relies on a combination of drugs to produce loss of consciousness, analgesia, and muscle relaxation, while producing and maintaining a lighter stage of anesthesia. Drugs used in balanced anesthesia include inhaled or parenteral anesthetics, ultrashort-acting barbiturates, neuromuscular blocking agents, benzodiazepines, and opioid analgesics.

15-2. Patients need to be given anesthesia in a controlled environment, such as the operating suite or critical care unit. A cardiac monitor, blood pressure monitor, and ventilator must be available for immediate use. Full resuscitation capability is mandatory.

15-3. First, the emulsion is a great medium for bacterial growth. Be aware of how infusion time must be monitored as a safeguard against bacterial growth. Second, the emulsion vehicle contains soybean oil, glycerol, and egg phosphatide. Assess for hypersensitivity to any of these elements before the drug is administered.

15-4. Bright-green urine.

15-5. Local anesthetic agents are relatively free of adverse effects if they are administered at an appropriate dosage and in the correct anatomic location. However, systemic and localized toxic reactions may occur, usually because of accidental intravascular or intrathecal injection or the administration of an excessive dose of the local anesthetic agent. Systemic reactions to local anesthetics primarily involve the central nervous system and the cardiovascular system.

15-6. Nondepolarizing NMJ blockers induce muscle flaccidity, whereas depolarizing NMJ blockers excite the muscle, promoting contraction until it can no longer receive neurocommunication and becomes paralyzed.

15-7. In discussing Mrs. Smith's prognosis, you need to remember that the patient may be paralyzed but not deaf. Because you do not know the outcome of the charge nurse's conversation, you may suggest moving the discussion to an environment where the patient cannot overhear the conversation.

15-8. Education of a patient undergoing surgical anesthesia with succinylcholine as an adjunctive therapy may focus on the patient's inability to speak, move, or breathe unassisted while using this drug. Reassure the patient that he or she will be monitored constantly for safety. Also, explain that uncomfortable aftereffects such as muscle ache can be relieved with acetaminophen.

CHAPTER 16: DRUGS RELIEVING ANXIETY AND PRODUCING SLEEP

16-1. Lorazepam intensifies the effects of GABA, a neurotransmitter that inhibits the nervous system.

16-2. Lorazepam decreases anxiety immediately, with some apparent effect after even one dose. The SSRIs require several weeks of treatment to take full effect.

16-3. Lorazepam is metabolized to an inactive metabolite, which can then be excreted renally. Other benzodiazepines are metabolized to active metabolites. With lorazepam, the liver does not have to do as much work to convert the drug to a form that can be eliminated.

16-4. Older adults are more at risk for sedation, ataxia, and confusion than younger adults. This combination places them at increased risk for falling in their homes.

16-5. Triazolam has a very quick onset but also a very short half-life. Because the effects of the drug wear off quickly, the patient may have problems with waking up early in the morning and not falling back asleep easily.

CHAPTER 17: DRUGS TREATING MOOD DISORDERS

17-1. Selective serotonin reuptake inhibitors (SSRIs), tricyclic antidepressants (TCAs), and monoamine oxidase inhibitors (MAOIs) are the three main classifications of antidepressants.

17-2. When depressed, a patient often lacks the energy to carry out plans for suicide. However, after beginning antidepressant therapy, a patient may experience increased energy before mood improves. Therefore, you must assess the patient for thoughts of self-harm and reassure the patient that the full effects of therapy have not yet occurred. Suicide precautions may have to be implemented to maintain patient safety.

17-3. It is important to continue antidepressant therapy even after symptoms of depression improve; otherwise, the depressive symptoms will come back.

17-4. Gastrointestinal distress is sometimes reported with sertraline therapy. This distress frequently lessens early on, as the patient's body adapts to the drug. Giving the drug with meals may also decrease gastrointestinal distress.

17-5. Adverse effects such as blurred vision, dry mouth, and constipation are the anticholinergic effects frequently associated with nortriptyline therapy.

17-6. The patient taking phenelzine must adhere to a strict diet that excludes foods high in tyramine, such as aged cheeses (especially blue, Camembert, Swiss, and Stilton), alcoholic beverages (especially Chianti wine and sherry), and some types of meats (especially liver, bologna, pepperoni, salami, and game).

17-7. Symptoms of an MAOI-induced hypertensive crisis are flushing of the face, occipital headache, sweating, suddenly elevated blood pressure, and fever.

17-8. Although lithium is still the first choice for treating bipolar disorder, anticonvulsants such as carbamazepine (Tegretol), valproic acid (Depakote), and gabapentin (Neurontin) are increasingly used as well.

17-9. A therapeutic range or level exists, sometimes called the therapeutic window of lithium therapy. In general, the serum concentration of lithium should be between 0.6 and 1.4 mEq/L.

17-10. Lithium toxicity usually presents as diarrhea, vomiting, unsteady gait, weakness, and slurred speech.

CHAPTER 18: DRUGS TREATING PSYCHOTIC DISORDERS AND DEMENTIA

18-1. Low-potency typical antipsychotic drugs are more likely to produce sedation and anticholinergic effects. High-potency typical antipsychotic drugs are more likely to produce EPS as an adverse effect.

18-2. EPS—extrapyramidal side effects—come from a relative lack of dopamine stimulation and relative excess of cholinergic stimulation. There are four major presentations of EPS: (1) Parkinson-like effects (pseudoparkinsonism), which are symptoms that are typically seen with Parkinson disease: cog-wheeling muscle rigidity, fine tremor, slow motor responses, shuffling gait, and a flat affect (a mask-like facial expression); (2) akathisia (a constant feeling of restlessness); (3) acute dystonia; and (4) tardive dyskinesia (involuntary lip smacking, chewing, mouth movements, tongue protrusion, blinking, grimacing, and involuntary muscle twitching of the limbs). Tardive dyskinesia, unlike the other EPS adverse effects, is usually permanent once it occurs.

18-3. Typical antipsychotics treat the positive symptoms of psychotic illness (delusions and hallucinations). Atypical antipsychotics treat the positive symptoms as well as the negative symptoms (flat or blunted emotions, lack of pleasure or interest in things [anhedonia], and limited speech). Atypical antipsychotics also produce very few adverse effects.

18-4. Acute dystonia is characterized by prolonged muscular contractions and spasms, especially in the neck (arching and twisting), the larynx and pharynx (contractions and spasms that may occlude the airway), back (arching), and eye (eye-rolling up toward the back of the head). Although all of the symptoms can be painful and require medical attention, airway occlusion can be life-threatening and constitutes a medical emergency.

18-5. Teach that the adverse effect is usually transient. Suggest that instead of taking two equal-sized doses daily, the larger dose or the entire daily dose could be taken at bedtime. Also, encourage the patient to be as active as possible during the daytime hours to help ward off sedation.

18-6. Rivastigmine is an acetylcholinesterase inhibitor, a drug that prevents the breakdown of acetylcholine. When acetylcholine is not broken down, its action on cortical cholinergic receptors and in the synapse is prolonged; neuronal transmission is also more effective. This increase in acetylcholine activity decreases the dementia found in mild to moderate Alzheimer disease.

CHAPTER 19: DRUGS TREATING SEIZURE DISORDERS

19-1. A seizure is hyperexcitation of the neurons in the brain producing changes in level of consciousness, involuntary muscle activity, or both. A convulsion is the jerky, involuntary muscle movement that can occur in a seizure.

19-2. Phenytoin slows the influx of sodium through the sodium channels into the cell. Sodium influx changes the negativity of the cell and produces an action potential. Slowing the influx of sodium lengthens the time between action potentials. Both seizures and some types of cardiac arrhythmias are caused by excessive firing of cells.

19-3. Diazepam or lorazepam.

19-4. Because the half-life of phenytoin lengthens considerably as the dose increases, it is easy to make too big a change in the blood drug level if the drug is not titrated in small amounts.

19-5. Phenytoin is highly protein bound. When serum protein (albumin) levels are low, more drug is free and active than would usually be expected from the dose. Because more drug is active, it is likely to cause more adverse effects.

19-6. Ethosuximide works by inhibiting the influx of calcium ions when they travel through a special set of channels, known as T-type calcium channels, in the hypothalamus, the site of absence seizure formation.

19-7. Benzodiazepines potentiate the effectiveness of the inhibitory neurotransmitter, GABA. Patients with seizures are believed to have a lack of GABA or an excess of glutamate, the opposing excitatory neurotransmitter.

CHAPTER 20: DRUGS AFFECTING MUSCLE SPASM AND SPASTICITY

20-1. A muscle spasm is defined as a sudden, violent, involuntary contraction of a muscle or group of muscles. Spasm is usually related to a localized skeletal muscle injury from acute trauma. Pain and interference with function attend muscle spasm, producing involuntary movement and distortion. Spasticity is a condition in which certain muscles are continuously contracted. This contraction causes stiffness or tightness of the muscles and may interfere with gait, movement, or speech. Damage to the portion of the brain or spinal cord that controls voluntary movement usually causes spasticity.

20-2. Cyclobenzaprine is chemically similar to amitriptyline. Combining these two drugs will increase anticholinergic effects. The patient should be monitored for symptoms such as dry mouth, blurred vision, constipation, and urinary retention. Because cyclobenzaprine and diazepam are both CNS depressants, the patient should be monitored for increased sedation. In the hospital, the bed should be in the lowest position with the side rails up. Caution the patient to call for help before attempting to ambulate. The sedative effects should be assessed before the patient drives a vehicle or performs tasks that require concentration.

20-3. Baclofen (Lioresal), diazepam (Valium), and dantrolene (Dantrium) can be used to manage spasm and spasticity. Dantrolene is generally reserved for patients with muscle spasticity.

20-4. Baclofen works at the spinal end of the upper motor neurons. Spasms caused by CVA or Parkinson disease involve lesional or functional impairment of basal ganglia, which are above the spinal motor neurons.

20-5. Symptoms suggesting hepatitis in the patient on long-term dantrolene therapy include loss of appetite, nausea or vomiting, yellowed skin or eyes, and changes in stool or urine color.

20-6. No, this drug would be a poor choice. This patient has an acute injury. Botulinum toxin is used to manage chronic pain that has not responded well to other medical or physical treatment. The patient needs quick relief, but the onset of action for botulinum toxin may take up to 2 weeks. Similarly, the duration of effect is up to 3 months, which is much longer than most acute musculoskeletal injuries last.

CHAPTER 21: DRUGS TREATING PARKINSON DISEASE AND OTHER MOVEMENT DISORDERS

21-1. Dopaminergics increase the amount of dopamine in the brain. Anticholinergics decrease the amount of acetylcholine in the brain. Both effects restore the necessary balanced antagonism of these two neurotransmitters.

21-2. A substantial amount of carbidopa is destroyed in the periphery of the body before it reaches the brain. Carbidopa decreases the amount of levodopa that is destroyed and increases the amount of levodopa that reaches the brain. Because more levodopa can pass the blood–brain barrier, a lower dose is needed to induce effects.

21-3. Neuroleptic malignant syndrome is characterized by rapid onset of marked rigidity, akinesia, tremor, and hyperpyrexia. It may occur if carbidopa-levodopa therapy is stopped abruptly.

21-4. A bradykinetic episode is associated with the eventual ineffectiveness of carbidopa-levodopa therapy. The episode, also called the on–off effect, is characterized by akinesia followed by a return of drug effectiveness. The patient is at risk for injury during these periods because hypotonia may occur.

21-5. Patients starting carbidopa-levodopa therapy should have a moderate amount of protein in divided portions throughout the day. They also should decrease their intake of pyridoxine, which is found in foods such as avocados, bananas, beef liver, oatmeal, halibut, chicken, pork, mashed potatoes, wheat germ, and sunflower seeds.

21-6. Throughout carbidopa-levodopa therapy, monitor patients for drug effectiveness, adverse effects, and the onset of new and progression of existing Parkinson symptoms.

21-7. Riluzole therapy aims to delay the need for tracheostomy or mechanical ventilation in the patient with ALS.

21-8. Some of the most frequent adverse effects of riluzole are asthenia, dizziness, and vertigo. These are also signs of ALS progression.

21-9. Dietary restrictions associated with riluzole therapy include caffeine, food high in fat, and charcoal-broiled foods.

21-10. Glatiramer is a synthetic drug that modifies the immune system by acting as a decoy for autoimmune antigens that destroy the myelin sheath in the nervous system. Interferon beta is a drug developed by recombinant DNA technology. It works by decreasing levels of interferon gamma and other proinflammatory cytokines and increasing production of nerve growth factor (NGF).

21-11. All of the current drugs used to manage MS are administered parenterally. Some patients fear injections, and others do not have the manual dexterity or visual skill to self-administer parenteral drugs.

CHAPTER 22: DRUGS STIMULATING THE CENTRAL NERVOUS SYSTEM

22-1.

Short-Acting	Intermediate-Acting	Long-Acting
Ritalin	Ritalin SR	Metadate CD
Methylin	Methylin ER	Concerta
Methylin Chewable	Metadate ER	Ritalin LA
Focalin		Adderall XR
Dexedrine		
Dextrostat		
Adderall		

22-2. "Have you noticed any changes in behavior since your last visit?"
"Has your child complained of nervousness, insomnia, dizziness, or palpitations?"
"Has your child been eating meals regularly?"
"Have you noticed any changes in sleep since your last visit?"
"Tell me about your child's intake of caffeine-rich products."
"Has your child had any behavior problems at school?"

Observations should include height and weight measurements, blood pressure and heart rate. Auscultate heart, lung, and bowel sounds. Palpate the thyroid. Coordinate periodic monitoring tests including ECG, CBC, thyroid function tests, and blood glucose.

22-3. To adequately assess the effectiveness of dextroamphetamine, ask questions such as, "How many sleep attacks has your mother had today, yesterday, and previous days?" "How many attacks per day was she having when you first brought her for treatment?" "Is your mother showing or complaining of any adverse effects, like hypertension, insomnia, irritability, hyperactivity, or psychosis?"

22-4. This patient describes caffeine withdrawal syndrome. Assess the difference between caffeine intake during the week and on weekends. Suggest that the patient decrease the amount of caffeine ingested during the week.

22-5. An important component of health promotion is encouraging and supporting the patient's commitment to weight loss. Remind the patient that sibutramine is only one component of weight loss strategy. Behavior modification and exercise are equally important to reach the patient's weight loss goal. It is also important to ensure that the patient understands that sibutramine may increase blood pressure and to make arrangements for serial checks of blood pressure.

22-6. Sibutramine works systemically by blocking the reuptake of norepinephrine, serotonin, and dopamine, resulting in a feeling of satiety. Orlistat works by inhibiting the absorption of fats from the GI tract. It does not have a systemic action.

Unit 6: Analgesic and Anti-inflammatory Drugs

CHAPTER 23: DRUGS TREATING SEVERE PAIN

23-1. Because morphine is a CNS depressant, it will suppress the respiratory drive and decrease the respiratory rate. When morphine is being used to treat acute pain, the patient will not have developed any tolerance to the effects of morphine. Therefore, giving morphine to someone who has respiratory depression will increase respiratory depression and may cause respiratory arrest.

23-2. Patients who have been receiving morphine regularly every day for a long period (e.g., as for chronic pain) will develop a tolerance to the respiratory depression that morphine may produce. They will not incur further respiratory depression from morphine. Patients with chronic pain who have a respiratory rate of 8 to 12 breaths/minute may receive their next dose of morphine.

23-3. Patients who abuse opioids or other CNS depressants may have cross-tolerance to the effects of morphine. For this reason, they may need a larger dose than other patients to achieve pain control.

23-4. A rescue dose is a dose of opioid used to treat breakthrough pain. It is ordered in addition to the baseline pharmacologic treatment for pain and

is about 10% to 30% of the opioid dose the patient receives in 24 hours.

23-5. The half-life of naloxone is very short compared with the half-life of morphine and other opiates. Therefore, the effect of naloxone will end, and the respiratory depression from the opiates may recur. Multiple doses of naloxone may be necessary so that the patient does not revert to severe respiratory depression.

23-6. Codeine acts directly on the medullary cough center to depress the cough reflex. It also has a drying effect on the mucous membranes and can increase the viscosity of secretions, which can contribute to respiratory depression or arrest because the patient would be unable to independently clear his or her airway.

CHAPTER 24: DRUGS TREATING MILD TO MODERATE PAIN, FEVER, INFLAMMATION, AND MIGRAINE HEADACHE

24-1. Inhibition of certain prostaglandins interrupts the inflammatory cycle, thus decreasing pain and fever.

24-2. There are two isoforms of prostaglandins: COX-1 and COX-2. COX-1 maintains the functioning of many cells of the body. COX-2 is found mainly in areas of inflammation. Use of drugs that are nonselective, such as the PSIs, results in inhibition of both types of COX. When COX-1 is inhibited, the cytoprotective mechanism of the body is altered, and the patient is at a higher risk for adverse effects.

24-3. The most potentially serious adverse effects are bone marrow depression, blood dyscrasias, renal dysfunction, and hepatic dysfunction. These reactions can be decreased by careful assessment of medical problems and medications that contradict their use. Obtaining baseline laboratory tests and monitoring them throughout therapy will also decrease adverse effects. Teaching the patient the signs and symptoms of potential adverse effects and the importance of contacting the health care provider is another intervention to decrease the severity of adverse effects.

24-4. COX-2 inhibitors preferentially inhibit COX-2, decreasing inflammation. Because they do not affect COX-1 as much, their cytoprotective mechanism is not altered, which results in a decreased risk for GI bleeding. The second major difference is that COX-2 inhibitors do not alter platelet aggregation.

24-5. The triptans decrease migraine pain by stimulating the 5-$HT_{1B/1D}$ receptors located on cranial blood vessels and sensory nerves of the trigeminal vascular system. The resultant vasoconstriction decreases the throbbing sensation in the head. Stimulating the 5-$HT_{1B/1D}$ receptors also inhibits the release of proinflammatory neuropeptides, resulting in decreased vascular inflammation.

24-6. The pharmacodynamics of the triptans is limited to stimulating the 5-$HT_{1B/1D}$ receptors. Ergotamine and dihydroergotamine also affect serotonergic, dopaminergic, and alpha-adrenergic receptors as well as stimulating uterine contraction and inducing nausea and vomiting.

CHAPTER 25: DRUGS TREATING ARTHRITIS AND GOUT

25-1. Salicylates, PSIs, and acetaminophen control only the symptoms of the disease. DMARDs have the advantage of actually halting the progression of inflammatory diseases and the potential damage they may cause.

25-2. The major disadvantage of DMARDs is the frequency of potentially serious adverse effects, such as depressed bone marrow function, hepatotoxicity, and renal toxicity. Another disadvantage is that most of the common DMARDs have a long period before results of the therapy can be noticed by the patient.

25-3. Joint destruction begins in the early stages of the disease, even before some patients have physical symptoms. Using DMARDs within 3 months of diagnosis halts the progression of the damage and ultimately can decrease the extent of damage.

25-4. The autoimmune and inflammatory processes of the body have many substances that continue the cycle. Multiple classes of drugs may be used because they have different mechanisms of action that can affect the immune response, the inflammatory response, or both responses at different sites of the cycle or affect different substances within the cycle.

25-5. Tumor necrosis factor (TNF) is a cytokine produced by macrophages and activated T cells, which play an important role in RA by mediating cytokines that cause inflammation and joint destruction.

25-6. TNF inhibitors should not be given to anyone with an active infection, and should be given very cautiously to an immunocompromised patient. The potential adverse effect common to all these drugs is an increased risk for serious infections. These drugs alter the immune and inflammatory response; thus, the patient may acquire a life-threatening infection.

25-7. Colchicine decreases the inflammatory process induced by gout; therefore, it is used in acute gout. Probenecid increases the excretion of uric acid. It is used as a prophylactic medication.

Unit 7: Cardiovascular and Renal System Drugs

CHAPTER 26: DRUGS AFFECTING CARDIAC RHYTHM

26-1. Ventricular arrhythmias (tachycardia and fibrillation) do not allow the ventricle to fill adequately with blood. The rapid contractions are also not effective at emptying the ventricle. Consequently, cardiac output decreases significantly. The body needs oxygenated blood to survive.

26-2. Proarrhythmia is the tendency of a drug to create a new arrhythmia or to exacerbate the arrhythmia it is supposed to be treating.

26-3. Antiarrhythmics alter the normal mechanisms that control heart rate and rhythm. Therefore, they can also cause an arrhythmia.

26-4. Class I depresses phase 0. Class II depresses phase 4 (depolarization). Class III produces a prolonged phase 3 (repolarization). Class IV depresses phase 4 (depolarization) and lengthens phases 1 and 2 of repolarization.

26-5. Amiodarone is only approved for use in life-threatening arrhythmias such as recurrent ventricular fibrillation or recurrent, hemodynamically unstable ventricular tachycardia. It is also used off label to treat atrial fibrillation

26-6. Several electrophysiologic effects occur with the administration of amiodarone. An increased cardiac

refractory period occurs, usually without influencing the resting membrane potential. Sinus rate decreases by 15% to 20%. The PR and QT intervals increase by about 10%. U waves appear and T waves are altered. These changes do not usually require discontinuation of amiodarone, although marked sinus bradycardia or sinus arrest and heart block can occur. QT prolongation can be associated with worsening of the arrhythmia, but this event is rare.

26-7. Amiodarone has a very long half-life. To quickly achieve a therapeutic level without waiting for steady state to occur, a loading dose is used. This quickly brings the drug into a therapeutic level. Because amiodarone is used for life-threatening arrhythmias, it is important to achieve a therapeutic effect as soon as possible so that the patient does not die.

26-8. Drink plenty of fluids and eat fresh fruits and vegetables. Include varied sources of fiber in the diet. Exercise if allowed by the physician. Discuss with physician the use of a stool softener (traps water in the stool).

CHAPTER 27: DRUGS AFFECTING BLOOD PRESSURE

27-1. Lifestyle changes of antihypertensive therapy include stopping smoking, controlling weight, limiting sodium intake, increasing potassium and calcium intake, restricting alcohol use, increasing aerobic exercise, and limiting cholesterol levels.

27-2. Thiazide diuretics are very effective in controlling hypertension and in preventing the sequelae that accompany uncontrolled hypertension. They are as effective as other drug classes; in some cases, they are more effective and less expensive. They should be the drug of first choice, unless there are other compelling reasons to use another drug class.

27-3. The ACE inhibitors prevent the conversion of angiotensin I to angiotensin II, which is a potent vasoconstrictor. By preventing vasoconstriction, ACE inhibitors decrease peripheral vascular resistance and therefore lower blood pressure. The effect of angiotensin II on aldosterone production is also blocked, preventing the sodium and fluid retention that aldosterone produces.

27-4. Aldosterone receptor blockers block the action of angiotensin II from all the different pathways where it is formed, not just the single substrate altered by ACE inhibitors. These drugs are effective in lowering blood pressure. In addition, they seem to block deleterious effects from angiotensin II at the end-organ stage. ARBs do not cause the chronic cough that ACE inhibitors cause, and they are better tolerated in some patients.

27-5. Clonidine decreases sympathetic outflow from the brain. Because of this effect, the drug is useful in preventing withdrawal from narcotics. The drug should not be prescribed to current narcotic abusers because it likely will not be used for blood pressure management but instead saved to prevent withdrawal or sold on the black market.

27-6. Hyperkalemia (elevated potassium).

27-7. The following are safety measures when administering nitroprusside: Always use an IV pump, preferably a volumetric pump, to infuse nitroprusside. Never allow the infusion solution to run by gravity. Monitor blood pressure constantly. Assess for signs of cyanide toxicity, thiocyanate toxicity, and methemoglobinemia. Do not infuse maximum dosage for longer than 10 minutes.

27-8. Dopamine increases renal perfusion. As the kidney becomes adequately perfused, it will resume its normal functioning and produce urine at a normal rate. Monitoring urinary output indicates whether the dose of dopamine is sufficient to adequately perfuse the kidneys. The systolic blood pressure should rise from dopamine administration. If the diastolic pressure rises greatly, or disproportionately, it indicates that the alpha-2 effects of dopamine are overriding the beta-2 and dopaminergic effects. The drug rate would need to be decreased if this effect occurred.

CHAPTER 28: DRUGS TREATING CONGESTIVE HEART FAILURE

28-1. Primary effects of digoxin include positive inotropic effect (increased force of contraction), negative chronotropic effect (decreased rate), and negative dromotropic effect (decreased speed of conduction).

28-2. Digitalization is initiated because the drug's half-life is long (30–40 hours). At normal dosing, it takes several days for digoxin to be in a therapeutic range. When a more rapid onset of action is desired, digitalization allows the therapeutic level to be achieved more quickly. Therapeutic levels will be achieved before the drug is in steady state (five half-lives).

28-3. Before giving digoxin, take the apical pulse for 1 full minute. If the pulse rate is less than 60 bpm, hold the dose of digoxin and notify the prescriber.

28-4. Digoxin is excreted renally. Therefore, serum drug levels will rise in the patient with decreased renal function above those normally expected for the dose administered. As a result, the patient is at greater risk for adverse effects. A smaller dose may be required.

28-5. Beta blockers block the effect of the sympathetic nervous system and cause vasodilation and decreased peripheral vascular resistance, which is helpful to patients with CHF. Beta blockers may also actually reverse the ventricular remodeling process that occurs in CHF by reducing left ventricular volumes and improving systolic function.

CHAPTER 29: DRUGS TREATING ANGINA

29-1. Limiting the duration of patch use prevents nitrate tolerance, which decreases the antianginal effects of the drug.

29-2. One every 5 minutes. Up to three tablets in 15 minutes may be given.

29-3. Nitroglycerin causes vasodilation, especially on the venous side. Vasodilation allows blood to pool in the venous beds, decreasing blood pressure. Verify that the patient is not hypotensive before administering the drug.

29-4. Vasodilation of the vessels in the head has occurred from exposure to nitroglycerin. Headache is a common adverse effect of vasodilation.

29-5. Nitroglycerin decreases preload and afterload. This effect decreases the energy the heart must use to eject blood, thus decreasing the oxygen needs of the heart. Additionally, the coronary vessels are dilated, increasing blood flow to the heart. Circulation is also redirected to use the smaller vessels more, improving blood flow to the heart.

CHAPTER 30: DRUGS AFFECTING LIPID LEVELS

30-1. High-density lipoprotein (HDL) cholesterol is believed to offer some protection against heart attack and is known as "good" cholesterol.

30-2. Elevated serum cholesterol levels lead to fatty deposits, or atherosclerosis, in the arteries. These deposits narrow the lumen of the vessel, increasing peripheral resistance and thus increasing blood pressure.

30-3. The patient is at risk for drug interactions because lovastatin is metabolized by the CYP3A4 hepatic pathway. If the patient is receiving other drugs that are also metabolized by CYP3A4, the metabolism of lovastatin is decreased, and increased drug levels will result. If the other drug therapy inhibits the CYP3A4 enzyme, metabolism of lovastatin will also be reduced.

30-4. Liver enzyme levels are frequently elevated from lipid-lowering drug therapy, regardless of the class of drug. If the levels rise enough, a dose adjustment (smaller dose) is required, or the drug therapy should be stopped.

30-5. Transient, moderately elevated CK levels (i.e., 3 to 10 times above the upper limit of normal) do not indicate serious muscle damage from lovastatin. If CK levels reach greater than 10 times the upper limit of normal and the patient has symptoms, therapy should be stopped. This is to prevent serious myopathy and rhabdomyolysis, which can be fatal.

CHAPTER 31: DRUGS AFFECTING COAGULATION

31-1. Heparin prevents fibrin formation. Warfarin interferes with the formation of prothrombin and factors VII, IX, and X.

31-2. An infusion control pump should be used to regulate the rate of heparin administration. Monitor activated partial thromboplastin time (aPTT) to prevent overdosage. Use general safety measures, such as placing the bed in a low position with the side rails up, to prevent patient falls. Assess the patient regularly for signs of bleeding.

31-3. The aPTT should be monitored while the patient is receiving heparin. A therapeutic aPTT value is 1.5 to 2 times greater than the given control. The prothrombin time (PT) is monitored while the patient is taking warfarin. PT is considered therapeutic when it is approximately 1.5 times the given control or the INR value is between 2 and 3.

31-4. Warfarin interferes with the synthesis of vitamin K–derived clotting factors. Increases in vitamin K intake will interfere with the action of warfarin if the increase occurs after the warfarin dosage has been titrated. Vitamin K does not affect the action of heparin.

31-5. You should check that each therapy is effective. Because both drugs are metabolized by the P-450 system, a drug interaction could occur that would decrease the effectiveness of one or the other drug.

31-6. An anticoagulant lengthens clotting time and prevents future blood clots; thrombolytics break down a formed clot.

31-7. Antihemophilic factor (AHF) would be administered before and after surgery until the appropriate level of factor VIII is obtained as determined by blood assays.

CHAPTER 32: DRUGS AFFECTING URINARY OUTPUT

32-1. Before thiazide therapy to treat hypertension is started, blood pressure, pulse, presence of edema, weight, and urinary output should be assessed.

32-2. Conditions treated by diuretic therapy include hypertension, CHF, pulmonary edema, peripheral edema (various causes), renal stones (thiazides), renal disease, increased intraocular pressure, and increased intra cranial pressure.

32-3. Fluid and electrolyte problems that are likely to occur in patients receiving thiazide or loop diuretics are hypokalemia, hyponatremia, hypochloremia, hypomagnesemia, hypercalcemia (thiazides), hypocalcemia (loop), hyperglycemia, hyperuricemia, and elevated cholesterol and triglyceride levels.

32-4. Loop diuretics work in the loop of Henle where more sodium is usually absorbed. Because loop diuretics promote more sodium loss than in the distal tubule, more potassium is lost.

32-5. Osmotic diuretics are different from thiazide or loop diuretics because they are composed of a sugar that passes through glomerular filtration but is not reabsorbed. The osmotic pressure that results pulls water into the vascular space and traps it until it is excreted in the urine.

32-6. Carbonic anhydrase inhibitors are used primarily to treat chronic open-angle glaucoma.

32-7. Blockade of the muscarinic receptors in the bladder restrict the bladder's ability to contract.

Unit 8: Hematopoietic and Immune System Drugs

CHAPTER 33: DRUGS AFFECTING HEMATOPOIESIS

33-1. Erythropoietin, thrombopoietin, G-CSF, GM-CSF, and interleukin are the principal polypeptides and glycoproteins involved in hematopoiesis.

33-2. The kidneys produce erythropoietin, which is responsible for stimulating the production of red blood cells. When the kidneys are not functioning fully, they do not produce normal amounts of erythropoietin, and so the patient becomes anemic.

33-3. The major risk is increased risk for infection, which can be fatal. This risk is increased in patients with neutropenia because neutrophils are the first line of defense against infection.

33-4. Platelets are fragments of large cells from the bone marrow called megakaryocytes. Thrombopoietin stimulates the production of megakaryocytes.

33-5. Fluid retention is the most common adverse effect of oprelvekin. Monitoring intake and output of fluids will indicate whether fluid retention is occurring. Additional fluid load can overburden the taxed heart and exacerbate the CHF, possibly causing pulmonary edema.

33-6. Thrombotic events can occur in CRF patients receiving epoetin alfa; the risk increases when attempting to raise the hemoglobin and hematocrit to normal levels. The usual target range is 30% to 36% for hematocrit.

CHAPTER 34: DRUGS AFFECTING THE IMMUNE RESPONSE

34-1. Cytokines enhance and accelerate the inflammatory response and other specific responses that destroy the invading antigen. Cytokines are

generally proinflammatory, but many also have antiviral, antiproliferative, and antineoplastic properties.

34-2. Interferons and interleukins are cytokines produced by activated lymphocytes.

34-3. Interferons suppress malignant cell replication and tumor growth.

34-4. The adverse effect profile of interleukin-2 is very similar to that of high-dose interferon, but is potentially more acute in onset and severe in intensity. Even severe adverse effects resolve when the agent is discontinued.

34-5. Rituximab is a type of monoclonal antibody that binds specifically to the CD20 antigen found on the surface of normal and malignant B lymphocytes and causes cell lysis. It produces immunosuppression through its effect on the B cells. All monoclonal antibodies achieve their desired target cell destruction by directly connecting to unique receptor sites on particular target cells, inducing inactivation or programmed cell death. Binding to the lymphocyte causes lymphocytic destruction and immune suppression, whereas binding to a CD20 molecule commonly found on malignant lymphocytes causes greater tumor cell death than normal lymphocyte death.

34-6. The most common adverse effects of rituximab are infusion-related reactions, including fever, flushing, chills, and rigors.

34-7. Cyclosporine is a potent immunosuppressant that suppresses some cell-mediated immune reactions and to a lesser extent humoral immunity. The exact mechanism of action is not known, but it is believed to be caused by specific, reversible inhibition of immunocompetent T lymphocytes.

34-8. Nephrotoxicity or hepatotoxicity may require the dose of cyclosporine to be reduced.

Unit 9: Antineoplastic Drugs

CHAPTER 35: DRUGS THAT ARE CELL CYCLE–SPECIFIC

35-1. The goals of chemotherapy are cure, control, and palliation.

35-2. The different strategies undertaken in the use of chemotherapeutic agents include adjuvant treatment, induction therapy, consolidation therapy, intensification, maintenance, neoadjuvant therapy, palliative therapy, and salvage therapy.

35-3. Malignant cells are characterized by uncontrolled cellular proliferation, decreased cellular differentiation, inappropriate ability to invade surrounding tissue, and ability to establish new growth at ectopic sites.

35-4. The following steps (in sequence) should be undertaken to clean up a chemotherapy spill:

- Put on a pair of powder-free latex gloves.
- Place an absorbent pad over the spill to contain it.
- Rinse the absorbed spill area with water.
- Clean the area with detergent.
- Dispose of all equipment used in clean-up as chemotherapy waste in a container designated for this purpose.

35-5. Health care workers can be exposed to chemotherapy through the following routes: skin and mucous membrane absorption, inhalation, and ingestion.

35-6. Vincristine's low myelosuppressive effect is the factor that makes it better than vinblastine for use with other antineoplastic drugs.

35-7. When extravasation occurs, the nurse (1) discontinues the infusion; (2) applies warm or cold compresses, as indicated; (3) administers the appropriate antidote, if known; (4) notifies the health care provider; (5) elevates and rests the affected extremity for 48 hours; (6) applies a sterile dressing over the site, allowing for visibility of the extravasated area; (7) avoids pressure to the site; (8) obtains a photograph of the site for baseline comparisons; (9) discusses with the health care provider the need for plastic surgery consultation if appropriate; (10) documents the patient's name and date/time of occurrence, name of drug, approximate volume of drug that infiltrated, needle gauge, site of extravasation, symptoms reported by the patient and assessed by the nurse, nursing measures implemented, health care provider notification, patient teaching given, and nurse's signature.

35-8. Hypotension occurs when etoposide is infused rapidly. The ideal infusion period should be at least 30 minutes to avoid this reaction.

35-9. The signs and symptoms of a hypersensitivity reaction include hypotension, bronchospasm (wheezing), tachycardia, facial flushing, and anxiety.

35-10. Before starting a paclitaxel infusion, the nurse checks for the correct setup of the infusion, such as the use of in-line filtration and non-DEHP containers and tubing. The patient should be taught about the possibility of a hypersensitivity reaction and the signs and symptoms to report immediately. The premedication regimen to prevent an infusion reaction consists of dexamethasone, 20 mg given 11 hours and 7 hours before the paclitaxel; an H2-receptor antagonist (e.g., cimetidine); and diphenhydramine, 50 mg given IV 30 minutes before infusion.

35-11. Any of the following neoplastic agents may potentially interact with St. John's wort: anastrozole (Arimedex), cyclophosphamide (Cytoxan), docetaxel (Taxotere), etoposide (VP-16), ifosfamide (Ifex), paclitaxel (Taxol), teniposide (VM-26), tretinoin (Retinoic acid), vinblastine (Velban), and vincristine (Oncovin).

CHAPTER 36: DRUGS THAT ARE CELL CYCLE–NONSPECIFIC

36-1. Anthracyclines are a class of red-pigmented antibiotics, namely doxorubicin, daunorubicin, and their analogues. Their major dose-limiting toxicity is cardiotoxicity.

36-2. The highly lipid-soluble cell cycle–nonspecific drugs are the nitrosoureas, which include carmustine, lomustine, and streptozocin. These drugs can cross the blood–brain barrier.

36-3. The antiemetic drug groups used to control acute emesis include serotonin antagonists, corticosteroids, phenothiazines, butyrophenones, cannabinoids, dopamine antagonists, and substituted benzamides.

36-4. Dexrazoxane (Zinecard) is a cardioprotectant that helps reduce the incidence and severity of cardiomopathy in women who have received a cumulative doxorubicin dose of 300 mg/m^2 and who could benefit from continued doxorubicin therapy. It is administered by slow IV push or IV drip over 15 minutes, and when it is com-

pleted, the doxorubicin flows so that both drugs are infused over 30 minutes.

36-5. Drugs used in combination therapy should be active when used alone, produce synergy with other drugs, differ in mechanism of action, differ in overlapping, and be given at consistent intervals in maximal doses.

36-6. Combination chemotherapy is superior to single-drug therapy because it kills a maximum number of cancer cells, has a high toxicity range tolerated by the patient, provides a broader range of coverage of resistant cells in the heterogenous tumor population, and is characterized by minimal or slow development of new resistant cancer cells.

Unit 10: Antimicrobial Drugs

CHAPTER 37: PRINCIPLES OF ANTIBIOTIC THERAPY

37-1. For antimicrobial therapy to be effective, the guiding principle is to use the right drug for the right bug.

37-2. Antimicrobials may be classified by the type of organism they affect or by their mechanism of action.

37-3. Antimicrobials work by inhibiting cell wall synthesis, inhibiting protein synthesis, inhibiting nucleic acid synthesis, disrupting the cell membrane permeability, inhibiting metabolic pathways, or inhibiting viral enzymes.

37-4. Selective toxicity means that the drug harms the pathogen but does not harm the host cell.

37-5. In the human host, many bacteria keep other microbes, such as fungus, in check. When the "good" bacteria are killed by antimicrobials, the nonsusceptible microbes can proliferate, causing an additional infection.

37-6. In the United States, the microbes that have developed substantial resistance include methicillin-resistant *Staphylococcus aureus* (MRSA), vancomycin-resistant *Enterococcus* (VRE), and multiple drug–resistant *Mycobacterium tuberculosis* (MDR-TB).

CHAPTER 38: ANTIBIOTICS AFFECTING THE BACTERIAL CELL WALL

38-1. Penicillins bind with penicillin-binding proteins located inside the bacterial cell wall. Binding at these sites alters the way the bacteria are able to build their cell walls by affecting the development of cross-bridges that give the cell wall its strength. As the cell wall weakens, the internal osmotic pressure of the bacteria changes to allow the cell to absorb water, swell, and then burst. The body's immune system completes the process of fighting the infection and cleans up debris from ruptured bacteria. Penicillins also "turn on" autolysin, an enzyme that actively promotes cell wall destruction.

38-2. Gram-negative bacteria have a cell wall envelope that actively keeps penicillin from entering the cell and binding to penicillin-binding proteins. Penicillins cannot work if they cannot bind to these proteins.

38-3. Penicillins are classified by their spectrum of activity. The narrow-spectrum penicillins can eradicate a limited number of bacteria, the penicillinase-resistant penicillins are effective against bacteria that produce penicillinase, the aminopenicillins are effective against most gram-positive bacteria, and the extended penicillins are specifically effective against *Pseudomonas* species.

38-4. Clavulanic acid, tazobactam, and sulbactam have very little antibacterial activity on their own. They fight beta-lactamase–producing bacteria by becoming "suicide agents." By binding to beta-lactamase's active site, they enable penicillin to reach its target site within the bacterial cytoplasmic membrane and destroy the bacteria.

38-5. Imipenem (Primaxin), meropenem (Merrem), and ertapenem (Invanz) are parenteral beta-lactam antibiotics. They are all broad-spectrum, with imipenem having the broadest spectrum of the three. Meropenem and ertapenem are administered as single agents, whereas imipenem is combined with cilastatin to reduce the potential for renal toxicity. Imipenem is indicated for severe resistant infections, especially nosocomial infections; meropenem is used for intra-abdominal infections and bacterial meningitis, whereas ertapenem is indicated to manage moderate to severe, complicated intra-abdominal infections, skin and skin structure infections, pyelonephritis, acute pelvic infections, and community-acquired pneumonia. They have similar contraindications, precautions, and adverse effects. Of the three, imipenem is most likely to cause seizures, especially in patients with pre-existing seizure disorders or insults to the brain such as head trauma. Ertapenem is the only carbapenem not indicated for use in children.

38-6. Cephalosporins can be grouped into four generations. As we progress from first- to fourth-generation drugs, they have increasing activity against gram-negative bacteria, increasing resistance to destruction by beta-lactamases, and increasing ability to reach the CSF.

38-7. Beta-lactam antibiotics include penicillins, cephalosporins, monobactams, and carbapenems. They are called beta-lactam antibiotics because they all contain a beta-lactam ring that is responsible for their antibacterial activity.

38-8. Vancomycin is reserved for serious infections because of its ability to cause serious adverse effects, especially ototoxicity and nephrotoxicity.

38-9. Daptomycin is the first of a new class of antibiotic that works in a totally different way than other antimicrobial drugs. At this time, no mechanism of resistance to daptomycin has been identified, there are no known transferable elements, or plasmids, that confer resistance, and cross-resistance has not been reported.

To keep bacteria from becoming resistant to daptomycin, use it only after other antibiotics have been unsuccessful.

CHAPTER 39: ANTIBIOTICS AFFECTING BACTERIAL PROTEIN SYNTHESIS

39-1. Tetracyclines have limited use because of emerging bacterial resistance. They are also associated with food interactions that decrease the absorption of the drug. They may not be used by pregnant or lactating women or children younger than 8 years because of their potential to damage primary teeth.

39-2. Aminoglycosides are used only in serious infections because of their potential to cause serious toxicities, including ototoxicity, nephrotoxicity, and neuromuscular blockade.

39-3. The most serious adverse effects of chloramphenicol therapy are irreversible bone marrow toxicity and life-threatening blood dyscrasias.

39-4. An antibiotic affects any bacterium within its spectrum. In the body, some bacteria are used to keep other organisms under control. When those bacteria are affected, organisms such as yeast can overgrow.

39-5. Patients receiving clindamycin therapy should be advised to stop the medication immediately if these symptoms occur and contact the provider. These symptoms may suggest antibiotic-associated colitis, also known as pseudomembranous colitis or *Clostridium difficile* colitis, which is associated with overgrowth of *C. difficile.*

39-6. Quinupristin/dalfopristin is a parenteral agent that is active against *E. faecium* but not *E. faecalis,* both of which may cause bacteremia. Linezolid is active against both *E. faecium* and *E. faecalis*. Additionally, linezolid is offered as both a parenteral or oral preparation. Because linezolid induces MAO inhibition, however, it has many more potential drug interactions in addition to food and beverage interactions.

CHAPTER 40: DRUGS THAT ARE MISCELLANEOUS ANTIBIOTICS

40-1. First-generation quinolones are used only to treat uncomplicated UTIs. Second-generation fluoroquinolones have better gram-negative and systemic activity. Third-generation fluoroquinolones have extended activity against gram-positive pathogens, but are less active than second-generation drugs against *Pseudomonas* species. In addition to having the spectrum of activity of third-generation fluoroquinolones, the fourth-generation drugs are also active against *Pseudomonas* species and anaerobic bacteria.

40-2. Fluoroquinolones inhibit DNA gyrase. This enzyme, essential for the replication of bacteria, has a counterpart in human cells, but the human enzyme is not affected by fluoroquinolones.

40-3. Ciprofloxacin should not be given to children younger than 18 years or to women who are pregnant or breast-feeding. Fluoroquinolones have caused cartilage deterioration in immature animals and may induce arthropathies in infants and children.

40-4. Compounds that contain aluminum, calcium, iron, magnesium, or zinc bind with ciprofloxacin. This affinity results in decreased absorption and bioavailability of ciprofloxacin.

40-5. Parenteral polymyxin B is used only in clinical situations in which patients have not responded to other less toxic drugs because of its potential to induce serious nephrotoxicity.

CHAPTER 41: DRUGS TREATING URINARY TRACT INFECTIONS

41-1. One of the most common uses for SMZ-TMP is prophylaxis and treatment of *Pneumocystis carinii* pneumonia (PCP). SMZ-TMP is frequently used for respiratory infections caused by *H. influenzae* or *S. pneumoniae.* In the respiratory tract, these microbes may cause bronchitis, sinusitis, or pneumonia. It is also an alternative treatment for *Legionella pneumophila* pneumonia. GI infections treated with SMZ-TMP include shigellosis and salmonella. SMZ-TMP concentrates in prostate and vaginal fluids and thus is useful in prostatitis and some types of vaginitis. SMZ-TMP is also effective for sexually transmitted diseases, such as acute gonococcal urethritis and oropharyngeal gonorrhea.

41-2. Sulfonamides interrupt the formation of folate, which is necessary for the microorganism's biosynthesis of DNA, RNA, and protein. If the microorganism does not rely on folate for this action, the drug is ineffective.

41-3. Antibiotics used to manage UTIs reach high concentration in serum; thus, they can be used for infections other than those of the urinary tract. Urinary tract antiseptics have a direct local action on urine and achieve only very low serum concentrations. Therefore, they are systemically ineffective and useful only in UTI.

41-4. UTIs cause several uncomfortable symptoms, including lower abdominal pain, dysuria, and a feeling of urgency. Phenazopyridine is an analgesic that decreases these symptoms in the bladder. It is generally used for a few days, until the antibiotic is able to decrease the bacterial count enough to decrease these symptoms.

CHAPTER 42: DRUGS TREATING MYCOBACTERIAL INFECTIONS

42-1. Patients with pre-existing hepatic disorders, renal insufficiency, or malnutrition, those who abuse drugs or alcohol, and those older than 35 years are at greatest risk for hepatitis resulting from isoniazid therapy.

42-2. Chemoprophylaxis consists of single-drug therapy with isoniazid to prevent active TB. The patient is asymptomatic, and the therapy continues for 6 to 12 months. Active TB therapy requires a multidrug regimen (usually isoniazid, rifampin, and pyrazinamide) and is used in patients with signs and symptoms of TB. Therapy may last up to 18 months.

42-3. TB bacilli have the ability to become resistant to all of the anti-TB drugs. Additionally, resistance develops because of the duration of therapy. Finally, multidrug resistance occurs because adherence for the complete duration of therapy is difficult. Patients repeatedly start and stop their drug therapies, allowing the bacillus to become resistant.

42-4. There are three major obstacles to successful therapy with rifampin. The first obstacle is adherence. Rifampin is given for up to 18 months to treat TB and for 12 months to treat leprosy. The second obstacle is the potential for serious adverse effects. Close monitoring and serial laboratory testing are necessary to ensure the safety of the patient. The third obstacle is the drug–drug interactions induced by rifampin. The patient must understand the importance of contacting the prescriber before taking any new medications, especially prescription medications.

42-5. All mycobacterial infections require lengthy treatment. Patients have difficulty adhering to long-term therapies, especially when the drug therapy does not make the patient feel different.

CHAPTER 43: DRUGS TREATING VIRAL AND FUNGAL DISEASES

43-1. Few effective antiviral drugs exist because a virus must replicate within the host cell. Drugs that affect the virus may also affect the host cell and do substantial harm.

43-2. Acyclovir is phosphorylated into its active form by the enzyme thymidine kinase. In its active form, acyclovir competes for a position in the DNA chain of the herpesvirus and terminates DNA synthesis.

43-3. Acyclovir should be given cautiously to patients with renal disease, seizures, and other neurologic disorders.

43-4. The interferons are used in managing hepatitis. The FDA approves each type of interferon for a specific subtype of virus; however, the interferons may also be used "off-label" for another subtype.

43-5. Amantadine and rimantadine are effective for the prophylaxis or management of influenza A, whereas oseltamivir and zanamivir are effective for both influenza A and B.

43-6. Although oseltamivir and zanamivir are useful to decrease the symptoms of influenza, they do not replace the need for a yearly influenza vaccination for patients who are immunocompromised.

43-7. Ribavirin is not generally used in adults because adult patients are usually not affected by RSV. Moreover, ribavirin is a teratogen and may produce testicular lesions.

43-8. Ribavirin is used to treat RSV, whereas palivizumab and RSV-IG are prophylactic drugs given to babies at risk for acquiring RSV.

43-9. Amphotericin B may produce nephrotoxicity; infusion reaction marked by headache, chills, fever, rigors, hypotension, bronchospasm, nausea and vomiting; electrolyte imbalances; and anemia.

43-10. Adverse effects of fluconazole therapy include elevated liver enzyme levels, hepatotoxicity, exfoliative skin disorders, and Stevens-Johnson syndrome.

43-11. Azole drugs that can be used to manage systemic fungal infections include fluconazole, itraconazole, ketoconazole, miconazole, and voriconazole.

CHAPTER 44: DRUGS TREATING HIV INFECTION AND AIDS

44-1. Blood testing is used to diagnose HIV. To detect antibodies to HIV, the patient may have an EIA, ELISA, rapid HIV test, or oral HIV test. If the patient tests positive with the EIA or ELISA, a WB test or other confirmatory test is performed to ensure accurate results. To test for presence of the virus itself, a PCR test may be done.

44-2. HIV has an affinity for CD4+ T cells. These cells are important for normal immune function. Destruction of these cells strips the person of protection against common organisms.

44-3. The CD4+ T-cell count is an indication of the current immunologic status of the patient. The CD4+ T-cell count indicates the amount of damage to the immune system. A viral load count reflects disease progression.

44-4. The HIV virus, like other viruses, has the ability to mutate and thus become resistant to a drug. Use of HAART attacks the virus during multiple stages of the viral replication process. This approach prolongs the time before the virus becomes resistant to a specific antiretroviral drug.

44-5. Anemia, granulocytopenia, and thrombocytopenia are adverse effects that indicate a need to stop zidovudine therapy.

44-6. Tests recommended before zidovudine therapy begins include CBC, blood chemistry profile, CD4+ T-cell count, and viral load. Renal and hepatic function tests should be considered if pre-existing damage is suspected.

44-7. Lifestyle, diet, and habit assessments and interventions that are important when initiating zidovudine therapy include highlighting the importance of adhering strictly to drug therapy; teaching that drug therapy does not affect the transmissibility of the disease; advising a high-carbohydrate, moderate-protein, and low-fat diet; taking zidovudine on an empty stomach; exploring the dangers of substance abuse during therapy and otherwise; and overcoming financial constraints to obtaining the prescribed drugs.

44-8. PIs work at the last stage of HIV replication. They prevent HIV from being successfully assembled and released from the infected CD4+ T cell.

44-9. Saquinavir is one of the most powerful PIs for fighting HIV. The potential for acquired drug resistance increases when saquinavir is taken incorrectly or indiscriminately. Resistance to saquinavir may eliminate use of many other PI drugs because cross-resistance may occur.

44-10. Although NNRTIs work at the same site as NRTIs, their mechanism of action is very different. NRTIs constrain HIV replication by incorporating into the elongating strand of viral DNA, which causes chain termination. NNRTIs do not incorporate into viral DNA; instead, they inhibit replication directly by binding noncompetitively to reverse transcriptase.

44-11. Entry inhibitors work by binding to gp41, thereby blocking its ability to bind to other cells. If the HIV virus cannot bind to a cell, it cannot enter the cell; thus, it cannot replicate.

44-12. Many infections that generally do little harm to humans may cause great morbidity and mortality in immunocompromised patients. In a person with a competent immune system, the infections are kept under control. In a person with an immunocompromised system, these minor microbes can create serious illness, blindness, and even death.

CHAPTER 45: DRUGS TREATING PARASITIC INFECTIONS

45-1. Vision examinations are important for patients receiving chloroquine because the drug has potential adverse ophthalmologic effects, including retinopathy. Retinopathy, which can lead to blindness, can progress even after the drug is discontinued.

45-2. Chloroquine is used cautiously in children because they are extremely susceptible to chloroquine toxicity. Fatalities have occurred with relatively small doses.

45-3. Baseline evaluations that should precede long-term antimalarial therapy include CBC, liver function tests, kidney function tests, eye examination, gross hearing evaluation, and ECG.

45-4. A patient with alcoholism should be monitored during antiparasitic therapy to detect hepatotoxicity. Many of the antiparasitic drugs have the potential for causing hepatic toxicity. Alcohol is also hepatotoxic. Therefore, patients with alcoholism may have an increased risk for the hepatic toxicity associated with these drugs.

45-5. Nurses and other health care providers should protect themselves when administering pentamidine because pentamidine frequently causes cough and bronchospasm during inhalation. Patients with immunodeficiency diseases are at high risk for respiratory diseases, such as tuberculosis. During

pentamidine therapy, these patients may cough and spread airborne pathogens.

45-6. Before administering pentamidine, evaluate the patient's baseline vital signs. Then with the patient supine, infuse pentamidine over 60 minutes. After the infusion, monitor the patient's blood pressure until it is stable.

45-7. The main reasons why lindane treatment does not succeed are failure to use the drug as directed and failure to treat all family members and other close contacts at the same time.

Unit 11: Respiratory System Drugs

CHAPTER 46: DRUGS AFFECTING THE UPPER RESPIRATORY SYSTEM

46-1. Dextromethorphan and narcotic antitussive drugs have the same efficacy in alleviating cough. Narcotic antitussives are more sedating and have more potential adverse effects and more drug–drug interactions.

46-2. Antihistamines block the antigen-antibody reaction. In the common cold or the flu, there is no allergic reaction, just an infection.

46-3. Fexofenadine is a second-generation antihistamine that does not easily pass the blood–brain barrier. This characteristic results in less sedation than is caused by first-generation antihistamines.

46-4. The advantage of inhaled antihistamines and steroids is that they act locally and are minimally absorbed, and thus induce few adverse effects.

46-5. Guaifenesin enhances the output of respiratory tract fluids by reducing the adhesiveness and surface tension of the respiratory fluids, allowing easier movement of the less viscous secretions. Thinner secretions result in a more productive cough. With a more productive cough, the frequency of coughing should decrease.

CHAPTER 47: DRUGS AFFECTING THE LOWER RESPIRATORY SYSTEM

47-1. Drugs can be grouped into mucolytic agents, such as acetylcysteine; bronchodilators, such as theophylline; and anti-inflammatory drugs, such as cromolyn sodium.

47-2. Theophylline acts by stimulating two prostaglandins, which results in smooth muscle relaxation in both the bronchi and vasculature. Beta-adrenergic agonists are sympathomimetic agents. That means the drugs mimic the action of norepinephrine. In the lungs, norepinephrine stimulates bronchodilation. Anticholinergic agents block the action of acetylcysteine. When acetylcysteine stimulates the lungs, bronchoconstriction occurs; thus, when its action is blocked, the bronchi do not constrict.

47-3. Beta-adrenergic agonists, such as albuterol, have the quickest onset of action. They are referred to as "rescue drugs."

47-4. Glucocorticosteroids are the most powerful anti-inflammatory agents.

47-5. Both drugs are effective in reducing inflammation. Glucocorticoid steroids given orally have the potential to cause more adverse effects because they are systemic. Steroids given by inhalation have a local action; thus, they cause fewer adverse effects.

47-6. Cromolyn sodium works by stabilizing the mast cell. When the mast cell ruptures in response to an antigen, bronchoconstrictive substances such as histamine, bradykinin, serotonin, and leukotrienes are released. By stabilizing the mast cell, the drug prevents release of these substances. Glucocorticoid steroids have a multitude of actions. In the lungs, they decrease the effectiveness of inflammatory cells, thus keeping the bronchioles open. Leukotriene antagonists block the ability of leukotrienes to bind to their receptor sites. Because leukotriene binding to these sites is what causes bronchoconstriction, bronchoconstriction is blocked.

47-7. The beta-adrenergic agonist inhaler should be used first because it has the fastest onset. It will open the bronchial tree, so that the other drugs can be dispersed further into the lungs to exert their action.

Unit 12: Gastrointestinal System Drugs

CHAPTER 48: DRUGS AFFECTING THE UPPER GASTROINTESTINAL TRACT

48-1. The cause of peptic ulcers is the bacterium *Helicobacter pylori*. Without treatment to kill these bacteria, the ulcer will almost always recur.

48-2. Highly acidic foods such as tomato juice and highly spiced foods may worsen GERD symptoms and may keep the patient from feeling relief of the pain and discomfort of GERD.

48-3. Omeprazole may interact with other drugs that also are metabolized through the cytochrome P-450 pathway (e.g., cyclosporine, disulfiram, and benzodiazepines). This interaction may produce elevated levels of these other drugs because their metabolism is decreased. Because omeprazole causes prolonged and substantial decreases in gastric acidity, drugs that depend on an acid environment for absorption may not be absorbed as well.

48-4. H_2 antagonists reduce gastric acid production by blocking histamine at the H_2 receptor site of parietal cells, resulting in a reduction in the hydrogen ion concentration and volume of gastric acid. H_1 antagonists are not effective at these sites and have no effect on gastric pH but are effective in relieving symptoms of allergic reactions. H_2 antagonists have no effect on the H_1 receptor sites.

48-5. Aluminum and magnesium are commonly combined in a preparation to balance the constipating effects of aluminum with the diarrheal effects of magnesium.

48-6. Patients with chronic renal failure tend to have elevated phosphate levels. Aluminum carbonate binds with the phosphate to return the patient's serum phosphate levels to normal.

48-7. The main adverse effects of orlistat are GI symptoms of oily spotting, flatus with discharge of stool, fecal urgency, fatty or oily stool, oily evacuation, increased defecation, and fecal incontinence.

48-8. Serotonin receptors of the 5-HT_3 type are located peripherally on the vagal nerve terminal and centrally in the chemoreceptor trigger zone. Stimulation of these receptors will bring on nausea and vomiting. During chemotherapy, special mucosal cells in the small intestine release serotonin, which stimulates these receptors. Ondansetron blocks these receptor sites, thus preventing nausea and vomiting.

CHAPTER 49: DRUGS AFFECTING THE LOWER GASTROINTESTINAL TRACT

49-1. Chew simethicone tablets thoroughly before swallowing. Shake suspension forms before measuring. Take after meals and at bedtime.

49-2. The unpleasant effects of atropine, such as dry mouth and tachycardia, discourage abuse of the drug for opioid effects.

49-3. Stool softeners.

49-4. No. The kidney that is not functioning optimally will not excrete magnesium. Hypermagnesemia may develop from the additional magnesium provided by magnesium hydroxide.

49-5. Lactulose pulls ammonia from the bloodstream into the digestive tract. Patients with severe hepatic disease have excessive ammonia in their blood. Lactulose will therefore decrease ammonia levels.

49-6. Alosetron is limited to women because insufficient data exist to support its use in men. Alosetron carries the risk for severe constipation and ischemic colitis, which is why it is limited to patients with severe symptoms of IBS in which diarrhea is the primary symptom.

Unit 13: Endocrine System Drugs

CHAPTER 50: DRUGS AFFECTING PITUITARY, THYROID, PARATHYROID, AND HYPOTHALAMIC FUNCTION

50-1. Calcium is used in many of the body's metabolic processes, including membrane transport processes, conduction of nerve impulses, muscle contraction, and blood clotting. Calcium levels are maintained within a narrow range by the interactions of parathyroid hormone, calcitonin, and vitamin D. These hormones alter calcium resorption from the intestine, affect osteoclast activity to alter the removal or deposit of calcium in bone, and affect the renal resorption of calcium.

50-2. A combination of neural and endocrine systems, originating in the hypothalamus, regulates central nervous system (CNS), autonomic nervous system (ANS), and endocrine functions. Major hypothalamic regulatory functions include somatic and visceral reactions, including temperature regulation, perspiration, GI activity, regulation of appetite and thirst, blood pressure, respiration, regulation of basic body rhythms (e.g., sleep and menstrual cycles), and complex behavioral and emotional reactions (e.g., sexual behavior and defensive reactions of fear and rage). To promote homeostasis, the hypothalamus transmits stimuli to the pituitary gland, causing hormonal release or hormonal inhibition. When stimulated by the hypothalamus, the pituitary gland releases vasopressin (ADH) to regulate water balance in the system or oxytocin to increase uterine contractions or stimulate milk let-down. The anterior pituitary releases various stimulating hormones that increase the activity of other endocrine glands in response to hypotdalamic releasing factors. These other endocrine glands regulate growth, development, and metabolism. The activity of both the hypothalamus and pituitary is carefully balanced through a series of negative feedback signals that maintain the levels of hormone present within an effective range.

50-3. Patients receiving somatropin will require it over the long term. It is administered only by injection. The patient or family needs to learn sterile technique and proper methods for reconstituting and storing the solution. In addition, they need to learn how to administer the injection and recognize the importance of rotating sites to prevent complications and ensure adequate absorption.

50-4. Signs and symptoms of hypothyroidism include lethargy, slowing of mental processes, neuropathies, decreased heart rate, decreased cardiac output, eyelid drooping, periorbital edema, enlarged tongue, decreased appetite, constipation, increased cholesterol levels, decreased deep tendon reflexes, decreased renal blood flow with decreased output, hypermenorrhea, decreased libido, pale and puffy skin, dry and brittle hair, brittle nails, and intolerance to cold.

50-5. Gallium can be extremely nephrotoxic. The patient will have to have renal function test results and serum electrolytes monitored closely. Renal failure can further complicate the patient's electrolyte disturbances. The patient needs to be well hydrated during the 5 days of treatment to flush the drug through the kidneys as quickly as possible.

50-6. Calcitonin, salmon is from an animal source, and there is a risk for allergic reaction, especially in patients with a known history of allergic reaction to animal products. A skin test should be administered before the drug is given. If no reaction is noted within 15 minutes of the skin test, the drug can be used. The patient should be evaluated periodically for any sign of the development of an allergic reaction and should be asked to report fever, rash, lethargy, or difficulty breathing.

CHAPTER 51: DRUGS AFFECTING CORTICOSTEROID LEVELS

51-1. The effects of glucocorticoids on metabolism are potent and varied. They include increased blood glucose concentrations, increased breakdown of protein and use of fatty acids for energy, and increased loss of calcium from bones.

51-2. Untreated acute adrenal insufficiency is life threatening. Signs and symptoms include hypoglycemia; anorexia, nausea, and vomiting; hypotension; fluid and electrolyte imbalance—dehydration, hyponatremia, and hyperkalemia; dehydration; and fatigue, weakness, and malaise. Untreated chronic adrenal insufficiency is not immediately life threatening but impairs the person's ability to cope with stress.

51-3. Cushing syndrome is a disease of adrenal hyperfunction. Chronic pharmacologic dosing of corticosteroids can lead to the same physiologic effects as adrenal hyperfunction. These effects are known as cushingoid characteristics and include fat stores in the face (moon face), glaucoma and cataract formation, hirsutism and masculinization, cervicodorsal fat (buffalo hump), extremity thinning and atrophy, abdominal striae, protuberant abdomen, truncal obesity, edema caused by sodium and fluid retention, and brittle bones. Any excess of corticosteroids, whether from endogenous or exogenous causes, can result in cushingoid characteristics.

51-4. Three major actions of the adrenal steroids are (1) metabolic effects on carbohydrate, protein, and fat metabolism; (2) anti-inflammatory and immunosuppressant effects; and

(3) sodium-retaining activity associated with potassium loss. The first two actions are classified as glucocorticoid actions, and the third is a mineralocorticoid action.

51-5. The two major clinical uses of adrenal steroids are replacement therapy in endocrine deficiency states and anti-inflammatory or immunosuppressive effects in nonendocrine states such as asthma or organ transplantation.

51-6. Exogenous administration of glucocorticoids suppresses the HPA axis, resulting in the adrenal glands losing their ability to synthesize cortisol and other glucocorticoids. Too abrupt cessation of glucocorticoid use may produce a withdrawal syndrome (i.e., hypotension, hypoglycemia, myalgia, arthralgia, and fatigue), leading to acute adrenal insufficiency (addisonian crisis), circulatory collapse, shock, and death.

51-7. Benefits of alternate-day therapy (ADT) are reduced adrenal suppression, reduced risk for growth retardation, and reduced overall toxicity and cushingoid changes. The likelihood of adrenal insufficiency is decreased because over the long interval between glucocorticoid doses, plasma glucocorticoids decline to a level that is low enough to permit some production of ACTH and some synthesis of cortisol by the adrenals. The disadvantages related to ADT include difficulty with patient adherence, potential for subtherapeutic plasma levels, and inconclusive data that adverse effects are substantially decreased.

51-8. Glucocorticoids interact with several types of drugs. Drugs that decrease the serum concentration of glucocorticoid drugs include barbiturates, hydantoins, and rifamycins. Monitor for therapeutic efficacy of glucocorticoid drugs if these other drugs are given concurrently. Glucocorticoid drugs may decrease the effects of anticholinesterase drugs, oral anticoagulants, and salicylates. Monitor the efficacy of those drugs when given concurrently with a glucocorticoid drug. When glucocorticoid drugs are given with oral contraceptives, monitor for possible steroid toxicity. Potassium-increasing diuretics enhance prednisone's potassium depletion.

51-9. Fludrocortisone is used in the treatment of primary (Addison disease) and secondary adrenocortical insufficiency. It also is used to treat salt-losing adrenogenital syndrome. An unlabeled use is the management of severe orthostatic hypotension. Fludrocortisone possesses both mineralocorticoid and glucocorticoid properties.

51-10. Patient teaching with fludrocortisone is just like patient teaching with the glucocorticoids because fludrocortisone has both mineralocorticoid and glucocorticoid properties. The patient receiving fludrocortisone is at risk for acute adrenal insufficiency when he or she experiences stressful situations during or after drug therapy. Moreover, the patient can develop adverse cardiovascular effects of hypertension, edema, congestive heart failure, and cardiomegaly from the mineralocorticoid actions of the drug. It is important to stress the importance of regular follow-up visits with the prescriber and prompt reporting of adverse effects of dizziness, severe or continuing headaches, swelling of the lower extremities or feet, and unusual weight gain.

51-11. The major clinical indication for the adrenal steroid inhibitors is Cushing syndrome, which is a rare disorder of adrenal cortical hyperfunction. The prototype inhibitor is aminoglutethimide. Aminoglutethimide suppresses the function of the adrenal cortex and thus reduces the amount of endogenous cortisol.

CHAPTER 52: DRUGS AFFECTING BLOOD GLUCOSE LEVELS

52-1. Insulin lowers blood glucose levels by allowing glucose to leave the bloodstream and enter the cells.

52-2. Glucagon helps regulate blood glucose levels. Falling blood glucose levels trigger the release of glucagon from the pancreas, as do sympathetic nerve impulses, exercise, infection, and trauma. In the liver, glucagon stimulates glycogenolysis and gluconeogenesis, resulting in a release of glucose into the blood. Glucagon helps to counterbalance the effect of insulin if insulin causes the blood glucose level to fall below normal.

52-3. A patient with type 1 diabetes mellitus has an absolute deficiency of endogenous insulin, and the disease can be controlled only by restoring insulin by injection. A patient with type 2 diabetes still has some natural insulin synthesis and secretion, but the cells are resistant to insulin. This patient's diabetes can usually be controlled by diet, exercise, and oral antidiabetic drug therapy, although insulin maybe required in some patients.

52-4. Insulin must be injected so that it bypasses the digestive system; peptides in the digestive enzymes of the GI tract will destroy the insulin molecule.

52-5. The effect of too much insulin would most likely be hypoglycemia and, in its most severe form, an insulin reaction. Early signs and symptoms are neurologic in nature and include irritability, tremors, headache, fatigue and malaise, diaphoresis, and tachycardia. A later symptom may be loss of consciousness.

52-6. Combining regular and NPH insulin provides an immediate onset of insulin (from the regular) to lower the current blood sugar level as well as a sustained effect (from the NPH) to maintain the glucose in a normal range throughout the day.

52-7. Regular, lispro, and aspart insulins can be used as sliding-scale coverage.

52-8. NPH is an intermediate-acting insulin. It is a suspension and is cloudy. Its pharmacokinetics include a definite peak and trough so that glucose control can vary. It is often dosed twice a day to achieve glucose control. Glargine is a long-acting insulin. It is not a suspension and is clear in appearance. Its pharmacokinetics do not include a peak and trough; hence, glucose control is more constant throughout the day. It is dosed once daily at bedtime.

52-9. Hypoglycemia.

52-10. Acarbose reduces the rate of digestion of complex carbohydrates. Less glucose is absorbed because the carbohydrates are not broken down into glucose molecules. Reduced absorption decreases the blood glucose level.

52-11. Glucagon is used to increase the blood glucose level of patients experiencing severe hypoglycemia. In addition to knowing the symptoms of hypoglycemia, the patient and family must be taught correct preparation and

administration techniques because it is given by the SC or IM route in the home setting. Furthermore, the family should be taught to provide supplemental carbohydrates as soon as possible after glucagon injection to restore liver glycogen and prevent secondary hypoglycemia.

CHAPTER 53: DRUGS AFFECTING MEN'S HEALTH AND SEXUALITY

53-1. The primary effects of testosterone are normal growth and development of the male sex organs and development and maintenance of the male secondary sexual characteristics (e.g., male hair distribution, hair texture and color, laryngeal enlargement and vocal cord thickening [voice deepening], and alterations in body musculature and fat distribution). Secondary effects of testosterone are retention of sodium, potassium, and phosphorus; decreased urinary excretion of calcium; stimulation of the growth of skeletal muscle tissue and enhancement of the growth of long bones in prepubes-cent boys; ossification of the epiphyseal growth plates; and stimulation ofthe production of red blood cells by enhancement of the production of erythropoietic-stimulating factor.

53-2. The main risk is premature ossification of the epiphyseal growth plate resulting in stunted growth.

53-3. When activated by nitric oxide, cGMP stimulates smooth muscle relaxation and allows the inflow of blood into the erectile tissue in the penis. Sildenafil inhibits the isoenzyme (phosphodiesterase [PDE] type 5) that metabolizes cGMP. The decrease in the metabolism of cGMP allows cGMP to remain active longer, promoting more smooth muscle relaxation and inflow of blood. This effect creates an improved and more sustained erection.

53-4. Finasteride is a pregnancy category X drug. Absorption through the skin is increased if the drug is crushed or broken.

53-5. Poor systemic absorption decreases the risk for adverse effects. The therapeutic effect is achieved without systemic absorption of topical minoxidil.

CHAPTER 54: DRUGS AFFECTING WOMEN'S HEALTH AND SEXUALITY

54-1. Progesterone is used to treat amenorrhea and abnormal uterine bleeding because after ovulation the ovarian follicle is transformed into the corpus luteum, which secretes a great deal of progesterone (and estrogens). This rise in progesterone prepares the endometrium for implantation. As progesterone levels (and estrogen levels) rise, production of FSH and LH decreases, preventing further ovulation. If fertilization does not occur, the corpus luteum disintegrates, and progesterone levels fall. Menstruation occurs. Thus, depending on the timing and duration of therapy, ovulation can be blocked or menses can be initiated.

54-2. The serious adverse effects of estrogen therapy are increased risk for endometrial cancer, possibly increased risk for breast cancer, increased risk for thromboembolic disorders (including thrombophlebitis, MI, and pulmonary embolus, or PE), gallbladder disease, and hypertension.

54-3. Raloxifene can achieve the same effects as estrogen on increasing bone mineral density and decreasing lipids. Raloxifene does not, however, have the same effects on uterine or breast tissue that estrogen does. Thus, the risk for endometrial and breast cancer is reduced. This distinction is especially important for women who have high risk factors for these cancers but who are also are at risk for or currently have osteoporosis.

54-4. If a dose of an oral contraceptive is missed, it should be taken as quickly as possible; two tablets may be taken on the same day. Two missed pills should be made up over 2 days. If three consecutive pills are missed, the patient should begin a new cycle either the day after the last pill was missed or 7 days after the last pill was taken. Another form of birth control should be used as a backup for at least 7 consecutive days of the new cycle and preferably for the rest of the cycle.

54-5. Instruct the patient to take alendronate at least 30 minutes before eating, drinking any beverage other than plain water, or taking any other medication. The patient should swallow the medicine with 6 to 8 oz (180–240 mL) of plain water and should not take it with coffee, juice, or mineral water. Instruct the patient not to lie down for at least 30 minutes after taking the medication.

CHAPTER 55: DRUGS AFFECTING UTERINE MOTILITY

55-1. Slow upward titration of oxytocin more closely resembles oxytocin excretion, which naturally induces labor. Additionally, doing so minimizes adverse fetal and maternal effects.

55-2. The three phases of oxytocin response are (1) the incremental phase (uterine activity increases evenly as the dose of oxytocin increases); (2) the stable phase (uterine activity remains constant even if the oxytocin dose increases because the myometrial receptor sites are already full); and (3) hyperstimulation (the dose continually increases, the frequency of contractions increases, but the uterine pressure decreases so that the contractions are less effective).

55-3. Water intoxication, which can be fatal.

55-4. Nursing assessments that may help to minimize adverse effects of oxytocin include maternal pulse rate, blood pressure, and fluid status; duration of contractions; time between contractions; fetal heart rate; and character of fetal movement.

55-5. Terbutaline is a beta agonist that selectively stimulates uterine receptors and stops uterine contractions.

55-6. If tachycardia, palpitations, and nervousness develop during terbutaline infusion, you should slow the infusion, or even stop it, and notify the physician or nurse midwife.

55-7. Magnesium sulfate is the drug of choice for treating or preventing seizures associated with preeclampsia, eclampsia, and pregnancy-induced hypertension. It is also used to treat preterm labor.

55-8. Calcium gluconate.

55-9. The most common maternal adverse effects are headache, hyporeflexia, weakness, thirst, flushing, and burning at the infusion site. The most common fetal or neonatal adverse effects are heart rate changes, neonatal hypotonia, and neonatal respiratory depression (possibly serious).

Index

Note: Page numbers followed by b indicate boxed material; those followed by f indicate figures; those followed by t indicate tables. Drugs are listed in **boldface** type under their generic names; trade names are listed in CAPITAL LETTERS.

A

B

C

D

E

F

H

I

M

N

O

P

Q

R

S

T

U

V

W

X

Y

Z